AF669520

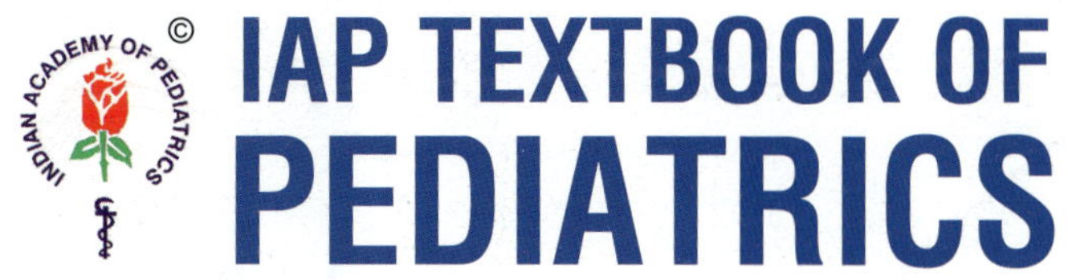
INDIAN ACADEMY OF PEDIATRICS
©
IAP TEXTBOOK OF
PEDIATRICS

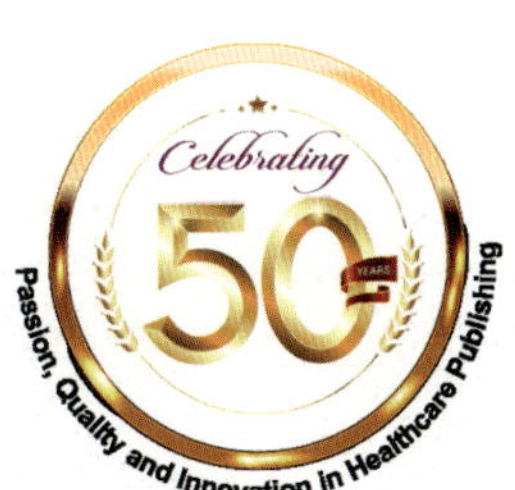
Celebrating
50
Passion, Quality and Innovation in Healthcare Publishing

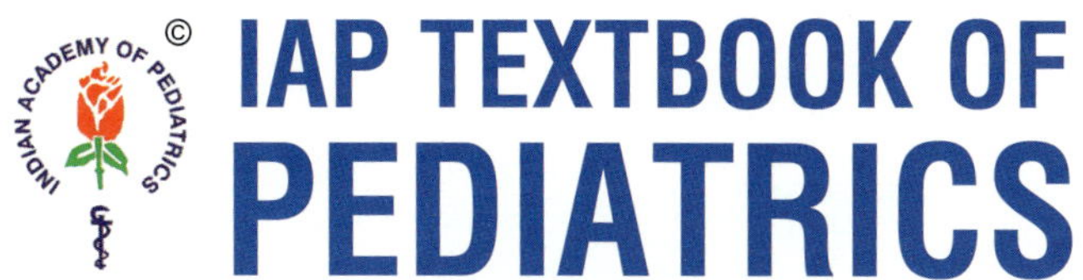

IAP TEXTBOOK OF PEDIATRICS

SEVENTH EDITION

Founder-Editor

A Parthasarathy
MD DCH DSc (Hon) FIAP
Senior Consultant Pediatrician, AP Child Care, Chennai
Former Distinguished Professor of Pediatrics
The Tamil Nadu Dr MGR Medical University
Retired Senior Clinical Professor of Pediatrics
Madras Medical College
Institute of Child Health and Hospital for Children
Chennai, Tamil Nadu

Editors-in-Chief

PSN Menon
MD MNANS FIAP
Consultant and Head
Department of Pediatrics
Jaber Al-Ahmed Armed Forces Hospital, Kuwait
Former Professor of Pediatrics
All India Institute of Medical Sciences
New Delhi

MKC Nair
MD MMedSc PhD DSc MBA FIAP
Vice-Chancellor
Kerala University of Health Sciences, Thrissur
Founder Director
Child Development Center
Government Medical College
Thiruvananthapuram, Kerala

Chief Academic Editors

Piyush Gupta
MD FNNF FIAP FAMS
Professor
Department of Pediatrics
University College of Medical Sciences and
Guru Teg Bahadur Hospital
New Delhi

Ritabrata Kundu
MD FIAP
Professor
Department of Pediatrics
Institute of Child Health
Kolkata, West Bengal

Executive Editor

Alok Gupta
MD FIAP
Pediatrician and Counselor
Pediatric Specialties Clinic, Jaipur
Former Assistant Professor (Pediatrics)
Mahatma Gandhi Medical College and Hospital
Jaipur, Rajasthan

Academic Editors

Abhay K Shah
MD DPed FIAP
Senior Consultant Pediatrician and Director
Children Hospital
Ahmedabad, Gujarat

Ashok Rai
MD PhD FIAP FIAMS FNNF FACI
Senior Consultant Pediatrician
Surya Superspecialty Hospital, Kilkari Institute of Child Health
Director, Indian Institute of Cerebral Palsy
and Handicapped Children
Varanasi, Uttar Pradesh

Dhanya Dharmapalan
MD PG Dip in PID (Oxford)
Consultant in Pediatrics and Pediatric
Infectious Diseases
Apollo Hospitals
Navi Mumbai, Maharashtra

Jaydeep Choudhury
DNB (Ped) MNAMS FIAP
Associate Professor
Department of Pediatrics
Institute of Child Health
Kolkata, West Bengal

K Nedunchelian
MD (Ped) DCH FIAP
Head (Research and Academics)
Senior Consultant Pediatrician
Mehta Multispecialty Hospitals India Pvt Ltd
Chennai, Tamil Nadu

P Ramachandran
MD (Ped) DNB (Ped)
Professor of Pediatrics and
Associate Dean (PG Studies)
Sri Ramachandra Institute of Higher
Education and Research
Chennai, Tamil Nadu

Ex-Officio Editorial Advisers

Digant D Shastri
MD (Ped) PGDHHM FIAP
Senior Consultant Pediatrician
Killol Children Hospital
Surat, Gujarat
President IAP 2019

Santosh T Soans
MD FIAP
Professor and Head
Chief Neonatal and Pediatric intensive Care Division
AJ Institute of Medical Sciences and Research Centre
Mangaluru, Karnataka
President IAP 2018

Bakul J Parekh
MD DCH FIAP
Professor of Pediatrics
Bakul Parekh Children's Hospital and
Multispecialty Centre
Mumbai, Maharashtra
President-Elect 2019

Remesh Kumar R
MD Dip Ped Env Health FIAP
Medical Superintendent and Chief Pediatrician
NSS Medical Mission Superspecialty Hospital
Pandalam, Kerala
Secretary General IAP 2018–19

Upendra S Kinjawadekar
MD DCH
Pediatrician
Kamlesh Mother and Child Hospital
Navi Mumbai, Maharashtra
Treasurer IAP 2018–19

Forewords

Digant D Shastri, Santosh T Soans

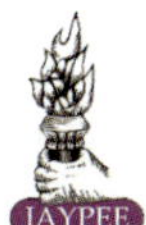

JAYPEE BROTHERS MEDICAL PUBLISHERS

The Health Sciences Publisher

New Delhi | London | Panama

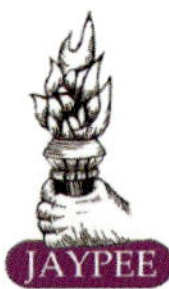

Jaypee Brothers Medical Publishers (P) Ltd.

Headquarters
Jaypee Brothers Medical Publishers (P) Ltd.
4838/24, Ansari Road, Daryaganj
New Delhi 110 002, India
Phone: +91-11-43574357
Fax: +91-11-43574314
Email: jaypee@jaypeebrothers.com

Overseas Offices

JP Medical Ltd.
83, Victoria Street, London
SW1H 0HW (UK)
Phone: +44 20 3170 8910
Fax: +44 (0)20 3008 6180
E-mail: info@jpmedpub.com

Jaypee-Highlights Medical Publishers Inc.
City of Knowledge, Bld. 235, 2nd Floor, Clayton
Panama City, Panama
Phone: +1 507-301-0496
Fax: +1 507-301-0499
E-mail: cservice@jphmedical.com

Jaypee Brothers Medical Publishers (P) Ltd.
Bhotahity, Kathmandu, Nepal
Phone: +977-9741283608
E-mail: kathmandu@jaypeebrothers.com

Website: www.jaypeebrothers.com
Website: www.jaypeedigital.com

IAP Textbook of Pediatrics

First Edition: 1999, 2000; Second Edition: 2002, 2003; Third Edition: 2006; Revised Reprint: 2007
Fourth Edition: 2009; Fifth Edition: 2013; Sixth Edition: 2016
Seventh Edition: **2019**

ISBN: 978-93-5270-801-7

Printed at: Replika Press Pvt. Ltd.

Dedicated to

The Future Adults of India whose Care and Nurture are our Goal, Concern and Commitment

IAP Presidents' Speak

The 6th edition of *IAP Textbook of Pediatrics* is an excellent combination of clinical pediatrics with recent advances in the field of child health.

The outstanding value of the textbook is due to its expert and authoritative contributors and every reader will be indebted to the dedicated authors for their hard work, knowledge, thoughtfulness and good judgment.

In the *Mahabharata*, Lord Krishna acted as the *sarathi* for chariot and guided *Partha (Arjuna)*. I congratulate Dr A Parthasarathy, who has performed a similar function of carrying forward the chariot of knowledge by editing *Maha* (Huge) *bharat*iya (Indian) *Textbook of Pediatrics* for guiding pediatricians.

Pramod Jog
President, IAP 2016

Ever since the introduction of its first edition, *IAP Textbook of Pediatrics* was a well-accepted desktop reference. This was because it had contributions from experts in their respective fields of interest and every new edition was revised and updated as per the then knowledge. The sixth edition with input from more than 250 national experts, has been revised with updated texts which are brief yet all-inclusive. In keeping with the times, Dr A Parthasarathy, *Editor-in-Chief*, appropriately supported by Drs MKC Nair, PSN Menon and Ritabrata Kundu along with many highly reputed editors have done a wonderful job of updating the chapters in this edition. Comprehensive revisions have ensured the most recent information on diagnosis and treatment of pediatric diseases based on the latest recommendations and methodologies. This edition will be priceless as a desktop reference for practitioners and an invaluable medical textbook for students.

S Sachidananda Kamath
President, IAP 2015

I welcome the 6th edition of *IAP Textbook of Pediatrics* produced with the efforts of highly experienced team under the brilliant leadership of Dr A Parathasarathy. I strongly recommend this book to every student, teacher, and practicing clinician in India who wants a reliable, up-to-date, comprehensive and very useful textbook. The chapters are underpinned by decades of experience of the authors and addresses both the general and specialized aspects of pediatrics. The editors and the authors are to be congratulated for providing us such a high standard textbook which is highly relevant for Indian pediatrics.

Vijay N Yewale
President, IAP 2014

Nelson is considered as the *Bible of Pediatrics*. If *Nelson's Textbook of Pediatrics* is the Bible, I can vouch that the *IAP Textbook of Pediatrics* is *Geeta Saar* of Pediatrics in India; the enlightenment delivered by a galaxy of pediatric expertise in India and chariot of knowledge driven by *Sarathi*—Parthasarathy. I am extremely privileged to be associated with this literary jewel of IAP's treasury in the past and proud that the *IAP Textbook of Pediatrics* is incarcinating into its 6th *avtaar*; the last 5 being extremely useful, disseminating optimum knowledge, comprehensively with clinical precision. The previous editions were at par with Nelson's standard and most popular amongst postgraduates and practitioners as well beyond being earning substantial revenues for IAP. I wish an infinite popularity to this 6th edition with compliments to all concerned editors and contributors.

Rohit C Agrawal
President, IAP 2012

It is my pleasure and privilege to write this message for the 6th edition of *IAP Textbook of Pediatrics*. The *IAP Textbook of Pediatrics* is the brain child of Dr A Parthasarathy and my hearty congratulations for all the editors. This book can be considered as an Indian counterpart of Nelson's Textbook of Pediatrics and I think this book will be a reference book for all academicians, practicing pediatricians and postgraduates as well. I wish that the new edition of the book should be released once in three years.

TU Sukumaran
President, IAP 2011

It gives me immense pleasure to see the 6th edition of *IAP Textbook of Pediatrics*. It is a result of efforts put in by a galaxy of experienced clinicians from across the country under the able leadership of Dr A Parthasarathy, Editor-in-Chief. I congratulate Dr Parthasarathy, editorial team, authors and publishers for their efforts to bring out this edition. This book is a very useful tool for students as well as practicing pediatricians to refer to for reliable and up-to-date information in pediatrics and is very relevant to our country. I strongly recommend this book to every student and practicing pediatrician in our country.

Deepak Ugra
President, IAP 2010

IAP Textbook of Pediatrics is an amalgam of knowledge, science, wisdom and expertise. It is a milestone in the history of IAP and Dr A Parthasarathy needs to be congratulated along with his worthy team for comprehensive 6th edition. True to eternal character, *Krishna* (Partha + sarathy), the only Hindu God, never had any weapon but only melodious flute for welfare of mankind, hence the creation of this *Textbook of Pediatrics*. It is meaningful to all readers and a token of pride and possession from a developing country. The contents are precise yet elaborate and cover all curative, preventive, social and national programs. I wish its longevity, consistency, regularity and periodic updating.

RK Agarwal
President, IAP 2008

The 6th edition of *IAP Textbook of Pediatrics* is a perfect book for all the pediatricians. The book has knowledge embedded by its expert and experienced authors and it will be helpful for the readers.

I congratulate all the contributors and editors who have worked immensely for preparing this textbook which will be a guide for pediatricians.

Naveen Thacker
Past President, IAP 2007

The entire team involved in the publication of the *IAP Textbook of Pediatrics*, 6th edition, deserves hearty congratulations for the tremendous effort and perseverance generated by them to make this publication a unique one. Hats-off to Dr A Parthasarathy for his leadership. We wish that this publication will continue to help the pediatricians of India and abroad.

Dilip Mukherjee
President, IAP 2002

The 6th edition of *IAP Textbook of Pediatrics* is very much relevant to Indian situation on etiology and management. It has relevant chapters on latest updates in pediatrics. It will be useful to undergraduate students as well as postgraduates and practicing pediatricians. My compliments to the editors, especially Dr A Parthasarathy for his untiring efforts in bringing out academy's first *Indian Textbook of Pediatrics* with all information, both clinically and newer updates. I am confident that pediatricians would find it very useful in day-to-day practice.

YC Mathur
President, IAP 2001

Indeed, it is a millennium gift to students and practitioners in a well-written and well-presented comprehensive format covering A to Z in pediatric care.

Swati Y Bhave
President, IAP 2000

Teachers of Pediatrics will find in this book guidelines for the course contents in undergraduate and postgraduate medical education. Medical students will find readable and reasonably detailed, yet concise information in this book, not only to complete the course and pass the final examination, but also to guide them during their clinical career as interns, house surgeons and medical practitioners.

T Jacob John
President, IAP 1999

Immense advancement has been made over the past decade in the field of pediatrics/pediatric subspecialties making necessitation of updating this book regularly. This book is not only a reference book for pediatricians in India but also is accepted by the academicians from the neighboring countries, postgraduate students and practicing pediatricians. There is a lot of unique features included in the 6th edition. This is the result of persistent hard work by Chief Editor, Dr A Parthasarathy and his team. Every chapter has been updated and re-written by the experts in their respective fields with great acumen. New chapters have been added keeping in mind the changing concept of pediatric care in the global scenario. I am sure that this book will become more and more popular and will be the desk reference for all those who are interested in the pediatrics and in its subspecialty. The book is a combination of current pediatric and what is stored for the future. It is a feather in the cap for IAP. I look forward to see many more editions at regular interval and become popular internationally.

MR Lokeshwar
President, IAP 1998

The 6th edition of this widely read text on pediatrics is an important landmark. Having been associated with this book since its inception, I have watched its progress. Each edition has been revised and updated to include rapid advances in knowledge and practice of pediatrics. Dr Parthasarathy and his team of editors, the contributors and Jaypee Brothers Medical Publishers deserve our gratitude for maintaining the high standards of its contents and excellent publication.

RN Srivastava
President, IAP 1996

This textbook has covered all aspects of child health contributed by reputed authors, in addition to National Health Programs. Thus, it has fulfilled all the criteria of a 'reader friendly' treatise.

Uday Bodhankar
President, IAP 1995

Contributors

A Balachandran
Pediatric Pulmonologist
Mehta Multispecialty Hospitals
India Pvt Ltd
Chennai, Tamil Nadu

A Parthasarathy
Senior Consultant Pediatrician
AP Child Care, Chennai
Former Distinguished Professor
of Pediatrics
The Tamil Nadu Dr MGR Medical
University
Retired Senior Clinical Professor
of Pediatrics
Madras Medical College
Institute of Child Health and Hospital for
Children, Chennai, Tamil Nadu

A Riyaz
Former Director, Professor and Head
Department of Pediatrics
Institute of Maternal and Child Health
Government Medical College
Kozhikode, Kerala

Abhay K Shah
Senior Consultant Pediatrician and
Director
Children Hospital
Ahmedabad, Gujarat

Abraham K Paul
Consultant Pediatrician
Cochin Hospital
Kochi, Kerala

Aditi Sharma
Senior Research Fellow
Division of Pediatric Nephrology
Department of Pediatrics
All India Institute of Medical Sciences
New Delhi

Aditi Sinha
Assistant Professor
Division of Pediatric Nephrology
Department of Pediatrics
All India Institute of Medical Sciences
New Delhi

AK Dutta
Professor and Head
Department of Pediatrics
School of Medical Sciences and Research
Sharda University
Greater Noida, Uttar Pradesh

Alok Gupta
Pediatrician and Counselor
Pediatric Specialties Clinic, Jaipur
Former Assistant Professor
(Pediatrics)
Mahatma Gandhi Medical
College and Hospital
Jaipur, Rajasthan

Amarjeet Chitkara
Director and Head
Department of Pediatrics
Max Superspeciality Hospital
New Delhi

Amita Trehan
Professor
Pediatric Hematology Oncology Unit
Department of Pediatrics
Postgraduate Institute of Medical
Education and Research
Chandigarh

Anita Saxena
Professor
Department of Cardiology
All India Institute of Medical Sciences
New Delhi

Anjali Tomar
Senior Resident
University College of Medical Sciences
and Guru Teg Bahadur Hospital
New Delhi

Anju Aggarwal
Professor Pediatrics
University College of Medical Sciences
and Guru Teg Bahadur Hospital
New Delhi

Anju Seth
Director Professor of Pediatrics
Lady Hardinge Medical College
New Delhi

Anju Virmani
Associate Director and Consultant
Pediatric Endocrinologist
MAX SMART and MAX Gurugram
RAINBOW; PENTAMED Hospitals
New Delhi

Anoop Verma
Consultant Pediatrician and Director
Swapnil Institute of Child Health
Raipur, Chhattisgarh

Anuj Singh
Senior Research Fellow
Department of Pediatrics
All India Institute of Medical Sciences
New Delhi

Anupam Sachdeva
Director
Pediatric Hematology, Oncology and
Bone Marrow Transplantation
Institute for Child Health
Sir Ganga Ram Hospital
New Delhi

Anupama S Borker
Head
Department of Medical and
Pediatric Oncology
Goa Medical College and Hospital
Bambolion, Goa

AP Dubey
Professor of Pediatrics
Guru Gobind Singh Indraprastha University
ESI-PGIMSR, New Delhi

Aparna Mukherjee
Early Career Fellow Wellcome Trust/
DBT India Alliance
Department of Pediatrics
All India Institute of Medical Sciences
New Delhi

Archana Kher
Consultant Pediatrician
Seven Hills Hospital, Mumbai
Professor Pediatrics (Retd)
Seth Gordhandas Sunderdas
Medical College and King Edward
Memorial Hospital
Mumbai, Maharashtra

Arun Bansal
Professor
Pediatric Critical Care Unit
Department of Pediatrics
Postgraduate Institute of Medical
Education and Research
Chandigarh

Arun Kumar Gupta
Professor and Head
Department of Radiodiagnosis
All India Institute of Medical Sciences
New Delhi

Arun Phatak
Professor of Pediatrics
KGP Children Hospital
Vadodara, Gujarat

Arushi G Saini
Pediatrician
Department of Pediatrics
Advanced Pediatrics Center
Postgraduate Institute of Medical
Education and Research (PGIMER)
Chandigarh

Arvind Bagga
Professor of Pediatrics
Division of Pediatric Nephrology
Department of Pediatrics
All India Institute of Medical Sciences
New Delhi

Ashish Bavdekar
Associate Professor
Consultant Pediatric Gastroenterologist
Department of Pediatrics
King Edward Memorial Hospital
Pune, Maharashtra

Ashok K Patwari
Former Director Professor
Department of Pediatrics
Lady Hardinge Medical College
New Delhi
Research Professor
International Health
Boston University School of
Public Health
Boston, USA

Ashok Kapse
Professor and Head
Department of Pediatrics
Mahavir Superspecialty Hospital
Surat, Gujarat

Ashok Kumar
Professor In-charge Neonatal Unit
Department of Pediatrics
Institute of Medical Sciences
Banaras Hindu University
Varanasi, Uttar Pradesh

Ashok Rai
Senior Consultant Pediatrician
Surya Superspecialty Hospital,
Kilkari Institute of Child Health
Director
Indian Institute of Cerebral Palsy and
Handicapped Children
Varanasi, Uttar Pradesh

(Col) ATK Rau
Senior Professor (Pediatrics)
Senior Consultant
(Pediatric Hematology-Oncology)
Principal and Dean
MVJ Medical College
Bengaluru, Karnataka

B Bhaskar Raju
Head
Department of Pediatric Gastroenterology
Dr Mehta Children's Hospital
Chennai, Tamil Nadu
Formerly Professor and Head
Department of Pediatric
Gastroenterology
Institute of Child Health and
Hospital for Children
Chennai, Tamil Nadu

Bakul J Parekh
Professor of Pediatrics
Bakul Parekh Children's Hospital and
Multispecialty Centre
Mumbai, Maharashtra
President-Elect 2019

Bala Ramachandran
Consultant and Head
Department of Intensive Care and
Emergency Medicine
Kanchi Kamakoti CHILDS Trust Hospital
Chennai, Tamil Nadu

Baldev S Prajapati
Professor of Pediatrics
GCS Medical College, Hospital and
Research Centre
Aakansha Children Hospital and
Postgraduate Institute
Ahmedabad, Gujarat

Balvir S Tomar
Professor and Head
Director
Institute of Pediatric Gastroenterology and Hepatology
MINS Medical College and Hospital and Chairman and Chancellor
NIMS University
Jaipur, Rajasthan

BD Gupta
Senior Consultant (Pediatrics)
Rajdadisa Hospital
Jodhpur, Rajasthan
Formerly Professor and Head
Department of Pediatrics
Superintendent
Umaid Hospital
Additional Principal
Dr SN Medical College
Jodhpur, Rajasthan

Bharat Agarwal
Professor Emeritus and
Former Head of Department
Department of Pediatric Hematology and Oncology
BJ Wadia Hospital for Children
Mumbai, Maharashtra

Bharat Mehra
Senior Resident
Department of Pediatrics
Dayanand Medical College and Hospital
Ludhiana, Punjab

Bibek Talukdar
Former Director-Professor
Pediatrics
Maulana Azad Medical College and Associated Chacha
Nehru Bal Chikitsalaya
New Delhi

Bikrant Bihari Lal
Assistant Professor
Department of Pediatric Hepatology
Institute of Liver and Biliary Sciences
New Delhi

BR Nammalwar
Professor of Pediatric Nephrology (Retd)
Institute of Child Health
Hospital for Children and
Director of Medical Education
Dr Mehta's Children's Hospital
Chennai, Tamil Nadu

Brijesh Arora
Professor and Head
Department of Pediatric Oncology
Tata Memorial Hospital
Mumbai, Maharashtra

C Thangadorai
Senior Clinical Professor of Pediatrics (Retd)
Madras Medical College
Chennai, Tamil Nadu

Chhaya A Divecha
Assistant Professor of Pediatrics
College of Medicine and Health Sciences
National University of Science and Technology
Sohar, Sultanate of Oman

Chhaya S Prasad
Developmental and Behavioral Pediatrician
Adolescent Health Expert
Director, ASHA—Centre for Autism and Intellectual Developmental Disorders
Chandigarh

D Nirmala
Professor and Head
Department of Pediatric Gastroenterology
Institute of Child Health and
Hospital for Children
Chennai, Tamil Nadu

D Vijayasekaran
Visiting Professor
Sree Balaji Medical College
Chennai, Tamil Nadu
Consultant and Pediatric Pulmonologist
Kanchi Kamakoti CHILDS Trust Hospital
and Apollo Children's Hospital
Professor of Pediatric Medicine and
Respiratory Diseases (Retd)
Madras Medical College
Chennai, Tamil Nadu

Deep Thacker
Executive Director
Child Health Foundation
Gandhidham, Gujarat

Deepa Bhaskaran
Assistant Professor
Developmental Pediatrics
Child Development Centre
Government Medical College
Thiruvananthapuram

Deepak Bansal
Professor
Hematology/Oncology Unit
Department of Pediatrics
Advanced Pediatrics Center
Postgraduate Institute of Medical Education and Research
Chandigarh

Deepak Ugra
Consultant Pediatrician
Lilavati Hospital and Research Centre
Hinduja Heathcare Surgicals
Visiting Pediatrician
Apollo Hospital
Mumbai, Maharashtra

Deepti Agrawal
National Programme Officer
Newborn and Child Health
Norway India Partnership Initiative
Jhpiego (John's Hopkins University Affiliate)
New Delhi

Devendra Mishra
Professor
Department of Pediatrics
Maulana Azad Medical College
New Delhi

Dhanya Dharmapalan
Consultant in Pediatrics and
Pediatric Infectious Diseases
Apollo Hospitals
Navi Mumbai, Maharashtra

Dheeraj Shah
Professor
Department of Pediatrics
University College of Medical Sciences
and Guru Teg Bahadur Hospital
New Delhi

Digant D Shastri
Senior Consultant Pediatrician
Killol Children Hospital
Surat, Gujarat
President IAP 2019

Dilip Mukherjee
Emeritus Professor of Pediatrics
Ramakrishna Mission Seva Pratishthan
Vivekananda Institute of Medical
Sciences
Kolkata, West Bengal

Divya Prabhat
Head
Department of ENT
Wadia Children Hospital
Jaslok, Bhatia and Raheja Fortis Hospital
Mumbai, Maharashtra

DK Agarwal
Professor and Head (Retd)
Department of Pediatrics
Banaras Hindu University
Varanasi, Uttar Pradesh
Secretary
Health Care and Research Association
for Adolescents
Noida, Uttar Pradesh

Gadadhar Sarangi
Former Professor and Director of
Post Graduate Studies
Department of Pediatrics
Hi-tech Medical College
Bhubaneswar, Odisha
Chairman
Baidyanath Memorial Hospital and
Research Center
Bhubaneswar, Odisha

Gauri Kapoor
Director and Head
Department of Pediatric
Hematology and Oncology
Rajiv Gandhi Cancer Institute and
Research Center, New Delhi

Geetha M
Clinical Professor
Pediatric Gastroenterology
Amrita Institute of Medical Sciences
Kochi, Kerala

George F Moolayil
Pediatrician and Consultant
(Medical Law)
KISCO Clinic
Kottayam, Kerala

H Paramesh
Chairman
Pediatric Pulmonologist and
Environmentalist
Lakeside Center for Health Promotion
Bengaluru, Karnataka
Visiting Professor
Divecha Center for Climate Change
Indian Institute of Science (IISc)
Bengaluru, Karnataka

Indira Agarwal
Professor
Christian Medical College
Vellore, Tamil Nadu

Jagdish Chandra
Director Professor
Department of Pediatrics
Lady Hardinge Medical College and
Kalawati Saran Children's Hospital
New Delhi

Jagdish Prasad Goyal
Additional Professor
Department of Pediatrics
All India Institute of Medical Sciences
Jodhpur, Rajasthan

Jai K Das
Assistant Professor
Division of Women and Child Health
Aga Khan University
Karachi, Pakistan

Jaya Shankar Kaushik
Associate Professor
Department of Pediatrics
Pandit Bhagwat Dayal Sharma
Postgraduate Institute of Medical
Sciences
Rohtak, Haryana

Jayakar Thomas
Professor and Head of Dermatology
Sree Balaji Medical College and Hospital
Chennai, Tamil Nadu

Jaydeep Choudhury
Associate Professor
Department of Pediatrics
Institute of Child Health
Kolkata, West Bengal

Jeeson C Unni
Senior Associate and Consultant
(Pediatrics)
Aster Medcity
Kochi, Kerala
Editor-in-chief
IAP Drug Formulary

Jitendra Meena
Pediatric Nephrology
Department of Pediatrics
All India Institute of Medical Sciences
New Delhi

JN Goswami
Pediatric Neurology and
Neurodevelopment Unit
Department of Pediatrics
Advanced Pediatrics Centre
Postgraduate Institute of Medical
Education and Research
Chandigarh

JN Sharma
Former Professor
Department of Pediatrics and Neonatology
Gauhati Medical College
Guwahati, Assam

Joseph L Mathew
Professor (Pediatric Pulmonology)
Advanced Pediatrics Centre
Postgraduate Institute of Medical Education and Research
Chandigarh

JP Dadhich
Technical Director
Breastfeeding Promotion Network of India (BPNI), New Delhi

Jugesh Chhatwal
Professor of Pediatrics
Christian Medical College
Ludhiana, Punjab

K Nagaraju
Professor of Allergy and Clinical Immunology
Senior Consultant in Paediatric Allergy and Clinical Immunology
Director
Saveetha Medical College
Apollo Children's Hospital
VN Allergy and Asthma Research Center
Chennai, Tamil Nadu

K Nedunchelian
Head (Research and Academics)
Senior Consultant Pediatrician
Mehta Multispecialty Hospitals
India Pvt Ltd
Chennai, Tamil Nadu

K Surendran
Surveillance Medical Officer
WHO National Polio Surveillance Project
Chennai, Tamil Nadu

Kakali Roy
Resident
Institute of Child Health
Kolkata, West Bengal

Kamer Singh Rana
Consultant
Commandant Military Hospital
Jabalpur, Madhya Pradesh

Kamran Afzal
Professor
Department of Pediatrics
Jawaharlal Nehru Medical College
Aligarh Muslim University
Aligarh, Uttar Pradesh

Kanishka Das
Professor and Head
Department of Pediatric Surgery
All India Institute of Medical Sciences
Bhubaneswar, Odisha

KE Elizabeth
Professor and Head
Department of Pediatrics
Sree Mookambika Institute of Medical Sciences
Kanyakumari, Tamil Nadu

Ketan Parikh
Consultant Pediatric Surgeon
Jaslok, SRCC Children Hospital, LH Hiranandani, Apollo (Navi Mumbai)
Seven Hills Medicity, Nanavati and Kohinoor Hospitals
Mumbai, Maharashtra

Kiran Aggarwal
Senior Consultant Pediatrician/Unit Head
Department of Pediatrics
Hindu Rao Hospital
New Delhi
Member, CWC and ICMR, New Delhi
Justice Gopal Singh Charitable Trust
New Delhi

Kishore Phadke
Director of Clinical Services
Head, Pediatric Nephrology
Rainbow Children's Hospital
Bengaluru, Karnataka

KN Agarwal
Professor of Pediatrics
Universal College of Medical Sciences and Teaching Hospital
Bhairahawa, Nepal

Krishna Mohan R
Consultant Pediatrician
Government Health Services Department
Taluk Hospital
Kozhikode, Kerala

Krishnendu Mondal
Pediatrician
Department of Pediatrics
Institute of Child Health
Kolkata, West Bengal

L Subramanyam
Pediatrician Pulmonologist
Mehta Hospitals
Mehta Multispeciality Hospital
India Pvt Ltd
Chennai, Tamil Nadu

Lalitha Kailas
Professor and Head
Department of Pediatrics
Sree Gokulam Medical College and Research Foundation
Thiruvananthapuram, Kerala

M Indra Shekhar Rao
Director
Division of Pediatrics and Neonatology
Navodaya Hospital for Women and Children, Medical Superintendent (Retd)
Professor and Head (Retd)
Department of Pediatrics
Institute of Child Health and Niloufer Hospital
Director Medical Education (Retd)
Government of Andhra Pradesh
Hyderabad, Telangana

M Jayashree
Professor and Chief
Pediatric Emergency and Intensive Care Units
Advanced Pediatrics Centre
Postgraduate Institute of Medical Education and Research
Chandigarh

Madhulika Kabra
Professor
Division of Genetics
Department of Pediatrics
All India Institute of Medical Sciences
New Delhi

Madhumati Otiv
Pediatric Intensivist
Program Director for ISCCM-IAP Certificate Course in Pediatric Intensive Care
King Edward Memorial Hospital
Pune, Maharashtra

Madhuri Kanitkar
Dean and Dy Commandant
Armed Forces Medical College
Pune, Maharashtra
Consultant
Department of Pediatric Nephrology
Rainbow Children's Hospital
Bengaluru, Karnataka

Malathi Sathiyasekaran
Consultant Pediatric Gastroenterologist
Kanchi Kamakoti CHILDS Trust Hospital
Chennai, Tamil Nadu

Maninder Dhaliwal
Consultant Pediatric Intensivist
Medanta—The Medicity
Gurugram, Haryana

Manju Mehta
Professor of Clinical Psychology (Retd)
Department of Psychiatry
All India Institute of Medical Sciences
New Delhi

Manorama Verma
Professor of Pediatrics (Retd)
Christian Medical College
Ludhiana, Punjab

Meena P Desai
Honorary Consultant
Division of Pediatric Endocrinology
Institute of Child Health
Bai Jerbai Wadia Hospital for Children
Mumbai, Maharashtra

Meenakshi N Mehta
Former Professor and Head
Department of Pediatrics
LTM Medical College and General Hospital
Mumbai, Maharashtra
Consultant Pediatrician, Head (Pediatrics) and Postgraduate Teacher
Mahatma Gandhi Memorial Hospital
Mumbai, Maharashtra

Milind S Tullu
Professor (Additional) of Pediatrics
Seth GS Medical College and KEM Hospital
Mumbai, Maharashtra

MKC Nair
Vice-Chancellor
Kerala University of Health Sciences
Thrissur
Founder Director
Child Development Center
Government Medical College
Thiruvananthapuram, Kerala

ML Kulkarni
Professor and Head
Department of Pediatrics
JJM Medical College
Davangere, Karnataka

Moinak Sen Sarma
Assistant Professor
Department of Pediatric Gastroenterology
Sanjay Gandhi Postgraduate Institute of Medical Sciences
Lucknow, Uttar Pradesh

Monjori Mitra
Associate Professor
Institute of Child Health
Kolkata, West Bengal, India

MR Lokeshwar
Consulting Pediatrician and Pediatric Hematologist/Oncologist
Lilavati Hospital and Research Centre
Mumbai, Maharashtra
Shushrusha Citizens Cooperative Hospital Ltd
Mumbai, Maharashtra

MS Mahadeviah
Hon Professor of Pediatrics
Kempegowda Institute of Medical Sciences
Bengaluru, Karnataka
Hon Medical Director
Spastics Society of Karnataka

Munni Ray
Additional Professor of Pediatrics
Advanced Pediatrics Centre
Postgraduate Institute of Medical Education and Research
Chandigarh

Narendra K Arora
Executive Director
Indian Society of Pediatrics
The INCLEN Trust International
New Delhi

Narendra Rathi
Consultant Pediatrician
Smile Institute of Child Health and Smile Child Development Centre
Akola, Maharashtra

Naveen Jain
Senior Consultant
Kerala Institute of Medical Sciences
Thiruvananthapuram, Kerala

Naveen Sankhyan
Assistant Professor
Department of Pediatrics
Advanced Pediatrics Center
Postgraduate Institute of Medical Education and Research
Chandigarh

Naveen Thacker
Director
Deep Children Hospital and Research Centre
Gandhidham, Gujarat

Neelam Mohan
Director
Department of Pediatric Gastroenterology,
Hepatology and Liver Transplantation
Medanta—The Medicity
Gurugram, Haryana

Niranjan Shendurnikar
Consultant Pediatrician
KG Patel Children Hospital
Vadodara, Gujarat

Nitin Shah
Honorary Pediatric Hematologist-Oncologist
Bai Jerbai Wadia Hospital for Children
Consultant Pediatrician
PD Hinduja National Hospital
Mumbai, Maharashtra

Nupur Ganguly
Associate Professor
Deputy Director—Academics
Institute of Child Health
Kolkata, West Bengal

P Leela Kumari
Assistant Professor
Department of Pediatrics
SAT Hospital
Government Medical College
Thiruvananthapuram, Kerala

P Raghupathy
Professor
Department of Pediatrics
(Pediatric Endocrinology)
Indira Gandhi Institute of Child Health
Bengaluru, Karnataka

P Ramachandran
Professor of Pediatrics and
Associate Dean (PG Studies)
Sri Ramachandra Institute of Higher Education and Research
Chennai, Tamil Nadu

PA Mohammed Kunju
Dean
Faculty of Medicine
University of Kerala
Professor and Head
Department of Pediatric Neurology
Government Medical College
Thiruvananthapuram, Kerala

Pallab Chatterjee
European Diplomate of Pediatric Pulmonology
Consultant Pediatrician
Apollo Gleneagles Hospital
Columbia Asia Hospital
Kolkata, West Bengal

Pankaj Hari
Professor
Department of Pediatrics
All India Institute of Medical Sciences
New Delhi

(Late) Panna Choudhury
Consultant Pediatrician (Retd)
Lok Nayak Hospital
New Delhi

Parang N Mehta
Consultant Pediatrician
Mehta Childcare
Surat, Gujarat

Parimalam Kumar
Professor and Head of Dermatology
Stanley Medical College
Government Stanley Hospital
Chennai, Tamil Nadu

Paul SS Russell
Professor (Psychiatry)
Child and Adolescent Psychiatry Unit
Christian Medical College
Vellore, Tamil Nadu

Payal Gupta
Fellow (Pediatric Ophthalmology)
Sadguru Netra Chikitsalaya
Chitrakoot, Madhya Pradesh

Piyush Gupta
Professor
Department of Pediatrics
University College of Medical Sciences and
Guru Teg Bahadur Hospital
New Delhi

PK Baskar
Senior Consultant
Sri Viveka Institute of Dental Health
Chairman
Baskar Dental Foundation
Chennai, Tamil Nadu

Pooja Balasubramanian
Pediatric Hematologist Oncologist
Asian Cancer Institute
Mumbai, Maharashtra

Pooja Dewan
Professor
University College of Medical Sciences
and Guru Teg Bahadur Hospital
New Delhi

PP Maiya
Former Professor of Pediatrics
Sagar Hospitals
Bengaluru, Karnataka

Prabir Maji
Assistant Professor
Department of Pediatric Hepatology
Institute of Liver and Biliary Sciences
New Delhi

Prajakta Joshi
Fellow in Pediatric Rheumatology
Jaslok Hospital and Research Center
Mumbai, Maharashtra

Pratibha Singhi
Director
Pediatric Neurology and Neurodevelopment
Medanta—The Medicity
Gurugram, Haryana
Former Head and Chief
Pediatric Neurology and Neurodevelopment
Department of Pediatrics
Advanced Pediatrics Centre
Postgraduate Institute of Medical Education and Research
Chandigarh

Pratima R Shah
Consulting Pediatrician and Neonatologist
Former Head and Professor
Department of Pediatrics
Sumandeep Medical College
Ankur Institute of Child Health
Ahmedabad, Gujarat

Praveen Khilnani
Clinical Director and Senior Consultant
Pediatric Critical Care and Pulmonology
Rainbow Children's Hospital
New Delhi

Prawin Kumar
Assistant Professor
Department of Pediatrics
All India Institute of Medical Sciences
Jodhpur, Rajasthan

Preeti Dabadghao
Professor
Department of Endocrinology
Sanjay Gandhi Postgraduate Institute of Medical Sciences
Lucknow, Uttar Pradesh

Prisca Colaco
Professor
Department of Pediatrics
Mahatma Gandhi Mission's Medical College
Navi Mumbai, Maharashtra

PSN Menon
Consultant and Head
Department of Pediatrics
Jaber Al-Ahmed Armed Forces Hospital
Kuwait
Former Professor of Pediatrics
All India Institute of Medical Sciences
New Delhi

Pukhraj Bafna (Padmashri)
Pediatrician and Adolescent Health Consultant
United Hospital, CDCRI
Rajnandgaon, Chhattisgarh

Purna A Kurkure
Chairman
Clinical Collegium for Oncology Services
Narayana Health Group
Head
Division of Pediatric Hemato-oncology and Bone Marrow Transplantation
SRCC Children's Hospital
Mumbai, Maharashtra

R Krishna Kumar
Clinical Professor and Head
Department of Pediatric Cardiology
Amrita Institute of Medical Sciences
Amrita Vishwa Vidyapeetham
Kochi, Kerala

Rachna Pasi
Senior Resident and PhD student
Department of Pediatrics
All India Institute of Medical Sciences
Rishikesh, Uttarakhand

Rajalakshmi Iyer
Senior Resident
DM Pediatric Critical Care
Advanced Pediatrics Centre
Postgraduate Institute of Medical Education and Research
Chandigarh

Rajeshwar Dayal
Professor and Head
Department of Pediatrics
SN Medical College
Agra, Uttar Pradesh

Rajiv Chandra Mathur
Consultant Pediatrician
Aditya Hospital
Hyderabad, Telangana

Rajniti Prasad
Professor and Head
Department of Pediatrics
Institute of Medical Sciences
Banaras Hindu University
Varanasi, Uttar Pradesh

Raju C Shah
Consulting Pediatrician and Neonatologist
Former Head and Professor
Department of Pediatrics
GCS Medical College
Ankur Institute of Child Health
Ahmedabad, Gujarat

Raju P Khubchandani
Senior Consultant
Pediatrics and Sectional Head
Pediatric Rheumatology
SRCC Childrens Hospital
Consultant Pediatrician
Jaslok Hospital and Research Center
Breach Candy Hospital
Mumbai, Maharashtra

Rakesh Lodha
Professor
Department of Pediatrics
All India Institute of Medical Sciences
New Delhi

Rakesh Manohar
Pediatrician
Department of Gastroenterology
Kanchi Kamakoti CHILDS Trust Hospital
Chennai, Tamil Nadu

Rakesh N Pillai
Program Officer
INCLEN Institute of Global Health (IIGH)
India Clinical Epidemiology Network
New Delhi

Ranjan Kumar Pejaver
Chief of Neonatology
Meenakshi Hospitals
Honorary Professor of Neonatology
Kempegowda Institute of Medical Sciences, Bengaluru, Karnataka

Rashmi Dalvi
Professor and Head
Department of Pediatrics
Senior Consultant
Pediatric Hematology Oncology
Bombay Hospital Institute of Medical Sciences
NH-SRCC Children's Hospital
Mumbai, Maharashtra

Rashmi Kumar
Professor and Head
Department of Pediatrics
King George's Medical University
Lucknow, Uttar Pradesh

RD Potdar
Pediatrician
Jeevak Children Hospital
Mumbai, Maharashtra

Rekha Hans
Assistant Professor
Department of Transfusion Medicine
Postgraduate Institute of Medical Education and Research, Chandigarh

Rekha Mittal
Additional Director
(Pediatric Neurology)
Madhukar Rainbow Children's Hospital
New Delhi

Remesh Kumar R
Medical Superintendent and Chief Pediatrician
NSS Medical Mission Superspecialty Hospital
Pandalam, Kerala
Secretary General IAP 2018–19

Rhishikesh Thakre
Director
Neo Clinic and Hospital
Aurangabad, Maharashtra

Richa Jain
Pediatric Hematology Oncology Unit
Department of Pediatrics
Postgraduate Institute of Medical Education and Research
Chandigarh

Ritabrata Kundu
Professor
Department of Pediatrics
Institute of Child Health
Kolkata, West Bengal

RK Agarwal
Consultant Pediatrician and Neonatologist
RK Hospital
Udaipur, Rajasthan

RK Anand
Emeritus Director
Department of Pediatrics and Neonatology
Jaslok Hospital and Research Centre
Mumbai, Maharashtra

RN Srivastava
Consultant Pediatric Nephrologist
Apollo Indraprastha Hospitals
New Delhi

Rohit C Agrawal
Consultant Pediatrician
Kohinoor Hospital and Chandra-Jyoti Children Hospital
Mumbai, Maharashtra

Ruchi N Nanavati
Professor and Head
Department of Neonatology
Seth Gordhandas Sunderdas Medical College and King Edward Memorial Hospital, Mumbai, Maharashtra

Ruchi Rai
Professor and Chief Consultant
Department of Neonatology
Superspeciality Pediatric Hospital and Postgraduate Teaching Institute
Noida, Gautam Budh Nagar

S Balasubramanian
Senior Consultant Pediatrician and Head
Department of Pediatrics
Kanchi Kamakoti CHILDS Trust Hospital
Chennai, Tamil Nadu

S Ramesh
Consultant Pediatrician
BRS Hospital
Chennai, Tamil Nadu

S Sachidananda Kamath
Director and Consultant Pediatrician
Welcare Hospital
Ernakulam, Kerala

S Srinivasan
Adjunct Professor of Pediatrics
Mehta's Hospital
Chennai, Tamil Nadu

S Venkat Reddy
Consultant Pediatrician
Navodaya Hospital for Women and Children
Secunderabad, Telangana

S Yamuna
Pediatrician and Adolescent Physician
Child and Adolescent Clinic
Chennai, Tamil Nadu

Sailesh Gupta
Pediatrician and Neonatologist
Ashna Childrens Hospital and Arushi Childcare Hospital
Mumbai, Maharashtra

Sandeep B Bavdekar
Visiting Consultant
Department of Pediatrics
TN Medical College and BYL Nair Charitable Hospital
Mumbai, Maharashtra

Santosh T Saons
Professor and Head
Chief Neonatal and Pediatric intensive Care Division
AJ Institute of Medical Sciences and Research Centre
Mangaluru, Karnataka
President IAP 2018

Satinder Aneja
Professor and Head
School of Medical Sciences and Research
Sharda University
Greater Noida, Uttar Pradesh

Satvik Bansal
Assistant Professor
Department of Pediatrics
Gajra Raja Medical College
Gwalior, Madhya Pradesh

Satya Prakash Yadav
Senior Consultant and Head
Pediatric Hemato-oncology and Bone Marrow Transplant Unit
Fortis Memorial Research Institute
Gurugram, Haryana

Saumil Gaur
Consultant
Department of Pediatric Nephrology
Rainbow Children's Hospital
Bengaluru, Karnataka

Savitri Shrivastava
Director
Department of Pediatric and Congenital Heart Disease
Fortis Escorts Heart Institute
New Delhi

Seema Alam
Professor and Head
Department of Pediatric Hepatology
Institute of Liver and Biliary Sciences
New Delhi

Shashi N Vani
Emeritus Professor of Pediatrics including Neonatology
PS Medical College and Sri Krishna Hospital, Gujarat
Retd Senior Professor and Head of Pediatrics including Neonatology
BJ Medical College and Civil Hospital
Ahmedabad, Gujarat

Shashidhararao Nagabhushana
Clinical Associate
CSI Hospital, Bengaluru
Visiting Consultant
Columbia Asia Hospital
Bengaluru, Karnataka

Sheffali Gulati
Professor
Department of Pediatrics
All India Institute of Medical Sciences
New Delhi
Chief, Child Neurology Division
Coordinator
DM Pediatric Neurology Programme
Faculty and In-charge
Centre of Excellence and Advanced Research for Childhood Neurodevelopmental Disorders

Sheila Bhave
Professor
Department of Pediatrics
King Edward Memorial Hospital and Research Centre
Pune, Maharashtra

Shruthi NM
Pediatrician
Division of Pediatric Neurology
Department of Pediatrics
All India Institute of Medical Sciences
New Delhi

Shubha Phadke
Professor and Head
Department of Medical Genetics
Sanjay Gandhi Postgraduate Institute of Medical Sciences
Lucknow, Uttar Pradesh

Somu Sivabalan
Consultant Pediatrician and Pulmonologist
Kanchi Kamakoti CHILDS Trust Hospital
Chennai, Tamil Nadu

Soonu Udani
Section Coordinator (Pediatrics)
PD Hinduja National Hospital and Medical Research Centre
Mumbai, Maharashtra

SR Banerjee
Head
Department of Pediatrics
Islamia Hospital
Kolkata, West Bengal

Srikanta Basu
Professor
Department of Paediatrics
Lady Hardinge Medical College and Kalawati Saran Children Hospital
New Delhi

Srinivas Sankaranarayanan
Consultant Pediatrician and Pediatric Gastroenterologist
Kanchi Kamakoti CHILDS Trust Hospital
Apollo Childrens Hospital
Chennai, Tamil Nadu

SS Kale
Consulting Pediatrician and
Director
Orbit Children Hospital and
Critical Care Unit
Akola, Maharashtra

Suchitra Ranjit
Head
Pediatric Intensive Care and Emergency
Services, Apollo Children's Hospital
Chennai, Tamil Nadu

Sukanta Chatterjee
Professor and Head
Department of Pediatrics
KPC Medical College
Jadavpur, Kolkata, West Bengal

Sumantra Kumar Raut
Senior Research Fellow
Division of Pediatric Nephrology
Department of Pediatrics
All India Institute of Medical Sciences
New Delhi

Sunanda K Reddy
Consultant
Developmental Pediatrics and
Community Health Chief NGO
Functionary
Centre for Applied Research and
Education on Neurodevelopmental
Impairments and Disability-related
Health Initiatives
New Delhi
Adjunct Faculty
South Asia Centre for Disability Inclusive
Development and Research
Hyderabad, Telangana

Suneeta Mittal
Director and Head
Obstetrics and Gynecology
Fortis Memorial Research Institute
Gurugram, Haryana

Sunil Dutt Sharma
Consultant Pediatric Intensivist
Surya Hospital
Jaipur, Rajasthan

Sunil Gomber
Director-Professor
Department of Pediatrics
University College of Medical Sciences
and Guru Teg Bahadur Hospital
New Delhi

Sunil Karande
Professor of Pediatrics and In-charge
Learning Disability Clinic
Department of Pediatrics
Seth GS Medical College and
KEM Hospital
Mumbai, Maharashtra

Sunit Singhi
Head
Department of Pediatrics
Medanta—The Medicity
Gurugram, Haryana
Former Professor and Head
Department of Pediatrics and
Advanced Pediatrics Centre
Postgraduate Institute of Medical
Education and Research
Chandigarh

Suresh Kumar S
Head
Department of Physiotherapy
Mehta Multispecialty Hospitals
India Pvt Ltd
Chennai, Tamil Nadu
President
Muscular Dystrophy Association India

Surjit Singh
Professor, Head (Pediatrics) and In-charge
Pediatric Allergy Immunology Unit
Advanced Pediatrics Centre
Postgraduate Institute of Medical
Education and Research
Chandigarh

Susan Uthup
Additional Professor and Chief
Department of Pediatric Nephrology
Sree Avittom Thirunal Hospital
Government Medical College
Thiruvananthapuram, Kerala
Honorary Consultant Pediatric
Nephrologist
Sree Chitra Thirunal Institute of Medical
Science and Technology
Thiruvananthapuram, Kerala

Sushil K Kabra
Professor
Department of Pediatrics
All India Institute of Medical Sciences
New Delhi

Sushila Russell
Lecturer in Clinical Psychology
Department of Psychiatry
Child and Adolescent Psychiatry Unit
Christian Medical College
Vellore, Tamil Nadu

Sushmita Banerjee
Consultant
Department of Pediatrics
Calcutta Medical Research Institute
Department of Nephrology
Institute of Child Health
Kolkata, West Bengal

Swarna Rekha Bhat
Former Professor Pediatrics and
Neonatology
St John's Medical College
Bengaluru, Karnataka

Swathi Chacham
Additional Professor
Department of Pediatrics
All India Institute of Medical Sciences
Rishikesh, Uttarakhand

Swati Kalra
Assistant Professor (Pediatrics)
Dr Baba Sahib Ambedkar Medical
College and Hospital
New Delhi

Swati Y Bhave
Adjunct Professor (Adolescent Medicine)
Dr DY Patil Medical College, Pimpri and
Dr DY Patil Vidyapeeth, Pune
Senior Consultant (Adolescent Pediatrics)
Head and In-charge
Adolescent Wellness Clinic, Jehangir
Hospital, Pune
Executive Director, Association of
Adolescent and Child Care in India
(AACCI), Mumbai
Maharashtra

T Jacob John
Emeritus Professor
Department of Virology
Christian Medical College and Hospital
Vellore, Tamil Nadu

T Ravikumar
Senior Consultant (Pediatrics)
Kanchi Kamakoti CHILDS Trust Hospital
Chennai, Tamil Nadu

Tanmay Amladi
Specialist Pediatrician
Grand Infinity Medical Center
Beirut Street, Al Muhaisnah 4
Dubai, UAE

Tanu Singhal
Consultant Pediatrics and
Infectious Diseases
Kokilaben Dhirubhai Ambani Hospital
and Medical Research Institute
Mumbai, Maharashtra

TU Sukumaran
Professor of Pediatrics
Pushpagiri Institute of Medical Sciences
Thiruvalla, Kerala

Tulika Seth
Additional Professor
Department of Hematology
All India Institute of Medical Sciences
New Delhi

Uday B Nadkarni
Consultant Pediatrician and
Neonatologist
Surya Mother and Child Care
Global Hospital, Sevenhills Hospital
Fortis Hospital, Maharashtra

Ujjal Poddar
Professor
Department of Pediatric
Gastroenterology
Sanjay Gandhi Postgraduate
Institute of Medical Sciences
Lucknow, Uttar Pradesh

Uma Ali
Head
Nephrology Division and PICU
Bai Jerbai Wadia Hospital for Children
Mumbai
Consultant Pediatrician
Lilavati Hospital, Mumbai
Jupiter Hospital
Thane, Maharashtra

Upendra S Kinjawadekar
Pediatrician
Kamlesh Mother and Child Hospital
Navi Mumbai, Maharashtra
Treasurer IAP 2018–19

Upreet Dhaliwal
Former Director-Professor
University College of Medical Sciences
New Delhi

Utpal Kant Singh
Professor and Head
Katihar Medical College
Katihar, Bihar
Professor and Head (Retd)
Nalanda Medical College
Patna, Bihar

Vaman Khadilkar
Pediatric Endcrinologist and PhD Guide
Health Sciences, Pune University
Jehangir Hospital, Pune
Bombay Hospital, Mumbai
Maharashtra

Vandhanaa Natarajan
Senior Resident
Department of Pediatrics
Institute of Child Health
Chennai, Tamil Nadu

Varinder Singh
Professor of Pediatrics
Lady Hardinge Medical College and
Associated Kalawati Saran Children's
Hospital, New Delhi

Ved Prakash Choudhry
Senior Consultant Hematology
Fortis Escorts Hospital
Faridabad, Haryana

VH Sankar
Additional Professor
Department of Pediatrics
SAT Hospital
Goverment Medical College
Thiruvananthapuram, Kerala

Vibhawari S Dani
Professor of Pediatrics and Dean (Retd)
Government Medical College
Nagpur, Maharashtra

Vijay N Yewale
Consultant Pediatrician and Head
Institute of Child Health
Apollo Hospitals
Navi Mumbai, Maharashtra

Vijayalakshmi Bhatia
Professor
Department of Endocrinology
Sanjay Gandhi Postgraduate Institute of
Medical Sciences
Lucknow, Uttar Pradesh

Vikram Datta
Director-Professor
Department of Neonatology
Lady Hardinge Medical College
New Delhi
President NQOCN, India

VR Ravikumar
Consultant Pediatric Surgeon
GKNM Hospital
Coimbatore, Tamil Nadu

VS Sankaranarayanan
Former Professor and Head
Department of Pediatric Gastroenterology
Madras Medical College and
Institute of Child Health and
Hospital for Children
The Tamil Nadu Dr MGR Medical University
Senior Consultant and Head
Department of Gastroenterology
Kanchi Kamakoti CHILDS Trust Hospital
Chennai, Tamil Nadu

YK Amdekar
Medical Director
BJ Wadia Hospital for Children
Mumbai, Maharasthtra

Zulfiqar A Bhutta
Robert Harding Chair in Global Child
Health and Policy
Co-Director
SickKids Centre for Global Child Health
Toronto, Canada
Professor and Founding Director
Centre of Excellence in Women and
Child Health
Aga Khan University
Karachi, Pakistan

Foreword

It gives me sense of honor and pleasure to write foreword for the seventh edition of *IAP Textbook of Pediatrics*.

As IAP president as well as an IAPian, I feel proud of the most prestigious publication of *Indian Academy of Pediatrics (IAP) Textbook of Pediatrics*. The project, which was conceived in 1997 during presidency of Dr A Parthasarathy, was completed in 1999 with the release of first edition of *IAP Textbook of Pediatrics*. Ever since then, it has progressed leaps and bounds. Over a period of 20 years' regularly a new edition is published, and what we see today is the 7th edition of *IAP Textbook of Pediatrics*. This speaks of the popularity of this publication and it has not only become learning textbook for undergraduate students in India but has received similar popularity in South Asian countries.

Going through the content of the book, I can confidently say that this is a *state of-the-art* textbook of pediatrics from Indian subcontinent origin having 21 Sections and nearly 239 Chapters and an Appendix, which covers the subject of pediatrics—from newborn care to adolescent health issues. This edition is a perfect blend of basic sciences and recent advances with comprehensive coverage of pediatric subspecialty also. It also covers various IAP guidelines and recommendations including the latest ACVIP recommendations.

My sincere compliments and congratulations to all the authors who as a part of their sincere efforts to disseminate the knowledge have contributed chapters for this prestigious publication. I wish to congratulate Dr A Parthasarathy (Founder Editor) and Drs PSN Menon and MKC Nair (Editors-in-Chief), the editorial team of Drs Piyush Gupta, Ritabrata Kundu, Alok Gupta and all members of the editorial team for this innovative concept.

I am sure that this book will be popular not only amongst undergraduate students but will be proved as useful reference material for postgraduate students, teaching faculties and practicing pediatricians.

I wish this landmark publication great success and I wish the readers an enriching, learning and pleasant reading experience.

Digant D Shastri
President 2019
Indian Academy of Pediatrics (IAP)

Foreword

One of the simple joys of life that I discovered only after becoming President, Indian Academy of Pediatrics (IAP) is the art of writing foreword for books. During the past year, I have been called upon to write a message for more books that I can perhaps keep track of. In a sense, I have found this aspect of my job very reassuring as it has reinforced my belief that the future of IAP should be built on the foundation of academics. It is time to go back to the basics. By calling itself an 'academy', IAP has a sworn obligation to adhere to its core function of disseminating scientific knowledge and professional expertise within the pediatric community of India. Doing so protects our organization health as well as relevance.

With membership touching 30,000, IAP has an unimaginably large talent pool of doctors which the organization should tap for furthering the cause of medicine through knowledge sharing. While I am impressed by the good number of books coming out, I feel that much more needs to be done. Bringing out a good book now and then will not add up to a large body of work. It is only when our output reaches an industrial scale will we be in a position to make a difference and say that our endeavor is thriving. I hope the present trend of compiling books on different topics will escalate gradually over the years and reach its critical mass required for explosive growth.

On our part, IAP has granted official patronage for a series of book projects, which includes *IAP Textbook of Pediatrics*. While perusing the contents of this book, I was astonished to see that the new edition has a total of 239 Chapters and an Appendix covering all aspects of child health. The editors of the book have roped in the best experts in each subject to give us a complete and reliable reference volume of nearly 1,500 pages. In fact, the word textbook itself is a misnomer; the right word is to call this book an encyclopedia! Compiling the book would have taken extraordinary effort and I congratulate the editorial board as well as the individual contributors for giving us a well-rounded work. I wish the reader a fruitful reading experience.

Santosh T Soans
President 2018
Indian Academy of Pediatrics (IAP)

Preface to the Seventh Edition

The editorial board dedicates the new revised and updated seventh edition of the *IAP Textbook of Pediatrics* to children and adolescents—the future citizens of India whose nurture and care are our goal, concern and commitment. It is our humble tribute to the Indian Academy of Pediatrics (IAP), which is the vanguard for the care of children of all hues and colors, at all ages and without barriers; that trained and fostered us as responsible professionals to care children with love and compassion.

The discipline of pediatrics has made substantial advances in the last decade in preventive and therapeutic care. New perspectives for care of children have been opened and many thrust areas requiring immediate or continued attention to decrease morbidity and mortality have been demarcated. These have provided fresh impetus to improve knowledge, harvest new information and continue the process of learning. The opportunities are infinite and it is for us to take advantage of these new frontiers. These developments have imposed the need for publication of an updated 7th edition of the book after a gap of three years. This was also inspired by the enthusiastic response to the previous editions from practicing pediatricians, postgraduates, undergraduates as well as faculty of departments of pediatrics throughout India and other SAARC countries.

It has been our endeavor to present the subject in a simplified and practical manner to provide adequate clinical guidance to pediatricians so that children derive the benefits of early diagnosis and optimal treatment. The basic simple and practical outline of the book is retained. We have tried our best to oversee that the "Art and Science" of clinical pediatrics maintains its central position without being dwarfed by newer technical advances.

The main focus of the new edition has now shifted to practicing pediatricians as against the original concept of undergraduates. The Indian Academy of Pediatrics currently has a membership of nearly 30,000 pediatricians and there is a felt need to continuously update our members, with the rapid advances in the field and the new national and global initiatives in the care of children.

The book represents a substantial revision and reorganization of the text based on a complete review of the field of pediatrics. This is not a watered-down version; efforts have also been made to keep a balance with incorporation of the curricular needs of the undergraduates, postgraduates and teachers in pediatrics. This edition has 239 Chapters arranged in 21 major sections. The entire contents of the textbook are reorganized to provide relevant clinical information and national priorities at one site. Inducting new experts in chosen fields made judicious balance of old and young authors. All the chapters have been thoroughly revised and updated in a lucid and readable style and have undergone a three-tier review and edit process. The Editorial Board and the Indian Academy of Pediatrics are indebted to those experts who made their valuable contributions without any remuneration or honorarium for their services.

Some of the thrust areas in the edition refer to felt needs of our country. It is our constant endeavor to inform, educate and update the reader about the current status of national community-oriented initiatives for children. We are justifiably proud of our achievements in preventive care with attainment of the status of polio-free nation among others, for more than six years. Strategies for incorporating newer technology and better coverage of immunization to contain communicable diseases and further reduction in disease burden, especially in the underprivileged areas of our society, hence, find a better thrust in this book. While we are able to combat infections at a better footing than before, the continued onslaught of newer infections and pandemics, especially from resistant microorganisms is our national priority. As pediatricians, our major commitment is to ensure a decrease in mortality and morbidity, especially among the under-fives. The book highlights the use of simple strategies to improve health status such as uniform growth charts and low-cost food supplements. More complex issues such as the increasing disease burden of new epidemics of noninfectious chronic diseases such as obesity, especially in the urban India and screening for congenital disorders in the newborns thus find adequate mention in this book, keeping in mind the changing concepts of pediatric care in the global scenario.

The Indian Academy of Pediatrics would like to place on record its appreciation to all the authors who have taken great pains to contribute and/or edit reader-friendly sections with practical guidelines amidst their busy professional and academic schedules. We are proud to inform you that we have inducted new authors in this edition of the textbook with valuable contributions. We welcome the new team members of the editorial board and gratefully acknowledge their efforts as a team. It is no exaggeration to record that they have devoted great deal of their time reviewing and editing the manuscripts. We do sincerely hope their efforts have made the book more concise and precise.

It is our earnest hope that this book will help in early diagnosis and efficient management leading to optimal outcome and improving the quality of patient care. Your valuable suggestions and comments are most welcome for improving the contents and quality of future editions.

A Parthasarathy
PSN Menon
MKC Nair
Piyush Gupta
Ritabrata Kundu

Preface to the First Edition

Pediatrics has grown and developed with significant milestones in preventive and therapeutic care over the past few decades. The WHO and UNICEF in their Primary Health Care (PHC) approach, have given due importance for effective child survival programs. So, the medical students need to be well oriented towards these approaches in pediatrics as the future middle level managers in primary health care.

Several luminaries in the Indian pediatric scenario have contributed their might in bringing out books for the undergraduate medical students. However, the rapid advances made in the various pediatric subspecialties have necessitated the updating of these books from time to time. Nevertheless, the need for a full-fledged textbook was felt for long. The Indian Academy of Pediatrics thought it fit to shoulder the responsibility of bringing out such a need-based textbook in pediatrics for medical students. Our erudite and enthusiastic editors and contributors made it possible at a record time. The Indian Academy of Pediatrics (IAP) owes its gratitude to all these experts for their worthy contribution.

The book has been divided into several sections. A few chapters included in this book are entirely newer concepts, which are not usually found in the conventional pediatric textbooks. It has also worthy annexures to the main contents. However, editing the text to suit the needs of medical students was a Himalayan task. The idea is to equip the medical students with adequate knowledge in pediatrics in order to make them confident to shoulder the responsibilities concerned with preventive and curative pediatrics. Thus, it is hoped that the practitioners of pediatric medicine will benefit from this book.

We are confident that the book will serve the needs of medical students, especially at a time when the Medical Council of India (MCI) has made pediatrics as a major examination. Thus, the publication of the book is not only timely but also out of necessity.

The Indian Academy of Pediatrics would like to place on record its appreciation to the senior editors, chapter editors, contributors and staff members of Indian Academy of Pediatrics (IAP), Central Secretariat, for help rendered in the creation of this book and M/s Jaypee Brothers Medical Publishers (P) Ltd, New Delhi, India, for their excellent cooperation in bringing out the 1st edition at record time.

A Parthasarathy
PSN Menon
MKC Nair

Acknowledgments

We are indebted to the President and Members of the Executive Board 1997 of the *Indian Academy of Pediatrics (IAP)* for the initiation and completion of the project of bringing out the first-ever *IAP Textbook of Pediatrics* for the medical students and practitioners. We are also grateful to the successive Presidents and Members of the Executive Boards 1998–2018 for their encouragement in sustaining the project towards the publication of the 7th edition.

Our sincere appreciations go to the various contributors and editors, past and present teachers of pediatrics who have contributed to the 7th edition and made the "Himalayan task" of production of the current edition a reality by their precise and updated texts. The Academy is indebted to all contributors, and members of the Production Department of M/s Jaypee Brothers Medical Publishers (P) Ltd, New Delhi, India, for their dedication, devotion and hard work.

The new contributions to the 7th edition by Drs Remesh Kumar R, Krishna Mohan, Satvik Bansal, Swati Chacham, Rachna Pasi, Ruchi Rai, Abhay K Shah, Aparna Mukherjee, Anuj Singh, Rakesh Lodha, Digant D Shastri, Jaya Shankar Kaushik, Jagdish Prasad Goyal, Prawin Kumar, Moinak Sen, Neelam Mohan, Aditi Sinha, Anju Seth, Vijayalakshmi Bhatia, Santosh T Soans, Maninder Dhaliwal, Pallabh Chatterjee, Sunil Dutt Sharma, Kiran Aggarwal, P Ramachandran, Pooja Dewan and Anjali Tomar are gratefully acknowledged.

The secretarial and organizational support of the staff at the Central Office of Indian Academy of Pediatrics, Mumbai, Maharashtra, India, and the guidance, cooperation and coordination provided by Drs Digant D Shastri, Santosh T Soans and Remesh Kumar R are gratefully acknowledged.

Our grateful thanks are due to Mr Shaji Jacob Ninan, Kuwait for the assistance rendered to the Dr PSN Menon (Editor-in-Chief) in editing, scrutinizing and proofreading of the chapters. Our special thanks are due to Mr N Asokan and for assisting Dr MKC Nair (Editor-in-Chief) at Thiruvananthapuram.

We would like to make a special mention of Ms Kritika Dua (Senior Development Editor), M/s Jaypee Brothers Medical Publishers (P) Ltd, New Delhi, India, for her untiring coordination efforts with more than 250 authors and members of the editorial board. But for her outstanding harmonization, it would not have been possible to publish this edition on schedule.

Our sincere and grateful thanks go to Shri Jitendar P Vij (Group Chairman), Mr Ankit Vij (Managing Director), Mr MS Mani (Group President), Ms Chetna Malhotra Vohra (Associate Director–Content Strategy), Ms Pooja Bhandari (Production Head), and other members of M/s Jaypee Brothers Medical Publishers (P) Ltd, New Delhi, India, for their untiring coordination efforts in the production of the 7th edition.

All attempts have been made to acknowledge the sources of information and illustrations. Inadvertent omission, if any, is regretted.

Editorial Board

Contents

SECTION 4 NUTRITION 159–216

SECTION 5 IMMUNITY, IMMUNIZATION AND INFECTIOUS DISEASES 217–418

SECTION 6 DISEASES OF CENTRAL NERVOUS SYSTEM 419–554

SECTION 7 DISEASES OF CARDIOVASCULAR SYSTEM 555–618

SECTION 8 DISEASES OF RESPIRATORY SYSTEM 619–666

SECTION 9 DISEASES OF GASTROINTESTINAL SYSTEM AND LIVER 667–792

SECTION 10 DISEASES OF KIDNEY AND URINARY TRACT 793–856

SECTION 11 DISEASES OF BLOOD 857–948

SECTION 12 PEDIATRIC MALIGNANCIES 949–988

SECTION 13 ENDOCRINOLOGY 989–1054

SECTION 14 GENETICS 1055–1100

SECTION 15 ADOLESCENT HEALTH 1101–1126

SECTION 19 COMMUNITY PEDIATRICS 1337–1404

SECTION 20 PEDIATRIC PROCEDURES 1405–1434

SECTION 21 PEDIATRIC THERAPEUTICS 1435–1530

Section 1

Basic Concepts of Child Care

1.1 Pediatrics: Yesterday, Today, and Tomorrow

YK Amdekar

INTRODUCTION

Care, survival, and development of children have always been our concern. The government of India and Indian Academy of Pediatrics (IAP) has undertaken several projects over last few decades to improve health of children, and it is time to introspect their impact on the ultimate goal.

DEMOGRAPHY

Due to a rapid rise in the population in India, which stands at 1.3 billion at present, there exists a shortage of health personnel and facilities. Though there has been a steady decline in infant mortality rate to 41/1,000 live births [National Family Health Survey (NFHS)-4, 2015–2016] *as compared to* 57 (2005–2006), and under NFHS-5, mortality rate to 50/1,000 live births *as compared to* 74 (2005–2006), it is still high and neonatal mortality rate has not changed much over years and is still stagnant at 28/1,000 live births. It means reduction in infant mortality is largely contributed by better performance in infants beyond the neonatal age of 28 days. Breastfeeding is initiated within first hour only in 41.6% of neonates and exclusive breastfeeding in first 6 months is practiced in 54.9% of infants. It suggests that there is a steady improvement in the abovementioned indicators, but it is still long way before we achieve our goals. Only 50% infants are on timely introduction of complementary feeds. This has not changed much over last few years. More than 60% of children do visit health facilities for common illnesses but even then, 35.7% (42.5% in *NFHS-3*) have remained underweight, 38.4% stunted, 21% wasted, 58.5% anemic with 5% having severe anemia. About 2–3% of children under 3 years of age suffer from acute severe malnutrition with 20–30% mortality in this group. Despite availability of free vaccines in Expanded Program on Immunization (EPI) program, there is *some* change over last decade in the number of fully vaccinated children that stands at 62%. Similarly, only 50.6% children use oral rehydration solution (ORS) during diarrheal episodes. Thus, health indices have *improved in* the last decade *but still need much more improvement.* It suggests that medical and paramedical personnel do not follow standard simple, cost-effective preventive measures, despite contact opportunity with the community.

DISEASE PROFILE

In the 1960s and 1970s, antibiotics and vaccines appeared to have controlled infectious diseases. However, infectious diseases have returned with a vengeance. Tripartite interaction between environment, microbes, and host status decides the outcome of infectious disease. There is a complex struggle for survival between humans and microbes, and microbes are exploiting the human behavior. Early and frequent exposures to infections, varying nutritional and immune status, lifestyle changes, global travel, and misuse of antibiotics have contributed to resurgence of old infections. Microbes have an inherent ability to mutate, change virulence, and acquire resistance to antibiotics. This has made the battle against infections more difficult. In addition, new organisms are being recognized. Forty new microbes have been recognized over the last 30 years. They include viruses such as rotavirus, Ebola virus, hantavirus, parvovirus B19, human T-lymphotropic viruses, types 1 and 2, hepatitis C and E, H5N1 avian strain of influenza, severe acute respiratory syndrome (SARS), human metapneumovirus, H1N1 swine reassortant influenza, bacteria such as *Legionella, Campylobacter jejuni,* toxin-producing staphylococci and streptococci, *Borrelia, Helicobacter pylori,* and parasites such as *Cryptosporidium* and *Cyclospora.* Changing epidemiology has been observed in dengue fever, leptospirosis, brucellosis, and rickettsial fever. Due to a breakdown in public health measures, there is resurgence of malaria and tuberculosis (TB). Coinfection with human immunodeficiency virus (HIV) has worsened the scenario of TB. Many malignant conditions are now being attributed to an infectious agent. Hepatocellular carcinoma induced by hepatitis B and C infections and cervical cancer due to human papilloma virus are some of the examples of infection-related malignancy. Many diseases of unknown etiology (Kawasaki syndrome, sarcoidosis, and diabetes) are suspected to be induced by infections.

Infections caused by antibiotic-resistant organisms are on the increase. Multidrug-resistant *Staphylococcus aureus*, first detected in 1961 in the United Kingdom, is now known both in nosocomial and community settings. *Streptococcus pneumoniae* has become resistant to penicillin almost all over the world; surprisingly, penicillin sensitivity is still maintained in India. Problem of resistance is mainly due to the misuse of antibiotics in human as well as veterinary medicine and also due to genetic mutation by bacteria. Empirical use of antibiotics, nonadherence to standard protocols by physicians, and noncompliant therapy by patients resulted in multidrug-resistant TB (MRTB), malaria, and typhoid in the community. "ESKAPE" pathogens are problem pathogens—*Enterococcus*, *S. aureus*, *Klebsiella*, *Acinetobacter*, *Pseudomonas*, and *Enterobacteriaceae* species—and are difficult to eradicate. In addition, methicillin and vancomycin-resistant *S. aureus*, coagulase-negative *staphylococci*, penicillin-resistant *pneumococci*, macrolide-resistant *streptococci*, multidrug-resistant *Salmonella* and *Shigella*, and extended spectrum beta-lactamase producing *enterococci* and *Acinetobacter* are also being reported more frequently.

Noninfective illnesses such as lifestyle diseases leading to metabolic syndrome consisting of hypertension, coronary heart disease and diabetes, asthma, malignancy, autism spectrum disorders, metabolic disorders, and immune deficiency disorders are being increasingly recognized. With a threat of epidemic of obesity, dual burden of malnutrition poses a stiff challenge.

It has been realized that vitamin D deficiency exists in significant proportion in all age groups despite the abundance of sunlight. This is because most children and adults are not exposed to sunlight due to change in lifestyle. Vitamin D deficiency has been attributed to recurrent infections, along with many other ailments being ascribed to it. Vitamin B12 deficiency is being reported especially in vegetarian families. Iron deficiency is universal in most of the children and women.

TECHNOLOGICAL ADVANCES

Etiological diagnosis of infections is possible today with modern culture techniques, such as BACTEC and polymerase chain reaction (PCR). Reversed transcription PCR is for amplification of ribonucleic acid (RNA), and real-time PCR allows quantitative measurement of deoxyribonucleic acid (DNA) or RNA. Southern blot is a method of probing a specific DNA sequence in a DNA sample. Western blot measures the antibodies against a specific protein as for HIV diagnosis. Gene therapy introducing a functional gene into a host genome, replacing abnormal gene, has been successful in cystic fibrosis, hemophilia, sickle-cell disease, and muscular dystrophy. Transfer of genes in brain using liposomes may prove to be useful for degenerative brain disorders. Inborn errors of metabolism can be diagnosed with certainty at birth, and cost-effective screening of common metabolic disorders is now feasible.

Availability of several immunological tests have opened new vista to diagnose otherwise fatal immune deficiency disorders. Imaging modalities have improved tremendously. Ultrasonography (USG) has undergone great advances over last five decades. Color Doppler, digital subtraction angiography, and transesophageal USG are some of the newer modalities. Computed tomography and magnetic resonance imaging (MRI) give anatomical diagnosis, while positron-emission tomography scan offers metabolic or functional profile. Many advances have taken place for better resolution and clarity, such as diffusion MRI scan, fluid-attenuated inversion recovery (FLAIR) image, MR angiography, and MR spectroscopy. Molecular diagnosis is increasingly available for many diseases though mutations are being recognized. Thus, negative molecular test may not completely rule out a specific disease as not all mutations have been known to science.

ADVANCES IN CURATIVE AND PREVENTIVE MANAGEMENT

Following a 40-year hiatus in discovering new classes of antibacterial compounds, three new classes of antibiotics have been brought into clinical use: (1) Cyclic lipopeptides (daptomycin), (2) glycylcyclines (tigecycline), and (3) oxazolidinones (linezolid). Bedaquiline and delamanid have been recently included in the treatment of MDRTB, and few other compounds are being researched. Other "new" antibiotics are merely chemically modified old molecules. With increasing antibiotic resistance, "phage" therapy needs to be revived.

Better drugs and improved understanding of their usage has modified outcome of malignant diseases. While minimal invasive surgery is fast replacing conventional open surgery, interventional radiology and cardiology provide better alternative to surgery in many conditions. Liver or kidney transplants are now available for such end-stage diseases, in addition to bone marrow transplant and heart transplant. Stem cell therapy is yet in infancy though many centers have come up with facility to bank stem cells collected right at birth. However, stem cells are required to be stored for even decades, and it is not sure whether such centers have adequate infrastructure for the same.

The 20th century saw development of many new vaccines. One-third infectious disease mortality can be prevented by vaccination. Indian EPI program covers only seven diseases unlike 12 or more diseases covered in national programs of many developed countries. Though a greater number of vaccines are being made available by the government in selective states, such as rotaviral vaccine, many newer vaccines are available in open market. Combination vaccines such as Hexaxim contain six vaccines in one injection. Poor coverage of susceptible population and non-affordability of non-EPI vaccines are the major hurdles. It is heartening that polio eradication efforts are nearing success. Till date, there has been just a single case of wild poliomyelitis reported in India in 2011. The time has come to phase out the oral polio vaccine (OPV) slowly over next few years and replace with inactivated polio vaccine (IPV). After eradication of smallpox from the world and polio from most of the countries of the world—including India, focus now has shifted to the eradication of measles. It may take several years before it is achieved mainly due to the logistic issues that are even more challenging than what we faced in polio eradication.

CHANGE IN CLINICAL PRACTICE

Before the advent of modern science, physicians healed their patients with commitment, concern, and compassion. They treated the child and family, not just the disease. As science developed, physicians started treating disease and not the child. Subsequently, they have learnt to treat diagnostic tests and not disease. Thus, modern clinical practice revolves around diagnostic tests, often without clinical correlation. Unfortunately, scientific advances have not translated into better health indices or quality of life for children at large. This is mainly because majority of children need simple approach to their common problems. Modern science cannot replace basic clinical bedside methods. For example, Kangaroo care and exclusive breastfeeding will save far more neonates than mechanical ventilation and modern facilities. ORS has saved many lives. Nutritional advice, growth monitoring, and immunization will contribute to better quality of life. Hence, priority in clinical practice should be implementation of basic care, and modern advances should be reserved only for most indicated situations.

CHANGE IN EDUCATIONAL REFORMS

Before the era of superspecialization and technological advance, pediatricians were well trained in the basics in clinical medicine. While superspecialization is a boon, it is expected that superspecialist is an excellent generalist. New generation of pediatrician has a challenging task of keeping abreast to scientific advances, but it should not be at the expense of basics. National Board of Examination has modified examination pattern that tests the candidates more thoroughly in actual life situations and hence training also has been suitably modified. This has been a better step forward in pediatric education.

PEDIATRICIANS MUST CHANGE

We need to change the focus from disease to health. We must combine the traditional wisdom with modern science. IAP has formulated guidelines for standard management of many common diseases that should be followed meticulously. Constant updating is necessary to keep up with the scientific advances, and they should be used selectively. Science will undergo frequent changes as nothing is constant, and ignorance is far more than knowledge. Hence, we need to learn, unlearn, and relearn.

BIBLIOGRAPHY

1. Cavazzana-Calvo M, Thrasher A, Mavilio F. The future of gene therapy. Nature. 2004;427(6977):779-81.
2. Gupta P, Shah D, Sachdev HP, et al. National workshop on development of guidelines for effective home based care and treatment of children suffering from severe acute malnutrition. Indian Pediatr. 2008;43:131-9.
3. National Family Health Survey. National Family Health Survey-4 (2015-16). [online] Available from http://rchiips.org/NFHS/factsheet_NFHS-4.html. [Accessed September, 2018].

1.2 History Elicitation

T Ravikumar

INTRODUCTION

The clinical interview and history elicitation are very important tools in the field of pediatric medicine. Though it is of much diagnostic value, the process of interaction with the parents and the child during history taking also has a therapeutic value. A pleasant and patient interaction is what any parent desires. There should be fewer distractions during the interview. It is good to use lay terms when talking to the parents and avoid medical terminologies as far as possible. While interviewing, the pediatrician should also observe the child to look for any clinical clues.

In pediatrics, the most important and distinct aspect is the fact that the person giving the history is usually not the patients (unless the child is about 4 or 5 years old). The parents are the usual source of information and, in certain cases, when caretakers (other than the parents) are bringing up the children, then they will be the source of information.

DEMOGRAPHY

Make a note of the name of the child, his or her age in years (with months and days), parents' names, address, date, and time of interview, informant's name and relationship to child, and their reliability (regarding the consistency of the information they provide).

Presenting Complaints

The main problem or complaint for which the child has been brought for medical attention should be recorded in the informant's own terms and should be recorded in chronological order with the duration of each complaint.

For example:

- Fever, 5 days
- Vomiting, 4 days
- Loose motions, 4 days
- Decreased urine output, 2 days
- Lethargy, 1 day
- Fast breathing, 1 day

HISTORY OF PRESENT ILLNESS

It is important to gather more information and elaborate on the specific presenting complaints. Find out the onset of the complaints (the time up to which the child was apparently well). The evolution of the problems should then flow in a clear, concise, temporal sequence, leading up to the present moment. They should be recorded in order of occurrence, and an account of any repeated episodes of symptoms (such as seizures or respiratory infections) should be given. Symptoms pertaining to complications expected for the presenting complaint, other symptoms that will help in detecting associated conditions and in differential diagnosis should be enquired. The details of treatment given so far and the response should be noted.

PAST HISTORY

Ask for the details of relevant past illness, knowledge of which will help you in diagnosis or management. History of occurrence of similar complaints in the past should be noted. For example, in a child with chronic suppurative lung disease or malnutrition, a history of previous exanthematous illness or whooping cough will help; in failure to thrive, a history of recurrent diarrhea; and in a child with fever and seizures, a history of febrile fits will be supportive. Past medication history will also be helpful, e.g. history of antiepileptic drugs or antituberculous (TB) drugs [history of red urine (rifampicin) while on treatment with anti-TB drugs]. Information on previous significant hospitalization, accident, or surgeries may also be helpful.

CONTACT HISTORY

History of contact with communicable diseases (e.g. TB and chickenpox) must be elicited with tact and patience. It is often denied and repeated probing with leading questions may be necessary.

ANTENATAL HISTORY

As many illnesses in children have their origin in the womb, it is important to get a good history about the period of pregnancy of the index child. A good guide for history elicitation would be the mnemonic of the three "Is" for the mother during pregnancy—illness, irradiation, and injections (i.e. drugs). Maternal illness such as syphilis, toxoplasmosis, acquired immune deficiency syndrome, rubella, cytomegalovirus, and herpes virus infections are associated with specific syndromes in the child. Folic acid supplementation during early pregnancy (the first trimester) prevents neural tube defects such as meningomyelocele.

BIRTH HISTORY

The actual events occurring during delivery must be enquired. The period of gestation, duration of labor, nature of delivery, drugs administered during labor, and any complications during delivery (such as cord around neck, low Apgar score) should be noted. The duration of every stage of labor (especially the second stage) is important as prolonged labor may result in fetal hypoxia. The normal first stage of labor, from the onset of labor pains to the rupture of membranes, is about 12–24 hours and 6–12 hours in a primigravida and multigravida, respectively. The second stage of labor, from the rupture of membranes to the delivery of the child, is about 1–2 hours in a primigravida and 0.5–1 hour in a multigravida. The third stage, which is the delivery of the placenta, lasts about 15 minutes.

POSTNATAL HISTORY

The neonate and its state after birth should be enquired. The term of the child, birth weight, cry, activity, and color immediately after birth should be noted. Presence of jaundice or cyanosis, resuscitation steps used (if any), and whether hospitalized after birth must be detailed. Poor cry and lethargy suggest perinatal depression. Paucity of movements of one side or a limb may suggest stroke or birth injury. The sucking effort of a child after delivery usually gives a clue to the neurological status of the child. All infants pass meconium within the first 24 hours; any delay would suggest cystic fibrosis, while absence of passage would indicate intentional obstruction or anal atresia. Most infants' void urine on the first day while all will void within 48 hour; any delay would point toward an obstruction or agenesis of the renal system.

DEVELOPMENT HISTORY

Development is one aspect of pediatrics that makes it unique as compared to adult medicine. The developmental milestones that a child attains are a good reflection of its physical and neurological maturity. They may be divided into gross motor (head control, rolling over, crawling, sitting, standing, walking, etc.), fine motor or adaptive (grasping reaching transferring object, scribbling, etc.), social (smile, recognition, response to calls, etc.), and language (cooing, babbling, saying syllables, vocabulary, etc.). Tailor the development history to the child's age. In the case of more than one child in the family, and if the other siblings are normal, the parents may be asked if the index child's development mirrored that of the other siblings. The pace of development differs from child to child. As the child grows older, the age range of attainment of specific developmental milestones usually widens. For example, a normal child may begin to sit without support between 5 months and 8 months as compared to a normal young infant developing social smile between 6 weeks and 8 weeks. Notice the range of normality becoming more in the older child. Always tabulate the attained milestones against the normal age for attainment of that milestone **(Table 1.2.1)**.

DIETETIC HISTORY

This history is highly problem-oriented and age-dependent. Details of the food and dietary patterns help in diagnosing protein-energy malnutrition and failure to thrive. In addition, it helps us to formulate a diet plan for nutritional rehabilitation of the child for a specific disease. The calculation of the dietary values of the food consumed should provide the actual value of proteins, calories, and fats and must mention whether it is sufficient in vitamins, minerals, and other micronutrients. Always state the approximate number of calories and proteins the child is getting for that age as compared to what is recommended **(Table 1.2.2)** which will help us to calculate the calorie and protein gap. Any problem such as feeding difficulty, regurgitation, or vomiting should be noted. Any possible natural toxins in the food consumed (fungal aflatoxins, copper, etc.) and feeding patterns during times of illness should also be mentioned. In young children, the complete breastfeeding history, including whether colostrum was given, duration of exclusive breastfeeding, weaning pattern, etc., must be elucidated. In children fed with other milk, it is important to note its dilution, mode of feeding (bottle-fed or cup and spoon-fed), frequency, and the amount consumed during each feeding.

FAMILY HISTORY

The health details of all the family members must be obtained. This includes their gender, present and past health status, treatment taken, and their proximity to the child. History of similar illness in the family must be looked for. History of stillbirths or abortions in the family should be noted (habitual abortions occur in maternal syphilis). The birth of abnormal children or children with illness in the family and the reasons for death, if any, of children or young adults in the family should be specifically enquired into. The consanguinity pattern with the degree of relationship may

Table 1.2.1: Normal developmental milestones.

Milestones	*Gross motor*	*Fine motor*	*Personal social*	*Language*
First month	Grasp reflex	Starts to smile		
Second month		Hands closed	Social smile	Cooing
Third month	Head mostly held up but still bobs forward	Hand open most often	Sustained social smile	Says "Aah"
Fourth month	Head held steady	Reaches for objects, grasps objects, and brings to mouth, hands in midline	Excited at sight of food	Laughs out aloud
Seventh month	Rolls over, creeping–crawling, sits with hands leaning forward	Reaches out and grasps larger objects, palmar grasp, transfers objects from hand to hand	Smiles at mirror	Babbling
Tenth month	Sits without support, cruises	Pincer grasp	Waves bye-bye	Says "Baba, mama"

Contd...

Contd…

Milestones	***Gross motor***	***Fine motor***	***Personal social***	***Language***
One year	Walks with one hand held	Releases objects to other person on request/gesture	Plays simple ball game	Says 2–3 words with meaning
Fifteen months	Walks alone, crawls upstairs	Makes tower of three cubes	Asks for objects by pointing	Follows simple commands
Eighteen months	Runs stiff, goes upstairs by holding the rails	Makes tower of four cubes, initiates vertical stroke scribbles	Feeds self. Dry by day	Speaks 10 words, identifies parts of the body
Two years	Runs well, walks upstairs and downstairs one foot at a time, jumps	Makes tower of seven cubes, initiates horizontal stoke	Handless spoon well and helps to undress	Puts sentence of three words
Two and half years	Goes upstairs with alternating feet	Makes tower of nine cubes	Helps put things away	Knows full name
Three years	Rides tricycle, stands momentarily on one foot	Draws circle, tower of 10 cubes, constructs bridge or three cubes	Dresses and undresses fully when helped with buttons, joins in play	Knows age and gender
Four years	Hops on one foot, throws ball overhead, climbs well	Draws cross and square, copies a bridge, constructs a gate of five cubes	Plays with several children with beginning of social interaction, goes to toilet alone	Tells story
Five years	Skips	Draws triangle	Dresses and undresses self. Asks question about meaning of words	Names 4 colors, repeats sentence of 10 syllables

Table 1.2.2: The recommended caloric and protein requirements.

Age	***Calories required/day***	***Protein/day***
1 month to 1 year	100–110 kcal/kg/day	2 g/day
1 year	1,000 kcal/day	20 g/day
2 years	1,100 kcal/day	20 g/day
3 years	1,200 kcal/day	20 g/day
4 years	1,300 kcal/day	30 g/day
5 years	1,400 kcal/day	30 g/day
6 years	1,500 kcal/day	30 g/day
7 years	1,600 kcal/day	40 g/day
8 years	1,700 kcal/day	40 g/day
9 years	1,800 kcal/day	40 g/day
10 years	1,900 kcal/day	40 g/day
11 years	2,000 kcal/day	50 g/day
12 years	2,100 kcal/day	50 g/day
Adolescent boy	2,500–3,000 kcal/day	70 g/day
Adolescent girl	2,200–2,400 kcal/day	65 g/day

be helpful for genetic disorders. The pedigree chart will help record the family history in a pictorial manner helping us to derive the inheritance pattern of an illness. Usually, three full generations should be recorded. Individuals of the same generations should be recorded in the same horizontal line and numbered from left to right using Arabic numerals. Males are usually placed on the left side of the pedigree and sibship listed in both orders. The maternal age at the time of child delivery is also important. Young mothers (less than 18 years) have more chances of preterm, intrauterine growth restriction babies, while older mothers (>32 years) have more chances of having children with Down syndrome and Klinefelter syndrome. In children with disease showing hereditary traits, an enquiry of a much wider circle of relatives must be made **(Tables 1.2.3 and 1.2.4)**.

SOCIOECONOMIC HISTORY

This has a bearing on the type of disease the child might be suffering from, and it also helps in planning rehabilitation and treatment options, in addition to helping in giving preventive advice. The following points are worth noting:

- *Type of family:* Joint or nuclear
- Occupation and employment history
- Per capita income (total income divided by the number or dependent family members)
- Type of housing, ventilation, toilet, and potable water facilities
- Psychiatric illness and substance abuse (alcoholism, drugs) in the family
- Marital stability
- Traditional beliefs and child-rearing practices.

IMMUNIZATION HISTORY

It is important to record the details of vaccines given to the child in chronological order. The vaccination schedule of the Indian Academy of Pediatrics or at least the Universal Immunization Program should be followed. Special vaccines

Table 1.2.3: Protein requirement and recommended dietary allowances.

For infants, boys, and girls age group	*Requirement (g protein/kg/day)*	*Body weight (kg)*	*Total daily requirement (g protein/day)*	*Requirement (g protein/kg/day)*	*Body weight (kg)*	*Total daily requirement (g protein/day)*
Infants (months)						
6–9	1.69	7.9	13.4			
9–12	1.69	8.8	14.9			
Preschool children (years)		*Boys*			*Girls*	
1–2	1.47	10.3	15.1	1.47	9.6	14.1
2–3	1.25	12.8	16.0	1.25	12.1	15.1
3–4	1.16	14.8	17.2	1.16	14.5	16.8
4–5	1.11	16.5	18.3	1.11	16.0	17.8
School children (years)		*Boys*			*Girls*	
5–6	1.09	18.2	19.8	1.09	17.7	19.3
6–7	1.15	20.4	23.5	1.15	20.0	23.0
7–8	1.17	22.7	26.6	1.17	22.3	26.1
8–9	1.18	25.2	29.7	1.18	25.0	29.5
9–10	1.18	28.0	33.0	1.18	27.6	32.6
Adolescents (years)		Boys			Girls	
10–11	1.18	30.8	36.3	1.18	31.2	36.8
11–12	1.16	34.1	39.6	1.15	34.8	40.0
12–13	1.15	38.0	43.7	1.14	39.0	44.5
13–14	1.15	43.3	49.8	1.13	43.4	49.0
14–15	1.14	48.0	54.7	1.12	47.1	52.8
15–16	1.13	51.5	58.2	1.09	49.4	53.8
16–17	1.12	54.3	60.8	1.07	51.3	54.9
17–18	1.10	56.5	62.2	1.06	52.8	56.0

Table 1.2.4: Calorie requirement and recommended dietary allowances.

Infants	0–6 months 6–12 months	5.4 8.4	500 670	92 80
Children	1–3 years	12.9	1,060	82
	4–6 years	18.1	1,350	75
	7–9 years	25.1	1,690	67
Boys	10–12 years	34.3	2,190	64
Girls	10–12 years	35.0	2,010	57
Boys	13–15 years	47.6	2,750	58
Girls	13–15 years	46.6	2,330	50
Boys	16–17 years	55.4	3,020	55
Girls	16–17 years	52.1	2,440	47

Source: ICMR. National Requirements and Recommended Dietary Allowances for Indians: A Report of the Expert Group of the Indian Council of Medical Research. Hyderabad: National Institute of Nutrition, ICMR; 2009.

(e.g. pulse polio vaccine) must also be enquired. Look for Bacillus Calmette Guerin scar at the outer aspect of the left arm at the insertion of the deltoid. If any vaccine has not been given, note the reason for not doing so.

HISTORY OF ALLERGIES

It is important to note down any known, specific drug or food allergies in the child.

BIBLIOGRAPHY

1. Barness LA. Pediatric history and physical examination. In: McMillan JA, DeAngelis CD, Feigin RD (Eds). Oski's pediatrics: principles and practice, 3rd ed. Philadelphia, PA: JB Lippincott Williams and Wilkins; 1999. pp. 39-52.
2. Gupta P. Clinical methods in pediatrics, 4th edition. New Delhi: CBS Publishers; 2017.
3. Harris R. The examination of children. In: Swash M (Ed). Hutchison's clinical methods, 20th edition. London: ELBS-WB Saunders Co.; 1995. pp. 365-86.
4. Rees PE. Evaluating the newborn infant: diagnostic approach. In: Pediatric clinical skills, 2nd edition. Philadelphia, PA: Churchill Livingstone; 1997. pp. 47-76.

1.3 Physical Examination

C Thangadorai

INTRODUCTION

The physical examination in a child is distinct in certain areas from that of an adult. In this discussion, only the facts that differ from that of an adult examination have been stated. As far as possible, no child should cry or get irritated while you are examining. *If a child cries when you examine it, then it is probably your fault.* This statement by John Apley sums up the care one should take while handling the child. Physical examination starts as the child and the attendant walk into the room. Even while eliciting history, an observant eye needs to be kept on the child to watch for clinical clues. There is no definite order to be followed while examining a child. Individualize the examination for every child. Do the invasive and potentially discomforting examinations at the end. Allow the child to be in its most comfortable position and place it in the mother's lap. Both the child and the mother must feel secure and confident about the examining doctor.

GENERAL EXAMINATION

Before starting general examination, analyze the history, and based on that, look for the specific features that would be relevant to the history which will help you to give a perfect diagnosis. Examining aimlessly is unhelpful, time consuming, and irritating to the child and parents. In general, examination must be thorough from head to foot. Always examine the child's throat irrespective of the complaint. The golden rule is *head to foot and back, but forget not the ear, throat, and urine.* The sensorium (e.g., stupor or unconscious in intracranial pathology), posture and attitude (e.g. frog-like and limp in a floppy infant), activity (e.g. apathetic in kwashiorkor), looks (e.g. acutely or chronically ill looking), and nutrition (i.e. marasmus, undernourished, or moderately nourished) need special mention.

Note the shape of the head **(Fig. 1.3.1)**, whether microcephaly, macrocephaly, plagiocephaly (asymmetrical due to lying of the normal infants with their heads persistently on one side), scaphocephaly [boat shaped with increased anteroposterior (AP) diameter due to premature closure of the sagittal suture], brachycephaly (decreased AP diameter), and oxycephaly (tower-shaped skull).

The size of the anterior fontanel (AF) (normal of about 2.5 cm × 2.5 cm) must be measured across the borders as shown in **Figure 1.3.2**. It normally closes by 9–18 months. Delayed closure is seen in rickets, hypothyroidism, hydrocephalus, Down syndrome, achondroplasia, and mucopolysaccharidosis. The AF in a quiet child usually shows a very slight depression from the surface and may pulsate. It is bulging when the child cries, and in hydrocephalus, intracranial hypertension, and pseudotumor cerebri (i.e., after drugs such as nalidixic acid, tetracyclines and steroids, and hypervitaminosis A). A sunken fontanel is a sign of dehydration. The posterior fontanel can be felt by running the finger along the sagittal suture to its junction with the lambdoid suture. It normally closes by 2–4 months of age. Ridging and overriding of sutures may normally be seen in the first few hours after birth, due to molding of the skull during delivery. It may also be seen in craniostenosis due to premature fusion of the sutures. Sutures normally get ossified by 6 months of age **(Fig. 1.3.3)**.

The Macewen's sign is useful in clinically detecting raised intracranial tension after the sutures have closed. It is the crack pot sound elicited by the percussion of the skull. Transillumination of the skull in a dark room is useful

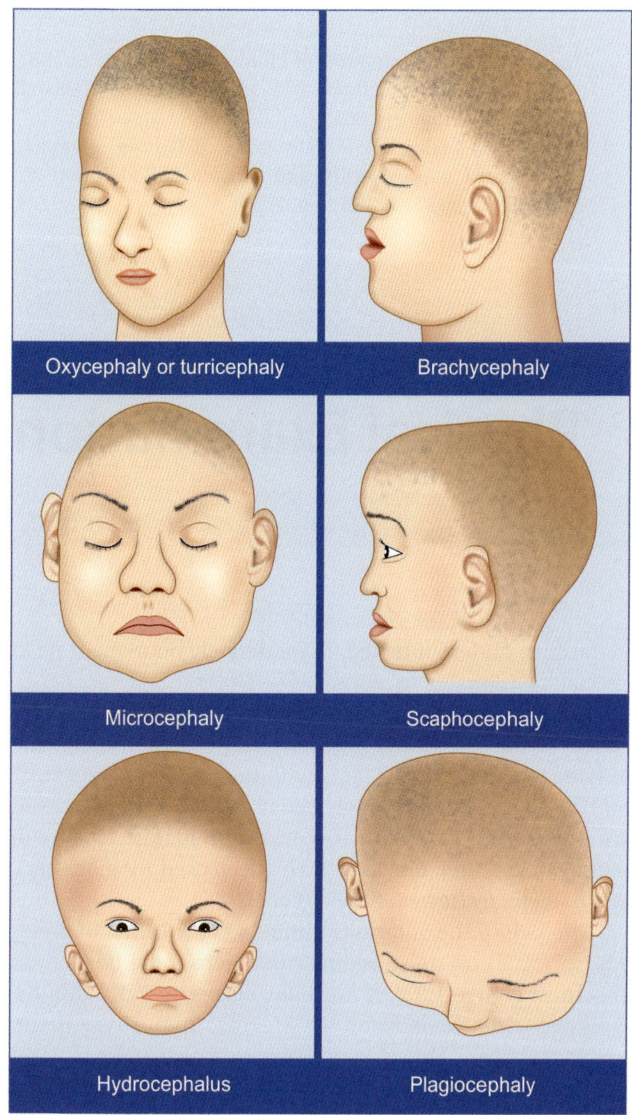

Fig. 1.3.1: The different shapes of the head.

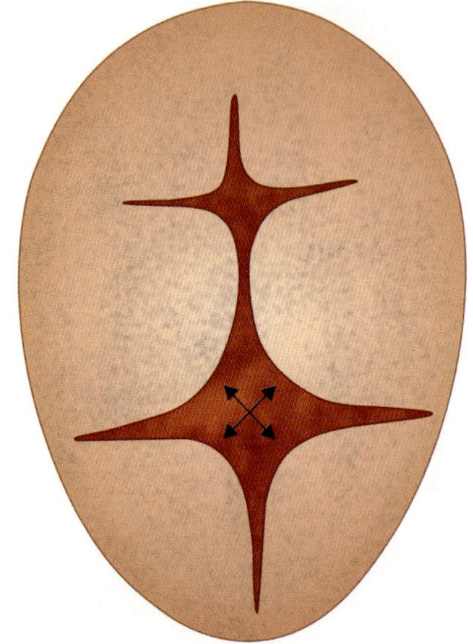

Fig. 1.3.2: The method of measuring the anterior fontanelle size.

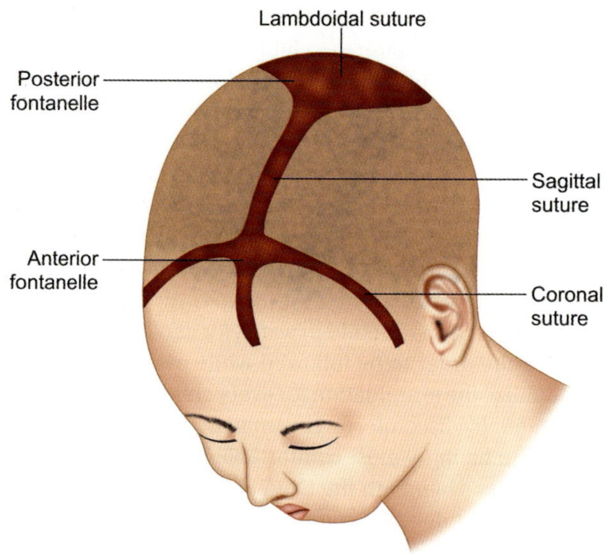

Fig. 1.3.3: The different cranial sutures at birth.

in children below 1 year, to detect subdural effusion or hematoma, if the translucency extends beyond 2 cm in the frontal and 1 cm in the occipital region.

The face must be observed for any dysmorphic features that may suggest chromosomal or developmental anomalies.

Table 1.3.1 shows some common abnormal features and a few conditions where they are seen. The interpalpebral line of the eyes, when continued horizontally backwards, normally divides the ears into the upper one third and the lower two thirds. If the line passes above the ears, it is suggestive of low set ears. The neck should be examined for lymph node enlargement, short neck (normal neck length:height ratio is 1:13), and low hairline (below C5). The examination should also include the hair (e.g. pale hair with "flag sign" in kwashiorkor), eyes (signs of vitamin A deficiency, icterus, pallor, etc.), ears (examine tympanic membrane for acute otitis media or chronic suppurative otitis media), oral cavity (with special reference to the dentition), extremities (limb deformities in skeletal dysplasia, widened wrists in rickets), nails (koilonychia in anemia), and skin (for pallor, icterus, scabies, impetigo, etc.). Fundus examination is important to make out papilledema, optic atrophy, or retinitis pigmentosa. The mouth is examined for the state of the gums, dental caries, and dentition. Delayed dentition may be familial or due to rickets or osteogenesis imperfecta.

Table 1.3.1: Some features to be looked for in the head and their associated conditions.

Features	***Important associated conditions***
Microcephaly	Familial, craniostenosis, intrauterine infections, trisomy 13 and 21 (Down syndrome)
Macrocephaly	Hydrocephalus, hydranencephaly, porencephaly, some neurodegenerative disorders such as metachromatic leukodystrophy, Alexander and Canavan disease, certain intrauterine infections
Frontal bossing	Rickets, congenital syphilis, mucopolysaccharidoses
Craniotabes (ping-pong skull)	Physiological (in preterm), rickets, congenital syphilis
Increased interpupillary distance (hypertelorism)	Genetic (racial), Down syndrome, Cri-du-chat syndrome, hypothyroidism
Proptosis (sclera is visible above and below the cornea)	Thyrotoxicosis, orbital leukemic deposits, orbital cellulites, arteriovenous aneurysm (pulsatile), cavernous sinus thrombosis, neurofibromatosis, Crouzon disease
Cataract	Idiopathic, traumatic, intrauterine infections, galactosemia, diabetes mellitus, Down syndrome
Mongoloid eyes (upward slant)	Down syndrome, racial, Prader-Willi syndrome
Antimongoloid slant (downward slant)	Turner syndrome, Cri-du-chat syndrome, Treacher-Collins syndrome
Depressed nasal bridges	Down syndrome, mucopolysaccharidoses, hypothyroidism, familial
Low set ears	Down syndrome, mucopolysaccharidoses, Turner syndrome, Potter facies (renal agenesis)
Facial puffiness	Renal disorder, kwashiorkor, congestive cardiac failures, angioneurotic edema, cavernous sinus thrombosis
Large tongue	Hypothyroidism, mucopolysaccharidoses, glycogen storage disorders, Down syndrome (relative)
Small mandible	Pierre Robin syndrome
Short neck	Turner syndrome, Down syndrome, mucopolysaccharidoses, hypothyroidism

The correct position for doing the ear, nose, and throat examination is shown in **Figure 1.3.4**, but this should be done preferably at the last. While examining lymph nodes, note the site, size, consistency, tenderness, warmth, matting, and scarring. Always remember to examine the drainage areas, for focus of sepsis, if there is any significant lymph node enlargement. In older children, discrete and nontender lymph node enlargement up to 1.5 cm in the cervical and inguinal region may not be significant.

The skin is examined **(Fig. 1.3.5)** by rolling a fold of loosely adherent skin on the abdominal wall between the thumb and forefinger to determine its consistency, the amount of subcutaneous tissue present, and the degree of hydration. Examination of the hips must always be carried out in younger children and infants, to look for dislocation. The Ortolani or Barlow procedure is done, and the typical clunk of the hip moving in and out of its socket is looked for. Infants and younger children do not exhibit classical pedal edema as they are confined to bed; hence sacral edema should be looked for in them.

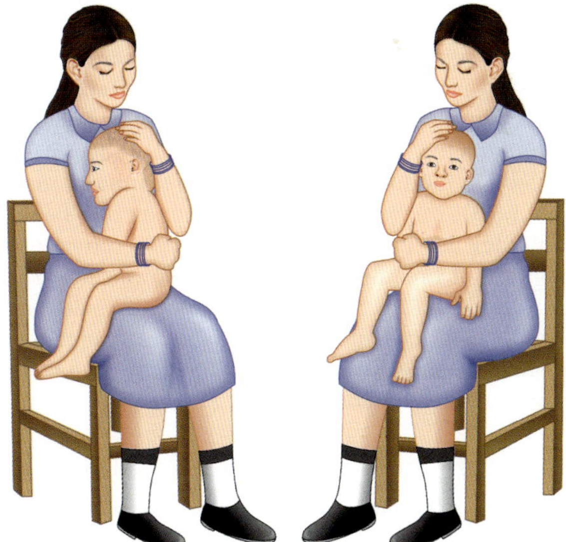

Fig. 1.3.4: Method of restraining a child for ENT examination. (ENT: ears, nose, and throat)

VITAL SIGNS

Temperature

Oral temperature should be taken in children older than 5 years, while in infants and younger children, the thermometer may be placed in the axilla. The groin or the rectum can also be used. The temperature in the axilla or the groin is about 0.5°C lower and the rectal temperature about 0.5°C higher than the oral temperature. The normal temperature in children is between 36.5°C and 37.5°C.

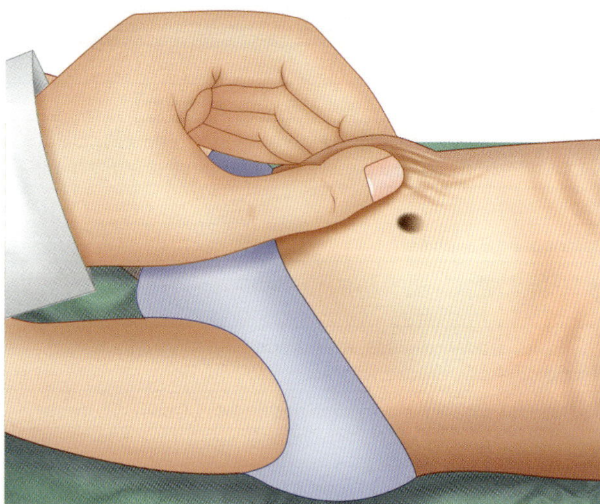

Fig. 1.3.5: Method of examining skin turgor in a child with dehydration.

Temperature above 41°C is hyperpyrexia. In conditions such as protein-energy malnutrition, where hypothermia is a problem, special low-reading thermometers (30–40°C) must be used.

Respiratory Rate

The rate of respiration in children is important for diagnosing respiratory disease and certain other nonrespiratory conditions such as acidosis and congestive cardiac failure. The rate varies in different age groups **(Table 1.3.2)**. However, for practical purposes, the guidelines offered in the reproductive and child health (RCH) program serve as a good guide to clinically suspect respiratory disease **(Table 1.3.3)**. The pattern of respiration must also be noted whether regular, irregular, Cheyne-Stokes respiration (the oscillation of breathing between apnea and hyperpnea with a crescendo-decrescendo pattern usually seen in the congestive cardiac failure, stages one and two, and rapid eye movement sleep), acidotic, etc. In children, the respiration is predominantly abdominothoracic.

Pulse Rate

The pulse is felt mainly over the radial artery at the wrist. The character, regularity, and volume must be observed. All the peripheral palpable vessels must be examined. The superficial temporal, carotid, brachial, radial, femoral, popliteal, posterior tibial, and dorsalis pedis arteries are easily accessible. In infants and very young children, it may not be possible to palpate the peripheral vessels, and in such situations, the heart rate must be counted by auscultation. The normal heart/pulse rates in the different age groups in children are given in **Table 1.3.4**. For practical purposes, heart rate more than 200/min in newborns, more than 150/min in infants, and more than 120/min in older children can be taken as significant tachycardia. The radial and femoral pulse must be palpated simultaneously to look for any radio-femoral delay. Remember, the heart rate in a struggling or crying child will be more.

Table 1.3.2: Normal respiratory rate in children of different age groups.

Age groups	*Normal respiratory rate (per minute)*
Newborn	40
1 year	30
5 years	20
10 years	18

Table 1.3.3: Tachypnea indicating significant respiratory disease (from Reproductive and Child Health program).

Age groups	*Normal respiratory rate (per minute)*
Below 2 months	60 or more
2–12 months	50 or more
12 months to 5 years	40 or more

Table 1.3.4: Normal heart rates in children of different age groups.

Age groups	*Normal heart rate (per minute)*
Newborn	140
1 year	110
3 years	100
8 years	90
10 years	80

Blood Pressure

Recording the blood pressure is one of the most important aspects in a pediatric examination. It is surprising, how often it is neglected. The correct size of the cuff must be used, i.e. the cuff should be two-thirds of the size of the arm. A large cuff will give an erroneously low reading, while a small cuff will give a high reading. In infants, the "flush method" may be used to check the pressure. Here, the child's arm is raised, and a tight bandage is applied up to the level of the cuff so as to empty the blood from the upper limb. Now, the cuff is inflated, and the bandage is removed so that the limb will be pale and bloodless. Deflate the cuff slowly and note the reading at which the skin flushes and the limb becomes red again. This corresponds approximately to the systolic pressure. In younger children, where auscultation at the cubital fossa is difficult, the systolic reading obtained by palpation may suffice. The Doppler technique of measuring blood pressure is more accurate and can be used in children, if available. For every pediatric examination, both the upper limb and lower limb pressures must be recorded to detect the coarctation of aorta, while in any child with a suspected cardiac illness, the pressure must be recorded in all four limbs. Normally, the pressure recorded in the lower limbs is about 10 mm Hg higher than the upper limbs. Reserve recording the pressure to the last in order not to irritate or scare the child. Normal blood pressure readings in children in the different age groups are given in **Table 1.3.5**. Normal blood pressure is defined as systolic and diastolic pressure, less than 90th percentile for that age and sex. Hypertension is defined as average systolic and/or diastolic blood pressure equal to or greater than the 95th percentile for that age and sex, on at least three occasions. As per the American Heart Association (pediatric advanced life support course) recommendations, a formula has been devised to calculate the 50th percentile of systolic pressure in children over the age of 2 years [90 + (2 × age in years)]. The lower limit of the systolic blood pressure has been approximated by the formula 70 + (2 × age in years). An observed fall of 10 mm Hg in systolic pressure suggests a shock.

Anthropometry

Measuring of various anthropometric data is essential for assessing the growth of the child and its nutritional status. It is also important for planning the diet and following up the child, especially while recuperating from an illness or during nutritional rehabilitation.

Weight

The child must be weighed during every examination. The weight of the child is also useful for calculating the right dosage of the drugs to be given. The newborn loses up to 10% of its weight during the first week but regains it in the next few days. The child doubles its birth weight by 4 months, triples it by 1 year, and increases it four times by 2 years. For calculating expected normal weight, the formula shown in **Table 1.3.5** may be used. While interpreting the weight of the child, the present weight must be compared to the expected weight for age, and the percentage must be calculated to find out which grade of nutrition the child falls under (as per **Tables 1.3.6 and 1.3.7**). Weight is recorded on a weighing scale which should be frequently checked with standard weights, and zero error must be adjusted before weighing.

Height

The height of the child is a good indicator of the chronicity of any debilitating illness. Height is ideally measured using Harpenden stadiometer. The child should stand against a wall with his bare feet touching each other, the heel, calf, buttock, upper back, and occiput touching the wall and the child looking straight ahead. A firm scale is pressed to the head to mark the point indicating height. The standing height can be measured for children more than 2 years old, while for younger children, the recumbent length should be measured using the infantometer **(Fig. 1.3.6)**.

In exceptions, such as a child with quadriplegic cerebral palsy where the height or length could not be measured, the length of various segments of the body is measured separately and added together to get the length. The formula shown in **Table 1.3.5** may be used for calculating the height for the age, or alternatively, the increase in height as shown in **Table 1.3.8** may be used for calculating the expected height.

While measuring the height, it is also important to measure the upper segment (from the vertex to the pubic symphysis) and the lower segment (from the pubic symphysis

Table 1.3.5: Formula for calculating expected normal weight.

Weight	*Kilograms*
At birth	3.25
3–12 months	(Age in months + 9)/2
1–6 years	(Age in years × 2) + 8
7–12 years	[(Age in years × 7) + 5]/2
Height	***Centimeters***
At birth	50
At 1 year	75
2–12 years	(Age in years × 6) + 77

Table 1.3.6: The Wellcome classification of nutritional status.

Nutritional status	*Expected weight for age (%)*	*Presence of edema*
Normal	More than 80	No
Undernutrition	60–80	No
Kwashiorkor	60–80	Yes
Marasmus	Less than 60	No
Marasmic kwashiorkor	Less than 60	Yes

Table 1.3.7: Indian Academy of Pediatrics—classification of nutritional status.

*Level of undernutrition**	*Expected weight for age (%)*
1°	60–69
2°	60–69
3°	50–59
4°	Less than 49

*The prefix "k" is added to indicate presence of edema.

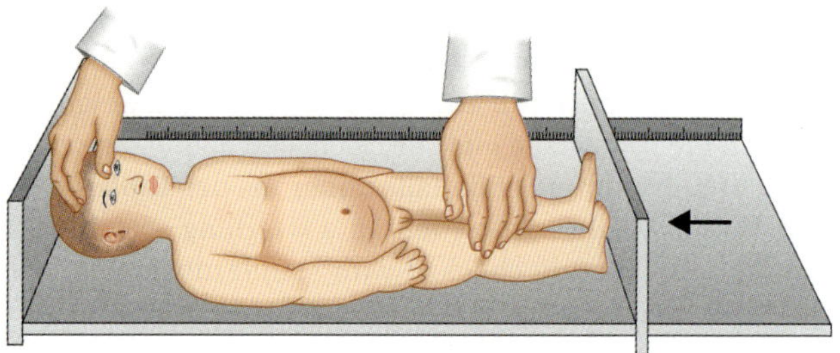

Fig. 1.3.6: The infantometer method of measuring the length of child.

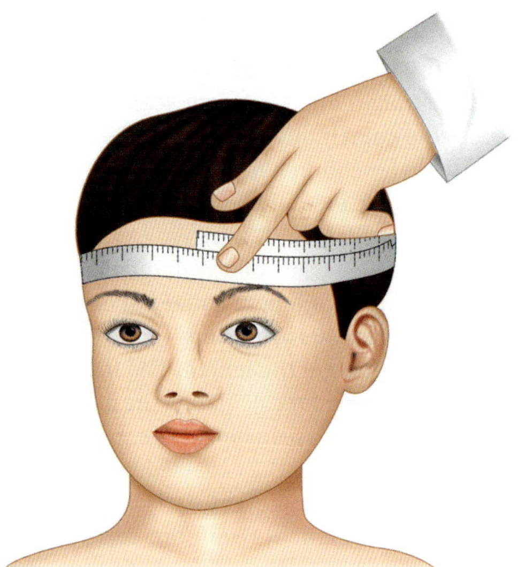

Fig. 1.3.7: Method of measuring the head circumference.

Table 1.3.8: Rate of increase in height in children.

Age	*Height*
At birth	50 cm
6 months	+12 cm (62 cm)
1 year	75 cm
2 years	85 cm (86–87 cm)
2–5 years	6–8 cm/year
5 years and above	5 cm/year

Table 1.3.9: Normal upper segment/lower segment ratio in children.

Age	*Upper segment/lower segment*
At birth	1.8/1
3–4 years	1.3/1
9 years	1/1
18 years	0.9/1

Table 1.3.10: Conditions with altered upper segment/lower segment ratio.

Upper segment/lower segment ratio	*Probable disorder*
Proportionate (normal ratio for age)	Delayed adolescence, hypopituitarism, constitutional dwarfism, nutritional dwarf
High ratio (upper segment > lower segment)	Hypothyroidism, chondrodystrophy, achondroplasia, Ellis-van Creveld syndrome, Turner syndrome
Low ratio (upper segment < lower segment)	Hurler syndrome, Morquio syndrome, hypogonadism

to the sole of the foot). The rate of growth of upper and lower segments varies with age as shown in **Table 1.3.9**. Hence, any difference in the proportion expected for that age may suggest the presence of specific growth disorders **(Table 1.3.10)**. Stature should also be defined with parent's height being considered, referred to as the midparental height.

For girls: Approximate projected adult height (in cm)

$$= \frac{\text{Mother's height} + (\text{Father's height} - 13)}{2}$$

For boys: Approximate projected adult height (in cm)

$$= \frac{(\text{Mother's height} + 13) + \text{Father's height}}{2}$$

Head Circumference

The size of the head is a good indicator of the size of its contents, namely the brain and the ventricles. Any abnormality in the head circumference should alert the doctor toward any problem with the brain or its related structures. Head circumference is measured with a nonstretchable tape passing through the maximum point of the external occupational protuberance posteriorly and a point just above the glabella anteriorly **(Fig. 1.3.7)**. It varies from 32 to 35 cm at 1 year, from 43 to 46 cm, and from 48 to 51 cm at 5 years. The expected head circumference for the age may be calculated from **Tables 1.3.11 and 1.3.12**. The adult head size is reached between 5 years and 6 years. Microcephaly is defined as head circumference, more than 3 standard deviations below the mean or less than the 5th percentile for the age and sex. Head size more than the 95th percentile for age suggests the macrocephaly.

Chest Circumference

This is measured at the level of the nipples **(Fig. 1.3.8)**. In the infant, the chest circumference is lesser than the head circumference by about 2.5 cm, and the two become equal by 1 year after which the chest circumferences exceed the head circumference. In undernutrition, the chest circumference

Table 1.3.11: Head circumference growth velocity.

Height for age	*Head circumference growth velocity*
Till 3 months	2 cm/month
3 months to 1 year	2 cm/3 months (1/3rd of initial velocity)
1–3 years	1 cm/6 months (1/12th of initial velocity)
3–5 years	1 cm/year (1/24th of initial velocity)

Table 1.3.12: Formula for estimating head circumference in the first year (after Dine et al.).

Normal range of head circumference in cm (5th–95th percentile)
$\frac{(\text{Length in cm} + 9.5) + 2.5}{2}$

remains lower than the head circumference even beyond 1.5 years, whereas in well-nourished children, the chest circumference may exceed the head circumference even before 1 year.

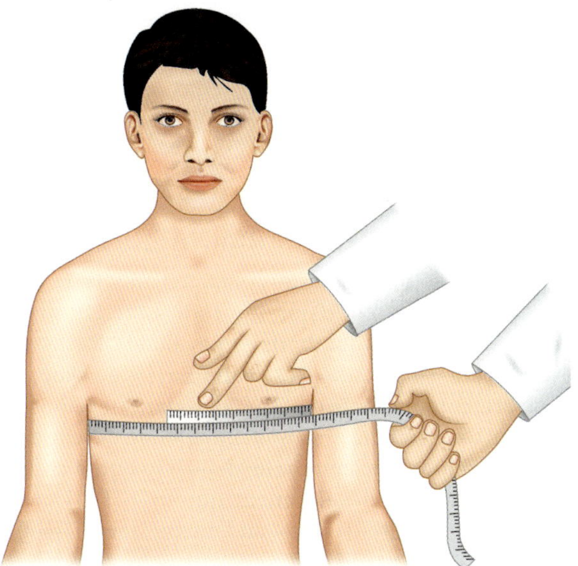

Fig. 1.3.8: Method of measuring the chest circumference.

Midarm Circumference

The midarm circumference (MAC) is taken as the name suggests, at the midpoint between the acromion and the olecranon with the arm hanging by the side of the body **(Fig. 1.3.9)**. It is useful to detect malnutrition in young children (1–4 years). Values more than 13.5 cm may be considered normal, while values less than 12.5 cm indicate significant wasting and undernutrition. Shakir tape is used for measuring MAC in the community and has color bands—green color indicates MAC is greater than 13.5 cm, yellow color a MAC between 13.5 cm and 12.5 cm, and red color a MAC lesser than 12.5 cm.

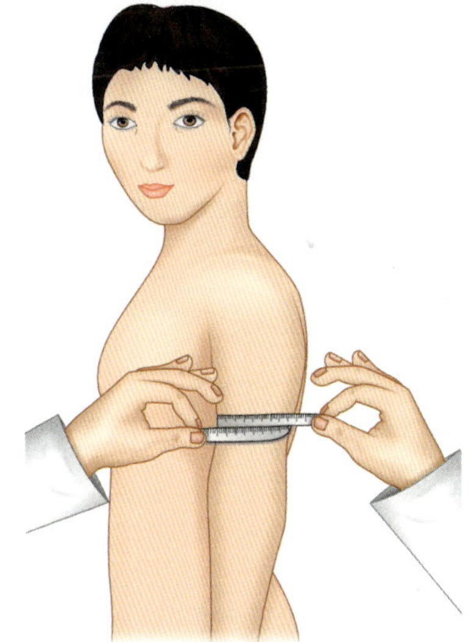

Fig. 1.3.9: Method of measuring the midarm circumference.

Arm Span

It is the distance between the tips of the middle fingers with both arms held wide open, that is, spread apart. Normally, in young children, it is 1-2 cm less than the length or height. It equals the height at 10 years, and after 10 years, it is from 1 cm to 2 cm more than the height. The increased arm span is seen in Marfan syndrome and homocystinuria.

Weight for Height

This is calculated as:

Weight for height (WFH) =

$$\left(\frac{\text{Weight of child}}{\text{Weight corresponding to height of child}}\right) \times 100$$

Values above 90% are normal, while those below 90% indicate malnutrition and above 120% indicate overweight.

Body Mass Index

It is calculated as:

$$\text{Body mass index (BMI)} = \left(\frac{\text{Weight in kg}}{(\text{Height in meter})^2}\right)$$

For adults, body mass index (BMI) of 18.5-24.99 is considered normal, 25-29.99 is overweight (preobese), above 30 is obese, and less than 18.5 is underweight—World Health Organization. BMI less than 16 is severe thinness, 16.00-16.99 is moderate thinness, 17.00-18.49 is mild thinness, 30.00-34.99 is obese class-I, 35.00-39.99 is obese class-II, and more than 40 is obese class-III. For children, BMI 85th–95th percentile is overweight, while greater than 95 percentiles is obesity.

Growth Patterns

See **Table 1.3.13**.

DEVELOPMENTAL EXAMINATION

Here, the developmental history obtained must be confirmed by examining the child for the milestones attained or lost. Many accepted methods are available for assessing development. Of this, the Gesell and Bayley developmental scales are commonly used. The Vadodara developmental screening tests and the Thiruvananthapuram developmental screening chart are useful for field assessment of children's development. The development quotient (DQ) must be calculated separately for motor and mental development.

$$DQ = \frac{\text{Developmental age}}{\text{Chronological age}} \times 100$$

Developmental evaluation is of special value in children with neurological diseases, such as neurodegenerative disorders, and chromosomal anomalies, such as Down syndrome. It is also useful for following up children with birth asphyxia or established cerebral palsy and mental retardation. The common developmental/primitive reflexes to be examined are shown in **Table 1.3.14**. The absence of appearance of the primitive reflexes at the expected time or their persistence beyond the time that they should normally disappear should lead to a suspicion of significant brain damage.

Table 1.3.13: Growth patterns.

Age	*Approximate daily weight gain (g)*	*Growth in length (cm/month)*	*Growth in head circumference (cm/month)*
0–3 months	30	3.5	2
3–6 months	20	2	1
6–9 months	15	1.5	0.5
9–12 months	12	1.5	0.5
1–3 years	8	1	0.25
4–6 years	8	3 cm/year	1 cm/year

Sexual Maturity Rating

Sexual maturity rating in boys and girls is shown in **Table 1.3.15**.

SYSTEMIC EXAMINATION

It is beyond the scope of this chapter to cover the examination of every system in detail; it can be obtained from any standard textbook of clinical examination. Here we attempted to give salient points in clinical examination, which are different in children when compared to adults.

Respiratory System

Inspect the chest wall for any deformities. Costochondral beading is seen in rickets (broad and dome shaped), in

Table 1.3.14: Primitive reflexes to be examined during developmental assessment.

Reflexes	*Age of appearance*	*Age of disappearance*
Stepping	Birth	6 weeks
Placing	Birth	6 weeks
Moro	Birth	3 months
Sucking and rooting	Birth	4 months while awake
Palmar grasp	Birth	6 months
Plantar grasp	Birth	10 months
Tonic neck	2 months	4–6 months
Landau	3 months	24 months
Neck righting	4 months	24 months
Parachute	9 months	Persists

Table 1.3.15: Sexual maturity rating (SMR) in boys/girls.

SMR stage	*Pubic hair (boys/girls)*	*Breasts*	*Penis*	*Testes*
1	Preadolescent	Preadolescent	Preadolescent	Preadolescent
2	Sparse, slightly pigmented	Breast and papilla elevated, areolar diameter increased	Slight enlargement	Enlarged scrotum, pink
3	Darker, beginning to curl	Breast and areola enlarged, no contour separation	Longer	Larger
4	Coarse, curly, abundant but less than adult	Areola and papilla form secondary mound	Larger	Larger, scrotum dark
5	Adult distribution, spreads to medial surface of thighs	Mature, nipple projects	Adult size	Adult size

scurvy (sharp due to posterior subluxation of the sternum), and in chondrodystrophy. Look for working of the accessory muscles of respiration, i.e. flaring of alae nasi, sternomastoid contraction, suprasternal and subcostal and intercostal retractions which would indicate dyspnea. Observe for indrawing of the lower ribs (Harrison's sulcus) which indicates chronic obstructive airway disease such as bronchial asthma. Vocal fremitus is rarely of value in young children. The grunting respiration in a child indicates severe respiratory disease. Percuss lightly in infants and small children, tap the chest wall directly rather than using another pleximeter finger. Due to the thin chest wall, the chest is more resonant than in adults. Before starting to auscultate, allow the child to play with your stethoscope, to allay its fears. Often it is less threatening to examine the back of the chest first. Due to the thin chest wall, breath sound is louder in children than in adults, and their character is more like the bronchial breathing of adults. This is called puerile breathing. Do not be disheartened with a crying child, as breath sounds can be auscultated better in them. Be careful to distinguish the conducted sounds from the upper respiratory tract as in laryngomalacia, upper respiratory tract infection, etc.

Cardiovascular System

In a neonate, the apical impulse is located slightly outside the midclavicular line in the fourth intercostal space. By 2 years, it comes to the midclavicular line in the fourth intercostal space and comes to the adult position, i.e. 5th intercostal space 1 cm medial to the midclavicular line between 4 years and 7 years. In infants, the right ventricles are dominant as compared to adults (where left ventricle is dominant). Due to the short neck of infants and young children, it is difficult to see the jugular venous pulse and pressure. Use a pediatric stethoscope with a small diaphragm to auscultate, as the intercostal spaces are narrow. It is preferable to auscultate the heart while the infant is comfortably sleeping or feeding from the mother. It is easier to hear the normal splitting of the heart sounds, and the P2 is louder in young children, i.e. less than 5 years. The functional systolic flow murmurs and venous hum are often heard in normal children.

Abdomen

The best place to examine the child's abdomen is the mother's lap, preferably while the child is feeding. Even if the child is struggling, it may be put on the mother's shoulder, and the abdomen is palpated from behind by "ballottement," i.e. palpation just when the child breathes, and the abdomen relaxes. Unlike adults, it is not necessary to fold the legs of the child while palpating the abdomen. Young children normally have a protuberant abdomen. Look for umbilical (which may be normally seen in infants) and inguinal hernia. The liver is normally palpable in children till the age of 4 years, i.e. up to 2 cm below the costal margin. In view of this, it is necessary to measure the span of the liver to figure out the actual enlargement. It is carried out by percussing the upper margin of dullness and by palpating the lower edge of the liver in the midclavicular line. The liver span ranges from about 4.5 cm to 5 cm at 1 week of age to approximately from 7 cm to 8 cm in males and from 6 cm to 6.5 cm in females by 12 years of age. The spleen may be normally palpable in infants, up to from 2 months to 3 months. Examine the genitalia and scrotum for hydrocele/hernia, intersex, phimosis, undescended testis, hypospadias, or epispadias. The anus is examined for anal excoriation and pinworms.

Nervous System

Neurological examination of the young child is quite difficult, especially sensory examination, and requires ingenuity on the part of the doctor to get the child's cooperation. Developmental screening and assessment of the primitive reflexes should be carried out as already mentioned. Much information regarding the neurological status of the child can be learnt by just observing the child, as the history is being elicited. Coordination is best tested by watching the child play. Orientation is best tested only in children above 4–5 years. Handedness becomes apparent at about 3 years of age. The signs of meningeal irritation, i.e. neck stiffness, Kernig's sign, Brudzinski's sign, must be looked for. They may not be present in infants and in the presence of severe undernutrition or overwhelming sepsis. Fundus may normally be pale in infants. Lifting the child gives a good idea about the muscle tone. If it is hypotonic, the child will slip through the hands. The plantar reflex may be extensor up to 1 year of age. But persistence of extensor plantar beyond 2 years is pathological. Tendon reflexes in young infants tend to be brisk. The deep tendon reflexes may be diagrammatically represented as shown in **Figure 1.3.10**, using the notations shown here:

0 = Absent
\+ = Sluggish
++ = Normal
+++ = Brisk
++++ = Exaggerated

History taking and clinical skill development in pediatrics are therefore to be learnt by the repeated exposure to case interviews and hands-on training in physical examination. The more a student gets this type of exposure, the more he can engage himself in self-analysis, which will help him carry out the clinical examination thoroughly.

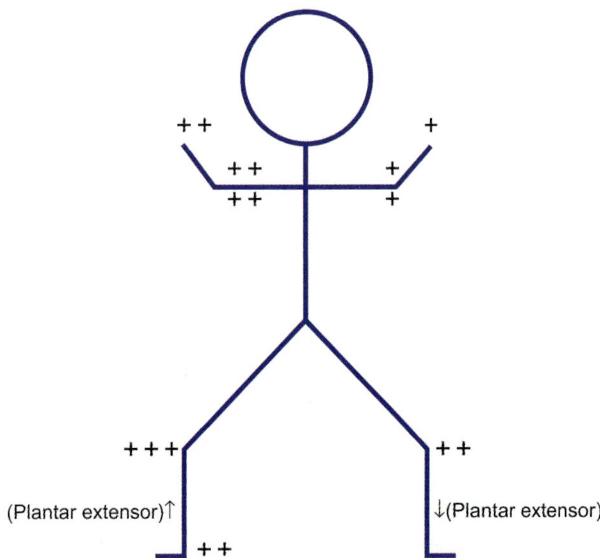

Fig. 1.3.10: Model diagrammatic representation of recording deep tendon reflexes.

PRACTICE OF DIFFERENTIAL DIAGNOSIS

During situations when the diagnosis of the child is not very clear (which may be the case quite often), it becomes necessary to make a set of most probable diagnoses. This is called differential diagnosis. This should be based on the history, clinical symptoms, and clinical signs that have been elicited. The differential diagnoses thus made will help us to plan out investigations toward proving or disproving each probable cause. Hence, to be of practical value, the list should be as short as possible and should only include the conditions that could reasonably explain most of the child's history, symptoms, and signs. The list should be given in descending order of probability of the various likely diagnoses, based on the positive and negative points toward each.

BIBLIOGRAPHY

1. Gupta P. Clinical methods in pediatrics, 4th edition. New Delhi: CBS Publishers; 2017.

1.4 Communication and Counseling

Parang N Mehta

INTRODUCTION

Communication skills are a core competence for clinicians. Good communication enhances patients' understanding and adherence to therapy and improves outcomes. Poor understanding of the disease and treatment issues by parents is associated with poor outcomes. Good communication and shared decision-making is essential for a positive patient experience. Poor communication puts patients at risk because of caregivers' lack of accurate information about the disease and treatment.

Communication is an important determinant of both patient satisfaction and complaints. It is everyone's responsibility to improve communication skills and provide time and place for it. In the current climate of suspicious and even hostile doctor-patient relationship, good communication can do a lot to establish and restore trust.

COMMUNICATION SKILLS

These are, quite simply, the skills that allow human beings to communicate effectively. For pediatricians, communication skills consist of:

- The ability to talk with parents. Not to parents, not at parents, but with them. Listening is an essential part; communication must be a two-way process. Good listening skills not only help in diagnosis, but also in judging what the family expects from the medical visit, and what treatment will be acceptable.
- The ability to communicate well enough with patients and parents to understand their concerns, problems, and beliefs and to elicit relevant information.
- The ability to explain the child's illness clearly, and in language that the parents can easily understand. The treatment options should be explained clearly and completely, so that they can make informed decisions about treatment.

- The ability to convince parents to follow a treatment plan. This is especially important when embarking on prolonged, expensive, difficult, or culturally unacceptable treatment for a child.
- The ability to establish a relationship with the parents and child, based on mutual respect and trust.
- The ability to let parents, and older children, understand that they have a say in their treatment decisions. Many people would like to participate in shared decision-making but need to be encouraged to do so.
- "Soft skills" such as being able to put all classes of parents at ease and being able to generate confidence. These components of a "good bedside manner" were once considered an important attribute of a successful practitioner.

THE IMPORTANCE OF COMMUNICATION AND COUNSELING SKILLS

The chief goals of communication are as follows:

- Creation of a good interpersonal relationship
- Facilitating exchange of information
- Including patients and parents in decision-making.

Communication skills contribute to a doctor's respect, a patient's belief, and adherence to treatment, among other advantages **(Box 1.4.1)**. A doctor with these skills is more likely to have happy, satisfied patients, than an equally technically competent doctor who does not bother about communication. Even if a pediatrician's diagnosis and treatment are accurate, thoroughly rational, and successful, poor communication leaves the parents unhappy and resentful. This is especially so with chronic or incurable diseases, which are associated with anxiety, stress, and uncertainty for the whole family.

Patients and parents do not have the knowledge to judge the quality of a doctor's examination, diagnosis, or prescription. Most complaints in health-care systems, both public and private, arise from poor communication. Parents are angered by the doctor's refusal to spend time with them, refusal to give explanations, and lack of courtesy and care. When these are followed by a poor treatment outcome, complaints, quarrels, and legal action are likely. Good communication can play a significant part in avoiding complaints and malpractice claims.

BARRIERS TO GOOD COMMUNICATION

The two most important barriers are not knowing what patients want from us **(Box 1.4.2)**, and not realizing the importance of good communication. Some other barriers are as follows:

- *Lack of time*: History taking, physical examination, and prescription writing are seen as essential parts of a clinical encounter. When time is short, it is the communication with parents that is sacrificed.
- *Arrogance:* Doctors expect patients and their parents to follow commands unquestioningly. Explanations are considered unnecessary.
- *Shyness:* Shyness, from the patient or the doctor, stands in the way of adequate information being exchanged.
- *Language and jargon:* Communication with people speaking different languages can be problematic and may need a special effort. If an interpreter is used, he should be given small bits of information to translate at a time, especially when the prescription is dealt with.
  Speaking in technical/medical language leaves the parents confused and uninformed and defeats the purpose of communication. It is important to talk in language that a nonmedical person can understand.
- *Deafness:* Speaking loudly, slowly, and distinctly helps parents with hearing impairment. Other useful measures are voice amplification devices, a quiet room, and the use of written communication.
- *Phones:* Phones are ubiquitous now, and calls can interrupt and hinder communication terribly.

INFORMATION NEEDS

When faced with a chronic/permanent condition, most parents want to know:

- What treatment can achieve for their child—Relief of symptoms, prolongation of life, shortening of the course of the disease, etc.
- Expected progress of the child during treatment

Box 1.4.1: Advantages of good communication.

- Facilitation of comprehension of medical information
- Better identification of patients' needs, perceptions, and expectations
- Patient satisfaction, leading to regular visits and referrals
- Feeling of empowerment and control
- Adherence to treatment plans
- Loyalty even if treatment is not immediately effective
- Less chances of complaints and legal action in the event of a mistake
- Doctors with good communication skills have better clinical and commercial success, less stress, and more job satisfaction

Box 1.4.2: What patients and parents want.

- Clarity and directness
- Listening
- Honesty
- More and better information about their illness, treatment plan, and expected outcome
- More openness about the hazards and side effects of treatment
- More information about the relief of symptoms and other concerns
- Advice on what they can do to help themselves
- Information on other treatments available
- A supportive, nonjudgmental, empathetic doctor

- What to expect by way of improvement, side effects, fresh problems, etc.
- Chances of complete cure
- Treatment options

Parents also often want to know about advertised alternative medicine. They have often invested time and effort in collecting such information and do not appreciate it being brushed off as nonsense. It is necessary to explain the unscientific and unproven nature of such "magic remedies."

In the private sector, information about likely costs of investigation and treatment should also be given. This preempts one of the major sources of conflict.

STRATEGIES FOR IMPROVING COMMUNICATION AND COUNSELING

- *Check what the parents know:* Many parents have faulty knowledge, acquired from magazines, lay books, and the internet.
- *Assess what the parents want to know:* Some parents want to know every little fact and detail about their child's condition. Others simply want a prescription and assurance.
- *Assess understanding:* Emotional distress, poor comprehension skills, language problems, etc. can hinder parents' comprehension. Understanding can be improved by giving time to absorb, and by repetition.
- *Listening skills:* Listening well is an essential part of communication. This requires the provision of adequate time and patience, and the willingness to listen to parents' concerns. A quiet room, lack of interruptions, provision of chairs for the parents, sitting at an appropriate distance, good eye contact, etc. are helpful.
- *Build confidence:* The parents' efforts and views deserve respect. A little specific praise for the parents' efforts helps significantly in building confidence and helping parents to cope. Some suggestions for future care improve their confidence that they will be able to manage the situation. Giving false hope is wrong, but information can be given in a positive manner.
- *Truth:* Parents deserve the truth, but the bald truth can be harsh and shocking. Disclosure must be tempered with common sense and empathy. Sometimes, the whole picture may need to be delivered in small parts spread out over two or more visits. However, withholding information leads to distrust.
- *Simplicity and clarity:* Many people do not comprehend words such as "growth" and "tumor." "Cancer" sounds shocking but may be necessary to drive home the problem to parents.
- *Be tolerant:* Blame, anger, a sudden outpouring of grief—these are common reactions. They should be met with understanding and support.

Table 1.4.3: Do's and don'ts of communication.

Do's	*Don'ts*
• Greet the child and parent by name • Smile • Sit down when talking • Try to talk in the patient's language • Direct the conversation to relevant directions • At the end of the consultation, ask if the parents have any questions • Engage the parents in a dialog • Give time for the parents to absorb and understand the content of your explanations, and then to ask questions	• Look at your watch frequently • Appear to be in a hurry • Use too many medical terms • Talk with your hand on the door handle, or foot outside the door • Interrupt all the time • Start examination and then write out a prescription before the main problem has been identified • Give long lectures as explanation • Ignore concerns mentioned by parents • Be dismissive of information the parents have come with from other sources

- *Empathy:* Parents of sick children are going through a difficult experience. They appreciate the fact that their doctor understands their situation and their difficulties.

Many other factors affect communication positively or negatively **(Table 1.4.3)**.

Good communication and counseling is an art that is acquired, developed, and improved by experience. Efforts in this direction will lead to better patient/parent satisfaction and perhaps better clinical outcomes. It is well to remember that compassion, explanation, and reassurance are valued by patients and their families as much as a diagnosis, treatment, and cure.

BIBLIOGRAPHY

1. Ammentorp J, Mainz J, Sabroe S. Patients' priorities and satisfaction with acute pediatric care. Arch Pediatr Adol Med. 2005;159:127-31.
2. Bartel DA, Engler AJ, Natale JE, et al. Working with families of suddenly and critically ill children. Arch Pediatr Adol Med. 2000;154:1127-33.
3. Bull SA, Hu XH, Hunkeler EM, et al. Discontinuation of use and switching of antidepressants: influence of patient-physician communication. JAMA. 2002;288:1403-9.
4. Fong J, Longnecker N. Doctor-patient communication: a review. Ochsner J. 2010;10:38-43.
5. Grocott A, McSherry W. The patient experience: informing practice through identification of meaningful communication from the patient's perspective. Healthcare. 2018;6:26.
6. Moore PJ, Adler NE, Robertson PA. Medical malpractice: the effect of doctor-patient relations on medical patient perceptions and malpractice intentions. West J Med. 2000;173:244-50.
7. Ranjan P, Kumari A, Chakrawarty A. How can doctors improve their communication skills? J Clin Diagn Res. 2015;9:JE01-4.

1.5 Legal and Ethical Issues in Pediatric Practice

George F Moolayil

INTRODUCTION

Doctor-patient relationship has undergone a sea of change from the olden times. Decades back, medical professionals were never questioned in their actions. If any death or other mishaps used to occur, it was attributed to the act of God and the public used to accept it without any adverse reactions. As the times have gone by, medical professionals are being viewed with suspicion and are being dragged into the court for genuine or frivolous reasons. Deterioration in moral values, increased value for materialistic things, commercialization of the profession, higher expectation of the patients, awareness of rights and privileges of the patients, increasing consumer activism, media sensationalism, undue interference by the politicians, etc. contribute to worsening of the doctor-patient relationship. It is prudent on the part of the doctor to understand what constitute medical negligence, and how to prevent it along with improvement in the doctor-patient relationship by good ethical practice.

MEDICAL NEGLIGENCE

Medical negligence has been divided into civil negligence and criminal negligence. In civil negligence, the affected party takes the doctor to the court for monetary compensation, whereas in criminal negligence, the prosecution is done by the State, and the punishment is usually fine or imprisonment.

Civil Negligence

A doctor can be found guilty under civil negligence by an act of omission or commission in a situation where he has failed to act in a manner which an ordinary professional of his standing would have been expected to act; or acted in a manner which an ordinary professional of his standing would not have been expected to act. The essential components of the modern tort of negligence propounded by Percy and Charlesworth are as follows:

- The existence of a duty to take care, which is owed by the defendant to the complainant
- The failure to attain that standard of care, prescribed by the law, thereby committing a breach of such duty
- Damage, which is both causally connected with such breach and recognized by the law, has been suffered by the complainant.

Standard of care is the standard of the ordinary skilled man exercising and professing to have that special skill at that time. A man need not possess the highest expert skill. It is a well-established law that it is sufficient, if he exercises the ordinary skill of an ordinary competent man exercising that particular art. He is not negligent, if he has acted in accordance with the practice accepted as proper by a responsible body of medical practitioners skilled in that art. Failure in attaining that average standard leads to a claim for civil negligence. Compensation can be claimed under law of contract, law of tort, or under Consumer Protection Act.

Criminal Negligence

The jurisprudential concept of negligence differs in civil and criminal law. What may be negligence in civil law may not necessarily be negligence in criminal law. For an act to amount to criminal negligence, the degree of negligence should be much higher, i.e. gross or of a very high degree. Negligence which is neither gross nor of a higher degree may provide ground for action in civil law but cannot form the basis for prosecution. To prosecute a medical professional for negligence under criminal law, it must be shown that the accused did something or failed to do something which in the given facts and circumstances no medical professional in his ordinary senses and prudence would have done or failed to do. The hazard taken by the accused doctor should be of such a nature that the injury which resulted was most likely imminent.

OTHER PENAL PROVISIONS

Action can be taken against the medical professionals under the Indian Medical Council Act for failure to follow the provisions of code of medical ethics or under infamous conduct. Penal action also can be taken against the doctors for failing to follow various other rules concerning medical professionals such as Prenatal Diagnostic Techniques, Drugs and Cosmetic Act, Transplantation of Human Organs Act, Biomedical Waste Act, Medical Termination of Pregnancy Act, etc.

PRECAUTIONS TO BE TAKEN DURING TREATMENT

In the practice of medical profession, some precautions must be taken to make the defense strong in cases of litigations. A doctor may be treating the patient in the correct manner.

However, many cases have been lost due to failure in proving the same in the judicial forums.

Documentation

A physician should document the following facts:

- Name, age, gender, religion, and address of the patient
- Date, month, and year along with the time of examination
- All relevant history including details of previous illness along with any history of drug allergy should be noted. If there is no history of drug allergy, it must be noted. If the patient develops allergy to a drug subsequently, the date of occurrence
- The complete examination details including the positive and relevant negative findings
- A record of investigations advised with reports
- A provisional diagnosis and a working diagnosis should be there before starting a line of management
- Final diagnosis
- Proper follow-up advice with review dates.

Informed Consent

Currently, the courts unanimously treat lack of informed consent as a matter of negligence of the doctor to disclose necessary information. Therefore, the doctor is duty bound to disclose the information as to the risk which can arise from the treatment of the patient. Risk is defined as exposure to a chance of an injury or loss. Most of the courts require the doctor to disclose information that other physician possess of the same skills or practicing in the same community would disclose in the same situation. Any person of sound mind who has attained the age of 18 years may give a legally valid consent. A consent given by a child under 12 years is invalid, between 12 years and 18 years is valid, if the court feels that the patient has understood the implication of the consent. In a situation, where there was no proper informed consent, and if some medically acceptable complication occurs as a treatment outcome, the doctor can be punished under medical negligence as it can be always claimed that if there was an awareness of the complications, the consent would not have been given, and hence, the doctor will be held responsible for the complications. However, in emergency or life-threatening situations, a doctor can proceed with treatment to save the life of a patient without waiting for the consent.

In a situation where the parents are not giving consent for a procedure that is essential for their ward, the doctor can proceed with the treatment in an emergency and in other situations can approach the court for overriding the decision of parents.

Life Support: Starting, Withholding, and Stopping

When a patient is brought in a condition requiring life support, it must be started even if the condition of the patient seems to be hopeless as not giving life support is an irreversible decision, whereas a decision to stop can be taken later also. In situations, where

- The relatives want to stop life support, but the doctor wants to continue;
- The doctor feels that there is no use in continuing life support, but relatives want to continue; and
- If both treating doctor and relatives want to discontinue life support.

An application must be made to the High Court that will refer the matter to an expert committee constituted for the purpose, and the committee will give its recommendations to the High Court. Inability to pay should not be a criterion for withholding or stopping life support. Recently the Supreme Court has given a judgment concerning passive euthanasia where an adult patient of sound mind can give advance directions refusing life support when required. The direction must be witnessed by two independent witnesses preferably in the presence of a judicial authority. However, this is not applicable to children.

Refusal of Treatment

A patient has a right to refuse the treatment. In situations, where there is a refusal of treatment, the consequences should be explained to the patients or parents in front of a witness, and it is better to get the refusal signed by them. The doctor has also got the right to refer the patients elsewhere if the treatment is refused. If the refusal involves the welfare of a minor or an unborn baby, the courts or even Child Rights Commission can override the objections of the parents. When a medical professional advances a plea that the patient did not give his consent to the treatment suggested by him, the burden is on him to prove that nonadministration of the treatment was because of the refusal to give consent thereto.

ETHICS IN PRACTICE AND GOOD DOCTOR–PATIENT RELATIONSHIP

A good ethical practice should have the following elements:

- *Standard:* A doctor should keep up high standard of behavior as prescribed in Code of Medical Ethics, 2002 of Indian Medical Council.
- *Choice:* The patient should be given the choice of treatment and doctor. If there is a request for reference, proper reference letter should be given.

- *Accessibility:* The patient should have accessibility to the best treatment in the hospital or referred to a higher center for better care, if necessary. The doctor will earn the respect of the patient and the relatives by doing so.
- *Nondiscrimination:* No discrimination should be shown to the patients based on religion, caste or social standing.
- *Transparency:* The doctor should be transparent with the patients and relatives on all possible matters. All matters regarding the bill, etc., should be explained, and there should not be any practice of dichotomy (receiving commission from scan centers, lab, etc., for sending the patient for investigations and for referrals).
- *Accountability:* The doctor should be accountable to the patient for the treatment.
- *Imparting information:* The parents and the relatives should be made aware of the condition of the patient. A proper communication can avoid misunderstandings later. Imparting of information should be done in a sensitive manner.
- *Quality of service:* Expectations on the part of the patients and relatives are quite high regarding the quality of medical service. Therefore a medical professional should update his medical knowledge by regular attendance at continuing medical education programs.
- *Dealing with complaints:* A medical professional should give serious consideration to complaints brought by the patients and relatives and do proper investigation on the complaints. If the complaint is genuine, an apology to pacify them is necessary, and if the complaint is due to some misunderstanding, the matter should be explained.

To conclude, a good doctor–patient relationship will decrease the adverse incidents in the practice of medical profession. A good understanding of the laws involving the medical profession and taking proper precautions will help the medical professional in dealing with litigations.

BIBLIOGRAPHY

1. Bag RK. Medical Negligence and Compensation, 2nd edition. 2014. 3rd revised reprint.
2. Lahoti RC. Jacob Mathew vs state of Punjab. KLT. 2005;3:967.
3. Supreme Court of India. Aruna Ramchandra Shanbaug vs Union of India & Ors. SC; March 7, 2011.

1.6 Research in Office Practice: Translating Clinical Information to Evidence-based Research

Narendra K Arora, Rakesh N Pillai

INTRODUCTION

Continuing success in child health was through high-quality research aimed for new knowledge architectures or for generating fresh interpretation of known facts and principles. Capabilities and goals of independent physicians and different actors of private clinics were integrated with medical research in order to solve many complex problems. This is practice-based research—meaning performance of research in physician's office. Presently, the majority of patients in India and developing countries are being treated in such private clinics. In 2013, these clinics in India were catering to 70% of urban and 63% of rural household health needs. If we assemble a cohort of 1,000 children, less than two are likely to receive treatment in a teaching hospital.

Major difference exists between physician office practices and teaching hospital practices. Patients seen in physician's office have a wide-spectrum of severity and differ significantly to that seen in hospitals most of them may be from marginalized groups and diverse locations. Such patient mix precludes generalization and application of results from studies that are mostly done in teaching hospitals. Equally, important is the frequently encountered psychosocial morbidity in primary care office practice but uncommon in hospital settings. On successful incorporation of robust clinical research into physician's office practices, many relevant practitioner queries could be resolved through locally relevant evidences to underpin clinical decisions. In addition, creating evidences in office setup is an opportunity to influence the behavior of future physicians for integrating research practices into day-to-day clinical practices.

Doing research in primary care office practice is important and has several advantages. A study sample represents the true population locally and prevalent problems; accurate character of the disease and natural history; research on psychosocial issues can be enabled; allows for health-care services research; large sample sizes can be accrued; and it helps to improve quality of care. In addition, physician's office engagement in the community will help to create knowledge basis for various transdisciplinary, high impact community interventions to foster the convergence of health, economics, and other nonhealth sectors. Office-based research makes a clinician feel "active;" prevents boredom of sitting in the outpatient department; and broadens the scope of physician beyond the basic service delivery; excitement of office-based research also includes intellectual stimulation, collaboration with academic colleagues, presentations in academic and scientific forums, and a sense of personal fulfillment. Office-based research has the potential for improving the effectiveness, efficiency, delivery, feasibility and reach of clinical care, and behavioral interventions. Equally important is the critical need to decipher deep and actionable knowledge of what drives human behavior in their individual and collective choices. Often perceived barriers for doing research at physician's office are lack of training and experience, lack of motivation and interest, time constrains and fear for increase in workload and difficulty in finding funds.

DEVELOPING RESEARCH IDEA

Many potential research topics can be identified from daily practice; however, knowledge, motivation, and perseverance are the key to translate them into viable research projects. Identifying and defining research problem is the first step to develop a research agenda. Advancement in technology and informatics infrastructures could be utilized for better management. It is important to understand few underlying philosophies which are essential to design such research projects. Research could be:

- *Empirical and theoretical research:* Documenting observations, experiences, and their analysis for specific conclusion falls under empirical research. Developing theory and abstracts-based on available evidences are grouped under theoretical research.
- *Basic and applied research:* Systematic enquiries to improve fundamental aspect of a phenomenon without specific application toward processes or products in mind is basic research, while applied research or action aims to find solutions or design interventions to solve a specific problem.
- *Descriptive and explanatory (analytic) research:* Surveys and fact-finding enquiries that aim to describe a situation, event, or a system fall under descriptive research. Researchers have no control over variables and report only what has happened or is happening. Explanatory research or analytical research aims to establish cause and effects relationships. It includes experimental research like clinical trials. The researchers analyze the facts or information for assessing or establishing these relationships.
- *Quantitative and qualitative research:* Use of numerical data that employs mathematical models, theories, and hypothesis is coined under quantitative research.

Qualitative research can provide rich information about any social processes in a specific setting.

Descriptive and analytic research is most commonly used in community and clinical practices; however, each school of thoughts has its own importance. For practicing physicians, it is important to distinguish between these study designs. Descriptive studies ask simpler questions about what is going on in the practice environment. For example:

- How many children with diarrhea have visible blood in my practice?
- What proportion of patients with cough longer than 10 days benefit from bronchodilator therapy?
- How many typhoid patients have I seen during March–June of the current year?

Analytic studies compare one or more interventions or exposures. For example:

- What is the duration of diarrhea, if antibiotic is not given versus given?
- How many doses of antipyretic are sufficient after diphtheria, pertussis (whooping cough), and tetanus shot?
- How is malnutrition associated with increased risk of infections?

The best ideas for research come from everyday clinical problems. When an idea comes, think, and reflect on this for a few days or weeks, and think it through your colleague(s). Broadly research questions should address the following four elements in the acronym PICO: patients, intervention (for intervention studies only), comparison group, and outcomes. Some also suggest for adding *T* for the time (thus making it PICOT). Once research questions are defined, it is important to think about how they will be answered. A good research question has four characteristics: Feasibility (availability of adequate number of subjects, technical expertise, availability of ancillary services and investigations, time, funds, and scope); interesting to the investigator (passion of physician is essential); newness (confirms or refutes previous findings in your settings, provides new insights to the subject); ethical and relevant (to your practice, scientific knowledge, policy, future research directions). In addition, few other aspects to be thought while framing a research study are illustrated in **Figure 1.6.1**.

SEARCHING LITERATURE AND ITS CRITICAL APPRAISAL

Next step in the process is to locate the best evidence that attempts to answer the research question identified. Not only literature review helps to fill knowledge gaps, it lets

Step 1	Step 2	Step 3	Step 4	Step 5	Step 6	Step 7
Identify research idea/ practice-based challenge or difficulty	Frame a research question (think in terms of PICO and T)	Frame the research hypothesis (null)	List out all primary and secondary objectives	Design the study methods and analysis plan with key variables	Plan the tools/ instruments for the study	Prepare a work plan with implementation strategies and a budget

Fig. 1.6.1: Illustrate key points to be thought while preparing a research. (PICO: patient population; intervention; comparison; outcome)

you demonstrate skills on information seeking and critical appraisals. Sometime, researchers quote Google and/or similar discussion forums to support their claims; however in research, preference are given to peer-reviewed scientific databases. There are a number of online information and electronic databases that the clinician may tap to find the evidence. "Medline" is the most commonly accessed resource through "PubMed." "Google Scholar" is another search engine to find current evidences to your scientific queries. There are several websites that are modeled to facilitate evidence-based medicine. These websites provide consolidated information on a wide range of clinically relevant areas and questions. Surfing in these websites could be enhanced through predecided key words or selected Medical Subject Headings terms. In addition, researchers need to create and maintain a bibliography of reviewed literatures. Tools like endnote are useful to create bibliographic libraries and manage search engines. If required, annotated bibliographies could be considered, which give an account of various research evidences available on a given topic.

The critical appraisal of the literature is an important step. Researchers need to think: whether the results of the manuscript are valid, was a representative sample of patients included, was follow-up complete, unbiased sample selection, etc. Standards for reporting literature reviews could guide physician to gain these critical appraisal skills. The literature should be relevant to the research question and the findings, valid and applicable to the setting or communities in which the physician is working. Study design and how the potential biases have been handled are critical factors determining the validity of the findings of an article. Findings of a study on the compliance of antitubercular therapy done in Latin America may not be applicable in Indian settings due to various social, cultural, and economic factors but do give an idea about the methods for studying the problem in your practice environment.

GENERATING HYPOTHESIS AND STUDY DESIGNS

All research questions should lead to formulation of hypotheses. A hypothesis is defined as "scientific reasoning for a phenomenon so as to design the study to prove or disprove it," which is formulated in one of two possible philosophies: inductive or deductive approach. Inductive methods are those where data (observations) is initially collected and analyzed to reach out to a hypothesis (theory), while deductive methods emphasize that theory comes first.

Every hypothesis has also four components: the research question, patient population and its description, study design to be applied and expected outcome. Good hypothesis will help researchers to select appropriate sample, design a data collection protocol (or in other words, appropriate research method), statistical test, and establish relationship between variables. Good hypothesis comes from experience and creativity which require thorough knowledge, review of literature and should satisfy following criteria: must be clear and precise, must be specific and use simple terms, should be capable of testing in a specific time, should state relationship between variables, and should be consistent with known facts.

Most of the practicing physicians will require consulting an academic colleague to choose the appropriate study design. Descriptive study designs include cross-sectional studies, case-control, case reports, and case series. Natural history of common childhood diseases can be easily researched through physician office. For example, card study is an observational design to collect and describe clinical problems, management, and outcomes at the point of primary care. Clinical trials are examples of analytic studies. Simple trials can be done in office practice.

At this point, it is important to understand the following three basic measures of disease frequency:

1. *Incidence rate*: It must take into account, the number of individuals in a population that become ill and the time periods (under risk) experienced by the members of the population during which these events occur. Most important dimension of incidence rate is time. The denominator could be considered a product of population by the average time period of observation for a member of the population. The denominator of the incidence rate is thus often referred to as a measure of person time.
2. *Cumulative incidence*: It is defined as the proportion of a fixed population that becomes diseased in a stated period of time. If risk is defined as the probability of an individual developing disease in a specified time interval,

then cumulative incidence is a measure of average risk. Like any proportion, its value varies between 0 and 1 and is dimensionless. It is not interpretable, however, without specification of the time period to which it applies. Case fatality rate is the cumulative incidence of death among those who develop an illness (it is therefore technically a proportion and not a rate). The time period for measuring case fatality is often unstated, but it is better to specify it. When unstated, presumably there is a short period of increased risk. For long periods of risk of death after disease onset, it is preferable to use the mortality rate among those with illness rather than case fatality rate.

3. *Prevalence:* Unlike incidence measures prevalence focuses on disease status. It may be defined as the proportion of a population that is affected by disease at a given point in time. The term point prevalence is sometimes used to mean the same thing. An individual that dies from an illness is thereby removed from the group that constitutes the numerator of the prevalence. Mortality from an illness decreases prevalence. Disease with large incidence rates may have low prevalence, if they are soon fatal or recovery occurs fast. For short-lived ailment like diarrhea, a more useful measure is period prevalence. Thus, period prevalence for acute diarrhea over a month in a village may be 10/200 = 50/1,000 population/month.

BARRIERS TO RESEARCH IN OFFICE PRACTICE AND SOME SOLUTIONS: FORMATION OF RESEARCH NETWORKS

There are difficulties in accomplishing good primary care research, such as perceived lack of time; translating potential research ideas into coherent research questions and proposals; training in research methods; obtaining ethical clearances; funding; analysis and writing of manuscripts; and working out research collaborations with academic colleagues. Loneliness of solo practitioners and emotional involvement with patients are additional barriers. This has restricted the opportunity for pediatricians and family physicians to improve the quality of care in office practices. During last two decades, there is worldwide movement to encourage and rope in clinicians in primary care to engage in the much-needed research. Research networks have been set up. Practice-based research network (PBRN) is a number of primary care clinics grouped together in a structure of a network for the purpose of performing research in the community.

Practice-based Research Network

Practice-based research network can be considered the research laboratory of the primary care setting. PBRN were initially set up as surveillance networks to report on common diseases and clinical problems or diseases of public health importance. Subsequently, these networks have been involved to answer and shed new light on the complex, adaptive processes of primary care practices and imperatives.

The key elements in a PBRN are participation of motivated practicing pediatricians, research projects, communication, and an academic framework. The design of such network studies have to be kept simple and easy; study duration should preferably be short with quick results to keep the motivation high, budgetary requirements need to be reasonable, and they should not have ethics-related complexity. The research coordinator is of critical significance; the person ought to have good research method knowledge, be able to carry network partners together, and accomplish the task with consistent implementation of quality assurance steps during execution of study protocol. Managing network brings with it some unique challenges as well. PBRN must receive approval from many ethics committees to conduct research in several locations and practice settings. In a network, there are issues of selection bias, sampling errors, and data collection standardization, which are method aspects that may not be easy to control in busy and varied practice settings.

Collecting research data in geographically dispersed network environment requires proactive efforts at coordination, accuracy, and timely transmission of data. Data collection must not put too much burden on the busy practitioner. Electronic data collection at the point of care is a feasible solution. It is important that data collection methods match the study design for accuracy and comfort.

AREAS OF RESEARCH

Office-based practitioners can answer many important clinical questions that are not necessarily important for those attending big hospitals. Some examples may include assessing severity of diarrhea and respiratory tract infections; determining indications for giving antibiotics in febrile child; when to order for investigations after a head concussion; assessing and managing first time pain abdomen which does not respond to antispasmodics; positive Mantoux test in a child with recently treated pulmonary tuberculosis; and many other such difficulties.

Sentinel surveillance; counting and characterizing clinical encounters; understanding primary care encounters; comparing approaches to manage patients; modifying patient or clinician behavior; conducting pragmatic clinical trials; comparing approaches to deliver services in practice, and monitoring outcomes are some of the broad areas where questions may be developed and research done. Studies such as these most often result from joint contributions of office-based physicians and hospital-based consultants, and have their major impact in community practice, where the results are most applicable.

Currently in India, much of the public health data is collected and analyzed from a unidisciplinary clinical and cross-sectional perspective. This requires convergence initiatives for assembling national and local government datasets, business, civil society, and academia for generating comprehensive information and to engage multisectoral approaches for attaining sustained economic and human development goals. One such advancement is the "whole-of-society-whole-of-government" (WoS-Wog) approach recommended and proposed by World Health Organization during the pandemic influenza preparedness in 2011. Using a WoS framework capabilities and goals of different actors has to be integrated in order to solve complex problems at the convergence of health and economics. Equally important is critical need to decipher deep and actionable knowledge of what drives human behavior in their individual and collective choices. Office practice by very nature is multidisciplinary and if role of markets, economic status of changing population, and social and cultural dimensions are also added, a "WoS" paradigm can be applied to address the core issues leading to disease, disability, and adverse economic consequences.

WHERE TO GET FUNDS FOR OFFICE-BASED RESEARCH?

Funding for practice-based research is definitely a major barrier but not that is impossible. Obtaining grants by individuals is more difficult compared to when PBRN approach for funding. Professional associations such as Indian Academy of Pediatrics may be able to facilitate and mobilize funds from donors, foundations, and government agencies. Collaboration with universities or medical schools is other option to generate resources. International agencies like the Agency for Health care Research and Quality support PBRN. The support from the industry is justified provided issues related to conflict of interest are taken care of and independence along with scientific rigor of the work are consistently maintained. With advancement in companies act, all companies in India are mandatorily required to spent 2% of their annual income under corporate social responsibility, which could be judiciously claimed by a practicing physician to chase his or her research dreams.

CONCLUSION

This is an era of shifting patient care from hospitals into the community and provides new and challenging opportunities to young and experienced alike for office-based research and improved education. Keeping in mind the methodological limitations and potential biases, office-based patient material represents the "real-world" situations and research findings have the possibility of wide community applicability to improve effectiveness, efficiency, and equity of care, particularly in resource constraint environments. Thus, it is recommended for transdisciplinary, high impact collaborative resear ch to foster the convergence of health, economics, and other nonhealth sectors. An advanced informatics, infrastructure could be created to improve health of people by enabling individuals, community organizations and networks, governments, and corporations to optimize decisions, so that their actions converge to enhance health and economic development of patients.

BIBLIOGRAPHY

1. Carey TS, Halladay JR, Donahue KE, Cykert S. Practice-based research networks (PBRNs) in the era of integrated delivery systems. The Journal of the American Board of Family Medicine. 2015;28(5):658-62.
2. Dubé L, Pingali P, and Webb P. Paths of convergence for agriculture, health and wealth. Proceedings of National Academy of Sciences of the United States of America (PNAS). 2012;109(31):12294-31.
3. European Medical Research Councils. Forward look - Implementation of Medical Research in Clinical Practice [Article in Internet]. Downloaded on 13th July 2015 from: http://www.esf.org/fileadmin/Public_documents/ Publications/Implem_MedReseach_ClinPractice.pdf.
4. Ipp M. Office-based research: A new era and new opportunities. Paediatr Child Health. 2002;7(7):445-6.
5. John M. Westfall. Card Studies for Observational Research in Practice. Ann Fam Med. 2011;9:63-8.
6. Lindbloom EJ, Ewigman BG, Hickner JM. Practice based research network: the laboratories of primary care research. Med Care. 2004;42:(4 suppl):III45-9.
7. Pace WD, Fagnan LJ, David WR. The Agency for Healthcare Research and Quality (AHRQ) Practice-based Research Network (PBRN) relationship: Delivering on an opportunity, challenges, and future direction. J Am Board Fam Med. 2011;24:489-92.
8. Prevent project team. Beyond Pandemics: A Whole of Society Approach to Disaster Preparedness. 2011. [Report in Internet] [Downloaded, on 07th May 2014, from: http://photos.state.gov/libraries/usun-rome/164264/PDF/tasw.pdf].
9. Rao PH. The Private Health Sector in India: A Framework for Improving the Quality of Care. ASCI Journal of Management. 2012;41(2):14-39.
10. Slora EJ, Harris DL, Bocain AB et al. Pediatric clinical research networks: Current status, common challenges, and potential solutions. Pediatrics. 2010;126:740-5.
11. Smith FO. Practice-based research: opportunities for the children. South Med J. 1991;84(4):479-82.
12. Taylor D. Health Science Writing Centre - University of Toronto. The literature review: A few tips on conducting it [Article in Internet]. Downloaded on 13th July 2015 from: http://www.writing.utoronto.ca/advice/specific-types-of-writing/literature-review.
13. Wasserman R, Slora E, Bocian A, et al. Pediatric research in office settings (PROS): A national practice-based research network to improve children's health care. Pediatrics. 1998;102:1350-7.

1.7 Media and Child Health: Handling Parents and Public

Remesh Kumar R, Krishna Mohan R

IMPACT OF MEDIA

In the present era of digital dominance, media is undoubtedly having a profound influence on our younger generation. Of course, children spend a good amount of their quality time with some form of media, television (TV), mobile, or social media. Media has got both positive and negative impacts in the childhood period.

Positive Effects

The educational programs in TV and internet help students in learning. Programs such as news and quiz help to update knowledge in current affairs. Social media platforms such as Facebook and WhatsApp help in group studies and project works. They also provide an excellent opportunity for children to showcase their creative works and ideas.

Negative Effects

Obesity: Increased TV viewing can lead to obesity, both directly and indirectly. More hours spent on TV viewing means less hours spent on exercise and other physical activities. Also, the various commercials on different unhealthy food products may lead to increased food consumption and overweight. Eating meals while watching TV is also a habit which should be discouraged.

Detrimental effects on academic performance: Increased TV and internet usage takes time away from reading and homework. Unsupervised TV viewing by children will have a deleterious effect on academic performance. Exposure to violence in films, TV programs, and videogames can negatively affect the mental and physical health of children. This increases the likelihood of aggressive and violent behavior in both short- and long-term contexts. Violence, substance abuse, and sex in media can have a harmful influence in the behavior and personality of the developing child.

Other negative impacts include language delay, eye strain, postural problems related to neck and head, and sleep disorders, such as insomnia and nightmares.

Role of parents (policy statement from American Academy of Pediatrics):

- Limit the amount of total entertainment screen time to <1-2 h/day after 2 years of age.
- Keep the TV set and internet-connected electronic devices out of the child's bedroom.
- Monitor what media your children are using and accessing, including any websites they are visiting and social media sites they may be using.
- Co-view TV, movies, and videos with children and teenagers, and use this as a way of discussing important family values.
- Model active parenting by establishing a family home use plan for all media. As part of the plan, enforce a mealtime and bedtime "curfew" for media devices, including cell phones. Establish reasonable but firm rules about cell phones, texting, internet, and social media use.

HANDLING PARENTS AND PUBLIC IN PEDIATRIC PRACTICE

Globally, media whether it is electronic, print, or internet plays a pivotal role in disseminating information to the public. The reporting by media can be biased at times and can either calm down or flare up the aggrieved parents and public alike, especially in situations such as a public health emergency. This may bring the credibility of the media information at stake, and the medical practitioner must dissect the parental perceptions on these news items and give them the best available opinion at the right time.

Types of Health News in Media

It is a known fact that media plays a tremendous influential role in public responses to health issues. It is usually during public health emergencies that demand for health information rapidly increases. In many occasions, public health officials often have the challenging task of both using the media to positively influence health practices and at the same time negating the rapid wildfire-like spread of untrue information.

Some of the positive impacts of both conventional as well as present-day social media include:

- Access to more health information, especially in developing countries.
- Mass dissemination of healthy practices effectively, such as advantages of hand washing, proper immunization schedule, etc.

- Updated knowledge on innovations and openings to newer frontiers in preventive health.
- More data easily available to health researchers.
- Helps patients in communicating effectively with others with similar health conditions.
- Helps in supporting health-related causes, such as donation toward treating poor patients, signing petition against harmful medical practices, etc.
- Patients can broadcast their experiences about a particular health-care provider, which makes them more accountable for the services they provide.

Despite all the virtues that media offers on health front, the policy makers and child health professionals always gauge the impact of negative information, many a time not evidence based, as quite ominous:

- Media, especially social media, often creates problems by spreading rumors during normal health events as well as health crisis situations.
- Knowingly or unknowingly, nonexperts can share health-related information which often creates confusion and panic. This leads to active dissemination of misinformation and medical myths.
- Media field is highly competitive. Often to attain the commercial goals of the media, even health news is twisted and converted into sensationalized stories. This act of fear mongering may turn dreadful in critical situations, such as epidemics, adverse events following immunization, etc.
- Extensive use of social media in health-related issues may lead to the breach of privacy, both for the patients as well as the treating doctors.
- News columns on health care and health policies are usually overwhelmingly negative, despite measurable improvement in both. Ultimately, this may tend public to be skeptical about national health programs.
- The tendency of the parents to find fault within the system even for trivial unanticipated sufferings of their wards in a medical care setting is often exploited by the media. Even before the genuinity of the incident could be verified by the appropriate authority, the media, who themselves always compete to flash any sensational breaking news, jump into the scene and make it viral. Further damage control is a herculean task.

The "Googling" Parents

In this digital era, all information related to health is literally available at our finger tips. It is not unusual for parents to have a preliminary web browsing of their child's symptoms before presenting to the doctor's cabin. But all our net browsing tools and apps are limited by their inability to reason and think. Though there is enormous health literature in the internet, most parents will not be able to filter it properly. Ultimately, the majority of them plunge into unnecessary worry and anxiety. For such parents, the consultant in the chamber naturally becomes only a tool to either confirm or refute the diagnosis provided by the "Google" doctor. It calls for much patience and skill from the pediatrician to reassure such "fussy" parents. Moreover, this internet-driven interpretation of symptoms can negatively affect the trust between doctor and patients.

Pitfalls in Media Usage in Child Health Issues

- The conversion of complex medical data into easily understandable public health messages continues to be an obstacle, even for most knowledgeable experts in the field.
- Media's tendency to overemphasize negative news creates unnecessary panic and confusion in society.
- There is no system to regularly censor health-related messages before being circulated through media.
- Even in the issues having overwhelming scientific consensus, the media at times fail to give clear positive messages. In the anti-vaccine propaganda against even expanded program on immunization vaccines, media often enjoys creating a verbal feud between public health officials and anti-vaccine campaigners rather than conveying definite positive messages supporting vaccines.
- The practitioner in their busy routines many a time tends to overlook the body language of the parents when certain newer modalities of investigations/treatment or new immunization schedule are advised.
- Lack of training of public health authorities to deal with media.

APPROACH FOR PROPER HANDLING OF IMPACT OF MEDIA

- *At the pediatrician's desk:*
  - The pediatrician should always be apprised about the happening in the society, especially the controversies and public dialogs on child health-related issues. This is sure to augment his/her preparedness to combat aggressive parents and calm them down with the scientific knowledge which is hitherto beyond the scope of a parent.
  - Always listen to the parents' perceptions about the disease/treatment protocols and the apprehensions about it, which they might have acquired through the media. May look absurd or silly, but this is of prime importance for providing an appropriate reply. Listening to the views of one parent is sure to help us to have a better preparedness when counseling yet another family with similar complaints.
  - Whenever a newer modality of treatment or investigation is advised, especially the ones which have captured public attention through media, the practitioner should be extra vigilant to convince the

parents about the need for the same. The doctor needs to anticipate the allied confusions which might have already cropped into their thoughts from the messages spread through media and be prepared to clear them with available quotes from the scientific updates of any sort.

- *Role of Indian Medical Association (IMA) and Indian Academy of Pediatrics (IAP):*
  - Professional and academic organizations, such as IMA and IAP, should have a media cell at national, state as well as district levels. An official spokesperson who is well trained in media interaction should be assigned to all these teams. At the earliest hint of any untoward public health issue, the media cell should go on a war footing to collect all evidences and information on the same. At the same time, the official spokesperson should go on air with the updated scientific knowledge on that sensitive issue which can be strengthened later with the information passed by his/her team.
  - It is ideal to have well-maintained websites for all professional medical organizations, with links to related websites.
  - The academic bodies should identify troublemakers in the society and media. Equally important is to locate trouble shooters who can deliver the goods with maximum results in such precarious situations.
- *Central and State Government initiatives:*
  - Public health authorities need to meet the media on a regular basis and communicate to ensure a balanced scientific reporting, especially with regard to national health programs.
  - Managing misinformation during health crisis situations such as an adverse effect following immunization and epidemics is very important. Ideally all public health agencies should be well equipped before a crisis with adequate strategies, educational material, and appropriate staff to counter misinformation and myths.
  - A censoring system to regularly monitor contents of health news dealt by mainstream as well as social media will be appropriate. Quacks and nonexperts without adequate scientific knowledge should be prevented from interacting with public on topics related to health.

BIBLIOGRAPHY

1. American Academy of Pediatrics. Policy statement: media use by children younger than 2 years. Pediatrics. 2011;128(5):1040-6.
2. Leask J, Hooker C, King C. Media coverage of health issues and how to work more effectively with journalists: A qualitative study. BMC Public Health. 2010;10:535.
3. Robotham J. Australia's media reporting of health and medical matters: A question of quality letter. Med J Aust. 2006;184:479-80.
4. WHO. Effective media communication during public health emergencies. In: WHO Handbook and Field Guide. WHO; 2005.

1.8 Child Health in South Asian Association for Regional Cooperation (SAARC) Countries

Zulfiqar A Bhutta, Jai K Das

INTRODUCTION

Although there has been a reduction in child mortality globally, annually around 5.6 million children die before reaching their fifth birthday, the majority within the neonatal period **(Fig. 1.8.1)**. During the neonatal period, preterm or low-birthweight birth, perinatal asphyxia, and sepsis are the leading causes of death, whereas infectious diseases including pneumonia, diarrhea, and malaria are the leading causes of death beyond the neonatal period. The majority (77%) of these deaths are taking place in Southern Asia and Sub-Saharan Africa. Southeast Asia including the majority of the South Asian Association for Regional Cooperation (SAARC) countries accounts for 31% of these deaths.

The SAARC region represents countries with overlapping World Health Organization and United Nations

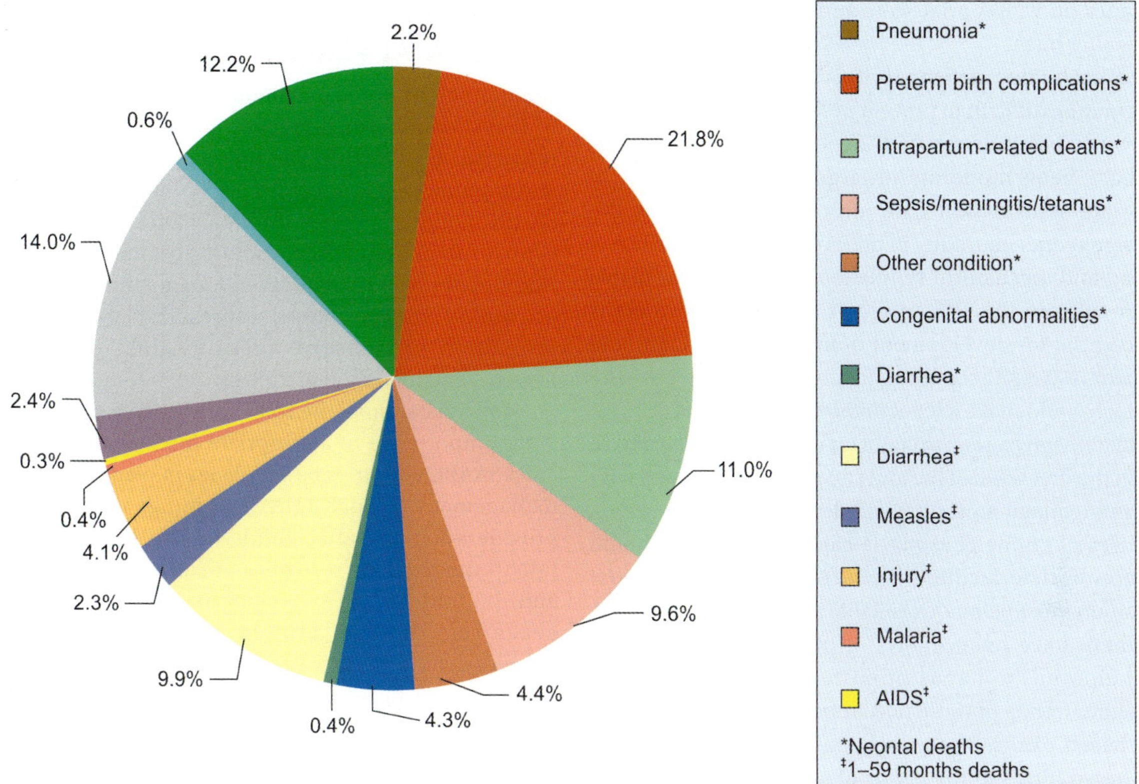

Fig. 1.8.1: Leading causes of death in children under 5 years of age in Southeast Asia. *Source:* Liu et al. 2015.

Table 1.8.1: Under-5 mortality rates.

	Value	
Country	***1990***	***2016***
Afghanistan	177	70
Pakistan	139	79
Bhutan	134	32
India	126	43
Bangladesh	144	34
Nepal	141	35
Maldives	94	9
Sri Lanka	21	9

Children's Fund regions and includes parts of Asia with the highest mortality rates. The combined population of SAARC countries is around 1.67 billion, representing approximately 23.5% of the total world's population. With the inclusion of Afghanistan, the region now houses countries with the highest child mortality rates in Asia. Of the eight SAARC countries, Afghanistan has the highest under-5 mortality rates (70), and Sri Lanka and the Maldives have the lowest under-5 mortality rate (9) **(Table 1.8.1)**.

In the year 2000, the millennium development goals (MDG) were set with specific targets for mortality reduction by two thirds by the year 2015; a recent countdown review indicates that out of the SAARC countries surveyed, India, Pakistan, and Afghanistan did not achieve MDG 4 goal, and these now face a challenge of achieving the sustainable development goals which is to end preventable deaths of newborns and children under 5 years of age by the year 2030, with all countries to reduce neonatal mortality to at least 12 deaths/1,000 live births and under-5 mortality to at least 25 deaths/1,000 live births.

COMMON NEONATAL PROBLEMS IN SOUTH ASIAN ASSOCIATION FOR REGIONAL COOPERATION COUNTRIES

Neonatal death accounts for around 60% of all infant deaths. The principal causes of neonatal mortality in the region include perinatal asphyxia, prematurity, and sepsis, and the majority of these deaths are preventable with existing interventions. These include appropriate care of the mother in pregnancy, skilled delivery, antenatal steroids in preterm labor, antibiotics for preterm premature rupture of membranes, and appropriate care during birth and in the first 48 hours after birth.

The exact burden of prematurity is unknown in the region. While it may be difficult to prevent prematurity, cost-effective care at birth and prevention of hypothermia are possible. There have been moderate-to-large-scale evaluations of appropriate skin-to-skin care after birth which has the potential to reduce mortality in preterm neonates. The use of surfactant and mechanical ventilation may only be available in larger cities in the private sector hospitals, but there is great potential for development of low-cost surfactant and equipment, especially continuous positive airway pressure units which could make a lot of difference to survival.

Perinatal asphyxia can account for up to half of all newborn deaths in the first week of life and can also be associated with significant neonatal morbidity and developmental disability. Many cases of perinatal asphyxia cannot be predicted, and hence appropriate facilities for recognition and neonatal resuscitation must be made available in all birthing facilities. While there have been efforts at promoting domiciliary resuscitation in the hands of birth attendants, there are encouraging trends of reduction in perinatal mortality with facility-based births. At the very basic level, encouraging facility-based births in the hands of skilled-birth attendants with appropriate basic equipment is a key intervention.

Although there have been remarkable reductions in neonatal tetanus, neonatal sepsis remains a major cause of morbidity and mortality in newborn, and although vertical transmission is possible, most of these infections are community acquired, and hence potentially preventable. A recent study to determine the causes and incidence of community-acquired serious infections among young children in South Asia showed that a cause could only be attributed to only 28% of episodes of which 16% were bacterial and 12% were viral. The leading pathogen was respiratory syncytial virus followed by *Ureaplasma* spp. Hand hygiene and the use of birth kits, followed by appropriate cord care, are important interventions to prevent infection. Emerging evidence from various SAARC countries indicates that the use of cord chlorhexidine is associated with significant reduction in the risk of neonatal omphalitis and sepsis. Given the high rates of infections in community settings and potential delays in recognition and referral, there is an increasing attention to community-based detection and management of potential neonatal infections and other problems. This includes the training of health-care providers in Integrated Management of Neonatal and Childhood Illness (IMNCI), as this approach can be used to recognize and treat serious infections at an early stage and impact outcomes.

COMMON PROBLEMS BEYOND NEONATAL PERIOD

Community-acquired pneumonia is one of the leading causes of death in children in the region [majorly due to *Haemophilus influenzae* type b (Hib) and pneumococcal infections]. Hib and pneumococcal vaccines are being rolled out in many SAARC countries either through national investments or Global Alliance for Vaccines and Immunization funding. Additional preventive interventions include strengthening of routine immunization, addressing low birth weight, promotion of exclusive breastfeeding, environmental hygiene, and reduction in exposure to indoor air pollution.

Notwithstanding, the role of preventive strategies, there is the importance of appropriate management. Currently, most SAARC countries have policies in place for appropriate management through IMNCI trainings of all health-care providers looking after children. The basic emphasis of IMNCI training is to recognize pneumonia at an early stage and the initiation of treatment at first or second level of health care. There is also the provision of referral in the event of deterioration or danger signs at presentation. Given the difficulties in referral in some instances, there is also an increasing focus on community-based care (detection and management of pneumonia), and preliminary findings from several studies in the region indicate promising outcomes.

Despite vast improvements in our understanding of the risk factors and strategies for the control of diarrheal disease as well as economic growth, diarrhea remains a leading cause of death in children in the SAARC region. Almost half of the childhood diarrhea deaths globally are in five countries of which two (India and Pakistan) are in the SAARC region. A major reason for poor progress is in this area is the relative lack of investment in large-scale water and sanitation projects and the fact that between 20% and 30% of the population still does not have access to improved and safe water, and over a third of the rural population practices open defecation. Prevention and treatment of dehydration is the key for successful management with provision of diet and zinc during the diarrheal episode helps not only to treat current episode but prevents malnutrition. A recent study to determine the etiology of diarrhea in low-resource settings suggested that viral diarrhea (36.4% of overall incidence) was more common than bacterial (25.0%) and parasitic diarrhea (3.5%). The 10 most common pathogens accounting for diarrhea included shigella, sapovirus, rotavirus, adenovirus, enterotoxigenic *Escherichia coli*, norovirus, astrovirus, *Campylobacter jejuni/coli*, *Cryptosporidium*, and typical enteropathogenic *E. coli.* Rotavirus infections account for almost a third of all diarrhea deaths; the newer rotavirus vaccines may offer a unique opportunity for prevention of severe diarrheal disease and mortality in the region and are being currently rolled out as part of the national immunization programs in many of the high-burden countries.

There is a high burden of typhoid fever in a few SAARC countries, and a current epidemic in Pakistan is showing worrisome trends as typhi blood culture isolates from these cases can be added to the list of bacterial pathogens of public health importance that have become extensively drug resistant. This is of greater public health concern, and it has the potential to spread worldwide, so greater efforts should be escalated to prevent typhoid through water-sanitation improvement, ensuring food safety and use of typhi vaccines in highly endemic areas.

ADDRESSING DETERMINANTS AND PUBLIC HEALTH OPTIONS

Maternal and child undernutrition is an important determinant of child mortality and long-term adverse outcomes including development. Given the high burden of low birth weight, stunting and wasting in the SAARC region, even among countries where mortality rates have improved, there is a much need to focus on these determinants. In addition to poverty and misdistribution of resources, the status of women in society, empowerment, ethnicity, and race play a critical role in existing inequities in care and access. Most people living in rural areas and urban slums live in abysmal conditions and have limited access to quality health-care services. Appropriate targeting, poverty alleviation strategies, such as conditional cash transfers, employment schemes, and good governance are essential elements in provoking change. An essential element in the quest for targeting the poor, especially in areas with the shortage of trained medical staff, is the strategy for task shifting and scaling up of interventions through lay workers and community health workers.

BIBLIOGRAPHY

1. Arifeen SE, Hoque DM, Akter T, et al. Effect of the integrated Management of Childhood Illness strategy on childhood mortality and nutrition in a rural area in Bangladesh: a cluster randomised trial. Lancet. 2009;374:393-403.
2. Baqui AH, Arifeen SE, Rosen HE, et al. Community-based validation of assessment of newborn illnesses by trained community health workers in Sylhet district of Bangladesh. Trop Med Int Health. 2009;14:1448-56.
3. Bhutta ZA, Black RE. Global maternal, newborn, and child health: so near and yet so far. N Engl J Med. 2013;369(23):2226-35.
4. Bhutta ZA, Chopra M, Axelson H, et al. Countdown to 2015 decade report (2000–10): taking stock of maternal, newborn, and child survival. Lancet. 2010;375:2032-44.
5. Bhutta ZA, Das JK, Bahl R, et al. Can available interventions end preventable deaths in mothers, newborn babies, and stillbirths, and at what cost? Lancet. 2014;384(9940):347-70.
6. Bhutta ZA, Das JK, Rizvi A, et al. Evidence-based interventions for improvement of maternal and child nutrition: what can be done and at what cost? Lancet. 2013;382(9890):452-77.
7. Darmstadt GL, Bhutta ZA, Cousens S, et al. Evidence-based, cost-effective interventions: how many newborn babies can we save? Lancet. 2005;365:977-88.
8. IGME (2017). Levels and trends in child mortality. Report 2017. Estimates developed by the UN Inter-Agency Group for Child Mortality Estimation. <http://www.childmortality.org/2017/files_v21/download/IGME%20report%202017%20child%20mortality%20final.pdf> [accessed July, 2018].
9. Klemm EJ, Shakoor S, Page AJ, et al. Emergence of an extensively drug-resistant *Salmonella enterica* serovar Typhi clone harboring a promiscuous plasmid encoding resistance to fluoroquinolones and third-generation cephalosporins. MBio. 2018;9(1):e00105-18.
10. Lassi ZS, Bhutta ZA. Community-based intervention packages for reducing maternal and neonatal morbidity and mortality and improving neonatal outcomes. Cochrane Database Syst Rev. 2015;3:CD007754.
11. Lazzerini M, Wanzira H. Oral zinc for treating diarrhea in children. Cochrane Database Syst Rev. 2016;(12):CD005436.
12. Liu L, Oza S, Hogan D, et al. global, regional, and national causes of child mortality in 2000–13, with projections to inform post-2015 priorities: an updated systematic analysis. Lancet. 2015;385(9966):430-40.
13. Saha SK, Schrag SJ, El Arifeen S, et al. Causes and incidence of community-acquired serious infections among young children in South Asia (ANISA): an observational cohort study. Lancet. 2018;392(10142):145-59.

Section 2

Care of the Newborn

2.1 Neonatal Nomenclature

Satvik Bansal

INTRODUCTION

There are several terms that are used about newborn infants and their care. This section will briefly summarize the commonly used terms in reference to the newborn infants.

- *Newborn/Neonate:* Any infant who is up to 28 days of life is termed a newborn or neonate.
- *Early neonatal period:* The period from birth up to 7 days of life is the early neonatal period.
- *Late neonatal period:* The period from day 7 up to day 28 of life is the late neonatal period.

GESTATIONAL AGE RELATED

Perinatal Period

The period from 28 weeks of fetal life up to the first 7 days after birth is the perinatal period.

Fetal Period

Early Fetal Period

This refers to a period of gestation up to 22 weeks. Usually, the fetus at this period weighs less than 500 g and has a crown-rump length (CRL) of less than 25 cm.

Intermediate Fetal Period

This refers to the period of gestation from 22 to 27 weeks of fetal life. The fetus usually weighs 500–999 g and has a CRL of 25 cm up to 35 cm.

Late Fetal Period

This refers to gestations greater than 27 weeks and the fetus usually weighs 1,000 g or more and has a CRL of at least 35 cm.

NEONATE

Term Neonate

A neonate born between 37 and 41 weeks of completed gestation is a term neonate.

Preterm Neonate

A neonate who is born before 37 weeks of completed gestation is a preterm neonate.

Post-term Neonate

A neonate who is born after 41 weeks of completed gestation is a post-term neonate.

BIRTH WEIGHT RELATED

Low Birth Weight

Any neonate who at birth has a weight of less than 2,500 g, irrespective of gestation, is a low-birth-weight (LBW) neonate.

Very Low Birth Weight

A neonate with a birth weight of less than 1,500 g is a very LBW neonate.

Extremely Low Birth Weight

A neonate with a birth weight less than 1,000 g is an extremely LBW neonate.

Small for Dates/Small for Gestation Age/ Intrauterine Growth Retardation

These are synonymous terms often used interchangeably and refer to a neonate whose birth weight is less than 10th centile or less than –2 standard deviation of the reference standard for a given gestational age.

Appropriate for Dates/Appropriate for Gestation Age

It refers to a neonate whose birth weight is between 10th and 90th centiles or between –2 and +2 standard deviation of the reference standard for a given gestational age.

Large for Dates/Large for Gestation Age

It refers to a neonate whose birth weight is greater than 90th centiles or greater than +2 standard deviation of the reference standard for a given gestational age.

2.2 Neonatal Resuscitation

Satvik Bansal

INTRODUCTION

The transition from fetus to neonate is smooth in most cases. Approximately, 10% of the babies born require some assistance, and only 1 to 2 babies/1,000 live births require the need for chest compressions with or without medications.

In recent times, neonatal resuscitation has been the subject of extensive research and review. After years of gathering evidence, many aspects of the neonatal resuscitation have been universally agreed upon. Still, discussions and debate in certain elements of resuscitation persists.

PERINATAL PHYSIOLOGY

A basic knowledge of fetal to extrauterine neonatal transition is essential in understanding the rationale behind resuscitation practices.

Changes in Thermoregulation

In fetal life, the body's core temperature is just slightly higher than the surroundings (0.5°C). This situation dramatically changes after birth, when the temperature gradient between newborn baby's core temperature and surroundings is much greater. The result is greater heat loss and a high risk for the development of hypothermia in the baby. So, in order to maintain body temperature, the newborn starts to generate heat from various metabolic processes and by the lipolysis of brown adipose tissue. Moreover, the preterm infants are at an increased risk of hypothermia as they have immature skin, a greater surface area to body weight ratio, and low brown-adipose-tissue stores.

Changes in Respiration

The physiological adjustments in respiration are the most important. Before birth, the lungs of the fetus are filled with fluid. After birth, this fluid is cleared, and the lungs expand for the effective air exchange. All these physiological adjustments generally require some time. As the infant takes the first few breaths, it causes expansion of the chest wall. This, in turn, generates negative intrathoracic pressure (around 50 mm Hg), which leads to the inflow of air into the alveoli and lung expansion. Now, there are several important circulatory transitions that occur secondary to the development of effective air exchange in the lungs. The pulmonary vascular pressures start to decrease, which reduces right to left shunting through the foramen ovale and ductus arteriosus. It also increases the venous return to left atrium leading to rise in left atrial pressure and further decreased right to left shunting from the foramen ovale.

Changes in Circulation

Fetal circulation is unique because gas exchange takes place in the placenta. In the fetal heart, the oxygenated blood returning via the umbilical vein is mixed with deoxygenated blood from the superior and inferior vena cava, and it is distributed differentially throughout the body. The blood returning from the placenta to the right atrium is channeled via the foramen ovale to the left atrium and ventricle and then to the ascending aorta, providing the brain with the most oxygenated blood. In fetal life, the lungs are fluid filled, have intrinsically high vascular resistance, and do not participate in gas exchange **(Fig. 2.2.1)**.

After birth, the low-resistance placental circulation is removed, which increases the overall systemic vascular resistance. Along with this, the pulmonary vascular resistance begins to fall as a result of pulmonary expansion, increased arterial and alveolar oxygen tension, and local vasodilators. These changes result in a dramatic increase in pulmonary blood flow **(Fig. 2.2.2)**. The result is the rise in oxyhemoglobin saturation gradually over the first 5 to 15 minutes of life, to 90% or greater, as the air spaces are cleared of fluid.

PRIMARY AND SECONDARY APNEA

The baby has to make a lot of transitions at the time of delivery and in a very short span of time as discussed above. Any adverse situation compromising fetal tissue perfusion and oxygenation may affect its ability to make these necessary transitions during and immediately after birth. Newborn initially responds to hypoxia by the cessation of respiration and ultimately depression of cardiac function. Perinatal stress results in an initial period of rapid breathing, followed by a period of primary apnea (no breathing or gasping). Usually, just proper stimulation and oxygenation are sufficient to recover from this state. If the period of hypoxia continues, the fetus will have an additional brief period of irregular gasps

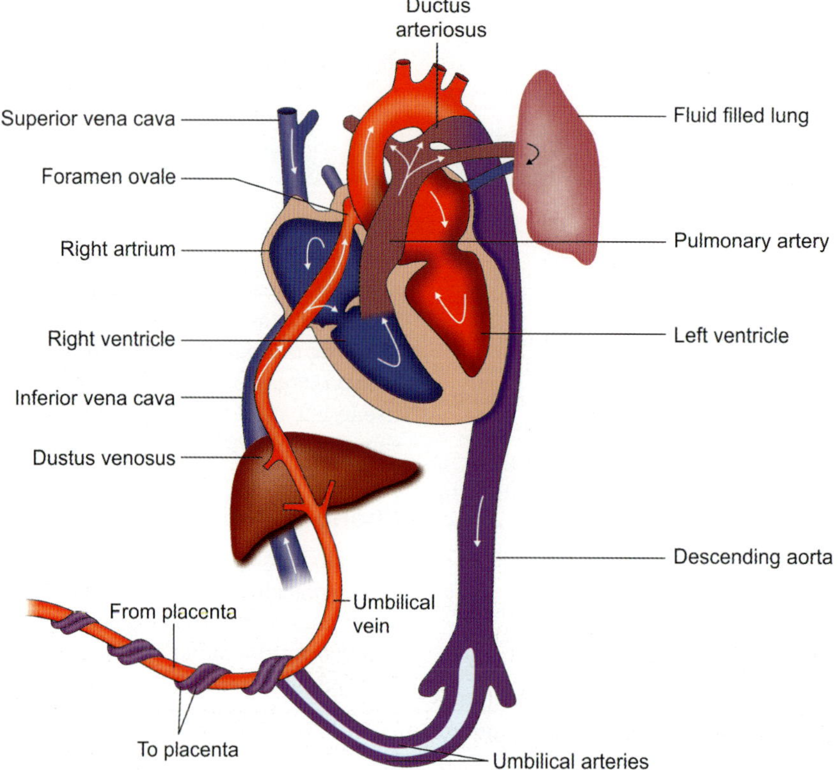

Fig. 2.2.1: Fetal circulation.

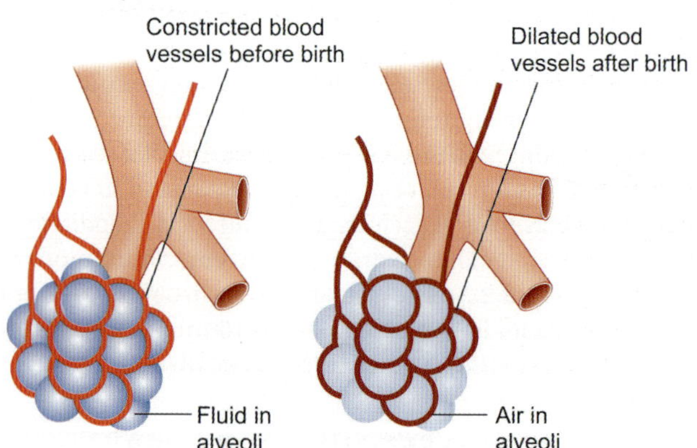

Fig. 2.2.2: Changes in pulmonary blood vessels after birth.

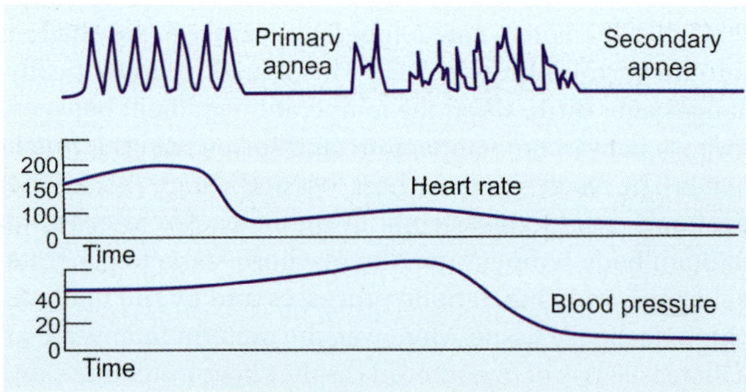

Fig. 2.2.3: Primary and secondary apnea.

and then will lapse into secondary apnea **(Fig. 2.2.3)**. During secondary apnea, stimulation will not restart the baby's breathing. Resuscitation with assisted ventilation and oxygen is required.

PREPARATION FOR RESUSCITATION

Risk Factors

It is very important to take a proper prenatal and intrapartum history and have knowledge of risk factors that can have a bearing on the baby. In most cases, it is possible to predict whether the baby may need extensive resuscitation, and this allows the resuscitation team to be better prepared and equipped. The most common risk factors include preterm birth, prolonged labor, meconium-stained amniotic fluid, pregnancy-induced hypertension, and nonreassuring fetal heart rate pattern. The complete list of significant risk factors is mentioned in **Table 2.2.1**.

Environment

It is important to have the temperature of the delivery room optimized. Necessary equipment **(Table 2.2.2)** must be

Table 2.2.1: Risk factors associated with need for neonatal resuscitation.

Prenatal risk factors
1. Gestational age less than 36 0/7 weeks or greater than or equal to 41 0/7 weeks 2. Preeclampsia or eclampsia 3. Intrauterine growth restriction 4. Multiple gestation 5. Fetal anemia 6. Polyhydramnios 7. Oligohydramnios 8. Fetal hydrops 9. Fetal macrosomia 10. Significant fetal malformations or anomalies 11. No antenatal visits
Intrapartum risk factors
1. Emergency cesarean delivery 2. Forceps or vacuum-assisted delivery 3. Breech or other abnormal presentation 4. Fetal distress (Category II or III fetal heart rate pattern) 5. Acute perinatal event (e.g. placental abruption, cord prolapse or abnormal fetal testing, or a scalp pH of 7.20 or less) 6. Maternal general anesthesia 7. Maternal magnesium therapy 8. Intrapartum bleeding 9. Chorioamnionitis 10. Shoulder dystocia 11. Meconium-stained amniotic fluid

Source: Adapted from American Academy of Pediatrics. AHA Textbook of Neonatal Resuscitation, 7th edition. Illinois: American Academy of Pediatrics/American Heart Association; 2016.

Table 2.2.2: Equipment for neonatal resuscitation.

Temperature	• Radiant warmer • Warm linen, shoulder roll • Cap • Plastic bag or plastic wrap (<32 weeks' gestation) • Thermal mattress (<32 weeks' gestation)
Airway	• Bulb syringe • 10 or 12 F suction catheter attached to wall suction • Meconium aspirator
Breathing	• Oxygen blender with flowmeter • Positive-pressure ventilation (PPV) device • Term- and preterm-sized masks • 5, 6, and 8 F feeding tube • Equipment to give free-flow oxygen with tubing • Pulse oximeter • Laryngoscope with size-0 and size-1 straight blades (size 00, optional) • Stylet (optional) • Endotracheal tubes (sizes 2.5, 3.0, 3.5) • CO_2 detector • Waterproof tape or tube-securing device • Scissors • Laryngeal mask (size 1) (optional)
Circulation	• Stethoscope • Electronic cardiac (ECG) monitor leads and ECG monitor • Epinephrine (1:10,000) • Normal saline • Supplies for placing emergency umbilical venous catheter (umbilical catheters, syringes, three-way stopcocks, blade)

(CO_2: carbon dioxide; ECG: electrocardiogram)

present and operating properly. As the need for significant intervention cannot always be predicted, it is recommended that ideally every delivery should be attended by at least one person who is trained in basic neonatal resuscitation. And, an advanced neonatal resuscitator should be immediately available, if need be.

Upon arrival in the delivery room, the resuscitator should not forget to introduce him or her first. Then he/she should obtain a short history of antenatal or intrapartum risk factors while preparing for the resuscitation. The checklist for preparation is given in **Table 2.2.3**.

ASSESSMENT AT BIRTH

The resuscitator should assess the answers to the following three questions:

1. Is the baby of term gestation?
2. Does the baby have a good tone?
3. Is the baby breathing regularly or crying?

If the answer to all the questions is "yes", then routine care should be given to the newborn. This includes drying the baby, maintaining normal temperature by placing the baby in skin-to-skin contact with the mother, and maintaining the airway that is, clearing the secretions if required and appropriate positioning. Cord clamping should be delayed by a minimum of 30 seconds. It is preferred that the newborn is not separated from the mother during routine care. The breastfeeding should be initiated as soon as possible. The breathing pattern and rate, activity of the baby, and color of the baby should be watched.

However, if the answer to any of the questions is "no", then the cord should be clamped, and the baby should be moved under a radiant warmer. Now, the baby should be managed according to the resuscitation algorithm **(Fig. 2.2.4)**.

INITIAL STEPS OF RESUSCITATION

Warm and Maintain Normal Temperature

It is very important to ensure that the infant remains warm. The American Heart Association (2015) recommendations clearly state, "admission temperature of newly born nonasphyxiated infants is a strong predictor of mortality at all gestational ages". The recommended range of normal temperature is between 36.5 and 37.5°C. Following strategies can be used in

Table 2.2.3: Preparation for resuscitation.

- The radiant warmer should be switched on at least 20 minutes before and put on manual mode
- Delivery room temperature should be more than 26°C
- Dry, warm blankets should be available
- Turn on the oxygen source or air–oxygen blend and adjust the flow to 5 to 8 L/min. Adjust the oxygen concentration to the desired initial level
- Test the self-inflating bag (if used) for pop-off control and leak
- Check that a proper-sized mask is present
- Make sure that the laryngoscope light is bright
- Check availability of an appropriate sized laryngoscope blade
    - no. 1 for full-term neonates
    - no. 0 for premature neonates
    - no. 00 for extremely low-birth-weight neonates
- Check availability of an appropriate ET tube for the expected birth weight
    - 3.5 mm for late preterm and full-term infants (>2,000 g)
    - 3.0 mm for premature infants (>1,000 to 2,000 g)
    - 2.5 mm for smaller infants
- An intubation stylet may be used (tip is kept at least 0.5 cm from the distal end of the tube)
- If there is any suggestion that extensive resuscitation may be needed, the following additional preparations are required:
    - Set up an umbilical catheterization tray for venous catheterization
    - Draw up 1:10,000 epinephrine and isotonic saline for catheter flush solution and volume replacement
    - Check that other potentially necessary drugs are present and ready for administration

(ET: endotracheal)

the delivery room—radiant warmer, exothermic mattresses, the use of plastic wrap, warm humidified gases, and increased room temperature. Extremely small infants may require a combination of the above-mentioned techniques.

Position

Infant should be placed supine with head in midline position and slight neck extension **(Fig. 2.2.5)**. This permits unrestricted air entry to the lungs. A rolled blanket or towel can be kept under the shoulders.

Clear Airway

Whenever required [in the cases of obvious obstruction or requirement of positive-pressure ventilation (PPV)], suctioning should always be done gently. Vigorous suctioning is harmful as apart from causing injury to the tissues, it may cause bradycardia or apnea. This happens because stimulation of posterior pharynx can generate a vagal response. Also, as a rule, mouth should be suctioned first, followed by nose.

Meconium-stained amniotic fluid: The recent guidelines do not consider meconium-stained liquor as a stand-alone criterion to stop routine care and start with initial steps of resuscitation. This means that babies born through meconium-stained amniotic fluid having good normal respiratory effort and tone should be given routine care, and not resuscitated.

Gentle clearing of meconium from the mouth and nose may be done.

However, if the respiratory efforts or tone is inappropriate, then baby is brought under a radiant warmer, and resuscitation algorithm is followed. The routine intubation for tracheal suction in non-vigorous babies is now not recommended, and the starting of PPV should not be delayed.

Dry and Stimulate

The baby should be gently dried using prewarmed sheets, and wet sheets should be removed immediately. Remember not to remove the vernix. In the cases of preterm babies, who are less than 32 weeks of gestation, it is recommended that they are covered in plastic wraps neck down without drying to prevent heat loss.

Some babies may require tactile stimulation to improve their breathing pattern or cry. Baby's trunk, back, or extremities can be rubbed gently. This is generally done while drying the baby. It is important to remember that overly vigorous stimulation is harmful as it may cause injury to the baby. Also, if the baby remains apneic despite gentle stimulation for few seconds, further time should not be wasted and initiate PPV considering the possibility of secondary apnea.

ASSESSMENT OF NEWBORN DURING RESUSCITATION

The initial steps of resuscitation and reevaluation of the baby should be completed within the first 60 seconds of life. The objective being that babies who are not improving should be given PPV latest by 1 min of life. This is termed as "the First Golden Minute".

The reevaluation after initials steps is based on heart rate and respiratory efforts. The indications for starting PPV include apnea, gasping, or heart rate less than 100. If there is labored breathing or persistent cyanosis, supplemental oxygen and continuous positive airway pressure (CPAP) should be considered.

After initiating PPV or supplementary oxygen administration, further reevaluation of the newborn consists of the assessment of heart rate, respiratory efforts, and oxygen saturation, as determined by pulse oximetry.

Assessment of Heart Rate

An improvement in the heart rate is considered the most sensitive indicator of successful resuscitation. The current recommendation is to use a 3-lead electrocardiogram, wherever possible. Other methods include chest auscultation and counting umbilical vessel pulsations.

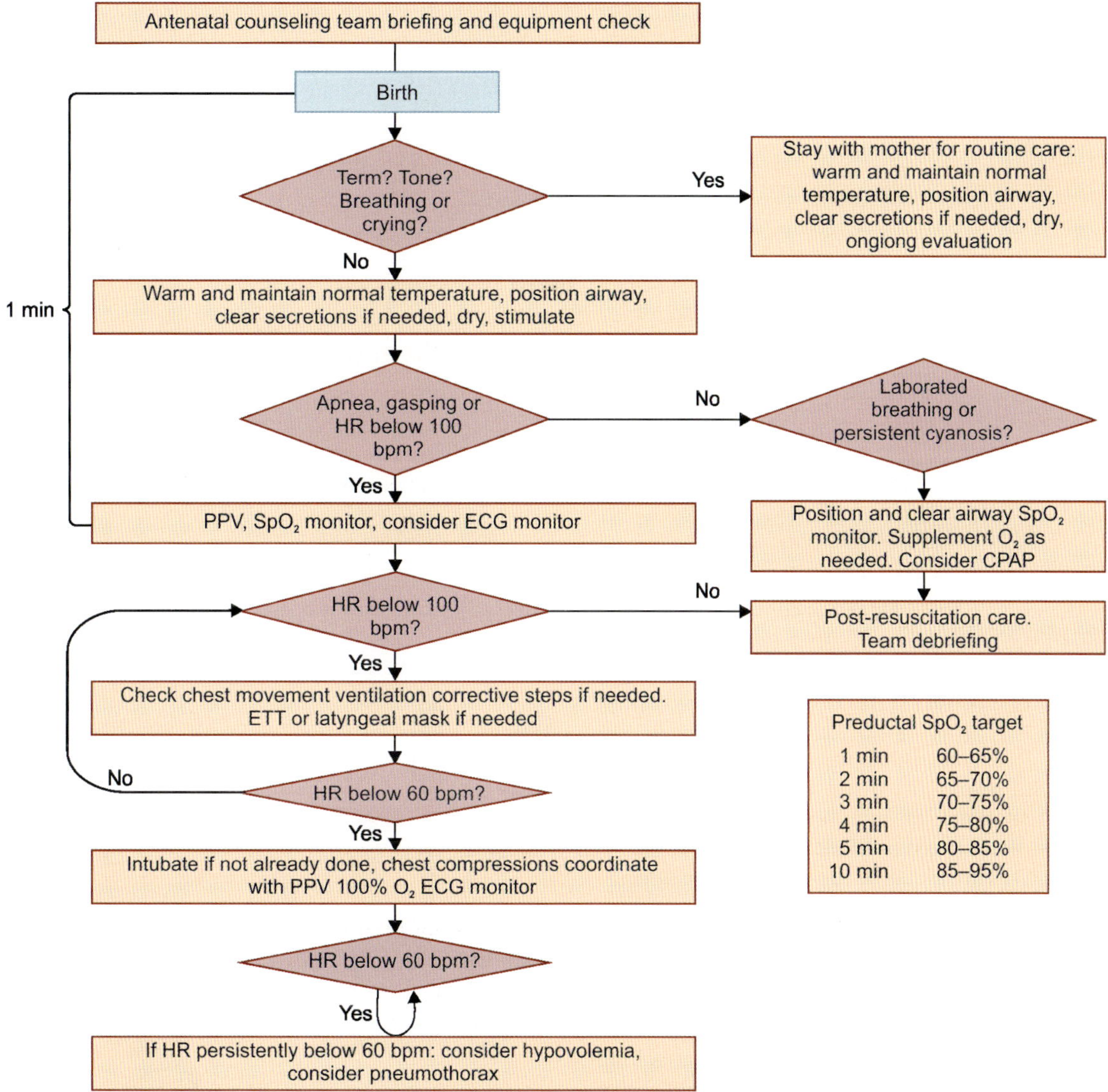

Fig. 2.2.4: Neonatal resuscitation algorithm.

Assessment of Need of Supplemental Oxygen

Both insufficient and excess of oxygen is harmful for the baby. And as cyanosis can be an unreliable indicator of oxygenation in a newborn, the use of pulse oximetry is recommended. So, when the baby is started on PPV or supplemental oxygen, pulse oximetry should be used wherever possible.

Administration of Oxygen

Term infants: The resuscitation should be started with room air. The supplemental oxygen may be administered and concentration titrated keeping the preductal oxygen saturation in the minute specific reference range **(Fig. 2.2.4)**.

Preterm infants: The resuscitation of newborn below 35 weeks of gestation should be initiated with low oxygen (<30%). The concentration of oxygen should be titrated as per preductal saturation. Different ranges have not been determined for preterm babies. In situations, where blended oxygen is not available, the use of room air is recommended to initiate resuscitation.

In both term and preterm infants, 100% oxygen is used if heart rate remains less than 60 bpm even after 90 seconds of resuscitation, or there is a need for chest compressions.

POSITIVE-PRESSURE VENTILATION

The indications of starting PPV during neonatal resuscitation can be any of the further given points.

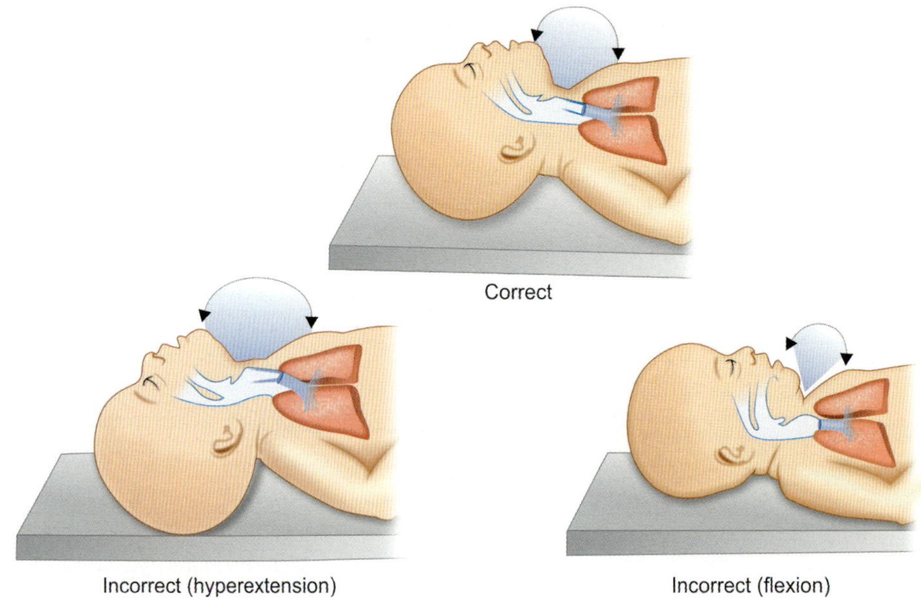

Fig. 2.2.5: Correct position of head and neck to keep the airway open.

- Inadequate respiratory efforts—apnea or gasping respiration
- Bradycardia—heart rate <100 bpm
- Newborns with respiratory distress, who are unable to maintain oxygenation in the minute specific range despite the use of free-flow oxygen or CPAP.

Three types of devices are available to ventilate a newborn:

1. Flow-inflating bag
2. Self-inflating bag
3. T-piece resuscitator

Self-inflating bag (200–750 mL) is the most commonly used device. It is easier to use, does not require a compressed gas source, and is portable. The bag has a site for attaching oxygen reservoir. It also has a pressure release "pop-off" valve which prevents barotrauma to the baby's lungs **(Fig. 2.2.6)**.

Alternate airways—endotracheal tube and laryngeal mask airway—can be used in certain cases **(Table 2.2.4)**.

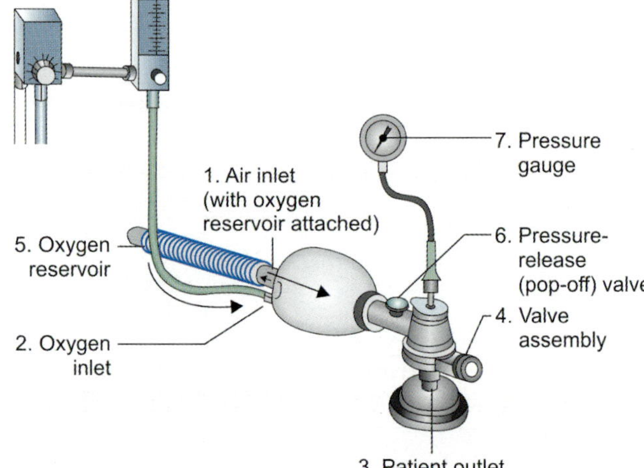

Fig. 2.2.6: Parts of a self-inflating bag.

The rationale behind the use of PPV is to force the gas into the lungs with some additional pressure which will open up the collapsed alveoli, and hence improve oxygenation. PPV should be started with higher peak pressures in the first few breaths. Once the lungs are inflated and functional residual capacity has been established, further ventilation can be continued at a lower peak pressure. There should not be excessive chest rise. This is essential so as to prevent damage to the lungs by PPV. In preterm babies, initial peak pressures of 20–25 cmH_2O are required, while full-term babies may require 30–40 cmH_2O in first few breaths. In babies with some respiratory pathologies, such as respiratory distress syndrome, congenital pneumonia or meconium aspiration, and others, higher pressures may be required to establish ventilation.

If the chest is not moving with each breath, and there are poor breath sounds, ventilation corrective measures should be initiated. There can be three possible reasons for ineffective ventilation:

1. Inadequate mask seal **(Fig. 2.2.7)**
2. Blocked airway
3. Inadequate pressure

The algorithm of *MR SOPA* should be followed **(Table 2.2.5)**.

Table 2.2.4: Indications for the use of alternate airways during neonatal resuscitation.

Endotracheal tube	***Laryngeal mask airway***
• Ineffective or prolonged face-mask ventilation • Chest compressions • Stabilization of a newborn with a suspected diaphragmatic hernia • Surfactant administration • Direct tracheal suction if the airway is obstructed by thick secretions	• Ineffective or prolonged face-mask ventilation • Tracheal intubation is unsuccessful

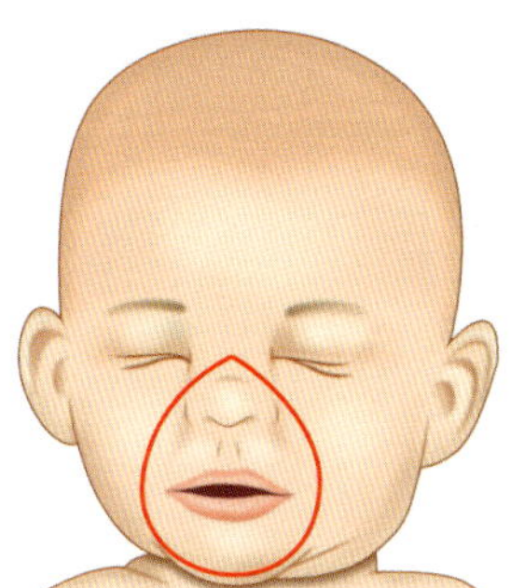

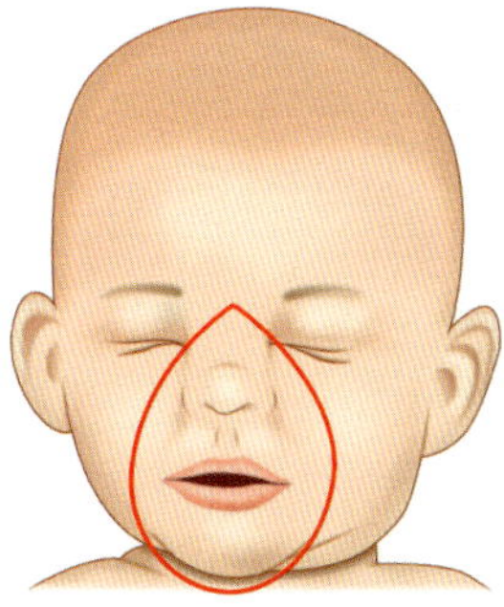

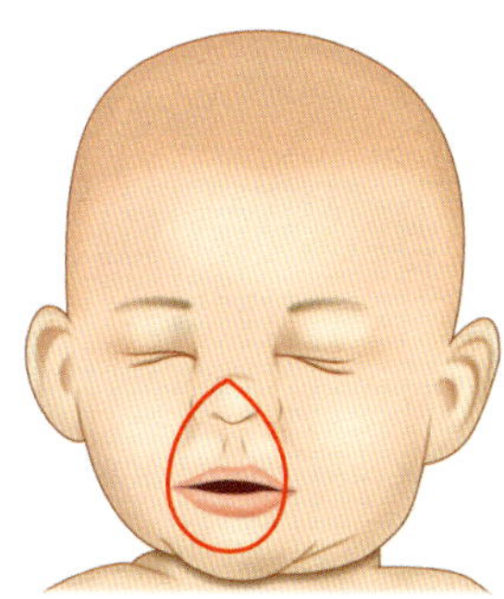

Fig. 2.2.7: Appropriate sized mask. The mask should cover the mouth and nose but not the eyes.

Once the effective ventilation is confirmed, PPV is continued at a rate of 40 to 60 breaths/min to maintain minute ventilation **(Fig. 2.2.8)**.

Once on PPV, the baby should be assessed after every 30 seconds. In general, before any betterment of respiratory efforts, there is improvement first in the heart rate, oxygen saturation, and tone of the baby. As the respiratory efforts of the baby improve, ventilatory breaths should be tapered. The PPV should be continued till there are regular, adequate spontaneous respiratory efforts with a heart rate of more than 100 bpm.

Table 2.2.5: Ventilation corrective algorithm.

M	Mask adjustment	Reapply the mask. Consider using the 2-hand technique
R	Reposition airway	Place head in "sniffing position" or slightly extended
S	Suction	Use bulb syringe or suction catheter
O	Open airway	Open the mouth and lift the jaw forward
P	Pressure increase	Increase pressure in 5–10 cmH_2O increments, maximum 40 cmH_2O
A	Alternate airway	Place and endotracheal tube or laryngeal mask airway

End-expiratory pressure: The evidence for the use of positive end-expiratory pressure (PEEP) in delivery room is not strong. The recent International Liaison Committee on Resuscitation guidelines suggest the use of approximately 5 cmH_2O PEEP, when PPV is administered to preterm infants.

Continuous positive airway pressure: There is now a clear recommendation that CPAP should be the treatment modality of choice for spontaneously breathing newborn with respiratory distress.

There is large evidence supporting the use of CPAP when compared with routine intubation and ventilation in such babies. The advantages include the reduction of combined outcome of death and/or bronchopulmonary dysplasia in preterm babies and reduced duration of mechanical ventilation.

Sustained inflation breaths: There is some evidence majorly from animal studies and some human trials that providing longer initial inflation breaths can be beneficial in establishing functional residual capacity and improving respiratory outcomes.

There is insufficient evidence on the safety of long-sustained inflation breaths and also on appropriate duration and pressures to be used while delivering them. The current guidelines do not recommend routine use of initial sustained inflation breaths greater than 5 seconds.

CHEST COMPRESSION

The chest compressions should be started, if the heart rate remains below 60 bpm after 30 seconds of PPV. It is important to ensure that the ventilation was effective by assessing the chest rise before moving on to the chest compressions.

It is advised to intubate the baby and administer 100% oxygen to the baby when starting chest compressions.

There are certain points to remember while giving chest compressions:

- The chest compressions should be given on the lower third of sternum.

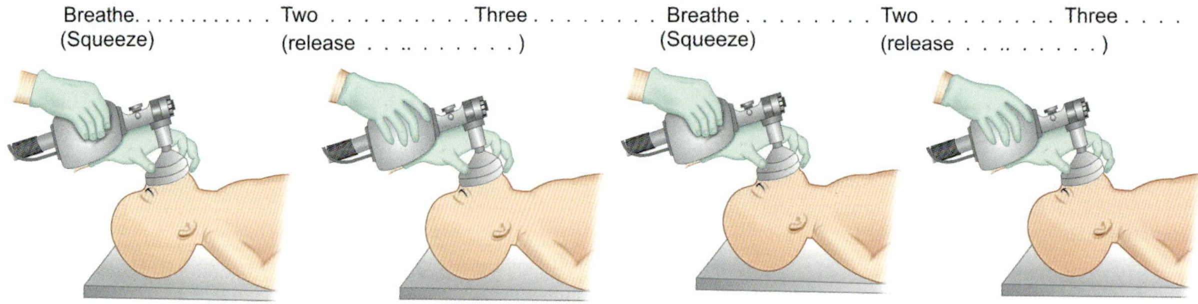

Fig. 2.2.8: Maintain the correct rate while giving positive-pressure ventilation.

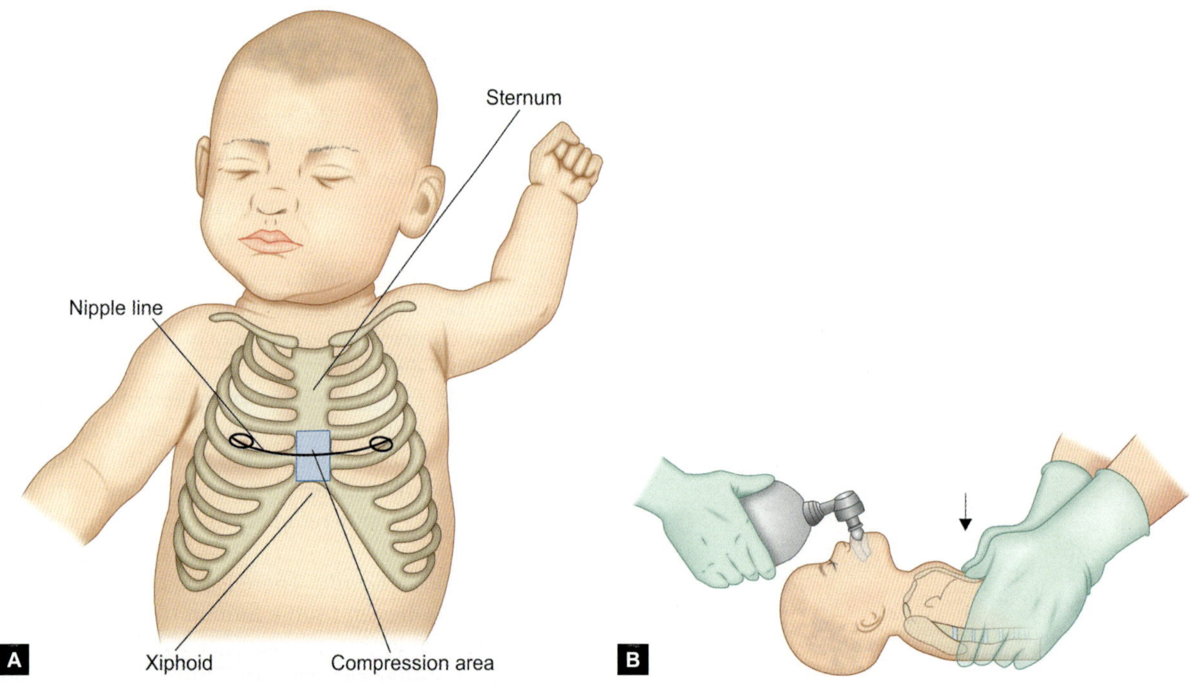

Figs. 2.2.9A and B: (A) Landmarks for chest compression; (B) Correct technique for chest compression.

- The chest wall should be compressed by around one third of the anteroposterior diameter of the chest **(Figs. 2.2.9A and B)**.
- There are two techniques to give compressions—thumb technique and two-finger technique. The thumb technique is preferred **(Table 2.2.6)**.
- Maintain proper coordination between compressions and ventilation to prevent their simultaneous delivery.
- It is essential to allow reexpansion of the chest, but the thumbs should not rise up from the chest wall.

The neonatal resuscitation guidelines recommend 3:1 ratio of compressions to ventilation. There should be a total of 120 events each minute (90 compressions and 30 ventilations). So, each event is given around half a second. In the cases where etiology of arrest is of cardiac origin, higher ratios (e.g. 15:2) may be considered.

Once chest compressions have begun regular assessments should be done after every 45–60 seconds. Once the heart rate becomes higher than 60 bpm, the chest compressions can be stopped.

MEDICATIONS

In conditions, when there is no improvement in heart rate, remains below 60 bpm, despite 1–2 min of chest compressions, the role of drugs should be considered **(Table 2.2.7)**. The following drugs are used in neonatal resuscitation.

- *Epinephrine hydrochloride*: It is a powerful adrenergic agent which increases the strength and the rate of cardiac contractions and causes peripheral vasoconstriction. The preferred route of administration is intravenous; however, it can be delivered through the intraosseous route or

Table 2.2.6: Techniques of giving chest compression.

Two-thumb technique	*Two-finger technique*
• Compressions are delivered with 2 thumbs, and the fingers encircle the chest while supporting the back • This is the *preferred technique* as it generates higher blood pressure and coronary perfusion with less rescuer fatigue	• Compressions are delivered by 2 fingers while a second hand supports the back

endotracheally (higher dose is required when given endotracheally). However, as there is a lack of supportive data for endotracheal epinephrine, this route may only be considered while establishing intravenous access. The heart rate should be checked about 1 min after giving epinephrine (longer if given endotracheally). The dose of epinephrine can be repeated after 3–5 min. If there is no response after two doses, while additional doses can be given other causes of depression should be sought out. There is no benefit of using higher doses.

- *Volume expansion*: Volume expansion is important in conditions of known or suspected blood loss. It can also be considered when the baby is not responding to any other resuscitative measures. An isotonic crystalloid solution or blood should be administered. The recommended dose is 10 mL/kg to be given over 5–10 min. The dose may be repeated. It is important to remember that volume expansion should not be done rapidly in preterm newborn for the risk of intraventricular hemorrhage.
- *Other drugs*: Intravenous administration of bicarbonate or other buffer solutions may be considered during prolonged arrests unresponsive to any other therapy. The European Resuscitation Council suggests a dose of 1–2 mmol/kg given slowly.

The easiest way to secure intravenous access in a baby undergoing resuscitation is the catheterizations of the umbilical vein. There are certain points to be kept in mind while catheterizing umbilical vein:

- Advance the catheter only up to 2–3 cm past the abdominal wall; this would be around 4–5 cm in total.
- There should be easy back flow of blood.
- Remember to flush the medications that are administered, because there will not be any flow in the vein subsequent to cord separation.

POSTRESUSCITATIVE CARE

Once adequate ventilation and circulation are established, the infant should be transferred to intensive care unit and kept under close monitoring **(Table 2.2.8)**.

Table 2.2.7: Medications used in neonatal resuscitation.

Drug	*Route*	*Dose (mL/kg)*	*Administration*
Epinephrine (1:10,000)	Intravenous or intraosseous	0.1–0.3	Flush with 0.5–1 mL normal saline
	Endotracheal	0.5–1	PPV breaths to distribute into lungs
Normal saline or O negative packed red cells (in suspected anemia)	Intravenous or intraosseous	10	Over 5–10 min. Caution in preterm newborns <30 weeks of gestation

Table 2.2.8: Postresuscitative care.

Monitoring and maintaining normal blood glucose values
The range of blood glucose concentration that is associated with the least brain injury following asphyxia and resuscitation has not yet been defined. However, hypoglycemia has been associated with an increased risk for brain injury, while increased glucose levels posthypoxic ischemic injury may be protective
Therapeutic hypothermia (33.5–34.5°C)
Term or near-term infants (more than 36 weeks' gestation) with evolving moderate-to-severe hypoxic-ischemic encephalopathy should, where possible, be offered therapeutic hypothermia. Both whole body cooling and selective head cooling are recommended. Cooling should be initiated and conducted under clearly defined protocols in an intensive care setting. It should be commenced within 6 hours of birth and continued for 72 hours of birth. The infants are slowly rewarmed over at least 4 hours. Presently, there is no evidence that cooling is effective, if started more than 6 hours after birth. There may be some associated adverse effects such as thrombocytopenia and need for inotropic support

Withholding and Discontinuing Resuscitation

As per medical ethics, not initiating resuscitation of a baby is equivalent to discontinuation of life-sustaining treatment during or after resuscitation.

- *At border of viability*: In general, in babies less than 25 weeks' gestation, the appropriateness of resuscitation should be determined by region-specific guidelines. Opinions may vary regarding using aggressive therapies. Variables affecting newborn survival should be kept in mind, such as the accuracy of gestational age assigned, chorioamnionitis, and the level of care available for the newborn at the delivery center.
- *Severely depressed at birth*: Non-improving Apgar score **(Table 2.2.9)** of 0 at 10 min is a strong predictor of the neonatal mortality and morbidity. It is considered reasonable to stop resuscitative efforts if even after 10 min, the heart rate remains undetectable. The variables such as optimal resuscitation, availability of advanced neonatal, special circumstances before delivery, and wishes expressed by the family should be considered.

Table 2.2.9: Apgar score.

Sign	*0*	*1*	*2*
Respiratory effort	Absent	Gasping	Good cry
Heart rate (bpm)	Absent	<100	>100
Color	Blue/pale	Pink body; blue extremities	Completely pink
Muscle tone	Limp	Some flexion of extremities	Active motion
Reflex*	No response	Grimace	Cry or active withdrawal

*Assessed by inserting catheter into the nose.

BIBLIOGRAPHY

1. Wyckoff MH, Aziz K, Escobedo MB, et al. Part 13: Neonatal resuscitation: 2015 American Heart Association guidelines update for cardiopulmonary resuscitation and emergency cardiovascular care. Circulation. 2015;132:S543-60.
2. Wyllie J, Bruinenberg J, Roehr CC, et al. European Resuscitation Council guidelines for resuscitation 2015. Resuscitation. 2015;95:249-63.
3. Wyllie J, Perlman JM, Kattwinkel J, et al. Part 7: Neonatal resuscitation: 2015 International Consensus on Cardiopulmonary Resuscitation and Emergency Cardiovascular Care Science With Treatment Recommendations. Resuscitation. 2015;95:e169-201.

2.3 Care of the Normal Newborn

B Vishnu Bhat

INTRODUCTION

Normal newborn is an infant born at term with birth weight greater than 2,500 g, without any asphyxia, major congenital malformations, or birth injuries.

NORMAL FEATURES IN NEWBORN

Anthropometry

The average birth weight of babies in India is 2,900 g. The length may vary from 47 cm to 52 cm and head circumference 33–37 cm. Generally, the head circumference is 2–3 cm more than chest circumference at birth, and they equal by 1 year after which chest circumference exceeds that of the head.

Respiration, Heart Rate and Blood Pressure

A newborn may have periodic breathing, and the normal rate may vary from 40/min to 60/min. The heart rate is usually 120–160 beats/min. The systolic blood pressure will vary from 40 mm Hg to 60 mm Hg and diastolic 25–40 mm Hg.

Skin Changes

Mongolian spots are bluish patches seen over the buttocks and back due to deposition of melanin pigment and disappear in 6 months to 2 years' time. Milia are tiny cream papules, which are inclusion cysts containing trapped keratinized stratum corneum, and usually resolve without treatment in 2–3 weeks. Erythema toxicum is erythematous papular, macular, or rarely pustular lesions present over the body surface because of eosinophilic infiltrate into the dermis. They usually appear 2 days after birth and disappear during the first week. Epstein's pearls are whitish papular lesions usually seen over the palate and sometimes over the prepuce and disappear after a few days. Small hemangioma may be seen over the body surface, which disappears within 2 years of life.

Physiologic Events

Physiologic jaundice usually appears after 2–3 days and disappears by 7–10 days of life and does not stain the palms and soles. Enlargement of the breast during first 3–7 days of life is known as mastitis neonatorum and does not require any treatment. This enlargement is related to maternal transfer of hormones. A female baby may have vaginal discharge and bleeding during that period, which is also hormone related and disappears within a few days. There may be molding of the head and caput succedaneum over the presenting part, which disappears within 2–3 days. Caput should be differentiated from cephalohematoma. The latter is due to the collection of blood under the periosteum, and hence does not cross the suture lines. It is usually noticed after 2 days of birth and disappears after 6–8 weeks. It usually does not require treatment.

Urine and Stool Passage

A newborn usually passes urine within 48 hours and meconium during the first 24 hours of life. If there is no distension of abdomen, delayed passage of urine usually indicates inadequate feeding. Distension of bladder in a male baby suggests posterior urethral valve. When there is a delay in passage of meconium, a soft rubber catheter should be passed into the rectum to confirm patency. The fingertip or thermometer should not be used for checking patency, since these may result in rectal injury. Prematurity, meconium plug, congenital megacolon, meconium ileus, and hypothyroidism may result in delayed passage of meconium. A baby may pass frequent yellow-colored watery to semisolid stools during first 3–7 days of life known as transitional stools. Some babies may pass stools once in 2–3 days. Hypothyroidism should be excluded in babies with constipation.

IMPORTANT EXAMINATION FINDINGS IN NEWBORN

Anterior and posterior fontanels are open at birth. Anterior fontanel can measure up to 3 × 3 cm at its widest points, though the size is very variable, and posterior fontanel is often open at this age. Large posterior fontanel or both anterior and posterior communicating is usually abnormal. In such cases, hypothyroidism, hydrocephalus, congenital rickets, etc. need to be excluded. Similarly, if anterior fontanel is very small, and there is ridging of suture lines, it may indicate craniosynostosis. Natal teeth may rarely be present. They may be loose and sometimes may result in injuries to mother's nipple, in that case, they may need to be extracted. Phimosis is normal during this period, but the meatus is visible when prepuce is retracted in more than 85% of the babies. Mucosal tags may be seen at the introitus in female babies.

Palpable liver 2–3 cm below the costal margin and palpable spleen tip are normal. Usually, both testes are in the bottom of the scrotum in term male babies. If the testes are not palpable or abnormally placed, it should be recorded and investigated. Sixty percent of the normal newborns have a systolic murmur (innocent murmur) at the age of 2 hours, but the incidence falls to around 1% by 24 hours age. Healthy term infants move between behavioral states, spending most time in quiet and active sleep. The undisturbed normal neonate lies predominantly in a flexed position with no lateral preference.

IMPORTANT NEONATAL REFLEXES

Rooting Reflex

Rooting reflex helps the baby to locate the mother's nipple without her directing the baby's mouth. The infant turns toward the point where the cheek is touched. When the corner of the mouth is touched, the lower lip is lowered, and the tongue is brought forward toward the contact **(Fig. 2.3.1)**. If the finger is moved away, the head turns to follow it.

Sucking and Swallowing Reflexes

These are elicited by introducing clean finger or mother's teat in the mouth. They disappear when voluntary control of feeding is achieved. They are decreased or absent when there is neurological depression, hypotonia, or immaturity. A baby would have usually crossed 34 weeks of gestation when he/she can feed directly from breast.

Moro Reflex

It is a vestibular reflex, which disappears by 3–5 months of age. It can be elicited by raising the shoulder for 45° from ground and then dropping by 30°. There will be abduction and extension of arms with opening of fingers. This is followed by flexion and adduction of arms **(Fig. 2.3.2)**. The reflex may be accompanied by crying, extension of trunk and neck with movements of legs. It is exaggerated when there is a cerebral irritation caused by hypoxia, infection, hyperbilirubinemia, etc. It is decreased with sedation, central nervous system depression, or prematurity. Asymmetrical response is seen with Erb's palsy, clavicle or humerus fracture, or shoulder dislocation.

Palmar Grasp Reflex

It is elicited by touching the baby's palm from the ulnar side with finger or any other suitable object **(Fig. 2.3.3)**. The fingers close and grasp the object. When the dorsum of the hand is touched, the fingers open. The grasp becomes stronger, if the head is turned to the opposite side, and the stimulating finger is moved toward the fingers. Similar reflex can be elicited in

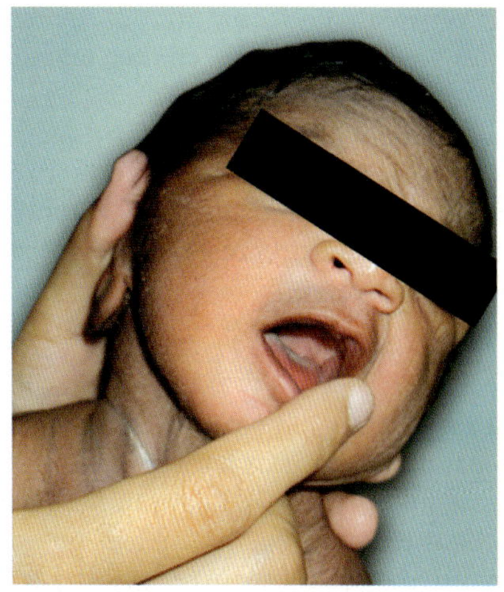

Fig. 2.3.1: Rooting reflex.

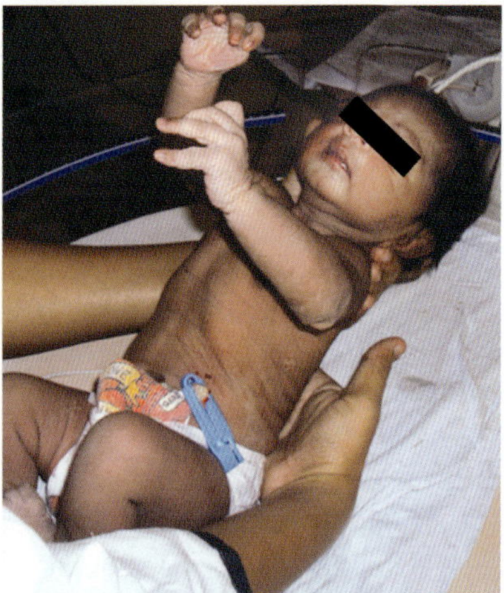

Fig. 2.3.2: Moro reflex.

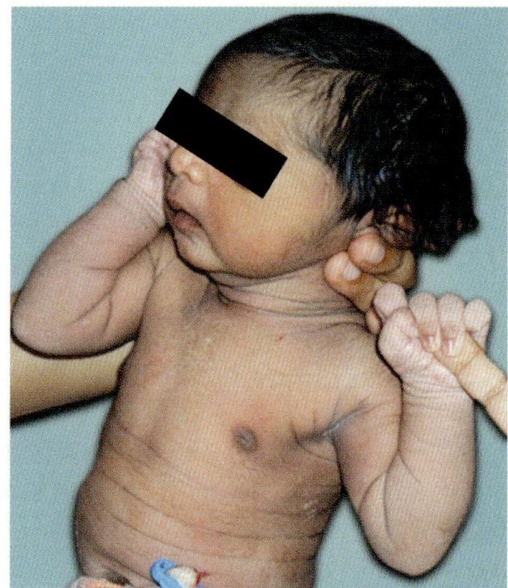

Fig. 2.3.3: Palmar grasp reflex.

the lower limb by stimulating the sole. Persistence of grasp after 3 months of age may indicate cerebral palsy.

MANAGEMENT

Temperature Maintenance and Monitoring

The normal body temperature of the newborn ranges from 36.5 to 37.5°C. Newborns are uniquely susceptible to hypothermia because they have a large body surface area, which causes heat loss and have reduced subcutaneous insulation. They are dependent on caregivers to keep them warm and dry. The temperature of the delivery room should be at least 26 ± 2°C and free from the draft of air. The infant should be received over the mother's abdomen or in prewarmed sterile linen and should be dried thoroughly from head to foot. The wet linen should be removed and replaced with a dry cloth. The baby should be made to wear cap and socks. Kangaroo care position is the most ideal. Skin-to-skin contact with the mother not only prevents hypothermia but also promotes breastfeeding and bonding. A bath is delayed until the temperature is stabilized. It is better, if baby bath is not given in hospital for fear of cross infection. Mother can be taught the simple technique of monitoring the baby's temperature by touching the periphery and observing for color change. Cold extremities with blue or pale color indicate inadequate warmth.

Cord and Eye Care

The umbilical stump should be cleaned with spirit and kept dry. The local application of antiseptics is not required. Usually, the stump will fall in 7–10 days' time. The eyes should be cleaned with sterile wet cotton. There is no need to instill antibiotic drops into eye except in areas with high incidence of vertically acquired conjunctivitis.

Feeding

Breastfeeding should be initiated soon after birth, and exclusive breastfeeding is advised till 6 months of age in normal term babies. A baby should receive 7–8 feeds a day during the first few weeks. The mother should be explained about the benefits of breastfeeding, and the family members are encouraged to support her. It is important not to separate the newborn from the mother without a justifiable reason. The initial alert period after birth is utilized to start breastfeeds, as babies tend to sleep a lot after that. Health workers caring for newborns should learn the signs of good attachment, which include mouth wide open, more areola seen above than below, chin touching the breast, and lower lip everted. Excessive weight loss of more than 8–10% in the first 3–4 days indicates inadequate breastfeeding or illness in the baby.

Vitamin K

All babies should receive vitamin K prophylaxis of 0.5 mg (for <1,000 g) to 1 mg (for >1,000 g) intramuscularly after birth to prevent hemorrhagic disease of the newborn.

Danger Signs

Mother should be informed about danger signs and the need to get medical advice as and when they are observed. Some of the danger signs are given in **Table 2.3.1**.

DISCHARGE PLANNING

It is ideal to discharge a normal newborn after 48–72 hours of life. The baby should be free of illness, significant jaundice, and the mother should be confident about breastfeeding. The baby should have received initial immunization with Bacillus Calmette-Guérin, oral polio, and hepatitis B vaccines and

Table 2.3.1: Danger signs in newborn.

- Poor sucking/cry
- Fever/hypothermia
- Respiratory distress
- Persistent vomiting
- Blood or bile-stained vomitus
- Abdominal distension
- Pallor
- Jaundice involving extremities
- Bleeding
- Convulsions
- Central cyanosis

have passed meconium and urine. If the baby is discharged early, he or she should be reviewed at home or hospital after 48 hours. Babies should be followed up and anthropometry recorded in a growth chart. The growth and development should be evaluated monthly during the first few months and 3 monthly thereafter.

KEY MESSAGES

- Temperature control and prevention of hypothermia is vital.
- Breastfeeding is initiated as soon as possible.
- All babies should receive vitamin K prophylaxis.
- Initial immunization should be given before discharge.
- Growth and development should be monitored during follow-up.
- Mother should be informed of the danger signs.

BIBLIOGRAPHY

1. Behrman RE, Kliegman RM, Jenson HB. Nelson Textbook of Pediatrics, 20th edition. Philadelphia, PA: Elsevier Saunders; 2015.
2. Bhat BV. Neonatal care. In: Parthasarathy A, Menon PS, Nair MK, Bhave SY, (Eds). Partha's Fundamentals of Pediatrics, 2nd edition. New Delhi: Jaypee Brothers Medical Publishers; 2013. pp. 21-38.
3. Cloherty JP, Echenwald EC, Stark AR. Manual of Neonatal Care, 7th edition. Philadelphia, PA: Lippincott Williams and Wilkins; 2012.
4. Illingworth RS. The Normal Child: Some Problems of the Early Years and Their Treatment, 10th edition. Edinburgh: Churchill Livingstone; 1997.
5. Rennie JM. Rennie and Roberton's Textbook of Neonatology, 5th edition. Philadelphia, PA: Elsevier Health Sciences; 2012.
6. Taeusch HW, Ballard RA, Gleason CA. Avery's Diseases of the Newborn, 10th edition. Philadelphia, PA: Elsevier Health Sciences; 2012.

2.4 Identification and Approach to a Sick Newborn

Swarna Rekha Bhat

INTRODUCTION

Early identification of a sick newborn is the key to successful management and improving neonatal outcome.

WHO IS A SICK NEWBORN?

A sick newborn may be described as one who is:

- Not feeding well
- Lethargic
- Has any systemic illness
- Has poor weight gain.

These are infants who require admission, additional support, such as oxygen, intravenous fluids, and constant monitoring. In addition, neonates who are preterm or low birth weight are also considered "sick" newborns as they require additional support and monitoring.

EVALUATING A SICK NEWBORN

History

Following history should be elicited to determine nature of illness and presence or absence of risk factors **(Table 2.4.1)**:

- Age of neonate in hours/days;
- Antenatal history to identify any risk factors;
- Intrapartum history to identify risk factors;
- Mode of delivery;
- Apgar score or crying or breathing immediately after delivery, need for resuscitation;

- *Feeding history:* Any feed given/is feeding adequate/is baby on breastfeeds;
- One should also elicit history suggestive of significant illness **(Table 2.4.2)**.

Examination

Examination of a sick neonate can provide useful clues to the etiology of sickness and provides a basis for the management plan. Important signs and their utility are summarized below.

Temperature Instability

Hypothermia (<36°C) could be due to environmental factors or because of sepsis. Hyperthermia is less common and could be environmental or a manifestation of sepsis.

Respiratory Distress

Breathing problems in a neonate can be tachypnea (respiratory rate >60/min), chest indrawing, stridor, or apnea.

Table 2.4.1: Risk factors: maternal and fetal.

Antenatal risk factors
• Maternal diabetes mellitus
• Pregnancy-induced hypertension (PIH); eclampsia
• Urinary tract infections (UTI)
• Any medical illness
• Rh negative mother
• Oligo- or polyhydramnios fetal
• Intrauterine growth retardation (IUGR)
• Abnormal ultrasonogram (USG)
• Abnormal Doppler study
• Preterm delivery intrapartum
• Premature rupture of membranes (PROM)
• Abnormal nonstress test (NST)
• Meconium-stained amniotic fluid (MSAF)
• Difficult delivery
• Operative delivery

Table 2.4.2: Features of significant illness on history.

Danger signs
• Lethargy
• Breathing difficulty or apnea
• Temperature instability
• Failure to pass urine/meconium in first 24–48 hours
• Vomiting
• Diarrhea
• Cyanosis
• Jaundice
• Abdominal distension
• Convulsions
• Bleeding
• Excessive weight loss

The severity of respiratory distress (RD) can be monitored using the RD score **(Table 2.4.3)**.

Cyanosis

The two most serious causes of cyanosis are congenital cyanotic heart disease and respiratory illness, such as RD syndrome, meconium aspiration syndrome, or pneumonia. However, simpler problems, such as polycythemia and hypoglycemia, can also present as cyanosis.

Shock

It can be due to fluid/blood loss, asphyxia, duct-dependent cardiac lesions, sepsis, or inborn errors of metabolism (IEM).

Pallor

Pallor may indicate anemia (due to blood loss or hemolysis) but may also indicate hypothermia, hypoxia, hypotension, and sepsis.

Convulsions

Any abnormal movement needs to be reported; jitteriness and sleep myoclonus needs to be differentiated from convulsions recognized. Subtle seizures are often missed; a high index of suspicion is needed to identify subtle seizures as these could mimic normal movements, such as blinking, staring, sucking, etc. Seizure can be a pointer for several illnesses, such as meningitis, intracranial bleeds, metabolic problems, and asphyxia.

Lethargic, Poor Feeding and Unresponsiveness

A sleeping neonate may appear lethargic. A simple method of determining whether a neonate is lethargic or sleeping is to observe if the neonate is responsive to stimulation. If a neonate does not change state during examination or handling, it indicates that the sensorium is not normal. The etiology of lethargy may range from simpler causes, such

Table 2.4.3: Respiratory distress score.

Features	***0***	***1***	***2***
Respiratory rate/min	<60	60–80	>80
Cyanosis	Nil	Nil on 40% O_2	Requires >40% O_2
Retractions	Nil	Mild	Moderate-to-severe
Grunting	Nil	Audible with stethoscope	Audible without stethoscope
Air entry	Normal	Decreased	Barely audible

as hypoglycemia and polycythemia, to more severe ones including sepsis, meningitis, intracranial bleed, and hypoxic brain injury. Neonates with IEM usually present with lethargy and poor feeding.

Excessive Crying, Irritability, and Restlessness

Inconsolable, excessive, and incessant crying may indicate severe illness. Stage I hypoxic-ischemic encephalopathy is one example of a central nervous system problem presenting as excessive crying. Pain, as in arthritis, sepsis, myocarditis, intracranial bleed, and hypoxia can all manifest as excessive cry and irritability in the initial stages of the illness.

Vomiting

A neonate presenting with vomiting may be having something as physiologic as regurgitation, or it could be due to an intestinal obstruction. Bilious vomiting and persistent vomiting associated with abdominal distension or lethargy indicate need for further evaluation and admission.

Abdominal Distension

Abdominal distension usually indicates a serious underlying problem such as sepsis, paralytic ileus, intestinal obstruction, or Hirschsprung's disease. It is uncommon for a well neonate to have abdominal distension. Occasionally, medications used for colic (e.g. antispasmodics) can lead to abdominal distension and constipation.

Bleeding

Bleeding can be from any site; it could be skin bleeds, mucosal bleeds [gastrointestinal (GI) bleed], or visceral bleed. The most common cause of GI bleed in a neonate is due to hemorrhagic disease of newborn. Skin bleeds usually indicate sepsis, disseminated intravascular coagulopathy, but in a well neonate, it could be due to thrombocytopenia. Intracranial bleed is a serious problem and is more common in preterm neonates.

Jaundice

Neonatal jaundice is often physiologic, but high bilirubin levels can be associated with neuronal damage. In neonates with persistent jaundice after 14 days, always check for color of stool. Pale-colored stool could indicate cholestatic jaundice, such as biliary atresia.

Inadequate Weight Gain

The most likely reason is poor milk intake; however, other more serious problems, which can present as poor weight gain include any systemic illness and IEM.

Assessment of Illness Severity

Severity of illness can be assessed at admission by assessing the physiologic alterations in the baby using the Score for Neonatal Acute Physiology and Perinatal Extension II. Details of this score have been provided in **Table 2.4.4**. The scores greater than 15 are usually associated with higher mortality.

Neonates who will require high-dependency care or shift to a tertiary center will include:

- Very low birth weight (<1,500 g) and extremely low birth weight (<1,000 g) neonates;
- Any neonate requiring ventilator support;
- Any sick neonate requiring constant monitoring (multiple seizures);
- A sick neonate requiring cardiovascular support (shock);
- Suspected or proven IEM.

Table 2.4.4: Score for neonatal acute physiology and perinatal extension II.

Parameter	*Value*	*Score*
Mean blood pressure	29 mm Hg	0
	20–29 mm Hg	9
	<20 mm Hg	19
Core temperature	>35.6°C	0
	35–35.6°C	8
	<35°C	15
Birth weight	999 g	0
	750–999 g	10
	<750 g	17
SGA < 3rd centile	No	0
	Yes	12
PaO_2/FiO_2 ratio	2.49	0
	1–2.49	5
	0.3–0.99	16
	<0.3	28
Lowest serum pH	7.19	0
	7.1–7.19	7
	<7.1	16
Urine output	>0.9 mL/kg/h	0
	0.1–0.9 mL/kg/h	5
	<0.1 mL/kg/h	18
Multiple seizures	No	0
	Yes	19
Apgar at 5 min	>7	0
	<7	18

(PaO_2/FiO_2: partial pressure arterial oxygen and fraction of inspired oxygen; SGA: small for gestation age)

Flowchart 2.4.1: Triaging sick neonates.

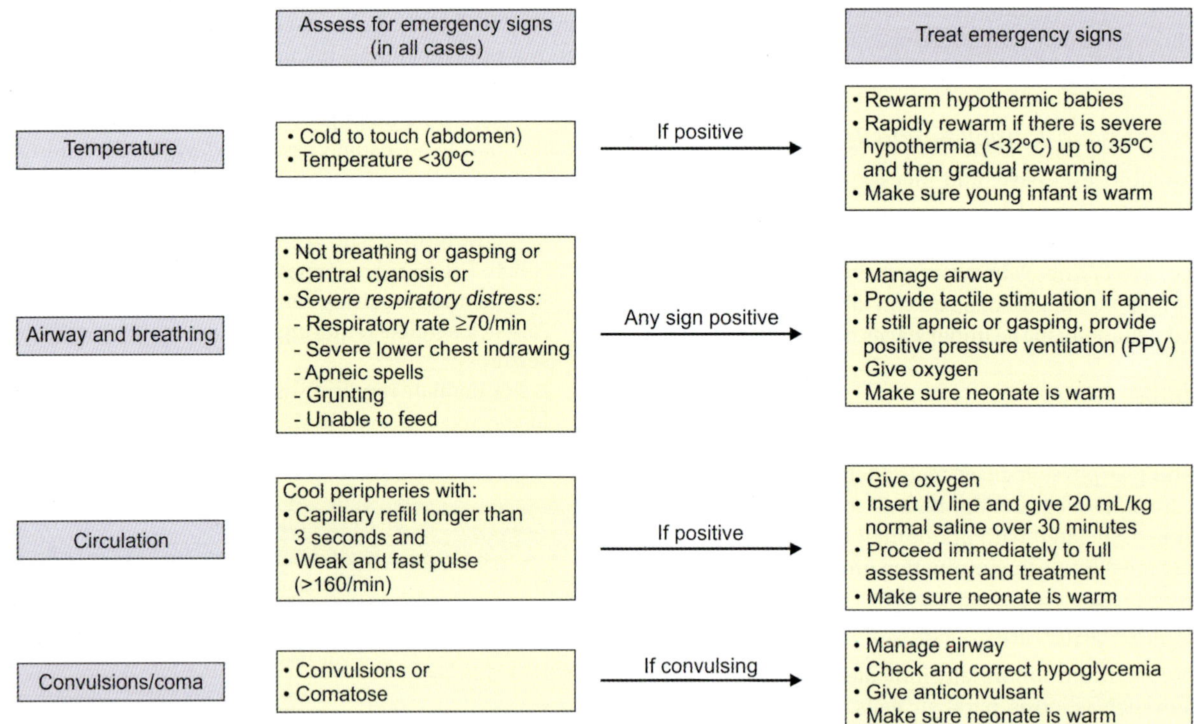

Triaging Sick Neonates

All neonates should be assessed for emergency signs:

- Assess for hypothermia. If present, arrange for rewarming of the baby.
- Check for severe respiratory problem, and if present, arrange to oxygenate or ventilate the baby.
- Determine if the child is in shock or has encephalopathy or convulsions, and if so, initiate urgent steps to manage.

The triaging process is outlined in **Flowchart 2.4.1**. Only after initiating emergency measures, proceed to investigate the neonate. Proceed to treat the neonate for underlying disorder based on the clinical examination and investigations.

GIVE EMERGENCY TREATMENT

Maintain Temperature

Place the neonate under a warmer and bring the temperature from 36.5°C to 37.5°C. Keep the baby dry; and the head, hands, and feet should be covered. Maintain the temperature within this range.

Maintain the Airway

Place the child in sniffing position. Place a shoulder roll under the shoulder to position the child. Clear the airway of secretions by suctioning the mouth first and then the nose.

Assist Breathing

Support the child's respiration, if there is distress. This can be done with noninvasive ventilation, provided by using nasal prongs, which can be placed just inside the nostrils and secured with a tape. The flow rate can maintained be around 1–2 L/min. The child could also be placed under an oxygen hood with an oxygen flow rate of 5–8 L/min. The oxygen can be monitored by a pulse oximeter targeting the saturation at 88–93%. Invasive ventilation may be needed for neonates with more severe distress.

If any sign is positive: Give treatment(s), call for help, and draw blood for emergency laboratory investigations (e.g. glucose).

Support Circulation

If the child is in shock, give an IV bolus of normal saline or ringer's lactate at the rate of 10 mL/kg over 20–30 minutes. Repeat if features of shock persist. Initiate dopamine in a dose of 5–20 µg/kg/min and dobutamine at 5–20 µg/kg/min, if the neonate remains in shock despite fluid boluses.

KEY MESSAGES

- Sick neonates should be triaged for emergency signs immediately at arrival to a health facility.
- Initiate emergency treatment first and then investigate.
- After stabilization, take detailed history and clinical examination to determine underlying etiology for sickness and then initiate appropriate specific treatment.

BIBLIOGRAPHY

1. Brousseau T, Shareiff DQ. Newborn emergencies: the first 30 days of life. Pediatr Clin North Am. 2006;53:69-84.
2. CRIB Investigators Group. The CRIB score: a tool for assessing initial neonatal risk and comparing performance of neonatal intensive care units. Lancet. 1993;342:193-8.
3. Lee KG. Identifying the high risk newborn. In: Cloherty JP, Eichenwald EC, Stark AR, (Eds). Manual of Neonatal Care, 6th edition. Lippincott Williams and Wilkins; 2008. pp. 41-58.
4. Munshi UK. Identifying the newborn who requires special care. In: McLnermy TK, (Ed). AAP Textbook of Pediatric Care. New Delhi: Jaypee Brothers Medical Publishers (P) Ltd.; 2009. pp. 666-73.
5. Richardson DK, Corcoran JD, Escobar GJ. SNAP-II and SNAPPE-II: simplified newborn illness severity and mortality risk scores. J Pediatr. 2001;138:92-100.
6. Sarkar PK. Evaluation of sick neonate. In: Guha DK, (Ed). Guha's Neonatology. Principles and Practice, 3rd edition. New Delhi: Jaypee Brothers Medical Publishers (P) Ltd.; 2005. pp. 481-7.
7. Singh M. Care of the Newborn, 5th edition. New Delhi: Sagar Publications; 1999.
8. Volpe JJ. Neurologic examination. In: Volpe JJ (Ed). Neurology of the Newborn, 5th edition. Philadelphia, PA: Saunders Elsevier; 2008. pp. 121-53.

2.5 Low Birth Weight

Vikram Datta

DEFINITION

Low birth weight (LBW) has been defined as a birth weight of less than 2,500 g. The prevalence of LBW in India has been reported to range from 21% to 33%. These infants have a very high risk of mortality compared to normal weight neonates. They also have a higher risk of neonatal morbidities, childhood growth failure, and developmental problems.

ETIOLOGY

A neonate may be LBW either due to being born prematurely (one third of all cases) or being intrauterine growth-retarded [birth weight less than 10th centile for gestational age—small for gestational age (SGA), two thirds of all cases]. The problems that these babies encounter are largely dependent on the cause of LBW. Various maternal risk factors contribute commonly to premature delivery and SGA neonates. The common causes are listed in **Table 2.5.1**.

Table 2.5.1: Etiology of low birth weight.

Preterm birth	***Fetal growth retardation***
Maternal • Preeclampsia • Chronic maternal conditions • Infection • Drug abuse • Premature rupture of membranes • Polyhydramnios • Iatrogenic placental • Placental dysfunction • Placenta previa • Abruptio placentae uterine • Incompetent cervix • Uterine malformation fetal • Multiple gestation • Malformations	*Maternal* • Anemia • Hypertension • Renal disease • Chronic illness • Addictions (alcohol and narcotics) fetal • Chromosomal disorders • Intrauterine infections (TORCH) • Congenital anomalies • Multiple gestation

[TORCH: Toxoplasmosis, other (syphilis, varicella-zoster, parvovirus B19), rubella, *Cytomegalovirus*, and herpes]

CLINICAL RECOGNITION OF LOW BIRTH WEIGHT TYPES

Low birth weight can be preterm or intrauterine growth-retarded (SGA). The clinical features, which help in recognition of these subtypes, are summarized here.

Ear Cartilage

The external ear or the pinna is soft and devoid of cartilage in preterm neonates, and hence, it does not recoil back promptly on being folded. In a term baby, there is instant recoil.

Breast Nodule

Breast nodule measures less than 5 mm in preterm neonates (also in growth-retarded newborns) and 5 mm or more in term babies.

Sole Creases

Anterior one third of the sole reveals a deep transverse skin crease in preterm neonates, and in term neonates, they are present over the anterior two-thirds.

External Genitalia

In males, the scrotum does not have rugae and testes are not descended into the scrotum. In female infants, the labia are widely separated, not covering the labia minora, resulting in the prominent appearance of the clitoris.

Skin

The skin of preterm neonate is thin, transparent, and gelatinous, whereas that of a term neonate is thick and keratinized.

Lanugo Hair

The back of the preterm babies has abundant growth of fine hair called lanugo, which are absent or sparse in term neonates.

Appearance

In addition, SGA infants have an emaciated look and loose folds of skin because of the lack of subcutaneous tissue. These are particularly prominent over the buttocks and thighs. They look alert and often plethoric.

PROBLEMS OF LOW BIRTH WEIGHT

Specific problems of the preterm infants include the following:
- Perinatal asphyxia
- Temperature instability
- Feeding problems due to absence of a coordinated sucking and swallowing reflex and absence of a mature intestinal peristaltic pattern
- Hyperbilirubinemia
- *Pulmonary diseases:* Apnea and respiratory distress syndrome
- *Metabolic disturbances:* Hypoglycemia, hypocalcemia, hyperkalemia, hypernatremia, hyponatremia, and hypomagnesemia
- Patent ductus arteriosus
- Increased susceptibility to infections
- Necrotizing enterocolitis
- Retinopathy of prematurity
- Intraventricular hemorrhage

Specific problems of SGA infants include the following:
- Perinatal asphyxia
- Meconium aspiration syndrome
- Infections
- Hypoglycemia
- Polycythemia
- Hypothermia
- Dysmorphology

MANAGEMENT OF LOW-BIRTH-WEIGHT BABIES

Delivery Room Management

The delivery room management consists of an expert resuscitation maintaining good thermoregulation, minimal handling and use of nasal continuous positive airway pressure, and intubation, when required for preterm births. LBW neonates who need care in a special care unit include those with birth weight less than 1,800 g, gestation less than 34 weeks, any neonate who is unable to feed from the breast and any sick neonate.

Thermoregulation

Low-birth-weight babies are more prone to develop hypothermia due to deficient heat regulatory mechanisms. Soon after delivery, the unclothed baby with the head and feet covered should be placed in between the breasts of the mother in skin-to-skin contact position (Kangaroo mother care). It not only maintains the temperature of the baby but also helps in the prompt initiation of breastfeeding. If the baby requires resuscitation or hospitalization, she may be placed under a servo-controlled radiant warmer with the temperature probe attached to the trunk of the baby. In the absence of a servo device, the baby should be covered with at least three to four layers of clothes, socks, mittens, and cap.

In a special care newborn unit, the infants may be kept warm using overhead radiant warmer or incubator. Regular monitoring of axillary temperature at least once every 6–8 hours should be carried out in all hospitalized babies. Devices that provide direct heating of the baby such as hot water bags, hot air blowers, and direct heaters should be avoided.

Fluids

If an LBW needs fluids, then in the first 48 hours after birth, neonates less than 1,250 g should be provided 5% dextrose and those more than 1,250 g should receive 10% dextrose. The fluid requirement volumes are given in **Table 2.5.2**. Sodium and potassium should be added after 48 hours or earlier, if there is more than 6% weight loss from the birth weight in the first 48 hours.

Table 2.5.2: Fluid requirements of neonates (mL/kg body weight).

Day of life	*Birth weight >1,500 g*	*Birth weight 1,000–1,500 g*
1	60	80
2	75	95
3	90	110
4	105	125
5	120	140
6	135	155
7 onwards	150	170

Enteral Feeding of the Low-Birth-Weight Neonate

The goal of nutritional management of the LBW infant should be to achieve full enteral nutrition as soon as possible. Breast milk is the best milk for the neonate, and the mother should be supported and counseled for the maintenance of regular lactation and the need for expression and its technique.

The guidelines for providing enteral feeds to the LBW neonate are summarized in **Table 2.5.3**. Neonates can undergo gradual transition from gastric feeding to spoon feeding and then onto breastfeeding. In infants less than 34 weeks, transition from tube to breast can be facilitated by allowing the infant to suck on empty breast of mother (nonnutritive sucking) before each gavage feeding session. Daily assessment of the sucking efforts of the neonate will provide indication of when and how fast the transit from one mode to another mode of feeding should be undertaken.

Monitoring for Feed Intolerance

The signs of feed intolerance are an increase in the abdominal girth by more than 2 cm from the baseline, vomiting of feeds, and a preferred residue of greater than 25–50%. The presence of such signs in the baby may prompt a cessation of feeding and initiating investigation into the cause of feed intolerance.

Vitamin and Mineral Supplementation

Supplementation should be started as soon as the infant is receiving at least 120–150 mL/kg of enteral feeds. All preterm should receive daily supplement of 400 IU of vitamin D, and 120–140 mg/kg/day (110–130 mg/100 kcal) of highly bioavailable calcium with 60–90 mg/kg/day (55–80 mg/100 kcal) of phosphate is recommended. At 4 weeks of age, iron supplements should be started in a dose of 2–3 mg/kg/day. At present, there is no evidence for routine zinc supplement or protein fortification of breast milk.

Table 2.5.3: Guidelines for the modes of feeding for low-birth-weight neonates.

Birth weight (g) **Gestation (week)** **Condition**	**<1,200** **<30**	**1,200–1,800** **30–34**	**>1,800** **>34**
Initial	Intravenous fluids; try gavage feeds, if not sick	Gavage	Breastfeeding; if unsatisfactory, give spoon or "paladai" feeds
After (1–3 days)	Gavage	Spoon or "paladai" feeds	Breastfeeding
Later (1–3 weeks)	Try spoon or "paladai" feeding	Breastfeeding	Breastfeeding
After some more time (4–6 weeks)	Breastfeeding	Breastfeeding	Breastfeeding

Fortification of Preterm Breast Milk

According to the Cochrane review, multicomponent human milk fortification leads to short-term increase in weight gain, linear growth, and head circumference growth. There is still insufficient evidence in contemporary literature to recommend routine fortification of human milk. The cost, greater risk of contamination, and theoretical risk of hypercalcemia are some factors, which are to be borne in mind before prescribing human milk fortifier to LBW infants.

Adequacy of Nutrition

The key measure of optimal feeding is the weight pattern of the baby. A preterm LBW baby loses up to 1–2% weight everyday amounting to 10% cumulative weight loss during the first week of life. Birth weight is regained between 10th and 14th day. The babies start gaining weight by the second week of life at the rate of about 15–20 g/day, and this is considered adequate. Excessive weight loss or inadequate weight gain indicates inadequate feeding, cold stress, excessive insensible water loss, or systemic illness (such as anemia, sepsis, late metabolic acidosis, etc.).

Immunization

All vaccines should be administered as per schedule, according to the chronological age irrespective of birth weight or period of gestation. Hepatitis B, Bacillus Calmette-Guérin, and birth dose of oral polio vaccine and can be safely and effectively given to LBW or preterm babies after stabilization.

premature infants. It will guide the parents to decide roughly on the outcome and whether to seek transfer to higher centers, if available.

Resuscitation

Resuscitation is not successful all the time. Discontinuation is justified, if there are no signs of life (no heart beat and no spontaneous respirations) after 10 minutes of full resuscitation. Parents should be informed, if possible about the progress and status of the baby at various steps. In major congenital abnormalities incompatible with life, discussion with parents is essential before taking decision to discontinue resuscitation. A concurrence of another colleague is ideal.

Withdrawal of Care

The same applies to question of parental request for withdrawal of care in babies receiving intensive care, having multiple organ systems involved, with remote possibility for ultimate survival, or likelihood of severe neurological sequelae is almost certain. Clinical indicators, laboratory investigations, and imaging studies showing bad prognostic signs should be documented and shown to parents. Decisions such as "do not resuscitate", "withdrawal of care", and "discharge against medical advice by parents" warrant due deliberation, proper documentation, and concurrence of authorized personnel and parents in black and white. Legal sanction for any of the above does not exist at present time!

Pregnancy Loss, Stillbirth, and Death of a Neonate

This is devastating to the family. There is a feeling of loss, guilt, shame, inadequacy, and anger in the parents. Compassionate counseling is required stressing on the point that neither of the parents is responsible for it. It may be essential that a diagnosis be arrived at in view of future pregnancies, even though it may not help in the current one. Especially, if genetic disorders or metabolic defects are suspected, investigations such as chromosomal analysis, autopsy, infantogram, clinical photographs, tissue biopsy, blood, and other body fluid analysis should be done. Informed consent of parents is needed for this. In cases of neonatal deaths, a meeting with the parents should be arranged after a few weeks when they would be more receptive having gone through the stages of bereavement, and the results of all investigations are available to have a more fruitful counseling. Future reproductive options, perinatal preventive strategies such as folic acid consumption, investigations, prenatal management as high-risk pregnancy, planning of delivery, and neonatal care could be discussed.

Visits by a social worker to the abode of the unfortunate couple at least during the first few months after the tragedy to counsel will be very beneficial.

Parental counseling is an important aspect of perinatal care. It should be given its due priority. It is ideal that every unit has a person who has had some formal training in counseling.

KEY MESSAGES

- Parents need counseling at several stages of perinatal period. It is the responsibility of care providers to support parents to make informed choices.
- Counseling should be conducted by trained personnel respecting the privacy of families.
- Counseling should be nonthreatening, nontechnical but supportive.

BIBLIOGRAPHY

1. American Academy of Pediatrics Committee on Fetus and Newborn. The initiation or withdrawal of treatment for high-risk newborns. Pediatrics. 1995;96:362-3.
2. Baker K, Kuhlman T, Magliaro B. Homeward bound: discharge teaching for parents of newborns with special needs. Nursing Clin North Am. 1989;24(3):655-64.
3. Freer Y, Lyon A, Stenson B, Russell C. BabyLink—improving communication among clinicians and with parents with babies in intensive care. Br J Healthcare Comput Inform Manag. 2005;22(2):34-6.
4. Harmon RJ, Glicken AD, Siegel RE. Neonatal loss in the intensive care nursery: effects of maternal grieving and a program for intervention. J Am Acad Child Psychiatry. 1984;23:68-71.
5. Leslie L, Harris LL, Douma C. End-of-life care in the NICU: a family-centered approach. NeoReviews. 2010;11:e194-9.
6. Munson D. Withdrawal of mechanical ventilation in pediatric and neonatal intensive care units. Pediatr Clin North Am. 2007;54:773-85.

2.7 Neonatal Hyperbilirubinemia

Rhishikesh Thakre

DEFINITION

Hyperbilirubinemia is a common neonatal problem. It is defined as an increased level of bilirubin in the circulation. A small proportion of these neonates develop jaundice that is significantly high to warrant treatment. Approximately, 60% of the term and 80% of the preterm babies develop jaundice during the first week of life. About 5% develop pathological jaundice. Studies suggest the possible impact of genetic polymorphisms on ethnic variation in the incidence and severity of jaundice.

ETIOPATHOGENESIS

Hyperbilirubinemia is the result of an imbalance between bilirubin production and its elimination. In majority, early neonatal jaundice is due to rise in unconjugated (indirect) bilirubin. The etiological basis for progressive hyperbilirubinemia is usually multifactorial. **Table 2.7.1** summarizes the important causes of unconjugated hyperbilirubinemia.

Table 2.7.1: Causes of indirect (unconjugated) hyperbilirubinemia.

- Physiological jaundice
- Breastfeeding jaundice, breast milk jaundice
- Increased production:
  - Blood group incompatibility (Rh, ABO, minor blood group)
  - RBC membrane defects (hereditary spherocytosis, elliptocytosis)
  - RBC enzyme defects (G6PD deficiency, pyruvate kinase deficiency)
- Disorders of bilirubin uptake
  - Gilbert's syndrome
- Disorders of conjugation
  - Crigler-Najjar types I and II, hypothyroidism, pyloric stenosis
- Enhanced enterohepatic circulation
  - Small or large bowel obstruction or ileus
- Idiopathic
- Others
  - Prematurity, sepsis, polycythemia, infant of diabetic mother, extravascular blood (cephalohematoma, bruising)

(G6PD: glucose-6-phosphate dehydrogenase; RBC: red blood cell; Rh: rhesus)

Physiological Jaundice

The functional immaturity in bilirubin metabolism, namely, increased enterohepatic circulation, increased fetal erythrocyte breakdown, decreased hepatic excretion, and immature hepatic conjugation predisposes to early jaundice which is transient, requiring no treatment. It usually appears after 24 hours, peaks between 3 and 5 days in term and 5–7 days in preterm and disappears by 2 weeks of life. The peak bilirubin is under 15 mg/dL.

Nonphysiologic Jaundice and Risk of Bilirubin Toxicity

Jaundice within 24 hours of life, peak bilirubin greater than 15 mg/dL, and persistence beyond 2 weeks are not physiologic and need to be investigated. The rate of rise of bilirubin greater than 0.5 mg/dL/h or bilirubin level greater than 25 mg/dL increases the risk of bilirubin toxicity in neonates. Bilirubin is a potential neurotoxin. Areas of the brain most commonly affected are the basal ganglia and brainstem nuclei for oculomotor and auditory function. Bilirubin toxicity or kernicterus can cause permanent sequelae, characterized by tetrad of choreoathetoid cerebral palsy, high frequency central hearing loss, vertical gaze palsy, and dental enamel hypoplasia.

CLINICAL ASSESSMENT

All newborns should be examined for jaundice at least once a day during the first 72 hours. Jaundice is assessed by inspecting the baby's skin, sclera, or mucous membranes preferably in natural light. The skin is blanched by digital pressure over bony parts to reveal underlying yellowing.

Newborns having jaundice should also be examined for bruising, cephalohematoma, lethargy, vomiting, excessive weight loss, pallor, plethora, and hepatosplenomegaly. Abnormality in tone, cry, or sensorium should alert to possibility of bilirubin neurotoxicity. In infants presenting with jaundice extending beyond 2 weeks, one must inquire for pale or white stools, which may indicate obstructive jaundice such as biliary atresia.

Assessment in Neonates Discharged Early

All newborns should be assessed for the presence of risk factors at the time of discharge **(Table 2.7.2)**. The more risk factors present, the greater the risk of severe hyperbilirubinemia, and the risk is extremely low, if risk factors are absent. If neonates are discharged within 24 hours, those with risk factors should be seen within 24–48 hours, and those without risk factors within 72 hours of discharge. If facilities are available, then serum bilirubin can be estimated by the use of transcutaneous bilirubinometer on each of these visits.

INVESTIGATIONS

In all neonates with jaundice that is not considered physiologic, investigations need to be done to assess the severity of jaundice (for planning treatment) and etiology of the jaundice. **Table 2.7.3** summarizes the important investigations that need to be done. Cord blood is collected for typing the baby's blood group, if mother's blood group is rhesus (Rh)-negative or O Rh-positive or blood group is not known. If an Rh-negative mother has an Rh-positive baby, the cord blood is subjected to direct Coombs test, total serum bilirubin (TSB), reticulocyte count, peripheral smear, and hemoglobin.

End-tidal carbon monoxide measurement in exhaled air may serve as indirect marker of ongoing hemolysis as equimolar concentrations of CO, and bilirubin are formed following the breakdown of red blood cell. Synthetic heme analogs and metalloporphyrins are competitive inhibitors of heme oxygenase, and their use has been proposed as an attractive alternative strategy for preventing or treating severe hyperbilirubinemia.

TREATMENT

Treatment of Indirect Hyperbilirubinemia

The decision-making in jaundice management is based on gestation, weight, well-being, and age of the infant. **Tables 2.7.4 and 2.7.5** provide guidelines of how to decide if an infant needs treatment—phototherapy (PT) or exchange transfusion (ET).

Table 2.7.2: Risk factors for significant hyperbilirubinemia.

- Primipara mother
- Visible jaundice at discharge
- Gestation <38 weeks
- History of jaundice requiring treatment in previous sibling
- ABO/Rh incompatibility
- Geographic prevalence for G6PD deficiency
- Weight loss at discharge >3%/day or >7% cumulative weight loss

(G6PD: glucose-6-phosphate dehydrogenase; Rh: rhesus)

Phototherapy

Phototherapy is the mainstay of treatment. When bilirubin is exposed to blue light (in the range of 420–480 nm), it undergoes change in structure to a product called lumirubin, which can be excreted in the urine without undergoing conjugation in the liver. The efficacy of PT depends on spectrum of light (460–480 nm), irradiance (8–30 μW/cm^2/nm), and surface area of infant's skin exposed to light. The choice of device depends upon the severity of jaundice. For majority of infants, standard PT (six special blue lights of Philips TL 52, 20 W each) is effective. When the bilirubin is rapidly rising or nearing ET range, intensive PT (using high-intensity light-emitting diodes) lights or double surface standard PT tubes are provided.

Administering PT: Phototherapy is administered continuously and interrupted only for nursing and feeding purpose. The infant is placed naked with genitalia and eyes covered. Close attention is paid to the infant's temperature, daily weight, and intake output. Breastfeeding is continued frequently. Hypoxia, hypothermia, hypoglycemia, acidosis, and sepsis need to be prevented, and if present, treated aggressively. Intravenous fluids are given only to infants who have inadequate oral intake, significant weight loss (>10%), or are dehydrated.

Monitoring: TSB is monitored every 4–12 hours, depending on patient's age and bilirubin level. PT should be stopped once serum bilirubin is 50 mmol/L or below the PT threshold **(Table 2.7.4)**. It should not be used to treat infants with conjugated hyperbilirubinemia because of the risk of bronze baby syndrome.

Exchange Transfusion

Exchange transfusion is indicated for infants whose bilirubin levels cross the threshold indicated in **Table 2.7.4** or those

Table 2.7.3: Investigations for significant hyperbilirubinemia.

- Total and direct bilirubin
- Mother and baby blood group
- Hemoglobin or PCV
- Peripheral blood smear (for RBC shape and evidence of hemolysis)
- Reticulocyte count
- Direct Coombs test (if mother is O or Rh-negative)
- G6PD assay

Sick infant with jaundice or prolonged jaundice (>3 weeks)

- Complete blood count, blood culture
- Urine examination and culture
- Evaluate for infection as indicated
- Urine for reducing substances
- Thyroid profile (T4, TSH)
- Evaluate for cholestasis (if direct bilirubin is elevated)

(G6PD: glucose-6-phosphate dehydrogenase; PCV: packed cell volume; RBC: red blood cell; Rh: rhesus; T4: thyroxine; TSH: thyroid-stimulating hormone)

Table 2.7.4: Treatment of indirect hyperbilirubinemia.

Age	*Phototherapy*		*Exchange transfusion*	
	Healthy newborns >35 weeks gestation (mg/dL)	*Newborns <35 weeks gestation (mg/dL)*	*Healthy newborns >35 weeks gestation (mg/dL)*	*Newborns <35 weeks gestation (mg/dL)*
Day 1	Any visible jaundice		15	10
Day 2	15	10	25	15
Day 3	18	15	25	20

who have clinical features of bilirubin encephalopathy. During ET, twice the infant's blood volume (160 mL/kg) is exchanged; this procedure can decrease the bilirubin level by approximately 50%. The procedure is invasive and carries a small risk of complications (1–5%)—fluid overload, infection, electrolyte imbalance, hypoglycemia, thrombocytopenia, thrombosis, and death.

Intravenous Immunoglobulin

Intravenous immunoglobulin 500 mg/kg is used when the serum bilirubin is rising despite intensive PT or the value is within the ET range in antibody-mediated hemolysis (Rh, ABO) settings.

Treatment of Direct Hyperbilirubinemia

Direct hyperbilirubinemia **(Table 2.7.5)** is defined as conjugated bilirubin level greater than 2 mg/dL or 15% of the TSB. It is an uncommon but potentially serious condition that indicates hepatobiliary dysfunction.

Evaluation should include total and direct bilirubin, urine examination and urine culture, evaluation for infection (as indicated), and thyroid profile. Further evaluation should be tailored with expert consultation to rule out surgical cause. Treatment is directed at the specific underlying cause if any and remains largely supportive with diet rich in calories, medium chain triglycerides, adequate proteins, and supplementation of fat and water-soluble vitamins. Early detection and diagnosis are important for successful treatment for a favorable prognosis.

PREVENTION

- Test during pregnancy for ABO and Rh blood types and provide appropriate prenatal care;
- Assess all infants for risk factors for jaundice prior to discharge and reevaluate on days 3–5 when the bilirubin level is highest;
- Inform parents to look for jaundice and report, if there are any concerns;

Table 2.7.5: Causes of conjugated (direct) hyperbilirubinemia.

- Bacterial sepsis
- *Neonatal hepatitis:*
  - Toxoplasmosis, cytomegalovirus, rubella, herpes, syphilis, parvovirus B19
- *Biliary obstruction:*
  - Biliary atresia, choledochal cyst, inspissated bile plug
- *Metabolic disease:*
  - Hypothyroidism, galactosemia, alpha-1-antitrypsin deficiency
- *Genetic disease:*
  - Dubin-Johnson syndrome, Rotor syndrome, cystic fibrosis, Alagille syndrome
- *Others:*
  - Drugs, cholestasis associated with total parenteral nutrition
- Idiopathic

- Provide appropriate support and advice to breastfeeding mothers;
- Follow-up neonates with severe jaundice for hearing loss and other neurodevelopmental sequelae.

PRACTICE POINTS AND TIPS

- Hyperbilirubinemia may develop both in the absence of identifiable risk factors and without clinically significant jaundice having been present at the time of discharge. Hence, clinicians should remain alert for jaundice during first postnatal week;
- Do not rely on visual inspection alone to estimate the bilirubin level in a baby with jaundice;
- Interpret bilirubin levels according to the infant's age in hours;
- Do not subtract conjugated bilirubin from TSB when making decisions.

KEY MESSAGES

- Neonatal hyperbilirubinemia is usually multifactorial in origin.
- The most common cause of neonatal hyperbilirubinemia is physiological jaundice, which is a diagnosis of exclusion.
- Conjugated hyperbilirubinemia is always pathological, and expert help should be sought early, especially to identify biliary atresia.
- Systematic approach in the form of clinical evaluation, assessment of risk factors, and interpreting bilirubin with age in hours paves way to rational management.

BIBLIOGRAPHY

1. American Academy of Pediatrics Subcommittee on Hyperbilirubinemia. Management of hyperbilirubinemia in the newborn infant 35 or more weeks of gestation. Pediatrics. 2004;114(1):297-316.

2. California Perinatal Quality Care Collaborative (CPQCC). Severe hyperbilirubinemia prevention (SHP) toolkit (Balasundaram M, Bhutani VK). [online] Available from: https://www.cpqcc.org/qi-tool-kits/severe-hyperbilirubinemia-prevention-shp. [Accessed September, 2018].
3. Guruprasad G, Chawla D, Aggarwal S. Management of neonatal hyperbilirubinemia, National Neonatology Forum of India. In: Kumar P (Ed). New Delhi: NNF clinical practice guidelines; 2010.
4. World Health Organization. WHO recommendations on newborn health: guidelines approved by the WHO Guidelines Review Committee. Geneva: World Health Organization; 2017.
5. Yaccha SK. Consensus report on neonatal cholestasis syndrome. Indian Pediatr. 2000;37:845-51.

2.8 Neonatal Infections

Naveen Jain

GLOBAL ESTIMATE OF NEONATAL SEPSIS

Sepsis is defined as a life-threatening organ dysfunction due to dysregulated host response to infection. It is a major killer of neonates. Recent population-based meta-analysis (from 12 middle- and high-income countries) reported an incidence of 2,202/100,000 live births and 11% mortality. Sepsis was 40 times commoner in middle-income than high-income countries, and the mortality was twice as higher. There are few estimates of incidence from the developing countries.

DEFINITION

Most of the neonatal infections are microbiologically unconfirmed. This is the reason for lack of consensus definitions and estimates. Definitions of sepsis would have to include clinical and laboratory markers in addition to microbiologic identification.

Recently, *three levels of definitions* were proposed based on the available test reports. These definitions were proposed for improved data collection, recognizing limitations at various levels of health care.

Level 1

Recognized pathogen identified using a validated method from a normally sterile site.

Level 2

Not meeting level 1 criteria, but three or more of clinical and laboratory criteria:

- Temperature ≥37.5 or <35.5°C or
- Tachycardia/New or more episodes of bradycardia or
- New apnea/Increased oxygen or ventilation needs
- Lethargy/Moving only when stimulated/Hypotonia
- Difficulty in feeding or abdominal distension
- Hypotension/Pallor/Poor perfusion
- Abnormal white blood cell (WBC) count/immature-to-total-neutrophil (IT) ratio >0.2
- Decreased platelet count
- Increased inflammatory marker—C-reactive protein (CRP) procalcitonin (PCT)
- Metabolic acidosis defined by a base.

Level 3

Not meeting level 1 or 2, but two or more of clinical:

- Temperature ≥37.5 or <35.5°C or
- Tachypnea or severe chest indrawing or grunting or cyanosis
- Change in level of activity
- History of feeding difficulty
- History of seizures.

In a more research-oriented accurate definition, sepsis in the newborn is defined, when it meets the following criteria:

- Any two clinical signs
- Any two laboratory signs
- In the presence of or as a result of suspect or proven infection (European Consensus Statement, 2010)
- *Any two clinical signs*:
  - *Temperature instability*:
    - Core temperature > 38.5 or <36°C
  - *Cardiovascular instability*:
    - Tachycardia (heart rate 180 beats/minutes) in the absence of external stimulus or pain or drugs, that is, "unexplained" increase in heart rate for 0.5–4 hours

- Bradycardia (heart rate 100 beats/minutes) for 0.5 hours in the absence of heart block, external vagal stimulus, and beta-blockers
- Rhythm disturbances
- Reduced blood pressure (BP) (systolic BP less than 65 mm Hg in the first week and less than 75 mm Hg between 1 week and 1 month)
- Mottled skin and impaired peripheral perfusion
- Decreased urine output (less than 1 mL/kg/h)

▪ *Respiratory instability*:
  - Apneic episodes
  - Respiratory rate greater than 2 standard deviation (>50 beats/minutes in the first week and 40 beats/minutes between 1 week and 1 month)
  - Increased oxygen need
  - Ventilation for acute process for causes other than neuromuscular or general anesthesia

▪ *Gastrointestinal*:
  - Feed intolerance, abdominal distension, and poor sucking

▪ Petechial rash or sclerema

▪ *Nonspecific*: Lethargy, irritability, and hypotonia.

- *Any two laboratory tests*:
  ▪ Abnormal leukocyte count (>20,000 × 10^9/L or <4,000 × 10^9/L)
  ▪ Immature-to-total-neutrophil ratio (>0.2)
  ▪ Platelet count less than 100,000 × 10^9/L
  ▪ C-reactive protein greater than 15 mg/L
  ▪ Procalcitonin greater than 2 ng/mL
  ▪ Metabolic acidosis; base excess greater than –10
  ▪ Blood sugar greater than 180 mg/dL or less than 45 mg/dL confirmed at least two times on age-appropriate infusions
- *Evidence of infection*:
  ▪ Proven [positive culture or microscopy or polymerase chain reaction (PCR)]
  ▪ Suspected (clinical syndrome such as perforation of viscous, petechial or purpuric rash, chest X-ray consistent with pneumonia or white cells in normally sterile fluid).

EPIDEMIOLOGY

Classically, sepsis has been differentiated into early onset neonatal sepsis (EONS) and late onset neonatal sepsis (LONS) based on onset before 72 hours of life or after. These two types of sepsis have different risk factors or settings. Knowledge of risk factors guides empiric antibiotic choices. In the developed world, the spectrum of microbes is distinct in the two settings. Most Indian studies have shown similar bugs and antibiotic resistance patterns in both EONS and LONS. This necessitates that antibiotic choices be based on regional microbiologic data and not be borrowed from studies published from the developed countries.

Risk Factors for Early-onset Neonatal Sepsis

- Maternal fever (>37.8°C) in the period from onset of labor to delivery;
- Prolonged rupture of membranes for more than 18 hours;
- Spontaneous preterm (<37 weeks) onset of labor;
- Preterm (<37 weeks) premature rupture of membranes;
- Maternal sepsis, urinary tract infection (UTI), or diarrhea within 7 days to the date of delivery;
- Clinical chorioamnionitis in the mother.

Risk Factors for Late-onset Neonatal Sepsis

- Low birth weight (LBW)
- Babies admitted to neonatal intensive care units and undergoing invasive procedures (ventilation, parenteral nutrition through central catheters, not feeding orally, admission to inadequately staffed units, and poor compliance to unit policy on prevention of infections).

ETIOLOGICAL AGENTS

Bacterial Infections

A recent study from three tertiary care centers in Delhi reported common pathogens and sensitivity pattern. The incidence of sepsis was 14.3% and 6% were culture positive. Gram-negative bugs were commonest—*Acinetobacter* (22%), *Klebsiella* (17%), and *Escherichia coli* (14%). Multidrug resistance was very common. A recent audit on antibiotic prescriptions in India noted that 70% of the antibiotic choices were empirical. Amikacin was the commonest prescribed antibiotic, and piperacillin/tazobactam was used more often in community-acquired infections. The use of meropenem was high. It appears that these antibiotic choices are reflection of high rates of antibiotic resistance to ampicillin and gentamicin.

Neonates are susceptible to infections. Fungal and viral infections are of great clinical importance in addition to sepsis caused by bacteria.

Fungi

Fungal infections are more common in babies weighing less than 1,500 g and are likely to be associated in babies with parenteral nutrition, central catheters, abdominal surgeries, broad-spectrum antibiotics, or steroids. Both *Candida albicans* and non-*albicans* are isolated. In a recent study on neonatal candidiasis, good susceptibility was reported to both fluconazole and amphotericin.

Viruses

Herpes infection should be considered in a baby with sepsis like syndrome (presenting after 1 week of life), if markers of bacterial infection are negative. Other viral infections that neonates can be exposed to include chickenpox, vertically transmitted rubella, and cytomegalovirus infections.

Parasites

Common parasitic infections that neonates can be exposed include toxoplasmosis, malaria, and syphilis.

CLINICAL FEATURES

Infection can be local or systemic.

Systemic Infections

Clinical features of systemic sepsis can be varied and nonspecific and have been described above under the definition of sepsis. In neonates with systemic signs of sepsis, presence of convulsions, neck retraction, or bulging fontanel must raise the possibility of meningitis. Neonates with septic arthritis or osteomyelitis may not have systemic symptoms and may present with painful limb movement and localized swelling with signs of inflammation.

Localized Infections

Infections of the eye (purulent discharge), umbilicus (pus discharge and/or erythema of surrounding skin), and pustules are superficial infections.

DIAGNOSIS

Neonatal sepsis is a serious disease and early diagnosis and treatment is crucial.

Blood Culture

The gold standard for diagnosis of neonatal sepsis is blood culture. Cultures are often negative in infected neonates due to the prior use of antibiotics, sampling issues, or poor laboratory resources. Yield of cultures can be improved by the collection of appropriate samples and enhanced faith of clinicians. The value of cultures is critical in guiding antibiotic changes in treatment failures and planning antibiotic policy for empiric therapy in that population.

Molecular Methods

The future of diagnostics in neonatal sepsis centers around molecular methods. These PCR-based tests have a rapid turnaround time for both detection of microbes (< 3–4 hours) and antibiotic resistance patterns. Detection of microbes is much higher than with cultures and is not affected by antibiotic use. The current limitations are high cost, availability of advanced laboratories, and false positives.

Biomarkers of Sepsis (Sepsis Screens)

Culture negative sepsis has prompted search for appropriate biomarkers. CRP is the best of the available tests that guides stopping of antibiotics. Serum PCT has shown promise in guiding antibiotic decisions. Other tests such as total WBC count and IT ratio are more universally available, but they do not have the ability to correctly confirm or exclude sepsis accurately.

C-Reactive Protein

C-reactive protein has value in ruling out infection. CRP rises late, and test done within 24 hours or beyond the suspicion of infection has greater sensitivity. Once started on antibiotics on clinical suspicion, negative CRP gives confidence to stop antibiotics.

Procalcitonin

Procalcitonin is a promising screening tool, but the cost and availability still limit its use. Algorithms based on PCT could decrease antibiotic overuse.

Hematological Indices

Total leukocyte count (TLC) has to be interpreted against age-specific normative data (Monroe, Zipurusky). The values as high as 24,000 and as low as 5,000 may be normal and do not suggest infection. IT ratio (>0.2) and absolute neutrophil counts have higher specificity but are often normal early in the course of infection.

Cerebrospinal Fluid Examination

Meningitis requires modifications in the choice of antibiotics, dose, and duration, and hence, cerebrospinal fluid examination must be performed in all symptomatic neonates or CRP/blood culture positive neonates on antibiotics. Cerebrospinal fluid cytology of greater than 30 cells (>50% polymorphs), with raised protein (>100 mg/dL), and/or sugar less than 30 mg/dL may suggest meningitis.

Urine Culture

It should be done in infants with failure to thrive, prolonged jaundice and fever, since these could be features of UTI. In all infants with obstructive uropathy who are ill, urine cultures should be done. Samples for cultures should be collected by suprapubic puncture.

Clinical Algorithms

Sepsis calculators (based on clinical information) have shown to reduce antibiotic use in EONS setting.

TREATMENT

Antibiotics

The indiscriminate use of broad-spectrum antibiotics without appropriate blood cultures and the practice of not stopping their use when no infection is documented have resulted in high antibiotic resistance rates amongst organisms isolated in India. Indian studies have shown amikacin to be the most effective first-line antibiotic in India. The National Treatment Guidelines for Antimicrobial Use in Infectious Diseases 2016 recommends the combination of ampicillin and Gentamicin as first line, and piperacillin-tazobactam and amikacin as second line if there is no improvement in 48–72 hours. In neonatal meningitis, cefotaxime and gentamicin are suggested second line. Some evidence suggests that the use of amikacin and piperacillin-tazobactam may have low failure rates. Piperacillin-tazobactam cannot be used if central nervous system is involved as it does not penetrate the cerebrospinal fluid barrier. There may be a justification in using cloxacillin if the incidence of *Staphylococcus* is high in a given setup. Antibiotics such as carbapenems and vancomycin should be treated as reserve drugs and be used only if the primary treatment plan fails.

The recommended duration of antibiotic therapy for uncomplicated culture positive neonatal sepsis (no meningitis, bone and joint or staphylococcal infections) is 7–10 days. Antibiotics may be stopped at 2–3 days in babies in whom these were started empirically, when cultures and CRP are negative and there is improvement symptomatically. In neonates with meningitis or staphylococcal sepsis, the duration of treatment may be 2–3 weeks and for up to 4–6 weeks in bone infections.

Adjunct Therapies in Treatment of Sepsis

Intravenous Immunoglobulins

There is no proven benefit of intravenous immunoglobulins in prevention or treatment of neonatal sepsis International Neonatal Immunotherapy Study. This expensive blood product is not without side effects. The expensive "off-label" use for expected benefits must be discouraged.

Granulocyte Colony Stimulating Factors or Granulocyte Monocyte Colony Stimulating Factors

The routine use of granulocyte colony stimulating factors or granulocyte monocyte colony stimulating factors is not recommended. When used in severely neutropenic neonates with proven sepsis, a survival benefit was demonstrated in some studies.

Single-volume Exchange Transfusion

A few studies (from India) have demonstrated good benefit in neonates with advanced sepsis—sclerema, persistent hypotension, coagulopathy, and metabolic acidosis. Concerns about the use of blood products have limited research in this direction.

Others

Pentoxifylline and recombinant human activated protein C have been tried but with no demonstrated benefits.

Supportive Care

Sepsis is a multiorgan disease that can result in death and disability. Antibiotics alone cannot change the outcome. Supportive care includes ventilation, inotropes, blood products, glucose, and acid-base monitoring and correction and is the most important determinant of outcome.

COMPLICATIONS

Sepsis remains the leading cause of neonatal mortality world over. In the acute phase, hypoglycemia, coagulopathy, organ failures such as pneumonia, pulmonary hypertension, shock due to myocardial dysfunction and capillary leaks, renal failure, and cholestatic jaundice are not uncommon with Gram-negative sepsis. Meningitis can result in complications such as hydrocephalus and developmental delay.

Prevention of Sepsis

Sepsis in the neonate can be prevented by promoting exclusive breastfeeding and simple hand hygiene and also by preventing applications on the umbilical cord during the first few days of life. Hospital-acquired infections can be minimized by good hand hygiene, promoting provision of breast milk to sick LBW neonates, good adherence to asepsis protocols, and strict antibiotic policy that limits its use, when required.

PRACTICE POINTS AND TIPS

- Use appropriate drug doses and schedules; refer drug formularies for right diluents, storage, interactions, and adverse events expected.
- *Storage of antibiotics*: Certain antibiotics such as ampicillin, gentamicin, and cefotaxime are so inexpensive (the disposable syringe costs more!) that keeping the vials for further use is only associated with risk of nosocomial sepsis. Some antibiotics such as meropenem and teicoplanin have a short shelf-life of less than 48 hours after reconstitution.
- Do not combine antibiotics with similar toxicities, for example, vancomycin and gentamicin.

- Be willing to de-escalate to a lower antibiotic, if culture suggests so.
- Stop antibiotics, if cultures, infection markers, and clinical signs allow. No benefit is known by completing a "course of 7–14 days".

BIBLIOGRAPHY

1. Autmizguine J, Tan S, Cohen-Wolkowiez M, et al. Antifungal susceptibility and clinical outcome in neonatal candidiasis. Pediatr Infect Dis J. 2018;37(9):923-9.
2. Cantey JB, Baird SD. Ending the culture of culture-negative sepsis in the neonatal ICU. Pediatrics. 2017;140(4):e20170044.
3. Fleischmann-Struzek C, Goldfarb DM, Schlattmann P, et al. The global burden of paediatric and neonatal sepsis: A systematic review. Lancet Respir Med. 2018;6(3):223-30.
4. Gandra S, Alvarez-Uria G, Murki S, et al. Point prevalence surveys of antimicrobial use among eight neonatal intensive care units in India: 2016. Int J Infect Dis. 2018;71:20–4.
5. Investigators of the Delhi Neonatal Infection Study (DeNIS) Collaboration. Characterisation and antimicrobial resistance of sepsis pathogens in neonates born in tertiary care centres in Delhi, India: a cohort study. Lancet Glob Health. 2016;4(10):e752-60.
6. Singer M, Deutschman CS, Seymour CW, et al. The third international consensus definitions for sepsis and septic shock (sepsis-3). JAMA. 2016;315(8):801-10.
7. Sinha M, Jupe J, Mack H, et al. Emerging technologies for molecular diagnosis of sepsis. Clin Microbiol Rev. 2018;31(2):e00089-17.
8. Tewari VV, Jain N. Monotherapy with amikacin or piperacillin–tazobactam empirically in neonates at risk for early-onset sepsis: A randomized controlled trial. J Trop Pediatr. 2014;60(4):297-302.
9. Vergnano S, Buttery J, Cailes B, et al. Neonatal infections: case definition and guidelines for data collection, analysis, and presentation of immunisation safety data. Vaccine. 2016;34(49):6038-46.
10. Xu L, Li Q, Mo Z, et al. Diagnostic value of C-reactive protein in neonatal sepsis: A meta-analysis. Eur J Inflamm. 2016;14(2):100-8.

2.9 Neonatal Seizures

Ruchi N Nanavati

INTRODUCTION

Seizures represent the most distinctive manifestation of neurological disease in the neonatal period. The tendency toward recurrent seizures and status epilepticus is far greater in the newborn period than at any other time of life. It is critical to recognize neonatal seizures, determine their etiology, and treat them as they usually relate to significant illness and seizures themselves and may be a cause of brain injury and potential long-term sequelae.

DEFINITION

Seizure is a paroxysmal alteration in neurological function, behavioral, motor, or autonomic.

EPIDEMIOLOGY

A population-based study of neonatal seizures revealed that the risk varied inversely with birth weight: 57.5/1,000 live births among very low-birth-weight (LBW) infants (<1,500 g) compared with 4.4/1,000 for infants with moderately LBW (1,500–2,499 g), and 2.8/1,000 for those with normal birth weight (2,500–3,999 g). Hypoxic ischemic encephalopathy (HIE), intracranial hemorrhage (ICH), intracranial infections, and developmental defects account for 80–85% of all the cases of normal saline (NS). Indian data is limited.

ETIOPATHOGENESIS

A seizure results from excessive synchronous electrical discharge of neurons produced by the inward migration of sodium ions (i.e. depolarization). The probable mechanisms for excessive depolarization are shown in **(Table 2.9.1)**.

Perinatal neuroanatomical and neurophysiological unique features determine neonatal seizure phenomena. The more advanced development within the limbic system with connections to the midbrain and brainstem explain the higher frequency of subtle features, while the balance of excitatory and inhibitory processes in the immature brain are weighed toward excitation with an excess of glutamatergic synapses over inhibitory synapses with gamma-aminobutyric

Table 2.9.1: Etiology of probable mechanisms for excessive depolarization.	
Probable mechanism	***Causes***
Failure of Na^{+}–K^{+} pump secondary to reduced energy production	Hypoxemia, ischemia, and hypoglycemia
Excess of excitatory neurotransmitter (GABA acts as an excitatory neurotransmitter due to elevated chloride levels in perinatal neurons)	Hypoxemia, ischemia, and hypoglycemia
Relative deficiency of inhibitory neurotransmitter	Pyridoxine dependency
Membrane alteration with increased Na^{+} influx	Hypocalcemia and hypomagnesemia

(GABA: gamma-aminobutyric acid)

acid acting as excitatory neurotransmitter. The threshold for seizure generation is lower in the developing brain than in the mature brain, but developing neurons are less vulnerable to injury from single prolonged seizures than are mature neurons. The electrical discharges readily generated in the neonatal brain do not propagate sufficiently due to inadequate myelination and thus lead to fragmentary seizures whose electrical activity may not spread to surface electroencephalography (EEG) electrodes. Best documented mechanisms for the occurrence of brain injury with repeated seizures are accompanied serious hypoventilation causing hypoxemia and hypercapnia, elevations of arterial blood pressure, disturbances of cerebral blood flow, decreased brain adenosine triphosphate and phosphocreatine concentrations, and increased release of excitatory amino acids. Dramatic fall in brain glucose within 5 minutes of onset of seizures with concomitant rise in brain lactate may interfere with deoxyribonucleic acid synthesis, glial proliferation, differentiation, and myelination. Evidence suggests that NS may predispose to impaired cognitive, behavioral functions, or susceptibility to epilepsy later in life. The most common etiologies are discussed below.

Perinatal Events

- Hypoxic ischemic encephalopathy;
- *Intracranial hemorrhage*: Germinal matrix intraventricular hemorrhage, subdural hemorrhage, primary subarachnoid hemorrhage (SAH: well baby with seizures);
- *Focal infarction:* Arterial/venous.

Metabolic

- *Hypoglycemia:* Preterm, LBW, infant of diabetic mother (IDM), sick baby
- *Hypocalcemia:* Early—preterm, asphyxia, IDM
- *Late:* Top feeding
- Hypomagnesemia
- Hypo/hypernatremia
- Pyridoxine dependency
- *Inborn errors of metabolism:* Disorders of amino acid metabolism, organic acidurias, peroxisomal diseases, mitochondrial disorders, disorders of glucose transport (glucose transporter protein type 1 deficiency), pyridoxine dependent seizures, folinic acid responsive seizures.

Infection

- Bacterial meningitis
- *Nonbacterial infections:* Toxoplasmosis, herpes simplex, coxsackie B, rubella, cytomegalovirus.

Congenital Malformations and Other Structural Lesions

- Cerebral cortical dysgenesis
- Lissencephaly, schizencephaly
- Neuronal migration disorders
- Pachygyria, polymicrogyria.

Miscellaneous

- Passive drug withdrawal
- Accidental injection of local anesthetic into fetal scalp
- Drug toxicity
- Polycythemia
- Hypertensive encephalopathy
- Neonatal epileptic syndromes.

Hypoxic Ischemic Encephalopathy

Hypoxic ischemic encephalopathy usually secondary to perinatal asphyxia is the single most common cause of NS in both full term and premature infants. The seizures generally start within 12–24 hours, increase in frequency over 24–36 hours, and usually burn out by days 4–5. Subtle seizures are most common followed by multifocal clonic and focal clonic seizures.

Hypoglycemia

The most common metabolic cause of NS is commonly seen in LBW infants, IDMs, and sick infants. The onset is usually the second postnatal day. The most critical determinant of neurologic symptoms is duration of hypoglycemia.

Neonatal Epileptic Syndromes

- *Benign familial NS:* Autosomal dominant disorder with primary generalized seizures on day 2 or 3 of life without any obvious risk factor. Seizures may recur and gradually resolve over weeks. Later epilepsy seen in <10%.
- *Benign idiopathic NS (fifth day fits):* Seizures, usually multifocal clonic often associated with apnea, onset

between days 4 and 6 of life in term infants with normal neurological state and diagnostic testing. Often, 80% leading to status epilepticus. Most seizures cease after 24 hours and in all patients within 2 weeks. Probably related to transient zinc deficiency. Long-term outcome favorable.

- *Early myoclonic encephalopathy:* Starts as focal motor fragmentary seizures and later evolve into typical infantile spasms. Usually associated with nonketotic hyperglycinemia. EEG reveals burst suppression pattern with poor long-term outcome.
- *Early infantile epileptic encephalopathy (Ohtahara syndrome):* Brief tonic spasms presenting between days 10 and 90 of life. Usually associated with structural disorders. EEG reveals burst suppression pattern with poor long-term outcome.

SEIZURE CLASSIFICATION

American Clinical Neurophysiology Society has described the following three types of neonatal seizures:

1. *Clinical only seizures*: No simultaneous EEG seizure
2. *Electroclinical seizure*: Clinical seizure coupled with simultaneous EEG seizure
3. *Electroencephalography only seizures*: Not associated with clinical seizure.

Numerous studies have indicated that about 80–90% of the electrographical seizures do not have associated clinical correlates and therefore would not be identified without continuous EEG (cEEG) monitoring. In addition, treatment with anticonvulsant medication may terminate clinical seizures but not necessarily electrical seizures, thereby further highlighting the importance of cEEG monitoring.

CLINICAL MANIFESTATIONS

Normal saline is difficult to recognize because they are brief, fragmentary, asymmetrical, lack the organization, and may be associated with non-motor phenomenon. Four patterns are described.

1. *Subtle seizures*: Most common subtype (50%) include broad spectrum of behavioral phenomena:
   - Ocular: Tonic horizontal deviation, ocular fixation, repetitive blinking
   - Oral-facial-lingual movements
   - Limb movements: Cycling, peddling
   - Autonomic phenomena: Tachycardia, bradycardia, irregular respiration, increased blood pressure
   - Apnea: Rarely the only manifestation, rarely lasts more than 10–20 seconds, initial tachycardia common.

   At bedside, subtle seizures are distinguished by their insensitivity to tactile stimulation or restrain and frequent association with autonomic effects.
2. *Clonic seizures*: Well-localized stereotypic and repetitive biphasic movements. May be unifocal, multifocal (progression from one part to another in nonordered fashion), or generalized, usually not associated with loss of consciousness. Primary generalized clonic seizures are extremely rare. They are provoked by metabolic disturbances, focal traumatic injury, SAH, and focal infarct. The most common cause of clonic seizures that remain unifocal is neonatal stroke. EEG reveals unifocal or multifocal abnormality and prognosis is good.
3. *Tonic seizures*: Characterized by sustained extension or flexion of axial or appendicular muscle group and resemble decerebrate or decorticate posture. May be focal or generalized, often associated with eye deviation or apnea and are most common in preterm with ICH or diffuse central nervous system (CNS) disease. Generalized tonic seizures may not be associated with time-synchronized EEG discharges. EEG may depict burst suppression pattern and prognosis is poor.
4. *Myoclonic seizures*: Characterized by synchronous single or multiple slow jerks and are associated with diffuse CNS pathology. Focal and multifocal myoclonic seizures are most commonly unassociated with while generalized myoclonic seizures are more likely to be associated with time-synchronized EEG discharges. EEG may reveal burst suppression or hypsarrhythmia pattern and prognosis is poor.

Neonatal seizures according to the time of onset are described in **(Table 2.9.2)**.

Nonepileptic Movements (Seizure Mimics)

Certain behavioral phenomena may be confused with NS.

- *Jitteriness* is characterized by tremulous movements (5–6/s) is stimulus sensitive, not associated with abnormal autonomic changes or eye movements and is terminated by passive flexion of extremity. EEG is normal.
- *Tremors* may be misidentified as clonic seizures. Tremors are reported in 50% of the healthy newborns and are hypothesized due to the immaturity of inhibitory neurons.

Table 2.9.2: Neonatal seizures and time of onset.

Time of onset	*Etiology*
<24 hours	HIE, severe birth trauma, congenital CNS anomalies, pyridoxine dependency, hypoglycemia, hypocalcemia, drug withdrawal, ICH
1–3 days	All above + Intracranial infections, subarachnoid hemorrhage, IEMs, benign familial neonatal seizures
>3 days	Late hypocalcemia, sepsis, meningitis, progressive hydrocephalus, epileptic syndromes, herpes encephalitis, IEMs

(CNS: central nervous system; HIE: hypoxic ischemic encephalopathy; ICH: intracranial hemorrhage; IEMs: inborn errors of metabolisms)

High amplitude tremors are more likely to be secondary to brain disorders.

- *Benign sleep neonatal myoclonus* usually presents in the first week and resolves spontaneously over weeks. It occurs during non-rapid eye movement sleep, abolishes on arousal, and never occurs during wakefulness. Neurological examination and EEG is normal. Transient dysmaturity of the brainstem reticular activating system is postulated. Anticonvulsants are not indicated. Long-term outcome is normal. Later epilepsy does not develop.
- *Hyperekplexia* is a rare autosomal dominant disorder characterized by hypertonia, hyperreflexia, and an exaggerated startle response. The mutation of inhibitory glycine receptor is described. Therapy with clonazepam/diazepam causes marked improvement.

INVESTIGATIONS

The following tests are required with first seizure episode:

- Blood sugar.
- Serum calcium, phosphorus, magnesium.
- Serum electrolytes.
- Cerebrospinal fluid analysis.
- Neuroimaging, especially with focal seizures.
- *Electroencephalography:* Continuous EEG, defined as >3 hours monitoring, is considered the gold standard for the diagnosis of NS. Ictal EEG is useful for the diagnosis of suspected seizures, while interictal EEG is useful for predicting long-term prognosis. Abnormal background activity indicates a high risk for long-term neurological sequelae. Amplitude integrated EEG, a bedside technique, is a useful initial complementary tool and is being increasingly used in neonatal intensive care units for neuromonitoring.

Additional Investigations

- *Neuroimaging:* Computed tomography scan is advisable when etiology is undetermined after first-line investigations and is especially good for hemorrhages and calcifications. Magnetic resonance imaging (MRI) provides better resolution of anatomy and details of function and perfusion with diffusion-weighted MRI, spectroscopy, and angiography. Neuroimaging has more value in prognostication.
- *Metabolic workup:* Inborn errors of metabolism should be suspected with family history of unexplained fetal/neonatal deaths; mental retardation; seizures occurring after introduction of feeds; or those associated with unexplained lethargy, coma, and vomiting. Initial workup includes arterial blood gases, blood ammonia, serum and urinary amino acids, serum lactate and pyruvate, and urinary reducing substances.
- Sepsis workup
- Toxoplasmosis, rubella cytomegalovirus, herpes simplex, and HIV screen
- Karyotyping
- Toxic drug screen
- As per suspected etiology.

TREATMENT

Normal saline is a medical emergency and mandates prompt treatment. World Health Organization (WHO) guidelines on NS recommend treatment of all clinical and electrographic seizures. A stepwise approach is shown in **(Flowchart 2.9.1)**.

Other Drugs Used in Resistant Seizures

- *Lidocaine:* Can be used as second-line therapy or for refractory neonatal seizures. The medication has good CNS penetration and acts as a CNS depressant. Dose—2 mg/kg IV bolus, then 6 mg/kg/hour drip, then titrate down by 2 mg/kg/hour every 12 hours until off. Because of the cumulative risk of toxicity, lidocaine must be stopped within 36 hours. Furthermore, the dose must be reduced in premature infants or if the newborn is undergoing therapeutic hypothermia, as clearance decreases during hypothermia. Lidocaine can cause arrhythmias and bradycardia. It should be avoided in newborns, who have congenital heart disease or have received other proarrhythmic drugs such as phenytoin.
- *Valproic acid:* As adjunctive or maintenance therapy, 20 mg/kg IV/per rectum/per os (PO) is followed by 5–10 mg/kg/day in two divided doses. Concern about hepatotoxicity, hyperammonemia, and hyperglycinemia limits its use.
- *Topiramate:* Blocker of the α-amino-3-hydroxy-5-methyl-4-isoxazolepropionic acid type of glutamate receptor. Shows promise in neonatal seizures because of its potential neuroprotective effect against injury caused by seizures. The higher volume of distribution compared with other drugs requires higher initial and maintenance doses of approximately 3 mg/kg.
- *Primidone, Carbamazepine, Lamotrigine, and Vigabatrin:* These have been tried in refractory seizures.
- *Pyridoxine:* Therapeutic trial of pyridoxine is warranted in refractory seizures. Pyridoxine dependency is diagnosed on rapid cessation of EEG seizures following 50–100 mg IV pyridoxine. Other drugs used in suspected metabolic causes are pyridoxal-5 phosphate, 30 mg/kg/day PO, folinic acid, 4 mg/kg/day PO, biotin 5–10 mg enterally or intravenously BD.

Detection and Treatment of Underlying Cause

Importance of history and physical examination to detect the cause of seizures cannot be overemphasized. Treatment of the underlying cause is essential.

Flowchart 2.9.1: Approach to neonatal seizures.

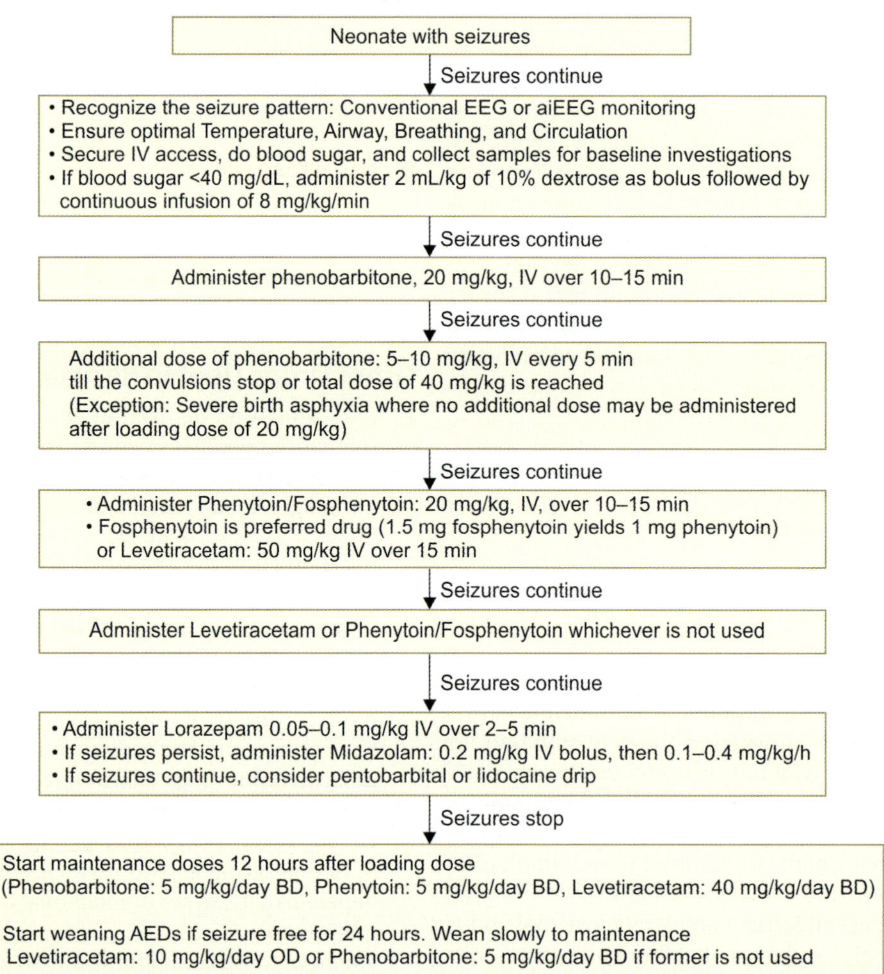

Calcium and magnesium: If hypocalcemia is present, administer 10% calcium gluconate IV 2 mL/kg (200 mg/kg). The electrocardiogram or at least cardiac rhythm by auscultation should be monitored during administration. Phenobarbitone can sometimes suppress the seizures of hypocalcemia; thus, a decrease in seizures after phenobarbitone administration does not rule out hypocalcemia as the cause. If hypomagnesemia is present, magnesium sulfate, 50%, is given intramuscularly in a dose of 0.2 mL/kg.

Long-term Therapy

A review by WHO recommends the consideration of weaning of anticonvulsant medication after 72 hours of treatment, if the neurological examination and/or EEG are normal. The possible adverse effects on developing CNS of continuing automated external defibrillators for several months have raised concerns. Attempts should be made to stop all antiepileptic drugs and wean the baby to only phenobarbitone or levetiracetam. Monotherapy is most appropriate. Recently, levetiracetam has shown promising results for long-term maintenance therapy. Neonatal neurological examination, etiology of neonatal seizures, and EEG findings are main determinants of the duration of antiseizure medication **(Flowchart 2.9.2)**.

PROGNOSIS

Prognosis mainly depends upon gestational age, nature and cause of seizures, neurological examination, EEG, and neuroimaging findings. Incidence of sequelae is different as per the etiology **(Table 2.9.3)**.

KEY MESSAGES

- The diagnosis of seizures requires a high index of suspicion, careful clinical observation, and cEEG monitoring.
- Continuous EEG monitoring, defined as more than 3 hours monitoring, is considered the gold standard for the

Flowchart 2.9.2: Long-term management of neonatal seizures.

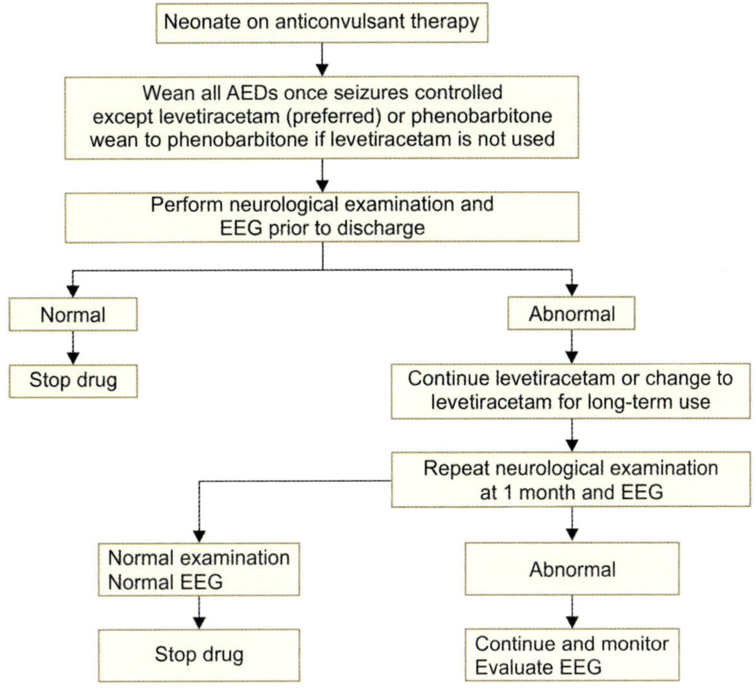

Table 2.9.3: Prognosis of neonatal seizures according to etiology.

Neurologic disease	***% Normal***
HIE	50
ICH with hemorrhagic infarct	<10
Primary SAH	90
Hypocalcemia—early	50
Hypocalcemia—late	100
Hypoglycemia	50
Bacterial meningitis	50
CNS malformation	0
Background EEG	***Neurosequelae***
Normal	<10
Severe abnormalities	≥90
Moderate abnormalities	~50

(EEG: electroencephalography; HIE: hypoxic ischemic encephalopathy; ICH: intracranial hemorrhage; SAH: subarachnoid hemorrhage)

diagnosis of NS as 80–90% of the electrographical seizures do not have associated clinical correlates and therefore would not be identified without cEEG monitoring.
- Neonatal seizures may predispose to cognitive, behavioral, or epileptic complications later in life.
- World Health Organization guidelines on NS recommend treatment of all clinical and electrographic seizures, and the goal of therapy is total or near total elimination of electrographic seizures and not merely elimination of clinical seizures.
- Phenobarbitone is preferred anticonvulsant for initial and maintenance therapy. Recently, levetiracetam has shown promising results for long-term maintenance therapy.
- Long-term prognostication should be guarded in recurrent or resistant seizures or those with EEG abnormalities.
- Topiramate and bumetanide causing inhibition of excitation at excitatory amino acid receptors with potent anticonvulsant and neuroprotective properties hold promising future.

BIBLIOGRAPHY

1. Laoria N. Controversies in diagnosis and management of neonatal seizures. Indian Pediatr. 2000;37:367-72.
2. Rennie JM. Seizures in the newborn. In: Rennie JM, Roberton NRC (Eds). Textbook of Neonatology, 3rd edition. Churchill Livingstone; 2000. pp. 1213-22.
3. Sansevere AJ. Neonatal seizures. In : Hansen AR, Eichenwald EC, Stark AR, Martin CR (Eds). Cloherty and Stark's Manual of Neonatal Care, 8th edition. Lippincott. 2016: pp. 813-45.
4. Tekgul H, Gauvreau K, Soul J, et al. The current etiologic profile and neurodevelopmental outcome of seizures in term newborn infants. Pediatrics. 2006.117:1270-80.
5. Volpe JJ. Neonatal seizures. In: Volpe JJ (Ed). Neurology of the Newborn, 6th edition. Philadelphia, PA: Saunders Elsevier; 2017. pp. 273-318.

2.10 Respiratory Distress

Ashok Kumar

DEFINITION

Respiratory distress (RD) in newborn is defined as one or more of the following features: respiratory rate greater than or equal to 60 per minute, chest retractions, and grunt.

ETIOPATHOGENESIS

Respiratory distress affects nearly 5–10% of all newborns. The etiology of RD depends on the age of onset of symptoms, gestational age, and maternal factors. **Table 2.10.1** summarizes the common causes of RD in newborn. The pathogenesis of the most common causes is outlined in this section.

Respiratory Distress Syndrome

The incidence is inversely related to the gestational age. Approximately 50% of the newborns delivered at 26–28 weeks of gestation develop RD syndrome (RDS), whereas the disease becomes infrequent after 34 weeks. Factors such as male gender, infants of diabetic mothers, multiple gestation, perinatal asphyxia, and cesarean section increase the risk of disease. It is caused by the deficiency of surfactant in the lungs, which is a composite mixture of phospholipids and proteins produced by type II epithelial cells of alveoli.

Table 2.10.1: Etiology of respiratory distress in newborn.

- *Respiratory system:*
  - Respiratory distress syndrome
  - Transient tachypnea of the newborn
  - Intrauterine pneumonia
  - Meconium aspiration syndrome
  - Pneumonia
  - Aspiration pneumonia
  - Air leak syndromes
  - *Surgical causes*: Tracheoesophageal fistula, diaphragmatic hernia, bilateral choanal atresia, and congenital lobar emphysema
- *Cardiovascular system:*
  - Congestive heart failure
- *Central nervous system:*
  - Perinatal asphyxia
  - Intracranial hemorrhage
- *Metabolic:*
  - Hypoglycemia
  - Metabolic acidosis
- *Miscellaneous:*
  - Hypothermia
  - Polycythemia

Transient Tachypnea of the Newborn

It is a benign, self-limiting, disorder, which commonly occurs in term and late preterm (34–36 weeks) newborns. It is caused by the delayed clearance of fetal lung fluid. The risk factors include poor respiratory effort at birth, cesarean delivery without the benefit of labor, multiple gestations, delayed cord clamping, male gender, and maternal diabetes.

Meconium Aspiration Syndrome

Meconium staining of amniotic fluid (MSAF) occurs in 10–15% of deliveries. Approximately, 5% of the babies born through MSAF develop meconium aspiration syndrome (MAS). It is common in term and post-term babies, especially those with intrauterine growth restriction.

CLINICAL FEATURES

In a newborn presenting within the first 6 hours of birth with RD, one should consider the possibilities of RDS, transient tachypnea of the newborn (TTN), MAS, congenital pneumonia, air leaks, or malformations as the etiology.

The neonates with RDS are preterm who present with tachypnea, chest retractions, expiratory grunt, cyanosis, and apneic spells. Neonates with TTN usually have mild-to-moderate RD with tachypnea, chest retractions, and flaring of alae nasi. However, the baby remains active and alert despite severe tachypnea. Quick recovery by 2–3 days helps to differentiate this condition from pneumonia or MAS. In MAS, RD develops soon after birth, manifesting as tachypnea, retractions, hyperinflated chest, and occasionally grunting. There is a history of meconium-stained amniotic fluid and/or meconium staining of the skin, and the babies are often born depressed at birth, requiring resuscitation in the delivery room. If there is history of chorioamnionitis in the mother, one may consider the possibility of congenital pneumonia. Air leak should be suspected in any newborn that has received positive-pressure ventilation at birth and would have features of decreased air entry and mediastinal shift to the opposite site. Chest X-ray is diagnostic. If facilities for transillumination are available, then air leak can be confirmed on the bedside by the bright transillumination on the side of the air leak. Suspect cardiac disease, if a newborn presents with RD and hepatomegaly, weak pulses, with or without cardiac murmurs, or cyanosis.

SURGICAL CAUSES OF RESPIRATORY DISTRESS

Suspect esophageal atresia (with/without tracheoesophageal fistula), if a newborn presents soon after birth with increased salivation and choking during feeds. Failure to pass a feeding tube into the stomach confirms the diagnosis. RD in a baby with scaphoid abdomen and a mediastinal shift should suggest diaphragmatic hernia. Bilateral choanal atresia presents as cyclic RD, particularly during feeding that disappears on crying or opening mouth, as it bypasses nasal obstruction. Inability to pass a catheter through nose into nasopharynx establishes the diagnosis.

Assessment of the Severity of Respiratory Distress

The severity of RD can be judged clinically by the *respiratory score* (Downe score) as given in **(Table 2.10.2)**. The score is used in babies who are breathing spontaneously, including those receiving continuous positive airway pressure (CPAP). A score of less than 5 indicates mild RD, a score of 5–8 moderate RD, and a score of greater than 8 severe RD.

DIAGNOSIS

Chest Skiagram

This is the most useful investigation that can help in the etiological diagnosis of RD in the newborn. In RDS, the radiological features include symmetrical fine reticulogranular pattern, reduced lung volume, diffuse haziness (ground-glass appearance), air bronchograms **(Fig. 2.10.1)**, and complete white out of the lungs in the late stages. In TTN, the chest X-ray shows normal or increased lung inflation, streaky perihilar infiltrates, and fluid in horizontal fissure **(Fig. 2.10.2)**. In MAS, the chest X-ray shows hyperinflation, coarse irregular opacities, and sometimes pneumothorax **(Fig. 2.10.3)**. Air leaks, esophageal atresia, and diaphragmatic hernia can all be diagnosed by typical radiological features. Pneumonia may show varying degrees of lung opacities and would have to be correlated clinically.

Table 2.10.2: Respiratory score (Downe score).

Score	*0*	*1*	*2*
Respiratory rate (per min)	40–60	60–80	>80
Oxygen requirement (%)	None	≤50	>50
Retractions	None	Mild-to-moderate	Severe
Grunting	None	With stimulation	At rest
Breath sounds	Normal	Decreased	Barely heard
Prematurity (weeks)	>34	30–34	<30

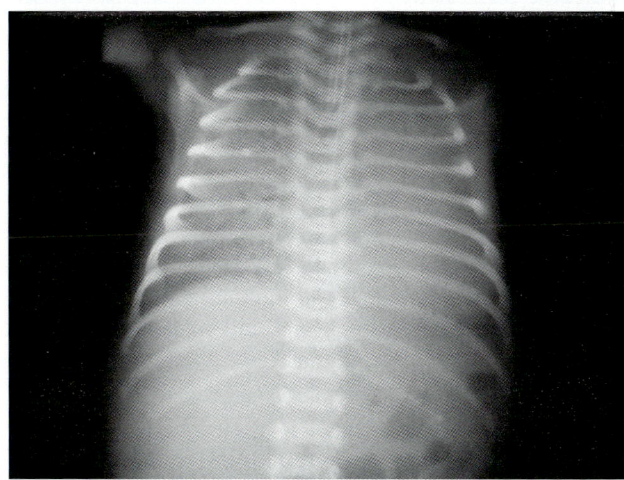

Fig. 2.10.1: Chest X-ray of respiratory distress syndrome (RDS) showing diffuse haziness, blurring of cardiac margins and air bronchogram.

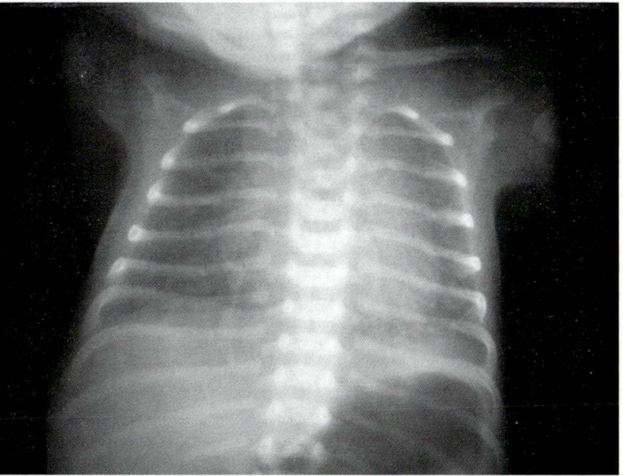

Fig. 2.10.2: Chest X-ray of transient tachypnea of the newborn (TTN) showing streaky perihilar infiltrates.

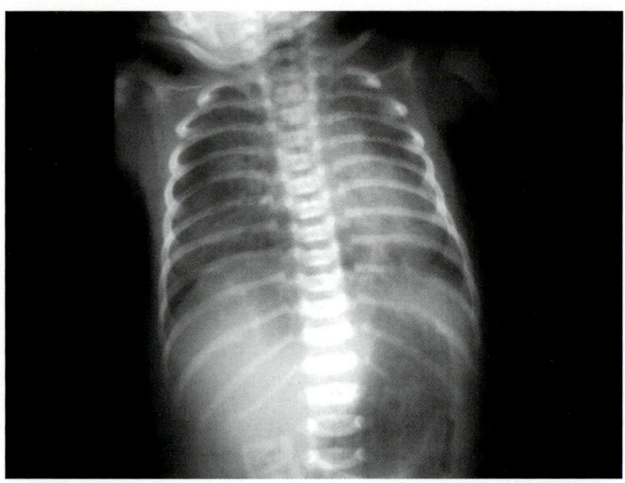

Fig. 2.10.3: Chest X-ray of meconium aspiration syndrome (MAS) showing patchy hyperaeration and heterogeneous opacities in the lung fields.

Shake Test

The test is based on the premise that if there are sufficient amounts of surfactant present in the amniotic fluid (or gastric aspirate taken within 30 minutes of birth), it would generate a stable foam layer at air-liquid interface when mixed with ethanol. Inadequate foam layer could suggest insufficient surfactant and an indirect support for the diagnosis of RDS.

Other Tests

In case, pneumonia is suspected then blood culture, C-reactive protein, total leukocyte count, and absolute neutrophil count should be done.

TREATMENT

Treatment is largely supportive. The infant should be nursed under a radiant warmer. Most newborns with severe RD are not usually capable of being fed orally and need to be initially kept on intravenous fluids.

Oxygenation

Provide oxygen by a headbox to maintain target oxygen saturations (SpO_2) in the 90–95%. Oxygen therapy must be monitored by a pulse oximeter to avoid hypoxia or hyperoxia, both of which are harmful to the baby.

Continuous Positive Airway Pressure

In neonates with RDS, CPAP is a simple, safe, and effective method to improve oxygenation. Being noninvasive, CPAP is the initial modality of choice in RDS. It works by preventing alveolar atelectasis, thereby reducing work of breathing. CPAP is utilized in spontaneously breathing babies. Intractable apnea is a contraindication for CPAP. Early CPAP use is more effective and may reduce the need of mechanical ventilation. CPAP is best delivered through short nasal prongs. Begin CPAP at 5–6 cm H_2O pressure (maximum 8 cm H_2O). Insert orogastric tube to prevent gastric distension from swallowed air (CPAP belly). The inability to maintain SpO_2 greater than 90% at 40–50% fraction of inspired oxygen (FiO_2) indicates the need for mechanical ventilation.

High Flow Nasal Cannula

High flow nasal cannula refers to the delivery of heated and humidified oxygen at high flows using small binasal prongs. High flows generate positive pressure in the nasopharynx which is transmitted to the lower airways and alveoli. It is easier to apply than CPAP and produces less nasal trauma. It can be used as an alternative to CPAP in mild-to-moderate RD.

Mechanical Ventilation

Mechanical ventilation should be considered in infants with RD who fail CPAP or have recurrent or intractable apnea or have the evidence of respiratory failure (blood gas revealing severe acidosis, pH < 7.25, $PaCO_2 > 55–60$ mm Hg, and $PaO_2 < 50$ mm Hg).

Surfactant Replacement Therapy

Surfactant replacement therapy (SRT) should be considered in neonates with RDS. Surfactant is instilled directly into the lungs through endotracheal tube. In symptomatic babies, early rescue therapy (within 2 hours) is better than delayed therapy. Prophylactic SRT (before the onset of RD) is indicated for newborns under 26 weeks' gestation and to those preterm who require intubation for stabilization in delivery room. Natural surfactants are better than synthetic preparations. The dose is 100–200 mg/kg. Single dose suffices for most infants. Dose may be repeated 6–12 hours later, if significant distress persists. Monitor baby carefully after SRT. Within a few minutes, there is an improvement in gas exchange, oxygen requirement comes down, and ventilator settings must be adjusted to prevent ventilator-induced lung injury. **Figure 2.10.4** shows radiological improvement in lung status after surfactant therapy.

Antibiotics

When pneumonia is suspected, appropriate antibiotics such as ampicillin/cephalosporin and an aminoglycoside should be initiated along with other supportive care.

COMPLICATIONS

Acute complications include air leaks, patent ductus arteriosus, intracranial hemorrhage, and infection. Long-term

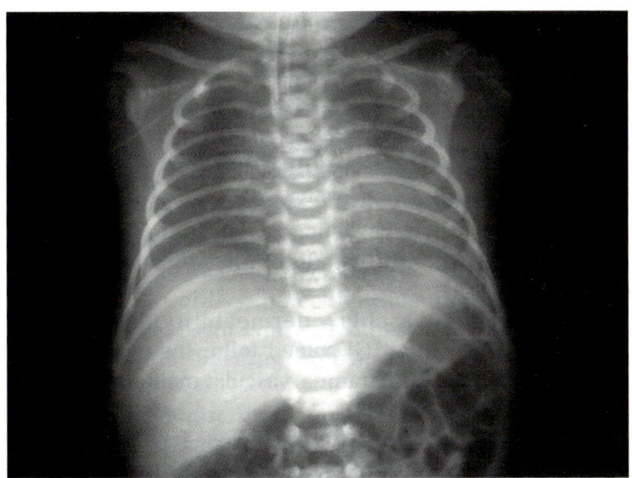

Fig. 2.10.4: Chest X-ray of the same baby as in Figure 2.10.1, showing considerable clearing of the lungs 5 hours after giving surfactant.

complications in preterm include retinopathy of prematurity, bronchopulmonary dysplasia, neurodevelopmental impairments, and other complications of prematurity.

PREVENTION OF RESPIRATORY DISTRESS SYNDROME

Respiratory distress syndrome can be prevented by using antenatal corticosteroids to pregnant women between 24 and 34 weeks of gestation with threatened preterm labor. A complete course consists of two doses of betamethasone (12 mg IM) at 24-hourly interval or four doses of dexamethasone (6 mg IM) at 12-hourly intervals. Multiple courses of steroids are not recommended in view of modest incremental benefit and real risk of brain damage to the fetus.

KEY MESSAGES

- The most common cause of RD is RDS in preterm newborns and TTN in late preterm and term newborns.
- Good supportive care improves outcome.
- Monitor oxygen therapy with a pulse oximetry. Unmonitored oxygen use is dangerous.
- Oxygen administration by hood is effective in mild RD.
- Continuous positive airway pressure is effective and cheap method to provide respiratory support in mild-to-moderate RD.
- Mechanical ventilation is the modality of choice for treating severe RD.
- Always obtain blood culture and sepsis screen before starting antibiotics.
- Single course of prenatal steroids between 24 and 34 weeks of gestation reduces the incidence of RDS by 50%.
- Surfactant replacement therapy is most effective, when it is given within 2 hours of the development of symptoms (early rescue therapy).

BIBLIOGRAPHY

1. Guha DK, Saili A, Bhat S, et al. Guha's Neonatology: Principles and Practice, 3rd edition. New Delhi: Jaypee Brothers Medical Publishers; 2005.
2. Sweet DS, Carnielli V, Greisen G, et al. European Consensus guidelines on the management of neonatal respiratory distress syndrome in preterm infants, 2010 update. Neonatology. 2010;97:402-17.
3. Warren JB, Anderson JM. Core concepts: respiratory distress syndrome. Neo Reviews. 2009;10:e351-61.
4. Welty S, Hansen TN, Corbet A. Respiratory distress in the preterm infant. In: Taeusch HW, Ballard RA, Gleason CA (Eds). Avery's Diseases of the Newborn, 8th edition. Philadelphia, PA: Saunders; 2005. pp. 687-703.

2.11 Bleeding Neonate

JN Sharma

INTRODUCTION

The hemorrhagic disorders in the newborn are a group of disorders with different etiologies, which have in common an abnormal tendency to bleed. The abnormal tendency to bleed is due to a defect in the mechanism of hemostasis. Severe bleeding, which is life-threatening and needs urgent intervention, is, however, uncommon in the newborn.

LABORATORY DIAGNOSIS

- *Essential investigations* for all cases include Hb and hematocrit (HCT) estimation, red cell morphology, total leukocyte count, differential leukocyte count, platelet count, and reticulocyte count. It should be remembered that the level of Hb and HCT immediately after acute blood loss does not decrease immediately. Hence, it should be repeated after 12 hours.
- *Apt and Downey test*: This test should be performed when there is only GI bleeding in a well neonate in the first 48 hours of life and is used to distinguish swallowed maternal blood from neonatal blood. One part of vomitus is mixed with five parts of distilled water and centrifuged. To the pink centrifuged supernatant fluid, add 1 mL of 1% sodium hydroxide and wait for 1–2 minutes. If the solution changes to yellow-brown color, it favors the possibility of swallowed maternal blood (HbA gets denatured by alkali while HbF stays pink). Two controls should be run alongside by taking two drops of blood each from a baby and an adult and repeating the procedure.
- *Screening tests* for hemorrhagic disorders include platelet count and examination of blood film for number, morphology and presence of platelet clumping, the bleeding time, prothrombin time (PT), activated partial thromboplastin time (APTT), and thrombin time.
- *Special tests* include prothrombin consumption test, coagulation factor assays, and platelet function tests. They are required to (1) identify the deficient coagulation factor, (2) determine the degree of deficiency, and (3) detect and quantitate immune inhibitors.
- A neonate who has a positive bleeding history or is having active bleeding should have a platelet count, bleeding time, PTT, and PT done. If the results are normal, a thrombin time and von Willebrand factor testing should be considered.
- The blood samples should be collected for coagulation studies as well as other investigations before blood transfusion.

Table 2.11.2 lists the differential diagnosis of coagulation disorders based on laboratory tests. **Table 2.11.3** lists the fetal and neonatal causes of thrombocytopenia.

MANAGEMENT

The management of a bleeding neonate includes supportive treatment with blood component therapy and identification and treatment of the cause.

Blood sample should be collected for the investigation. Then all babies should be given vitamin K, 2 mg IV or subcutaneous (SC), if not given earlier. Naturally occurring vitamin K_1 or K_2 is preferred because of its rapid action and lack of any risk of producing hyperbilirubinemia. An X-ray, plain picture abdomen (erect posture), should be obtained to exclude GI perforation or other surgical conditions in cases with GI bleeding.

Table 2.11.2: Differential diagnosis of coagulation disorders based on laboratory tests.

Abnormality	***Diagnosis***
Long PTT + normal PT + normal platelets + normal bleeding	Factors VIII, IX, XI, XII deficiency
Long PTT + normal PT + normal platelets + long bleeding time	von Willebrand disease
Long PTT + long PT + normal platelets	Vitamin K deficiency
Long PTT + long PT + decreased platelets	DIC or generalized coagulopathy
Normal PTT + long PT	Factor VII deficiency
Normal PTT + normal PT + normal platelets + normal bleeding time + bleeding especially umbilicus	Factor XIII deficiency
Normal PTT + normal PT + low platelets	ITP, aplasia, leukemia, etc.
Many petechiae and normal platelets	HSV, CMV, infections

(CMV: cytomegalovirus; DIC: disseminated intravascular coagulopathy; HSV: herpes simplex virus; ITP: idiopathic thrombocytopenic purpura; PT: prothrombin time; PTT: partial thromboplastin time)

Infant in Shock

- If the baby has clinical signs of shock or if estimated blood loss exceeds 20% of the blood volume, an immediate blood transfusion should be given.
- The infant in shock requires a rapid transfusion of 15–20 mL/kg of uncross-matched O negative blood or 10–20 mL/kg of normal saline over 5–15 minutes. If there are no signs of recovery from shock, another bolus should be given over 15–20 minutes.
- The BP and central venous pressure (CVP) should be monitored. The aim is to achieve BP > 40 mm Hg (in term infants) and CVP < 8 cmH_2O.
- If necessary, a further transfusion should be given cross-matched against maternal blood, 10–30 mL/kg over 2–3 hours accompanied by 1–2 mg/kg furosemide IV.
- In the cases with severe anemia due to prolonged slow bleeding, partial exchange transfusion is recommended to avoid circulatory overload.
- Monitoring of vital signs, estimation of concurrent blood loss, Hb, and HCT should be done to determine the need for subsequent transfusion.

Infant not in Shock

- The infant may need a transfusion with packed red cells 10 mL/kg over 2–3 hours with 2 mg/kg furosemide IV to raise Hb to 10–12 g/dL. It needs to be mentioned that 10 mL/kg of packed red cells will raise Hb by 2–3 g/dL or the HCT by 10%.

Table 2.11.3: Causes of fetal and neonatal thrombocytopenia.

Time of onset	*Possible etiology*
Fetal thrombocytopenia	• Alloimmune thrombocytopenia • Congenital infections (e.g. CMV, *Toxoplasma*, rubella, HIV) • Aneuploidy (trisomy 13, 18, 21) • Autoimmune thrombocytopenia (ITP, SLE, severe Rh hemolytic disease)
Early-onset neonatal thrombocytopenia (<72 hours)	• Placental insufficiency (PET, IUGR, diabetes) • Perinatal asphyxia • Perinatal infections (e.g. *Escherichia coli*, Group B streptococci, *Haemophilus influenzae*) • DIC • Alloimmune thrombocytopenia • Autoimmune thrombocytopenia (maternal ITP, SLE) • Congenital infections (e.g. CMV, *Toxoplasma*, rubella, HIV) • Thrombosis (e.g. aortic, renal vein) • Kasabach-Merritt syndrome • Metabolic diseases (e.g. propionic and methylmalonic acidemia) • Congenital inherited syndromes (e.g. TAR, CAMT)
Late-onset neonatal thrombocytopenia (>72 hours)	• Late-onset sepsis • NEC • Congenital infections (e.g. CMV, *Toxoplasma*, rubella, HIV)

(CMAT: congenital amegakaryocytic thrombocytopenia; CMV: cytomegalovirus; DIC: disseminated intravascular coagulopathy; HIV: human immunodeficiency virus; ITP: idiopathic thrombocytopenic purpura; IUGR: intrauterine growth restriction; NEC: necrotizing enterocolitis; PET: positron emission tomography; Rh: rhesus; SLE: systemic lupus erythematosus; TAR: thrombocytopenia with absent radii)

- All critically ill infants with weight less than 1,500 g should be given IV fresh frozen plasma (FFP), 10 mL/kg, if PT and PTT are prolonged.
- Platelet transfusion should be given when platelet count is less than 20,000/mm^3.

TREATMENT OF SOME SPECIFIC CAUSES OF BLEEDING

Hemorrhagic Disease of Newborn

Classical HDN should be treated with vitamin K (K_1 or K_2) in the dose of 1–2 mg/kg IV or SC. It is followed by a dramatic response with the correction of coagulation abnormalities within 24 hours. The dose for early HDN is vitamin K_1 2 mg IV at birth and for late HDN 1 mg intramuscular every month till the underlying disorder is controlled.

For life-threatening bleeding, vitamin K therapy should be followed 10–20 mL/kg of FFP. If there is evidence of shock, immediate blood transfusion is life-saving.

Alloimmune Thrombocytopenia

Therapeutic interventions include platelet transfusion and administration of IV immunoglobulin (IVIg). Platelet transfusion is indicated when platelet count is less than 30 × 10^9/L. In infants with no bleeding but platelet counts between 30 and 50 × 10^9/L, use of IVIg in the dose of 1 g/kg/day on 2 consecutive days can effectively raise the platelet count.

Autoimmune Thrombocytopenia

The mother should be advised prednisolone 10–20 mg four times daily for 10–14 days or IVIg prior to delivery. The baby should be delivered by lower segment cesarean section, if fetal scalp platelet count is less than 50 × 10^9/L. Postnatally, the neonate should be treated with platelet transfusion, steroid (2 mg/kg/day short course), or IVIg (1 g/kg/day × 2 days).

Disseminated Intravascular Coagulation

The principles of treatment include:

- Treatment of the trigger factor that caused DIC
- Restoration of normal hemostasis by the correction of shock, acidosis, and hypoxia
- Replacement of the coagulation factors and platelets
- Inhibition of the clotting process.

Congenital Deficiency of Coagulation Factors

Fresh frozen plasma, 10–15 mL/kg bodyweight is enough to stop bleeding. If higher plasma concentration of factors is desired, then factor concentrate or cryoprecipitate should be used.

Giant Hemangioma with Kasabach-Merritt Syndrome

It is treated with platelet transfusion, clotting factors, prednisolone, and alpha interferon. Spontaneous involution of the hemangioma may take 1–2 years. Surgical excision is reserved for intractable cases.

KEY MESSAGES

- Coagulation factors do not cross the placenta. The coagulation mechanism is handicapped in the newborn due to physiological deficiency of vitamin K-dependent coagulation factors, resulting in prolongation of PT and PTT, however, not necessarily associated with clinical bleeding.
- Bleeding is more common and severe in preterm and low-birth-weight infants due to exaggeration of this deficiency state with or without superimposed problems, for example, sepsis, asphyxia, etc.
- The most common cause of bleeding neonate is classical HDN, which can be prevented. Hence, all neonates should receive one dose of vitamin K after birth as a prophylactic measure.

BIBLIOGRAPHY

1. Andrew M, Paes B, Milner R, et al. Development of the coagulation system in the full term infant. Blood. 1987;70: 165-72.
2. Andrew M, Paes B, Milner R, et al. Development of the human coagulation system in the healthy premature infant. Blood. 1988;72:1651-7.
3. Arasan DG. Approach to bleeding neonate. Indian J Pract Pediatr. 2010;12:401-11.
4. Homans A. Thrombocytopenia in the neonate. Pediatr Clin North Am. 1996;43:737-53.
5. Jadav D, Chandra J. Petechial rash in neonates: management algorithm. J Neonatol. 2008;22:19-27.
6. Kuhle S, Mitchell L, Massicotte P, et al. Hemostatic disorders of newborn. In: Taeusch HW, Ballard RA, Gleason EA (Eds). Avery's Diseases of the Newborn, 8th edition. Philadelphia, PA: Elsevier Saunders; 2003.
7. Pramanik AK. The bleeding neonate. In: Singh M (Ed). Medical Emergencies in Children, 3rd edition. New Delhi: Sagar Publications; 2000.
8. Roberts I, Murray NA. Neonatal thrombocytopenia: causes and management. Arch Dis Child Fetal Neonatal Ed. 2003;88:F359-64.
9. Roy AD. Bleeding neonate. In: Sharma JN (Ed).Manual of Care of Critical newborn, 2nd edition. New Delhi: Peepee Publishers; 2011.
10. Singh M. Bleeding Disorders: Care of the Newborn, 7th edition. New Delhi: Sagar Publication; 2010.

2.12 Hypoxic–Ischemic Encephalopathy and Intracranial Hemorrhage

Swathi Chacham, Rachna Pasi

HYPOXIC–ISCHEMIC ENCEPHALOPATHY

Introduction

Perinatal asphyxia is an important etiological factor for neonatal mortality. It accounts for nearly 20% of neonatal deaths in India, and all the asphyxia-related deaths (97.8%) occur in the first week of life of which most of them (70%) die in the first 24 hours (day 0).

Definitions

World Health Organization defined asphyxia as failure to initiate or sustain respiration after birth.

Moderate asphyxia: It is defined as slow gasping breathing or an Apgar score of 4–6 at 5 minutes of age.

Severe asphyxia: It is considered when there is no breathing or an Apgar score of 0–3 at 5 minutes of age. Essentially, it is a state of diminished gas exchange resulting in hypoxemia, hypercarbia, and fetal acidosis during intranatal period.

Fetal acidosis: It is defined as umbilical arterial blood pH < 7.0.

Hypoxic-ischemic encephalopathy (HIE): It refers to altered neurobehavioral response of the neonate along with manifestations of brainstem dysfunction with objective evidence of HI etiology.

Incidence

In India, the incidence of HIE varies from 2% to 16.2% in community-based studies with a significantly high case fatality rates (38.5–74%). Moreover, a large hospital-based study reported that 2.8% and 5.6% of all live births had moderate and severe asphyxia, respectively, with a lower case fatality rate (8.7%). The incidence is inversely proportional to gestational age (GA) and birth weight (BW). It is high in pregnancies complicated with diabetes, pregnancy-induced hypertension, and abruptio placentae.

Etiology

Asphyxia can result from either prenatal or natal insults in term newborns, which reduce gas exchange through the placenta resulting in impaired oxygenation and reduced elimination of CO_2 and hydrogen (H^+). Structural abnormalities of respiratory, cardiovascular, and central nervous system (CNS) can result in postpartum asphyxia. Broadly, asphyxia is multifactorial resulting from maternal, placental, fetal, and neonatal causes as shown in **Table 2.12.1**.

Pathogenesis

Transient hypoxemia may occur during normal labor due to uterine contractions, cord compression, and maternal dehydration. This results in limited O_2 reserve in the majority of the neonates after the normal labor. Hypoxia-ischemia results in varied physiologic and biochemical changes. Following transient asphyxia, heart rate (HR) initially increases and decreases later, while blood pressure (BP) and central venous pressure (CVP) increase. However, cardiac output (CO) remains unaltered. Subsequently, there is redistribution of CO, resulting in enhanced blood flow to the brain, heart, and adrenal glands (diving reflex). But this phenomenon does not occur when there is complete cessation of blood flow as in placental abruption, resulting in characteristic ischemic lesions in subcortical white matter and brainstem nuclei. When asphyxia is prolonged, cerebral autoregulation and CO_2 responsiveness are lost leading to impaired cerebral perfusion. This will be further handicapped by hypotension and decreased CO. As cerebral blood flow (CBF) is decreased, glucose production is impaired, which leads to anaerobic metabolism and cellular energy failure. This is coupled with enhanced glucose utilization by the brain, depleted glycogen stores, phosphocreatine, and adenosine triphosphate (ATP). Thus, prolonged asphyxia leads to diffuse injury involving both cortical and subcortical structures, with specific predilection to neuronal populations susceptible to HI injury.

Table 2.12.1: Etiological factors for perinatal asphyxia.

Maternal factors	Pregnancy-induced hypertension, essential hypertension, renal failure (acute or chronic), shock, hypotension, infection (including chorioamnionitis), bronchial asthma, congenital or acquired heart disease, diabetes, maternal vascular disease, and cocaine abuse
Placental factors	Abruptio placentae, placenta previa, infarction, fibrosis or hydrops fetalis, ruptured uterus
Umbilical cord factors	Entanglement, true knot, compression, prolapse, vasa previa
Fetal factors	Fetal anemia (fetomaternal hemorrhage), infection, cardiomyopathy, hydrops fetalis, cardiovascular insufficiency
Neonatal factors	PPHN, cyanotic congenital heart disease, cardiomyopathy, cardiogenic shock/septic shock, respiratory failure occurring from meconium aspiration syndrome, neonatal pneumonia, pneumothorax

(PPHN: persistent pulmonary hypertension of the newborn)

The pathognomonic feature of HIE is cellular dysfunction due to impaired oxidative phosphorylation and ATP production. As energy failure sets in, ion pump function is diminished causing intracellular accumulation of ions, such as Na^+, Cl^-, H_2O, and Ca^{2+}, and buildup of extracellular K^+ along with excitatory neurotransmitters, such as glutamate. This energy failure may be a result of both primary and secondary HI insults, and secondary energy failure sets in 6 to 24 hours after the triggering insult. Similarly, cell death can be both necrotic and apoptotic occurring either instantly or later.

Immediate neuronal death (necrosis): This is a result of ion pump failure and intracellular osmotic overload.

Delayed neuronal death (apoptosis): This is a manifestation of uninhibited enzyme and secondary mediator activation within the cell (e.g. proteases, lipases, and caspases), impairment of electron transport system in mitochondria, leukotrienes, free radicals, and nitric oxide production.

Reperfusion injury: Not only the ischemic insult causes neuronal dysfunction but also the reperfusion of ischemic tissue results in neuronal injury by releasing oxygen free radicals, such as hydroxyl, hydrogen peroxide, and superoxide, which can damage deoxyribonucleic acid, ribonucleic acid, lipids, proteins, and blood-brain barrier. Moreover, this may lead to the activation of inflammatory cascade with the release of tumor necrosis factor α and interleukin 1-β release. HIE can affect any major organ and lead to multisystem involvement as shown in **Table 2.12.2**.

Diagnosis

Clinical Features

History of maternal, placental, fetal morbidities can lead to asphyxia along with assessment of fetal wellbeing with

Table 2.12.2: Possible impacts of perinatal asphyxia.

CNS	Hypoxic-ischemic encephalopathy, intracranial hemorrhage, seizures, long-term neurological sequelae
Cardiac	Myocardial dysfunction, valvular dysfunction, rhythm abnormalities, congestive cardiac failure
Renal	Hematuria, acute tubular necrosis, renal vein thrombosis
Gastrointestinal	Necrotizing enterocolitis, hepatic dysfunction
Hematological	Thrombocytopenia, DIC/coagulation abnormalities
Pulmonary	Respiratory failure, apnea, meconium aspiration, surfactant depletion, pulmonary hypertension
Metabolic	Hypoglycemia, acidosis, hypocalcemia, hyponatremia (SIADH or renal involvement)

(CNS: central nervous system; DIC: disseminated intravascular coagulation; SIADH: syndrome of inappropriate antidiuretic hormone secretion)

the help of antenatal ultrasound, biophysical profile, and nonstress test. Fetal bradycardia (HR < 60/minutes), delivery details, and need for positive pressure ventilation for >1 minute or delayed first cry for >5 minutes and low Apgar score should be evaluated. Apgar score more than 6 at 5 minutes rules out perinatal asphyxia to a major extent.

Neurologic Signs

Hypoxic-ischemic encephalopathy is classified as mild, moderate, or severe, according to Levene's classification, (as shown in **Table 2.12.3**), and staging of 1, 2, and 3 is given by Sarnat and Sarnat. All the three categories of HIE—mild, moderate, and severe—have altered consciousness. Asphyxiated term neonates have characteristic differential hypotonia in the early stages of HIE. Upper limbs are more affected than lower limbs, and proximal musculature is more involved than the distal musculature. Thus, abnormal scarf sign is seen. Active tone assessment reveals poor flexor muscle tone during traction response. Fifty percent of the neonates with HIE manifest seizures usually within 24 hours after the HI insult. Subtle seizures are more frequent, followed by tonic or clonic. They occur in moderate or severe encephalopathy. They need to be distinguished from jitteriness or clonus, which are easily controlled by pressure application over the affected limb(s). As seizures are often subtle with electrographic changes, they need to be differentiated from seizure mimics. Thus, electroencephalogram (EEG) is an essential tool to confirm the seizure activity. Similarly, the features of raised intracranial pressure (ICP), due to extensive cortical necrosis, can also occur suggesting poor prognosis.

Differential Diagnosis

Maternal anesthesia, trauma, infection, central nervous system, or cardiac malformations.

Laboratory Evaluation

The evaluation of cardiovascular system, CNS, and renal injury is an essential part of the management of asphyxiated neonates as given in **(Table 2.12.4)**.

Table 2.12.3: Levene's classification of hypoxic-ischemic encephalopathy.

Feature	*Mild Grade I*	*Moderate Grade II*	*Severe Grade III*
Consciousness	Irritable	Lethargy	Comatose
Tone	Normal	Hypotonia	Flaccid
Seizures	No	Yes	Prolonged
Sucking	Weak suck	Weak suck/ Unable to suck	Unable to suck
Heart rate	Tachycardia	Bradycardia	Variable

Neuroimaging: As shown in **Table 2.12.4**, following neuroimaging modalities are recommended in evaluating neonates with asphyxia. In general, EEG, computed tomography (CT), and cranial ultrasound do not help a great deal in the acute management of the baby. Their utility is essentially for prognostication.

Cranial ultrasound: It is a simple, noninvasive, nonionizing bedside tool which demonstrates diminished gray-white matter differentiation and shrunk ventricles. Although not very useful in term neonates, it can demonstrate intraventricular hemorrhage (IVH) in preterm neonates associated with asphyxia.

Computed tomography: CT scan in term neonates with acute stage of HIE *shows* generalized low attenuation of brain parenchyma. It can also depict hemorrhage and cerebral edema and should be reserved if other modalities are not available as it poses the risk of ionizing radiation.

Magnetic resonance imaging (MRI) brain: Ideal investigation to delineate the degree of brain injury, although time consuming and poses practical problems with sedation in neonates. Moreover, it is a costly investigation to perform. However, MRI brain can reveal various neuropathologoical changes that occur in HIE as mentioned in **Table 2.12.5**.

Other newer neuroimaging modalities include diffusion-weighted imaging, proton magnetic resonance (MR) spectroscopy (*proton-MRS* or *H-MRS*), susceptibility-weighted imaging, MR angiography, or venography which aid in detecting vascular abnormalities associated with asphyxia.

Electroencephalogram

It can demonstrate seizures, differentiate seizures from seizure mimics and helps to assess the efficacy of antiepileptic drugs. Various types of EEG that are seen in asphyxia include burst suppression, discontinuous, low-voltage, or isoelectric patterns. These carry poor prognosis. Amplitude EEG (aEEG) can also be used as a bedside tool. EEG aids in monitoring newer therapies, such as cerebral hypothermia. However,

Table 2.12.4: Laboratory evaluation of asphyxia.

CNS	Serum CK-BB, S-100, NSE
CVS	CK-MB, Cardiac troponin I (ctni), cardiac troponin T (ctnt),
Renal	Blood urea nitrogen (BUN) and serum Cr, Fractional excretion of Na^+ (fena), Urine levels of β2-microglobulin
Brain imaging	Cranial ultrasound, CT, MRI brain, conventional T1- and T2-weighted MRI sequences, diffusion-weighted imaging (DWI), proton magnetic resonance spectroscopy (*proton-MRS* or *H-MRS*), Susceptibility-weighted imaging, magnetic resonance (MR) angiography or venography
EEG	EEG, integrated aEEG

aEEG may not be available in the majority of the centers in the developing countries, and EEG is cumbersome to do in sick neonates. Thus, they have predominant role in prognostication than in management.

Treatment

The management of HIE is multidimensional as enlisted in **Table 2.12.6**.

Transfer the baby to neonatal intensive care unit: Neonates with severe asphyxia (Apgar score <3 at 1 minute or requiring prolonged positive pressure ventilation for >5 minutes) need to be transferred to neonatal intensive care unit for observation and treatment.

Vital signs monitoring: Neonates with perinatal asphyxia need frequent monitoring of vitals including respiration, HR, BP, capillary refill time, temperature, and oxygen saturation, along with urine output monitoring. Also the blood gas monitoring helps to maintain adequate oxygenation.

Metabolic monitoring: Check blood sugar, hematocrit, calcium, and electrolytes—blood sugar monitoring (2, 6, 12, 24, 48, and 72 hours of age) for hypo or hyperglycemia. Maintain blood sugar above 60 mg/dL, but not exceeding 100 mg/dL. Hematocrit measurement to pick up anemia or polycythemia (once daily in the initial few days) and hematocrit should be maintained >40% in ventilated neonates. It is also necessary to treat polycythemia. Blood gas analysis to detect metabolic acidosis, hypoxia, hyperoxia, and respiratory failure. Hyperoxia, hypocarbia, and hyperglycemia are equally harmful to asphyxiated neonates and need to optimize these parameters in the initial 48–72 hours following asphyxia. Serum sodium, potassium, and calcium should be measured once daily. Hypocalcemia can reduce cardiac contractility and precipitate seizures. Calcium should be supplemented at 4 mL/kg/day of 10% calcium gluconate for 1–2 days either as a continuous infusion or as 1:1 diluted boluses, slowly under cardiac monitoring.

Optimum oxygenation and ventilation: Neonates with respiratory failure require supplemental oxygen and assisted ventilation. Oxygenation in spontaneously breathing neonate can be achieved with the oxygen hood or nasal prongs. Apnea, inadequate spontaneous respirations, or hypoxia or hypercarbia necessitate assisted ventilation. pH should be maintained above 7.30. The target PaO_2 is 80–100 Torr in term neonates and 60–80 Torr in preterm infants. Both hypoxia and hyperoxia should be avoided using pulse oximeter. Hyperoxia reduces CBF and causes free radical injury. The target $PaCO_2$ value is 40–45 Torr. As CO_2 is a potent cerebral vasodilator, hypercapnia leads to "steal phenomenon", and hypocapnia causes further cerebral hypoperfusion.

Volume expanders: Volume expansion using normal saline (or Ringer lactate), 10 mL/kg over 5–10 minutes, is recommended when there is of prolonged capillary refill time (>3 seconds) and metabolic acidosis and can be repeated as per the need. It is important to note that decreased vascular tone in asphyxia may lead to reduced preload and relative hypovolemia. Hence, maintaining adequate perfusion is vital in asphyxiated neonates.

Thermoregulation: Avoid hyperthermia and passive cooling by switching the warmer off can be used to provide hypothermia.

Maintain adequate perfusion: Ensuring normal perfusion is of critical importance in management. The markers of normal perfusion are normal BP, capillary refill time of less than 3 seconds, normal urine output, and absence of metabolic acidosis.

Intravenous fluids: Avoid both hypovolemia and hypervolemia as they are at risk of developing syndrome of inappropriate antidiuretic hormone secretion. Fluid restriction to two thirds of the maintenance fluid is advised in the presence of renal failure and is shown to reduce cerebral edema.

Vasopressors: Dopamine and dobutamine are the drugs of choice and can be started with 3–5 μg/kg/minute and need to be increased as per the clinical requirement, the maximum dose being 20 μg/kg/minute.

Treatment of Seizures

Phenobarbitone is the drug of choice for seizures given as a loading dose of 20 mg/kg, intravenously, over 20 minutes. If seizures persist, additional doses of 5–10 mg/kg can be given; if there is no response, phenytoin sodium, dose of 15–20 mg/kg intravenously over 20 minute; and if available, fosphenytoin can be used. Maintenance therapy is started 12–24 hours later

Table 2.12.5: Neuropathology seen in asphyxia.

- Selective neuronal necrosis
- Periventricular white matter injury
- Bilateral parasagittal cortical and subcortical white matter injury
- Focal or multifocal cortical necrosis/cystic encephalomalacia/ulegyria
- Diffuse cerebral cortical necrosis
- Injury of brainstem, thalamus, and basal ganglia

Table 2.12.6: Management of neonatal asphyxia.

- Transfer to neonatal intensive care unit
- *Temperature monitoring*: therapeutic hypothermia (33–34°C)
- Blood sugar, hematocrit and acid–base balance and metabolic monitoring
- *Fluid supplementation:* 2/3rd restriction
- Management of shock/hypotension, vasopressors
- Management of seizures
- Oxygenation and ventilation

in a dose of 3–5 mg/kg/day, BD for phenobarbitone and 4–8 mg/kg, every eighth hourly for phenytoin. Although seizures are often refractory in HIE, either of these anticonvulsants are effective in most of the cases. Infrequent, transient, mild seizures not compromising cardiopulmonary status need no treatment. For uncontrolled seizures, lorazepam can be given at 0.05–0.1 mg/kg/dose intravenously. Newer anticonvulsants, such as levetiracetam, can be used intravenously which is safe in neonates. However, neonates should be investigated for other metabolic causes, such as hypocalcemia, hypomagnesemia, hypoglycemia, hyponatremia, hypernatremia, and polycythemia, which may also coexist.

Newer Modalities of Therapy

Many neuroprotective treatment modalities, including drugs and therapeutic hypothermia, have been projected in experimental trials including animals and humans. However, their utility is high in the early phase of HI injury and in moderate, severe HIE. Western literature reports efficacy and safety of therapeutic hypothermia comprising total body cooling and selective head cooling up to 33°–34°C. It is useful in neonates of ≥36-week gestation and more than or equal to 2,000-g BW. It needs to be initiated within 6 hours of life and continued till 72 hours of life, guided by EEG. It acts by reducing neuronal metabolism and shown to improve neurodevelopmental outcome and has become standard of care in developed nations. Few of the centers in India also are implementing this therapeutic modality with varying success. However, it needs to be used as per standard guidelines to avoid serious complications.

Outcome and Prevention

Neurodevelopmental sequelae correspond closely with the staging or severity of HIE. Moreover, the neonate's diagnosis is based on its worst HIE grade during the course of management. It has been noted that HIE grade I has no long-term impairments, and 20% of HIE grade II have long-term neurological morbidities. On the other hand, 50–70% HIE grade III neonates may die or have severe long-term motor, cognitive, and sensory impairments. Optimum antenatal, intrapartum, and postnatal monitoring can aid in prevention of HIE.

INTRACRANIAL HEMORRHAGE

Introduction

Intracranial hemorrhage (ICH) is an important cause for morbidity and mortality in neonates. As neonatal brain is at risk of potential damage by maternal, fetal, and neonatal factors, ICH can have devastating effect on the developing brain with its long-term neurological sequelae. ICH can manifest either as intraparenchymal bleed or extraparenchymal bleed. It can be classified as subdural, epidural, subarachnoid, intraventricular, and intraparenchymal hemorrhage (IPH), as shown in **Table 2.12.7**. They have varying etiopathology, clinical manifestations, and prognosis as per the severity and GA with an overlap among the various types.

Table 2.12.7: Classification of intracranial hemorrhage and their determinants in neonates.

Type of hemorrhage	*Location*	*Predisposing factors*	*Management*	*Outcome*
SDH	(Intracranial, extraparenchymal) Amidst dura and arachnoid	Bleeding disorders, clotting disorders, instrumental delivery, difficult labor	Prompt correction of anemia, hypovolemia and hypotension, seizures, surgical intervention for large SDH	Good for small SDH
SAH	Underneath the arachnoid mater	Bleeding disorders, clotting disorders, instrumental delivery, difficult labor	Prompt correction of anemia, hypovolemia and hypotension, seizures, surgical intervention for large SDH	Good for small SAH
GMH/IVH	Germinal matrix in the caudothalamic groove	Prematurity, RDS, PDA, shock, acidosis, reperfusion injury, rapid administration of hyperosmolar fluids, pneumothorax, ET suctioning, frequent intubations, hypo/hypercapnia	Prompt correction of anemia, hypovolemia and hypotension, seizures, follow-up for hydrocephalus	Grades I and II have good prognosis and Grades III and IV: likely to develop posthemorrhagic hydrocephalus
IPH	Cerebral hemorrhage and cerebellar hemorrhage	Arteriovenous malformation, aneurysm, coagulation disorders: hemophilia, thrombocytopenia, reperfusion injury in HIE	Prompt correction of anemia, hypovolemia and hypotension, seizures	Focal cerebellar hemorrhage: good prognosis

(ET: endotracheal intubation; GMH/IVH: germinal matrix hemorrhage/intraventricular hemorrhage; HIE: hypoxic–ischemic encephalopathy; IPH: intraparenchymal hemorrhage; PDA: patent ductus arteriosus; RSD: respiratory distress syndrome; SAH: subarachnoid hemorrhage; SDH: subdural hemorrhage)

Incidence

The incidence ranges from 2% to >30% in neonates and instrumental deliveries carry higher risk over cesarean section.

Subdural Hemorrhage and Epidural Hemorrhage

Etiopathology

The basic pathology in subdural hemorrhage (SDH) is bleeding into the subdural space due to rupture of the draining veins and sinuses in it. This results in blood accumulation below the dura and above subarachnoid villi. The process of delivery and tractional forces on head during labor can precipitate SDH by tearing off dural sinuses in falx cerebri or the tentorium cerebelli, and hence, these are the common sites of small SDH. Similarly, posterior fossa SDH can occur due to ripping of the transverse sinus, inferior sagittal sinus, straight sinus, or vein of Galen. A severe form of SDH can result from rupture of the occipital sinus during breech presentation due to occipital osteodiastasis.

Supratentorial space SDH is a manifestation of tearing off the superficial bridging veins in the cerebral cortex. Major predisposing factors for SDH comprise instrumented delivery, bleeding/clotting disorders, fetal macrocephaly, unfavorable pelvis, abnormal presentations, and prolonged or precipitous delivery or birth injury.

The incidence is higher in vaginal deliveries when compared to cesarean deliveries with 2.9/10,000 spontaneous deliveries in contrast to 8–9.8/10,000 in vacuum and forceps deliveries, respectively. The incidence is higher 21.3/10,000 when both vacuum and forceps are used. Recent studies report a higher prevalence of asymptomatic, small SDH (up to 45%).

Clinical Manifestations

A major proportion of SDH can be small, asymptomatic, and can resolve without sequelae. Depending on the location and severity of injury, it can manifest soon after birth or within 24–48 hours of life with features of ICP and compression of the underlying brain parenchyma. Frequent clinical features consist of altered sensorium, apnea, irregular respirations, opisthotonus posture, and seizures. Bulging of fontanel and sutural separation can also be there. Hemodynamic instability, shock, and anemia can occur due to large hemorrhage. It can often accompany subarachnoid hemorrhage (SAH), and in long run, SDH can lead to chronic subdural effusion and hydrocephalus.

Diagnosis

Subdural hemorrhage can be diagnosed based on history, clinical manifestations, and confirmed by neuroimaging. While CT and MRI are usual definitive modalities that can demonstrate SDH, ultrasound head is readily available, noninvasive, although less specific. MRI is superior and sensitive to delineate the extent of SDH. CT head will aid in both early diagnosis and in follow-up for the evolution of hydrocephalus or subdural effusion and requires less time to perform the procedure. Along with neuroimaging, other investigations necessary to diagnose bleeding/clotting disorder and sepsis are required.

Management and Outcome

The mainstay of treatment is supportive and symptomatic. Large SDH mandate immediate stabilization with fluids, blood, inotropes, and ventilatory support as per the requirement. In all the neonates with suspected SDH, immediate CT head should be performed followed by the opinion of neurosurgery team. The neonate needs close follow-up for subsequent complications, such as chronic subdural effusion and hydrocephalus. Usual prognosis in small SDH is good when there is no underlying neuronal damage and requirement for surgical intervention.

Epidural Hemorrhage

Epidural hemorrhage (EH) is more common in infants and children than neonates and is often associated with birth injury as in instrumented delivery. It has been described that 50% of them are accompanied by a skull fracture or large cephalohematoma requiring drainage of the hemorrhage, and isolated EH carries good prognosis.

Subarachnoid Hemorrhage

Etiopathology

Subarachnoid hemorrhage manifests frequently in neonatal period. It has been described as primary SAH and SAH secondary to IVH. Primary SAH is often unnoticed as it is clinically asymptomatic. As with SDH, usual process of normal labor can result in a small SAH due to the tearing of veins of subarachnoid villi. The reported prevalence of SAH is 1.3/10,000 spontaneous vaginal deliveries and instrumental deliveries, such as vacuum or forceps, have higher prevalence rate.

Subarachnoid hemorrhage can also occur due to the spreading of germinal matrix hemorrhage (GMH)//IVH into subarachnoid space in premature neonates. Similarly, SAH can develop as a progression of SDH, IPH, or rarely in term neonates manifest as subpial hemorrhage due to birth injury.

Clinical Features

Similar to SDH, SAH predominantly manifests with features of acute volume depletion due to blood loss and raised ICH.

Frequent neurological features include altered mental status, irritability, and seizures.

Diagnosis

Any neonate presenting with seizures, altered mental status, and focal neurologic deficits necessitates evaluation for SAH by neuroimaging with MRI brain or CT head for definitive diagnosis. MRI is preferred over CT brain as it poses no risk of radiation and delineates the depth of hemorrhage and underlying pathology accurately. EEG is necessary to diagnose subtle seizures.

Management and Outcome

As with SDH, the first line of management is supportive and symptomatic including management of raised ICP, volume depletion, anemia, and seizures. Prognosis depends on extent and location of the hemorrhage. The outcome is good for small SAH, although large SAH can have long-term neurological morbidities, especially when coupled with perinatal asphyxia. Hence, it is vital to have periodic clinical and radiological follow-up in neonates with large SAH.

Intraventricular Hemorrhage

Etiopathology

Most frequently manifesting ICH in preterm neonates is GMH/IVH. Although less common in term neonates, it leads to significant long-term neurological morbidity. The incidence is 25–30% in very-low-BW (VLBW) neonates and <32 weeks' GA. In the preterm newborn, GMH/IVH arises from the delicate, vulnerable involuting vessels in caudothalamic groove, which occupy the subependymal germinal matrix. Germinal matrix is situated near the ventricles and produces neurons and glial cells in growing fetus. The blood vessels of this germinal matrix are deficient in basement membrane, which predisposes them for rupture in the face of abnormal CBF autoregulation. The ependymal germinal matrix is extremely vascularized receiving its blood supply from anterior choroidal vessels, anterior, and the middle cerebral arteries. And hence, hemorrhage in this location can be localized to the germinal matrix or may spread into the lateral ventricles, and IVH can become unilateral or bilateral. These risk factors are enlisted in **Table 2.12.8**.

The predisposing factors for GMH/IVH include the factors occurring within the blood vessels (more frequent and preventable) and factors external to the blood vessels. Chorioamnionitis increases risk of IVH by 1.6-folds. Low BW, prematurity, male sex, and respiratory distress syndrome are important risk factors. In contrast, prenatal steroids reduce the incidence of IVH by reducing the risk of respiratory distress syndrome, duration of ventilation, and balancing the vasodilatory effect of hypercarbia. Rapid alterations in CBF and cerebral venous pressure due to reperfusion following ischemia predispose to GMH/IVH. Moreover, neonates with patent ductus arteriosus, asynchrony on ventilator, high positive end expiratory pressure in ventilator setting, tracheal suctioning, pneumothorax, anemia, and hypoglycemia can predispose to IVH.

Table 2.12.8: Causes of germinal matrix hemorrhage/intraventricular hemorrhage in premature neonates.

Prenatal factors	Failure to administer antenatal steroids, chorioamnionitis, inflammation of amniotic sac, and abruption
Intrapartum factors	Prolonged labor, obstructed labor, instrumental delivery
Postnatal factors	Fast infusion of colloids, hyperosmolar solutions (sodium bicarbonate), normal saline in preterm, hypertension, transportation, genetic factors, acidosis, respiratory distress with hypo or hypercapnia
Systemic factors	Bleeding, clotting disorders

As with other types of ICH, prolonged labor, instrumental delivery leads to higher incidence of GMH/IVH in premature neonates. Preterm neonates have pressure-passive circulation, which plays a key role in the development of IVH. Moreover, platelet and clotting factor disorders can predispose to IVH as with other forms of ICH. Grading of IVH is given by Papile and Volpe. As per severity, Grade 1 is small, Grade 2 is moderate, and Grade 3 is severe.

Intraventricular hemorrhage is less frequent in term neonates as germinal matrix involutes beyond 34 weeks of GA (complete involution by 36 weeks GA), decreasing risk of GMH. Primary IVH in term neonates arises from choroid plexus, hemorrhagic thalamic infarction, venous sinus thrombosis **(Fig. 2.12.1)**, or from subependymal germinal matrix remnants. It is predominantly due to traumatic delivery, perinatal asphyxia.

Clinical Presentation

In the preterm newborn, GMH/IVH can remain clinically silent and noted by periodic ultrasound head. Most of them manifest by 72 hours of life necessitating the performance of head ultrasound in the first week of life (3–4 days) in neonates <32 weeks GA. Severe IVH can manifest with bulging fontanel, altered consciousness, decreased spontaneous activity and tone, along with subtle seizures, ocular movements, and features of blood loss. Sudden pallor in an otherwise normal preterm neonate should prompt the diagnosis of IVH. It can be a catastrophic presentation with features of shock, neurologic deterioration, and tonic seizures. However, in term neonates, IVH can manifest with irritability, seizures, apnea, vomiting, and bulging fontanel, which can be associated with ventriculomegaly.

Diagnosis

The mainstay of diagnosis of GMH/IVH is ultrasound head in the premature neonates. Neonates <32 weeks' GA and VLBW newborns need ultrasound head performed by 1, 4, and 8 weeks. Neonates >32 weeks with predisposing factors also need screening. It needs to be done early by 24 hours in very sick neonates.

Management and Outcome

The management is predominantly supportive and symptomatic along with management of complications. Periventricular hemorrhagic infarction (PVHI) and posthemorrhagic ventricular dilation (PVD) are the two principal complications of GMH/IVH. Larger and severe IVH have higher predisposition to these complications. PVHI was thought to be an expansion of severe IVH and hence referred to as grade IV IVH. However, some authors denote PVHI as separate lesion from IVH. Asphyxia, acidosis, prematurity, patent ductus arteriosus, need for assisted ventilation, pulmonary hemorrhage, and pneumothorax and need for vasopressors are predisposing factors for PVHI. Another complication following IVH is posthemorrhagic hydrocephalus/progressive PVD, which can manifest weeks after the occurrence of GMH/IVH. The principal mechanism for PVD includes reduced cerebrospinal fluid resorption or aqueductal obstruction. About 50–75% of IVH survivors manifest with cognitive disturbances, cerebral palsy (CP), or hydrocephalus.

Prevention

Prenatal steroid are used in preterm labor of less than 34 weeks gestation and can prevent IVH along with HMD. Also avoiding other risk factors for IVH can prevent it to some extent.

Intraparenchymal Hemorrhage

Etiopathology

Cerebellar hemorrhage is the commonest form of IPH, and primary cerebral hemorrhage is rare and occurs due to tearing of arteriovenous malformation, aneurysm, or due to bleeding or coagulation disorder. It often occurs due to the expansion of GMH/IVH, SAH, SDH, reperfusion injury in HIE, hemorrhagic venous infarction, or venous sinus thrombosis **(Figs. 2.12.2 to 2.12.4)**. It can be a complication of extracorporeal membrane oxygenation therapy. Cerebellar hemorrhage is frequently seen in preterm neonates, which may go unnoticed by ultrasound, and MRI is the best imaging modality to diagnose it.

Clinical Presentation

The manifestations are similar to other ICH. Small IPH can be silent, and large hemorrhage can have seizures, altered sensorium, and features of blood loss.

Diagnosis

Although MRI is the diagnostic modality of choice, ultrasound head is a useful bedside tool. Moreover, CT is useful due to easy availability, and MR angiography/venography can diagnose underlying vascular abnormalities, venous sinus thrombosis, or arterial emboli.

Management and Outcome

As with other ICH, immediate management is symptomatic and supportive. Large hemorrhage mandate neurosurgical

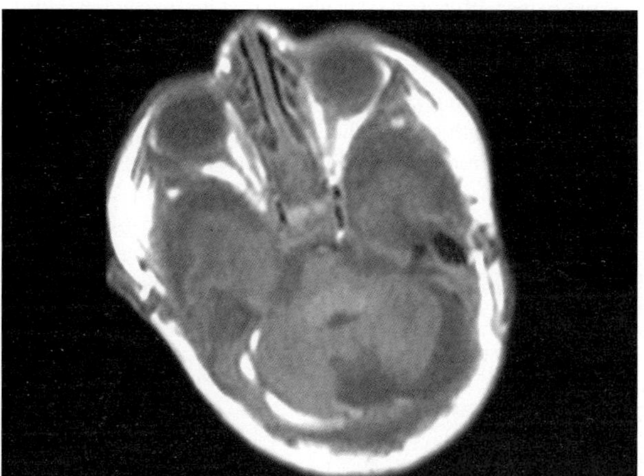

Fig. 2.12.1: MRI image axial T1W along the posterior fossa, showing distended right transverse sinus with hyperintense luminal signal, suggestive of subacute thrombus: right transverse sinus thrombosis. (MRI: magnetic resonance imaging; T1W: T1-weighted)

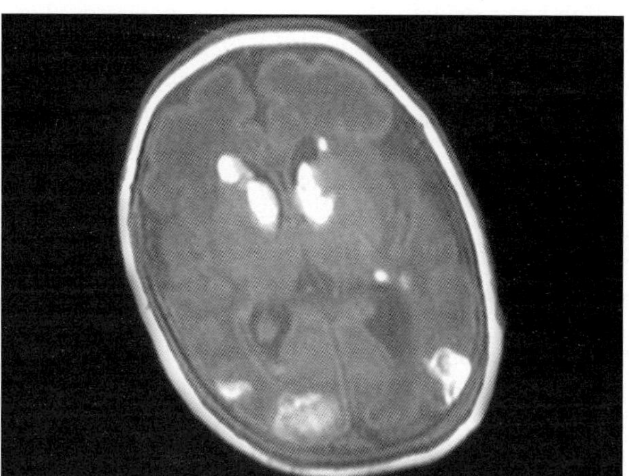

Fig. 2.12.2: MRI axial T1W image along the body of lateral ventricle, demonstrating bilateral intraventricular hemorrhage and parenchymal hemorrhages in bilateral (B/L) temporal, right occipital, and in the deep white matter associated with subacute hemorrhagic foci in (B/L) basal ganglia, thalamus, and cerebral hemispheres (abnormal T1 hyperintensities) mildly increased enhancement along the basal cisterns. (MRI: magnetic resonance imaging; T1W: T1-weighted)

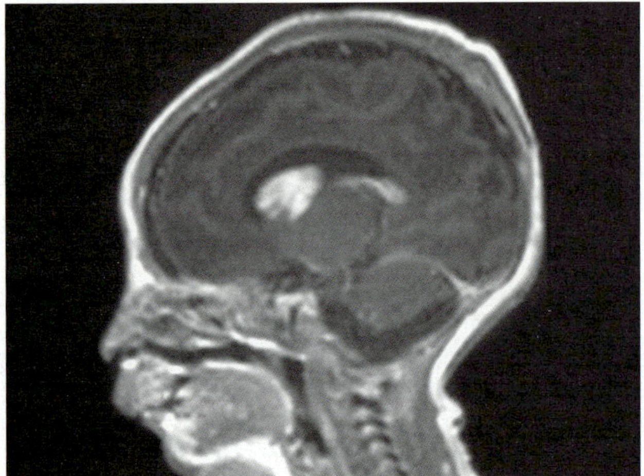

Fig. 2.12.3: MRI sagittal view revealing intraventricular hemorrhage. (MRI: Magnetic resonance imaging)

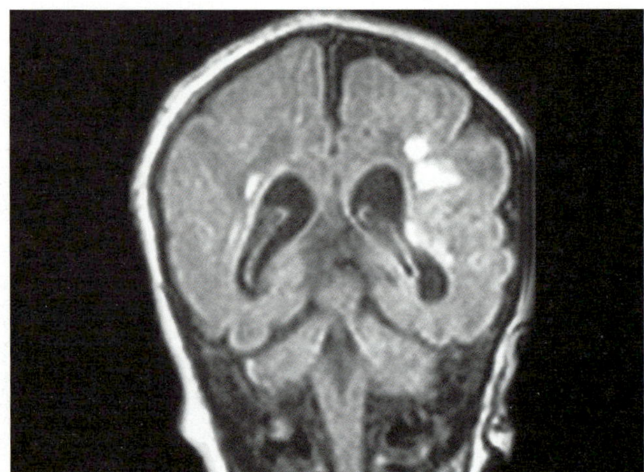

Fig. 2.12.4: MRI coronal view depicting intraparenchymal hemorrhages. (MRI: magnetic resonance imaging)

involvement. Moreover, the treatment of predisposing factors is equally essential. Large IPH can lead to hydrocephalus and long-term neuromorbidity. Serial head circumference monitoring coupled with neuroimaging aids in early detection of complications. The outcome is based upon the size and the site of IPH, along with GA. Usually, small hemorrhages have no long-term neuromorbidity, while larger ones can lead to epilepsy, CP, and cognitive disturbances.

Periventricular Leukomalacia/ White Matter Injury

Periventricular leukomalacia (PVL) is a neuropathological finding seen principally in premature neonates due to hypoxia, ischemia, and inherent susceptibility of white matter of cerebral cortex in preterm neonates enhanced by inflammation or infection. This leads to significant motor, sensory, and cognitive disturbances in childhood. MRI is the diagnostic modality of choice to depict PVL.

KEY MESSAGES

- Perinatal asphyxia is preventable with adequate prenatal, intranatal, and postnatal monitoring.
- It is an important etiological factor for long-term motor, cognitive, and sensory impairment.
- Therapeutic hypothermia is a novel, promising modality to be implemented in the developing countries with stringent protocols, after cost-benefit analysis.
- Intracranial hemorrhage is more frequent in instrumental deliveries in contrast to cesarean deliveries.
- Grades III and IV IVHs have significant long-term neurological sequelae.
- Prenatal steroids have proven role in reducing the incidence of IVH by decreasing the incidence and severity of hyaline membrane disease.

BIBLIOGRAPHY

1. Aggarwal R, Deorari A, Paul VK. Post-Resuscitation Management of Asphyxiated Neonates. New Delhi: WHO Collaboration Centre/All India Institute of Medical Sciences; 2007.
2. Bruschettini M, Romantsik O, Zappettini S, et al. Heparin for the prevention of intraventricular haemorrhage in preterm infants. Cochrane Database Syst Rev.2016;(5):CD011718.
3. Chacham S, Nagasravani J, Reddy UN. Acute renal failure in neonates with perinatal asphyxia and its correlation with HIE staging: a prospective case control study. J Neurol Neurobiol. 2016;2(2).
4. Hansen AR, Soul JS. Perinatal asphyxia and hypoxic-ischemic encephalopathy. In: Cloherty and Stark's Manual of Neonatal Care, 8th edition. Philadelphia: Wolters Kluwer; 2017. pp. 761-89, 790-811.
5. Levene MI. The asphyxiated newborn infant. In: Levene MI, Lilford RJ (Eds). Fetal and Neonatal Neurology and Neurosurgary. Edinburgh: Churchil Livingstone; 1995. pp. 405-26.
6. Sankar MJ, Neogi SB, Sharma J, et al. State of newborn health in India. J Perinatol. 2016;36:S3-8.
7. Shah NA, Wusthoff CJ. Intracranial hemorrhage in the neonate. Neonatal Netw. 2016;35(2):67-72.
8. Volpe JJ. Intracranial hemorrhage: subdural, primary subarachnoid, cerebellar, intraventricular (term infant), and miscellaneous. In: Neurology of the Newborn, 5th edition. Philadelphia, PA: Saunders Elsevier; 2008. pp. 483-516.
9. Zulfiqar ST, Bhutta A, Ramji S, et al. Global application of therapeutic hypothermia to treat perinatal asphyxial encephalopathy. Int Health. 2010;2(2):79-81.

2.13 Necrotizing Enterocolitis

Ruchi Rai

INTRODUCTION

Necrotizing enterocolitis (NEC) is a disease condition, which is characterized by acute bowel inflammation ultimately, leading to necrosis. It primarily affects the preterm babies, although it can also be less commonly seen in term neonates. It is one of the commonest gastrointestinal emergencies seen in neonates. Approximately 7–10% of preterm babies born with a birth weight less than 1,500 g develop NEC. The incidence varies inversely with the birth weight and the gestation; so, the smallest and the most premature babies are at highest risk. As more and more preterm babies are surviving due to advances in neonatal care, the incidence of NEC is also increasing.

PATHOGENESIS

The pathogenesis of NEC is complex and multifactorial. All factors ultimately lead to oxidative stress, inflammation, and bowel necrosis. The etiology of the disease is not very clear, but the following factors seem to be involved and play a role in pathogenesis, although none have been supported by definite evidence.

- *Genetic predisposition.*
- *Intestinal immaturity:* In preterm babies, the gastrointestinal system is immature in terms of motility, digestion, absorption, immune defenses, barrier functions, and circulatory regulation as well as microvascular tone. This makes the gut of preemies vulnerable to ischemia and necrosis.
- *Prematurity:* The most strongly associated factor is prematurity. The age of onset of NEC is inversely proportional to the weight and gestation of the baby at birth. So, the term babies have onset of symptoms much earlier than the preterm babies.
- *Enteral feeding:* Almost universally, all the babies who develop NEC have been fed. It is hypothesized that osmolar stress due to feeds may act as a potential stress. The rapid advancement of feeds also may lead to abnormal vascular regulation of the gut. The activation of gut hormones may play a role. Feeding with human milk seems to have a protective role for NEC, whereas feeding with bovine milk increases the risk of NEC.
- *Bowel ischemia:* Blood flow in splanchnic circulation is compromised in situations of stress in newborns to maintain blood flow to the vital organs, such as brain and heart. As a result, bowel ischemia and tissue necrosis ensue.
- *Bacterial colonization and proinflammatory responses:* Though none of the bacterial or viral species have been specifically incriminated in the pathogenesis, the gut microflora definitely plays an important role. They are likely to cross the compromised gut barrier and release endotoxins and cytokines, leading to inflammation. Inflammatory mediators, such as platelet-activating factor, lipopolysaccharides, and tumor necrosis factor-, have been suspected to play a significant role.
- *Risk factors:* Many risk factors such as perinatal asphyxia, sepsis, polycythemia, umbilical catheterization, rapid increase in feeds, shock, and administration of indomethacin have been associated with the development of NEC.

CLINICAL PRESENTATION

Like most other diseases in neonates, NEC does not have specific signs and symptoms. A close observation for early signs and symptoms is crucial to suspect the disease. Premature infants develop NEC around the second week of life, whereas the term babies manifest earlier. A baby with NEC may present with the following signs:

- *Systemic:* Lethargy, temperature instability, apnea, shock, irritability, and respiratory distress.
- *Abdominal:* Distention, gastric residuals, vomiting, blood in stools, abdominal wall erythema, and bilious aspirates. **Figure 2.13.1** shows a neonate with NEC having abdominal distention.

Modified Bell staging has been used for diagnosing and staging the disease **(Table 2.13.1)**.

INVESTIGATIONS

A high level of suspicion with a clinically high-risk setting is the mainstay for diagnosing NEC. But certain supportive laboratory investigations may be of help.

Blood investigations: Clinical biomarkers have been unsuccessful in predicting as well as diagnosing NEC. The typical triad of persistent acidosis, thrombocytopenia, and refractory hyponatremia is the characteristic of babies with NEC.

Stool: It may sometimes show occult blood, but this is not routinely done.

Radiology: X-ray of the abdomen may show features of ileus, such as dilated bowel loops **(Fig. 2.13.2)**. There may be bowel wall edema, pneumatosis intestinalis (gas in bowel wall) **(Fig. 2.13.3)**, presence of hepatobiliary gas, or if the disease has advanced to intestinal perforation, there is pneumoperitoneum **(Fig. 2.13.4)**. Pneumatosis intestinalis or portal venous gas are considered diagnostic of NEC but is seen in only some babies.

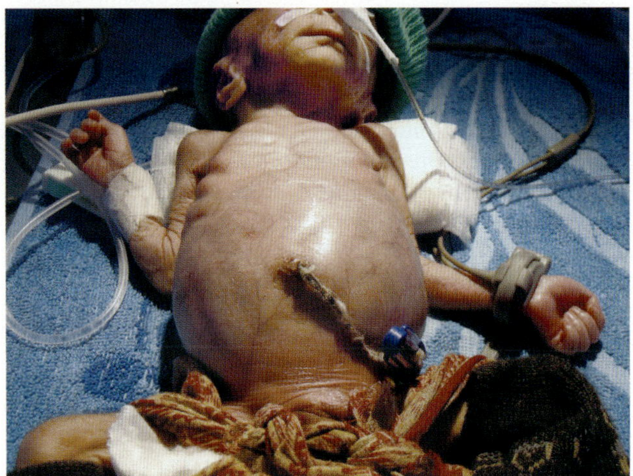

Fig. 2.13.1: NEC with abdominal distention. (NEC: Necrotizing enterocolitis)

Ultrasound abdomen is a good tool to diagnose bowel necrosis. It has the benefit that it does not expose the baby to harmful radiations due to repeated X-rays, and it is easily available at the bedside. Ultrasound can detect pneumatosis intestinalis and portal venous gas earlier than X-ray. Color Doppler is very sensitive in detecting bowel necrosis.

MANAGEMENT

No specific treatment approach is well defined.

Supportive: Supportive care during the disease can make significant difference in the morbidity and mortality, and it remains the mainstay of the disease, while the disease is evolving. This includes maintenance of temperature, circulation, fluid and electrolyte balance, acid-base status, treatment of anemia, and thrombocytopenia along with close monitoring of the vitals.

Nutrition: The baby should be kept nil per oral and should be started on parenteral nutrition if possible, especially in babies with stages II and III. This will take care of the nutrition till the baby can be fed enterally.

Decompression of the bowel: Bowel must be given rest, an orogastric tube should be kept in situ for regular decompression of the bowel, and abdominal girth should be monitored.

Antimicrobials: As sepsis is one of the hypothesized factors leading to NEC, the babies must be started on broad-spectrum antibiotics after a blood culture sample has been withdrawn.

Table 2.13.1: Modified Bell staging for NEC.

Stage		***Systemic signs***	***Intestinal signs***	***Radiological signs***	***Treatment***
I Suspected NEC	A	Temperature instability, apnea, lethargy, bradycardia	Increased pre-feed residue, mild abdominal distention, emesis, stool positive for blood	Normal or mild dilation of intestinal loops	NPO antibiotics × 3 days
	B	Same as I A	Same as I A + bleeding per rectum	Same as I A	Same as I A
II Definite NEC	A Mildly ill	Same as above	Same as above + absent bowel sounds, abdominal tenderness	Ileus, pneumatosis intestinalis	NPO, antibiotics × 7–10 days
	B Moderately ill	Same as above + acidosis, thrombocytopenia	Same as above + definite abdominal tenderness, ascites, abdominal cellulitis, or right lower quadrant mass	Same as above + portal venous gas, ascites	NPO, antibiotics × 14 days
III Advanced NEC	A Severely ill, bowel intact	Same as above + hypotension, bradycardia, apnea needing ventilatory support, acidosis, DIC, neutropenia	Same as above	Same as above + definite ascites	• NPO, antibiotics × 14 days • Inotropes, ventilator support, fluid resuscitation, paracentesis
	B Severely ill, bowel perforated	Same as III A	Same as III A	Same as III A + pneumoperitoneum	Same as III A + surgery

(DIC: disseminated intravascular coagulation; NEC: necrotizing enterocolitis; NPO: nil per oral)

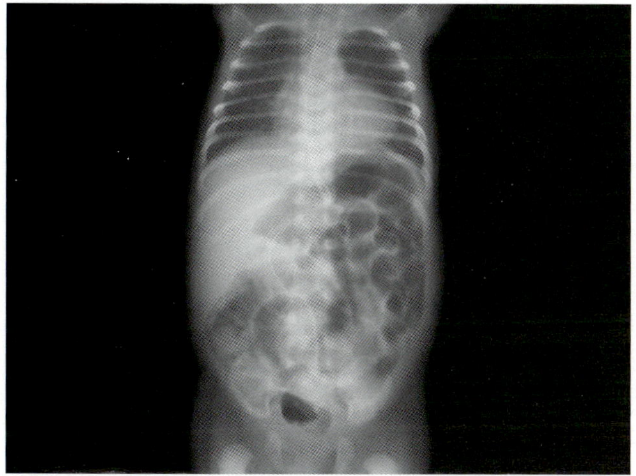

Fig. 2.13.2: X ray of the abdomen showing dilated bowel loops (Bell stage I).

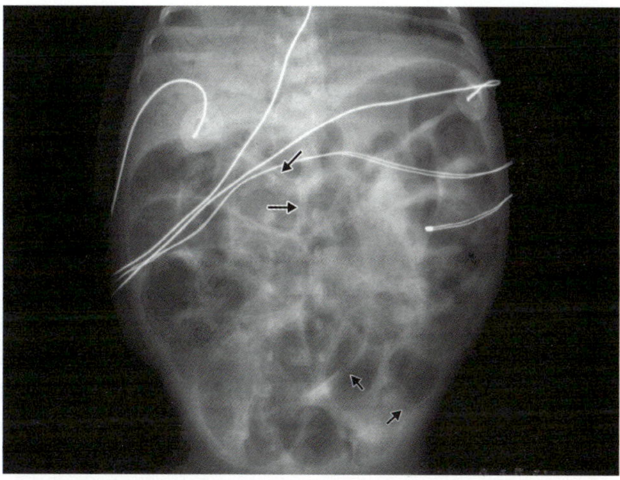

Fig. 2.13.3: Bell stage II showing pneumatosis intestinalis (arrows).

Clindamycin or metronidazole should be added for anaerobic coverage.

Surgical intervention: This may be needed in 30–50% of the babies. It may be in the form of open laparotomy or insertion of a peritoneal drain. The choice and the timing of the surgical intervention remain controversial. Many recent studies have shown no definite difference in the outcomes in babies who had undergone laparotomy compared to those in whom a drain was inserted.

PREVENTION

All interventions, which may prevent or reduce the risk of development of NEC, must be followed. Prevention is the most effective method to reduce NEC.

- *Feeding with human milk:* Human milk has immune-protective and anti-inflammatory factors, such as immunoglobulins, lactoferrin, lysozyme, etc.
- *Infection control practices:* It should be strictly adhered to in the neonatal intensive care unit, to prevent any hospital-acquired infection. Prolonged empirical use of antibiotics should also be strongly discouraged.
- *Feeding:* It should be gradually increased.
- *Pre/probiotics:* Many studies showing varying results have been conducted to assess the protective role of pre/probiotics in preterm babies for NEC. Some studies have found probiotics to be protective; in these studies, enteral probiotics supplementation significantly reduced the incidence of severe NEC (stage II or more). Probiotics preparations containing either lactobacillus alone or in combination with *Bifidobacterium* were found to be effective.
- *Antenatal steroids:* Administration of prenatal steroids to the pregnant mothers has been found to have a protective role for the development of NEC in preterm babies by enhancing the gut maturity.

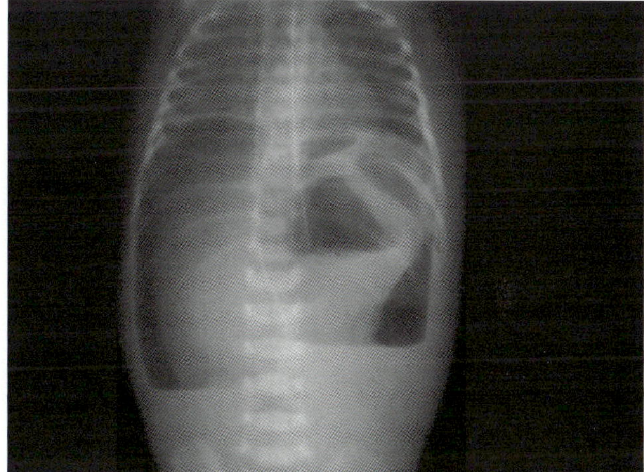

Fig. 2.13.4: Bell stage III showing pneumoperitoneum.

OUTCOME

Despite the advancement in neonatal care and diagnostic modalities, etiology of NEC is still poorly understood; specific treatment strategies are lacking, and the morbidity and mortality remain high. The mortality in babies developing NEC may be around 30%. The survivors have a high risk of developing dreaded complications, such as short bowel syndrome, intestinal strictures, and partial bowel obstruction. The neurodevelopmental outcomes in the survivors of NEC are also worse than their matched controls.

BIBLIOGRAPHY

1. AlFaleh K, Anabrees J. Probiotics for prevention of necrotizing enterocolitis in preterm infants. Cochrane Database Syst Rev. 2014;(4):CD005496.
2. Caplan MS. Neonatal necrotising enterocolitis: clinical observation, pathophysiology and prevention. In: Martin RJ, Fanaroff AA, Walsh CM (Eds). Neonatal-Perinatal Medicine: Diseases of Fetus and Infant, 9th edition. Missouri: Elsevier Mosby; 2011. pp. 1431-42.
3. Deshpande G, Jape G, Rao S, et al. Benefits of probiotics in preterm neonates in low-income and medium-income countries: a systematic review of randomised controlled trials. BMJ Open. 2017;7(12):e017638.
4. Premkumar MH. Necrotising enterocolitis. In: Clohery JP, Eichenwald EC, Hansen AR, Stark AR (Eds). Manual of Neonatal Care, 7th edition. Philadelphia, PA: Lippincott Williams & Wilkins; 2012. pp. 340-349.
5. Rao SC, Basani L, Simmer K, et al. Peritoneal drainage versus laparotomy as initial surgical treatment for perforated necrotizing enterocolitis or spontaneous intestinal perforation in preterm low birth weight infants. Cochrane Database Syst Rev. 2011;(6):CD006182.
6. Sharma S, Young C, Neu J. Necrotising enterocolitis. In: Neu J, Polin RA (Eds). Gastroenterology and Nutrition: Neonatology Questions and Controversies, 2nd edition. Philadelphia, PA: Elseviers Saunders; 2012. pp. 217-26.

Section 3

Growth and Development

3.1 Growth and Development: Basic Concepts

Dilip Mukherjee

INTRODUCTION

Growth denotes an increase in size of an individual due to increase in the number and diameter of the cells, and development denotes functional maturity of the child. Growth and development are not synonymous but they are assessed simultaneously. The growth performance in a child should be coupled with the assessment of the development to get an idea of the child's performance in overall growth. Growth and development begin at conception and end at maturity. They are unique characteristics of children and any obstacle in this process at any stage can possibly result in aberration of growth and/or development.

While growth is a continuous process, the rate or velocity of growth is variable. Any description of growth categorized into ages will not capture the beginnings or ends of epochs of growth. These epochs are more physiologically divided into the following growth phases:

- Intrauterine or prenatal growth, i.e. growth from conception till birth
- Infantile growth spurt (0–1 years)
- Midgrowth spurt (6–8 years)
- Adolescent growth spurt (onset of puberty to young adult life)

ASSESSMENT OF GROWTH AND DEVELOPMENT

Growth can be measured in terms of

- Physical anthropometry (e.g. weight, height, circumferences of head, chest, and waist)
- Assessment of tissue growth (e.g. skinfold thickness and measurement of muscle mass)
- Bone age (radiological by appearance center of ossification and fusion of the various epiphyseal centers)
- Dental age (by counting the number of erupted teeth)
- Biochemical and histological means

Development can be studied under motor (gross and fine motor), linguistic, adaptive, and personal social behavior category.

Physical Anthropometry

Physical anthropometry should be done in every child from birth till maturity at regular intervals. The methods of assessment are given in Chapters 3.2 and 3.4. It needs to be emphasized that the growth measurement needs to be done meticulously with absolute precision and recorded, so as to allow us on subsequent visit, to ascertain whether the child has grown optimally. The measurements should preferably be done by the same person on calibrated checked equipment to avoid personal human errors.

Weight

The weighting scales best suited are those, which are designed on balance arm principle. The accuracy up to 0.1 kg is acceptable. For smaller babies, machines of more accuracy are required as 0.1 kg forms a higher percentage of total body weight. More recently, many electronic weighing scales giving accuracy up to 0.1 kg have been made available.

The weighing scales should be checked for accuracy using known weight periodically. The beam scales are better for all purposes than spring weighing scales, i.e. bathroom scales, as the spring may get expanded due to repeated use, may get rusted, and the variation of temperature may give false reading.

A special type of new weighing scale is recently devised in Japan, which, in addition to the weight of an individual, also notes body mass index (BMI) and the amount of subcutaneous fat.

Length (Crown-Heel Length)

Until 24 months of age, length in recumbency is measured using an infantometer (Chapters 1.3 and 3.2). The length is recorded in centimeters up to one decimal point.

Height

After the age of 2 years, standing height is recorded by a stadiometer. The details have been provided in the Chapters 1.3 and 3.2. For community survey, portable types of anthropometric rods are also used. For recording stature (height), the subject should remove his/her socks and shoes and stand perfectly straight with arms relaxed by his/her sides and ankles and knees together. Before measurement starts, a gentle pressure may be applied over the spine with one hand, while other hand adjusts the sliding headpiece over the anthropometric rod. The subject's head is positioned in Frankfort plane [a line passing through the inferior margin of the orbit (orbitale) and upper margin of external auditory meatus (portion)].

Sitting Height (Crown-rump Length)

For recording sitting height, the subject is made to sit on a table or other convenient hard surface so that his/her head lies in Frankfort plane. The back should be straight, thighs horizontal and comfortably positioned. The feet should be supported on the foot board, and hands should be rest comfortably on the subject's lap. To ensure that the subject's back is fully extended, the observer may run his/her index finger up the spine applying pressure to the lumber and sacral regions, causing the subject to set up a reflex action. The head board should be lowered and made to touch the head of the subject, and the reading should be recorded to the nearest completed unit.

Body Proportions

The total body length is divided into two segments. The upper segment (US) is from head to symphysis pubis and lower segment (LS) from symphysis pubis to the toes. The US-to-LS ratio is 1.7:1 at birth. By 6–7 years, it reaches 1:1. If the ratio is infantile after 1 year of age, it suggests short limb dwarfism due to bone disorders, such as rickets and hypothyroidism.

Body Circumferences

The details of measuring head and midarm circumference (MAC) are given in Chapter 1.3. It should be kept in mind that upper arm circumference can be measured both in flexed and extended positions and also either at the maximum circumference of biceps muscle or midpoint, as the difference between the two is negligible.

Chest circumference for boys, prepubertal girls, and men can be recorded at the level of nipples during normal breathing. It is recorded to the nearest 0.1 cm.

Age-Independent Anthropometry

Midarm Circumference

As the MAC is relatively constant between 16.5 cm and 17.5 cm in 1–5 years of age, this measurement may be considered as an age-independent variable up to 5 years of age. Any child whose MAC is less than 12.5 cm up to 5 years of age is considered malnourished. Shakir's tape also measures the MAC. A bangle of 4 cm in diameter, used in field studies, is not a reliable method (Bangle test).

Weight for Height

The degree of wasting can be measured by comparing the child's weight with that of the expected for a healthy child of the same height. The combinations of these measurements have been used to distinguish different types of malnutrition. Waterlow suggested that weight for height can be used to distinguish between malnutrition of recent origin, i.e. wasting and malnutrition due to a considerable period of month, i.e. stunting. In chronic malnutrition, the child is stunted with the weight for the age and height for the age being low. In acute malnutrition, height for age is normal but weight for age is low (wasting). In nutritional dwarf (short stature), the weight/height is equal; the child may pass off as a normal child of lower age if the chronological age is not known. These have been discussed in Chapter 4.4, Malnutrition.

Midarm-to-Head Circumference

It is a simple and useful criterion for the detection of malnutrition. A ratio 0.280–0.314 indicates early malnutrition, 0.250–0.279 moderate, and less than 0.249 denotes severe malnutrition.

Quetelet's Index

It is based on the relationship between weight and height and is expressed as weight (kg)/height (cm) × 100. Normal value varies from 0.14 to 0.16. In gross malnutrition, it is less than 0.14. It is a quite reliable ratio for assessing malnutrition.

Mid-upper Arm to Height Ratio

It is also a very good indicator of nutritional status. A ratio of less than 0.29 indicates gross malnutrition, while the normal value ranges from 0.32 to 0.33.

Body Mass Index

$$\text{BMI} = \frac{\text{Weight (kg)}}{\text{Height}^2\ (\text{m}^2)}$$

Body mass index (BMI) is similar to Quetlet's index, except that the values are in SI units. BMI values can be used to draw standardized percentile curves in children and adolescents. It is especially useful for defining obesity. BMI values above the 95th percentile for age are usually used to define obesity.

Ponderal Index

$$\text{PI} = \frac{\text{Height (cm)}}{\text{Cube root of body weight (kg)}}$$

Ponderal index (PI) is similar to BMI and used in defining newborn with intrauterine growth retardation.

Tissue Growth

This measurement is done for special purposes and is not used in routine clinical practice. It is measured with a special caliper and skinfold caliper.

Triceps Skinfold Thickness

The skinfold is picked up over the posterior surface of the triceps muscle, 1 cm above the mark on a vertical line passing upward between bony point identified for taking measurement, maintaining a pressure of 10 g/mm^2 on the caliper and freeing the skinfold from the underlying muscle with left hand between thumb, index, and middle finger and holding caliper with the other hand. The reading is recorded to the nearest 0.1 mm, maintaining the pressure of caliper as before.

Biceps Skinfold Thickness

For recording biceps, the child is made to stand erect, facing the observer with arm on side, and palm facing forward. The skinfold is picked up over the belly of biceps and 1 cm above the line marked for the upper arm circumference and triceps skinfold on a vertical line joining antecubital fossa to the head of humerus. The caliper is applied at the marked level, and the reading is recorded to 0.1 mm.

Bone Age or Skeletal Maturity

The appearance and fusion of various epiphyseal centers follow a definite sequence related to chronologic age from birth to maturity. Radiological examination of felt wrist and elbow is usually considered for bone age assessment. X-ray of the lower end of femur and talus is used for the assessment of maturity of newborn babies. The details of appearance and fusion of various centers are given in subsequent sections.

Dental Development

The eruption of teeth follows a definite sequence. The eruption of temporary of deciduous teeth begins at about 6 months with upper or lower central incisor. By 1 year of age, 4–8 teeth are present. The permanent teeth begin to erupt at 6 years. The details of dental development are provided in subsequent chapters.

ASSESSMENT OF DEVELOPMENT

Development refers to qualitative and quantitative changes and acquisition of a variety of competencies for functioning optimally in a social milieu. Further, development is a continuous process from birth to maturity. It depends on maturation and myelination of brain; unless that has occurred, no amount of practice can make the child learn that skill. The process of development is an interaction between the child and his/her required environment. It may be stressed that besides 10% prevalence of development delay, the early identification remains difficult. Although severe disorders can be recognized, in infancy, it is usual to diagnose speech impairment, hyperactivity, or emotional disorders before the age of 3 or 4 years, and learning disabilities are rarely recognized before children start schooling. If one can diagnose early stage development delay in early stages of growth, the intervention can minimize long-term quantum of disability.

It takes a long time, great patience, and perseverance to assess the development of a child. It should be done with cooperation of the child and parents. The development is assessed by Gesell's method, Denver Development Screening Test, Bayley Scale of Infant Development, Brazelton Neonatal Behavioral Assessment Scale, Baroda Scale, Thiruvananthapuram Development Screening Chart, and others **(Table 3.1.1)**. The detailed discussion on development assessment is given in Chapters 3.5 and 3.6.

GROWTH STUDIES

Four types of growth studies are as follows:
1. Cross-sectional study
2. Longitudinal study
3. Linked cross-sectional study
4. Linked longitudinal study

Cross-sectional Study

This is a very convenient, easy, less time-consuming, and economical method to study physical anthropometric growth. For example, healthy children of each age group and gender (minimum being 200 at each point) are measured for their weight, height, and other parameters are recorded, and an average is found out. These groups of children are studied just once in 20 years to develop national norms.

Linear or Longitudinal Study

In this study, a group of children is followed through time and measured at regular intervals. The same child is measured sequentially, and this provides the strength and richness of individual variation as seen in real life. Longitudinal measurements reflect changing environments and shifting hormonal profiles, such as in puberty. The growth spurts are more clearly appreciated and less blunted in contrast to that with cross-sectional studies. Velocity curves can only be constructed through longitudinal observations. The longitudinal records are also useful to store valuable information, such as the effect of nutrition, illness, and sociocultural changes.

Table 3.1.1: Development screening test that can be used for children less than 3 years.

S. No.	Name of the test	Age range	Domains of development identified	Administration time (in minutes)
I	Developmental Observation Card	0–1 year	Social smile, head holding, sitting, and standing	3
II	Thiruvananthapuram Development Screening Chart	0–2 years	Personal social, fine motor, language, and gross motor	5
III	Baroda Development Screening Test	0–2.5 years	Gross motor, fine motor, cognitive, and language	10
IV	Denver Developmental Screening Test	2 weeks to 6 years	Personal social, fine motor, language, and gross motor	20
V	Gesell Development Schedules	4 weeks to 6 years	Language, fine and gross motor, cognitive, and personal social	Not specified
VI	Receptive-Expressive Emergent Language Scale	0–3 years	Receptive language and expressive language	20
VII	Vineland Adaptive Behavior Scale	0–19 years	Communication, daily living skills, socialization, and motor skills	25
VIII	STYCAR Vision Test	6 months to 7 years	Integrity of vision	20
IX	STYCAR Hearing Test	6 months to 7 years	Integrity of hearing	20
X	Checklist for Autism in Toddlers	18–36 months	Screening for autism	10

(STYCAR: screening test for young children and retardates)

Linked Cross-sectional Study

In some longitudinal studies, not all of the subjects can be followed up for the duration of the study due to dropouts. If we consider this a longitudinal study, we are then left with only a small number. If, on the other hand, we use appropriate mathematical constructs, we will be able to incorporate a large portion of the data in the remaining children, thereby enhancing the quality of the study.

The linked cross-sectional study is a compromise between a cross-sectional study and a pure longitudinal study. It is less expensive and time-consuming, when compared to a longitudinal study. We should be able to obtain efficient estimates with minimal variance of anthropometric measurements.

Linked Longitudinal Study

A linked longitudinal study is one, which comprises several relatively small longitudinal studies, which can be joined up to form a larger whole. Observers working separately but simultaneously study the individual components. These components are then amalgamated into a continuous data set simulating a true longitudinal study.

The greatest advantage of this study is the compression of time whilst retaining reasonable longitudinal quality.

PERCENTILES AND *Z*-SCORES

Concept of Percentiles

While making various calculations, the use of terms such as mean or average and standard deviation (SD) are well known. While expressing the growth, the term percentile or centile is often used. This may be used. This may be explained in a simple way, for example, the height of 100 1-year-old normal children is not exactly the same. They are arranged in such a way that the shortest is number 1 and the tallest is number 100. The rows of children are thus made. The mean of each number is worked out. The child at number 1 is the 1st percentile, number 10 is the 10th centile, number 50 is the 50th centile, and so on. The child on the 10th centile on height chart means that 9 children are less in height and 90 children are more in height. The 50th centile is the median value and is also termed the standard value. Accepted range for normal is between the third percentile and the 97th percentile.

The SD charts are based on the distribution of data above and below a mean value. The average normal range falls above and below 2 SD expressed as 2 SD ± 1 SD is equal to the 84th centile and –1 SD is equal to the 16th centile. A total of ±2 SD corresponds to the 97th centile and –2 SD corresponds to the third centile. The mean ± SD curves are useful for quantifying the degree of retardation exactly.

Z-scores

Z-Scores or SD scores are the measures of dispersion from the median value. *Z*-scores are helpful to compare the child's height and weight with a reference population. The World Health Organization (WHO) recognizes that *Z*-scores are a reliable and convenient method to describe the states of nutrition and is an apt descriptor of malnutrition. *Z*-Scores can be used for a variety of auxologic parameters—weight for age, height for age, weight for height, and BMI. The formula to calculate *Z*-score is as follows:

$$\text{Z-score} = \frac{\text{Observed value - Median value of the reference population}}{\text{SD value of reference population}}$$

While percentiles convey similar information about auxologic parameters, *Z*-scores are more useful for mathematical analysis. *Z*-Score data can be used to calculate mean, median, and SDs or other summary statistics. *Z*-Score conversion from raw values of auxologic data ensures data is on a linear scale; data then becomes directly comparable across all age groups. Another major advantage of *Z*-score conversion is gender independence. When using age and gender-specific reference data, *Z*-scores allow comparison between auxologic parameters in males and females.

It is worth noting how percentiles and *Z*-scores are interchangeable. For a growth chart, the upper and lower ends of a percentile chart at the 98th and 2nd centiles represent approximate *Z*-scores of +2.0 and –2.0. In a normal distribution curve (such as weight), the 98th and 2nd centiles therefore represent the upper and lower cutoffs of the normal distribution. Some growth charts utilize wider dispersion data—the 99.6th and 0.4th centiles. These represent *Z*-scores of +2.67 and –2.67, respectively. A wider dispersion indicates that any measurement plotted outside such extreme values is usually abnormal. In countries where growth hormone (GH) is licensed for administration in short children who were born small for gestation age (SGA), a height *Z*-score of –2.5 is used as a cutoff. Therefore, growth charts that utilize the 0.4th centile (–2.67 SD) would be useful in understanding if a child's height measurements were short enough to receive GH treatment as per the SGA license.

GROWTH CHARTS

Growth chart is the most important tool in the assessment of growth of an individual child. A standard chart contains weight for age, height for age, and weight for height. The head circumference is included for first 3 years of life. They depict mean, ±SD, or percentile values at each age. The available charts are discussed in Chapters 3.2 and 3.3.

Velocity Growth Charts

These charts are developed by the long-term longitudinal studies. Velocity charts show the rate of change, which could be due to chronic illness, nutrition, or GH deficiency. Different countries may use their own growth charts. In Great Britain, Tanner's growth charts are used. In India, Indian Academy of Pediatrics has published revised growth charts for 5–18-year-old children, in 2016. Presently, the WHO growth charts are being preferred, especially for children less than 5 years of age. This is discussed in Chapter 3.3.

BIBLIOGRAPHY

1. Agarwal DK, Agarwal KN. Physical growth in Indian affluent children (Birth to 6 years). Indian Pediatr. 1994;31(4):377-413.
2. Agarwal DK, Agarwal KN, Upadhyay SK, et al. Physical and sexual growth pattern of affluent Indian children from 5 to 18 years of age. Indian Pediatr. 1990;29(10):1203-82.
3. Falkner F, Tanner JM. Human Growth, 2nd edition. New York, NY: Plenum; 1986.
4. Khadilkar VV. Revised Indian Academy of Pediatrics 2015 growth charts for 5 to 18 years old Indian children. In: IAP Textbook of Pediatrics, 6th edition. New Delhi: Jaypee Brothers Medical Publishers (P) Ltd.; 2016. pp. 96-109.
5. Khadilkar VV, Khadilkar AV, Choudhury P, et al. IAP growth monitoring guidelines for children from birth to 18 years. Mumbai: Indian Academy of Pediatrics; 2005.
6. Mukherjee D, Nair MKC. Growth and Development. New Delhi: Jaypee Brothers Medical Publishers (P) Ltd.; 2008.
7. Tanner JM. Growth at Adolescence, 2nd edition. Oxford: Blackwell Scientific Publication; 1962.
8. Tanner JM. Physical growth and development. In: Forfar JO, Arneil GC (Eds). Textbook of Pediatrics, 2nd edition. London: Churchill Livingstone; 1978. pp. 249-303.
9. Tanner JM, Whitehouse RH, Cameroon N, et al. Assessment of Skeletal Maturity and Prediction of Adult Height, 2nd edition. London: Academic Press; 1983.

3.2 Growth: Birth to Puberty

KN Agarwal

DEFINITION

Growth is a continuous process commencing at conception and progressing at a varying pace till its near completion about two decades later. The process of "growth" is accompanied with increase in body size and/or mass at varying rates. It is multifactorial and complex, but still remarkably predictable. Boys and girls grow differently, and each child has his or her distinct growth pattern. Growth charts (curves) are used to measure growth.

The distance growth curve **(Fig. 3.2.1)** is a measure of size over time; it records height, weight, and/or skull circumference as a function of age and gets higher with age.

The velocity growth curve measures the rate of growth at a given time for a body feature (such as height or weight). The height velocity curve is highest in infancy, up to 2 years of age, with more consistent annual growth afterward, and increases again at puberty **(*see* Fig. 3.2.1)**.

Any faltering in growth process may indicate disease. Therefore, frequent and accurate growth assessment is of primary importance.

FACTORS INFLUENCING GROWTH

Growth is influenced by interaction of both genetic and environmental factors. Children generally grow to their genetic height potential with little outside assistance. What parents can do to help their child's optimal growth and development is to create the best possible environment for their growth to take place.

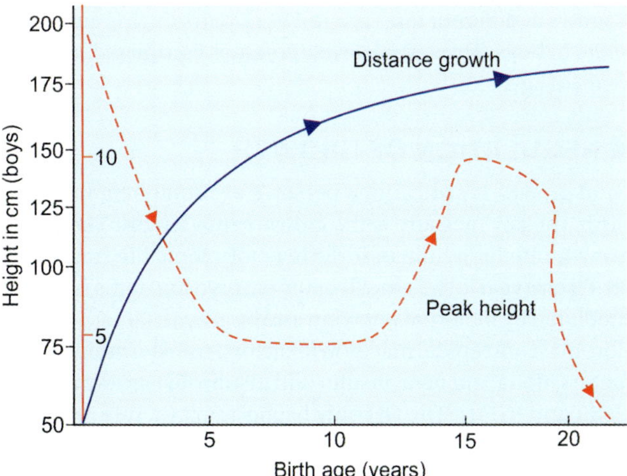

Fig. 3.2.1: Distance growth curve. Increase in height with age in boys (birth to 18 years). The broken line is velocity height curve with peak height velocity.

Genetic Factors

Racial Influence

Growth potential of children of different races varies despite of similar environments. Asians tend to be smaller than Europeans, while Afro-Americans are taller than White Americans.

Parental Influence

Tall parents tend to have taller children. The midparental height reflects the genetic potential for growth for an individual.

Gender

With same genetic potential and environment, boys tend to be taller and heavier than girls. The difference is obvious from early childhood and gets more pronounced during puberty.

Genetic Disorders

Certain genetic disorders can adversely influence growth. These include chromosomal disorders (e.g. Down syndrome and Turner syndrome) and genetic mutations (e.g. mucopolysaccharidosis).

ENVIRONMENTAL FACTORS

Prenatal Growth

The size at birth is primarily influenced by maternal health and uterine environment. Common causes of fetal growth retardation in India are maternal malnutrition and anemia. Disorders leading to placental insufficiency, such as pregnancy-induced hypertension, multiple pregnancies, chronic systemic disorders, and maternal tobacco/alcohol abuse are other important causes of fetal growth retardation.

Maternal diabetes, by stimulatory insulin production in the fetus, is an important cause of excessive intrauterine growth leading to a large for date baby.

Postnatal Growth

- *Nutrition*: During the first 2 years of life, undernutrition has far-reaching consequences; growth deficit that occurs during this period is never fully recoverable.
- *Chronic systemic diseases*: Chronic disorders, especially congenital heart disease, recurrent pneumonia, persistent diarrhea, recurrent urinary tract infection, tuberculosis, etc., lead to growth failure by causing catabolism and poor nutrition intake. This may become irreversible if there is inadequate disease-free period to allow catch-up growth.
- *Hormonal influences*: After first 6–8 months of life, the growth hormone (GH) and thyroxine deficiency, and in addition to these hormones during puberty, the sex hormones have also an important role in induction of the pubertal growth spurt.
- *Emotional factors*: Emotional deprivation, anxiety, and insecurity influence the neurochemical regulation of GH and may affect a child's growth.

IMPORTANCE OF GROWTH ASSESSMENT

Pediatricians should remember that the first thing that springs to most parents' minds when they hear the phrase "physical growth" used in the context of child development is height. Height or how tall a child grows can easily be measured. It is by no means the only facet of physical growth in children. In addition to height, the development of gross motor skills, fine motor skills and coordination are all important indicators of physical growth.

- Growth is a fundamental characteristic of childhood.
- Despite being influenced by many factors, it remains remarkably predictable.
- Normal growth is an indicator of optimum health.
- Deviation from the normal pattern is indicative of a pathological process.
- Periodic assessment facilitates early detection of growth faltering, which may be the first manifestation of undernutrition/infection/disease.

GROWTH PATTERN OF DIFFERENT BODY SYSTEMS

The various growth periods are shown in **Table 3.2.1**.

Table 3.2.1: Growth periods.

- *Embryo*: Implantation to 8 weeks of gestation
- *Fetus*: 9th week of gestation to birth
- *Infant*: Birth to 1 year of age
- *Toddler*: 1–3 years of age
- *Preschool*: 3–5 years of age
- *School age*: 5–12 years
- *Adolescence*: 10–19 years

General Body

The general body growth is rapid during fetal life and first 1–2 years of age. The growth velocity slows later during mid-childhood and accelerates once again during puberty (***see* Fig. 3.2.1**). The limbs and arms grow faster than the trunk so that body proportions undergo marked variation as an infant grows into an adolescent.

Brain (Head Circumference–Brain Size)

Brain growth occurs very rapidly during fetal life and infancy. Although brain cell formation is almost complete before birth, brain maturation continues after birth. The brain of the newborn is not yet fully developed. It contains about 100 billion brain cells that have yet to be connected into functioning networks. But brain development up to age one is more rapid and extensive than was previously realized. At birth, the brain of the infant is 25% of the adult size. At the age of 1 year, the brain has grown to 75% of its adult size and to 80% by age three, reaching 90% by age seven. The influence of the early environment on brain development is crucial. Infants exposed to good nutrition, toys, and playmates have better brain function at age 12 than those raised in a less stimulating environment. The rapid brain growth is reflected by an increase in head circumference.

LYMPHOID TISSUE GROWTH

The growth of lymphoid tissue is the highest during mid-childhood when children are often observed to have enlarged tonsils and lymph nodes, maximum being at 8–9 years of age, and later decreases in size.

REPRODUCTIVE (SEXUAL) DEVELOPMENT

It grows at different rates around 9–11 years in girls and 11–13 years in boys. The sexual development is completed by 19–20 years of age.

REGULATION OF GROWTH

Fetal growth is critical to a person's eventual height. Before birth, the key measure is the crown-rump length. The fastest growth rate for a human is during embryonic life (rate being 50–60 cm/year). The growth of the embryo and fetus is mainly mediated by maternal nutrition and by growth factors, such as fibroblast and epidermal growth factors, transforming growth factors alpha and beta, insulin and insulin-like growth factors (IGFI and IGFII). The GH only begins to play a role in growth in the final weeks before birth.

The three components of postnatal growth, which are infancy, childhood, and puberty, represent different modes of growth regulation.

The growth rate during infancy is rapid but sharply decelerating and is principally dependent on nutrition. The GH and thyroxine have an increasingly important role from 1 year of age. During the first 2 years, the infants establish their own growth trajectory (pathways); later from about 2 years of age to the onset of puberty, growth occurs in relatively constant annual increments.

CLINICAL APPLICATIONS

Physical growth begins to slow at around age 1 year. As growth slows, children need fewer calories and parents may notice a decrease in appetite. Two-year-old children can have very erratic eating habits that sometimes make parents anxious. It appears that some children eat virtually nothing yet continue to grow and thrive. Actually, they eat little 1 day and then make up for it by eating everything in sight the next day.

Rapid early growth in low-birth-weight or healthy full-term infants (centile crossing) is associated with later fatness, obesity, hypertension, hypercholesterolemia, and insulin resistance; the key risk factors for coronary vascular disease. Buyken et al. showed that breastfeeding reduces these risks.

Early growth and the brain in undernutrition and/or anemia induce structural changes. Studies show that the impact of undernutrition in brain growth induces structural changes (loss of frontal lobe asymmetry); impairs higher mental functions; and there is persistence of soft neurological signs. Maternal anemia (iron deficiency) affects development of neurotransmitters irreversibly.

Puberty is fueled by the secretion of GH and sex steroids. Puberty is the process of physical maturation from child to adult. The timing of this growth spurt is extremely variable. At puberty, a second growth spurt occurs, being earlier in girls by 1.0–2.0 years than in boys, giving rise on the average, to a difference in adult height between men and women of about 14–15 cm.

GROWTH ASSESSMENT IN INFANCY AND CHILDHOOD

Length

It is measured on an infantometer in children too young to stand until 2 years of age.

Height

It is measured on an anthropometric rod or a stadiometer if the child can stand (>2 years of age). In general, length in normal term infants increases about 30% by 5 months of age and more than 50% by 12 months of age. Infants grow about 25 cm during the first year, and the height at 4 years is about the double of the birth length. In boys, half the adult height is attained at around 2 years of age, while in girls, height at 19 months is about half the adult height. Some small-for-gestational-age infants tend to be shorter throughout the life than infants whose size is appropriate for their gestational age.

TOOLS FOR ANTHROPOMETRY

Length on an Infantometer

Infant lying straight with his shoulders and buttocks flat against the measuring surface, eyes looking up, second person holds head to touch the head piece, align the body and extend both legs by one hand on knees, and bring the foot piece firmly against the heels. Record the length to the nearest 0.1 cm **(Fig. 3.2.2)** (*see* Chapters 1.3 and 3.1).

Height

It is measured standing for a child with minimum clothing without shoes and socks, standing with feet parallel on an even platform, stretching fullest, arms hanging on the sides, and occiput, shoulder blades, buttocks, and heels touching the rod. The head is held erect with lower border of the eye orbit in the same horizontal plane as the external canal of the ear (Frankfort plane). The headpiece is lowered to touch the top of the head **(Fig. 3.2.3)**.

Weight

Infant/child should be naked or in minimal clothing. Ideal is to use sliding beam balance scale or electronic scale **(Figs. 3.2.4 and 3.2.5)**. Weighing scale is checked for zero, center the infant on the scale tray and weigh to the nearest 10 g; older child is weighed standing to the nearest 50 g.

HEAD CIRCUMFERENCE

This is measured over the most prominent part of the occipital and just above the supraorbital ridges, using a flexible, nonstretchable tape. Position the tape just above the

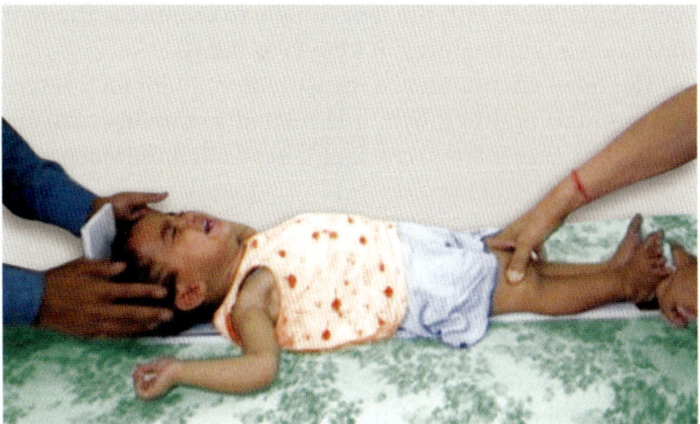

Fig. 3.2.2: Infantometer for length: help of two measurers is required.

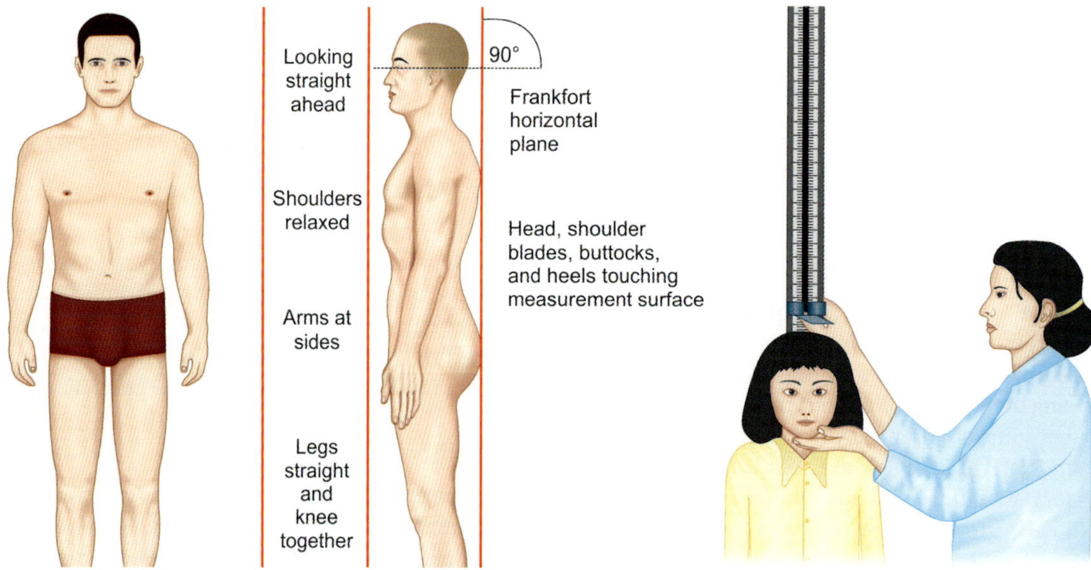

Fig. 3.2.3: Stadiometer for height measure: note the position.

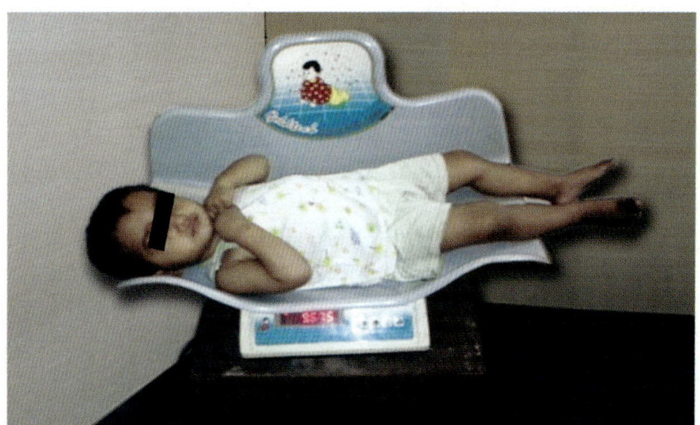

Fig. 3.2.4: Electronic weighing scale.

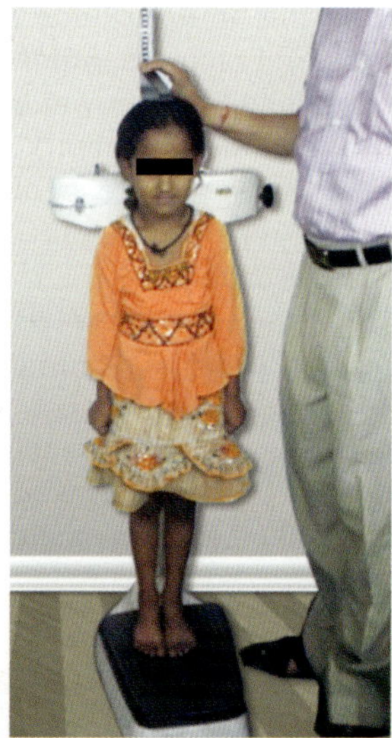

Fig. 3.2.5: Scale to measure height and weight.

eyebrows, above the ears, and around the biggest part on the back of the head. Pull the tape snugly to compress the hair and take reading nearest to 0.1 cm **(Fig. 3.2.6)**.

The head circumference measurement in infancy serves as a guide to brain growth; it is related to intelligence and cognition. Large infants have larger head circumference.

Anterior Fontanel

Anterior fontanel (AF) is a diamond-shaped open gap situated in midline at the junction of the coronal and sagittal sutures (size around 2 × 2 cm) that close by 18 months (range 10–18 months). Small or closed AF at an earlier age is a warning sign, i.e. microcephaly. Large AF may be present in hydrocephalus, hypothyroidism, Down syndrome, achondroplasia, osteogenesis imperfecta, and mucopolysaccharidosis.

Posterior Fontanel

Posterior fontanel (PF), placed between the intersection of the occipital and parietal bones, closes within 6–8 weeks of life. An open PF in later life is noted in congenital hypothyroidism.

MIDARM CIRCUMFERENCE

This is measured on the left upper arm midway between the acromion and olecranon processes. It measures 9.8 cm at birth, 14.5 cm around 1 year with slow increase from 14.8 to 16.2 cm between 1 and 5 years of age.

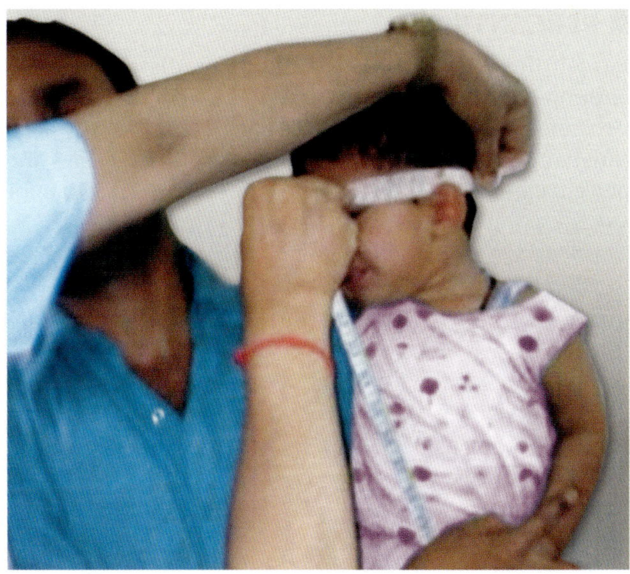

Fig. 3.2.6: Crossover technique to measure head circumference by fiberglass tape.

In field surveys, it helps in diagnosis of mal/undernutrition: a value more than 13.5 cm is taken as normal nourished, 12.5–13.4 cm as borderline, 11.5–12.4 cm as mild-to-moderate undernutrition, and less than 11.5 cm as severe undernutrition, between the ages of 6 months and 5 years.

CHEST CIRCUMFERENCE

At birth, chest circumference is 3 cm less than the head circumference. It equals or exceeds head circumference by 10–12 months of age. In prepubertal children, it is recorded at the level of nipples.

ARM SPAN

Measure outstretched arms, from fingertip to fingertip. In children of European origin, the arm span should approximate the height (intermediate-length arms). The Asians have proportionally shorter arms than Europeans, and Africans have significantly longer arms.

Upper and Lower Segments

Lower Segment

Measure from the symphysis pubis to the floor.

Upper Segment

Subtract the lower segment (LS) from the height. The upper segment (US)/LS ratio is calculated by dividing the US by the LS. In children of European origin, this ratio is about 1.7 at birth and decreases to 1 at about age 10, where it remains throughout adulthood. The Asians have proportionally shorter legs (therefore, larger US/LS ratio), and Africans have longer legs (therefore lower US/LS ratio).

Body Mass Index

Body mass index (BMI) is the ratio of weight in kilogram to the square of height in meters (wt/ht^2). This is a good indicator of variability of energy status. If more than 95th centile, it suggests obesity and less than 5th centile, undernutrition (thin). In adolescents, calculate with the weight and height values in relation to the sexual maturity. The BMI values for Indian children are different than the National Center for Health Statistics (NCHS)—BMI values.

Skinfold Thickness

Around 50% of body fat is located under the skin. The measurement of triceps and biceps skinfold thickness (SFT) gives the estimate of peripheral fat, and subscapular and suprailiac SFT indicates the amount of central fat. The Lange's or Harpenden's skinfold calipers are used. The measurements are done as follows:

- *Biceps*: At the midpoint of their muscle belly, a point generally opposite/at the level of the nipple;
- *Triceps*: Between the tip of olecranon process of ulna (elbow) and the acromion process of the scapula (shoulder), a point is marked on the back of the arm;
- *Subscapular*: Below inferior angle of scapula 45° to vertical;
- *Suprailiac*: Above iliac crest in midaxillary line (approximately 2.5 cm above hip bone).

WAIST-TO-HIP RATIO

Waist-to-hip ratio (WHR): Waist circumference is measured over the highest palpable points of the iliac crests, by a fiber glass tape. Hip circumference is measured around the maximum extension of the buttocks.

- Waist-to-hip ratio index of 0.7 for women and 0.9 for men have been shown to correlate strongly with general health and fertility.
- Women within the 0.7 range have optimal levels of estrogens and are less susceptible to major diseases, such as diabetes, cardiovascular disorders, and ovarian cancers.
- Men with WHR around 0.9, similarly, have been shown to be more healthy and fertile with less prevalence of prostate and testicular cancers.

WAIST-TO-HEIGHT RATIO

Values less than 0.5 exclude central obesity, but values more than 0.5 indicate central obesity, even in children with normal weight and height. Waist-to-height ratio may predict cardiometabolic risk in normal weight as well as in overweight/obese children, according to the results obtained from the Bogalusa Heart Study (2011).

GROWTH CHARTS

Growth charts consist of a series of percentile curves. It means graphical representation of growth reference standards and consists of a series of percentile curves that illustrate the distribution of body measurements in the study population **(Figs. 3.2.7 to 3.2.12)**.

PERCENTILES

Percentiles describe the frequency distribution of anthropometric parameters, such as weight, height, skull circumference, BMI, etc. The 50th percentile is the average (median) line for the given population. It describes the percentage of children expected to be on or below that line, for

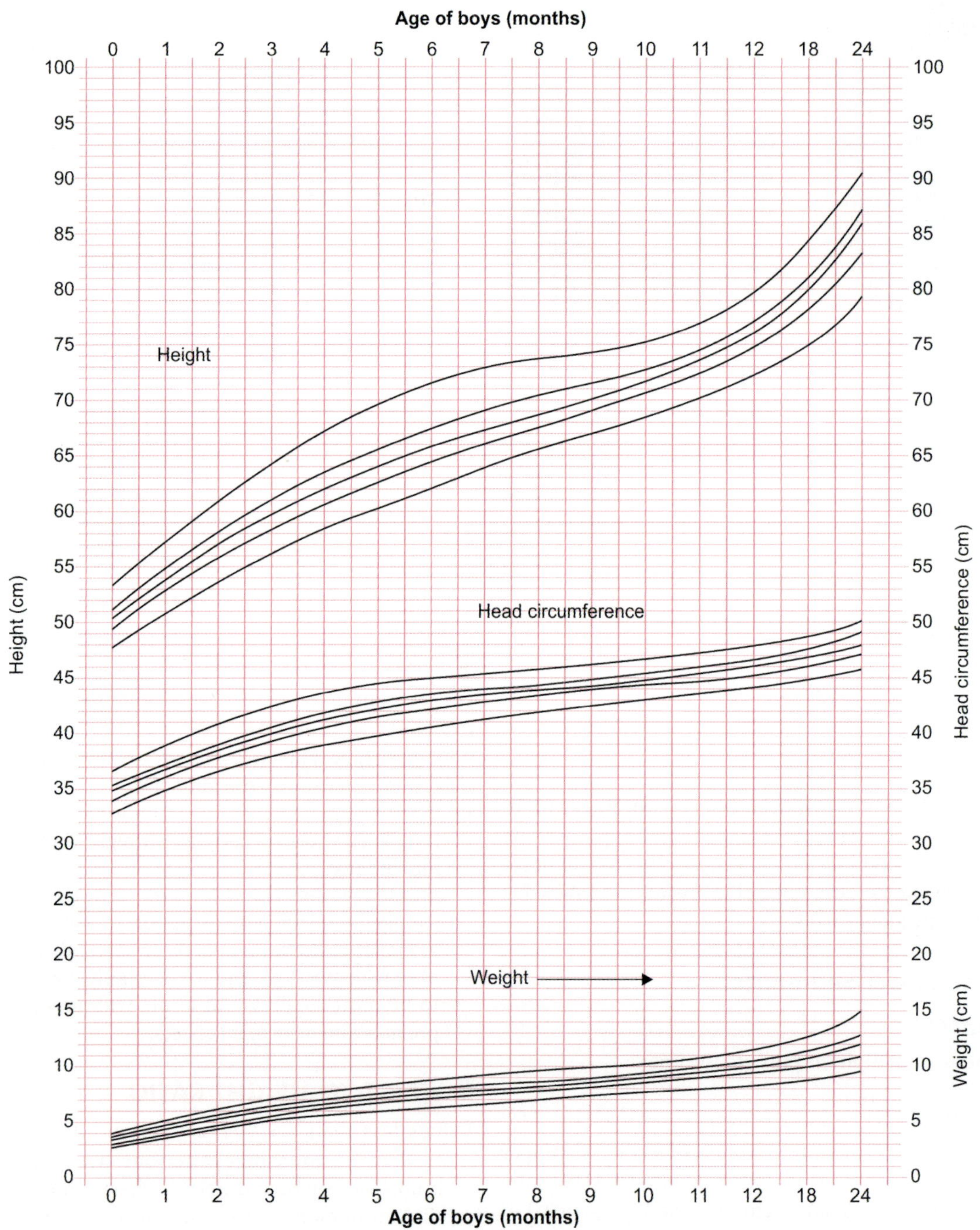

Fig. 3.2.7: Height, weight, and head circumference percentiles for boys (0–24 months).
Source: Agarwal DK, Agarwal KN. Physical growth in affluent Indian children (birth to 6 years). Indian Pediatr. 1994;31:377-413.

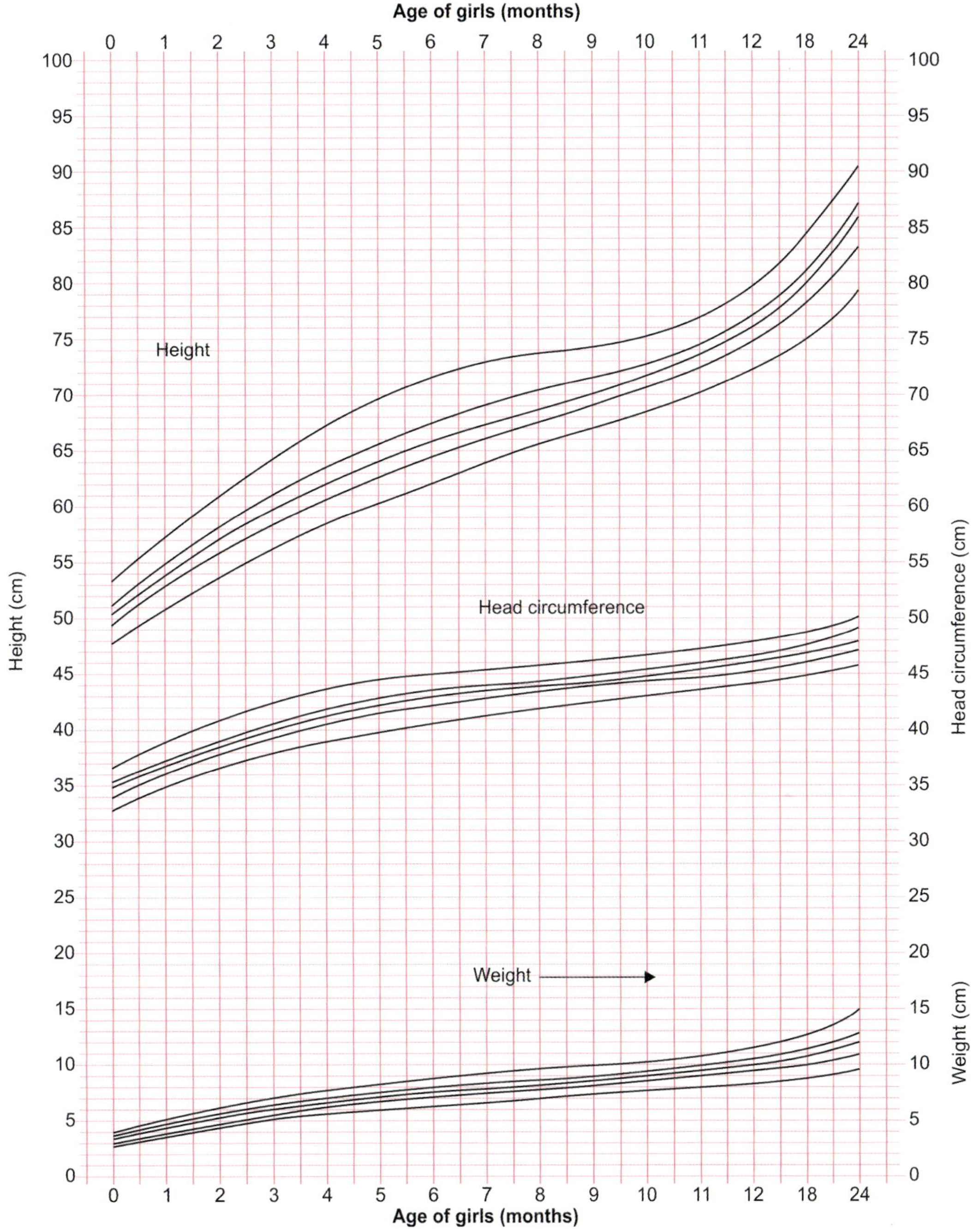

Fig. 3.2.8: Height, weight, and head circumference percentiles for girls (0–24 months).
Source: Agarwal DK, Agarwal KN. Physical growth in affluent Indian children (birth to 6 years). Indian Pediatr. 1994;31:377-413.

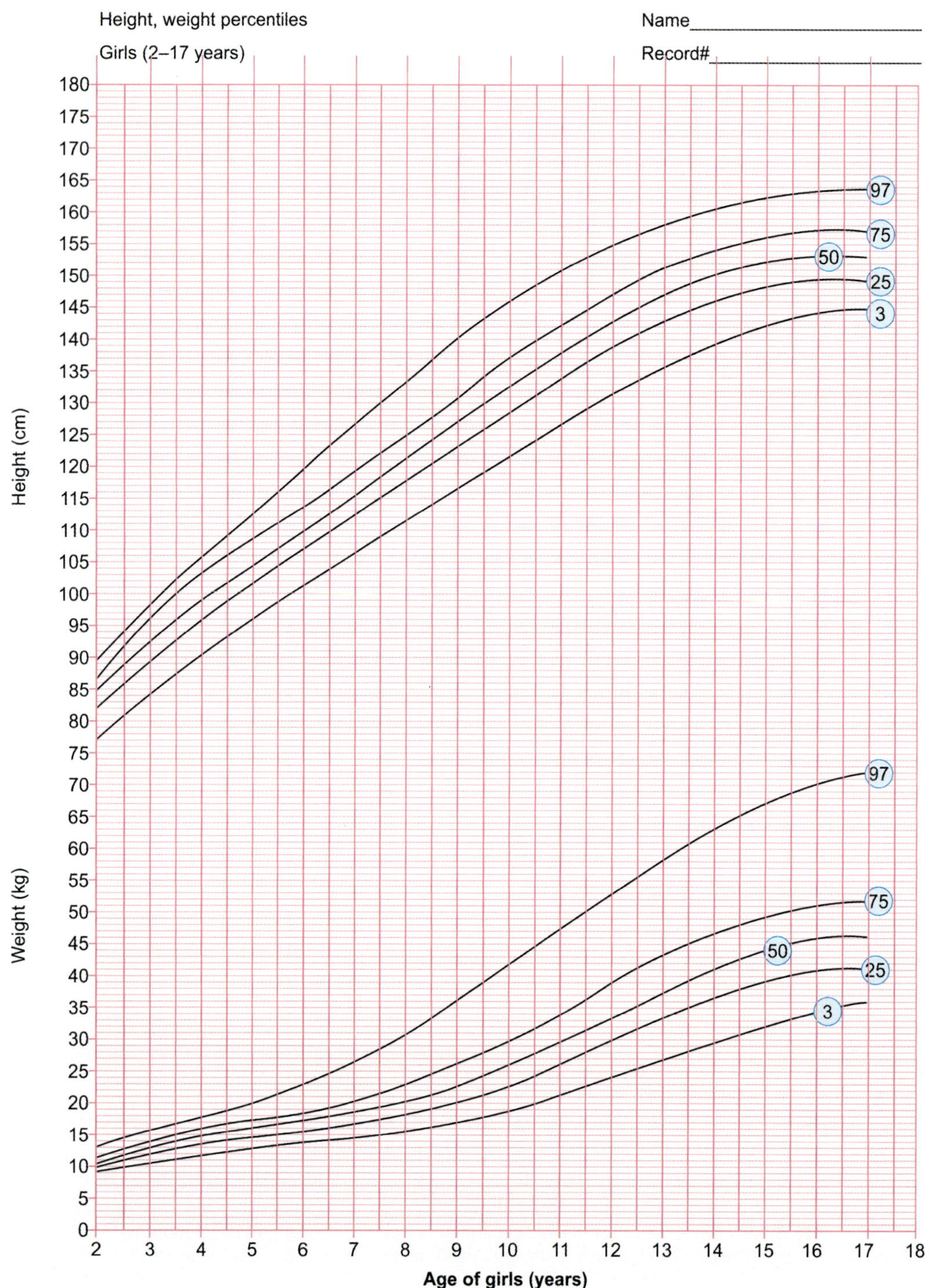

Fig. 3.2.9: The growth curves (data) for height and weight for girls from 2 to 17 years.

Source: Agarwal KN, Agarwal DK, Upadhaya SK, et al. Physical and sexual growth pattern of affluent Indian children from 5 to 18 years of age. Indian Pediatr. 1992;92:1203-82; Agarwal DK, Agarwal KN. Physical growth in affluent Indian children (birth to 6 years). Indian Pediatr. 1994;31:377-413; Agarwal KN, Saxena A, Bansal AK, et al. Physical growth assessment in adolescence. Indian Pediatr. 2001;38:1217-35.

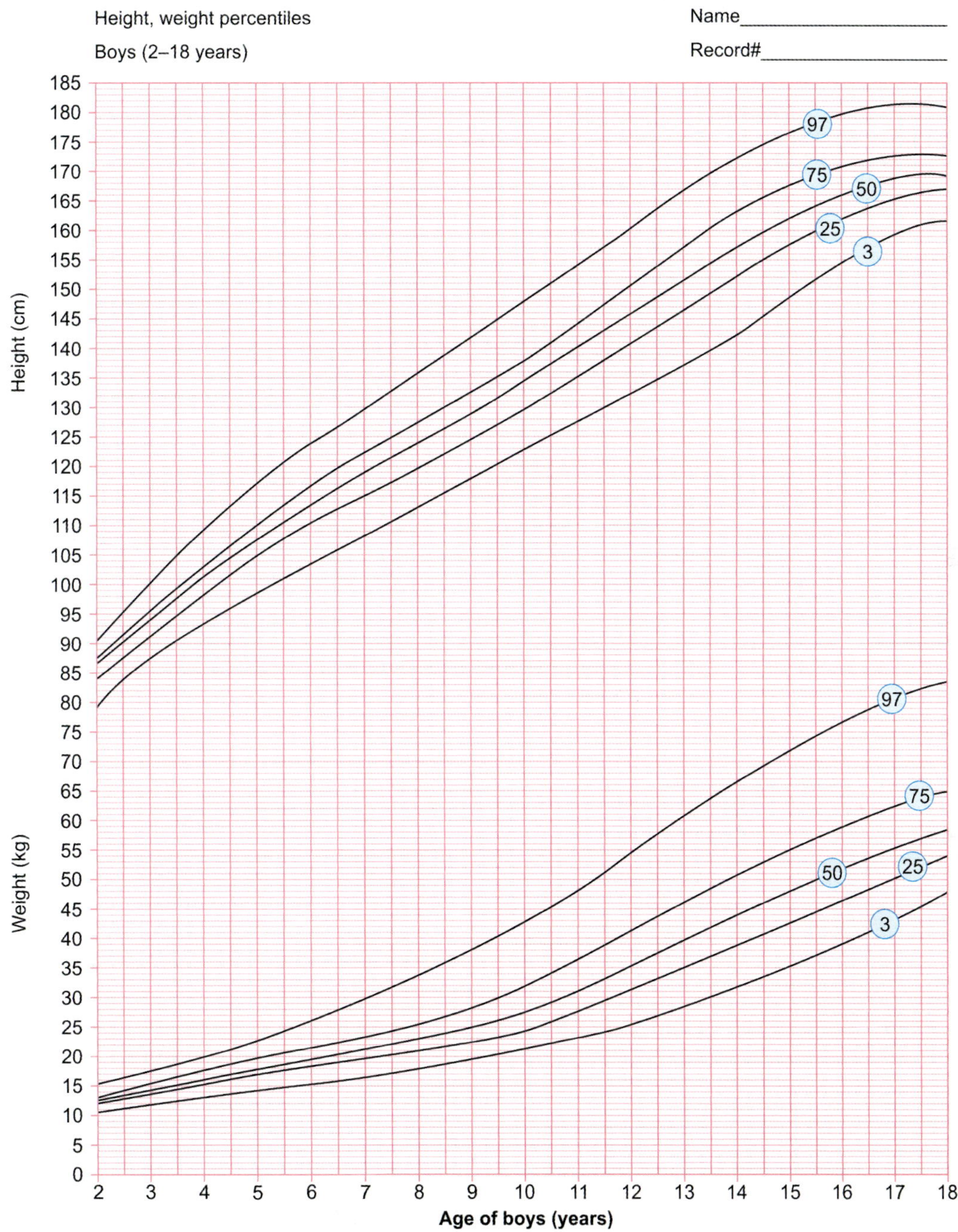

Fig. 3.2.10: The growth curves (data) for height and weight for boys from 2 to 17 years.

Source: Agarwal KN, Agarwal DK, Upadhaya SK, et al. Physical and sexual growth pattern of affluent Indian children from 5 to 18 years of age. Indian Pediatr. 1992;92:1203-82; Agarwal DK, Agarwal KN. Physical growth in affluent Indian children (birth to 6 years). Indian Pediatr. 1994;31:377-413; Agarwal KN, Saxena A, Bansal AK, et al. Physical growth assessment in adolescence. Indian Pediatr. 2001;38:1217-35.

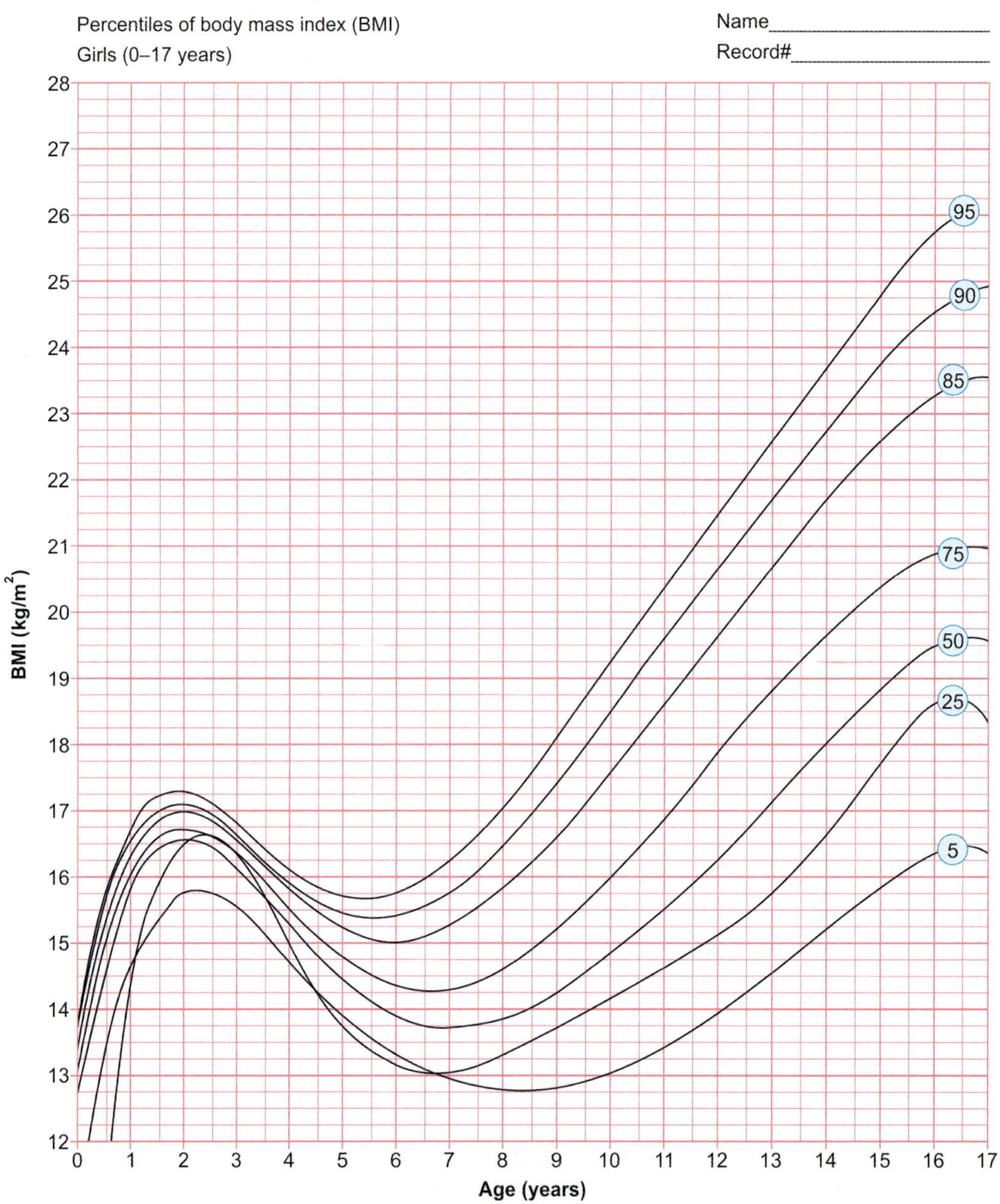

Fig. 3.2.11: The growth curves (data) for body mass index for girls from birth to 17 years.

Source: Agarwal KN, Agarwal DK, Upadhaya SK, et al. Physical and sexual growth pattern of affluent Indian children from 5 to 18 years of age. Indian Pediatr. 1992;92:1203-82; Agarwal DK, Agarwal KN. Physical growth in affluent Indian children (birth to 6 years). Indian Pediatr. 1994;31:377-413; Agarwal KN, Saxena A, Bansal AK, et al. Physical growth assessment in adolescence. Indian Pediatr. 2001;38:1217-35.

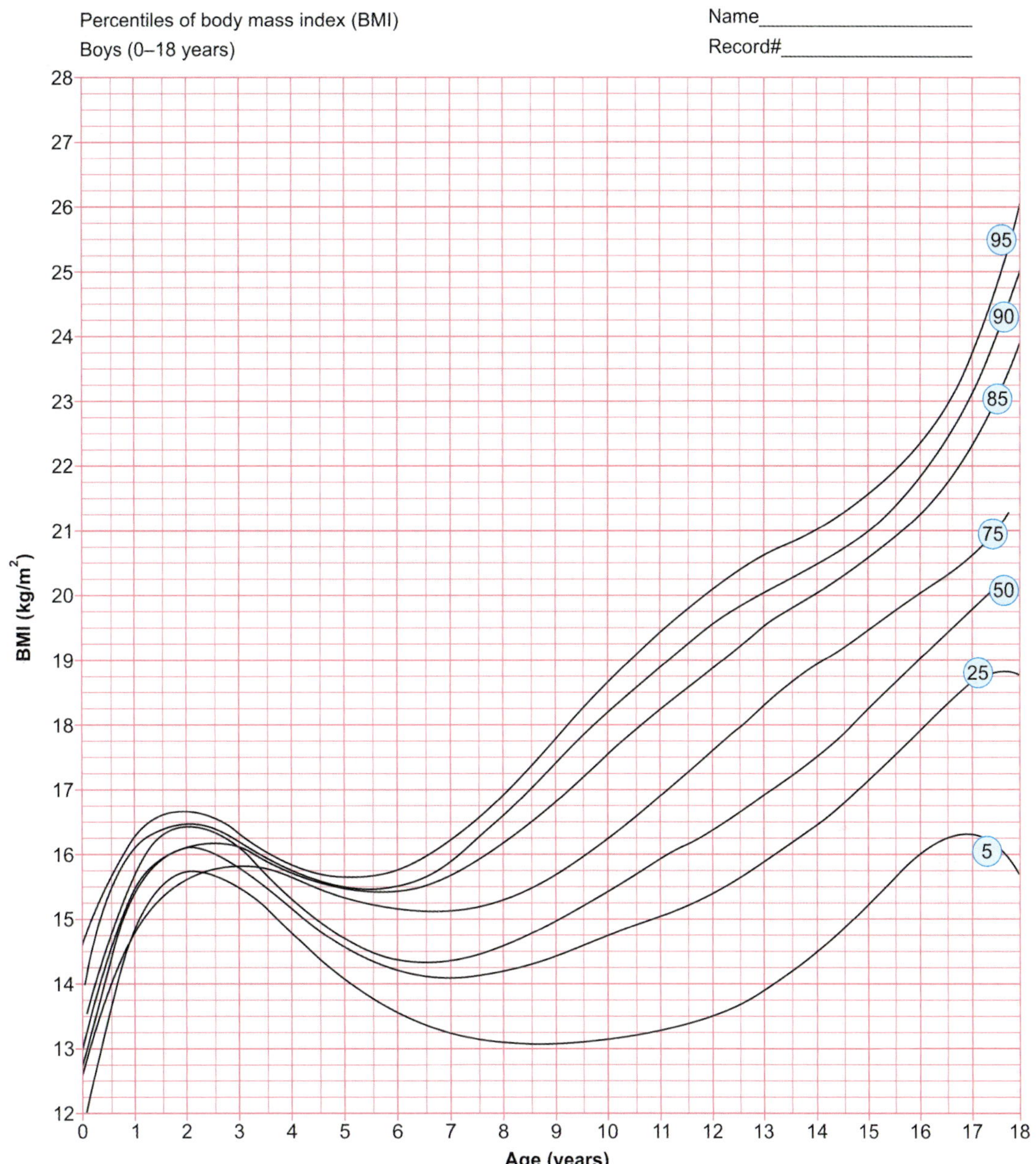

Fig. 3.2.12: The growth curves (data) for body mass index for boys from birth to 17 years.

Source: Agarwal KN, Agarwal DK, Upadhaya SK, et al. Physical and sexual growth pattern of affluent Indian children from 5 to 18 years of age. Indian Pediatr. 1992;92:1203-82; Agarwal DK, Agarwal KN. Physical growth in affluent Indian children (birth to 6 years). Indian Pediatr. 1994;31:377-413; Agarwal KN, Saxena A, Bansal AK, et al. Physical growth assessment in adolescence. Indian Pediatr. 2001;38:1217-35.

example, the 50th centile means that 49% of the observations are below and 50% above that observation. A child's growth parameters may be on the centile line or between two centile lines. Conventionally, for all parameters, the 3rd and 97th percentiles are the lowest, and highest in 94% of observations. Any child with parameters below or above these limits or those who cross percentiles after 2 years of age needs careful evaluation.

Examples

- If height and weight are consistently on the 60th percentile line until a child is 5 years old, and then if the height has dropped to the 30th percentile at age 6, it might indicate that there is a growth problem (catch down-retardation of growth) because the child is not following his or her previous growth pattern. This indicates disease.
- A boy with height in the 40th percentile and weight in the 85th percentile (he is taller than 40% of the kids of his age, but weighs more than 85% of kids of his age)—this might be a health problem (overweight/obesity). On the other hand, if he is in the 85th percentile for height and weight and follows that pattern consistently over time, it usually means that he is a normal child, just larger than average.

Z-scores

It is calculated as below:

$$\text{Z-score} = \frac{\text{Observed value - Median reference}}{\text{SD of reference population}}$$

A value of −2 *Z*-score corresponds to the 3rd percentile. *Z* scores are labeled as 1, 2, 3, −1, −2, and −3. These indicate how far points are above or below the mean (*Z*-score 0). A range of ±2 *Z* scores includes 95.4% of all observations and is the conventionally accepted limits of normality.

Choice of Growth Curve for Indian Children

Table 3.2.2 provides the summary of the details of physical growth in Indian children related to weight and height gain. **Table 3.2.3** provides a summary of the changes in head circumference at different ages in children.

The data on affluent Indian children were collected during 1989-1991 by the Nutrition Foundation of India from birth to 5 years (seven states); only full term with birth weight more than or equal to 2,500 g (boys 433 and girls 346) were followed during the first year of life at 3, 6, 9, and 12 months of age with minimum of three readings for every infant (cohort I). In cohort II, from 12 months to 5 years of age, 1,011 boys and 874 girls were followed on their birthday and 6 monthly with minimum of three measurements for each child up to 72 months of age. Children had received exclusive breast milk for 3-4 months of life in cohorts I and II (as prevalent in those years).

Table 3.2.2: Growth pattern in infancy and early childhood: summary of changes in weight and height.

Anthropometric measures of normal full-term newborns
• *Birth weight:* 2.5–4.0 kg • *Length:* 50 cm (approximately) • *Head circumference:* 34–35 cm
Weight gain
Neonates generally lose 5%–8% (maximum being 10%) weight during first 2–3 days of life, which is regained by the 10th day. *Average daily weight gain during*
• *First 3 months:* 30 g • *3–6 months:* 20 g (birth weight doubles by 5–6 months of age) • *6–9 months:* 15 g • *9–12 months:* 12 g (birth weight triples by the first birthday) • *1–3 years:* 8 g (around 3 kg/year). Birth weight quadruples by 2 years of age • *4–6 years:* 6 g (around 2 kg/year); this rate of gain continues till the onset of puberty
Length/height gain (height velocity)
• *Birth to 3 months:* 3.5 cm/month • *3–6 months:* 2.0 cm/month • *6–9 months:* 1.5 cm/month • *9–12 months:* 1.2 cm/month • *1–3 years:* 1.0 cm/month • *4–6 years:* 5 cm/year (at 4 years = 100 cm; double of birth length)
Gains in length
• *During the first year of life:* 25 cm • *During the second year of life:* 12.5 cm • *During the third year of life:* 7.5–10 cm • 7 cm/year at 3–4 years • 6 cm/year at 5–6 years • 5 cm/year till puberty • In immediate prepubertal period, growth velocity slows down before the pubertal spurt begins (adrenarche)
Abnormal growth
• Less than 7 cm/year for less than 4 years of age • Less than 6 cm/year for 4–6 years • Less than 4.5 cm/year for 6 years–onset of puberty

Table 3.2.3: Summary of changes in head circumference.

At birth	35 cm
Birth to 3 months	2 cm/month
3–6 months	1 cm/month
6–9 months	0.5 cm/month
9–12 months	0.25 cm/month
On first birthday	46–47 cm, 35% increase from birth size
At 2 years age	48 cm
At 5 years	50–51 cm
12 years	52 cm

The Indian Council of Medical Research (ICMR) cross-sectional data for physical growth and sexual development for 5–17 years in girls and 5–18 years in boys (9 states, 23 schools, 12,893 boys, and 10,941 girls), on affluent Indian children, were collected during 1989–1991. These two data sets were collected around the same time on the affluent Indian children—"birth to adolescence." These data sets on physical growth and sexual development (birth to 18 years of age) continue to serve as the baseline reference data for assessing physical growth and sexual development, assessed by the same measurers at all centers for seeing secular trend in height and percentile of children becoming overweight and obese. These "growth charts" **(*see* Figs. 3.2.7 to 3.2.12; Tables 3.2.4 to 3.2.13)** give height, weight, skull circumference, and BMI for age and gender.

World Health Organization Multicenter Growth Reference Study (See also Chapter 3.3)

The World Health Organization (WHO) growth data, in India, were collected from South Delhi area and pooled in the international data. The WHO Multicenter Growth Reference Study (MGRS) was undertaken between 1997 and 2003 to generate new growth curves for assessing the growth of infants and young children around the world. The MGRS collected primary growth data and related information from approximately 8,500 children from widely different ethnic backgrounds and cultural settings (Brazil, Ghana, India, Norway, Oman, and the United States). The new growth curves are expected to provide a single international standard that represents the best description of physiological growth for all children from birth to 5 years of age and to establish the breastfed infant as the normative model for growth and development. These growth charts depart from the growth reference model in several ways. Children from the six countries provided the data measurements, which were not representative of their country of residence, and were selected on the basis of sociodemographic criteria and child's nutrition as per the WHO guidelines.

Comparing Agarwal and Khadilkar Data Sets (See also Chapters 3 and 4)

Comparing Agarwal et al. school data ICMR against recently available Khadilkar et al. data set, the changes in height vary from 1% to 2.5% among boys and 1% to 3% in girls. The median final height in boys is higher by 0.7 cm but the 97th percentile is higher by 1.7 cm, whereas in girls, the median is same but the 97th percentile is higher by 2.4 cm. The changes in weight vary from 20% to 29% among boys and 18% to 25% among girls. Therefore, Khadilkar et al. data showed marginal secular trend for height with marked increase in obesity, which is in line with the data from the Western countries, such as the United Kingdom. Their observations are similar to those recently published by Marwaha et al. Khadilkar and Marwaha data sets of school children have important health implications, alarming increase in obesity, which needs immediate action to control or prevent and create nationwide awareness.

Table 3.2.4: Weight (kg) percentiles for girls (birth to 6 years of age): affluent Indians.

	Percentiles								
Age (months)	***3rd***	***5th***	***10th***	***25th***	***50th***	***75th***	***90th***	***95th***	***97th***
0	2.6	2.6	2.7	2.9	3.1	3.4	3.7	3.8	3.9
3	4.4	4.5	4.8	5.2	5.6	6.0	6.4	6.6	6.7
6	5.6	5.7	5.9	6.4	6.9	7.4	7.9	8.2	8.4
9	6.9	7.0	7.3	7.5	8.0	8.5	8.9	9.2	9.5
12	7.8	8.0	8.2	8.6	9.1	9.7	10.0	10.4	10.6
18	8.7	9.0	9.5	10.0	10.5	11.4	11.8	12.1	12.4
24	9.4	9.6	10.0	10.9	11.6	12.2	13.0	13.5	13.9
30	9.9	10.2	10.6	11.7	12.5	13.0	13.9	14.4	14.8
36	10.5	10.8	11.4	12.4	13.4	14.2	15.0	15.7	16.4
42	11.4	11.8	12.1	13.2	14.2	15.2	16.5	17.2	17.8
48	11.9	12.2	12.9	13.9	15.0	16.5	17.5	18.2	18.9
54	12.9	13.3	14.0	14.8	16.0	17.5	18.7	19.7	20.0
60	13.4	13.9	14.5	15.4	17.0	18.4	19.9	20.0	21.0
66	14.2	14.9	15.6	16.2	17.9	19.2	20.1	21.0	21.4

Table 3.2.10: Weight (kg) percentiles for girls (6–17 years): affluent Indians.

Age (years)	*Percentiles*					
	3rd	*5th*	*25th*	*50th*	*75th*	*97th*
6.0	14.1	15.2	16.4	17.8	19.2	23.7
6.5	14.4	15.5	16.9	18.3	19.9	25.4
7.0	14.8	15.8	17.3	19.0	20.9	27.5
7.5	15.3	16.2	18.0	19.9	22.2	29.8
8.0	15.9	16.4	18.7	20.8	23.6	32.3
8.5	16.4	16.8	19.6	22.0	25.3	34.9
9.0	17.1	17.6	20.7	23.5	27.2	37.7
9.5	18.3	18.5	22.1	25.1	29.3	40.5
10.0	19.5	19.7	23.6	26.9	31.4	43.4
10.5	20.9	21.0	25.3	28.9	33.7	46.4
11.0	22.3	22.4	27.1	30.9	36.0	49.3
11.5	23.7	24.0	28.9	32.9	38.4	52.2
12.0	25.1	25.6	30.8	35.0	40.7	55.1
12.5	26.5	27.2	32.6	37.1	42.9	57.9
13.0	27.9	28.9	34.5	39.1	45.1	60.7
13.5	29.3	30.6	36.2	41.0	47.1	63.2
14.0	30.7	32.1	37.8	42.7	48.9	65.7
14.5	32.1	33.6	39.3	44.3	50.5	67.9
15.0	33.4	35.0	40.6	45.7	51.8	70.0
15.5	34.6	36.2	41.7	46.8	52.9	71.8
16.0	35.7	37.3	42.5	47.7	53.6	73.3
16.5	36.7	38.1	43.0	48.2	54.0	74.6
17.0	37.6	38.7	43.3	48.4	53.9	75.6

Table 3.2.11: Height (cm) percentiles for girls (6–17 years): affluent Indians.

Age (years)	*Percentiles*					
	3rd	*5th*	*25th*	*50th*	*75th*	*97th*
6.0	102.1	104.5	108.8	112.5	115.9	123.3
6.5	104.5	107.0	111.1	114.9	118.4	126.0
7.0	107.1	109.4	113.7	117.4	121.3	129.3
7.5	109.7	111.6	116.4	120.3	124.4	132.8
8.0	112.3	113.9	119.3	123.2	127.5	136.4
8.5	115.0	116.2	122.2	126.2	130.7	139.8
9.0	117.8	118.8	125.1	129.2	133.8	143.1
9.5	120.6	121.4	128.0	132.3	136.9	146.2
10.0	123.4	124.1	130.8	135.2	139.8	149.0
10.5	126.1	126.9	133.7	138.1	142.7	151.7
11.0	128.8	129.7	136.4	140.9	145.4	154.2
11.5	131.4	132.4	139.0	143.5	147.9	156.5
12.0	133.9	135.0	141.5	146.0	150.3	158.5
12.5	136.3	137.5	143.8	148.3	152.5	160.4
13.0	138.5	139.8	145.9	150.4	154.4	162.1
13.5	140.6	141.9	147.8	152.2	156.2	163.5
14.0	142.4	143.8	149.4	153.8	157.6	164.7
14.5	144.1	145.4	150.8	155.1	158.8	165.8
15.0	145.5	146.6	151.8	156.0	159.7	166.5
15.5	146.6	147.5	152.6	156.6	160.4	167.1
16.0	147.5	148.0	152.9	156.8	160.4	167.4
16.5	148.0	148.1	152.9	156.5	160.5	167.6
17.0	148.3	148.5	153.0	157.0	160.5	168.0

Redoing the curves in response to increasing weight alone will have the effect of "normalizing" the weight gains you are seeing at the higher end of the scale since the definition of "normal" weight will shift to the right, potentially putting more children who today are classified as overweight into the normal weight category. At the bottom of the scale, some children who are today classified as normal weight will be classified as underweight. On both the high and low ends of the scale, creating new reference curves with these changes may not be beneficial from a public health perspective.

Second, Khadilkar et al. data line for 3rd centile flattens after 14 years of age (Agarwal et al. and Marwaha et al.). Third, it is important to take lesson from the "methods including the data source in construction of the Centers for Disease Control and Prevention 2,000 growth charts," as weight data from the National Health and Nutrition Examination Survey (NHANES) III (1988–1994) were excluded from the weight for age and BMI-for-age curves because of a secular trend in body weight that occurred between NHANES II (1976–1980) and NHANES III.

RECOMMENDATIONS

Presently, the choice remains using Indian Academy of Pediatrics recommended 2007 growth charts based on data (birth to 18 years of age) by Agarwal et al. This was also recommended in growth chart evaluation study by Khadgawat et al. The WHO curves may be used up to 2 years of age to assess growth as practiced in the United States. It is important to note that in spite of unprecedented economic growth since 1991, Indian women remain short by 5.5 cm as compared to the average height, in 54 developing countries.

Table 3.2.12: Weight (kg) percentiles for boys (6–18 years): affluent Indians.

Age (years)	Percentiles					
	3rd	5th	25th	50th	75th	97th
6.0	15.2	15.7	18.0	19.0	20.7	25.4
6.5	15.7	16.4	18.6	20.0	21.9	27.7
7.0	16.2	16.9	19.4	21.0	22.9	29.7
7.5	16.8	17.5	20.0	22.0	23.9	31.6
8.0	17.5	18.0	20.7	22.6	25.0	33.5
8.5	18.2	18.6	21.3	23.5	26.3	35.5
9.0	19.2	19.4	22.0	24.4	27.7	37.7
9.5	19.9	20.2	22.9	25.6	29.4	40.1
10.0	20.9	21.2	24.1	27.0	31.3	42.7
10.5	21.9	22.3	25.5	28.7	33.4	45.4
11.0	22.9	23.5	27.1	30.6	35.6	48.2
11.5	24.1	24.9	28.9	32.7	37.9	51.1
12.0	25.3	26.3	30.7	34.8	40.3	54.1
12.5	26.7	27.8	32.7	37.1	42.7	57.1
13.0	28.1	29.3	34.7	39.4	45.1	60.0
13.5	29.6	31.0	36.8	41.8	47.6	63.0
14.0	31.2	32.7	38.8	44.1	50.0	65.9
14.5	32.9	34.5	40.9	46.3	52.4	68.7
15.0	34.6	36.3	42.8	48.5	54.6	71.4
15.5	36.5	38.1	44.7	50.5	56.8	73.9
16.0	38.5	40.0	46.5	52.4	58.8	76.3
16.5	40.6	41.9	48.1	54.0	60.6	78.5
17.0	42.8	43.9	50.0	55.5	62.3	80.5
17.5	45.2	45.8	52.0	57.2	63.7	82.2
18.0	47.6	47.8	54.0	58.6	64.9	83.6

Table 3.2.13: Height (cm) percentiles for boys (6–18 years): affluent Indians.

Age (years)	Percentiles					
	3rd	5th	25th	50th	75th	97th
6.0	103.7	105.5	112.0	114.2	118.0	125.9
6.5	106.1	107.5	113.5	117.3	120.7	128.4
7.0	108.5	109.8	115.9	119.7	123.0	130.8
7.5	110.9	111.3	117.8	121.6	125.2	133.2
8.0	113.3	114.4	119.7	123.6	127.4	135.8
8.5	115.2	116.2	121.9	125.7	129.8	138.5
9.0	118.0	118.5	124.2	128.2	132.5	141.4
9.5	120.3	120.9	126.7	130.8	135.3	144.5
10.0	122.7	123.4	129.4	133.6	138.3	147.7
10.5	125.1	125.9	132.4	136.6	141.5	151.0
11.0	127.5	128.5	135.6	139.6	144.7	154.3
11.5	129.9	131.1	138.0	142.7	147.9	157.5
12.0	132.4	133.8	141.0	145.8	151.1	160.8
12.5	134.9	136.5	143.9	148.9	154.2	163.9
13.0	137.4	139.2	146.8	152.0	157.3	166.9
13.5	140.0	141.8	149.7	154.9	160.2	169.7
14.0	142.6	144.5	152.4	157.6	162.9	172.7
14.5	145.2	147.2	155.0	160.2	164.4	174.7
15.0	148.0	149.8	157.4	162.5	167.7	176.8
15.5	150.8	152.4	159.6	164.6	169.6	178.5
16.0	153.6	154.9	161.6	166.3	171.2	179.8
16.5	156.6	157.4	163.3	167.7	172.4	180.7
17.0	159.6	159.8	165.0	168.7	173.1	181.2
17.5	162.7	163.1	167.5	169.3	173.4	181.1
18.0	161.0	163.5	168.8	169.8	173.4	181.6

The Indian affluent children at 18 years of age are still shorter than the NCHS/WHO data. Thus, we must examine our children in nationally collected growth data sets, as calculated BMI values are also different as compared to the WHO/NCHS values.

BIBLIOGRAPHY

1. Agarwal DK, Agarwal KN. Physical growth in affluent Indian children (birth to 6 years). Indian Pediatr. 1994;31:377-413.
2. Agarwal KN. The growth infancy to adolescence, 3rd edition. New Delhi: CBS Publishers; 2015. pp. 1-30, 115-144.
3. Agarwal KN, Agarwal DK, Upadhaya SK, et al. Physical and sexual growth pattern of affluent Indian children from 5 to 18 years of age. Indian Pediatr. 1992;92:1203-82.
4. Buyken A, Karaolis Danckert N, Renner T, et al. Effects of breastfeeding on trajectories of body fat and BMI throughout childhood. Obesity (Silver Spring). 2008;16:389-95.
5. Gupta P. Anthropometry: assessment of growth. In: Gupta P (Ed). Clinical methods in pediatrics, 2nd edition. New Delhi: CBS Publishers; 2011. pp. 58-110.
6. Khadgawat R, Dabadghao P, Mehrotra RN, et al. Growth charts for evaluation of Indian children. Indian Pediatr. 1998;35:859-65.
7. Khadilkar VV, Khadilkar AV, Cole TJ, et al. Cross sectional growth curves for height, weight, and body mass index for affluent Indian children, 2007. Indian Pediatr. 2009;46:477-85.
8. Kuczmarsi RJ, Ogden CL, Guo SS, et al. 2000 CDC growth charts for the United States: methods and development. Vital Health Stat 11. 2002;(246):1-190.
9. Marwaha RK, Tandon N, Ganie MA, et al. Nationwide reference data for height, weight and body mass index of Indian school children. Natl Med J India. 2011;24:269-77.
10. WHO Multicenteric Growth Reference Study Group. WHO child growth standards based on length/height, weight and age. Acta Pediatr Suppl. 2006;450:76-85.

3.3 World Health Organization Under-5 Growth Standards 2006

Vaman Khadilkar

INTRODUCTION

Growth charts are an essential component of the pediatric tool kit. Their value resides in helping us to determine the degree to which physiological needs for growth and development are met during the critical childhood period. Beyond their usefulness in assessing children's nutritional status, many governments and United Nation agencies rely on growth charts to measure the general well-being of populations, formulate health and related policies, plan interventions, and monitor their effectiveness.

The relative magnitude of different measures of nutritional status is affected by the choice of reference charts used. In April 2006, World Health Organization (WHO) released child growth standards for children up to the age of 5 years, to provide a multiethnic benchmark for breastfed children. The standards are derived from children who were raised in environments that minimized constraints to growth, such as poor diet and infection. In addition, their mothers followed healthy practices, such as breastfeeding and not smoking during and after pregnancy. Because WHO standards depict physiological human growth under optimal environmental conditions, they provide an improved tool for assessing growth. These charts thus are prescriptive standards and not descriptive references.

These standards provide an opportunity to redefine and revitalize actions to promote optimal child growth, foster the adoption of "best practices," such as incorporating height and body mass index (BMI) to assess the dual burden of under- and overnutrition (stunting and overweight), and provide coherence between national and international infant feeding guidelines that recommend breastfeeding as the optimal source of nutrition during infancy. Thus, these charts are recommended for assessing the pattern of infant growth and harmonize growth assessment systems within and between the countries.

An important feature of the study that makes it attractive as a basis for an internationally applicable standard is that it included children from a diverse set of countries: Brazil, Ghana, India, Norway, Oman, and the United States. By selecting privileged, healthy populations, the study reduced the impact of environmental variation. Another key characteristic of the new standards is that they explicitly identify breastfeeding as the biological norm and establish the breastfed child as the normative model for growth and development.

The method used to construct the WHO standards generally relied on the Box-Cox power exponential distribution and the final selected models simplified to the least means square model.

WHY NEW GROWTH CHARTS?

The linear growth patterns of these highly selected, healthy infants were strikingly similar between countries, supporting the view that they represent a standard against which the growth of all children can be assessed, wherever, they live and, however, they are fed. Government of India has given a directive to use WHO growth charts for all children under the age of 5 years, and Indian Academy of Pediatrics has accepted these standards for children under 5-years-old.

WHERE TO GET WHO GROWTH CHARTS?

The list of charts available is as follows:
- Length or/height-for-age
- Weight-for-age
- Weight-for-length
- Weight-for-height
  - Body mass index-for-age
  - Head circumference-for-age
  - Arm circumference-for-age
  - Subscapular skinfold-for-age
  - Triceps skinfold-for-age
  - Motor development milestones

World Health Organization growth charts can be downloaded from *http://www.who.int/childgrowth/standards/en/*.

INTERPRETATION OF WHO CHARTS AND CUT OFFS

Doctors and health-care workers find it difficult to interpret various cutoffs for the diagnosis of underweight, overweight, stunting, wasting, etc. These have therefore been clearly spelt out in the new WHO multicenter growth reference study and are given in **Tables 3.3.1 and 3.3.2**. These make it easy for

Table 3.3.1: Correlation between percentiles and *Z*-scores for World Health Organization charts.

Z-score	*Exact percentiles*	*Rounded percentiles*
0	50	50
–1	15.9	15
–2	2.3	3
–3	0.1	1
1	84.1	85
2	97.7	97
3	99.9	99

Table 3.3.2: Growth parameters and their interpretation for the World Health Organization charts.

Z-score (percentile)	*Length/height-for-age*	*Weight-for-age*	*BMI-for-age*
>3 (99)	May be abnormal	May be abnormal (use BMI)	Obese
>2 (97)	Normal	Use BMI	Overweight
>1 (85)	Normal	Use BMI	Risk of overweight
0 (50)	Normal	Use BMI	Normal
<-1 (15)	Normal	Normal	Normal
<-2 (3)	Stunted	Underweight	Wasted
<-3 (1)	Severely stunted	Severely underweight	Severely wasted

(BMI: body mass index)

Table 3.3.3: Weight (kg) by age of boys and girls aged 0–2 years (World Health Organization).

Age in months	*Percentiles for boys*							*Percentiles for girls*						
	3rd	*5th*	*25th*	*50th*	*75th*	*95th*	*97th*	*3rd*	*5th*	*25th*	*50th*	*75th*	*95th*	*97th*
0	2.5	2.6	3.0	3.3	3.7	4.2	4.3	2.4	2.5	2.9	3.2	3.6	4.0	4.2
3	5.1	5.2	5.9	6.4	6.9	7.7	7.9	4.6	4.7	5.4	5.8	6.4	7.2	7.4
6	6.4	6.6	7.4	7.9	8.5	9.5	9.7	5.8	6.0	6.7	7.3	7.9	8.9	9.2
9	7.2	7.4	8.3	8.9	9.6	10.6	10.9	6.6	6.8	7.6	8.2	8.9	10.1	10.4
12	7.8	8.1	9.0	9.6	10.4	11.5	11.8	7.1	7.3	8.2	8.9	9.7	11.0	11.3
15	8.4	8.6	9.6	10.3	11.1	12.3	12.7	7.7	7.9	8.8	9.6	10.4	11.8	12.2
18	8.9	9.1	10.1	10.9	11.8	13.1	13.5	8.2	8.4	9.4	10.2	11.1	12.6	13.0
21	9.3	9.6	10.7	11.5	12.5	13.9	14.3	8.7	8.9	10.0	10.9	11.8	13.4	13.8
24	9.8	10.1	11.3	12.2	13.1	14.7	15.1	9.2	9.4	10.6	11.5	12.5	14.2	14.6

Table 3.3.4: Weight (kg) by age percentiles of boys and girls aged 2–5 years (World Health Organization).

Age		*Percentiles for boys*							*Percentiles for girls*						
Years	*Months*	*3rd*	*5th*	*25th*	*50th*	*75th*	*95th*	*97th*	*3rd*	*5th*	*25th*	*50th*	*75th*	*95th*	*97th*
2	0	9.8	10.1	11.3	12.2	13.1	14.7	15.1	9.2	9.4	10.6	11.5	12.5	14.2	14.6
2	6	10.7	11.0	12.3	13.3	14.4	16.2	16.6	10.1	10.4	11.7	12.7	13.8	15.7	16.2
3	0	11.4	11.8	13.2	14.3	15.6	17.5	18.0	11.0	11.3	12.7	13.9	15.1	17.3	17.8
3	6	12.2	12.5	14.1	15.3	16.7	18.9	19.4	11.8	12.1	13.7	15.0	16.4	18.8	19.5
4	0	12.9	13.3	15.0	16.3	17.8	20.2	20.9	12.5	12.9	14.7	16.1	17.7	20.4	21.1
4	6	13.6	14.0	15.9	17.3	19.0	21.6	22.3	13.2	13.7	15.6	17.2	18.9	22.0	22.8
5	0	14.3	14.7	16.7	18.3	20.1	23.0	23.8	14.0	14.4	16.5	18.2	20.2	23.5	24.4

the practicing pediatrician and health-care worker to follow as a guideline for management and referral **(Tables 3.3.3 to 3.3.8 and Figs. 3.3.1 to 3.3.5)**. It is important to note that the overweight and obesity BMI cutoffs for children under the age of 5 years (above +1 or the 85th percentile is risk for overweight, +2 or the 97th percentile is overweight, and above +3 or the 99th percentile is obese) are higher than those for older children (above +1 or the 85th percentile is overweight,

Table 3.3.5: Weight (kg) by age of boys and girls aged 5–10 years (World Health Organization).

Age (years)	Percentiles								
	3rd	5th	15th	25th	50th	75th	85th	95th	97th
Boys									
5	14.3	14.7		16.7	18.3	20.1		23.0	23.8
6	16.1	16.6	17.9	18.8	20.5	22.5	23.6	25.8	26.7
7	17.9	18.4	19.9	20.9	22.9	25.2	26.5	29.1	30.1
8	19.8	20.4	22.0	23.1	25.4	28.1	29.7	32.7	34.0
9	21.6	22.3	24.2	25.4	28.1	31.3	33.2	36.9	38.6
10	23.6	24.4	26.6	28.0	31.2	34.9	37.3	41.9	43.9
Girls									
5	14.0	14.4		16.5	18.2	20.2		23.5	24.4
6	15.5	16.0	17.4	18.3	20.2	22.4	23.7	26.2	27.3
7	17.0	17.6	19.2	20.2	22.4	24.9	26.5	29.5	30.8
8	18.9	19.5	21.3	22.5	25.0	28.0	29.8	33.4	34.9
9	21.1	21.8	23.9	25.3	28.2	31.7	33.9	38.1	40.0
10	23.7	24.5	26.9	28.5	31.9	35.9	38.5	43.5	45.7

Table 3.3.6: Length (cm) by age of boys and girls aged 0–2 years (World Health Organization).

Age (months)	Percentiles for boys							Percentiles for girls						
	3rd	5th	25th	50th	75th	95th	97th	3rd	5th	25th	50th	75th	95th	97th
0	46.3	46.8	48.6	49.9	51.2	53.0	53.4	45.6	46.1	47.9	49.1	50.4	52.2	52.7
3	57.6	58.1	60.1	61.4	62.8	64.8	65.3	55.8	56.3	58.4	59.8	61.2	63.3	63.8
6	63.6	64.1	66.2	67.6	69.1	71.1	71.6	61.5	62.0	64.2	65.7	67.3	69.5	70.0
9	67.7	68.3	70.5	72.0	73.5	75.7	76.2	65.6	66.2	68.5	70.1	71.8	74.1	74.7
12	71.3	71.8	74.1	75.7	77.4	79.7	80.2	69.2	69.8	72.3	74.0	75.8	78.3	78.9
15	74.4	75.0	77.4	79.1	80.9	83.3	83.9	72.4	73.0	75.7	77.5	79.4	82.0	82.7
18	77.2	77.8	80.4	82.3	84.1	86.7	87.3	75.2	75.9	78.7	80.7	82.7	85.5	86.2
21	79.7	80.4	83.2	85.1	87.1	89.9	90.5	77.9	78.6	81.6	83.7	85.7	88.7	89.4
24	82.1	82.8	85.8	87.8	89.9	92.8	93.6	80.3	81.1	84.2	86.4	88.6	91.7	92.5

Table 3.3.7: Height-for-age percentiles for boys and girls 2–5 years of age (World Health Organization).

Age		Percentiles for boys							Percentiles for girls						
Years	Months	3rd	5th	25th	50th	75th	95th	97th	3rd	5th	25th	50th	75th	95th	97th
2	0	81.4	82.1	85.1	87.1	89.2	92.1	92.9	79.6	80.4	83.5	85.7	87.9	91.0	91.8
2	6	85.5	86.3	89.6	91.9	94.2	97.5	98.3	84.0	84.9	88.3	90.7	93.1	96.5	97.3
3	0	89.1	90.0	93.6	96.1	98.6	102.2	103.1	87.9	88.8	92.5	95.1	97.6	101.3	102.2
3	6	92.4	93.3	97.2	99.9	102.5	106.4	107.3	91.4	92.4	96.3	99.0	101.8	105.7	106.7
4	0	95.4	96.4	100.5	103.3	106.2	110.2	111.2	94.6	95.6	99.8	102.7	105.6	109.8	110.8
4	6	98.4	99.4	103.7	106.7	109.6	113.9	115.0	97.6	98.7	103.1	106.2	109.2	113.6	114.7
5	0	101.2	102.3	106.8	110.0	113.1	117.6	118.7	100.5	101.6	106.2	109.4	112.6	117.2	118.4

Table 3.3.8: Height (cm) by age of boys and girls aged 5–10 years (World Health Organization).

	Height-for-age percentiles								
Age (years)	***3rd***	***5th***	***15th***	***25th***	***50th***	***75th***	***85th***	***95th***	***97th***
Boys									
5	101.2	102.3		106.8	110.0	113.1		117.6	118.7
6	106.7	107.8	110.8	112.6	116.0	119.3	121.1	124.1	125.2
7	111.8	113.0	116.3	118.2	121.7	125.3	127.2	130.4	131.7
8	116.6	118.0	121.4	123.5	127.3	131.1	133.1	136.6	137.9
9	121.3	122.7	126.3	128.5	132.6	136.6	138.8	142.5	143.9
10	125.8	127.3	131.2	133.5	137.8	142.1	144.4	148.3	149.8
Girls									
5	100.5	101.6		106.2	109.4	112.6		117.2	118.4
6	105.5	106.7	109.8	111.7	115.1	118.6	120.4	123.5	124.8
7	110.5	111.8	115.1	117.1	120.8	124.5	126.5	129.8	131.1
8	115.7	117.0	120.5	122.6	126.6	130.5	132.6	136.1	137.5
9	121.0	122.4	126.2	128.4	132.5	136.6	138.8	142.5	144.0
10	126.6	128.1	132.0	134.3	138.6	143.0	145.3	149.2	150.7

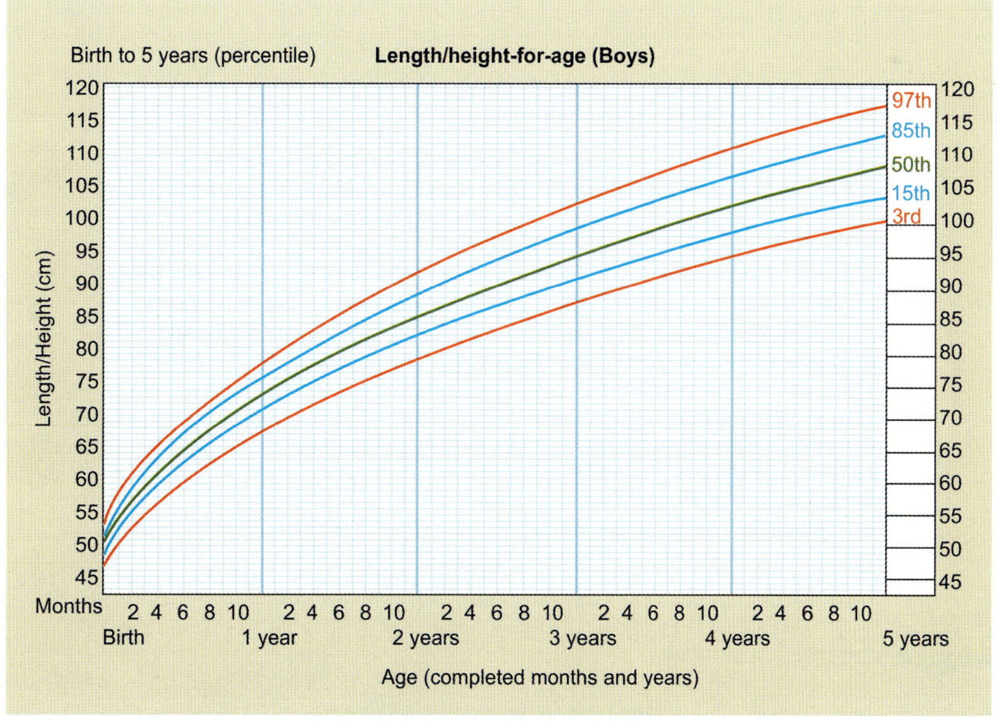

Fig. 3.3.1: Length/height-for-age (boys) (birth to 5 years, percentile).
Source: WHO multicenter growth reference study group. WHO child growth standards based on length/height, weight, and age. Acta Paediatr Suppl. 2006;450:76-85.

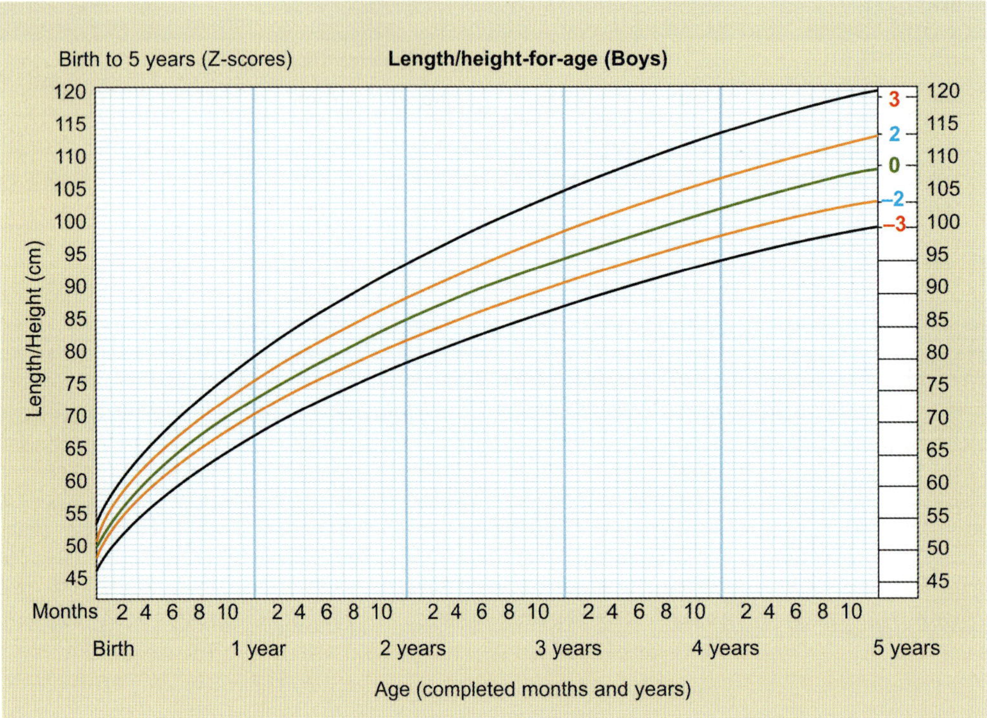

Fig. 3.3.2: Length/height-for-age (boys) (birth to 5 years, *Z*-scores).
Source: WHO multicenter growth reference study group. WHO child growth standards based on length/height, weight, and age. Acta Paediatr Suppl. 2006;450:76-85.

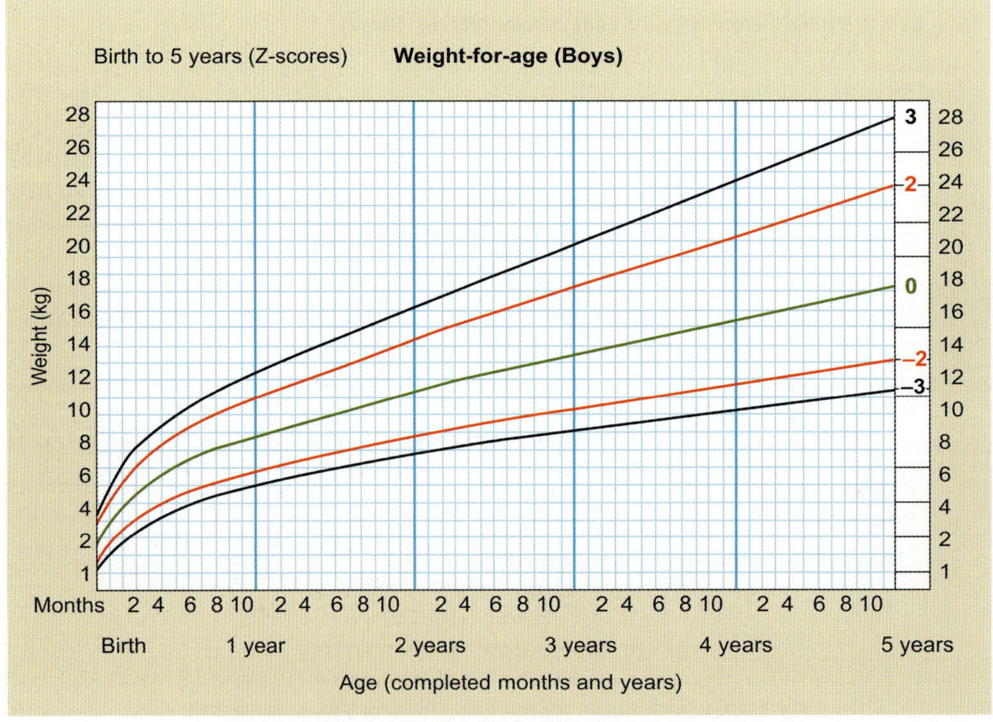

Fig. 3.3.3: Weight-for-age (boys) (birth to 5 years, *Z*-scores).
Source: WHO multicenter growth reference study group. WHO child growth standards based on length/height, weight, and age. Acta Paediatr Suppl. 2006;450:76-85.

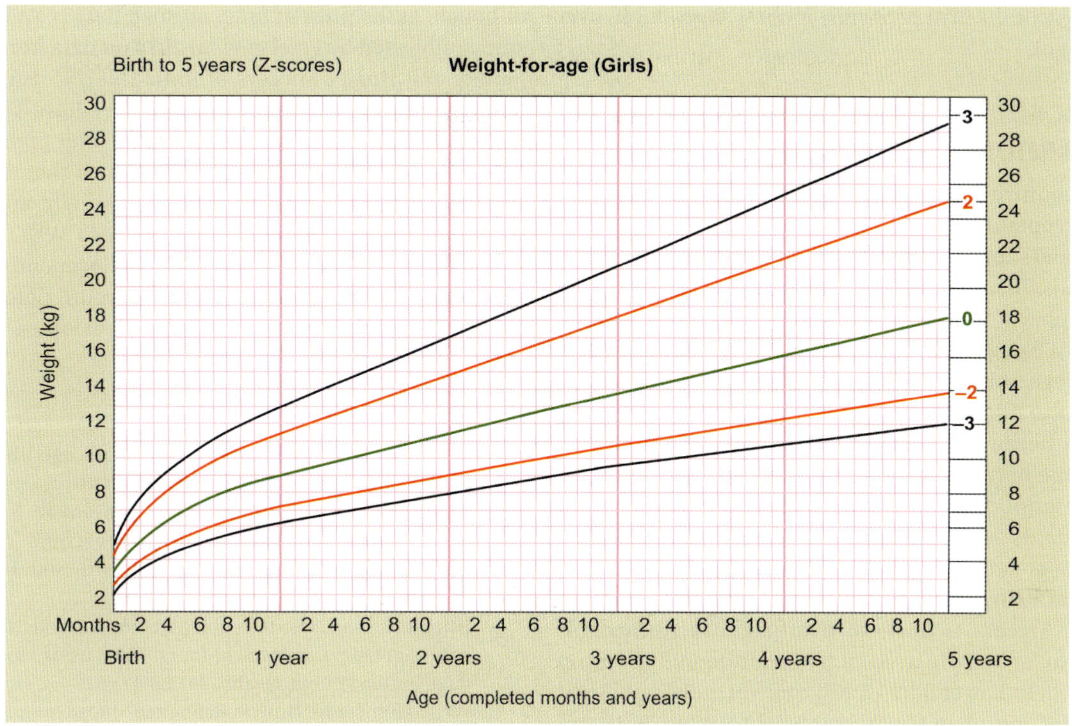

Fig. 3.3.4: Weight-for-age (girls) (birth to 5 years, *Z*-scores).

Source: WHO multicenter growth reference study group. WHO child growth standards based on length/height, weight, and age. Acta Paediatr Suppl. 2006;450:76-85.

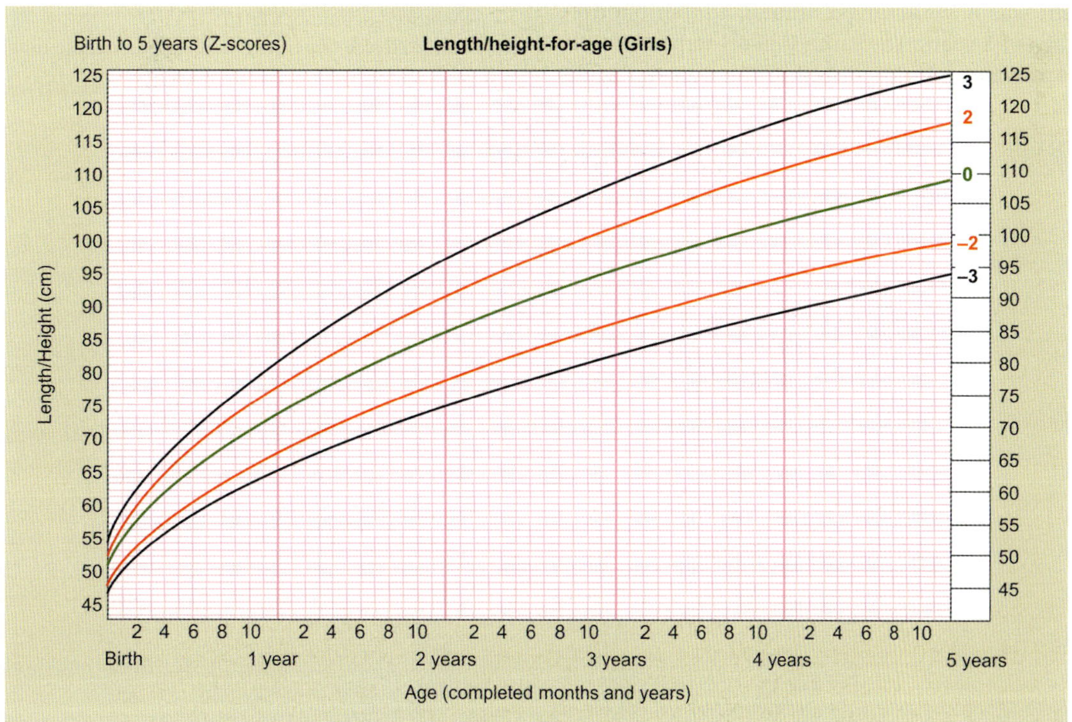

Fig. 3.3.5: Length/height-for-age (girls) (birth to 5 years, *Z*-scores).

Source: WHO multicenter growth reference study group. WHO child growth standards based on length/height, weight, and age. Acta Paediatr Suppl. 2006;450:76-85.

and above +2 or the 97th percentile is obese for children over 5 years of age).

APPLICABILITY OF WHO CHARTS IN INDIA AND AROUND THE WORLD

Different countries have adopted different policies on the use and acceptability of WHO growth charts. In the United States, Centers for Disease Control and Prevention (CDC) recommends the use of WHO charts up to the age of 2 years and CDC charts from 2 years to 19 years. In the United Kingdom, WHO growth charts are used for children up to 4 years of age, and thereafter, the British charts are used. The reason to adopt WHO growth charts for use in young children is because it establishes the growth of breastfed infants as the norm for growth; the WHO standards provide a better description of physiological growth in infancy, and WHO standards are based on a high-quality study designed explicitly for creating growth charts.

In India, using WHO growth charts for children under the age of 5 years is likely to overdiagnose stunting or underweight, or both. In a recent multicentric study done on 1,493 affluent Indian children on all zones of India, published by the author, the mean *z*-scores for height, weight, BMI, and weight-for-height [-0.75 (1.1), -0.59 (1.1), -0.19 (1.22), and -0.26 (1.18), respectively] were much below the WHO 2006 standards. The overall incidence of stunting was 13.6% and underweight was 8.5% amongst affluent Indian children under the age of 5 years. The same is likely to be higher in rural areas and in underprivileged urban areas of India, although, at the present time, no such data is available. In a study published by Patel et al. in 2014 on data from National Family and Health Surveys of India (NFHS) using 133,540 children under the age of 5 years, they have shown that Indian children are much shorter and lighter than the WHO 2006 standards. The study has also shown that the pattern of growth both in terms of height and weight are different in Indian children, when compared with WHO norms. It may therefore be more logical to use a lower cutoff of WHO standards (i.e. using the first rather than 3rd percentile) for referral to specialized centers in the developing countries, such as India.

BIBLIOGRAPHY

1. de Onis M. Growth curves for school age children and adolescents. Indian Pediatr. 2009;46(6):464-5.
2. Khadilkar VV, Khadilkar AV, Chiplonkar SA. Growth performance of affluent Indian preschool children: a comparison with the new WHO growth standard. Indian Pediatr. 2010;47(10):869-72.
3. Patel R, Unisa S. Construction of national standards of growth curves of height and weight for children using cross sectional data. Indian J Public Health. 2014;58(2):929.
4. WHO Multicentre Growth Reference Study Group. WHO child growth standards based on length/height, weight, and age. Acta Paediatr Suppl. 2006;450:76-85.
5. World Health Organization. Growth charts. [online] Available from http://www.cdc.gov/growthcharts/who_charts.htm. [Accessed September, 2018].
6. World Health Organization. Training course on child growth assessment. Geneva: WHO; 2008.

3.4 Revised Indian Academy of Pediatrics 2015 Growth Charts for 5–18 Years Old Indian Children

Vaman Khadilkar

INTRODUCTION

In 2006, the World Health Organization (WHO) published the first global growth standards for children under the age of 5 years, and Government of India and Indian Academy of Pediatrics (IAP) have adopted these standards for use in under five Indian children.

In older children, however, growth patterns differ among different populations of the world as nutritional, environmental, genetic factors, and timing of puberty seem to play a major role not only in the attainment of final height but also in the characteristics of the growth curves. Data from Asian countries such as China, Japan, Korea, and Saudi Arabia have shown that the growth of older non-European children is different, especially after puberty with a relatively attenuated pubertal growth spurt. Hence, it is necessary to have country-specific modern updated growth charts to monitor the growth of children beyond 5 years of age.

In January 2015, Indian Academy of Pediatrics (IAP) published revised growth charts for 5- to 18-year-old Indian children to replace earlier IAP charts. The growth references used in the old IAP charts were based on data collected in 1989, which is now nearly three decades old and hence outdated. The pattern of growth of a population changes with time; hence, it is recommended that references should be updated regularly so that they reflect current growth patterns of children and are representative of secular trends, especially in a country such as India where major changes in nutritional status of children have been witnessed.

PROCESS OF CONSTRUCTING INDIAN ACADEMY OF PEDIATRICS 2015 GROWTH CHARTS

The revised IAP 2015 growth charts have been produced from anthropometric data collected over last 10 years (2005–2014) on apparently healthy 87,022 (males 54,086, females 32,936) Indian children between the age of 5 and 18 years from upper and upper middle socioeconomic classes. These children are believed to express their genetic potential to their best as nutritional constraints are less, whereas data from lower socioeconomic class is likely to represent suboptimal growth. Data from 14 cities, that is, Agartala, Ahmedabad, Chandigarh, Chennai, Delhi, Hyderabad, Kochi, Kolkata, Madurai, Mumbai, Mysore, Pune, Raipur, and Surat, representing all five zones of India were included in these charts.

However, when data are collected from upper middle and upper socioeconomic classes, there are likely to be more overweight children in the study population; thus, there is a risk of normalizing higher weights. To reduce this impact of unhealthy weights (overweight and obesity) on growth curves, WHO recommends removing subjects that are above +2 standard deviation for weight for height in cross-sectional data. A total of 1.7% children with unhealthy weights were removed from analysis before producing the IAP 2015 growth charts taking care not to "normalize" overweight and obesity.

The most widely accepted Cole's least means square (LMS) method was used to compute smoothed growth curves for height, weight, and body mass index (BMI). For height and weight, the 3rd, 10th, 25th, 50th, 75th, 90th, and 97th percentiles were generated. For BMI, however, using International Obesity Task Force (IOTF) approach, the 3rd, 5th, 10th, 25th, 50th, 23 adult equivalent (as overweight cutoff) and 27 adult equivalent (as obesity cutoff) percentiles were generated as these are more appropriate cutoffs for overweight and obesity for Asian Indian population. As Indians are more prone to develop metabolic syndrome and other complications of obesity at a lower BMI as compared to the Caucasian population, lower BMI cutoffs are necessary (for overweight 23 instead of 25, and for obesity 27 instead of 30). IAP 2015 BMI charts are designed to show childhood equivalent of these cutoffs.

HEIGHT, WEIGHT, AND BODY MASS INDEX CHARTS

Figures 3.4.1 and 3.4.2 show IAP 2015 charts for height and weight for boys and girls from 5 to 18 years, respectively.

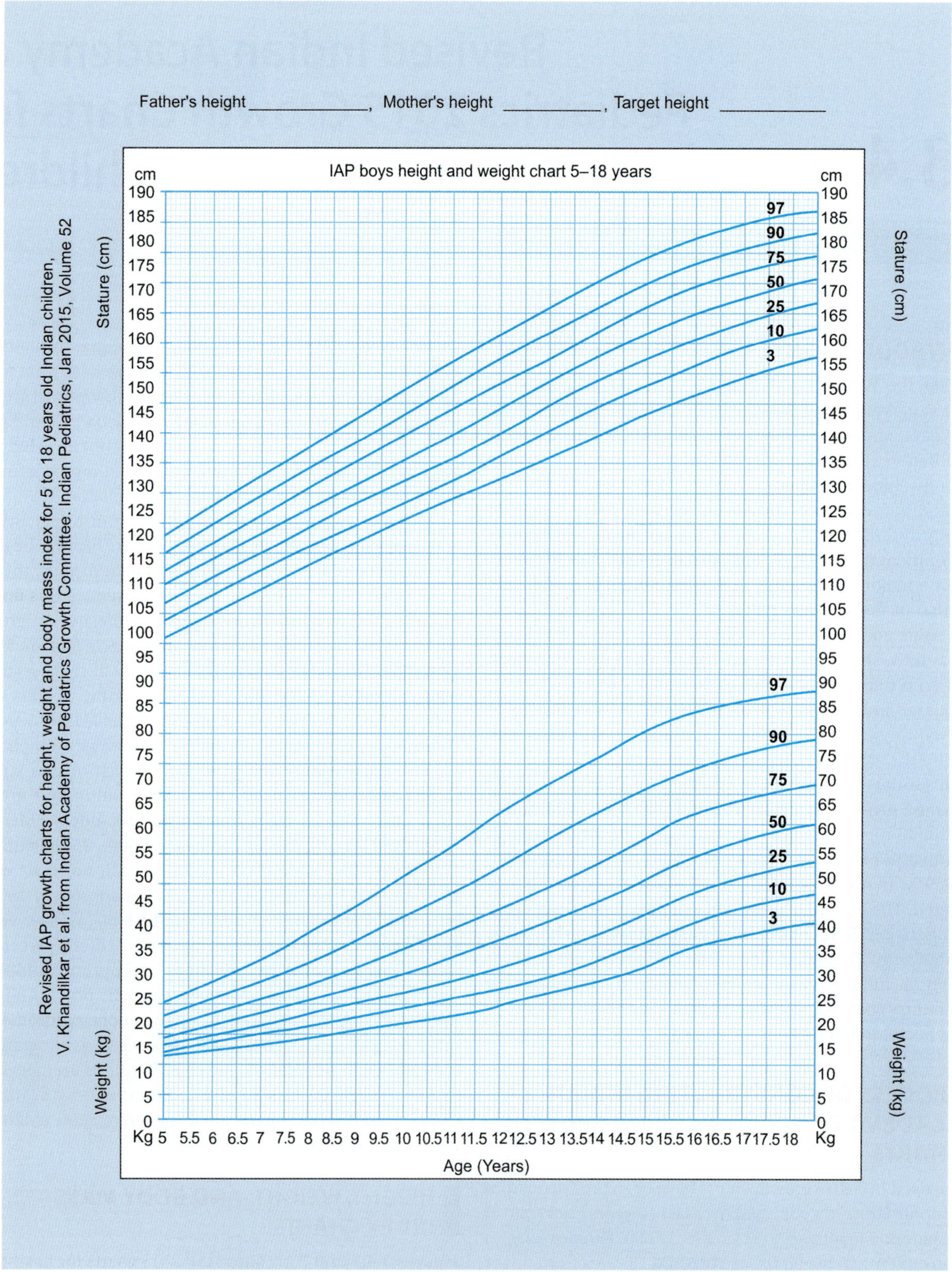

Father's height ____________, Mother's height __________, Target height ___________

IAP boys height and weight chart 5–18 years

Stature (cm)

Weight (kg)

Age (Years)

Kg 5 5.5 6 6.5 7 7.5 8 8.5 9 9.5 10 10.5 11 11.5 12 12.5 13 13.5 14 14.5 15 15.5 16 16.5 17 17.5 18 Kg

Percentiles: 97, 90, 75, 50, 25, 10, 3

Revised IAP growth charts for height, weight and body mass index for 5 to 18 years old Indian children, V. Khandilkar et al. from Indian Academy of Pediatrics Growth Committee. Indian Pediatrics, Jan 2015, Volume 52

Fig. 3.4.1: IAP 2015 charts for height and weight for boys from 5 to 18 years. (IAP: Indian Academy of Pediatrics)

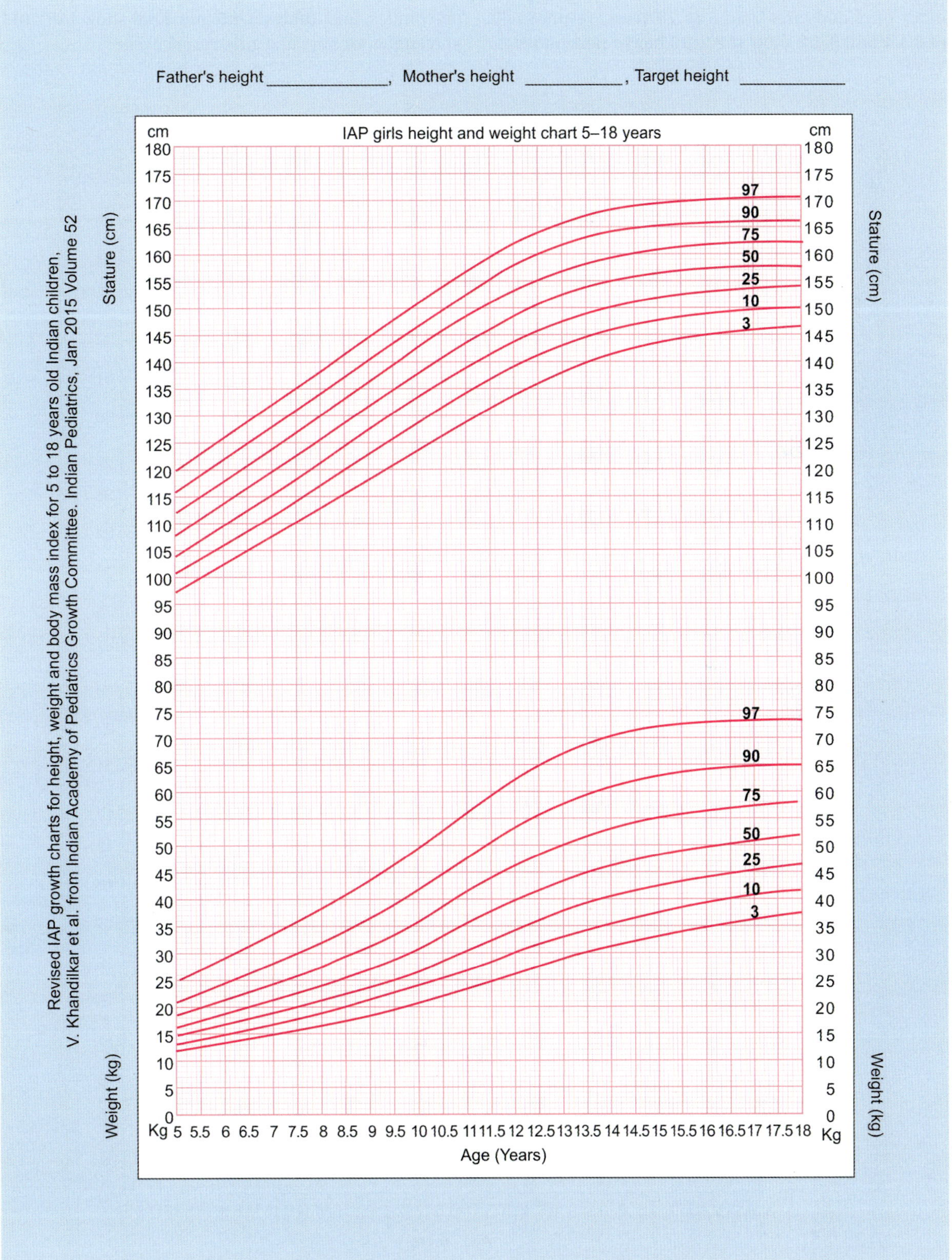

Fig. 3.4.2: Indian Academy of Pediatrics (IAP) 2015 charts for height and weight for girls from 5 to 18 years.

Figures 3.4.3 and 3.4.4 show the IAP 2015 BMI percentile charts for boys and girls from 5 to 18 years, respectively. **Tables 3.4.1 and 3.4.2** show IAP 2015 height percentiles for boys and girls. **Tables 3.4.3 and 3.4.4** show IAP 2015 weight percentiles, and **Tables 3.4.5 and 3.4.6** show IAP 2015 BMI percentiles for boys and girls, respectively.

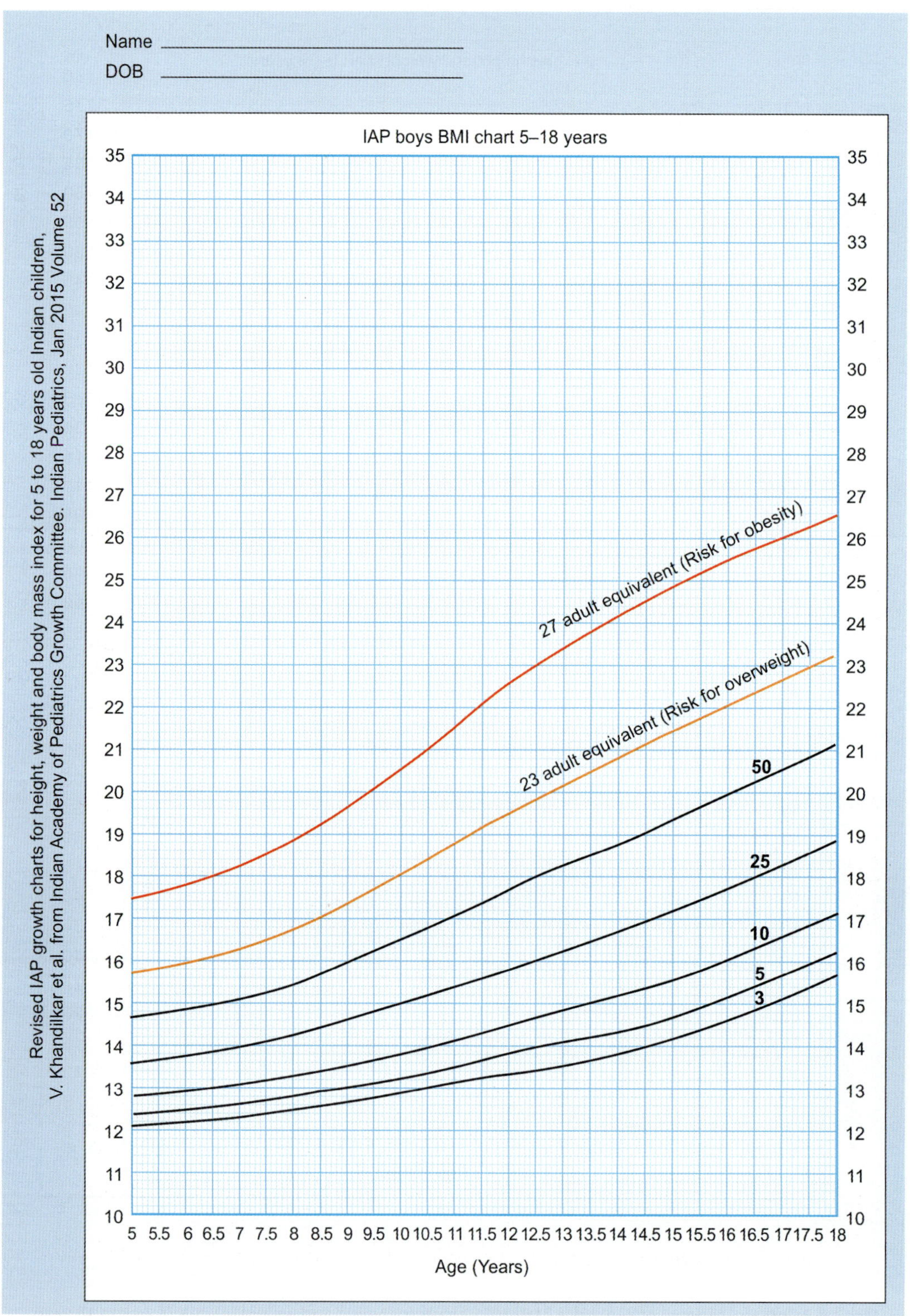

Fig. 3.4.3: Indian Academy of Pediatrics 2015 body mass index percentile chart for boys from 5 to 18 years.

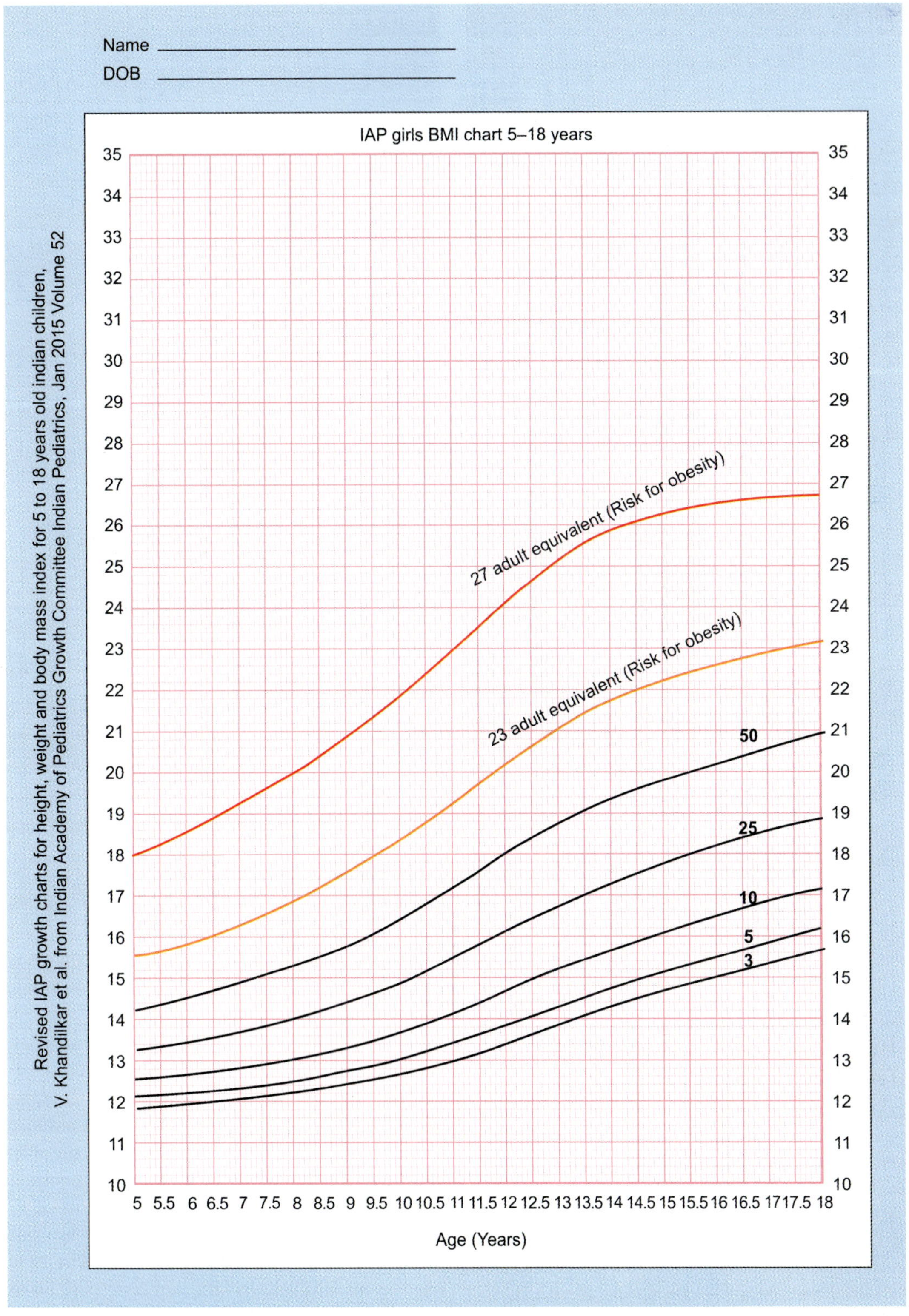

Fig. 3.4.4: Indian Academy of Pediatrics 2015 body mass index percentile chart for girls from 5 to 18 years.

Table 3.4.1: Boys height in centimeters and standard deviations.

Age	3	10	25	50	75	90	97	SD
5	99.0	102.3	105.6	108.9	112.4	115.9	119.4	5.7
5.5	101.6	105.0	108.4	111.9	115.4	119.0	122.7	5.3
6	104.2	107.7	111.2	114.8	118.5	122.2	126.0	5.6
6.5	106.8	110.4	114.0	117.8	121.6	125.4	129.3	5.5
7	109.3	113.0	116.8	120.7	124.6	128.6	132.6	5.9
7.5	111.8	115.7	119.6	123.5	127.6	131.7	135.9	5.7
8	114.3	118.2	122.3	126.4	130.5	134.8	139.1	6.3
8.5	116.7	120.8	124.9	129.1	133.4	137.8	142.2	6.1
9	119.0	123.2	127.5	131.8	136.3	140.7	145.3	6.4
9.5	121.3	125.6	130.0	134.5	139.1	143.7	148.3	6.4
10	123.6	128.1	132.6	137.2	141.9	146.6	151.4	6.8
10.5	125.9	130.5	135.2	139.9	144.7	149.5	154.4	6.5
11	128.2	133.0	137.8	142.7	147.6	152.5	157.5	7.6
11.5	130.7	135.6	140.6	145.5	150.5	155.6	160.6	7.3
12	133.2	138.3	143.3	148.4	153.5	158.6	163.7	8.1
12.5	135.7	141.0	146.2	151.4	156.5	161.7	166.8	7.9
13	138.3	143.7	149.0	154.3	159.5	164.7	169.9	9.0
13.5	140.9	146.4	151.8	157.2	162.4	167.6	172.7	8.4
14	143.4	149.0	154.5	159.9	165.1	170.3	175.4	9.0
14.5	145.8	151.5	157.0	162.3	167.6	172.7	177.7	7.8
15	148.0	153.7	159.2	164.5	169.7	174.8	179.7	7.9
15.5	150.0	155.7	161.2	166.5	171.6	176.5	181.4	6.6
16	151.8	157.4	162.9	168.1	173.1	178.0	182.7	7.2
16.5	153.4	159.1	164.5	169.6	174.5	179.3	183.8	6.7
17	155.0	160.6	165.9	171.0	175.8	180.4	184.8	6.9
17.5	156.6	162.1	167.3	172.3	177.0	181.5	185.8	6.1
18	158.1	163.6	168.7	173.6	178.2	182.5	186.7	6.9

(SD: standard deviation)

Table 3.4.2: Girls height in centimeters and standard deviations.

Age	3	10	25	50	75	90	97	SD
5	97.2	100.5	103.9	107.5	111.3	115.2	119.3	5.4
5.5	99.8	103.2	106.8	110.5	114.4	118.3	122.5	5.7
6	102.3	106.0	109.7	113.5	117.4	121.5	125.6	5.8
6.5	104.9	108.7	112.5	116.5	120.5	124.6	128.7	5.5
7	107.4	111.4	115.4	119.4	123.5	127.7	131.9	6.1
7.5	110.0	114.1	118.2	122.4	126.6	130.8	135.0	6.0
8	112.6	116.8	121.1	125.4	129.6	133.9	138.1	6.2
8.5	115.2	119.6	124.0	128.4	132.7	137.0	141.3	6.8
9	117.8	122.4	126.9	131.4	135.8	140.2	144.5	6.9
9.5	120.5	125.2	129.9	134.4	138.9	143.3	147.6	6.6
10	123.3	128.1	132.8	137.4	142.0	146.4	150.8	7.8
10.5	126.1	130.9	135.7	140.4	145.0	149.5	153.9	7.3
11	128.8	133.7	138.6	143.3	147.9	152.4	156.8	7.9
11.5	131.5	136.4	141.2	145.9	150.6	155.1	159.6	7.1
12	134.0	138.9	143.7	148.4	153.0	157.5	162.0	7.0
12.5	136.3	141.1	145.8	150.5	155.1	159.6	164.1	6.7
13	138.2	142.9	147.6	152.2	156.8	161.3	165.9	6.9
13.5	139.9	144.5	149.1	153.6	158.2	162.7	167.2	6.0
14	141.3	145.8	150.2	154.7	159.2	163.7	168.2	6.6
14.5	142.4	146.8	151.1	155.5	160.0	164.5	169.0	5.9
15	143.3	147.5	151.8	156.1	160.5	165.0	169.5	6.6
15.5	144.1	148.1	152.3	156.6	160.9	165.3	169.8	5.9
16	144.7	148.6	152.7	156.9	161.2	165.6	170.1	6.1
16.5	145.2	149.1	153.1	157.2	161.4	165.7	170.2	6.4
17	145.7	149.5	153.4	157.4	161.6	165.9	170.4	6.5
17.5	146.2	149.8	153.6	157.6	161.7	166.0	170.5	6.7
18	146.6	150.2	153.9	157.8	161.9	166.1	170.6	6.6

(SD: standard deviation)

HIGHLIGHTS OF INDIAN ACADEMY OF PEDIATRICS 2015 GROWTH CHARTS

The revised IAP 2015 growth charts for 5- to 18-year-old Indian children thus represent the most modern, contemporary updated growth charts for use in Indian children. As compared to the previous IAP charts, boys and girls are taller at all ages. At 18 years, average boys' height is 2.8 cm higher, and the 97th percentile is 5 cm higher; for girls, these figures are 0.8 cm and 2.6 cm. Thus, there is a secular trend in height, which underlines the importance of updating growth charts, especially in a developing nation, such as India.

Weight charts show higher weights for both boys and girls at all ages suggesting improved nutritional status, but there is no difference in the 3rd percentile as compared to 1989 data thus suggesting a widespread in weight distribution. By adopting, the approach as suggested by the WHO, weight percentiles have been lowered in comparison to the recently published weight charts on affluent Indian children, thus reducing the impact of unhealthy weights on weight charts.

Body mass index charts presented are based on the same method as suggested by the IOTF. The 23 and 27 adult equivalent cutoffs lines (and not 25 and 30 Eq as suggested for Caucasian population), for overweight and obesity, respectively, are more appropriate for use in Asian children as Asians are known to have more adiposity and increased

Table 3.4.3: Boys weight in kilograms and standard deviations.

Age	*3*	*10*	*25*	*50*	*75*	*90*	*97*	*SD*
5	13.2	14.3	15.6	17.1	19.0	21.3	24.2	3.2
5.5	13.8	15.0	16.5	18.2	20.3	22.9	26.1	2.9
6	14.5	15.8	17.4	19.3	21.7	24.6	28.3	3.6
6.5	15.3	16.8	18.6	20.7	23.3	26.6	30.8	3.8
7	16.0	17.6	19.6	21.9	24.9	28.6	33.4	4.2
7.5	16.7	18.5	20.7	23.3	26.6	30.8	36.2	4.9
8	17.5	19.5	21.9	24.8	28.5	33.2	39.4	5.7
8.5	18.3	20.5	23.2	26.4	30.5	35.7	42.6	6.5
9	19.1	21.5	24.3	27.9	32.3	38.0	45.5	6.3
9.5	19.9	22.4	25.6	29.4	34.3	40.5	48.6	7.0
10	20.7	23.5	26.9	31.1	36.3	43.0	51.8	7.9
10.5	21.6	24.6	28.3	32.8	38.5	45.8	55.2	8.3
11	22.6	25.9	29.8	34.7	40.9	48.7	58.7	8.9
11.5	23.8	27.3	31.6	36.9	43.5	51.8	62.5	9.3
12	24.9	28.7	33.3	39.0	46.0	54.8	66.1	10.0
12.5	26.1	30.2	35.1	41.2	48.6	57.8	69.5	10.6
13	27.5	31.8	37.0	43.3	51.1	60.7	72.6	11.3
13.5	29.0	33.6	39.1	45.7	53.8	63.6	75.6	11.4
14	30.7	35.5	41.3	48.2	56.4	66.3	78.3	12.1
14.5	32.6	37.7	43.7	50.8	59.1	69.1	80.9	11.6
15	34.5	39.8	45.9	53.1	61.6	71.5	83.1	12.1
15.5	36.1	41.6	47.9	55.2	63.6	73.4	84.7	11.2
16	37.5	43.1	49.5	56.8	65.2	74.8	85.8	12.2
16.5	38.7	44.4	50.9	58.2	66.6	76.1	86.8	12.6
17	39.8	45.6	52.1	59.5	67.8	77.1	87.5	12.3
17.5	40.8	46.7	53.2	60.6	68.7	77.8	88.0	12.3
18	41.8	47.7	54.3	61.6	69.7	78.6	88.4	11.3

(SD: standard deviation)

Table 3.4.4: Girls weight in kilograms and standard deviations.

Age	*3*	*10*	*25*	*50*	*75*	*90*	*97*	*SD*
5	12.3	13.4	14.8	16.4	18.5	21.3	25.0	2.5
5.5	13.0	14.3	15.7	17.6	19.9	22.9	27.0	3.5
6	13.7	15.1	16.7	18.7	21.3	24.6	29.1	3.4
6.5	14.4	15.9	17.7	19.9	22.7	26.3	31.2	4.1
7	15.1	16.8	18.7	21.2	24.2	28.2	33.4	4.4
7.5	15.9	17.7	19.9	22.5	25.9	30.1	35.7	4.8
8	16.7	18.7	21.1	24.0	27.6	32.2	38.1	5.2
8.5	17.5	19.7	22.3	25.5	29.5	34.4	40.7	6.4
9	18.5	20.9	23.7	27.2	31.5	36.7	43.4	6.4
9.5	19.5	22.1	25.3	29.0	33.6	39.3	46.3	6.9
10	20.7	23.5	26.9	31.0	36.0	42.0	49.4	7.7
10.5	22.0	25.1	28.8	33.2	38.4	44.8	52.6	8.3
11	23.3	26.7	30.7	35.4	41.0	47.7	55.9	8.5
11.5	24.8	28.4	32.6	37.6	43.6	50.6	59.1	9.1
12	26.2	30.0	34.5	39.8	46.0	53.4	62.1	9.0
12.5	27.6	31.6	36.3	41.8	48.2	55.8	64.8	9.7
13	28.9	33.1	37.9	43.6	50.2	57.9	67.1	9.4
13.5	30.2	34.4	39.4	45.1	51.8	59.7	69.0	9.8
14	31.3	35.6	40.6	46.4	53.2	61.1	70.4	9.6
14.5	32.3	36.6	41.7	47.5	54.3	62.2	71.4	9.4
15	33.1	37.5	42.5	48.4	55.1	62.9	72.1	9.6
15.5	34.0	38.3	43.3	49.1	55.8	63.5	72.5	8.7
16	34.7	39.1	44.0	49.7	56.3	64.0	72.8	8.7
16.5	35.5	39.8	44.7	50.3	56.9	64.4	73.1	9.2
17	36.2	40.5	45.3	50.9	57.3	64.7	73.3	8.8
17.5	36.9	41.1	46.0	51.5	57.8	65.0	73.4	9.5
18	37.6	41.8	46.6	52.0	58.2	65.3	73.5	10.2

(SD: standard deviation)

cardiometabolic risk at a lower BMI. These 23 and 27 adult equivalent cutoffs are very close to IOTFs extended 23 and 27 cutoffs in both sexes.

Comparing the final height and weight data with recent international studies from China, Saudi Arabia, WHO, and Centers for Disease Control and Prevention, it is noted that Indian children are growing almost at par with Chinese and Saudi Arabian children but are still shorter and lighter than their Caucasian counterparts. Indian children's stature seems to be comparable to Caucasian children until the onset of pubertal years; however, the growth spurt after puberty is attenuated in Indian children in both sexes, the effect being more pronounced in girls. Thus, the average difference in height between Caucasian girls and Indian girls from 5 to 11 years of age is only about 1 cm; however, this gap widens to 6 cm at 18 years. Similar figures in boys are 1 cm from the age of 5 to 12.5 years and 3.5 cm at 18 years. Interestingly, Chinese children show a very similar growth pattern suggesting that this is a characteristic of Asian children. These findings are of particular relevance in interpreting target height and predicting final adult height based on prediction equations, thus stressing the need for ethnic-specific growth charts.

Since the inceptions of these charts, they have been used as reference in several publications and to pick up children with overweight and obesity at par with the IOTF extended Asian standard cutoffs. They have also been shown to pick

Table 3.4.5: Boys body mass index percentiles and standard deviations.

Age	3	5	10	25	50	23 Eq (71)	27 Eq (90)	SD
5.0	12.1	12.4	12.8	13.6	14.7	15.7	17.5	1.6
5.5	12.2	12.4	12.9	13.7	14.8	15.8	17.6	1.5
6.0	12.2	12.5	12.9	13.7	14.9	16.0	17.8	1.8
6.5	12.3	12.5	13.0	13.8	15.0	16.1	18.0	1.8
7.0	12.3	12.6	13.1	13.9	15.1	16.3	18.2	1.9
7.5	12.4	12.7	13.2	14.1	15.3	16.5	18.5	2.2
8.0	12.5	12.8	13.3	14.2	15.5	16.7	18.8	2.5
8.5	12.6	12.9	13.4	14.4	15.7	17.0	19.2	2.8
9.0	12.7	13.0	13.5	14.5	15.9	17.3	19.6	2.6
9.5	12.8	13.1	13.7	14.7	16.2	17.6	20.1	2.8
10.0	12.9	13.2	13.8	14.9	16.4	18.0	20.5	3.1
10.5	13	13.3	14.0	15.1	16.7	18.3	21.0	3.2
11.0	13.1	13.5	14.1	15.4	17.0	18.7	21.5	3.2
11.5	13.2	13.6	14.3	15.6	17.3	19.1	22.1	3.3
12.0	13.3	13.8	14.5	15.8	17.7	19.5	22.6	3.4
12.5	13.5	13.9	14.6	16.0	17.9	19.8	23.0	3.6
13.0	13.6	14.0	14.8	16.3	18.2	20.2	23.4	3.5
13.5	13.7	14.2	14.9	16.5	18.5	20.5	23.8	3.7
14.0	13.8	14.3	15.1	16.7	18.7	20.8	24.2	3.7
14.5	14	14.5	15.3	16.9	19.0	21.1	24.5	3.5
15.0	14.2	14.7	15.5	17.2	19.3	21.4	24.9	3.7
15.5	14.4	14.9	15.8	17.4	19.6	21.7	25.2	3.4
16.0	14.6	15.1	16.0	17.7	19.9	22.0	25.5	3.7
16.5	14.9	15.4	16.3	18.0	20.2	22.4	25.8	3.8
17.0	15.1	15.6	16.6	18.3	20.5	22.6	26.0	3.8
17.5	15.4	15.9	16.8	18.6	20.8	22.9	26.3	3.6
18.0	15.6	16.2	17.1	18.9	21.1	23.2	26.6	3.2

(SD: standard deviation)

Table 3.4.6: Girls body mass index percentiles and standard deviations.

Age	3	5	10	25	50	23 Eq (75)	27 Eq (95)	SD
5	11.9	12.1	12.5	13.3	14.3	15.5	18	1.4
5.5	11.9	12.2	12.6	13.4	14.4	15.7	18.3	1.7
6	12.0	12.2	12.7	13.5	14.5	15.9	18.6	1.7
6.5	12.1	12.3	12.8	13.6	14.7	16.1	18.9	2.0
7	12.1	12.4	12.8	13.7	14.9	16.4	19.3	2.1
7.5	12.2	12.5	12.9	13.9	15.1	16.6	19.7	2.2
8	12.3	12.6	13.1	14	15.3	16.9	20.1	2.3
8.5	12.3	12.7	13.2	14.2	15.6	17.2	20.5	2.7
9	12.4	12.8	13.3	14.4	15.8	17.6	21	2.7
9.5	12.5	12.9	13.5	14.6	16.1	18	21.4	2.8
10	12.7	13.1	13.7	14.9	16.5	18.4	21.9	2.9
10.5	12.8	13.2	13.9	15.2	16.8	18.8	22.5	3.1
11	13	13.4	14.1	15.5	17.2	19.3	23	3.1
11.5	13.2	13.7	14.4	15.8	17.6	19.8	23.6	3.3
12	13.4	13.9	14.7	16.1	18	20.2	24.1	3.2
12.5	13.7	14.2	15	16.5	18.4	20.7	24.7	3.3
13	13.9	14.4	15.2	16.8	18.8	21.1	25.2	3.2
13.5	14.1	14.6	15.5	17.1	19.1	21.5	25.6	3.5
14	14.3	14.9	15.7	17.3	19.4	21.8	25.9	3.4
14.5	14.5	15.1	16	17.6	19.7	22	26.2	3.3
15	14.7	15.2	16.1	17.8	19.9	22.3	26.3	3.4
15.5	14.9	15.4	16.3	18	20.1	22.4	26.4	3.1
16	15	15.6	16.5	18.2	20.3	22.6	26.5	3.1
16.5	15.2	15.8	16.7	18.4	20.4	22.8	26.6	3.2
17	15.4	16	16.9	18.6	20.6	22.9	26.7	3.0
17.5	15.5	16.1	17.1	18.7	20.8	23.1	26.7	3.1
18	15.7	16.3	17.3	18.9	21	23.2	26.8	3.6

(SD: standard deviation)

up overweight, obesity as well as underweight children with more accuracy as compared to the old IAP charts.

These growth charts can be downloaded from the IAP website: *http://www.iapinidia.org*. LMS values are computed at monthly intervals and are available for research purpose from the author.

The revised IAP 2015 growth charts are recommended by IAP for use in children from 5 to 18 years to replace the old IAP growth charts. For younger children, IAP recommends use of WHO 2006 growth standards.

BIBLIOGRAPHY

1. Agarwal DK, Agarwal KN, Upadhyay SK, et al. Physical and sexual growth pattern of affluent Indian children from 5–18 years of age. Indian Pediatr. 1992;29:1203-82.
2. Chudasama RK, Eshwar TKM, Thakrar D, et al. Prevalence and comparison of obesity, overweight, and thinness by different growth standards among affluent school children (8–18 years) in Rajkot. J Mahatma Gandhi Inst Med Sci. 2017;22:99-104.
3. Cole TJ, Lobstein T. Extended international (IOTF) body mass index cutoffs for thinness, overweight and obesity. Pediatr Obes. 2012;7:284-94.

4. Haq I, Raja MW, Ahmad MM. A comparison of the 2015 Indian Academy of Pediatrics, International Obesity Task Force and World Health Organization growth references among 5-18-year-old children. Ann Trop Med Public Health. 2017;10:1814-9.
5. Indian Academy of Pediatrics Growth Charts Committee; Khadilkar V, Yadav S, Agrawal KK, et al. Revised IAP growth charts for height, weight and body mass index for 5- to 18-year-old Indian children. Indian Pediatr. 2015;52(1):47-55.
6. Khadilkar VV, Khadilkar AV, Borade AB, et al. Body mass index cutoffs for screening for childhood overweight and obesity in Indian children. Indian Pediatr. 2012;49:29-34.
7. Khadilkar VV, Khadilkar AV, Choudhury P, et al. IAP growth monitoring guidelines for children from birth to 18 years. Indian Pediatr. 2007;44:187-97.
8. Khadilkar VV, Khadilkar AV, Cole TJ, et al. Cross sectional growth curves for height, weight and body mass index for affluent Indian children, 2007. Indian Pediatr. 2009;46:47789.
9. Khadilkar VV, Khadilkar AV, Cole TJ, et al. Overweight and obesity prevalence and body mass index trends in Indian children. Int J Pediatr Obes. 2011;6:216-24.
10. Marwaha RK, Tandon N, Ganie MA, et al. Nationwide reference data for height, weight and body mass index of Indian schoolchildren. Natl Med J India. 2011;24:269-77.

3.5 Growth and Sexual Development in Puberty

KN Agarwal

DEFINITION

Puberty is the growth process associated with the appearance of both primary and secondary sexual characteristics in children. The changes encompass aspects of sexuality and somatic growth, together with cognitive development. Pubescent children are those in whom secondary sexual characters and early genital changes are appearing. The World Health Organization (WHO) defines adolescents as individuals in the age group of 10–19 years. The various physiological developments are as follows:

- Adolescent growth spurt
- Change in body composition (muscle/fat)
- Skeletal maturity

The time of onset and the rate of sexual development have individual variability but the sequence of events remains the same. From a biological perspective, puberty is the stage of physical maturation; in which, an individual becomes physiologically capable of sexual reproduction. The biological changes that occur during puberty include several neurosecretory factors and/or hormones, all of which modulate somatic growth, the development of the sex glands and their endocrine as well as exocrine secretions. The resultant increase in sex steroid production will ensure the appearance and maintenance of sexual characteristics and the capacity for reproduction. It is essentially the activation of the hypothalamic-pituitary-gonadal axis that induces and enhances the progressive ovarian and testicular sex hormone secretion that are responsible for the profound biological, morphological, and psychological changes to which the adolescent is subjected.

INITIATION OF PUBERTY

- It occurs between 8 years and 14 years of age in girls and between 9 years and 15 years of age in boys.
- *Girls*: Breast enlargement, occasionally initially unilateral, is the first obvious sign of puberty and occurs between 10 years and 11 years of age.
- *Boys*: Testicular volume increases from 2.0 mL to more than 4.0 mL or testes length from 2.0 cm to 3.2 cm between 12 years and 13 years of age; 1 year later penile and scrotal enlargements occur.

Growth Spurt

- Period extends for 4 years in girls and 6 years in boys to cross "sexual maturity stages."
- Height gain is 27–29 cm in boys and 24–26 cm in girls.
- Weight gain in both is around 25–30 kg.

ENDOCRINAL CONTROL OF PUBERTY

For 2 years before puberty, there is a rise in levels of adrenal androgens (adrenarche) that can sometimes result in the early appearance of pubic hair and spots.

The initial event of puberty is an increase in pulsatile release of gonadotropin-releasing hormone (GnRH). Therefore, the initiation of the pubertal process itself requires both changes in trans-synaptic communication and the activation of glia-to-neuron signaling pathways. While neurons that utilize excitatory and inhibitory amino acids as transmitters represent major players in the trans-synaptic control of puberty, glial cells utilize a combination of trophic factors and small cell-signaling molecules to regulate neuronal function and, thus, promote sexual development. A coordinated increase in glutamatergic transmission accompanied by a decrease in inhibitory GABAergic tone appears to initiate the trans-synaptic cascade of events leading to the pubertal increase in GnRH release.

In response to GnRH stimulation, pituitary releases luteinizing hormone (LH) and follicle-stimulating hormone (FSH). In males, LH stimulation is responsible for testosterone production, while FSH causes maturation of sperms. In females, both LH and FSH are required for the production of estradiol, while FSH is also required for ovulation.

DIFFERENCES BETWEEN BOYS AND GIRLS

For boys, testosterone is the principal sex hormone. It induces the characterization known as virilization. A substantial product of testosterone metabolism in males is estradiol, though levels rise later and more slowly than in girls. The male "growth spurt" also begins later, accelerates more slowly, and lasts longer before the epiphysis fuse. Although boys are on average similar in height or 2 cm shorter than girls before puberty begins, adult men are, on average, about 13 cm taller than women. The growth spurt occurs later in boys than in girls because testosterone is a poor stimulator to growth hormone (GH) responsiveness than estradiol in girls. Testosterone is required in relatively higher concentration to produce the same growth effect.

The hormone that dominates female development is an estrogen called estradiol, which rises earlier and reaches higher levels in women than in men. It promotes growth of breasts and uterus and is responsible for the pubertal growth spurt, epiphysis maturation and closure.

Girls attain reproductive maturity about 4 years after the first physical changes of puberty appear. In contrast, boys accelerate more slowly but continue to grow for about 6 years after the first visible pubertal change.

Normal Puberty in Girls

The first sign of ovarian estradiol secretion is breast development "thelarche" [breast budding, B2, or sexual maturity rating (SMR)2] with "growth in height" **(Fig. 3.5.1 and Table 3.5.1)**. Estradiol being a good stimulator of "GH" doubles the growth velocity. The maximum height velocity [peak height velocity (PHV) = 9–10 cm/year] coincides with B3. Thus, growth spurt occurs early in female puberty, following B2 by 1 year. Height velocity reduces to 4 cm/year at menarche. The growth in the postmenarche period is limited as girls can gain 5–6 cm in linear growth, only.

Puberty is associated with change in body shape, such as hip growth, increase in body fat from 16% to 28%, and reduction in lean body mass from 80% to 72%.

- Menarche follows PHV by 14–18 months or usually occurs about 2–3 years after the start of breast development (thelarche). The age of menarche is around 12–13 years (12.6 years in Indian girls).

Estradiol is the main hormone in females influencing the pubertal development, i.e. breast and genitals, and promotes uterine maturation and fat deposition in typical female contours, while androgens from adrenals and ovaries are responsible for pubic and axillary hair and the typical body odor and acne.

Normal Puberty in Boys

The first sign of puberty is testicular enlargement, which usually occurs between ages of 12 and 13 years. The prepubertal testis

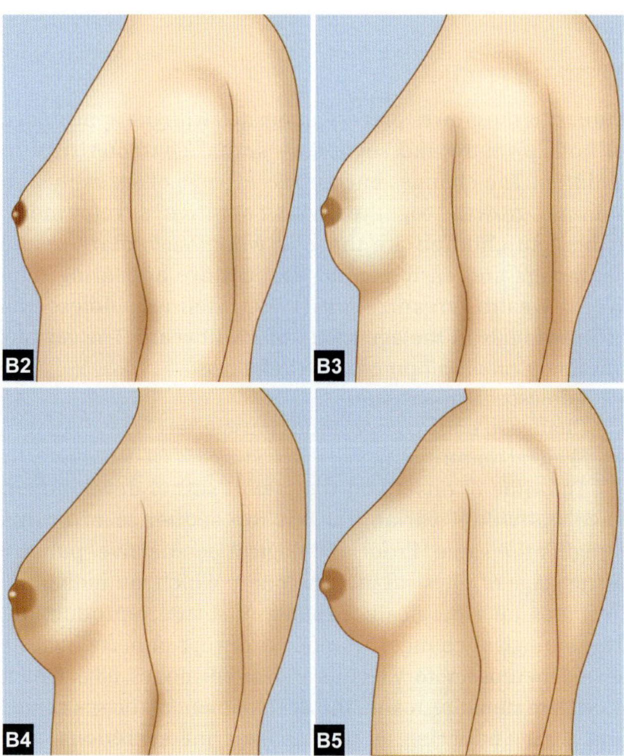

Fig. 3.5.1: Development of breast (stages B2–B5) during puberty in girls.

Table 3.5.1: Stages of normal puberty (Tanner stages) in girls for breast, pubic hair, and in relation to the peak height velocity (values in parenthesis are for Indian girls).

Tanner stage	***Breast***	***Pubic hair (mean age = 13.6 years)***	***Growth height***	***Other features***	***Undernourished rural girl (India)***
Stage 1 (B1)	*Prepubertal:* Elevation of *papilla* only	Prepubertal villus *hair* only	*Basal level*: 5–6 cm/year	*Adrenarche:* Ovaries grow and enlarge	*Height* was lower by 15.3 cm vs affluent girl
Stage 2 (B2)	*Breast bud* appears under an enlarged areola. Milk ducts begin to grow (mean age 10.2 years)	Sparse *hair* along labia (in 22%)	*Accelerated growth*: About 7–8 cm/year	*Clitoral* enlargement with *labial* pigmentation, *uterine* enlargement, increase in *vaginal* length, *menarche* attained in 10%	*Breast* development delayed by 2.2 years
Stage 3 (B3)	Breast tissue grows beyond areola but without contour separation. The areola begins to darken in color. The milk ducts give rise to milk glands that also begin to grow (mean age 11.6 years)	Hair coarser and pigmented: spreads across pubes (becoming thicker, curly, and darker in 92%)	*Peak velocity:* About 8 cm/year	*Axillary hair + in majority acne and menarche attained in 20% (total 30%)*	*Peak height velocity not observed Height gain 24–26 cm*; early life deficit not corrected
Stage 4 (B4)	*Projection of areola*: Papilla forms a secondary mound (mean age 13.6 years)	Adult pattern but without spread to medial thigh, growing faster and already forming sexual pubic triangle (in 98.8%)	*Deceleration*: Less than 7 cm/year	*Menarche:* Mean age = 12.6 years. Regular periods (around 14 years) menarche attained in total = 90%	*Menarche* delayed by 0.82 years
Stage 5 (B5)	Adult breast contour with projection of nipple only (mean age 14.5 years)	Adult triangle is already developed. Hair is thick and often curly with spread to medial thigh but not up linea alba (100%)	Cessation of growth at around 16 years	Adult genitalia menarche in all girls	Total period of growth in puberty shortened

Source: Agarwal KN, Saxena A, Bansal AK, et al. Physical growth assessment in adolescence. Indian Pediatr. 2001;38:1217-35.

is about 2 mL in volume with puberty taken to begin when a volume of around 4 mL is attained. The rapid pubertal growth occurs once testes are more than 6 mL. Actually, testicular growth starts as early as 10 years of age, associated with the enlargement of seminiferous tubules, epididymis, seminal vesicles, and prostate. Prader *testicular orchidometer* **(Fig. 3.5.2)** is used to measure testicular volume.

Penile and scrotal enlargements occur typically about a year after testicular enlargement is noticed. Pubic hair appears at a similar time **(Fig. 3.5.3 and Table 3.5.2)**.

- A greater and later growth spurt occurs in boys and ultimately achieves an average 12.6 cm with greater height in adult men. The growth spurt in boys is an average 2 years later than girls in SMR stages 3 and 4.

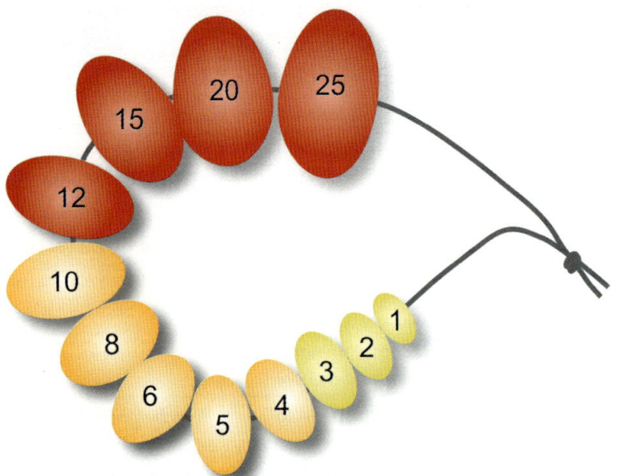

Fig. 3.5.2: Prader testicular orchidometer.

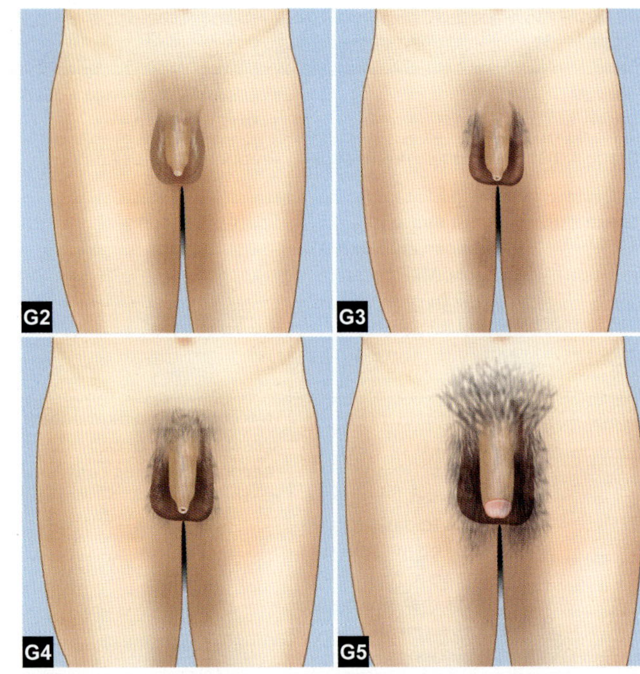

Fig. 3.5.3: Genital development in boys in sexual maturity stages (G2–G5).

Table 3.5.2: Genital development and growth in boys during puberty (the values in parenthesis are for Indian boys).

Tanner stage	***Genitalia***	***Pubic hair***	***Growth—height***	***Other***	***Undernourished rural boy (India)***
Stage 1(G1)	*Prepubertal*: Testes less than 2.5 cm or less than 2–0 mL	Villus hair only	Basal height velocity 5–6 cm/year	*Adrenarche*	Height at 13 years was short by 13.6 cm vs affluent Indian boy
Stage 2(G2)	• Thinning and reddening of scrotal skin (mean age 11.3 years). • Testes 2.5–3.2 cm or 4 mL	Sparse growth at base of penis (60%)	As above	Total body fat 16–18%	
Stage 3(G3)	• Growth of *penis* (mean age 12.8 years). • *Testes* 3.3–4.0 cm or 6–8 mL	*Thicker hair*: Spreads to mons pubis (97%)	*Accelerated growth*: 7–8 cm/year	• Gynecomastia voice • Break increase in muscle mass	Genital development delayed by 1.54 years
Stage 4(G4)	• Growth of penis and glans with darkening of scrotum (mean age 14.1 years) • Testes 4.1–4.5 cm or 10–12 mL	Adult but no spread to medial thigh (99%)	*Peak velocity* about 10.0 cm/year	• Axillary hair • Voice change • Acne	• *Delayed appearance*: axillary hair by 0.65 year; pubic hair by 0.82 year • No peak height velocity noted
Stage 5 (G5)	• Adult genitalia (mean age 16.4 years) • Testes greater than 4.5 cm or 12 mL (adult volume 18 mL)	Adult with spread to medial thigh but not linea alba	Deceleration and cessation (about 17 years)	• *Facial hair* (mean age 14.8 years) • Muscle mass increases further and beyond stage 5	Total weight gain only 38% as compared to affluent Indian boy

- *Face*: 25% of the total height of the mandible ramus occurs between 12 and 20 years of age.
- *Eyes*: Growth in axial diameters results in a tendency to "myopia" in adolescence.
- *Voice*: Growth of larynx, pharynx, and lungs leads to typical voice.

MUSCLE GROWTH

The body takes on a more muscular and angular shape because of testosterone. This generally begins around age 12.5 years when testosterone causes muscle mass to increase. The greatest effect can usually be seen in the upper chest and shoulder muscles. Testosterone also causes bones to lengthen, giving young men a heavier bone structure and longer arms and legs. At the end of puberty, adult men have heavier bones and nearly twice as much skeletal muscle. Some of the bone growths (e.g. shoulder width and jaw) are disproportionately greater, resulting in noticeably different male and female skeletal shapes. The average adult male has about 15% of the lean body mass, of an average female, and about 50% less of the body fat. Muscle growth can continue even after boys are biologically adult. The peak of the so-called strength spurt, the rate of muscle growth, is attained about 1 year after a male experiences his peak growth rate.

BODY ODOR AND ACNE

Rising levels of androgens can change the fatty acid composition of perspiration, resulting in a more "adult" body odor. As in girls, another androgen effect is increased secretion of oil (sebum) from the skin and the resultant variable amounts of acne. Acne cannot be prevented or curtailed easily, but it fully disappears at the end of puberty.

FACTORS AFFECTING PUBERTY

The genetic factors account for half of the variation of pubertal timing; the association of timing is strongest between mothers and daughters. The environment factors are clearly important as well; puberty occurs later in children raised at higher altitudes and in undernourished children (***see* Tables 3.5.1 and 3.5.2**). It is advanced in obese children.

LATE PUBERTY

- When a boy or girl has passed the usual age of onset of puberty by 2–3 years with no physical or hormonal signs.
- Puberty may be delayed for several years and can still occur normally—constitutional delay, a variation of healthy physical development. Delay of puberty may also occur due to undernutrition (malnutrition, cystic fibrosis, and anorexia nervosa), many forms of systemic diseases (thalassemia and chronic renal failure) or defects of the reproductive system (hypogonadism and polycystic ovarian disease) or the body's responsiveness to sex hormones.
- Constitutional growth delay is the most common cause in boys (>50%). The most common cause in girls is Turner syndrome (>80% girls have pathological cause of delayed puberty).

Pointers for Delayed Puberty

Girls

- No breast development by 13 years;
- No menarche by 3 years after breast development;
- Menarche not attained by 16 years.

Boys

- No testicular enlargement by the age of 14 years;
- Pubic hair absent by the age of 15 years;
- More than 5 years between the start and the completion of growth of the genitalia.

Precocious Puberty

Precocious puberty is defined as the onset of secondary sexual characteristics before the age of 8 years in girls (although some sources lower this to 7 years) and 9 years in boys. It is five times more common in girls. The precocious puberty is usually a benign central process in girls but in boys a pathological peripheral cause should be excluded (found in 50%).

Benign variants may manifest as breast development in girls aged less than 3 years, which spontaneously regresses, and pubic hair in both boys and girls aged less than 7 years due to adrenal androgen secretion in middle childhood (polycystic ovary syndrome—recommend follow-up).

In central precocious puberty, the puberty process starts too soon. Although they begin earlier than they should, the pattern and timing of the steps in the process are otherwise normal. For the majority of children, with this condition, there is no underlying medical problem and no identifiable reason for the early puberty.

GROWTH PATTERN AND ACHIEVEMENT DURING PUBERTY

Changes Under Sex Hormone Effects

Growth begins in distal parts, such as feet and hands, which also stop growing first. It is followed by the growth of arms, legs, trunk, and chest. The growth of trunk changes—upper segment/lower segment ratio becomes 1.1 at 10–11 years, 0.98–1 at 13–14 years, and 1–1.1 at the completion of puberty.

Pelvic inlet is wider in girls (wider hips) with more growth of acetabula. In contrast, boys have greater stature and broader shoulders.

Height and Weight Gains in Puberty (Duration 4–6 Years)

- At 10.5 years, boys and girls have similar height
- At 11–12.5 years, girls are taller by 2.0 cm
- At 14 years, boys are taller by 5 cm
- At 16 years, boys are taller by 12.5 cm
- The height velocity is given in relation to sexual maturity in **Tables 3.5.1 and 3.5.2**
- Total weight gain is around 25–30 kg during puberty. The peak weight velocity follows PHV
- *Bone growth*: 50% completed during the first month of life to puberty onset, 30% in puberty, and 20% in late adolescence to adult. Girls mature earlier than boys, grow for a shorter time, and ultimately have shorter overall bone lengths by about 7%.

ESSENTIAL MEASUREMENTS TO ASSESS SEXUAL DEVELOPMENT AND GROWTH IN PUBERTY

Assess sexual maturity as per Tanner classification **(Tables 3.5.1 and 3.5.2; Figs. 3.5.4 and 3.5.5)**. The variability in time of onset and progression of puberty, which relates to somatic growth rather than chronological age, requires assessment

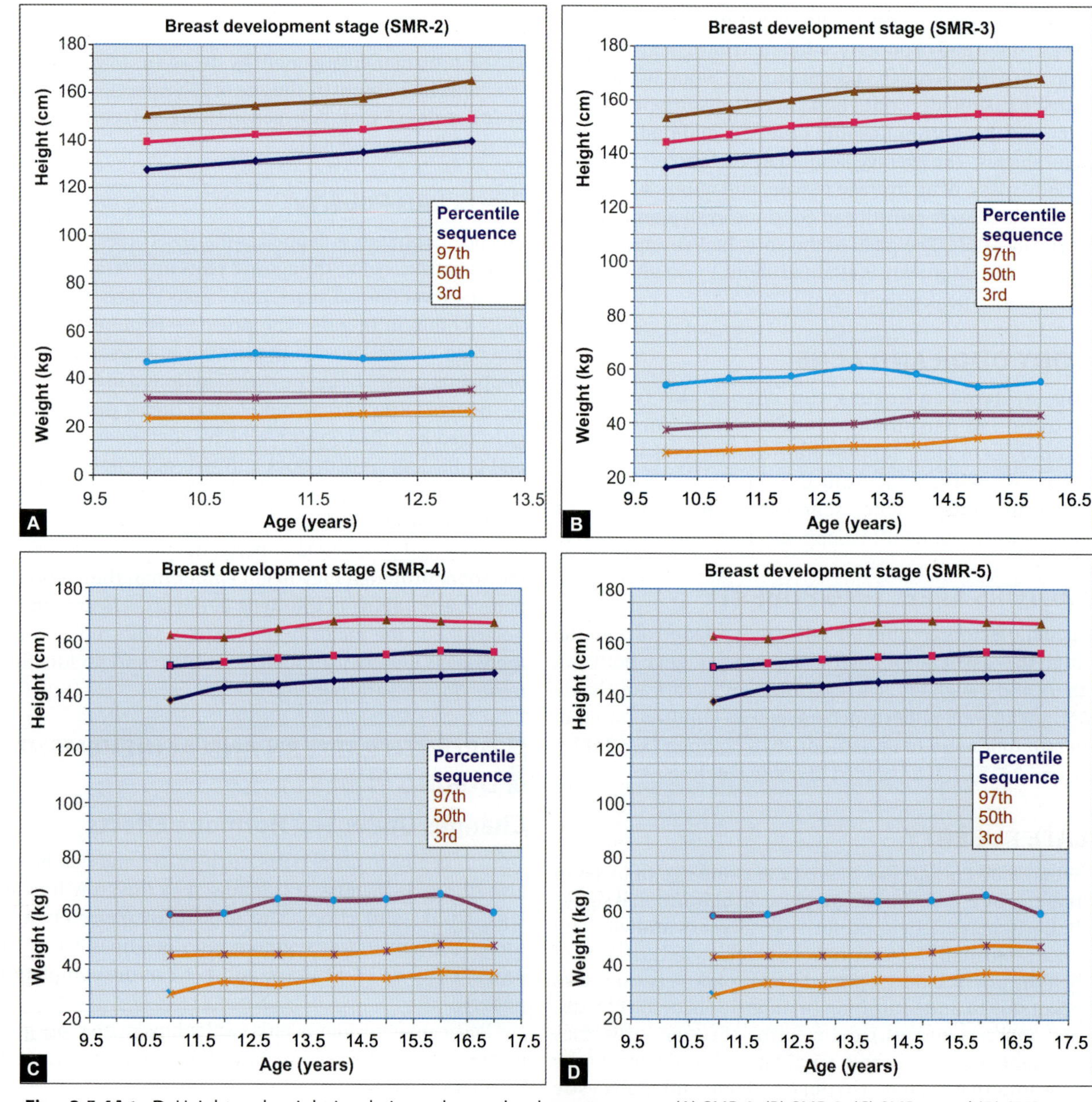

Figs. 3.5.4A to D: Height and weight in relation to breast development stages: (A) SMR-2; (B) SMR-3; (C) SMR-4; and (D) SMR-5. (SMR: sexual maturity rating)

Source: Agarwal KN, Saxena A, Bansal AK, et al. Physical growth assessment in adolescence. Indian Pediatr. 2001;38:1217-35.

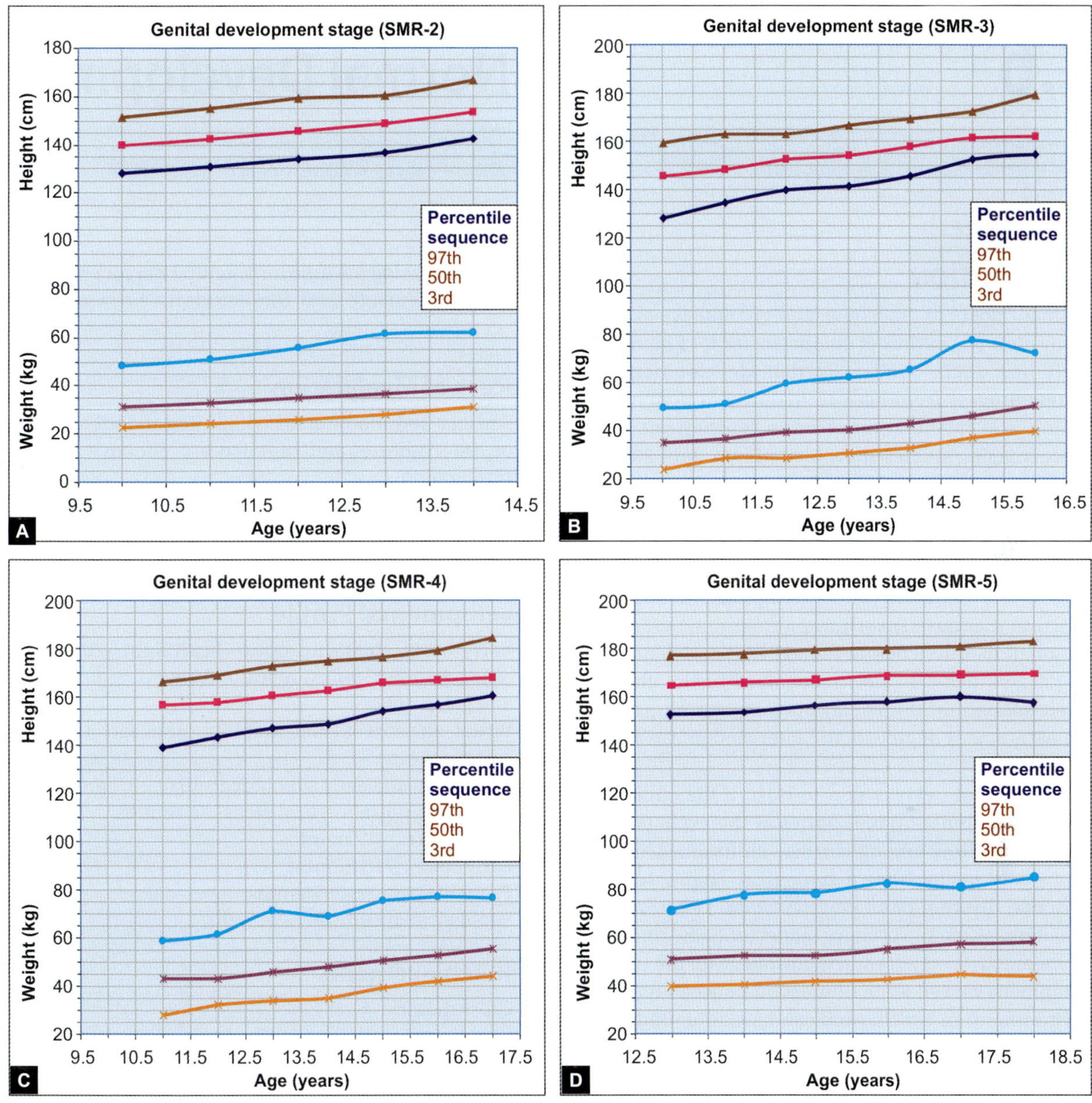

Figs. 3.5.5A to D: Height and weight in relation to genital development stages: (A) SMR-2; (B) SMR-3; (C) SMR-4; and (D) SMR-5. (SMR: sexual maturity rating)

Source: Agarwal KN, Saxena A, Bansal AK, et al. Physical growth assessment in adolescence. Indian Pediatr. 2001;38:1217-35.

of stage of sexual maturation. The necessity to undress the teenager has seriously curtailed the assessment by experts, the best approach is to give Tanner stages as diagram to children, and they make self-assessment *in a lighted closed room.*

- The height, weight, body mass index, and skin fold thickness values for age in relation to "sexual maturity" are described (Agarwal et al., 2001).
- Waist/hip ratio less than 0.8 in women and less than 0.9 in men indicates good health, values over and above suggest overweight/obesity).
- Waist-to-height ratio less than 0.5, no central obesity versus more than or equal to 0.5, central obesity present.

BIBLIOGRAPHY

1. Agarwal DK. The somatic growth and sexual development. In: Agarwal KN (Ed). The growth infancy to adolescence, 3rd edition. New Delhi: CBS Publishers; 2015. pp. 31-42.
2. Agarwal KN, Agarwal DK, Upadhaya SK, et al. Physical and sexual growth pattern of affluent Indian children from 5–18 years of age. Indian Pediatr. 1992;29:1203-82.
3. Agarwal KN, Saxena A, Bansal AK, et al. Physical growth assessment in adolescence. Indian Pediatr. 2001;38:1217-35.
4. Duke PM, Litt IF, Gross RT. Adolescents' self-assessment of sexual maturation. Pediatrics. 1980;66:918-20.
5. Tanner JM. Growth in adolescence, 2nd edition. Oxford: Blackwell Scientific Publication; 1962.

3.6 Normal Development

DK Agarwal

INTRODUCTION

Development refers to qualitative and quantitative changes and acquisition of a variety of competencies for functioning optimally in a social milieu. Further, development is a continuous process from birth to maturity. It depends on maturation and myelination of brain (current magnetic resonance imaging studies show it continues until 25 years of age). Unless that has occurred, no amount of practice can make the child learn that skill. It may be stressed that in addition to 10% prevalence of developmental delay, the early identification of such problems remains difficult. Although severe disorders can be recognized in infancy, it is unusual to diagnose speech impairment, hyperactivity, or emotional disorders before the age of 3 or 4 years, and learning disabilities are rarely recognized before children start their schooling. If one can diagnose developmental delay in early stages of growth, the intervention can reduce long-term sequel.

Developmental delay is said to exist, if the child does not reach developmental milestones at the expected age, i.e. broad variation among normal children. Although the delay may occur from a biological factor, such as chromosomal disorder or an environmental factor, such as maternal depression, the primary model for pathogenesis of developmental delay is a transactional one, with the process of development viewed as an interaction between the child and environment; in which, each can have profound effect on the other.

BRAIN GROWTH AND DEVELOPMENT

Brain growth is important to receive stimuli and take body functions. The process of brain growth and acquisition of developmental processes is summarized as follows.

Process of Brain Growth

- In the ectoderm, notochord develops to form a neural groove—neural tube (cavity with overlying neural crest) forms in 18–24 days.
- *Error:* Results in spina bifida, anencephaly, etc.
- Few weeks after the conception to cellular level through adolescence, brain continues to grow and myelinate.
  - Cells inside the tube form central nervous system
  - Cells outside and the ectoderm form autonomic nervous system.

Process of Myelination

- Sensory and motor areas within first month to first year of life—training and practice are effective only after myelination.
- Maximum myelination occurs by 6 years of life.
- Prefrontal cortex is not myelinated until close to the completion of adolescence growth (25 years of age).

Developmental Profile

- Early brain stem and cord—birth:light reflex, startle reflex, Babinski reflex, reflex movement, reflex birth cry, and grasp reflex
- Visual, auditory, tactile, mobility, language, and manual competences
- Brain stem and early subcortical areas—2.5 months
- Midbrain and subcortical areas—7 months
- Initial cortex—12 months
- Early cortex—18 months
- Primitive cortex—36 months
- Sophisticated cortex—72 months.

Skill Achievements

- Gross motor
- Fine motor
- Language
- Cognitive
- Self-help
- Social

The developmental pattern from birth to first birthday is given in **Figure 3.6.1**. Normal development is given in **Table 3.6.1** for the developmental abilities at various ages.

ASSESSMENT OF NORMAL DEVELOPMENT

The developmental history and physical findings should be compared with the achievements listed for normal children. For preterm, one must take their corrected age into account. If one finds any "warning sign," take note of the points in history and physical examination and define the type of impairment,

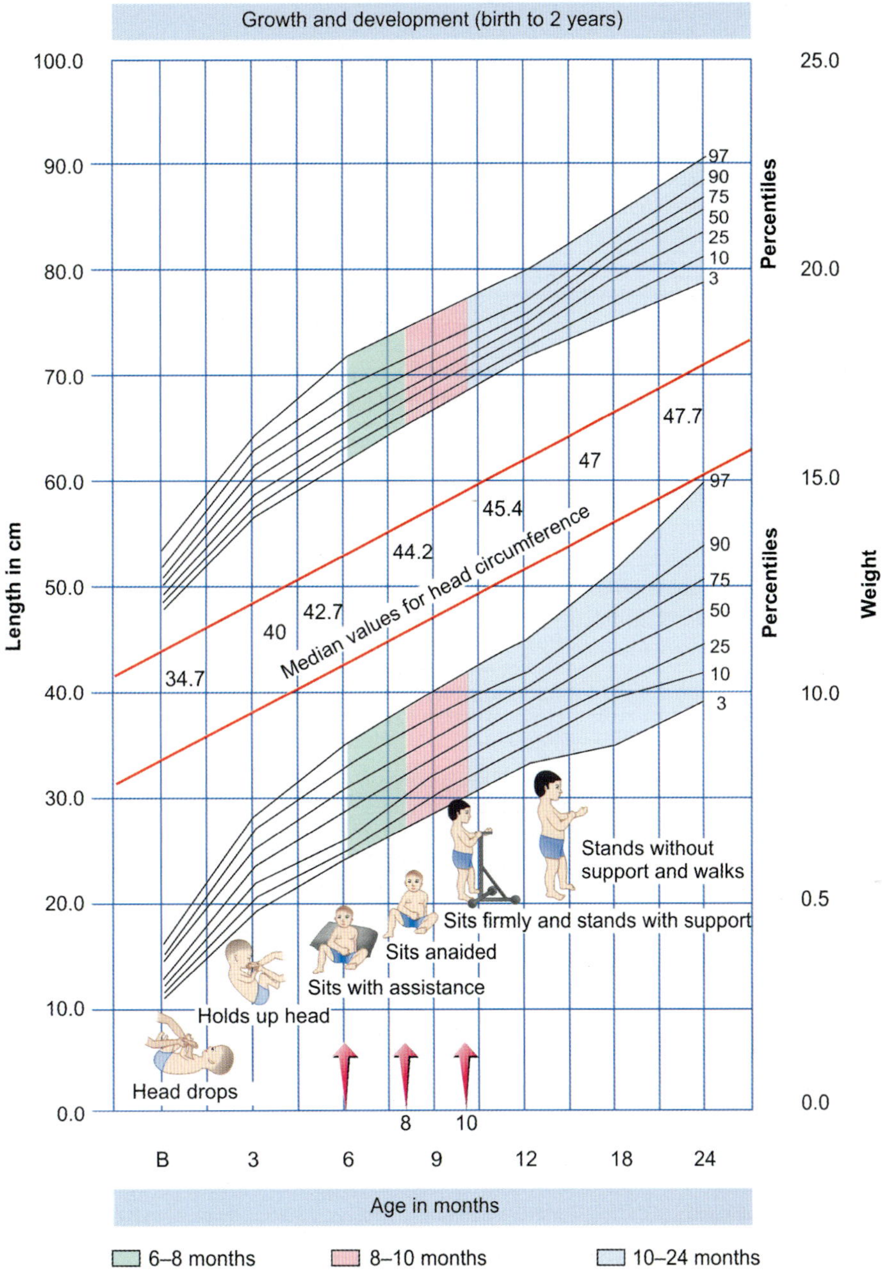

Fig. 3.6.1: Growth and development in first 2 years of life.

Source: Agarwal DK, Agarwal KN. Physical growth in Indian affluent children (birth-6 years). Indian Pediatr. 1994;31:377-413.

disability, or any handicap. The children may be observed for their activities as follows.

Preschool Age

- Play, climbing stairs, speech, hand (for adaptive behavior), and feeding;
- Posture, walking, play, and manipulation with toys (tests for vision);
- *Performance*: Understanding, matching color, concentration, and visual acuity;
- *Comprehension of language*: To point to body parts, objects in books, to pick named toys, and accept commands appropriate to age.

Table 3.6.1: Developmental abilities and warning signs at various ages.

Areas Personal/social	***Language Hearings and speech***	***Adaptive***	***Gross Motor***	***Warning Signs***
6 weeks old				
Smiles, coos responsively	Stills to mother's voice, startles at sudden noise	Follows face 90° stares intently	Primitive reflexes + head In line with trunk when lifted	• None is elicited • Abnormal Moro's • Persistent squint
6–9 months old				
6 months—enjoys bath, playing boo, and chew on items. 9 months—show objects to mother, mirror image	6 month produces babbling sounds ma ma, ba ba. Smiles when spoken to, makes noises to attract attention; by 9 months words doll, toy	6 to 7 months—change grasp palmar to index, transfers objects hand to mouth. 9 months—pincer grasp foot regard. Fixes pellet of paper, follows fallen object	6 months—bears some weight on legs, rolling over, in prone head up, weight of hands. 7 months—crawls and pulls to stand	• Slow social responses • Absence of babble • Persistence of hand pats regard • Abnormal voluntary hand grasp • Persistent primitive reflexes
12 months old				
Comes when called, finds hidden objects, waves bye-bye, gives toys on request	Understands some words, uses "mama, dada" with meaning "No"	Throws objects, watches them fall, picks up crumbs from floor. Pincer grasp, shakes head, bangs two bricks together	Shuffling gait like a bear, cruises round holding on to furniture, walks one hand held, pivots when sitting	• No tuneful babble • Hold objects close to eyes • Immature gait • No sitting
18 months old				
Cup: Lifts, drinks, and puts down, self-spoon-feeding, pulls at dirty nappy, does dusting, sweeping	Points to 3 body parts, obeys single commands, says six words, jargons echoes, speech	Neat pincer picking of threads pins, scribbles using fisted grasp, turns 2 or more pages at a time, builds tower of 3–4 (2.5 cm) cubes	Walks well, carries toys, climbs stairs, climbs into chair	• Drools no words • Absent pincer grasp • Does not walk
2–2.5 years				
Plays alone, tantrums, demanding; day by day, puts on shoes, socks, and pants; turns door handles; uses spoon and fork	Phrases of 2–3 words, gives name, 50 words+, naming games, has inner language	Turns one page at a time, imitates a straight line in both vertical and horizontal and a circle, unscrews lids, makes tower of 6–8 cubes	Pushes tricycle with feet, walks downstairs 2 feet per tread; runs, kicks ball jumps on the spot	• No speech • Unsteady on feet
3–3.5 years				
Goes toilet unassisted, dresses/undresses with minimum assistance. Knows some nursery rhymes, *handles spoon/knife* and fork, plays with peers	Gives full name, sex, counts to 10, 3–5 word sentences	Mature pen grasp, copies + and 0; correctly matches two or more colors; threads large beads; makes tower of 9	Stands on one leg for a few seconds, peddles tricycle, stairs adult style for ascent, jumps of bottom step	• No phrases • Persistent daytime wetting/soiling • Clumsy
4–5 years				
Wipes own bottom, eats using knife and fork, dresses—except for tie and laces, imaginative play, plays in groups, shares toys, obeys rules	Gives address/age/telephone no, counts up to 10 by 4 years, 20 by 5 years, knows 3 coins, grammatical speech asks meaning of abstract words	Matches 4 colors, copies cross, square, and by 5 a triangle; draws a recognizable man	4 years, climbs trees and ladder, enjoys ball games 5 years, hops, skip jumps off 3 steps, catches a ball	• Socially isolated • Unintelligible or ungrammatical speech • Unable to tell name or address

School Age

- Test for reading, arithmetic functions, such as +, –, ×, ÷, writing name, age, address, drawing a picture to test application, concentration, and organizational skills;
- Test deafness and physical examination;
- Vision by 3–5 years age of 6/6 (adult) capability;
- Intelligence assessment.

Various tests which can be used for developmental screening are already detailed in Chapters 3.1 and 3.7.

BIBLIOGRAPHY

1. Agarwal DK Awashthi A, Upadhyay SK, et al. Growth, behavior, development and intelligence in rural children between 1-3 years of age of life. Indian Pediatrics. 1992;29:467-80.
2. Bhatia VP, Katiyar GP, Agarwal KN. Effect of intrauterine utritional deprivation on neuromotor behavior of the newborn. Acta Paediatr Scand. 1979;68:561-6.
3. Kleigman, et al. (Eds). Nelson's Textbook of Pediatrics: Part II Growth Development and Behavior. Publ Elsevier Inc. 2011. pp 26-39.
4. The Early Years Foundation Stage (2012). Child Development Overview. [Online] Available from: http:// webarchie. nationalarchieves.gov_uk/2013401151715. [Accessed September, 2018].
5. Upadhay SK Saran A, Agarwal DK, et al. Growth and behavior development in rural infants in relation to malnutrition and nutrition. Indian Pediatrics 1992; 29:595-606.

3.7 Developmental Delay

MKC Nair, Deepa Bhaskaran

DEFINITION

Developmental delay exists when a child does not reach developmental milestones at the expected age (with the adequate provision for the broad variation among normal children). Developmental delays may occur in any or all the major areas of child development: gross motor, fine motor, language, and social. Identification of developmental delay is useful for introducing early intervention programs, with the objective of reducing childhood disability. Developmental prediction is not always possible, as we may go wrong often. By doing developmental assessment, we can only opine on present status in relation to age and average performance of other children of same age. We cannot accurately predict future intelligence, delayed maturation effect, and long-term effects of emotional deprivation.

EPIDEMIOLOGY

Statistics from different sources indicate that in India, 3.8% of the population has some form of disability, and the same was found to be more common among children of the lowest socioeconomic class families when compared with the next-to-lowest class families. A state-wide study revealed 2.5% prevalence of developmental delay using Thiruvananthapuram Developmental Screening Chart (TDSC 0–3) and 2.8% speech and language delay using Language Evaluation Scale Thiruvananthapuram (0–3). A district-wide study of children below 6 years revealed that 3.08% children had two or more item delay using TDSC 0–6. Among the screen positives (item delay cases) evaluated in detail, the majority had developmental delay alone (50%), speech and language delay (25%), multiple disabilities (23%), intellectual disability (17%), cerebral palsy (8%), hearing impairment (5%), seizure disorders (4%), visual impairment (3%), neuromuscular disorders (1%), and autism (1%) using appropriate tools. The presence of biological risk factors for developmental delay, such as low birth weight, birth asphyxia, poor home environment, and alternate child-care services, has highlighted the need for simple cost-effective community model for promoting early child development.

ETIOPATHOGENESIS

Child development is a dynamic process optimally utilizing the genetic potential of the baby, within the context of the available environment, enabling achievement of full potential. Severe forms of disability are less common and are often due to congenital, genetic, metabolic causes or intrauterine infections, and need-specific preventive strategies. Experience of a developmental evaluation clinic has shown that nearly 50% of babies referred for developmental evaluation had developmental delay without a specific clinical diagnosis. Delayed cry at birth, increasing age of the child, presence of feeding problems, assisted delivery, and birth injury were found to be associated with increasingly abnormal developmental test.

A risk factor is something that increases the likelihood of getting a disease or condition. The risk factors can be classified as follows:

- *Established risk:* These include medical disorders that can lead to developmental delay. It includes Down syndrome, hydrocephalus, cerebral palsy, hearing impairment, visual impairment, and other congenital anomalies.
- *Environmental risk:* This includes limited environmental factors, which put a child at risk for developmental delay. The various factors are a very young mother, extreme poverty, low socioeconomic status, single parent, etc.
- *Biological risk:* These include factors, such as prematurity, low birth weight, neonatal hypothermia, asphyxia, hypoglycemia, hyperbilirubinemia, and convulsions. These are factors which operate in the prenatal, natal, and postnatal periods.
- *No apparent risk:* Developmental delays also occur in infants without any apparent risks. In not more than 10% of cerebral palsy cases, perinatal asphyxia could be attributed as the true cause.

Advances in perinatal care have improved the survival chances of low-birth-weight babies, thus adding to the burden of developmental delay. It has been shown that 40% reduction in poor performance could be achieved among neonatal nursery graduates by Child Development Center (CDC) model early stimulation. Which "high-risk" newborns require periodic screening ideally needs to be determined locally. It must also be remembered that many babies not considered "high risk" may also manifest developmental problems as they grow. These babies would obviously not been seen during "high-risk" focused follow-up screening.

DEVELOPMENTAL ASSESSMENT

Developmental screening of all babies particularly graduates of neonatal intensive care unit, including vision and hearing domain, is important in identification of potentially handicapping conditions that may be prevented or ameliorated if addressed early. A screening test is only meant to identify children who might have a delay and who need further developmental evaluation.

Birth to One Year

Developmental Observation Card

The developmental observation card is a simple developmental card that can be used by parents to identify delay.

- *Completed 2 months:* Social smile—baby smiling back in response to smile.
- *Completed 4 months:* Holds head steady—keeping head steady when baby is held upright.
- *Completed 8 months:* Sits alone—baby can sit alone with back straight, no support.
- *Completed 12 months:* Stands alone—baby can stand bearing weight on both legs with minimal support.

Child Development Center Grading for Motor Milestones

Head holding grading (assessed at completed 4 months):

- *Grade 0:* No head holding at all;
- *Grade I:* Head erect and steady momentarily **(Fig. 3.7.1)**;
- *Grade II:* Dorsal suspension—lifts head along with body **(Fig. 3.7.2)**;
- *Grade III:* Prone position—elevates on arms, lifting chest **(Fig. 3.7.3)**;
- *Grade IV:* Holds head steady while mother moves around **(Fig. 3.7.4)**;
- *Grade V:* Head balanced always **(Fig. 3.7.5)**.

Sitting grading (assessed at completed 8 months):

- *Grade 0:* No sitting at all;
- *Grade I:* Sits momentarily **(Fig. 3.7.6)**;
- *Grade II:* Sits 30 seconds or more leaning forward **(Fig. 3.7.7)**;

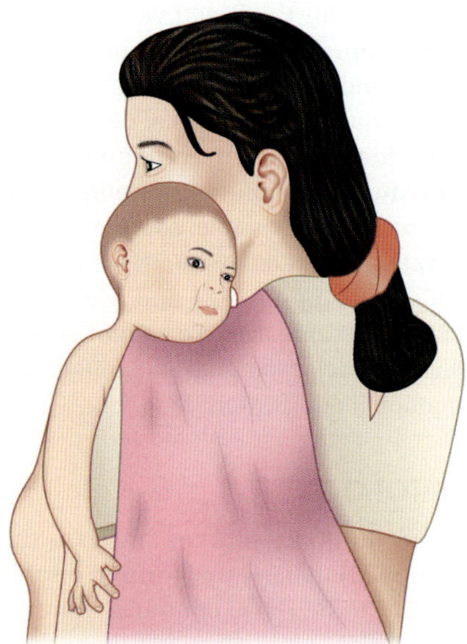

Fig. 3.7.1: Head holding Grade I.

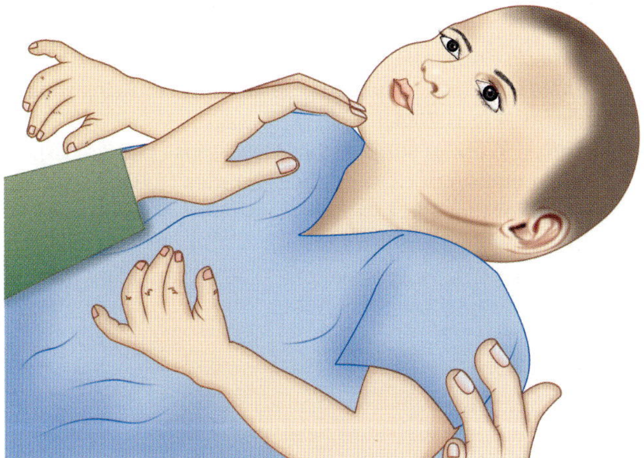

Fig. 3.7.2: Head holding grade II.

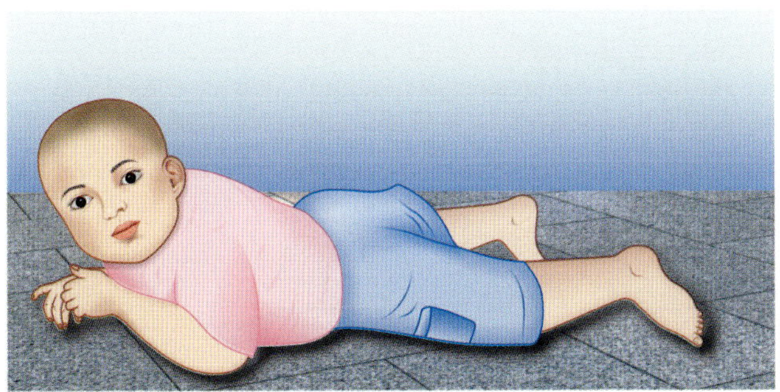

Fig. 3.7.3: Head holding grade III.

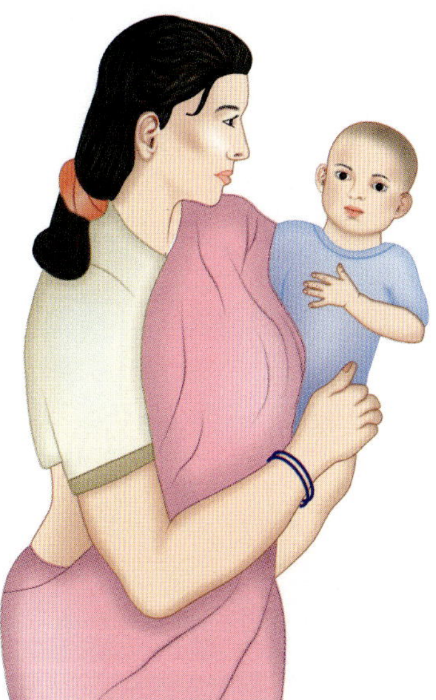

Fig. 3.7.4: Head holding grade IV.

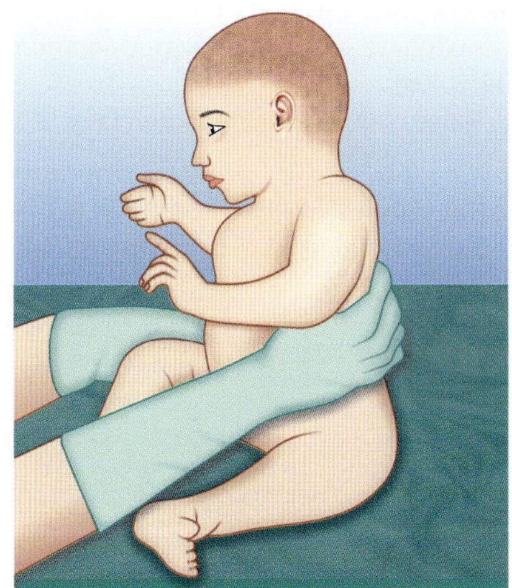

Fig.3.7.5: Head holding grade V.

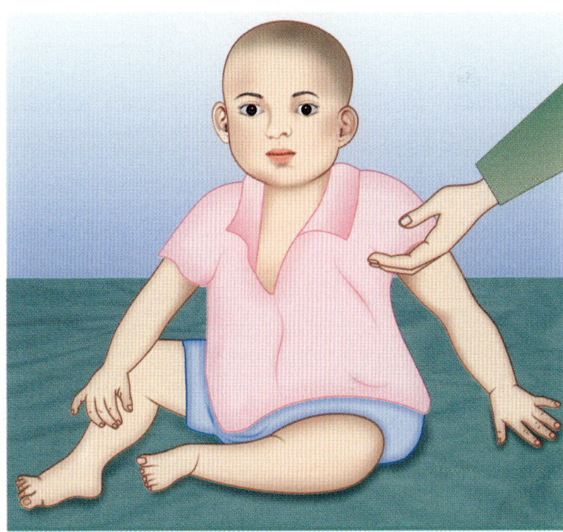

Fig. 3.7.6: Sitting grade I.

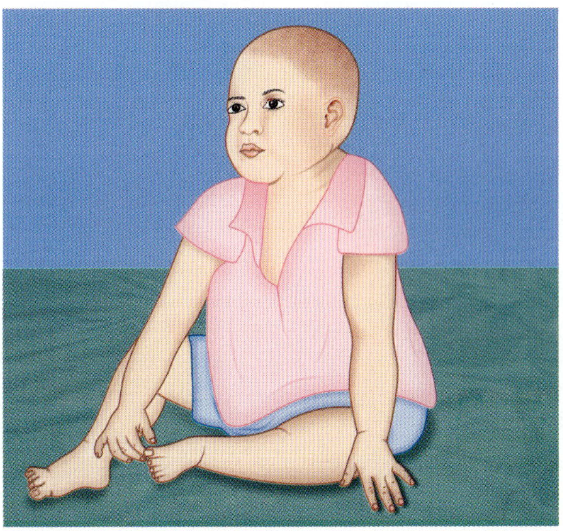

Fig. 3.7.7: Sitting grade II.

- *Grade III:* Sits with the child's back straight **(Fig. 3.7.8)**;
- *Grade IV:* While sitting, can turn around and manipulate a toy **(Fig. 3.7.9)**;
- *Grade V:* Raises self to sitting position **(Fig. 3.7.10)**.

Standing grading (assessed at completed 12 months):

- *Grade 0:* Not standing well;
- *Grade I:* Stands holding on to furniture momentarily **(Fig. 3.7.11)**;
- *Grade II:* Takes few steps with both hands supported **(Fig. 3.7.12)**;
- *Grade III:* Can stand alone with legs apart **(Fig. 3.7.13)**;
- *Grade IV:* Comes to standing position by throwing weight on arms **(Fig. 3.7.14)**;
- *Grade V:* Without support takes few steps **(Fig. 3.7.15)**.
- (Interpretation of CDC grading—grades III, IV, and V are normal for that age.)

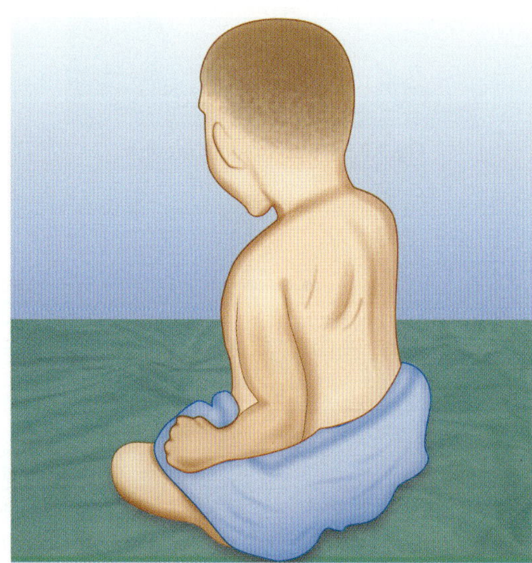

Fig. 3.7.8: Sitting grade III.

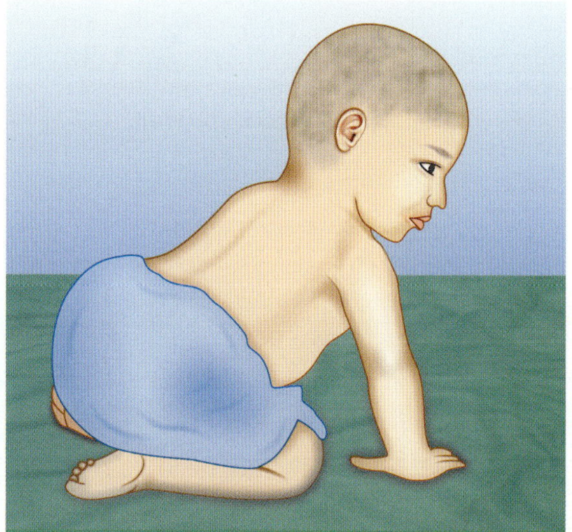

Fig. 3.7.10: Sitting grade V.

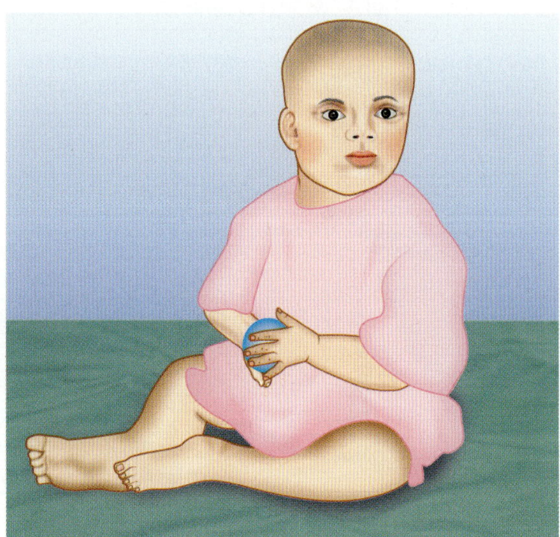

Fig. 3.7.9: Sitting grade IV.

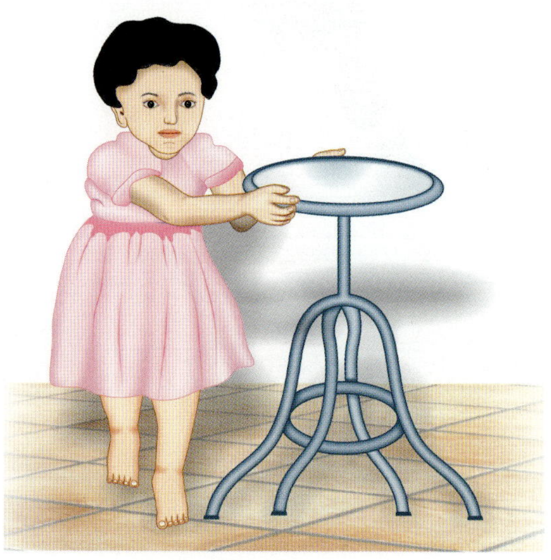

Fig. 3.7.11: Standing grade I.

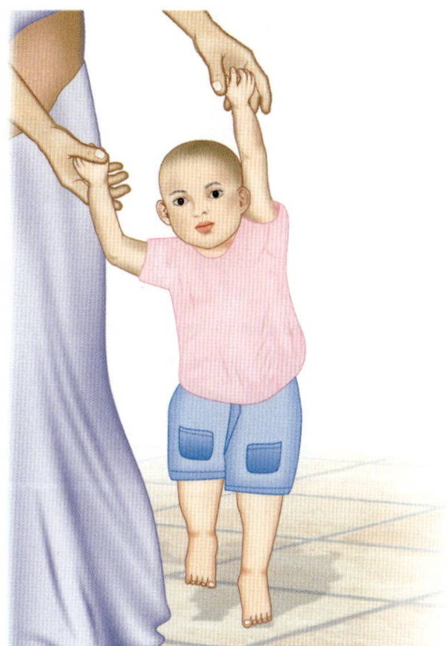

Fig. 3.7.12: Standing grade II.

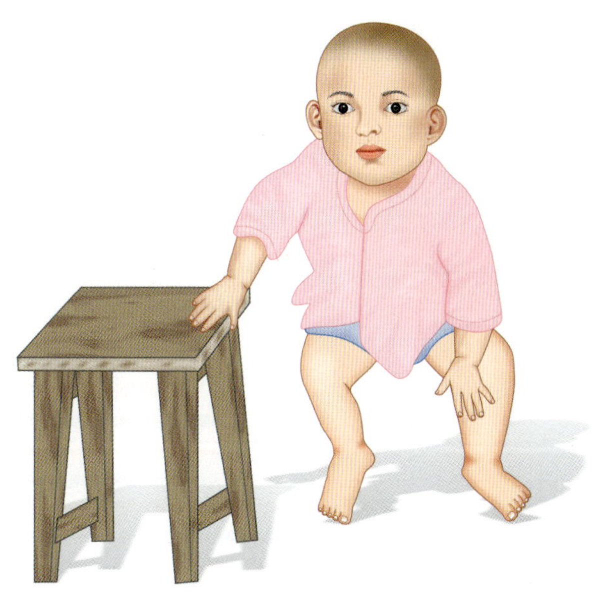

Fig.3.7.14: Standing grade IV.

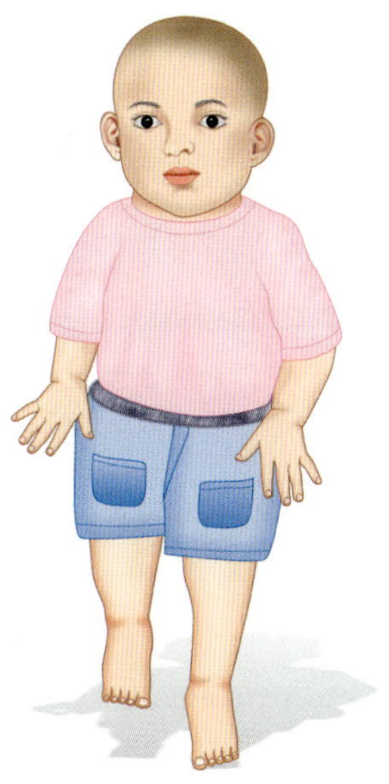

Fig. 3.7.13: Standing grade III.

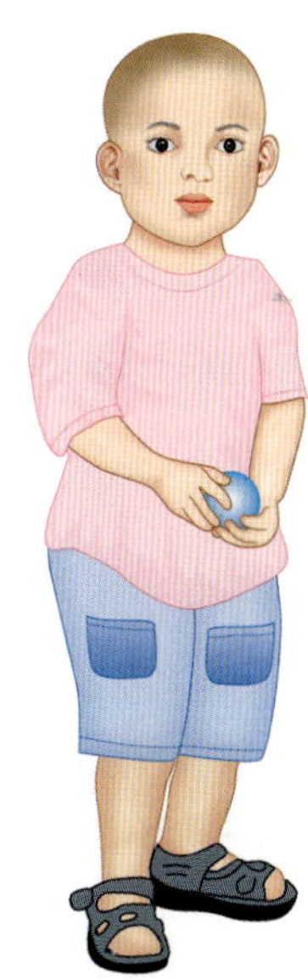

Fig.3.7.15: Standing grade V.

Birth to 2 Years

Thiruvananthapuram Developmental Screening Chart (0–3 years and 3–6 years) (Figs. 3.7.16 and 3.7.17; Table 3.7.1)

This is a simple developmental screening test for babies below 6 years that can be used in large-scale community.

Developmental screening programs can be done in the community by "anganwadi" workers and other health workers using TDSC. The left end of each horizontal dark line represents the age at which 3% of children passed the item, and the right end represents the age at which 97% of the children passed the item. A vertical line is drawn, or a pencil is kept vertically, at the level of the chronological age of the child being tested. If the child fails to achieve any item

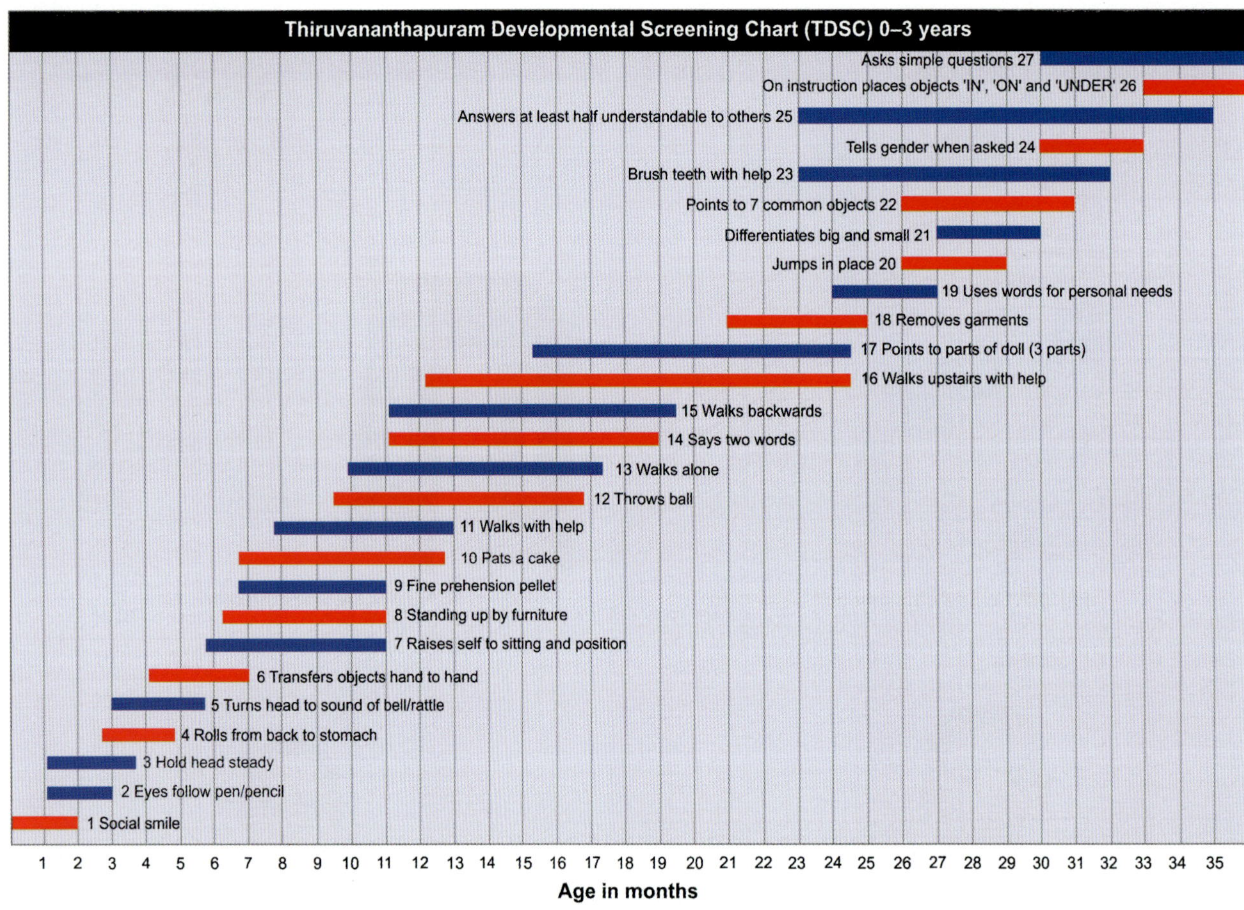

Fig. 3.7.16: Thiruvananthapuram Developmental Screening Chart (TDSC: 0–3 years).

that falls short on the left side of the vertical line, the child is considered to have a developmental delay.

LANGUAGE EVALUATION SCALE THIRUVANANTHAPURAM (0–3 YEARS) (FIG. 3.7.18)

This is a simple language screening tool for babies below 3 years to identify delay in language development in the community or developmental clinic, to provide simple language stimulation by mother and other care givers. The left end of each horizontal dark line represents the age at which 3% of children passed the item, and the right end represents the age at which 97% of the children passed the item. A vertical line is drawn, or a pencil is kept vertically, at the level of the chronological age of the child being tested. If the child fails to achieve any item that falls short on the left side of the vertical line, the child is considered to have a language delay.

Two to Four Years

Developmental Assessment Tool for Anganwadi

Developmental assessment tool for anganwadi is a short, psychometrically strong, and norm-referenced developmental scale with partial criterion, referencing to identify toddlers at "anganwadi" who are at risk for developing developmental delays and differentiate those who already have developed delays at 2.5 years for appropriate interventions. In addition, it is recommended that regular developmental assessments be conducted on the beneficiaries of "anganwadi" every year at three more key ages of 3.5, 4.5, and 5.5 years to institute early intervention when required **(Fig. 3.7.19)**.

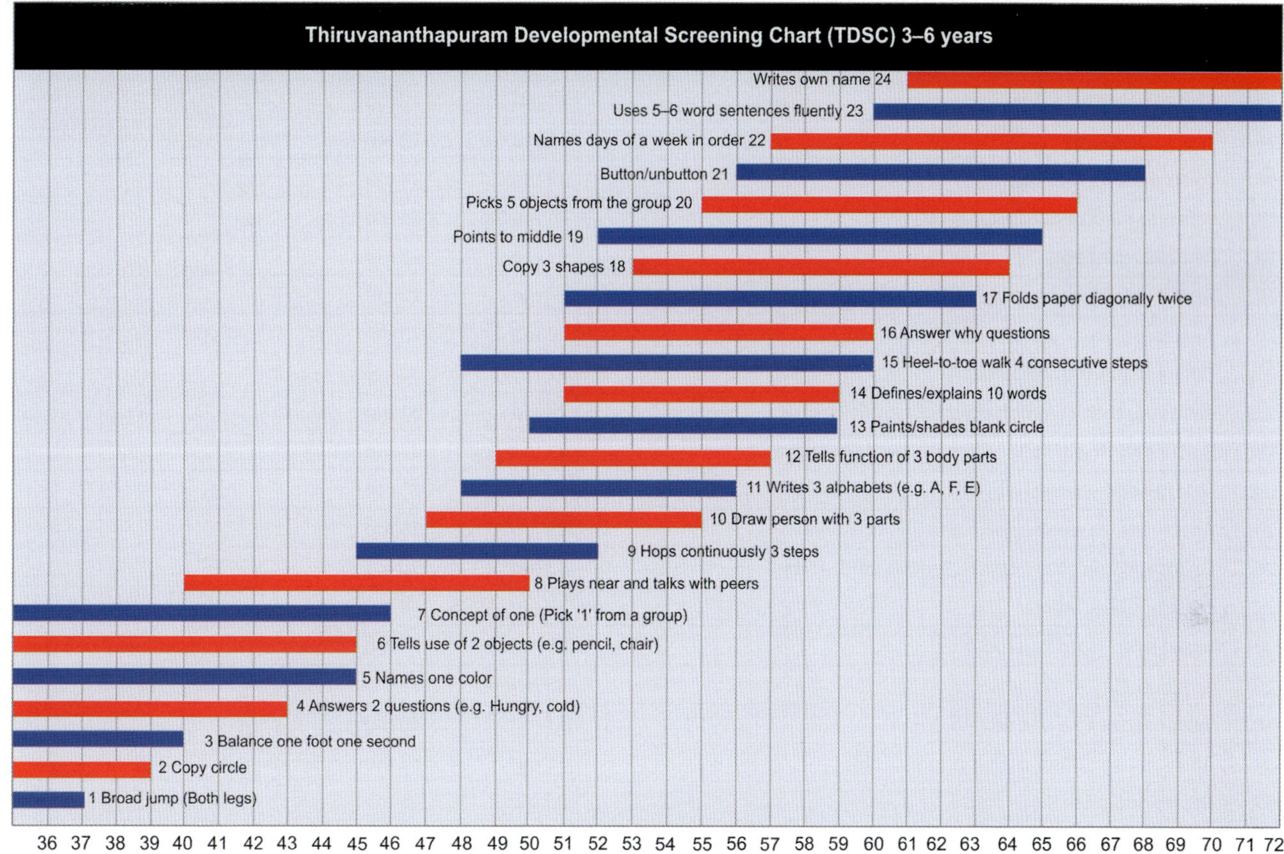

Fig. 3.7.17: Thiruvananthapuram Developmental Screening Chart (TDSC: 3–6 years).
Source: Nair MKC, Nair GH, Mini AO, Indulekha S, Letha S, Russell PS. Development and validation of language evaluation scale Trivandrum for children aged 0-3 years--LEST (0-3). Indian Pediatr. 2013;50(5):463-7.

Table 3.7.1: Test items used in Thiruvananthapuram Developmental Screening Chart (0–6 year).

	Items	*Lower limit*	*Upper limit*
1.	Social smile	1 d	2 mo
2.	Eyes follow pen/pencil	1 mo 3 d	3 mo
3.	Holds head steady	1 mo 3 d	3 mo 24 d
4.	Rolls from back to stomach	2 mo 21 d	4 mo 24 d
5.	Turns head to sound of bell/rattle	3 mo	5 mo 24 d
6.	Transfers objects hand to hand	4 mo 3 d	7 mo
7.	Raises self to sitting position	5 mo 24 d	11 mo
8.	Standing up by furniture	6 mo 9 d	11 mo
9.	Fine prehension pellet	6 mo 24 d	11 mo
10.	Pats a cake	6 mo 24 d	12 mo 21 d
11.	Walks with help	7 mo 24 d	13 mo
12.	Throws ball	9 mo 15 d	16 mo 24 d
13.	Walks alone	9 mo 27 d	17 mo 12 d

Contd...

Contd...

	Items	**Lower limit**	**Upper limit**
14.	Says two words	11 mo 6 d	19 mo
15.	Walks backwards	11 mo 6 d	19 mo 15 d
16.	Walks upstairs with help	12 mo 6 d	24 mo 15 d
17.	Points to parts of doll (three parts)	15 mo 9 d	24 mo 15 d
18.	Removes garments	21 mo	25 mo
19.	Uses words for personal needs	24 mo	27 mo
20.	Jumps in place	26 mo	29 mo
21.	Differentiates big and small	27 mo	30 mo
22.	Points to seven common objects	26 mo	31 mo
23.	Brushes teeth with help	23 mo	32 mo
24.	Tells gender when asked	30 mo	33 mo
25.	Answers at least half understandable to others	23 mo	35 mo
26.	On instruction, places objects "in," "on," and "under"	33 mo	36 mo
27.	Asks simple questions	30 mo	36 mo
28.	Broad jump (both legs together)	35 mo	37 mo
29.	Copies circle	35 mo	39 mo
30.	Balances one foot one second	35 mo	40 mo
31.	Answers two questions (e.g. hungry, cold)	35 mo	43 mo
32.	Names one color	35 mo	45 mo
33.	Tells use of two objects (e.g., pencil, chair)	35 mo	45 mo
34.	Concept of one (pick one from a group)	35 mo	46 mo
35.	Plays near and talk with peers	45 mo	50 mo
36.	Hops continuously three steps	45 mo	52 mo
37.	Draws person with three parts	47 mo	55 mo
38.	Writes three alphabets (e.g. A, F, E)	48 mo	56 mo
39.	Tells function of three body parts	49 mo	57 mo
40.	Paints/shades blank circle	50 mo	59 mo
41.	Defines/explains 10 words	51 mo	59 mo
42.	Heel-to-toe walk four consecutive steps	48 mo	60 mo
43.	Answers why questions	51 mo	60 mo
44.	Folds paper diagonally twice	51 mo	63 mo
45.	Copy three shapes	53 mo	64 mo
46.	Points to middle	52 mo	65 mo
47.	Picks five objects from the group	55 mo	66 mo
48.	Button/unbutton	56 mo	68 mo
49.	Names days of a week in order	57 mo	70 mo
50.	Uses 5- to 6-word sentences fluently	60 mo	72 mo
51.	Writes own name	61 mo	72 mo

(d: Day/Days; mo: Month/Months)

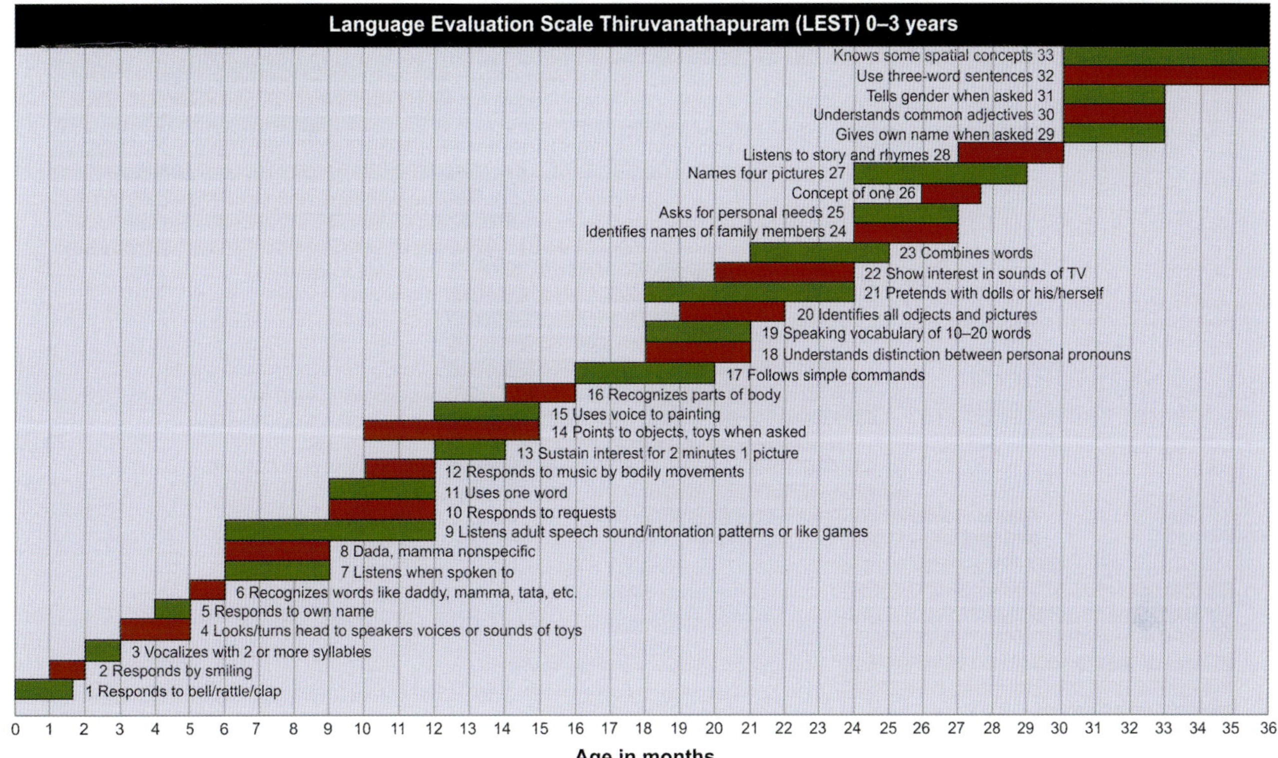

Fig. 3.7.18: Language Evaluation Scale Thiruvananthapuram (LEST 0–3 years).
Source: Nair MKC, Nair GH, Mini AO, Indulekha S, Letha S, Russell PS. Development and validation of language evaluation scale Trivandrum for children aged 0-3 years--LEST (0-3). Indian Pediatr. 2013;50(5):463-7.

Four to Six Years

Nursery Evaluation Scale Thiruvananthapuram—Abridged (Table 3.7.2)

Assessment of a preschool child in a clinic setting by a developmental pediatrician or psychologist using Denver Developmental Screening Test (DDST) II would help identify children with developmental delay. But in a borderline case, what is more important is to understand the level of skill development in the child as compared to other children of the same age (percentile position), so that appropriate item-based interventions can be offered. Nursery Evaluation Scale Thiruvananthapuram—Abridged is such a simple tool that consists of skill-based items in the areas of gross motor, fine motor, cognitive, personal social, expressive language, and receptive language to give an overall assessment of the child.

Denver Developmental Screening Test II

This instrument was designed to be a quick and simple screening tool to be used in clinical settings by persons with little training in developmental assessment. The test comprises of 125 items, divided into four categories:

1. Gross motor,
2. Fine motor/adaptive,
3. Language, and
4. Personal social.

The items are arranged in chronological order according to the ages at which most children pass them. The test items are represented on the form by a bar that spans the age at which 25%, 50%, 75%, and 90% of the standardization sample passed that item. The child's age is drawn as a vertical line on the chart, and the examiner administers the items bisected by the line. The child's performance is rated "pass," "caution," or "delay" depending on where the age line is drawn across the bar. The total number of delays or cautions determines the rating of DDST as normal, questionable, or abnormal.

Developmental Assessment Scale for Indian Infants

This is the gold standard test used for developmental evaluation, developed by Pramila Pathak, and is based on Bayley scales of infant development. Developmental

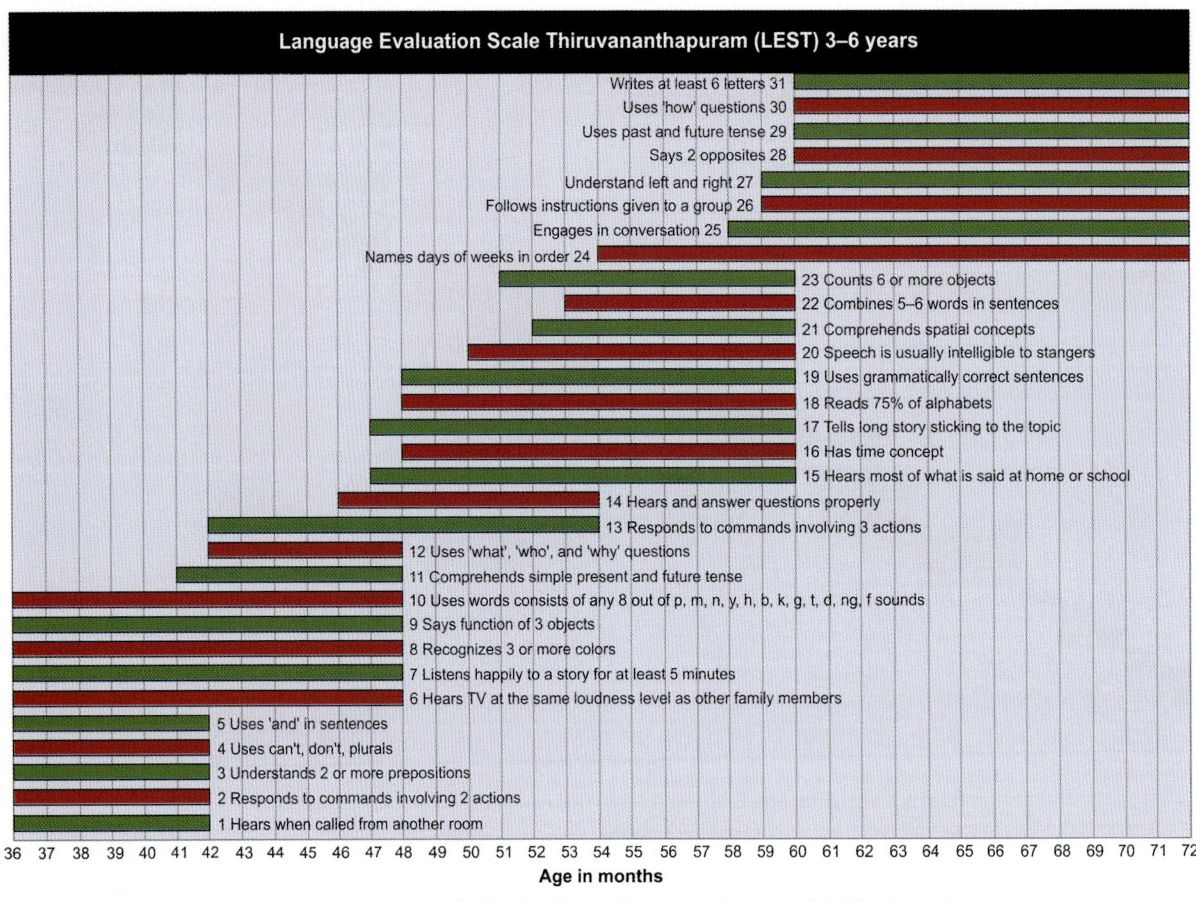

Fig. 3.7.19: Language Evaluation Scale Thiruvananthapuram (LEST 3–6 years)
Source: Nair MKC, Harikumaran Nair GS, George B, et al. Language Evaluation Scale Trivandrum (LEST 3-6 years) development and validation. Indian Pediatr. 2016;53(3):257-8.

Assessment Scale for Indian Infants consists of two scales, namely, mental scale and motor scale. The results of administration of mental scale are expressed as a standard score, the mental development index, and that of the motor scale as the psychomotor development index.

NEUROLOGICAL EVALUATION

Although it is easy to diagnose a given case of cerebral palsy, when it comes to follow-up of high-risk babies, a system of neurological examination that allows detection and recording of subtle neurological abnormalities that may disappear at the end of the first year (called transient abnormalities) or persist even beyond that (persistent abnormalities) is needed. Amiel-Tison has provided us with a comprehensive system of neurological evaluation for the first 5 years of life that gives us a framework for instituting physical therapy program. In the Amiel-Tison method of neurological evaluation, the presence of tone abnormalities is identified by measuring the following angles **(*see* Table 3.7.1)**.

Adductor Angle

With the infant lying supine, the legs are extended and gently pulled as far apart as possible. The angle formed by the legs at this point is called the adductor angle. Asymmetry between the right and the left leg should be noted **(Fig. 3.7.20)**.

Heel to Ear

With the infant lying supine, the legs are held together and pressed as far as possible, toward the ear. The pelvis must not be lifted from the table. The angle is represented by the arc extending from the infant's heel to the table. The increased

Table 3.7.2: Nursery Evaluation Scale Thiruvananthapuram—Abridged.

Items	*3rd, 50th, and 97th percentile age placements in months*		
	3rd percentile	***50th percentile***	***97th percentile***
Gross motor development			
1. Heel-to-toe walk eight steps	61	68	72
2. Stands on one foot 10 s	48	57	66
3. Walk on 20-cm elevated balanced beam	64	69	72
4. Catches a soft ball with one hand	53	64	68
Fine motor development			
5. Paints shape	50	56	59
6. Tears simple shape	53	64	68
7. Copies diamond shape	63	66	72
8. Prints A E F	48	53	56
9. Threads 10 beads in 1 min	50	57	65
10. Draws picture with three parts (excluding draw a man)	56	61	66
Cognitive development			
11. Picks specific number of objects (5)	55	64	66
12. Builds pyramid of 10 blocks	54	66	71
13. Arranges objects according to width and length	53	63	69
14. Puts numbers 1–10 in a sequence	48	54	59
15. Names positions of objects	46	52	65
16. Completes a simple maze	50	56	60
17. Names days of a week in order	57	65	70
18. Reads 10 printed words	61	68	72
Personal social development			
19. Buttons and unbuttons dress	56	63	68
20. Washes hands and mouth when directed	42	45	48
Expressive language development			
21. Names function associated with three body parts	49	52	57
22. Tells materials out of which objects are made of	53	60	66
Receptive language development			
23. Points to hard/soft/rough/smooth	51	59	63
24. Points to middle	52	60	65
25. Points to absurdities in a picture	51	57	62
26. Puts together five parts picture	58	68	72

resistance on one side is an indication of asymmetry, but it might be difficult to apply equal pressure to both sides **(Fig. 3.7.21)**.

Popliteal Angle

The thighs are flexed laterally at the hip along both sides of the abdomen. While holding the infant in this position, the examiner presses the lower leg as far as possible toward the thigh. The popliteal angle, which is formed by the calf and the thigh, is estimated in both legs simultaneously.

In contrast to the maneuvers described above, it is easier to apply equal pressure to both sides when examining the popliteal angle. Therefore, the estimation of asymmetry is more objective. Significant asymmetry is indicated by a difference of 10°–20° between the right and left angles **(Fig. 3.7.22)**.

Dorsiflexion Angle of the Foot

The examiner holds the infant's leg straight and flexes the foot toward the leg. This is accomplished by applying pressure with the thumb to the sole of the foot. The dorsiflexion angle is formed by the dorsum of the foot and the anterior aspect of the leg **(Fig. 3.7.23)**.

Scarf Sign

The infant is held in a semireclining position, supported by the examiner's palm. At the same time, the examiner takes the infant's hand and pulls the arm as far as possible, across the chest toward the opposite shoulder. Four positions are possible in describing the position of the elbow in relationship to the umbilicus **(Fig. 3.7.24 and Table 3.7.3)**.

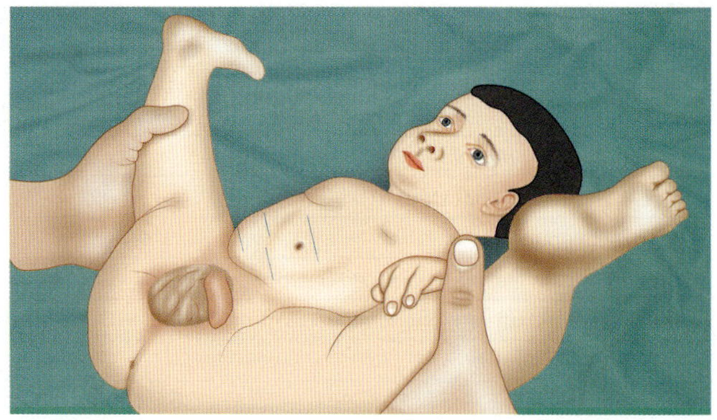

Fig. 3.7.22: Popliteal angle.

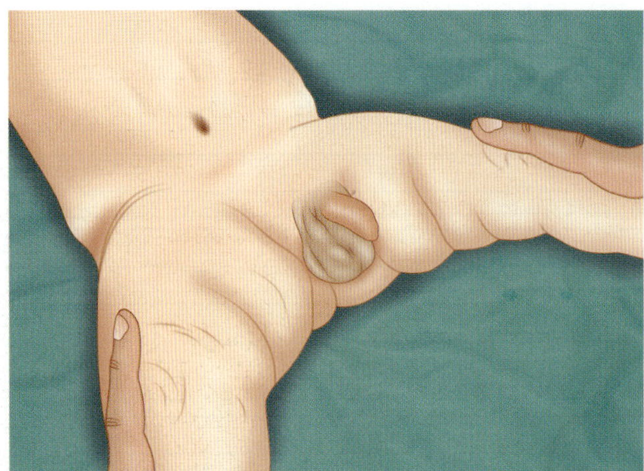

Fig. 3.7.20: Adductor angle.

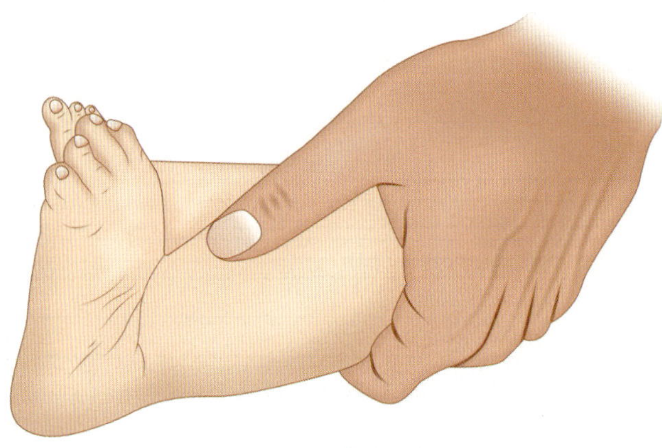

Fig. 3.7.23: Dorsiflexion angle.

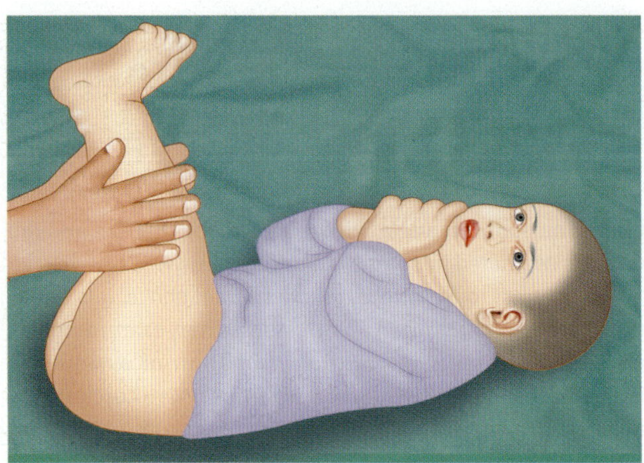

Fig. 3.7.21: Heel-to-ear angle.

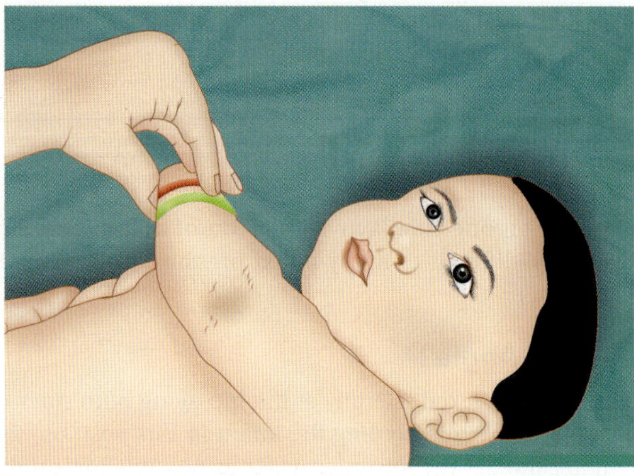

Fig. 3.7.24: Scarf sign.

Table 3.7.3: Neurological assessment.

	Angles in degrees			
Angle	***1–3 months***	***4–6 months***	***7–9 months***	***10–12 months***
Adductor	40–80	70–110	100–150	130–150
Heel-to-ear	80–100	90–130	120–150	140–170
Popliteal	80–100	90–130	120–150	140–170
Dorsiflexion	45	45	45	45
Scarf sign	Elbow not cross midline	Elbow cross midline	Elbow reaches axilla	Elbow beyond axilla

DEVELOPMENTAL THERAPY

Therapy Based on Passive Exercises

Out of the items assessed in the Amiel-Tison method, the angles give an important clue for the therapy and stimulation part of intervention. A limitation in angles indicates hypertonia, and wide angle indicates hypotonia in most cases. In such instances, stimulation becomes effective only after normalizing the muscle tone. The purpose of passive therapy is essentially to reduce these deformities by constant effort of the mother in a playful manner. Home therapy based on Amiel-Tison passive angles is a simple concept which does not aim to hasten developmental milestones, but aims to prevent:

- Mental subnormality by better mother–infant interaction;
- Joint stiffening by repeated passive movements;
- Contractures by repetitive passive movements;
- Muscle wasting and fibrosis;
- Helplessness in parents.

Therapy Based on Motor Milestones

Head Holding/Neck Control

- Stimulating the child to hold the head by carrying the child in an upright position by supporting the infant's head, as and when possible.
- While playing and talking with the child, lift the child by supporting his upper arm and chest, thereby stimulating him to lift and hold his head.
- The child must be made to lie on his stomach and is guided on his elbow (a roll or round pillow can be used if necessary). Encourage the child to lift and hold his head by showing a colorful toy.
- Stimulate the child in prone position guiding on his hand on the surface, encourage the child to lift and hold his head, and then rotate laterally showing a colorful toy.

Sitting

- Encourage the child to sit by putting him in an arm chair in a sitting position supporting him with pillows, as and when possible.
- While playing and talking with the child, encourage the child to sit with a wide base (thighs apart), supporting at the pelvis with a downward force.
- During play, the child can be encouraged to sit in side-sitting position on both sides by supporting himself on the hand to the side toward which he is sitting.
- Guide the child to support on his hand and knees (four-point kneeling/quadruped position) during play. A roll or pillow can be used, if necessary. Then slowly guide him to sit on one of his sides supported by the same hand. Help the child to maintain this position for a while. Then guide him again on to his hands and knees and then gradually to side sitting on the other side.
- Baby walker can also be used to stimulate and improve sitting.

Standing

- Guide the child on to both his knees during play. Finally, support him at the pelvis. If necessary, give support to the upper part of his body. Gradually, the support can be withdrawn, and the child can be made to support himself by holding on to a low stool. This position can be maintained by directing the child's attention to any play activity.
- From lying on the back position (supine position), stimulate the child to sit and gradually to the standing position during play time.
- First, guide the child to both his knees, while he is supporting himself on a low stool with both hands. While directing his attention to a colorful toy through play, slowly help him to raise one leg to make him stand on one foot (leg straight), the other on the knee (half standing position), and help the child to maintain this position while playing and talking with him. This position can be repeated on the other side. Meanwhile, depending on the child's ability, stimulate him to pull to standing position by himself, supporting on the stool.
- Encourage the child to stand, as and when possible, first with support then gradually withdrawing the support as per the child's ability. A baby walker will also serve the purpose of developing standing and walking skills.

BIBLIOGRAPHY

1. Indian Pediatrics (2009). Supplement issue on child development: Indian Pediatrics. [online] Available from: http://www.indianpediatrics.net/suppl2009/supple.htm. [Accessed September, 2018].
2. Malhi P, Singhi P. Screening young children for delayed development. Indian Pediatr. 1999;36(6):569-77.
3. Nair MKC. Developmental pediatrics, 1st edition. Delhi: Noble Vision (Medical Book Publishers); 2017.
4. Nair MKC, Babu G, Sabarinathan. CDC grading for head holding sitting and standing. Indian J Pract Pediatr. 1995;3(1):534.
5. Nair MKC, Harikumaran Nair GS, Beena M, et al. CDC Kerala 16: early detection of developmental delay/disability among children below 6 y—a district model. Indian J Pediatr. 2014;81(Suppl 2):S151-5.
6. Nair MKC, Jain N, Murkhi S, et al. The high risk newborn. New Delhi: Jaypee Brothers Medical Publishers (P) Ltd; 2007.
7. Nair MKC, Mathews S, George B, et al. Early stimulation: CDC Trivandrum model. Indian J Pediatr. 1992;59(6):663-7.
8. Nair MKC, Nair GS, George B, et al. Development and validation of Thiruvananthapuram Development Screening Chart for children aged 0-6 years [TDSC (0-6)]. Indian J Pediatr. 2013;80(Suppl 2):S248-55.
9. Nair MKC, Nair GH, Mini AO, et al. Development and Validation of Language Evaluation Scale Thiruvananthapuram for children of 0-3 years—LEST (0-3). Indian Pediatr. 2013;50(5):463-7.
10. Nair MKC, Princly P, Leena ML, et al. CDC Kerala 17: early detection of developmental delay/disability among children below 3 y in Kerala—a cross sectional survey. Indian J Pediatr. 2014;81(Suppl 2):S156-60.
11. Nair MKC, Russell P. Illingworth's the development of the infant and young child: normal and abnormal, 10th edition. Gurugram: Reed Elsevier Private Limited; 2012.

3.8 Failure to Thrive

Madhulika Kabra

INTRODUCTION

Failure to thrive (FTT) is a common and often perplexing concern for parents and pediatricians. Pathophysiologically, FTT is a state of caloric insufficiency without an apparent etiology. It is a descriptive term used for children whose attained weight or rate of weight gain is significantly below their age, gender, and ethnicity matched controls. Though primarily weight is affected, linear growth and head circumference may also get affected if the insult is prolonged and severe.

Failure to thrive is not a specific diagnosis, but a physical sign indicating that the child is not receiving adequate nutrition affecting optimal growth and development. A pediatrician's responsibility is to work up the child in stepwise manner based on the history and examination and to identify the cause of inadequate nutrition ruling out an underlying organic cause but at the same time keeping in mind that the etiology may be multifactorial. The traditional concept of "organic" versus "nonorganic" FTT is no longer preferred but may still be referred to by some health professionals.

DEFINITION

Failure to thrive is sustained weight loss, failure to gain weight, or a persistent fall in weight from the child's normal centile (**Fig. 3.8.1**). This definition excludes transient weight loss associated with acute illness. It includes a child whose weight is below the 3rd or 5th percentile for age on more than one consecutive evaluation or if the weight drops below two major percentiles. It also includes a child whose weight is less than 80% of the ideal weight for age and also a child whose weight is below the 3rd or 5th percentile for the weight-for-length. Following these definitions strictly may not always be easy as serial measurements may be required and action during the first visit may be confusing, though the last two definitions may facilitate diagnosis, but the child may not qualify the specific definition though subjectively malnourished. Commonly used criteria are shown in **Table 3.8.1**.

Persistence of FTT may not only lead to long-term complications related to physical growth but also development and behavior.

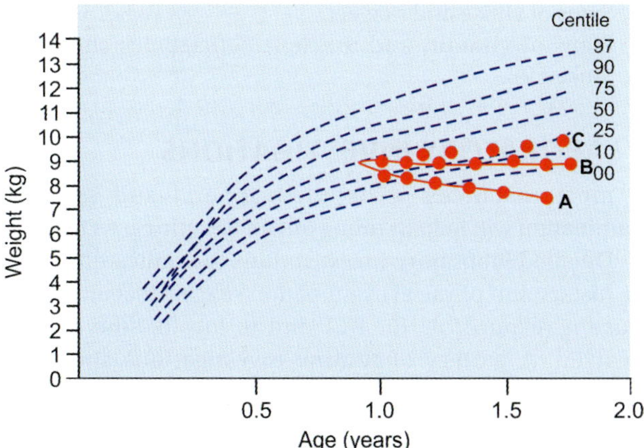

Fig. 3.8.1: Failure to thrive—(A) weight loss, (B) static weight, and (C) falloff in weight gain.

Table 3.8.1: Definition of failure to thrive.
Attained growth
• Weight <3rd percentile on standard growth chart • Weight for height <5th percentile on standard growth chart • Weight 20% or more below ideal weight for height
Rate of growth
• Less than 20 g/day from birth to 3 months of age • Less than 15 g/day from 3 months to 6 months of age • Falloff from previously established growth curve • Downward crossing of >2 major percentiles

Important points to remember are as follows:
- Label of FTT should not be given, based on a single observation, that is, failure to gain weight or weight loss should be observed over a period of time.
- Small size alone is not an adequate criterion for confirming FTT, as constitutional and genetic factors may result in short stature.

ETIOLOGY

As discussed above, the traditional classification of dividing the causes of FTT as organic and nonorganic is probably not very appropriate. Whether the condition is primarily organic or nonorganic in origin, all children who fail to thrive suffer the physical and psychological consequences of malnutrition and are at a significant risk for long-term physical and psychodevelopmental sequelae. **Table 3.8.2** summarizes the causes of FTT.

Organic diseases are responsible for less than 20% of the cases with FTT. It should be recognized that environmental deprivation can coexist with and complicate organic FTT. For example, a child with cerebral palsy or multiple congenital malformations is likely to be environmentally deprived due to lack of care. Organic causes of FTT are most commonly gastrointestinal or neurologic.

Table 3.8.2: Causes of inadequate weight gain.
Inadequate intake and inappropriate feeding practices
Nonavailability of food: • Misperceptions about diet and feeding practices • Errors in formula reconstitution • Dysfunctional parent–child interaction, child abuse, and neglect • Behavioral feeding problem • Mechanical problems with sucking, swallowing, and feeding • Primary neurological diseases • Chronic systemic disease resulting in anorexia, food refusal, and neurological problems
Reduced absorption or digestion
• Pancreatic insufficiency—cystic fibrosis • Damage to villus surface—celiac disease
Excessive loss
• Persistent vomiting • Gastroesophageal reflux disease • Gastrointestinal obstruction • Increased intracranial pressure • Renal losses—renal tubular acidosis • Diabetes mellitus • Inborn errors of metabolism
Increased caloric requirements
• Congenital heart disease • Chronic respiratory disease • Neoplasm • Hyperthyroidism • Chronic or recurrent infection
Altered growth potential or regulation
• Chromosomal abnormalities • Endocrinopathies

DIAGNOSIS

History and physical examination is the mainstay for the diagnosis of FTT. It should be emphasized that extensive laboratory investigations have no role in the diagnosis unless assessment suggests a probable organic cause and localizes the pathology to a particular system. Before labeling an infant as FTT, one should exclude normal variants of growth. These include infant with small parents, constitutional delay, and prematurely born babies.

HISTORY

Ideally, both parents should be present during the interview, and parent-child and parent-parent interaction must be critically assessed.

Antenatal, Natal, and Perinatal History

Apart from the details of pregnancy, delivery and perinatal details, some points need special mention.

- Was the child born of unplanned pregnancy? Did the parents consider medical termination of pregnancy? Children born of unplanned pregnancy tend to be emotionally deprived.
- Was it a preterm delivery? If growth parameters are not corrected for gestational age, these children may be erroneously labeled as FTT.
- Intrauterine growth retardation is another risk factor for FTT. Symmetrical intrauterine growth restriction children have a worse prognosis in this regard.
- History suggestive of exposure to intrauterine infections.

Growth Data

Evaluation of growth pattern is the most important aspect. Review child's present and past growth parameters. This is only possible if parents have maintained a growth chart or previous growth status is known. In situations where previous record is not available, it is advisable to follow the child for weight gain.

Dietary History

A detailed dietary history, both past and present, should be elicited to evaluate caloric and protein intake.

Social and Family History

A detailed social and family history provides useful clues for diagnosis of nonorganic FTT. Following factors need special evaluation:

- Lack of "support systems:" Relatives and friends;
- Financial constraints;
- Psychiatric problems or drug abuse in family;
- Marital problems and parental discord;
- Serious illness or death in family.

Detailed Evaluation of Developmental Milestones

These are provided in the earlier chapters.

PHYSICAL EXAMINATION

Physical examination should be thorough and complete. Detailed anthropometry should include length/height, weight, head circumference, upper/lower segment ratio, skinfold thickness, and mid-upper arm circumference.

- Routine and thorough general and systemic examination is a must, as it gives clues to do specific investigations.
- Detailed neurodevelopmental assessment should be performed.
- Specific behavior patterns should be looked for. These may give a positive clue for nonorganic FTT. These include unusual watchfulness, decreased vocalization, lack of cuddliness, head banging, rocking movements, rumination.
- Signs of abuse and neglect.
- Signs of vitamin and nutrient deficiencies should be looked for.

LABORATORY INVESTIGATIONS

In most instances, a detailed general and systemic examination will help in ruling out an organic cause for FTT.

Detailed laboratory investigations are indicated, only if the history and physical examination suggest that an organic cause is responsible for FTT and to localize the systems involved. A battery of routine investigations should be avoided because they are unproductive in most instances, expensive, and may be misleading and diverting attention. The following investigations are considered adequate for initial evaluation:

- Complete blood count with erythrocyte sedimentation rate
- Urine and stool examination
- Urine culture and sensitivity
- Tuberculin test
- Blood urea and serum creatinine
  - *Specific tests*: Workup for inborn errors of metabolism, karyotyping, sweat test, celiac serology, endoscopy, etc. may be considered if indicated based on history and examination.
  - Radiological investigations are not routinely indicated, unless the child needs evaluation for tuberculosis or physical abuse. Determination of bone age may be required in some cases. More invasive diagnostic procedures are called for, when a specific diagnosis is suspected.

Treatment

The major goals of management are nutritional rehabilitation, treating an organic cause if detected, and addressing psychosocial and developmental issues involved. Individual management of these has been discussed in detail in the subsequent chapters.

The first decision that one must take is whether the child requires hospitalization or not. Indications for hospitalization are as follows:

- Weight for height less than 70% of the median;
- Detailed evaluation for a suspected organic disorder;
- Suspected abuse or neglect;
- Nonresponse to outpatient management.

Nutritional repletion is the major aim of the treatment of FTT, even if the underlying cause is organic which can be managed in parallel. Associated problems due to an organic/nonorganic cause, such as anorexia, nausea, emesis, pain, or malaise, may cause poor eating or aversive feeding behaviors. The response of anxious family members may further potentiate psychogenic issues.

After the careful history, examination and investigations as indicated, management may be planned as follows:

- Start management of the underlying organic cause in parallel if identified.
- Careful, structured observation of the child's eating or feeding behavior and of how he or she interacts with family members during meals. Observe the following:
  - Does the child exhibit hunger and is attracted to food?
  - Is the child comfortable through the mealtimes for a developmentally appropriate length of time?
  - Any difficulty in chewing or swallowing food?
  - Any indications of aversive eating or abnormal behaviors, such as tantrums, gagging, injuring self or others?
  - Does the child induce emesis or retain food in the mouth for long periods?
- An experienced dietician should always be involved in planning and supervising diet. Unless there is a strong suspicion of an organic cause, which must be managed in parallel, one should proceed directly for a 2-week trial feeding. Daily monitoring during this period is extremely important. Nutrition monitoring record includes daily weight and the total calories consumed during the last 24 hours against expected. Every effort should be made to feed the child orally. If oral feeding is inadequate, tube feeding may be tried for short periods. Altering food textures, preparations, spacing meal times, etc. may help generate interest in feeding.
- Help of a child psychologist may be sought if indicated. Organization of a program of intensive environmental stimulation and affection is also needed. Every attempt should be made to see that parents are actively involved in the management. Initial treatment may include procedures, such as decreasing oromotor hypersensitivity, and working with the family to develop child-specific behavioral interventions, such as positive reinforcement for desired eating behaviors and extinction procedures to eliminate undesired behaviors. Punishment of undesired behaviors should be explicitly avoided.
- At the end of 2 weeks of trial feeding, the child is reassessed. A good intake during the feeding trial, and a good response in terms of weight gain, suggests that the primary problem was nutritional deprivation usually associated with emotional deprivation. It is perfectly justified to undertake detailed investigations in the child with FTT who fails to respond to a 2-week trial feeding. However, by this time, the physician usually has an idea of the diagnostic possibilities, and he/she can tailor the investigations accordingly.

PROGNOSIS

Most children with FTT have good growth recovery in all domains provided optimal care is taken for nutritional supplementation and emotional support. The overall prognosis for intellectual and behavioral recovery is variable and less certain.

BIBLIOGRAPHY

1. Bergman P, Graham J. An approach to "failure to thrive". Aust Fam Physician. 2005;34(9):725-9.
2. Corbett SS, Drewett RF. To what extent is failure to thrive in infancy associated with poorer cognitive development? A review and meta-analysis. J Child Psychol Psychiatr. 2004;45:641-54.
3. Goh LH, How CH, Ng KH. Failure to thrive in babies and toddlers. Singapore Med J. 2016;57(6):287-91.
4. Hank DA, Jeisel SH. Failure to thrive. Pediatr Clin North Am. 1998;35:1187-205.
5. Jaffe AC. Failure to thrive: current clinical concepts. Pediatr Rev. 2011;32(3):100-7.
6. Maggioni A, Lifshitz F. Nutritional management of failure to thrive. Pediatr Clin North Am. 1995;42(4):791-810.
7. Nangia S, Tiwari S. Failure to thrive. Indian J Pediatr. 2013;80(7):585-9.
8. Overby KJ. Failure to thrive. In: Rudolph AM (Ed). Rudolph's Pediatrics, 20th edition. Stamford: Appleton and Lange; 1996. pp. 39.
9. Suri M, Kabra M, Aggarwal A, et al. Failure to thrive. Indian J Pediatr. 1994;8.

Disclaimer: The views expressed by the individual authors about the "growth curves" are their own and do not reflect the official position/stand of the Editors or Indian Academy of Pediatrics.

Section 4

Nutrition

4.1 Infant and Young Child Feeding

RK Anand

We know that shamefully large numbers of children in both wealthy and poverty-stricken regions suffer malnutrition: the malnutrition of excess amounts of inappropriate foods and the malnutrition of insufficient nutritious foods. As adults, we should feel embarrassed that so many small children are so poorly fed. We can change this situation, if we want to and many people are already working to this end. Good nutrition for children harmonizes with good nutrition for adults...and it would be good for the world if we worked to this end.

—**Gabrielle Palmer**

INTRODUCTION

While adequate nutrition is important throughout the childhood, it is crucial during the first 5 years of a child's life, particularly so, in the first 2–3 years when rapid growth occurs and when the child is entirely dependent on the mother and the family for food.

OPTIMAL INFANT AND YOUNG CHILD FEEDING

Optimal infant and young child feeding (IYCF) is an evidence-based measure for improving child nutrition and child survival. The "World Health Organization (WHO)/ United Nations Children's Fund (UNICEF) Global Strategy for Infant and Young Child Feeding and the National Guidelines on Infant and Young Child Feeding 2010" recommended by the IYCF subspecialty chapter of the Indian Academy of Pediatrics stress that for proper growth and development, infants should be exclusively breastfed with no other food or drink—not even water, in the first 6 months of life (*see* Chapter 4.2). This must be followed by the sequential addition of nutritionally adequate, preferably homemade semisolid, and solid foods to complement (not to replace) breast milk, till the child is gradually able to eat normal family food after 1 year while breastfeeding is continued up to 24 months of age or beyond **(Fig. 4.1.1)**. Adequate nutrition for adolescent girls, pregnant, and lactating mothers is also important for child nutrition.

The period after 6 months, when other foods are added is also referred to as weaning. Some wrongly interpret it as weaning the baby away from the breast. Complementary feeding is a better term than weaning.

COMPLEMENTARY FEEDING

It is the process of giving a child other food while continuing breastfeeding, when her or his nutritional demands can no longer be fulfilled by breastfeeding alone. Appropriate

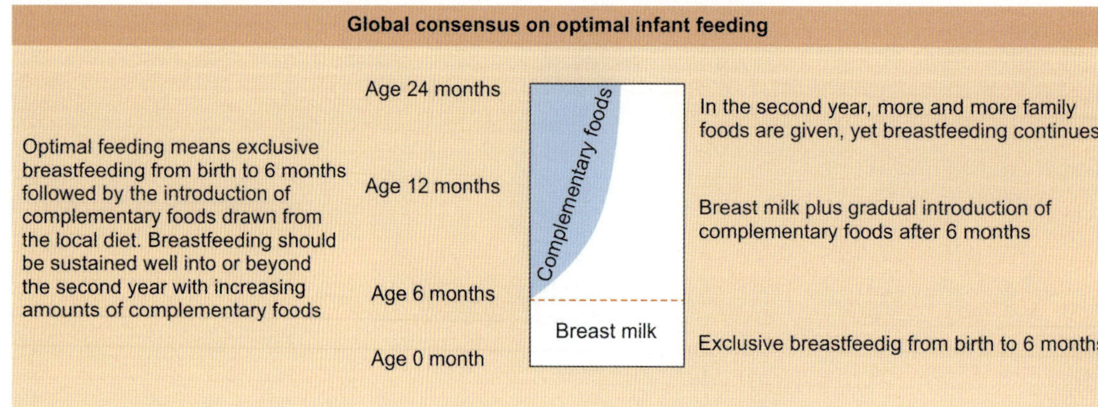

Fig. 4.1.1: Optimal infant and young child feeding.

complementary feeding should be timely, culturally acceptable, nutritionally adequate, safe, and responsive.

Timely Feeding

It is recommended that infants must be exclusively breastfed for 6 months, and adequate complementary foods should be added after that. Complementary feeding indicators in India are far from satisfactory. According to the National Family Health Survey 4 (NFHS-4), the introduction of complementary feeding along with continued breastfeeding in children of 6–8 months is only 42.7%.

Addition of anything other than breast milk before 6 months is fraught with danger for the following reasons:

- Addition of foods and other liquids (including water, soup, juice, rice water, *dal* water, etc.) interfere with optimal breastfeeding. They may fill up the child's stomach and quench the thirst and, consequently, may lead to less suckling at the breast with reduced milk production.
- Increased risk of allergic disorders due to allergens passing through the not-yet-fully-mature gut of the infant. It takes about 6 months after birth for the intestine to become reasonably mature.
- The tongue-thrust reflex is active before 6 months. Infants tend to push out with the tongue anything other than liquids.
- Breastfeeding has significant impact on cognitive growth.
- Foods other than breast milk may result in more gastrointestinal and other infections and malnutrition. They may put an unnecessary load on the kidney and lead to obesity, hypertension, and coronary artery disease later in life.
- Breastfed children have less risk of sudden infant death syndrome, types 1 and 2 diabetes, high cholesterol, and inflammatory bowel disease. It has been seen that there is increased risk of development of Crohn's disease and ulcerative colitis in children who have not been breastfed.
- Less frequent suckling also increases the possibility of the mother becoming pregnant again.
- Breastfeeding also protects mother against stress, postpartum depression, breast and ovarian cancer.

Nutritionally Adequate Complementary Feeding

To be nutritionally adequate, the complementary foods should contain all food groups—the staple, proteins, vitamins, and minerals **(Fig. 4.1.2; Tables 4.1.1 and 4.1.2)**.

After 6 months, add homemade porridge or a fruit, such as ripe banana. Porridge can be made with the staple cereal used by the family, such as whole-wheat flour (*atta*), rice, semolina (*suji* or *rawa*), broken wheat, *ragi* (*nachni*), or millet. Breast milk or any other milk can be used to make the porridge. Pieces of *chapatti* could also be soaked in milk, mashed properly, and passed through a sieve, to provide a soft semisolid food for the infant. Sugar and cream (*malai*) can be added to make it energy dense.

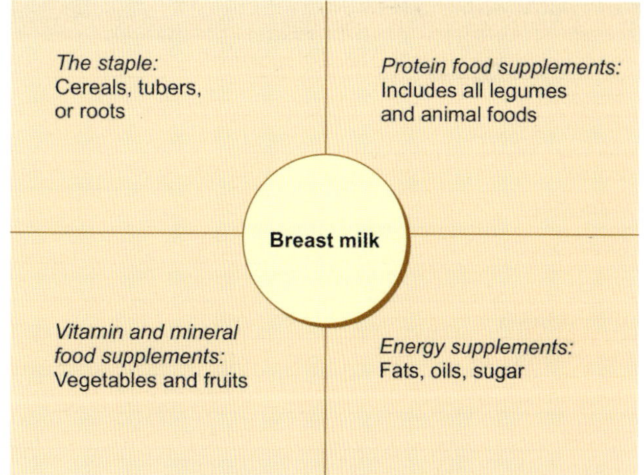

Fig. 4.1.2: Food square for the young child.
Source: Elizabeth KE. Current concepts on nutritional requirements of infants and children. Indian J Pract Pediatr. 2011;13(1):5-11.

Boiled or well-cooked mashed vegetables (pumpkin, peas, cauliflower, carrots, leafy vegetables, sweet and other potato, beet, tomato) should be added to provide vitamins and iron. Also, offer other seasonal fruits. Gradually, introduce *khichdi* with ghee, butter, or oil, *seera* or *halwa, upma, poha, dhokla, idli, dosa, pongal, and missi roti* (*paratha* made with a batter of wheat flour, gram flour, spices, and *dal*). If foods of animal origin are acceptable to the family, the same may be given to the child.

Start with only one food at a time. Wait for a week before introducing another food so that we know whether the child is tolerating it. Infants should be offered food, fruits, or milk feed every 2–3 hours. The child should be encouraged but not forced to eat. Some children tend to choke a little while learning to eat. Parents may be told not to get scared but to be with the child to ward off any trouble. When children are helped to use a spoon, let it be dipped into a preparation, such as *shrikhand or phirni.* A bit will stick to the spoon and give children the joy of getting something into their mouth on their own.

A child eating well around 7 months or so may suddenly become disinterested in eating. The parents should be told not to panic but to try some new preparation. In any case, children should never be forced to eat more than what they want. Even if half a spoon is left in the bowl and the child is not interested to eat any more, the parents should respect the child's appetite. Water can be given once the child starts taking foods other than breast milk and fruits. It should be offered from an ordinary glass. Children learn to sip from the glass within a few days.

Table 4.1.1: Foods rich in iron.

Foods rich in iron (mg/100 g of edible portion)			
Vegetables		*Cereals*	
Cauliflower leaves	40	Ragi	3.9
Chaulai	22.9	Maize flour	2.3
Muli leaves	18	Barley	1.67
Suva ni bhaji	17.4	Rawa	1.6
Pudina	15.6	*Dry fruits*	
Arvi pan green	10	Black sesame seeds	56.7
Carrot leaves	8.8	Sesame seeds	9.3
Green onion	7.43	Coconut (dry)	7.8
Kothmir	1.42	Cashew nuts (*kaju*)	5.81
Spinach	1.14	Almonds	5.09
Arvi pan black	0.98	Walnut	2.64
Sargava pan	0.85	*Singdana*	2.5
Milk and its products		*Pulses*	
Mawa-khoa	5.8	Soybean	10.4
Cheese	2.1	Moth bean (Turkish gram)	9.5
Sugars		Black-eyed beans (*chauli*)	8.6
Jaggery	2.64	Red lentils (*masoor*)	7.86
Sago	1.3	Dried green peas	7.05
Meat		Bengal gram (*channa dal*)	5.3
Liver (sheep)	6.3	Red kidney beans (*rajma*)	5.1
Egg (hen)	2.1	Green gram dal (*mung*)	4.4
Cereals		*Mung* bean	3.9
Rice flakes (*poha*)	20	Black gram (*urad* dal)	3.8
Pearl millet (*bajra*)	8	Pigeon peas (*tuvar* dal)	2.7
Rice puffed (*mamra*)	6.6		
Wheat flour	4.9	Poppy seeds	15.9
Sorghum bicolor (*jowar*)	4.1		
Vermicelli-sev (wheat *sev*)	2		

Few general guidelines about the nutritive value of foods are as follows:

- To retain the nutrients, vegetables including potatoes should be scraped instead of peeling them. The water in which rice or vegetables have been boiled for cooking should be used and not thrown away. The vegetables should not be overcooked. Children should be encouraged to get used to the taste of properly washed raw vegetables from an early age. In general, some amounts of spices are good for health. Most children can tolerate moderate amount of spices used for cooking in most homes.
- Dry fruits are good, but they must also be rationed, partly because they are expensive and more so because some of these, such as dates, figs, and raisins, can remain stuck between the teeth leading to caries. Foods that may lead to choking in children should be avoided in those below 3 years. The examples of these foods are—raw carrots, roasted grams, peanuts, other nuts, popcorn, hard candies, berries, and whole grapes.
- Foods, such as *idli* and *parathas*, made from whole-wheat flour should be preferred to white bread.

Avoidable Foods

In families with a strong history of allergy, peanuts and other nuts should be avoided. If any member of the family is known to react adversely to a particular food, avoid that as well. Also fried foods, foods containing too much sugar, artificial sweeteners, monosodium glutamate (MSG, *ajinomoto*), and high intake of salt should be avoided.

Table 4.1.2: Foods rich in calcium and zinc.

Foods rich in calcium (mg/100 g of edible portion)		***Foods rich in zinc (mg/100 g of edible portion)***	
Milk products and dry fruits		Gingelly seeds	12.2
Sesame seeds	1,450	Bengal gram (*desi*)	6.1
Cheese	790	Cashew nut	5.99
Khoya	650	Safflower seeds	5.2
Coconut (dry)	400	Mustard seeds	4.8
Black sesame seeds	300	Cowpea	4.6
Almond	230	Omum seeds	4.52
Milk (buffalo)	210	Red kidney bean (*rajma*)	4.5
Curd	149	Soybean black	4.4
Pistachios	140	Poppy seeds	4.34
Milk (cow)	120	Groundnut	3.9
Watermelon seeds	100	Samai almond	3.7
Walnut	100	Betel leaves	3.44
Cereal and pulses		Soybean white	3.4
Finger millet (ragi)	344	Black gram (whole)	3.3
Red kidney beans (*rajma*)	260	Coriander seeds	3.26
Soybean	240	Sorghum bicolor (*bajra*)	3.1
Turkish gram (*moth*)	202	Lentil dal	3.1
Chickpeas	202	Red gram (whole)	3.1
Black gram (*urad* dal)	154	Fenugreek seeds	3.08
Vlung	124	Black gram (dal)	3
Pigeon peas (*tuvar* dal)	73	Green gram (whole)	3
Bengal gram (*channa* dal)	56	*Sanwa* millet	3
Cashew nuts	50	Garbanzo beans (*kabuli*)	2.9
Poppy seeds	1,584	Cardamom	2.81
Almond	230	Maize (dry)	2.8

As recommended by the National Institute of Nutrition, the following points need to be kept in mind:

- The recipes for complementary foods should be based on locally available foodstuffs.
- The cooking methods must be simple.
- The cost should be minimal.
- The recipes should be acceptable in taste and consistency.
- Gradually, the child should be introduced to healthy foods eaten by the rest of the family.

Consistency of Complementary Foods (Fig. 4.1.3)

- To provide more calories from smaller volumes, food must be thick in consistency—thick enough to stay on the spoon without running off when the spoon is tilted.
- Foods, such as nuts, which can pose choking hazard, should be avoided. Introduce lumpy or granular foods and new tastes by about 9–10 months. Missing this age may lead to fussy eating later. Avoid using mixers to make the food too smooth.
- Three to four teaspoons of roasted groundnut powder can be added to the daily diet of the infant. The meal can also be made energy dense by adding ghee, butter, oil, and sugar or jaggery.

Ready-to-use Infant Weaning Foods

Table 4.1.3 gives the different ingredients from which weaning foods can be prepared in bulk and kept ready at hand for feeding infants. For that powder the ingredients individually, mix them in the proportion suggested, and store in air-tight containers.

Finger Millet (Ragi, Nachni) Infant Food

Use 45 g of finger millet, (*ragi*) prepared as given here instead of bajra in the earlier formula. Soak finger millet (*ragi*) in water overnight. Drain the water, spread the grains on a plate, and allow them to germinate by covering with a damp cloth for 1 day. Dry the germinated finger millet (*ragi*) under the sun and roast till it develops a malted flavor. Powder and store in an airtight tin.

Methods of Feeding

When required, take suitable amounts (say 3 tablespoons) of any one of the above ready-to-use infant food and mix with a small amount of hot water. Add more sugar or jaggery, if required, before feeding.

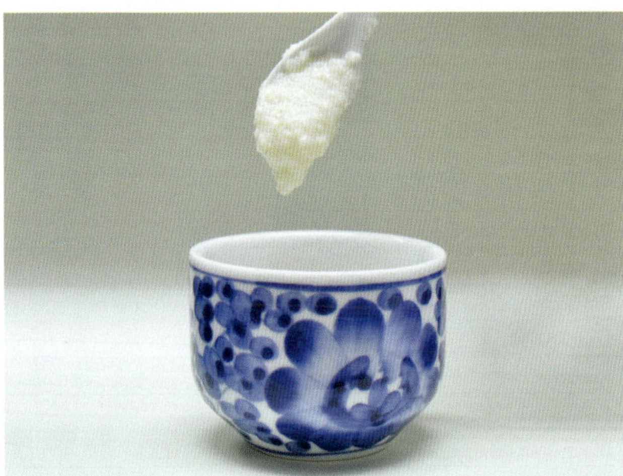

Fig. 4.1.3: Consistency of complementary food.

Table 4.1.3: Ready-to-use infant weaning foods.

Food	*Amount*
Pearl millet (*bajra*), (dehusked, roasted)	3 tablespoons
Roasted green gram dal (or any other dal)	1.5 tablespoon
Roasted groundnut	3/4th tablespoon
Roasted decorticated sesame (gingelly) seeds	1 tablespoon
Sugar	2 tablespoons

Amount and Frequency of Food to be Offered (Table 4.1.4)

This depends on the capacity or the size of the child's stomach, which is usually 30 mL/kg of the child's body weight. A child who weighs 8 kg will have a stomach capacity of 240 mL, about one large full cup and cannot be expected to eat more than that at one meal. Parents may not realize that a child of 1 year needs about 1,000 cal each day—almost half of what an adult may take. So, some guidance to parents may be given in this respect. After that, children should be left to decide how much they want to consume. A good guide that children were having optimum quantity of food is their level of activity and weight gain.

Safe Complementary Feeding

All utensils used for feeding must be washed thoroughly. There is no need to sterilize the utensils. Eating by hand need not be discouraged. Finger foods, which the child can hold and chew, may be given. However, the hands of the caregiver and the child must be washed thoroughly with soap and water before and after eating. Microbial contamination of complementary foods is more in hot weather. It is slower, if the food is refrigerated. When that is not possible, the food should be eaten within 2 hours of its preparation. Even if the food is kept in the refrigerator, it should be consumed within a day or two.

Responsive Feeding (Fig. 4.1.4)

While feeding young children, the caregivers should provide psychosocial stimulation to the child through age-appropriate play and praise. Children sitting on the lap of a caregiver or eating with loved ones learn to enjoy eating. Self-feeding must be encouraged even if the child makes a mess **(Fig. 4.1.5)**. Forced feeding, threatening, and punishment interfere with the development of proper feeding habits. Distractions during meals and feeding in front of the television or smartphone, etc. should be avoided.

Table 4.1.4: Amount of food to be offered.

Age	*Texture*	*Frequency*	*Average amount of each meal*
6–8 months	Start with thick porridge, well-mashed foods	2–3 meals per day plus frequent breastfeeding	Start with 2–3 tablespoons full
9–11 months	Finely chopped or mashed foods and foods that baby can pick up	3–4 meals along with breastfeeding. Depending on appetite, offer 1–2 snacks	1/2 of a 250 mL cup or bowl
12–23 months	Family food chopped or mashed, if necessary. As per appetite, offer 1–2 snacks	3–4 meals plus breastfeeding. Depending on appetite, offer 1–2 snacks	3/4 to one 250 mL cup or bowl
If baby is not breastfed, give in addition: 1–2 cups of milk per day and 1–2 extra meals per day.			

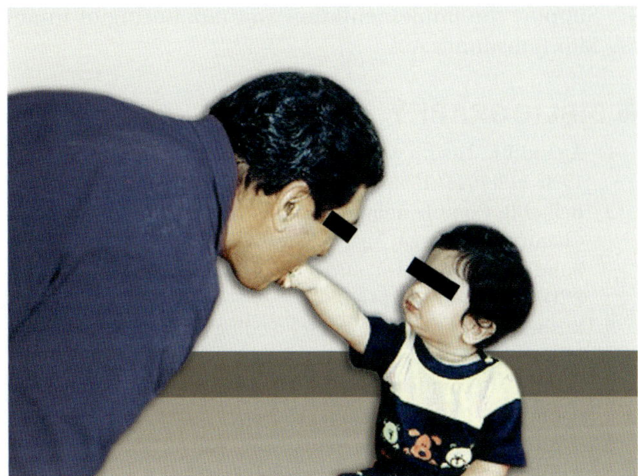

Fig. 4.1.4: Responsive feeding.

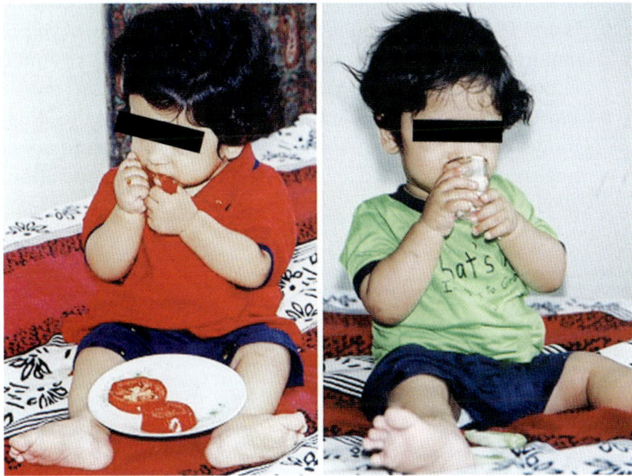

Fig. 4.1.5: Self-feeding.

Feeding during and after Illness

The appetite during an illness may go down. However, even sick babies continue to breastfeed quite often. They should be encouraged to take enough liquids and small quantities of nutrient-rich food that they like to eat. After the illness, the nutrient intake can be increased by adding one or two extra meals in the daily diet for about a month by offering nutritious snacks between meals, by giving extra amount at each meal and continuing breastfeeding.

Junk and Commercial Nutrition Supplements

Commercial ready-made cereals, though convenient to use, are not preferred over homemade foods. In addition to the high cost, the smooth consistency of such products may make the children get so used to them that they may not accept homemade foods. Families must be equipped with means and knowledge to feed their children without the need for processed foods. All effort must be made to ensure that government policies protect public health before private profits.

Tinned food, juices, cold drinks, packaged drinks and packaged wafers, health drinks, nutrition supplements promoted for "picky eaters," bakery products, and drinks with low nutrient value, such as tea, coffee, and sugary drinks, should be avoided.

Picky Eaters

Of late, a nutritional supplement is being aggressively promoted for so-called picky eaters for better growth and height. Before the parents start using such a product, they should be given the following information:

- An infant grows rapidly in the early months of life. In the second year, the growth will be slower; the appetite may decrease and vary from day to day. Between 15 months and 3 years, the child often passes through a phase of negativism and does the opposite of what the parents want. If the child is unwell, the appetite may suffer even more, though the mother's milk is often not refused.
- Keeping the earlier point in mind, the child should not be forced to eat. Of course, various healthy food options must be offered at frequent intervals. Allow children to eat with their hands even if it turns out to be a messy affair. Then let them learn to use the spoon. The parents may fill the spoon off and on or may offer the child some food with a separate spoon, while gradually encouraging the child to eat independently.
- Parents need not get upset if the child does not eat "nourishing" foods for a few days. Children have their moods; for some days, they may eat less of certain foods, but if left to themselves, they may start eating the same again after a gap of few days.
- Children, who are small at birth, may not weigh as much as their peers. The parents should be told that so long the child follows the growth curve, they should be happy. In fact, if these children are given food or products too high in calories and become obese, they become potential candidates for developing diabetes and cardiovascular diseases.
- Make sure the child is not anemic and does not have urinary or any other infection responsible for anorexia.
- Convey to the parents that the product promoted for "picky eaters" is expensive, not wholesome and comes in the way of the child developing healthy food habits. Moreover, one may get a false sense of security while the underlying causes for fussy eating mentioned earlier are missed.

KEY MESSAGES FOR OPTIMUM INFANT AND YOUNG CHILD FEEDING

- Initiate breastfeeding as early as possible after birth, preferably within 1 hour.
- Except for any essential medicine or supplements, practice exclusive breastfeeding from birth to 6 months of age and introduce complementary foods at 6 months (180 days).
- Continue frequent on-demand breastfeeding until 2 years of age or beyond.
- Start complementary foods at 6 months of age with small amount. Increase the quantity and frequency as the child gets older, while maintaining frequent breastfeeding.
- Gradually, increase food consistency and ensure that all nutrient needs of the child are met.
- Practice responsive feeding by applying the principles of psychosocial care.
- Practice good hygiene by handwashing with soap and water before preparing food and feeding the child and after using the toilet.
- Increase fluid intake during illness including more frequent breastfeeding and encourage the child to eat soft favorite foods. After illness, encourage the child to eat more often.
- Ensure adequate nutrition, including control of anemia in infants, young children, adolescent girls, and pregnant and lactating mothers. Vitamin and mineral supplements must be given, if required.
- Support the implementation and monitoring of Infant Milk Substitutes Act.

BIBLIOGRAPHY

1. Anand RK. Health workers and the baby food industry. BMJ. 1996; 312(7046):1556-7.
2. Bellad R. Complementary feeding. In: Bharadva K, Tiwari S, Chaturvedi P, BangA, Agarwal RK (Eds). Feeding fundamentals: handbook on infant and young child nutrition. Jaipur: PEDICON; 2011. pp. 141-8.
3. Kushwaha KP. Complementary feeding of breastfed children. In: Anand RK, Kumta NB, Kushwaha KP, Gupta A (Eds). The science of infant feeding. New Delhi: Jaypee Brothers Medical Publishers (P) Ltd; 2002. pp. 117-34.
4. National Institute of Nutrition. Low-cost Nutritious Supplements, 2nd edition. Hyderabad; 2000.
5. Palmer G. Complementary feeding: nutrition, culture and politics. Great Britain: Pinter and Martin Ltd.; 2011.
6. Wiessinger D, West D, Pitman T. The womanly art of breastfeeding, 8th edition. New York: Ballantine Book; 2010.
7. World Health Organization. Complementary feeding of young children in developing countries: a review of current scientific knowledge. Geneva: World Health Organization; 1998.
8. World Health Organization. Infant and young child feeding: model chapter for textbooks for medical students and allied health professionals. Geneva: World Health Organization; 2009.

4.2 Breastfeeding

JP Dadhich

The provision has been made for infants to be feed upon their mother's milk. They find their food and their mother at the same time. It is complete nourishment for them, body and soul. It is their first introduction to the great truth that man's true relationship with the world is that of personal love and not that of the mechanical law of causation.

—Rabindranath Tagore

INTRODUCTION

Optimal infant and young child feeding (IYCF) practices are critical for child nutrition and survival. Breastfeeding is a vital component of IYCF. The "global strategy for IYCF" states that "breastfeeding is an unequalled way of providing ideal food for the healthy growth and development of infants; it is also an integral part of the reproductive process with important implications for the health of mothers. As a global public health recommendation, infants should be exclusively breastfed for the first 6 months of life to achieve optimal growth, development and health. Thereafter, to meet their evolving nutritional requirements, infants should receive nutritionally adequate and safe complementary foods while breastfeeding continues for up to 2 years of age or beyond." Presently, when global efforts are on to achieve better nutritional status and survival for children enshrined in the sustainable development goals, breastfeeding emerges as a very effective intervention to achieve these targets.

DEFINITIONS RELATED TO BREASTFEEDING

Various definitions used in the context of breastfeeding are summarized in **Table 4.2.1**.

Recommendations for Breastfeeding

Child health and nutrition programs across the world (including India) conform to these guidelines based on the global recommendations. These recommendations are based on the available scientific evidence; some of which are defined as follows:

Initiation of Breastfeeding Immediately after Birth, Preferably within 1 Hour

Early initiation has been documented to improve neonatal survival, and protective against the infection-specific mortality among newborn infants. Early initiation of breastfeeding helps to develop a bond between a mother and her baby. Early initiation is extremely important to establish successful and sustained lactation. It stimulates uterine contractions and expulsion of placenta. The practice of delaying breastfeeding after birth and giving something else, i.e. prelacteal feeds, expose the infant to infections and lead to problems in establishing a successful lactation. Scientific evidence suggests that earlier the initiation of breastfeeding, more are the chances of survival of neonate.

Table 4.2.1: Definitions related to infant feeding.

- *Exclusive breastfeeding*: Giving a baby no other food or drink, including water, in addition to breastfeeding apart from syrup/ drops of vitamins, minerals, and medicines (expressed breast milk is also permitted)
- *Predominant breastfeeding*: Giving small amounts of water in addition to breastfeeding
- *Partial breastfeeding*: Giving a baby some breastfeeds and some artificial feeds, either milk or cereal, or other food
- *Bottle feeding*: Feeding a baby from a bottle, whatever is in the bottle, including expressed breast milk
- *Cup feeding*: Feeding a baby from cup (*Katori, Paladai*, etc.) whatever is in the cup including breast milk
- *Artificial feeding*: Feeding a baby on any kind of artificial milk, such as animal milk, tinned milk, etc. and not breastfeeding at all
- *Complementary feeding*: Giving other foods and liquids in addition to breast milk or nonhuman milk
- *Replacement feeding*: Process of feeding a child who is receiving no breast milk with a diet that provides all nutrients the infants need until the age at which they can be fully fed on family foods

Source: Adapted from Infant and young child feeding counseling: a training course, the "4 in 1 course" (integrated course on breastfeeding, complementary feeding and infant feeding and HIV). New Delhi: Breastfeeding Promotion Network of India (BPNI); 2015.

After cesarean section, some delay in initiation of breastfeeding may be unavoidable due to the condition of the mother or infant. After cesarean section with spinal anesthesia, breastfeeding can often be initiated immediately. With general anesthesia, breastfeeding can be initiated within a few hours as soon as the mother regains consciousness.

Exclusive Breastfeeding for the First 6 Months

Exclusive breastfeeding is recommended for the first 6 months of life as breast milk contains all the necessary nutrients, which are sufficient to sustain appropriate growth and development of a healthy term infant. There is sufficient evidence that a significant number of under-6-month deaths in resource-poor countries could be prevented through the achievement of 90% coverage with exclusive breastfeeding for 6 months. Any supplementation during the first 6 months will expose infant to infections and decrease breast milk output.

Appropriate and Adequate Complementary Feeding after 6 Months of Age while Continuing Breastfeeding

Additional foods are needed at this stage to complement the breast milk to sustain the growth and development of the infant. Along with the breastfeeding, children aged 6–24 months should be fed from three or more different food groups, two to three times a day (see more details in Chapter 4.1).

Continued Breastfeeding up to the Age of 2 Years or Beyond

Breastfeeding along with other foods remains an important and safe source of high-quality protein, energy, and other nutrients, such as vitamin A and vitamin C, between 6 and 24 months of life. It is, therefore, crucial in preventing undernutrition and morbidities. It can provide about one third of energy needs, half of protein, and 75% of the vitamin A requirements of a child of this age **(Fig. 4.2.1)**. Thus, breast milk helps a child to get enough energy and high-quality nutrients from breastfeeding during the second year of life. These nutrients may not be easily available from the family diet. Continuing to breastfeed during the second year can help to prevent malnutrition and vitamin deficiencies.

STATUS OF BREASTFEEDING PRACTICES IN INDIA

The status of breastfeeding and complementary feeding practices is very dismal in India.

According to the National Family Health Survey-4, only 41.6% of children are breastfed within the first hour of birth and about 81% initiate breastfeeding within the first day of life.

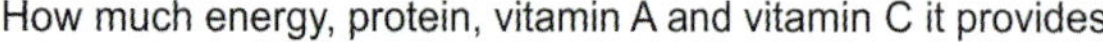

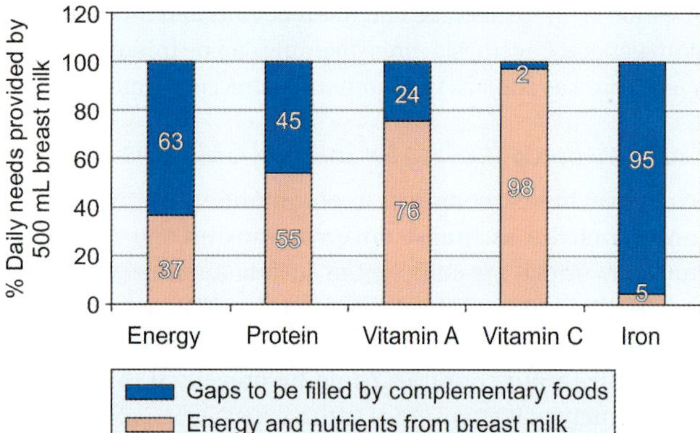

Fig. 4.2.1: Nutrition provided by breast milk in the second year of life.

Source: Reproduced with permission from Infant and Young Child Feeding counseling—a training course, the "4 in 1 course" (integrated course on breastfeeding, complementary feeding and infant feeding and HIV). New Delhi: Breastfeeding Promotion Network of India (BPNI); 2015.

Timely initiation of breastfeeding has been found particularly low in women with no schooling, babies delivered at home, and in deliveries conducted by a *dai* (traditional midwife). Twenty-one percent of newborn infants receive prelacteal feeds, such as milk other than breast milk, honey, sugar or glucose water, and plain water. The exclusive breastfeeding rate up to the age of 6 months is only 54.9%. Exclusive breastfeeding rapidly declines from the first month to the sixth month.

Possible reasons for suboptimal breastfeeding are primarily due to the lack of proper information to mothers, inadequate healthcare support, inability of the healthcare providers to help mothers experiencing breastfeeding difficulty, aggressive promotion of baby foods by the commercial industry, and lack of proper support structures at the community and at workplace, which includes maternity entitlements and crèches. Cultural beliefs also appear to be important, for example, breastfeeding initiation is delayed because of the belief that mother's milk does not "come" at the time of childbirth but flows 2–3 days later.

NUTRITIONAL COMPOSITION OF BREAST MILK

The breast milk contains all the macronutrients (carbohydrates, proteins, and fats), micronutrients, such as vitamins and minerals, and adequate water to meet the requirements of a healthy term infant for the first 6 months of life. Apart from the nutrients, breast milk provides a variety of bioactive factors, which protect the infant against infection and modulate the composition of the indigenous intestinal microbiota. Breast milk also contains some factors to help in digestion and absorption of nutrients.

Fats

The mature human breast milk contains 3.2–3.8 g/dL of fats. Fats provide 50% of the total energy content of the breast milk. Breast milk fat in immediate postpartum period contains fat needed for gray matter development and in later months, fat, which is needed for myelination. Breast milk fat has steady higher level of cholesterol than animal milks and formula. Breastfed babies have significantly higher total cholesterol and low-density lipoprotein (LDL) cholesterol compared to mixed fed babies in the first 6 months of life with improving high-density lipoprotein cholesterol/LDL cholesterol ratio at 6 months. High-cholesterol intake in infancy may have a beneficial long-term programming effect on the synthesis of cholesterol by downregulation of hepatic enzymes. Human milk contains essential fatty acids and $n - 3$ fatty acids (docosahexaenoic acid and eicosapentaenoic acid), which are needed for a baby's growing brain and eyes and for healthy blood vessels. Human milk contains the enzyme lipase, which helps to digest fat. Thus, the fat in breast milk is more completely digested and more efficiently used by a baby's body than the fat in cow's milk or formula. The lipase in breast milk is called bile salt-stimulated lipase because it starts working in the intestine in the presence of bile salts. The lipase is not active in the breast or in the stomach before the milk mixes with bile.

Carbohydrates

Lactose is the main carbohydrate in human breast milk and provides about 50% of its energy content. Breast milk also contains oligosaccharides, such as glucose, galactose, *N*-acetylglucosamine, and sialic acid. These oligosaccharides attach to the epithelial cell surface in the intestines and prevent adhesion of microorganisms, thereby preventing their growth.

Proteins

Proteins in breast milk provide amino acids for growth and anti-infective factors. Mature breast milk contains 0.9 g/dL of protein, while colostrum contains 2.3 g/dL. The breast milk protein contains more whey protein and less casein. Due to high whey to casein ratio, the breast milk forms softer curds which are easier to digest.

In human milk, much of the whey protein consists of anti-infective proteins, which help to protect a baby against infection. The anti-infective proteins in human milk include lactoferrin (which binds iron and prevents the growth of bacteria which need iron) and lysozyme (which kills bacteria) as well as antibodies [immunoglobulin (Ig), mostly IgA]. Animal milk and formula may lack the amino acid cystine, and formula may lack taurine which newborns need especially for brain growth. Human infant is ill equipped to handle phenylalanine and tyrosine, two amino acids that are in high concentration in the animal milk in comparison to breast milk.

DYNAMIC COMPOSITION OF BREAST MILK

The composition of breast milk is not always the same. It varies according to the age of the baby, and from the beginning to the end of a feed. It also varies between feeds and may be different at different times of the day.

Colostrum

The milk produced during the first few days after the delivery is known as colostrum which is a special, thick, sticky, bright lemony yellowish fluid. It is secreted in small quantities for first 3–4 days of life. Although it is in small quantities, it is sufficient to meet the needs of the newborn baby. Colostrum contains more protein than later milk. Colostrum is considered the first immunization for newborn, as it is rich in the anti-infective factors that help protect the baby against diarrhea, respiratory and other infections. Colostrum contains more epidermal growth factors in comparison to mature breast milk, which help a baby's immature intestine to develop after birth. This helps to prevent the baby from developing allergies and intolerance to other foods. Colostrum helps to clean baby's intestine, which is important to prevent jaundice in the newborn. Colostrum is also rich in vitamin A.

Transitional Milk

During the transition from colostrum to the mature milk, the amount of Ig, proteins, vitamin A and vitamin E decreases, and amount of lactose, fats, energy, and water-soluble vitamins increases.

Mature Milk

After a few days, colostrum changes into mature milk. Mature milk is in large amounts, and the breasts feel full, hard, and heavy. Some people call this as the milk "coming in."

Foremilk is the bluish milk that is produced early in a feed. It is produced in larger amounts, and it provides plenty of protein, lactose, and other nutrients. Because a baby gets large amounts of foremilk, he or she gets all the water that he or she needs from it. Hindmilk is the whiter milk that is produced later in a feed. It contains more fat than foremilk. This fat provides much of the energy of a breastfeed. Therefore, it is important not to take a baby off a breast too quickly, not until he or she leaves the breast on her/his own.

BENEFITS OF BREASTFEEDING

The benefits of breastfeeding for infant, mother, and community include:

- Breastfeeding provides all the nutrients a baby needs for the first 6 months of life, after which it continues to provide a major portion of the infant's nutrition along with appropriate family foods. It provides almost half of the nutritional requirements between 6 months and 12 months of age, and up to one-third between 12 months and 24 months of age.
- Breast milk is easily digested by the baby.
- Breast milk contains antibodies and other factors, which protect the baby against diarrhea and other infections.
- Breast milk contains enough water which is sufficient even for very dry and hot climates.
- Breast milk is clean, safe, and cheap.
- Breastfeeding provides a perfect opportunity for building a close bond between mother and baby.
- It helps the mother by reducing the postdelivery bleeding and thus preventing anemia.
- Breastfed babies are less prone to have diabetes, heart disease, eczema, asthma, rheumatoid arthritis, and other allergic disorders later in life.
- Breastfeeding enhances brain development, visual development, and visual acuity leading to learning readiness.
- Breastfeeding has contraceptive effect for the mother, if she exclusively breastfeeds her infant for first 6 months.
- Mothers have a lower risk of breast and ovarian cancers.
- Breastfeeding costs less in terms of healthcare expenses as breastfed infants get ill less often.
- Breastfeeding protects the environment.

Risks of Formula Feeding

Infant formula, which is generally used as an artificial substitute for human breast milk, is time consuming, less nutritious, and expensive. It is also fraught with innumerable risks for the infants and children in comparison with the breastfeeding. Some of these risks are depicted in **Table 4.2.2.**

Science of Milk Transfer

Understanding the structure of breast and the process of breast milk production and transfer to the infant is useful to provide effective skilled help to the lactating mother.

ANATOMY OF THE BREAST

The human breast consists of the nipple and areola, mammary tissue, the soft tissue including supporting connective tissue and fat, blood and lymphatic vessels, and nerves **(Fig. 4.2.2)**.

The nipple is the area from which the milk comes out of the breast through multiple small openings. This area of breast is very richly supplied with nerves. The nerve endings in the nipple are important to provide stimulus for the hormonal reflexes important for production and release of the milk from breast. The areola is the dark skin surrounding the nipple. The milk ducts beneath the areola are filled with milk and become wider during a feed. Areola is an important anatomical landmark as it is important to ensure that majority of areola is in baby's mouth during the feed to achieve an effective suckling. The mammary tissue is composed of alveoli, which are small sacs, made up of millions of milk-secreting cells.

Milk produced in the alveoli is carried toward the nipple via tubular structures called ducts. These ducts open outside at the nipple area. The alveoli are surrounded by myoepithelial tissue, which helps in pushing the milk present in the alveoli toward nipple.

Table 4.2.2: Risks of formula feeding.

• Increased risk for infection from inherent and subsequent contamination of formula with microbes, such as *Enterobacter sakazakii* and *Salmonella*
• Increased risk of acute respiratory infections, diarrhea, otitis media, and ear infections
• Increased risk of necrotizing enterocolitis
• Increased risk of asthma and other allergies
• Increased risk of chronic diseases, such as type 1 diabetes, ulcerative colitis, and Crohn's disease
• Increased risk of cardiovascular disease, increased blood pressure, obesity, altered blood cholesterol levels, and atherosclerosis in later adulthood
• Increased risk of side effects of environmental contaminants and harmful chemicals such as melamine and bisphenol A

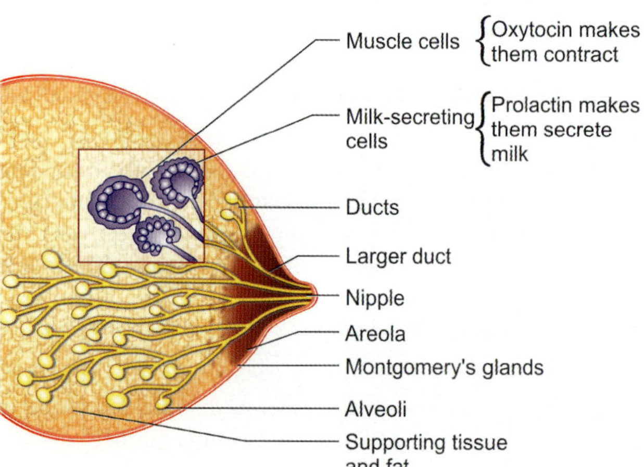

Fig. 4.2.2: Anatomy of the breast.

Source: Reproduced with permission from World Health Organization. Infant and young child feeding: model chapter for textbooks for medical students and allied health professionals. Geneva: WHO Press; 2009.

PHYSIOLOGY OF LACTATION

Production of Breast Milk

Production of the breast milk is controlled by the hormone prolactin. When a baby suckles at the breast, sensory impulses go from the nipple to the brain. In response, the anterior part of the pituitary gland at the base of the brain secretes prolactin. Prolactin goes in the blood to the breast and makes the milk-secreting cells produce milk. This process is known as the prolactin reflex **(Fig. 4.2.3)**. From this, it is evident that milk production is dependent on the suckling stimulus. If the baby suckles more, the breast will produce more milk. For the same reason, if a mother has two babies, breast milk production increases accordingly. Prolactin is present in the blood for about 30 minutes after the baby finishes the feed. It makes the breast produce milk for the next feed. More prolactin is produced at night due to the inhibition of dopaminergic drive during sleep, so breastfeeding at night is especially helpful for keeping up the milk supply. Prolactin suppresses ovulation, so breastfeeding can help to delay a new pregnancy.

Flow of Breast Milk

When a baby suckles, sensory impulses go from the nipple to the brain. In response, the posterior part of the pituitary gland at the base of the brain secretes the hormone oxytocin. Oxytocin goes in the blood to the breast and makes the muscle

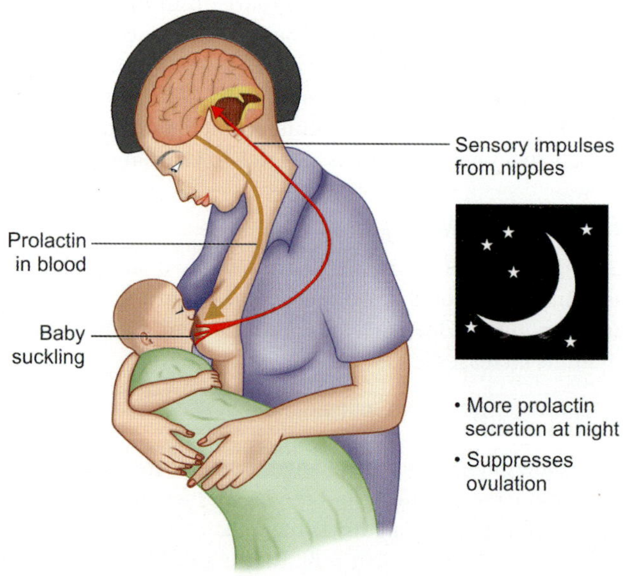

Fig. 4.2.3: Prolactin reflex.

Source: Reproduced with permission from World Health Organization. Infant and young child feeding: model chapter for textbooks for medical students and allied health professionals. Geneva: WHO Press; 2009.

cells around the alveoli contract. This makes the milk, which has collected in the alveoli, flow along the ducts toward nipple. It makes the milk in the breast flow for this feed **(Fig. 4.2.4)**. Sometimes the milk is ejected in fine streams. This is the oxytocin reflex or the milk ejection reflex. Oxytocin can start working before a baby suckles, when a mother expects a feed. The oxytocin reflex is positively affected by mother's sensations and feelings, such as thinking lovingly about the baby; touching, smelling, or seeing the baby; or hearing the baby cry. If the oxytocin reflex does not work well, the baby may have difficulty in getting the milk. This may happen, if the mother is emotionally disturbed or experiencing pain and discomfort. In such a condition, mother needs support to make her physically and/or emotionally comfortable to make the oxytocin reflex work again and let the milk flow.

Signs of an active oxytocin reflex are a tingling sensation in the breast before or during a feed, milk flowing from breasts when mother thinks of the baby or hears him/her crying, milk flowing from the other breast when the baby is suckling, milk flowing from the breast in streams, if suckling is interrupted, and uterine pain or a flow of blood from the uterus during the feed. However, the absence of these signs does not indicate an inadequate oxytocin reflex.

Breast Milk Inhibitor

Breast milk production is also controlled within the breast itself. Sometimes one breast stops making milk, while the other breast continues to make milk although oxytocin and prolactin go equally to both breasts. There is a substance in breast milk, which can reduce or inhibit milk production. If a lot of milk is left in a breast, the inhibitor stops the cells from secreting any more. If suckling or expression removes breast milk, the inhibitor is also removed, and the breast makes more milk.

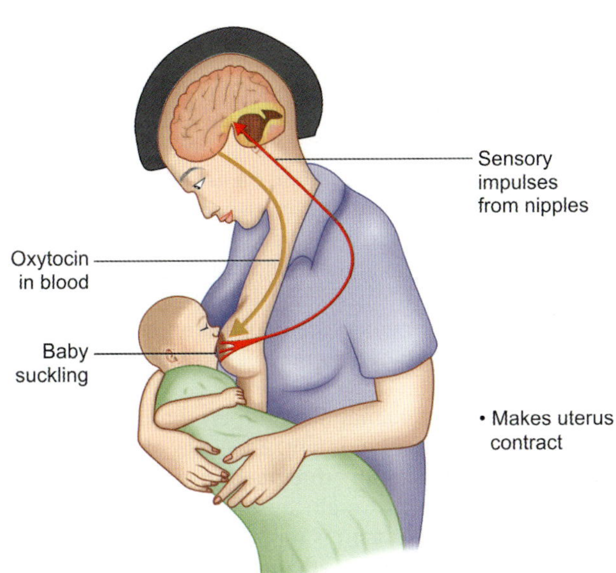

Fig. 4.2.4: Oxytocin reflex.

Source: Reproduced with permission from World Health Organization (WHO). Infant and young child feeding (IYCF); model chapter for textbooks for medical students and allied health professionals. Geneva: WHO Press; 2009.

Positioning and Attaching the Baby at the Breast

For effective milk transfer from mother to the infant, good breastfeeding skills including proper positioning of the baby and good attachment at the breast are required.

Positioning

A woman can feed her baby in any comfortable position, such as sitting, lying, or even standing. If the baby suckles properly from the breast, he or she will get sufficient milk. However, for a good attachment on breast, some basic principle need to be observed for relative positioning of the baby while breastfeeding. These are as follows:

- Baby turned toward mother, and his or her ears, shoulder, and buttock are in a straight line
- His face should face the breast with nose opposite the nipple.
- Mother should hold the baby close to her.
- In a newborn, she should support his bottom with hand, and not just his head and shoulders.
- The mother should be explained how to support the breast with her hand while offering it to the baby:
  - With her fingers and palm placed on her chest wall below the breast so that her first finger forms a support at the base of the breast.
  - With her thumb placed on the top of the breast so that it is easier for her baby to attach well.
  - She should not hold her breast too near to the nipple.

The mother should be explained how to bring the baby to the breast:

- Touch baby's lips with her nipple;
- Wait until baby's mouth is wide open;
- Move the baby quickly onto the breast from below.

Attachment

This is important how baby's mouth is attached to mother's breast for a successful suckling **(Figs. 4.2.5 and 4.2.6)**. In good suckling position, baby is suckling with nipple and a larger breast tissue having in his or her mouth. In poor suckling position, baby is suckling with nipple only or nipple with a small breast tissue in his or her mouth.

The signs of good suckling attachment are as follows:

- The baby's chin touches the breast;
- His mouth is wide open;

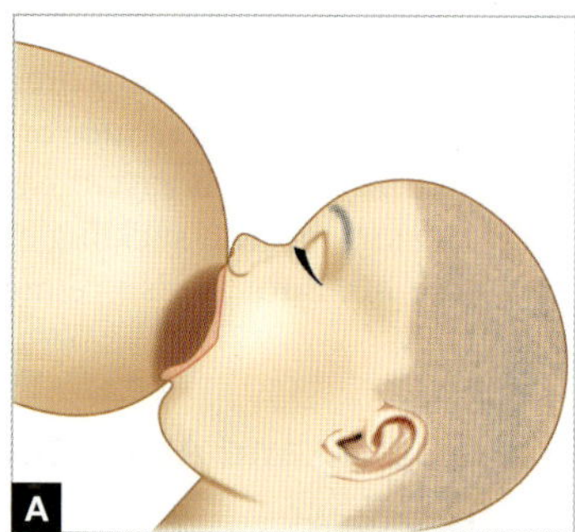

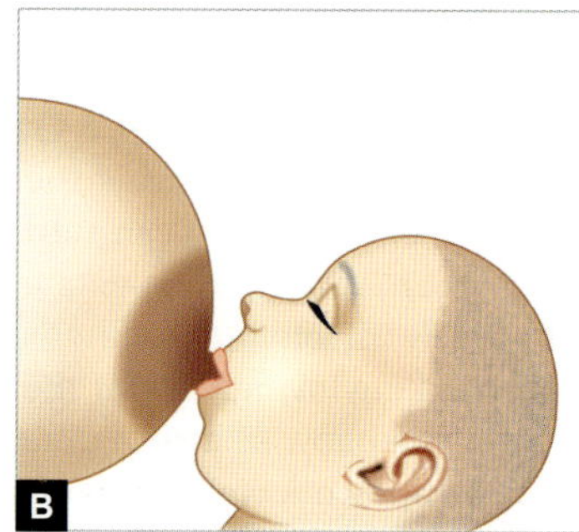

Figs. 4.2.5A and B: (A) Good and (B) poor attachment. External signs.
Source: Reproduced with permission from World Health Organization (WHO). Infant and young child feeding (IYCF); model chapter for textbooks for medical students and allied health professionals. Geneva: WHO Press; 2009.

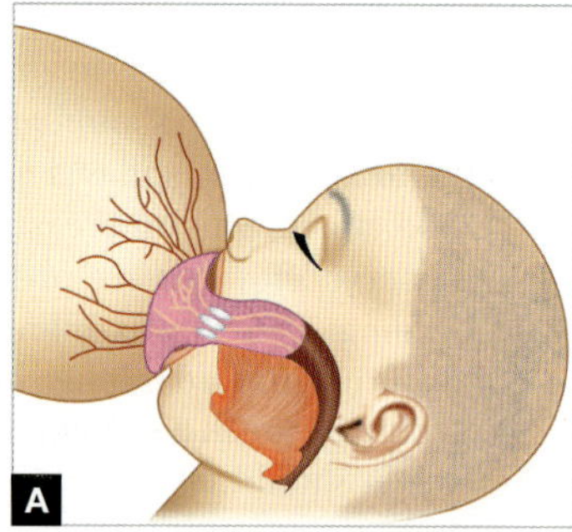

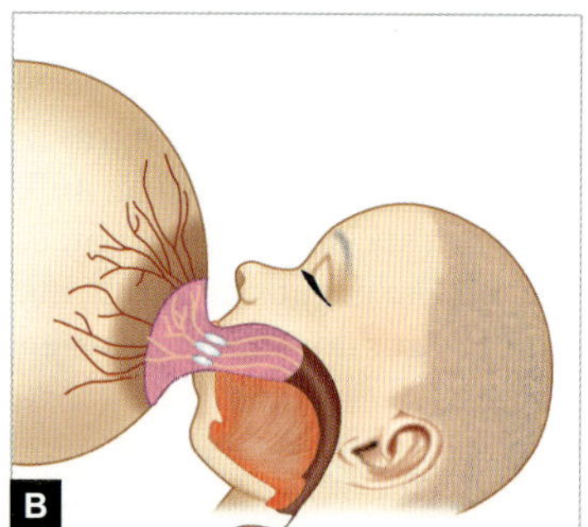

Figs. 4.2.6A and B: (A) Good attachment and (B) poor attachment inside the infant's mouth.
Source: Reproduced with permission from World Health Organization. Infant and young child feeding: model chapter for textbooks for medical students and allied health professionals. Geneva: WHO Press; 2009.

- His lower lip is turned outwards;
- One can see more of the areola above his or her mouth and less below. This shows that he or she is reaching with his tongue under the lactiferous sinuses to press out the milk.

Poor attachment may lead to pain and damage to mother's nipple, and she may develop sores or fissures in nipple. It may also lead to engorgement of the breast due to improper milk removal. The baby remains hungry and frustrated that leads to refusal to suck. Ultimately, it leads to the production of less milk in the breast; baby is not able to feed properly, leading to weight loss. Common causes of poor attachment are use of feeding bottle, inexperience of mother, and lack of skilled support.

Practices for Successful Breastfeeding

To ensure adequate milk production and flow for 6 months of exclusive breastfeeding and thereafter continued breastfeeding, certain practices are very important.

- The infant should be fed as frequently and for as long as he or she wants to, during both day and night. The suckling should be allowed until the infant spontaneously releases the nipple. This is called demand feeding. Restricting length of the breastfeeding session may result in the baby getting less of the energy-rich hindmilk. The 24-h average intake of milk is about 800 mL/day during the first 6 months.
- At the time of delivery, before breastfeeding is initiated, no prelacteal feed should be given to the infant. Apart from having the harmful effects on the infant, such as risk of infection, such a practice may interfere in the establishment of breastfeeding. Later, in the first 6 months of life, no supplementary feed, such as other milks, should be given to the infant. This may lead to a decreased supply of breast milk.
- Sometimes, mother may have the perception that her milk is not sufficient for her infant. Adequacy of breastfeeding may be ascertained by documenting, if the infant has regained the birth weight by 2 weeks of age, and the cumulative weight gain is more than 500 g in a month, and the infant is passing adequate urine at least six times a day, while on exclusive breastfeeding.

Hospital Practices and Breastfeeding

Maternity homes and healthcare practices should support exclusive breastfeeding during the first 6 months of life and continued breastfeeding along with appropriate complementary feeds thereafter. To motivate maternity facilities to practice 10 steps to successful breastfeeding, the World Health Organization (WHO) and the United Nations Children's Fund launched the baby-friendly hospital initiative (BFHI) in 1991. The initiative is a global effort for improving the role of maternity services to enable mothers to breastfeed babies for the best start in life. It aims at improving the care of pregnant women, mothers, and newborns at health facilities that provide maternity services for protecting, promoting, and supporting breastfeeding. The BFHI package was relaunched in 2009 with an updated version which included new evidence and specifically addressed infant feeding in women living with human immunodeficiency virus (HIV). In 2018, BFHI package has been further revised, which is based on the 2017 WHO guideline on protecting, promoting, and supporting breastfeeding in facilities providing maternity and newborn services, and an implementation guidance has been published. The key to successful breastfeeding lies in the prenatal priming of the expectant mother about the undisputed facts of benefits of breastfeeding the newborn child within 1 hour of birth and addressing all the issues which may delay or prevent the initiation of breastfeeding the newborn. The elders in the family should also be taken in confidence about breastfeeding soon after the birth.

Components of Baby-friendly Hospital Initiative

Ten steps to successful breastfeeding have been regrouped under two headings, critical management procedures and key clinical practices and given in **Table 4.2.3**.

Table 4.2.3: Ten steps of baby-friendly hospital initiative (revised 2018).

Step no.	***Description***
Critical management procedures	
1a.	Comply fully with the International Code of Marketing of Breast-milk Substitutes and relevant World Health Assembly resolutions
1b.	Have a written infant feeding policy that is routinely communicated to staff and parents
1c.	Establish ongoing monitoring and data-management systems
2.	Ensure that the members of the staff have sufficient knowledge, competence, and skills to support breastfeeding
Key clinical practices	
3.	Discuss the importance and management of breastfeeding with pregnant women and their families
4.	Facilitate immediate and uninterrupted skin-to-skin contact and support mothers to initiate breastfeeding as soon as possible after birth
5.	Support mothers to initiate and maintain breastfeeding and manage common difficulties
6.	Do not provide breastfed newborns any food or fluids other than breast milk, unless medically indicated
7.	Enable mothers and their infants to remain together and to practice rooming-in 24 hours a day
8.	Support mothers to recognize and respond to their infants' cues for feeding
9.	Counsel mothers on the use and risks of feeding bottles, teats, and pacifiers
10.	Coordinate discharge so that parents and their infants have timely access to ongoing support and care

Breastfeeding the Preterm Babies

The nutritional management plays a large role in the immediate survival and subsequent growth, and development of the preterm infants. The optimal diet for premature infants should support growth at intrauterine rates without imposing stress on the infant's immature metabolic and excretory functions and ensures healthy short-term and long-term outcomes. Breast milk produced during early postpartum period offers nutritional advantage because of its higher protein and electrolyte concentrations. Preterm infant fed preterm milk demonstrates increase in weight, length, and head circumference as well as retention rates of various nutrients comparable to those for the fetus of similar postconception age. Fat absorption in preterm babies fed their own mother's milk is significantly higher in comparison to infants fed cow's milk formula. Long-chain polyunsaturated fatty acids, which are important for mental and visual development, are also higher in human milk.

Preterm infants fed breast milk have lesser incidence of necrotizing enterocolitis in comparison to feeding with formula milk. Even if the disease occurs in infants fed with breast milk, the course of disease is less severe, and the prevalence of intestinal perforation is lower. This is due to various protective factors in breast milk, such as Ig, erythropoietin, interleukin-10, epidermal growth factor, platelet-activating factor, acetylhydrolase, and oligosaccharides, which are in greater quantity than in term milk. These factors may prevent intestinal attachment of enteropathogens by acting as receptor homologues resulting in the suppression of enteral colonization with harmful microorganisms. Breast milk also prevents a host of neonatal infections, a leading cause of neonatal mortality across the globe. The use of human milk can be adopted as an important healthcare intervention in neonatal units.

Breast Conditions and Difficulties in Breastfeeding

There are several common breast conditions which sometimes cause difficulties with breastfeeding. Management of these conditions is important both to relieve the mother and to enable successful breastfeeding. The difficulties in breastfeeding can be overcome by careful guidance, reassurance, and encouragement to the mother during prenatal period to prepare for breastfeeding and by providing skilled counseling after birth.

Flat Nipple

Many a times, mother becomes apprehensive that a flat nipple is a hindrance in successful breastfeeding. However, in a good suckling attachment, the infant takes the nipple and the breast tissue underlying the areola into his mouth to form a "teat." The anatomical nipple only forms about one third of the "teat" of breast tissue in the baby's mouth. This is therefore evident that the shape of the nipple is immaterial for successful suckling. The nipple is just a guide to show where the baby must take the breast. A woman with flat nipples should be reassured that she has normal nipples, even if they look short provided her nipples protract easily.

Inverted Nipple

Sometimes, a nipple does not protract, and on attempting to pull out the nipple, it goes deeper into the breast. The condition is known as inverted nipple **(Figs. 4.2.7A and B)**. The mother needs support in such a situation. She should be reassured that with some help she will be able to breastfeed her infant successfully. Help is most important soon after delivery when the baby starts breastfeeding.

A mother with the inverted nipple may be helped with the syringe method as follows **(Fig. 4.2.8)**:
- Cut the nozzle end of a disposable syringe (10–20 mL).
- Introduce the piston from the ragged cut end side.
- Ask the mother to apply the smooth side of the syringe on the nipple and gently pull out the piston and let her wait for a minute.

Nipple would then protrude into the syringe. Ask the mother to slowly release the suction and put the baby to breast; at this time, it helps the nipple to erect out, and baby is able to suckle in the proper position.
- After feeding, the nipple may retract back but doing it each time before feeding over a period of few days will help to solve the problem.

Engorgement of Breasts

If breasts are not emptied, the milk gets collected in the breast leading to engorgement. The engorged breast is tight, shiny (because of edema), and painful. Moreover, the milk may stop flowing. The factors, which cause engorgement of breasts, are as follows:
- Giving prelacteal feeds to the baby
- Delayed initiation of breastfeeds
- Long intervals between feeds
- Early removal of the baby from the breast
- Bottle-feeding and any other restrictions on breastfeeding.

Engorgement of the breast can be prevented by avoiding

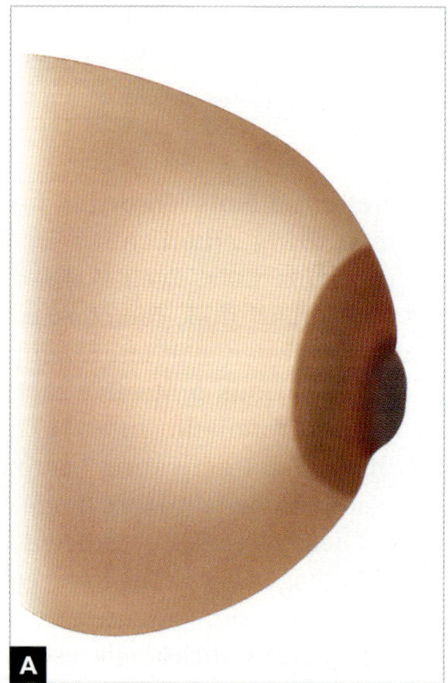

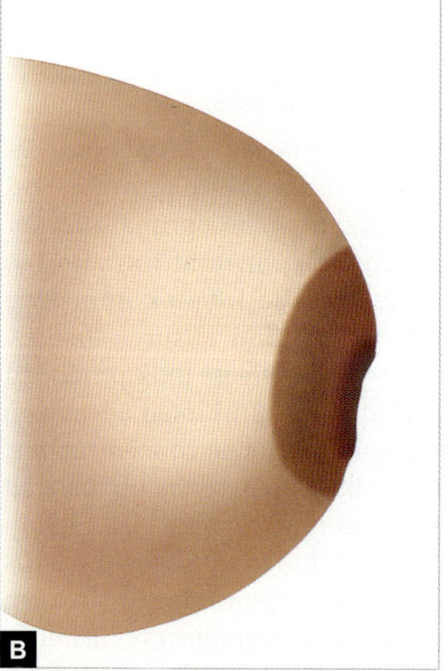

Figs. 4.2.7A and B: (A) Flat and (B) inverted nipple.
Source: Adapted with permission from Gupta A, Kushwaha KP, Sobti JC, et al. Breastfeeding and complementary feeding. New Delhi: Breastfeeding Promotion Network of India (BPNI); 2001.

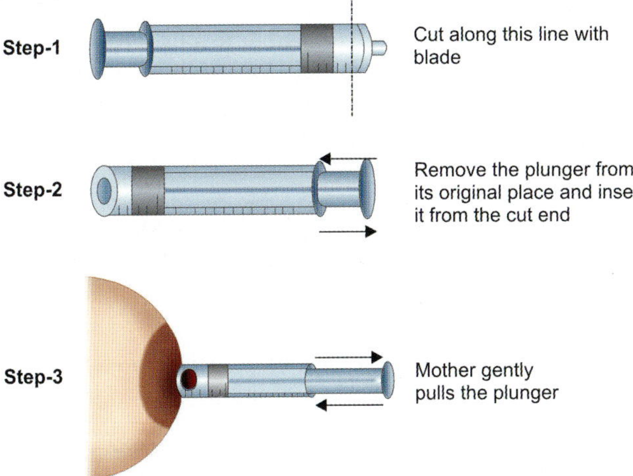

Fig. 4.2.8: Syringe method for correction of inverted nipple.
Source: Adapted from: Infant and young child feeding counseling—a training course, the "4 in 1 course" (integrated course on breastfeeding, complementary feeding and infant feeding and HIV). New Delhi: Breastfeeding Promotion Network of India (BPNI); 2015.

factors mentioned earlier. If the baby can suckle, he or she should feed frequently. If pain and tightness of the breast does not allow suckling, expressed milk may be given to the infant with cup/spoon. Once the mother feels comfortable, she should be advised again to breastfeed the infant on demand. Applying cold compress may reduce edema of the breasts. Engorged breasts may cause mild fever, which subsides spontaneously within a day or two.

Mastitis and Abscess

Mastitis is an inflammation of the breast; which makes it red, hot, tender and swollen. The mother feels sick, has fever, and severe pain in breast. Mastitis usually affects a part of the breast and usually unilateral. Mastitis may develop in an engorged breast, or it may follow a condition called blocked duct. Mastitis must be treated promptly and adequately. If treatment is delayed or incomplete, there is an increased risk of developing breast abscess. An abscess is when a collection of pus forms in part of the breast. The most important part of treatment is supportive counseling and improved drainage of milk from the affected part of the breast. The mother needs clear information and guidance about all measures needed for treatment, how to continue breastfeeding or expressing milk from the affected breast. This is important to help the mother to improve infant's attachment at the breast with frequent unrestricted breastfeeding. If necessary, express breast milk by hand or with a pump until suckling is resumed. Antibiotic should be given, if laboratory tests indicate infection, symptoms are severe, or symptoms do not improve after 12–24 hours of improved milk removal. Pain should be treated with an analgesic and warm packs to the breast. Incision and drainage should be done, if abscess develops.

Sore and Cracked Nipples

The most common cause of sore nipples is poor attachment in which the infant pulls the nipple in and out as he or she sucks and rubs the skin of the breast against his or her mouth. If the baby continues to suckle in this way, it damages the nipple skin and causes a crack or fissure. Oral thrush in the infant's mouth is another important cause of sore nipple but it usually develops when a baby is few weeks old. The situation is very painful for the mother. If a mother has sore or cracked nipples, improving infant's attachment to the breast relieves the pain. Medicated creams are best avoided as they may worsen the soreness. Hindmilk, which is rich in fat, should be applied on the nipple after feeding. For oral thrush, 1% gentian violet or Clotrimazole mouth paint 1% should be applied over the nipple as well as inside the baby's mouth every 4–6 hours for 5–7 days.

Breastfeeding and Maternal Illness

Maternal illnesses can have adverse effects on lactation. A sick woman may perceive that her milk supply has gone down because of illness. She may also believe that her milk will make the baby ill. These factors may lead to the discontinuation of breastfeeding. Minor illnesses, such as cold and other mild viral infection, which are self-limiting, should not prevent a mother to continue breastfeeding. However, major illness requires a more careful approach. The potential role of breastfeeding in the transmission of infections must also be acknowledged, and appropriate precautions should be taken. If the mother has tuberculosis, the mother-infant dyad should be treated together, and breastfeeding should be continued. Similarly, in the case of hepatitis (A, B, and C), breastfeeding can continue normally as the risk of transmission by breastfeeding is very low. In HIV-positive mother, mother should be provided with counseling and support for appropriate infant feeding practice. With adequate and appropriate antiretroviral drugs to mother and infant, exclusive breastfeeding for first 6 months of life is now the preferred recommendation in India.

Certain maternal drugs may affect the breastfed infant adversely as they are secreted in the breast milk. Breastfeeding should be avoided, if mother is consuming cytotoxic drugs, such as cyclophosphamide, methotrexate, and doxorubicin, radioactive compounds, such as gallium 67, indium 111, iodine 131, and technetium 99m.

Infant Feeding during Emergencies

In disasters and emergencies, such as earthquakes, floods, typhoons, and tsunami, breastfeeding is the safest, often the only reliable choice for infants and young children. It provides adequate and appropriate nutrition to the affected infants in a situation where child survival is a key issue. In disasters, infants are more likely to become ill and die from malnutrition. Uncontrolled distribution of breast milk substitutes during disasters may lead to early and unnecessary cessation of breastfeeding. For the vast majority of infants, emphasis should be on protecting, promoting and supporting breastfeeding, and ensuring timely, safe, and appropriate complementary feeding.

Protecting Breastfeeding from Commercial Influence

During last many decades, extensive promotion by the infant food manufacturing companies through advertisements, free samples, gifts to mothers, and health workers has led to convince them that formula feeding is as good as breastfeeding. This has also made a dent in the confidence of lactating women in her capacity to optimally breastfeed and has contributed to the decline of breastfeeding rates. Recognizing this trend, the Indian Parliament enacted the "infant milk substitutes (IMSs), feeding bottles and infant foods (regulation of production, supply and distribution) Act 1992 IMS Act". The IMS Act was further amended in the year 2003. The IMS Act controls marketing and promotion of IMSs, infant foods, and feeding bottles. Some salient features of the IMS Act include:

- It bans any kind of promotion or advertisement of IMSs, infant foods, and feeding bottles to the public, including electronic and print media.
- It prohibits providing free samples of IMS, infant foods and feeding bottles, and gifts to any one including pregnant women, mothers of infants, and members of the families.
- It prohibits donation of free or subsidized supplies of IMS, infant foods, and feeding bottles for health-care institutions except donations to the orphanages.
- It prohibits display of posters of IMSs, infant foods, and feeding bottles at healthcare facilities, hospitals, and health centers.
- It prescribes rules for information on the containers and labels of IMSs and infant foods, including a specific statement in English and local languages that "mother's milk is best for the baby" in capital letters.
- It prohibits having pictures of infants or women or phrases designed to increase the sale of the product on the labels of the products.
- It prohibits any contact of employers manufacturing and distributing company with pregnant women even for providing educational material to them.
- It prohibits direct or indirect financial inducement or gift to health worker or to any members of his family by the producer, supplier or distributor of the IMS, infant foods, and feeding bottles.
- The IMS Act also prohibits offering or giving any contribution or pecuniary benefit to a health worker or any association thereof including funding of seminar, meeting, conference, educational course, contests, fellowship, research work, or sponsorship, etc. by the manufacturers, supplier, or distributors of the products mentioned earlier.
- It prescribes standards for the IMS, infant foods, and feeding bottles.

BIBLIOGRAPHY

1. American Academy of Pediatrics. Section on breastfeeding: breastfeeding and the use of human milk. Pediatrics. 2012;129:e827-41.
2. Anand RK, Kumta NB, Kushwaha KP, et al. The science of infant feeding. New Delhi: Jaypee Brothers Medical Publishers; 2002.
3. Breastfeeding Promotion Network of India. Infant and young child feeding counseling—a training course, the "4 in 1 course" (integrated course on breastfeeding, complementary feeding and infant feeding and HIV). New Delhi: Breastfeeding Promotion Network of India; 2015.
4. Butte NF, Lopez-Alarcon MG, Garza C. Nutrient adequacy of exclusive breastfeeding for the term infant during the first six months of life. Geneva: World Health Organization; 2002.
5. World Health Organization. (2013). Long-term effects of breastfeeding: a systematic review (Horta BL, Victora CG). [online] Available from: http://apps.who.int/iris/bitstream/10665/79198/1/9789241505307.eng.pdf. [Accessed September, 2018].
6. Infant and Young Child Feeding Chapter, Indian Academy of Pediatrics. Infant and young child feeding guidelines: 2010. Indian Pediatr. 2010;47:995-1004.
7. Lawrence RA, Lawrence RM. Breastfeeding in modern medicine. In: Breastfeeding: a guide for the medical profession, 5th edition. St Louis: Mosby; 1999.
8. Ministry of Women and Child Development, Food and Nutrition Board, Government of India. National guidelines on infant and young child feeding, 2nd edition. New Delhi: Food and Nutrition Board; 2006.
9. Ministry of Women and Child Development, Government of India. (2003). The Infant Milk Substitutes, Feeding Bottles and Infant Foods (Regulation of Production, Supply and Distribution) Amendment Act, 2003. [online] Available from: http://wcd.nic.in/IMSamendact 2003.pdf. [Accessed September, 2018].
10. World Health Organization, United Nations Children's Fund. Global strategy for infant and young child feeding. [online]. Available from: http://www.who.int/nutrition/publications/gs_infant_feeding_text_eng.pdf. [Accessed September, 2018].
11. World Health Organization. (2018). Implementation guidance: protecting, promoting and supporting breastfeeding in facilities providing maternity and newborn services—the revised baby-friendly hospital initiative. [online] Available from: http://www.who.int/nutrition/publications/infantfeeding/bfhi-implementation/en/. [Accessed September, 2018].

4.3 Human Milk Banking

RK Agarwal

INTRODUCTION

History of breastfeeding dates back since evolution in mammalians (around 4200 BC) on this mother earth. Each mammalian milk is species specific and perfectly suited for their offspring.

Millennium Development Goals 4 aimed to reduce under-five child mortality by two thirds by 2015. To accelerate the progress on child survival, there is a heightened global interest in increasing the rates of optimal infant and young child feeding practices, especially the human milk for the first 6 months. The under-5 mortality rate (U5MR) for India was estimated at 50 for the year of 2015–16 (National Family Health Survey 2015–16). Infant mortality rate (IMR) in India has registered a decline from 58 in 2005 to 41 in 2015–16. World Health Organization (WHO) estimates that 53% of the acute pneumonia and 55% of the diarrhea deaths are attributable to poor feeding practices during the first 6 months of life. WHO and United Nations Children's Fund made a joint statement in 1980: "Where it is not possible for the biological mother to breastfeed, the first alternative, if available, should be the use of human milk from other sources. Human milk banks should be made available in appropriate situations."

Breastfeeding is the best method of infant feeding because human milk is uniquely suited to the human infant. All mothers should be encouraged to breastfeed their infants.

When a mother, for some reason, is unable to feed her infant directly, her breast milk should be expressed and fed to her infant. If mother's own milk is unavailable or insufficient, the next best option is to use pasteurized donor human milk (PDHM). In India, the burden of low-birth-weight (LBW) babies is about 20–30% with significant mortality and morbidities. Feeding these babies with breast milk can significantly reduce the risk of infections.

Though "wet nursing" had been in practice since mythological ages, modern human milk banking is in its infancy in India. The first human milk bank in Asia was established by Armida Fernandez in 1989 in Mumbai. Currently, the number of human milk banks has grown to nearly 50 in India, and Rajasthan leads with 18 banks. Brazil has the largest network of 210 banks in the world. Its strategy includes innovative measures, such as training postmen to provide information on breastfeeding to pregnant women and using firefighters to collect surplus milk for donation from lactating women. One of the major reasons for slow growth and loss of interest in human milk banking was the promotion of milk formula by the industry.

LOCATION OF HUMAN MILK BANKING

Human milk banks are primarily focused to provide donor milk to high-risk newborns. Thus, a location near or even inside the boundaries of neonatal unit is desirable. Postnatal wards are most suited for the purpose as the number of donors is likely to be in large number, where counselors can encourage them to donate milk. Certain nongovernmental organizations (NGOs) that take care of abandoned babies should have a human milk bank in their facility. Presence of human milk banks in the neonatal intensive care units (NICUs) is associated with elevated rates of exclusive breastfeeding rates in very-low-birth-weight (VLBW) babies.

THE RECIPIENTS

Pasteurized donor human milk can be prescribed on priority for:

- Preterm babies and sick babies;
- Babies of mothers with postpartum illnesses;
- Babies whose mothers have lactation failure till their milk output improves.

Therapeutic benefits are noted in short gut syndrome, sepsis, and postsurgical gut healing in omphalocele, gastroschisis, bowel obstruction, and intestinal fistulas. In extremely preterm infants given exclusive diets of preterm formula versus human milk, there was a significantly greater duration of parenteral nutrition and higher rate of surgical necrotizing enterocolitis (NEC) in infants receiving preterm formula. It is possible to do gut priming exclusively with human milk.

If PDHM supplies are sufficient, donor milk may be supplied for:

- *Absent or insufficient lactation*: Mothers with multiple births, who cannot secrete adequate breast milk for their neonates initially;
- For babies of nonlactating mothers who adopt neonates, and if induced, lactation is not possible;
- Abandoned neonate and sick neonates;
- Temporary interruption of breastfeeding;

- Infant at health risk from breast milk of the biological mother;
- Babies whose mother died in the immediate postpartum period.

INFRASTRUCTURE

There are no standard recommendations. The average requirement is a room of 250 ft^2 which can accommodate the equipment required for milk banking, a work area for the technician as well as some storage space for records and administration and area for counseling donors, etc. Privacy is of paramount importance for the area of breast milk expression. Provision of music or television and crèche for her baby help in reducing stress of donors. Teaching videos of Kangaroo mother care, expression of breast milk, and advantages of breast milk feeding can be shown.

Equipment

Pasteurizer (Shaker Waterbath)

It is essential to have a device to carry out heat treatment of donor milk at the recommended temperature of 62.5°C for 30 minutes (Holder pasteurization). A conventional pasteurizer is extremely expensive and of dairy-industry size and is not suitable for a human milk banks. A well-accepted alternative is the use of a shaker waterbath with a microprocessor-controlled temperature regulator, an electronic timer device, and a shaker speed controller. The milk in the container is boiled through the steam and hot water in the water-shaker bath. To avoid coagulation of the milk and to distribute heat evenly, the tray on which the stainless steel containers are placed is shaken wobbled. This shaker waterbath should be double walled and made of steel. The size of the shaker waterbath varies according to the need of the milk bank with the tray capacity varying from 9 to 24 flasks or stainless steel containers of 200–400 mL capacity.

Effect of Pasteurization on Human Milk

Pasteurization (62.5°C for 30 minutes) does affect *some* of the nutritional, immunologic, and the other components of human milk. This heat treatment reliably eliminates all the functional white blood cells and bacteria, inactivates human immunodeficiency virus (HIV) and human T-lymphotropic virus (HTLV), cytomegalovirus, and will eliminate or significantly decrease the titers of most other viruses. Immunologic factors are variously affected by heat treatment. Most of the secretory immunoglobulin A (IgA), bifid growth factor, and lysozymes remain (0% to 30%) destroyed; lipids are unaffected but 57% of the lactoferrin and 34% of the immunoglobulin G are destroyed well.

Holder pasteurization does not appear to influence nitrogen absorption or retention in LBW infants. Most enzymes, growth factors, vitamins, and minerals are unchanged or minimally decreased. Heat treatment of donor milk appears to foster more rapid growth of intestinal epithelial cells by inactivating heat-labile inhibitory cytokines, allowing heat-stable epidermal growth factor to act. Freezing inactivates milk cells and most viruses but does not appear to affect the nutritional or anti-infective quality of the milk.

Deep Freezer

A deep freezer to store the milk at –20°C is essential. It is desirable to order a deep freezer with a digital display of the temperature with an alarm setting.

- First deep freezer is for storage of milk awaiting culture—used for storage of the milk till the postpasteurization milk culture reports are available. This freezer should be locked always, so that no milk is accidentally used till the culture reports are available.
- The second deep freezer is used for the storage of the pasteurized milk once the culture reports are negative and the milk is considered safe for disbursement.

Refrigerators are required to store the milk till the whole day's collection is over, and the milk is ready to be mixed and pooled for further processing. It is also required for thawing the milk before being dispatched.

Hot Air Oven or Autoclave

A hot air oven or autoclave in the milk bank is essential for sterilizing the containers used for collection from donors, containers for pasteurizing and storing the milk, as well as the test tubes needed for sending milk culture samples to the microbiology laboratory.

Breast Milk Pumps

For milk banking, hospital grade electric pumps are preferred as they result in better volumes of expressed milks and are relatively painless and comfortable to use. There is no major difference in the types of electrical breast pumps. If there are cost constraints, manually operated breast milk pumps can be used. They can be reused with chemical sterilization. Simultaneous breast expression in breastfeeding women is more efficacious than sequential breast expression. Breast pumps can be a source of infection. They should be cleaned properly. Detachable parts should be sterilized as per manufacturer's instructions.

Containers

For collection and storing the collected milk, single-use hard plastic containers of polycarbonates, Pyrex, or propylene are used; however, cylindrical, wide-mouthed stainless steel containers of 200 mL capacities with tight-fitting or screwed caps are equally effective. They are easily available, durable, easy to clean, and autoclave. There is no significant decrease in nutrient composition on storage; however, cellular components are reduced. Polythene milk bags are not suitable as they are fragile, associated with loss of lipids and vitamins, and there is a risk of contamination.

Generator or Uninterrupted Power Supply

Every milk bank should have a centralized source of uninterrupted power supply in the form of a generator, UPS or inverter, to run the deep freezers and refrigerators in case of electricity failure.

Milk Analyzer

It is desirable to have macronutrient analysis of breast milk to estimate the calorie, protein, and fat of a milk sample, using infrared spectroscopy technology, in teaching hospitals as a step toward lacto-engineering.

ADMINISTRATIVE STAFF

Milk banks should have a panel from pediatrics, neonatology, microbiology, nutrition, lactation management, public health and food technology, milk bank officer (usually a doctor), lactation management nurses (for counseling mothers and assisting expression of breast milk), technician (for pasteurization of breast milk and microbiological surveillance), attendant (for collecting, sterilization of the containers and maintaining hygiene), receptionist (for record keeping and public relations), and a microbiologist (for microbiology testing and infection-control policies).

General Guidelines for Staff

- Hygienic practices, such as proper hand wash; donning gowns, mask, gloves; trimming nails; and locking long hairs should be maintained.
- Gloves should be worn and changed between handling raw and heat-treated milk.
- Standard operating procedures of the bank (which should be displayed at proper places) should be adhered to.
- Staff should undergo regular health checks and be immunized against hepatitis B virus (HBV).

Banks should have an operational objective of ensuring full traceability from individual donation to recipient and maintaining a record of all storage and processing conditions.

DONOR POPULATION

The donor population is formed by healthy lactating mothers with healthy babies, who are voluntarily willing to give their extra breast milk for other babies without compromising the nutritional needs of their own baby. The donors are not paid for their donations in India. It can include mothers attending well-baby clinics, mothers whose babies are in NICU, mothers who have lost their babies but are willing to donate the milk, or lactating working staff in the hospital, and motivated mothers from the community.

Maximum donor population should be reached by spreading awareness and mass communication. NGOs, social clubs, and senior female students can play a good role in it.

Who Can Donate?

Those lactating women can donate who

- Are in good health and not regularly on medications or herbal supplements (except for prenatal vitamins, human insulin, thyroid replacement hormones, nasal sprays, asthma inhalers, topical treatments, eye drops, progestin-only or low-dose-estrogen birth control products);
- Willing to undergo blood testing for screening of infections;
- Has enough milk after feeding her baby satisfactorily.

Who Cannot Donate?

A donor is disqualified, if she:

- Uses illegal drugs or tobacco products or nicotine replacement therapy;
- Regularly takes more than two ounces of alcohol or equivalent or three caffeinated drinks per day;
- Has a positive blood test result for HIV, HTLV, hepatitis B or C, or syphilis;
- Has a sexual partner having high-risk behavior or suffering from HBV, HIV, hepatitis C virus, and venereal diseases in last 12 months;
- Has received organ or tissue transplant, any blood transfusion, or blood product within the prior 12 months;
- Is taking radioactive or other drugs or has chemical environmental exposure or over-the-counter prescriptions or megadoses of vitamins, which are known to be toxic to the neonate and excreted in breast milk;
- Has mastitis or fungal infections of the nipple or areola, reactivation of herpes simplex or varicella zoster infections in the mammary or thoracic region.

COLLECTION OF BREAST MILK

After checking the suitability for donation, getting written informed consent, history taking, physical examination, and sampling for lab tests, the donor mother is sent to designate breast milk collection area. The breast milk is collected by trained staff after the method of breast milk expression is chosen by the donor. Although home collection of the breast milk is being practiced in some countries abroad, but the experts felt that due to the risk of contamination and difficulty in tracking, it is better avoided at present in our country; however, milk collection camps can be practiced under proper supervision.

Washing the breast with simple water before expression is as good as washing with disinfectant. There is no rationale in discarding the first few milliliters of foremilk to reduce the infection rate. The breast milk may be expressed with the help of breast pumps either electrical or manual. Donation should be collected in properly labeled sterile container.

Processing

All batches of the collected raw breast milk should be refrigerated immediately in preprocess refrigerator till the serological report comes negative. Fresh raw milk should not be added to the frozen milk since this can result in defreezing with hydrolysis of triglycerides. While mixing fresh raw breast milk to frozen raw breast milk, previously collected from the same donor, it should be chilled before adding to frozen milk. But for sick or preterm babies, it is advisable to use a new container for each pumping.

Microbiological screening of donated milk is done before (if there is no cost constraint) and as soon as possible after pasteurization. Prepasteurization microbiology can result in the wastage of milk to the tune of 30% in some cases. Even after pasteurization, the end toxins of organisms are still present in the milk in some cases, but they have not been found to have any clinical effect on the baby. A bacterial count of 10^5 or more in raw breast milk can be considered as an indicator of the milk's poor quality. Based on this and on the theoretical concern that heavily contaminated milk with specific bacteria (e.g., *Staphylococcus aureus*, *Escherichia coli*) may contain enterotoxins and thermostable enzymes even after pasteurization, expert panel selected 10^5 CFU/mL for total bacterial count, 10^4 CFU/mL for *Enterobacteriaceae* and *S. aureus* as threshold values which are in consonance with milk banks operating in other parts of the world.

No growth is acceptable in postpasteurization microbiology cultures. Whole pasteurized batch of culture positive container of processed milk should be discarded. Before pasteurization, pooling and mixing may be carried out, from multiple donors to ease the process of processing and storage.

Storage

Pasteurized milk awaiting culture report should be kept in separate freezer area taking precaution not to disburse it till the culture is negative. Culture negative processed milk should be kept at –20°C in tightly sealed container with clear mention of expiry date and other relevant data on the label. It can be preserved for 4–6 months. Random cultures of preserved milk before disbursal can aid quality assurance.

Disbursal

Pasteurized donor human milk should be disbursed on the requisition from NICU after informed consent from recipient's parents. It should be done on "First-in-first-out" basis from the storage.

Frozen PDHM should be thawed by either defrosting the milk rapidly in a waterbath at a temperature not exceeding 37°C or under running lukewarm water. It should never be thawed in the microwave as this result in reduction in the IgA content of the milk. Milk should not be refrozen after being thawed as this increases the hydrolysis of the triglycerides in the milk. While bringing to room temperature, it should be gently agitated to make a homogeneous mixture before use and be used preferably within 3–4 hours to prevent contamination. Preterm baby should preferably get PDHM from preterm donors.

Labeling and Record Keeping

Proper labeling at all levels is mandatory, from sterile container for the collection of donation, pooling vessel, pasteurization container to storage containers. Labels should be water resistant and read clearly names and identification number of donors and dates of pasteurization batch numbers. Record keeping at all levels should be meticulous for donor record file containing consent form, donor's data and screening reports, and pasteurization batch files; and for PDHM disbursal record file, containing relevant data including recipient consent form.

As incubation period for most infection varies from a few weeks to 6 months and the appearance of symptoms is faster in infants and children, there seems to be no rationale for keeping records beyond 5 years, unless one is working in an area where milk kinship issue is of paramount importance. In India, the blood bank records are preserved for a minimum period of 5 years.

Economic Implications

There has been a definite cost effectiveness of using banked human milk in NICUs observed in western countries largely by reduction in the rate of NEC. In a country, such as ours, the cost of running a milk bank with potential cost saving due to the reduction in NEC and sepsis rate and, ultimately, the duration of hospital stay have not been adequately evaluated, but given the high incidence of sepsis and a large burden of premature births, this intervention is likely to result in substantial saving for the nation.

CONCLUSION

Artificial formula will never provide the broad range of benefits of human milk. Given the high rate of preterm births in the country and level of malnutrition that ensues in the postnatal growth in such babies after birth, there is an urgent need for establishing milk banks across the country, especially in the large NICUs of all hospitals. The author is of the opinion that human milk banks be opened in all 707 (2018) districts of India to help in reducing Neonatal Mortality rate, IMR, and U5MR. It only requires a pediatrician and pathologist and very little budget.

BIBLIOGRAPHY

1. Arnold LD. The cost-effectiveness of using banked donor milk in the neonatal intensive care unit: prevention of necrotizing enterocolitis. J Hum Lact. 2002;18(2):172-7.
2. Arslanoglu S, Moro GE, Bellu R, et al. Presence of human milk bank is associated with elevated rate of exclusive breastfeeding in VLBW infants. J Perinat Med. 2013;41(2):129-31.
3. Bharadva K, Tiwari S, Mishra S, et al.; Infant and Young Child Feeding Chapter; Indian Academy of Pediatric. Human milk banking guidelines. Indian Pediatr. 2014;51:469-74.
4. International Institute for Population Sciences (2015). National Family Health Survey-4. [online] Available from: http://rchiips.org/NFHS/pdf/NFHS4/India.pdf. [Accessed September, 2018].
5. Israel-Ballard K, Chantry C, Dewey K, et al. Viral, nutritional, and bacterial safety of flash-heated and pretoria-pasteurized breast milk to prevent mother-to-child transmission of HIV in resource-poor countries: a pilot study. J Acquir Immune Defic Syndr. 2005;40(2):175-81.
6. Morera Pons S, Castellote Bargallo AI, Lopez Sabater MC. Evaluation by high-performance liquid chromatography of the hydrolysis of human milk triacylglycerides during storage at low temperatures. J Chromatogr A. 1998;823(1-2):467-74.
7. Nash C, Amir L. Human milk banking: a review. Retrieved from: http://www.breastfeedingindia.com/breastfeeding/human_milk_banks.html-top. [Accessed September, 2018].
8. Simmer K, Hartmann B. The known and unknowns of human milk banking. Early Hum Dev. 2009;85(11):701-4.
9. Wight NE. Donor human milk for preterm infants. J Perinatol. 2001;21(4):249-54.

4.4 Malnutrition

Meenakshi N Mehta

INTRODUCTION

"Underlying every other condition is malnutrition, due to both calorie and protein deficiency. Though poverty is the main contributing cause, it is greatly aggravated by lack of proper dietary knowledge" **(Fig. 4.4.1)**.

Adequate nutrition is essential in early childhood to ensure healthy growth, proper organ formation and function, a strong immune system and neurological, and cognitive development. Good nutrition allows children to survive, grow, develop, learn, play, participate, and contribute, while malnutrition robs children of their futures and lives, young lives hanging in the balance. Nutrition has increasingly been recognized as a basic pillar for social and economic developments. Economic growth and human development require well-nourished populations who can learn new skills, think critically, and contribute to their communities. Child malnutrition impacts cognitive function and contributes to poverty through impeding individual's ability to lead productive lives. Malnutrition is the gravest single threat to the world's public health. Protein energy malnutrition (PEM) is one of the most widely spread health and nutritional problems of the developing countries. Annually, undernutrition kills or disables millions of children. It is estimated that more than half of under-5 deaths are attributable to under nutrition. It often causes disease and disability in the survivors and prevents millions from reaching their full potential **(Fig. 4.4.2)**.

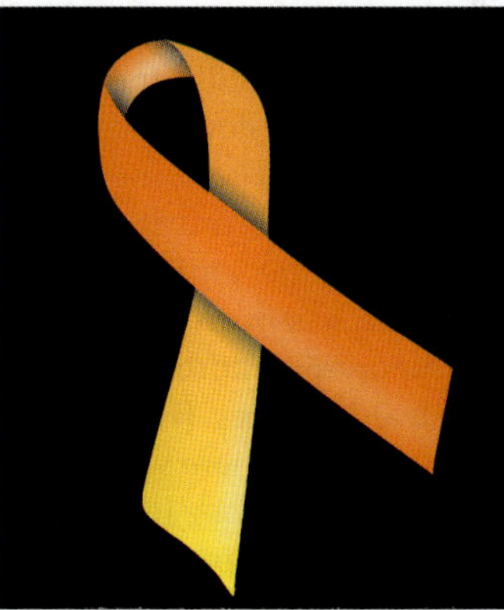

Fig. 4.4.1: The orange ribbon—an awareness ribbon for malnutrition.

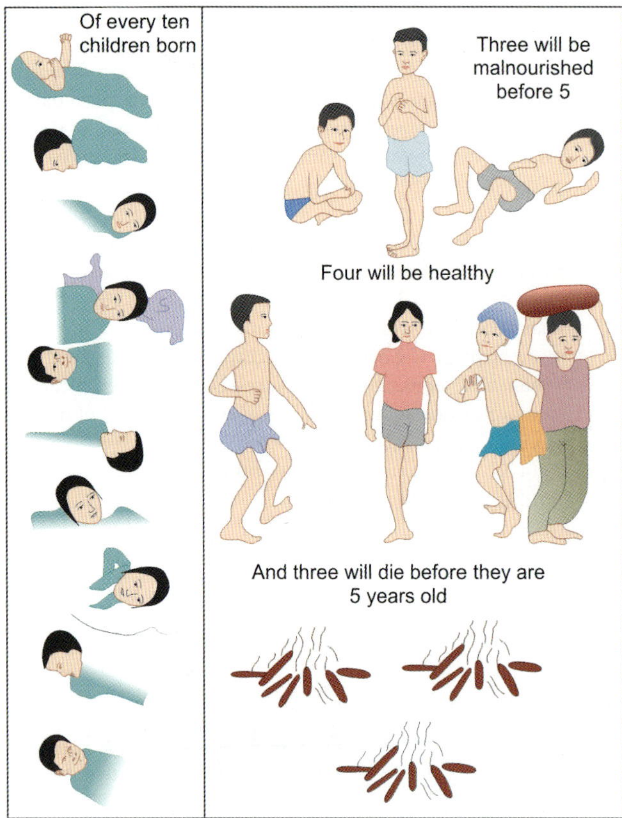

Fig. 4.4.2: Morbidity and mortality.

MAGNITUDE OF THE PROBLEM

Globally in 2017, of the under-5 children (<5 years old) wasting affected 7.5% or 51 million, with 16 million severally wasted. Stunting affected an estimated 22.2% or 151 million, and an estimated 5.6% or 38.3 million were overweight. Of these, more than half stunted and overweight and the two-thirds of wasted live in Asia, whereas one third of the stunted and one fourth each of the overweight and wasted live in Africa. By economy while only about half of all the children under-5 live in the lower middle-income countries, two thirds of all stunted and three-fourths of all wasted children live there.

In India, childhood undernutrition accounts for 45% of under-5 mortality alone and remains a key public health problem. There has been hardly any difference in the proportion of under-5 children with wasting between National Family Health Survey (NHFS)-3 (2005–06) and NHFS-4 (2015–16); however, there was a wasting reduction in prevalence of stunting by about 10% at the national level. Maximum prevalence of wasting was seen in Jharkhand (29%) and minimum in Kerala (15.7%). Similarly, stunting was maximum nearly half (48.3%) in Bihar and least in Kerala. Even after 35 years of the launch of the Integrated Child Development Services scheme, the problem of undernutrition still continues and the reduction in the prevalence is relatively unimpressive **(Figs. 4.4.3 to 4.4.6)**.

These alarming statistics have dire consequences for morbidity, mortality, productivity, and economic growth. The prevalence of malnutrition in India varies state-wise with the highest in Madhya Pradesh, Jharkhand, and Bihar; and the lowest in Mizoram, Sikkim, Manipur, Kerala, Punjab and Goa, although the rate is still considerably higher than that of the developed nations. It is more in rural areas and generally in those who are poor.

The PEM has higher incidence in nutritionally vulnerable groups: young children between 6 months to 2 years, women during pregnancy and lactation, and the elderly age group, as the nutritional requirements are larger relative to their body size than in older children and adults. The damage caused by malnutrition in the intrauterine life or in the first 2 years of life may be due to impairment in the developing brain.

DEFINITIONS AND CLASSIFICATIONS

The World Health Organization (WHO) defines PEM as range of pathological conditions arising from coincidental lack in varying proportions of proteins and calories, occurring most frequently in infants and young children, and commonly associated with infection. The extent of weight loss and growth rate varies with severity of PEM—in early stages, there is failure to maintain weight or growth rate, but as it becomes progressive, there is loss of weight associated with loss of subcutaneous fat and muscle mass with dysfunction of many vital organs, which leads to a variety of clinical features. With increasing severity, there is increasing failure in the homeostatic mechanisms of the body and damage to the immune defences which may result in infections, shock, and death.

Protein energy malnutrition is a generalized syndrome complex and it is very difficult to classify it using a single parameter. A large number of classifications using anthropometric, clinical, and biochemical parameters have been proposed. Nutritional anthropometry is a valuable index of assessment of nutritional status of children and mothers. Among the most studied are weight, length or height, arm circumference, skinfold thickness, and head circumference.

Since Gomez first proposed classification based on weight for age (WFA), standard WFA measurement used was Harvard growth standard, 50th centile being 100%, many classifications have been suggested **(Table 4.4.1)**. In 2009, WHO recommended new growth standards replacing the earlier National Centre for Health Statistics reference charts.

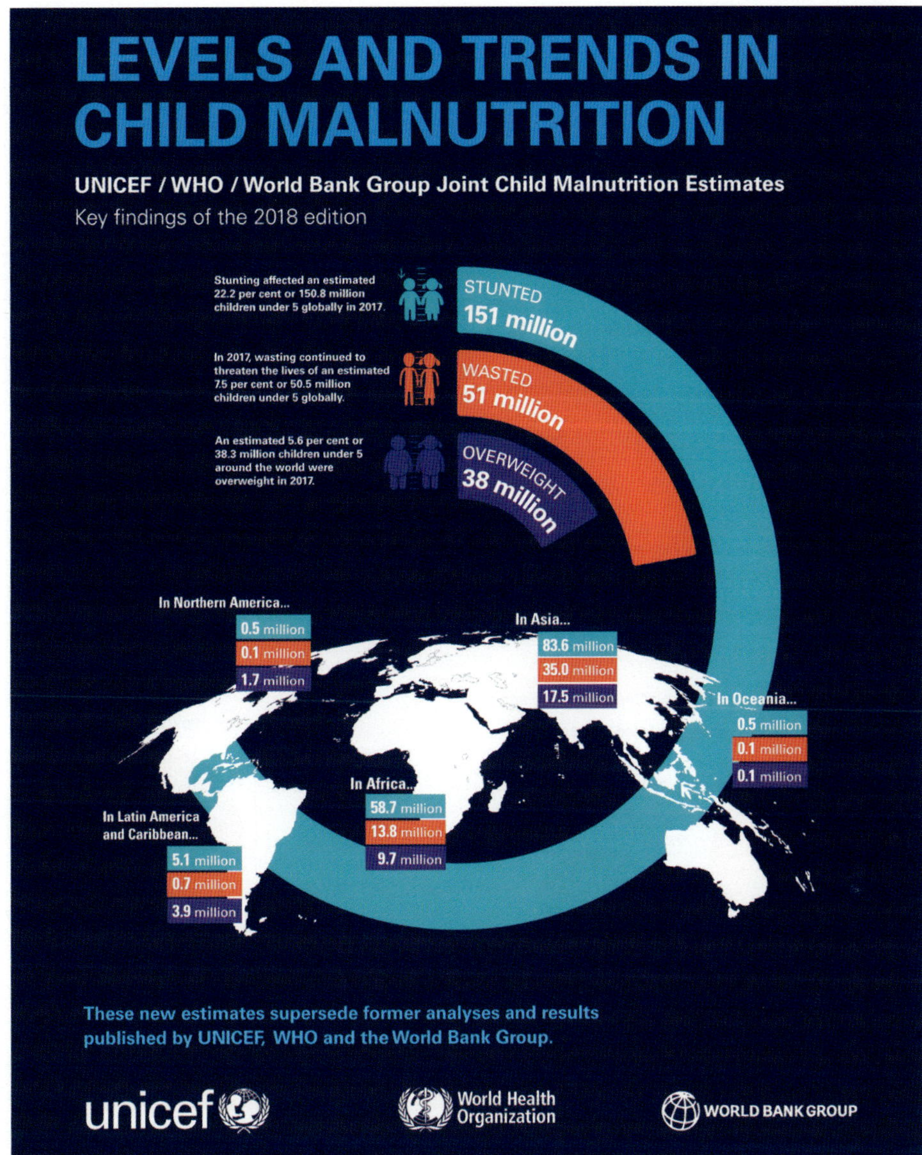

Fig. 4.4.3: UNICEF/WHO/World Bank Group. Joint child malnutrition estimates—Key global findings in 2017 (2018 edition).

Table 4.4.2 presents the diagnostic criteria for severe acute malnutrition (SAM) based on WHO growth standards. Moderate malnutrition is defined when the weight for length or height is between -2SD and -3SD, or when the mid-arm circumference (MAC) is between 11.5 cm and 12.5 cm.

ACUTE VERSUS CHRONIC DEFICIENCY

Weight and arm circumference are affected within a short duration of inadequate nutrient intake and ill-health, while height and head circumference do not change so rapidly. A slowing in the rate of growth indicated by poor gain in height would take at least 6 months to manifest itself, while a slowing of weight gain or loss can be demonstrated within a month. A child can lose weight but not height.

Anthropometric parameters can be classified into two main groups—(1) the age-dependent and (2) age-independent criteria if child's age is not known.

Age-dependent Criteria

- Weight for age expressed as percentage of the median value, Z (SD) score or as percentiles.
- Height for age compares child's height with the expected height or length for a healthy child of the same age.

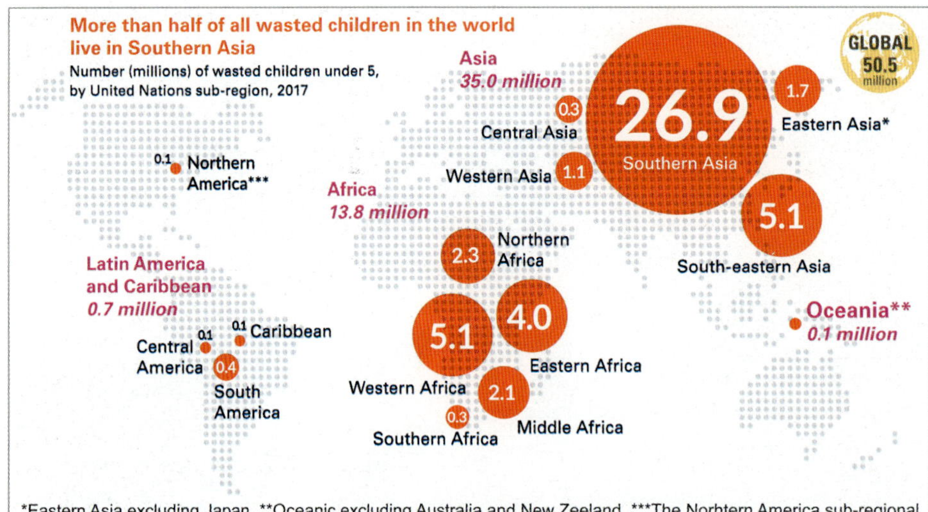

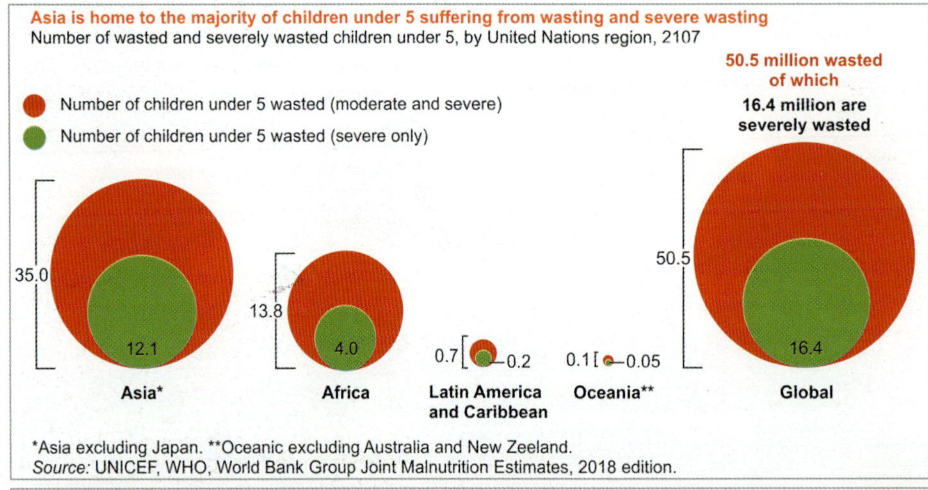

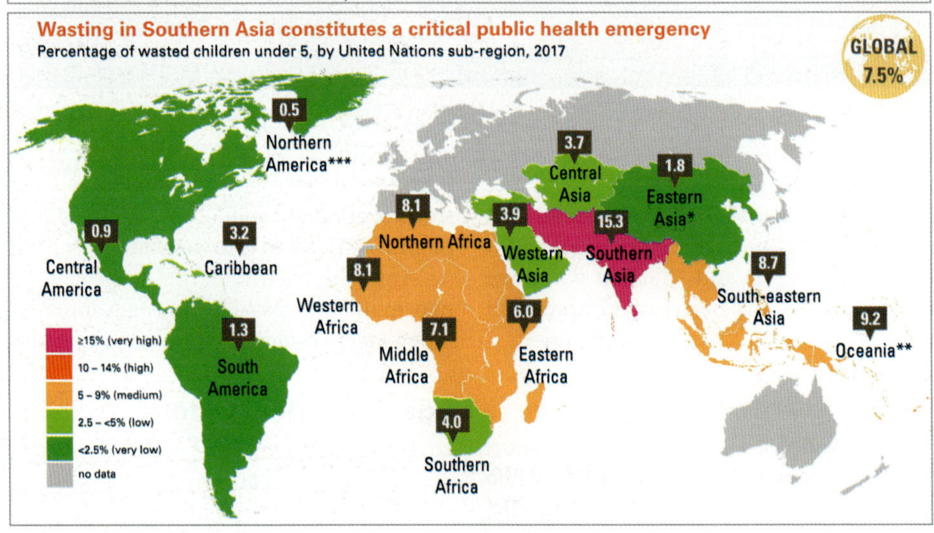

Fig. 4.4.4: Severe wasting prevalence—global-wise.

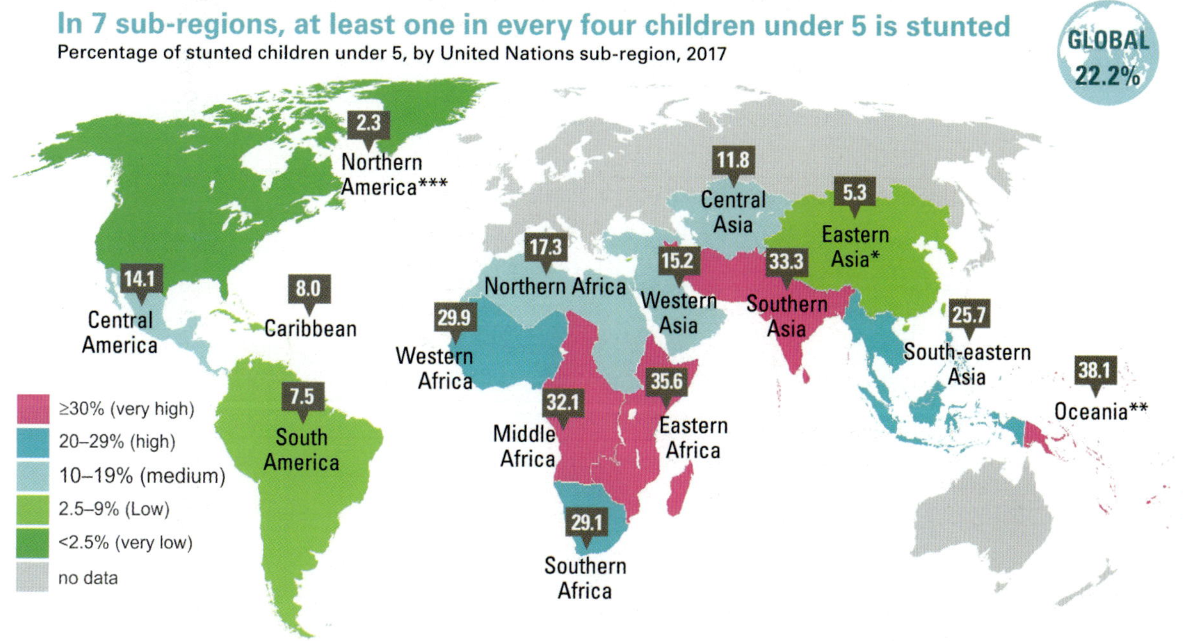

Fig. 4.4.5: Stunting prevalence.

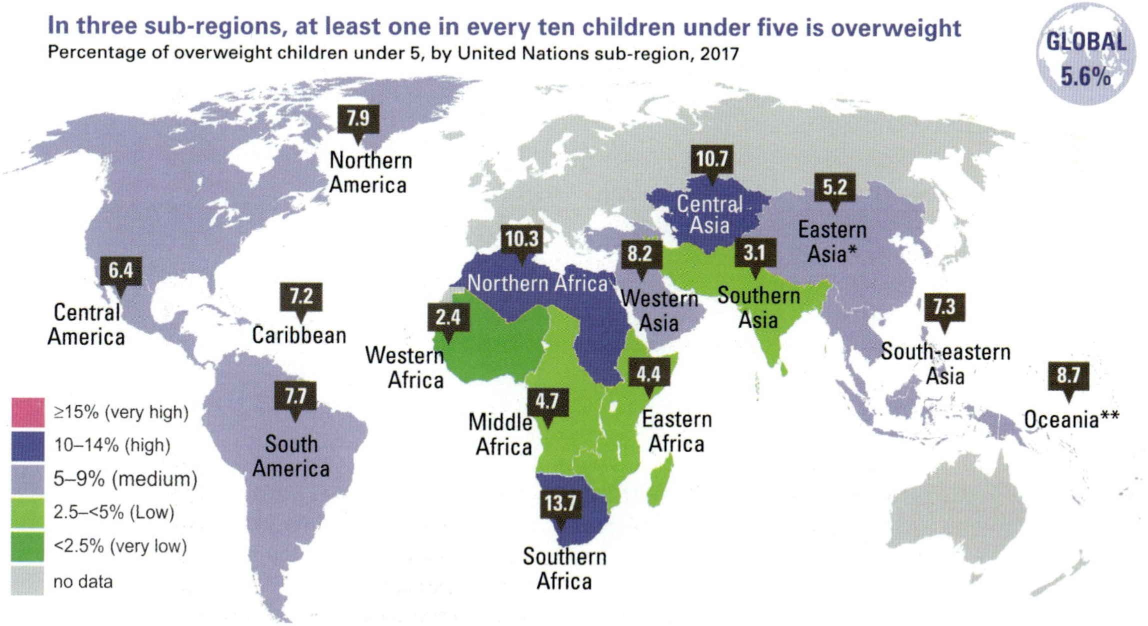

Fig. 4.4.6: Overweight prevalence.

Age-independent Criteria

- *Mid-upper arm circumference (MUAC) or MAC*: Between 1 and 5 years, the MUAC is relatively constant between 16.5 and 17.5 cm. Any child in this group whose MUAC is less than 12.5 cm is classified as undernourished. MUAC is a useful method of screening large number of children during nutritional emergencies but is less useful in long-term growth monitoring programs.

Table 4.4.1: Classification of malnutrition.

Classification	***Definition***	***Grading***	
Gomez	Weight below percentage of median value WFA	Mild (Grade 1)	75–90% WFA
		Moderate (Grade 2)	60–74% WFA
		Severe (Grade 3)	<60% WFA
Waterlow	*Z*-scores (SD) below median WFH	Mild	80–90% WFH
		Moderate	70–80% WFH
		Severe	<70% WFH
WHO (wasting)	*Z*-scores (SD) below median WFH	Moderate	*Z*-score < −2
		Severe	*Z*-score < −3
WHO (stunting)	*Z*-scores (SD) below median WFA	Moderate	*Z*-score < −2
		Severe	*Z*-score < −3
Kanawati	MUAC divided by occipitofrontal head circumference	Mild	<0.31
		Moderate	<0.28
		Severe	<0.25
Cole	*Z*-scores of BMI for age	Grade 1	BMI for age *Z*-score < −1
		Grade 2	BMI for age *Z*-score < −2
		Grade 3	BMI for age *Z*-score < −3
Jelliffe	Percentage of standard weight for age (50th centile of Harvard standard)	Normal	>90%
		Grade 1	80–90%
		Grade 2	70–79%
		Grade 3	60–69%
		Grade 4	<60%
Arnold	Mid-arm circumference	Normal	>13.5 cm
		Mild–moderate	12.5–13.4 cm
		Severe PEM	<12.5 cm
Welcome	• Presence or absence of edema • Weight or age percentage of expected	<80%	Edema absent (underweight)
		60–80%	Edema present (Kwashiorkor)
		<60%	Edema absent (Marasmus), Edema present (Marasmic kwashiorkor)c
		<60%	

(BMI: body mass index; HFA: height for age; MUAC: mid and upper arm circumference; SD: standard deviation; WFA: weight for age; WFH: weight for height; WHO: World Health Organization)

Table 4.4.2: Diagnostic criteria for severe acute malnutrition in children of age 6–60 months.

Indicator	***Measure***	***Cutoff***
Severe wasting	Weight for height	<–3 SD
Severe stunting	Height or age	<–3 SD
Severe undernutrition	Weight or age	<–3 SD
Severe wasting	Midarm circumference	<115 mm
Bilateral edema	Clinical signs	

(SD: standard deviation)

- *Weight for height (WFH)*: The degree of wasting is assessed by comparing the child's weight with the expected weight of a healthy child of same height. Combinations of these measurements have been suggested sometimes to distinguish types of malnutrition. For example, Waterlow proposed that weight or height allows one to distinguish between children who have suffered malnutrition in the past from those who are currently experiencing malnutrition. In chronic malnutrition, the child is stunted, i.e. her or his WFA and height for age are low. In acute malnutrition, however, her or his height for age is appropriate, but she or he is wasted (low WFH and age). Thus, weight and height measurements together are useful to understand the dynamics of malnutrition, distinguishing between current malnutrition and long-term or chronic malnutrition.

- *Quack stick*: Quacker's MAC measuring stick is a height-measuring rod calibrated in MUAC rather than height, values of 80% of expected MUAC for height are marked on the stick at corresponding height levels, and the child is made to stand in front of this stick.
- His/her nutritional status is easily read as 50%, 60%, 70%, or 80% of the standard. If a child is taller than his/her circumference level on the stick, he/she is considered malnourished **(Fig. 4.4.7)**.

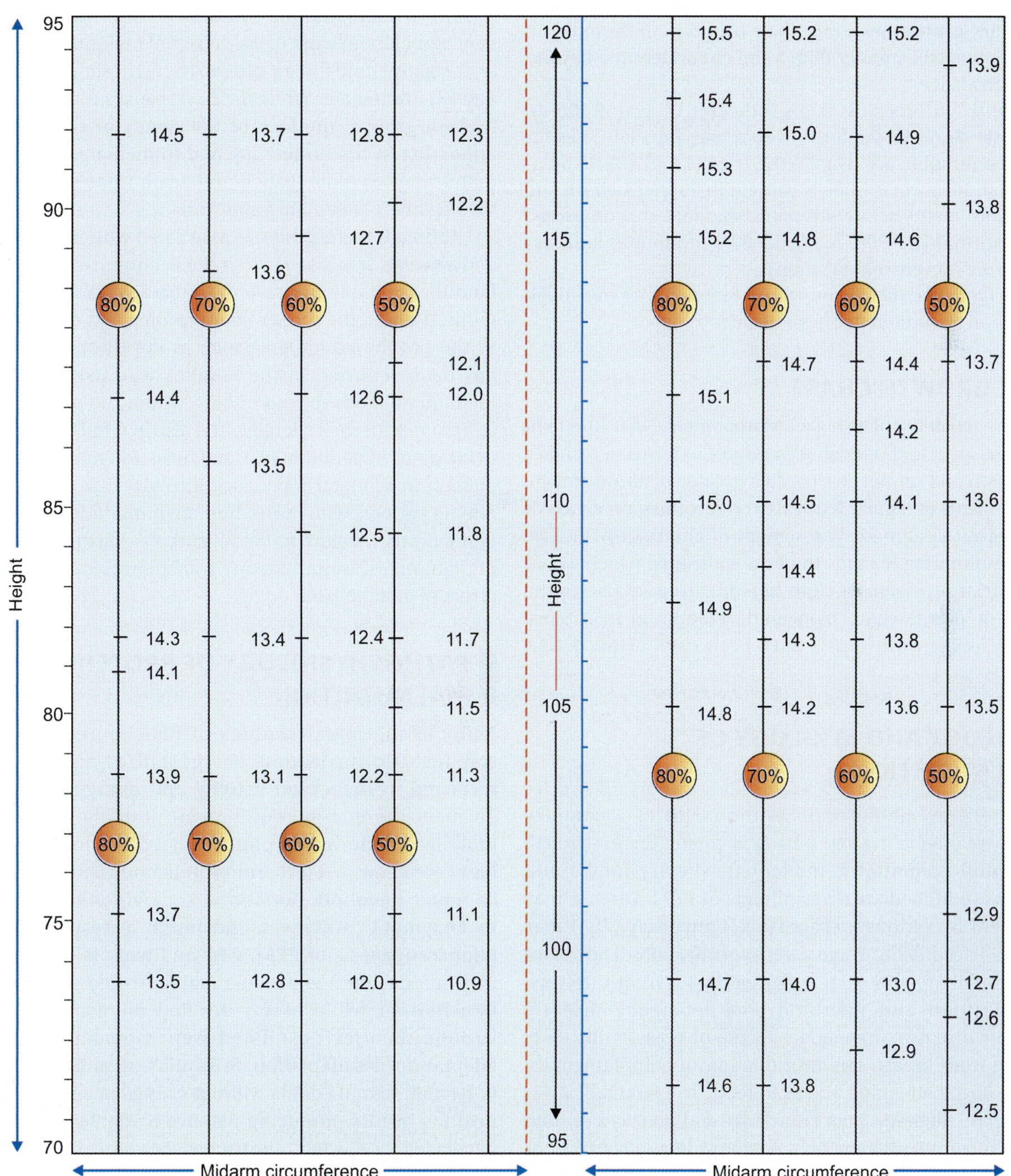

Fig. 4.4.7: Quack stick: Modified for Indian children.

- *Mid-arm circumference to head circumference ratio*: A ratio of 0.280–0.314 indicates mild malnutrition, 0.250–0.279 indicates moderate PEM, and less than 0.249 indicates severe PEM.
- *Mid-arm/height ratio*: Less than 0.29 indicates gross malnutrition (normal 0.32–0.33).
- *Chest/head circumference ratio*: Chest circumference becomes equal to head circumference at 1 year, and after 2 years it becomes more than head circumference. In PEM, it is still smaller than head circumference beyond 2 years of age.
- *Skinfold thickness*: It is an indicator of availability of caloric stores in the form of subcutaneous fat. Sites for measurements are usually the triceps and subscapular region. Its normal value is present in Tanner's chart, and measurements below 90% of the standard are considered subnormal (80–90% mild, 60–80% moderate, and less than 60% severe malnutrition).
- *Mid-thigh and calf circumference*: Standards for mid-thigh and calf circumference have been developed.

THE GROWTH CHART

While the reliability of a single anthropometric measurement may be suspect and difficult to interpret in terms of a child's past growth and cannot give predictive value of future growth, measurements at regular intervals and recording on a growth chart permit systematic assessment of child's growth. The idea of monitoring the growth of the individual which would be useful in provision of child health care gave rise to the concept of "growth chart" pioneered by Morley in 1959. Since then, various growth charts have been used **(Figs. 4.4.8A and B)**.

ECOLOGY AND ETIOLOGY OF MALNUTRITION

Protein energy malnutrition is the result of a complex interplay of interacting and related factors in the individual, family, and community. Inadequate dietary intake and diseases are immediate determinants of PEM. Disease may affect PEM by various mechanisms. Conversely, PEM may increase susceptibility to and severity of infections. The causes in individual are anorexia, increased losses from intestine, malabsorption and micronutrient deficiency disease, infectious diseases, inadequate intake of breast milk, early weaning from breast, late introduction of complementary feeding, and inadequate access to food. The familial causes are maternal illiteracy, poor knowledge and practices of child rearing, maternal malnutrition, overcrowding, poverty, poor living and sanitary conditions, unemployment, alcoholism, or debt. The community causes include national poverty, poor educational status, inadequate medical facilities, poor access to health services, cultural practices and beliefs, marginalizing of girls and women, natural and man-made disasters, poor rainfall or excess rain, or poor facilities for storage and transport, and hoarding and black marketing. The community and national causes have direct impact on the family and individual child. Thus, PEM is an end result of many ecological problems **(Flowchart 4.4.1, Figs. 4.4.9 to 4.4.12)**.

The United Nations Children's Fund has suggested a conceptual framework of the causes of malnutrition (positive and negative) and three main causes: (1) basic, (2) underlying, and (3) immediate. While the basic causes remain the same in both groups, the lack or deficiency of resources start appearing in the underlying and immediate causes finally manifesting as malnutrition and death **(Flowchart 4.4.2)** in the negative conceptual framework.

Although malnutrition is associated with the lack of food and poverty, it is also seen in the economically advantaged families probably because of the lack of awareness in the mothers about the proper infant feeding and child nutrition. In the developed nations, such as the United States, PEM has been reported in the families who use unusual and inadequate foods to feed infants, whom the parents believe to be at risk for milk allergies, and also in families who believe in fad diets. In addition, PEM has been noted in chronically ill patients in neonatal or pediatric intensive care units as well as among patients with burns, human immunodeficiency virus, cystic fibrosis, failure to thrive, chronic diarrhea syndromes, malignancies, bone marrow transplantation, and inborn errors of metabolism.

PATHOPHYSIOLOGY OF PROTEIN ENERGY MALNUTRITION

Many of the manifestations of PEM represent adaptive responses to inadequate energy and/or protein intakes, resulting in decreased activity and energy expenditure. To meet the energy requirement, initially fat stores are mobilized, followed by protein catabolism for maintaining basal metabolism. Furthermore, micronutrients are essential in many metabolic functions as components, cofactors in enzymatic processes and immune response. In the etiopathogenesis of PEM, why and what is it that among children destined to become malnourished; some develop kwashiorkor while others develop marasmus. Amongst various theories postulated were Gopalan's theory on adaptation/dysadaptation, Srikantia's on antidiuretic effect of ferritin, loss of edema without change in serum albumin, noxious insults producing reactive oxidative free radicals, decreased Na, K, adenosine triphosphatase activity, depressed cellular protein synthesis, etc. The latest theory, postulated by Golden, suggests deficiency of type I (functional nutrients), such as zinc, and type II nutrients, such as phosphorus,

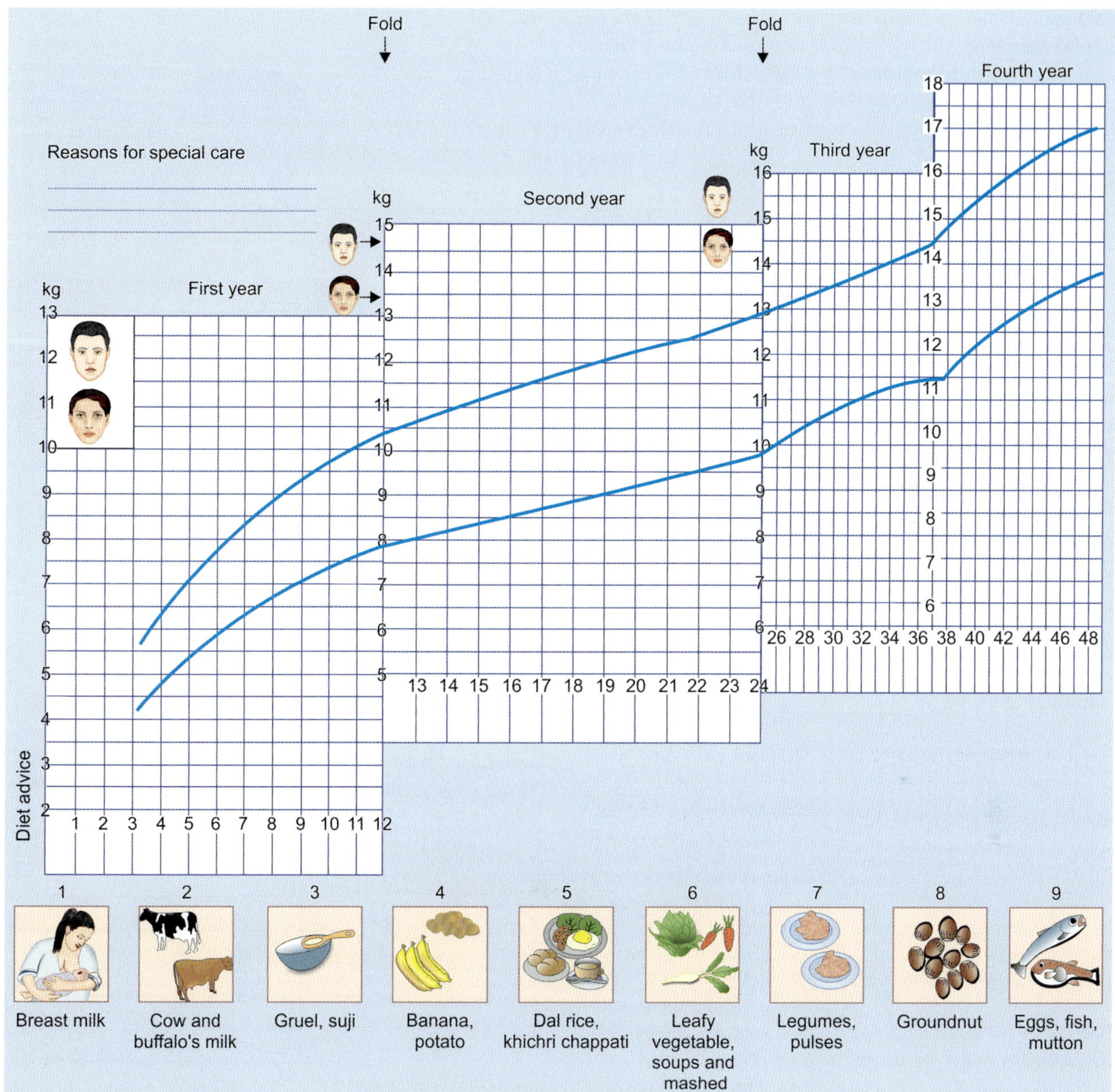

Fig. 4.4.8A: Prototype of growth chart—front view

magnesium, manganese, copper, and vitamins D and C, in the diets of malnourished children due to decrease in appetite. No amount of additional energy as lipids or carbohydrates would enhance convalescence of PEM, unless these specific nutrients are supplied in the balanced form.

CLINICAL MANIFESTATIONS

The clinical manifestations of malnutrition depend on the severity and duration of nutritional deprivation, the age of the undernourished subject, relative lack of different proximate principles of food and micronutrients and the associated infection. Nutritional marasmus and kwashiorkor are two different extreme forms of a continuous process of malnutrition. Nutritional marasmus results from predominant energy deficiency, whereas kwashiorkor is due to predominant protein deficiency though some energy deficiency may coexist.

Occasionally, patients who are initially marasmic may develop edema due to protein loss when the individual is known as marasmic kwashiorkor. In clinical practice, such

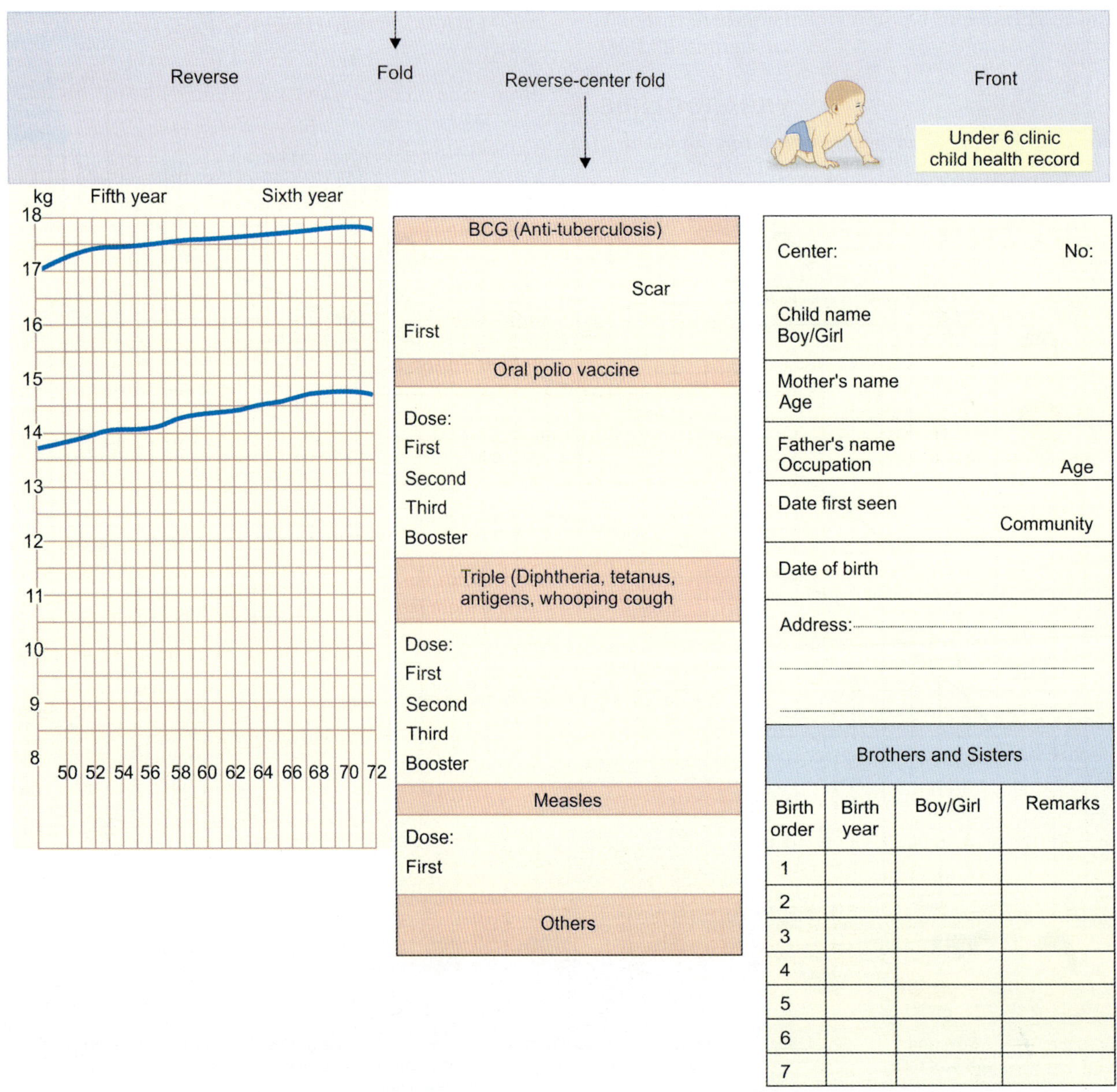

Fig. 4.4.8B: Prototype of growth chart—rear view

extremes account only for a small proportion of cases of malnutrition. A majority has mild to moderate deficiency with varied clinical manifestations, and this range is known as PEM. Malnutrition can be compared to an iceberg, while only the tips of the iceberg, i.e. the severe forms are seen by the health workers **(Fig. 4.4.13)**. Those hidden in the community constitute a vast majority of children suffering from mild and moderate forms of PEM. They are not brought for any medical attention and are at a high risk of deterioration and progress to severe forms if uncared for prolonged period. PEM impairs resistance to infection and may present with its varied manifestations. Mild degrees of PEM lead to growth retardation, frank malnutrition, if prolonged may cause mental retardation.

Initial responses to nutritional deprivation are of two types: (1) dynamic children, who remain active but fail to gain weight and later length, and (2) sedentary children, who maintain their growth initially by limiting their activities but ultimately fail to grow. Two thirds of malnourished children do not present with any clinical signs and are diagnosed by anthropometry.

Flowchart 4.4.1: Ecology of protein energy malnutrition (PEM).

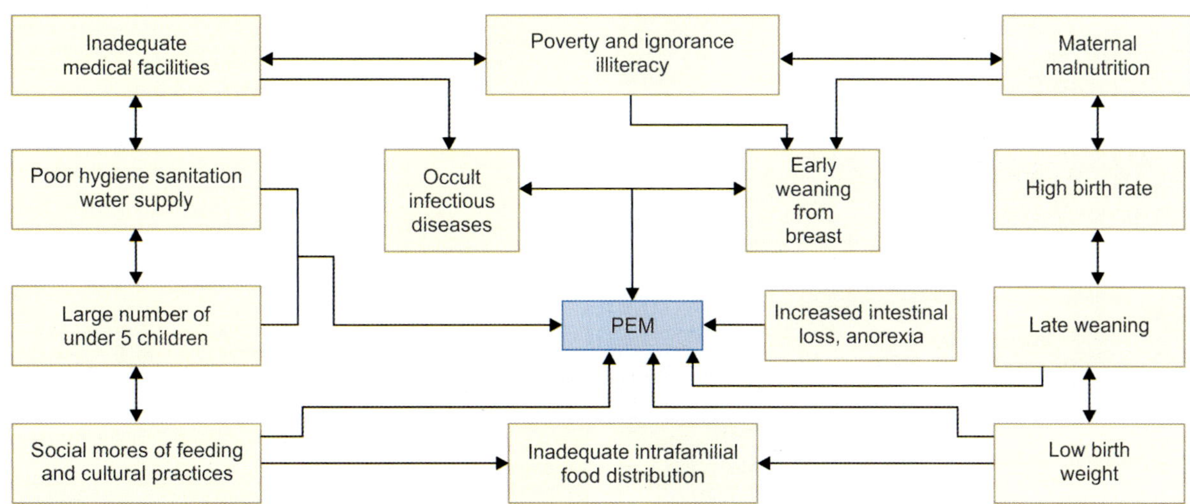

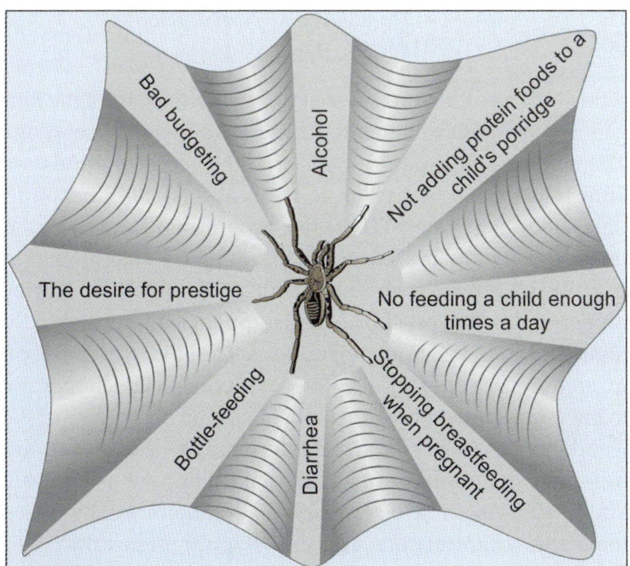

Fig. 4.4.9: Socioeconomical and biological determinants of protein energy malnutrition (PEM).

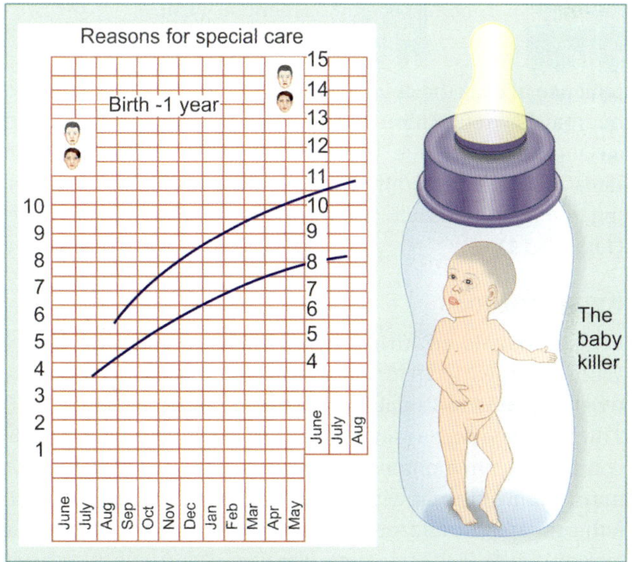

Fig. 4.4.10: Mortality related to bottle-feeding.

Marasmus

Marasmus can develop in the first few months of life, commonly from birth to 2 years. It results, if the baby is fed with diluted milk from buffalo, cow, goat, or even tin milk without offering breast milk or any other food. Marasmus is characterized by failure to gain weight and irritability, followed by weight loss and listlessness until emaciation results. It is diagnosed by the gross loss of subcutaneous fat, and the infant seems to have only skin and bones, ribs become visible, and costochondral junctions look prominent. There is a conspicuous absence of edema. Growth retardation is severe and obvious. The head appears disproportionately large with very little hair. Weight is less than 60% of the expected weight; muscles may be atrophied leading to hypotonia. The child is conscious, alert but apathetic and in extreme cases, is also disinterested in surroundings and sits listless for long hours. The facial pads of the fat are last to go; when the child looks like a wizened old man. Anemia is moderate and may be associated with vitamin deficiencies, infections and infestations, and electrolyte imbalance. In the early stages, the child's appetite is good, and he readily accepts what is offered. However, in advanced stages, there is loss of appetite and it requires a lot of tact and

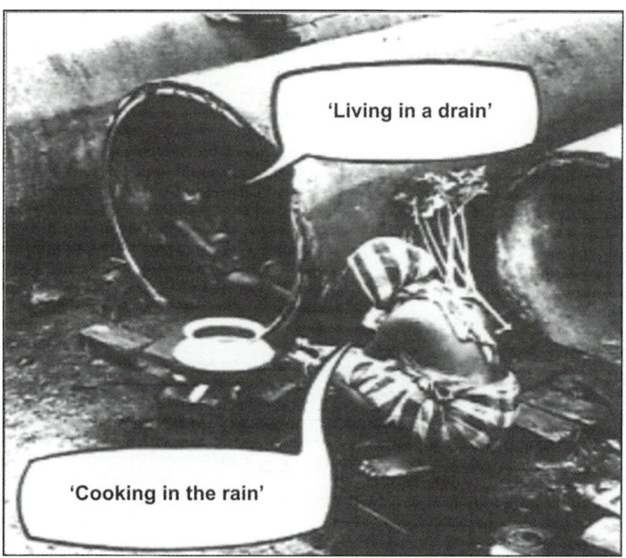

Fig. 4.4.11: Socioeconomical milieu of protein energy malnutrition (PEM).

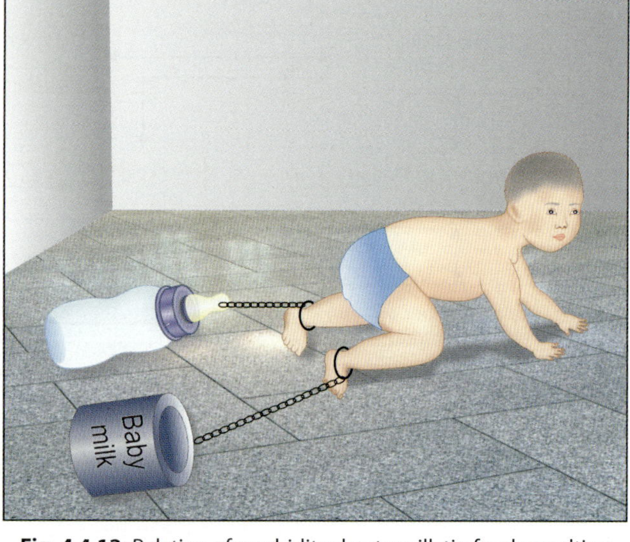

Fig. 4.4.12: Relation of morbidity due to milk tin foods resulting into severe protein energy malnutrition.

patience to coax the child to eat. Infants are often constipated but may have starvation diarrhea with frequent small mucoid stools. The abdomen may be distended or flat with the intestinal pattern readily visible. As the condition progresses, the temperature usually becomes subnormal and pulse slows **(Fig. 4.4.14)**.

Kwashiorkor

Kwashiorkor is an African word was suggested by Cicely Williams in early 1930s, meaning "the disease that occurs when the child is displaced from the breast by another child." The age incidence is later than that of marasmus, and this condition is uncommon under the age of 1 year. Kwashiorkor may initially present with vague manifestations that include lethargy, apathy, and/or irritability. When advanced, there is lack of growth, lack of stamina, loss of muscle tissue, increased susceptibility to infections, vomiting, diarrhea, anorexia, flabby subcutaneous tissues, and edema. The edema usually develops early and may mask the failure to gain weight. It is often present in internal organs before it is recognized in the face and limbs.

Edema is characteristically pitting. It usually occurs first around the eyes, then above the ankles and above dorsum of the feet. In the later stages, the whole face, hands, and body may be edematous, but ascites is rarely due to kwashiorkor alone. Edema is mainly due to tissue wasting, together with low plasma osmotic pressure caused by low serum albumin levels. The child is listless, lethargic, apathetic, and miserable; her/his moaning cry is characteristic. The hair changes are variable. Hair may be thin, dry, brittle, and lusterless. These become straight and hypopigmented (grayish-white or reddish-brown). During recovery, the growing part of the hair gets approximately pigmented and gives appearance of "flag." The skin changes are not constant, and manifestations are known as dermatosis **(Figs. 4.4.15A and B)**. Skin becomes darkened in irritated areas, but in contrast to pellagra, it does not occur in areas exposed to sunlight. Depigmentation may occur after desquamation in these areas, or it may be generalized. The skin lesions appear as large areas of erythema, followed by hyperkeratosis. The epidermis peels off in large scales, exposing a raw area underneath which is prone to infection. It resembles old paint flaking off the surface of the wood, hence called "flaky paint dermatosis." The lesions are moist and common on areas exposed to continuous pressure and irritation. In severe cases, petechiae or ecchymoses may appear. Alternate areas of hypopigmentation and hyperpigmentation give a resemblance to pavement, and this is known as "pavement dermatosis" or when skin changes are seen in a particular mosaic form, as "mosaic dermatosis." Liver may be enlarged and fatty. There may be associated infections in the form of diarrhea, respiratory infections, urinary tract infections, and vitamin deficiencies, especially vitamin A, thiamine, riboflavin, and niacin. Eventually, there is stupor, coma, and death.

Marasmic Kwashiorkor

Children with severe muscle and fat wasting but with presence of edema are called marasmic kwashiorkor. This syndrome is seen in children who have marasmus but suddenly develop edema due to increased deficiency of protein than before. Thus, the clinical features are those of both marasmus and

Flowchart 4.4.2: The United Nations Children's Fund conceptual framework.

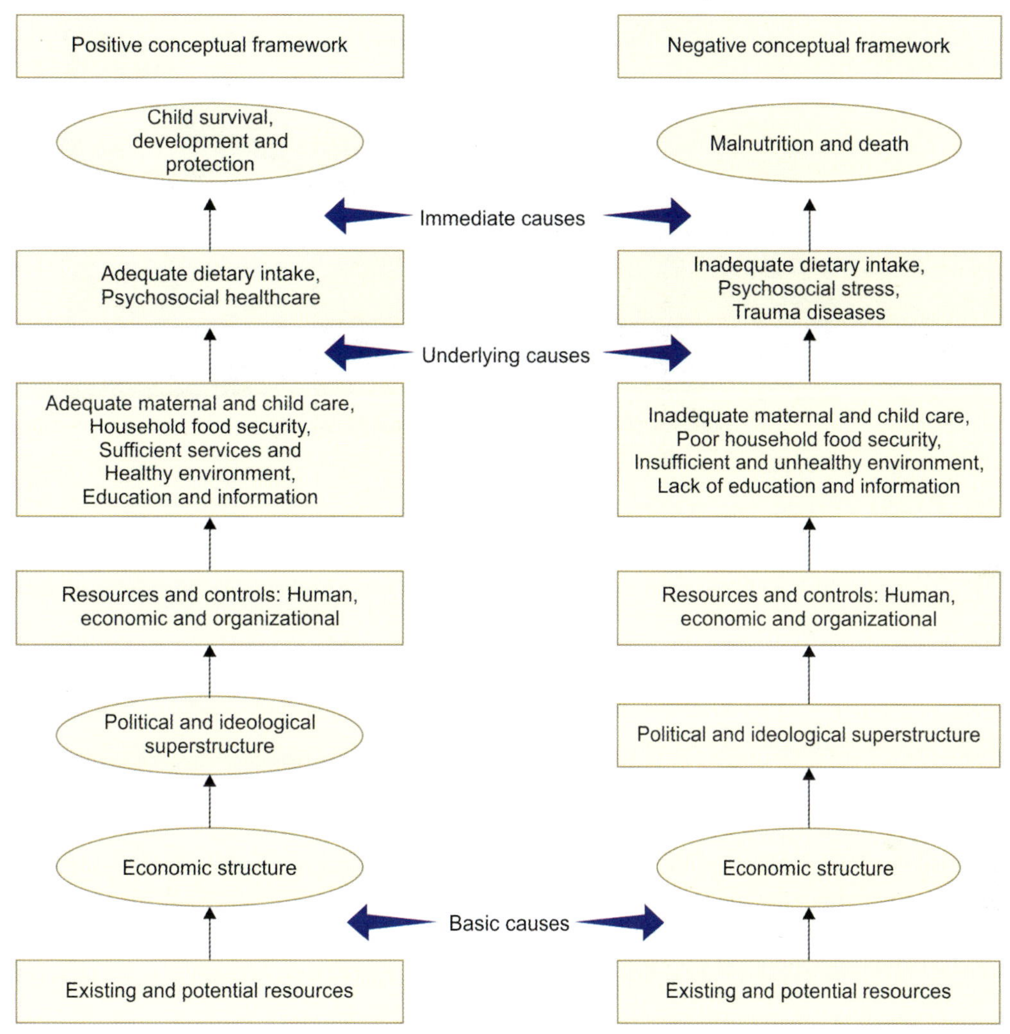

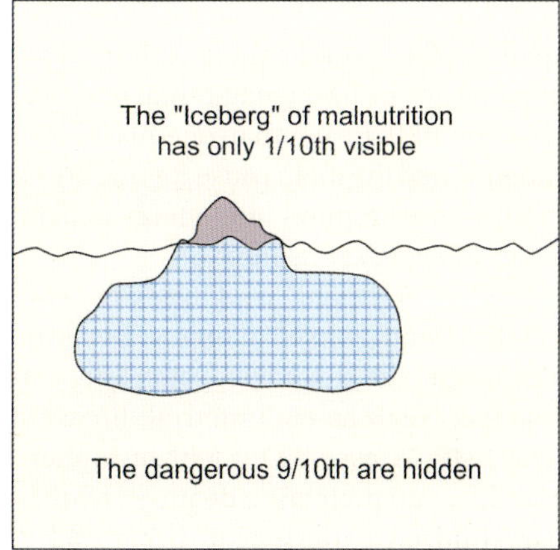

Fig. 4.4.13: The "iceberg" of malnutrition.

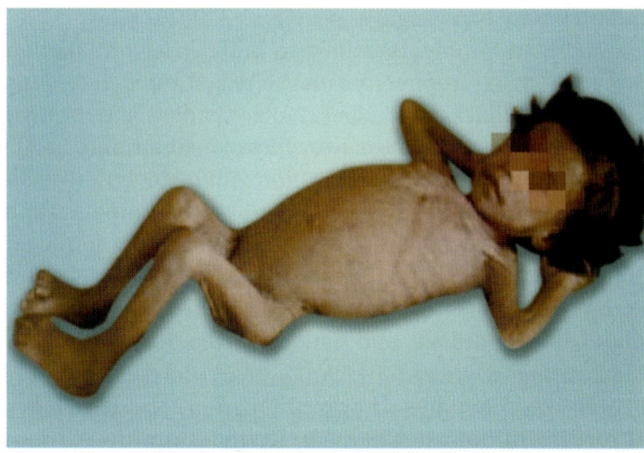

Fig. 4.4.14: Marasmus.

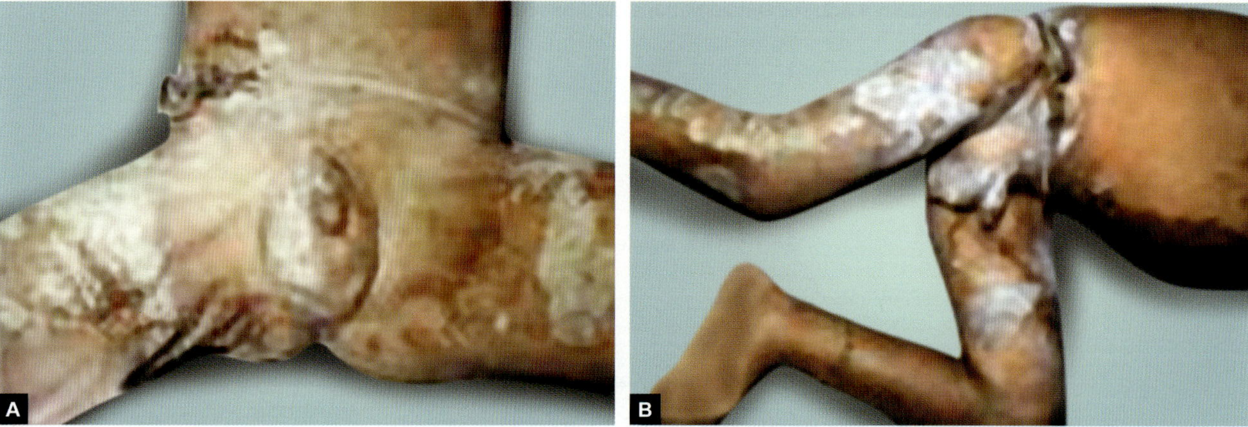

Figs. 4.4.15A and B: Dermatosis of kwashiorkor.

kwashiorkor **(Fig. 4.4.16)**. Anemia may be moderate, and one or more vitamin deficiencies may be evident. The usual differentiating features of marasmus and kwashiorkor are summarized in **Table 4.4.3**.

Overnutrition and Obesity

Once considered a problem of high income countries, overweight obesity are now on the rise in the low- and middle-income countries, particularly in urban settings. In developing countries with emerging economics, the rate of increase of childhood overweight and obesity has been more than 30% higher than that of the developed countries, and worldwide obesity has more than doubled since 1980. Most of the world population lives in countries where overweight and obesity kill more people than underweight. Worldwide in 2017, 38 million or 5.6% children under age 5 were overweight. Eastern Europe and Central Asia had the highest overweight prevalence in 2017 with 14.8 affected, followed by the Middle East and North Africa at 10.9% and North America at 7.9%. In India 2% were overweight as per NFHS-4 (2015–16).

There are problems unique to India. The combination of people living in poverty and the recent rapid economic globalization have led to rapid changes in diets and lifestyle, resulting in coemergence of two types of malnutrition, i.e. (1) undernutrition and (2) overnutrition. Although underweight and malnutrition are rampant in poor families, urbanization with increased consumption of food with higher fat and sugar content of "fast food," along with sedentary lifestyles, i.e. TV, computers, lack of space for outdoor games, exercise with improved technology, and transport (cars, trains, etc.) has unknowingly increased overweight and obesity, especially in well-to-do families. However, micronutrient deficiency is present in both of them, i.e. in undernutrition and in overnutrition. In general, the average Indian diet remains largely deficient in green leafy vegetable, milk and milk products, and thus, micronutrient such as vitamin A, iron, and iodine remain deficient in all children with improper diet. Overweight and obesity are defined by the World Bank as age and gender specific. Body mass index (BMI) greater than or equal to 25 is overweight, and BMI greater than or equal to 30 is obesity, or BMI greater than or equal to 85–95% is overweight, and BMI greater than or equal to 95% is obesity. As already mentioned the main cause for obesity is imbalance between energy consumption and energy expenditure with higher practice of energy consumption.

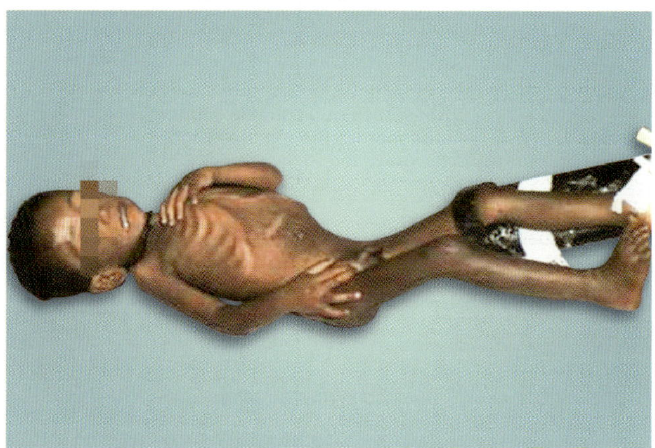

Fig. 4.4.16: Marasmic kwashiorkor.

Overeating, overweight, and obesity lead to many diseases, such as early onset diabetes, heart disease and stroke, musculoskeletal disorders, especially osteoarthritis and some cancer, such as endometrial, breast, and colon. Childhood obesity is associated with a higher chance of obesity, disability, and premature death. In addition to future risks, obese children experienced breathing difficulties, increased risk of fractures, hypertension and early markers of cardiovascular disease, insulin resistance, and psychological

Table 4.4.3: Differences between marasmus and kwashiorkor.

	Marasmus	***Kwashiorkor***
A. Usual age	0–3 years	1–3 years
B. *Essential features*:		
1. Edema	None	*Lower legs, sometimes face or generalized
2. Wasting	*Gross loss of subcutaneous fat "All skin and bone"	Sometimes hidden, sometimes fat blubbery
3. Muscle wasting	Obvious	Sometimes hidden
4. Growth retardation	Obvious	Sometimes hidden
5. Mental changes	Usually, apathetic quiet	Usually irritable moaning, also apathetic
C. *Variable features*:		
1. Appetite	Usually good	Usually poor
2. Diarrhea	Often (past or present)	Often (past or present)
3. Skin changes	Seldom	Often diffuse depigmentation, occasionally flaky paint or enamel dermatosis
4. Hair changes	Seldom	Often sparse, straight silky, dyspigmentation, gray, or reddish
D. *Biochemistry/pathology*:		
1. Serum albumin	Usually normal (or low)	*Low
2. Urinary urea per g creatinine	Usually normal (or low)	*Low
3. Urinary hydroxyproline per g creatinine	*Low	*Low
4. Serum essential amino acid index	*Low	*Low
5. Anemia	Uncommon	*Common
6. Liver biopsy	*Normal or atrophic	*Fatty changes

*These are the most characteristic or useful distinguishing features.

effects. The treatment of overweight and obesity in children and adolescents requires a multidisciplinary, multiphase approach. Overall obesity is a preventable disorder.

Multiple Nutritional Deficiencies

The nutritional deficiencies are generally multiple, and anemia due to deficiencies of iron, vitamin $B_{12,}$ or folate may be associated. Anemia may be hypochromic microcytic, macrocytic, or normocytic normochromic. Deficiencies of vitamin B-complex factors, especially ariboflavinosis, vitamin A (manifesting as keratomalacia and xerophthalmia), and vitamin C occur commonly. Since growth gets arrested in severe PEM, rickets may become manifest only when the child starts growing with nutritional rehabilitation.

Electrolyte Imbalances

Potassium

The total body potassium may be markedly decreased in PEM. The loss is due partly to the cellular breakdown but more so by the loss in diarrheal stools.

Other Electrolytes

There is also deficit of total body sodium, calcium, phosphorus, magnesium, and chloride. The body sodium is 93% of the expected values. There is a significant loss of magnesium from the cells, levels being significantly low in children with moderate and severe malnutrition, and in children with marked linear growth retardation.

Endocrine Changes

Growth hormone, plasma cortisol levels, thyroid stimulating hormone and T4 levels may be raised in PEM, while insulin levels and T3 levels are reduced both in marasmus and kwashiorkor.

Infection and Immunity

Infectious disease worsens, when malnutrition is present and conversely, malnutrition usually weakens resistance to various infections which are more serious in a malnourished host than in a well-nourished child. Malnourished children with PEM have recurrent episodes of acute infections or chronic insidious infections which may go undetected unless carefully looked for. Thus, recurrent diarrheal diseases, lower respiratory tract infections, and occult urinary tract infection are common and have high mortality. Measles is usually a preceding illness. Tuberculosis and malaria must be always ruled out, and intestinal parasitosis, such as ascariasis, hookworm, and giardiasis, must be treated. Septicemia, especially in infants and toddlers, may be life threatening.

Regarding humoral immunity immunoglobulin (Ig) G, IgM, and secretory IgA, blood concentrations are not significantly affected in mild and moderate forms of PEM and show a good response when challenged with bacterial and viral vaccines but is depressed in severe forms of PEM with infections. The cell-mediated immunity (CMI) is impaired in all grades of malnutrition except in Grade I. It is severely impaired in grades III and IV, PEM, and kwashiorkor. This explains a high incidence of Gram-negative bacterial infections and serious morbidity, and high mortality to viral infection, such as herpes simplex and measles. Due to depressed CMI, the tuberculin skin test is often negative in marasmus and kwashiorkor, in spite of active tuberculosis. Following dietary treatment of 4–6 weeks, the CMI might improve and the skin test may become positive. Serum C-reactive protein and C3 complement levels are depressed in severe malnutrition but rise in presence of infections and thus, behave as acute phase reactants.

COMPLICATIONS

The complications of PEM are usually seen with severe malnutrition. They are dehydration, hypothermia, hypoglycemia, infections, anemia, xerophthalmia, congestive heart failure, hypomagnesemia, hypocalcemia, zinc, copper, chromium, and manganese deficiency and deficiencies of vitamins.

LONG-TERM CONSEQUENCES

Malnourished children are more susceptible to disease, have a reduced capacity to learn, have deficits in cognitive function, less likely to perform well in school, and are likely to drop out. The evidence suggests that undernutrition has pervasive effects on immediate health and survival as well as on subsequent performance. These include not only acute effects on morbidity and mortality but also long-term effects on cognitive and social development, physical work capacity, productivity, and economic growth. The magnitude of both the acute and the long-term effects is considerable. Survivors of undernutrition have deficits in height and weight that persist beyond adolescence into adulthood. These may be accompanied by deficit in frame size as well as muscle circumference and strength. The implications of these deficits with respect to the work capacity of both men and women and to women's reproductive performance are obvious. Once in the job market, their productivity is low. For the economy as a whole, this translates into losses of nearly 3% of gross domestic product. All these place India's large population, the basis of its much-awaited demographic dividend, at a growing disadvantage in today's globalizing world. These deficits are related to the severity of PEM and can be decreased probably by a combination of dietary and behavioral interventions, coupled with improvements to the overall quality of home and/or school environment. Such interventions appear to be much more effective, if instituted in early life.

MANAGEMENT

The management of PEM depends on nutritional status, degree of hypermetabolism, expected duration of illness, and associated complications. The goals are to minimize weight loss, maintain body mass, and encourage body mass repletion or growth. The principles of management are as follows:

- The patient is evaluated for the severity, presence of systemic infections, other nutritional, micronutrients deficits, anemia and fluid, and electrolyte disturbances.
- The intake of food is promoted by all available means. Locally available, culturally acceptable, and affordable foods are advised.
- Complications of malnutrition and sequelae are prevented by careful surveillance and prompt remedial action.
- Possible epidemiological factors for malnutrition are considered and attempt is made to eliminate these as far as possible.

Mild-to-moderate PEM is best managed at home. Majority of cases of severe PEM are associated with some of the complications listed above and hence are best managed in hospital.

Domiciliary or Community Management

This is recommended for mild-to-moderate PEM and those uncomplicated severe PEM who have fairly good appetite, normal body temperature, who are conscious and active, and without evidence of serious infection. These children are managed at home by parents under observation and supervision. They are monitored through weekly visits by paramedicals or visits to the hospital or at a nutritional rehabilitation center every week. The main goal of treatment is to provide adequate calories to replace losses, to build up nutrition, and to promote growth. Caution must be taken to gradually build up the calories and proteins. The expected calories and proteins are calculated on the present weight. Once this is achieved, then over the next 7 days, calories and proteins are calculated of the average weight. After that, over the 2 weeks, the diet (calories and proteins) are increased for the expected weight for that age. It takes about 6 months to achieve this target.

The examples are cereal pulse combinations—double or triple mixes, such as *dal* rice, *khichdi*, with seasonal green leafy and yellow orange vegetables, root vegetables with sugar, jaggery; thick butter milk based diets, milk based diets, either of them supplemented with proteins, such as ground nut, soya, and amylase-based food formulations. Emphasis must be laid on adding enough oil/*ghee*/butter to the diet to increase calories and palatability. The energy recommended is 80–100 kcal/kg/day and protein 0.70–1.0 g/kg/day, stepped up gradually to 120–150 kcal/kg/day and protein 2–3 g/kg/day of high biological value.

Basically, these should be from locally available, seasonal, and affordable food sources, commonly consumed by the family. The diet should be liquid, semisolid, or solid depending on the child's acceptability and appetite. Frequent small feeds are encouraged, increased gradually rather than one or two major bulky meals. Nonvegetarian articles, such as egg, fish, chicken, meat, etc. are recommended for those whose cultural, religious practices permit them. Zinc is added when child improves weight. Parents are educated about proper cooking, clean drinking water, sanitation, and personal hygiene. Some basic advice is also given for the management of common problems, such as diarrhea by oral rehydration solution, of anemia with oral iron and folic acid, vitamin deficiencies, infestations, and infection as well as immunization.

Severe Malnutrition

The management of uncomplicated SAM using simple, ready-to-use therapeutic foods (RUTFs)—fortified with all essential nutrients, such as zinc, potassium, magnesium, and phosphate with low levels of sodium, protein, and iron, with community-based care is encouraging and worthwhile. With these diets, children recover their appetite. Home-based management has the advantage of easier access by rural population, promoting early intervention in the disease, improving coverage rates, and preventing nosocomial infections. The limited hospital staff can focus on inpatient complicated cases.

The risk of death rises progressively with worsening nutritional status. However, over 80% malnutrition deaths occur in mild to moderately malnourished children as these greatly outnumber children with severe malnutrition.

Hence, for better child survival, intervention is necessary for management of mild and moderately malnourished children in addition to that of severely malnourished children. Hence, there is an urgent need to identify these malnourished children timely and plan the treatment based on the need of an individual child.

Case fatality rates in children with severe malnutrition have remained unchanged at 20–30% over the past five decades. Infections, including diarrheal dehydration and electrolyte disturbances are common in severely malnourished children and found to be the poor prognostic factors. According to the WHO, a death rate of more than 20% is considered unacceptable in the management of severely malnourished children, 11–20% is poor, 5–10% is moderate, 1–4% is good, and less than 1% is excellent. Appropriate feeding, micronutrient supplementation, broad-spectrum antibiotic therapy, less use of intravenous fluids for rehydration, and careful management of complications are factors that can reduce death, morbidity, and cost of treating these children. On the basis of these factors, WHO have prepared guidelines for the inpatient case management of severe malnutrition. Not all severely malnourished children need hospitalization **(Table 4.4.4)**. Majority of the children usually have some complications, they need hospitalization for critical care and intense monitoring.

The management of SAM can be achieved by the following three ways and in three phases **(Fig. 4.4.17)**:

1. *Three ways:*
   i. Traditional nutrition therapy (community-based management of SAM);
   ii. Hospital-based therapy using F-75 and F-100 diets;
   iii. Initial stabilization in hospital using F-75 diet and rehabilitation at home using RUTF.
2. *Three phases:*
   i. *Phase 1:* Phase of resuscitation. The initial or acute phase (0–7 days) when the child is being treated for complications, dietary therapy is started simultaneously.
   ii. *Phase 2:* Phase of restoration or recovery (1–2 weeks) when the child will increase dietary intake and gain weight.
   iii. *Phase 3:* Phase of rehabilitation and follow-up (2–26 weeks) which may be after discharge.

Table 4.4.4: Indications for hospitalization in severe malnutrition.

- Hypothermia
- Infection
- Fluid and electrolyte imbalance
- Convulsions
- Unconsciousness
- Jaundice, purpura
- Raised liver enzymes
- Severe anemia and congestive cardiac failure
- Xerophthalmia
- Severe dermatosis
- Extreme weight deficit
- Bleeding
- Marked hepatomegaly
- Persistent vomiting
- Severe anorexia
- Distended tender abdomen
- Age less than 1 year

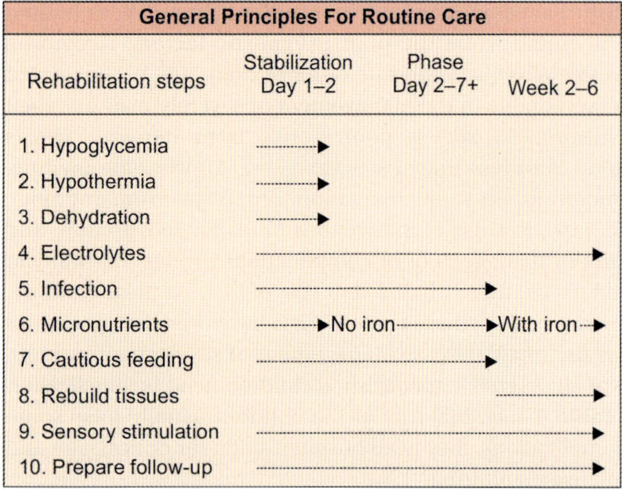

Fig. 4.4.17: Stepwise management of severe malnutrition. *Source:* The World Health Organization.

Phase I: Resuscitation or Stabilization and Treatment of Complications

Dehydration: Cautious management to avoid over hydration.

- *Severe/shock:* Intravenous Ringer lactate 20–30 mL/kg in 1 hour, followed by 70 mL/kg over the next 2 hour, followed by 0.45% glucose saline/Isolyte-P as maintenance fluid. Total fluid and sodium not to exceed 75% of allowance.
- *Mild:* Oral rehydration solution—hypoosmolar/preferably ReSoMal 5 mL/kg every 30 minutes—orally/by nasogastric tube (ReSoMal: 45 mmol sodium, 40 mmol potassium, and 3 mmol magnesium).

Electrolyte imbalance:

- *Potassium:* 2–5 mmol/kg/day;
- *Magnesium:* 0.3–0.6 mmol/kg/day or 50% $MgSO_4$, intramuscularly 0.3 mL/kg (2 mL maximum) OD. It is common medical term.
- *Sodium:* Restrict salt, no diuretics.

Hypoglycemia:

- Ten percent glucose 1–2 mL/kg intravenously bolus, followed by 10% dextrose in N/5 saline as maintenance for 24 hour. If 10% intravenous glucose not available, give 10% sucrose (1 full teaspoonful sugar in 3.5 tablespoonful of water) orally/by nasogastric tube then every 30 minutes for 2 hours;
- Early and frequent feeding.

Hypothermia: Warm bed and room, keep the baby with mother, double clothing, and cover head and feet. Treat hypoglycemia and sepsis. Start feeds early.

Septicemia: Intravenous ampicillin 50 mg/kg, 6 hourly for 2 days, gentamicin 7.5 mg/kg intramuscularly/intravenously. If no improvement, add chloramphenicol/cephalosporin. If anorexia persists, continue antibiotics for 10 days. Give metronidazole 7.5 mg/kg 8 hourly for 7 days for potential anaerobic infections.

Congestive heart failure: This mostly occurs due to fluid overload (e.g., overuse of intravenous fluids, unmonitored blood transfusion) or due to severe anemia. When congestive heart failure is due to fluid overload, administer frusemide 1–2 mg/kg and reduce/stop fluid infusion. Avoid digitalis. Diuretics should never be used to correct edema in case of edematous malnutrition.

Anemia: If hemoglobin is less than 5 g/dL, give packed cells transfusion 5–10 mL/kg. Iron should be started only after resolution of infection (2–3 weeks).

Micronutrients:

- *Iron*: Oral ferrous sulfate or fumarate syrup 4 mg (elemental)/kg;
- *Calcium gluconate—intravenous*: 1–2 mL/kg or oral calcium lactate powder—3 g/day;
- *Zinc*: 2 mg/kg/day;
- *Copper*: 20 µg/kg/day;
- *Chromium*: 0.2 µg/kg/day;
- *Manganese*: 10 µg/kg/day;
- *Vitamin A*: 100,000 IU for age less than 1 year and 50,000 IU for age less than 6 months
- *Vitamin D*: Rickets—oral vitamin D
- *Other vitamins*: B-complex, vitamin K (5 mg weekly).

Phase II: Restoration

After the initial phase of resuscitation, there is improvement in child's condition with return of appetite, beginning of loss of edema and return of smile. During this phase the aim is to make the child gain weight and restore WFH.

Dietary management of severe PEM: In the initial stabilization phase, because of child's fragile physiological and metabolic state, great caution is required in dietary intervention of SAM children. The rule of "go slow, rather than hurry" is appropriate. Feeding is designed to provide 75–80 cal/kg/day and proteins 0.7 g/kg/day. Each feed should be small, gradually increased, of low osmolality, and lactose offered at frequent intervals, according to the child's tolerance **(Table 4.4.5)**. Breastfeeding should be continued and Starter formulas, such as F-75 (milk-based containing 75 cal/100 mL and 0.9 g/100 mL protein and fluid volume 130 mL/kg) are satisfactory for most children **(Table 4.4.6)**. Very weak children or those with anorexia may be fed with spoon, dropper, or nasogastric tube.

As per the child's progress and response to the treatment of complications by the end of 1 week, the calories and proteins may be stepped up to 100 cal/kg and proteins 1–1.5 g/kg/

Table 4.4.5: Feeding schedule.

Days	*Frequency (hourly)*	*Volume/kg/feed (mL)*	*Volume/kg/day (mL)*
1–2	2	11	130
3–5	3	16	130
6–7+	4	22	130

Table 4.4.6: Composition of F-75 starter formula.

	F-75						
Type of milk	*Milk (g)*	*Eggs (g)*	*Sugar (g)*	*Oil (g)*	*Cereal powder (g)**	*CMV† (red scoop = 6 g)*	*Water (mL)*
Dry skim milk	25	0	70	27	35	2	Up to 1,000
Dry whole milk	35	0	70	20	35	2	Up to 1,000
Fresh cow milk	280	0	65	20	35	2	Up to 1,000
Fresh goat milk	280	0	65	20	40	2	Up to 1,000
Whole eggs	0	80	70	20	40	2	Up to 1,000
Egg yolks	0	50	70	15	40	2	Up to 1,000

*Cereal powder should be cooked for around 10 min and then the other ingredients be added.
†CMV special mineral and vitamin mix adapted to severe acute malnutrition treatment.
(CMV: combined mineral vitamin mix)

Table 4.4.7: Composition of F-100 catch-up formula.

	F-100					
Type of milk	*Milk (g)*	*Eggs (g)*	*Sugar (g)*	*Oil (g)*	*CMV* (red scoop = 6 g)*	*Water (mL)*
Dry skim milk	80	0	50	60	2	Up to 1,000
Dry whole milk	110	0	50	30	2	Up to 1,000
Fresh cow milk	900	0	50	25	2	Up to 1,000
Fresh goat milk	900	0	50	25	2	Up to 1,000
Whole eggs	0	220	90	35	2	Up to 1,000
Egg yolks	0	170	90	10	2	Up to 1,000

*CMV special mineral mix adapted to severe acute malnutrition.
(CMV: combined mineral vitamin mix)

day. Minerals and vitamins are also added. In the phase of restoration, the principle is to increase weight and catch up growth as the child's appetite has regained.

The calories and proteins (preferably 50% should have high biological value, for example, milk, chicken, meat, or egg) are stepped up gradually, approximately from 25 cal/kg/day on every other day, to 100–120 cal/kg/day, and proteins 1–2 g/kg/day based on patient's changing weight.

F-100 formulas (skimmed milk/fresh egg based) are used in inpatients only **(Table 4.4.7)**. Diets/RUTF based on cereal pulse, (rice, *moong dal*) combinations, fortified with oil, jaggery, and seasonal vegetables, or buttermilk-based diets added with whey, soy/casein, fine roasted powdered groundnut protein and sugar, and oil are recommended and can be prepared and fed as RUTF. A typical recipe RUTF (peanut based) **(Table 4.4.8)** can also be given. Occasionally, children with secondary lactose intolerance do not tolerate milk-based feeds. Depending on the severity, either the amount of milk may be diminished in the diet by replacing with other articles, such as rice, egg, curds, etc. In severe lactose intolerance, milk will have to be temporarily completely omitted and replaced by cereals, pulses—rice, *dal*, soya, rice gruel, egg, soy milk, chicken gruel/rice, curds and rice, etc. **(Table 4.4.9)**.

Phase III: High Energy Feeding

By now, the child has progressed well with return of appetite, tolerance to high energy, and protein feeds. In this phase,

Table 4.4.8: Composition of peanut butter based ready-to-use therapeutic food.

Ingredients	***Contents (% by weight)***
Full fat milk powder	30
Sugar	28
Vegetable oil	15
Peanut butter	25
Fortified with micronutrients (sodium, potassium, calcium, phosphorous, magnesium, iron, zinc, copper, selenium, iodine, vitamin A, vitamin D, vitamin E, vitamin K, vitamin B_1, vitamin B_2, vitamin B_6, vitamin B_{12}, vitamin C, folic acid, niacin, pantothenic acid, biotin)	1.6
Energy	520–550 kcal/100 g
Proteins	10–12% of total energy
Fat	45–60% of total energy

Table 4.4.9: Diet for lactose intolerance (of varying severity).

Name	***Constituents***	***Calories***	***Proteins***
Low lactose diet			
Dried skimmed milk	• Skimmed milk (60 g) • Sucrose (12 g) • Vegetable oil (15 g)	400	20
Milk and rice	• Milk (75 mL) • Rice (5 g) • Sugar (25 g) • Water (100 mL)	79	3
Lactose free diet			
Rice and egg	• Rice (50 g) • Glucose (45 g) • Egg (one) • Oil (30 g)	710	10
Cereal pulse	• Rice (50 g) • Green gram pulse (25 g) • Jaggery (50 g) • Oil (25 g)	715	9.2
Soya rice gruel	• Rice (25 g) • Soybean (25g) • Glucose (50 g) • Oil (35 g)	715	12.5
Chicken gruel	• Chicken (100 g) • Glucose (40 g) • Oil (50 g) • Water (1 L)	720	26

emphasis is on intensive feeding to restore lost weight, catch up growth, and recover emotionally and physically. The calories are gradually increased from 150 to 180 cal/kg/day and proteins 1.5–2.5/3 g/kg/day. Milk is gradually withdrawn, semisolids and solids are introduced. Ideally, this phase extends from 6 weeks to 26 weeks to give the child his/her immune system, the best chance to recover before being challenged to home environment, if the child is in hospital (if not already discharged) or a nutritional rehabilitation unit.

Phase IV: Transfer to Family Diet or Phase of Rehabilitation

By now, as the child is accustomed to semisolid or solid diet. The child and parents are encouraged and taught to make

Table 4.4.10: Energy-rich foods.			
Name	***Ingredients***	***Calories/100 g***	***Proteins/100 g***
Besan mix/ladoo Panjiri	Bengal gram flour, Wheat flour Jaggery, ghee (1 part of each)	500	9
Sooji (Rawa) Kheer	• Toned milk (750 mL) • Sugar (100 g) • Sooji (25 g) • Oil (5 g)	1432	28.4
Hyderabad mix	• Whole wheat (40 g) • Bengal gram (16 g) • Groundnuts (10 g) • Jaggery (20 g)	330/86	11.3/86
Shakti Ahar	• Roasted peanut (10 g) • Roasted wheat (40 g) • Roasted gram (20 g) • Jaggery (30 g)	390	11.4

Table 4.4.11: Discharge from hospital.	
No definite guidelines Attainment of 75%, 80–90%	• Criteria vary from hospital to hospital: Of weight/age • Difficult to attain and associated with high morbidity and mortality
General guidelines	• Acute problems are over • Appetite has returned • Oral dietary intake adequate • Weight gain has started
Prolonged hospitalization	• Risks of acquiring nosocomial infection • Cost of hospital therapy increases • Inconvenience to family and loss of daily wages
Premature discharge	• Incomplete recovery, morbidity, recurrence of illness, rarely death 10–30%
Follow-up after discharge	• Continued supervision is vital for sustained and complete recovery • Prevent recurrence

Note: Along with medical and nutritional management providing care and stimulation is vital.

the child share family diet. Additional supplements can be offered as shown in **Table 4.4.10**. The discharge criteria of severely malnourished child may vary and are summarized in **Table 4.4.11**.

During recovery and follow-up, tender loving care should be provided. Provide a cheerful stimulating environment in form of structured play therapy 15–30 minutes/day. Physical activity should be encouraged as soon as possible. Mother should be involved in caring for the baby as far as possible (e.g., comforting, feeding, bathing, and play).

Dietary diversification still remains the most appropriate way forward, though supplementation and fortification should also be considered potential solutions to fill nutritional gaps.

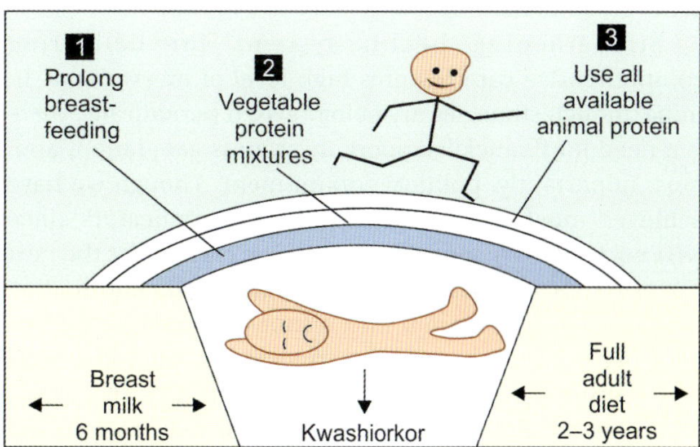

Fig. 4.4.18: Prevention of protein energy malnutrition (PEM).

PREVENTION OF PROTEIN ENERGY MALNUTRITION (FIG. 4.4.18)

Prevention requires a coordinated approach of many disciplines: nutrition, agriculture, food technology, education, health administration, social services, nongovernmental organizations, community, and religion. A strong political commitment is must for tackling malnutrition in the country.

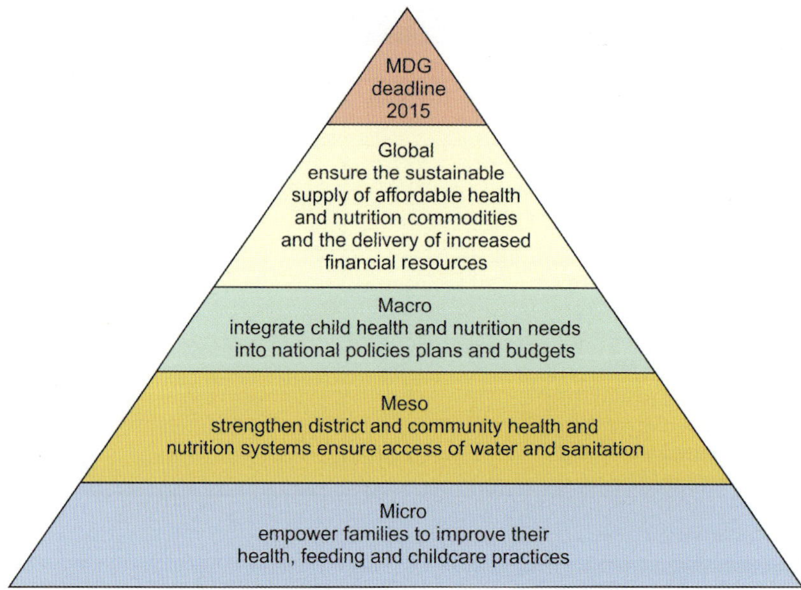

Fig. 4.4.19: Action from micro to global level.
(MDGs: Millennium development goals)

Nutrition should be a priority at national and sub-national levels as it is central for human, social and economic development. As the World Bank advocated nutrition needs to be repositioned in national development, if the *millennium development goals* (MDGs) were to be achieved. To achieve the MDG target i.e. halving the proportion of underweight children between 1990 and 2015, it involved effort at micro, meso, macro, and global levels as well as partnerships among all sectors of the society **(Fig. 4.4.19)**. Despite India's progress in launching and scaling up programs aimed at achieving optimal child nutrition over the last decade, India fell short of the 2015 MDGs.

Strengthening health systems for delivering comprehensive care requires high level of investments. In India, though strategies are being revised periodically, there is a need for financial support, awareness generation, and, most importantly, political commitment. Though we have achieved much more in terms of health indicators since NHFS-3 (2005–06), long time period has elapsed for the next survey NHFS-4. Such surveys act as major health information tools which help to act and react responsibly and quickly. The poor performing states are still lagging behind. Identifying core reasons through research is essential. The challenges identified require committed action and may be resolved by progressive and imaginative programs. The actions at the national level need to be directed toward meeting these challenges in a rational, coordinated, and unbiased manner with total commitment toward achieving the desired goals.

BIBLIOGRAPHY

1. Addis Ababa Ethiopian Federal Ministry of Health. (2007). Protocol for the management of severe malnutrition. [online] Available from www.files.ennonline.net/attachments/897/ethiopia-sam-guideline-march-2007.pdf. [Accessed September, 2018].
2. Golden MH. Evolution of nutritional management of acute malnutrition. Indian Pediatr. 2010;47(8):667-78.
3. International Institute for Population Sciences. National Family Health Survey 2015–2016 (NFHS-4). New Delhi: Ministry of Health and Family Welfare, Govt. of India; 2017.
4. Wikipedia. Malnutrition in children. [online] Available from: www.en.wikipedia.org/wiki/Malnutrition_in_children. [Accessed September, 2018].
5. Wikipedia. Malnutrition in India. . [online] Available from: www.en.wikipedia.org/wiki/Malnutrition_in_India. [Accessed September, 2018].
6. Morris SS, Cogill B, Uauy R. Effective international action against undernutrition—why has it proven so difficult and what can be done to accelerate progress. Lancet. 2008;371(9612):608-21.
7. Raj M, Kumar K. Obesity in children and adolescents. Indian J Med Res. 2010;132(5):598-607.
8. Sachdev HPS, Kapil U, Vir S. Consensus statement: national consensus workshop on management of SAM children through medical nutrition therapy. Indian Pediatr. 2010;47(8):661-5.
9. The World Bank. (2018). Joint child malnutrition estimates—UNICEF/WHO/World Bank. [online] Available from: www.data.worldbank.org/child-malnutrition. [Accessed September, 2018].
10. United Nations Children's Fund. (2015). Childinfo—monitoring the situation of children and women. [online] Available from: www.childinfo.org/undernutrition_underweight.php. [Accessed September, 2018]

4.5 Water-soluble Vitamins

Dheeraj Shah

INTRODUCTION

Water-soluble vitamins include all vitamins in B-complex group [thiamine (vitamin B_1), riboflavin (vitamin B_2), niacin (vitamin B_3), pyridoxine (vitamin B_6), cobalamin (vitamin B_{12}), folate, biotin, pantothenic acid, choline, inositol] and ascorbic acid (vitamin C). These vitamins act as coenzymes in many inter-related metabolic pathways. As these vitamins are water-soluble and heat-labile, large amounts are lost from the ingredients, if they are repeatedly washed, and when the cooking water is discarded. These vitamins are not stored for prolonged period in the body; significant toxicities at therapeutic doses are uncommon.

VITAMIN B COMPLEX

Thiamine

The active form of this vitamin acts as a cofactor for enzymes involved in carbohydrate catabolism, nucleic acid synthesis, and nerve conduction.

Dietary Sources

Rice, wheat, legumes, fortified flours, fish, and meat are good sources of thiamine. Polished rice is depleted of thiamine. It can be retained in rice by steaming the rice in the husk before milling (parboiling).

Deficiency State

Malnutrition, gastrointestinal disorders, such as malabsorption, blind loops, and short bowel, and chronic debilitation conditions, such as malignancies, are common causes of deficiency. Fatigue, irritability, poor mental concentration, anorexia, and nausea are the early manifestations of deficiency. A full-fledged deficiency state (*beriberi*) manifests as peripheral neuropathy, resulting in tingling, paresthesia, leg cramps, hyporeflexia, ataxia, and lack of coordination. Cardiac manifestations include cardiomegaly and congestive heart failure. Central nervous system (CNS) involvement occurs late in disease and is characterized by psychic disturbances, optic atrophy, hoarseness, raised intracranial pressure, and coma.

Treatment

Oral administration of thiamine is sufficient in mild-to-moderate deficiency states. Children with cardiac and CNS manifestations should be given 10 mg of thiamine intramuscularly or intravenously daily for the 1st week, followed by 3–5 mg/day orally for 6–12 weeks. Most children show dramatic improvement to oral or parenteral thiamine.

Riboflavin

Majority of this vitamin in tissues is found in the form of coenzyme flavin adenine dinucleotide, which participates in oxidation–reduction reactions in numerous metabolic pathways and in energy production via the respiratory chain.

Dietary Sources

This includes milk and its products, eggs, fortified cereals and grains, and liver. Vegan diets are poor sources.

Deficiency State

Ariboflavinosis is characterized by glossitis, angular cheilosis, keratitis, conjunctivitis, photophobia, corneal vascularization, and seborrheic dermatitis. Malnutrition, malabsorption, and gastrointestinal infections commonly precipitate the deficiency.

Treatment

Oral administration of riboflavin (3–10 mg/day) as a part of vitamin B-complex mix rapidly corrects the deficiency and controls the associated symptoms.

Niacin

Niacin is a component of the coenzymes nicotinamide adenine dinucleotide (NAD) and nicotinamide adenine dinucleotide phosphate (NADP), which are important for many redox reactions involved in carbohydrate metabolism, fatty acid synthesis, and steroid synthesis.

Dietary Sources

Niacin is rapidly absorbed from the stomach or the intestine. Good sources are fish, meat, cereals, legumes, milk, and green leafy vegetables. Predominantly maize-eating populations suffer from niacin deficiency.

Deficiency State

The classical triad of niacin deficiency (*pellagra*) is diarrhea, dermatitis, and dementia. Certain inborn errors of tryptophan metabolism (carcinoid syndrome, Hartnup disease) are also associated with niacin deficiency. Skin lesions of pellagra start as symmetric erythematous areas, resembling sunburn. These lesions are distributed on hands and feet in a "glove-and-stocking" pattern and are sometimes present over the neck (Casals necklace). Infants and young children often do not develop classical deficiency signs, and present with irritability, fatigue, anorexia, and scaly skin.

Treatment

Oral administration of niacin (50–200 mg/day) as a part of vitamin B-complex mix is indicated for pellagra. Severe cases may require intravenous administration. Sun exposure should be avoided during active skin lesions, and soothing agents are applied.

Pyridoxine

Pyridoxine (vitamin B_6) is a component of pyridoxine hydrochloride, pyridoxal and pyridoxamine cofactors in metabolism of carbohydrates, amino acids, steroids, and nucleic acids.

Dietary Sources

Poultry, meat, fish, fortified cereals, and bananas are good sources of pyridoxine. Drugs inhibiting pyridoxine activity (e.g., isoniazid, oral contraceptives, penicillamine, and phenytoin) may precipitate the deficiency.

Deficiency State

Early symptoms or signs are electroencephalography abnormalities, irritability, and vomiting. Seizures, failure to thrive, skin lesions, and microcytic anemia may occur in severe deficiency states.

Treatment

Oral administration of 10–100 mg/day is sufficient for correcting the deficiency and dependency. Intramuscular or intravenous administration of 100 mg pyridoxine is administered in the case of seizures. Treatment should be followed by ensuring adequate dietary consumption.

Folate and Vitamin B_{12}

Folate is involved in a variety of reactions involved in amino acid and nucleotide metabolism. Vitamin B_{12} (cobalamin) is required as a cofactor for methyl group transfer from a folic acid cofactor to form methionine. The unmethylated folate cofactor then participates in single carbon reactions for nucleic acid synthesis. Thus, some B_{12} and folic deficiency symptoms are similar.

Dietary Sources

Legumes, fortified cereals, citrus fruits, and leafy vegetables are good sources of folate. On the other hand, vitamin B_{12} is found only in foods from animal sources. Organ meats, sea foods, egg yolk, fish, and poultry are rich sources of vitamin B_{12}. Vegetarians get their requirements mainly from fortified cereals and milk.

Deficiency State

Megaloblastic anemia results from either (or combined) folate or vitamin B_{12} deficiency. Maternal folate deficiency increases the risk of neural tube defects in the fetus. Vitamin B_{12} also may result in neurological manifestations, such as irritability, poor attention span, hypotonia, abnormal movements, and peripheral neuropathy progressing, to subacute combined degeneration. Hyperpigmentation of knuckles is another commonly observed sign of vitamin B_{12} deficiency.

Treatment

Megaloblastic anemia due to folate deficiency requires oral administration of 0.5–1 mg/day of folic acid until a definite hematologic response has occurred. Intramuscular or intravenous administration of single dose of 1,000 µg of vitamin B_{12} is adequate for achieving hematological response in vitamin B_{12} deficiencies. Repeated doses are required for those with severe deficiency, neurological manifestations, or malabsorption. A combined treatment is required, if the blood levels for both are not available.

Others

Biotin

Biotin (found in a variety of vegetarian and nonvegetarian foodstuffs) deficiency causes scaly periorificial dermatitis, alopecia, hypotonia, and apathy.

Pantothenic Acid

Pantothenic acid (found in seafood, organ meats, egg yolk, legumes, and milk) deficiency causes muscle cramps and burning feet syndrome; clinical deficiency is extremely rare.

Choline and Inositol

Though important for normal body functions, these are not known to be associated with any specific deficiency syndromes.

VITAMIN C (ASCORBIC ACID)

Vitamin C has an important role in collagen synthesis, the synthesis of steroid hormones, neurotransmitters, and bile acids. It increases the gastrointestinal absorption of iron and has an important antioxidant activity.

Dietary Sources

Citrus fruits, tomatoes, capsicum, and green leafy vegetables are good sources of vitamin C. Breast milk is a good source of vitamin C, but children consuming animal milk are at risk of deficiency.

Deficiency State

Scurvy, resulting from severe vitamin C deficiency, manifests as gum bleeding, petechial hemorrhages, painful and swollen bones, and poor wound healing. Children having scurvy often have other nutrient deficiencies including severe malnutrition, anemia, and vitamin B-complex deficiency. The diagnosis of scurvy is usually made by radiographs, the changes being most prominent at the knee **(Fig. 4.5.1)**. The shafts of the long bones have a typical ground-glass appearance with thin and dense cortex (pencil thinning). Metaphyseal changes are characterized by thickened bands (white line of Frankel) with a zone of destruction underneath (Trummerfeld zone). Ends of the white lines often end abruptly into a spur (Pelkan's spur). Epiphyses are also outlined by dense line giving the appearance of a ring (Wimberger's ring). Subperiosteal hemorrhages may complicate the disease causing periosteal elevation and underlying calcifications.

Treatment

Oral administration of vitamin C (100–200 mg/day) results in complete recovery. Resolution of clinical symptoms is rapid, whereas bony changes and subperiosteal hemorrhages take more time to recover. Treatment must be followed by ensuring adequate dietary vitamin C to prevent recurrence.

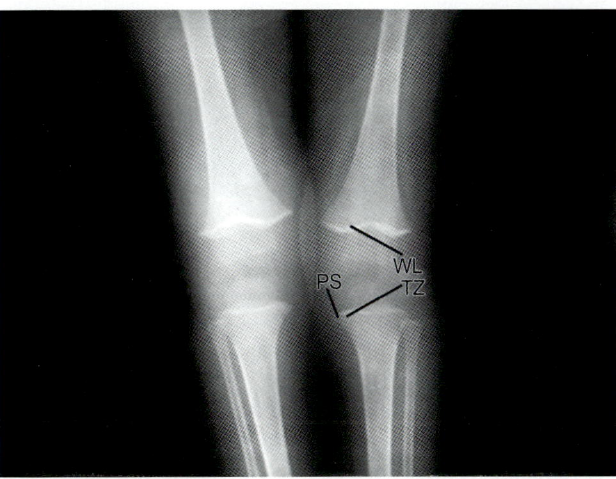

Fig. 4.5.1: Bony changes of scurvy at knee.
(PS: Pelkan's spur; TZ: Trummerfeld zone; WL: white line)

BIBLIOGRAPHY

1. Allen LH. Causes of vitamin B_{12} and folate deficiency. Food Nutr Bull. 2008;29(2 Suppl):S20-34.
2. Black MM. Effects of vitamin B_{12} and folate deficiency on brain development in children. Food Nutr Bull. 2008;29(2 Suppl):S126-31.
3. Brickley M, Ives R. Skeletal manifestations of infantile scurvy. Am J Phys Anthropol. 2006;129:163-72.
4. Kauffman G, Coats D, Seab S, et al. Thiamine deficiency in ill children. Am J Clin Nutr. 2011;94:616-7.
5. Rasmussen SA, Fernhoff PM, Scanlon KS. Vitamin B12 deficiency in children and adolescents. J Pediatr. 2001;138:10-7.
6. Sachdev HPS, Shah D. Vitamin B complex deficiency and excess. In: Kliegman RM, Stanton B, Geme JS, Schor N, Behrman RE (Eds). Nelson Textbook of Pediatrics, 19th edition. New York: Saunders (Elsevier Inc.); 2011.
7. Shah D, Sachdev HPS. Vitamin C (ascorbic acid). In: Kliegman RM, Stanton B, Geme JS, Schor N, Behrman RE (Eds). Nelson Textbook of Pediatrics, 19th edition. New York: Saunders (Elsevier Inc.); 2011.
8. Suskind DL. Nutritional deficiencies during normal growth. Pediatr Clin North Am. 2009;56:1035-53.

4.6 Fat-soluble Vitamins

(Late) Panna Choudhury

VITAMIN A

Vitamin A is a generic descriptor of retinoids that exhibit qualitatively the activity of all *trans* retinol compounds. Retinol signifies vitamin A alcohol and is found in the foods of animal origin only. Some carotenoids, found in plants, bacteria, algae, and fungi, can be converted into retinol and are called provitamin A. The carotenoid with the highest vitamin A activity is beta-carotene. Beta-carotene yields two molecules of retinol. Retinol is esterified in the mucosal cell with palmitic acid. Retinyl palmitate is stored in the liver. Being fat-soluble, retinol mobilized from the liver must be bound in serum to retinol binding protein (RBP), which is synthesized in the liver. RBP also protects retinol from oxidation and releases it to specific receptor sites on the surface of the target cell. Zinc deficiency impairs synthesis of RBP, which affects retinol transport from the liver to the blood and other tissues.

PHYSIOLOGY

Retinol is the predominant circulating form of vitamin A in the blood. In response to tissue demand, it is released from the liver in a 1:1 ratio with RBP. In the blood, this complex combines with transthyretin. Specific receptors on target cell surfaces or nuclei bind this complex or its active metabolites, thereby regulating many critical functions in the body, including vision, growth, and hematopoiesis. It is often termed as anti-infective vitamin for its role in maintaining epithelial tissue integrity and immune competence. However, the key to most of these functions is the role of vitamin A in regulating the expression of several hundred genes and cell differentiation, practically for every cell in the body. The importance of vitamin A in functioning of the retina for vision has been well established. Visual pigment in rods is called rhodopsin, which is composed of a protein called opsin and a pigment, 11-*cis* retinine (vitamin A). Rhodopsin is light sensitive and when light falls on eyes, rhodopsin splits and 11-*cis* retinine is converted to 11-*trans* retinine. This initiates an electrochemical signal to be carried to the brain where visual images are constructed. In vitamin A deficiency, the threshold for stimulating rods is raised, thus, affecting the vision under dim light.

Quantification of vitamin A is expressed in various ways. One international unit (IU) equals 0.3 µg retinol and 0.6 µg of beta-carotene (1 µg retinol will equal 3.31 IU).

DIETARY SOURCES

Rich sources of vitamin A include fish liver oils, whole milk, and milk products, such as butter, cheese, and egg yolk. Carotenoids are plentiful in fruits and vegetables that are green or deep yellow or orange in color, such as green leafy vegetables, carrots, tomatoes, sweet potatoes, papaya, and mango. Food fortified with vitamin A is an important source. Breastfeeding protects children during infancy.

VITAMIN A DEFICIENCY

Indian Council of Medical Research (ICMR) has recommended daily intake of vitamin A as retinol equivalent to 350 µg for infants, 400 µg for preschool children, and 600 µg for school children and adolescents. Deficiency of vitamin A can occur from deficient diet, decreased absorption due to chronic intestinal disorders or reduced storage in liver diseases. Vitamin A deficiency leads to impaired vision in addition to many ocular and extraocular lesions. Vitamin A deficiency was also believed to be associated with higher mortality and morbidity in children. However, recent evidence has not substantiated the mortality reduction claim of vitamin A supplementation. A large trial covering one million children in Uttar Pradesh has not found significant difference in mortality rates between children who received the massive dose of vitamin A and those who did not.

Clinical Features of Deficiency State

Ocular Lesions

These affect the posterior segment of eye initially with impairment of dark adaptation and night blindness. Often, the mother of the infant notices that, the child takes considerable time to adjust to dim light or darkness (twilight blindness). Xerosis of conjunctiva is usually the first sign that can be seen on examination. The conjunctiva becomes dry, lusterless, wrinkled, and dirty brown in color. These changes are most obvious in the interpalpebral bulbar conjunctiva. Conjunctival xerosis may lead to formation of the so-called Bitot's spot, which consists of almost a triangular area, usually about the temporal aspect of the limbus covered by a fine, white foamy or greasy substance. It is composed of heaped-up, sloughed-off keratinized cells and saprophytic

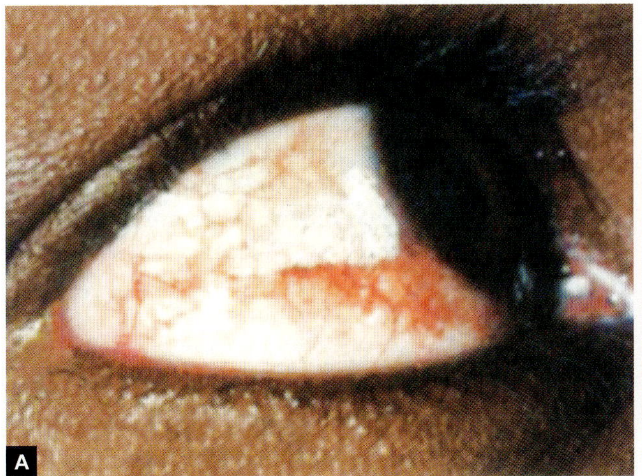

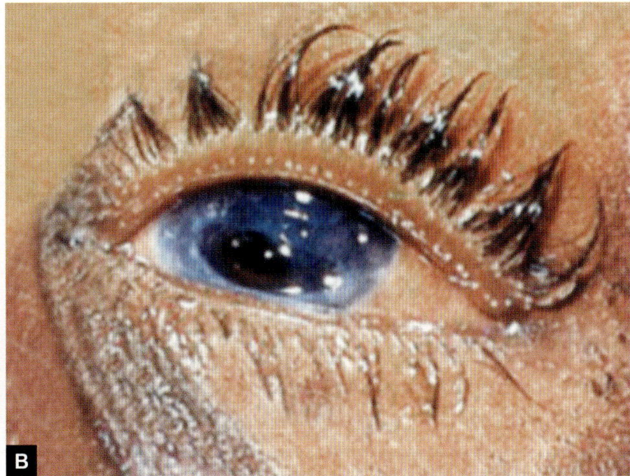

Figs. 4.6.1A and B: (A) Bitot's spots. (B) Corneal xerosis.

bacilli, which collect on conjunctival surface **(Fig. 4.6.1A)**. Corneal xerosis reflects more advanced deficiency **(Fig. 4.6.1B)**. Keratomalacia is seen in the late stage and consists of softening, necrosis, and ulceration of the cornea. Once cornea gets involved, photophobia accompanies the clinical profile. World Health Organization (WHO) has proposed a classification for xerophthalmia **(Table 4.6.1)**.

Extraocular Lesions

These include dry, scaly skin, especially over the outer aspect of the limbs, called follicular hyperkeratosis, toad skin or phrynoderma. Increased susceptibility to infections due to squamous metaplasia of respiratory, urinary and vaginal tract epithelium; renal and vesical calculus may occur more often in such subjects.

Table 4.6.1: World Health Organization classification for xerophthalmia.

Classification	***Primary signs***
X1A	Conjunctival xerosis
X1B	Bitot's spots
X2	Corneal xerosis
X3A	Corneal ulceration
X3B	Keratomalacia
	Secondary signs
XN	Night blindness
XF	Fundal changes
XS	Corneal scarring

Diagnosis of Vitamin A Deficiency

In the presence of clinical manifestations, diagnosis is not difficult. Dark adaptation tests can be used to assess early stage of vitamin A deficiency. Serum retinol level below 20 µg/dL is indicative of vitamin A deficiency state. Conjunctival impression cytology is a noninvasive technique that assesses vitamin A status by detecting early losses of vitamin A-dependent, mucus-secreting goblet cells, and early metaplasia of the epithelium.

Prevention of Vitamin A Deficiency

It is heartening that prevalence of clinical signs of vitamin A deficiency has declined drastically. There is virtual disappearance of keratomalacia. Survey of the National Nutrition Monitoring Bureau showed that prevalence of Bitot's spots had declined in 2006 compared with 1985 from 1.8% to 0.7%. Prevalence of Bitot's spots of 0.5% and more (conventional cutoff to define public health problem) is mostly limited to population groups in backward areas. However, subclinical vitamin A deficiency may still be a significant problem.

Prevention of vitamin A deficiency can be achieved by making available the recommended daily allowances of vitamin A to all children. According to the National Program for Prevention of Blindness, children in the age group of 6–11 months should receive 100,000 IU (30 mg) of vitamin A orally (preferably during measles immunization), and other children between 1 and 5 years should receive 200,000 IU (60 mg) vitamin A every 6 months in the target areas. Infants who are not breastfed should also receive a dose of 50,000 IU (15 mg) at 2 months of age. Considering that India is endowed with various varieties of fruits, and green leafy vegetables, which are rich sources of beta-carotene, vitamin A deficiency is easily preventable. Daily intake of 100 g of leafy vegetables is an efficient way to meet the requirement of vitamin A.

Fortification of commonly eaten foods with vitamin A can be an effective prophylactic measure.

Treatment of Vitamin A Deficiency

For treatment of xerophthalmia, according to WHO guidelines, 200,000 IU vitamin should be given orally on presentation, the following day, and whenever possible, 1–4 weeks later. Infants aged between 6 months and 12 months should receive a half dose, and infants less than 6 months should receive one quarter the dose, following the same schedule. Children with severe malnutrition, recurrent diarrhea, pneumonia, and severe infections should also receive full treatment course of vitamin A. Cochrane review showed that vitamin A megadoses (200,000 IU on each day for 2 days) lowered the number of deaths from measles in hospitalized children under the age of 2 years.

HYPERVITAMINOSIS A

Signs of toxicity may appear with massive doses (e.g., 300,000 IU) or with large doses over a long period (e.g., over 20,000 IU/day). Child may have nausea, vomiting, drowsiness, papilledema, and symptoms suggestive of raised intracranial tension. This syndrome is known as pseudotumor cerebri. In chronic cases, marked anorexia, failure to thrive, alopecia, seborrheic dermatitis, hepatomegaly, and tender bone swelling may develop. Radiographic examination may show hyperostosis of the shafts of long bones. Symptoms subside on withdrawal of the vitamin. However, beta-carotene ingestion is seemingly without toxicity. With chronic high consumption, the skin but not the sclera is stained yellow orange, which is benign and reversible.

VITAMIN D

Antirachitic properties of vitamin D are the result of small structural changes, under the influence of ultraviolet irradiation in a number of steroids related to cholesterol. However, only ergosterol and 7-dehydrocholesterol have practical importance. Ergosterol is of plant origin, and on irradiation, it transforms to vitamin D_2 (calciferol). The 7-dehydrocholesterol is normally present under the skin, and on exposure to ultraviolet rays of the sunlight, it converts to vitamin D_3 or cholecalciferol. The latter is converted to 25-hydroxycalciferol in the liver and is further converted to 1,25-dihydroxycholecalciferol, which is specifically helpful in promoting synthesis of "calcium transport protein" in the intestinal wall. Parathyroid hormone (PTH) controls the production of 1,25-dihydroxycholecalciferol, the metabolically active form of vitamin D. Quantification of vitamin D is expressed as 1 µg will equal 40 IU.

SOURCES

Vitamin D, unlike other vitamins, is not abundantly available in foodstuffs. Rich source of vitamin D is fish liver oil and to some extent, it is available in butter and egg. Milk provides minimal amounts of vitamin D (0.1 µg/dL). Cutaneous synthesis is an important source of vitamin D, but efficiency of the process is affected, if ultraviolet rays are cutoff by haze, windowpane, oblique rays, etc. Pigmented skin also requires more sunlight exposure to be effective.

DAILY REQUIREMENT

The normal daily requirement of vitamin D for infants and children is 400 IU (10 µg). In Indians, due to our skin pigment and modest pattern of clothing, 45–60 minutes of direct sun exposure to face, neck, forearms, and hands in summer and 150–180 minutes to face and hands in winters should provide adequate dermal vitamin D production. Considering the rampant vitamin D deficiency and the vulnerability to its serious consequences during infancy, the current recommendations by the Indian Academy of Pediatrics and Global Consensus Group suggest daily supplementation of 400 IU/day for all infants beginning in the first few days of life. The Indian Academy of Pediatrics also recommends routine vitamin D supplementation to all children up to 12 years of age. However, there are no recommendations on routine vitamin D supplementation by the ICMR or any other governmental agency.

VITAMIN D DEFICIENCY

Infants are more prone to vitamin D deficiency, as natural diet of infants such as milk, cereals, vegetables, and fruits are deficient in vitamin D. This gets aggravated, if there is also lack of access to sunlight. In a study from Delhi, clinical vitamin D deficiency was noted in 11.5% apparently healthy schoolgirls, whereas biochemical hypovitaminosis D (serum 25-hydroxyvitamin D <50 nmol/L) was seen in 90.8% of girls. Vitamin D deficiency also occurs in presence of malabsorption, liver, and kidney diseases. Rickets, a metabolic disorder of growing bone leading to bony deformities, when results from vitamin D deficiency are known as nutritional rickets.

Biochemical Changes

Vitamin D deficiency causes decreased absorption of calcium from gut. The resulting hypocalcemia leads to increase in PTH secretion. This helps in release of calcium from bone. PTH also reduces the excretion of calcium by kidneys and renal tubular reabsorption of phosphate. As a result, the serum calcium level tends to become normal, while the serum phosphate level falls. After sometime, this compensatory mechanism fails and both calcium and phosphorus levels fall. Since calcium phosphate is necessary for deposition of calcium in growing bones, decrease in blood levels of calcium, phosphorus, or both, interferes with the calcification of the osteoid tissue. Serum alkaline phosphatase level also gets increased due to increase in osteoblastic activity.

Pathology of Rickets

The epiphyseal plate is a narrow well-defined strip from where cartilage cells grow in parallel column toward the metaphysis. After initial proliferation, the old cartilage cells degenerate and disappear, leaving spaces into which the blood vessels and osteoblasts of the shaft can penetrate. Calcium is deposited in the zone of degenerating cartilage, which is then called "zone of preparatory calcification." In rickets, the cartilage cells go on multiplying giving rise to a broad, irregular cartilaginous zone. The process of degeneration and calcification becomes incomplete, leading to softness of the bone. Rapidly growing cartilage cells, particularly, affect the costochondral junctions and the end of long bones. There is also defective mineralization in the subperiosteal bone. In long-standing cases, the bones under stress may become deformed or even have pathological fractures. Supplementation of vitamin D restores the normal development of bone with calcification starting at the zone of preparatory calcification, which in radiography would be seen as a thin dense line near the epiphysis.

Clinical Features

Rickets is a disease of growing bones and its incidence is particularly high between 4 and 18 months. Skeletal deformities are the most striking feature of rickets. One of the early signs of rickets is craniotabes. In this condition, on pressing occipital or posterior part of parietal bone, a sensation, such as pressing a ping-pong ball, can be felt. It results from the thinning out of inner table of the skull due to absorption of noncalcified osteoid tissue. Fontanel may remain wider than normal and close late. Other early evidences of osseous changes are palpable enlargement of costochondral junctions, i.e. rachitic rosary and widening of the wrists **(Fig. 4.6.2)** and ankles.

Signs of advanced rickets can be easily recognized. Bossing of skull generally starts after the age of 6 months. It occurs due to heaping up of osteoid tissue in the frontal and parietal regions, so that the skull appears square-like or box-like shape. In thorax, the sternum is pushed forward producing a "pigeon chest." A horizontal depression known as Harrison's groove, corresponding to costal insertion of the diaphragm develops. The chest deformities decrease the lung resilience and predispose the child to intercurrent infections. Bending of the spine backward (kyphosis) and laterally (scoliosis) may occur. Pelvis may become softened, and the promontory of the sacrum is pushed anteriorly and the acetabulum inward, resulting in a narrowed pelvic inlet. This is helped by lax ligaments. Deformity of the pelvis in a female results in difficulty during labor at a later stage. Long bones of the legs get deformed when the child starts bearing weight and is thus, usually seen after the age of 1 year. Bending of the femur, tibia, and fibula result in the deformities as "bow-legs" or "knock-knees." Coxa vara and greenstick fractures may also occur. All deformities of bones result in rachitic dwarfism. Dentition may be delayed, and disordered eruption of temporary teeth occurs. In children between 8 months and 18 months, permanent teeth, which are undergoing calcification, may be affected.

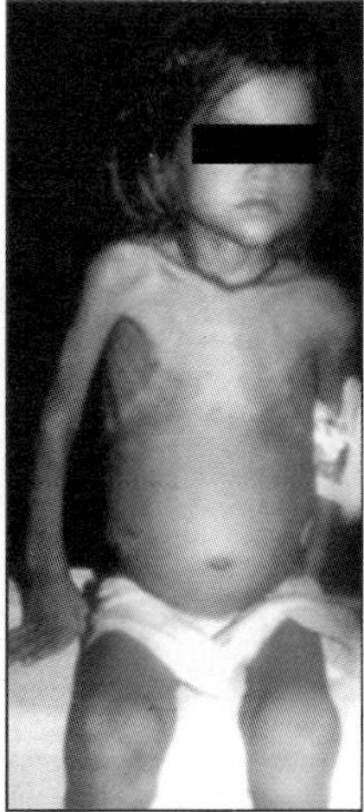

Fig. 4.6.2: Case of rickets showing widening of wrists and beading of ribs on chest.

In addition to skeletal deformities, there is a generalized hypotonia with delay in motor development. The abdomen is protuberant, and generalized flabbiness of muscles may result into visceroptosis with downward displacement of spleen and liver.

Diagnosis

The diagnosis of rickets is based on the clinical features, biochemical findings, and characteristic radiological picture. The serum calcium level may be normal or low, the serum phosphorus level is below 4 mg/dL, and the serum alkaline phosphatase is usually elevated. Radiological changes are best seen in the lower end of radius and ulna. Skiagram of the wrist shows widening, cupping, and fraying of the epiphyses in contrast to the normally sharply demarcated and slightly convex epiphyseal line **(Figs. 4.6.3A and B)**. The density of shafts decreases with prominent trabeculae. There is an increase in distance between concave epiphyseal line and the ends of metacarpals. Greenstick fractures, expansion of bone

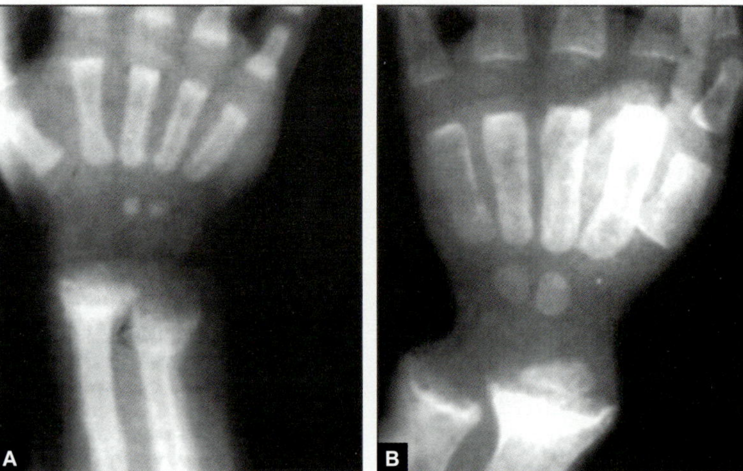

Figs. 4.6.3A and B: (A) Florid rickets showing cupping, fraying, and widening of metaphysis of distal end of radius and ulna; (B) Healing rickets showing zone of calcification at the distal end of radius and ulna; also seen at the periosteal calcification of metaphysis.

ends, and bending of bones may be evident on radiographs. Periosteum may be raised due to excess of osteoid lying under the periosteum.

Differential Diagnosis of Rickets

Nutritional rickets should be differentiated from the other types of rickets and chondrodystrophy. Other conditions producing bony deformities may, sometimes, need consideration. Craniotabes and a large head apart from rickets occur in hydrocephalus, congenital syphilis, and osteogenesis imperfecta. Enlargement of costochondral junctions may also be seen in scurvy and chondrodystrophy.

Management

Vitamin D (cholecalciferol) is given in a dose of 1,000 IU for newborns up to 1 month of age, 2,000 IU for infants, and 5,000–10,000 IU for older children orally daily. If there is no sign of healing line in skiagram taken 3–4 weeks after therapy, the same dose can be repeated. If there is no response within 3–4 weeks of the second dose, investigations for refractory rickets should be initiated. Rickets can also be treated with single large dose of 60,000 (older infants) to 120,000 IU (older children) orally (stosstherapy), with a repeat dose, if necessary, after 2 months. Therapy with single large doses ranging from 150,000 to 600,000 IU may be effective, costless and can be given under direct observation. However, it is not recommended below 3 months of age, due to fear of toxicity including hypercalcemia. After the healing of rickets, normal daily requirement of calcium (50–75 mg daily) and vitamin D (400/600 IU daily) should be ensured. Deformities of bones are corrected by orthopedic measures. Normalization of vitamin D status may not occur even 12 weeks of single dose stosstherapy; it is necessary to check the vitamin D status following therapy.

HYPERVITAMINOSIS D

High dose of vitamin D given over a long period may cause anorexia, vomiting, hypotonia, irritability, polydipsia, and polyuria. Hypercalcemia and hypercalciuria are also present. Radiological examination reveals evidence of metastatic calcification and osteoporosis of long bones.

VITAMIN E

Vitamin E is a group of closely related, naturally occurring fat-soluble compound of which tocopherol is functionally the most potent. It is active as an antioxidant and probably involved in the metabolism of nucleic acids. It is widely present in most foods. One milligram of alpha-tocopherol provides 1.5 IU activity of vitamin E. The deficiency of vitamin E is rare. The most common causes are diarrhea and poor intake of food. Deficiency may result in areflexia, ataxia, muscle weakness, and dysarthria. In premature infant, low levels of vitamin E are associated with hemolytic anemia, hyperbilirubinemia, and intraventricular hemorrhage. This responds quickly to 5–25 mg of vitamin E therapy. Generally, infants should receive 3 mg of alpha-tocopherol daily.

VITAMIN K

Vitamin K is a naphthoquinone derivative. Absence or failure of its absorption from the intestine leads to hypoprothrombinemia and decreased synthesis of some coagulation factors (VII, IX, and X). The normal requirement of vitamin K is met by bacterial synthesis in the intestine.

In addition, it is also found in high concentration in a wide variety of foods and vegetables, such as spinach, cabbage, peas, tomatoes, soybean, and liver.

The deficiency of vitamin K can occur in malabsorption states, biliary obstruction, after oral antibiotic therapy, or in newborn before colonization of the guts. In general, vitamin K deficiency or hypoprothrombinemia should be considered in all patients with hemorrhagic disturbances. Hemorrhagic disease of the newborn is one of the most common manifestations. The bleeding is variable and can occur anywhere, though, most common is gastrointestinal bleeding. A daily dose of 1–2 mg of vitamin K orally is sufficient for treatment. In severe deficiency state, 5 mg of aqueous vitamin K can be given parenterally.

BIBLIOGRAPHY

1. Arlappa N, Laxmaiah A, Balakrishna N, et al. Clinical and subclinical vitamin A deficiency among rural pre-school children of Maharashtra, India. Ann Hum Biol. 2008;35:606-14.
2. Awasthi S, Peto R, Read S, et al. Vitamin A supplementation every 6 months with retinol in 1 million pre-school children in north India: DEVTA, a cluster-randomised trial. Lancet. 2013;38:1469-77.
3. Gupta P, Dewan P, Shah D, et al. Vitamin D supplementation for treatment and prevention of pneumonia in under-five children: a randomized double-blind placebo controlled trial. Indian Pediatr. 2016;53(11):967-76.
4. Holick MF, Binkley NC, Bischoff-Ferrari HA, et al. Evaluation, treatment, and prevention of vitamin D deficiency: an Endocrine Society clinical practice guideline. J Clin Endocrinol Metab. 2011;7:1911-30.
5. Huiming Y, Chaomin W, Meng M. Vitamin A for treating measles in children. Cochrane Database Syst Rev. 2005;(4):CD001479.
6. Huynh J, Lu T, Liew D, et al. Vitamin D in newborns. A randomised controlled trial comparing daily and single oral bolus vitamin D in infants. J Paediatr Child Health. 2017;2:163-9.
7. Indian Council of Medical Research. Dietary guidelines for Indians. New Delhi: Indian Council of Medical Research; 2010.
8. Khadilkar A, Khadilkar V, Chinnappa J, et al. Indian Academy of Pediatrics 'Guideline for Vitamin D and Calcium in Children' Committee. Prevention and treatment of vitamin D and calcium deficiency in children and adolescents: Indian Academy of Pediatrics (IAP) Guidelines. Indian Pediatr. 2017;54:567-73.
9. Munns CF, Shaw N, Kiely M, et al. Global Consensus Recommendations on Prevention and Management of Nutritional Rickets. J Clin Endocrinol Metab. 2016;101:394-415.
10. Wagner CL, Greer FR, American Academy of Pediatrics Committee on Nutrition: Prevention of rickets and vitamin D deficiency in infants, children, and adolescents. Pediatrics. 2008;122:1142-52.

4.7 Trace Elements

KE Elizabeth, P Leela Kumari

INTRODUCTION

Trace elements are minerals required only in minute amount for living organisms for normal body function and growth and are included under micronutrients. These are present in concentrations less than 0.01% body dry weight. World Health Organization (WHO) expert consultation has categorized nutritionally significant trace elements into three groups:

1. *Essential trace elements*: Iron, iodine, zinc, selenium, copper, molybdenum, and chromium
2. *Elements which are probably essential*: Manganese, silicon, nickel, boron, and vanadium
3. *Potentially toxic elements*: Fluorine, lead, cadmium, mercury, arsenic, aluminum, lithium, and tin.

EPIDEMIOLOGY

Trace elements deficiencies are common in growing children and pregnant women because of the increased requirement. A balanced diet that includes all the food groups can supply all the trace elements. Infant and young child feeding practices, especially in the –9 to +24 months that corresponds to the first 1,000 days of life, are crucial in preventing deficiency and ensuring enough stores of trace elements. Trace elements deficiencies occur usually in those with undernutrition, picky eaters, low-birth-weight (LBW) babies, and in those on exclusion diets and total parenteral nutrition (TPN). Excess intake of dietary fiber, phytates, and oxalates reduce trace element absorption. Both deficiency and excess of trace elements can affect normal body functions. Recent epidemiological surveys and animal studies have revealed the significant role of trace elements in human health and have highlighted the association of trace element deficiency state with reduced antioxidant potential, leading to accelerated aging, early onset of cancer, atherosclerosis and lifestyle-related diseases, growth retardation, and immunological abnormalities.

Various aspects related to trace elements are summarized in **Table 4.7.1**.

Table 4.7.1: Sources, functions, deficiencies, clinical features, requirements, and toxicity of the various trace elements.

TE	***Sources***	***Functions***	***Deficiency***	***Clinical features***	***Requirement***	***Remarks and toxicity***
Iron	Heme 7–35% and nonheme 2–20% Fish, meat, liver 3 Gs: grams, grains, greens Jaggery/ molasses, asafetida, turmeric, dates, watermelon Cooking in iron vessels	Constituent of myoglobin and enzymes, role in oxygen transport For physical stamina, learning ability and myelination Also known as the "energy mineral"	LBW, excess of cow's milk, blood loss, hookworm, whipworm, malabsorption poor intake, increased demand	Pallor, dyspnea, CCF, irritability, lack of concentration, pica, koilonychia *Investigation*: S. iron (50–150 µg/dL), iron-binding capacity (100–400 µg/dL) S. ferritin (50–250 ng/mL), transferrin saturation <15%, blood smear hypochromic microcytic anemia, MCV, MCH, MCHC reduced, and RDW increased	*Prophylaxis*: 2–3 mg/kg/day; children 10–20 mg/day, pregnancy and lactation 60 mg/day *Treatment oral*: 4–6 mg/kg/day for 3–4 months; *injection*: Weight in kg × deficit in g/dL × 2.5 + 25%, iron sucrose IV/IM *Packed red cell transfusion*: 5–10 mL/kg; always treat the cause	Oxalate, phytates, Zn, coffee/tea inhibit absorption. Vitamin C, cobalt, lime juice and acid medium increase absorption. *Toxicity:* Chronic-hemosiderosis, hemochromatosis. *Acute*: GI upset, stages of quiescent phase, metabolic derangement, hepatic failure and strictures. Gastric lavage with soda bicarbonate and desferrioxamine. IV Desferal 50 mg/kg followed by 10 mg/kg/h × 24 h serum iron >1,800 µg/dL is fatal
Iodine	Seafoods, drinking water (two-thirds requirement), iodized salts	Constituent of thyroxine, for metabolic control, modulation of estrogen and fetal health	Low content in water, especially mountainous areas, excessive intake of brassica species, cabbage, cauliflower	Endemic goiter, hypothyroidism, stillbirth, CNS defect *Investigation*: Urinary iodine, PBI, T3, T4, TSH, iodine uptake study	50–150 µg/day	Iodized salt to contain 15 µg/g (15 ppm); up to 30 ppm added to tackle loss. Excess can cause iodism, reversible dermatitis and cobalt deficiency/excess, iron deficiency, manganese excess and fluorine excess may aggravate goiter
Copper	Liver, fish, meat, oyster, legumes, competes with Zn and Mo for absorption	Constituents of enzymes, ceruloplasmin, and hormone function, role in hemopoiesis, essential for Zn, iron and vitamin C function, bone Also called twin mineral of iron	LBW, preterm TPN, PEM, nephrotic syndrome, Menkes kinky hair syndrome is an X-linked metabolic disturbance of copper metabolism characterized by mental retardation, abnormal hair texture, hypocupremia (<65 µg/dL) and low circulating ceruloplasmin (<20 mg/dL)	Hypochromic anemia, neutropenia, hypopigmented hair, bony defects *Investigation*: S. Cu 75–150 µg/dL S. ceruloplasmin 10–50 µg/dL	1–2 mg/day	*Toxicity*: Indian childhood cirrhosis, hepatitis, cirrhosis, Coomb's negative hemolytic anemia, Zn deficiency, Cu deposition occurs in Wilson's disease

Contd...

Contd...

TE	***Sources***	***Functions***	***Deficiency***	***Clinical features***	***Requirement***	***Remarks and toxicity***
Zinc	Liver, beef, oyster, cereals, nuts, grapes	Constituents of enzymes, role in protein and nucleic acid synthesis, epithelial repair, fluid electrolyte transport, taste function, immunity	PEM, TPN, hepatitis, nephrotic syndrome, acrodermatitis enteropathica, especially as a genetic defect	Growth retardation, anorexia, gonadal atrophy, alopecia, dermatitis, diarrhea, reduced taste sensation *Investigation*: S. Zn 60–150 µg/dL, Zn in hair	5–15 mg/day Treatment: Diarrhea—ORS and Zn—2–6 months: 10 mg/day and >6 months: 20 mg/day × 2 weeks Dose 1–2 mg/kg/day up to 150-mg elemental zinc	Phytates reduce absorption, excess reduces iron and copper levels. Used as adjuvant in Wilson's disease Toxicity: GI upset, Cu deficiency
Chromium	Yeast, liver cereals, nuts, cocoa, pepper	Facilitates insulin action and weight loss, helps to prevent diabetes	PEM, TPN	Hyperglycemia, encephalopathy. *Investigation*: S. Cr 0.02 µg/dL	10 µg/day *Treatment*: Single dose 180 µg in hyperglycemia	*Toxicity*: Renal failure, dermatitis
Fluorine	Drinking water, seafoods, tea, cheese	Constituent of bone and teeth	Poor water content	Dental caries	1–5 mg/day drinking water up to 1 ppm	*Excess*: Dental and skeletal fluorosis, genu valgum with excess in drinking water and sorghum intake, >2–3 ppm in drinking water needs defluoridation by alum and/or by reverse osmosis (OS)
Selenium	Meat groups, green, garlic	Antioxidant, cofactor of enzyme function, maintains liver integrity	PEM, TPN, poor soil content	Keshan cardiomyopathy, arthritis, myalgia, growth retardation, liver necrosis, risk of liver cancer Kashin Beck disease (endemic osteoarthropathy) *Investigation*: S. Se 13 µg/dL	100 µg/day	Dental caries, alopecia, garlic odor in breath
Manganese	Cereals, legumes, greens, tea	Component of superoxide dismutase, role in oxidative phosphorylation	TPN	Growth retardation, reddening of hair, increased prothrombin time *Investigation*: S. Mn 0.06 µg/dL	1–5 mg/day	Iron decreases Mn absorption *Toxicity*: Encephalitis, goiter, cardiomyopathy, cholestasis
Nickel	Chocolate	Component of urease, and nickel plasmin, stabilizes membranes	TPN	*Investigation*: S. nickel 0.02 µg/dL	Not known	*Excess*: Dermatitis, liver necrosis, nasal and lung cancers
Silicon		Crosslinkage of collagen, helps in bone formation	TPN	Growth retardation, defective bone growth	Not known	*Excess*: Granuloma and fibrosis of lung Silicosis, urolithiasis

Contd...

Contd...

TE	Sources	Functions	Deficiency	Clinical features	Requirement	Remarks and toxicity
Vanadium	Protein-rich food	Regulation of enzyme Na^+/K = ATPase. adenylate cyclase, and protein kinase	PEM	Deficiency associated with nutritional edema	Not known	
Molybdenum	Legumes and green leafy vegetables, liver	Molybdenum containing enzymes in humans are xanthine oxidase/ dehydrogenase, aldehyde oxidase and sulfite oxidase		Molybdenum deficiency coexisting with selenium deficiency may be obligatory for the development of Keshan disease, tachycardia, central scotoma, irritability, coma, and probably increased incidence of mouth and esophageal cancers	2–3 µg/kg/day	Excess may unmask hyperuricemia, gout and genu valgum. Abnormally, high level leads to copper deficiency

(CNS: central nervous system; IM: intramuscular; IV: intravenous; LBW: low-birth-weight; MCH: mean corpuscular hemoglobin; MCHC: mean corpuscular hemoglobin concentration; MCV: mean corpuscular volume; ORS: oral rehydration salts; OS: osmosis; PBI: protein-bound iodide; PEM: protein energy malnutrition; RDW: red cell distribution width; S.: serum; TE: trace element; TPN: total parenteral number; TSH: thyroid-stimulating hormone)

DIAGNOSIS

Except for iron, iodine, zinc, and selenium, specific features of deficiency may not occur and, in most of the cases, it is subclinical deficiency. Therefore, clinical diagnosis is often difficult. Recent advances in analytical technologies, such as atomic absorption spectrometry, have made it possible to measure these elements precisely and to determine deficiency as well as excess. A high index of suspicion and therapeutic response to supplementation helps in clinching the diagnosis. Methods currently used for diagnosis include:

- Measurement of trace elements in samples, such as serum, erythrocytes, leucocytes, hair, urine, and other body fluids
- Measurement of activity of enzymes containing trace elements, for example, 5′ nucleotidase (zinc), thyroid hormone (iodine), and glutathione peroxidase (selenium)
- Function tests, for example, taste test (zinc), electroretinogram (zinc)
- Analysis of daily intake (of theoretical importance)
- Observing the response to supplementation.

TRACE ELEMENT DEFICIENCIES OF PUBLIC HEALTH IMPORTANCE

A three-pronged approach is suggested to tackle deficiency, namely dietary diversity, specific supplementation, and food fortification.

IRON DEFICIENCY AND IRON-DEFICIENCY ANEMIA

Iron deficiency (ID) is the most common micronutrient deficiency worldwide; it is a major public health problem. The current global prevalence of anemia (WHO report, 2015) is 42.6% in children, 38% in pregnant women, and 29.4% in all women of reproductive age group (WRA). In India, the recent family health survey (National Family Health Survey-4, 2015–16) reported anemia as a severe public health problem: >40% prevalence in all vulnerable age groups, 58.4% in children of age 6–59 months, 53.1% in WRA, 50.3% in pregnant women, and 23% in men. Iron is needed in human body for hemoglobin and myoglobin synthesis. It is a cofactor of many enzymes and is required for a wide spectrum of biologic functions. It is needed for brain growth, maturation, and for neurotransmitter synthesis and metabolism. It is needed for immunity and cell maturation and differentiation. Literature evidences reveal that early ID can lead to irreversible changes in the growing brain. Anemia during pregnancy is associated with poor maternal and fetal outcome.

The stages of ID are prelatent stage, latent stage, and frank ID. Iron insufficiency leads to iron depletion, ID and ID anemia (IDA), reduced physical stamina, lack of concentration and learning ability, pica, and koilonychia. Pica includes eating disorders, such as geophagia (mud), amylophagia (eating raw rice), and pagophagia (ice cubes). IDA is an added risk factor

Table 4.7.2: Hemoglobin levels to diagnose anemia (WHO, 2008).

Age group	*No anemia*	*Mild*	*Moderate*	*Severe*
6–60 months	≥11 g/dL	10–10.9	7–9.9	<7
5–11 years	≥11.5	11–11.4	8–10.9	<8
12–14 years	≥12	11–11.9	8–10.9	<8
WRA	≥12	11–11.9	8–10.9	<8
Pregnant women	≥11 g/dL	10–10.9	7–9.9	<7

(WRA: women in the reproductive age group)

for breath-holding spell, febrile fit, and hypercyanotic blue spell in children with cyanotic heart diseases.

Investigations for iron deficiency include hemoglobin estimation **(Table 4.7.2)**, red cell indices: low mean corpuscular volume, mean corpuscular hemoglobin (MCH), MCH concentration, blood picture showing microcytic hypochromic red blood cells, with increased red cell distribution width, total iron binding capacity >450 μg/dL, transferrin saturation <16%. The most accurate biochemical test for ID is serum ferritin (*N*: >15 μg/L). Point-of-care hemoglobin estimation is recommended to be digital hemoglobinometer, instead of Sahli's or color scale method.

In 2013, the Anemia Control Programme was renamed as National Iron Plus Initiative programme and was revised in 2018. This includes the life-cycle approach: (1) biweekly 20 mg elemental iron and 100 μg of folic acid as syrup for infants of 6-23 months; (2) biweekly 20 mg elemental iron and 100 μg of folic acid and biannual deworming of preschool children of 24-60 months; (3) weekly supplementation of 45 mg elemental iron and 400 μg of folic acid for children of 6-10 years and biannual deworming; (4) weekly 60 mg elemental iron 500 μg folic acid and biannual deworming in adolescents (10-19 years); (5) weekly supplementation 100 mg elemental iron 500 μg folic acid for women in the reproductive age group (WRA) (15-49 years); and (6) Daily IFA for pregnant mothers from 14 weeks for 180 days till delivery and daily IFA for lactating mothers for 180 days postpartum. Recently, enteric-coated iron folic acid tablets have been changed to sugar-coated tablets to increase bioavailability. Higher doses are found to be counterproductive. Hence, the *National Expert Group Technical consultation of prevention and treatment of India, 2018* has recommended to reduce elemental iron from 100 to 60 mg.

The distribution of double (iodine and iron) fortified salt (DFS) as a public health measure to tackle anemia is under trial in selected districts of Uttar Pradesh. The other measures recommended are to popularize dietary diversity to include a variety of food items rich in non-heme and heme iron, food fortifications such as infant cereal with iron, use of sprinklers containing iron, to encourage cooking one item daily in iron vessel, avoiding anti-nutrients to iron such as tannins in tea, polyphenols in *Amla* along with iron rich food, encouraging intake of vitamin C and vitamin C rich items such as guava, lemon juice with food and undertake iron supplementation throughout the life-cycle as per the National Iron Plus Initiative (NIPI).

IODINE-DEFICIENCY DISORDERS

Iodine is one of the essential trace elements needed for normal human growth and development. It is needed for the synthesis of thyroid hormone. About two thirds of this is generally derived from the drinking water and one third from diet. Iodine deficiency is a preventable cause of mental deficiency. Iodine-deficiency disorders (IDD) can affect children's mental health and survival. Severe iodine deficiency during pregnancy can lead to stillbirths, abortions, and cretinism. Its daily requirement is 150 μg. Universal iodization of salt ensuring potassium iodate 15 ppm (15 μg/g) is recommended in India. Salt-testing kits are made available to ensure optimum iodization. In commercial, iodized salt up to 30-50 ppm is added to cover losses. DFS contains potassium iodate and ferrous sulfate to tackle IDA and IDD. Urinary iodine excretion is reduced in deficiency. Urinary iodine can be tested using dipstick or laboratory method. Excretion less than 100 μg/L indicates iodine deficiency, 50-100 mild, 20-50 moderate, and less than 20 indicates severe deficiency. Goiter is an indication of previous deficiency state, and the rates more than 5% in prepubertal children indicates endemic goiter: 5-20% mild, 20-30% moderate, and >30% severe. *Grade 0*: goiter not visible or palpable, *Grade 1*: goiter palpable, and *Grade 2*: both visible and palpable (WHO staging).

Recommended daily intake is 90 μg for preschool children, 120 μg for school children (6-12 years), 150 μg for adolescents and adults, and 250 μg for pregnant and lactating women. Certain substances (goitrogens) can adversely affect the iodine utilization. These are thiocyanates, flavonoids, disulfides, phthalates, and biphenyls, and these are found in abundance in certain tubers and vegetables, such as tapioca, cabbage, and cauliflower.

The healthy human body contains 15-20 mg of iodine, of which about 70-80% is concentrated in the thyroid gland and is utilized for thyroid hormone synthesis which is essential for normal growth and development.

The spectrum of IDD includes:

- *Fetus*: Abortions, still birth, congenital abnormalities, cretinism, mental deficiency
- *Neonate*: Neonatal hypothyroidism, mental deficiency
- *Childhood and adolescence*: Goiter, hypothyroidism, dwarfism, mental retardation, poor school performance.

ZINC DEFICIENCY

Zinc is an essential trace element and a component of many proteins and metalloproteins, and is needed for many biologic functions in human body. It is found in almost all tissues and body fluids. It is a component of many enzymes,

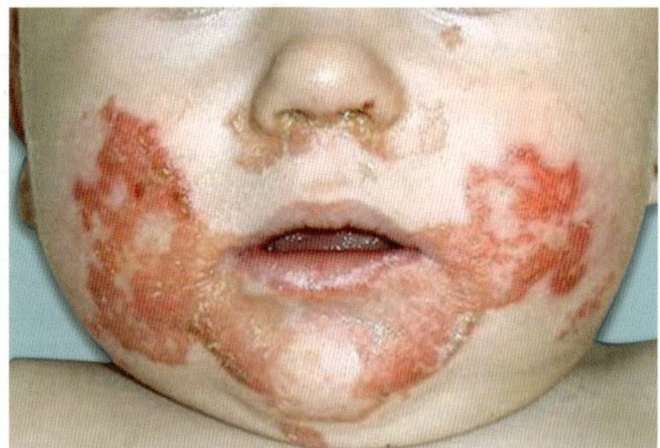

Fig. 4.7.1: Symmetrical periorificial lesions in zinc deficiency due to acrodermatitis enteropathica (note that overall growth is normal).

such as nicotinamide adenine dinucleotide dehydrogenase, ribonucleic acid (RNA) and deoxyribonucleic acid polymerases, superoxide dismutase, carbonic anhydrase, etc. Hence, zinc is needed for cell multiplication and growth, fertility, protein and fat synthesis, immunity, protection against free radicals, etc. It is needed for several body functions, such as vision, insulin function, taste perception, anti-inflammatory functions, etc.

It is needed for myelination, neurotransmitter metabolism [gamma-aminobutyric acid (GABA)], and for cognitive function in the brain. It is an intracellular signaling molecule and plays an important role in cell-mediated immunity and protection from oxidative stress.

Zinc deficiency is estimated to be widespread. The initial cases of zinc deficiency in human were reported in the early 1960s with delayed sexual development and short stature. Subclinical zinc deficiency is more common than overt. It is useful in the treatment of Wilson's disease, as it opposes copper absorption. Zinc supplementation is found to result in better catch-up growth in LBW and protein energy malnutrition. In field settings, oral rehydration salts and Zn are promoted for diarrhea control and prevention of diarrhea, as Zn results in repair of mucosa, replenishment of brush border enzymes, fluid regulation, and improvement of taste. The 20-mg zinc sulfate tablets are recommended in diarrhea, 1/2 tablet in 2–6 months old, and 1 tablet in >6 months old for 14 days. In those less than 2-month-old, it can be prescribed, whenever indicated. Along with diarrhea, skin changes are also seen in acrodermatitis enteropathica (AE), which is symmetrical and periorificial **(Fig. 4.7.1)**. Nutritional dermatosis noted in severe malnutrition may be more extensive and associated with growth failure. AE is an autosomal recessive metabolic disorder affecting the uptake of zinc through the mucous membrane.

OTHER TRACE ELEMENTS

Boron is essential for healthy bones and utilization of vitamin D and calcium in the body. Cobalt is an essential component of vitamin B_{12}; it increases iron absorption and iodine utilization. Deficiency produces anemia and goiter and excess can also lead to goiter and cardiomyopathy. Germanium is said to be the secret behind the health benefits of garlic, ginseng, and mushrooms. Fluorine is not considered an essential mineral by some as humans do not require it for growth or to sustain life. However, it prevents dental caries, and primary action occurs topically. Strontium is involved in the utilization of calcium. It promotes calcium uptake into bone at moderate dietary levels but has rachitogenic action at higher dietary levels. Arsenic, bromine, cadmium, silicon, tungsten, and vanadium have biochemical roles as structural or functional cofactors in other organisms. Arsenic is thought to promote nail and hair growth. Excess residue of arsenic found in cow's milk may be toxic to skin, central nervous system, and respiratory tract. Mercury is toxic to enzymes and RNA. Excess can lead to Minamata disease in fetus and acrodynia in others.

KEY MESSAGES

- Most of the trace elements are essential or probably essential, but a few are potentially toxic.
- Trace elements are required only in minute quantities and are present in selected food items.
- Deficiency of these micronutrients causes various pathologic effects in human body. Excess can also cause serious adverse reactions in body. So optimum trace element balance in body is essential.
- Optimum trace element balance should be considered in TPN and food fortification.
- Trace element deficiencies should be diagnosed in the early phase and corrected.
- Along with optimum dietary intake recommendations, factors influencing the absorption and bioavailability should be considered.

BIBLIOGRAPHY

1. Elizabeth KE. Vitamins, minerals and micronutrients. In: Elizabeth KE (Ed). Nutrition and child development, 5th edition. Hyderabad: Paras Medical Publisher; 2015. pp. 98-120.
2. National Family Health Survey-4. Key findings from NFHS-4 fact sheets for key indicators based on final data—Kerala, 2015-16. [online] Available from: rchiips.org/NFHS/factsheet_NFHS-4.shtml. [Accessed September, 2018].
3. WHO. Trace elements in human nutrition and health. In: Report of a WHO Expert Committee. Geneva: WHO; 1996.
4. Williams AF. Pediatric nutrition. In: Gibney MJ, Elia M, Ljungqvist O, Dowsett J, (Eds). Clinical nutrition. Oxford: Blackwell Science; 2006. pp. 379-427.
5. World Health Organization. Hemoglobin concentrations for the diagnosis of anemia and assessment of severity. World Health Organization; 2011.
6. World Health Organization. The global prevalence of anemia in 2011. WHO report. World Health Organization; 2015.
7. World Health Organization. Vitamin and mineral requirements in human nutrition, 2nd edition. Geneva: WHO; 2005.

Section 5

Immunity, Immunization and Infectious Diseases

5.1 Basics of Immune System

Naveen Thacker, Deep Thacker

INTRODUCTION

Our environment contains a huge range of pathogenic microbes and toxic substances that challenge the host by a very broad selection of pathogenic mechanisms. It requires a vigorous and vigilant immune system to keep the body free from pathogens. Immune system is a collection of mechanisms within an organism that protects against disease by eliminating pathological microbes and toxic or allergenic proteins.

The immune system consists of major lymphoid organs such as spleen and lymph nodes as well as smaller lymphoid tissues lining the mucosal entry points of the body like the airway (adenoids and tonsils) and gut-associated lymphoid tissue. The immune cells are found in the reticuloendothelial system of many organs and in circulation. There is a constant traffic of these cells from one point to the other in the body, which helps disseminate immune message throughout the body.

BASICS OF IMMUNE SYSTEM IN CHILDREN

There are three levels of defense mechanisms for protection against pathogens:

1. The first line of defense mechanism (nonspecific) is the *physical barrier* (skin and mucous membrane).
2. If a pathogen breaches these barriers, the *innate immune system* provides an immediate, but nonspecific response **(Table 5.1.1)**.
3. However, if pathogens successfully evade the innate response, vertebrates possess a third layer of protection, the *adaptive immune system*, which is activated by the innate response. Here, the immune system adapts its response during an infection to improve its recognition of the pathogen. This improved response is then retained after the pathogen has been eliminated, in the form of an immunological memory, and allows the adaptive immune system to mount faster and stronger attacks each time the same pathogen is encountered **(Table 5.1.1)**.

Table 5.1.1: Comparison of innate and adaptive immunity.

Nonspecific immunity (innate)	*Specific immunity (adaptive)*
Its response is "antigen independent"	Its response is "antigen dependent"
There is an "immediate" response	There is a "lag time" between exposure and maximal response
It is "not antigen specific"	It is "antigen specific"
Exposure does not result in the induction of memory cells	Exposure results in the induction of memory cells
Some of its cellular components or their products may aid "specific immunity"	Some of its products may aid "nonspecific immunity"

ACQUIRED IMMUNITY

Acquired immunity has two components: (1) Humoral immunity and (2) cellular immunity.

1. *Humoral immunity* is mediated by circulating *immunoglobulin antibodies* in the blood. Immunoglobulin is produced by *B-lymphocytes*, and they activate the complement system, attack, and neutralize antigens. Humoral immunity is the major defense system against bacterial infections.
2. *Cellular immunity* is mediated by *T-lymphocytes*. It is responsible for delayed allergic reactions and rejection of the foreign tissue transplants. It constitutes a major defense against infections due to viruses, fungi, and a few bacteria such as the tubercle *Bacillus*. It also plays an important role in protection against tumors.

COMPONENTS OF THE IMMUNE SYSTEM

The immune system consists of T-lymphocytes, B-lymphocytes, natural killer (NK) cells, dendritic cells (DCs), phagocytic cells, and complement proteins **(Fig. 5.1.1)**.

T-lymphocytes

Cellular immunity is mediated by T-lymphocytes which are derived from the thymus. In the blood, T-cells constitute

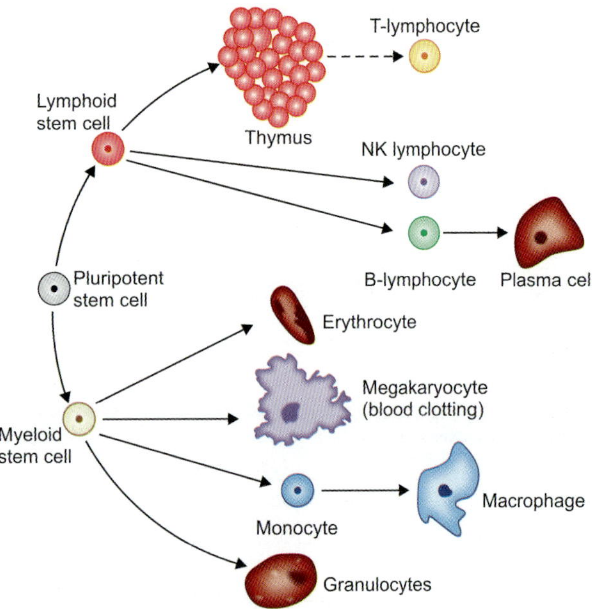

Fig. 5.1.1: Origin of immune cells.

60–70% of the peripheral lymphocytes. Each T-cell can recognize a specific cell-bound antigen by an antigen-specific T-cell receptor called TCR. Subpopulations of lymphocytes may be identified by surface markers as well as by functional abilities. Markers on the surface of the lymphocytes are assigned CD (clusters of differentiation) numbers on the basis of their reactions to a panel of monoclonal antibodies.

There are three major types of T-cells: (1) Cytotoxic T-cells, (2) helper T-cells, and (3) memory T-cells. Most *cytotoxic T-cells* display the glycoprotein CD8 and the *helper T-cells* display the glycoprotein CD4. These proteins are closely associated with the TCRs and may function as coreceptors. CD4 is expressed on approximately 60% of the mature T-cells, whereas CD8 is expressed on about 30% of the T-cells. Thus in a normal healthy person, the CD4 to CD8 ratio is about 2:1.

There are two subtypes of the helper T-cells depending on the cytokines they produce on activation. *T-helper 1 cells* secrete interleukin (IL)-2 and gamma interferon which promote cytotoxic T-cell or delayed hypersensitivity types of responses. *T-helper 2 (TH2) cells* secrete IL-4 and IL-5 and interact primarily with B-cells in relation to humoral immunity and allergic sensitization. Cytotoxic T-cells recognize foreign or self-altered antigen on the surface and destroy them. This mechanism may play a role in the rejection of transplanted tissues, detection of virus-infected cells, and surveillance against malignancy.

Clinical Significance

- Normal newborn infants are also capable of mounting antigen-specific T-cell responses at birth, as evidenced by the vigorous tuberculin reactivity a few weeks after bacillus Calmette-Guérin vaccination even on the first day of life.
- Patients with severe defects of T-lymphocyte number and/or function, such as severe combined immune deficiency and thymic aplasia (DiGeorge syndrome), show an increased susceptibility to infections due to *Candida*, cytomegalovirus, and *Pneumocystis carinii*. They also have higher incidence of malignancies, if they survive infections.
- Human immunodeficiency virus (HIV) selectively binds to the cells expressing CD4 molecules on their surface, primarily helper T-cells (CD4 cells) leading to the progressive depletion of these cells.

B-lymphocytes

B-cells are derived from *bursa of Fabricius* in birds (hence, the name B-cells). But in mammals, as there is no bursa, the transformation occurs in bursal equivalents, i.e. fetal liver and, after birth, the bone marrow. B-lymphocytes constitute 10–20% of the circulating peripheral lymphocyte population. B-cells can bind to antigens directly, but they must contact helper T-cells to produce full activation and antibody production. It is the TH2 subtype that is mainly involved. The activated B-cells proliferate and transform into plasma cells. The plasma cells secrete large quantities of antibodies into the general circulation. Circulating antibodies protect their host by binding to and neutralizing some protein toxins, by blocking the attachment of some viruses and bacteria to cells, by opsonizing bacteria, and by activating complement.

As with T-cells, each B-cell receptor has unique antigen specificity, derived in part from the somatic rearrangements of immunoglobulin genes. Thus the presence of rearranged immunoglobulin genes in a lymphoid cell is used as a molecular marker of B-lineage cells. B-cells also possess several other molecules that are essential for B-cell function. These include complement receptors, Fc receptors, and CD19.

B-lymphocytes produce five different classes of immunoglobulins called IgG, IgA, IgM, IgE, and IgD.

1. *Immunoglobulin G* is the most abundant of all immunoglobulins found in plasma and plays a major role in the prevention of infections. It crosses the placenta and thus is the primary defense against infections in the first few weeks of life in the neonate.
2. *Immunoglobulin M* is the first antibody to be produced after an antigenic stimulation and is especially important in the initial period of primary immune response. The fetus can synthesize IgM in utero starting from 20 weeks of gestation.
3. *Immunoglobulin A* is the secretory immunoglobulin which is secreted by the B-cells and protects the mucosal surfaces of the gastrointestinal, respiratory and genitourinary tracts, and the breast.

4. *Immunoglobulin E* is found in low concentrations in the serum. The normal biological role of the IgE antibody is not clear. It is probably important in defense against parasitic infestations. Generally, an elevated level of IgE is found in the patients suffering from atopic diseases.
5. *Immunoglobulin D* is found in small amounts in serum and also on the surface of the lymphocytes.

Clinical Significance

- Patients with immune deficiency syndromes involving B-lymphocytes, viz. X-linked agammaglobulinemia, suffer from recurrent pyogenic infections primarily involving the sinopulmonary tract. These defects usually manifest after 6 months of life when the passively transferred maternal IgG antibodies level begins to decline.
- The capacity to produce specific antibodies to protein antigens is intact at the time of birth. However, normal infants cannot produce antibodies to polysaccharide antigens until usually after 2 years of life. But if the polysaccharide antigen is conjugated to a protein carrier, as in the conjugate *Haemophilus influenza* type b (Hib) and *Streptococcus pneumoniae* vaccines, the child less than 2 years of age can produce the immune response.
- Complement receptor 21 (CD21) is also the receptor for the Epstein-Barr virus (EBV) and hence B-cells are readily infected by EBV.
- Clusters of differentiation 19, a signal-transducing molecule, is B-cell restricted and appears early in B-cell differentiation. It is therefore useful in the identification of B-cell tumors.

Sequence of Events on Exposure to an Antigen (Fig. 5.1.2)

The ability to recognize the antigen is innate and develops without exposure to the antigen. Stem cells differentiate into many million different T- and B-lymphocytes, each with the ability to respond to particular antigen.

In the primary immune response, native antigen is carried to a lymph node and taken up by specialized cells called follicular DCs. Virgin B-cells, bearing surface Ig, specific for that antigen then bind to this antigen. This antigenic adherence stimulates the B-cells to differentiate into antibody-producing plasma cells. Initially, these plasma cells produce IgM. Later, a switchover in the production of immunoglobulins takes place and plasma cells start producing IgG class of immunoglobulins. When the stimulus is removed, the B-cell division and differentiation stops, but the circulating pool of B-lymphocytes still contains a large population of memory cells. During reexposure to the same antigen (secondary immune response), immediate and extensive divisions of the B-cells with IgG receptors take place and large quantity of IgG antibodies are produced. These antibodies combine with the antigen.

Macrophages

Macrophages are a part of mononuclear phagocyte system. The functions carried out by macrophages in the immune response are as follows:
- They are required to process and present antigen to immunocompetent T-cells.
- They produce a variety of cytokines such as IL-1 and tumor necrosis factor and thus exert modulatory effect on inflammatory response.
- They are the effector cells of some forms of cell-mediated immunity, e.g. delayed hypersensitivity reaction.

The enzymes in macrophages include lysozymes, cathepsins, acid hydrolases, and neutral proteases. They can secrete digestive enzymes, complement component, arachidonic acid metabolites, enzyme inhibitors, interferons, and chemotactic factors in its environment.

Clinically, the deficiency of phagocyte function is acquired secondary to systemic illnesses, viz. diabetes mellitus, malnutrition, and neoplasia; in which, the defects of chemotaxis may contribute to susceptibility to infections. The most common congenital deficiency is chronic granulomatous disease. *Staphylococcus*, gram-negative rods, and fungi are troublesome for these individuals who suffer from skin, periorificial, and deep organ infections.

Natural Killer Cells

Approximately 10–15% of the peripheral blood lymphocytes do not bear TCR or cell-surface immunoglobulins. These cells are endowed with an innate ability to lyse a variety of tumor cells and virally infected cells without prior sensitization. Hence, they are called NK cells. Two cell-surface molecules, CD16 and CD56, are widely used to identify NK cells.

Cytokines

These are the substances that regulate the immunologic, inflammatory, and reparative host responses and comprise previously designated lymphokines (lymphocyte derived), monokines (monocyte derived), and several other polypeptides.

Complement System

The cell-killing effects of innate and acquired immunity are mediated in part by a system of plasma enzymes originally named the complement system. Complement activation occurs in two phases, viz. the activation of C3 component followed by activation of the attack or lytic sequence. The critical event is a cleavage of C3 by complement-derived enzymes termed *C3 convertases*. The major fragment (C3b) of activated C3 mediates a number of vital biological activities.

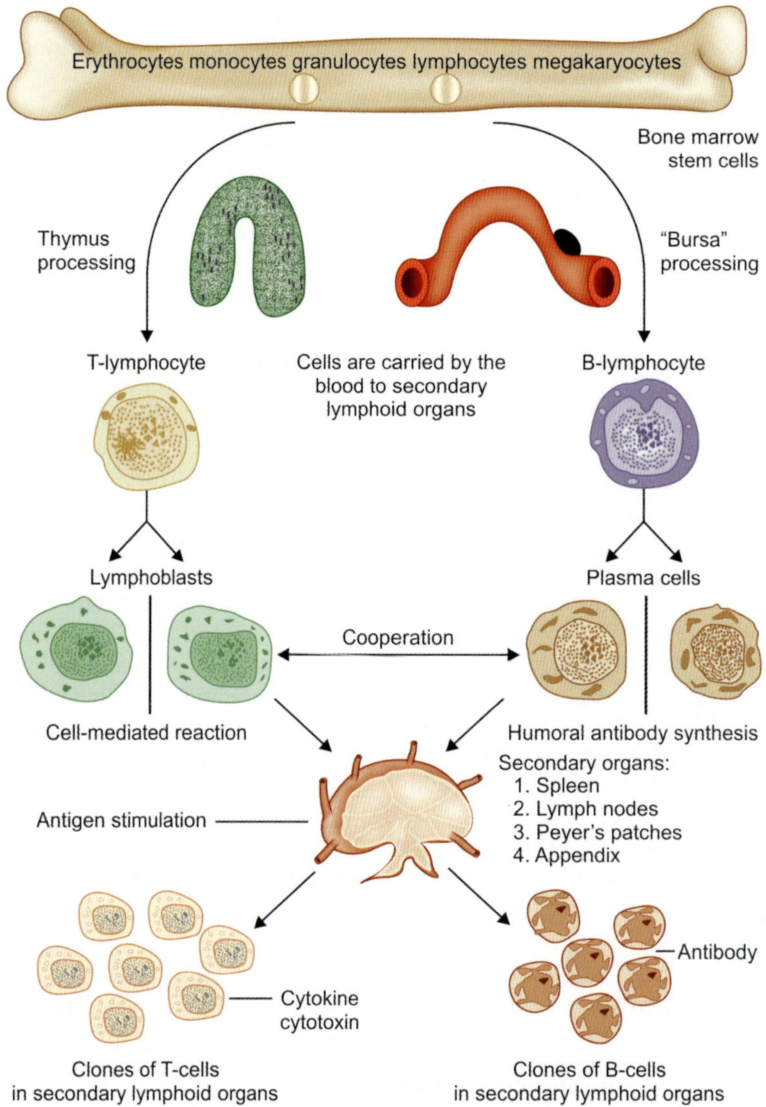

Fig. 5.1.2: Cellular and humoral immunity.

Two different pathways or enzyme cascades activate the system: (1) the *classic pathway,* triggered by immune complexes, and (2) the *alternative or properdin pathway,* triggered by contact with various viruses, bacteria, fungi, and tumor cells. These proteins have two functions:

1. They help killing invading organisms by opsonization, chemotaxis, and eventual lysis of the cells.
2. They serve in part as a bridge between innate to acquired immunity by activating B-cells.

Antigen-presenting Cells and Dendritic Cells

Antigen-presenting cells (APCs) are the cells that capture antigens by endocytosis or phagocytosis, process them into small peptides, display them at their surface through major histocompatibility complex (MHC) molecules, and provide costimulation signals that act synergistically to activate antigen-specific T-cells. Antigen-presenting cells include B-cells, macrophages, and DCs, although only the DCs are capable of activating naive T-cells.

Dendritic cells are major APCs in the body in addition to the B-cells and the macrophages. The major role of these cells is to identify dangers, which is done by the special receptors on the APC named Toll-like receptors (TLRs).

Antigens are taken up by immature DCs activated by the local inflammation, which provides the signals required for their migration to draining lymph nodes. During this migration, DCs mature and their surface expression of molecules changes. DCs sense "danger signals" through their TLRs and respond by a modulation of their surface or secreted molecules. Simultaneously, antigens are processed into small fragments and displayed at the cell surface in the grooves of *MHC-human leukocyte antigen (HLA)* molecules in humans. As a rule, MHC class I molecules present peptides from antigens that are produced within infected cells, whereas phagocytosed antigens are displayed on MHC class II molecules. Thus mature DCs reaching the T-cell zone of lymph nodes display MHC-peptide complexes and high levels of costimulation molecules at their surface. CD4+ T-cells recognize antigenic peptides displayed by class II MHC molecules, whereas CD8+ T-cells bind to class I MHC-peptide complexes.

Antigen-specific TCRs may only bind to specific MHC molecules (e.g. HLA-A2), which differ among individuals and populations. Consequently, T-cell responses are highly variable within a population.

IMMUNE RESPONSE

The response mounted by the body is called immune response, and it consists of producing either proteins called antibodies as in *humoral response* or specific cells as in *cellular response*. Both these with the help from other cells such as neutrophils, monocytes, macrophages as well as chemicals like complements and other cytokines elaborated by immune cells lead to the ultimate clearance of the invading organism. The immune response is both specific and highly effective, e.g. anti-measles antibodies do not react with varicella virus and vice versa.

Antigen has specific site to which the antibody binds is called epitope. There are multiple epitopes on the same antigen, and there are multiple antigens on the same organism. Accordingly, the immune system mounts multiple antibodies to the same organism. Only some of these antibodies are actually protective in nature and the rest are not useful in this sense. In general, viruses contain lesser number of antigens than bacteria, fungi, or parasites.

Specific Immunity

This is the most important arm of immune system as proved by the fact that defects in this pathway are often life threatening in nature. Except for the transplacental transfer of immunoglobulin, which offers protection to the newborn for a temporary period of time, it is not fully active at birth and develops gradually after birth on repeated exposure to the microbes in the surrounding. It can be divided into *natural versus acquired, passive versus active, and humoral versus cellular*.

The most important cells of this arm include the B-lymphocytes, T-lymphocytes, and their various subsets. On activation by an antigen the B-cells proliferate and get converted to plasma cells, which in turn produce the antibodies. Approximately 10% of the lymphocytes in the blood consist of B-cells, and they reside mostly in the peripheral lymphoid organs. For the effective production of antibodies, B-cells need help from T-helper cells.

On the other hand, T-cells lead to cellular response and mature in thymus. The cellular response involves the T-cells, macrophages, and lymphokines, which are secreted by the lymphocytes and act as signal for communication between many of these immune cells.

Humoral Immune Response

This arm is mediated by the production of antibodies against the specific antigens on the microbes. The antibodies consist of heavy chains and light chains. There are two types of light chains: lambda and kappa chains, whereas there are five different types of heavy chains which identify the five types of immunoglobulins, IgG, IgM, IgA, IgD, and IgE. Of this, IgG, IgM, and IgA are protective against pathogens. IgE may play a role against parasites and is also involved in allergies.

During acute infection, IgM antibodies appear within a few days, peak at around 7–10 days and disappear in next few months to undetected levels. Hence, the presence of IgM indicates recent infection. Similarly, IgM being a large molecule is not transferred transplacentally in a newborn. Hence, the presence of IgM antibodies indicates congenital infection in the newborn. The IgM response is usually seen in primary response. It is short lived, and the titers of the antibodies are lower.

Immunoglobulin G response usually picks up along with IgM, or after a few days, peaks it around 2–3 weeks, and lasts for a very long time. It is usually seen best during the secondary response, classically seen on reexposure, and the titers are very high.

Immunoglobulin A response depends upon the route and the type of infection. Serum IgA is seen in organisms that invade from mucosa, whereas surface IgA is classically seen with localized mucosal infections such as in cholera, respiratory syncytial virus infection, etc.

Primary versus Secondary Immune Response

When the antigen is introduced for the first time, the immune system responds primarily after a lag phase of up to 10 days. On reintroduction of the same antigen, there is no lag phase and the immune system responds by producing antibodies immediately, and this is called secondary response. There are some basic differences in both these responses. Primary response has lag phase, is of predominantly IgM type, is short lived, and the titers are low. As compared, the secondary response is almost immediate, is of IgG type, is long lasting, and the titers are very high. These differences are more with the antigens stimulating both B-cells and T-cells.

Sometimes, there is a *negative phase* where there is transient drop in the antibody levels immediately after the infection. The significance of this negative phase is not well known. Repeated exposure of the same antigen leads to more maturation of the immune response with better affinity and avidity of the antibodies, and a longer time till anamnestic response occurs. Affinity is the force with which the antigen-binding site on the antibody bonds with the epitopes and such combined forces lead to avidity. High-affinity and avidity antibodies are very useful in controlling infections.

T-cell-dependent Immune Response

Certain antigens, mainly proteins, induce both B-cell and T-cell stimulation leading to what is called T-cell-dependent immune response, whereas large molecular antigens like polysaccharides induce only B-cell response as they are incapable of inducing T-cell response on their own.

The *T-cell-dependent response* is usually prompt with higher titers, IgG type, and longer lasting. It also shows booster effects with repeated exposure. Infants of 6 weeks of age onward are capable of T-cell-dependent responses. Lastly, IgA antibodies are also produced in such response which probably helps in providing mucosal protection and eradicating the carrier state. As compared to this, T-cell-independent response being only B-cell mediated. It is predominantly IgM type with low titers. The response is short lived and does not lead to boosting, and such vaccines are actually revaccination rather than boosters when given repeatedly which produces the same type of response every time the antigen is introduced. Lastly, IgA is not produced, and hence, there is no local mucosal protection with this type of antigens.

A T-cell-independent antigen like polysaccharide can be converted to T-cell-dependent antigen by the technique of conjugation where a carrier protein is conjugated with the polysaccharide. When this conjugated moiety is presented to the T-cell, it recognizes the protein carrier as an antigen and leads to internalization of the whole complex, which leads to the T-cell now responding even to the carbohydrate antigen of the complex, producing T-cell response to the polysaccharide. This technique is very useful in producing vaccines such as conjugated Hib, pneumococcal, typhoid, and meningococcal vaccines.

Cell-mediated Immunity

This type of immunity is transferable by the lymphocytes and not by antibodies and is mediated via T-cells. T-cell lymphocyte is a very important cell in the immune response. It has many subsets which carry out different functions. These cells are in circulation and in the lymphatic vessels. There are three essential subsets: helper T-cells, suppressor T-cells, and cytotoxic T-cells. T-helper cells are CD4 positive and help the B-lymphocytes proliferate and produce antibodies.

T-suppressor cells suppress various immune responses, and cytotoxic T-cells lead to the lysis of the infected macrophages and cancer cells. Both the suppressor and cytotoxic T-cells are CD8 positive. T-cell response is very important for T-cell-dependent humoral response as discussed before and for immunity against certain organisms which are essentially intercellular pathogens such as *Mycobacterium tuberculosis, Mycobacterium leprae,* fungal infections, etc. They are also important in surveillance against malignant cells. The patients with T-cell deficiency suffer from opportunistic infections which are intracellular like tuberculosis and fungal infection as well as peculiar cancers such as Kaposi's sarcoma in an HIV-infected person. T-cells communicate with one another and with other types of cells through the production and release of substances called lymphokines.

Passive Immunity

Passive immunity is specific immunity which is transferred passively to the recipient. It gives ready-made immunoglobulins, which helps to fight infection immediately. However, it is for a temporary period, and it wanes after few weeks to few months depending upon the half-life of the transferred immunoglobulins. In addition to the natural transplacental passive transfer of the immunoglobulins in the newborn, the other examples of the passive immunity are infusing immunoglobulins in the person to protect him for a specific disease.

Transplacental Passive Immunity

The most common form of passive immunity is that given to the newborn from the mother. Immunoglobulins are transferred predominantly in the last trimester and are mainly of IgG type. This means that at birth the child will have similar type of antibody pattern as the mother. This protects the child for first few months till the time she/he develops her/his own immunity after repeated exposure to various antigens after birth. The protection offered by transplacental passive immunity depends on the half-life of the specific antibody, e.g. the antibody against poliomyelitis does not protect child for more than 4–6 weeks (the time of starting the polio vaccination in the baby), whereas the anti-measles antibody protects the child till 6–9 months (the reason for delaying the measles vaccine till 9 months). Not only does the passive immunity protect the child against the specific diseases, it also interferes with the immune response to the concerned vaccine, if given in the presence of maternal antibody such as for measles as discussed before.

Acquired Passive Immunity

Immunoglobulins can be passively transferred by giving immunoglobulin preparation intramuscularly (IM) or intravenously (IV). It can also be done inadvertently by infusing blood and blood products which will also infuse immune globulins which may interfere with some live vaccines such as measles vaccine. There are three types of preparations which will lead to passive transfer of the immune globulins. They are (1) pooled human immunoglobulin preparation, (2) homologous hyperimmune globulin, and (3) heterologous hyperimmune globulin preparation.

Pooled Human Immunoglobulins

This is prepared by pooled plasma from more than 100 healthy donors and fractionation of this plasma to produce the final product, which is available as IM as well as IV preparation. As it contains a variety of antibodies, it is ideally suitable for replacement therapy in congenital and acquired immune deficiency with antibody deficiency. It is also used in many autoimmune disorders. It is also used for passive prophylaxis for measles or hepatitis A infection.

Homologous Hyperimmune Globulins

This is obtained by pooling plasma from specific donors who have high titers of a specific antibody either due to repeated past natural exposure or due to vaccination. This preparation serves to protect against a specific disease. Of course, it will also have other types of antibodies, albeit to a lesser extent. They are used for prophylaxis of diseases such as hepatitis B, tetanus, varicella, or rabies.

Heterologous Hyperimmune Globulins

These were used in past to prevent diseases, such as rabies or tetanus. It is obtained from animals mainly horse or rabbit, who are hyperimmunized by repeated vaccination against the concerned disease and then collecting plasma which is fractionated to obtain pure product. Being an animal product, it can lead to severe allergic reactions including anaphylaxis, anaphylactoid reactions, or serum sickness.

Active Immunity

Active immunity is developed by stimulating the immune system by antigens which can lead to specific humoral or cellular immune response, or both. It can happen in two ways, either by exposure to the wild pathogen naturally where the immunity develops after the person suffers from the disease which has chances of morbidity and even mortality; or by exposure to the antigens given as vaccines where the person has least morbidity and the person becomes immune without much suffering. Not all the natural diseases lead to protective immunity like in natural tetanus or typhoid where repeated clinical courses are known unless vaccination is done. Most of the time, natural disease leads to strong protective immunity which probably lasts lifelong, e.g. in measles or varicella. Vaccination on the other hand is the introduction of antigens with the purpose of inducing immune response without leading to clinical disease.

ACKNOWLEDGMENTS

Parts of this chapter including the figures are adapted from Chapter 20.1 "Basics of Immune System in Children" by Keya R Lahiri and Roshani N Taori from the 4th edition of the *IAP Textbook of Pediatrics*.

BIBLIOGRAPHY

1. Chaplin DD. Overview of the immune response. J Allergy Clin Immunol. 2010;125:S3-23.
2. Lahiri KR, Taori RN. Basics of immune system in children. In: Parthasarathy A, Menon PSN, Nair MKC (Eds). IAP Textbook of Pediatrics, 4th edition. New Delhi: Jaypee Brothers Medical Publishers (P) Ltd; 2009. pp. 1080-4.
3. Paul Y, Vashishtha VM. Immunology of vaccines: basics and beyond. In: Vashishtha VM, Kalra A, Thacker N (Eds). FAQs on Immunization, 1st edition. New Delhi: Jaypee Brothers Medical Publishers (P) Ltd; 2011. pp. 3-23.
4. Shah NK, Thacker N. General principles of vaccination. In: Thacker N, Shah NK (Eds). Immunization in Clinical Practice. New Delhi: Jaypee Brothers Medical Publishers (P) Ltd; 2005. pp. 1-5.

5.2 Primary Immunodeficiency Disorders

Tanu Singhal

INTRODUCTION

Primary immunodeficiency disorders (PIDs) are inheritable genetic disorders that disrupt immune cells either quantitatively or qualitatively in the performance of their functions. They occur at an incidence of 1 in 2,000 live births and are often underdiagnosed or diagnosed late. Early diagnosis, correct classification, and appropriate treatment is essential to reduce morbidity and mortality. More than 150 PIDs have been described; this section gives a bird's eye view of the common ones.

Primary immunodeficiency disorders are broadly classified as:

- Humoral immunodeficiencies
- Cellular immunodeficiencies
- Combined humoral and cellular immunodeficiencies
- Disorders of phagocyte function
- Disorders of the complement system.

HUMORAL IMMUNODEFICIENCIES

These are the most common PIDs and account for half of all cases.

Agammaglobulinemia

The earliest recognized immunodeficiency disorder, *Bruton's agammaglobulinemia* (X-linked inheritance), is characterized by severe depletion of circulating β-cells and very low levels of immunoglobulin G (IgG), IgM, and IgA. Another variant is inherited autosomal recessive. Most children present by late infancy with severe and recurrent ear, nose, and throat (ENT) as well as airway infections and susceptibility to severe enteroviral meningitis. Treatment consists of lifelong immunoglobulin replacement therapy and antibiotic therapy. Live vaccines, such as oral polio vaccine, are absolutely contraindicated in these children and their close contacts.

Class-switch Immunoglobulin Deficiencies

Class-switch immunoglobulin deficiencies (earlier known as hyper-IgM syndromes and now reclassified as combined immunodeficiencies) are characterized by low levels of IgG and IgA and normal or high levels of IgM. There is associated T-cell deficiency and neutropenia and propensity for severe pneumocystis infections in addition to respiratory bacterial infections.

Common Variable Immunodeficiency

Common variable immunodeficiency is characterized by levels of IgG below two standard deviations of normal, in the presence of decreased IgA and/or IgM levels, recurrent infections, impaired response to immunization, exclusion of defined causes of hypogammaglobulinemia, and an age above 2 years. These patients present in late childhood or young adulthood with recurrent ENT and airway infections, granulomatous inflammation of the lungs and gastrointestinal tract, chronic diarrhea, hematological malignancies, and endocrine growth problems.

Transient Hypogammaglobulinemia of Infancy

Transient hypogammaglobulinemia of infancy is characterized by delay in the production of immunoglobulins after disappearance of maternal immunoglobulins. Many cases are asymptomatic; others may have recurrent airway infections, severe sepsis, meningitis, recurrent diarrhea, oral candidiasis, and severe varicella infection. Antibody levels normalize by 2 years in most. Treatment consisting mainly of antibiotic prophylaxis and immunoglobulin replacement is indicated only in those with severe infections.

Selective Immunoglobulin A Deficiency, Specific Immunoglobulin G2 Subclass Deficiency, and Specific Antipolysaccharide Deficiency

Selective IgA deficiency, specific IgG2 subclass deficiency, and specific antipolysaccharide deficiency (SPAD) are the most common immunodeficiency disorders and usually occur in combination. The SPAD is diagnosed by impaired response to pneumococcal polysaccharide vaccine in children above 2 years and should be suspected in the setting of repeated infections when all other immunodeficiencies are ruled out. These disorders may be asymptomatic or present with recurrent airway infections and in IgA deficiency with chronic diarrhea due to giardiasis.

CELLULAR IMMUNODEFICIENCIES

Disorder of Interferon-γ or Interleukin-12 Axis

Disorder of interferon-γ (IFN-γ) or interleukin-12 axis presents with disseminated infections due to bacillus Calmette-Guérin, nontuberculous mycobacteria, *Mycobacterium tuberculosis, Salmonella typhi*, nontyphoidal *Salmonella*, or severe herpes virus infections. All the screening tests for B- and T-cell functions are normal. Markedly elevated serum IFN-γ levels may be used as a screening test. Treatment involves regular administration of subcutaneous IFN-γ or in some cases with hematopoietic stem cell transplant (HSCT).

Chronic Mucocutaneous Candidiasis

Chronic mucocutaneous candidiasis is characterized by recurrent candidiasis of skin, nails, and mucous membranes, and in some with autoimmune endocrinopathy. Systemic or invasive candidiasis is rare. Treatment is with prolonged administration of antifungal agents.

Natural Killer Cell Defects

Natural killer (NK) cell defects are characterized by severe susceptibility to herpes viral infections (cytomegalovirus, Epstein-Barr virus (EBV), varicella zoster virus, and herpes simplex virus). These patients benefit with chemoprophylaxis with antiviral drugs.

Idiopathic CD4 Lymphocytopenia

Idiopathic CD4 lymphocytopenia is an illness characterized by opportunistic infections in patients with a CD4 count less than 300 cells/μL and absence of human immunodeficiency virus (HIV) by serologic and molecular tests.

Management is by antimicrobial prophylaxis.

COMBINED IMMUNODEFICIENCIES

Severe Combined Immunodeficiency

Severe combined immunodeficiency (SCID) is a group of syndromes of differing genetic basis characterized by complete lack of specific lymphocyte-dependent adaptive immunity. These children present in the first few months of life with recurrent, persistent, severe and disseminated bacterial, viral, or fungal infections and failure to thrive, diarrhea, and rashes. There is absence of lymphoid tissue and no thymic shadow on the radiograph. There is severe lymphopenia and depletion of all lymphocyte subpopulations with panhypogammaglobulinemia. Severe combined immunodeficiency is a medical emergency, and patients need to be referred for HSCT to a specialist center as soon as possible.

Wiskott-Aldrich Syndrome

Wiskott-Aldrich syndrome is characterized by eczema, bleeding complications due to thrombocytopenia with small platelet size, recurrent and severe infections, autoimmune disease, and tendency for EBV-related lymphoma. Treatment options include gammaglobulin replacement, antibiotic prophylaxis, splenectomy, and finally best medical treatment.

Ataxia Telangiectasia

Ataxia telangiectasia-related disorders are characterized by ocular telangiectasia, ataxia, and recurrent severe bacterial respiratory infections. There is an increased tendency for malignancy owing to chromosomal fragility. The presence of acanthocytes in the peripheral smear is a diagnostic pointer.

DiGeorge Syndrome

DiGeorge syndrome is characterized by thymic hypoplasia, hypoparathyroidism, and structural cardiac defects. The immune deficiency is variable, and very severe lymphopenia is rare.

PHAGOCYTE DEFECTS

Chronic Granulomatous Disease

The most prominent defect of phagocyte function is *chronic granulomatous disease* occurring at a rate of 1:200,000 births, mostly inherited as X-linked recessive inheritance, and is due to the defect in the neutrophil oxidative burst. It is characterized by recurrent skin, soft tissue and lymph node infections, and granulomatous abscesses in internal organs. Commonly implicated organisms are *Staphylococcus aureus, Aspergillus, Serratia, Nocardia, Candida*, and *Burkholderia*. In India, it is commonly misdiagnosed as tuberculosis due to the presence of granulomas on histopathology. Diagnosis is by the estimation of neutrophil oxidase activity, and treatment includes cotrimoxazole prophylaxis, itraconazole prophylaxis, use of IFN-γ, and finally HSCT.

Chédiak-Higashi Syndrome

Chédiak-Higashi syndrome presents with recurrent infections of skin, respiratory tract with oculocutaneous albinism, neurologic defects, and propensity to develop an immunoproliferative disease.

Leukocyte Adhesion Deficiency

Leukocyte adhesion deficiency (LAD 1 and 2) presents with delayed separation of umbilical cord (LAD 1), recurrent cellulitis and abscesses with the absence of pus formation, severe periodontitis, and characteristic facies (LAD 2). There

complicated, expensive, and not readily available. It is crucial to develop regional referral centers that can evaluate and treat patients with primary immune deficiency disorders.

BIBLIOGRAPHY

1. Bonilla FA, Bernstein IL, Khan DA, et al. Practice parameter for the diagnosis and management of primary immunodeficiency. Ann Allergy Asthma Immunol. 2005;94:S1-63.
2. Desai M, Currimbhoy Z (2010). Primary immunodeficiency disorders in India. Electronic Publication. [online] Available from: http://sites.google.com/site/mmdesai007/. [Accessed October, 2018].
3. Driessen G, Van der Burg M. Educational paper: primary antibody deficiencies. Eur J Pediatr. 2011;170:693-702.
4. Morimoto Y, Routes JM. Immunodeficiency overview. Prim Care. 2008;35:159-73.

5.3 The Principles and Practice of Immunization

T Jacob John

ACTIVE IMMUNIZATION

The induction of immune response by the deliberate inoculation of appropriate immunogen(s) in the form of a vaccine is termed as active immunization or simply immunization or vaccination. In practice, this term applies to the inoculation of vaccine, regardless of the success or failure of inducing the desired immune response.

PASSIVE IMMUNIZATION

The injection of preformed antibodies to a specific antigen, in the form of "antiserum" or "immune globulin," is termed as passive immunization. The term "gammaglobulin" is used to denote that the product is not "hyperimmune" to any specific antigen but contains antibodies to all common antigens encountered by adults from whom plasma had been collected for its extraction. The physiological transfer of immunoglobulins across the placenta to the fetus from the mother provides natural passive immunity to the infant.

ANTISERA AND IMMUNE GLOBULINS

Antisera prepared in horses against tetanus toxin, diphtheria toxin, rabies virus, and snake venom is widely used in India. Horse serum may cause hypersensitivity reactions including anaphylaxis and serum sickness. The active principle is immunoglobulins; hence, unwanted components such as albumin may be removed and more concentrated "hyperimmune" equine immunoglobulins may be prepared. Even with such preparations, hypersensitivity remains a problem. The fragment crystallizable (Fc) part of immunoglobulins are responsible for such responses and removing Fc portion while preserving the antigen-binding fragment portion has become the standard practice in presenting equine hyperimmune immunoglobulins against rabies and hepatitis B viruses (HBVs).

Homologous products prepared from pooled human plasma are safer and more potent, but also more expensive. Human immune globulins against tetanus, rabies, and HBV are available in India; elsewhere other preparations are available, e.g. *varicella-zoster* immune globulin. Apart from these antigen-specific products, human gammaglobulin preparations are available for intramuscular (IM) and intravenous injection either as replacement in hypogammaglobulinemia or for therapeutic purposes in certain specific autoimmune disorders.

IMMUNE SYSTEM AND RESPONSES

A network of cells with the functions of detection of any microbial (foreign) elements and of specific immune responses to them, and organized within specific tissues (lymph nodes, spleen, thymus, bone marrow, and several submucosal tissues), constitute the immune system. These cells include dendritic cells and macrophages that recognize and interact with pathogen-associated molecular patterns (PAMP) or detect and ingest microbes, and process and present the immunogenic epitopes to T- and B-lymphocytes; T- and B-cells are thus stimulated to respond. T-cells have subsets. CD4-positive T-helper (Th) cells of Th-1 pathway regulate cell-mediated immunity (CMI) through cytotoxic lymphocytes, which are CD8 positive. Th-2 pathway regulates antibody production by B-cells and their activated progeny called plasma cells. Th-17 cells modulate autoimmunity (antibody-related). Humoral immunity is mediated through immunoglobulins (antibodies) which belong to class IgM, IgG, IgA, IgD, and IgE. When stimulated, B-cells transform into plasma cells and secrete antibodies. After adequate stimulation of the regulatory (T-cells) and effector cells (T- and B-cells), memory cells (T- and B-cells) survive for very long periods, ready to respond rapidly to the same immunogens, if reintroduced (anamnestic response).

Microbial infection is the prototype of immune stimulation; many vaccines contain attenuated infectious organisms. Being intracellularly placed, they tend to be strong inducers of CMI in addition to humoral immunity. To nonreplicating antigens (killed microbes/subunits containing PAMP), the initial response is weak and slow (mainly IgM), but the immune system gets "primed," ready for anamnestic (booster) responses (mainly IgG) that are greater and brisker than primary response. Such vaccines require one or two priming doses and one or more boosting doses (prime-boost principle).

Protein antigens stimulate T-cells to regulate immune responses, resulting in sequential secretion of IgM, IgA, and IgG by plasma cells and in development of memory cells. Polysaccharide antigens are T-cell independent but can directly stimulate B-cells and induce only IgM secretion without establishing memory cells. B-cells mature to directly respond in this manner only after the child is about 2 years old.

Mucosal immunization (with live-attenuated viruses or bacteria) induces mucosal (secretory) IgA responses in addition to systemic immunity. Mucosal protection from infection is mediated through several factors, and local/secretory IgA is only one of them. Humoral IgG, IgM, and IgA do reach mucosal surfaces by passive transport (or spill over) and mediate microbial binding or viral neutralization.

Most immune responses (natural and vaccine-induced) are not necessarily protective against infection, but prevent disease when exposed. When reinfected, immune persons shed less quantum of pathogen for shorter duration than in the nonimmune, resulting in less transmission and epidemiological herd effect (less frequency of disease even in the unvaccinated); this is the basis of vaccination in public health, in which every individual need not be targeted for immunization.

VACCINES IN CURRENT USE

The vaccines licensed in India include live-attenuated bacteria (bacillus Calmette-Guérin or BCG; *Salmonella typhi* Ty21a), live-attenuated viruses (oral polio vaccine or OPV, trivalent, monovalent types 1, 2, and 3; and bivalent 1 and 3; measles, mumps, rubella, varicella, Japanese encephalitis, rotavirus, and hepatitis A), killed bacteria (*Bordetella pertussis*, killed *Vibrio cholerae*), polysaccharides (pneumococcal capsular antigens with 23 serotypes; *S. typhi* Vi; meningococcal capsular antigens), protein-conjugated polysaccharides (*Haemophilus influenzae* type b, Hib) antigen conjugated with different proteins; pneumococcal conjugated antigens of 10 or 13 serotypes, conjugated meningococcal vaccine, conjugated *S. typhi* Vi, killed viruses (rabies, polioviruses, hepatitis A, Japanese encephalitis, influenza, and Kyasanur Forest disease), structural subunits (HBV, human papilloma virus), or antigen components (acellular pertussis). Killed poliovirus vaccine is also called inactivated polio vaccine (IPV). Many are presented in combinations such as diphtheria pertussis tetanus (DPT), measles and rubella (MR), measles, mumps, and rubella (MMR), MMR with varicella, DPT-HBV, DPT-Hib, DPT-HBV-Hib (pentavalent), and DPT-HBV-Hib-IPV (hexavalent).

Immunization Schedules

Refer to "Chapter 5.4 Rationale of Immunization Schedules" for details of National Immunization Schedule and Indian Academy of Pediatrics (IAP) Immunization Timetable.

LOGISTICS OF IMMUNIZATION

Immunization in Preventive Medicine and Public Health Modes

Pediatricians immunize children in healthcare setting, choosing vaccines after risk assessment and with concurrence of parents, with cost borne by parents. The IAP immunization schedule illustrates the choice of vaccines in preventive medicine mode. The Immunization Division under Ministry of Health provides a selected subset of licensed vaccines and provides them free of charge, under Universal Immunization Program (UIP). The purpose of UIP is to control target diseases, in many cases taking advantage of herd effect (reduced incidence in unvaccinated segment of population). Elimination of wild polioviruses through intensive immunization was achieved in 2011 and so certified in 2014, illustrating the power of immunization in public health. Currently, measles is targeted for elimination. As MR vaccine is used, rubella will also be eliminated when vaccine coverage reaches the level required for achieving zero transmission of measles virus. However, the goal is to eliminate congenital rubella infection and the national program is called "measles elimination and rubella control."

Supply of Vaccines

Vaccines are allowed to be marketed in India, only after licensing by the National Regulatory Authority (Drugs Controller General of India, DCGI). Every batch of vaccine manufactured in India or imported is checked for quality assurance by the Central Research Institute (at Kasauli) of the Directorate General of Health Services. All UIP vaccines are centrally purchased by the Department of Family Welfare and distributed to the governments of all states and union territories. Pediatricians are allowed to collect all UIP vaccines from the local area health authority without any charge, to be given to children according to the national schedule. Vaccine utilization must be accounted for by returning the list of beneficiaries. Although UIP has this policy, in some places, the local officers face difficulties in accounting for vaccines shared with the private sector.

Vaccines outside the UIP list (and those on the UIP list) are available for purchase from various vaccine distributors.

Cold Chain

All vaccines are susceptible to loss of potency, when exposed to warm temperatures, but are very stable at 2–8°C. Lyophilized vaccines (BCG, measles, and MMR) and nonadjuvanted liquid vaccines (OPV) are also stable when frozen. Adjuvanted vaccines (DPT and HBV) lose potency, when frozen. If they accidentally freeze, they should be rejected. Vaccines should be used within their date of expiry.

The system of transporting, distributing, and storing vaccines from the manufacturer right up to the point of use under refrigeration is referred to as the cold chain. In clinics, vaccines must be stored in a refrigerator, which maintains the inside temperature between 4°C and 8°C. If temperature falls below 3°C, there is a chance for some vaccines to freeze solid. Where vaccines are maintained in the cold chain in clinics, multidose vials can be used to reduce cost. Partially used vials of vaccines allowed under "open vial policy" must be maintained under cold conditions for later use. However, care should be taken to disinfect the top before puncturing the vial.

Reconstituted lyophilized vaccines (BCG, measles, MMR, varicella, and Hib) should be used immediately after reconstitution; open vial policy does not apply to them. Multidose BCG or measles vaccine may be used over a few hours, preferably 4 hours but maximum 6 hours; during the interim, they should not be frozen, but kept cold and not exposed to bright light. Any leftover contents must be discarded after 6 hours.

Techniques of Vaccination

Every pediatrician must familiarize oneself with the descriptive leaflet supplied by the vaccine manufacturer and also with the techniques of inoculation, side effects, and contraindications, if any.

When OPV is given, the nose of the infant should not be pinched in order to make the infant open the mouth. Instead, a slight pressure may be applied on both the cheeks, between upper and lower jaws, using the thumb and a finger. There is no need to withhold breastfeeding for long periods before or after giving OPV; in practice, a gap of 10–15 minutes is usually observed to breastfeed after OPV.

Bacillus Calmette–Guérin must be given intradermally; the preferred site is the lateral aspect of the convex region of the left shoulder. IPV given as fractional dose intradermally the site should be the right shoulder, so that by recall of site the vaccine could be identified. In infancy, IM injections are given in the anterolateral aspect of the thigh. Subcutaneous (SC) injections may be given into the tissue targeted by pinching the skinfold over the muscle. Hepatitis B viruses, or indeed any vaccine, should not be given in the gluteus. In older children, the deltoid muscle is often chosen for IM injections and the thigh, deltoid, or triceps region for SC injections.

There is no need to warm the vaccine vial in the hands before it is drawn in the syringe or given in the mouth. Frozen OPV needs to be just thawed before giving.

Adverse Reactions and Contraindications

All licensed vaccines except OPV are virtually/completely safe products. However, many vaccines do cause some adverse reactions, most of which are temporary, self-limited, and inconsequential. Specific contraindications are very few. Minor illnesses are not a contraindication to giving any vaccine. However, if the nature of illness is not clear, caution must be exercised in order to avoid the vaccine from being blamed for the worsening of an illness. Immunization is better postponed when there is any illness that requires treatment, unless access to the infant is difficult later or there is an outbreak of illness, e.g. measles. Every clinic or hospital visit or admission must be used as an opportunity to assess the immunization needs of the child and to offer any pending doses.

No gastrointestinal or systemic reactions occur after giving OPV. Mild diarrhea may occur after feeding rotavirus vaccine. On rare occasions, vaccine-associated paralytic polio (VAPP) has been documented, either in the vaccine recipient or in contacts in the vicinity. Its frequency in India appears to be more common than previously thought; adults are not at risk in India, since virtually all the adults are immune due to prior asymptomatic infections. Since hypogammaglobulinemia has been noted as a risk factor for VAPP, the recommendation is to give the noninfectious IPV to immunodeficient children and any of their family members. Oral polio vaccine is usually given to infants born to human immunodeficiency virus (HIV)-infected mothers whether or not they themselves are HIV infected without problems. Bacillus Calmette-Guérin is contraindicated in infants known to be HIV infected. In practice, many infected but untested infants get BCG but do not come to any harm.

Diphtheria pertussis tetanus vaccine causes local inflammation and fever in a proportion of vaccines. Paracetamol is advised only after fever develops but not prophylactically, as it may reduce immune response. If any neurological reactions other than febrile convulsions are observed within days after DPT, the infant must be carefully assessed for any preexisting disease process. There is no evidence that DPT per se causes any neurological illness; in specific instances of difficulty, expert opinion must be obtained and discussed with the family before continuing or discontinuing further doses of DPT. In such a situation, one option is to offer DPT containing acellular P component.

The immunization clinic staff must be trained to recognize vasovagal syncopal attacks and anaphylaxis in vaccinated infants/children. While it is true that rural health workers vaccinate at convenient places in the villages where there are no facilities for resuscitation, the immunization clinic must be equipped to handle such events. Any serious event, not recognized as the usual side reaction of the vaccine, must be reported to the local area health authority. Any illness occurring within a month after vaccination is to be considered adverse event following immunization (AEFI). Serious AEFI includes illness requiring hospitalization, which may result in chronic disability or death. In UIP, serious AEFI must be reported to the district immunization officer; AEFI following non-UIP vaccines should be reported also to the DCGI. This rule does not mean that such events are caused by the vaccine. On the other hand, it is in the best interests of the child and also to detect any problem with vaccine quality.

EFFECT OF IMMUNIZATION ON DISEASE EPIDEMIOLOGY

Herd Effect and Herd Immunity

Only the immunized child is directly benefitted; the unimmunized peers remain fully susceptible to infection and disease, when exposed. However, as increasing proportions of children in a community are immunized against a disease, the transmission/circulation of the infectious agent may be retarded; hence, the incidence of disease may decline even in the unimmunized segment of the childhood population. This benefit is confined to vaccines against human-to-human transmitted pathogens. This phenomenon is called the herd effect. Immunization in public health mode takes advantage of herd effect for disease control. Elimination is extreme control; global level of elimination is eradication.

The term *herd immunity* refers to the proportion of individuals in the population that have immunity due to immunization (and also due to natural infection, if so defined for investigational purpose). As immunization coverage increases, herd immunity increases and herd effect may become manifest. Herd effect can be recognized, only if the incidence of disease is measured before, during, and after the immunization activities.

Method and Purpose of Pulse Immunization

An epidemic of an infectious disease reaches a peak and declines rapidly because of the very high herd immunity consequent upon the epidemic spread of the agent. The transmission may be interrupted soon after an epidemic. Only when sufficient numbers of susceptible children accumulate over time, the agent will reestablish itself in the community. This principle is applied in pulse immunization using live vaccines. When a large proportion of susceptible children are vaccinated in a short period of time, an epidemic is simulated. The consequent "herd effect" may result in break of transmission of the agent. For epidemic-prone diseases with more than 1 year of interepidemic intervals such as poliomyelitis and measles, the pulsing of the vaccine at annual intervals has been shown to be effective in disease control. The term pulse immunization is given to denote the repetitive campaigns at chosen intervals.

The herd effect of pulse immunization would be higher than the same volume of vaccine is given routinely throughout the year. In other words, better herd effect for the same herd immunity is achieved with annual pulse immunization. In the developing countries where the transmission of polioviruses was not interrupted in spite of high coverage with the routine use of OPV, pulse method was applied to interrupt it. Since measles virus is very contagious, it will be virtually impossible to interrupt its transmission without resorting to pulsing of vaccine at intervals that are shorter than the regional interepidemic intervals.

BIBLIOGRAPHY

1. Indian Academy of Pediatrics (2014). Indian Academy of Pediatrics (IAP) Recommended Immunization Schedule for Children Aged 0 through 18 years—India, 2014 and Updates on Immunization. [online] Available from: http://www.iapindia.org/immunization/immunization-schedule. [Accessed October, 2018].
2. John TJ, Samuel R. Herd immunity and herd effect: new insights and definitions. Eur J Epidemiol 2000;16:601-6.
3. World Health Organization (2014). Global and vaccine safety. [online] Available from: http://www.who.int/immunization_safety/publications/aefi/en/. [Accessed October, 2018].
4. World Health Organization South East Asia Region. [online] Available from: http://whoindia.org/en/Section6/Section284/Section286_508.htm. [Accessed October, 2018].

5.4 Rationale of Selection of Vaccines in National Immunization Program and Indian Academy of Pediatrics Immunization Timetable

Vijay N Yewale, Alok Gupta

RATIONALE OF THE SELECTION OF A VACCINATION SCHEDULE

The following factors are considered in the selection of a vaccination schedule:

- Age-specific burden of disease
- Age-specific immunologic response to vaccines
- Potential interference with the immune response by passively transferred maternal antibodies
- Age-specific risks of vaccine-associated complications
- Programmatic feasibility.

The basic schedule of 6-10-14 weeks for the primary doses of diphtheria, tetanus toxoids, and pertussis (DTP) and polio is followed by some developing countries including India due to high burden of disease from pertussis in very young infants. Most of the developed countries, such as the United States, use schedules (2-4-6 months) that start later in infancy and have longer intervals between doses. For killed vaccines, such as diphtheria, pertussis, and tetanus (DPT), *Haemophilus influenzae* type B (Hib), pneumococcal conjugate vaccine (PCV), and hepatitis B (HepB) which are administered as early as birth/6 weeks, the first dose acts only as a priming dose while subsequent doses provide an immune response even in presence of maternal antibodies. Booster dose at 18 months is required for sustaining the immunity. As the age of commencement of vaccination advances, the number of doses reduces for some antigens (e.g. two doses at 6-12 months, followed by a booster dose and 1-2 doses between 12 months and 23 months for Hib and PCV). Live vaccines are even more susceptible to maternal antibodies as compared to killed vaccines. However, bacillus Calmette-Guérin (BCG) vaccine may be given at the time of birth as the maternal antibodies actually enhance T-cell responses. Oral polio vaccine (OPV) may be given at birth as there is no maternal immunoglobulin A (IgA) in the gut to neutralize the virus. Furthermore, measles vaccine, if given at the age of 6 months (in an outbreak situation) may work by inducing T-cell immunity.

The World Health Organization (WHO) encourages countries to select vaccination schedules that are epidemiologically relevant, immunologically effective, operationally feasible, and socially acceptable. The expanded program on immunization (EPI) against six most common, preventable childhood diseases, viz. DPT, polio, tuberculosis, and measles, was launched by the WHO in 1974. The WHO recommendations are usually followed by the national governments who are member states of the United Nations.

IMMUNIZATION PROGRAM OF INDIA

The National Immunization Schedule (NIS) is prepared by the Ministry of Health and Family Welfare, it makes vaccines available free of cost and delivered through various central/state government agencies, health workers, and private practitioners. The National Technical Advisory Group on Immunization (NTAGI) is a group of experts from the Government of India (GoI), state governments, academic institutions, development partners, and professional organizations, who meet on an annual basis to discuss the technical and policy issues pertaining to the program and advice on the introduction of newer vaccines based on the available disease burden data. Any major immunization decision is first discussed by the NTAGI, and the recommendations given are then considered by the Program Division within the Ministry. Indian Academy of Pediatrics (IAP) is also represented through its national president who is an important member of this committee. The vaccines licensing authority in India, i.e. the National Regulatory Authority, is the Drugs Controller General of India (DCGI) approved by the WHO.

THE NATIONAL IMMUNIZATION SCHEDULE

The NIS is designed on the five criteria—(1) epidemiological relevance, (2) immunological appropriateness, (3) technical feasibility, (4) economic viability, and (5) sociocultural acceptability **(Table 5.4.1)**.

Table 5.4.1: National Immunization Schedule (NIS) for infants, children and pregnant women.

Vaccine	*When to give*	*Dose*	*Route*	*Site*
For pregnant women				
TT-1	Early in pregnancy	0.5 mL	Intramuscular	Upper arm
TT-2	4 weeks after TT-1*	0.5 mL	Intramuscular	Upper arm
TT-Booster	If received 2 TT doses in a pregancy within the last 3 years*	0.5 mL	Intramuscular	Upper arm
For infants				
BCG	At birth or as early as possible till one year of age	0.1 mL (0.05 mL until 1 month age)	Intradermal	Left upper arm
Hepatitis B—Birth dose	At birth or as early as possible within the first 24 h	0.5	Intramuscular	Anterolateral side of mid-thigh
OPV-0	At birth or as early as possible within the first 15 days	2 drops	Oral	Oral
OPV 1, 2 and 3	At 6 weeeks, 10 weeks and 14 weeks (can be given till 5 years of age)	2 drops	Oral	Oral
Pentavalent 1, 2 and 3	At 6 weeks, 10 weeks, and 14 weeks (can be given till one year of age)	0.5 mL	Intramuscular	Anterolateral side of midthigh
Rotavirus#	At 6 weeks, 10 weeks, and 14 weeks (can be given till one year of age)	5 drops	Oral	Oral
IPV	Two fractional doses at 6 and 14 weeks of age	0.1 mL	Intradermal two fractional dose	*Intradermal*: Right upper arm
Measles/MR 1st Dose$	9 completed months to 12 months. (can be given till 5 years of age)	0.5 mL	Subcutaneous	Right upper arm
JE-1**	9 completed months to 12 months.	0.5 mL	Subcutaneous	Left upper arm
Vitamin A (1st dose)	At 9 completed months with measles-Rubella	1 mL (1 lakh IU)	Oral	Oral
For children				
DPT booster-1	16–24 months	0.5 mL	Intramuscular	Anterolateral side of midthigh
Measles/MR 2nd dose$	16–24 months	0.5 mL	Subcutaneous	Right upper arm
OPV Booster	16–24 months	2 drops	Oral	Oral
JE-2	16–24 months	0.5 mL	Subcutaneous	Left upper arm
Vitamin A*** (2nd to 9th dose)	16–18 months. Then one dose every 6 months up to the age of 5 years	2 mL (2 lakh IU)	Oral	Oral
DPT Booster-2	5–6 years	0.5 mL	Intramuscular	Upper arm
TT	10 years and 16 years	0.5 mL	Intramuscular	Upper arm

*Give TT-2 Booster doses before 36 weeks of pregnancy. However, give these even if more than 36 weeks have passed. Give TT to a woman in labor, if she has not previously received TT.

**JE Vaccine is introduced in select endemic districts after the campaign.

***The 2nd to 9th dose of Vitamin A can be administered to children 1–5 years old during bilannual rounds, in collaboration with ICDS.

#Phased introduction, at present in Andhra Pradesh, Haryana, Himachal Pradesh and Orissa from 2016 & expanded in Madhya Pradesh, Assam, Rajasthan, and Tripura in February 2017 and planned in Tamil Nadu and Uttar Pradesh in 2017.

$Phased introduction, at present, in five states namely Karnataka, Tamil Nadu, Goa, Lakshadweep and Puducherry. (As of Feb 2017).

IMMUNIZATION COVERAGE IN INDIA

The National Family Health Survey IV (NFHS IV), conducted in 2015–2016, showed that there was a significant improvement of fully immunized children from 43.5% to 62% nationally.

The findings on immunization coverage of the NFHS IV are summarized in **Table 5.4.2**.

INDIAN ACADEMY OF PEDIATRICS IMMUNIZATION TIMETABLE

The IAP is an independent body which is committed to provide unbiased, rational, ethical, practical, and yet balanced guidelines to its members on the various issues related to immunization in India. The recommendations made by the IAP are the "best individual practice schedule" for a given child, while the NIS of the GoI is meant for the public at large. Therefore, these recommendations go beyond the national immunization program (NIP) and cater primarily to pediatricians in office practice **(Table 5.4.3)**.

General Instructions

Footnotes: Recommended immunization schedule for persons aged 0 year through 18 years—IAP, 2016.

- Vaccination at birth means as early as possible within 24–72 hours after birth or at least not later than 1 week after birth.
  - Whenever multiple vaccinations are to be given simultaneously, they should be given within 24 hours, if simultaneous administration is not feasible due to some reasons.
- The recommended age in weeks/months/years means completed weeks/months/years.
- Any dose not administered at the recommended age should be administered at a subsequent visit, when indicated and feasible.
- The use of a combination vaccine generally is preferred over separate injections of its equivalent component vaccines.
  - When two or more live parenteral/intranasal vaccines are not administered on the same day, they should be given at least 28 days (4 weeks) apart; this rule does not apply to live oral vaccines.
- Any interval can be kept between live and inactivated vaccines.
- If given less than 4 weeks apart, the vaccine given second should be repeated.
  - The minimum interval between two doses of same inactivated vaccines is usually 4 weeks (exception rabies). However, any interval can be kept between doses of different inactivated vaccines. Vaccine doses administered up to 4 days before the minimum interval or age can be counted as valid (exception rabies). If the vaccine is administered more than 5 days before minimum period, it is counted as invalid dose.
- Any number of antigens can be given on the same day.
- Changing needles between drawing vaccine into the syringe and injecting it into the child is not necessary.
  - Once the protective cap on a single-dose vial has been removed, the vaccine should be discarded at the end of the immunization session because it may not be possible to determine if the rubber seal has been punctured.
- Different vaccines should not be mixed in the same syringe unless specifically licensed and labeled for such use.
- Patients should be observed for an allergic reaction for 15–20 minutes after receiving immunization(s).
- When necessary, two vaccines can be given in the same limb at a single visit.
- The anterolateral aspect of the thigh is the preferred site for two simultaneous intramuscular (IM) injections because of its greater muscle mass.

Table 5.4.2: Immunization coverage of the NFHS IV.

NFHS IV	*Urban*	*Rural*	*NFHS*	*III*
Children age 12–23 months fully immunized (BCG, measles, and 3 doses each of polio and DPT) (%)	63.9	61.3	62.0	43.5
Children age 12–23 months who have received BCG (%)	93.2	91.4	91.9	78.2
Children age 12–23 months who have received 3 doses of polio vaccine (%)	73.4	72.6	72.8	78.2
Children age 12–23 months who have received 3 doses of DPT vaccine (%)	80.2	77.7	78.4	55.3
Children age 12–23 months who have received measles vaccine (%)	83.2	80.3	81.1	58.8
Children age 12–23 months who have received 3 doses of hepatitis B vaccine (%)	63.3	62.5	62.8	na
Children age 9–59 months who have received vitamin A dose in last 6 months (%)	62.9	59.1	60.2	16.5
Children age 12–23 months who received most of the vaccination in public health facility (%)	82.1	94.2	90.7	82.0
Children age 12–23 months who received most of the vaccination in private health facility (%)	16.7	3.4	7.2	10.5

(NFHS IV: The National Family Health Survey IV)

Table 5.4.3: IAP Recommended immunization schedule for children aged 0-18 years (with range), 2018–2019.

	Birth	6 weeks	10 weeks	14 weeks	6 months	9 months	12 months	13 months	15 months	16–18 months	2–3 years	4–6 years	9–14 years	15–18 years
BCG	BCG													
Hepatitis B	HB 1	HB 2	HB 3	HB* 4										
Polio	OPV 0	IPV** 1	IPV** 2	IPV** 3						IPV*** B1				
DTwP/DTaP		DTP 1	DTP 2	DTP 3						DTP B1		DTP B2		
HiB		HiB 1	HiB 2	HiB 3						HIB B1				
Pneumococcal		PCV 1	PCV 2	PCV 3					PCV B1				PCV	
Rotavirus		Rota 1	Rota 2	Rota 3****										
MMR						MMR 1			MMR 2			MMR3/MMRV		
Varicella									Varicella 1			Varicella 2		
Hepatitis A							Hep A1			Hep A2*****				
Typhoid					TCV#									
Influenza							Influenza (yearly)******							
Meningococcal						MCV 1	MCV 2				MCV			
JE							JE 1	JE 2						
Tdap													Tdap	Td
HPV##													HPV 1 and 2	HPV 1,2,3
Cholera									Cholera 1 and 2					

Legend (color)	Meaning
Yellow	Range of recommended age for all children
Green	Range of recommended age for catch-up immunization
Blue	Range of recommended age for high-risk children/area
White	Not recommended

*Fourth dose of Hepatitis B permissible for combination vaccines only

**In case IPV is not available or feasible, the child should be offered bOPV (3 doses). In such cases, give two fractional doses of IPV at 6 weeks and 14 weeks

***b-OPV, if IPV booster (standalone or combination) not feasible

****Third dose not required for RV 1. Catcth-up up to 1 year of age in UIP schedule

*****Live attenuated Hepatitis A vaccine: Single dose only

******Begin influenza vaccination after 6 months of age, about 2–4 weeks before season; give 2 doses at the interval of 4 weeks during first year and then single dose yearly till 5 years of age

#TCV: typhoid conjugate vaccine; ##HPV: human papilloma virus

Meningococcal vaccine (MCV): 9 months through 23 months: 2 doses, at least 3 months apart; 2 years through 55 years: single dose only

Japanese encephalitis (JE): For individuals living in endemic areas and for travelers to JE endemic areas provided their expected stay is for a minimum period of 4 weeks

HPV: 2 doses at 6 months interval 9–14 years age; 3 doses (at 0, 1–2 and 6 months) 15 years or older and immunocompromised

Cholera vaccine: Two doses 2 weeks apart for >1 year old; for individuals living in high endemic areas and traveling to areas where risk of transmission is very high

- The distance separating the two injections is arbitrary but should be at least 1 inch so that the local reactions are unlikely to overlap.
  - Although most experts recommend aspiration by gently pulling back on the syringe before the injection is given, there are no data to document the necessity for this procedure. If blood appears after negative pressure, the needle should be withdrawn and another site should be selected using a new needle.
  - A previous immunization with a dose that was less than the standard dose or one administered by a nonstandard route should not be counted, and the person should be reimmunized as appropriate for age.

RATIONALE OF BACILLUS CALMETTE-GUÉRIN AT BIRTH

Childhood tuberculosis in India is believed to constitute 15-20% of all tuberculosis cases. Bacillus Calmette-Guérin vaccine is the only effective vaccine available against tuberculosis. Bacillus Calmette-Guérin has an efficacy of 50-80% for prevention of miliary and meningeal forms of the disease. Protective efficacy for pulmonary tuberculosis is 50%. For programmatic convenience and to capture all those delivered in the institutions or healthcare facilities, BCG is advised at birth and the maternal antibodies actually enhance T-cell responses.

Routine Vaccination

It should be given at birth or at first contact.

Catch-up Vaccination

It can be given up to 5 years of age.

RATIONALE OF ZERO AND MULTIPLE DOSES OF ORAL POLIO VACCINE

Oral polio vaccine is recommended at birth for routine immunization at 6 weeks, 10 weeks, and 14 weeks; 18–24 months and at 5 years; and on all national immunization days (NIDs) and sub-NIDs. Data from the composite of Vellore studies in the 1970s and 1980s suggests that seroconversion rates after three doses of OPV average 65%, 96%, and 63% for types I, II, and III, respectively. Therefore, multiple doses of OPV are necessary before 90–95% of children develop immune responses to all three poliovirus types. The zero dose of OPV is given at birth to initiate early immunization against polio as there are no maternal IgA in the gut, the vaccine virus is not neutralized, and the risk of vaccine-associated paralytic poliomyelitis (VAPP) is minimized due to the presence of maternal antibodies.

RATIONALE BEHIND ORAL POLIO VACCINE AND INACTIVATED POLIO VACCINE COMBINATION

The IAP Committee on Immunization (IAPCOI) and the Advisory Committee on Vaccines and Immunization Practices (ACVIP) recommend three primary doses of inactivated polio vaccine (IPV) at 6 weeks, 10 weeks, and 14 weeks, followed by two doses of OPV at 6 months and 9 months, another dose (booster) of IPV at 15–18 months, and OPV at 5 years. The recommendation for combined use of OPV and IPV is for the following reasons:

- *Excellent and highly predictable immunogenicity, efficacy, and safety of IPV:* The seroconversion rates of IPV are 90–100% after two doses given after the age of 2 months and at 2 months interval or in the EPI schedule of three doses at 6 weeks, 10 weeks, and 14 weeks and can be used in combination with diphtheria, tetanus combined with whole-cell pertussis (DTwP)/diphtheria, tetanus with acellular pertussis (DTaP), Hib, and HepB vaccines without compromising seroconversion or increasing side effects.
- Better mucosal immunity of OPV and IPV combination schedule as compared to IPV alone.
- The incidence of VAPP has been estimated at four cases per million (1/1000,000) birth cohort per year in countries using OPV. The risk of VAPP with the combined OPV and IPV schedule is extremely low as the child is receiving birth dose of OPV at the time when he/she is already protected against VAPP by maternal antibodies. Subsequent protection from VAPP is by IPV. If we adopt an all IPV schedule, without the birth dose of OPV, the child may still be at a small risk for VAPP through exposure to the OPV virus through contacts or environment before the child receives its first dose of IPV.
- Oral polio vaccine and IPV used simultaneously in combination in the trials in Gambia, Oman, and Thailand, and Pakistan have shown higher levels of seropositivity as compared to all OPV or IPV alone schedules. In the Gaza Strip, combined IPV and OPV use reduced the incidence of paralytic polio from 10 to less than 2 cases per 100,000 persons in the first 3 years, and it further reduced to 0.16 per 100,000 cases in the next 5 years.

Routine Vaccination

Recommended schedule: Birth dose of OPV, three primary doses of IPV at 6 weeks, 10 weeks, and 14 weeks, followed by two doses of OPV at 6 months and 9 months; another dose (booster) of IPV at 15–18 months and OPV at 5 years.

- Birth dose of OPV usually does not lead to VAPP.
- Oral polio vaccine in place of IPV, if IPV is unfeasible, minimum three doses. Additional doses of OPV on all supplementary immunization activities (SIAs).
- *Inactivated polio vaccine:* Minimum age 6 weeks.
- *Inactivated polio vaccine*: Two instead of three doses can also be used if primary series started at 8 weeks, and the interval between the doses is kept 8 weeks.

No child should leave your facility without polio immunization (IPV or OPV), if indicated by the schedule!

Catch-up Vaccination

Inactivated polio vaccine catch-up schedule: Two doses at 2 months apart, followed by a booster after 6 months of previous dose.

Catch-up is recommended till 5 years of age as of now.

RATIONALE OF RECOMMENDING DIPHTHERIA, TETANUS COMBINED WITH WHOLE-CELL PERTUSSIS AND DIPHTHERIA, TETANUS WITH ACELLULAR PERTUSSIS

The ACVIP unequivocally endorses the continued use of DTwP vaccine in EPI because of its proven efficacy and safety. DTaP vaccine is not more efficacious than DTwP vaccine but has fewer adverse effects. Serious adverse effects are rare phenomena even with the whole-cell vaccine unlike popular belief. The parents should be made aware of these facts and be asked to decide on the choice of the DTP vaccine they wish to immunize their child with. The DTwP vaccine should be preferred in the primary series as well as booster doses at

18–24 months and 5 years. However, DTaP may be used as booster doses if reactogenicity is an issue provided resources permit. The DTaP vaccines may be preferred to DTwP vaccines in those children with history of severe adverse effects following DTwP vaccines or children with neurologic disorders, if resources permit. The schedule is same as with DTwP vaccines. Like DTwP vaccines, DTaP vaccines must not be used in children age of 7 years or older because of increased reactogenicity. DTaP, if used, should contain three or more components of acellular pertussis (aP).

Routine Vaccination

Minimum age: Six weeks.

Recommended schedule: Three primary doses at 6 weeks, 10 weeks, and 14 weeks and two boosters at 15–18 months and 5 years.

- The first booster (fourth dose) may be administered as early as age 12 months, provided at least 6 months have elapsed since the third dose.
- Diphtheria, tetanus with acellular pertussis vaccine/ combinations should preferably be avoided for the primary series.
- Diphtheria, tetanus with acellular pertussis may be preferred to DTwP in children with history of severe adverse effects after previous dose/s of DTwP or children with neurologic disorders.
- First and second boosters may also be of DTwP. However, considering a higher reactogenicity, DTaP can be considered for the boosters. If any "aP" containing vaccine is used, it must, at least, have three or more components in the product.

Catch-up Vaccination

Catch-up schedule: The second childhood booster is not required if the last dose has been given beyond the age of 4 years.

Catch-up below 1 year: Three primary doses at 4-week interval.

Catch-up (1–7 years): Three doses of DTwP/DTaP at 0 month, 1 month, and 6 months.

Catch-up above 7 years: Tetanus-diphtheria-acellular pertussis (Tdap), tetanus and diphtheria toxoids (Td), and Td at 0 month, 1 month, and 6 months.

RATIONALE OF TETANUS-DIPHTHERIA-ACELLULAR PERTUSSIS AT 10 YEARS

Tetanus-diphtheria-acellular pertussis is the acronym for the collective vaccine preventing tetanus, diphtheria, and pertussis recommended for adolescents and adults with reduced concentration of diphtheria and pertussis toxoids to prevent adverse effects. There is no data on the incidence of adolescent and adult pertussis in India but is perceived to be significant, especially in those states where childhood immunization coverage is good, and reduced natural circulation of pertussis has led to infrequent adolescent boosting. A safe and efficacious vaccine is available. The ACVIP, therefore, recommends offering Tdap vaccine instead of Td/TT vaccine in all children and adolescents who can afford to use the vaccine at 10 years.

Routine Vaccination

Recommended schedule: One dose of Tdap to all adolescents aged 11 through 12 years.

Minimum age: Seven years [Adacel® is approved for 11–64-year old by the Advisory Committee on Immunization Practices (ACIP) and 4–64-year old by the Food and Drug Administration (FDA), while Boostrix® for 10-year old and older by the ACIP and 4 years of age and older by the FDA in the United States].

Tetanus-diphtheria-acellular pertussis during pregnancy: One dose of Tdap vaccine to pregnant mothers/adolescents during each pregnancy (preferred during 27 through 36 weeks gestation) regardless of number of years from prior Td or Tdap vaccination.

Catch-up Vaccination

Catch-up above 7 years: Tdap/Td at 0 month, 1 month, and 6 months.

Persons aged 7 through 10 years, who are not fully immunized with the childhood DTwP/DTaP vaccine series, should receive Tdap vaccine as the first dose in the catch-up series; if additional doses are needed, use Td vaccine. For these children, an adolescent Tdap vaccine should not be given for dose two and three.

Persons aged 11 through 18 years who have not received Tdap vaccine should receive a dose, followed by Td booster doses every 10 years thereafter.

Tetanus-diphtheria-acellular pertussis vaccine can be administered once regardless of the interval since the last Td vaccine.

RATIONALE OF MEASLES VACCINE AT 9 MONTHS

The immunogenicity and efficacy are best when the measles vaccine is administered beyond the age of 12 months. However, in India, a significant proportion of measles cases occur below the age of 12 months. Hence, in order to achieve the best balance between early protection and high seroconversion, completed 9 months of age has been recommended as the appropriate age for measles vaccination in India. In case of an outbreak, however, the vaccine can be given to infants as

administration of a single dose of the polysaccharide vaccine in the age group of 2–15 years would be highly cost-effective. The typhoid Vi-PS vaccine is a polysaccharide, and hence, unlike a protein antigen is not capable of inducing T-cell-dependent immune response and cannot be used below the age of 2 years. The immunity wanes over 3 years due to the lack of T-cell-dependent memory response with the polysaccharide antigen. However, the phenomenon of hyporesponsiveness following repeated doses of a polysaccharide antigen is not observed with the typhoid polysaccharide antigen, and hence, revaccination is recommended every 3 years starting at 2 years of age.

Indian Academy of Pediatrics has approved the use of two typhoid conjugate vaccines, Typbar-TCV and PedaTyph®, for the prevention of typhoid fever in pediatric population. A single dose of the vaccine at 9–12 months of age is recommended for primary schedule. World Health Organization does not recommend maintaining an interval of least 4 weeks between typhoid conjugate vaccine and MMR vaccine. For children vaccinated before the age of 2 years, a booster dose is recommended.

A child with a history of suspected/confirmed enteric fever may be vaccinated 4 weeks after recovery, if there is no history of vaccine administration in the past 3 years. The need for revaccination following a booster of Typbar-TCV® has not been determined yet.

Routine Vaccination

Both Vi-PS conjugate and Vi-PS vaccines are available.

Minimum ages:
- *Vi-PS (Typbar-TCV®)*: Six months
- *Vi-PS vaccines*: Two years.

Vaccination Schedule

Typhoid conjugate vaccines: Single dose at 9–12 through 23 months and a booster during the second year of life.

Vi-PS vaccines: Single dose at 2 years, revaccination every 3 years.

Currently, two typhoid conjugate vaccines, Typbar-TCV® and PedaTyph®, are available in Indian market. Primary dose of conjugate vaccine should follow a booster at 2 years of age.

Typbar-TCV® is preferred over Vi-PS for booster.

Typhoid revaccination is done every 3 years, if Vi-PS vaccine is used.

No evidence of hyporesponsiveness on repeated revaccination of Vi-PS vaccine so far.

Need of revaccination following a booster of Typbar-TCV® not yet determined.

Catch-up Vaccination

Recommended throughout the adolescent period, i.e. 18 years.

Vi conjugate typhoid vaccine should be preferred over Vi-PS vaccine wherever feasible owing to generation of superior immune responses with the former. Only a single dose of either of the two available conjugate vaccines, i.e. Typbar-TCV® and PedaTyph®, is recommended for children above 2 years of age. The need of the booster doses is not yet determined.

RATIONALE OF TWO DOSES FOR VARICELLA VACCINE

The varicella vaccines are licensed for age 12 months and above. However, the risk of breakthrough varicella is lower if given 15 months onward. Hence, the ACVIP recommends administration of varicella vaccine in children aged 15 months or older. After a single dose of varicella vaccine, approximately 15% of vaccines remain at risk of developing a breakthrough varicella disease. These varicella infections in immunized population may raise concern regarding vaccine efficacy and a misunderstanding by physicians or parents who may lose faith in vaccination. Because immunized children who experience breakthrough disease are coinfected with both wild and vaccine strains of varicella virus, they may be at increased risk of zoster from the reactivated wild-type strain later in life compared with vaccine recipients who do not experience breakthrough disease. Two doses of varicella vaccine offer superior individual protection as compared to a single dose. The risk of breakthrough disease is 3.3-fold less when two doses are administered.

The ACVIP now recommends two doses of varicella vaccine for children of all age groups. For primary immunization, the first dose should be given at the age of 15 months and the second dose at 4–6 years. However, the immune response to the vaccine when given at 3 months interval is same as that when given at a longer interval of 4–6 years.

Routine Vaccination

Minimum age: Twelve months.

Administer the first dose at age 15 through 18 months and the second dose at age 4 through 6 years.

The second dose may be administered before age of 4 years, provided at least 3 months have elapsed since the first dose. If the second dose was administered at least 4 weeks after the first dose, it can be accepted as valid.

The risk of breakthrough varicella is lower if given 15 months onward.

Catch-up Vaccination

Ensure that all persons aged 7 through 18 years without "evidence of immunity" gets two doses of the vaccine.

For children aged 12 months through 12 years, the recommended minimum interval between doses is 3 months.

However, if the second dose was administered at least 4 weeks after the first dose, it can be accepted as valid.

For persons aged 13 years and older, the minimum interval between doses is 4 weeks.

For persons without evidence of immunity, administer two doses if not previously vaccinated or the second dose, if only one dose has been administered.

"Evidence of immunity" to varicella includes any of the following:

- Documentation of age-appropriate vaccination with a varicella vaccine
- Laboratory evidence of immunity or laboratory confirmation of disease
- Diagnosis or verification of a history of varicella disease by a healthcare provider
- Diagnosis or verification of a history of herpes zoster by a healthcare provider.

RATIONALE OF FIRST DOSE OF HEPATITIS A AT 12 MONTHS AND TWO DOSES OF HEPATITIS A

All hepatitis A (HepA) vaccines are licensed for use in children aged 1 year or older. In its earlier publications, the committee had recommended initiation of HepA vaccination at the age of 18 months so that interference with maternal antibodies is minimized. However, new data suggests decline in the adult seropositivity rates especially in those belonging to the high socioeconomic status. Consequently, babies may be born with no maternal antibodies. Immunogenicity studies also show that antibody titers achieved with vaccination at 12 months are comparable to those achieved at 18 months to 2 years. In light of these facts, the committee now recommends initiating HepA vaccine at the age of 12 months. For catch-up vaccination, prevaccination screening for HepA antibody is recommended in children older than 10 years as at this age the estimated seropositive rates exceed 50%.

Two doses of killed HepA vaccine at 6 months apart are recommended. Single dose of live-attenuated H2-strain vaccine is sufficient for long-term protection.

Routine Vaccination

Minimum age: Twelve months.

Killed HepA vaccine: Start the two doses of HepA vaccine series for children aged 12 through 23 months and separate the two doses by 6–18 months.

Live-attenuated H2-strain HepA vaccine: Single dose starting at 12 months and through 23 months of age.

Catch-up Vaccination

Either of the two vaccines can be used in "catch-up" schedule beyond 2 years of age.

Administer two doses for killed vaccine at least 6 months apart to unvaccinated persons.

Only single dose of live-attenuated H2-strain vaccine.

For catch-up vaccination, prevaccination screening for HepA antibody is recommended in children older than 10 years as at this age the estimated seropositive rates exceed 50%.

RATIONALE FOR INCLUSION OF NEWLY LICENSED VACCINES

Rotavirus Vaccine (Oral)

Diarrhea is the second leading cause of deaths in under-five children. About 25–40% of hospitalized diarrhea is caused by rotavirus (RV). In India alone, RV causes more than 120,000 deaths annually, 450,000 hospitalizations, 5 million clinic visits, and 25 million diarrheal episodes in under-five children. A study from India showed that the RV detection rates were the greatest among children aged 6–23 months and 13.3% of RV infections involved children aged less than 6 months. The study also documents the early incidence of RV disease in India. The most common types of strains were G2P[4] (25.7% of strains), G1P[8] (22.1%), and G9P[8] (8.5%); G12 strains were seen in combination with types P[4], P[6], and P[8], and together comprised 6.5% of strains. Human monovalent live vaccine (RV1) and bovine human pentavalent (RV5) live vaccine are available in India and administered orally in a two-dose or three-dose schedule, respectively. Both the vaccines have demonstrated, though less as compared to the developed nations, acceptable efficacy and significant impact on reduction in RV diarrhea episodes in the developing countries of Africa and Asia. Recently, indigenously developed neonatal human live-attenuated RV monovalent (strain 116E) vaccine has been developed, which has shown promising results and is used in three-dose schedule (6–10–14 weeks), similar to RV5.

The minimum age to administer any of the three available vaccines is 6 weeks; however, ACVIP advises RV1 (GlaxoSmithKline) to be given at 10 weeks and 14 weeks for better immune response. The maximum age for the commencement of the first dose of any oral RV vaccine is 14 weeks and 6 days, and last dose should not be given after 8 months and 0 day. All available oral RV vaccines should not be initiated (first dose) in infants aged 15 weeks, 0 day, and older.

The ACVIP acknowledges the morbidity and mortality burden of RV and need for an RV vaccine. Such a vaccine would be most needed in the NIP as the disease consequences are the most serious in the underprivileged. Given the minimal impact that water and sanitation measures have had on the burden of RV in the developing areas, there is wide agreement that effective vaccination represents the most promising prevention strategy against the disease.

Routine Vaccination

Minimum age: 6 weeks for both RV1 (Rotarix) and RV5 (RotaTeq).

Only two doses of RV1 are recommended at present.

Rotavirus 1 should preferably be employed in 10 weeks and 14 weeks schedule, instead of 6 weeks and 10 weeks; the former schedule is found to be far more immunogenic than the latter.

Rotavirus 5 should be employed in a three-dose 6 weeks, 10 weeks, and 14 weeks schedule. If any dose in series was RV5 or vaccine product is unknown for any dose in the series, a total of three doses of RV vaccine should be administered.

Catch-up Vaccination

The maximum age for the first dose in the series is 14 weeks, 6 days.

Vaccination should not be initiated for infants aged 15 weeks, 0 day, or older.

The maximum age for the final dose in the series is 8 months, 0 day.

Pneumococcal Vaccines

Streptococcus pneumoniae is responsible for 15–50% of all episodes of community-acquired pneumonia, 30–50% of all cases of acute otitis media, and a significant proportion of bacterial meningitis and bacteremia. It is estimated that 50% of the 2 million deaths due to pneumonia globally every year are attributable to *S. pneumoniae.* According to a recent publication, seven serotypes (1, 5, 6A, 6B, 14, 19F, and 23F) (PCV7) were the most common globally. World Health Organization, in 2007, recommended PCV in the NIP of any country with under-five mortality rate (U5MR) of more than 50/1,000 live births or absolute child deaths of greater than 50,000/year. With U5MR of 72/1,000 live births and nearly 2 million under-five deaths per year, India merits to include PCV in NIP with high priority. Now PCV7 has been replaced by PCV10 and PCV13 having 10 and 13, respectively, of the most common serotypes causing infection globally.

Following three priming doses of PCV at 6 weeks, 10 weeks, and 14 weeks, it is important to give a single booster dose between 12 months and 15 months to maintain the antibody titers above the minimum required for protection against the invasive pneumococcal disease. Pneumococcal conjugate vaccine is not recommended routinely in a healthy child above 5 years, as most of the invasive pneumococcal disease is seen below the age of 5 years. Pneumococcal conjugate vaccine 13 is also licensed to prevent pneumococcal disease in adults over 50 years of age.

There is another type of pneumococcal vaccine, the nonconjugate 23 valent polysaccharide pneumococcal vaccine (PPSV23) which is recommended only for the high-risk group (HRG) persons in addition to routine PCV doses. Since PPSV does not elicit a good immune response below the age of 2 years, it is not recommended for children below 2 years of age for routine immunization. PPSV is reserved for the HRG persons above 2 years in addition to routine PCV vaccination. Because of the hyporesponsiveness phenomenon associated with repeated doses of the polysaccharide vaccines, not more than two doses are recommended at any time in life, and the vaccine is recommended for use only in persons at risk for pneumococcal disease.

Routine Vaccination

Minimum Age: 6 weeks.

Both PCV10 and PCV13 are licensed for children from 6 weeks to 5 years of age (although the exact labeling details may differ by country). In addition, PCV13 is licensed for the prevention of pneumococcal diseases in adults more than 50 years of age.

Primary schedule (for both PCV10 and PCV13): Three primary doses at 6 weeks, 10 weeks, and 14 weeks with a booster at age 12 through 15 months.

Catch-up Vaccination

Administer one dose of PCV13 or PCV10 to all healthy children aged 24 through 59 months, who are not completely vaccinated for their age.

For PCV13: Catch-up in 6–12 months—two doses 4 weeks apart and one booster, 12–23 months—two doses 8 weeks apart, and 24 months and above—single dose.

For PCV10: Catch-up in 6–12 months—two doses 4 weeks apart and one booster, 12 months to 5 years—two doses 8 weeks apart.

Vaccination of persons with high-risk conditions is as follows:

- Pneumococcal conjugate vaccine and PPSV both are used in certain HRG of children.
- For children aged 24 through 71 months with certain underlying medical conditions, administer one dose of PCV13, if three doses of PCV were received previously, or administer two doses of PCV13 at least 8 weeks apart, if fewer than three doses of PCV were received previously.
- A single dose of PCV13 may be administered to previously unvaccinated children aged 6 through 18 years who have anatomic or functional asplenia (including sickle cell disease), human immunodeficiency virus (HIV) infection or an immunocompromising condition, cochlear implant or cerebrospinal fluid (CSF) leak.
- Administer PPSV23 at least 8 weeks after the last dose of PCV to children aged 2 years or older with certain underlying medical conditions.

- An additional dose of PPSV should be administered after 5 years to children with anatomic/functional asplenia or an immunocompromising condition.
- Polysaccharide pneumococcal vaccine should never be used alone for prevention of pneumococcal diseases amongst high-risk individuals.
- Children with following medical conditions for which PPSV23 and PCV are indicated in the age group 24 through 71 months.
- Immunocompetent children with chronic heart disease (particularly cyanotic congenital heart disease and cardiac failure), chronic lung disease (including asthma if treated with high-dose oral corticosteroid therapy), diabetes mellitus, CSF leaks, or cochlear implant.
- Children with anatomic or functional asplenia (including sickle cell disease and other hemoglobinopathies, congenital or acquired asplenia, or splenic dysfunction).
- *Children with immunocompromising conditions*: HIV infection, chronic renal failure, and nephrotic syndrome; diseases associated with treatment with immunosuppressive drugs or radiation therapy, including malignant neoplasm, leukemia, lymphomas and Hodgkin's disease or solid organ transplantation, congenital immunodeficiency.

Human Papillomavirus Vaccine

Infection with human papillomavirus (HPV) is an obligatory cause of cervical cancer. In India, high-risk HPV types were found in 97% of cervical cancers. Types 16 and 18 account for 70% of the cases of invasive cervical cancer globally. A meta-analysis of HPV type distribution from India showed that in invasive cervical carcinoma (ICC), HPV16 was the predominant type (64.8%), followed by HPV18, 45, 33, 35, 58, 59, and 31. The estimated HPV16/18 positive fraction was 78.9% in women with ICC (87.7% in North and 77.2% in South India), 61.5% with high squamous intraepithelial lesion, 30.8% with low squamous intraepithelial lesion, and 3.9% in women with normal cytology/histology. It is estimated that HPV16/18 vaccines will provide over 75% protection against ICC in South Asia. Oncogenic HPV serotypes have also been implicated in causation of anal, vulvar, vaginal, penile, and oropharyngeal cancers. In addition, nononcogenic HPV serotypes 6 and 11 are responsible for more than 90% of anogenital warts and most recurrent respiratory papillomatosis.

Clinical trials of the two HPV vaccines conducted in India prior to licensure demonstrated high immunogenicity and a good safety profile, confirming the findings reported in other countries. These have been approved by the DCGI for general use. The ACVIP recommends offering HPV vaccine to all women in the abovementioned schedule. Since protection is seen only when the vaccine is given before infection with HPV, the vaccine should preferably be given prior to sexual debut. The vaccine should preferably be introduced to parents as a cervical cancer preventing vaccine and not as a vaccine against a sexually transmitted infection. Though HPV vaccines are of public health importance, cervical cancer prevention is not a public health priority, and the programmatic feasibility and economic sustainability need to be given due consideration before including the HPV vaccine in NIP.

Minimum age: Nine years.

Human papilloma virus 4 (Gardasil) and HPV2 (Cervarix) are licensed and available.

Only two doses of either of the two HPV vaccines (HPV4 and HPV2) for adolescent/preadolescent girls aged 9–14 years.

For girls 15 years and older and immunocompromised individuals, three doses are recommended.

For two-dose schedule, the minimum interval between doses should be 6 months.

Either HPV4 (0 month, 2 months, and 6 months) or HPV2 (0 month, 1 month, and 6 months) is recommended in a three-dose series for females aged 15 years and older.

Human papilloma virus 4 can also be given in a three-dose series for males aged 11 years or 12 years, but not yet licensed for use in males in India.

For three-dose schedule, administer the second dose 1–2 months after the first dose and the third dose 6 months after the first dose (at least 24 weeks after the first dose).

RATIONALE OF VACCINES IN SPECIAL SITUATIONS

Japanese Encephalitis Vaccine

In India, Japanese encephalitis (JE) is believed to be responsible for approximately 2,000–3,000 clinical cases and 500–600 deaths every year. Highly endemic states include West Bengal, Bihar, Karnataka, Tamil Nadu, Andhra Pradesh, Assam, Uttar Pradesh, Manipur, and Goa. Indian Academy of Pediatrics Committee on Immunization recommends that the government should implement universal immunization with this vaccine in all children in JE endemic states. The SA-14-14-2 vaccine appears best suited for this purpose. A recent study from Philippines showed acceptable efficacy and safety of this vaccine when coadministered with the measles vaccine at 9 months. Along with all infants, all susceptible children up to the age of 15 years should be administered catch-up vaccination.

It is recommended only for individuals living in endemic areas.

The vaccine should be offered to the children residing in rural areas only and those planning to visit endemic areas (depending upon the duration of stay).

Three types of new generation JE vaccines are licensed in India: One, live-attenuated, cell culture-derived SA-14-14-2, and two inactivated JE vaccines, namely "Vero cell culture-derived SA-14-14-2 JE vaccine" (JEEV® by BE India) and "culture-derived, 821564XY, JE vaccine" (JENVAC® by Bharat Biotech).

Live-attenuated, cell culture-derived SA14142 minimum age: Eight months.

Two-dose schedule, first dose at 9 months along with measles vaccine and second at 16–18 months along with DTP booster; not available in private market for office use.

Inactivated cell culture-derived SA-14-14-2 (JEEV® by BE India) minimum age: One year (USFDA—2 months).

Primary immunization schedule: Two doses of 0.25 mL each administered IM on days 0 and 28 for children aged 1–3 years.

Two doses of 0.5 mL for children greater than 3 years and adults aged 18 years.

Need of boosters still undetermined.

Inactivated Vero cell culture-derived Kolar strain, 821564XY, JE vaccine (JENVAC® by Bharat Biotech)

Minimum age: One year.

Primary immunization schedule: Two doses of 0.5 mL each administered IM at 4 weeks interval.

Need of boosters still undetermined.

Cholera Vaccine

Cholera cases are reported from almost all states, the predominant strain being *Vibrio cholerae* O1, and *V. cholerae* O139 is an emerging strain. The variant whole-cell/recombinant B subunit vaccine first developed and licensed in Vietnam comprises only killed whole-cell *V. cholerae* O1 (classical and El Tor) and *V. cholerae* O139. This inexpensive oral vaccine without buffer and cold chain requirements administered as two doses 2 weeks apart has been demonstrated to have 50% efficacy for up to 3 years after vaccination. This vaccine is now manufactured and licensed in India for children above the age of 1 year.

The inclusion of new killed whole-cell oral cholera vaccine in the NIS is being considered by the policy makers in those areas where cholera is highly endemic, particularly, the states of West Bengal and Orissa. For office practice purposes, the cholera vaccine remains a vaccine to be used in special circumstances. These include travel to residence in a highly endemic area and circumstances where there is risk of an outbreak, such as during pilgrimages like *Kumbh mela*, etc. Protection starts 2 weeks after receipt of the second dose.

Minimum age: One year [killed whole-cell *V. cholerae vaccine* (Shanchol)].

Not recommended for routine use in healthy individuals, recommended only for the vaccination of persons residing in highly endemic areas and traveling to areas where risk of transmission is very high, such as *Kumbh mela*, etc.

Two doses 2 weeks apart for greater than 1 year old.

Influenza Vaccine

Till 2009, pandemic data on morbidity and mortality of influenza in India was very limited. A handful of studies showed that influenza contributed to 5–10% of all acute respiratory tract infections. The course of influenza is mild and self-limited. However, serious complications leading to morbidity and death occur, especially, in those with underlying chronic illnesses. The H1N1 2009 virus caused deaths in young children, adolescents, and nearly 25–30% of the deaths occurred in those without any underlying risk factors. In the current scenario wherein we are in the postpandemic phase, the IAPCOI recommends using the influenza vaccine in all children with risk factors and also wherein the vaccine is desired/requested by parents (discussing with them the benefits and limitations of the vaccine).

Minimum age: Six months for trivalent inactivated influenza vaccine (TIV).

Recommended only for the vaccination of persons with certain high-risk conditions.

First-time vaccination: 6 months to below 9 years: Two doses 1 month apart; 9 years and above—single dose.

Annual revaccination with single dose.

Dosage (TIV): Aged 6–35 months 0.25 mL; 3 years and above: 0.5 mL.

For children aged 6 months through 8 years: Administer two doses (separated by at least 4 weeks) to children who are receiving influenza vaccine for the first time.

All the currently available TIVs in the country contain the "Swine flu" or "A (H1N1)" antigen, no need to vaccinate separately.

Best time to vaccinate is as follows:

- As soon as the new vaccine is released and available in the market
- Just before the onset of rainy season.

Meningococcal Vaccine

In a comprehensive study of epidemiology of meningococcal disease in India, prevalence of meningitis was 1.5–3.3% of all acute hospital admissions in children. Contribution of meningococcus to this is just 1.9%. Unconjugated meningococcal polysaccharide vaccine is either bivalent (A and C) or quadrivalent (A, C, Y, and W135) and contains 50 µg of each of the individual polysaccharides, available in lyophilized form, reconstituted with sterile water and stored at 2–8°C. These "T-cell-independent" vaccines do not induce immunological memory, and the response in children younger than 2 years is poor; hence, these are indicated for adults and children older than 2 years (only under special circumstances in children from 3 months to 2 years of age). The conjugate vaccines are preferred but currently unavailable in India. At present only the quadrivalent and bivalent polysaccharide vaccines are available.

Recommended only for certain HRG of children, during outbreaks and international travelers including students going for study abroad and travelers to Hajj and sub-Sahara Africa.

Both meningococcal conjugate vaccines [Quadrivalent MenACWY-D, Menactra® by Sanofi Pasteur and monovalent group A, serogroup A meningococcal polysaccharide–tetanus toxoid conjugate vaccine (PsA–TT), MenAfriVac® by Serum Institute of India] and polysaccharide vaccines (bi- and quadrivalent) are licensed in India. PsA–TT is not freely available in market.

Conjugate vaccines are preferred over polysaccharide vaccines due to their potential for herd protection and their increased immunogenicity, particularly in children less than 2 years of age.

As of today, quadrivalent conjugate and polysaccharide vaccines are recommended only for children 2 years and above. Monovalent group A conjugate vaccine, PsA–TT, can be used in children above 1 year of age.

Rabies Vaccine

Rabies is a fatal disease and vaccination is the only effective tool to reduce the burden. The currently available vaccines are the modern tissue culture vaccines (MTCVs) and include purified chick embryo cell (PCEC) vaccine, human diploid cell vaccine (HDCV), purified Vero cell rabies vaccine (PVRV), and purified duck embryo vaccine (PDEV). Rabies vaccine is recommended as postprophylaxis in any significant contact with a warm blooded animal and as preprophylaxis in those with high-risk of rabies exposure.

- Practically, all children need vaccination against rabies.
- Following two situations included in "high-risk category of children" for rabies vaccination and should be offered "preexposure prophylaxis (PreEP)."
- Children having pets in home.
- Children perceived with higher threat of being bitten by dogs such as hostelers, risk of stray dog menace while going outdoor.
- Only MTCVs and IM routes are recommended for both postexposure prophylaxis (PEP) and PreEP in office practice.

Postexposure prophylaxis is recommended following a significant contact with dogs, cats, cows, buffaloes, sheep, goats, pigs, donkeys, horses, camels, foxes, jackals, monkeys, mongoose, squirrel, bears, and others. Domestic rodent (rat) bites do not require PEP in India.

Postexposure Prophylaxis

Modern tissue culture vaccines are recommended for all category II and III bites.

Dose: 1.0 mL IM in anterolateral thigh or deltoid (never in gluteal region) for HDCV, PCEC vaccine, PDEV, 0.5 mL for PVRV. Intradermal administration is not recommended in individual practice.

Schedule: 0, 3, 7, 14, and 30 with day "0" being the day of commencement of vaccination. A sixth dose on day 90 is optional and may be offered to patients with severe debility or those who are immunosuppressed.

Rabies immunoglobulin (RIG) along with rabies vaccines are recommended in all category III bites.

Equine RIG (dose 40 U/kg) can be used if human RIG is not available.

Pre-exposure Prophylaxis

Three doses are given IM in deltoid/anterolateral thigh on days 0, 7, and 28 (day 21 may be used if time is limited but day 28 preferred).

For pre-exposure at any point of time after completed (and documented) PreEP or PEP, two doses are given on days 0 and 3.

Rabies immunoglobulin is not required during preexposure therapy.

INTRODUCTION OF A NEW VACCINE IN NATIONAL IMMUNIZATION PROGRAM

There are several factors that determine introduction of a new vaccine in NIP for public use that include burden of disease, cost-effectiveness of a vaccination program, suitability of vaccine product available in the world market, safety and efficacy of the vaccine, and programmatic issues. Although inclusion of a new vaccine in NIS adds the cost of vaccine and logistics to the health budget of a country, it also results in savings by reduction of the disease burden. Still, the decision to include a new vaccine in national schedule is not straightforward as there are numerous issues in prioritizing investments of an NIP. These issues need to be tackled systematically, providing best possible immunization schedule as per the needs and resources of the country.

BIBLIOGRAPHY

1. Bhatla N, Lal N, Bao YP, et al. A meta-analysis of human papillomavirus type distribution in women from South Asia—implications for vaccination. Vaccine. 2008;26(23):2811-7.
2. Hadler SC, Dietz V, Okwo-Bele JM, et al. Immunization in developing countries. In: Plotkin SA, Orenstein WA, Offit PA (Eds). Vaccines, 5th edition. Philadelphia, PA: Saunders; 2008. pp. 1541-72.

3. Indian Academy of Pediatrics (2015). The definitive guide to vaccination in India. [online] Available from: http://acvip.org/professional/index.php [Accessed October, 2018].
4. UNICEF/WHO (2006). Pneumonia—the forgotten killer of children. [online] Available from: http://www.childinfo.org/files/Pneumonia_The_Forgotten_Killer_of_Children.pdf. [Accessed October, 2018].
5. World Health Organization (2006). Global immunization data. [online] Available from: http://www.who.int/immunization/newsroom/Global_Immunization_Data.pdf [Accessed October, 2018].
6. World Health Organization (2015). Immunization surveillance, assessment and monitoring. [online] Available from: http://www.who.int/immunization/monitoring_surveillance/en/ [Accessed October, 2018].
7. Pneumococcal conjugate vaccine for childhood immunization—WHO position paper. Wkly Epidemiol Rec. 2007;82(12):93-104.
8. Yewale V, Choudhury P, Thacker N (2011). IAP guide book on immunization. [online] Available from: http://www.iapindia.org/files/IAP%20Immunization%20Guide%20Book_2009_2010.pdf [Accessed October, 2018].

5.4.1 POLIO ENDGAME: GLOBAL AND NATIONAL PERSPECTIVES

K Surendran, A Parthasarathy

GLOBAL PERSPECTIVE

Smallpox was successfully eradicated and certified in 1980. Subsequent to this historical success, the 41st World Health Assembly, in May 1988, passed a resolution calling for the Global Polio Eradication by the year 2000. Tremendous progress has been made since then. There were 125 countries endemic for polio in 1988, which had been reduced to three, viz. Pakistan, Afghanistan, and Nigeria. It was estimated that nearly 350,000 children were affected due to polio in the year 1988. Currently, there are 13 wild polio virus (WPV) cases globally (as on July 24, 2018), and these are detected in Afghanistan (10 cases) and Pakistan (three cases), respectively. All these 13 WPV cases reported are of P1 serotype. The last global WPV P2 serotype was reported from Aligarh, India, in October 1999, and WPV P3 serotype was reported from Nigeria in November 2012.

Global Polio Eradication Initiatives envisaged the following strategies:

- At least 90% routine immunization (RI) coverage
- Mass campaign [national immunization days (NIDs) and sub-NIDs (SNIDs)]
- Acute flaccid paralysis (AFP) surveillance
- Mop-up immunization response.

Migration of people is a major risk factor for the spread of polio virus transmission, both globally and nationally.

Continued use of oral polio vaccine (OPV) at global level poses two known risks, viz.

1. Vaccine-derived polio virus (VDPV)
2. Vaccine-associated paralytic poliomyelitis (VAPP).

More than 90% of circulating VDPV (cVDPV) cases and 40% of VAPP cases are due to type 2 polio virus. During the period 2000–2018, there were 923 cases of cVDPV reported in 26 countries (as on July 24, 2018) **(Fig. 5.4.1.1)**.

The other polio eradication challenges are as follows:

- Maintaining population immunity
- Sustaining AFP surveillance
- Readiness to respond to importation
- Minimizing risk.

World Health Organization (WHO) executive board passed resolution in January 2012 for endorsing eventual replacement of trivalent OPV (tOPV) with bivalent OPV (bOPV) globally, and member states should start preparing appropriate policies, potentially as early as 2014–2015. To mitigate the risk associated with OPV type 2 withdrawal, introduction of at least one dose of inactivated polio vaccine (IPV) should be administered to all infants under National Immunization Schedule (NIS). World Health Organization certified that WPV type 2 was globally eradicated on September 20, 2015. The globally synchronized cessation of tOPV was successfully implemented during April 18–May 1, 2016 replacing tOPV with bOPV. The cessation of bOPV use is globally planned during 2019–2020 **(Fig. 5.4.1.2)**.

NATIONAL PERSPECTIVE

Government of India (GOI) initiated mass OPV campaign, popularly called pulse polio immunization program during 1995–1996 targeting children in the age group 0–3 years. Subsequently, the target age group was revised to include 0–5 years in the years 1996–1997 onward. World Health Organization in collaboration with GOI had initiated National Polio Surveillance Project (NPSP) in 1997 with network of Surveillance Medical Officers to establish and strengthen AFP surveillance system across the country. This syndromic AFP surveillance had enabled to map WPV transmission geographical areas accurately.

India Expert Advisory Group on poliomyelitis, comprising both national and international experts, periodically reviews polio eradication strategies. India Expert Advisory Group recommends on strategies for stopping wild polio transmission and polio certification process including NIDs and SNIDs for the country. It was estimated that approximately 200,000 paralytic poliomyelitis cases occurred before OPV introduction in RI during 1978 **(Fig. 5.4.1.3)**.

Based on evident information, monovalent OPV [(mOPV) type 1 ($mOPV_1$)] elicited better immune response than tOPV. Monovalent OPV_1 was introduced in India during April 2005, to control polio outbreaks, particularly in Uttar Pradesh and Bihar. Subsequently, mOPV type 3 was introduced to improve

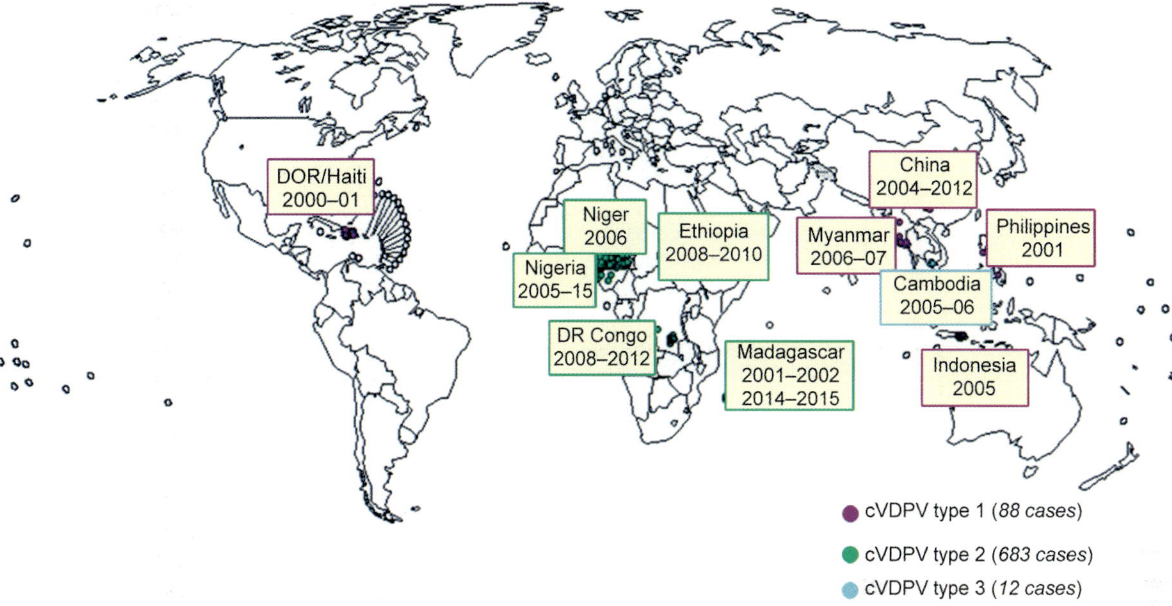

Fig. 5.4.1.1: A total of 923 cases of circulating vaccine-derived polio virus, 2000–2018 in 26 countries (as on July 24, 2018).
Source: World Health Organization.

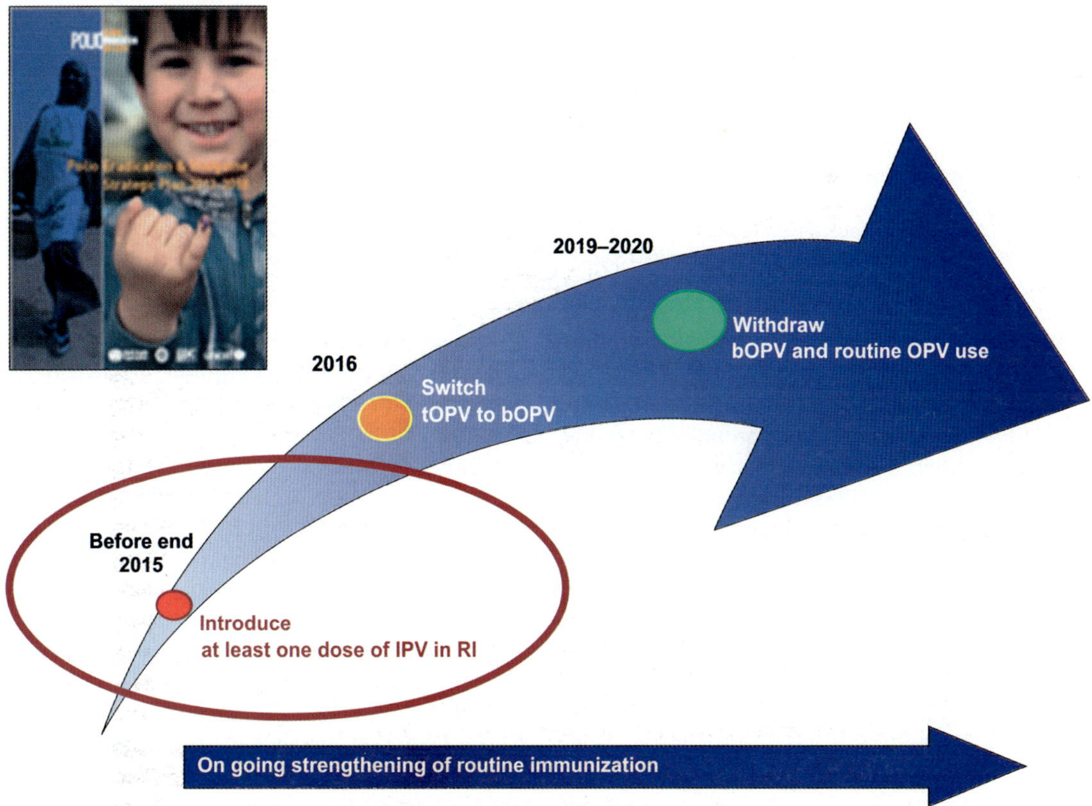

Fig. 5.4.1.2: The polio endgame strategy.
(bOPV: bivalent oral polio vaccine; IPV: inactivated polio vaccine; OPV: oral polio vaccine;
RI: routine immunization; tOPV: trivalent oral polio vaccine)

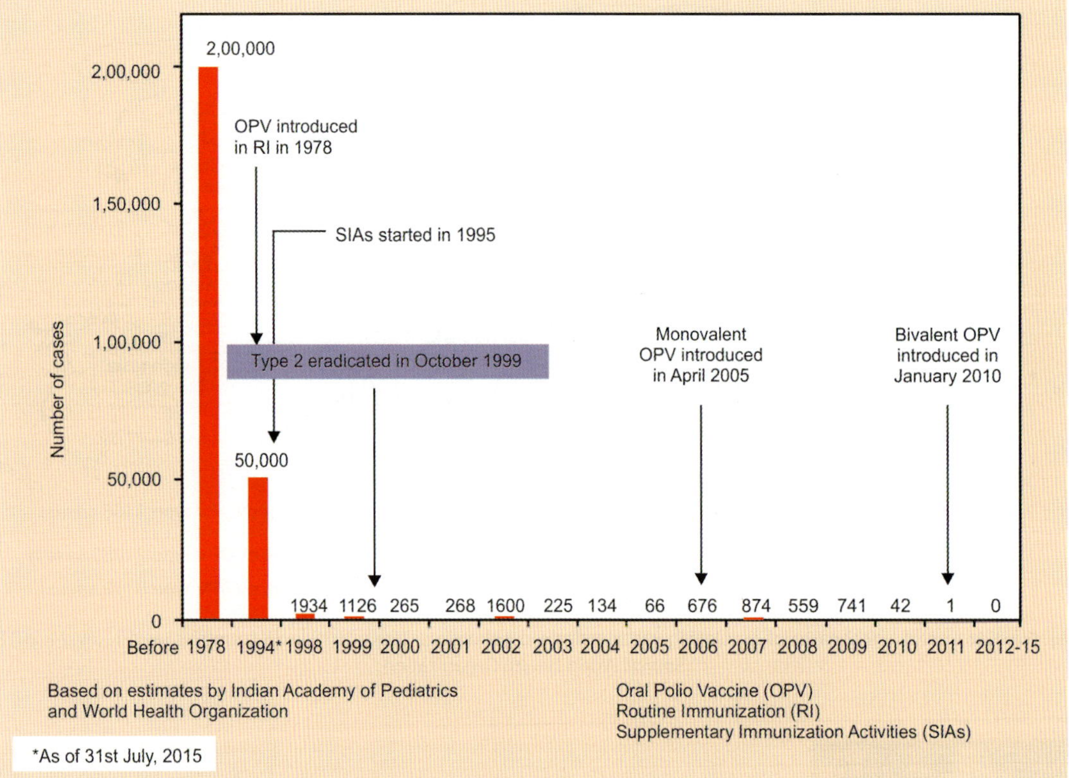

Fig. 5.4.1.3: History of polio in India (1978–2018*) (data as on July 28, 2018).

*Here is a brief overview of key events in the history of polio in India.

- India historically has had the highest estimated burden of paralytic polio in the world. In the late 1970s the annual polio burden was estimated to be more than 200,000 cases per year.
- Oral polio vaccine was introduced as part of the childhood RI in 1978. Polio substantially decreased after RI was introduced.
- Supplementary immunization activities began in India in 1995 as mass vaccination campaigns with tOPV.
- Wild Polio Virus Type 2 was last detected in 1999.
- In 2005, monovalent vaccines, first for type 1 and then for type 3 polio, were introduced in SIAs.

(OPV: oral polio vaccine; RI: routine immunization; SIA: supplementary immunization activity)

serotype-specific herd immunity in wild polio P3 serotype transmission areas. Bivalent OPV was introduced in selected states in India during the year 2010.

Migration of people was identified as one of the major risk factors for polio virus spread. Government of India in collaboration with WHO-NPSP initiated migrant sites and high-risk areas (HRAs) and high-risk groups (HRGs) with settled population mapping since December 2008. These low population immunity areas were targeted during supplementary immunization activities (SIAs) and strengthening RI coverage. Hard-to-reach Kosi riverine areas and 107 high-risk blocks in Uttar Pradesh and Bihar were identified and targeted for quality SIA coverage. After aggressive initiation of polio eradication strategies, polio incidence dramatically declined over the years 1995–2011.

Environmental surveillance for polio is carried out through sewage sampling in Mumbai since 2001. This supplementary surveillance is functional at 41 sites in eight states, and it is under process of expansion to other geographical areas.

Any WPV (in a case or in the environment) from any source will be considered a public health emergency and responded with urgent mop-up immunization campaigns.

All states in India have developed Emergency Preparedness and Response Plan against polio virus importation. Aggressive and emergency mop-up immunization response will target 0–5-year age group cohort. IR will be carried out within 10 days of WPV case confirmation. An outbreak simulation exercise is conducted on an annual basis to ensure adequate preparedness.

India had reported the last WPV type 1 case in Howrah (West Bengal) on January 13, 2011 (onset of paralysis). During the Polio Summit (February 25–26, 2012) in New Delhi, WHO declared that India is no longer polio endemic country. South East Asian Region of WHO was certified as polio free on March 27, 2014. This was a remarkable success of India's polio eradication initiative **(Fig. 5.4.1.4)**.

India had reported VDPV cases during the years 2014 (three cases), 2015 (two cases), and 2016 (one case),

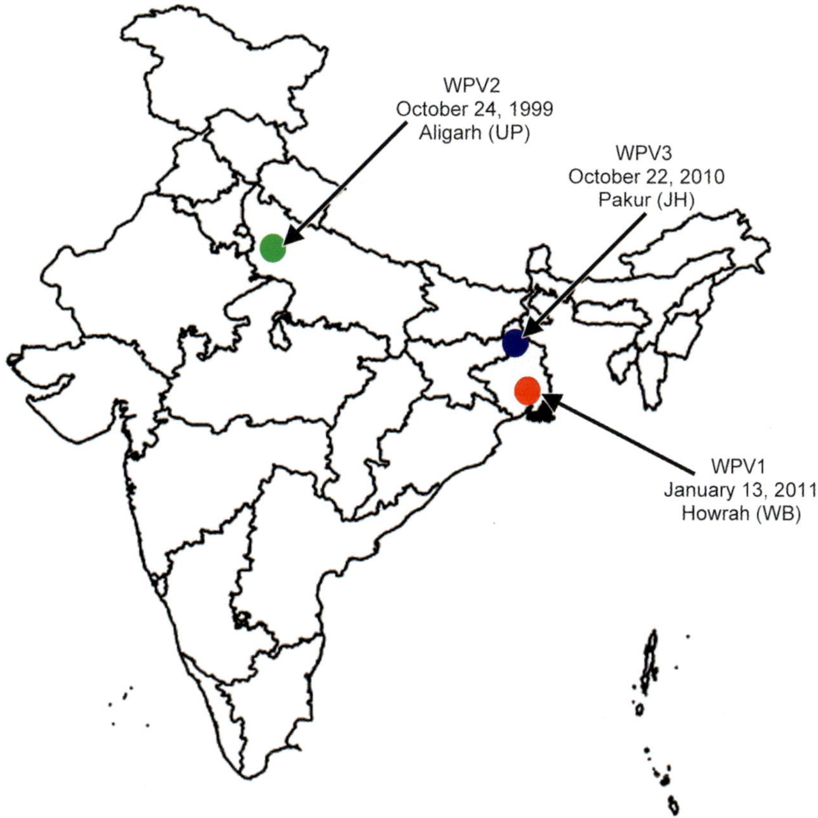

Fig. 5.4.1.4: Location of WPV cases by type, India.
(GOI: Government of India; JH: Jharkhand; NPSP: National Polio Surveillance Project; UP: Uttar Pradesh; WB: West Bengal; WPV: wild polio virus)
Source: GOI-WHO (NPSP).

respectively **(Fig. 5.4.1.5)**. There are no VDPV cases reported for the years 2017 and 2018 (till July 20, 2018).

In India, the evaluated RI coverage (National Family Health Survey, 2015–2016) showed that 62% were fully immunized against six vaccine preventable diseases. Sustaining high levels of population immunity against polio is critical to prevent emergence of cVDPV.

India Expert Advisory Group in 2018 had proposed the following polio endgame actions in India:

- To sustain certification standard AFP surveillance
- Expansion of existing environmental surveillance from 41 sites in eight states
- High RI coverage with bOPV and fractional IPV (fIPV) in all states
- Trivalent oral polio vaccine to bOPV switch successfully completed on April 25, 2016
- One round of bOPV, NID and two rounds of bOPV SNID will be conducted during the years 2019 and 2020
- Country should have emergency preparedness plan to respond to polio outbreaks.

Government of India has made it mandatory for all inbound and outbound international travelers to the following eight polio-affected countries (Pakistan, Afghanistan, Nigeria, Kenya, Ethiopia, Somalia, Syria, and Cameroon) from March 1, 2014 with one dose of OPV, irrespective of age. Valid certificate issued by the district immunization officer is essential for visa processing. This certificate is valid for 1-year period from the date of OPV vaccination.

Polio eradication in India was accomplished by sheer professionalism involving all categories of government staff, volunteers of private sector, and international service organizations, viz. WHO, United Nations Children's Fund, Centers for Disease Control and Prevention, Rotary International and Professional Organizations, such as Indian Academy of Pediatrics, Indian Medical Association, etc. The most geographically inaccessible terrains were reached by the committed polio vaccination team, particularly in Bihar and Uttar Pradesh. Special microplans were evolved for these hard-to-reach areas, and implementation was closely monitored. The intelligent strategy of replacing tOPV by mOPV and bOPV 1 and 3 in SNID and mop-ups had succeeded in interrupting polio transmission in India.

Routine immunization was strengthened in all poor coverage states. Special immunization campaigns, such as

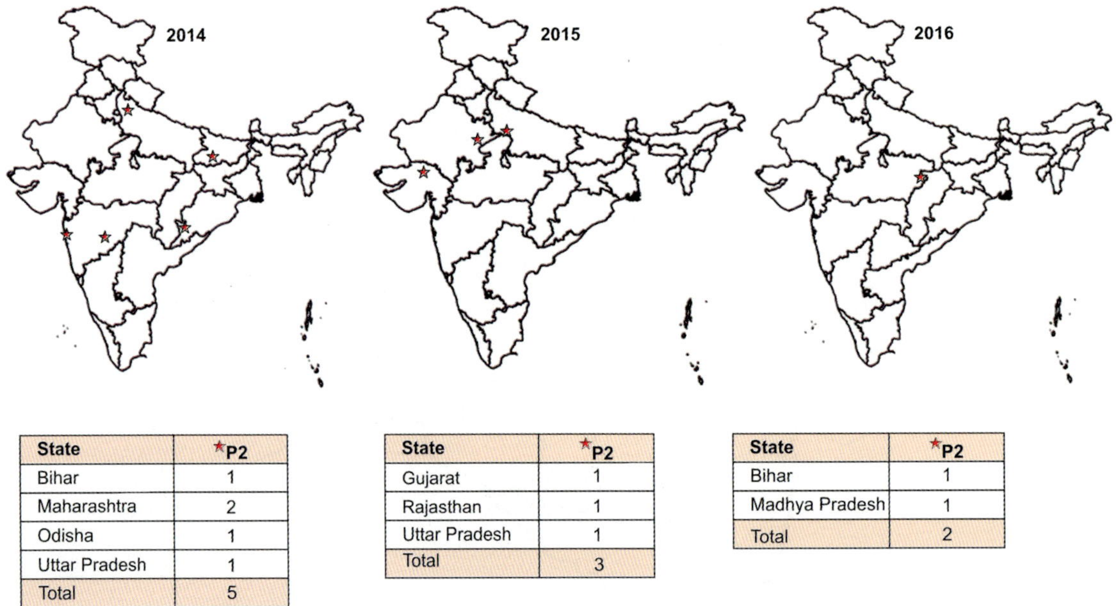

State	*P2
Bihar	1
Maharashtra	2
Odisha	1
Uttar Pradesh	1
Total	5

State	*P2
Gujarat	1
Rajasthan	1
Uttar Pradesh	1
Total	3

State	*P2
Bihar	1
Madhya Pradesh	1
Total	2

Fig. 5.4.1.5: Location of VDPV cases by type, India. Data as on July 20, 2018. (VDPV: vaccine-derived polio virus)

Mission Indradhanush and Gram Swaraj Abhiyan, targeted low immunization coverage districts across the country. The quality AFP surveillance system with timely polio laboratory results was guiding India's polio eradication efforts. All the above factors coupled with focused hard work were critical for the phenomenal polio eradication success and certification in India.

TOWARD POLIO ENDGAME

Comprehensive polio endgame strategy will involve the following:

Global

- Global tOPV to bOPV switch successfully completed in April 2016 in all 155 OPV-using countries
- Eventual cessation of bOPV use
- Inactivated polio vaccine was introduced in all OPV-using countries as a prerequisite prior to tOPV to bOPV switch.
- Sustaining high levels of population immunity through RI coverage with focus on HRAs and HRGs
- Sustaining standard AFP surveillance system
- Protect population against WPV and cVDPV
- Immunization of children at border areas during SIA campaign.

India

- National Switch tOPV to bOPV was meticulously implemented on April 25, 2016
- Introduction of two fIPV doses at 6 weeks and 14 weeks of age under NIS to protect children against type 2 VDPV
- Eventual cessation of bOPV use at appropriate period of time with successful implementation of the "New Strategy" for RI
- Sustaining high RI coverage in all the states of India inclusive of migrant sites
- Maintaining high levels of mucosal immunity and thus offering "Herd Protection" at the community
- Eradication of both WPV and VDPV paralysis with the implementation of revised polio eradication strategy
- Maintaining sensitive AFP surveillance and expanding environmental surveillance.

BIBLIOGRAPHY

1. Global Immunization Vision and Strategy (GIVS). 2006–2015, WHO & UNICEF.
2. Immunization Handbook for Medical Officers, 2017. Ministry of Health and Family Welfare, Govt. of India.
3. Operational Guidelines for tOPV to bOPV SWITCH, 2016 Ministry of Health and Family Welfare, Govt. of India.
4. Polio Eradication and End Game Strategic Plan. 2013–2018 (Available from www.who.int).
5. Pulse Polio Immunization Programme: Operational Guidelines (February, 2006). Ministry of Health and Family Welfare, Govt. of India.
6. Securing a Lasting World Free of all Polio Viruses Annual Report. 2017 (Available from www.polioeradication.org).
7. South East Asian Polio Free Regional Certification, 2014 (Available from *www.who.int*)
8. Surveillance of Acute Flaccid Paralysis: Field Guide, 3rd edition (September, 2005) Ministry of Health and Family Welfare, Govt. of India (Available from *www.npspindia.org*)

The Indian Academy of Pediatrics Advisory Committee on Vaccines and Immunization Practices has published a new set immunization schedule (2018–19) and an update on immunization for children 0 to 18 years. Readers are advised to go through the details provided in the Appendix at the end of the textbook.

5.5 Universal Immunization Program in India

Tanmay Amladi

INTRODUCTION

Delivering effective and safe vaccines through an efficient system is one of the most cost-effective public health interventions. Immunization programs aim to reduce mortality and morbidity due to vaccine preventable diseases (VPDs), particularly, for children.

Following the World Health Organization (WHO) recommendation, India Introduced six vaccines under the expanded program on immunization (EPI) in 1978 to reduce child mortality. These included bacillus Calmette-Guérin, tetanus toxoid (TT), diphtheria-pertussis-tetanus (DPT) vaccine, diphtheria-tetanus (DT) vaccine, poliomyelitis, and typhoid vaccines. Subsequently, in 1985, the Government of India (GoI) included measles vaccine in the national immunization schedule and launched the universal immunization program (UIP) and the national technology mission on immunization to achieve more than 85% immunization coverage of all infants and pregnant women by the year 1990. This was an undertaking of the immunization division of Ministry of Health and Family Welfare (MoHFW), GoI.

India's immunization program is one of the largest in the world in terms of quantities of vaccines used, number of beneficiaries, number of immunization sessions organized, and the geographical area covered. In India, in the National Immunization Program (NIP), since 1985, the target populations are infants under 1 year of age and pregnant women. Infants receive vaccines against six killer diseases, viz. tuberculosis, poliomyelitis, diphtheria, pertussis, tetanus, and measles; and pregnant women and the newborn are protected with TT, respectively.

IMMUNIZATION DIVISION OF THE MINISTRY OF HEALTH AND FAMILY WELFARE

Immunization division is a part of the Reproductive Child Health Program under National Rural Health Mission (NRHM) and is placed under the immunization division of the MoHFW, Nirman Bhavan, New Delhi. This division provides all the technical assistance required to undertake the activities under UIP.

The key roles of this division include the following:
- Activities related to routine immunization (RI), campaigns such as polio, measles, and Japanese encephalitis (*see* Bibliography)
- Monitoring adverse events following immunization (AEFI)
- Vaccine and cold chain logistics
- Strategic communication related to immunization program
- Trainings related to immunization program
- Facilitation of the national technical advisory group on immunization (NTAGI) to review and recommend its views on various technical and programmatic issues related to immunization, such as new vaccine introduction, etc.
- Reviewing and sharing the learnings of the program with state and district program officers

The division also works closely with all development partners and other stakeholders. The organogram of the UIP in the central government is depicted in **Flowchart 5.5.1**.

Flowchart 5.5.1: The organogram of the UIP in Government of India.

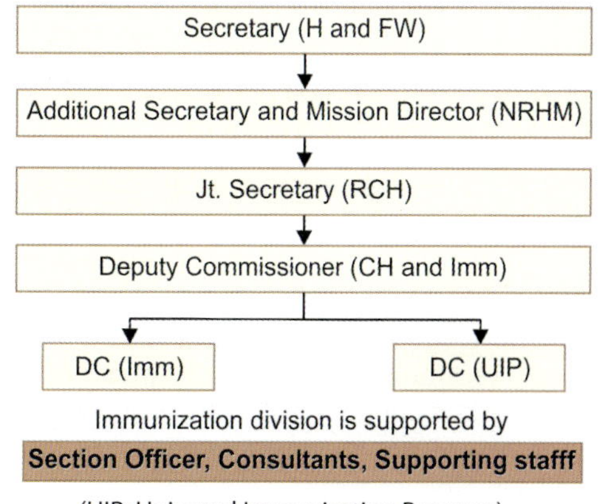

(UIP: Universal Immunization Program).

EVOLUTION OF THE UNIVERSAL IMMUNIZATION PROGRAM

- 1978—EPI
  - Mostly urban area based—Limited reach
- 1985—Universal program of immunization
  - For reduction of mortality and morbidity of six VPDs
  - Indigenous vaccine production capacity enhanced
  - Cold chain established
  - Phased implementation—All districts covered by 1989–1990
  - Monitoring and reevaluation system implemented
- 1986—Technology mission on immunization
  - Monitoring under Prime Minister's Office 20-point program
  - Coverage of infants monitored
- 1992—Child survival and safe motherhood
  - Included both UIP and safe motherhood program
- 1997—Reproductive and child health—1
- 2005—NRHM

The NTAGI recommends from time to time on issues such as addition of newer vaccines and allied issues in the NIP. Since 1997, the single disease surveillance, viz. acute flaccid paralysis (AFP) surveillance as part of Indian polio eradication initiative (IPEI) by National Polio Surveillance Project (NPSP) has been carried out to find the impact of pulse polio immunization (PPI) on polio eradication. The India Experts Advisory Group (IEAG) in collaboration with NPSP makes recommendations on the strategies for PPI through national immunization days (NIDs) and sub-NIDs in polio hyperendemic regions and for the whole country during PPI.

Subsequently since 2001–2002, the integrated disease surveillance project (IDSP) has also been introduced to focus attention on VPDs and other notifiable infectious diseases from remote reporting sites, private health facilities, and the sentinel centers throughout the country in the specially designed "reporting format" to enable the GoI to make evidence-based recommendations on introduction of newer vaccines based on epidemiological data available.

VACCINES UNDER UNIVERSAL IMMUNIZATION PROGRAM

Under UIP, the following vaccines are available to all target population in India and provided through government centers:

- Bacillus Calmette-Guérin
- Diphtheria, tetanus, poliomyelitis (DTP)
- Oral polio vaccine (OPV) (refer to Chapter 5.4.1 for recent developments on poliomyelitis and its prevention)
- Measles
- Hepatitis B (HB)
- Tetanus toxoid
- Japanese encephalitis vaccine (in hyperendemic areas)
- *Haemophilus influenzae* type B (Hib) containing pentavalent vaccine (DTP + HB + Hib)

Diseases Protected by Vaccination under Universal Immunization Program

- Tuberculosis
- Diphtheria
- Pertussis
- Tetanus
- Poliomyelitis
- Measles
- Hepatitis B
- Japanese encephalitis
- Meningitis and pneumonitis caused by Hib

VACCINE-PREVENTABLE DISEASES SURVEILLANCE

Vaccine preventable diseases surveillance system is needed to create evidence-based planning and deployment of effective interventions.

India has different surveillance models for this; the IDSP is one such project. It is a case-based surveillance system for early detection of outbreaks using recognized early warning signs. Other sentinel surveillance systems that fall under different vertical national health programs contribute to the other aspects—control, elimination, and eradication. One more exemplary surveillance system is the NPSP which has performed exceedingly well in polio (and measles) surveillance in India. The WHO and NPSP provide technical training support for AFP and measles surveillance.

INTRODUCTION OF ADDITIONAL VACCINES IN THE NATIONAL IMMUNIZATION PROGRAM IN INDIA—HISTORICAL PERSPECTIVES

Hepatitis B Vaccine

Hepatitis B vaccination was introduced in UIP in the financial year 2002–2003 as a pilot in 33 districts and 15 cities and was further expanded to all the districts of 10 states, namely, Andhra Pradesh, Himachal Pradesh, Jammu and Kashmir, Karnataka, Kerala, Madhya Pradesh, Maharashtra, Punjab, Tamil Nadu, and West Bengal. Following the recommendation of NTAGI, it has been decided to provide HB vaccination all over the country.

Measles Vaccine—Second Dose

Measles immunization directly contributes to the reduction of under-five child mortality and hence to the achievement of millennium development goal number 4. In order to accelerate the reduction of measles-related morbidity and mortality, second opportunity for measles vaccination is being implemented. The NTAGI has recommended the introduction of another dose of measles vaccine through measles supplementary immunization activity for states where evaluated coverage for measles vaccine is less than 80%. For the remaining states where coverage is more than 80%, NTAGI recommended a second dose through RI. The 14 states with measles coverage of less than or equal to 80%, viz. Arunachal Pradesh, Assam, Bihar, Chhattisgarh, Gujarat, Haryana, Jharkhand, Madhya Pradesh, Manipur, Meghalaya, Nagaland, Rajasthan, Tripura, and Uttar Pradesh, are being covered through, in a phased manner followed by the introduction of second dose at 16–24 months in RI.

Japanese B Encephalitis Vaccine

Japanese B encephalitis (JE) vaccination was started in 2006 in a campaign approach in JE hyperendemic areas to cover 109 endemic districts in phased manner, using SA 14-14-2 vaccine imported from China. Single dose of JE vaccine was given to all children between 1 year and 15 years of age through campaigns followed by one dose at 16–24 months under RI to cover the newer cohort. By the end of 2009–2010, 90 districts have been covered under the JE vaccination program, and the remaining 19 districts are being covered in 2010–2011. In addition, in 2010–2011, recampaign has been planned in nine districts—seven in Uttar Pradesh and two in Assam—in view of their low coverage as per the coverage evaluation survey (CES) conducted in 2008. The JE vaccine is being integrated into RI in the districts where campaign had already been conducted to immunize the new cohort of children by vaccinating with single doses at 16–24 months.

India Polio Eradication Initiative

Refer to Chapter 5.4.1, Polio Endgame: Global and National Perspectives.

Implementation of Routine Immunization under Universal Immunization Program

Routine immunization targets to vaccinate 26 million neonates per year with all primary doses and approximately 100 million children between 1 year and 5 years of age with booster doses of UIP vaccines. In addition, 30 million pregnant women are targeted for TT vaccination every year. To vaccinate this cohort of 156 million beneficiaries, approximately 9 million immunization sessions are conducted annually, the majority being at the village level.

As per the coverage survey of 2009, 89.8% of vaccination in India is being provided through the public sector (53% from outreach sessions held through Anganwadi centers and subcenters, etc.), while private sector contributes to 8.7%.

Accredited social health activist (ASHA) and Anganwadi worker (AWW) support auxiliary nurse midwifes (ANMs) by mobilizing eligible children to session sites. To ensure potent and safe vaccine delivery, a network of approximately 27,000 cold chain points have been created across the country where vaccines are stored appropriately.

COMPONENTS OF UNIVERSAL IMMUNIZATION PROGRAM

Strategy and Policy

National Health Policy (2002) is directed toward achieving an acceptable, affordable, and sustainable standard of health through an appropriate health system. Provision of universal immunization of children against VPDs is one of the major goals under this policy.

The country's 5-year plan also puts emphasis on reduction in maternal and infant mortality rates as major maternal and child health indicators. The country developed a comprehensive multiyear strategic plan for immunization in 2005 with an addendum in 2010 to achieve these targets of improving access and utilization of immunization in the country. This document is a national strategy document to guide development of UIP plans at national and state levels. Currently, development of next multiyear plan is under process. The MoHFW also revised the national vaccine policy in 2011.

The goal of this vaccine policy is to guide decision-making in order to develop a long-term plan to strengthen the UIP. This policy addresses issues of vaccine security, management, regulation guidelines, vaccine research and development, and product development. To ensure informed decision-making for any modification in UIP schedule or inclusion of new vaccines, there is an NTAGI, which comprises a number of technical experts, national program leaders and managers, representatives from development partners, and professional bodies.

The NTAGI has made the following recommendations subsequent to introduction of new vaccines like HB since 2002–2003:

- Introduction of at birth dose of HB vaccine.
- Introduction of second dose for measles at 15–18 months of age.
- Introduction of diphtheria, tetanus, whole-cell pertussis (DTwP)-HB-Hib vaccine—a combination of diphtheria and TT, whole-cell pertussis vaccine, and vaccines against HB and Hib—(penta-combo-vaccine, pentavac) in pilot project areas of the country where the routine DTwP coverage is more than 85%.
- Initially 10 such states were selected for pentavac introduction and the union cabinet nod was also

obtained. Due to logistic reasons, currently, the pentavac introduction is restricted to the states of Kerala and Tamil Nadu from October 2011, which strategy will be expanded to the other eight states in a phased manner aiming at national roll out in future.
- The second DTwP booster at 5 years in place of DT vaccine.
- National technical advisory group on immunization has also discussed and recommended in principle the introduction of pneumococcal conjugate vaccine, rotavirus, and human papilloma virus vaccines in the NIP with aid from global alliance for vaccines and immunization (GAVI) in future in a phased manner.

However, the recommendations and strategies on polio vaccines are exclusively made by India Expert Advisory Group on Polio Eradication in collaboration with NPSP.

The immunization coverage has seen an improvement over the years. However, there is further need for improvement especially in DPT3 and OPV3 coverage and reducing dropouts (refer to Chapter 5.6). To strengthen RI, some newer initiatives have been introduced as part of the state program implementation plan. These initiatives are provision of auto-disable (AD) syringe to ensure injection safety.

Cold Chain System, Vaccines, and Logistics

India has built a vast cold chain infrastructure to ensure that only potent and effective vaccines reach millions of beneficiaries across the country.

Equipment

The GoI procures and supplies all UIP vaccines along with the diluents and syringes to all the states quarterly based on indents and from there to primary health centers (PHCs) and community health centers (CHCs) monthly. This then necessarily involves forecasting, scheduling, and supplying as per the need and maintaining the cold chain properly in the process. States can store vaccines up to a maximum of 3 months and PHCs up to maximum 1 month.

Injections and Safe Disposal of Injection Equipment

To prevent infections such as human immunodeficiency virus, HB, and hepatitis C, etc. that can be transmitted through shared needles or recycled ones, the GoI endeavors to provide continuous and adequate supply of safe injection equipment such as AD syringes, reconstitution syringes, hub cutters, and waste disposal bags. Disposal of immunization waste is done strictly as per the central pollution control board guidelines for disposal of biohazardous waste material. The principles are as follows:
- Segregation of waste at source (at the session site)
- Transportation to the PHC or CHC
- Treatment of sharps in sharp pits and treated plastic waste through proper recycling
- Provision of funds to states to procure hub cutters, black and red plastic bags, and construction of sharp pits in PHCs and CHCs

Sequence

- The vaccines are supplied by manufacturers directly to four government medical store depots (GMSDs) (at Karnal, Mumbai, Chennai, and Kolkata) and state and regional vaccine stores.
- The GMSDs supply to the states and regional vaccine stores; state and regional vaccine stores supply vaccines to divisional vaccine stores and district.
- The vaccines are further supplied to last cold chain points that are usually situated in PHCs and CHCs.
- Transportation of vaccines from state/regional stores is done in cold boxes using insulated vans.
- Vaccine carriers with ice-packs are used to transport vaccines from PHCs to outreach sessions inside villages.

Personnel

- In the states, there are state cold chain officers who are in charge to ensure smooth functioning of all cold chain equipment in the state.
- At regional, divisional, and district levels, there are cold chain technicians whose responsibility is to maintain and repair cold chain equipment as per standards. They have been provided with training and tool kits for performing installation, maintenance, and repair activities. Maintenance funds for the equipment come from the state under the aegis of NRHM.
- At the PHCs and CHCs, cold chain handlers who are health personnel (pharmacists, multipurpose health workers, etc.) are responsible for proper storage and handling of vaccines and daily upkeep of ice-lined refrigerators (ILRs) and deep freezers (DFs), including temperature charting on regular basis.

Periodic Evaluation

The performance and efficiency of the cold chain system at different levels is monitored continuously, through supervisory visits and review meetings.

Adverse Effects Following Immunization Surveillance in India

The AEFI surveillance system started in 1988. In 2005, the national AEFI guidelines were disseminated, and in 2007, state and district-level AEFI committees were formed.

The national AEFI committee was formed in 2008 and guidelines formulated and disseminated by 2010. Over the next 2 years, standard operating procedures were printed and widely circulated, and the AEFI secretariat was established under the immunization technical support unit to strengthen and coordinate all activities of the AEFI surveillance.

The Indian National Regulatory Authority assessment was passed successfully in 2012, and in 2013, the national AEFI committee was revised with to include a broader range of expertise such as in pharmacology, forensic medicine, pathology, immunology, epidemiology, communication, etc., along with pediatricians and other experts in the field of immunization.

Strategic Communication

Use of all media including posters and hoardings, radio, television, newspapers and magazines, websites, social networking sites has been a focal point for the GoI to achieve its goals of UIP.

Development of the Routine Immunization Logo (Fig. 5.5.1)

The new logo depicts a baby holding a syringe, indicating RI on the baby's right, gives RI its distinct identity. The purple color has been used to avoid the use of pink and yellow which are polio vaccine potency marking colors, to avoid confusion.

Immunization Trainings

The following training programs are conducted in India under the auspices of the UIP **(Table 5.5.1)**.

In the year of intensification of RI in 2012–2013, the GoI has supported the training of approximately 1,250,000 frontline workers (ANMs, lady health visitor, AWWs, and ASHAs) in nine high-priority states—Uttar Pradesh, Madhya Pradesh, Rajasthan, Bihar, Chhattisgarh, Jharkhand, Haryana, Gujarat, and West Bengal.

The objective is to motivate and strengthen the capacity of frontline workers to reduce dropouts and left-outs and improve the quality of services.

Cold chain technicians at various levels are trained on repair and maintenance of ILRs and DFs, of walk in coolers

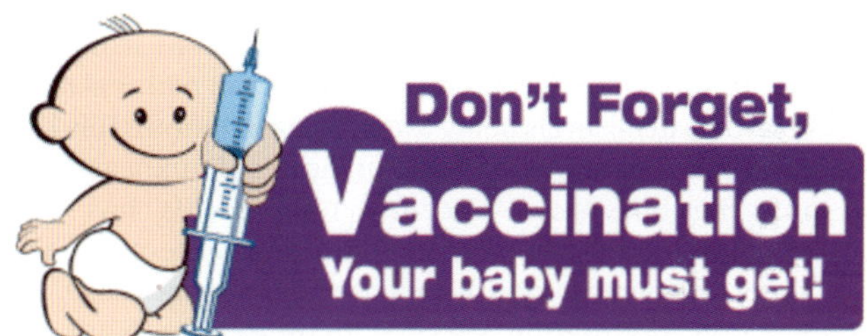

Fig. 5.5.1: Routine immunization logo.

Table 5.5.1: Training programs conducted under UIP, GoI.

S. no.	*Name of training*	*Duration (day)*	*Level/Venue*	*Participants*	*Training module*	*Evaluation*
1.	Immunization training for medical officers (since 2009–2010)	3	State/ Regional/ District	All contractual and regular medical officers including AYUSH	Immunization handbook for medical officers (revised 2011), Department of Health and Family Welfare, MoHFW, GoI	Conducted in 2012–2013
2.	Immunization training of health workers (since 2006 and from 2012 using revised version)	2	District level	All female and male multipurpose health workers and their supervisors	Immunization handbook for health workers (revised 2011), Department of Health and Family Welfare, MoHFW, GoI	Conducted in 2009
3.	Training of vaccine and cold chain handlers (since 2010–2011)	2	District level	All health workers (pharmacists/staff nurses/ ANMs/LHVs/male MPWs, etc.) in charge of handling vaccines and cold chain equipment at all vaccine stores (state/region/districts/ hospitals/PHCs/CHCs)	Handbook for vaccine and cold chain handlers (revised 2011), Department of Health and Family Welfare, MoHFW, GoI	Conducted in 2012–2013
4.	Training of state, district, and block data entry operators (ongoing)	1	State level	Immunization program data entry operators at state, district, and block levels	–	–

(ANM: auxiliary nurse midwifes; AYUSH: Ayurveda, Yoga and Naturopathy, Unani, Siddha, and Homeopathy; CHC: community health center; GoI: Government of India; LHV: lady health visitor; MoHFW: Ministry of Health and Family Welfare; MPW: multipurpose health; UIP: Universal Immunization Program)

and walk in freezers and generator sets, on installation and maintenance of solar refrigerators, and also on repair of voltage stabilizers.

New training courses under development include induction training for state immunization officers and training on effective cold chain and vaccine management.

The GoI has set up the National Cold Chain and Vaccine Management Resource Center at the National Institute of Health and Family Welfare, New Delhi, and also the National Cold Chain Training Center at State Health Transport Organization, Pune, Maharashtra.

Monitoring and Evaluation of Universal Immunization Program

This occurs at three levels:

1. The regular computerized reporting system from the health subcenter to PHC, district, state, and national level with data at all levels being available each month; this has been made possible with help of the health management information system—recently, the MoHFW has also implemented mother and child tracking system to track every pregnant woman and child under 5 years of age.
2. Periodic population surveys including the National Family Health Survey, district-level health survey, annual health survey, and United Nations Children's Fund CES.
3. In between surveys and administrative reporting, GoI conducted targeted studies and surveys to evaluate the performance of various components under UIP, viz. volume management activation tool/enterprise volume system management, postintroduction evaluation, and Microsoft certified technology specialist.

Reviewing is done monthly at PHC and district level, less frequently at state and national levels.

SUMMARY

Thus UIP in India and the IPEI have achieved remarkable success in eliminating the six killer diseases which were targeted in 1985 with the launch of UIP. However, reemergence of VPDs like diphtheria and pertussis in certain regions of the country is causing concern. There is reemergence of certain eliminated VPDs and NTAGI is looking forward strengthening the UIP coverage of routine vaccines and to the introduction of newer vaccines in the NIP with aid from GAVI funded and supported by Melinda and Gates foundation, United States Agency for International Development, Rockefeller Foundation, global vaccine manufacturers, etc. The laudable objective of GAVI—"all vaccines for ALL children of the world"—will be the future achievement of the global immunization program which will become a reality rather than a dream, ensuing equity of the affluent as well as the downtrodden children and pregnant women of the international society.

BIBLIOGRAPHY

1. Ministry of Health and Family Welfare (2011). Annual Report of the Ministry of Health and Family Welfare, Govt. of India. [online]. Available from: http://mohfw.nic.in/showfile.php?lid=767 [Accessed October, 2018].
2. WHO (1997). National Polio Surveillance Project. [online]. Available from: www.npsp.com [Accessed October, 2018].
3. World Health Organization (2013). Global Polio Eradication Initiative. [online] Available from: www.polioeradication.org [Accessed October, 2018].
4. Yewale V, Choudhury P, Thacker N. Immunization schedules, individual vaccines. In: Yewale V, Choudhury P, Thacker N (Eds). IAP Guidebook on Immunization 2011. Mumbai: Indian Academy of Pediatrics; 2011. pp. 47-50.

The Indian Academy of Pediatrics Advisory Committee on Vaccines and Immunization Practices has published a new set immunization schedule (2018-19) and an update on immunization for children 0 to 18 years. Readers are advised to go through the details provided in the Appendix at the end of the textbook.

5.6 Non UIP Vaccines in India

Anju Aggarwal

INTRODUCTION

Vaccines are included in the immunization schedule of a country based on the World Health Organization (WHO) recommendations, which takes into consideration the epidemiology, cost-effectiveness, and availability of the vaccines in that country along with the scientific evidence of efficacy or immunogenicity of a particular vaccine in the country. In the last decade, several new vaccines have been developed and are available in India apart from the basic vaccines included in the national immunization schedule (NIS) under universal immunization program. Indian Academy of Pediatrics (IAP) Advisory Committee on Vaccination and Immunization Practices (IAP-ACVIP) periodically reviews the need for these vaccines and recommends their use. Physicians should be able to counsel the parents regarding the efficacy and importance of these vaccines in the present health situation.

This chapter includes a brief description of these vaccines. In fact, almost all these vaccines are included in the Expanded Program on Immunization (EPI) national schedules of several developed countries. In India, almost all these vaccines find a place in the IAP-ACVIP Immunization Timetable 2016 for routine use.

PNEUMOCOCCAL VACCINE

Currently two types of pneumococcal vaccines are marketed in India: conjugate [13-valent pneumococcal conjugate vaccine (PCV13), 10-valent pneumococcal conjugate vaccine (PCV10)] and nonconjugate or polysaccharide [23-valent nonconjugate capsular polysaccharide vaccine (PPSV23)] pneumococcal vaccines. Conjugate pneumococcal vaccine 13-valent is now included in the immunization schedule of many districts in India, with a plan that it will be included in the National Immunization Program of India.

Nonconjugate Capsular Polysaccharide Vaccine

A PPSV23 is available for use in children above 2 years of age who belong to the "high-risk group" and for use in older children, adolescents, and adults, routinely. This vaccine covers most of the prevalent strains of *Pneumococcus* causing disease. It is given as a single dose of 0.5 mL subcutaneously (SC) or intramuscular (IM) in children, more than 2 years of age. The vaccine being a capsular polysaccharide is not immunogenic in children of less than 2 years of age. At present, the vaccine is recommended in children with sickle cell disease, functional and anatomic asplenia, nephrotic syndrome, patients with cerebrospinal fluid leak, and children with malignancies and human immunodeficiency virus infection.

Polysaccharide vaccine fails to elicit a protective immune response in children less than 2 years, even though 80% of the pneumococcal disease occurs in children less than 2 years of age. Hence, the use of conjugated vaccines is preferred.

7-Valent Pneumococcal Conjugate Vaccine

This was the first pneumococcal conjugate vaccine. It contained seven purified capsular polysaccharides of *Streptococcus pneumoniae* coupled with a nontoxic variant of diphtheria to cross-reacting material 197. It had serotypes 4, 6B, 9V, 14, 18C, 19F, and 23F, responsible for 85% of invasive disease and 65% of otitis media in the western countries. It covers only 50% of the prevalent strains in India. Dose is 0.5 mL IM. Schedule is same as diphtheria, pertussis, and tetanus (DPT) at 6 weeks, 10 weeks, and 14 weeks with a booster at 15–18 months. After 6 months, two doses are required. Single dose is required after 2 years. 7-valent pneumococcal conjugate vaccine has been replaced by PCV13 since 2011.

13-Valent Pneumococcal Conjugate Vaccine

A 13-valent conjugate pneumococcal vaccine is now available, which covers about 70% of strains worldwide and India. It has 1, 5, 7F, 3, 6A, and 19A in addition to the 7-valent vaccine. Schedule of immunization is the same. Routine use is not recommended in children above 5 years. Details of the schedule to be followed in various ages and situations should be as per recommendation of IAP and American Academy of Pediatrics.

10-Valent Pneumococcal Conjugate Vaccine

This 10-valent pneumococcal vaccine has 1, 5, and 7F strains in addition to the 7-valent strains. This vaccine has been proved to be immunogenic when used in the EPI schedule in European countries and covers up to 70% of the prevalent strains in a given geographical area. The vaccine is available and can be used in the same schedule as PCV13.

Both PCV10 and PCV13 are licensed for use in children 6 weeks to 5 years. PCV13 is now recommended for use in adults 50 years of age and above.

TETANUS WITH LOW DOSE OF DIPHTHERIA AND ACELLULAR PERTUSSIS VACCINE (TETANUS-DIPHTHERIA-ACELLULAR PERTUSSIS)

Immunity following primary/booster diphtheria, tetanus, and pertussis (DTP/diphtheria, tetanus, and acellular pertussis (DTaP) vaccination wanes over 5–10 years. Standard strength DTP and DTaP vaccines cannot be used in children above 7 years due to increased reactogenicity. Tetanus-diphtheria-acellular pertussis (Tdap) vaccine contains lower doses of diphtheria and acellular pertussis components and hence can be used in children above 7 years. Systemic side effects are rarely seen. A dose of this vaccine can be given at 10–11 years of age as DTP booster. A single dose is recommended after 7 years, if the child has not received the vaccine before. This vaccine is now routinely recommended as a single booster to be followed by boosters of tetanus and diphtheria vaccine at intervals of 10 years by the IAP-ACVIP in view of reemerging pertussis and diphtheria in certain regions of the country. The IAP now suggests single dose of Tdap in pregnancy during third trimester (preferred 26–27 weeks) regardless of previous immunization with Tdap. This protects the young infant from pertussis till 6–8 weeks of life.

TYPHOID VACCINE

Typhoid vaccine was included in the NIS till 1987 but discontinued because the vaccine had lot of side effects. Now typhoid is occurring in younger age groups, and there is emergence of multiple drug resistance. Hence, there is a need for typhoid vaccines. Two types of typhoid vaccines are now available.

Vi-Polysaccharide Typhoid Vaccine

The Vi antigen of *Salmonella typhi* is a capsular antigen with known virulence property of the organism and is available as injectable vaccine containing 25-mg purified Vi-capsular polysaccharide (Vi-PS) per dose. The dose is 0.5 mL IM in the deltoid region above the age of 2 years with revaccination every 3 years. The efficacy of the vaccine varies from 64% to 72% in various studies. Adverse reactions include pain, erythema, and induration at the local site and rarely fever. All the reactions are of mild nature and self-limiting.

Conjugated Typhoid Vaccines

The limitations of the polysaccharide typhoid vaccine include the following:

- Noneffectiveness below the age of 2 years.
- Limited efficacy (of around 60%).
- T-cell-independent response, which lacks immune memory.
- It is not boostable.

Conjugation of the Vi antigen with a protein carrier is hence desirable, as it would induce a T-cell-dependent immune response.

Vi-Polysaccharide Vaccines Conjugated with Tetanus Toxoid

There are two conjugate vaccines developed in India using tetanus toxoid as the carrier protein. One contains 25 μg/0.5 mL and another 5 μg/0.5 mL of Vi-PS antigen.

Recommendations for Use

Vi-capsular polysaccharide vaccine: IAP-ACVIP recommends the administration of the currently available Vi-PS vaccine 0.5 mL IM every 3 years beginning at the age of 2 years. A child with history of suspected/confirmed enteric fever might be vaccinated 4 weeks after recovery, if he/she has not received the vaccine in the past 3 years.

Considering the typhoid epidemiology in the country and analyzing the available data of the vaccine, IAP recommends the use of new conjugate vaccine below 1 year of age, preferably between 9 months and 12 months (minimum age 6 months). Since the incompatibility data with measles vaccine is not available, there should be an interval of at least 4 weeks either before or after the former. The initial dose should be followed by a booster dose in the second year. Only one dose is required if started above 2 years.

INACTIVATED POLIO VACCINE

This vaccine is prepared from the virus of the original Salk strain grown in monkey's kidney, human diploid, or Vero cell line and is inactivated by formalin. At present, it is available as an enhanced potency inactivated poliovirus vaccine (eIPV) containing 40, 8, and 32 D antigen units against types I, II, and III polioviruses, respectively, in 0.5 mL of the vaccine.

Dosage and Schedule

Three doses of 0.5 mL IM along with DPT vaccine can be given according to the DPT schedule (6 weeks, 10 weeks, and 14 weeks). The booster dose is recommended along with DPT at 15–18 months. As a catch-up vaccine in children less than 5 years of age completing the primary immunization with oral polio vaccine (OPV), two doses of IPV 4–8 weeks apart may be given. The efficacy of the enhanced potency IPV is over 90–100% in various studies. The IAP-ACVIP recommends IPV at 6, 10, and 14 weeks or as a compromised IPV schedule at 6 weeks and 14 weeks followed by a single booster at 18 months and OPV at 0 month, 6 months, 9 months, and the annual pulse polio immunization doses in addition. In view of shortage of IPV, a fractional dose 0.1 mL of IPV is given intradermally at two sites at 6 weeks and 14 weeks in some states in government setups.

Adverse Effects

Local minor adverse reactions include pain, swelling, and erythema, which are self-limiting.

HEPATITIS A VACCINE

There are two types of hepatitis A vaccines now available: inactivated and live-attenuated formulations.

Inactivated Hepatitis A Vaccine

This contains formaldehyde inactivated hepatitis A virus derived from HM175 or GBM strain adsorbed onto aluminum hydroxide.

Dose and Schedule

Hepatitis A vaccine is given in a prime boost schedule, viz. the priming dose on elected date "0," followed by a single booster at 6-month interval. The IAP-ACVIP now recommends the vaccine to be given at 12 months of age routinely for optimal protection in view of waning maternal antibodies in infants. Dose is 0.5 mL IM containing 750 enzyme-linked immunosorbent assay units in children.

Adverse Effects

Adverse reactions are minimal and include self-limiting local reactions at injection site. It can be given after 1 year in children as a routine vaccine.

Live-attenuated Hepatitis A Vaccine

The vaccine is derived from the H2 strain of the virus attenuated after serial passage in human diploid cell. It has been in use in China since the 1990s in mass vaccination programs. The vaccine meets requirements of the Chinese Drug Authority and WHO. It is also licensed and available in India. The recommended dose is 1 mL SC in children aged 1–15 years. Immunogenicity studies with single dose show seroconversion rates of more than 98%, 2 months after vaccination and persistence of protective antibodies in more than 80% of vaccines at 10-year follow-up. Two immunogenicity studies from India in 143 and 505 children, respectively, have demonstrated greater than 95% seroconversion with single dose of the live-attenuated vaccine with persistence of antibodies on follow-up.

VARICELLA VACCINE

Varicella vaccines are derived from the original Oka strain, but the virus contents may vary from one manufacturer to another. The recommended dose is 0.5 mL by SC route, and the minimum infectious virus content should be 1,000 plaque-forming units. It is available as lyophilized vaccine. It should be protected from light and needs to be used within 30 minutes of its reconstitution. It may be given with all other childhood vaccines.

The IAP-ACVIP recommends offering the vaccine to all healthy children with no prior history of varicella with special emphasis in all children belonging to certain high-risk groups. Varicella vaccine is licensed for 12 months and above. However, the risk of breakthrough varicella is lower if given 15 months onward. Hence, the IAP Committee on Immunization recommends the administration of varicella vaccine in children aged 15 months or older. After a single dose of varicella vaccine, approximately 15% of vaccines remain at risk of developing breakthrough varicella disease. Two doses of varicella vaccine offer superior individual protection as compared to a single dose. It is now recommended two doses of varicella vaccine for children with all age groups. For primary immunization, the first dose should be given at the age of 15 months and second dose at 4–6 years. For catch-up vaccination, children below the age of 13 years should receive two doses 3 months apart, and those aged 13 years or more should receive two doses at interval of 4–8 weeks.

A combined measles, mumps, and rubella (MMR) and varicella vaccine is also licensed in India. It has an efficacy of 95–100%. It is recommended in 4- to 6-year age group, as there is a chance of increased incidence of febrile seizure if it is used below 2 years.

HUMAN PAPILLOMAVIRUS VACCINE

Human papillomavirus (HPV) serotypes 16 and 18 are implicated in 70% of cervical cancers globally. Types 6 and 11 are known to cause 90% of anogenital warts.

Two HPV vaccines have been licensed globally, a quadrivalent and a bivalent vaccine. Both are manufactured by recombinant deoxyribonucleic acid technology that produces noninfectious virus like particles comprising the HPV L1 protein, the major capsid protein of HPV. Quadrivalent vaccine available in India is a mixture of L1 proteins of HPV serotypes 16, 18, 6, and 11 with aluminum containing adjuvant. The bivalent vaccine is a mixture of L1 proteins of HPV serotypes 16 and 18 with ASO4 as an adjuvant.

The IAP-ACVIP recommends offering HPV vaccine to all females in the schedules. Since protection is seen only when the vaccine is given before infection with HPV, the vaccine should be given prior to sexual debut. Both the vaccines are equally efficacious and safe for protection against cervical cancer and percutaneous lesions as of currently available data. The quadrivalent vaccine additionally protects against anogenital warts.

The vaccines should be stored at 2–8°C and must not be frozen. The dose is 0.5 mL by IM route in deltoid. The vaccine can be given to females above 9 years age. Two doses of either vaccine are recommended at 0 month and 6 months in 9- to 14-year age group. From 15 years onward, three doses at 0 month, 2 months, and 6 months are recommended with quadrivalent vaccine (minimum interval between first and second dose is 4 weeks and second and third dose is 12 weeks) and 0 month, 1 month, and 6 months with the bivalent vaccine.

Both the vaccine formulations are now recommended in women up to 45 years of age. Pregnancy is a contraindication. Preferably the vaccine should be administered in naive adolescent girls and young women, where microabrasions following sexual activity facilitating invasion of the virus in the vaginal epithelium have occurred preferably in cervical intraepithelial neoplasia (CIN) stages 1 and 2 only. Cervical intraepithelial neoplasia stage 3 is considered to be precancerous, and the vaccine is contraindicated at this stage. Hence, a prevaccination screening for evidence of precancerous stage is ideal and recommended in married women prior to administration of HPV vaccine.

A 9-valent HPV vaccine has been approved in the United States in December 2014 and will be available in India by 2019.

ROTAVIRUS VACCINES

Currently, the live-attenuated oral rotavirus vaccines are available.

1. *Monovalent vaccine (RV1)*: It is an attenuated human rotavirus vaccine derived from human rotavirus strain 89-12 that contains GIP8 strain. It is available as a lyophilized vaccine to be reconstituted with a diluent. First dose can be given at 6 weeks (not later than 12 weeks). Second dose is given 4 weeks later. The two-dose schedule should be completed by 16 weeks and not later than 32 weeks.
2. *Pentavalent human-bovine reassortant vaccine (RV 5)*: Pentavalent human-bovine reassortant vaccine contains five reassortants between the bovine WC23 strain and human G1, G2, G3, G4, and P1A8 rotavirus strain. Recommended schedule is three oral doses at 2 months, 4 months, and 6 months. First dose is to be started at 6–12 weeks with subsequent doses at the interval of 4–8 weeks, and all the recommended doses should be completed before 32 weeks. It is available as a liquid formulation and should not be frozen or injected.
3. *Indian neonatal rotavirus live vaccine, 116 E:* This vaccine developed in India is a live, naturally attenuated vaccine containing monovalent, bovine-human reassortant strain characterized as G9P10, with the VP4 of bovine rotavirus origin, and all other segments of human rotavirus origin. The vaccine strain was isolated from asymptomatic infants, with mild diarrhea by Indian researchers in 1985 at All India Institute of Medical Sciences, New Delhi. Follow-up of these infants indicated that they were protected against severe rotavirus diarrhea for up to 2 years. This strain was sent for vaccine development to the NIH by Department of Biotechnology—India and later transferred to Bharat Biotech International Limited in 2001 for further development. This vaccine is licensed in India. The recommended schedule is three oral doses.

The first dose of rotavirus vaccines should be given at 6 weeks and not later than 14 weeks and 6 days. The final dose (second for RV1 or third dose for the rest) should be completed by 32 weeks.

All these vaccines have an efficacy of 85–98% against severe rotavirus gastroenteritis and 42–60% against hospitalization from diarrhea of any cause. These vaccines have been recommended by the WHO to be included in the routine schedule in countries where more than 10% of under-five deaths are due to diarrhea. It is a public health vaccine. National Technical Advisory Group on Immunization has recommended the inclusion of this vaccine in the National Immunization Programme with Global Alliance for Vaccines and Immunization aid.

MEASLES, MUMPS, AND RUBELLA VACCINE

This is a live-attenuated vaccine. The vaccine is available as combined vaccine with MMR vaccine. The IAP-ACVIP recommends three doses of MMR vaccine at 9 months, 12–15 months, and at 4–6 years. It is a very safe vaccine. Minor allergic reactions, febrile seizure, rash, pruritus, and encephalopathy have been reported.

Measles Rubella Vaccine

In 2018, Government of India has introduced measles and rubella vaccine. It is a freeze-dried vaccine, given in dose of 0.5 mL SC or IM. All children 9 months to 15 years are to be immunized with this vaccine to bring down the incidence of measles and rubella.

VACCINES RECOMMENDED UNDER SPECIAL CIRCUMSTANCES

Rabies Vaccine

Four types of tissue culture vaccines are available: (1) Human diploid cell vaccine, (2) purified chick embryo vaccine, purified Verocell rabies vaccine, and (3) purified duck embryo vaccine.

Postexposure Prophylaxis

All tissue culture vaccines are given in five doses on 0 day, 3 days, 7 days, 14 days, or 28 days. The vaccine is given IM in the deltoid region or in anterolateral aspect of thigh in infants. The vaccine is not given in gluteal region. The dose is same, irrespective of age, viz. 2.5 IU/dose in 1 mL or 0.5 mL as recommended by the manufacturer. Intradermal schedules have been recommended at government centers.

Pre-exposure Prophylaxis

This is indicated in persons at high-risk of exposure, e.g. laboratory staff working with rabies virus, veterinarians, animal handlers, and wildlife officers. Even children who are exposed to stray dogs are candidates for pre-exposure prophylaxis. Three doses on 0 day, 7 days, and 28 days are recommended with reinforcing doses given if the antirabies antibody titer falls below 0.5 IU/mL. If persons who have received full course of pre- or postexposure prophylaxis get an animal bite at any point of time, two doses on day 0 and day 3 are recommended.

Rabies Immunoglobulin and Rabies Monoclonal Antibody

Rabies immunoglobulin (RIG) contains specific antirabies antibodies that neutralize the rabies virus and provide

cold chain equipment should be used/operated without a voltage stabilizer.

Cold Boxes (Coolers)

Cold boxes are big insulated boxes with ice packs. They are mainly used for the transportation of vaccines from district store to the primary health center (PHC). In emergency, they can also be used to store vaccines and frozen ice packs. Before placing vaccines in the cold boxes, first put fully frozen ice packs at the bottom and sides of the cold box. The vials of DPT, DT, hep B, and TT vaccines should not be placed in direct contact with frozen ice packs, place it in cartoon or plastic bag.

Vaccine Carriers

It is used by health workers for carrying vaccines (16–20 vials) to subcenters or to villages. They maintain the cold chain during transport from the PHC for 1 day's use in the field. The inside temperature is maintained between +2°C and –8°C with four frozen ice packs for 1 day (if not opened frequently) **(Table 5.7.2)**.

Domestic Refrigerator

The majority of the vaccination service providers in private sector use domestic refrigerator to store the vaccines. The domestic refrigerator is designed and built to store fresh or frozen food and drinks and not for the special storage temperature need of vaccines. They do not have accurate temperature controlling system, and hence, it can place the safety of vaccines at risk. For vaccine storage, the domestic refrigerator has following drawbacks:

- Temperature varies significantly every time the door is opened.
- Temperature rises during defrosting in cycle in cyclic defrost and frost-free refrigerator.
- Cabinet temperature is easily affected by ambient temperature.
- Temperature setting using dial is crude and inaccurate.

However, if domestic refrigerator is the only alternative to store the vaccines in that, it is acceptable to store vaccines provided that the refrigerator and freezer compartments have separate external doors. There are two types of domestic refrigerators: (1) frost-free refrigerator and (2) manual and cyclic defrost refrigerator. The frost-free refrigerators have no heating cycles but have low level warming cycles, and hence, it provides more uniform temperatures than manual and cyclic defrost models and may be more suitable for vaccine storage. The manual and cyclic defrost model refrigerator and bar refrigerator (dormitory style) should not be used to store the vaccine as they have wide fluctuations in the temperature in the internal compartment. Safe vaccine storage is possible in domestic refrigerators if the following points are observed:

- Store vaccine in a dedicated refrigerator, especially for biologics. Do not store food or drink in vaccine refrigerators.
- The refrigerator compartment temperatures is maintained between 2°C and 8°C, and freezer compartment temperatures maintained at or below 5°F (–15°C).
- The door seals are in good condition and are sealing tightly.
- The door closes properly automatically on leaving it free.
- The refrigerator has separate freezer compartment.
- The refrigerator compressor is quiet.
- The refrigerator is free from any coolant or water leak.
- Vaccination clinic staff is well aware about vaccine storage plans.

If the above criteria cannot be met with that, one should go for purpose-built refrigerator for storing the vaccine.

Table 5.7.2: Summary of cold chain equipment used under expanded program on immunization.

Equipment	*Temperature*	*Storage capacity*	*Holdover time*
Electrical			
Deep freezer	–15°C to –25°C	200 ice packs or OPV stock for 3 months	43°C for 18 hours
			32°C for 22 hours
ILR	+2°C to +8°C	BCG, DPT, DT, TT, measles, hep B vaccine stock for 3 months	43°C for 18 hours
			32°C for 22 hours
Nonelectrical			
Cold box (large)	+2°C to +8°C	All vaccines stored for transport or in case of power failure	43°C for 6.5 days
			32°C for 10 hours
Vaccine carrier	+2°C to +8°C	All vaccines carried for 12 hours	43°C for 34 hours
			32°C for 51 hours

(BCG: bacillus Calmette–Guérin; DPT: diphtheria, pertussis, and tetanus; DT: diphtheria and tetanus; Hep B: hepatitis B; ILR: ice-lined refrigerator; OPV: oral poliomyelitis vaccine; TT: tetanus toxoid)

Tips for Better Vaccine Storage in Domestic Refrigerators (Table 5.7.3)

- *Placement of refrigerator:* Refrigerator should be placed away from exposure to direct sunlight, away from heat, and with restricted accessibility only to the vaccination staff so as to minimize unnecessary door opening and preventing accidental switch off of power supply.
- *Recognize individual vaccine refrigerator:* Before starting storing the vaccines, identify which are the cold and warm areas in refrigerator.
- *Stabilize the temperature of the refrigerator before stocking:* The refrigerator temperature needs to be stabilized before start using for vaccine storage.
- *Monitoring temperatures inside the refrigerators:* Monitor internal temperature regularly with thermometer—preferably Celsius digital minimum/maximum thermometer. Place the thermometer in a central location within the storage compartment **(Fig. 5.7.4)**.
- *Safeguard the power source:* Ensure the power source is marked clearly in a way to prevent the refrigerator from being accidentally unplugged or turned off **(Fig. 5.7.5)**.

Table 5.7.3: Periodic maintenance plan for vaccine refrigerator.

Daily	*Weekly*	*Every fortnight*
• Check to make sure the doors are closed and sealed	• Check for ice buildup in the freezer and defrost if >0.5 cm frost has accumulated	• Clean the coils and the motor • Defrost and clean the refrigerator and freezer compartments • Adjust the thermostat if necessary

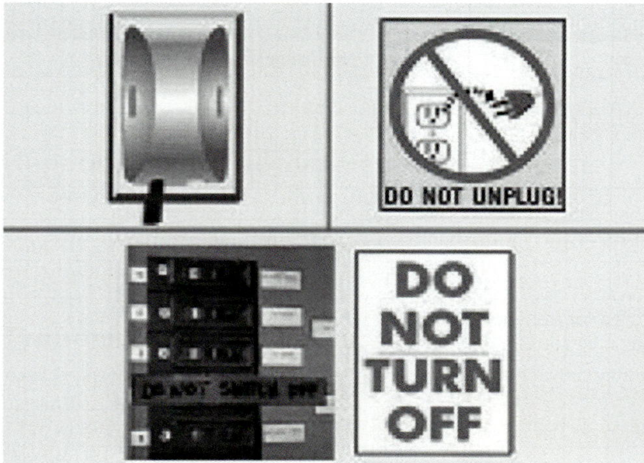

Fig. 5.7.5: Safeguard the power source.

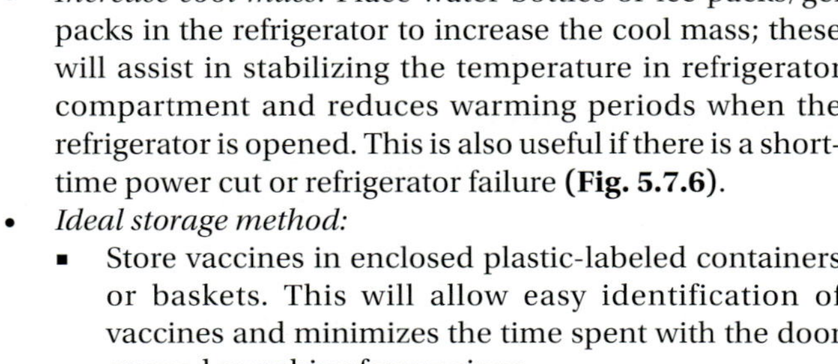

- *Increase cool mass:* Place water bottles or ice packs/gel packs in the refrigerator to increase the cool mass; these will assist in stabilizing the temperature in refrigerator compartment and reduces warming periods when the refrigerator is opened. This is also useful if there is a short-time power cut or refrigerator failure **(Fig. 5.7.6)**.
- *Ideal storage method:*
  - Store vaccines in enclosed plastic-labeled containers or baskets. This will allow easy identification of vaccines and minimizes the time spent with the door opened searching for vaccines.
  - Store vaccines in original packing as it can provide some protection from very short-term fluctuations.
  - Do not crowd the vaccines by overfilling the shelves. Allow space between containers and gap of at least

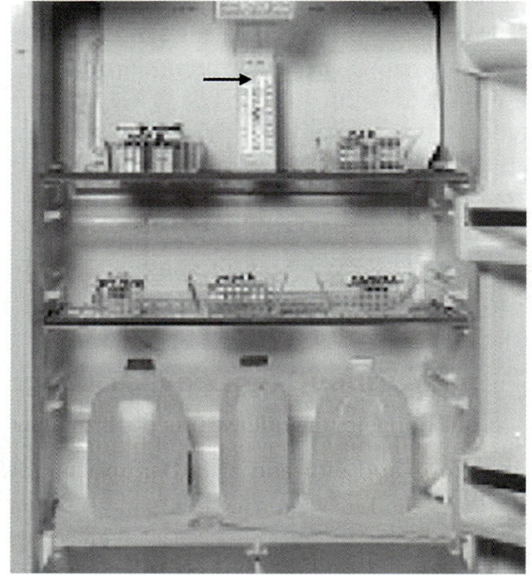

Fig. 5.7.4: Temperature monitoring.

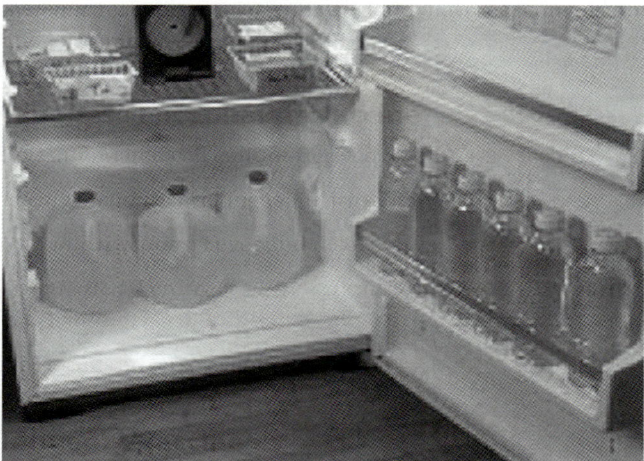

Fig. 5.7.6: Water bottles to increase cool mass.

4 cm from all refrigerator walls to allow free air circulation.

- Never store any vaccine in the door of the refrigerator.
- Place freeze-tolerant vaccines (measles, mumps, rubella, OPV, and bacillus Calmette-Guérin) in the top shelf and freeze-sensitive vaccines (diphtheria, tetanus, pertussis-containing vaccines; *Haemophilus influenzae* type B, pneumococcal, influenza, hepatitis, inactivated polio vaccine, and some varicella vaccines) on the middle shelf (**Figs. 5.7.7 and 5.7.8**).

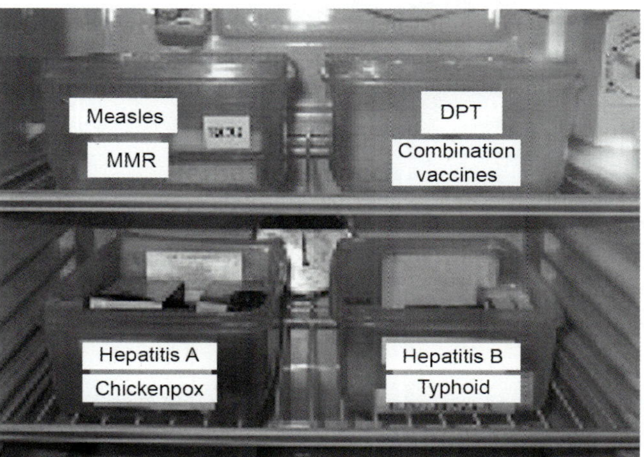

Fig. 5.7.7: Vaccine storage pattern.

- *Keep the door closed as much as possible:*
  - Reducing door opening helps to keep internal temperatures stable.
  - Vaccine refrigerators should have a sticker to remind staff of avoiding unnecessary door opening.
  - Stick a basic map of vaccine locations outside of the refrigerator door so staff can go "straight" to the vaccine when the door is opened.
  - Do not open the door fully while using, keep it to minimum sufficient for the need.
- *Training and assigning staff:*
  - Good vaccine storage and handling depends on knowledge and habits of the staff.
  - Training ensures that everyone handling vaccines knows how to protect them.
  - Ensure that one person is responsible for adjusting refrigerator controls and who is responsible for cold chain management to enable consistency.
- *Maintenance of the vaccine refrigerator:*
  - Report breakdowns immediately and arrange for alternative storage for vaccines while the refrigerator is repaired (**Table 5.7.3**).
  - Defrost refrigerator regularly. This also aids in the efficient functioning of refrigerator.
- *Power failure:*
  - During a power failure of 4 hours or less, the refrigerator door should be kept closed.

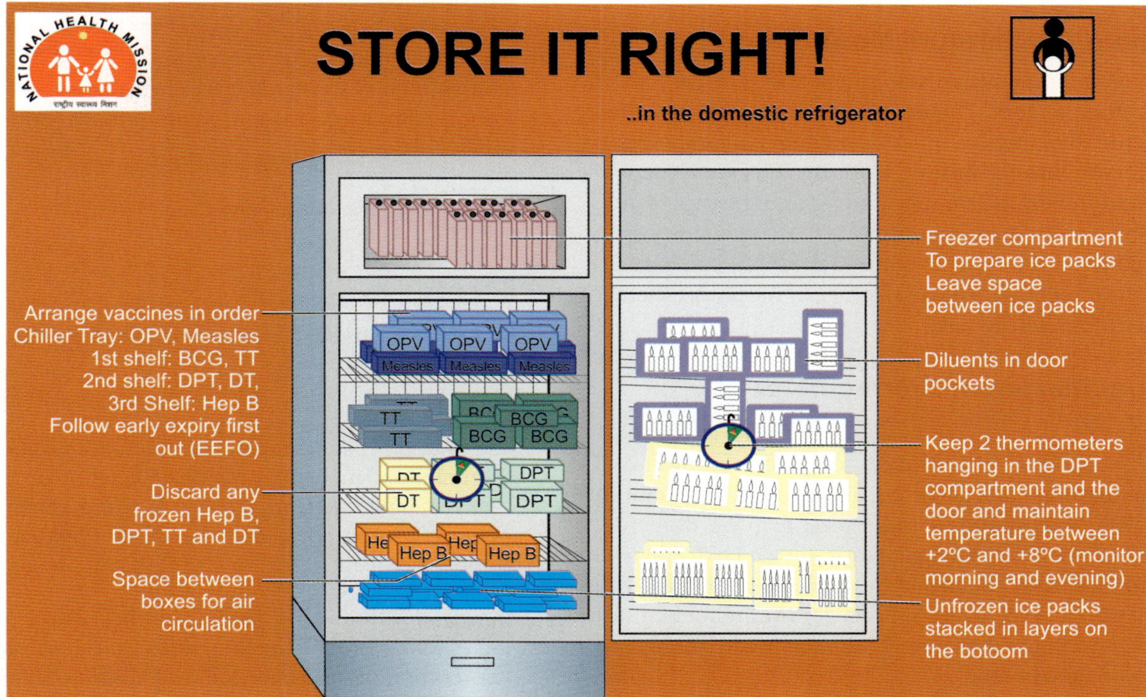

Fig. 5.7.8: Storage protocol in domestic fridge.

- If the backup generator facility is lacking, identify an available unit at another nearby site.
- If a refrigerator with a backup generator has not been located or is not working and for power failures more than 4 hours, store vaccines in a cooler with conditioned icepacks/gel packs.

Purpose-built Vaccine Refrigerator

Purpose-built vaccine refrigerator is preferred refrigerator for vaccine storage. It is used by hospitals, pharmacies, and larger general practices. It has the following advantages over the domestic refrigerator **(Fig. 5.7.9)**:

- Do not require to modify for vaccine storage.
- Programmed to maintain an internal temperature between 2°C and 8°C.
- Cabinet temperature is not affected by ambient temperature and is stable and uniform.
- Evaporator operates at 2–8°C, preventing vaccine from freezing.
- Defrost cycle allowing defrosting without rise in cabinet temperature.
- Even distribution of temperature because of ongoing air circulation.
- Have external temperature reading display, maximum/minimum temperature continuous display, and an out-of-range temperature alarm.
- *Good temperature recovery*: When the fridge is open to access the vaccines.

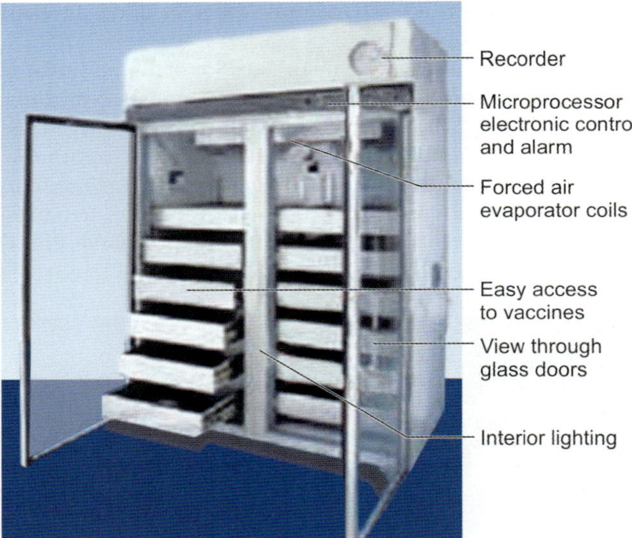

Fig. 5.7.9: Purpose-built vaccine refrigerator.

Cold Chain Temperature Monitoring

Monitoring of temperature is a critical and integral part of any cold chain system. The expensive equipment installed may become meaningless unless a meticulous temperature record documents its proper working. In every vaccine storage equipment, the temperature should be monitored. Temperature should be recorded at least two times in a day and plotted on a chart to show high/low excursions. To measure the temperature during storage of vaccines, different type of thermometers is used.

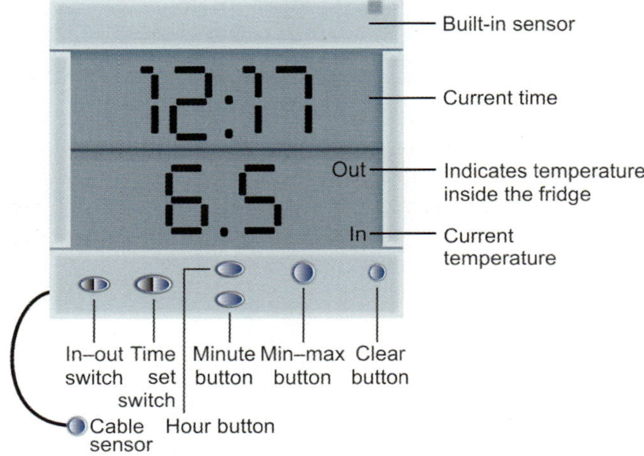

Fig. 5.7.10: Minimum/maximum thermometer.

Minimum/Maximum Thermometer (Fig. 5.7.10)

It shows the current temperature and the minimum and maximum temperatures achieved. Temperature fluctuations outside the recommended range can also be detected. Available in fluid-filled and digital forms of which digital type with a probe is most effective type. Place the probe directly in contact with a vaccine vial or package. Thermometer must be reset regularly; the thermometer battery must be checked and replaced time to time.

- *Dial thermometer:* They are the most common but not the most accurate. They only indicate the temperature at the time they are read. Temperature fluctuations outside the recommended range may not be detected.
- *Stem (Alcohol) thermometer:* It is more sensitive and accurate compared to dial thermometer as it records temperature from +50°C to –30°C. It can be used in ILR and deep freezers.
- *Digital thermometer:* These are the most accurate constant monitors and also offer alarm to safeguard against damage from refrigerator malfunction. To get accurate reading, place the temperature probe in proper location.

Data Loggers

This temperature chart recording system can record temperatures over a long period of time as well as providing visual and audio alarms. Loggers use a similar measuring principle to chart as recorders but record the data electronically.

The objective of data logging is to build up a "temperature map" of the vaccine storage areas within the refrigerator to identify the safest areas and the most dangerous areas for vaccine storage, particularly for looking for areas where vaccine could freeze.

Each logger is a self-contained miniature computer. Once programmed via a computer, loggers are disconnected from the computer and placed in the vaccine refrigerator in close proximity to the temperature probe. The logger then operates independently on its own battery until the recording is downloaded to the computer.

Vaccine Vial Monitor

A VVM is a label containing a heat-sensitive material, which is placed on a vaccine vial to register cumulative heat exposure over time **(Fig. 5.7.11)**. A VVM enables the health worker to know whether vaccine has been damaged by exposure to heat. The VVM is a circle with a small square inside it, which is lighter in color than surroundings. The inner square of VVM is made of heat-sensitive material that is lighter in color at the starting point. The combined effect of time and temperature causes the inner square of the VVM to darken gradually. The color change is irreversible. A direct relationship exists between the rate of color change and temperature. Thus lower the temperature, slower the color change; and higher the temperature, faster the color change.

Thus VVM gives information about the heat exposure over a period of time that affects vaccine potency. It does not give information about other factors responsible for vaccine degradation like light. Vaccine vial monitors are not substitutes for expiry dates. If the inner square is lighter than the outer ring, the vaccine can be used, whereas if inner square matches or has darker color than outer ring, the vaccine should be discarded **(Fig. 5.7.12)**.

VACCINE HANDLING PERSONNEL

Designated Vaccine Coordinators Staff

Each vaccination clinic should designate one staff member to be the primary vaccine coordinator and another staff member as a backup in case the primary coordinator is unavailable. The designated person will be responsible for ensuring that all vaccines are handled correctly, that procedures are documented, and that all personnel receive appropriate cold chain training. Designated vaccine coordinators should be fully trained in routine and urgent vaccine storage and handling protocols.

Other Staff

All staff members should be familiar with the policies and procedures for vaccine storage and handling. This especially includes staff members, such as receptionists who accept vaccine shipments. Written policies and procedure documents should be available near the vaccine storage units for easy reference.

Fig. 5.7.11: Vaccine vial monitor.

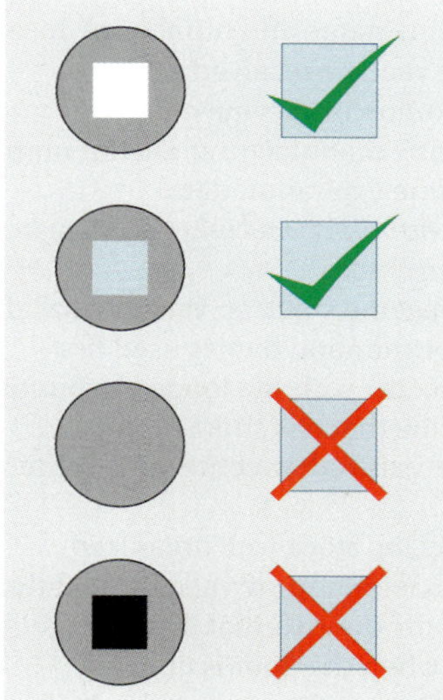

Fig. 5.7.12: Decision to use vaccine/s based on VVM sensitivity. (VVM: vaccine vial monitor)

Training Personnel

All staff that handle or administer vaccines should be trained in proper vaccine storage and handling practices. All staff should be trained to have an understanding of the importance of cold chain maintenance and basic practices so that they are aware of their responsibilities to the cold chain. Staff who monitor and record vaccine storage unit temperatures should immediately report inappropriate storage conditions (including exposure to inappropriate temperature or light exposures) to the designated vaccine coordinator.

EFFICIENT VACCINE MANAGEMENT PROTOCOLS

Routine Vaccine Storage and Handling Protocols

Routine protocols should include all aspects of day-to-day vaccine management, from ordering vaccines, controlling inventory, handling vaccines, and monitoring storage conditions. It should include the following four elements:

1. *Ordering and accepting vaccine deliveries*:
   - Order vaccines to maintain an adequate stock to meet the needs of the vaccination unit.
   - Ensure that the "ordered vaccine stock" is delivered when the Immunization Clinic is open. Vaccine shipments should be delivered when staff is available to unpack and store.
   - Store vaccines at the recommended temperatures, immediately on arrival—refrigerated vaccines between 2°C and 8°C and frozen vaccines between –50°C and 15°C.
   - *Maintain a vaccine inventory log including as under*:
     - Vaccine name and number of doses received
     - Date vaccine received
     - Condition of vaccine on arrival
     - Vaccine manufacturer and lot number
     - Vaccine expiration date.
2. *Storing and handling vaccines* (as discussed above)
3. *Managing inventory*:
   - Rotate vaccine stock so vaccine and diluent with the shortest expiration date is used first.
   - Place vaccine with the longest expiration date behind the vaccine that has short expiry.
   - Remove expired vaccine and diluent from usable stock.
   - Keep vaccine stock well organized.
   - Stick a basic map of vaccine locations outside the refrigerator door so that staff can go "straight" to the vaccine when the door is opened.
   - Inspect the storage unit daily. A physical inspection helps to ensure vaccines, and thermometers are placed appropriately within the unit.
   - Dispose of all vaccine materials using medical waste disposal procedures.
4. *Managing potentially compromised vaccines*:
   - Identify and isolate all potentially compromised vaccines and diluents.
   - Label these vaccines "DO NOT USE" and store separately from uncompromised vaccines and diluents in the recommended temperature range.
   - Contact vaccine manufacturers and/or state immunization program for appropriate actions that should be followed for all potentially compromised vaccines and diluents.

Emergency Vaccine Retrieval and Storage

Various situations, such as equipment failures, power outages, or natural disasters, may compromise vaccine storage conditions, and it is important that all the staff involved in the immunization activity is aware of the probable adverse effect of such situations on vaccine storage conditions. Ensure that all staff has appropriate training so that they understand the urgent vaccine storage and handling protocols and their responsibility in maintaining the cold chain. Emergency vaccine retrieval and storage plan should include the following components:

- Designate an alternate site where vaccines and diluents can be safely stored. While choosing an alternate site, consider availability of types of storage unit(s), temperature monitoring capabilities, and backup generator.
- Obtain and store an adequate packing containers and materials (e.g. frozen or refrigerated gel packs, bubble wrap) in the facility that will be needed to pack vaccines for safe transport.
- Include written directions for packing vaccines and diluents for transport. A calibrated thermometer should be placed in each packing container near the vaccine.
- Incorporate written procedures for managing potentially compromised vaccines.
- Include contact information for vaccine manufacturers and/or the immunization program.

BIBLIOGRAPHY

1. Centers for Disease Control. Vaccine management, recommendations for handling and storage of selected biologicals. Atlanta, GA: Department of Health & Human Services; 1991.
2. Centers for Disease Control. Safety of vaccines affected by a power outage. In: Quick clinical notes, disaster management and response. Atlanta: CDC; 2004. pp. 62-3.
3. Department of Health and Ageing. Strive for 5: national vaccine storage guidelines. Canberra: Department of Health and Aging, Australian Government; 2013.
4. Galazka A, Milstien J, Zaffran M. Thermostability of vaccines. Geneva: WHO (Global Programme for Vaccines and Immunization); 1998.

5. Gupta SK, Shastri DD. Cold chain and vaccine storage. In: Shah NK, Agrawal R, Sukumaran TU, Vashishtha VM (Eds). IAP textbook of vaccines, 1st edition. New Delhi: Jaypee Brothers Medical Publishers (P) Ltd.; 2014. pp. 89-99.
6. Ketan B, Jariwala V, Kirit S. Target-5: guide to vaccine storage and handling, 1st edition. Gujarat: IAP Surat Publication; 2006.
7. Shastri DD. Vaccine storage and handling. In: Parthasarathy A (Ed). IAP textbook of pediatrics, 6th edition. New Delhi: Jaypee Brothers Medical Publishers (P) Ltd.; 2013. pp. 1-5.
8. Shastri DD. Vaccine storage and handling. In: Parthasarathy A (Ed). IAP textbook of pediatrics infectious diseases, 1st edition. New Delhi: Jaypee Brothers Medical Publishers (P) Ltd.; 2013. pp. 493-501.
9. World Health Organization. Getting started with VVMs. VVM for all, technical session on vaccine vial monitors. Geneva: WHO; 2002.
10. World Health Organization. Immunization in practice (WHO/EPI/PHW/84.01 to 84.07). Geneva: WHO; 2014.

5.8 Adverse Events Following Immunization

M Indra Shekhar Rao, A Parthasarathy, S Venkat Reddy

INTRODUCTION

Immunization is a major contributor to the success story of child health in the last century, which has enhanced and improved the child survival all over the world. Vaccines used in National Immunization Programs (NIP) are extremely safe and effective. Several scientific, ethical, and statutory obligations are fulfilled by the manufacturers and elaborate field trials regarding safety and protection offered by individual vaccines are established before they are recommended for routine use. However, no vaccine is perfectly safe and adverse events can occur following immunization.

The adverse event following immunization (AEFI) is defined as *a medical incident that takes place after immunization, causes concern and is believed to be caused by the immunization.* Any untoward medical occurrence which follows immunization and which does not necessarily have a causal relationship with the use of the vaccine is clubbed under AEFI.

The vaccines are foreign for human bodies, given to healthy infants and children. In the natural process of developing immunity, a vaccine may cause fever, erythema, local pain, etc. In addition, there is a slight risk of foreign body reaction to the components in the vaccines. These factors are likely to cause some concerns in the caregivers/parents. Whatever the cause, an AEFI may upset people to an extent that they may refuse further vaccination for their children. This makes it more likely for the children to get a vaccine preventable disease (VPD), become seriously ill, disabled, and risk death.

Adverse event following immunization surveillance, therefore, helps to preserve public confidence in the immunization program. A reported adverse event can be true adverse event or an event coincidental to the immunization. The AEFIs are classified into five categories.

Immunization can cause adverse events from the inherent properties of vaccine (*vaccine reaction*), which comprises vaccine product-related reactions and vaccine quality defect-related reactions. Some error in immunization process (*program error*) such as contaminated vaccine, diluent, reuse of disposable syringe or needle, and reuse of reconstituted vaccine. The event may be unrelated to the immunization but have temporal association (*coincidental event*). This can cause anxiety-related reactions can arise from fear or pain of the injection rather than the vaccine itself, e.g. fainting, hyperventilation, vomiting, and convulsions. In some cases, the cause of AEFI remains unknown **(Table 5.8.1)**.

Vaccine reactions can be classified into two groups:

1. *Minor reactions*
   - Usually occur within a few hours of injection.
   - Resolve after short period of time and pose little danger.
   - Local (includes pain, swelling, or redness at the site of injection).
   - Systemic (includes fever, malaise, muscle pain, headache, or loss of appetite).

2. *Severe reactions*
   - Usually do not result in long-term problems.
   - Can be disabling.
   - Are rarely life threatening.
   - Include seizures and allergic reactions caused by the body's reaction to a particular component in a vaccine.

The adverse event following the immunization may be anticipated and not severe enough to cause discomfort for a long duration of time [e.g. pain or fever after diphtheria, tetanus, and pertussis (DTP) vaccination], whereas a severe or a rare event following the vaccine may be in the form of unexpected anaphylactic shock or induction of active disease following measles or oral polio vaccine, respectively. Hypothetical type of reaction may be related to vaccine scares which have causal relationship relating to the issues which are of controversial nature occurring in vaccinated children.

The common vaccine reactions are due to the immune response of the host and sometimes due to vaccine components (e.g. aluminum adjuvant and preservatives). A successful vaccine reduces these reactions to a minimum while inducing the best possible immunity. These anticipated reactions occur within a day or two of immunization and are listed in **Table 5.8.2**.

Another notable component of AEFI is due to program errors that would result from errors and accidents in vaccine preparation, handling, or administration **(Table 5.8.3)**. The identification and correction of these errors are of great importance which would otherwise lead to a cluster of other events associated with immunization. The most common program error is iatrogenic infection as a result of nonsterile injection, e.g. sterile abscess, which may have a systemic effect or blood-borne infection (e.g. human immunodeficiency virus and hepatitis B).

Table 5.8.1: Classification of AEFI.

Types of AEFI	*Definition and characteristics*
Vaccine reactions	Event caused by individual response to the vaccine
Immunization error	Event caused by an error in vaccine preparation, handling, storage, or administration
Coincidental event	Event that happens after immunization but not caused by the vaccine or its administration
Immunization anxiety	Event from anxiety about or pain from the injection itself rather than the vaccine
Unknown	Event's cause cannot be determined

(AEFI: adverse events following immunization)
Source: World Health Organization. Immunization Safety Surveillance: Guidelines for managers of immunization programmes on reporting and investigation adverse events following immunization. Manila: World Health Organization; 1999. p. 2.

Table 5.8.2: Common, minor vaccine reactions, and treatment.

Vaccine	*Local reaction (pain, swelling, redness)*	*Fever >38°C*	*Irritability, malaise, and systemic symptoms*
BCG	90–95%	–	–
Hib	5–15%	2–10%	–
Hepatitis B	• *Adults*: 15% • *Children*: 5%	1–6%	–
Measles/MMR/MR	10%	5–15%	5% (Rash)
Oral polio vaccine	–	<1%	<1%
Tetanus/DT/Td	10%	10%	25%
Pneumococcal conjugate	~20%	~20%	~20%
Pertussis (DTwP)	Up to 50%	Up to 50%	Up to 55%
Treatment	• Cold sponging at injection site • Oral paracetamol	• Give extra fluids • Wear cool clothing • Tepid sponge or bath • Oral paracetamol	Give extra oral fluids

(BCG: bacillus Calmette–Guérin; DT/Td: tetanus-diphtheria vaccine; DTP/DTwP: diphtheria, tetanus, and pertussis; Hib: *Haemophilus influenzae* type b; MMR: measles, mumps, and rubella; MR: measles and rubella virus vaccine)
Source: World Health Organization. Immunization Safety Surveillance: Guidelines for managers of immunization programmes on reporting and investigation adverse events following immunization. Manila: World Health Organization; 1999. p. 10.

Table 5.8.3: Program errors leading to adverse events.

Nonsterile injections: • Reuse of disposable syringe or needles • Improperly sterilized syringe or needles • Contaminated vaccine or diluents • Reuse of reconstituted vaccine at subsequent session	• Local injection site reactions (e.g. abscess, swelling, cellulitis, and induration) • Sepsis • Toxic shock syndrome • Blood-borne transmission of disease, e.g. hepatitis B, HIV • Death
Vaccine prepared incorrectly: • Vaccine reconstituted with incorrect diluent • Drugs substituted for vaccine or diluent	• Vaccine ineffective • Effect of drug, e.g. insulin, oxytocin, etc.
Immunization injected at wrong site: • Subcutaneous instead of intradermal for BCG • Too superficial for toxoid vaccine (DTP, DT, TT) • Buttocks	• Local reaction or injection site abscess • Local reaction or injection site abscess • Sciatic nerve damage
Vaccine transported/stored incorrectly: • Freezing vaccine during transport • Failure to keep vaccine in cold chain	• Increased local reaction from frozen vaccine • Ineffective vaccine
Contraindications ignored	Avoidable severe reaction

(BCG: bacillus Calmette–Guérin; DT: diphtheria-tetanus vaccine; DTP: diphtheria, tetanus, and pertussis; HIV: human immunodeficiency virus; TT: tetanus toxoid)

Source: World Health Organization. Immunization Safety Surveillance: Guidelines for managers of immunization programmes on reporting and investigation adverse events following immunization. Manila: World Health Organization; 1999. p. 30.

Each vaccine administered in the immunization program has specific complications most of which are anticipated and mild. Some of them are serious adverse reactions, which always have to be expected and immediate remedial measures have to be given as described here.

VACCINATION COMPLICATIONS AND THEIR MANAGEMENT

Bacillus Calmette–Guérin

Local Adverse Reactions

- Persistent discharging sinus at the site of vaccination.
- *Regional axillary lymphadenitis*:
  - Below 2 cm—no treatment
  - Fluctuant, more than 2 cm—treatment with isonicotinic hydrazide for 3–6 months/excision
- *Bacillus Calmette-Guérin complex (local lymphadenitis + positive Mantoux reaction + paratracheal lymph node)*: Treat with rifampicin (R), pyrazinamide (Z), and isoniazid (H) [RHZ (2 months)] plus R + H [RH (4 months)].
  Systemic reactions: Disseminated infection, tuberculous osteomyelitis, scrofuloderma—treat these like tuberculosis.

Diphtheria, Tetanus, and (Whole-cell) Pertussis Vaccine

Adverse Reactions

- Incessant cry (more than 3 hours)
- Febrile convulsions
- Hyperpyrexia
- Hypotonic hyporesponsive episode (HHE, shock-like state)
- Acute encephalopathy
- Anaphylactic shock

Diphtheria, Tetanus, and (Acellular) Pertussis Vaccine

Adverse events such as pain or swelling are minimal with above vaccine.

Clinical features of anaphylaxis: These involve multiple body systems (skin, respiration, and circulation).

- Itchy, urticarial rash, and facial flushing
- Progressive edema involving face, mouth, and body parts
- *Respiratory symptoms*: Sneezing, coughing, wheezing, and airway obstruction
- Hypotension and shock.

Oral Polio Vaccine

- Adverse event following immunization almost none
- Very rarely vaccine-associated paralytic poliomyelitis

Inactivated Polio Vaccine

- *Local reactions*: Erythema and induration if the patient is sensitive to streptomycin/neomycin. She/he might develop hypersensitive reactions as inactivated polio vaccine contains these as preservatives.

- *Systemic reactions*: Transient arthralgia, rarely agitation, somnolence, and convulsions.

Measles

Anticipated reaction: Local pain, tenderness, and measles-like illness 7–12 days after vaccination.

Treatment: Paracetamol.

Adverse reactions:
- Toxic shock syndrome (TSS)
- Thrombocytopenic purpura may occur at 1 per 30,000 vaccines

Toxic Shock Syndrome

Measles vaccine does not contain any preservatives. When measles vaccine cap is punctured, it allows bacterial growth, especially staphylococci which can cause TSS due to the exotoxins liberated by it. This can happen due to usage of unsterile syringes, needles, and using a vaccine vial beyond 4 hours after reconstitution. It can occur after 30 minutes to few hours after vaccination and the child presents with fever, vomiting, diarrhea, and shock.

Treatment: It should be treated as medical emergency. Child should be resuscitated with intravenous (IV) fluids (ringers lactate and normal saline), and treated with antibiotics (cloxacillin 100–200 mg/kg/day in divided doses), steroids, antipyretics, and supportive therapy.

Measles, Mumps, and Rubella Vaccine

Anticipated reactions: Mild fever, rash, and febrile seizures.

Mumps Component

Adverse reactions: Fever, rarely encephalopathy, seizures, Guillain-Barré syndrome (GBS), parotid swelling, hemolytic uremic syndrome, and aseptic meningitis.

Rubella Component

Adverse reactions: Arthralgia, lymphadenopathy, fever, and sore throat; rarely thrombocytopenia and peripheral neuropathy.

Hepatitis B Vaccine and Hepatitis A Vaccine

Local reactions: Soreness at the site of injection.

Systemic reactions: Mild fever, myalgia, arthralgia, and rarely anaphylaxis.

Typhoid Vi Antigen Vaccine

Local reaction: Mild pain and swelling for 1 day.

Vi-polysaccharide conjugate vaccine conjugated with tetanus toxoid (TT) (pedatyph, Vi-TT).

No major local or systemic side effects are seen.

Vi-polysaccharide conjugate vaccine conjugated with TT (typbar, typhoid conjugate vaccine).

Adverse effects: Pain at injection site and fever.

Tetanus Toxoid

Systemic reactions: Frequent TT injections can lead on to increased severity of local and systemic reactions due to binding of the toxoid with the preformed antitoxin leading on to immune complex-mediated reactions (swollen limbs and Arthus type 2 reactions).

Haemophilus influenzae Type B Vaccine

Local reactions: Mild redness, pain, and swelling.

Varicella Vaccine

Local reactions: Pain, redness, swelling at injection site.

Systemic reactions: Varicella-like rash in around 5% of the vaccines.

Rabies Tissue Culture Vaccine

Local reactions: Soreness.

Systemic reactions: Headache, fever.

Meningococcal Vaccine (Quadrivalent)

Local reactions: Pain and swelling at injection site.

Systemic reactions: GBS is possible but unproven risk in adolescents.

Pneumococcal Vaccine

Local reactions: Swelling, redness, and pain.

Systemic reactions: Fever, vomiting and diarrhea, convulsion, and HHE rarely.

Japanese Encephalitis Vaccine

Live attenuated cell culture-derived SA 14-14-2 vaccine.

Local reactions: Swelling, pain, irritability.

Systemic reactions: Fever and rash.

Inactivated Vero cell culture-derived SA 14-14-2 Japanese encephalitis vaccine.

No serious adverse event.

Influenza Vaccine

Trivalent influenza vaccines

Local reactions: Pain and swelling

Systemic reactions: Fever, malaise, myalgia

The slightly increased risk of GBS after trivalent influenza vaccine has not been associated with statistically significant increase in hospital admission because of GBS. Vaccine is preferably avoided in those with history of GBS and should be administered with caution in those with egg allergy if benefits of vaccine are more than the risks of side effects.

Rotavirus Vaccine

Systemic reactions: Mild undesirable side effects such as fever, vomiting, irritability, and rash may occur. The risk of intussusception with rotavirus is not increased as with placebo group.

Human Papillomavirus Vaccine

Common Side Effects

- Pain, redness, or swelling in the arm where the shot was given
- Fever
- Headache or feeling tired
- Nausea
- Muscle or joint pain

Brief fainting spells and related symptoms (such as jerking movements) can happen after any medical procedure, including vaccination. Sitting or lying down for about 15 minutes after a vaccination can help prevent fainting and injuries caused by falls.

On very rare occasions, severe (anaphylactic) allergic reactions may occur after vaccination. People with severe allergies to any component of a vaccine should not receive that vaccine.

HOW TO MANAGE AN ANAPHYLAXIS AFTER A VACCINE?

Emergency Management of Anaphylaxis

- Administer epinephrine (1:1,000 solution) 0.01 mL/kg/dose (maximum 0.5 mL) intramuscular in anterolateral thigh.
- Set up IV access.
- Lay patient flat and elevate legs, if tolerated. Give high flow oxygen and airway/ventilation, if needed.
- If hypotensive, set up additional wide-bore access and give IV normal saline 20 mL/kg under pressure over 1–2 minutes.
- Intramuscular adrenaline may be repeated after 3–5 minutes, if required.
- Oral antihistaminics may be given to ameliorate skin symptoms, but IV antihistaminics are not recommended. Oral or injectable corticosteroids equivalent to prednisone 1–2 mg/kg may be given, but benefit is yet unproven.

VACCINES AND CONTRAINDICATIONS

It is often difficult to prove definite cause-effect relationship between the act of vaccination and subsequent complication. The following guidelines as well as the list of contraindications for vaccinations will help in deciding vaccine administration **(Table 5.8.4)**.

GUIDELINES FOR SAFE VACCINATION

Always ensure safe injection practices for safe health by using disposable syringes.

- Select proper vaccine and follow manufacturer's instructions (dose/route/administration).
- Maintain cold chain.

Table 5.8.4: Vaccines and contraindications.

Avoid: Live vaccine	• Immunodeficient individuals • Immunosuppressant therapy • Chronic debilitating illness (till recovery)
Avoid: DTP (1st dose)	• Progressive neurological disease • Uncontrolled seizure disorder (postpone till control)
Avoid: Rubella vaccine	• During pregnancy
Avoid: Measles vaccine/should not be given	• If person is sensitive to egg protein
Delay: Live vaccine	• Measles/MMR for 6 weeks following immunoglobulin therapy • Severe febrile illness
Discontinue DTP	• In case of severe postvaccinial reactions
Do not stop vaccination in	• Malnutrition • Moderate fever • Respiratory infections • Mild diarrhea • Any benign ailment

(DTP: diphtheria, tetanus, and pertussis; MMR, measles, mumps, and rubella)

Source: Bhatia R, Ichhpujani RL. Immunization against infectious disease. London: HMSO; 1996. pp. 20-60.

- Inform the parents regarding vaccine benefits and their anticipated reactions.
- Obtain written or at least oral consent before vaccination.
- Keep the child under observation for 30 minutes after vaccination. Be equipped and geared up to treat any untoward reactions.
- Have always resuscitation kit ready.
- Use desired injection procedure, i.e. load the vaccine into appropriate syringe size.
- Do not mix vaccines in single syringe unless approved for such use. Use different syringes for different vaccines. Use different sites for injection.
- Always use anterolateral aspect of thigh in young children and deltoid area for older children for injections. Never use gluteal region in children.
- Avoid fomentation/vigorous rubbing after vaccination. Firm pressure for a few minutes is sufficient.
- Document every vaccination procedure in the immunization card and keep a copy of it.
- Complete the vaccination schedule as per immunization calendar. Remind the parents regarding next date.
- There is no need to restart immunization of multidose vaccine, e.g. Hib, DTP, etc. if the child is not brought for immunization on suggested date. Instead just continue and complete the schedule.

PREVENTION AND TREATMENT OF VACCINE REACTION

It is mandatory for the person administering the vaccine to have sufficient knowledge regarding vaccines and expected side effects and to inform parents thoroughly regarding such adverse effects, which may however occur very rarely. It is also essential to be prepared and to always have a "kit" with lifesaving drugs and equipment at each place of vaccination. Advice on managing the common reactions as well as the instructions to return to the clinic if there are more serious symptoms should be given to parents. This will help to reassure parents about immunization and prepare them for common reactions. Program errors are easily preventable. Identification and correction of these errors are of great importance. World Health Organization (WHO) guidelines to avoid program errors are as follows:

- Vaccines must be reconstituted only with the diluents supplied by the manufacturer.
- Reconstituted vaccines must be discarded at the end of each immunization session and never retained.
- No other drugs or substances should be stored in the refrigerator of the immunization center.
- Immunization workers must be adequately trained and closely supervised to ensure that proper procedures are being followed.
- Careful epidemiological investigation of an AEFI is needed to pinpoint the cause and to correct immunization practices.

REPORTING ADVERSE EVENT FOLLOWING IMMUNIZATION

The reportable AEFI must include any death or serious event believed by the public or health worker to be caused by immunization **(Table 5.8.5)**.

Table 5.8.5: List of reportable adverse event following immunization (AEFI).*

Time period	*Type of adverse effects*
Occurring within 24 hours of immunization	• Anaphylactoid reaction (acute hypersensitivity reaction) • Anaphylaxis • Persistent (more than 3 hours) inconsolable screaming and crying • HHE
Occurring within 5 days of immunization	• TSS • Severe local reaction • Sepsis • Injection site abscess (bacterial/sterile)
Occurring within 15 days of immunization	• Seizures, including febrile seizures (6–12 days for measles/MMR; 0–2 days for DTP) Encephalopathy (6–12 days for measles/MMR; 0–2 days for DTP)
Occurring within 3 months of immunization	• Acute flaccid paralysis (4–30 days for OPV recipient; 4–75 days for contact) Brachial neuritis (2–28 days after tetanus containing vaccine)
Occurring within 1 month and 12 months	• Thrombocytopenia (15–35 days after measles/MMR) • Lymphadenitis and disseminated BCG infection after BCG immunization • Osteitis/osteomyelitis
No time limit	• Any death, hospitalization, or other severe and unusual events that are thought by health workers or the public to be related to immunization

(BCG: bacillus Calmette–Guérin; DTP: diphtheria, tetanus, and pertussis; HHE: hypotonic hyporesponsive episode; MMR: measles, mumps, and rubella vaccine; OPV: oral polio vaccine; TSS: toxic shock syndrome)

Source: World Health Organization. Immunization Safety Surveillance: Guidelines for managers of immunization programs on reporting and investigation adverse events following immunization. Manila: World Health Organization; 1999. pp. 23-6.

The minor common reactions such as local reactions, fever, and self-limiting systemic symptoms need not be reported. It is important for the persons administering the vaccine to advise the parent/patient at the time of immunization that these reactions are expected and advise them how to manage these common reactions (e.g. paracetamol to treat fever). For more serious problems, the patient should be advised to return or to seek medical attention and to allow detection of AEFI. More importantly, they should be advised not to delay treatment of a coincidental illness falsely attributed as vaccine reaction. Severe local reactions, especially if occurring in clusters, should be reported, as they can be markers for program errors or for problems with specific vaccine lots.

CHANNELS AND TIMELINE FOR REPORTING SERIOUS ADVERSE EVENT FOLLOWING IMMUNIZATION (PRIVATE)

Private sectors contribute to about 20% of total immunization and also provide vaccines not available in government sector. Hence, AEFI from this sector are also reported and investigated as per the laid down national guidelines. Also the AEFI reporting from private sector will provide vital information on the safety of new and underutilized vaccines in India. Once a serious AEFI happens in the private sector at a clinic of pediatricians in the rural area, she/he should immediately inform medical officer (MO) in-charge of nearest primary health center (PHC) or other health facility. In the urban area, either she/he can inform MO in-charge of nearest urban health center or to the "District Immunization Officer (DIO)." By all channels, the information should reach DIO as soon as possible. The private practitioners (including pediatricians) should use the "First Information Report (FIR)" form for reporting serious AEFI cases to the district officials. Once an AEFI is reported from private sector, the DIO, and district AEFI committee members would then investigate the reported AEFI case. The pediatricians should help the investigation team in collection of all the related information. Indian Academy of Pediatrics (IAP) through its IAP Advisory Committee on Vaccines and Immunization Practices has resolved to collaborate with the national AEFI program by suggesting the following measures—Integrate IAP Disease Surveillance Project (IDSURV) with AEFI reporting for a web-based and integrated voice recording reporting (already incorporated: *www.idsurv.org*). The IDSURV program is fine-tuned to automatically send information to the concerned DIO/state immunization officer for prompt action.

Serious Adverse Event Following Immunization Cases (Government)

When to Report? Who Should Report?

- Minor AEFI are to be reported by the village health nurse (VHN) to the MO of PHC in the monthly reports who will include the report from all VHNs in the monthly report to the district headquarters authority.
- Pediatricians can report any AEFI case to the PHC/community health center MOs (in rural area) or may directly report to DIO **(Flowchart 5.8.1)**.
- The DIO reports this in the monthly report to the state and the state to the Government of India as per the timeline for monthly report.

The report should contain the following details at a minimum as per standard operating procedure:

- Description of the event
- Timing of the event in relation to immunization
- Vaccines given
- Patients identifying details

This is called FIR. The routine vaccination program should continue while awaiting the completion of the reporting and investigation.

Communicating with the Media

The media plays an important role in public perception. The media is more interested in stories that will attract attention; hence, there is tendency to dramatize and personalize the event. It is easy for the media to create sense of panic and outrage about the events which are unrelated to immunization (coincidental). The guiding principle while dealing with media must be that one should show empathy and caring, honesty and openness, and dedication and commitment; whenever possible, positive terms like immunization safety or vaccine safety should be used. Key messages have to be prepared before media contact, and they should include some of these facts:

- That benefit of immunization in preventing disease is well proven.
- It is very risky not to immunize (risk of disease and complications).
- Vaccine preventable diseases caused millions of deaths and/or disability before the introduction of vaccines and that situation would return without continued use of vaccines.
- Vaccines do cause reactions, but these are rarely serious and hardly ever cause long-term problems.
- Immunization safety is of paramount importance, and any suspicion of a problem is investigated (advantage of well-established immunization safety surveillance).
- The AEFI is currently being investigated but is likely to be coincidental due to a local problem (depending on type of event), and the immunization program must continue to keep the population safe from diseases.

Flowchart 5.8.1: Channels and timeline for reporting serious AEFI cases.

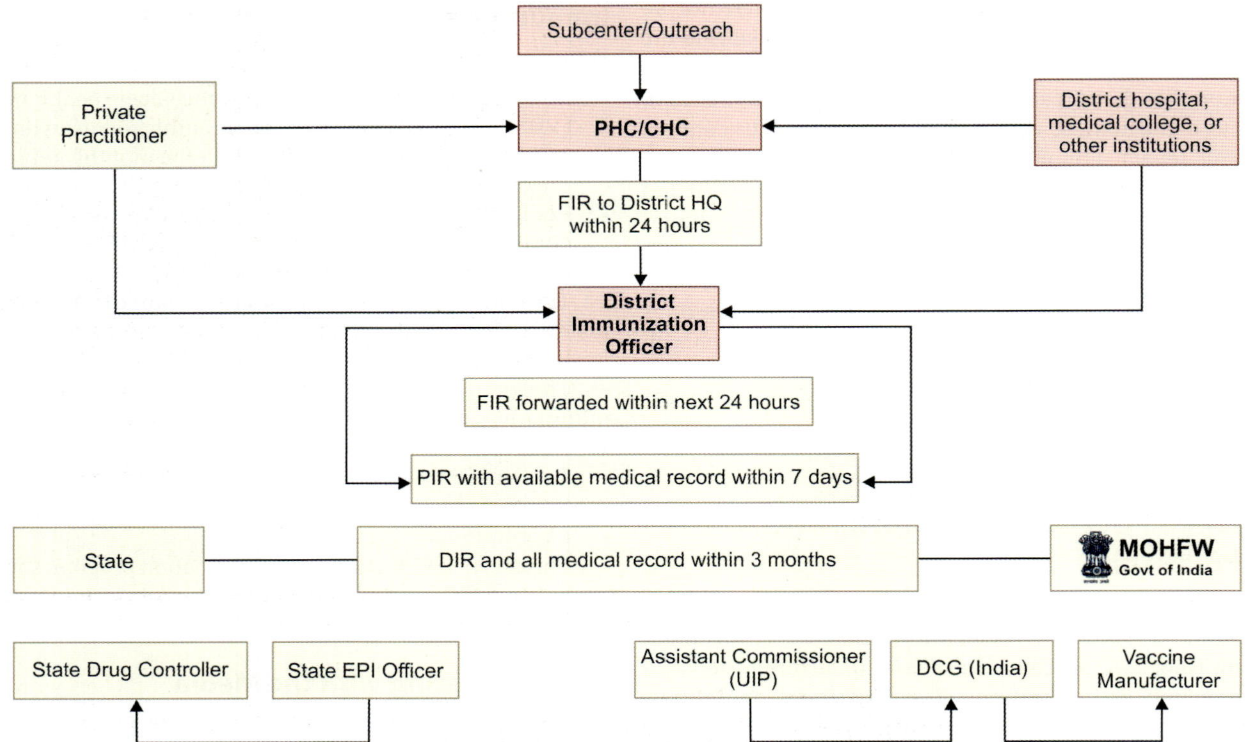

(AEFI: Adverse Event Following Immunization; DCG: Drug Controller General; DIR: Domestic Incident Report; EPI: Expanded Program Immunization; FIR: First Information Report; HQ: Headquarter; MOHFW: Ministry of Health and Family Welfare; PHC/CHC: Primary Health Center/Community Health Center; PIR: Program Information Report; UIP: Universal Immunization Program)

CONTROVERSIES IN VACCINE SAFETY

Vaccines and Autism

Over the past decade, there has been tremendous controversy on the relationship between vaccines, particularly measles, mumps, and rubella (MMR) and autism/autistic spectrum disorder (ASD). Review of all currently available evidence does not support any causal relationship between MMR vaccine and autism.

Safety of Thiomersal

Thiomersal (50% ethylmercury) is a preservative in inactivated vaccines, particularly in multidose vials which has been linked in the past to ASD and neurodevelopmental disorders. Consequently, most of the vaccine preparations available in the developed nations are thiomersal free. Systematic review of evidence however has not supported any causal association between thiomersal and neurotoxic effects. Therefore, in developing nations where multidose vials significantly bring down vaccine costs and cold chain space requirement, the benefits of thiomersal far outweigh any possible risks.

VACCINE-ASSOCIATED ADVERSE EVENT REPORTING SYSTEM

A system for reporting vaccine-associated adverse event reporting system (VAERS) is crucial in any immunization program, so as to pick up previously unrecognized adverse effects and generate further data on vaccine safety. A robust system for reporting VAERS exists in most developed countries including the United States. However, such a system is currently not available in India. Pediatricians are encouraged to report VAERS to the IAP immunization website *www.iapcoi.com*. Events that should be reported include all serious adverse effects, irrespective of causal association, nonserious adverse events that are unexpected in nature, severity, frequency or outcome, vaccine failures, and all usage in pregnancy.

Vaccine injury compensation: In certain countries, there is the National Childhood Vaccine Injury Compensation Program to provide compensation for certain AEFI. Vaccine Injury Compensation Program is a "no-fault" system to compensate individuals whose injuries may have been caused by any routinely recommended childhood vaccines. Vaccine Injury Compensation Program is separate from VAERS.

CONCLUSION

The immunization focus as established by the WHO has the objective "to eliminate sickness and death caused by VPDs through the development of strong, sustainable NIP, capable of delivering high-quality vaccines in a safe and effective way to all children." Safe and efficient immunization practices with thorough knowledge of the vaccines, well-maintained cold chain, proper parent education, and efficient resuscitation equipment are vital components essential to make immunization most cost-effective public health tool in child survival programs.

BIBLIOGRAPHY

1. Chitkara AJ, Thacker N, Vashishtha VM, et al. Adverse event following immunization (AEFI) surveillance in India, position paper of Indian Academy of Pediatrics. Indian Pediatr. 2013;50(8):739-41.
2. Indian Academy of Pediatrics. IAP Guide Book on Immunization. Mumbai: Indian Academy of Pediatrics; 2011. pp. 43-6.
3. Rao I. Vaccination complications, their management and contraindications. Paediatr Clin India. 2001;36:30-5.
4. Rao MIS. Adverse events following immunization. In: Parthasarathy A, Lokeshwar MR, Shah NK (Eds). Immunization Digest, 1st edition. New Delhi: Jaypee Brothers Medical Publishers (P) Ltd; 2004. pp. 59-62.
5. Rao MIS. Adverse events following immunization. In: Thacker N, Shah KN (Eds). Immunization in clinical practice. New Delhi: Jaypee Brothers Medical Publishers (P) Ltd; 2005. pp. 37-46.
6. Salisbury DM, Begg TM. Immunisation against infectious disease—1996 Edward Jenner Bicentenary Edition. Commun Dis Rep Wkly. 1996;6(39):339.
7. WHO. (2014). AEFI Module. [online] Available from: http://www.wpro.who.int/immunization/documents/polioendgame/training_mod6_aefi_monitoring.pdf [Accessed October, 2018].
8. World Health Organization. Immunization Safety Surveillance: guidelines for managers of immunization programmes on reporting and investigation adverse events following immunization. Manila: World Health Organization; 1999.

5.9 Future Vaccines, Adjuvants, and Immunization Techniques

Bharat Mehra, Amarjeet Chitkara

INTRODUCTION

Anecdotal evidence of vaccination does exist since the 11th century, but it was the landmark observation of Edward Jenner and Louis Pasteur about 200 years ago, which started the success story of vaccination. Though attenuation and inactivation remain the cornerstones of modern vaccinology, the rapid advancements in the field of immunology, structural biology, systems biology, and bioinformatics have led to the development of newer, effective, and highly safe vaccines. The synthetic microbial antigens, expression of protective antigens in live vectors and plants, antigen sparing adjuvants that manipulate the desired immune response in the host, alternate modes of delivery, high productivity, and thermostability are some of the exciting developments which shall not only revolutionize the prevention of infectious diseases but also target the noninfectious ailments like malignancy and degenerative diseases. Translational research shall further expedite the development of safe vaccines. The advances in vaccinology with its innumerable applications has led all the stakeholders to adopt "call to action for the new decade of vaccines" emphasizing the need of intensified research and funding, advocacy at all levels for not only equity in distribution and access to vaccines but also ensure its consumption. The argument that vaccines create wealth and prevent unnecessary deaths has to be percolated at all levels to ensure global health.

TARGETING NEW DISEASES

Recent Advances Affecting Vaccine Development

The empirical approach of selecting a vaccine antigen had an inherent problem of longer gestation period till it could be available for mass usage and was associated with a high failure rate as well as safety concerns. Genomics have changed the concept of antigen selection by the reverse vaccinology. The genomic details of a pathogen help to identify the potential vaccine antigen that can be protective and further enhanced using an adjuvant to steer the immune response in the desired direction. Meningococcal B protection, which has eluded the researchers till now, has become feasible. The rapid development of influenza vaccine is another example of reverse vaccinology.

The detailed atomic configuration of an antigen by structural biology shall further help to identify the specific epitopes determining viral entry into the cell or the virulence and can be used as vaccine antigen. Such efforts are being made for a new measles vaccine.

Systems biology is another emerging discipline, which based on cytokine and immunological responses, can identify markers, which can predict safety and efficacy of a vaccine using modeling techniques. These developments have helped to identify numerous potential vaccine antigens but have complicated the issue of selecting the best.

The antigens being targeted today are not only the virulence factors but also those having a crucial role in pathogenesis of disease and the survival of bacteria and viruses in the host. Pneumococcal adhesin antigen is being looked upon as a potential candidate for a multiserotype protection with a high herd effect. Glyco-conjugation of polysaccharide antigen has already revolutionized protection against *Haemophilus influenzae* type b, meningococcal, and pneumococcal organisms and is being further exploited for group A and B *Streptococcus* and *Staphylococcus aureus*.

The first marvel of genetic engineering in vaccinology has been the hepatitis B vaccine made from yeast carrying the surface antigen gene. Subsequently, recombinant proteins as effective immunizing agents have been enabled by gene insertion in yeast, *Escherichia coli*, and Chinese hamster ovary cells for Lyme disease, cytomegalovirus (CMV), and pertussis. Vectored vaccines are live recombinants using pathogenic viruses or bacteria to deliver vaccine antigens, which have met with reasonable success for diseases, such as Japanese encephalitis, dengue (yellow fever virus vector), and respiratory syncytial virus (RSV) (human parainfluenza virus-3). The vectors serve as a carrier for the pathogenic gene and have the advantage of simulating a natural infection and stimulating both humoral and cell-mediated immunity (CMI) effectively. The vectored approach has also the potential for therapeutic vaccines for cancer, e.g. fowl poxvirus encoding prostate specific antigen for prostatic cancer. The preferred vector candidates are poxviruses, adenovirus, yellow fever, and bacillus Calmette-Guerin. The strategy is being used for much work on human immunodeficiency virus (HIV) and malaria vaccines. Virus-like particles produced in vitro by assembly of viral proteins are highly immunogenic and the basis for the human papilloma virus (HPV) vaccines available today. Severe acute respiratory syndrome vaccine is being developed on the same premise. Cell culture techniques in use since 1950 are being further refined and offer the advantage of attenuation (many live viral vaccines), cold adaptation live attenuated influenza vaccine (LAIV), single clone selection with highest efficacy and lowest virulence, rapid and high productivity, and reassortment, i.e. mixing ribonucleic acid (RNA) segments of attenuated strain with the protective antigen from the wild strain (pandemic influenza and rotavirus vaccines).

Deoxyribonucleic Acid and Ribonucleic Acid Vaccines

Deoxyribonucleic acid (DNA) vaccines are bacterial plasmids containing viral or nonviral genes that get integrated with the host-cell DNA and encode for the surface proteins of the pathogen, which are carried to the cell surface and incite immune response in the body. The first-generation DNA vaccines, though safe and well tolerated, failed miserably because of erratic immunogenicity. The second-generation DNA vaccines formulated with plasmids encoded with carefully designed antigens, delivered effectively by needle-free approaches, such as electroporation, particle bombardment, dermal patches, and simultaneous incorporation of genes encoding for molecular adjuvants, such as cytokines, chemokines, or costimulatory factors, such as granulocyte-macrophage colony-stimulating factor have renewed interest in this platform. The second-generation DNA vaccines lead to a high antigen expression and a directed and predictable immune response. Currently, there are 43 ongoing clinical trials, majority being for HIV and cancer. The other targets being evaluated are influenza, hepatitis B virus (HBV), hepatitis C virus (HCV), malaria, and HPV. Safe, stable, cheaper, and unaffected by maternal antibodies, there are concerns about genomic integration and anti-DNA immune responses, but these have not been substantiated in many nonhuman primate studies till now. Ribonucleic acid vaccines prepared with tumor antigens are highly immunogenic and have potential use in cancer immunotherapy. The DNA vaccines undergoing trials, at present, are targeted for cancers (breast, ovarian, cervical, lymphoma), HIV treatment, malaria (*Plasmodium falciparum*), hepatitis B, and influenza.

Transgenic Approaches

The euphoria of developing edible vaccines in the form of locally available fruits or other plant parts for oral use, providing mucosal immunity about two decades back was short lived. The difficulties of standardization, regulatory affairs, and the potential risk of contaminating food chain halted further progress. However, there has been a renewed interest in plant-made vaccines utilizing plants like tobacco which are not staple foods and using recombinant protein synthesis as used in yeast, bacteria, and mammalian cells. The proteins are highly purified and used as vaccine antigen. The two closest products have been a veterinary vaccine for Newcastle disease virus and the most recent attempts to express the protective antigens of various influenza viruses including H5N1 in tobacco plant *Nicotiana benthamiana* using an agrobacterium-mediated transient expression system yielding a purified vaccine within 3 weeks of viral sequence release and have completed phase II human trials in the United States of America. However, regulatory permissions would be delayed for such novel products.

NEWER ADJUVANTS

Live vaccines mimic a natural infection and induce strong immunological response without unacceptable adverse events. However, the inactivated vaccines, be it subunits, peptides, polysaccharides, or DNA plasmids, need adjuvants to enhance immunogenicity. The conventional alum adjuvant though safe had its limitations of reactogenicity, incompatibility with certain antigens, and a narrow spectrum of only TH2 stimulation (humoral). Newer adjuvants, such as MF59, ASO_4, lipidated peptides, and the most recent lecithin nanoparticles, appear to be promising to overcome these limitations. Molecular adjuvants, which are plasmid encoded vectors, are another novel approach to target specific regional antigen presenting cells and are being tried for DNA vaccines **(Table 5.9.1)**.

Table 5.9.1: Newer adjuvants and the immunological characteristics.

Adjuvant	*Immunological characteristics*	*Usage in vaccines*
Alum (aluminum salt)	Depot and proinflammatory effects	Many vaccines (e.g. DTaP–hepatitis B)
MF59 oil-in-water emulsion	Local proinflammatory effects and immune-cell activation	Influenza and pandemic influenza
AS03 oil-in-water emulsion	Local proinflammatory effects and immune-cell activation	Influenza and pandemic influenza
AS02 oil-in-water emulsion containing MPL and Q-21	Induces antibody and cell-mediated immune response	Malaria vaccine candidate
AS04 (combination of aluminum salts and MPL)	Strong antibody and cell-mediated immune response, and Toll-like receptor 4 dependent	HPV vaccine
CG sites	Toll-like receptor 9 agonist	Hepatitis B, cancer, and malaria
IC31 (oligonucleotides plus KLKL5 bacterial peptide)	Toll-like receptor 9 agonist	Influenza and tuberculosis
GLA synthetic lipid A	Activates Toll-like receptor 4 receptors and induces Th1 CD4 helper cells with broad humoral response	Tuberculosis, leishmaniasis, and malaria

(CD4: cluster of differentiation 4; DTaP: diphtheria, tetanus, and acellular pertussis; GLA: glucopyranosyl lipid adjuvant; HPV: human papilloma virus; KLKL5: kallikrein-like protein 5; MPL: monophosphoryl lipid A)

Source: Rappuoli R, Black S, Lambert PH. Vaccine discovery and translation of new vaccine technology. Lancet. 2011;378(9788):360-8.

ADVANCES IN IMMUNOLOGY AND VACCINOLOGY

Immunology and vaccinology have a long intertwined relationship. Both have had a different pace of development, and often vaccinology has lagged behind. The success of vaccines till now has rested on high avidity, long-lasting protective antibodies. The role of CMI, especially for chronic diseases, such as HIV, tuberculosis, HCV, HBV, malaria, and cancer, mucosal immunity and interaction between mucosal and systemic immunity (many respiratory and enteric pathogens), has given the necessary fillip to the development of vaccines regulating these pathways for a higher efficacy. Respiratory syncytial virus disease can worsen with a vaccine that only enhances humoral response without adequately stimulating T-cell responses. The most recent studies on Toll-like receptors (TLRs) mediated stimulation of innate immunity and neuroregulation of host defenses, newer adjuvants capable of inducing CMI, availability of laboratory assessment of CMI by enzyme-linked immunosorbent spot tests and tetramer staining, systems biology techniques to study innate immunity have further opened exciting opportunities in vaccinology. The impact of T-regulatory cells on pathogens evading immune response has been another recent development. One can foresee vectored, DNA and RNA vaccines, synthetic peptides using adjuvants, such as lecithin nanoparticles, lipid-in-water emulsions, TLR agonists, liposomes, and cytokines, to selectively guide host TH1 and/or TH2 for effective protection against many infectious and noninfectious diseases. Therapeutic vaccines for chronic infections by cell-mediated immunity viral load for HCV, HPV (E6, E7 oncogenes), and HIV (gag and tat genes) appear feasible in future.

VACCINES IN THE PIPELINE

Though vaccines against 25 infectious diseases have been licensed, the future vaccine list is gradually expanding. The vaccine candidates are in varying stages of development. Human immunodeficiency virus, malaria, and tuberculosis remain elusive, while a chimeric dengue vaccine-tetravalent dengue vaccine (CYD-TDV) was licensed for use in five countries. The CYD-TDV is a moderately performing vaccine licensed for age 9 years and above as in younger children it may lead to severe disease on reinfection. Many novel antigens from cancer cells and autoimmune disorders are being targeted for specific immune responses to prevent/treat disease and improve survival **(Table 5.9.2)**.

Table 5.9.2: Vaccines in the pipeline showing technology and disease targeted.

Vaccine/technology	*Targeted disease*
Live vaccines: • Virus variant • Recombinant virus • Recombinant viral vector • Bacterial using recombinant bacterial vector	• ROTA/RSV • HSV/polio HIV using vaccinia/adenovirus, Ebola, allergy, and CMV using alphavirus • *Salmonella typhi, Vibrio cholerae, Shigella flexneri, Streptococcus gordonii, Listeria monocytogenes*, BCG
Inactivated vaccines: • Recombinant polypeptide based • B-cell epitope based • T-cell epitope based • Conjugated polysaccharide based • DNA based • Nucleic acid–based viral vector	• HIV and HSV • Malaria • HBV and HIV • Group-B strep • Influenza, HBV, and HIV • *Flavivirus*
Vaccines for non-infections	Glioblastoma, autoimmunity, multiple myeloma diabetes, allergy, Alzheimer, hypercholesterolemia, fertility, pancreatic cancer, non-small cell lung cancer, HIV, melanoma, and prostate cancer

(BCG: bacillus Calmette–Guerin; CMV: cytomegalovirus; DNA: deoxyribonucleic acid; HBV: hepatitis B virus; HIV: human immunodeficiency virus; HSV: herpes simplex virus; ROTA: rotavirus; RSV: respiratory syncytial virus)

Source: Plotkin SA, Orenstein WA, Offit PA. Vaccines, 6th edition. Philadelphia, PA: Elsevier; 2015.

Targeting New Age Groups

Conventionally, vaccines have been primarily used for infants and children, but the future needs demand universal immunization of adolescents and adult population, especially targeted for diphtheria, tetanus toxoids, and pertussis because of the changing epidemiology of herpes simplex virus, HPV, CMV, and influenza. A structured vaccination schedule may be desirable. The concerns of an aging population will merit a similar program for elderly, e.g. zoster, influenza, pneumococcal, cancer, and degenerative diseases, such as Alzheimer disease. Vaccination during pregnancy is done to prevent vertical transmission of infections (Guillain–Barré syndrome and HIV), ensure high levels of protective antibodies in neonate, especially for RSV, pneumococcal infection, pertussis and to protect the pregnant women against diseases, such as influenza, compounded by various ethical issues merits consideration in future. Protection against nosocomial infections and bioterrorism are areas where lots of new vaccines are being targeted.

COMBINATION VACCINES

The ever-increasing list of not only available but also desirable vaccines for children will result in babies becoming pin cushions. Introduction of new vaccines shall become challenging in such a scenario. To simplify the immunization schedule, it is imperative that age appropriate combination vaccines are made available to simplify schedule, better compliance and coverage with feasible costs and logistics. However, there are multiple technical challenges in maintaining immunogenicity and safety of different antigens in combination vaccines. The need to combine pneumococcal and meningococcal vaccines to existing diphtheria-tetanus-pertussis combinations is being explored. To address these immunogenicity and safety issues, different carrier proteins, such as protein D, diphtheria toxin, CRM197, peptides containing T-helper cell epitopes, novel adjuvants, and developing in vitro assays for potency, are being researched.

Targeting Newer Routes of Administration

Since most pathogens invade through the epithelia (skin, mucosa) or blood (cuts and abrasions, insect bites), same routes have been conventionally used for vaccination guided by the fact that most of the immune system is within or close to these entry portals. Because of the physical and chemical barriers posed by the skin and mucosa, the mainstay has been the parenteral route, which is painful and poses a big challenge to mass vaccination. It is now an established fact that mucosal immunity is highly important for protection against many pathogens. Recent developments in immunology, biotechnology, pharmacology, microbiology, and biomedical engineering have opened new vistas in alternative routes of immunization, chiefly the nasal and painless cutaneous administration.

Nasal administration has been found effective for LAIV, RSV, group-B meningococcal, and human parainfluenza virus-3 (HPIV-3). The nasal-associated lymphoid tissue elicits a strong mucosal secretory immunoglobulin A (IgA) and systemic IgG response. The secretory IgA can also be detected in other mucosal sites following nasal administration. Attempts are in progress to develop highly safe and immunogenic nasal vaccines by optimizing antigenic formulation and novel adjuvants and mass administration by inhalational devices.

Painless cutaneous administration by microneedles containing transdermal patches shall soon revolutionize the vaccination practices. The microneedles just pierce the stratum corneum without reaching the pain receptors in the dermis. The breach in skin helps deliver antigen and/or the adjuvant to the abundant dendritic cells and Langerhans cells in the dermis. Several studies using various formulations of influenza vaccine have demonstrated a dose sparing, stable formulation, and early and directed immune response better than the intramuscular administration. Electroporation, jet propulsion, and ultrasonic (sonophoresis) are other methods being evaluated but are cost intensive. Oral administration of inactivated vaccines and rectal or vaginal administration are other areas of future research (**Figs. 5.9.1 and 5.9.2**; *www.path.org*).

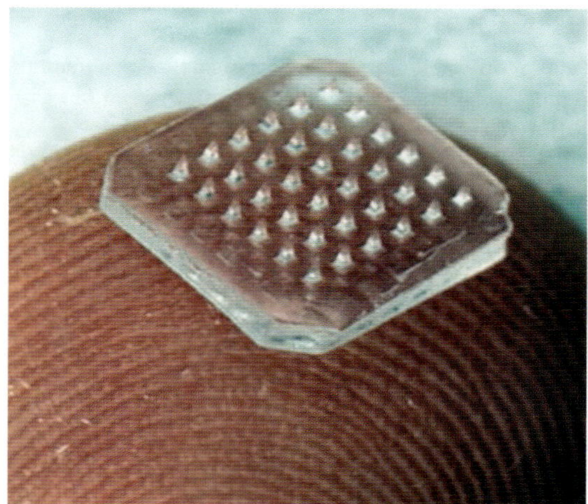

Fig. 5.9.1: Microneedle patch.

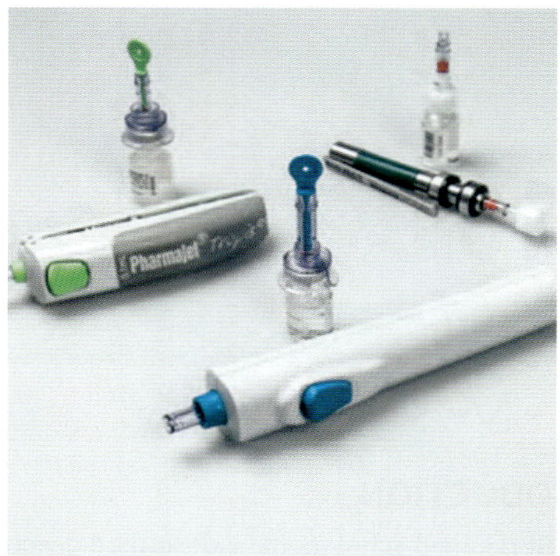

Fig. 5.9.2: Needle-free devices.

TARGETING SAFETY AND EFFICACY CONCERNS

New vaccine development is highly cost intensive and has a long gestation period till licensing. The stringent regulatory approach to guard against the remotest adverse event puts the industry on the back foot. Translational studies can help identify the early predictors of success by the assessment of early events after vaccination, such as inflammatory biomarkers and innate immunity activation within 1–5 days of vaccination. The safety concerns in the preclinical stage can be addressed using bioinformatics and systems biology to avoid vaccine antigens that can mimic human antigens (proteins and polysaccharide) and cause autoimmunity. Microarray technology can effectively demonstrate immune stimulation at the site of injection within hours of administration. The vaccine formulations with extensive nonspecific immune stimulation are best avoided. Identification of specific genetic risk factors for adverse events is being studied to further ensure safety. This "bench-to-bedside" methodology can expedite rapid development of safe and effective vaccines in the near future. The challenges of postlicensure assessment of vaccine safety and effectiveness are also likely to be addressed by availability of large computer databases, comprehensive surveillance networks, and genomic information of the population.

TARGETING CHALLENGES

Vaccines are perfect interventions that prevent morbidity and mortality, yet its introduction into public health is a herculean task especially in a developing country. The availability, cost, its sustainability, safety and efficacy concerns, regulatory constraints, logistics of access, and political will are the major impediments. In countries with a high disease burden, some trade-off for safety may be acceptable, but it may erode the already meager public confidence in the vaccination program. This decade shall clearly witness unprecedented development in vaccines, and a highly consistent advocacy by all the stakeholders is necessary to promote a simple idea "vaccines save lives, prevent suffering, and create wealth."

BIBLIOGRAPHY

1. Bachmann MF, Jennings GT. Vaccine delivery: a matter of size, geometry, kinetics and molecular patterns. Nat Rev Immunol. 2010;10(11):787-96.
2. Bitter C, Zimmermann KS, Surber C. Nasal drug delivery in humans. Curr Probl Dermatol. 2011;40:20-35.
3. Ferraro B, Morrow MP, Hutnick NA, et al. Clinical applications of DNA vaccines: current progress. Clin Infect Dis. 2011;53(3): 296-302.
4. Hegde NR, Kaveri SV, Bayry J. Recent advances in administration of vaccine for infectious diseases: microneedles as painless delivery device for mass vaccination. Drug Discov Today. 2011;16(23-24):1061-8.
5. Moxon ER, Das P, Greenwood B, et al. A call to action for the new decade of vaccines. Lancet. 2011;378(9788):298-302.
6. Plotkin SA. Vaccines: past, present and future. Nat Med. 2005;11(4 Suppl.):S5-11.
7. Poland GA, Jacobson RM, Ovsyannikova IG. Trends affecting the future of vaccine development and delivery: the role of demographics, regulatory science, the anti-vaccine movement and vaccinomics. Vaccine. 2009;27(25-26):3240-4.
8. Rappudi R, Black S, Lambert PH. Vaccine delivery and translation of new vaccine technology. Lancet. 2011;378(9788): 360-8.
9. WHO. (2016). Weekly Epidemiological Record. Dengue vaccine: WHO position paper. [online] Available from: http://www.who.int/wer/2016/wer9130/en/ [Accessed October, 2018].
10. WHO. (2018). Revised SAGE recommendation on use of dengue vaccine. [online] Available from: www.who.int/immunization/diseases/dengue/revised_SAGE...dengue_vaccines.../en [Accessed October, 2018].

5.10 Controversies in Immunization

Abhay Shah

INTRODUCTION

Health and medical scholars have described vaccination as one of the top 10 achievements of public health in the 20th century. The reduction in global morbidity and mortality over the past century because of routine childhood immunizations is quite dramatic. Vaccines are responsible for many global public health successes, such as the eradication of smallpox, elimination of polio, and significant reductions in other serious infections like diphtheria, measles etc. Thus vaccines have been among the most successful and most cost-effective medical technologies ever developed.

Despite such phenomenal success story, it is surprising that mandates for a safe and effective preventive modality of vaccinating an individual should generate a controversy. Opposition to vaccination has existed as long as vaccination itself. Critics of vaccination have taken a variety of positions, including opposition to the smallpox vaccine in England and the United States in the mid-to-late 1800s, and the resulting anti-vaccination leagues as well as more recent vaccination controversies such as those surrounding the safety and efficacy of the diphtheria, tetanus, and pertussis (DTP) immunization, the measles, mumps, and rubella (MMR) vaccine, and the use of a mercury-containing preservative called thimerosal.

Vaccines are generally victims of their own success. Much of that controversy focuses on the true safety and efficacy of the vaccines. Other aspects of controversy focus on the politics and legality of mandates of any sort. Ironically, as the numbers of cases of vaccine-preventable infectious diseases are falling, the controversies relating to vaccine safety are growing. Controversies can afflict the positive acceptance of immunization, decrease the coverage and uptake, and finally threaten the health of children and adults.

The vaccine controversy is based on a dispute over various issues, such as their safety, morality, effectiveness, breakthrough infections, misconceptions related to vaccines, dynamics of vaccine recommendations, mandatory vaccinations, ethical and other vaccine-related issues. There are number of misconceptions hovering around vaccination practices and vaccines as well.

VACCINE SAFETY

Let us not forget that no vaccine is 100% effective or safe. All vaccines carry some risk of adverse reactions. However, majority of adverse reactions to the routinely recommended vaccines are minor and are related to pain, erythema, or inflammation at the injection site. These local reactions are common and may occur in up to 50% of vaccines. Systemic symptoms, such as fever, headache, irritability, or diminished activity, are less common; the frequency of systemic symptoms is vaccine specific. Rarely, moderate-to-severe reactions to vaccines, such as febrile seizures and allergic reactions, occur at a frequency of 1 per thousands or millions of doses administered. The risks of moderate-to-severe vaccine reactions are carefully weighed against the benefits that vaccines produce in preventing serious and life-threatening illnesses in the vast majority of the general population. There is a small but vocal anti-vaccine movement concerned about vaccine safety that may affect vaccination efforts in the developed as well as other parts of the globe. A small number of highly publicized claims unsubstantiated by valid data, regarding vaccine adverse events, have further heightened the suspicion that some or all vaccines may cause unacceptable adverse events. **Table 5.10.1** outlines the summary of the risks and benefits for six recommended pediatric vaccine antigens.

Table 5.10.1: Summary of the risks and benefits for six recommended pediatric vaccine antigens.

MMR	***MMR vaccine***
Risk from disease: • *Measles* – Pneumonia: 1 in 20 – Encephalitis: 1 in 2,000 – Death: 1 in 3,000 • *Mumps* – Encephalitis: 1 in 300 • *Rubella* – *Congenital rubella syndrome*: 1 in 4 (if woman infected during first trimester)	*Risk from vaccine*: *Encephalitis or severe allergic reaction*: 1 in 1,000,000
DTP	***DTP vaccine***
Risk from disease: • *Diphtheria* – *Death*: 1 in 20 • *Tetanus* – *Death*: 3 in 100 • *Pertussis* – *Pneumonia*: 1 in 8 – *Encephalitis*: 1 in 20 – *Death*: 1 in 200	*Risk from DTP vaccine*: • *Continuous crying, then full recovery*: 1 in 100 • *Convulsions or shock, then full recovery (hypotonic/ hyporesponsive episode)*: 1 in 1,750 • *Acute encephalopathy*: 0 to 10.5 in 1,000,000

Note: Risk expressed as number of adverse events per persons with disease or number of adverse events per vaccinated persons.
Source: Maldonado YV. Current Controversies in Immunization. JAMA. 2002;285:24.

Recent efforts to improve vaccine safety have led to a heightened awareness of the possible adverse effects of routine vaccine administration, especially to infants and young children. These changes include recent recommendations regarding the elimination of the mercury-based preservative thimerosal from vaccines, and the withdrawal of a rotavirus vaccine from the United States market because of early postlicensure surveillance demonstrating an increased risk of intussusception associated with the first dose of this vaccine to young infants. Although these were rational and necessary policy changes, they have spurred some anxiety among those concerned about vaccine safety.

One must always look at both risks and benefits and try to weigh risk and benefits involved with a particular intervention. Even one serious adverse effect in a million doses of vaccine cannot be justified if there is no benefit from the vaccination. If there were no vaccines, there would be many more cases of disease, and along with them, more serious side effects and more deaths.

VACCINE EFFECTIVENESS

It is also important to remember that no vaccine achieves 100% efficacy, so even among vaccinated individuals, a few will remain susceptible to infection in the event of exposure. In this situation, cohorts of vaccinated and unvaccinated susceptible individuals may serve as a focus for disease outbreaks after exposure. It is therefore difficult for public health officials and health-care practitioners to convey to the public a sense of urgency regarding vaccination. In addition, importation of vaccine-preventable illnesses is a constant concern in this era of global travel. Sometimes we may experience breakthrough infection cases as well.

A *breakthrough infection* is a case of illness in which a vaccinated individual becomes sick from the same illness that the vaccine is meant to prevent. Breakthrough infections have been identified in individuals immunized against a variety of different diseases including mumps, varicella (chicken pox), and Influenza. Such breakthrough infections will create controversy and reduce the confidence and subsequently vaccine acceptance. It is important to discuss these issues with the parents.

Causes of breakthrough infections include improper administration or storage of vaccines, mutations in viruses, waning immunity, compromised hosts, antibody blocking etc. For these reasons, vaccines are rarely 100% effective. For example, the common flu vaccine is estimated to provide immunity to the flu in 58% of recipients. The measles vaccine fails to provide immunity to 2% of children that receive the vaccine. However, if herd immunity exists, it typically prevents individuals who are ineffectively vaccinated from contracting the disease. One of the most important and well-established distinct advantages of vaccination is its success in prevention of severe diseases and complications. The classical examples are varicella vaccine where two doses provide 100% protection against severe varicella and bacillus Calmette–Guérin imparts nearly 100% protection against hematogenous spread of tuberculosis in an otherwise immunocompetent child.

Controversies Related to Vaccine Recommendations

Vaccine recommendations are going to be a dynamic process. The recommendations are changing as per the available scientific evidences, new researches, and clinical trial along with postlicensure data. However, too frequent changes in the recommendations can cause confusions and controversy.

Many vaccines require multiple doses for maximum effectiveness, either to produce enough initial immune response or to boost response that fades over time. Over the past two decades, the recommended vaccination schedule has grown rapidly and become more complicated as many new vaccines have been developed. Vaccine mandates, their target population, vaccine schedules, and types of vaccines used have been an immense sources for controversies. Too frequent changes in vaccine recommendations, though scientifically substantiated, have found to be counterproductive as far as vaccine acceptance is concerned.

Vaccine recommendations are different in the developing and developed countries. In the developing countries, vaccine recommendations also consider the level of health-care access, the cost of vaccines, and issues with vaccine availability and storage. For example, inadequate availability of inactivated polio vaccine has posed a challenge to our polio end game program. The disparity in the recommendations in developing and developed world has been a source of controversy for handful people. Similarly, dispute and controversies prevail due to disparity in the recommendations for public and private sectors. The anti-vaccine lobby has a strong perception that unnecessary vaccines are pushed without much health benefits only for mere financial gain.

Some of the recent controversies that created a lot of interest and anxiety are diphtheria, tetanus whole-cell pertussis (DTwP) versus diphtheria, tetanus, acellular pertussis (DTaP), two doses of chickenpox in place of one dose, three doses of MMR in place of two doses of measles containing vaccines, routine use of flu vaccine, etc.

Diphtheria, Tetanus Whole-cell Pertussis versus Diphtheria, Tetanus, Acellular Pertussis

The success story of pertussis control by these vaccines has suffered a setback since 2000 when despite high vaccine coverage there has been resurgence especially in infants, adolescents, and adults. The recently witnessed large-scale outbreaks in the developed countries have initiated a vigorous debate on the efficacy of vaccines, the immunization schedule, and the demographic factors. The outbreaks have been reported from Australia, New Zealand, the United Kingdom, and the USA; the most notable and analyzed have been in the Queensland 2009–2011 (Australia), California 2010, and Washington 2012 (USA). The common feature has been the exclusive use of acellular pertussis (aP) vaccine in all these places and a peak seen in 7–14 years of age. These outbreaks are enough to doubt the efficacy of aP vaccine.

But it is a known fact that a well-manufactured whole-cell vaccine is slightly better than a well-manufactured aP vaccine with somewhat long duration of protection, and at the same time, it has more reactogenicity. The replacement of DTwP vaccines by DTaP has been a fine balance between the modest efficacy and the significantly reduced reactogenicity to overcome the poor acceptance of DTwP vaccine. The World Health Organization also has not condemned the aP-containing vaccines nor has it insisted on any vaccine nor made any comments about the number of components in aP vaccines and their effectiveness.

Influenza Vaccine

There has been a great deal of dispute regarding efficacy of influenza vaccine and recommendation for its routine use. Influenza vaccine is the major preventative measure to modify the morbidity and mortality risk from influenza. Vaccine efficacy varies from year to year and directly relates to whether the included vaccine viral components reflect the circulating strains. Because of antigenic drift, it is difficult to predict the circulating strains of influenza A and B from year to year. Sometimes predictions are wrong, and the vaccine is less efficacious than predicted. Pandemics present a different set of problems as people demand vaccines that are in short supply.

Measles, Mumps, and Rubella Vaccine

India has already launched a measles–rubella (MR) elimination initiative, one of the world's largest vaccination campaigns against measles, a major childhood killer disease, and congenital rubella syndrome, responsible for irreversible birth defects. As an MR elimination initiative, in place of standalone measles vaccine, MR combination vaccine is recommended at 9 months in public sectors in India. However, IAP recommends MMR vaccine instead of MR at 9 months to safeguard against mumps. Regarding the timing of administration of MMR vaccine, the IAP Advisory Committee on Vaccination and Immunization Practices (ACVIP) believes the vaccine should be given early to have much higher coverage than introducing it late at the time of first booster of DTP. However, this early immunization will be less immunogenic due to interference by maternal antibodies. The IAP ACVIP recommends three doses of MMR at 9 months, 15 months, and 4–5 years. Thus the recommendations of MMR at 9 months and three doses of MMR, though based on scientific evidence, has been an area of dispute and dialogs.

MORTALITY ASSOCIATED WITH VACCINATION

Deaths following vaccination have had a negative impact on vaccination programs particularly in the low- and middle-income countries implementing large-scale infant vaccination programs even when investigations do not find evidence of a causal relationship. In a review of reports of death following vaccination submitted to the Vaccine Adverse Event Reporting System (VAERS) from the early 1990s, the Institute of Medicine concluded that most were coincidental, not causally associated. Vaccine Adverse Event Reporting System received 2,149 death reports (reports of death after any vaccination from July 1, 1997 to December 31, 2013), most [*n* = 1,469 (68.4%)] in children. Most common causes of death, among 1,244 child reports, included sudden infant death syndrome (SIDS) [*n* = 544 (44%)], asphyxia [*n* = 74 (6.0%)], septicemia [*n* = 61 (4.9%)], and pneumonia [*n* = 57 (4.6%)]. Among 526 adult reports, most common causes of death included diseases of the circulatory [*n* = 247 (46.9%)] and respiratory systems [*n* = 77 (14.6%)], certain infections and parasitic diseases [*n* = 62 (11.8%)], and malignant neoplasms [*n* = 20 (3.8%)]. In majority of cases, when, after careful investigation, an event is felt to be a genuine vaccine-related event, it is most frequently found to be a programmatic error, not related to vaccine itself.

However, it is important to remember that in a rarest of the rare instance a causal relationship between vaccination and death can be established or a plausible theoretical risk exists; these include anaphylaxis, intussusception, Guillain-Barré syndrome, yellow fever vaccine-associated viscerotropic disease, and syncope after vaccination leading to head trauma and subsequent death.

Misconceptions Related to Immunization (Table 5.10.2)

An important misconception regarding vaccination is the perceived association of a variety of systemic adverse events linked to specific vaccines or to vaccine administration in general. In most cases, these associations are based on anecdotal reports or data not sufficiently stringent to support the association. Some common misconceptions are elaborated here.

- Vaccines cause many harmful side effects, illnesses, and even death. Vaccines are very safe, despite implications to the contrary in many anti-vaccine publications. Most vaccine adverse events are minor and temporary, such as a sore arm or mild fever. These can often be controlled by taking paracetamol after vaccination. More serious adverse events and/or death occur rarely and are so rare that risk cannot be accurately assessed.
- A claim has been made that increased rates of diabetes mellitus in the general pediatric population are due to increased exposure to vaccine antigens in childhood. Scientifically rigorous studies have refuted this hypothesis.
- Another hypothesis linking measles immunization to the development of autism has been the subject of intense international controversy. However, rigorous analysis of the incidence of autism relative to the timing of introduction of measles vaccine into populations has failed to demonstrate any temporal association between these two events. The alleged association between the combined MMR vaccine and autism, developed into a "controversy," as despite sound epidemiological studies showing no excess of autism onsets after MMR vaccine, there remained a vocal lobby that did not accept the evidence. It's important to know that the average age of an autism diagnosis is the same in both children who have received the MMR vaccine and children who have not received the vaccine.
- Diphtheria-tetanus-pertussis vaccine and SIDS.

If you consider that most SIDS deaths occur during the age range when three shots of DTP are given, you would expect DTP shots to precede a fair number of SIDS deaths simply by chance. In fact, when several well-controlled studies were conducted during the 1980s, the investigators found, nearly unanimously, that the number of SIDS deaths temporally associated with DTP vaccination was within the range expected to occur by chance. In other words, the SIDS deaths would have occurred even if no vaccinations had been given.

VACCINE REFUSALS—ANTI-VACCINE CAMPAIGNING

The reasons why scientific evidence on vaccine safety and effectiveness is rejected by the so-called "anti-vaxxers" are complex and varied. The most common perceptions are:

- Distrust of the scientific "establishment" who generally promotes vaccination, based on careful risk-benefit analyses.
- Suspicion that those conducting vaccine safety studies are in the pay of the pharmaceutical industry.
- Personal belief that their child will be damaged by a vaccine.
- Pseudoscientific beliefs that vaccination is unnatural, and it is better for a child to experience the real disease.
- Getting a disease provides immunity forever and vaccinations might not provide lifelong protection.
- Nonscientific notion that giving several vaccines to a young child can overload the immune system, despite

Table 5.10.2: Myths and truths related to immunization.

Vaccine	*Myths*	*Truth*
HPV	• Giving girls HPV vaccine implies tacit consent to engage in sexual activity • Giving girls this vaccine will confer a false sense of protection from sexually transmitted infections and will lead to sexual disinhibition • Children already have too many vaccinations on the immunization schedule • Long-term side effects of HPV vaccine are unknown • The vaccine's enduring effectiveness is unknown and booster shots may be required	• HPV vaccine is highly efficacious for prevention of cervical cancer • It provides 99–100% efficacy against vaccine type viruses
Whole-cell DPT vaccine	Implicated as a cause of sudden infant death and other serious chronic conditions	• Causes high fever, irritability, and occasional benign febrile seizures • Highly efficacious
OPV	Causes paralysis	• Causes VAPP but its incidence is very less • OPV has been instrumental in polio elimination
Rotavirus vaccine	Causes intussusception	The initial vaccine Rota shield was licensed in August 1999 and withdrawn months later due to a slight increase in the risk of intussusception in the immunized population But new vaccines are shown to be 90% effective for the prevention of severe disease, and there is no increased risk of intussusception
Measles–mumps–rubella vaccine	Can lead to autism in children	There are number of published statements "refuting all causal relationships" between the vaccine and autism.
Chickenpox vaccine	It is better to have a disease and get permanent immunity	Chickenpox is a mild illness but at times it can have complications and serious disease with a possibility of scarring and secondary bacterial infections; second, social and financial implications of children missing a week of school and parents staying home from work is huge from a global perspective
Thimerosal-containing vaccines	It has been linked to brain damage	No causal association established between early exposure to mercury from thimerosal-containing vaccines and any deficit in neuropsychological function in children 7–10 years of age
Flu vaccine	Prevents cold	Protects against influenza
Pneumococcal vaccine	Prevents all pneumonia	Prevents pneumococcal disease spectrum illnesses Serodiversity and seroprevalence are important considerations

(DPT: diphtheria-tetanus-pertussis; HPV: human papilloma virus; OPV: Oral polio vaccine; VAPP: Vaccine-associated paralytic poliomyelitis)

strong scientific arguments against the immune overload hypothesis and epidemiological studies showing no increased risk of infections after multiple vaccinations.

TRANSPARENCY IN RESEARCH FUNDED BY PHARMACEUTICAL COMPANIES

The vaccine development and research process includes diverse experts many scientific and social disciplines, including public health, epidemiology, immunology, and statistics, and from pharmaceutical companies. These stakeholders may have conflicting priorities and motives, which contributes to various ethical discussions. Hiding unfavorable safety results in a trial is not an option. As part of the licensing process, manufactures must also submit a risk management plan that identifies possible risks of their product, including any potential prelicensure safety signals, together with a mitigation strategy to reduce the risk. For example, when the second generation of rotavirus vaccines was licensed, manufacturers were required to conduct large postmarketing studies to assess the risk of intussusception, as this rare side effect was the cause of the withdrawal of the first licensed rotavirus vaccine.

While it is important to convey the huge benefits of vaccination, it is also necessary to honestly acknowledge that the absolute safety of a new vaccine can only be confirmed after it has been given to hundreds of thousands of individuals and that the decision to vaccinate is a risk-benefit judgment that requires full informed consent.

Conflict of Interest

Vaccine recommendations are always dynamic and most of the time substantiated by scientific evidences. However, they are unfortunately read as a conspiracy to push vaccines unnecessarily for financial rewards by enriching pharmaceutical makers who make vaccines. Such perceived "conflict of interest" will adversely affect the vaccination programs.

SHOULD VACCINATION BE MANDATORY?

Mandatory vaccination is again an area of controversy. Making vaccination compulsory by law is often seen as a way of improving compliance and dealing with the problem of vaccine hesitancy or refusal. While individual freedom of choice is an important principle, those who refuse vaccination not only pose a risk to themselves but also to others.

To make sure children are being vaccinated, most countries have some sort of vaccination policy, although the details vary widely. Some nations like to focus on education and leave the choice of vaccination up to the individual, while other countries offer financial incentives for vaccinating children. In the countries, such as the United States and Australia, compulsory vaccination has contributed to the success of immunization programs, but the balance between individual freedoms and public benefits is a fine judgment and not all countries can make the same decision. In countries, such as Sweden, Norway, Denmark, the Netherlands, and the United Kingdom, compulsory immunization is unlikely to be acceptable and indeed high coverage has been achieved through other approaches. Ten nations that have made vaccinations mandatory for one or the other vaccines are Slovenia, Belgium, Latvia, the United States, Australia, Italy, Germany, Romania, France, and Canada.

PARENTAL, MEDIA, AND PUBLIC PERCEPTION

Parental Perception about Immunization

Policies that mandate immunization have always been controversial. Anxiety and fear are commonly seen before immunization. For routine childhood immunizations, many parents have fears about both short- and long-term side effects. Parental worries change as the rate of vaccination in the community changes. When most children are vaccinated, parents worry more about side effects than they do about disease. Because of these worries, immunization rates go down. As immunization rates go down, disease rates go up, and parents worry less about side effects of vaccination and more about the complications of the diseases. Immunization rates then go up. Better education of parents and health providers would result in a change in the attitude of the population in regard to vaccinations.

Media and Public Perception

Unfortunately, rare adverse events and theoretical concerns tend to make more headlines than the remarkable success story of vaccinations. These problems are then seized on by vaccine opponents and spread online through the web. The result will be vaccine refusal and/or vaccination acceptances with doubts. An implacable rejection of vaccination, despite strong evidence of its safety, is damaging. For example, in the case of the MMR controversy, sustained interest in the alleged association by the British media with its extensive coverage and scant attention to the actual scientific evidence resulted in a critical fall in MMR vaccine coverage in the United Kingdom.

A Way Forward

We must develop methods and means to derive our own data through well-planned epidemiological surveillance. The lessons from the past events and experiences must be analyzed and interpreted to guide immunization efforts. The systemic efforts are needed to generate evidence for deciding to or not to introduce new antigens in immunization schedule. Once it is introduced we must put all the efforts to know the impact that the vaccine has produced. There have been significant changes to the regulatory framework in recent years, which have ensured that manufacturers of any medicinal product, including vaccines, operate in a more transparent manner, with improved systems for detection of adverse events.

CONCLUSION

Vaccines are responsible for many global public health successes. Thus vaccines have been among the most successful and most cost-effective medical technologies ever developed. In spite of such phenomenal success story, such a safe and effective preventive modality of vaccinating an individual has generated lots of controversy. Majority of time controversy focuses on the true safety and efficacy of the vaccines. It is critical that pediatricians remain up to date on vaccine efficacy and safety and serve as advocates for timely administration. The media have aggressively focused on controversies regarding immunizations, often with little regard for science. This focus has resulted in increased parental anxiety, confusion, and, at times, refusal to vaccinate.

Scientist, researchers, epidemiologists must continue to provide data proving safety, efficacy and cost-effectiveness of vaccines so that all the proven and perceived concerns regarding childhood immunizations can be scientifically addressed. It is important to be emphasized that any small risk is dramatically outweighed by the advantages to the child and to society.

BIBLIOGRAPHY

1. Centers for Disease Control and Prevention. Notice to readers: summary of the joint statement on thimerosain vaccines. MMWR Morb Mortal Wkly Rep. 2000;49:622-31.
2. Centers for Disease Control and Prevention. Ten great public health achievements—United States, 1900–1999. MMWR Morb Mortal Wkly Rep. 1999;48:241-3.
3. Centers for Disease Control and Prevention. Withdrawal of rotavirus vaccine recommendation. MMWR Morb Mortal Wkly Rep. 1999;48:1007.
4. Dales L, Hammer SJ, Smith NJ. Time trends in autism and in MMR immunization coverage in California. JAMA. 2001;285:1183-5.
5. Global Advisory Committee on Vaccine Safety, 12–13 June 2013. Wkly Epidemiol Rec. 2013;88:301-12.
6. Graves PM, Barriga KJ, Norris JM, et al. Lack of association between early childhood immunizations and beta-cell autoimmunity. Diabetes Care. 1999;22:1694-7.
7. Moro PL, Arana J, Cano M, et al. Deaths reported to the Vaccine Adverse Event Reporting System, United States, 1997–2013. Clin Infect Dis. 2015;61:980-7.
8. National Immunization Program. Six common misconceptions about vaccination and how to respond to them. [online]. Available from: http://www.cdc.gov/nip/publications/6mishome.htm [Accessed October, 2018].
9. Taylor B, Miller E, Lingam R, et al. Measles, mumps, and rubella vaccination and bowel problems or developmental regression in children with autism: population study. BMJ. 2002;324:393-6.
10. World Health Organization. Global vaccine safety—six common misconceptions about immunization. [online] Available from: http://www.who.int/vaccine_safety/initiative/detection/immunization_misconceptions/en/ [Accessed October, 2018].

5.11 Fever and Fever of Unknown Origin

PP Maiya

"Humanity has but three great enemies: fever, famine, and war; of these by far the greatest, by far the most terrible, is fever".
—Sir William Oscar

INTRODUCTION

Fever in children is one of the most common manifestations of an illness, which makes parents seek medical attention early. Fever occurs when various infectious and noninfectious processes interact with the host's defense mechanism. It is important that all children with fever are carefully assessed to find the cause. Nevertheless, the cause remains undetermined in a significant percentage of cases, leading to the designation of FWF (fever without focus) and FUO (fever of unknown origin). But even with the etiology being determined, fever remains the overriding source of anxiety.

DEFINITION

Fever should always be measured by a clinical thermometer, not by mere touching, and documented. Fever may be defined in both physiological and clinical terms:

Physiologically, fever is an interleukin-1 (IL-1) mediated elevation of the thermoregulatory set point of the hypothalamic center.

Clinically, fever is a body temperature of 1°C (1.8°F) or greater above the mean at the site of temperature recording.

- Rectal temperature greater than 38.0°C (100.4°F)
- Oral temperature greater than 37.6°C
- Axillary temperature greater than 37.4°C

The normal body temperature is maintained between a range of 36.8 ± 0.4°C (98.2 ± 0.7°F) with a circadian rhythm of lowest temperature at 6:00 am (37.2°C or 98.9°F) and highest temperature of 37.7°C or 99.9°F at 4:00 pm.

Phases of Fever

Fever is characterized by three phases:

1. Phase of temperature rise is often characterized by discomfort and is the result of decreased heat loss through vasoconstriction and increased heat production through shivering. The patient feels cold and the skin also feels cold to the touch.
2. Phase of temperature stabilization (fastigium) occurs at the new level of the thermoregulatory set point. Heat production and heat loss are balanced as in normal health, but at the higher hypothalamic set point. A flushed or pink appearance signifies that the fever has peaked. Once this phase is reached, the child usually feels comfortable without shivering.
3. Phase of falling temperature or defervescence occurs either by lysis (falling gradually within 2–3 days to a normal level) or by crisis (falling within a few hours to a normal level).

MECHANISM OF FEVER

The fever reaction is a series of cellular events that begins peripherally and ends centrally with a resetting of body's temperature set point. Unlike hyperthermia fever does not represent a failure of temperature control, but rather an upward shift of the regulated temperature, as a result of body's exposure to infecting microorganisms, immune complexes, and other sources of inflammation. Various mediators, such as cytokines, tumor necrosis factor, IL-1, and IL-6, stimulate prostaglandin E2 (PGE2) production in the anterior hypothalamus, which then brings about rise in the temperature set point by a variety of physiological mechanisms including activation of cyclic adenosine monophosphate. When this happens, signals are sent to various efferent nerves innervating peripheral blood vessels to conserve heat. The vasoconstriction causes the feeling of chills, which may lead to rigors with sudden elevation of body temperature. Also, the thermoregulatory center sends signal to cerebral cortex to initiate behavioral changes, such as seeking warm environment, extra clothing, and flexed posture. All these mechanisms act to elevate the core body temperature so that the blood bathing neurons in the anterior hypothalamus is warm and matches with the new temperature set point. **Flowchart 5.11.1** summarizes the pathogenesis of fever.

Flowchart 5.11.1: Pathogenesis of fever.

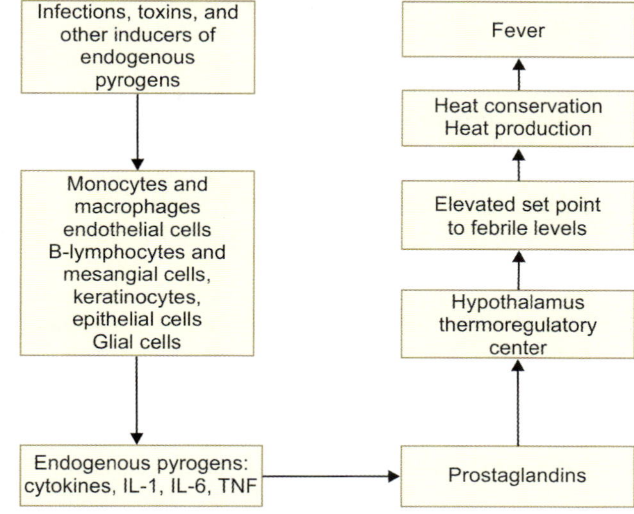

(IL: interleukin; TNF: tumor necrosis factor)

Patterns of Fever

Patterns of fever include the type of onset (insidious or abrupt), variation in temperature degree during a 24-hour period and during the entire episode of illness, cycle of fever, and response to therapy.

- *Continuous fever*: Continuous or sustained fever is characterized by a persistent elevation of body temperature with fluctuation not more than of 1°C (1.5°F) during a 24-hour period, but never touches the baseline. Normal diurnal fluctuation temperature is usually absent or insignificant, e.g. typhoid fever and malignant falciparum malaria.
- *Remittent fever*: Remittent fever is characterized by a fall in temperature each day but not to a normal level. Fluctuation is more than 2°C without touching the baseline. This is the most common type of fever in pediatric practice and is not specific to any disease. Diurnal variation is usually present, particularly if the fever is infectious in origin, e.g. most viral or bacterial diseases.
- *Intermittent fever*: In intermittent fever, the temperature returns to normal each day, usually in the morning and peaks in the afternoon. This is the second most common type of fever encountered in clinical practice, e.g. malaria, lymphoma, and endocarditis.
- *Hectic or septic fever* occurs when remittent or intermittent fever shows a very large difference between the peak and the nadir, e.g. Kawasaki disease and pyogenic infection.
- *Undulant fever* describes a gradual increase in temperature that remains high for a few days and then gradually decreases to normal level.
- *Prolonged fever* describes a single illness in which duration of fever exceeds that expected for this illness, for example greater than 10 days for a viral upper respiratory tract infection.
- *Recurrent fever* is an illness involving the same organ (e.g. urinary tract) or multiple-organ systems in which fever recurs at irregular intervals, e.g. familial Mediterranean fever.

- *Periodic fever* is characterized by episodes of fever recurring at regular or irregular intervals. Each episode is followed by one to several days and weeks or months of normal temperature. Examples are seen in malaria (termed *tertian* when the febrile spike occurs every third day and *quartan* when the spike occurs every fourth day) and brucellosis.
- *Relapsing fever (RF)* is the term usually applied to recurrent fevers caused by numerous species of *Borrelia* and transmitted by lice (louse-borne RF) or ticks (tick-borne RF).
- *Pel-Ebstein fever* described by Pel and Ebstein in 1887 was originally thought to be characteristic of Hodgkin's lymphoma. The pattern consists of recurrent episodes of fever lasting 3–10 days, followed by an afebrile period of similar duration.

Manifestations during fever include symptoms, such as chills (rigor), myalgia, headache, anorexia, excessive sleep, fatigue, thirst, delirium, and scanty urine (oliguria). Commonly observed clinical signs include the following:

- Tachycardia, with the pulse rate rising 10 beats/min for every 1°C temperature elevation.
- Tachypnea, during fever there is an increase of respiratory rate by approximately 2.5 breaths/min, for each 1°C elevation of body temperature, occasionally associated with grunting.
- In pneumonia and malaria, the temperature effect on the respiratory rate is even higher at 3.7 breaths/min/°C.
- Initial phase of fever is accompanied by a rise in blood pressure and a decrease in glomerular filtration rate (GFR). Sustained fever is associated with a fall in blood pressure and a slight increase in the GFR.
- Accentuation or appearance of a functional murmur and third heart sound.

CLASSIFICATION OF FEVER SYNDROMES

Fever with Focus

The majority of febrile episodes in children are associated with infections. The diagnosis is made by identifying the focus, e.g. ear discharge in otitis media, cough and respiratory distress in respiratory infections, vomiting, diarrhea, jaundice in gastrointestinal (GI) infections, convulsions and focal neurological deficit in central nervous system infections, joint swelling in collagen vascular diseases or sepsis.

Majority of the children presenting with acute fever are due to viral infections. Many a times, one may find difficulty in differentiating between viral and bacterial infections. **Table 5.11.1** gives clues to differentiate between viral and bacterial infections.

Table 5.11.1: Clinical differentiation between viral and bacterial infections.

Viral infections	*Bacterial infections*
Abrupt onset	Insidious onset
Duration 3–5 days	May last for more than 7 days
Prodrome usually present	No prodrome
Rash is very common	Rash is less common
Seasonal variations	No seasonal variation
Investigations are usually normal	Elevated WBC counts, CRP positive and culture positivity
No localizing findings	May have systemic localization and organomegaly
Mostly self-limiting	Require antibiotic therapy

(CRP: C-reactive protein; WBC: white blood cell)

Fever without Focus

The term "Fever without Focus" refers to fever of acute onset and short duration (less than 1 week) without any localizing symptoms or any clinical signs on physical examination. Following conditions are important causes of FWF:

- Acute viral fever
- Septicemia or bacteremia
- Vaccine associated fever
- Urinary tract infection
- Sinusitis
- Occult bacteremia
- Prodrome of conditions like infectious mononucleosis, Kawasaki's disease, etc.

Fever with Nonspecific Signs

When the duration of fever is yet less than 2 weeks at presentation and child manifests with hepatomegaly, splenomegaly, rash, jaundice, or lymphadenopathy, specific investigations for anicteric or icteric hepatitis, enteric fever, malaria, and infectious mononucleosis may provide clues to diagnosis. Assess the epidemiological details suggestive of dengue fever and leptospirosis, etc.

Fever Complicating Chronic Illness

A child who has fever persisting for over 2 weeks may have a chronic disease to be investigated for lymphomas or leukemia. Childhood tuberculosis (TB) may present in a similar way.

TREATMENT OF FEVER

The main objective is to make the child comfortable and not just bring the temperature down to a "normal range." It has to be remembered that the degree of fever does not correlate with the severity of illness.

Whether or not to treat elevated temperature is a common question. To determine an answer, one must first identify the cause of fever, degree of fever, and then establish goals of therapy. In patients with fever of less than 40°C, there is no benefit of antipyretic therapy. The use of antipyretics will alter the pattern of fever, which may mask the diagnosis. The goal of the treatment is to correct fluid deficit and ensure that the child's fluid intake is adequate. The knowledge that fever is an important immunological defense mechanism has always been used to support the arguments against treating fever. There is enough evidence to support this view that uncomplicated fever is relatively harmless. Fever has physiological benefits to the human body which include the following:

- Increases immune response by increased production of interferons, B-cell proliferation, and increased bactericidal effect of polymorphonuclear cells
- Improves nutrition of cells with protective influence on their activity
- Growth and virulence of several bacteria, such as malaria, syphilis is impaired
- Augments hepatic synthesis of acute phase reactants.

There are situations where fever can be harmful in young children if not treated, e.g. debilitating children with systemic infections. It is common experience that fever often makes child uncomfortable, increases metabolic rate, O_2 consumption, and CO_2 production. It also increases demands on cardiopulmonary system. Therefore, the administration of antipyretics becomes necessary in children.

Antipyretic Therapy—Indications

- Fever >101°F
- Children known to have febrile convulsions
- Shivering
- Children with heart disease.

Characteristics of an Ideal Antipyretic

- Gives rapid result and be effective in reducing fever by at least 1°C (1.8°F)
- Be available in liquid and suppository form
- To have low rate of side effects in therapeutic doses and low toxicity when taken in overdose
- To have low incidence of interaction with other medications and rarely contraindication in pediatric doses.

Supportive Therapy

Physical therapy is often used to promote loss of heat in high-grade fever, which includes the following:

- Removes excess clothing or blankets and keep the child in well-ventilated room
- Encourages taking extra fluid to compensate for increased insensible fluid loss and to maintain blood flow necessary for heat dissipation
- Discourages vigorous activities
- *Tepid sponging*: It is a cheap, easy, and safe physical measure to reduce body temperature. Studies have found that tepid sponging is effective in the first 30 min. Following is the effect of sponging with water at different temperatures:
    - Tap water 20 min 0.2°C
    - Lukewarm 15 min 0.8°C
    - Cold water 20 min 0.1°C
- Some studies have found tepid sponging for 20 min is ineffective and recommended 2–4 hours of therapy
- Rapid cooling methods, such as ice baths, alcohol rub down, and cool water enemas, should be avoided

Drug Therapy

Most of the drugs used as antipyretics reduce levels of prostaglandins synthesis in brain and thus sets the thermostat back to normal. The pharmacological therapy includes different classes of drugs with antipyretic analgesic, antipyretic or analgesic effects only. Commonly used antipyretics in children include paracetamol (PCM), ibuprofen, and mefenamic acid. Drugs, such as Aspirin and Nimesulide, are generally being avoided in children.

Paracetamol (Acetaminophen)

Paracetamol is an active metabolite of acetanilide and phenacetin. Currently, PCM is the most commonly used antipyretic and analgesic drug in pediatric practice. It is available in oral, rectal suppositories, and intravenous (IV) preparations.

Dose: Oral dose is 15 mg/kg/dose, and IV dose 10 mg/kg/dose. Following administration of a therapeutic dose, fever begins to fall in about 30 min, a nadir is reached in about 2 hours, and recurrence of fever is observed in 3–4 hours. A peak plasma level is reached in about 30 min.

Adverse reactions of PCM: These include GI symptoms, such as vomiting and abdominal pain, dermatological symptoms, such as urticarial, erythema multiforme type of reaction. Other manifestations include worsening of bronchospasm and hypothermia.

Ibuprofen

It is a propionic acid derivative with a comparable antipyretic efficacy with PCM or aspirin. (Ibuprofen in a dose of 6 mg/kg has equal efficacy with 8–12 mg/kg of PCM.)

Dose: 5–10 mg/kg/dose. It is metabolized in the liver and can lead to gastric ulceration, hemorrhage, and perforation.

Mefenamic Acid

It is a potent inhibitor of cyclooxygenase with both central and peripheral actions. It has been reported to have longer duration of action and therefore more effective than ibuprofen. It has a high rate of fecal excretion and therefore causes diarrhea, other GI effects, and nephrotoxicity, if used, more than a week.

Dose: 4–12 mg/kg/dose.

FEVER OF UNKNOWN ORIGIN

Fever of unknown origin in children remains one of the most challenging clinical evaluations for pediatricians. It indicates a persistently febrile child without a cause even after reasonable evaluation including laboratory investigations. Unlike adults, there is no strict timeframe to diagnose FUO in children. The causes of FUO in children are infective, rheumatological, malignancy, and some cases remain undiagnosed.

Fever of unknown origin can be further categorized into four types:

1. *Classic FUO*: The child should have a temperature greater than 38.3°C for a duration of greater than 3 weeks and should have been evaluated on at least three outpatient department visits or 3 days of inpatient stay, e.g. infection, malignancy, inflammatory disease, etc.
2. *Nosocomial FUO*: Temperature of more than 38.3°C developing on several occasions in a hospitalized patient who is receiving acute care and in whom infection was not manifest at admission. Three days of investigations, including at least 2 days incubation of cultures, are the minimum requirement for this diagnosis.
3. *Neutropenic FUO*: Temperature of 38.3°C on several occasions in a patient whose neutrophil count is less than 500/cells/mm^3. The diagnosis of neutropenic FUO is invoked if a specific cause is not identified after 3 days of investigations including at least 2 days incubation of culture.
4. *Human immunodeficiency virus (HIV)-associated FUO*: Temperature of 38.0°C on several occasions over a period of more than 4 weeks for outpatient or 3 days for hospitalized patient with HIV infection. The diagnosis is invoked if appropriate investigations over 3 days including 2 days incubation of culture reveal no organism.

Etiology

Incidence of disease causing FUO varies depending upon the age of the child. In children less than 6 years of age most common is infective cause accounting for 65% followed by neoplastic 8% and autoimmune 8%. In the age group between 7 years and 12 years, infective causes account for 38%, neoplastic 4%, and autoimmune 23%. All these are identified by history, physical examination, or simple laboratory studies. Tuberculosis is common and diagnosis can be established by appropriate investigations. Second most common are autoimmune diseases, such as juvenile rheumatoid arthritis or inflammatory bowel disease. Relatively small numbers are malignant; most commonly, leukemia and lymphoma are other causes of FUO **(Table 5.11.2)**.

Table 5.11.2: Etiology of fever of unknown origin.

Infectious cause	*Fungal disease*	*Local septic infections*	*Noninfectious cause*
Specific infection: *Bacterial:* • Salmonella • Tuberculosis • Brucellosis • Yersiniosis • Meningococcemia • *Bartonella henselae* (Cat-scratch disease) • Rat bite fever (*Streptobacillus moniliformis*) • Actinomycosis • Mycoplasma pneumonia *Spirochetal:* • *Borrelia burgdorferi* • Relapsing fever • Leptospirosis • Syphilis *Parasitic disease:* • Amebiasis • Babesiosis • Malaria • Toxoplasmosis • Visceral larva migrans (Toxocara)	• Blastomycosis • Coccidioidomycosis • Histoplasmosis • Chlamydial • Lymphogranuloma venereum • Psittacosis *Rickettsial:* • Q-fever • Rocky mountain • Spotted fever • Tick-borne typhus *Viruses:* • CMV • Hepatitis • HIV • Epstein-Barr virus	• Dental abscess • Hepatic abscess • Subphrenic abscess • Bronchiectasis • Sinusitis • Mastoiditis • Cholangitis • Infective endocarditis • Osteomyelitis • Pneumonia • Pyelonephritis *Local infection without pus formation:* • UTI • Phlebitis • Diverticulitis *Endocrine:* • Thyrotoxicosis • Addison disease • Diabetes insipidus *Granulomatous diseases:* • Crohn disease • Granulomatous hepatitis • Sarcoidosis	*Collagen vascular disorder:* • JRA • Behçet disease • Juvenile dermatomyositis • SLE • Rheumatic fever *Neoplastic:* • Leukemia • Lymphoma • Neuroblastoma • Wilms tumor *Metabolic:* • Gout • Porphyria *Hypersensitive reaction:* • Serum sickness • Drug fever • Familial Mediterranean fever *Miscellaneous:* • Poisoning • Factitious fever malingering • Hemophagocytic syndromes • Inflammatory bowel disease • Kawasaki disease • Kikuchi-Fujimoto disease

(CMV: cytomegalovirus; HIV: human immunodeficiency virus; JRA: juvenile rheumatoid arthritis; SLE: systemic lupus erythematosus; UTI: urinary tract infection)

Etiology of FUO can be classified into infective causes and noninfective causes. **Table 5.11.2** lists the etiology for FUO.

Diagnostic Approach to Fever of Unknown Origin

The diagnostic approach for each child has to be individualized. It has to be kept in mind that in most cases, the cause of FUO is a familiar disease with an uncommon presentation, rather than a rare disease. For most patients, diagnostic evaluation may be initiated on an outpatient basis. However, young infants, children who appear toxic or chronically ill, and children who have been febrile for a prolonged period should be hospitalized for evaluation. Hospitalization helps in documenting the fever, exploring the history further, repeating the physical examination, and maintaining constant observation along with laboratory evaluation.

History

Carefully taken and detailed history is the most important tool in the diagnosis of FUO.

- *Age*: Neonates and young children are susceptible to specific organisms, such as *Listeria monocytogenes*, and group B *Streptococcus*. Connective tissue disorders are four times more common in children who are more than 6 years old.
- *Sex*: Chronic granulomatous disease and Bruton's agammaglobulinemia is restricted to boys. Pelvic inflammatory disease occurs more often in females.
- History of fever in the family members or neighbors may point toward infectious cause of fever.
- Contact with TB and past history of exanthematous illness may suggest the possibility of TB.
- Pets in the house raise the possibility of toxoplasmosis, visceral larva migrans, and cat-scratch disease.
- History of pica, ingestion of dirt provide clue for toxocara or toxoplasma.
- Note should be made about the presence of epidemics in the community, such as dengue, enteroviral, and leptospira infections, for considering appropriate diagnosis.
- Take details regarding travel to areas with endemic illnesses.
- Recent history of surgery suggests possibility of occult infection.
- Medication history should be looked into and should include over the counter preparation, topical agents, including atropine (atropine induced fever).
- Genetic background of the patient is important for conditions like Riley-Day syndrome.

Physical Examination and Clues to the Diagnosis of Fever of Unknown Origin

Careful and meticulous physical examination is mandatory in all children with FUO. Repetitive examinations, preferable daily examination is important to pick-up subtle or new signs, which appear during the course of illness and help in identifying the etiology.

Following are the clinical parameters, which give clues to the diagnosis:

- *Temperature*: Temperature pattern during hospitalization may give clues to the diagnosis, e.g.
  - *Intermittent*: Malaria, acute pyelonephritis
  - *Continuous*: Typhoid, miliary TB, subacute bacterial endocarditis (SABE), and pneumonia periodic/undulating-Hodgkin and brucellosis
- *Pulse rate*: Relative bradycardia (typhoid, meningitis, dengue, and Weil's disease)
- *Anemia*: Malaria, kala-azar, SABE, acute lymphoblastic leukemia (ALL), chronic disease
- *Lymph node*: All lymph nodes should be described and recorded
  - *Generalized lymphadenopathy*: Hodgkin's disease, ALL, secondary syphilis
  - *Localized lymphadenopathy*: Glandular fever, Kawasaki disease, Kikuchi-Fujimoto disease
- *Jaundice*: Infectious hepatitis, Weil's disease, malaria, and liver abscess infectious mononucleosis
- *Skin rash*: Viral exanthematous illnesses, such as measles and varicella, meningococcemia, dengue, septicemia, SABE, and rickettsial illness
- *Clubbing*: Lung abscess, bronchiectasis, SABE, and liver abscess
- *Arthritis*: Rheumatic fever, SABE, meningococcemia, leukemia
- *Bony tenderness*: Arthritis, leukemia
- *Eye examination*: Uveitis suggests sarcoidosis, juvenile idiopathic arthritis, systemic lupus erythematosus, Kawasaki disease, Behçet disease, and vasculitis. Chorioretinitis suggests cytomegalovirus, toxoplasmosis, and syphilis. Proptosis suggests an orbital tumor, thyrotoxicosis, metastasis (neuroblastoma), orbital infection, Wegener granulomatosis, or pseudotumor
- *Fundus*: Choroid tubercles in TB
- *Cardiovascular system*: This should be examined for murmurs daily
- *Musculoskeletal system*: Point tenderness over a bone can suggest occult osteomyelitis or bone marrow invasion from neoplastic disease. Generalized muscle tenderness suggests dermatomyositis, Kawasaki disease, or mycoplasma or arboviral infection

Investigations

Investigations should be appropriate and based on clinical history and physical findings. Further investigation depends upon the child **(Table 5.11.3)**.

Routine investigations should include total and differential counts, peripheral smear, erythrocyte sedimentation rate (ESR),

Table 5.11.3: Investigations for FUO.

Routine workup
• Complete blood count with differential count; peripheral blood swear • C-reactive protein; ESR; ferritin; procalcitonin • Blood cultures • Renal and hepatic function tests; LDH • Urine: routine and microscopy examination with culture • Throat swab culture • Mantoux test • Cardiologic evaluation with echocardiography • Abdominal ultrasound • Chest X-ray (to rule out infiltrates, effusions, or enlarged hilar lymph nodes) • HIV serology
Categorical workup
Infectious diseases: • Specific antibody or molecular test for EBV, CMV, *Toxoplasma*, *Parvovirus*, HIV, *Salmonella*, *Brucella*, *Bartonella*, *Yersinia*, *Borrelia*, *Leishmania* • Blood culture—aerobic and anaerobic • Cerebrospinal fluid culture if indicated • Thick and thin blood smears for malaria • FDG-PET/CT whole-body scanning to diagnose infectious and noninfectious inflammatory foci • Whole-body Tc-99m MDP bone scan for suspected bone infection • Head MRI for suspected central nervous system infections
Oncologic diseases: • Bone marrow biopsy and aspiration • Lymph node biopsy • Uric acid for suspected leukemia and lymphoma (consider tumor lysis syndrome) • Chest–abdomen–pelvic CT scan for suspected masses (or pyogenic collections) and related enlarged lymph nodes • PET/CT in order to detect neoplasms, infections, and inflammation • Lymphangiography to localize retroperitoneal, aortic, and iliac lymph nodes • 24-hour urine collection for total catecholamines, vanillyl mandelic acid, and metanephrines, monitoring for suspected pheochromocytoma
Autoimmune/Rheumatological: • Autoimmune workup (RA factor, ANA factors) • Thyroid function tests
Immunodeficiency: • Immunoglobulins and lymphocyte surface marker analysis for humoral and cellular immunodeficiencies • Assessment of neutrophil function
Gastrointestinal: • Upper GI series and barium enema to detect changes or abnormalities in esophagus, stomach, duodenum, and colon • ASCA, ANCA, LKM, ASMA antibodies for suspected inflammatory GI disorders • Exploratory laparotomy

(ANA: anti-nuclear antibody; ANCA: anti-neutrophil cytoplasmic antibodies; ASCA: anti-*Saccharomyces cerevisiae* antibodies; ASMA: antismooth muscle antibody; CMV: cytomegalovirus; CRP: C-reactive protein; CSF: cerebrospinal fluid; CT: computed tomography; EBV: Epstein–Barr virus; ESR: erythrocyte sedimentation rate; FDG-PET: fluorodeoxyglucose positron emission tomography; GI: gastrointestinal; HIV: human immunodeficiency virus; LDH: lactate dehydrogenase; LKM: liver-kidney microsomal; MDP: methylene diphosphonate; MRI: magnetic resonance imaging; RA: rheumatoid arthritis; Tc-99m: technetium-99m)

urine analysis, and blood culture. Total count greater than 11,000/mm^3 has a high likelihood of bacterial infection. Peripheral eosinophilia provides clue to parasitic infestation, immunodeficiency disorder, or occult malignancies. Direct smear examination with Giemsa or Wright stain reveals organisms of malaria, toxoplasma, RF, etc. Erythrocyte sedimentation rate exceeding 30 mm/hour indicates inflammation and needs for further evaluation. Erythrocyte sedimentation rate greater than 100 mm/hour may suggest TB, Kawasaki's disease, autoimmune or malignant diseases. Procalcitonin, a precursor to the hormone calcitonin, is a biomarker for bacterial infection. Levels more than 2.0 ng/mL are highly suggestive of systemic bacterial infection. Blood culture should include aerobic and anaerobic cultures. Chest X-ray should be initial investigation. X-ray of the sinuses, mastoids, or GI tract may be indicated by specific history or physical findings. Other investigations, such as ultrasonography, computed tomography scan, bone marrow examination, must precede stepwise. Lumbar puncture is necessary in young infant or child with meningeal signs and altered mental status.

Isotope scans with technetium-99m, gallium citrate, and indium-111 labeled leukocytes help in localizing inflammatory processes. 18F-fluorodeoxyglucose positron emission tomography, in which radiolabeled glucose marks foci of increased glucose metabolism, has been used successfully in oncology diagnostics and can also be used to diagnose infectious and noninfectious inflammatory foci. Bronchoscopy, laparoscopy, GI endoscopy, and mediastinoscopy may be warranted on individual merits of the case. Lymphangiography is resorted to localize aortic, iliac, and retroperitoneal lymph nodes. Exploratory laparotomy performed when all the other diagnostic procedures fail.

TREATMENT

As far as possible any treatment for FUO should be started only when sufficient grounds for diagnosis are available. Mild antipyretics are given for the patient comfort. Empirical trial with antibiotics should not be started. It may mask the diagnosis of infective endocarditis, osteomyelitis or meningitis. Exception may be of antituberculosis treatment (ATT) in a critically ill child with possible disseminated TB. Here also efforts should be made to bacteriologically diagnose TB and ATT should be discontinued if any other diagnosis is established. In general observation of the temperature pattern, repeated clinical examination, careful laboratory evaluation, and interpretation of the results might throw a light on the diagnosis. Specific treatment depends on the diagnosis.

BIBLIOGRAPHY

1. Attard L. Overview of fever of unknown origin in adult and paediatric patients. Clin Exp Rheumatol. 2018;36:S10-24.
2. Chandra J. Antipyretics in children. Indian J Pediatr. 2002;69:69-74.
3. Chandrashekhar PH. Pyrexia of unknown origin. Arch Int Med. 1994;154:841-9.
4. Cunha BA. Fever of unknown origin. Infect Dis Clin North Am. 1996;10:111-27.
5. El-Radhi AS, Carroll J, Klein N. Fever. Clinical manual of fever in children. Pediatrics. 2009:1-25.
6. Long SS. Distinguishing among prolonged recurrent and periodic fever syndromes. Pediatr Clin North Am. 2005;52:811-35.
7. Lorin MI. Fever of unknown origin. In: McMillan JA, Feigin RD, DeAngelis C, Jones DM (Eds). Oski's principles and practice of pediatrics. Philadelphia, PA: Lippincott Williams and Wilkins; 1999. pp. 848-50.
8. Lorin MI. Pathogenesis of fever and its treatment. In: McMillan JA, Feigin RD, DeAngelis C, Jones DM (Eds). Oski's Principles and Practice of Pediatrics. Philadelphia, PA: Lippincott Williams and Wilkins; 1999. pp. 851-8.
9. Robinson MJ, Roberton DM. FUO. Pract Pediatr. 1995;3:301-4.
10. Singh M. Fever of acute onset. A practical approach. IAP J Pract Pediatr. 2002;4:85-90.

5.12 Approach to a Child with Fever and Skin Rash

Jayakar Thomas, Parimalam Kumar

INTRODUCTION

Skin rash in a child with fever is always a cause for great concern. They can be caused by a drug reaction, an infection, or an allergic reaction **(Table 5.12.1)**. The skin can only react to injury in a few ways, and many different agents can cause rashes that look the same. Often, the symptoms in addition to the rash help make the diagnosis, such as a history of insect bites, exposure to other ill children or adults, recent use of medication, environmental exposure, or prior immunizations.

Most rashes caused by viruses do not harm the child and go away over time without any treatment. However, some childhood rashes have serious or even life-threatening causes. A physician should be familiar with these rashes. Many rashes can look the same, making it difficult to know the exact diagnosis. About 10% of all febrile children have a dermatological problem. The approach to such a situation is a challenge, and in clinical practice, physicians "lean" on their eyes in no other situation more than they do when confronted by an acutely ill child with fever and a skin eruption.

The morphology of the skin lesions may contribute reasonably to its cause in relation to the fever. It is common to see more than one type of morphology at a given point of time. Drug reactions are classical examples of such presentation. At times the lesions go through stages, and in such cases, the presenting lesion along with relevant evidence from the history on evolution will help clinch the diagnosis. Yet others may start in a particular form and continue the same morphology, as in measles and rubella. Therefore, it is mandatory that the physician familiarizes himself/herself with a sound knowledge of the morphology of skin lesions in the different disorders. Definitions of these patterns are given in the chapter on skin diseases in children.

Some examples are shown in **Tables 5.12.1 and 5.12.2**. These are only guidelines and should not be considered as complete and comprehensive.

Table 5.12.1: Some examples of skin rashes in a febrile child.

Allergy
• Urticaria • Drug rash • Allergic vasculitis
Infection
• Measles • Varicella • Dengue fever • Typhoid • Rubella • Herpes zoster (disseminated) • Scarlet fever • Meningococcemia
Other illnesses
• Kawasaki's disease (KD) • Systemic lupus erythematosus (SLE) • Erythema multiforme • Toxic epidermal necrolysis (TEN) • Staphylococcal scalded skin syndrome (SSSS) • Erythema marginatum (EM) • Erythema infectiosum • Dermatomyositis • Hand foot and mouth disease (HFMD)

DIAGNOSTIC APPROACH

An algorithmic or stereotyped approach to a child with fever and skin rash would not sound meaningful. Prudence, however, demands a systematic approach. It will comprise the following:

- Careful history taking
- Astute clinical examination
- Relevant laboratory workup

In history taking with regard to the fever, the points to be considered include the following:

- Duration of fever
- Variation with time of day
- Drug intake
- Itching/burning/pain
- Other symptoms

With regard to the skin rash, the points to be considered include the following:

- Distribution of rash
- Morphology or pattern of skin rash
- Evolution
- Prodrome, if any.

Clinical examination will include the following:

- Grade of fever
- Pattern of fever
- Type of skin lesions
- Configuration
- Arrangement
- Distribution
- Site of first appearance
- Evolution
- Tenderness
- Mucosal involvement
- Involvement of palms/soles hair/nails
- Other systems

Laboratory workup, in terms of essential investigations, includes the following:

- Complete hemogram
- Urine microbiology
- Blood biochemistry
- Smear examination from skin lesion

Table 5.12.2: Examples of various types of rashes and their possible etiology.

Macules, papules, and blisters	***Macules and blisters***	***Macules only***
• Drug rash • Hand foot and mouth disease (HFMD) • Systemic lupus erythematosus (SLE) • Erysipelas • Meningococcemia • Bacterial endocarditis	• Erythema multiforme • Toxic epidermal necrolysis (TEN) • Staphylococcal scalded skin syndrome (SSSS) • Varicella	• Dermatomyositis • Urticaria • Allergic vasculitis • Scarlet fever • Kawasaki's disease • Erythema infectiosum • Measles • Rubella • Erythema marginatum • Typhoid

- Gram/Leishman/acid-fast bacteria staining
- Dark field microscopy
- Lupus erythematosus (LE) cell test
- Blood serology
- Skin biopsy

Many childhood diseases have bacterial or viral causes and include a rash of some type. As study continues and more vaccines become available, these diseases become less of a threat to the child's long-term health. A rash of any kind should be taken seriously, however, and may require a laboratory workup for evaluation.

Since the viral and bacterial disorders are described elsewhere, this chapter will deal with the more serious life-threatening and vascular drug rashes.

LIFE-THREATENING VASCULAR REACTIONS AND DRUG RASHES

Life-threatening rashes are uncommon, and the child usually appears quite ill if he or she has a life-threatening rash. Fever and petechiae are the common symptoms. These two symptoms are present with many rashes and are often signs of a more serious condition. Children can develop petechiae from a number of causes. It is not unusual for forceful coughing or vomiting to cause petechiae on the face and chest. Petechiae with fever are more concerning, although most of these children have a viral illness that does not require any therapy. A small percentage (2–7%) may have diseases that need immediate evaluation.

Petechiae are red dots on the skin that do not fade when pressure is applied. The dots represent bleeding from the capillaries leaving a small and temporary blood blister in the skin. Examples include toxic epidermal necrolysis (TEN), erythema multiforme, and staphylococcal scalded skin syndrome (SSSS). These are briefly discussed here.

Toxic Epidermal Necrolysis

- The process seems to be immune complex mediated.
- Septicemia, gastrointestinal hemorrhage, leukopenia, pneumonia, fluid and/or electrolyte imbalance, and renal insufficiency are the major complications that contribute to a mortality rate of approximately 15–40%.
- Physical examination may show the following:
    - Pyrexia may be present.
    - Skin lesions may begin as hot, tender, erythematous morbilliform, or discrete macules that rapidly coalesce and become patches of loose skin. These patches may wrinkle, slide laterally, and separate with slight pressure (Nikolsky sign).
    - The oral mucosa, especially, is susceptible to inflammation, blistering, and erosion. The vaginal tract epithelium also may be involved.
    - Eye involvement may result in bilateral purulent conjunctivitis, which manifests as edema, crusting, and ulceration with pain and photophobia.
    - Pulmonary involvement leads to bronchopneumonia in approximately 30% of all cases. Many patients require ventilator support because of respiratory failure.
- *Differential diagnosis*: Stevens-Johnson syndrome and SSSS.
- No definitive or specific emergent laboratory tests are indicated.
- Basic laboratory tests may be helpful in planning symptomatic or supportive therapy.
- No specific definitive therapies for TEN exist; therefore, intensive care is supportive. Care is given to minimize fluid and electrolyte loss and prevent secondary infection.
- Discontinuation of the offending agent (if identified) should be immediate.
- Intensive care or critical care specialists should be consulted, depending on severity of disease. Ophthalmologists may manage ocular manifestations and help to prevent sequelae. Further inpatient care includes continuance of supportive care and meticulous wound care to prevent secondary infection. Transfer to intensive care unit or burn unit may be necessary for those patients with the involvement of a large body surface area or with hemodynamic instability. Numerous complications appear to be unfavorable prognostic signs.

Erythema Multiforme

- A reaction of the skin to different causes, such as viral infections (commonly herpes simplex), bacterial, mycotic or parasitic infections drugs, or systemic diseases (rheumatic fever, systemic LE, etc.).
- Exhibited clinically as characteristic erythematous iris-shaped papules.
- The characteristic lesions are also known as target lesions.
- The eruption begins rapidly with varying degrees of constitutional symptoms.
- The mucous membranes are severely involved, and there are severe general constitutional symptoms.
- Skin lesions may be pruritic or painful.
- Mouth lesions are painful and tender.
- All attempts must be made to rule out occult viral, fungal, and bacterial infections.
- Systemic corticosteroids are usually given (prednisolone 50–80 mg daily in divided doses, quickly tapered), but their effectiveness has not been established by controlled studies.

Staphylococcal Scalded Skin Syndrome

- Staphylococcal scalded skin syndrome is a toxin-mediated epidermolytic disease characterized by erythema and widespread detachment of the superficial layers of the epidermis, resembling the effects of scalding.

- Nikolsky sign is positive.
- Mucous membranes are usually uninvolved.
- Investigations include Gram staining.
  - *Bullous impetigo*: Findings include pus in bullae and clumps of gram-positive cocci within polymorphonuclear leukocytes.
  - *Generalized SSSS*: Gram-positive cocci are only observed at colonized site, not in areas of epidermolysis.
- Bacterial culture may be yielding.
- For a newborn, hospitalization and treatment with intravenous cloxacillin, 200 mg/kg body weight/day divided in every 4 hours, are preferable.
- Hospitalize infants with extensive sloughing of skin or if parental compliance to treatment is questioned.
- With reliable home care and mild involvement, cloxacillin, 30–50 mg/kg body weight/day, can be given orally.
- Topical care includes baths or compresses, and sisomicin/mupirocin ointment.
- The reader is reminded that the above description is narrated only as guidelines and is advised to refer to other standard books of dermatology for more comprehensive information.

5.13 Malaria

Krishnendu Mondal, Ritabrata Kundu

INTRODUCTION

Malaria is a major public health problem of the developing countries. About 1.5 million cases of malaria are reported annually of which nearly 50% is due to *Plasmodium falciparum* which is rising in recent years. The magnitude of the problem is further enhanced by resistance of *P. falciparum* to standard antimalarial drugs, particularly chloroquine. The important contributing factors to drug resistance are population movement, infrastructure deficiency, deforestation, unplanned development, drug pressure, and haphazard use of drugs. Drug pressure is the single-most important factor in the development of resistance followed by presumptive antimalarial treatment.

ETIOLOGY

Malaria is caused by the protozoan parasite of the genus *Plasmodium* through bite of female anopheles mosquito. The four *Plasmodium* species that infect humans are *P. falciparum*, *P. vivax*, *P. ovale*, and *P. malariae* of which the first two are the main causative agents in our country.

CLINICAL FEATURES

Fever is the most important feature of malaria. The symptom complex is nonspecific and may mimic other diseases with fever. Fever is often accompanied by headache, nausea, vomiting, aches and pains in muscles and joints, chills, and lassitude. In endemic areas, the diagnosis of malaria on the basis of symptoms alone invariably leads to overdiagnosis due to their nonspecificity. If not diagnosed in time, the parasite burden, particularly in falciparum malaria, may increase, leading to severe malaria often in a few hours. Severe malaria if left untreated has mortality nearly up to 100%, but timely adequate supportive care and specific antimalarial therapy can reduce around 80% of deaths.

Severe malaria is characterized by one or more of the following clinical or laboratory features:

- Impaired consciousness or nonarousable coma
- Prostration so that the patient is unable to walk or sit up without assistance
- Failure to feed
- Multiple convulsions, more than two episodes in 24 hours
- Deep breathing, respiratory distress (acidotic breathing)
- Circulatory collapse or shock, systolic blood pressure less than 50 mm Hg in children
- Clinical jaundice plus evidence of other vital organ dysfunction
- Hemoglobinuria
- Abnormal spontaneous bleeding
- Pulmonary edema (radiological).

The laboratory features include:

- Hypoglycemia (blood glucose < 40 mg/dL)
- Metabolic acidosis (plasma bicarbonate < 15 mmol/L)

- Severe normocytic anemia [hemoglobin < 5 g/dL, packed cell volume (PCV) < 15%]
- Hyperparasitemia (>2% or 100,000/mL)
- Renal impairment (serum creatinine > 3 mg/dL)
- Hyperlactatemia (lactate > 5 mmol/L).

Though all manifestations of severe malaria may be seen in children, the most common are cerebral malaria, severe anemia, respiratory distress due to acidosis, and hypoglycemia. Convulsions are common in children and symptoms preceding coma are very brief, i.e. 1–2 days. Generalized seizures are the most common features of cerebral malaria in children. Repeated seizures more than two in 24-hour period may occur. The most common neurological feature is symmetrical upper motor neuron lesions. Severe anemia with hepatomegaly, gallop rhythm, and heart failure is common. Indrawing of lower chest wall without any localizing sign in the chest suggests metabolic acidosis and is seen in malaria with severe anemia and dehydration. Hypoglycemia often presents with convulsions or coma.

DIAGNOSIS OF MALARIA

All efforts should be made to diagnose malaria before commencing treatment. However, in complicated malaria or malaria with danger signs, presumptive treatment may be started after collecting blood for examination.

Microscopic Diagnosis

Light microscopy of well-stained thick and thin films by a skilled microscopist has remained the "gold standard" for diagnosis. Thick films are nearly 10 times more sensitive for the diagnosis of malaria as larger amount of blood is there in a given area compared to thin films. Species identification is better with thin films as morphology of the parasite and red blood cells (RBCs) is well preserved.

Sample collection should be done as soon as malaria is suspected. It can be collected any time irrespective of fever and not necessarily only at the height of fever. Collection should be before administration of antimalarials which causes detection of parasites difficult due to its morphologic alteration.

Rapid Diagnostic Tests

These are immunochromatographic tests to detect *Plasmodium*-specific antigens in blood sample. They employ monoclonal antibodies directed against targeted parasite antigens. In our country, where falciparum and vivax malaria parasites cocirculate, typically occurring as a single species infection, a rapid diagnostic test (RDT) which can detect both falciparum and vivax malaria and distinguish between them is warranted.

Laboratory confirmation of malaria is an essential component of disease management. Expert microscopic diagnosis is available in central levels of healthcare system, such as metro cities but is often unreliable or unavailable in areas with poor health facilities. So, RDT will be useful in the following situations in our country:

- In faraway communities with poor healthcare facilities where microscopic diagnosis is not available and in areas where laboratory service is inadequate, of an unacceptable standard or not available at odd hours.
- In places where quality microscopy is available, RDT and microscopy can run in parallel. RDT will provide rapid or screening diagnosis, whereas microscopy is reserved for resolution of confusing cases, confirmation of negative result in RDT with high clinical suspicion of malaria.
- In some cases of severe and complicated malaria, peripheral parasitemia may be negative due to sequestration, but RDT is expected to provide evidence of antigenemia.

Other Methods of Diagnosis

Other diagnostic methods, namely microscopy using fluorochromes on centrifuged blood specimens, molecular probes, polymerase chain reaction, and serology, are available. Unfortunately, they are not suitable for routine disease management and do not have wide field application. Their use is currently for only research and epidemiological purposes.

MANAGEMENT OF UNCOMPLICATED MALARIA IN CHILDREN

Malaria in children has some unique features. Young children below 5 years of age, whose passive immunity wanes and have not developed sufficient immunity of their own, are most vulnerable. Falciparum malaria can be rapidly progressive leading to rapid clinical deterioration; hence, this group needs constant monitoring. Children can tolerate antimalarial drugs better than adults and their symptoms resolve more quickly following successful treatment.

Malaria parasite develops resistance to drugs randomly due to de novo genetic mutations. Nonimmune patients of our country are infected with large number of parasites, and if they receive inadequate treatment, they become potent sources of de novo resistance. Here lies the importance of prescribing highly effective treatment regimen in hyperparasitemic patients and ensuring good adherence to prescribed drugs.

It has been noted that monotherapy in the case of resistant falciparum malaria invariably results in failure. Sulfadoxine-pyrimethamine (SP) introduced following chloroquine resistance was ineffective in the early 1980s. Similarly, mefloquine (MQ) introduced as monotherapy took only 4–5 years to report resistance. So to counter the threat of resistance of falciparum to monotherapy, the World

Box 5.13.4: Recommended treatment of complicated and severe malaria.

Drug dosage

Quinine salt 20 mg salt/kg (loading dose) diluted in 10 mL of isotonic fluid/kg by infusion over 4 hours.

Then give a maintenance dose of 10 mg salt/kg every 8 hours, calculated from beginning of previous infusion, until the patient can swallow, then quinine tablets, 10 mg salt/kg 8 hourly to complete a 7-day course of treatment (including both parenteral and oral). Tetracycline or doxycycline or clindamycin is added to quinine as soon as the patient is able to swallow and should be continued for 7 days.

Tetracycline (above 8 years) or doxycycline (above 8 years) to be given for 7 days 4 mg/kg/dose 4 times daily or 3.5 mg/kg once a day, respectively. Clindamycin to be given 20 mg/kg/day in 2 divided doses for 7 days.

If controlled IV infusion cannot be administered then quinine salt can be given in the same dosages by IM injection in the anterior thigh (not in buttock).

The dose of quinine should be divided between two sites, half the dose in each anterior thigh. If possible, IM quinine should be diluted in normal saline to a concentration of 60–100 mg salt/mL. (Quinine is usually available as 300 mg salt/mL.) Tetracycline or doxycycline or clindamycin should be added as above.

Or

Artesunate 2.4 mg/kg IV stat then at 12 and 24 hours, then once a day.

Once the patient is able to swallow oral medication, complete the treatment by giving a course of:

- Artemether plus lumefantrine in northeastern states as shown in **Box 5.13.3.**
- Artesunate plus sulfadoxine–pyrimethamine in all states other than northeastern states of India as shown in **Box 5.13.2.**

Or

Artemether 3.2 mg/kg (loading dose) IM, followed by 1.6 mg/kg daily. Once the patient is able to swallow oral medication, complete the treatment by giving a course of:

- Artemether plus lumefantrine in northeastern states as shown in **Box 5.13.3.**
- Artesunate plus sulfadoxine–pyrimethamine in all states other than northeastern states of India as shown in **Box 5.13.2.**

I. Parenteral treatment in severe malaria should be continued at least for 24 hours irrespective of patient's ability to tolerate oral medication earlier than 24 hours.
II. Loading dose of quinine should not be used if the patient has received quinine, quinidine, or mefloquine within the preceding 12 hours. Alternatively loading dose can be administered as 7 mg salt/kg by IV infusion pump over 30 minutes, followed immediately by 10 mg salt/kg diluted in 10 mL isotonic fluid/kg by IV infusion over 4 hours.
III. Quinine should not be given by bolus or push injection. Infusion rate should not exceed 5 mg salt/kg/hour.
IV. If there is no clinical improvement after 48 hours of parenteral therapy, the maintenance dose of quinine should be reduced by one third to one half, i.e. 5–7 mg salt/kg.
V. Quinine should not be given subcutaneously as this may cause skin necrosis.
VI. Artesunate, 60 mg per ampoule is dissolved in 0.6 mL of 5% sodium bicarbonate diluted to 3–5 mL with 5% dextrose and given immediately by IV bolus (push injection).
VII. Artemether is dispensed in 1 mL ampoule containing 80 mg of artemether in peanut oil.
VIII. Mefloquine should be avoided in cerebral malaria due to neuropsychiatric complications associated with it.
IX. According to the latest WHO guideline, children weighing <20 kg should receive a higher dose of artesunate (3 mg/kg bw per dose) than larger children (2.4 mg/kg bw per dose) to ensure equivalent exposure to the drug.

(bw: body weight; IM: intramuscular; IV: intravenous; WHO: World Health Organization)

reduction of parasites per asexual cycle. They have the broadest time window of antimalarial effects from ring forms to early schizonts. Thus, they can stop parasite maturation, particularly from the less pathogenic circulating ring stages to the more pathogenic cytoadherent stages.

Artemisinin also has an excellent safety profile, and the cost of therapy as compared to quinine is almost similar.

There are no reports of resistance to artemisinin at present, but declining sensitivity to quinine has been reported from some Southeast Asian countries like Thailand.

Randomized trials comparing AS and quinine from Southeast Asia show clear evidence of benefit with AS.

However, artemisinin should be used when rate-controlled IV infusion of quinine is not possible; patients have contraindications to quinine use and evidence of inadequate response or resistance to quinine noted. Simultaneous use of quinine and artemisinin is not indicated as it may be harmful, and there is no added advantage. In limited studies available, AS has been found to be better than artemether.

Supportive Management

- Rapid clinical assessment with respect to level of consciousness (use Blantyre coma scale), blood pressure, rate and depth of respiration, anemia, state of hydration, and temperature.
- Good nursing care with proper positioning, meticulous attention to airways, eyes, mucosa, and skin should be done.
- For unconscious child, nasogastric tube is to be inserted to reduce the risk of aspiration.
- Oxygen therapy and respiratory support should be given if necessary.
- In case of shock resuscitate with normal saline or Ringer lactate by bolus infusion, avoid under or overhydration.

- Hyperpyrexia should be treated with tepid sponging, fanning, and paracetamol.
- Close monitoring of the vital signs preferably every 4 hours to be done till the patient is out of danger. Also maintain intake output chart and watch for hemoglobinuria.
- Monitoring of the response to treatment is essential. Blood smear examination every 6–12 hours for parasitemia for first 48 hours is needed.
- In case of artemisinin derivatives, parasite count usually comes down within 5–6 hours of starting therapy. Asexual parasitemia generally disappears after 72 hours of therapy.
- In case of quinine, parasite count may remain unchanged or even rise in first 18–24 hours which should not be taken as an indicator of quinine resistance. However, parasite count should fall after 24 hours of quinine therapy and should disappear within five days.

MANAGEMENT OF COMPLICATIONS OF MALARIA

Of the various complications of falciparum malaria, the common and important ones in children are as follows:

- Cerebral malaria
- Severe anemia
- Respiratory distress (acidosis)
- Hypoglycemia

Cerebral Malaria

Initial presentation is usually fever followed by inability to eat or drink. The progression to coma or convulsion is usually very rapid within 1 day or 2 days. Convulsions may be very subtle with nystagmus, salivation, or twitching of an isolated part of the body. Effort should be given to exclude other treatable causes of coma (e.g. bacterial meningitis, hypoglycemia). Patients should be given good nursing care, convulsions should be treated with diazepam/midazolam, and avoid harmful adjuvant treatment such as corticosteroids, mannitol, adrenaline, and phenobarbitone.

Severe Anemia

Children with hyperparasitemia due to acute destruction of red cells may develop severe anemia. Packed red cell transfusion should be given cautiously when PCV is 12% or less, or hemoglobin is below 4 g%. Transfusion should also be considered in patients with less severe anemia in the presence of respiratory distress (acidosis), impaired consciousness, or hyperparasitemia (>20% of RBCs infected).

Lactic Acidosis

Deep breathing with indrawing of lower chest wall without any localizing chest signs suggests lactic acidosis. It usually accompanies cerebral malaria, anemia, or dehydration. Correct hypovolemia, treat anemia, and prevent seizures. Monitor acid-base status, blood glucose, and urea and electrolyte level.

Hypoglycemia

It is common in children below 3 years, especially with hyperparasitemia or with convulsion. It also occurs in patients treated with quinine. Manifestations are similar to those of cerebral malaria, so it can be easily overlooked. Monitor blood sugar every 4–6 hours. If facilities to monitor blood glucose are not available, assume hypoglycemia in symptomatic patient and treat accordingly. Correct hypoglycemia with IV dextrose (25% dextrose 2–4 mL/kg by bolus), and it should be followed by slow infusion of 5% dextrose containing fluid to prevent recurrence.

PREVENTION OF MALARIA

- Awareness
- Avoid being bitten by mosquito with effective by vector control:
  - Insecticide-treated nets
  - Long sleeves and pants
  - Insect repellents
- Chemoprophylaxis

  It is indicated in high *P. falciparum* endemic areas.

  Short-term chemoprophylaxis (till 6 weeks): It should start 2 days before coming to the malarias are and should be continued 4 weeks after leaving area.

  Long-term chemoprophylaxis (more than 6 weeks): MQ 5 mg/kg weekly (250 mg) to be administered 2 weeks before coming to the malarias are and should be continued 4 weeks after leaving the area.

BIBLIOGRAPHY

1. National Institute of Malaria Research. Guidelines for diagnosis and treatment of malaria in India. New Delhi: National Institute of Malaria Research; 2009.
2. World Health Organization. Guidelines for the Treatment of Malaria, 2nd edition. Geneva: World Health Organization; 2010.

5.14 Kala-Azar (Visceral Leishmaniasis)

Utpal Kant Singh, Rajniti Prasad

INTRODUCTION

Leishmaniasis refers to a diverse group of diseases that may affect viscera, skin, or mucous membranes caused by infection due to parasites of genus *Leishmania*. Kala-azar (visceral leishmaniasis) is a chronic infection of reticuloendothelial system characterized by intermittent fever, hepatosplenomegaly, cachexia, and anemia. In India, etiological agent is a protozoal parasite, *Leishmania donovani*, a hemoflagellate. Transmission occurs by the bite of infected sand fly. Parasitization of reticuloendothelial system, such as spleen, liver, lymph node, and bone marrow, accounts for the salient features of the disease.

EPIDEMIOLOGY

Kala-azar is distributed worldwide with about 12 million people infected and about 1.5 million new cases each year [World Health Organization (WHO)]. Fifty percent of these cases are children. In India, it is endemic in Bihar, West Bengal, Odisha, Assam, Sikkim, and Eastern Uttar Pradesh, but sporadic cases have been reported from different parts of the country. Furthermore, *L. donovani* has emerged as an opportunistic pathogen of human immunodeficiency virus-infected children. Human beings are the only reservoir of infection in India. Kala-azar does not usually occur above 600 m altitude. The disease is more or less confined to rural areas, especially those along rivers (Ganga-Brahmaputra) and lakes. Its epidemic is known to follow famine and war. In recent years, it no longer remains restricted to its known geographical belt, thereby altering its epidemiological scenario.

CLINICAL FEATURES

The incubation period is 2–6 months, but there may be wide variations between 2 weeks and 2 years. A large majority of the cases have insidious onset though acute onset may rarely be seen with high fever and rapidly enlarging spleen. Persistent, mild-to-moderate, intermittent pyrexia with enlargement of spleen in 2–4 weeks' time is the characteristic feature. Liver enlargement occurs rather slowly. Fever, hepatosplenomegaly, and pallor are seen in more than 95% of cases. Malnutrition in association with pigmentation of skin, polymorphic waxy nonulcerating nodules and sparse, falling, and brittle hairs are the additional manifestations. Appetite is however good. Rarely it may present as bleeding, epistaxis, hematemesis, melena, and retinal hemorrhage.

The serious complications may occur in kala-azar and include pneumonia, dysentery, severe hemorrhage, agranulocytosis, acute glomerulonephritis, amyloidosis, papilledema, jaundice, and cancrum oris. Cancrum oris, also called gangrenous stomatitis, is characterized by gangrene of the cheek and adjacent structures and is believed to be caused by an organism, *Treponema vincentii*. This organism is capable of producing rapid tissue destruction in debilitated patient.

DIAGNOSIS

The diagnosis of kala-azar is usually clear from clinical manifestations. However, chronic cases need to be differentiated from tropical splenomegaly, malaria, Hodgkin disease, leukemia, tuberculosis, and hemolytic anemia. At times, cirrhosis and storage diseases also warrant exclusion. When the onset is typhoid-like, kala-azar should be differentiated from enteric fever, septicemia, miliary tuberculosis, brucellosis, and hepatic amebiasis. Kala-azar with malaria-like onset needs differentiation from malaria, urinary tract infection, and tuberculosis.

Laboratory Diagnosis

The diagnosis of kala-azar is substantiated by direct demonstration of amastigote form of parasites in blood, bone marrow, spleen, liver and lymph node aspirates, or promastigote forms in culture of aspirated materials in Novy-MacNeal-Nicolle media and modified USMARAO media. The splenic aspiration and smear examination is the most sensitive (95–98%) method. Prior assessment of coagulation profile including platelet count and international normalized ratio (INR) are essential as this procedure may lead to splenic hemorrhage and if massive may lead to death. The contraindications of splenic aspiration are INR more than 2.5 and platelet count less than 40,000/mm^3. Bone marrow aspiration is usually without any risk and positive in 75–85% of cases. Lymph node aspiration and liver biopsy are positive in 60% and 50% of cases, respectively. The peripheral smear in kala-azar usually shows anemia, thrombocytopenia, leukopenia with neutropenia, marked eosinopenia, and relative lymphocytosis and monocytosis. The ratio of WBC to RBC may be altered from 1:750 to 1:2,000–1:10,000.

Serological Tests

- *Aldehyde test (Napier test):* It is simple and nonspecific test for kala-azar. The increase in immunoglobulin is the basis of this test. The sensitivity of this test is 35–94% with poor specificity. False-positive reactions may occur in children with cirrhosis, malaria, and multiple myeloma. In this test, one or two drops of formalin (40%) are added to 1–2 mL of patient's serum in a test tube. The egg white jellification of serum with opacification within 2–20 min indicates strongly positive reaction and within 24 hours weakly positive.
- *Others serological tests*: Tests which detect antileishmania antibodies may be positive for a long time even after cure or in healthy individuals living in endemic areas due to asymptomatic infection. Direct agglutination test (DAT) is very useful in diagnosis and epidemiological studies, whereas enzyme-linked immunosorbent assay helps to follow the disease during and after therapy. Direct agglutination test measures antileishmania antibody titers using freeze-dried antigen. It is simple, cheap, and effective. A titer of 1:1,600 or above is taken as positive. Its sensitivity is 94.8% and specificity 85.9%. The K39 dipstick test is highly specific for diagnosis of visceral leishmaniasis. It detects antibodies to a specific 39 amino acid sequence (K39) and easy to perform. Its sensitivity is 93.95% and specificity 90.6%.
- *Deoxyribonucleic detection:* The minicircle sequence of kinetoplast deoxyribonucleic is unique and species specific. Polymerase chain reaction offers the best approach to parasite detection and characterization by amplifying sequence found in minicircle of *Leishmania*.

MANAGEMENT

The specific treatment consists of administration of antileishmanial drug. In the last decade, a lot of new parenteral drugs have been tried and found to be effective, but the availability of an oral antileishmanial drug has revolutionized therapy.

Pentavalent antimonials, especially sodium stibogluconate (SSG), were commonly used previously for treatment of kala-azar despite a gradual increase in resistance against them. World Health Organization has recommended that SSG should be used in a dose of 20 mg/kg/day (maximum 850 mg) intramuscular (IM) once daily for 30 days but duration may be extended up to 40 days in nonresponders. Approximately 60–80% of injected drug undergoes renal excretion within 6 hours; hence, toxicity is very low. Children tolerate this drug better than adults. Toxic effects of SSG include hypersensitivity, arthralgia, myalgia, hepatitis, renal dysfunction, myocarditis, and rarely pancreatitis. Unfortunately, the majority of patients in endemic areas are resistant to SSG.

Amphotericin B, an antifungal antibiotic, which acts by binding to and inhibiting synthesis of sterol in the membrane of parasites creating multiple holes, is very effective.

Government of India has recommended amphotericin as first-line drug in treatment of visceral leishmaniasis. The dose is 0.5–1 mg/kg intravenous (IV) with 5% dextrose over 6 hours daily or alternate day till a cumulative dose of 7.5–20 mg/kg. Toxic effects include anaphylaxis, thrombocytopenia, convulsions, chills, fever, thrombophlebitis, anemia, hypokalemia, renal, liver, and cardiac damage. Thus, all patients should be monitored clinically and for electrolyte disturbances particularly hypokalemia.

Recently, three new lipid associated formulations of amphotericin B have been found to be very effective. They are liposomal amphotericin B, cholesterol dispersion amphotericin B, and amphotericin B lipid complex of which the former is approved by US Food and Drug Administration. The dose of liposomal amphotericin B is 3 mg/kg IV on days 1–5, day 14, and day 21. The main disadvantage is high cost of therapy but it achieves a higher concentration in reticuloendothelial system with more targeted response and no appreciable toxicities. The latest regimen of liposomal amphotericin B is 10 mg/kg intravenously as single dose with proper monitoring of adverse events associated with infusion.

Aminosidine is an effective (95%) and well-tolerated antileishmanial drug. The dose is 15 mg/kg/day IM for 21 days. Some authors recommend this drug as first-line antileishmanial drug in endemic areas of kala-azar. Miltefosine, a phosphocholine analog, which was developed as antimalignant drug has shown to be highly active against *L. donovani* and cure rate is more than 95% in India. It is given orally in a dose of 2.5 mg/kg/day OD or BD for 28 days. Side effects are transient and reversible and include gastrointestinal disturbances, hepatic, and renal dysfunction. It is cheap, safe, very effective, and easy to administer.

Combination therapy using SSG, amphotericin B, miltefosine, and aminosidine in various doses and schedules is under phase III trial and observed to be highly effective but final recommendation is yet to come.

Splenectomy needs to be reserved for cases with poor response to conventional antileishmanial drug and massive splenomegaly. It should be followed by SSG, 20 mg/kg/day IM for 20–40 days and penicillin prophylaxis. Prior to splenectomy, children must be vaccinated against *Meningococcus*, *Pneumococcus*, and *Haemophilus influenzae*.

Monitoring of Therapy

Children on antileishmanial therapy should be monitored clinically (fever), hematologically (hemoglobin, total leukocyte count, differential leukocyte count), biochemically (C-reactive protein) by splenic size and parasitological index.

PROPHYLAXIS

The sheet anchor of prevention is control of sand fly and early detection and treatment of kala-azar cases. Spraying of houses and breeding places such as crevices in the walls with residual insecticides and use of mosquito nets during night are very effective. Kala-azar vaccine, based on combination of leishmanial antigen and bacillus Calmette–Guérin vaccine, is round the corner.

BIBLIOGRAPHY

1. Bhattacharya SK, Sur D, Karbwang J. Childhood visceral leishmaniasis. Indian J Med Res. 2006;123:353-6.
2. Murray HW, Berman JD, Davies CR, et al. Advances in leishmaniasis. Lancet. 2005;366:1561-77.
3. Prasad R, Kumar R, Jaiswal BP, et al. Miltefosine: an oral drug for visceral leishmaniasis. Indian J Pediatr. 2004;71:143-4.
4. Singh UK, Prasad R, Mishra OP, et al. Miltefosine versus amphotericin B in children with visceral leishmaniasis: a prospective, multicentric, observational study. Indian J Pediatr. 2006;73:1077-80.
5. Singh UK, Prasad R, Jaiswal BP, et al. Amphotericin B therapy in children with visceral leishmaniasis: daily versus alternate day, a randomized trial. J Trop Pediatr. 2010;56:321-4.

5.15 Dengue Illnesses

Ashok Kapse

INTRODUCTION

Dengue is a vector-borne disease which is transmitted among humans by Aedes group of mosquitoes. From unapparent infection, undifferentiated mild febrile condition to life-threatening dengue hemorrhagic fever (DHF)-dengue shock syndrome (DSS) and severe organopathy; the disease exhibits diverse clinical presentations. A systemic and dynamic viral disease dengue is known for its unpredictable clinical evolution and outcome.

The first clinically recognized dengue epidemics occurred almost simultaneously in Asia, Africa, and North America in the 17th century. The first clinical description dates back to 1780 in an epidemic in Philadelphia. Benjamin Rush depicted detailed clinical picture and because of the symptoms of myalgia and arthralgia coined the term "break bone fever." Barring Antarctica outbreaks of dengue-like illness continued erupting from almost all subcontinents during 18th and 19th century. The first virologically proved epidemic of dengue fever (DF) in India occurred in Calcutta and eastern coast of India in 1963-1964.

Right up to the mid-20th century, dengue was considered as a mild febrile illness; however by mid-1950, dengue underwent an enigmatic evolution; Southeast Asian countries experienced epidemics of a life-threatening disease associated with dengue viruses (DENVs). Patients with new affliction exhibited two potentially deadly expressions: bleeding diathesis and shock. A new name DHF-DSS was coined for this novel entity; by 1975, it had become a leading cause of hospitalization and death among children in many countries.

In the 1980s, DHF had first big intrusion into other Asian countries: India, Sri Lanka, Maldives Islands, Bangladesh, and Pakistan experienced their major DHF epidemics. With its hot and humid mosquito-friendly climate, India soon became a favorite place for dengue outbreaks, DHF started simmering in various parts of India however first major wide-spread epidemics of DHF/DSS occurred in 1996 involving areas around Delhi and then it spread to all over the country. Hyperendemicity (circulation of multiple serotypes) favoring severe DHF outbreaks have become frequent occurrence. The recent epidemics in Sri Lanka and India were consequence of hyperendemicity. End of the 20th century witnessed further geographical expansion of dengue viruses; consequentially, DHF which was missing from the Pacific region and the Americas made its appearance in there also.

This rapidly expanding dengue has emerged as a threat to public health across the globe (**Figs. 5.15.1A and B**); as per World Health Organization (WHO) estimation, nearly 100 million DENV infections occur annually all over the world;

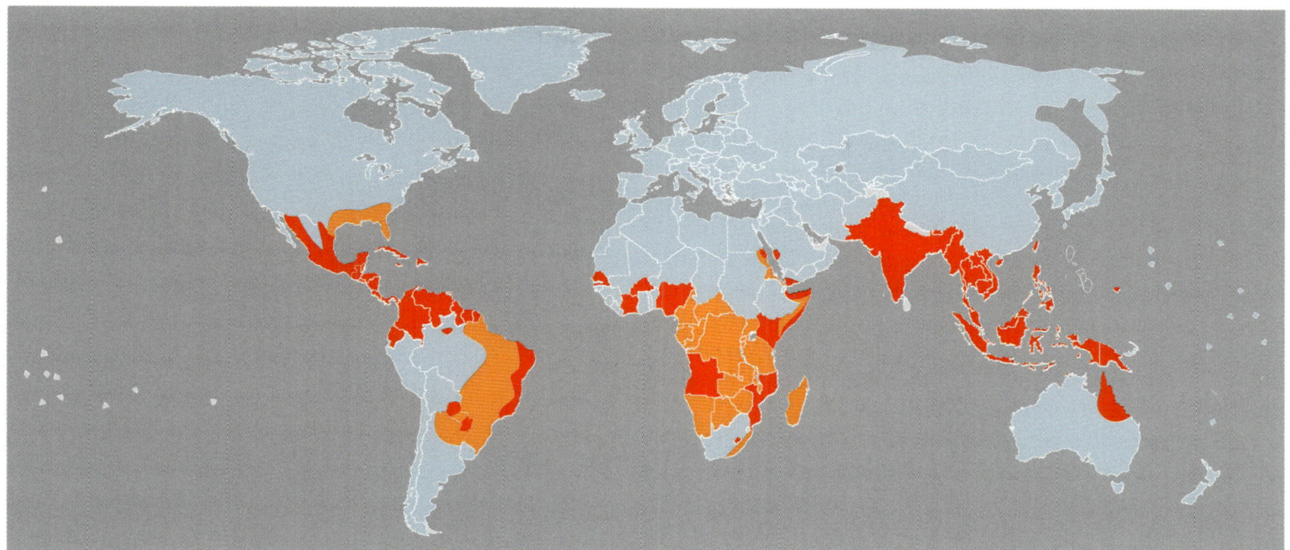

Fig. 5.15.1: Current global status.

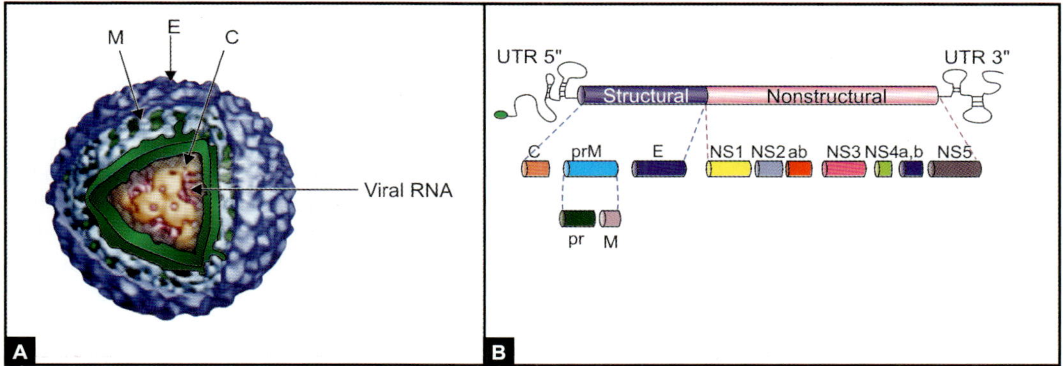

Figs. 5.15.2A and B: Dengue virus.

these infections culminate into 500,000 hospitalizations and over 20,000 deaths. India is bearing a big brunt of dengue onslaught; a recent study conducted at the Oxford University estimated that India had the largest number of dengue cases, with about 33 million apparent and another 100 million asymptomatic infections occurring annually.

TRANSMISSION

Dengue illnesses are caused by the four closely linked yet antigenically diverse serotypes. Viruses belong to the genus *Flavivirus* and family Flaviviridae.

Dengue Viruses

Dengue viruses are small spherical single-stranded ribonucleic acid (RNA) viruses with a lipid envelope (**Fig. 5.15.2**).

The viral genome encodes for three structural proteins: C is the capsid protein, M is the membrane protein, and E is the envelope glycoprotein. Antibodies to E protein determine the viral neutralizing activity. The differential amino acid sequence of the E proteins separates DENV into four serotypes which are designated as DEN-1, DEN-2, DEN-3, and DEN-4. Based on phylogenetic differences, each serotype has following genotypes:

- Dengue viruses-1: three
- Dengue viruses-2: two (one nonhuman primate)
- Dengue viruses-3: four
- Dengue viruses-4: four (one nonhuman primate)

Recently, a fifth variant of dengue virus (DENV-5) has been isolated in October 2013. This new serotype follows the sylvatic cycle unlike the other four serotypes which follow the human cycle. The likely cause of emergence of the new serotype could be genetic recombination, natural selection, and genetic bottlenecks. There is no indication of the presence of DENV-5 in India till date.

Certain serotypes and genotypes within each serotype considered to have more virulence than the others and have been linked to outbreaks of severe disease. Studies indicate that certain DENV strains like DENV-2 and DENV-3 have more commonly been associated with DHF as compared to DF. In general, Asian genotypes appear to be more virulent than American and the South Pacific genotypes. Phylogenetic analyses showed that the Native American DENV-2 genotype was associated only with DF, whereas the Asian DENV-2 genotypes were more correlated with DHF cases. Variation in nucleotide sequence is the likely explanation for the genotype-dependent divergent severity.

Viral genome also encodes for seven nonstructural (NS) proteins: NS1, NS2a, NS2b, NS3, NS4a, NS4b, and NS5.

Nonstructural proteins of DENV are involved in RNA replication, RNA assembly, and in viral protein processing. In addition to their roles in viral replication, some NS proteins such as NS1 also play a role in modifying host immune system. NS1 is the only NS protein with a soluble form that can be measured in circulation; this particular property is utilized for diagnostic purpose.

Infection with one dengue serotype generally provides lifelong immunity to that virus; however, there is no cross-protective immunity to the other serotypes; consequentially, person living in a dengue endemic area is vulnerable to be infected with all four dengue serotypes during his life time. Concept of lifelong homotypic immunity has recently been challenged in couple of current studies, Waggoner et al. and Forshey et al., working differently documented second homotypic infections; these findings have significant bearing on vaccine induced protection.

Vector

Dengue viruses are arthropod-borne viruses, and they employ two mosquitoes, *Aedes aegypti* and *Aedes albopictus*, as vectors to perpetuate infection cycle. These mosquitoes do not only carry the virus but also serve to amplify their replication.

Aedes aegypti, the principal vector **(Fig. 5.15.3)**, is a small, black-and-white, exceedingly adaptable, tropical mosquito. Over the years, mosquito has become highly domesticated; it prefers to lay its eggs in artificial containers commonly found in and around homes, for example flower vases, old automobile tires, buckets that collect rainwater, and trash in general. Black-colored plastic water storage drums, cement cisterns, and even septic tanks, are most favored breeding sites and hence are notorious in producing large numbers of adult mosquitoes near human dwellings.

The adult mosquitoes prefer to rest indoors and like to feed on humans during daylight hours. There are two peaks of feeding activity, early morning from 9 hours to 13 hours and in the afternoon from 15 hours to 17 hours; however, these are exceptionally adaptable mosquitoes and could effectively change their feeding habits as per needs. The female mosquitoes are very apprehensive feeders, and they would discontinue the feeding process at the slightest disturbance, however, would return to the same or a different person for completion of feeding a few moments later. Because of this behavior, female *A. aegypti* will often feed on several persons for completion of a single blood meal and, if infective, may transmit dengue virus to multiple persons in a short time. Therefore, it is not uncommon to observe that several members of the same household or several children from same school would be falling sick with dengue fever within a short time frame, implying that all of them were infected by a single infective mosquito. This particular behavior of *A. aegypti* makes it an exceedingly efficient epidemic vector. The female *Aedes* mosquito deposits eggs singly on damp surfaces just above the waterline. Under optimal conditions, the adult emerges in 7 days. The eggs can withstand desiccation (can remain in a viable dry condition) for more than a year and emerge within 24 hours once it comes in contact with water. This poses a big hurdle in prevention and control of dengue.

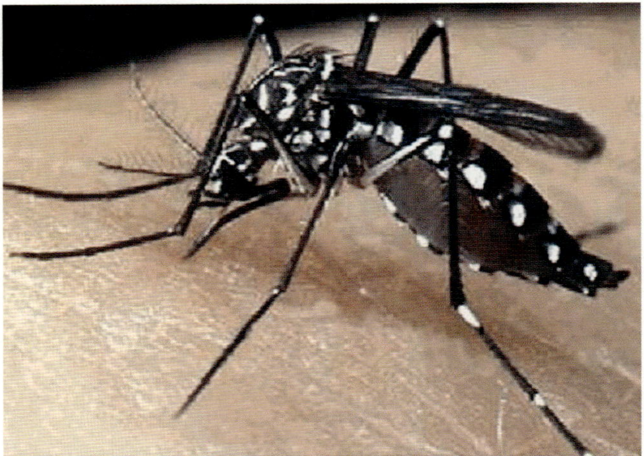

Fig. 5.15.3: *Aedes aegypti.*

Following an infective mosquito bite **(Fig. 5.15.4)**, the virus undergoes an incubation period of around 4–7 days, before person turns symptomatic mainly febrile. During this acute febrile period, which may be as short as 2 days or as long as 10 days, dengue viruses circulate in the peripheral blood. Other *A. aegypti* mosquitoes become infective when they bite and suck blood from such a febrile viremic person. Humans can be infectious to mosquitoes from 1.5 days prior to the onset of symptoms to around 5 days after the commencement of symptoms. Dengue viruses need around 8–12 days for development in mosquitoes before they become

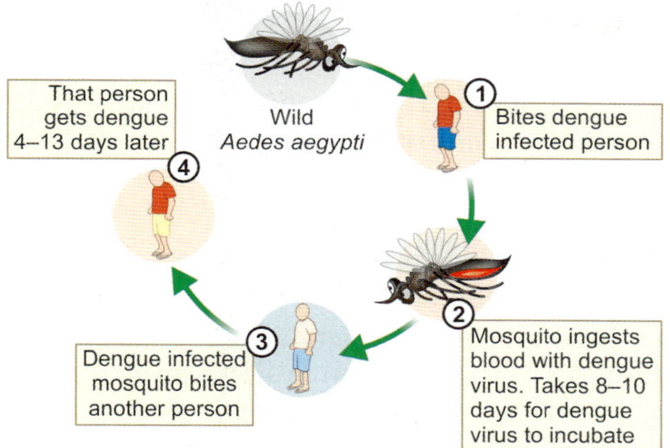

Fig. 5.15.4: Dengue transmission cycle.

infective; this period is termed as extrinsic incubation period. These infected mosquitoes would transmit the virus to other persons during their subsequent blood meal. Level of plasma viremia required to infect vector mosquitoes differed between serotypes; it is 10-fold lower for DENV-1 and DENV-2 compared to DENV-3 and DENV-4.

Climatic changes have direct bearing on dengue epidemiology. The changes in temperature and humidity affect the biology and ecology of the vectors and consequently the risk of virus transmission. An increase in temperature translates into better transmission potential. A temperature rise of 1–2°C could result in an increase in the vulnerable population by several hundred million annually as per a WHO estimate. Following are few of the reasons for such occurrence:

- In warm water, the mosquito larvae take a shorter time to mature, and consequently, there is a greater capacity to produce more offsprings during the transmission period.
- In hot and humid conditions, mosquitoes feed more frequently and digest blood faster, and thereby facilitate dengue transmission.
- The extrinsic incubation period of the virus within the vector gets shorter in hot and humid climate, thus proportionately increase the number of infected mosquitoes.

Though dengue primarily spreads through the mosquito bite, transovarial transmission is also a significant and efficient mechanism for the maintenance of the disease, a recent Brazilian study using reverse transcription polymerase chain reaction (RT-PCR) demonstrated all four DENV serotypes in larval samples. Rarely dengue could transmit through blood transfusion and organ transplantation. There are also reports of congenital dengue infections occurring in neonates born to mothers infected very late in pregnancy.

Victims

Reasons for Recent Rise in Dengue and Dengue Hemorrhagic Fever

Major global demographic changes like marked population growth has driven unplanned urbanization, which in turn has culminated into substandard housing, inadequate water supply needing water storage, and a poor waste management system; all these demographic factors have favorably influenced dengue vector growth.

Movement of a viremic person introduces a new virus into a susceptible population. The markedly increased air travels allow the movement of the virus, different serotypes, strains, and even genotypes from one region to another; generated hyperendemicity facilitates DHF outbreaks.

Dengue Fever vis-a-vis Dengue Hemorrhagic Fever

The first infection with any of the dengue virus in a dengue virgin body produces mild self-limiting febrile illness recognized as dengue fever. During subsequent infection with other dengue serotype some of the patients develop severe life-threatening disease the DHF.

There are various theories put forward for such outcome; antibody-dependant enhancement of infection is the most favored of all.

Antibody-dependant Enhancement

Dengue hemorrhagic fever usually occurs in two clinical settings: secondary dengue infection at any age and primary dengue infection in an infant. In past, few years lots of advances have been made in the understanding of DENV biology yet pathogenesis explaining DHF in two different set of patients is still an intriguing puzzle. Various factors—including total viral virulence, virus burden, host immune response, and genetic predisposition, have been implicated as risk factors for DHF, yet all these factors fail to explain occurrence of DHF in both clinical settings.

In majority of human studies preexistence of nonneutralizing antibodies either from previous infection or transplacentally acquired (mother-to-child transmission) is the most consistently documented risk factor for DHF.

Neutralizing antibodies to DENV are responsible for serotype specific protection. Antibodies against E, pre-M proteins, and to NS1 are capable of neutralizing DENV and providing protection against dengue infection. Infection with one DENV serotype generally results in lifelong immunity to infecting serotype.

Initial infection also produces heterotypic neutralizing antibodies as well nonneutralizing antibodies. Heterotypic neutralizing antibodies do provide protection against other serotypes for some time; however, they are short lived and disappear after few months. During a secondary infection with a different serotype, the presence of heterotypic nonneutralizing antibodies forms complexes with dengue viruses; these complexes facilitate enhanced cellular infection, this phenomenon has been called antibody-dependent enhancement.

Antibody-dependent enhancement theory proficiently elucidates observed occurrence of DHF in both clinical settings that is primary infection in infants and during secondary infection at any age.

PATHOPHYSIOLOGY

Transient increase in vascular permeability and a hemorrhagic diathesis are the underlying mechanistic causes for the manifestations of severe dengue.

Vascular Leak

Transient increase in vascular permeability is the cardinal feature of dengue illnesses, this increased permeability results into leakage of fluid into the interstitium. Extravasation is selective, and fluid primarily seeps out into serous cavities such as peritoneum, pleura, and pericardium, generalized edema is exceptional. The vascular leak is observed to occur from postcapillary venules. Leakage starts few hours before the defervescence and may herald the onset of severe disease. Typically, vascular leak is transitory, yet the extent and volume of leak is the most important determinant of severity of dengue illness.

Prolonged and voluminous leakage results into hemoconcentration and hypovolemia; unattended it may culminate into shock, multiorgan failure, and death; fortunately, it is infrequent and in majority of the patient's vascular permeability spontaneously resolves. After a while (few hours to few days), the extravasated fluid gets reabsorbed and the patient quickly recovers. Children are prone for intense leakage; more permeable vasculature is the basis behind this phenomenon.

Mechanism for Vascular Leak

The pathophysiological mechanisms **(Fig. 5.15.5)** underlying the capillary leak are poorly understood. Luminal surface of the vascular endothelium has a layer of glycocalyx. Layer incorporates into it glycosaminoglycans (GAGs) which are complex, negatively charged polysaccharides. This layer creates both a size selective physical barrier that only allows the passage of certain molecules between the fibers and an electrostatic barrier that limits the access of negatively charged molecules to the underlying cellular transport mechanisms. Rather than the endothelial cellular structures, it is the glycocalyx layer that determines molecule selectivity. Recent research points toward an alteration in the function of the endothelial glycocalyx during dengue infection. Usual size-dependent sieving mechanism is well preserved while the selective restriction based on negative charge is significantly impaired. Research is being directed to identify various factors responsible for vascular leak, few implicated factors are cytokine tsunami, emergence of NS1 as viral toxin, mast cell products, and inflammatory lipid mediators.

Cytokine Tsunami

Coincident with defervescence there is sudden surge of cytokines (cytokine tsunami) in symptomatic secondary dengue infections. Levels of these proinflammatory and immunosuppressive cytokines are shown to be higher in patients with DHF as compared with dengue fever; the levels of these cytokines are also found to be greatly elevated during critical phase of the disease. Cytokine levels are increased in many other diseases, e.g. severe influenza, yet those levels are much lower compared to DHF.

This cytokine tsunami is believed to be responsible for pathognomonic DHF vasculopathy. Chemokine (C-C motif) ligand 2, a protein that reduces tight junctions of vascular endothelium cells, is found to be consistently high in DHF/DSS patients. Proinflammatory cytokines like tumor necrosis factor (TNF) were thought to be produced by highly cross-reactive T cells; however, recent studies suggest that DENV-specific T cells could in fact be protective, and instead, it is likely that other hematopoietic cells that are directly infected with the DENV such as dendritic cells, monocytes, and macrophages could be the predominant source of these cytokines.

Nonstructural 1: A Viral Toxin

Nonstructural 1 is a 50 kDa glycoprotein that is secreted from dengue-infected cells and can be detected in the patient's serum from early in the disease through to several days after defervescence. NS1 may play a role in the pathogenesis of severe disease, as higher levels have been detected in dengue shock patients.

In a hospital-based study, free NS1 levels in plasma correlated with viremia levels and were higher in patients with DHF than in those with DF. An elevated free sNS1 level (600 ng/mL) within 72 h of illness onset identified patients at risk for developing DHF. Quantitative estimation of NS1 may prove to be useful prognostic tool for dengue illnesses.

Nonstructural 1 has been implicated in the pathogenesis of vascular leak. NS1, along with the viral E protein, can bind to heparan sulfate, one of the major GAGs in the glycocalyx of the endothelial cell layer. The adherence of NS1 and of the DENV E protein to the glycocalyx, and the resulting damage, could alter the permeability properties of the microvascular layer; alterations to microvascular layer contribute to the

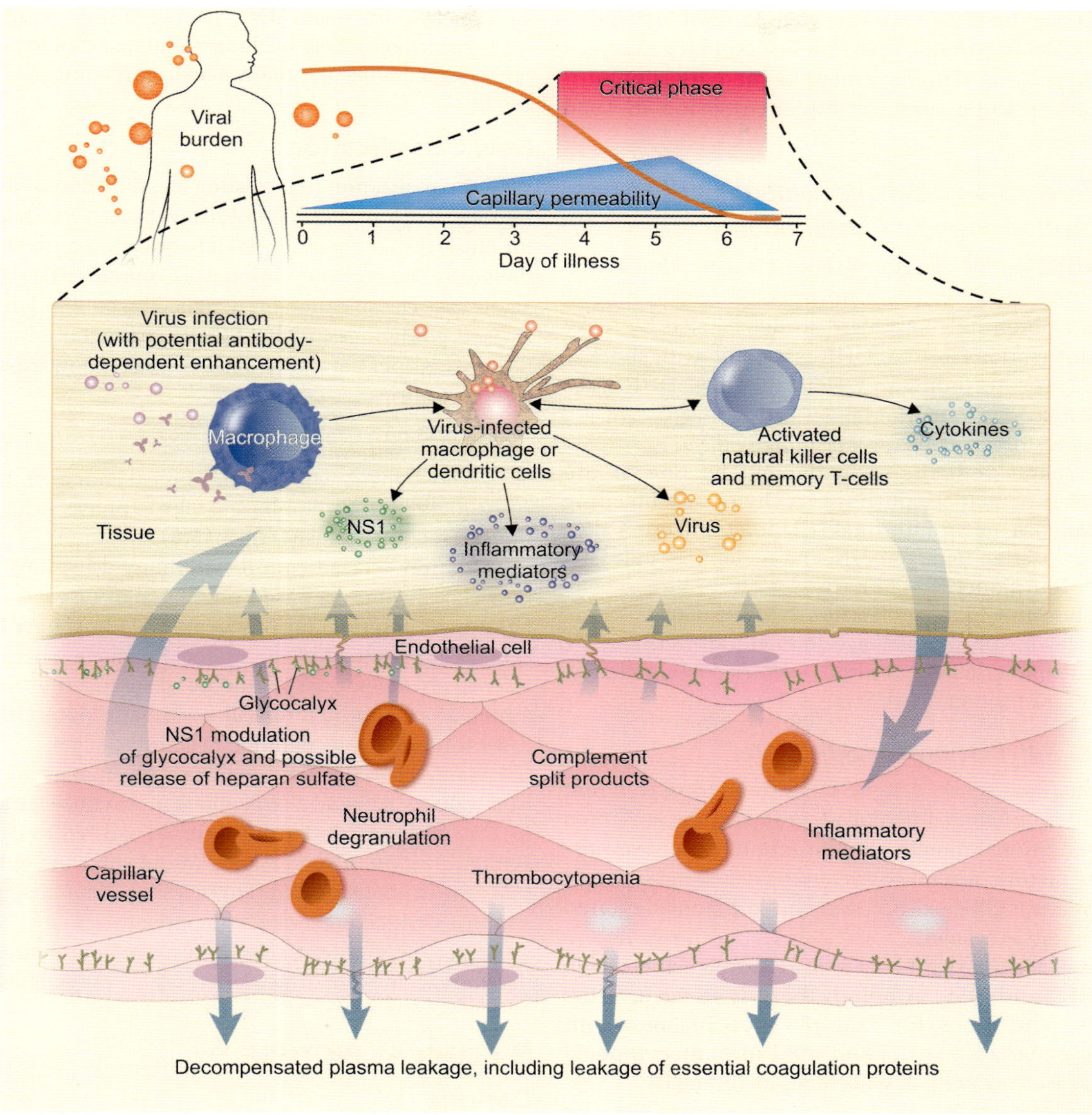

Fig. 5.15.5: Dengue pathogenesis.

characteristic vascular leak. Increased urinary heparan sulfate excretion has been detected in children with severe infection and urinary levels of heparin sulfate correlates with extent of vascular leak.

In a recent study, researcher has observed that NS1 behaves like a pathogen-associated molecular pattern. NS1 directly activated human peripheral blood mononuclear cells via Toll-like receptor 4 (TLR4), which leads to generation of proinflammatory cytokines and chemokines that are responsible for vascular leak. The process of leakage was prevented by a TLR4 antagonist and by anti-TLR4 antibody treatment. Their results suggest NS1 as a viral toxin akin to bacterial lipopolysaccharide endotoxin. Research also highlights TLR4 antagonists as a possible therapeutic option.

DISEASE CLASSIFICATION

Old Classification

Way back in 1974, WHO constituted a Technical Advisory Committee which met in Manila, Philippines. Committee classified dengue illnesses into DF/DHF/DSS. This classification to a large extent was based on the pioneering studies done at the Children's Hospital, Bangkok, Thailand, in the early 1960s. In 1980, WHO published first guidelines for the clinical case management of dengue illnesses; the guidelines underwent subsequent revision in 1986 and 1997.

Dengue Fever vis-a-vis Dengue Hemorrhagic Fever: Central Theme in Previous Classification

The center theme in dengue disease classification is the differentiation between DF, a nonspecific febrile illness, and DHF, a potentially serious disorder caused by leaky vasculopathy (serious form of DHF associated with shock is labeled as DSS). According to WHO guidelines, DHF cases must fulfill following four criteria:

1. Fever or history of acute fever lasting 2–7 days
2. Hemorrhagic tendencies evidenced by one of the following: petechiae, purpura, ecchymoses; bleeding from mucosa, gastrointestinal (GI) tract, injection sites or other location hematemesis, and melena; or at least a positive tourniquet test (TT)
3. Thrombocytopenia (platelets less than 100,000)
4. Evidences for plasma leakage in DHF: More than 20% rise in hematocrit, fluid in serous cavities documented by X-ray, or ultrasonogram (USG).

Difficulties with Previous Classification

Over the last few years, dengue has extended to different parts of the globe and to different age groups. Clinicians often observed additional dengue manifestations other than the established picture; several physicians have felt and reported difficulties in using the existing system. Commonly reported difficulties were as follows:

- The classification rigorously tries to distinguish between DF, DHF, and DSS, although there is much overlap between the three, for example bleeding or occult bleeding tendency (+TT) and mild thrombocytopenia could as well occur in all syndromes including DF.
- Documentation of all four requirements for the WHO definition of DHF (fever, hemorrhage, thrombocytopenia, and signs of plasma leakage) needs frequent assessment of packed-cell volume and platelet counts which may not always be available or feasible; moreover, a properly fluid managed patient from early stage of disease may not show 20% rise in hematocrit despite vascular leak.
- Tourniquet test is an integral part of the existing diagnostic scheme; however, test fails to differentiate DHF from DF; in addition to this, test is neither sensitive nor specific for dengue illnesses, many children with non dengue febrile illnesses may also have positive tests.
- The DF/DHF/DSS classification fails to include severe dengue disease associated with organ involvement such as hepatitis, encephalitis, and myocarditis.
- Finally, the term DHF places undue emphasis on hemorrhage when the danger sign that should be watched for and managed is plasma leakage leading to shock.

New Classification

With the realization that existing classification of the disease into DF, DHF, and DSS may not always be universally applicable for clinical management, WHO convened a meet of global dengue experts in 2008 in Geneva. Committee recommended a new case classification for dengue illnesses and put forward revised guidelines in 2009 for the management of dengue illnesses. As per new guidelines, disease is now classified into three categories:

1. Dengue
2. Dengue with warning signs
3. Severe dengue whereas the clinical course of the disease is divided in three phases: febrile phase, critical phase, and recovery phase **(Fig. 5.15.6)**.

This new classification has many advantages. As the new classification is based on degree of disease severity, it has a high potential for practical use **(Flowchart 5.15.1)**. It is of great help to clinician in deciding as to where and how intensively the patient should be observed and treated. It is anticipatory and includes all severe and potentially severe cases through the recognition of warning signs.

As new classification can be used even in primary health-care settings, it would also facilitate more consistent reporting in the national and international surveillance system; standardization of surveillance would solve the old problem that arose from using different case classifications in different countries, which prevented comparisons.

It also has potential to be an end-point measure for dengue vaccine and drug trials.

CLINICAL PICTURE

Dengue

Febrile Phase

Following a short incubation period of 2–7 days, there is an abrupt onset of high-grade fever. Fever typically associated with headache, retro-orbital pain, photophobia, backache, myalgia, and arthralgia. Aches and pains assume more severity in older children and adolescence justifying its nick name as break bone fever.

During fever, whole body is invariably covered with bleachable erythematous flush **(Fig. 5.15.7)**. With suffused and swollen face, injected eyes, reddened ears, crimson malar area, swollen, and purplish lips, patients assume a measly look **(Fig. 5.15.8)**. The flush deepens with advancing disease. In few of these patients, a classical maculopapular exanthem **(Fig. 5.15.9)** may erupt on the top of erythematous flush.

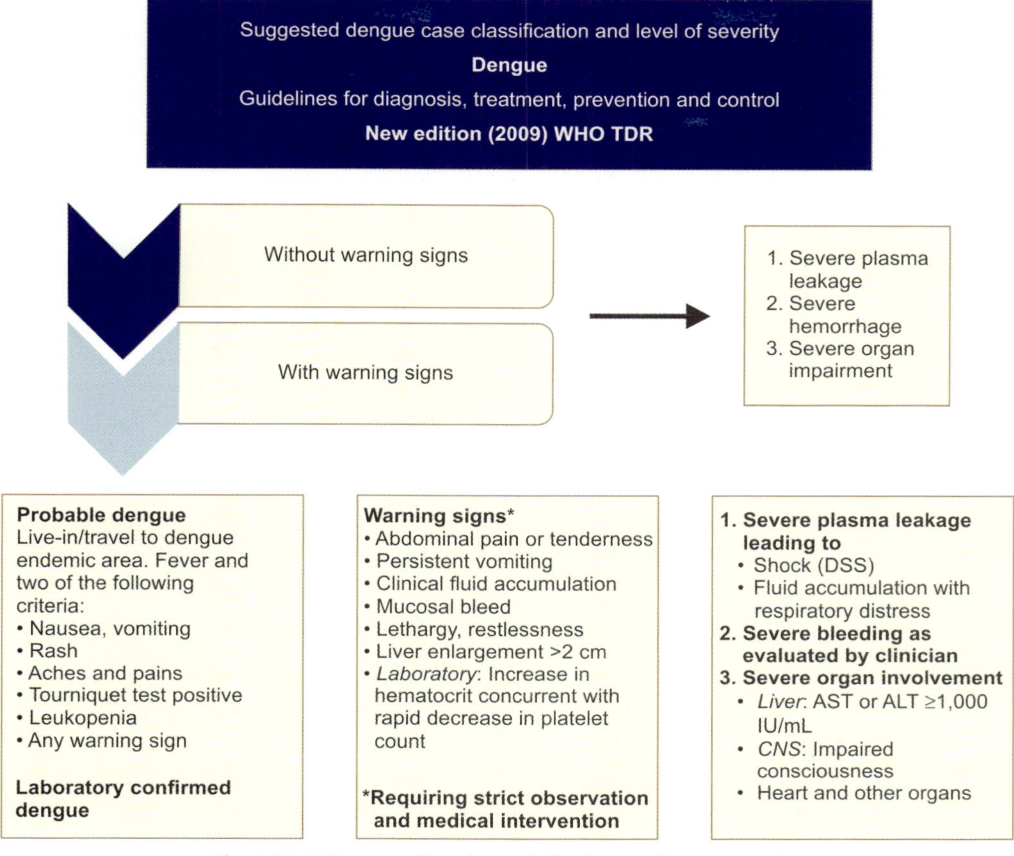

Fig. 5.15.6: Dengue clinical case definition by disease severity.

Mild hemorrhagic manifestations such as petechiae (**Fig. 5.15.10**) and mucosal membrane bleeding (e.g. nose and gums, conjunctiva) may be seen **(Fig. 5.15.11)**; however, massive GI bleeding commonly reported in adults is sporadic in children. Some patients may have sore throat, injected pharynx, and conjunctival injection; however, catarrh a typical characteristic of respiratory viruses is generally missing. Anorexia, nausea, and vomiting are frequent and usually lead to dehydration.

In the early febrile phase of the disease, it may not always be possible to differentiate dengue from nondengue febrile diseases. A positive TT indicating bleeding tendency increases the probability of dengue diagnosis **(Fig. 5.15.12)**.

Early leukopenia, atypical lymphocytosis, and mild thrombocytopenia are some of the commonly observed hematological changes during febrile phase of dengue illness.

An acute febrile illness in a dengue endemic area exhibiting any two of the above clinical features is enough basis for suspecting dengue illness. After a variable febrile period of 2–7 days, most of the dengue fever patient's makes a smooth and complete recovery and attains normal well-being.

Dengue with Warning Signs

In a small number of patient's, disease deteriorates with defervescence and may pass into critical phase. These patients before passing into critical phase generally forewarn with certain set of clinical sign-symptoms designated as warning signs. Roll of these warning signs include abdominal pain, persistent vomiting, lethargy and restlessness, mucosal bleeding (epistaxis, hematemesis, gum bleeding, menorrhagia, metrorrhagia and conjunctival bleeding), hepatic enlargement, scanty urine, lipothymia (postural hypotension), clinical signs of fluid accumulation (ascites, effusion, edema) **(Fig. 5.15.13)**, and rising hematocrit with progressive thrombocytopenia.

Triad of intense abdominal pain, lethargy, and mucosal bleeding correlates best with disease severity.

Abdominal Pain

Intense abdominal pain indicates that the patient is already in shock or may soon develop it. It has a high positive predictive value for plasma leakage and consequent

Flowchart 5.15.1: Organization of clinical management.

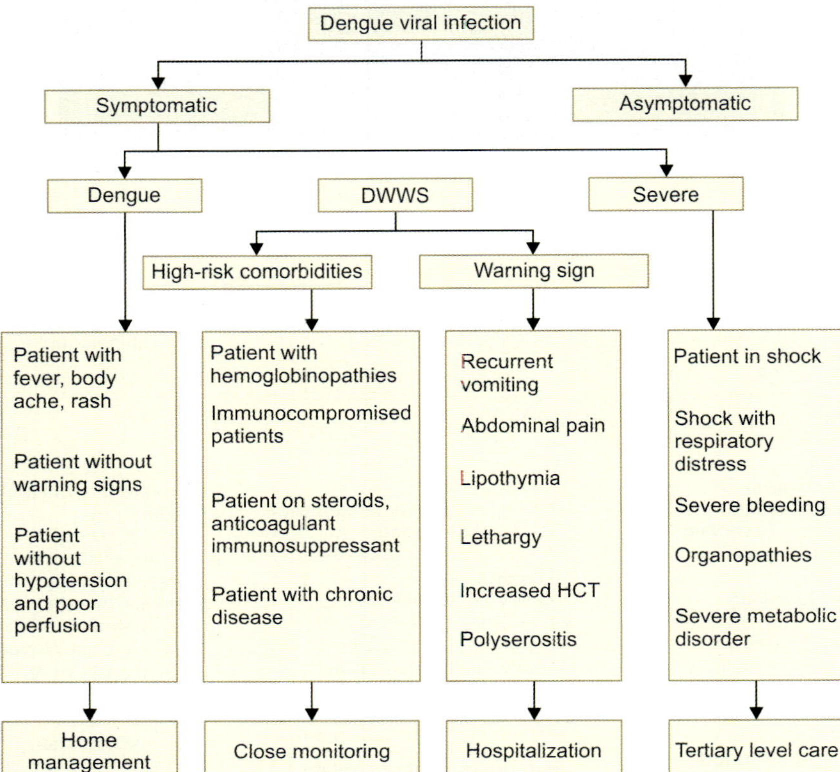

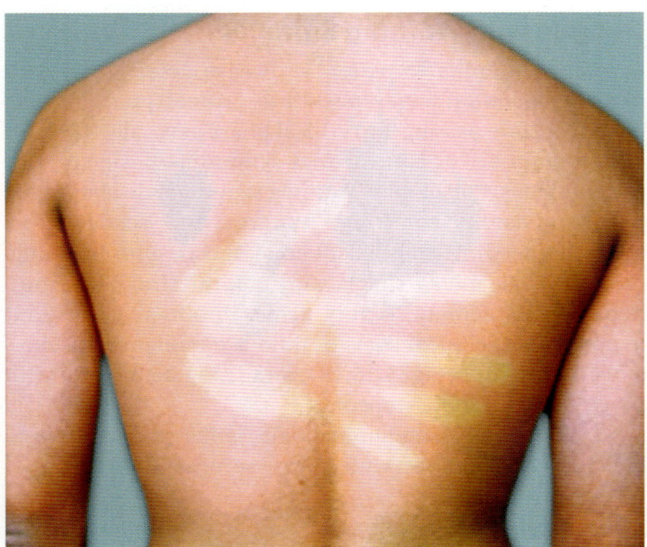

Fig. 5.15.7: Blanchable erythematous flush.

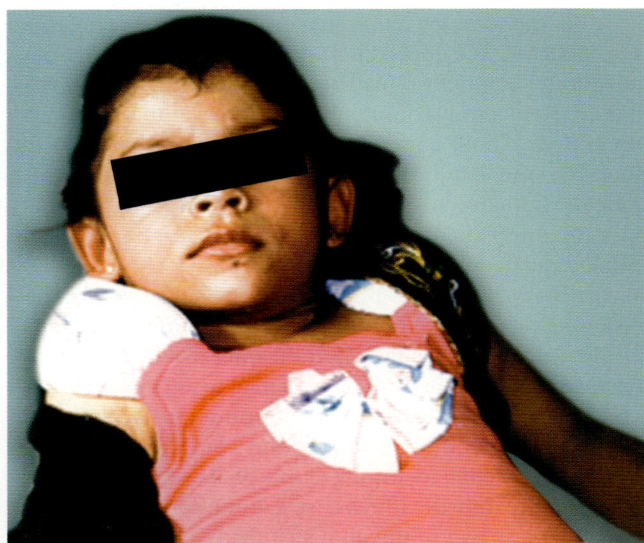

Fig. 5.15.8: Dengue facies (measely look).

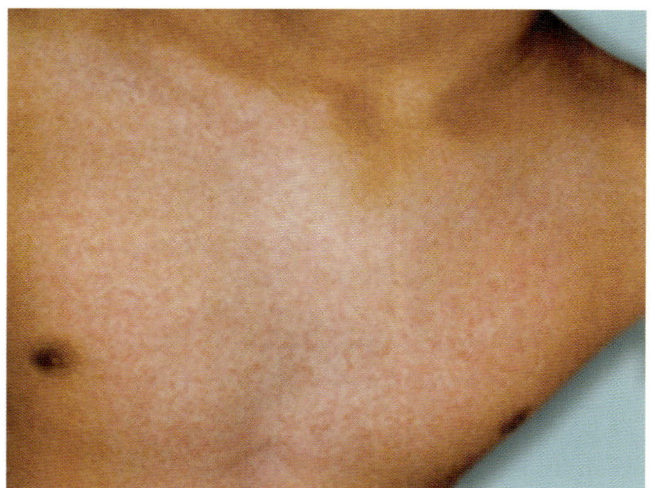

Fig. 5.15.9: Maculopapular rash.

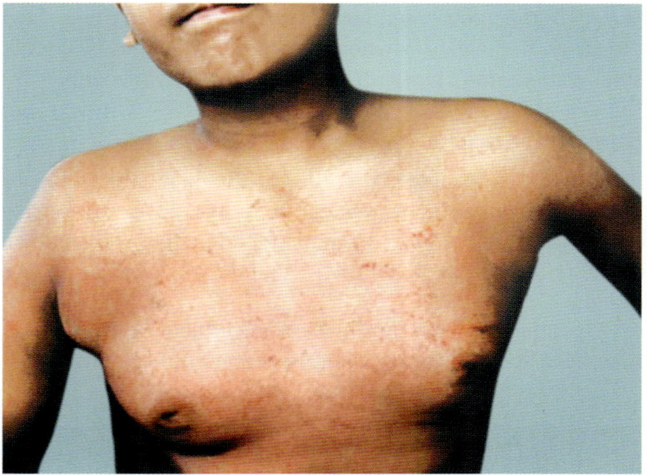

Fig. 5.15.10: Dengue purpuric rash.

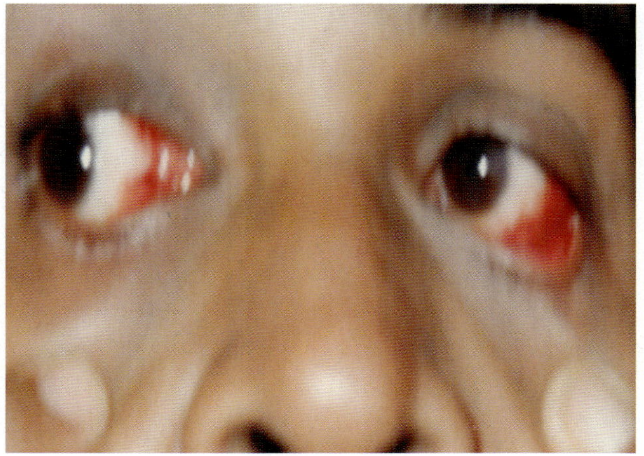

Fig. 5.15.11: Minor bleed (conjunctival hemorrhage).

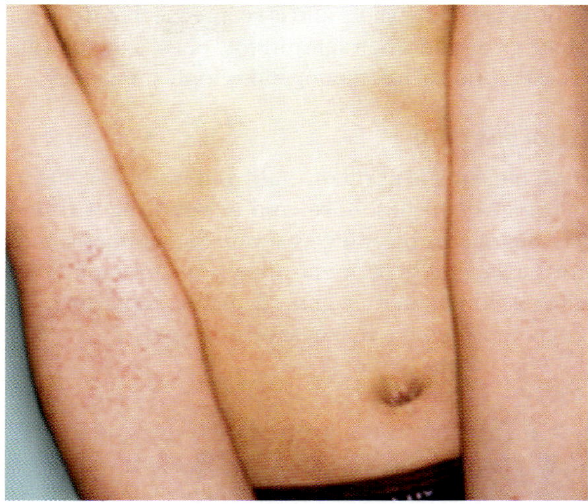

Fig. 5.15.12: Positive TT.
(TT: Tourniquet test)

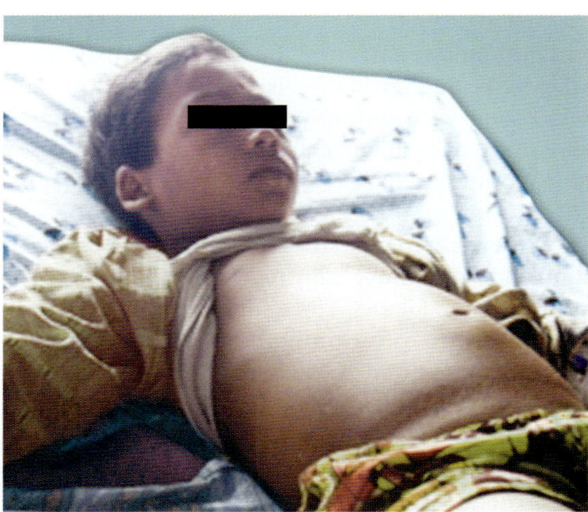

Fig. 5.15.13: Clinical ascitis.

shock. Pain could be located to either epigastrium or right hypochondrium.

The intense epigastric pain is generated as reflex pain caused by leakage of large amount of fluid into the retroperitoneal region, the collected "fluid masses" in pararenal and perirenal areas demonstrated by USG, irritate the nerve plexuses of the region. The fluid masses are demonstrated only in dengue shock patients, showing a clear association between the accumulation of fluid in the retroperitoneal region and dengue shock.

Right hypochondric pain is a consequence of plasma leakage into gallbladder wall and is well demonstrated on abdominal USG as gallbladder wall edema.

Leakage may also occur in the bowel wall under the serous layer; the sharp increase in its volume due to accumulated fluid causes severe abdominal pain in any location. The pain could be located anywhere and is so intense that it can mimic acute surgical abdomen conditions, such as appendicitis, cholecystitis, bowel infarction, and ectopic pregnancy.

Mucosal Bleeding

Mucosal bleeding is normally mild and mostly occurs in the gums (gingivorrhagia), nose, and as vomiting with bloody streaks. Significant bleeding as severe hematemesis, melena, metrorrhagia, and hypermenorrhea is uncommon. Mucosal bleeding accompanied by hemodynamic impairment of the patient is considered a sign of severe dengue.

Lethargy

Altered mentation in the form of drowsiness (lethargy) or irritability (restlessness) is always a dreadful warning sign. Both are manifestations of cerebral hypoxia induced by the hypovolemia caused by plasma leakage.

Rising Hemoconcentration and Thrombocytopenia

Rise in hemoconcentration occurs as consequence of vascular leak; degree of rise is proportionate to amount of leak. Along with hemodynamic evaluation increasing hematocrit hematopoietic cell transplantation constitutes a valuable monitoring tool.

Thrombocytopenia in dengue has multiple causes; however, megakaryocytic arrest due to direct dengue viral infection and immunologically mediated platelet destruction are two important factors. The antibodies are formed against viral proteins, and these antibodies via molecular mimicry turn into autoantibodies and cross-react with platelet proteins, fibrinogen, and some of the endothelial vascular proteins.

In the dengue patients, thrombocytopenia has a wide range and follows a unique self-recoverable time course. With megakaryocytic arrest platelet count start dropping around the fourth day of sickness, the fall continues next few days attaining nadir by the seventh day to eighth day. Self-recovery starts around day 9 of sickness which typically completes between the 10th day and the 12th day. Although thrombocytopenia per se is not a determinant of shock or bleeding tendency, the progressive decline in platelet count is an excellent marker of increasing patient severity, especially when accompanied by increasing hematocrit.

As initial clinical features are indistinguishable between severe and nonsevere dengue; therefore, it is essential that patient should be frequently monitored for warning signs for recognizing progression to the critical phase. Presence of these warning signs should alert clinician for intense hemodynamic monitoring and prompt fluid therapy to improve patient outcome.

Polyserositis

Fluid leakage in dengue patients is selective; fluid primarily leaks into various serous cavities such as peritoneum pleura and pericardium **(Fig. 5.15.14)**, generalized edema is by and large a consequence of excessive or wrong (hypotonic) fluid therapy. Significant fluid collection is clinically noticeable however a small leakage could be shown only on USG. A small amount of fluid, undetected clinically and shown only on USG, does not constitute warning sign.

Critical Phase (Fig. 5.15.15)

In some of the patients, around the time of defervescence, an increase in capillary permeability sets in. Extravasations of plasma, through these leaky capillaries result into hypovolemia and progressive hemoconcentration. A parallel drop in platelets and progressive leukopenia usually precedes plasma leakage. Together these changes mark the beginning of the critical phase. Patients in this phase would display variety of the above-mentioned warning signs. In majority of the cases, the leak is transient lasting for a few hours, once it stops patient quickly stabilizes and completely recovers.

Severe Dengue

Patients with prolonged and prolific leak are likely to deteriorate; poorly managed leaky patients may progressively pass into hypovolemia, hypotension, and shock. Since these patients are at risk of fatality, they are regarded as severe dengue.

Over the last few years, it was realized that dengue illness may have serious manifestations which could be unrelated

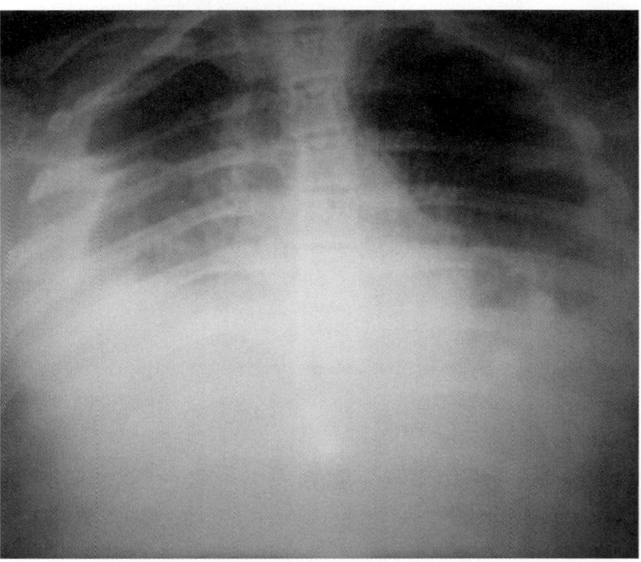

Fig. 5.15.14: Ascitis with bilateral pleural effusion.

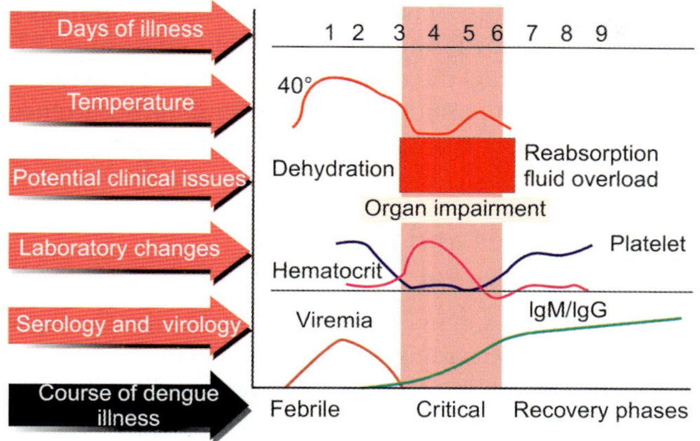

Fig. 5.15.15: Course of dengue illness.

to vascular leak phenomenon and shock. Severe bleeding and organopathies, such as hepatitis, myocarditis, and encephalitis, are some of the notable serious manifestations observed with dengue illnesses which too are potentially fatal. A new category, severe dengue is created to include these serious manifestations.

Category includes four types of dengue patients:

1. Patients with severe plasma leakage:
   - Shock [cold clammy peripheries, prolonged capillary refill time (CRT), narrow pulse pressure, fall in systolic pressure]
   - Fluid accumulation in serous cavities resulting into respiratory distress
2. Patients with profuse bleeding
3. Patients with significant organ involvement:
   - Hepatic involvement (transaminases >1,000)
   - Patients with neurological involvement
4. Patients with cardiac involvement.

Dengue Shock

In general shock develops in the peridefervescence period on the fourth or fifth day of the disease. Extravasating plasma initially produces hypovolemia; a poorly managed such patient could progress to shock. To maintain normal systolic pressure, body initially tries to compensate with peripheral vasoconstriction and tachycardia. Peripheral vasoconstriction reduces skin perfusion, resulting in cold extremities and delayed CRT. A normal systolic pressure under such situation may falsely underestimate the critical state of the patient. With persistent hypovolemia, the diastolic pressure rises, that in turn results in narrowing of pulse pressure and drop in mean arterial pressure; therefore, a narrow pulse pressure, even with normal systolic pressure, is a vital indicator of critically deranged hemodynamic status in a dengue patient. In the light of the above, narrative dengue patient is supposed to be in shock if his pulse pressure (i.e. the difference between the systolic and diastolic pressures) is less than or equal to 20 mm Hg or if has rapid and weak pulse and at least has two signs of poor capillary perfusion (cold limbs, delayed capillary refill > 2 s, mottled skin).

In the most advanced stage of shock, both the pressures systolic as well diastolic drop and may disappear abruptly. Prolonged shock and hypoxia lead to metabolic acidosis, multiorgan failure, and disseminated intravascular coagulation (DIC), a difficult clinical situation to manage. Surprisingly, a dengue patient may remain conscious and eloquent till late stage of shock.

In patients with massive leak, extravasated fluid collects primarily into serous cavities such as peritoneum, pleura, and pericardium **(Fig. 5.15.14)**. Large ascites and pleural effusions create respiratory distress; this situation where patient has developed respiratory distress and still needs intravenous (IV) fluids for shock is one of the trickiest clinical management **(Fig. 5.15.15)**.

Recovery Phase

Vascular leak stops within 2–3 days, and plasma which had extravasated during the leaky phase starts returning to circulation. An increase in urine output is an earliest indicator of plasma intravasation. Hemodynamic changes such as bounding pulse, wide pulse pressure, and rise in blood pressure accompany excessive urination. Hemoconcentration resolves, it may drop even below the baseline due to dilutional effect. Appetite and patient's wellbeing improve. Platelets start rising and become normal by around the 10th day of sickness. Typically, effusions are slow to resolve and may take a few more days for complete clearance.

Respiratory Distress in Recovery Phase

Patients with profound leak usually need massive resuscitative fluid therapy to maintain hemodynamics during critical phase. With the resolution of vascular leak all the extravasated fluid returns into vascular compartment. This returning fluid may compromise cardiac function and manifest as tachycardia, tachypnea, muffling of heart sounds, and basal rales; the problem is particularly augmented in patients given blood products and colloids. The pre-existing pleural effusion and ascites **(Figs. 5.15.13 and 5.15.14)** further add to respiratory compromise. This phase may last for few hours (12–36). During this period, the patient is hemodynamically unstable and needs intense monitoring. *Patient may need oxygen support, assisted ventilation, and decongestive (diuretics) therapy to relieve respiratory distress.*

During this stage of disease, severe dengue patient is hemodynamically still unstable; he regularly needs close clinical monitoring and even intensive therapy; this is against the tenet of recovery; therefore, author has reservations naming this stage of illness as recovery phase. In severe dengue, recovery would be considered only after uneventful passage of this stage of disease. It should better be named as congestive or regurgitation phase.

Convalescence

Termination of the illness is swift and is usually marked by a distinctive acral exanthem; a bright red confluent petechial rash **(Fig. 5.15.16)** erupts along the lateral margins of soles and palms termed as confluent petechial rash. Ascending upwards and medially rash assumes a less confluent character. In some cases, there are small round areas of clear skin giving it a name of isles of white in the red sea or annular petechial rash **(Fig. 5.15.17)**. Peripheral pruritis, asthenia, and transient bradycardia are few other inconsequential clinical findings noted during convalescence.

Major Bleeding

There are multiple causes for major bleeding in dengue. Severe prolonged shock with consequent combinations of hypoxia, metabolic acidosis, *multiorgan failure*, and consumptive coagulopathy is the commonest cause for major bleeding.

Inadvertent administration of acetylsalicylic acid (aspirin), nonsteroidal anti-inflammatory medications or anticoagulants is one of the important yet an avoidable factor for severe bleeding.

Some of the patients may not have vascular leak yet may present with severe bleeding. An ill understood vague vasculopathy is believed to be the underlying cause for such manifestation. Condition finds place as severe dengue in revised WHO classification.

Severe dengue has lots of hemostatic changes; coagulopathy in the form of elevated prothrombin time (PT) and activated partial thromboplastin time (aPTT), increased fibrinolysis, and thrombocytopenia are common occurrence; nevertheless, these changes are usually not enough to cause severe bleeding.

Organopathies and Expanded Dengue Syndrome

In recent outbreaks, dengue infection is shown to be associated with hepatitis, myocarditis, encephalitis, and many other life-threatening afflictions; most of these serious disorders may occur in febrile phase of the disease and is devoid of severe plasma leakage or shock. This vicious organ impairment is by itself a criterion for severe dengue. Clinical manifestations, evaluations, and management of these conditions in dengue are like situations when these organs are affected by other primary viruses.

Hepatitis

Liver is commonly involved in dengue viral infection, involvement clinically manifests as hepatomegaly and elevated transaminases. Changes generally parallel the disease severity. Enzymes elevation starts around the third day of the disease and peak on the seventh or eighth day and returns to normal values over 3–8 weeks. In contrast to viral hepatitis, the elevation in the level of serum glutamic oxaloacetic transaminase enzyme is normally greater than the elevation in the level of serum glutamic pyruvic transaminase in dengue patients. Fortunately, severe hepatitis is uncommon in children.

Fig. 5.15.16: Confluent petechial rash.

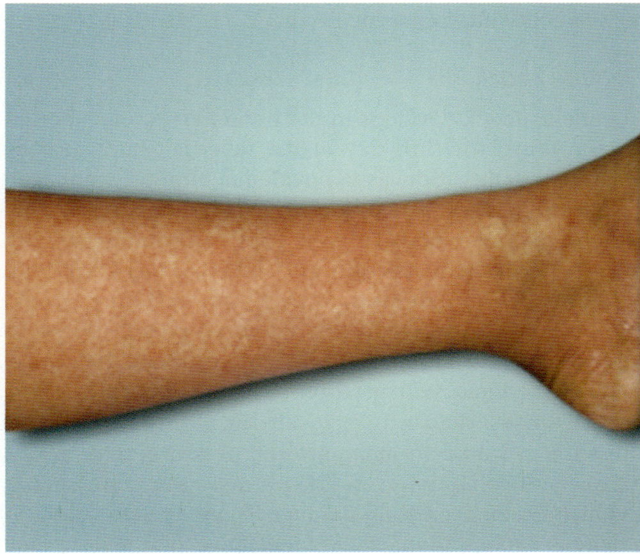

Fig. 5.15.17: Annular petechial rash.

Cardiac Complications

Transient benign bradycardia was known to occur with dengue illnesses; however, recent Indian subcontinent outbreaks displayed serious cardiac afflictions with dengue viral infections. Myocarditis from dengue is mainly expressed by changes in heart rhythm (tachyarrhythmias and bradyarrhythmias, and T-wave and ST-segment inversion) and ventricular dysfunction (reduction of left ventricular ejection fraction). Global hypokinesia, low ejection fraction, and elevated cardiac enzymes are noted in some of the recent studies. Fortunately, the majority of changes are transient and reversible.

Neurological Complications

Encephalitis, myelitis and meningitis are the most important neuroinvasive diseases associated with dengue. The neurological symptoms are diverse and related to the location of the lesion. Headache, alteration of consciousness, irritability, insomnia, seizures, and focal neurological deficit are the most common symptoms observed during the acute dengue. Neurological events are more common in children, are seen early in the febrile phase, and most of the manifestations are unrelated to the perfusion status. The symptoms of dengue infection (myalgias, diarrhea, joint or abdominal pain, rash, and bleedings) may be absent in cases presenting with neurological involvement; hence, a clinician must keep a high-suspicion index for possibility of dengue in any neurological patient presenting during dengue outbreak.

The neuropathogenesis of DENV infection is still poorly understood. Current research suggests that some of the dengue viruses', especially DEN-2 and DEN-3 has strong neurotropism and can cause encephalitis due to direct viral invasion of the brain. Cerebrospinal fluid examination in dengue encephalitis can show presence of the virus or its NS1 antigen, or the presence of immunoglobulin M (IgM)-specific antibodies.

Neuromuscular Disorders

Like other viral infections, autoimmune reaction in nervous system can follow in dengue infection. Guillain-Barré syndrome (GBS), neuromyelitis optica and optic neuritis, and acute disseminated encephalomyelitis are some of the reported immunological dysfunction in dengue infection.

The three major complications: (1) myositis, (2) hypokalemic paralysis, and (3) GBS manifest with flaccid quadriparesis. Occasionally, these complications may even be life-threatening. Dengue is also associated with many infrequent but disabling complications such as plexopathies and mononeuropathies.

Hemophagocytic Lymphohistiocytosis

Hemophagocytic lymphohistiocytosis (HLH) is a rare, potentially fatal medical condition that can occur after a patient has an infection. While HLH is most commonly associated with Epstein-Barr virus infections, it has also been recognized as a complication of dengue. Patients of dengue-associated HLH had longer duration of fever and were more likely to have anemia, hepatomegaly, and elevated liver transaminases. Complication prolongs hospital stay and adds to dengue severity. Dengue patient developing hepatic injury and anemia in absence of significant bleeding and should alert to the possibility of HLH.

Dengue in Infants

As in older children and adults', dengue infection can cause a wide spectrum of outcomes in infants. The burden of severe dengue lies predominantly in infants 4–9 months of age. Compared to older children upper respiratory tract symptoms (cough, nasal congestion, runny nose, dyspnea), GI symptoms (vomiting, diarrhea), and febrile convulsions are more common in infantile dengue. During the febrile stage, it is difficult to differentiate between dengue and other common infections of infancy such as pneumonia, meningoencephalitis, measles, and rotavirus infections; erythroderma is a useful clue to dengue suspicion.

Around the time of defervescence which may be earlier in infants, an increase in capillary permeability, in parallel with increasing hematocrit levels, become apparent in most dengue infants. The period of clinical plasma leakage usually lasts 24–48 hours. Organomegaly such as liver and splenic enlargement is more frequent in infants than older children. Plasma leakage tends to be generalized and manifests as palpebral and peripheral edema; hydroelectrolytic disorders are rather frequent. Shock in young children is expressed mainly as hypothermia, restlessness or lethargy, cold extremities, and tachycardia. Systolic pressure tends to decline later.

Dengue in Neonates

Vertical dengue infection transmission from pregnant women to their fetus can occur. Effect of dengue infection on fetus and newborn should be carefully examined to access capillary leakage and bleeding tendency. Clinical manifestations of vertically infected neonates vary from mild illness, such as fever with petechial rash, thrombocytopenia, and hepatomegaly, to severe illness with pleural effusion, gastric bleeding, circulatory failure, massive intracerebral hemorrhage.

Timing of maternal infection is important; peripartum maternal infection may increase the likelihood of symptomatic disease in the newborn. Antibodies to the dengue virus in the dengue-infected mother can cross the placenta and can cause severe dengue in newborn infants. Initial presentation may be confused with bacterial sepsis therefore during the times of dengue outbreak clinician must keep high-suspicion index for disease possibility in the neonates of dengue-infected mothers.

CLINICAL MANAGEMENT

Proper management of dengue illnesses incorporates following principles:

- Suspicion and reporting of the disease
- Assessments and management of early febrile phase
- Initiating and maintaining oral rehydration treatment on the patient's first contact with health-care services
- Identifying patients with warning signs who need close observation
- Identifying patients with warning signs who need IV fluid
- Recognizing early critical phase and initiating timely fluid therapy
- Monitoring and recording vital hemodynamic signs (temperature, heart rate, respiration rate, blood pressure, pulse quality, and urine output)
- Recognizing and managing severe dengue (shock, massive bleeding, and severe organ impairment) promptly and adequately.

Suspicion of Disease

As majority of dengue patients present with undifferentiated febrile illness, therefore clinician should have a high-suspicion index. A febrile patient residing in endemic area fitting into dengue clinical case definition should immediately arouse suspicion for dengue illness. *Any suspected dengue patient should immediately be reported to public health authorities, so that proper measures could be taken to prevent further spread of disease.*

Assessments and Management of Febrile Phase

Hydration Status

Suspected patient should be thoroughly assessed for hydration status: history of voiding (frequency, amount, and color), quantity of oral intake, excessive diaphoresis, and history of diarrhea and vomiting should be frequently asked. *Vascular leak is a major dengue complication that occurs during peridefervescence period hence date and timing of onset of fever needs special noting.*

Physical Examination

Detecting signs of dehydration and hypotension is important aim of clinical examination. Scanty urine, giddiness, inability to walk unsupported, and narrow pulse pressure is some of the significant clinical findings of ongoing vascular leak. Signs of pleural and peritoneal effusion (dull percussion note, abdominal pain, and distension) are important clinical evidences for vascular leakage. Enlarged and tender liver with or without icterus may be suggestive of liver impairment. Abnormal mentation, impaired consciousness, and convulsions may suggest early neurological dysfunction. Massive hemorrhage and mucosal bleed would be clinically apparent; however, diligent search is needed to find out petechiae, purpura, and ecchymoses. A TT should always be performed; positive test suggests underlying bleeding tendency and augments probability of dengue diagnosis.

During the early febrile phase, it is often not possible to predict clinically which patient will progress to severe dengue. Various severe manifestations may unfold as the disease progresses to the critical phase. The warning signs are good indicators of a higher risk of developing severe dengue; therefore, all ambulatory patients should be evaluated daily at the health-care unit to monitor, warning signs, and disease progression. It is important to educate patients and their family members on the warning signs and disease severity.

Laboratory Diagnosis

Complete Blood Count

A hematocrit test in the early febrile phase establishes the patient's own baseline value which serves as reference figure for any change occurring during further course of disease. A decreasing white blood cell count increases the probability of a dengue diagnosis. Rapid and sequential fall in platelet count points to disease progression; progressive rise in hematocrit in consecutive samples suggests evolution to critical phase (DHF) of disease.

Confirmatory Diagnosis (Fig. 5.15.18)

Early and accurate diagnosis of dengue is important for confirmation of infection, medical care of the patient, and differential diagnosis of other infectious diseases; *however, when dengue is suspected, do not wait for laboratory diagnosis to initiate treatment.*

Diagnosis of dengue infection could be direct by viral isolation, viral genome detection (through RT-PCR or real-time RT-PCR), or detection of a dengue antigen. Viral isolation and viral genome detection are restricted to a few referral laboratories only and largely inaccessible for clinical uses. An indirect detection could be achieved by demonstrating antibodies; unfortunately, as antibodies appear late in the course of the disease, antibody-based detection is futile in early phase of disease.

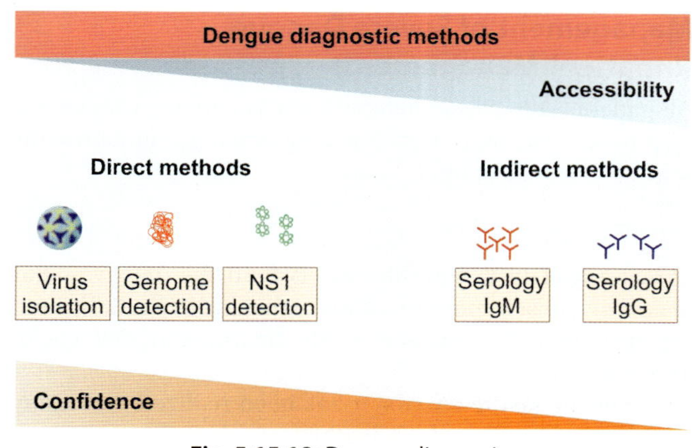

Fig. 5.15.18: Dengue diagnosis.

Table 5.15.1: Model for dengue diagnostic organization.

Diagnostic tests	*Primary care*	*District-regional care*	*Reference centers*
Virus isolation			X
Viral genome detection			X
Antigen detection	X	X	X
– ELISA	X	X	X
– Rapid strips	X	X	X
Serology	X	X	X
– ELISA	X	X	X
– Rapid strips	X	X	X

Nonstructural 1 Antigen

Detection of NS1 antigen through enzyme-linked immunosorbent assay (ELISA) has emerged as the most important diagnostic tests for dengue. NS1 a soluble antigen of dengue virus appears in patient's blood as early as second day of illness and may persist all through the viremic phase that is febrile period of the disease. NS1 carries a high sensitivity and specificity for dengue diagnosis, particularly when elicited by ELISA. In secondary dengue infection, exceptionally NS1 may be falsely undetectable as IgG antibodies from first infection may form antigen (NS1) antibody complexes and leaves hardly any free NS1 antigen to be detected.

Immunoglobulin M Antibodies

Detection of IgM antibodies against dengue is concurrent with the disappearance of viremia and fever. Primary infection is characterized by detectable levels of IgM antibodies by day 5 or day 6 after onset of fever; levels peak at about 14–15 days and can remain high up to 30–60 days later, and then decline gradually over time. IgM antibody capture ELISA (MAC-ELISA) is a fast and simple test used for the detection of IgM antibodies.

Immunoglobulin G Antibodies

Immunoglobulin G antibodies against dengue are elevated after the eighth or ninth day of the onset of fever and are detectable for life. In secondary infection, very high levels of IgG antibodies against dengue are observed from the second or third day of fever. IgM antibody levels can be less elevated in secondary infections and are sometimes not detectable.

The presence of IgG antibodies in serum generally indicates past infection. However, the presence of high IgG antibody titer in a serum sample, or a four-fold or greater increase in the antibody titer in paired serum samples obtained from a case of clinically suspected dengue, indicates recent infection or confirmed infection, respectively. This approach has special utility in cases of secondary infection where in IgM antibodies levels may be undetectable. IgG ELISA is the most commonly used test that detects the presence of IgG antibodies and even determines its titer.

Rapid Immunochromatographic Tests

Currently, many commercial kits offer immunochromatographic tests using rapid strips that detect NS1, IgM, and IgG antibodies, these tests have become handy as they can provide early and quick diagnosis. Tests are especially useful in peripheries where ELISA or other methods are unavailable. Regrettably, these rapid tests are inconsistent and offer differing degrees of sensitivity and specificity, and therefore, their results are not trusted for dengue diagnosis **(Table 5.15.1)**.

Ultrasonogram

Clinical signs of fluid leakage may not be apparent in mild cases; a decubitus X-ray chest used to be employed by past clinicians for demonstrating mild pleural effusion; however, sonography has made things more convenient; it can demonstrate smallest amount of extravasated fluid in any of the serous cavity. Gallbladder edema is a consistent sonological finding in dengue illnesses.

Out-Patient Management

Dengue patients without any warning signs, underlying chronic disorder, or vulnerable social conditions could be very well treated as out-patients; however, all these patients need close clinical observations right through during the febrile period and 2–3 days beyond the defervescence.

Outpatient treatment of dengue entails two important aspects:

1. Management of hydration and
2. Management of fever.

Parents or care takers should be given following instructions:

- Give a set goal to parents for child's fluid intake [100–150 mL/kg body weight (BW)]. Adequate fluid intake may reduce the number of hospitalizations. Fluids could be oral rehydration solution, water, milk, buttermilk, fruit juices, etc.
- Instruct parents to collect child's urine and compare the output against fluid intake; passing scanty urine with adequate oral fluid intake should alert clinician for vascular leak.
- Do not use aspirin, ibuprofen, mefenamic acid, nimesulide, or other nonsteroidal anti-inflammatory drugs for fever or pain as these drugs interfere with platelet functioning. Solely use paracetamol for pain and fever.
- Inform parents for warning signs, viz. scanty urine, giddiness, restlessness, anxiety, vomiting severe abdominal pain, cold extremities, and hemorrhage.
- Assess for warning signs, as has been earlier stated a handbill in patient's own language describing warning signs should be an integral part of dengue prescription.
- Any patient exhibiting warning signs should be carefully assessed for impending shock, e.g. poor volume pulse, narrowing of pulse pressure, and fall in blood pressure. Patient with these symptoms need immediate hospitalization for intensive IV fluid therapy.
- Defervescence is the time when crucial pathophysiology changes start in dengue illnesses; hence, any child deteriorating or failing to improve with subsidence of fever should be carefully assessed for progression to critical phase.
- Instruct the care-givers that the patient should be brought to hospital, immediately if any of the following symptoms emerge around the time of defervescence: deterioration or no clinical improvement, severe abdominal pain, persistent vomiting, cold and clammy extremities, lethargy or irritability/restlessness, bleeding (e.g. black stools or coffee-ground vomiting), not passing urine for more than 6 hours.

Management of Patients with Warning Signs

Majority patients without warning signs would tolerate oral fluids; however, patients with warning signs may need IV fluid therapy. Patients exhibiting warning signs need transient hospitalization for observation and treatment. Normal saline or Ringer's lactate with or without dextrose given at maintenance rate generally suffice in most of the patients. Switch quickly over to oral fluids as soon as patients tolerate. Patients should remain under close medical supervision for at least 2–3 days beyond defervescence.

Management of Severe Dengue (Inpatient Management)

All patients with severe dengue such as patients with shock, respiratory distress, profuse bleeding, and organ impairments require hospitalization.

Intravenous Fluid Therapy

In majority of the dengue illnesses IV fluid therapy of vascular leak is the most important aspect of management. Early fluid replacement is the mainstay for the treatment of this type of severe dengue.

Over the last few years, it has been realized that many of the complications and deaths were due to overzealous fluid management leading to fluid overload, and it was comprehended that dengue vascular leak could be managed with lesser fluid therapy. In 2009, WHO came out with new set of guidelines; according to new guidelines correction of shock is undertaken with boluses of (10 mL/kg BW) isotonic fluid while replacement is done with much smaller doses.

Choice of Fluid

Two common types of IV fluids currently used in dengue shock are crystalloids and colloids. Theoretically, colloid solutions offer some advantages over crystalloid solutions, as they provide volume expansion over and above the actual fluid volume infused. The colloid molecules increase plasma oncotic pressure and reverse the net flux of fluid out of the intravascular compartment. Moreover, pathophysiological studies indicate that there is preferential leakage of relatively small plasma proteins (e.g. albumin) as compared with larger molecules like globulins, thus implies that resuscitation with colloid preparations of larger molecular weights may offer therapeutic advantages. Unfortunately, these theoretical advantages have not been substantiated in clinical studies. A recent meta-analysis observed that colloids does decrease the hematocrit and pulse rates of children with DSS after the first 2 hours of fluid resuscitation; however, these changes were transient, and no significant advantage was found over crystalloids in reducing the recurrence of shock, the need for rescue colloids, the total amount of fluids, the need for diuretics, and in reducing mortality. *Consensus is crystalloids should be used for initial resuscitation while colloid boluses are reserved for patients presenting with hypotensive shock, recurrent shock, and refractory hypotensive shock.*

Management Plan

Patients with severe dengue need urgent hospitalization and emergency treatment. Patient should be hospitalized only at a place where proper intensive care and blood transfusion facilities are available.

Currently IV fluid therapy is separated as fluid resuscitation and fluid replacement.

Fluid Resuscitation

Fluid resuscitation is a strategy in which larger volumes of fluids (e.g. 10–20 mL boluses) are administered for a limited period under close monitoring. Goals for this resuscitation are to improve central and peripheral circulation and end organ perfusion.

Fluid Replacement

Following resuscitation, further plasma losses are continually replaced with IV fluid over next 24–48 hours; however, recommendation for this fluid as per new concept is much smaller; replacement fluid should be just enough to maintain effective circulation and perfusion. *Only isotonic fluids must be used for resuscitation as well replacement, hypotonic fluids have no place in dengue management.*

Compensated Shock (Flowchart 5.15.2)

Patient presenting with narrowed pulse pressure (20 or < 20), tachycardia, increased CRT, poor volume peripheral pulses, cold, and/or mottled peripheries is considered to be in compensated shock importantly patient would have normal systolic blood pressure.

Start IV fluid resuscitation with isotonic crystalloid solutions at a rate of 10 mL/kg/h over first hour. End of the bolus reassess the patient's hemodynamic condition. Further management depends on the patient's condition, if he improves, IV fluids should be gradually tapered to 5–7 mL/kg/h for next 1–2 hours, then to 3–5 mL/kg/h for further 2–4 hours, then to 2–3 mL/kg/h all through the management **(Fig. 5.15.19)**. Patient with stable hemodynamic status may need only maintenance fluid therapy for next 24–48 hours however a frequent and close monitoring is imperative during this period.

Monitoring

Frequent and thorough monitoring is foundation for successful dengue management. Monitoring has two important aspects: hemodynamic evaluation and hematocrit measurement *(H-2 assessment)*. Regular hemodynamic evaluation at short interval is must. Hematocrit check is needed only if hemodynamics are unstable (i.e. shock persists).

Flowchart 5.15.2: Fluid management in compensated shock.

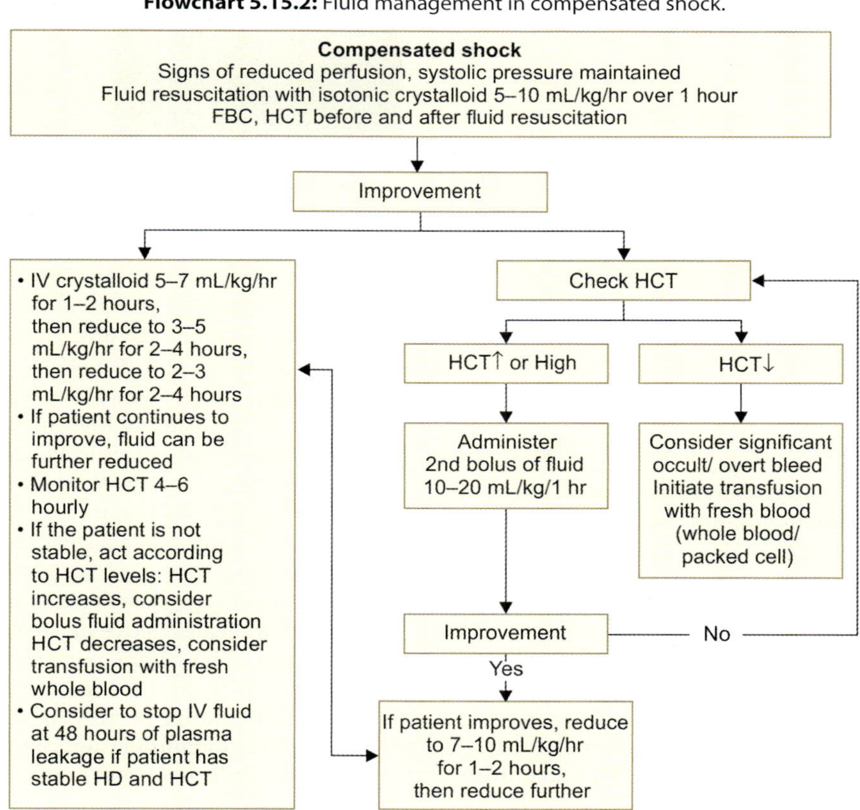

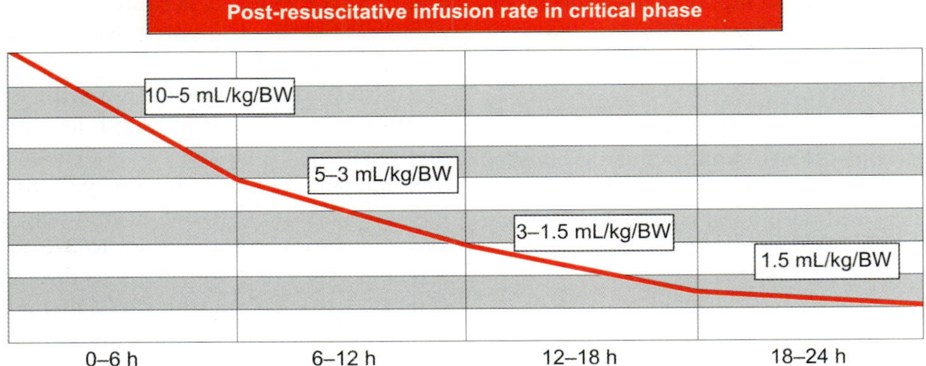

Fig. 5.15.19: Post-resuscitative infusion rate in critical phase.

Hemodynamic Evaluation

Holding a patient's hand and feet can give vital hemodynamic information (CCTVR: C-color, C-CRT, T-temperature, V-volume of pulse, R-rate of pulse) **(Fig. 5.15.20)**. In addition to CCTVR appraisal, measurements of blood pressure, urinary output, and evaluation of mentation complete hemodynamic check.

Peripheral pulses: A nicely perceptible peripheral pulse is a sign of adequate perfusion. Imperceptible or feeble peripheral lower limb pulses (posterior tibial and dorsalis pedis) particularly during replacement fluid therapy indicate higher fluid requirement.

Pulse pressure: Dengue shock is unusual in the term that a slow leak occurs over several days; this permits compensatory mechanisms to come into play. Before the development of overt cardiovascular collapse, the diastolic pressure rises to meet the systolic pressure, and the pulse pressure narrows; therefore, narrowing of the pulse pressure is the most significant parameter for defining dengue shock and maintaining pulse pressure of more than 20 mm Hg is one of the most important goal for IV fluid therapy. A narrow pulse pressure less than 20° mm Hg is an indication for stepping up IV fluid rate.

Urine Output

Maintaining fluid input output chart is very important. Urine output gives vital information about end organ perfusion; it should be checked hourly till the patient is out of shock and there after 4–6 hourly until patient is out of risk. In a shocked patient continuous bladder catheter enables correct monitoring of urine output. An acceptable urine output would be above 0.5 mL/kg/h.

Hematocrit

Hematocrit assessment has significant importance in the dengue shock management; however, *it is always dictated by hemodynamic status*; in an unstable patient, it should be monitored before and after every fluid bolus. About 4–6 hourly assessment is good enough once patient is stabilized and is on replacement therapy. *Hematocrit should always be interpreted along with hemodynamics*; following are the explanations for certain clinical situations:

- A rising or persistently high hematocrit together with stable hemodynamic status and adequate urine output does not require extra IV fluid. In this situation, it is expected that the hematocrit will start to fall within the next 24 hours as the plasma leakage stops.
- A rising or persistently high hematocrit together with unstable vital signs (particularly narrowing of the pulse pressure) indicates active plasma leakage and the need for a further bolus of fluid replacement.
- A falling hematocrit together with unstable vital signs (particularly, narrowing of the pulse pressure, tachycardia, metabolic acidosis, poor urine output) indicates significant occult hemorrhage and the need for urgent blood transfusion.

Pearls in clinical examination of dengue patients

The "5-in-1 maneuver" magic touch - CCTV-R

Hold the patient's hand to evaluate peripheral perfusion.

Save life in 30 s by recognizing shock

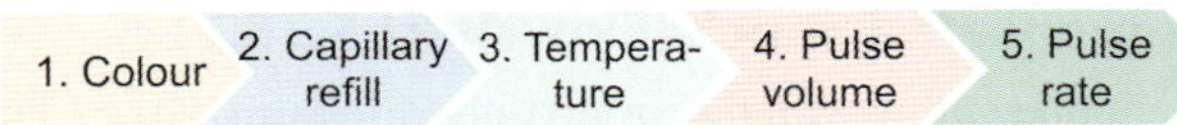

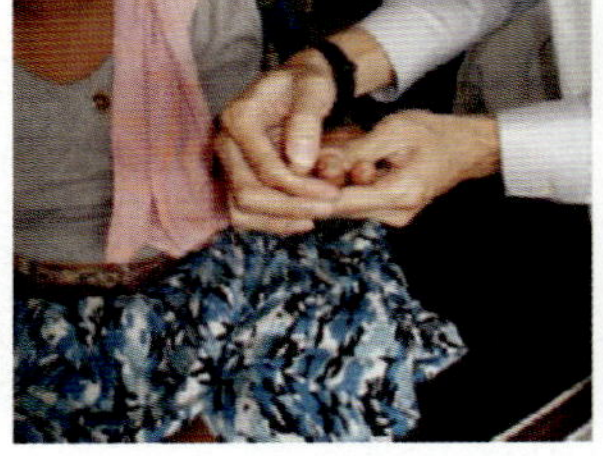

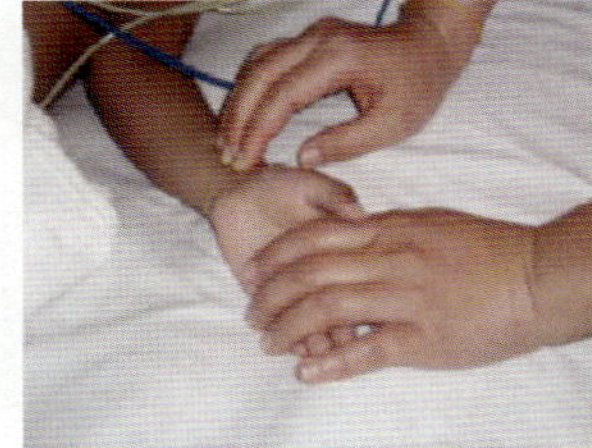

Fig. 5.15.20: Pearl in clinical examination.

- Decrease in hematocrit together with stable hemodynamic status and adequate urine output indicates hemodilution and/or intravasation of fluids suggestive of stopping of further IV fluids.

Hemodynamically unstable patient needs hematocrit assessment. In patients with high or rising hematocrit, repeat a second bolus of crystalloid solution at a rate of 10–20 mL/kg/h over an hour. After this second bolus, if there is improvement, reduce the rate to 7–10 mL/kg/h for next 1–2 hours, and then continue to taper as suggested above.

Recurrent Shock

Recurrences of shock in a properly managed and monitored case are uncommon but could occur; such patients may need further boluses during next 24–48 hours. A fall in hematocrit in a hemodynamically unstable patient denotes internal bleeding; a timely blood transfusion is the most important intervention in this situation.

Hypotensive Shock (Flowchart 5.15.3)

Patient with low systolic pressure poor, cold clammy extremities, poor or imperceptible peripheral pulses, prolonged CRT, and abnormal mentation is in hypotensive shock. A more aggressive approach is needed for such patients. An initial resuscitative bolus of 20 mL/kg BW of crystalloid is pushed over 30 minutes to quickly rescue patient from shock. *Patient who has been in hypotensive shock for prolonged time would be better off with colloids.* If patient improves, a further bolus

Flowchart 5.15.3: Fluid management in hypotensive shock.

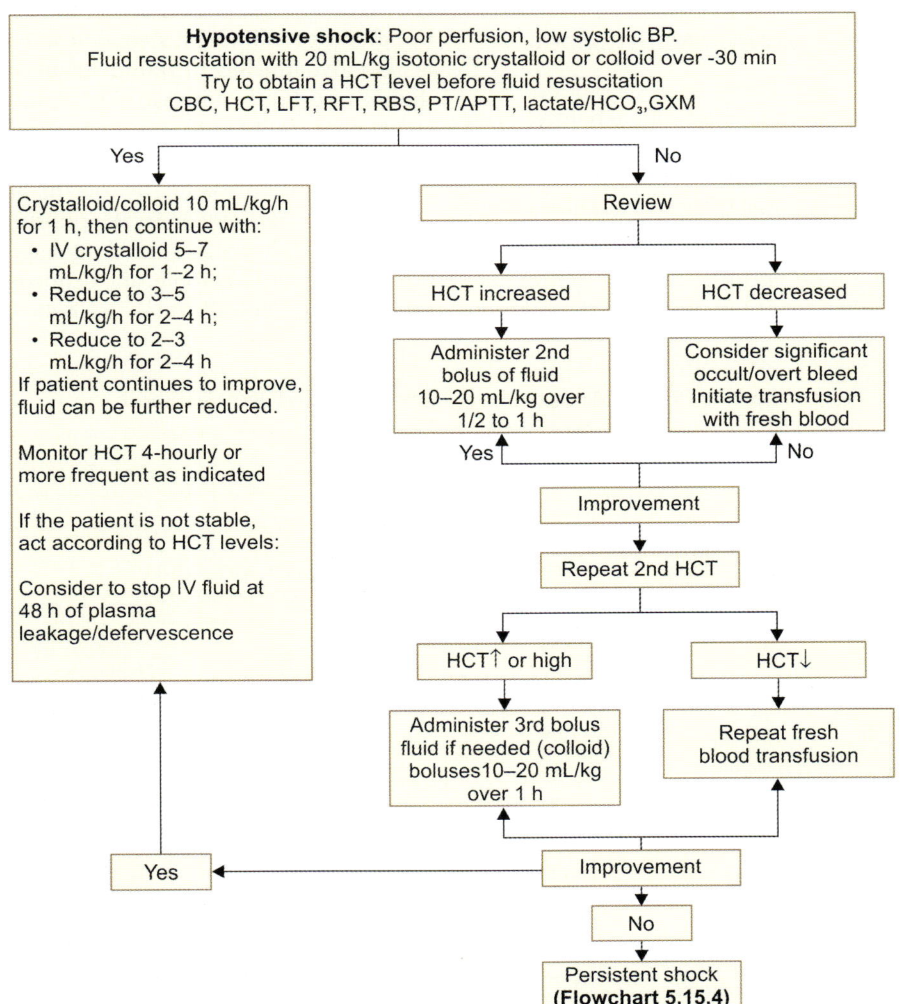

of IV fluid (crystalloid/colloid) 10 mL/kg/h is infused over next 1 hour. In a hemodynamically stable patient, fluid is gradually tapered over following 6–8 hours. Further fluid replacement for subsequent 24–48 hours is like compensated shock.

Persistent Hypotensive Shock

Patient who remains hemodynamically unstable after first bolus needs hematocrit review. If the hematocrit has risen compared to the baseline value; a second bolus of colloid solutions at 10–20 mL/kg is pushed over next 30–60 minutes. Third bolus is repeated if patient is still unstable and has high hematocrit. Patient who remains unstable even after third crystalloid bolus (persistent shock) should be infused with a colloid bolus in a dose of 10 mL/kg of BW, another colloid bolus may be considered if patient is still not out of shock. An improved patient after colloid infusion should be put on tapering crystalloid infusion as mentioned above.

Fluid-unresponsive Persistent Hypotensive Shock (Flowchart 5.15.4)

A patient who fails to improve even after colloid boluses need considerations for possible following conditions: myocardial dysfunction, marked hypoalbuminemia, metabolic compromises (metabolic acidosis, hypoglycemia), occult bleeding, and organopathies.

Patient need special investigations: Liver function test including serum proteins, renal function test, coagulation profile (PT, aPTT, fibrinogen, D-dimers), arterial-blood gas (ABG) with electrolytes, and echocardiography.

Such patient are specifically vulnerable for bleeding; therefore, if patient has low fibrinogen (less than 100 mg/dL), consider transfusion of cryoprecipitates (1 U/10 kg). Patient with prolonged PT and aPTT (more than 1.5 times the standard reference values) with normal fibrinogen (>100 mg) should be infused with fresh-frozen plasma (10 mL/kg).

Fresh plasma and/or 5% albumin boluses have found to be an effective treatment in fluid-unresponsive dengue shock patients. In myocardial dysfunction, an inotrops preferably a dobutamine infusion may prove helpful.

Intense Monitoring

Dengue shock has a dynamic clinical course; intense anticipatory monitoring for likely complications is crucial for good outcome. Frequency of assessment is generally dictated by patient's condition; it should be at least hourly till patient is hemodynamically unstable. Regular monitoring (no less than 4 hourly) is mandatory even in a hemodynamically stable patient till fluid regurgitation is complete and patient is totally out of risk. Frequent assessment of CCTVR, blood pressure, pulse pressure, heart rate, abdominal girth, and urinary output are obligatory. Monitoring of arterial or venous blood gases, other organ functions such as renal profile, liver profile, coagulation profile, and echocardiography should be performed as per individual case indication.

Flowchart 5.15.4: Management of fluid-unresponsive persistent shock.

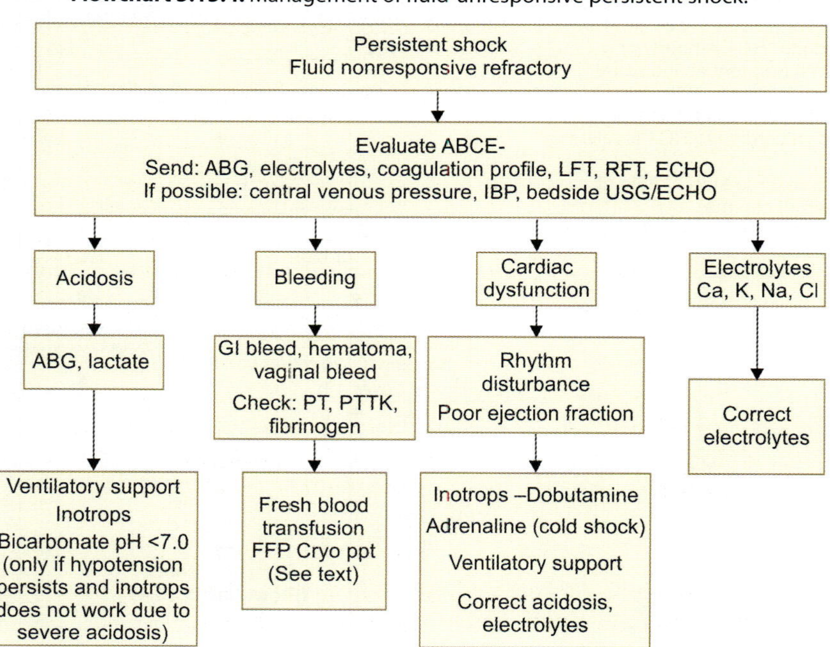

Mechanical Ventilation

Patients with respiratory distress with ongoing plasma leakage, myocardial dysfunction, central nervous system involvement are likely to benefit with mechanical ventilation; it facilitates more liberal fluid management in situation of ongoing plasma leak and helps in prevention of pulmonary edema. Reduction in work of breathing decreases myocardial workload and improves cardiac output.

Vasopressors and Inotrops

In a severe fluid-unresponsive hypotensive dengue shock, vasopressors and inotrops may be used as supportive measure to improve outcome. Patients with myocardial dysfunction intrinsic or because of aggressive fluid therapy and pulmonary edema are likely to be benefited with inotrops. Dobutamine is preferred inotrops for cardiac dysfunction; however, in late stages of cold hypotensive shock, other drugs such as adrenaline and nor adrenaline need to be considered.

It should be well understood that primary pathology in dengue shock is vascular leakage, and therefore, appropriate fluid therapy is the mainstay in managing dengue shock; vasopressors and inotrops are just a temporary supportive measure and never a substitute to appropriate fluid therapy.

Recovery Phase

Sudden increase in urinary output is earliest indication that vascular leakage and critical phase is about to end. Changes in hemodynamics such as, bounding peripheral pulses, widening of pulse pressure, and normalization of blood pressure, are soon to follow and herald the recovery phase. Large amount of fluid which had leaked out during critical phase is bound to intravasate during recovery phase of the disease therefore for next few hours patient would have vascular congestion; this is the time to stop fluid infusion as continuation of IV fluids at this stage of disease would result into fluid overload.

Criteria for Discharge

Patient should remain under medical supervision for at least 48 hours beyond full recovery, a regular monitoring of hemodynamics is mandatory during this period. Following conditions should be met before patient could be discharged from hospital: patient should be afebrile without antipyretics for 48 hours, should have feeling of wellbeing and good appetite, hemodynamics including urine output are normal, no evidence for bleeding and respiratory distress, and has stable hematocrit and rising trend for platelets.

COMPLICATIONS

There could be multiple complications, yet a duo of bleeding and respiratory distress is life-threatening and common enough to be anticipated in every severe dengue disease.

Hemorrhagic Complications

Minor Bleed

Minor mucosal bleeding in form of epistaxis, gum bleed, conjunctival hemorrhages may occur in any patient with dengue illness; most of these patients remain stable and do not need any intervention beyond fluid resuscitation/ replacement. Such bleeds rapidly improve during the recovery phase.

Major Bleed

Clinically significant bleeding necessitating intervention is uncommon in dengue illnesses in pediatric age group. In pediatric patients' major bleeding is almost always secondary to persistent refractory hypotensive shock culminating into multiorgan dysfunction, acidosis, and consequential DIC.

Major GI bleed could occur in a child who has been treated with nonsteroidal anti-inflammatory agents or who has been on anticoagulant therapy. Iatrogenic trauma in the form of intramuscular injection and nasogastric tube insertion could provoke significant hemorrhage.

There are reports of unusual bleeding in hemodynamically stable patients with some of the dengue outbreaks; etiopathogenesis of such events is believed to be undetermined vasculopathy.

Recognizing Major Bleed

Gastrointestinal tract is the commonest site for major internal bleeding. A major GI bleed may take hours before it manifests as melena, but it would immediately destabilize hemodynamics in a critically placed dengue shock patient. Shock with decrease in baseline hematocrit before fluid resuscitation or decreasing hematocrit after fluid resuscitation in an unstable hemodynamic dengue patient are valuable indicators of internal bleeding; these findings should be taken as an urgent signal for blood transfusion.

International standards for sepsis management recommends hematocrit levels of less than 30% (7 g/dL) as an indication for blood transfusion. *This recommendation is unsuitable for severe dengue for the simple reason that before bleeding hematocrit level in dengue patient goes phenomenally up owing to vascular leakage.* With bleeding hematocrit falls but even after the drop hematocrit level may not to be as low as in the absence of plasma leakage. For this obvious reason, it could be dangerous to abide by that recommendation for prescribing red blood cell transfusion in a dengue patient.

Plan for Treatment of Major Bleed

Infuse 10 mL/kg of fresh-packed red cells or 20 mL/kg of fresh whole blood at an appropriate rate. Observe the clinical response: improvement in hematocrit, hemodynamic status,

Flowchart 5.15.5: Management of dengue shock with respiratory distress.

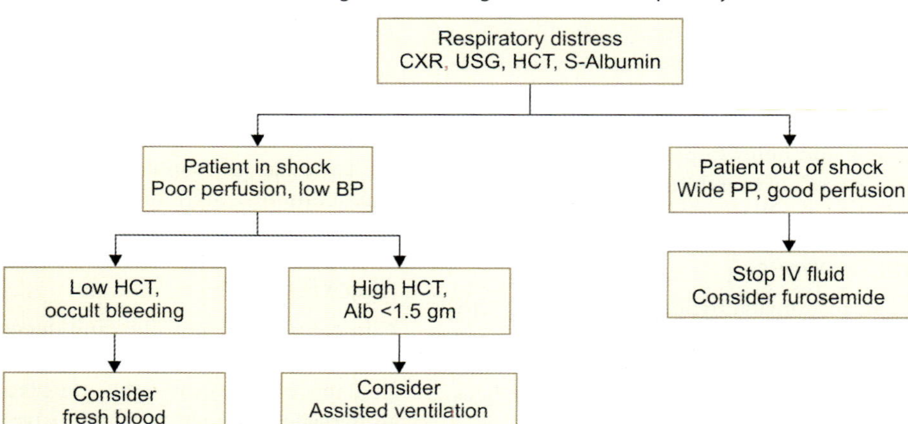

and acid-base balance is an indicator of successful therapy. A repeat transfusion is indicated in case of inadequate rise in hematocrit and poor clinical response. Stored blood loses 2,3-diphosphoglycerate, which in turn impedes the oxygen-releasing capacity of hemoglobin and results into functional tissue hypoxia; therefore, it is pertinent to use only fresh whole blood or fresh red cells in the management of dengue shock.

Respiratory Distress (Flowchart 5.15.5)

Causes

Polyserositis (severe ascites, pleural effusions, and pericardial effusion) due to fluid overload is the commonest cause for respiratory distress. Acute pulmonary edema, acute respiratory distress syndrome, and severe metabolic acidosis from severe shock are other notable causes of respiratory distress.

Fluid Overload

Causes for fluid overload **(Fig. 5.15.21)** are as follows:

- Excessive and/or too rapid IV fluids ignoring proper hemodynamic evaluation
- Erroneous use of hypotonic rather than isotonic crystalloid solutions
- Inadvertent continuation of IV fluids even after leakage has stopped
- Administration of large volumes of IV fluids instead of blood in patients with unrecognized severe bleeding
- Over use of colloids
- *Inappropriate transfusion of blood products*: fresh-frozen plasma, platelet concentrates, and cryoprecipitates
- Comorbid conditions such as congenital heart disease, chronic lung, and renal diseases.

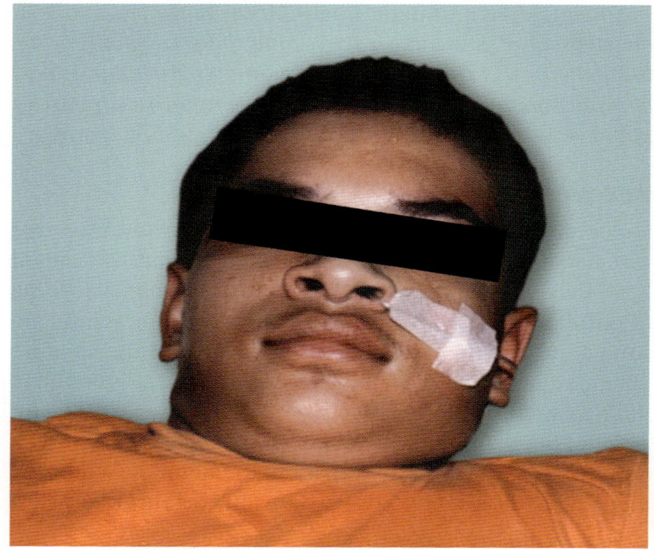

Fig. 5.15.21: Puffy edematous face (fluid overload).

Clinical Features

Tachypnea, dyspnea, wheezing, chest wall in-drawing, jugular engorgement, wide pulse pressure, basal crepitations, and tachycardia are some of the early signs of fluid overload.

Tense ascites and pleural effusions may cause severe respiratory embarrassment. Cough with frothy pink sputum herald the inception of pulmonary edema and congestive heart failure (CHF).

Cardiopulmonary Evaluation

Patients need detailed clinicoinvestigative cardiopulmonary evaluation. Arterial-blood gases, chest X-ray, electrocardiogram, echocardiogram, and cardiac enzymes need constant monitoring.

Management

Patient with respiratory distress mandatorily need oxygen supplementation; patient with respiratory failure may even require assisted ventilation.

Remaining management of fluid overload is dictated by hemodynamics, hematocrit, and phase of the disease.

- Intravenous fluids should be decreased and discontinued if plasma leakage has ceased and patient has normal hemodynamic status: pulse and peripheral perfusion (CRT) are normal, systolic pressure and pulse pressure (>30) are normal, hematocrit has decreased, urine output is adequate, and no fever for more than 24–48 hours (without the use of antipyretics).
- A patient with fluid overload occasionally may need diuretic therapy; few doses of furosemide would resolve their respiratory distress. Monitoring of serum potassium and correcting the ensuing hypokalemia is important for patients treated with Furosemide.
- Reduce the IV fluid if the patient is in critical phase but has stable hemodynamic status. *Never use diuretics during the plasma leakage phase, as they may lead to intravascular volume depletion.*
- Patient of fluid overload, who still is in shock and has low or normal hematocrit levels, may have occult hemorrhage. Such a patient needs urgent blood transfusion.
- Exceptional patient of severe dengue may have a very large vascular leak causing massive polyserositis; such patient may develop significant respiratory distress although has elevated hematocrit and is still in shock and need continuous fluid resuscitation. These patients develop severe hypoalbunemia which prevents hemodynamic stabilization because of very poor oncotic pressure; infusion of albumin or fresh-frozen plasma would restore the biochemical imbalance and stabilize the hemodynamics.

Thrombocytopenia and Platelet Transfusion

Thrombocytopenia is a regular and striking accompaniment of dengue so much that for a laymen dengue is synonymous with platelet deficiency. Characteristically, platelet levels match with disease severity; however, they do not have any impact on shock, bleeding, or other serious manifestations of disease. Therefore, there is *no place for prophylactic platelet replacement therapy irrespective of level of thrombocytopenia*. Prophylactic transfusion with platelets, on the contrary increases the risk of fluid overload and consequent respiratory distress.

Exceptionally platelet transfusion could be considered in case of uncontrolled bleeding due to persistent shock still transfusion should be undertaken only after adequately correcting coagulopathy. Patient of dengue who need to undergo cesarean section or other emergency surgery which entail risk of bleeding, the minimum platelet count should be more than 50,000 mm^3, and for undergoing eye surgery and neurosurgery, the platelet count should be at least more than 100,000 mm^3; prophylactic platelet transfusion is justified in such situations.

Patients with have profound thrombocytopenia (platelet count <10,000 mm^3) must adhere to strict bed rest and be protected from trauma and risk of bleeding. Thrombocytopenia in dengue is transitory and follows a fixed time bound relationship with disease. It doesn't need correction by corticosteroids or any other medication. Drug such as IV immunoglobulin is huge monetary waste; they do not make any difference in duration of thrombocytopenia or in antiplatelet antibody levels.

Dyselectrolytemia and Metabolic Disturbances

Possibilities of electrolyte disturbances such as hyponatremia, hypokalemia, hyperkalemia, hyperchloremia, serum calcium imbalances, and metabolic acidosis should be kept in mind while treating dengue shock. Dyselectrolytemia is rare and occurs due either to incorrect uses of hypotonic solutions for resuscitation and replacement or diarrhea vomiting resulting into GI electrolyte losses.

Regular blood sugar monitoring is necessary as both hypoglycemia and hyperglycemia could occur and destabilize a precariously positioned hemodynamics.

DENGUE MORTALITY: REASONS AND PREVENTION

Failing to Appreciate that Patient is Passing in Critical Phase of Disease

In a febrile illness parents and treating physician gets relieved when temperature subsides. Dengue is a unique situation where in critical manifestations evolve with defervescence, patient quickly deteriorates during this period; failure to appreciate this deterioration may lend patient into dengue shock. Late detection and delayed therapeutic intervention of shock is one of the commonest causes of dengue fatality.

It is crucial for treating clinician to regularly assess every patient for warning signs during peridefervescence period. Patient displaying any kind of warning signs at defervescence should immediately alert treating physician for possible development of shock; a probable mortality could be averted by timely hospitalizing such patient for IV fluid therapy.

Failure to Appreciate Internal Bleeding

Although major clinical hemorrhage are uncommon in pediatric dengue, rarely however occult massive GI bleed may prove life threatening. As has already been stated above falling hematocrit in a hemodynamically destabilized patient should alert clinician for such an eventuality and a timely blood transfusion would save a patient. Pulmonary and intracranial bleeding are rare however usually terminal events.

Failure to Appreciate Vascular Congestion

Inappropriate continuation of IV fluid in the wake of intravasation of leaked out fluid would cause cardiac overload and consequential CHF and death. Falling hematocrit with increased urinary output is a pointer to intravasation of leaked out fluid and should be taken as signal to terminate IV fluid therapy.

Even though a complex disease DHF exhibits a set clinical pattern and observes a fixed time bound course of events. Awareness and familiarity with its course greatly facilitates diagnosis-making and proper therapy. With appropriate IV fluid management and frequent monitoring, mortality in dengue shock could be greatly minimized.

Dengue Vaccine

Efforts to develop a vaccine against dengue have been ongoing for decades. The biggest challenge has been to find out a tetravalent vaccine which could simultaneously induce long lasting protective immunity against all four viruses. The first vaccine recommended for use is chimeric yellow fever virus-DENV-tetravalent dengue vaccine (marketed as Dengvaxia) a live, attenuated tetravalent product developed by Sanofi Pasteur. Following two phase 3 clinical trials published in 2014, Dengvaxia was licensed in December 2015. Expert opinion and a position paper on Dengvaxia were issued by WHO in 2016.

Even at the time of licensing, vaccine was besieged with couple of serious problems: (1) The vaccine had a poor efficacy and safety in younger children; there was an increase in hospital admissions due to dengue between 2 years and 5 years of age in vaccinated children; therefore, the vaccine was approved only for people aged 9–45 years. (2) Vaccine had poor serological responses against dengue strain-2, particularly in Southeast Asian trials.

In 2016, some experts warned that the increased risk of hospital admission was a serious safety concern: Maíra Aguiar and colleagues argued that "ethically no one should have been put under risk by receiving this vaccine."

Prompted by WHO Sanofi had to come out with supplemental data that clearly showed an augmented risk of severe dengue in vaccinated population, particularly if they were dengue seronegative at the time of vaccination, irrespective of their age.

A supplemental statement from WHO on December 22, 2017, verifies that overall Dengvaxia reduces the risk of confirmed severe dengue and hospital admissions; however, among seronegative recipients regardless of age at vaccination—there was a higher risk of severe dengue disease and hospital admission compared with unvaccinated controls. Thus, in seronegative individuals, the vaccine seems to enhance the severity of subsequent dengue infection.

Dengvaxia is not yet licensed for use in India.

BIBLIOGRAPHY

1. Bandyopadhyay S, Lum LCS, Kroeger A. Classifying dengue: a review of the difficulties in using the WHO case classification for dengue haemorrhagic fever. Trop Med Int Health. 2006;11,8:1238-55.
2. Government of India. National guidelines for clinical management of dengue fever. J Indian Med Assoc. 2015;113(12).
3. Halstead SB. Seminar: dengue. Lancet. 2007;370:1644-52.
4. Jacqueline LD, Harris E, Bridget W, et al. The WHO dengue classification and case definitions: time for a reassessment. Lancet. 2006;368:170-3.
5. Jose G. Severe dengue: the need for new case definitions. Lancet Infect Dis. 2006;6:297-302.
6. Kapse AS. A study of an epidemic of dengue at Surat; clinico-investigative analysis. In: Environment and health in developing countries. New Delhi: APH Publishing; 1998. pp. 339-50.
7. Pan American Health Organization: Dengue: guidelines for patient care in the region of the Americas. Washington, DC: PAHO; 2016. ISBN 978-92-75-11890-0.
8. Sharon LR, Michelle DV, Marissa MA. The use of colloids and crystalloids in pediatric dengue shock syndrome: a systematic review and meta-analysis. BMC Infect Dis. 2011;11:52.
9. WHO, TDR. Dengue: guidelines for diagnosis, treatment, prevention and control. Geneva: WHO; 2009.
10. Wills BA, Nguyen MD, Loan HT, et al. Comparison of three fluid solutions for resuscitation in dengue shock syndrome. N Engl J Med. 2005;353:877-89.

5.16 Chikungunya Fever

Rajniti Prasad

INTRODUCTION

Chikungunya fever is caused by an alpha virus and spread by bite of *Aedes aegypti* mosquito. The name derives from *kungunyala*, which means, "to dry up or become contorted," i.e. bent posture of patients. It has caused numerous outbreaks and epidemics in both Africa and South East Asia, involving thousands of children.

CHIKUNGUNYA VIRUS

Chikungunya virus (CHIKV), a positive stranded, enveloped ribonucleic acid virus, is a member of the *Alphavirus* genus and belongs to the Togaviridae family. Genetic analysis based on partial *E1* envelope glycoprotein gene sequences showed presence of three distinct phylogroups. The first contained all isolates from West Africa; second comprised all Central, Southern, and Eastern African strains; and the third contained isolates from Asia.

EPIDEMIOLOGY

Chikungunya virus is commonly transmitted to humans through the bite of infected mosquitoes of the *Aedes* genus, which usually bite during daylight hours. In Africa, CHIKV appears to be maintained in sylvatic cycle involving wild primates such as monkeys that may serve as reservoir of the virus. The secondary attack rate is 4–45%.

Aedes aegypti, *Aedes albopictus*, and *Aedes polynesiensis* are commonly involved in the transmission of virus, although *Culex* has also been reported for some transmission. *A. aegypti*, the principal vector of CHIKV in India, is anthropophilic, endophagic, and bites during the daytime. It mainly breeds in man-made discarded containers where rainwater accumulates. The recent epidemic in India suggested that Asian tiger mosquito was responsible for spread. The mutation in the envelope protein gene (*E1-A226V*) was reported in some strains of CHIKV. This mutation is responsible for CHIKV adaptation to the Asian tiger mosquito. With the global climate warming, CHIKV could expand to new geographic locations.

PATHOGENESIS

Chikungunya virus replicates primarily in fibroblasts and macrophages but can replicate in various human cells, including epithelial and endothelial cells. Viral entry occurs through a power of hydrogen (pH)-dependent, endocytic pathway. It is highly cytopathic and induces apoptosis of infected cells. In humans, CHIKV produces symptoms after 48 hours of mosquito bite. Patients have high viral load in blood during the first 2 days of illness. Viremia declines around day 3 or day 4 and usually disappears by day 5. Hemagglutination inhibition and neutralizing antibodies can usually be detected after day 5. Clinical or silent infection is thought to confer lifelong immunity. A recent study has suggested CHIKV tropism for muscular satellite cells, which can act as small reservoirs for virus or virus-encoded components or both for longer periods.

CLINICAL MANIFESTATIONS

Chikungunya fever is characterized by the triad of abrupt onset fever, rashes, and arthralgia followed by other constitutional symptoms. The incubation period is usually 2–3 days (range 1–12 days). All age groups are affected, including newborns but full-blown disease is common in adults. Fever rises abruptly, often reaching 39–40°C accompanied by intermittent shaking chills. This acute phase lasts for 2–3 days. The temperature may remit for 1–2 days, after a gap of 4–10 days, resulting in a "saddle back" fever curve.

Arthralgia is polyarticular, migratory, and predominantly affects the small joints of hands, wrists, ankles, and feet with lesser involvement of larger joints **(Fig. 5.16.1)**. In acute stage, patients complain bitterly of pain, when asked to move and assume an attitude of flexion. Pain on movement is worse in the morning, improved by mild exercise and exacerbated by strenuous exercise. Swelling may occur but fluid accumulation is uncommon. Patients with mild articular manifestation are usually symptom-free within a few weeks, but severe cases require months to resolve entirely.

Cutaneous manifestations include flushing of the face and trunk. This is usually followed by maculopapular rash. Trunks and limbs are commonly involved, but face, palms, and soles may also show lesions. Rashes may simply fade or desquamate. Petechiae may occur alone or in association with rash and observed during the acute stage of illness and convalescence. Pigmentary changes have been reported to be the most common cutaneous finding (42%), followed by maculopapular eruption (33%) and intertriginous

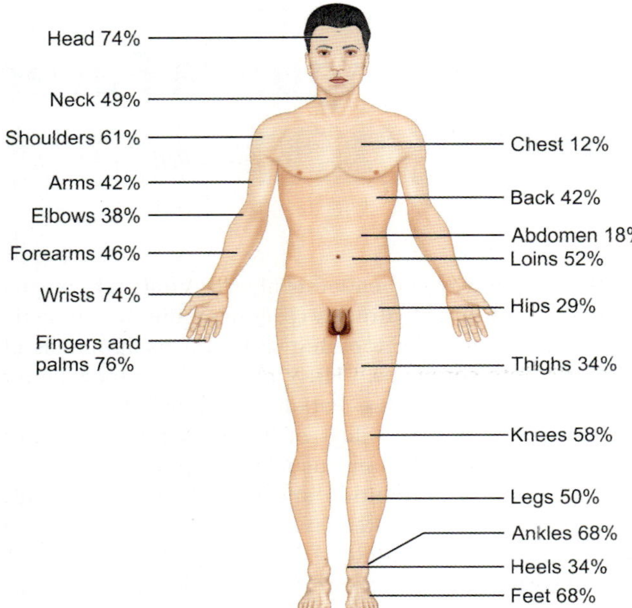

Figure 5.16.1: Frequency of pain and arthritis by location during acute stage.

aphthous—such as ulcers (21.37%). Exacerbation of existing psoriasis and unmasking of undiagnosed Hansen's disease may occur. Rash usually lasts for 1–7 days.

Iridocyclitis and retinitis are the most common ocular manifestations associated with chikungunya fever, with a typically benign clinical course. Less frequent ocular lesions include episcleritis. Other rare manifestations include meningoencephalitis, fulminant hepatitis, and mild hemorrhagic manifestations.

Most symptomatic patients (93.7%) complain of a chronic stage of the disease, which is characterized by pains in joints, bones, or both. This persisting pain may be continuous or discontinuous with alternation of clinical remission and relapses (58.7%). Some infected individuals may also have fever at this stage.

LABORATORY DIAGNOSIS

Some patients show leukopenia with mildly decreased platelet count. Elevated levels of aspartate aminotransferase and C-reactive protein are also seen. However, virus isolation is the most definitive tests in first week. Recently, reverse transcription polymerase chain reaction (RT-PCR) technique for diagnosis has been developed using nested primer pairs amplifying specific components of three structural gene regions. PCR results can be available within 1–2 days.

Serologic diagnosis can be made by the demonstration of fourfold increase in antibody in acute and convalescent sera or demonstrating immunoglobulin M (IgM) antibodies specific for CHIKV. A commonly used test is the IgM antibody capture enzyme-linked immunosorbent assay (MAC-ELISA). Results of MAC-ELISA can be available within 2–3 days. Cross-reaction with other flavivirus antibodies, such as O'nyongnyong and Semliki, may occur in MAC-ELISA; however, the latter viruses are relatively rare in South East Asia. A positive virus culture supplemented with neutralization is taken as definitive proof for the presence of CHIKV.

MANAGEMENT

There is no specific treatment for chikungunya fever. The illness is usually self-limiting and resolves with time. Supportive care with rest is recommended during the acute joint symptoms. Movement and mild exercise tend to improve stiffness and morning arthralgia, but heavy exercise may exacerbate rheumatic symptoms. Nonaspirin and nonsteroidal anti-inflammatory drugs (NSAIDs) are recommended. In unresolved arthritis refractory to NSAID, chloroquine (10 mg/kg/day) has proved to be useful. Chloroquine inhibits viral replication by blocking pH-dependent endocytosis of CHIKV into host cells. Although chloroquine blocks CHIKV replication, therapeutic (antiviral) index of chloroquine in cell cultures is rather narrow. Thus one should be cautious when planning the use of chloroquine as an antiviral treatment in infected individuals.

Self-resolution occurs with cutaneous lesions. Patients with hyperpigmentation may be treated with sunscreens and topical steroids. All patients with only centrofacial involvement usually show complete clearance during follow-up by 3 weeks. Patients with more diffuse involvement show a slower resolution. Aphthous ulcers usually heal over 7–10 days with local cleaning and topical antimicrobials to prevent secondary infection. Iridocyclitis and retinitis have a typically benign clinical course. All the patients respond well to the treatment with preservation of good vision.

Infected persons should be protected from further mosquito exposure (staying indoors and/or under mosquito net during the first few days of illness), so that they do not contribute to the transmission cycle.

VACCINE

The current live vaccine (Lot 1-85, TSI-GSD-218) was developed in the United States in Army Medical Research Institute of Infectious Diseases and was produced at the Salk Institute, from GMK strain 15,561 by serial passage in Medical Research Council-5 cells. The results of phase I and phase II trials strongly suggest that live vaccine is safe and well tolerated and produces no severe or frequent symptoms than found in placebo recipients.

PREVENTION

Prevention is entirely dependent upon taking steps to avoid mosquito bites, which includes wearing full sleeve clothes and elimination of mosquito breeding sites. The use of mosquito coils, repellents, electric vapor mats during the daytime, and permethrin treated mosquito nets during sleep prevents transmission of disease. Drainage of water from coolers, tanks, barrels, drums, and buckets and empty coolers, when not in use, prevents mosquito breeding.

Active surveillance by health workers of cases should be undertaken. This will help in identifying the affected areas, so that control measures may be initiated. Vector surveillance should also be done and will help in initiating early control measures and assess the impact of the measures taken. Education of people about the disease, mode of transmission, availability of treatment and adoption of control measures are important for prevention of disease.

BIBLIOGRAPHY

1. Centers for Disease Control and Prevention (2006). Chikungunya fever fact sheet: CDC Division of Vector Borne Infectious Diseases. [online] Available from: http://www.cdc.gov/ncidod/chikungunya/chickfact.htm.2006. [Accessed September, 2018].
2. Chhabra M, Mittal V, Bhattacharya D, et al. Chikungunya fever: a re-emerging viral infection. Indian J Med Microbiol. 2008;26:5-12.
3. Inamadar AC, Palit A, Sampagavi VV, et al. Cutaneous manifestations of chikungunya fever: observations made during a recent outbreak in south India. Intern J Dermatol. 2008;47:154-9.
4. Lahariya C, Pradhan SK. Emergence of chikungunya virus in Indian subcontinent after 32 years: a review. J Vect Borne Dis. 2006;43:151-60.
5. Mahendradas P, Ranganna SK, Shetty R, et al. Ocular manifestations associated with chikungunya. Ophthalmology. 2008;115(2):287-91.
6. Mohan A. Chikungunya fever: clinical manifestations and management. Indian J Med Res. 2006;124:471-4.
7. Parola P, Lamballerie X, Jourdan J, et al. Novel Chikungunya virus variant in travelers returning from Indian Ocean Islands. Emerg Infect Dis. 2006;12:1493-9.
8. Pialoux G, Gauzere BA, Strobel M. Chikungunya virus infection: review through an epidemic. Med Mal Infect. 2006;36: 253-63.
9. Queyriaux B, Simon F, Grandadam M, et al. Clinical burden of chikungunya virus infection. Lancet Infect Dis. 2008;1:2-3.

5.17 Poliomyelitis

AK Dutta

INTRODUCTION

Poliomyelitis is a highly infectious crippling and often-fatal disease caused by any of the three serotypes of z, e.g. types 1, 2, and 3, which mainly affects children under 5 years of age. It is most often recognized by acute onset flaccid paralysis of the limbs. The condition was considered in the past as one of the most feared infectious disease because of the permanent residual paralysis and disability. However, with the intelligent use of the available polio vaccines, the disease has become a rarity with only three countries of the world, e.g. Pakistan, Afghanistan, and Nigeria, as the only endemic countries in the world. However, there is always threat of spread of the disease from these countries, and in 2013-2014, several countries in African horn have been affected with fresh cases of poliomyelitis from Nigeria. At present, vaccine-associated paralytic poliomyelitis (VAPP) and vaccine-derived poliovirus (VDPV) are occurring in many countries. World Health Organization (WHO) aims at eradicating both wild as well as vaccine virus causing poliomyelitis.

EPIDEMIOLOGY

Poliovirus is highly communicable disease for which human is the only reservoir. It multiplies in the intestine and is spread via fecal-oral route. The average incubation period is 7–10 days (range 4–35 days). The maximum excretion of virus occurs just before the onset of paralysis and during the first 2 weeks after the onset of paralysis. However, the virus is excreted intermittently for up to 2 months after infection.

Polio cases have decreased by over 99% since 1988, from an estimated 350,000 cases to 359 in 2014 globally. In

2018, only two countries (Afghanistan and Pakistan) in the world remain polio-endemic. Till the end of June 2018, only 13 cases of poliomyelitis have been reported and all are with poliovirus type 1, 10 cases from Afghanistan and three cases from Pakistan. However, cases of circulating VDPV (cVDPV) are still occurring in many countries of the world with poor immunization coverage. Almost all cVDPV cases are occurring with type 2 oral polio vaccine (OPV) virus.

ETIOPATHOGENESIS

Poliomyelitis is caused by three antigenically distinct serotypes (type 1, 2, and 3) of polioviruses. The polioviruses are nonenveloped, positive-stranded ribonucleic acid viruses, and belong to the genus *Enterovirus* in the family Picornaviridae. These viruses can remain active for several days at room temperature and can be stored indefinitely frozen at –20°C. It is rapidly inactivated by heat, chlorine, and ultraviolet light. Wild-type 2 and 3 poliovirus has been eradicated from the world and only type 1 wild poliovirus is causing disease. However, cVDPV in almost all the cases and 60% of VAPP cases are caused due to type 2 poliovirus. Polioviruses enter the intestine by fecal-oral route of transmission through contaminated water and food. The primary site of replication is small intestine and regional lymph nodes. Poliovirus probably accesses the central nervous system through peripheral nerves and primarily infects motor neuron cells in the spinal cord (the anterior horn cells) and the medulla oblongata.

CLINICAL MANIFESTATIONS

In 90–95% of infected individuals, poliovirus infection is unapparent. In the remaining 5–10% of individuals infected by poliovirus, one of the following three syndromes may occur:

1. *Abortive polio*: This occurs in 4–8% of infections and is characterized by a minor illness with low-grade fever, sore throat, vomiting, abdominal pain, loss of appetite, and malaise. Recovery is rapid and complete; there is no paralysis.
2. *Nonparalytic polio*: It occurs in 1–2% of infections and is characterized by headache and neck, back, and leg stiffness, which occurs several days after the prodrome (fever, malaise, etc.). Presentation resembles other causes of aseptic meningitis and recovers within 2–10 days.
3. *Paralytic polio*: This form occurs in 0.5–1% of infections (i.e. one case of paralysis in every 100–200 infected children). Symptoms often occur in two phases, minor and major, and are often separated by several days without symptoms. The minor phase consists of symptoms similar to those of abortive poliomyelitis. The major phase of illness begins with muscle pain, spasms, and the fever. This is followed by rapid onset of flaccid paralysis that is usually complete within 72 hours.

There are mainly three types of paralytic poliomyelitis:

1. *Spinal paralytic poliomyelitis* is the most common form of paralytic poliomyelitis, seen in approximately 80% of paralytic cases. It results from a lower motor neuron lesion of the anterior horn of the spinal cord and affects the muscles of the legs, arms, and/or trunk. The affected muscles are flaccid (lower motor neuron type) and reflexes are diminished. There is no sensory involvement. Paralysis is often asymmetrical, affecting legs more often than arms. Paralytic manifestation in extremities begins proximally and progresses to involve distal muscle groups (i.e. descending paralysis). Severe cases may develop quadriplegia and paralysis of the trunk, abdominal, and thoracic muscles. Residual flaccid paralysis is usually present after 60 days.
2. *Bulbar polio* accounts up to 2% of paralytic cases and results from a cranial nerve lesion, resulting in respiratory insufficiency and difficulty in swallowing, nasal regurgitation, and difficulty in phonation.
3. *Bulbospinal polio* accounts for approximately up to 20% of paralytic cases, which is a combination of both spinal and bulbar component.
4. In rare cases, an *encephalitic type of poliomyelitis* has been reported.

RESIDUAL PARALYSIS

As the acute phase of illness (0–4 weeks) subsides, the recovery begins in paralyzed muscles. The extent of recovery is variable depending upon the extent of damage caused to the neurons by the virus. Maximum neurological recovery of the paralyzed muscle takes place in the first 6 months of the illness but slow recovery continues up to 2 years. After 2 years, no more recovery is expected and the child is said to have "postpolio residual paralysis," which remains as such throughout life.

VACCINE-ASSOCIATED PARALYTIC POLIOMYELITIS

In some of the recipients of OPV (in <1%), genetic changes in *VP1* gene of vaccine virus take place, and the vaccine virus becomes virulent and causes paralysis in the same recipient or among close contacts who are not immune. Approximately one case of VAPP occurs after 2.3 million of first doses and after 12 million subsequent doses. According to WHO, approximately 500 cases/year occur in the world out of which 75 cases are from India. VAPP is clinically indistinguishable from paralysis due to wild poliovirus.

VACCINE-DERIVED POLIOVIRUS

It is a derivative of Sabin strain from OPV, which exhibits about 1–15% genetic changes in the *VP1* gene and usually transmits disease to nonimmune individual. The strain has potential for human infection and paralysis including sustained circulation and spreading disease in other countries through human travel and is a serious threat to spread of the disease in various countries of the world. In the last 5 years, more than 500 cases of cVDPV type 2 disease have occurred in various countries, which were declared polio free. This mutant strain is of three types as described in the following subsections.

Circulating Vaccine-derived Poliovirus

This emerges in areas with poor OPV coverage and chances of sustained person-to-person spread. WHO considers cVDPV as serious threat to polio eradication process. In 2018, till the end of April 2018, a total of 35 cases of cVDPV have been reported from democratic republic of Congo and Syrian Arab Republic where no case of wild poliovirus has been reported. Somalia and Kenya are other two outbreak countries for cVDPV as per WHO. Several other countries in Africa and Middle East are at risk for cVDPV.

Immunodeficient-associated Vaccine-derived Poliovirus

This strain is isolated from persons with primary immune deficiency states who exhibit prolonged infection after OPV exposure. These strains can persist for over 20 years.

Ambiguous Vaccine-derived Poliovirus

This strain is clinical isolate from nonimmunocompromised individual or environmental isolation from unidentified source.

DIFFERENTIAL DIAGNOSIS

The differential diagnosis of abortive and nonparalytic polio includes other viral fevers. Paralytic poliomyelitis needs differentiation from other causes of acute flaccid paralysis (AFP). Paralytic poliomyelitis, Guillain–Barré syndrome, traumatic neuritis, and transverse myelitis represent the most common causes of AFP, but the complete differential diagnosis includes numerous etiologies (hypokalemia, encephalitis, meningitis and other enterovirus infections, polymyositis, peripheral neuritis, myasthenia and other myopathies, etc.). Distinguishing characteristic of paralytic polio are asymmetric, AFP, mostly involving proximal muscles with fever and muscular pain at onset, rapid progression from onset to maximum paralysis (usually < 4 days), intact sensory nerve function, and most often, residual paralysis or weakness after 60 days.

Salient features of differentiation are summarized in **Table 5.17.1**.

DIAGNOSIS

Characteristic clinical presentation of acute lower motor neuron type of asymmetrical paralysis of proximal limb

Table 5.17.1: Differential diagnosis of paralytic poliomyelitis.

Signs and symptoms	*Polio*	*GBS*	*Transverse myelitis*	*Traumatic neuritis*
Fever at onset	High, present	Not common	Rarely present	Present
Flaccidity	Asymmetrical and proximal	Symmetrical and distal	Symmetrical lower limbs	Asymmetrical limb
DTR	Decreased or absent	Absent	Absent in LL early, hyperreflexia late	Decreased or absent
Sensation	Myalgia, no sensory loss	Cramps, tingling hypoanesthesia of palms and soles	Loss of sensation with sensory level	Pain in gluteal region
Cranial nerves involvement	Only in bulbar and bulbospinal	Often present VII, IV, X, XI, XII	Absent	Absent
CSF: WBCs, protein	• High WBCs • Normal or slight increase in protein	<10 WBCs High protein	Normal or slight increase in protein	Normal protein
Bladder dysfunction	Absent	Transient	Present	Never
NCV—3rd week	• Abnormal • Anterior horn cell disease	Abnormal demyelination	No diagnostic value	Abnormal in sciatic nerve
EMG—3rd week	Abnormal	Normal	Normal	Normal

(CSF: cerebrospinal fluid; DTR: deep tendon reflexes; EMG: electromyography; GBS: Guillain–Barré syndrome; LL: lower limbs; NCV: nerve conduction velocity; WBCs: white blood cells)

muscles without any sensory involvement is highly suggestive of poliomyelitis. However, all cases of AFP should be investigated by sending a stool sample for isolation of virus.

Stool for Virus Isolation

Recommended in every case of AFP. Virus usually can be found in the feces from onset to up to 8 or more weeks after paralysis, with the highest probability of detection during the first 2 weeks after onset. Isolation of wild poliovirus from stool is the recommended method for laboratory confirmation of paralytic poliomyelitis. Two stool specimens are collected from each case for laboratory confirmation.

Adequate stool specimen is defined as two specimens collected at least 24 hours apart within 14 days of onset of paralysis. Each sample should have volume (8–10 g or thumb size) and sent to a WHO-accredited laboratory in good condition with no desiccation, leakage, and maintaining cold chain.

TREATMENT

The aim of treatment is to promote recovery, to minimize residual muscle paralysis and disability. Treatment of the child with paralytic poliomyelitis varies with the stage of illness and the severity of paralysis. Children with bulbospinal polio and respiratory paralysis would require hospitalization. In acute stage, children with isolated limb/limbs paralysis should be advised complete rest, proper positioning of the affected limb, and passive range of movement at the joints. Massage and intramuscular injection should be avoided during acute phase of illness. The child should be made to lie on firm bed and maintain limbs in neutral position. The child should lie with trunk and hip straight with slight flexion (5–10°) at knees and feet at right angle at ankle joint. This position can be maintained with pillows, rolled towels, or sand bags. The support should also be given on lateral sides of limb/limbs to prevent external rotation. Warm moist fomentations and passive range of movements of all the joints of affected limb/limbs should be given.

As the acute phase of illness subsides, recovery in muscle power is helped by giving physiotherapy in the form of active exercises aimed at strengthening weak muscle groups, improvement of functional skills of the child, helping ambulation, and prevention of deformities. Physiotherapy plays an important role in the management of children during recovery and postpolio residual paralysis stage. Some children with fixed deformities and contractures may require orthopedic surgery.

STRATEGIES FOR POLIO ERADICATION INCLUDING ENDGAME STRATEGY

In May 1988, the World Health Assembly committed the member nations of the WHO to achieving the goal of global eradication of poliomyelitis. Since most of the countries in the world have been declared as polio free, the endgame strategy has been defined now by the WHO Strategic Advisory Group on Polio Eradication as complete eradication and containment of all wild, vaccine, and Sabin poliovirus disease from the world. The details of the strategy would be discussed in the chapter on polio vaccine. The detail timeline is given in **Figure 5.17.1**. For the eradication of poliomyelitis from the world, the strategies include:

- Continuation of mass polio vaccination to susceptible individuals in national immunization days (NID) and sub-NID (SNID).
- Maximum coverage of infants in routine immunization.
- Excellent clinical and virological surveillance of AFP.
- Inclusion of either one dose of inactivated polio vaccine (IPV) along with the third dose of diphtheria-pertussis-tetanus (DPT) and OPV to all children or two fractional intradermal (one-fifth) dose of IPV at 6 weeks and 14 weeks.
- Switching of trivalent OPV (TOPV) to bivalent OPV (BOPV containing types 1 and 3 only) 6 months after the introduction of IPV (already done in all OPV-using countries in the world, in April 2016).
- In the country, this strategy would prevent cVDPV type 2 responsible for almost all cVDPV and also most of the VAPP cases (caused by type 2 virus).
- Stoppage of BOPV by 2019 and continuing IPV thereafter till 2022 and then the strategy would be decided.
- Environmental surveillance for both wild and Sabin virus circulation in the community.

Please refer to Chapter 5.4.1, Polio Endgame: Global and National Perspectives, for more details.

PREVENTION OF POLIOMYELITIS

Polio Vaccines

There are currently two effective polio vaccines, the IPV, which was the first vaccine to become available in 1955, and the live-attenuated OPV, which was licensed in 1959.

Oral Polio Vaccine

Induces both circulating antibody and intestinal immunity, and by secondary spread, probably protects susceptible contacts. The seroconversion after three doses of OPV has been reported to be more than 95% in the developed countries but data from the developing countries has shown wide variation in seroconversion and protective efficacy with rates

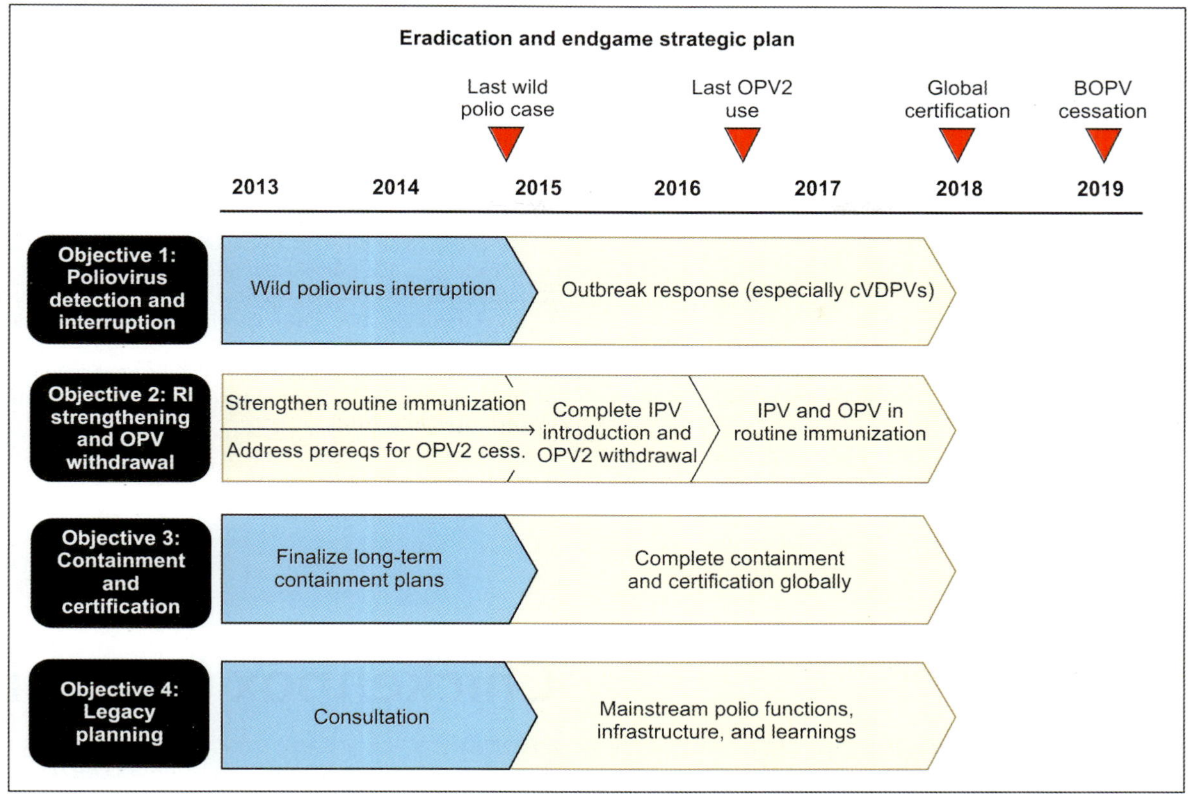

Fig. 5.17.1: Polio eradication and endgame strategic plan. (IPV: inactivated polio vaccine; OPV: oral polio vaccine)

varying from 70% against types 1 and 3 and approximately 90% for type 2 strains. Presently, only BOPV (containing types 1 and 3 Sabin live-attenuated strain) is available in the world. Type 2 OPV is now not used anywhere in the world.

Dosage, Administration, and Formulation

Oral polio vaccine is formulated as a bivalent vaccine, containing antigens for poliovirus serotypes (1–3). Bivalent vaccine is used for both routine immunizations as well as for NID and SNID.

Oral polio vaccine should be administered orally, that is, directly into the mouth. Each single dose consists of two drops of live OPV. OPV is given at birth followed by three more doses at 6 weeks, 10 weeks, and 14 weeks and at 16–18 months as per National Immunization Schedule of India. In addition, BOPV doses are recommended as per recommendations regarding NID or SNID from time to time.

Oral polio vaccine is one of the most heat-sensitive vaccines in common use. The vaccine should be stored at 2–8°C at all times. Unopened vials of OPV may be stored for up to 6 months at –20°C. The potency is monitored with color changes in vaccine vial monitor.

Trivalent OPV has been discontinued in 2016 and there has been switch to BOPV (types 1 and 3). This strategy was adopted to prevent cVDPV by augmenting the immunity induced by earlier doses of TOPV. By 2019, it is expected that if there is no case of poliomyelitis in the world, there shall be complete cessation of OPV and at least one dose of IPV will be given to each child till 2024.

Inactivated Polio Vaccine

Inactivated polio vaccine also known as Salk vaccine is a mixture of the three polioviruses made by harvesting cell culture supernatants and submitting them to inactivation by formalin. When used as primary vaccination of infants, the vaccine produces seroconversion in 90–95% of children. IPV is relatively heat stable. Risk of vaccine-associated paralysis is nonexistent with IPV and can be safely used in immunocompromised individuals. Three doses are recommended as primary schedule at 6, weeks 10 weeks, and 14 weeks, followed by booster doses at 18 months and 5 years by Indian Academy of Pediatrics. However, in National Immunization Schedule, two fractional doses of

IPV (one-fifth) of intramuscular dose at 6 weeks and 14 weeks along with pentavalent vaccine and BOPV are used for routine immunization. Studies have shown that two doses of intradermal IPV is not inferior to single dose of intramuscular dose.

BIBLIOGRAPHY

1. Child Health Division, Department of Family Welfare. Surveillance of AFP: A Field Guide (Red Book), 3rd edition. New Delhi: Ministry of Family Welfare, Govt. of India, Nirman Bhavan; 2005.
2. Dutta AK. Poliomyelitis. In: Parthasarathy A, Menon PSN, Gupta P, Nair MK (Eds). IAP Textbook of Pediatrics. New Delhi: Jaypee Brothers Medical Publishers (P) Ltd.; 2013. pp. 350-61.
3. Nathanson N, Kew OM. From emergence to eradication—the epidemiology of poliomyelitis deconstructed. Am J Epidemiol. 2010;172:1213-29.
4. National Polio Surveillance Project. [online] Available from: http/www.npspindia.org [Accessed October, 2018].
5. Plotkin SA, Vidor E. Polio vaccine-inactivated. In: Plotkin SA, Orenstein WA, Offit PA (Eds). Vaccine, 5th edition. Philadelphia, PA: Saunders; 2008.
6. Simoes EA. Poliovirus. In: Kliegman RM, Jenson HB, Stanton BE (Eds). Nelson Text Book of Pediatrics, 19th edition. Philadelphia, PA: Elsevier/Saunders; 2011.
7. Sutter RW, Kew OM, Cochi SL. Polio vaccine-live. In: Plotkin SA, Orenstein WA, Offit PA (Eds). Vaccine, 5th edition. Philadelphia, PA: Saunders; 2008.
8. World Health Organization. Global polio eradication initiative. [online] Available from: http/www.polioeradication.org. [Accessed July, 2018].

5.18 Chickenpox (Varicella)

Lalitha Kailas

INTRODUCTION

Chickenpox is a common childhood disease, caused by the *Varicella zoster* virus (VZV). Though generally considered as a benign self-limited infection, this can cause severe illness especially in newborns, immunocompromised children, and elderly patients. The incidence of the disease has now markedly decreased as varicella vaccine has become more widely used.

EPIDEMIOLOGY

Chickenpox is worldwide in distribution; epidemics do not have any definite periodicity. Most of the children are affected by 15 years of age. Within household contacts, transmission rate is 65–86%; more casual contacts such as occurring in a class room are associated with lower attack rates among susceptible children.

ETIOLOGY

Varicella zoster virus is a double-stranded DNA virus, a member of the herpes virus family. Humans are the only reservoir for VZV and cause primary, latent, and recurrent infections. Primary infection causes chickenpox and results in a lifelong latent infection of sensory ganglion neurons. Reactivation of latent infection causes localized form of the disease known as herpes zoster (shingles), which is not common in children.

PATHOGENESIS

The virus present in the respiratory secretions and in the fluid of skin lesions of an affected child is transmitted either by airborne or by direct contact. Viral replication occurs initially in the respiratory tract, followed by subclinical viremia. Host immune responses limit viral replication and facilitate recovery from infection. In immunocompromised children, however, viral replication continues with resultant injury to lungs, brain, and other organs. Virus is transported in a retrograde manner through sensory axons to the dorsal route ganglia through the spinal cord and establishes a latent infection; subsequent reactivation of this lesion results in herpes zoster. Maximum period of infectivity is from 2 days prior to the onset of rash till all the lesions have crusted, which is usually 5 days after the onset of rash. Chickenpox is highly contagious with secondary household attack rate of more than 90% in susceptible individuals.

CLINICAL FEATURES

The illness usually begins 14–16 days after exposure, although the incubation period can range from 10 days to 21 days. The prodromal period starts as mild fever, headache, generalized body ache, and tiredness. Fever is usually moderate ranging from 38°C to 39°C. After 2–3 days, the rash appears, initially as maculopapular, which evolves into vesicles filled with clear fluid, which becomes cloudy and umbilicated, described as "dew drops on rose petals" **(Fig. 5.18.1)**. The rash is intensely pruritic, and distribution is typically central or centripetal. Lesions also occur in the oral mucosa, pharynx, conjunctiva, and genitalia. New lesions appear for 1–7 days. While the initial lesions are crusting, new crops form on the trunk and then extremities. *Simultaneous presence of lesions in various stages of evolution is characteristic of varicella.* The lesions vary in number, from 10 to 1,500, and the crests completely fall off within 1–2 weeks leaving behind hypo- or hyperpigmented marks that persist for days to weeks. Scarring is unusual unless the lesions are secondarily infected or scabs are removed prematurely.

Herpes zoster occurs due to reactivation of latent VZV infection and is uncommon in childhood and is characterized by clustered vesicular lesions on erythematous base, distributed over one or two dermatomes. Unlike in adults, severity is less except in immunocompromised children **(Fig. 5.18.2)**.

Breakthrough Varicella

Breakthrough varicella occurs in a vaccinated child when exposed to varicella virus, usually 2–5 years following vaccination. Generally, it is mild with less than 50 skin lesions, predominantly maculopapular rather than vesicular rash, low or no fever, shorter (4–6 days) duration of illness, and generally less contagious.

COMPLICATIONS

Complications of varicella are not common; uneventful recovery is the rule except in immunocompromised persons.

Bacterial Infections

Secondary bacterial infections of skin (cellulitis and abscess) occur most commonly due to *Staphylococcus aureus* and *Streptococcus pyogenes*, which can lead to complications such as necrotizing fasciitis, septicemia, septic arthritis, and even toxic shock syndrome occasionally.

Neurologic Complications

Encephalitis and cerebellar ataxia are the common neurologic complications encountered, usually manifest 2–6 days after the onset of rash, but may occur in the incubation period also. Cerebellar ataxia can appear as late as 21 days also. Condition is benign and with complete recovery within 2–4 weeks. Encephalitis is more serious and occurs in 0.1–0.25% of persons with the disease with the mortality established between 5% and 20%. Other complications include transverse myelitis, Guillain-Baré syndrome, and optic neuritis.

Respiratory Complications

Varicella pneumonia is a severe complication, which is more common among immunocompromised children, and it sets in during first 6 days after the onset of rash.

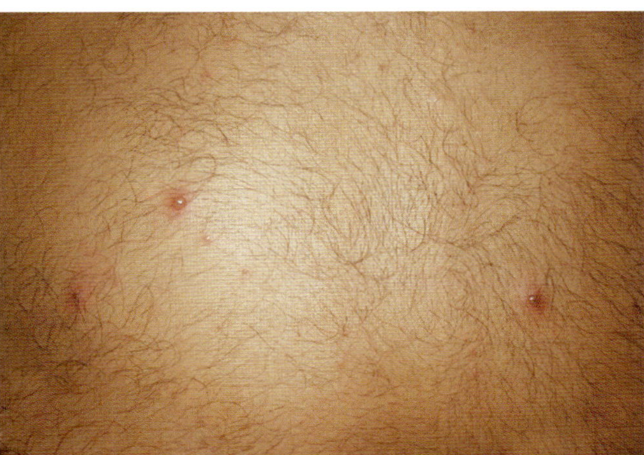

Fig. 5.18.1: Varicella rashes as "dew drops on rose petals".

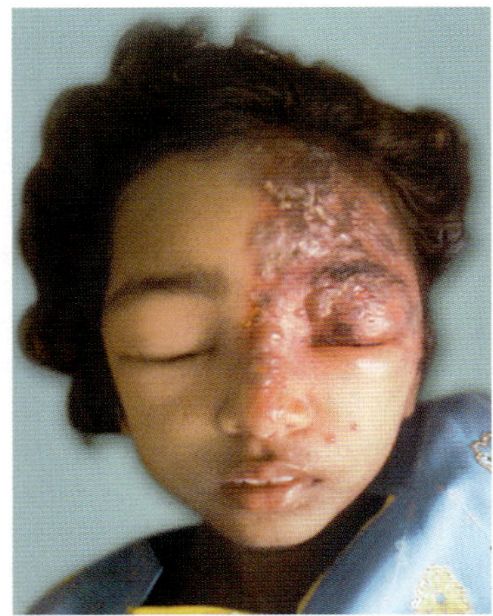

Fig. 5.18.2: Herpes zoster.

Other Complications

These include purpura fulminans, central nervous system vasculitis, autoimmune thrombocytopenia, and Reye syndrome.

Progressive varicella is a dreaded complication, which follows primary varicella infection in children with congenital cellular immune deficiency, malignancy, HIV, after organ transplantation, or those on chronic steroid therapy. It is characterized by severe visceral organ involvement, coagulopathy, and hemorrhage; and lesions will continue to develop for a longer time.

Varicella Embryopathy

Chickenpox in pregnancy is associated with increased risk of fetal malformations, especially if infection occurs in the first or second trimester. The incidence of congenital varicella syndrome following gestational varicella in the first 20 weeks is approximately 2% and is characterized by cicatricial skin scarring in a dermatomal fashion, limb hypoplasia, and ocular and brain abnormalities (microcephaly, seizures, mental retardation, etc.).

Neonatal Varicella

Varicella is associated with high mortality in newborn. The risk in newborn is dependent on the amount of maternal antibody that the fetus has acquired transplacental before birth. If there is 1 week or more intervals between maternal chickenpox and delivery, it is likely that newborn received sufficient antibody to VZV to ameliorate neonatal infection. Alternatively, if interval was less than 1 week, the newborn is unlikely to have enough VZV antibodies, and neonatal chickenpox may be exceptionally severe.

DIAGNOSIS

Diagnosis is clinical and not usually difficult in a typical case. Often a history of exposure to the disease is helpful in reaching the diagnosis. Chickenpox should be differentiated from other exanthemata such as herpes simplex, enteroviral infections, insect bites, and drug reactions.

Laboratory abnormalities include leukopenia in the initial 72 hours, followed by relative lymphocytosis. Although multinucleated giant cells can be detected with nonspecific stains (Tzanck smear), they have poor sensitivity and do not differentiate VZV from herpes simplex viral infections. VZV can be identified quickly by direct fluorescence assay of cells from cutaneous lesions and by polymerase chain reaction amplification testing. VZV immunoglobulin G (IgG) antibodies can be detected by several methods, and a fourfold increase in IgG antibodies is also confirmatory of acute infections. Testing for VZV IgM antibodies is not useful for clinical diagnosis as the kits available are generally unreliable.

MANAGEMENT

Management is symptomatic and includes antipyretics, antipruritic agents, and good hygiene. Antiviral treatment modifies the course of both varicella and herpes zoster. There is controversy in treating uncomplicated varicella in a healthy child. For healthy children <12 years, varicella is typically self-limited, and antiviral therapy is not routinely recommended as per American Academy of Pediatrics (AAP) as most of the viral replication stops by 72 hours after the onset of rash. AAP recommends treatment only in high-risk individuals such as unvaccinated children >13 years, those with chronic cutaneous/pulmonary diseases, secondary cases in household contacts, and children on oral/inhaled steroids. Acyclovir is the drug of choice; 20 mg/kg/dose four times a day for 5 days. Treatment should be initiated within 24 hours of onset of the disease to get maximum effectiveness. Intravenous (IV) acyclovir is indicated in severe varicella, neonates, and in immunocompromised individuals in a dose of 10 mg/kg 8 hourly for 7–10 days. Valacyclovir—20 mg/kg/dose three times for 5 days is also licensed for the treatment of varicella in children aged 2–18 years.

PREVENTION

Active Immunization

Varicella is a vaccine-preventable disease. Varicella vaccine, a live-attenuated vaccine, is recommended as two-dose regimen at all ages. For primary immunization, the first dose should be given at the age of 15 months and second dose at the age of 5–6 years. For catch-up vaccination, children below the age of 13 years should receive two doses at 3 months apart and above 13 years of age, two doses at 4–8-week interval. No booster is recommended.

Postexposure Prophylaxis

Vaccine given within 3–5 days of exposure (as soon as possible preferably) is effective in preventing or modifying varicella, especially in a household setting. Oral acyclovir, administered late in the incubation period, beginning 7 days after exposure may prevent/modify subsequent varicella in a healthy child.

Varicella zoster immunoglobulin (VZIG) is recommended for postexposure prophylaxis for susceptible individuals with significant contact with varicella or herpes zoster. Immunocompromised children and newborns of mothers with varicella within 5 days before delivery and 2 days after delivery should be protected with passive immunization. VZIG should be given as soon as possible but not later than 96 hours after exposure. The dose is 1.25 U/10 kg (maximum 625 U) body weight administered intramuscularly. The currently available VZIG is for IV use and administered at a dose of 0.2–1 mL/kg. If VZIG is not available, IVIG can be considered as an alternative in the dose of 400 mg/kg once.

BIBLIOGRAPHY

1. American Academy of Pediatrics. Varicella-zoster virus infections. In: Kimberlin DW (Ed). Red Book: 2015 report of the Committee on Infectious Diseases, 30th edition. Elk Grove Village: American Academy of Pediatrics; 2015. pp. 846.
2. LaRussa PS, Marin M. Varicella zoster virus. In: Kliegman RM, Jenson HB, Behrman RE, Stanton BF (Eds). Nelson Textbook of Pediatrics, 20th edition. New Delhi: Elsevier; 2015. pp. 1580-3.
3. UpToDate. (2018). Treatment of varicella (Albrecht MA). [online] Available from: https://www.uptodate.com/contents/treatment-of-varicella-chickenpox-infection. [Accessed September, 2018].
4. Vashishta VM, Choudhary P, Kalra A, et al. Indian Academy of Pediatrics (IAP) recommended immunization schedule for children aged 0 through 18 years—India, 2016 and updates on immunization. Indian Pediatr. 2014;51(10):785-800.
5. Whitely R. Chickenpox and herpes zoster. In: Bennett JE, Dolin R, Blaser MJ (Eds). Mandell, Douglas and Bennett's principle and Practice of Infectious Diseases, 8th edition. Philadelphia: Elsevier, Saunders; 2014. pp. 1731-3.

5.19 Measles

AP Dubey

INTRODUCTION

Measles is a contagious disease characterized by catarrhal symptoms, followed by appearance of a typical rash. The incidence of measles has come down world over with effective immunization, but still it is a major cause of preventable blindness and the leading vaccine-preventable killer in children. India contributes 27% of the global measles deaths.

The World Health Organization (WHO) has started the Measles Surveillance Project in India from 2007. Measles vaccination resulted in 84% drop in measles deaths between 2000 and 2016 worldwide. In 2016, about 85% of the world's children received one dose of measles vaccine by their first birthday through routine health services—up from 72% in 2000. During 2000–2016, measles vaccination prevented an estimated 20.4 million deaths making measles vaccine one of the best buys in public health. In 2016, there were 89,780 measles deaths globally—marking the first year measles deaths have fallen below 100,000 per year. The 11 member states of WHO South-East Asia Region committed to eliminate measles by 2020. In phased manner, the Government of India is working on this goal and has introduced two-dose strategy for measles vaccine in the routine immunization. Molecular epidemiology of measles in India has been considerably growing and would be useful for understanding the circulation of wild-type measles in pre- and postelimination period.

ETIOLOGY

Measles is caused by a RNA virus, of genus *Morbillivirus*, of the family Paramyxoviridae. Only one serotype of measles is known.

Measles is seen in early childhood in the developing countries. The disease usually occurs in infants below 3 years of age. Infants are usually protected till the age of 4–6 months due to immunity acquired transplacentally from mother. Usually these antibodies are undetectable by the age of 9 months but antibodies may persist up to 12 months of age. The disease runs a mild course in healthy children, whereas the disease is severe in malnourished children. Transmission occurs either by direct contact or droplet spray. The period of infectivity is 4 days before and 4 days after the appearance of rash. It is rarely subclinical. It is highly contagious, and secondary attack rate is approximately 90% in susceptible household contacts.

PATHOGENESIS

Measles virus enters the human body through the respiratory epithelium of the nasopharynx. The virus replicates initially in these cells including the epithelial cells lining the buccal mucosa and conjunctiva. Later it spreads to the regional lymph nodes. Further replication of the virus leads to the primary viremia with seeding of the cells of the reticuloendothelial system. Infection of these cells leads to the secondary viremia, whereby the measles virus is disseminated throughout the body, coincident with the clinical manifestations of the disease. Measles causes immunosuppression, which may persist for weeks to months and predisposes individuals to severe bacterial infection.

CLINICAL MANIFESTATIONS

The clinical course of measles can be divided into four stages:
1. Incubation period
2. Prodromal stage
3. Catarrhal stage
4. Postmeasles stage of complications

The *incubation period* ranges from 10 days to 12 days. In the later part of incubation period, the child shows prodromal symptoms, which last for 2–4 days and consist of fever, malaise, coryza, and tracheobronchitis.

At the end of *prodromal phase*, the child gets fever, which may be high grade. Koplik's spots, which are pathognomonic sign of measles, are seen on days 2–3 of fever. These are grayish white or bluish white dots with reddish areola. Occasionally they are hemorrhagic, mostly seen on buccal mucosa opposite lower molars but may be seen all over the buccal mucosa. Conjunctival congestion and photophobia are also classical of measles, which occur before Koplik's spots appear. Temperature rises abruptly as rash appears and often reaches 40°C or higher.

Rash appears on 4th–6th days of fever. It starts as faint erythematous maculopapular rash on upper lateral aspect of neck and typically behind the ears and increasingly involves face then spreading on to trunks and then to legs and arms over the next 3–4 days. By the time rash appears on feet, it starts disappearing from face and fades down in the same pattern. Temperature also suddenly normalizes, once rash starts fading and child suddenly looks well from sick look. The severity of disease is directly related to the extent and confluence of rash. In severe cases, rash may become hemorrhagic. The rash fades in the next 3–4 days. As the rash disappears, it leaves behind the brownish desquamation and brownish discoloration characteristic of postmeasles state and disappears in 7–10 days.

COMPLICATIONS

Measles can affect various systems in the body resulting in following complications:

- *Respiratory system:* Postmeasles bronchopneumonia, empyema, mediastinal and subcutaneous emphysema, and flaring of pulmonary tuberculosis;
- *Gastrointestinal tract:* Diarrheal episodes are quite common after measles;
- *Ear-nose-throat:* Otitis media;
- *Central nervous system:* Measles encephalitis and encephalopathy;
- *Subacute sclerosing panencephalitis:* It is a degenerative disease of the brain caused by a persistent infection with measles virus. It can manifest several years (usually 7 years) after measles infection. The patient develops progressive personality changes, developmental retardation, myoclonic seizures, and motor disability. Measles virus has been isolated from the brain tissue of such patients. Their sera and cerebrospinal fluid show a high titer of measles-specific antibodies;
- *Eye:* Keratitis;
- *Cancrum oris (Noma) and stomatitis*;
- *Systemic:* Acute malnutrition, secondary bacterial infections, such as septicemia with *Streptococcus*, etc.

PROGNOSIS

In the developing countries, measles has a devastating course with a mortality of 1–3% and may go up during epidemics up to 5–15% with a high rate of complications.

MANAGEMENT

Management is mainly supportive. The child may be given antipyretics, fluids, and antihistamines during acute phase. No antiviral therapy is available. The child may be isolated for the period of infectivity. There is inverse correlation between serum retinol concentration and measles severity. A single dose of vitamin A 100,000 U orally for children, 6–12 months of age and 200,000 U orally for more than 1 year of age children reduces mortality. Antibiotics may be indicated if there is evidence of otitis media or bacterial pneumonia.

PREVENTION

Isolation of the patient from 7th day of exposure to 5 days after rash appearance is recommended.

Measles Vaccine

Measles can be effectively prevented by *measles vaccine*. The newborn baby is protected by transplacentally acquired maternal antibodies. The antibody gradually wanes and the infant becomes susceptible to measles starting from 6 months of age. By 9–12 months of age, most infants become susceptible. At this age, live-attenuated measles vaccine offers good protection. Vaccine that is not reconstituted remains viable for 2 years at 2–8°C, but once reconstituted, it should be used within 4 hours as vaccine does not contain any preservative or antibiotic.

Measles vaccine is a potent and effective vaccine with a seroconversion rate of 95–98%. As per National Immunization Program in India and EPI policy, first dose of measles vaccine is given as *measles and rubella* vaccine at 9 months of age as 0.5 mL subcutaneous injection, followed by a second dose at 15–18 months of age. The highly infectious nature of measles virus requires maintenance of very high levels of population immunity through high routine coverage. Measles remains widespread in India because of delayed implementation of mass vaccination campaigns.

Measles, mumps, and rubella (MMR) vaccine contains MMR vaccine. The global recommendation now is two doses for MMR vaccine—the first dose at 15 months and the second at 4–6 years. It will be ideal to administer the second dose at 5th year along with diphtheria, tetanus, pertussis booster and oral polio vaccine. Indian Academy of Pediatrics Advisory Committee on Vaccination and Immunization Practices recommends three-dose MMR vaccines at 9 months, 15 months, and at 4–6 years.

Measles vaccine is contraindicated in pregnancy, children with primary immunodeficiency, untreated tuberculosis, cancer, organ transplantation or those receiving long-term immunosuppressive therapy, or severely immunocompromised HIV-infected children.

Postexposure Prophylaxis

For a child, less than 6 months of age (mother usually immune in India), there is no need for prophylaxis as child is already protected from passively transferred maternal antibodies.

- For a child of 6–12 months age, if unimmunized, vaccinate with measles vaccine within 72 hours.
- For a child more than 12 months age, if unimmunized, vaccinate with measles or MMR vaccine within 72 hours of exposure.
- For immunocompromised child, give 0.5 mL/kg immunoglobulin (maximum 15 mL) intramuscular irrespective of immunity status.

BIBLIOGRAPHY

1. Bhargava I. Measles. In: Control of Measles, Mumps and Rubella, 1st edition. New Delhi: BI Churchill Livingstone; 1995.
2. Centers for Disease Control and Prevention. Epidemiology and Prevention of Vaccine-preventable Diseases, 10th edition. Georgia: Department of Health and Human Services, CDC; 2007.
3. WHO SEARO. (2018). India EPI Fact Sheets, 2018, countryfact sheet. Geneva: WHO SEARO; 2018.

5.20 Mumps

Jaydeep Choudhury

INTRODUCTION

Mumps is an acute viral infection, which is characterized by swelling of one or more of the salivary glands, most commonly the parotid glands. It generally occurs in children and young adults. The salivary glands, the pancreas, the testes or ovary, the brain, the breast, the liver, the joints, and the heart are the organs which are usually affected by the virus. About one-third of infections do not cause clinically apparent cervical gland swelling and manifest only as respiratory infection.

ETIOLOGY

Mumps virus is a ribonucleic acid virus of the genus *Paramyxovirus* in the family Paramyxoviridae. Only one serotype of mumps virus is known.

EPIDEMIOLOGY

The mumps virus is endemic worldwide, it also occurs in small epidemics. The only known host is the human. In unimmunized population, epidemics tend to occur every 2–5 years, throughout the year but often with a peak in late winter or early spring.

ETIOPATHOGENESIS

The mumps virus is transmitted by infected respiratory tract secretions such as saliva, through airborne droplets, by direct contact, fomites contaminated by saliva, and possibly by urine. The secondary infection rates in susceptible populations have been as high as 80%. The period of maximum communicability extends from 1–2 days before the onset of symptoms to 5 days thereafter. The incubation period is 2–4 weeks, average 16–18 days. The virus proliferates in the upper respiratory tract epithelium and then enters circulation. Viremia occurs after 12–25 days and lasts for 3–5 days. During viremia, the virus spreads to multiple tissues. It then localizes in glandular and neural tissue. Infection with the virus or immunization is thought to confer lifelong immunity.

CLINICAL FEATURES

Symptoms begin acutely with fever, malaise, and headache to be followed parotitis, which is the most common manifestation and occurs in 30–40% of infected persons. It may involve one or both the glands. Earache, jaw tenderness with chewing, and dry mouth are among the presenting complaints that worsen over the next several days. Sucking a sour stimulus produces significant worsening of the pain. The swelling is at the angle of the jaw and obliterates the angle, often extending to the lower portion of the ear, which may be lifted upward and outward. Defervescence and resolution of parotid tenderness takes about a week. The orifice of the Stensen's duct is commonly red and swollen.

The submaxillary and sublingual glands are involved less often and may be without parotid swelling. Presternal pitting edema has been described due to lymphatic obstruction.

Other than parotitis, orchitis is the second common feature in adolescent and postpubertal males but uncommon in prepubescent males. Epididymo-orchitis, bilateral in 30%, usually occurs 1–2 weeks after parotitis, but it may occur without parotitis. Symptoms begin abruptly with testicular swelling and tenderness and associated nausea, vomiting, and headache. The testicle may enlarge three or four times and become very tender. Some degree of atrophy develops in nearly half of the affected organs, but sterility is uncommon. Oophoritis in girls is much uncommon and may cause lower abdominal pain but does not lead to sterility.

The central nervous system (CNS) involvement, both in children and adults, is characterized by aseptic meningitis that occurs in 1–10% of patients. Meningeal symptoms may develop anytime between a week before and several weeks after the parotitis. Pleocytosis of cerebrospinal fluid (CSF) with lymphocytic predominance of about 500 cells is usual, but total white cell counts may rise to over 2,000 in the spinal fluid. CSF glucose is usually normal but may be low at times and the protein is normal or slightly elevated. These findings revert to normal after about a week and sequels are uncommon.

Encephalitis is rare, but it can be very serious with seizures and cortical blindness. Recovery is usually complete. Occasionally meningitis or encephalitis may occur without manifest parotitis. Aqueductal stenosis and hydrocephalus have been associated with mumps infection. Other CNS problems include transverse myelitis, cerebellar ataxia, facial palsy, and Guillain-Barré syndrome (GBS).

Mumps pancreatitis may be present with pain abdomen, but diagnosis is difficult as serum amylase is elevated both in parotitis and pancreatitis, but serum lipase is normal in former and elevated in later.

WHO (2016) Mumps Case Definition

Clinical case definition: Acute onset of unilateral or bilateral tender, self-limited swelling of the parotid or other salivary gland, lasting 2 or more days, and without other apparent cause.

Laboratory criteria for diagnosis:
- Isolation of mumps virus from a clinical specimen *OR*
- Seroconversion or significant (at least fourfold) rise in serum mumps immunoglobulin G *OR*
- Positive serological test for mumps-specific immunoglobulin M antibodies.

Case definition:
- *Clinical case:* A case that meets the clinical case definition.
- *Laboratory confirmed:* A case that meets the clinical case definition and is laboratory confirmed.
- *Epidemiologically confirmed:* A case that meets the clinical case definition and is linked epidemiologically to a laboratory confirmed case.

COMPLICATIONS

Central nervous system is commonly affected by mumps infection, and it is also the most common site of mumps affection after the salivary glands. Usually it presents as benign aseptic meningitis, seen in about 10% cases. But it may also present as meningoencephalitis. Other manifestations include ataxia, acute disseminated encephalomyelitis, auditory nerve involvement, and GB syndrome.

Pancreatitis is a manifestation of mumps and occurs in approximately 5% of the patients. Infection with mumps virus has been implicated as a possible cause of juvenile onset of diabetes but causal link has not been proven.

There is no evidence of impairment of fertility in postpubertal girls with oophoritis. Other complications include myocarditis, deafness—unilateral or bilateral (transient or permanent), arthritis, optic neuritis, and thyroiditis have been reported.

Deafness caused by mumps virus may be unilateral in about 80%. It may be associated with vestibular reactions. Onset is usually sudden and results in permanent hearing impairment.

Electrocardiogram changes typical of myocarditis are seen in 3–15% of patients with mumps. Usually there is complete recovery.

Arthralgia, arthritis, and nephritis are other less common complications.

DIAGNOSIS

Virus Isolation

Mumps virus can be isolated in cell culture inoculated with buccal swab, throat washing, saliva, or CSF.

Serologic Tests

These are rarely done, but it is possible to identify infection acutely by detecting antibodies to the "S" antigen by complement fixation antibody titers which rise in the first week of illness, and "V" antigen by complement fixation antibody titers that follow with a rise several weeks later and may persist at low levels for years. Neutralizing and hemagglutination inhibiting antibodies appear during convalescence.

MANAGEMENT

There is no specific treatment. The majority of cases resolve within 2 weeks. Symptomatic and supportive treatment includes simple analgesics, such as paracetamol. Mumps immunoglobulin treatment is of no value.

PROGNOSIS

Mumps is a self-limited disease, and prognosis is generally good in children.

PREVENTION

The live-attenuated mumps virus vaccine strains include Leningrad-Zagreb, Leningrad-3, Jeryl-Lynn, RIT 4385, or Urabe AM9 strains and are grown in chick embryo or human diploid cell cultures. The measles, mumps, and rubella (MMR) vaccines are supplied in lyophilized form and should be frozen for long-term storage. In the clinic, these vaccines can be stored at 2–8°C. The vaccines should be protected from light. Reconstituted vaccine should be stored at 2–8°C, protected from light, and used within 4–6 hours. Immunization is indicated at 9 months and 15 months of age in combination with measles and rubella vaccination. The dose is 0.5 mL subcutaneously. The vaccine can be given along with all other childhood vaccines except bacillus Calmette-Guérin (BCG) vaccine. The virus does not spread from vaccinee to contacts. Mumps-containing vaccines should be given at least 2 weeks before or 3 months after administration of immunoglobulins or blood transfusion. There is theoretical possibility that antibody will neutralize vaccine virus and interfere with seroconversion.

Patients who have received high dose of corticosteroid (greater than 2 mg/kg/day or greater than 20 mg/day of prednisolone or equivalent) for 14 days or more and who are otherwise not immunocompromised, mumps-containing vaccines should be given at least 1 month after the discontinuation of corticosteroid.

Mumps vaccine is live-attenuated vaccine, available as a part of the combined MMR vaccine. As per Indian Academy of Pediatrics, Advisory Committee on Vaccines and Immunization Practices guidelines, three doses for MMR vaccines are recommended, the first dose at 9 months, the second at 15–18 months, and the third at 4–6 years of age. Those who have missed MMR vaccine, two doses of catch-up vaccine may be given at any age at 8-week interval.

BIBLIOGRAPHY

1. American Academy of Pediatrics. Mumps. In: Red Book 2009: report of the Committee on Infectious Diseases, 28th edition. New Delhi: Jaypee Brothers Medical Publishers; 2009. pp. 468-72.
2. Atkinson W, Homborsky J, McIntyre L, et al. Epidemiology and Prevention of Vaccine-preventable Diseases, 10th edition. Washington, DC: Department of Health and Human Services, Centers for Disease Control and Prevention; 2007. pp. 149-54.
3. Choudhury J. Mumps. In: Parthasarathy A, Menon PSN, Gupta P, Nair MKC, (Eds). IAP Textbook of Pediatrics, 5th edition. New Delhi: Jaypee Brothers Medical Publishers; 2013. pp. 241-3.
4. Caroll KC, Hobden JA, Miller S, et al. Mumps virus infections. In: Brooks GF, Morse SA, Caroll KC, Mietzner TA, Butel JS, (Eds). Jawetz, Melnick and Adelberg's Medical Microbiology, 25th edition. New York: McGraw Hill Medical; 2010. pp. 563-5.
5. Vashishtha VM, Choudhary J, Jog P, et al. Indian Academy of Pediatrics (IAP) recommended immunization schedule for children aged 0 through 18 years—India, 2014 and updates on immunization. Indian Pediatr. 2016;51:785-800.
6. World Health Organization. Recommended surveillance standard of mumps. [Online] Available from: www.who.int/immunization. [Accessed September, 2018].

5.21 Rubella

Nupur Ganguly

INTRODUCTION

The name "*Rubella*" is derived from the Latin, meaning *little red*. The disease was first described by German physicians in the mid-18th century; hence, it is also known as *German measles*. This disease is often mild and attacks pass unnoticed as trivial infection. The disease may last 1–3 days with children recover faster than adults. Its importance lies in its teratogenic effects. Infection during early pregnancy may cause fetal death or congenital rubella syndrome (CRS).

EPIDEMIOLOGY

Humans are the only natural host of rubella virus. The virus is transmitted by aerosol droplets from person to person and transplacentally causing CRS. Volunteer studies have shown that the virus remains in the nasopharynx from 7 days before to 14 days after the onset of rash. It replicates in the mucosal cells of upper respiratory tract and spreads to the regional lymph nodes, especially the posterior auricular and the suboccipital group. Small number of infants with congenital rubella can continue to shed the virus in nasopharyngeal secretions and urine and can transmit infection to susceptible contacts.

Secondary attack rate is 50–60% in family contacts and almost 100% in closed populations, such as institutions or military barracks.

Reliable statistics on CRS are rare in the developing countries. The World Health Organization (WHO) estimates that worldwide more than 100,000 children are born with CRS each year, and most of them are in the developing countries. Data regarding the prevalence of rubella in India is scarce. Serosurveys have shown that 8–47% of women are susceptible to rubella infection.

ETIOLOGY

The rubella virus is a cubical, medium-sized (70 nm) virus. It is a ribonucleic acid (RNA) virus of the genus *Rubivirus* in the family Togaviridae. A capsid protein surrounds the viral RNA. The virus has two transmembrane proteins, E1 and E2. Only one serotype has been identified.

CLINICAL MANIFESTATIONS

The incubation period is 14–21 days. Initial prodromal symptoms include malaise, headache, mild catarrhal symptoms, and low-grade fever. Most characteristic features are retroauricular, posterior cervical and suboccipital lymphadenopathy. Discrete rose-colored spots on the soft palate (Forchheimer spots) may be seen in approximately 20% patients before the onset of skin rash. Skin rash is mostly discrete maculopapular but quite variable in size and confluence. It starts on face and spreads rapidly over trunk. Progression is so fast that by the third day it usually clears up without significant desquamation. Occasionally conjunctivitis is seen. In women and young girls, arthralgia and polyarthritis may occur. Any joint can be involved but small joints of hand are affected most frequently lasting for few days to few weeks and leaves no sequelae.

Congenital Rubella Syndrome

In pregnant women, rubella virus can cross the placenta and infect the developing embryo or the fetus resulting in various congenital malformations. The exact nature and extent of these malformations depend on the gestational age of the affected fetus. The risk for congenital defects is greatest with primary maternal infection. Congenital defects occur in about 90% infants if maternal infection occurs before 11 weeks of pregnancy and about 10–20% by the end of the first trimester. CRS may result in spontaneous abortion or birth of a severely malformed baby. Maternal infection after 16th week is associated with low-risk of congenital defects.

Classically, the CRS includes a triad of malformations, cataract, sensorineural hearing loss, and congenital heart disease. It may also be a disease with multisystemic involvement, a wide spectrum of clinical expression, and long postnatal period of active infection with shedding of viruses. It can also lead to intrauterine growth retardation, microphthalmia, microcephaly, and mental and motor retardation **(Table 5.21.1)**.

Though the exact burden of CRS in India is not known, it is one of the most important causes of preventable blindness and deafness in the country.

DIAGNOSIS

Confirmation is by serology or viral culture. Virus can be isolated from throat and urine from 1 week before to 2 weeks after the onset of rash. Congenital rubella is associated with

Table 5.21.1: Main clinical manifestations of congenital rubella syndrome.

General: • Fetal loss (spontaneous abortion and stillbirths) • Low birth weight • Micrognathia
Ears and central nervous system: • *Sensorineural deafness*: Unilateral or bilateral • Central auditory deafness • Mental retardation • Speech defects
Cardiovascular system: • Patent ductus arteriosus • Pulmonary arterial stenosis • Ventricular septal defect
Eyes: • Retinopathy • *Cataracts*: Pearly, dense, nuclear; 50% bilateral; always accompanied by retinopathy • Microphthalmos
Transient neonatal manifestations: • Thrombocytopenia which may manifest as purpura • Hepatosplenomegaly • Meningoencephalitis • Bony radiolucencies
Late emerging or developmental: • Late-onset interstitial pneumonitis, at age 3–12 months • Chronic diarrhea • Insulin-dependent diabetes mellitus
Thyroid dysfunction

low platelet counts, abnormal liver function tests, hemolytic anemia, pleocytosis, and very high immunoglobulin M antibody titer. X-ray shows pneumonitis, bone metaphyseal longitudinal lucencies in CRS.

DIFFERENTIAL DIAGNOSIS

It is often confused with mild variety of scarlet fever or rubeola. Other viral illnesses, such as roseola infantum, infectious mononucleosis, enteroviral infection, and drug rash, closely resemble rubella.

PROGNOSIS

The prognosis of childhood rubella is good, that of congenital rubella varies with the gestational age at the time of infection and organ involved.

TREATMENT

No specific antiviral therapy is available for rubella. Antipyretics are used for symptomatic relief.

PREVENTION

Congenital rubella syndrome is a significant public health problem and is entirely preventable by ensuring vaccination of prepubertal girls with rubella-containing vaccine (RCV). Rubella vaccination induces seroconversion rates of 95% or higher after the administration of a single dose. Hence, it is an excellent candidate for the prevention of CRS. The WHO rubella vaccine position paper recommends that countries take advantage of the measles platform to introduce RCV as either measles and rubella (MR) or measles-mumps-rubella (MMR) vaccine. Countries should give RCV in the routine schedule at the same age as they currently give the first dose of measles-containing vaccine (MCV). WHO global recommendations for rubella also recommends regular follow-up campaigns with MR-containing vaccines, in the countries with MCV1 coverage less than 90–95%; efforts to reach women of childbearing age; and surveillance for rubella and CRS.

Special care should be taken in reproductive females to avoid pregnancy for 3 months after MMR vaccination. However, inadvertent vaccination during pregnancy is not an indication for termination of pregnancy.

BIBLIOGRAPHY

1. Cutts FT, Robertson SE, Diaz-Ortega JL, et al. Control of rubella and congenital rubella syndrome (CRS) in developing countries, Part 1: Burden of disease from CRS. Bull World Health Organ. 1997;75(1):55-68.
2. Dewan P, Gupta P. Burden of congenital rubella syndrome (CRS) in India: a systematic review. Indian Pediatr. 2012;49(5):377-99.
3. Levin MJ, Weinberg A. Infections: viral and rickettsial. In: Hay WW, Levin MJ, Sondheimer JM, Deterding DR (Eds). Current Diagnosis and Treatment: Pediatrics, 20th edition. New York: McGraw-Hill Medical; 2009. pp. 1107-47.
4. Mason WH. Rubella. In: Kliegman RM, Jenson HB, Behrman RE, Stanton BF (Eds). Nelson Textbook of Pediatrics, 18th edition. Philadelphia: Elsevier; 2007. pp. 1337-41.
5. Sharma H, Chowdhari S, Raina TR, et al. Sero-surveillance to assess immunity to rubella and assessment of immunogenicity and safety of a single dose of rubella vaccine in school girls. Indian J Community Med. 2010;35(1):134-7.

5.22 Rabies

Krishnendu Mondal, Ritabrata Kundu

INTRODUCTION

Rabies is primarily a zoonotic disease which is transmitted to human usually by bite of an infected animal, mainly dogs. Other common household animals responsible include cats, cattle, and pigs, and among wild animals are mongoose and jackals. Two interrelated cycles—sylvatic and urban—maintain the disease, and dogs are the main reservoirs for urban cycle. With deforestation and increased urbanization, the urban cycle dependent on stray dog population has become the main force in maintaining and spreading rabies. Human rabies is highly endemic throughout the mainland of India with islands of Andaman and Nicobar in the east and Lakshadweep in the west being rabies free.

EPIDEMIOLOGY

According to World Health Organization (WHO), there are about 17 million animal bite cases in India per year of which nearly 20,000 deaths occur due to rabies. Unfortunately, most of the rabies deaths (about 35%) are in children.

Short stature of children leads to more bites in the upper part of the body which leads to shorter time for the virus to reach the brain. Playful nature and tendency to tease animals make them more vulnerable. Softer skin results in more severe injury, and finally they do not inform about the injuries because of the fear of painful injections.

Bites by domestic and peridomestic rabid mammals can cause the disease, but bites by house rats, squirrels, and rabbits usually do not transmit rabies.

Other than bites and scratch from infected animals, licks on broken skin, or intact mucous membrane may transmit rabies. Rare causes of transmission include aerosol transmission in bat-infested caves and human-to-human transmission by organ transplant (corneal transplant).

ETIOPATHOGENESIS

Rabies virus is a single-stranded ribonucleic acid virus belonging to the genus *Lyssavirus* in the family Rhabdoviridae. It is a neurotropic virus having a phospholipid envelop. The virus is rapidly inactivated by oxidizing agents, quaternary ammonium compounds, soap, and detergents.

Once it enters the human body, it replicates in muscles in and around wounds. Then as it gains access to the nerve endings, it ascends passively in the axoplasm of the nerves. On reaching dorsal root ganglia, there is further replication and the virus traverses further to the anterior horn cells of spinal cord. Once the central nervous system is involved, there is rapid and extensive replication of the virus. The incubation period of rabies in human is highly variable, as brief as 4 days to as long as 3 years (average 3 weeks to 3 months). Early initiation of the disease may be related to the size of viral inoculum, bites in head and neck region due to close proximity to brain, and in hands due to excessive innervation.

CLINICAL FEATURES

There are two distinct clinical forms:

1. *Furious rabies or encephalitic type* accounting for 80% of cases.
2. *Dumb rabies or paralytic type* accounting for 20% of cases. In both the types, initial presentation may be nonspecific with generalized malaise, headache, and fever. Some may complain of numbness or tingling sensation at the bite site. In furious type, symptoms are related to spasm of the gullet with hydrophobia, aerophobia, dysphagia, and other aggressiveness which ultimately leads to coma and death usually due to respiratory failure.

In contrast, the paralytic type starts with ascending paralysis from lower limbs. The patient lives longer with gradual involvement of abdominal muscles, upper limbs, and respiratory muscle leading to death due to respiratory failure.

DIAGNOSIS

Diagnosis of rabies is mainly clinical. Laboratory tests may be required in atypical cases:

- Antemortem diagnosis is by detection of virus or viral antigen in saliva or cerebrospinal fluid. Viral nucleic acids may be detected in infected tissue by reverse transcriptase-polymerase chain reaction analysis.
- Serological assays to detect antibodies to rabies virus are used for diagnostic, epidemiological, and to assess immunological response following vaccination.
- Postmortem diagnosis by demonstration of Negri bodies in brain tissue is pathognomonic of rabies.

MANAGEMENT

Once symptoms of rabies have developed neither rabies vaccine nor rabies immunoglobulin (RIG) will improve prognosis, and there is no specific treatment. In rabies endemic country, such as India, every animal bite is suspicious and treatment should be started immediately. As the incubation period in rabies is long, it is possible to institute prophylactic postexposure treatment early enough before the virus reaches the nervous system. Before starting treatment, it is important to categorize the exposure according to WHO recommendations **(Table 5.22.1)**.

General Considerations in Postexposure Prophylaxis

History of bite by a rabies vaccinated animal is not always a guarantee that the animal is not rabid. Animal vaccine failure does occur, and considering the fatal nature of the disease, it is prudent to start prophylaxis. Provoked bites are also not a guarantee that the animal is not rabid. After starting the vaccination, the schedule may be modified in cases where the animal is suspected not being rabid (i.e. vaccinated animal)—if it remains healthy throughout an observation period of 10 days by converting postexposure prophylaxis (PEP) to pre-exposure prophylaxis, by omitting the vaccine dose on day 14 and administrating on day 28 as per Essen schedule. However, this observation is valid for bites only by dogs and cats as natural history of rabies following bites by other mammals is not fully understood. Bites by all wild animals including mongooses should be treated at category III exposure. Bat rabies is not conclusively proved in India; hence, exposure to bats does not warrant treatment.

Table 5.22.1: Categories of exposure and use of rabies biologicals.

Category	*Type of exposure*	*Recommended postexposure prophylaxis*
I	• Touching, feeding of animals, or licks on intact skin • Contact of intact skin with secretions or excretion of rabid animal/human case	No prophylaxis if history is reliable
II	Minor scratches or abrasions without bleeding or nibbling of uncovered skin	Wound treatment and antirabies vaccine
III	Single or multiple transdermal bites or licks on broken skin or contamination of mucous membrane with saliva (i.e. licks)	Wound treatment plus rabies immunoglobulin plus antirabies vaccine

Treatment should be started as early as possible following exposure, but persons who present even months after exposure should be dealt with the same manner as recent exposure. Also infancy is not a contraindication for PEP.

Postexposure Prophylaxis

The PEP has three modalities which are of equal importance and should be followed meticulously.

1. *Management of wound*
2. *Passive immunization*: Rabies immunoglobulin
3. *Active immunization*: Antirabies vaccine (ARV).

Management of Wound

As the virus remains localized in the site of bite for sometime, wound toileting should be done even if the patient presents late. Immediate washing and flushing the wound with soap and water or water alone is essential. It should be followed by disinfection with ethanol or iodine (tincture or aqueous solutions). Suturing of the wound should be avoided, but if it is necessary, loose sutures are applied following infiltration of RIG. Administer tetanus toxoid or tetanus immunoglobulin or both as the condition demands.

Passive Immunization: Rabies Immunoglobulin

Two types of rabies immunoglobulin (RIG)—equine RIG (ERIG) and human RIG (HRIG), are available. Antiserum of equine origin requires preadministration sensitivity testing as per manufacturer's instructions as anaphylactic shock may occur. HRIG does not require prior sensitivity testing. ERIG and HRIG are available in concentration of 300 IU/mL and 150 IU/mL, respectively. The total dose of ERIG and HRIG are 40 IU/kg and 20 IU/kg with a maximum of 3,000 IU and 1,500 IU, respectively.

The total calculated dose should be infiltrated into and around the wounds. Remaining amount, if any, must be administered by deep intramuscular (IM) injection at a site distant from the vaccine site. In case of multiple wounds, if total dose is not sufficient to infiltrate all wounds, it may be diluted in normal saline as many folds to permit complete infiltration. If RIG is not administered along with vaccine, it can be started up to the seventh day following vaccination; thereafter, the vaccine itself elicits an adequate antibody response.

Rabies immunoglobulin should never be administered at the same anatomical site or in the same syringe as vaccine. Transient tenderness at injection site or mild fever occurs following RIG therapy does not require any treatment. RIG should never be used intravenously.

Active Immunization: Antirabies Vaccine

Active immunization against rabies is by administration of either cell culture rabies vaccines or purified duck embryo vaccine (PDEV). The different vaccines available in our country are as follows:

Cell culture vaccines (CCVs):

- Human diploid cell vaccine (HDCV)
- Purified chick embryo cell vaccine
- Purified vero-cell rabies vaccine.

Purified duck embryo vaccine: All CCVs are in freeze-dried (lyophilized) form and should be stored and transported at temperature range of 2–8°C. Freezing does not damage lyophilized vaccine but PDEV is in liquid suspension form which should never be frozen but kept between 2°C and 8°C. Lyophilized vaccine should be administered after reconstitution with the diluents provided immediately prior to use. Under no circumstances, reconstituted vaccine should be kept for more than 6–8 hours.

Side effects of CCV are minimal with local pain and tenderness at injection site. Systemic effects include fever, urticaria, malaise, and rarely lymphadenopathy.

Interswitching between different CCVs is not recommended; however, under unavoidable conditions, different brands may be used to complete PEP. All CCVs and PDEV should have potency (antigen content) above 2.5 IU/dose.

Vaccine Regimen

Rabies vaccine may be used either by IM regimen or intradermal (ID) regimen.

Intramuscular Regimen

The dosage of all CCVs is same irrespective of the age or body weight of the child. The vaccine should not be administered in gluteal region as fat impairs absorption of antigen with impaired immune response. In infants and smaller children, anterolateral aspect of thigh and older children deltoid region is the ideal site of vaccination.

Two schedules of vaccination can be followed which are mentioned below but the former is currently in vogue in India.

1. *Essen schedule*: Five-dose IM regimen (1-1-1-1-1) given as a single injection on day 0, day 3, day 7, day 14, and day 28.
2. *Zagreb schedule*: Five-dose IM regimen (2-0-1-0-1) given as two doses on day 0 on either deltoids or anterolateral thigh followed by one dose on day 7 and one on day 21.

Intradermal Regimen

This regimen requires considerably less amount of vaccine. It reduces the volume of vaccine required and vaccine cost by 60–80%. Vaccines which are approved by Drug Controller General of India should be used. All the vaccines mentioned previously are approved except HDCV and PDEV for ID use.

Vaccines should be stored at 2–8°C after reconstitution and should be used within 8 hours. If the vaccine intended for ID use is accidentally administered intramuscularly or subcutaneously, a fresh dose should be administered intradermally at a nearby site. Dose of 0.1 mL of vaccine, irrespective of reconstituted volume, is administered intradermally per site. This regimen also requires trained staff and will be economically viable where multiple cases are available. Two regimens are currently used which are as follows:

1. *Updated Thai red cross schedule (2-2-2-0-2):* Two doses of 0.1 mL of vaccine at different sites (one on each deltoid area) administered intradermally on day 0, day 3, day 7, and day 28. Day 0 is the first day of vaccination and not the day of rabies exposure.
2. *Thai red cross schedule (2-2-2-0-1-1):* This schedule is same as the previous one excepting a single dose administered on day 28 and day 90.

Former schedule is preferred as the chances of dropouts are much higher in later.

Postexposure Therapy for Previously Vaccinated

A child who has received full postexposure or pre-exposure prophylaxis may be given two booster doses either by IM regimen or ID regimen on day 0 and day 3, irrespective of the time elapsed between initial vaccination and subsequent exposure. Proper wound management must be followed, but they do not require treatment with RIG.

Postexposure Prophylaxis of Immunocompromised Children

They also merit RIG and ARV. Immunocompromised with category II exposure should receive RIG in addition to full postexposure vaccination.

Pre-exposure Vaccination of Children

Children constitute special risk group for rabies exposure, and the disease (rabies) is uniformly fatal. Hence, active consideration should be given to vaccinate children in endemic country like India where children very often come in contact with stray and pet dogs. Vaccine is usually administered from 3 years of age when they start playing in streets and parks.

Vaccine Schedule

- *Intramuscular schedule:* Three doses of vaccine on day 0, day 3, and day 28.

- *Intradermal schedule:* Three dose of vaccine (0.1 mL single dose) on day 0, day 7, and day 28.

Recently, Indian Academy of Pediatrics has recommended preexposure prophylaxis routinely for children who are of high-risk category. They include children having pets at home or who are perceived with higher threat of being bitten by dogs such as hostellers.

BIBLIOGRAPHY

1. American Academy of Pediatrics. Rabies. In: Pickering LK, Baker CJ, Kimberlin DW, Long SS, (Eds). Red Book: 2009 report of the Committee on Infectious Diseases, 28th edition. Elk Grove Village, IL: American Academy of Pediatrics; 2009. pp. 552-9.
2. Kundu R, Ganguly N, Ghosh TK. IAP protocol on infectious diseases in children. Kolkata: IAP Infectious Diseases Chapter; 2008. pp. 57-71.

5.23 Pediatric Human Immunodeficiency Virus Infection and Acquired Immunodeficiency Syndrome

Chhaya A Divecha, Milind S Tullu

INTRODUCTION

Acquired immunodeficiency syndrome (AIDS) is caused by human immunodeficiency virus (HIV), HIV-1 and 2. Children constitute 6% of global HIV disease burden, 9% of new HIV infections, and 11% of AIDS-related deaths and have rapid progression and a high mortality. The disease has now become a chronic disorder due to availability of antiretroviral (ARV) therapy (ART) and drugs to treat opportunistic infections (OIs). HIV infection is not only a medical disorder but also has social implications (especially in children, due to demise of parents) and economic consequences.

EPIDEMIOLOGY

World/Global Scenario

As per the United Nations Program on HIV/AIDS report on global AIDS epidemic, there were 36.7 million adults and children living with HIV or AIDS in 2016, of which 2.1 million were children below 15 years of age. In 2016, an estimated 1.8 million people became newly infected while 160,000 children contracted HIV (mainly through transmission of the virus from their mothers during pregnancy, delivery, or while breastfeeding). Annual AIDS-related deaths have reduced from 1.9 million in 2005 to 1.0 million in 2016 (a decline of 48%). Childhood AIDS-related deaths have also reduced from 210,000 in 2010 to 120,000 in 2016. Of the 2.1 million children living with HIV in 2016, about 920,000 children under age 15 (43%) were receiving ART, up from about 640,000 in 2012, 350,000 in 2009 and 85,000 in 2005. In the Asia and Pacific region, there were 5.1 million people living with HIV in 2016, of which 190,000 were children. Of these, 15,000 children were newly infected and 11,000 children died due to AIDS. There were 1.8 million orphans (1–17 years of age) due to AIDS in 2016 in the Asia and Pacific region.

Indian Scenario

India has the third largest population of patients with HIV/AIDS. In 1986, the first known case of HIV was reported amongst the female sex workers in Chennai. As of 2016, 2.1 million people in India are living with HIV of which 49% are on ARV treatment. There were 80,000 new infections and 62,000 AIDS-related deaths in 2016. Of the total infected, an estimated 40% are females and 6.5% are children. The adult HIV prevalence in India has declined from estimated level of

0.41% in year 2000 to 0.3% in 2016. HIV is more common in north-eastern and southern states of India. As of 2014-2015, the HIV prevalence figures in various Indian states were 0.29% for antenatal attendees, 9.9% in intravenous drug users, 4.3% in men having sex with men, 2.2% in female sex workers, and 7.2% in transgender people.

Modes of Human Immunodeficiency Virus Transmission

Human immunodeficiency virus infection occurs through sexual contact, parenteral exposure to infected blood or blood products, sharing of needles by drug users, or vertical transmission from the mother to child. The route of infection in pediatric population is mostly through vertical transmission. Most new adult and adolescent HIV infections occur through heterosexual transmission. As per 2009–2010 figures from India, heterosexual transmission accounts for 87.1% cases, parent-to-child transmission 5.4%, injecting drug use 1.6%, homosexual transmission 1.5%, blood or blood products use 1%, and unknown route in 3.3% cases. Rate of transmission from mother to child varies from 12% to 30% with figures as high as 50% reported from Africa. Effective perinatal treatment of HIV-infected mothers with ARV drugs has decreased these rates to below 2%. The vertical transmission can occur during intrauterine (5–10%), intrapartum (10–15%), or breastfeeding (5–20%) periods.

The overall risk of transmission without breastfeeding is about 15–25%. With breastfeeding of 6-month duration, the risk is about 20–35% and with breastfeeding of 18–24 months, the risk increases to 30–45%. Mixed feeding also increases this risk of transmission. The mechanism of intrapartum transmission is exposure to infected blood and cervicovaginal secretions during birth. Risk factors increasing the rate of vertical transmission include preterm delivery (less than 34 weeks), low maternal antenatal cluster of differentiation (CD) 4 count, high maternal viral load, symptomatic disease in mothers, more than 4-hour duration of ruptured membranes, intrapartum hemorrhage, and birth weight less than 2,500 g. Elective cesarean section delivery can decrease HIV transmission.

ETIOPATHOGENESIS

Etiology

The HIV-1 and HIV-2 belong to the Retroviridae family (genus *Lentivirus*). The HIV-1 genome contains two copies of single-stranded ribonucleic acid (RNA). At either ends of the genome, exist the "long terminal repeats," which contain the regulation and expression genes of HIV. The HIV genome includes three major regions: GAG region (encodes the viral core proteins including p24); POL region (encodes the viral enzymes including reverse transcriptase and protease); and ENV region (encodes viral envelope proteins gp120 and gp41). The gp120 glycoprotein carries the binding site for CD4 molecule. The viral tropism for CD4+ T cells reduces the effectiveness of the host immune system. Other CD4-bearing cells include macrophages and microglial cells. After viral attachment, the gp120 and CD4 molecule undergo conformational changes, with the gp41 interacting with fusion receptor on cell surface. Viral fusion with the cell membrane occurs, allowing entry of viral RNA into cell cytoplasm. Viral DNA copies are transcribed from virion RNA (viral reverse transcriptase enzyme) with duplication of the DNA copies producing double-stranded circular DNA, which is transported into host cell nucleus and gets integrated into chromosomal DNA (referred to as "provirus" which has the advantage of latency or dormancy for long period). The proviral DNA encodes production of viral RNA leading to synthesis of viral proteins required for viral assembly. The virus-specific protease is important for HIV-1 viral assembly. The HIV-1 reverse transcriptase is error prone leading to multiple mutations, thus creating wide genetic variation in the isolates. HIV-1 transcription is followed by translation. The RNA genome is incorporated into newly formed viral capsid with generation of new virus particles, which then bud off from the host cell to infect other cells.

Pathogenesis

The HIV is lymphotropic in nature. When the mucosa serves as the portal of entry, initial cells to be infected are the dendritic cells, which transport the virus to lymphoid tissues. In lymph nodes, the virus binds to cells expressing CD4+, primarily the helper T-lymphocytes (CD4+ T cells) and cells of monocyte-macrophage lineage. The infected CD4+ lymphocytes get activated in lymph nodes and proliferate (causing generalized lymphadenopathy). When HIV replication reaches a threshold (usually within a month), a burst of viremia occurs leading to flu-like illness (fever, rash, lymphadenopathy, arthralgia, etc.). A complex immune (cellular and humoral) response is mounted by the immune system of host leading to control of the viremic episode in next 2–4 months and the patients enter a clinically silent latent phase. The long period of clinical latency (up to 8–12 years) does not indicate viral latency but has very high virus turnover and depletion of CD4+ lymphocytes. Viral replication in infected monocytes may suggest their role as reservoirs of HIV and as effectors of tissue damage. CD8 T cells play an important role in containing the infection. During states of immunologic quiescence, a complex interaction of cytokines leads to a constant level of viral expression (especially in lymph nodes). With the progression of the disease, there is increase in viral replication and progressive decline in CD4 cell counts ultimately compromising immunity and leading to OIs. The progression of the disease is related to gradual disruption of lymph nodes with loss of its ability to restrict the virus; the virus thus recirculates producing high level of viremia and a rapid decline of CD4+ T cells (during later stages). When compared with adults, the disease progression is more rapid in children, the immune system is more immature with higher CD4 counts, and high viremia in perinatally transmitted HIV leads to rapid progression in infants. Lymphopenia is usually only seen in older children or those with end-stage disease. Infections such as invasive bacterial infections and *Pneumocystis carinii* (*Jiroveci*) pneumonia (PCP) are more common in children while malignancies such as Kaposi's sarcoma are more common in adults.

Clinical Patterns

Three clinical patterns of HIV disease have been described in children [prior to availability of the highly active ART (HAART)].

1. *Rapid progressors or rapid disease course (15–25%):* In these, the onset of AIDS occurs within the first few months of life with a median survival time of 6–9 months (if left untreated). OIs and neurological manifestations are common. In resource-poor countries, most of HIV-infected newborns will have this rapidly progressing disease.
2. *Short-term progressors or slower progression (60–80%):* The majority of those infected perinatally (intrapartum) have a median survival time of 6 years with slower progression. HIV-related illnesses develop by 3–4 years progressing to AIDS by 6–7 years. They present clinically with recurrent bacterial infections, failure to thrive, and lymphocytic interstitial pneumona (LIP).
3. *Long-term progressors or long-term survivors (less than 5%):* Few of those perinatally infected have minimal or no progression of disease with relatively normal CD4 counts and very low viral loads for longer than 8 years. Possible mechanisms for this delay in disease manifestations include effective humoral immunity and/or cytotoxic T-lymphocytic responses, host genetic factors, and infection with attenuated or defective virus.

CLINICAL FEATURES

The HIV infection is a disease with various clinical manifestations of varying severity. Important manifestations occurring in infancy and childhood include lymphadenopathy, hepatosplenomegaly, failure to thrive, chronic or recurrent diarrhea, recurrent pneumonia, oral thrush, recurrent otitis media, tuberculosis (TB), PCP, pyrexia of unknown origin, etc. Recurrent bacterial infections, chronic parotid swelling, Lymphocytic interstitial pneumonia, and early onset progressive neurologic deterioration are manifestations seen more commonly in children as compared to adults.

The World Health Organization Clinical Staging of Human Immunodeficiency Virus/Acquired Immunodeficiency Syndrome in Children below 15 Years

This system is used in children proven to have HIV infection to decide the severity and also to determine the need for ART. Only the common or important manifestations are mentioned below and readers are referred to the original World Health Organization (WHO) document for a complete list.

- *Clinical stage 1:* Asymptomatic or persistent generalized lymphadenopathy.
- *Clinical stage 2 (mild):* Unexplained persistent hepatosplenomegaly, persistent parotid enlargement, herpes zoster, recurrent or chronic upper respiratory tract infections, etc.
- *Clinical stage 3 (advanced):* Unexplained moderate malnutrition or wasting, persistent diarrhea, persistent fever, persistent oral candidiasis, lymph node or pulmonary TB, recurrent bacterial pneumonia, bronchiectasis, unexplained anemia or neutropenia or thrombocytopenia, etc.
- *Clinical stage 4 (severe):* Unexplained severe malnutrition or wasting, PCP, recurrent severe bacterial infections, esophageal or tracheobronchial or lung candidiasis, extrapulmonary TB, cytomegalovirus (CMV) organ infection, central nervous system (CNS) toxoplasmosis, HIV encephalopathy or cardiomyopathy or nephropathy, etc.

Immune Classification

The immune classification is based on absolute CD4 lymphocyte count or the percentage of CD4 cells. CD4 counts are relatively high in infancy and reduce steadily up to 6 years of age. WHO immunological classification for established HIV infection (2007) defines age-related CD4 values. Below 11 months of age, the CD4% cutoffs for mild, advanced, and severe immunodeficiency are 30–35%, 25–29%, and less than 25%, respectively. In children of 12–35 months of age, the cutoffs for mild, advanced, and severe immunodeficiencies are 25–30%, 20–24%, and less than 20%, respectively. For those between 36 months and 59 months, the cutoffs for mild, advanced, and severe immunodeficiencies are 20–25%, 15–19%, and less than 15%, respectively. Above 5 years of age, absolute CD4 counts are used (cutoffs for mild, advanced, and severe immunodeficiencies are 350–499 cells/mm^3, 200–349 cells/mm^3, and less than 200 cells/mm^3 or less than 15%, respectively).

Opportunistic Infections

With gradual deterioration of the immune system, children are at a high risk for infections from bacteria, viruses, fungi, and protozoa. These opportunistic infection (OIs) need to be diagnosed and treated early to prevent morbidity and mortality. Young children generally have primary infection and owing to lack of prior immunity, the infections often have a more fulminant course. Some important OIs are discussed here. Other OIs are summarized in **Table 5.23.1**. **Table 5.23.2** enlists the drugs used for primary and secondary prophylaxis for OIs.

Recurrent Bacterial Infections

About 20% of AIDS-defining illnesses in children are due to recurrent bacterial infections caused by *Streptococcus*

Table 5.23.1: Opportunistic infections in HIV infection: clinical manifestations, diagnosis, and treatment.

Infectious agent	*Clinical features*	*Diagnostic test(s)*	*Treatment*
Pneumocystis carinii (Jiroveci)	Manifests with fever, cough, breathlessness, cyanosis, tachypnea, fine rales, etc.	Demonstration of trophozoite (Wright stain) on specimen obtained by BAL or in sputum or tracheal secretion/ lung biopsy. Chest radiograph shows interstitial infiltrates or diffuse alveolar disease. High level of lactate dehydrogenase	TMP-SMX *Alternatives:* • Pentamidine, primaquine/ clindamycin • Dapsone/Trimethoprim • Steroids (adjuvant therapy)
Mycobacterium tuberculosis	Organ-specific manifestations	Demonstration of organism, specific histopathological features, and supportive evidence in the form of contact tracing, chest radiograph, and Mantoux test (>5 mm positive)	Antituberculous therapy (with extended duration, if required)
MAC nontuberculous, especially with CD4 count below 100 cells/mm^3 (*M. avium, M. intracellulare, M. paratuberculosis*)	• Isolated lymphadenitis or disseminated (involvement of lungs, liver, spleen, bone marrow, and GI tract) • Recurrent fever, malaise, weight loss, night sweats, chronic diarrhea, recurrent abdominal pain, etc.)	• Isolation of organism or culture (blood/biopsy) with typical histopathological features on biopsy of lymph node, bone marrow, or other tissues • Species differentiation by DNA probe assays • Associated laboratory features such as disproportionate anemia, neutropenia, leukopenia, and raised alkaline phosphatase	• Clarithromycin or azithromycin and ethambutol • Combination of 2 or more drugs for at least 18 months • Disseminated disease needs 3–4 drugs. Third drug (rifabutin) or alternative (levofloxacin/ciprofloxacin and/or amikacin, streptomycin) given till improvement followed by 2 drugs
HSV	• Neonates (HSV2 commoner) and manifestations are in CNS, skin, or mouth • Postneonatal period, common manifestations are gingivostomatitis, genital ulcers, HSV encephalitis, or systemic disease	• Clinical diagnosis by typical ulcers • Isolation of virus in culture • Detection of HSV 1 or 2 antigens from skin or mucosal scrapings by IF technique • HSV-DNA in CSF by PCR (especially in HSV encephalitis) • Rising titers of HSV-1 and 2 antibodies	Acyclovir *Neonatal period:* • 21 days for CNS involvement and disseminated disease • 14 days for skin, eye, and mouth involvement *Postneonatal period:* • 21 days for disseminated/CNS disease • 7–14 days for mild gingivostomatitis and genital herpes
VZV	Severe infection, mucosal involvement, visceral dissemination (pneumonitis, hepatitis, encephalitis, retinitis), recurrent, persistent, and chronic infections	Clinical picture is classical. Tzanck smear (cell scrapings), VZV antigen (lesions) viral isolation (culture)	Isolation and oral/IV acyclovir for 7–14 days Use foscarnet in cases resistant to acyclovir
CMV (usually with severe CD4 depletion below 50 cells/mm^3) 8–10% of pediatric AIDS-defining illness	CMV retinitis, GI involvement, colitis, esophagitis, liver, lungs, pancreas, and CNS	• *Fundoscopy*: Yellowish white area of retinal necrosis with perivascular exudates and hemorrhage at the periphery • GI—Mucosal biopsy and demonstration of CMV inclusion bodies • *Endoscopy*: Small confluent ulcers	Ganciclovir for 14–21 days or foscarnet. Followed by lifelong maintenance therapy with ganciclovir

Contd...

Contd…

Infectious agent	***Clinical features***	***Diagnostic test(s)***	***Treatment***
Cryptococcus neoformans	• Subacute or chronic • Meningoencephalitis • Others—joints, bones, skin, and lungs	CSF: Elevated opening pressure, India ink preparation, rapid cryptococcal antigen assay (serum or CSF) and culture	• *Induction therapy*: Amphotericin B with flucytosine/fluconazole for 2 weeks • *Consolidation therapy*: Fluconazole for 8 weeks • *Maintenance therapy*: Secondary prophylaxis with fluconazole*
Histoplasmosis	Acute pneumonia/ meningitis/disseminated disease (when CD4 < 150 cells/mm^3) manifesting as failure to thrive, progressive fever, hepatosplenomegaly, lymphadenopathy, pneumonitis	• Recovery in culture (sputum, BAL, blood, bone marrow, etc.) • Wright stain of peripheral blood leukocytes shows fungal elements • Antigen detection, antibodies and PCR	• *Induction*: Amphotericin B • *Consolidation*: Itraconazole for 12 months
Penicilliosis	• Persistent fever, anemia, thrombocytopenia, hepatomegaly, generalized lymphadenopathy, translucent umbilicated papules • Seen in north-eastern parts of India	Isolation from blood, bone marrow, or sterile sites. Wright staining of skin scrapings	• *Induction therapy*: Amphotericin B for 2 weeks • *Consolidation therapy*: Itraconazole for 10 weeks • *Maintenance therapy*: Secondary prophylaxis with itraconazole
Toxoplasma gondii	Commonly asymptomatic CNS toxoplasmosis (meningitis with/without chorioretinitis)	CT scan brain (ring-enhancing lesions in basal ganglia, corticomedullary junction, intracranial granulomas and calcification). IgG antibodies in CSF	• Pyrimethamine-sulfadiazine (with folinic acid) • Alternative drugs—clindamycin, azithromycin, and TMP-SMX • Steroids may be added in severe chorioretinitis or CNS lesions with mass effect
Recurrent bacterial infections	Bacteremia, pneumonia, meningitis, osteomyelitis, sinusitis and skin, ear, and upper respiratory infections	• Relevant investigations to be carried out depending upon the site of infection. • All efforts should be made to isolate the causative organism	Appropriate antimicrobial therapy
Isospora belli and *Cyclospora*	Rarer causes of chronic diarrhea	Stool examination demonstrating the acid-fast oocyst, IF, and ELISA	TMP–SMX
Cryptosporidia	• Diarrhea (acute/persistent) • Other complications: Severe malabsorption, hepatitis, pancreatitis, cholangitis	Stool examination demonstrating the acid-fast oocyst, IF, and ELISA	• Fluid resuscitation • Nitazoxanide or azithromycin
Microsporidia	Chronic diarrhea with weight loss	Stool examination demonstrating the acid-fast oocyst, IF, and ELISA	Albendazole or nitazoxanide

*In children aged less than 2 years with successfully treated cryptococcal disease, antifungal maintenance treatment should NOT be discontinued. In HIV-infected children aged between 2 years and 5 years with successfully treated cryptococcal disease (meningeal and nonmeningeal), discontinuation of antifungal treatment maintenance is recommended, if the child is stable and adherent to ART and antifungal maintenance treatment for at least one year and with a CD4 cell count percentage greater than 25% or absolute count greater than 750 cells/mm^3 (two measurements 6 months apart).

(AIDS: acquired immunodeficiency syndrome; BAL: bronchoalveolar lavage; CD: cluster of differentiation; CMV: cytomegalovirus; CNS: central nervous system; CSF: cerebrospinal fluid; CT: computed tomography; DNA: deoxyribonucleic acid; ELISA: enzyme-linked immunosorbent assay; GI: gastrointestinal; HIV: human immunodeficiency virus; HSV: herpes simplex virus; IF: immunofluorescence; IgG: immunoglobulin G; IgM: immunoglobulin M; LA: latex agglutination; MAC: *Mycobacterium avium complex*; PCR: polymerase chain reaction; TMP-SMX: trimethoprim-sulfamethoxazole; VZV: varicella/herpes zoster virus)

Table 5.23.2: Primary and secondary prophylaxis for opportunistic infections in HIV-infected infants and children.

Pathogen	***Agents used for primary prophylaxis***	***Agents used for secondary prophylaxis***
Pneumocystis carinii (*Jiroveci*)	TMP-SMX or *Alternatives*: Dapsone/atovaquone/ aerosolized pentamidine/doxycycline	TMP-SMX or dapsone
Mycobacterium tuberculosis	Isoniazid	IPT for an additional 6 months after successful completion of treatment for TB
Mycobacterium avium complex	• Clarithromycin or azithromycin. Indications: CD4 counts (cells/mm^3) below 50 in > 6 years age, below 75 in 2–6 years of age, below 500 in 1–2 years of age and below 750 in < 1 year of age) Or • WHO clinical stage 4 (irrespective if CD4 count)	Clarithromycin plus ethambutol Or Azithromycin plus ethambutol
Toxoplasma gondii	• TMP-SMX used for PCP prophylaxis also protects against toxoplasmosis • Prevent exposure to cat feces, proper handwashing, and avoid ingestion of uncooked/raw meat	Sulfadiazine plus pyrimethamine plus leucovorin Or Clindamycin plus pyrimethamine plus leucovorin
CMV	Valganciclovir in HIV-infected children with severe immunosuppression (CD4 < 50 cells/mm^3 in > 6 years; CD4% < 5% in children < 6 years)	Ganciclovir or valganciclovir
Candidiasis	Not recommended	Fluconazole or itraconazole
Cryptococcus neoformans	Not recommended	Fluconazole
Histoplasma capsulatum	Itraconazole	Itraconazole
Penicillium marneffei	Not recommended	Itraconazole
HSV	Not recommended	Oral acyclovir for frequent or severe orolabial or genital recurrences Or Post-treatment in lesions of neonatal CNS, skin, eye, and mouth (6 months)
Varicella/*Herpes zoster* virus	Varicella immunoglobulin within 96 hours of exposure	–
Recurrent bacterial infections (at least 2 documented serious episodes within 1 year)	Not recommended	IVIG every 2–4 weeks
Cryptosporidium parvum, Isospora belli, Microsporidia, Cyclospora	CPT also protects against *Isospora* and *Cyclospora*	Secondary prophylaxis with cotrimoxazole (5 mg/kg/day of TMP) is recommended to prevent relapse

(CD4: cluster of differentiation 4; CMV: cytomegalovirus; CNS: central nervous system; CPT: cotrimoxazole prophylaxis; HIV: human immunodeficiency virus; HSV: herpes simplex virus; IPT: isoniazid preventive therapy; IVIG: intravenous immunoglobulin; PCP: *Pneumocystis carinii* (*Jiroveci*) pneumonia; SMX: sulfamethoxazole; TB: tuberculosis; TMP: trimethoprim; WHO: World Health Organization).

pneumoniae, *Haemophilus influenzae*, *Staphylococcus*, pneumococcus, *Escherichia coli*, *Salmonella*, *Enterococcus*, *Pseudomonas aeruginosa*, etc. Common serious infections include bacteremia, sepsis, bacterial pneumonia, etc. which account for more than half of the infections in HIV-infected children. Also, meningitis, urinary-tract infections, abscesses, and bone or joint infection may be seen. Milder recurrent infections (otitis media, sinusitis, skin or soft tissue infections, etc.) are also commonly seen and may become chronic. These infections are essentially similar to those in children uninfected with HIV; however, the disease may be chronic or severe and the duration of the treatment may need to be prolonged.

Tuberculosis

Up to 48% of HIV-infected children have been diagnosed with culture-positive TB, with disease being severe, extrapulmonary, drug-resistant, and associated with atypical mycobacteria. All forms of TB are seen in HIV-infected children including pulmonary, lymph node, and extrapulmonary TB (including TB meningitis or disseminated TB) **(Fig. 5.23.1)**. The diagnosis of TB in HIV-infected patients should be preferably made by Xpert *Mycobacterium tuberculosis* (MTB)/rifampicin (RIF) testing and drug sensitivity should be performed in culturepositive specimens, especially for treatment of relapses and failures. A Mantoux (tuberculin) test reaction of 5 mm or more is considered positive in HIV-infected children. TB should be suspected and evaluated in HIV-infected children with fever, poor weight gain, or current cough or history of TB contact. If the evaluation is negative, isoniazid preventive therapy (IPT) should be given irrespective of their age. IPT (10 mg/kg/day for 6 months) should be offered to HIV-infected children above 12 months of age who are unlikely to have active TB on symptom-based screening and without TB contact as a part of HIV prevention and care. However, in those below 12 months of age, only those with TB contact with negative evaluation of TB (on investigations) should receive 6 months of IPT. All HIV-infected children should receive IPT for an additional 6 months after successful completion of treatment for TB. Treatment of TB is with standard antituberculous therapy (ATT) with prolongation of the duration (if necessary). The emergence of multidrug-resistant TB has necessitated use of second-line drugs. In children with active disease, ART has to be started at the earliest, within 2 months of intensive ATT irrespective of clinical staging and CD4 counts. In those with severe immunosuppression (CD4 counts < 50 cells/mm^3), ART may be started within 2 weeks of beginning the antituberculous management. RIF reduces level of protease inhibitors (PIs) and nonnucleoside reverse transcriptase inhibitors (NNRTIs) and thus, dose adjustments are required in concomitant use with efavirenz (EFV) and nevirapine (NVP).

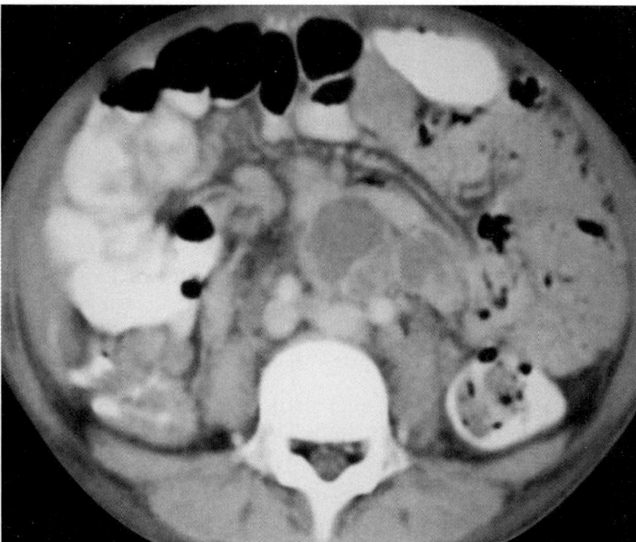

Fig. 5.23.1: *Computed tomographic scan of abdomen:* Multiple enlarged conglomerated peripherally enhancing and necrotic lymph nodes (para-aortic, peripancreatic, periportal, and mesenteric) in an HIV-infected child with abdominal tuberculosis.
(HIV: human immunodeficiency virus).

P. Carinii (Jiroveci) Pneumonia

This is the most common OI in infants (mortality rate up to 35%). The highest occurrence is at age of 3–6 months (highest mortality rate in children below 1 year). The infant presents with acute onset fever, dyspnea, tachypnea, cough, cyanosis, and marked hypoxia. Insidious onset of cough and dyspnea may be seen in older children. The risk of new infection or activation of latent infection increases when CD4 counts fall below 200 cells/mm^3 (or < 14%). The radiographic findings include interstitial infiltrates or diffuse alveolar disease (which progresses rapidly). Nodular lesions, streaky or lobar infiltrates, or pleural effusions may be seen. Presumptive diagnosis is supported by clinical manifestations, radiological findings, hypoxia on arterial blood gas, and high lactate dehydrogenase. Diagnosis is confirmed by demonstration of *P. carinii (Jiroveci)* in induced sputum or bronchoalveolar lavage, transbronchial biopsy by fiber-optic bronchoscopy, or open lung biopsy with appropriate staining. Treatment is with intravenous cotrimoxazole [trimethoprim (TMP)–sulfamethoxazole (SMX)] (15–20 mg/kg/day of TMP and 75–100 mg/kg/day of SMX every 6 hourly) with adjunctive corticosteroids (prednisolone or dexamethasone) if the partial pressure of arterial oxygen (PaO_2) is less than 70 mm Hg (in room air). The therapy can be completed for 21 days with oral TMP–SMX replacing the intravenous drug after clinical improvement. Cotrimoxazole (TMP–SMX) prophylaxis reduces the incidence of PCP infection (6 mg/kg/day of TMP). TMP–SMX also protects against development of infections by other bacteria, malaria, isospora, cyclospora as well as toxoplasmosis along with reducing the mortality in HIV-infected children. The 2015 WHO guidelines for cotrimoxazole use states that the drug should be started in all HIV-exposed infants and children at 4–6 weeks of age after birth and continued till HIV infection is definitely excluded or till risk of HIV infection ends (to be continued for 2 years in high malaria transmission regions). It is recommended for all infants, children, and adolescents with HIV, irrespective of clinical and immunological conditions, priority being in all children below 5 years of age (regardless of CD4 cell count or clinical stage) and children with severe or advanced HIV clinical disease (WHO—clinical stage 3 or 4) and/or those with CD4 < 350 cells/mm^3. Based on prevalence of malaria and serious bacterial infections, cotrimoxazole prophylaxis should be continued until adulthood in high prevalence areas, whereas in low prevalence areas, it may be discontinued in those 5 years of age or older who are clinically stable and/or virologically suppressed on ART for at least 6 months and CD4 > 350 cells/mm^3. In those HIV-infected children with TB coinfection, PCP prophylaxis should be initiated regardless of the CD4 counts and discontinued as per age appropriate criteria. Children with previous infection with PCP should be administered secondary prophylaxis similar to the primary prophylaxis; the general recommendation is that secondary cotrimoxazole prophylaxis should not be discontinued, irrespective of clinical and immune response to ART.

Candidiasis

Candidiasis is the most common fungal infection in HIV-infected children. Oral thrush is the most common presentation and its recurrence in infants older than 8 weeks of age is a clinical indicator for HIV. Esophageal candidiasis is an AIDS-defining condition and common in those with CD4 counts less than 100 cells/mm^3, neutropenia, high viral load, and coexisting oropharyngeal candidiasis. Also, extended antibiotic duration predisposes these individuals to systemic candidiasis, with severe presentation such as shock, sepsis, or endophthalmitis. Oral nystatin suspension or clotrimazole (4–6 hourly for 1–2 weeks) can be used for the treatment of oral thrush (with oral fluconazole, ketoconazole, or itraconazole used for resistant infection). Esophageal candidiasis requires treatment with intravenous fluconazole, which may be converted to oral formulation once child can swallow food. Systemic candidiasis is managed with intravenous amphotericin B or fluconazole (or flucytosine in severe invasive disease) for 14–21 days after clinical resolution and last positive blood culture.

Organ-specific Manifestations

Pulmonary or Respiratory Tract

Recurrent upper and lower respiratory tract infections (pneumonia) are common, and complications such as invasive sinusitis and mastoiditis may also occur. Bronchiectasis with recurrent secondary infections may be seen (**Fig. 5.23.2**). In addition to PCP, *S. pneumoniae*, *Haemophilus influenza*, *P. aeruginosa*, pathogens, such as viruses (CMV) and fungi (*Aspergillus*, *Histoplasma*, or *Cryptococcus*), can be the causes of lung disease. As stated earlier, pulmonary and extrapulmonary TB is an important association. *Lymphocytic interstitial pneumonia (LIP)*, a noninfectious lymphoproliferative condition due to HIV-related immune deficiency, can occur in up to 25% of HIV-infected children. It is a chronic process with progressive alveolar capillary block due infiltration of lymphoid cells in the lung interstitial parenchyma, alveolar septae and lymphatics along with pulmonary lymphoid tissue hyperplasia. Its onset is around 2–3 years of age with slow progression. Lymphocytic interstitial pneumonia manifests with insidious onset of cough, tachypnea, fatigue, clubbing, and hypoxia with minimal rales or normal auscultatory findings. Hepatosplenomegaly, generalized non-matted symmetrical lymphadenopathy, and parotid enlargement may occur. Chest radiograph shows chronic diffuse bilateral reticulonodular infiltrates (predominantly lower zones) with hilar/mediastinal lymphadenopathy. Serum immunoglobulin [immunoglobulin G (IgG)] levels more than 2,500 mg/dL have been observed. High-resolution computed tomography has value in confirming the interstitial involvement, monitoring the extent and severity of the disease. Lung biopsy is diagnostic but not commonly practiced in children. The treatment of severe disease is with systemic corticosteroids (2–4 weeks with gradual tapering).

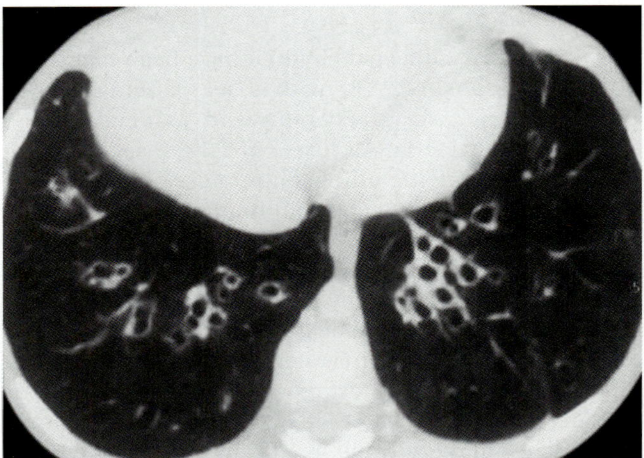

Fig. 5.23.2: *High-resolution computed tomographic scan of chest.* Note the bilateral bronchiectatic changes in a HIV-infected child. (HIV: human immunodeficiency virus).

Central Nervous System

Human immunodeficiency virus is a neurotropic virus leading to primary CNS involvement. The incidence in perinatally infected children is 50–90% in developing countries (median age of onset at 19 months). Neurological manifestations can be caused by the HIV itself, OIs, tumors, or drugs. The manifestations vary and range from developmental delay to progressive encephalopathy with loss or arrest of developmental milestones, impaired brain growth (acquired microcephaly), symmetric motor perilesional edema (tuberculoma) in an HIV-infected child, dysfunction, marked apathy, spasticity, hyperreflexia, abnormal plantar reflex, gait disturbance, loss of language or motor skills, neuropsychiatric manifestations, etc. Older patients can have scholastic backwardness, cognitive deterioration, behavioral problems, and learning disabilities. Neuroimaging reveals cerebral atrophy, increased ventricular size, basal ganglia calcifications, leukomalacia, etc. **(Fig. 5.23.3)**. HIV encephalopathy needs early initiation of treatment with HAART with drugs penetrating well in the CNS [zidovudine (ZDV), stavudine (d4T), and EFV]. Focal neurologic signs and seizures may imply a comorbid pathologic process (CNS tumor, OI, or stroke). CNS infections with TB **(Fig. 5.23.4)**, *Toxoplasma*, CMV, John Cunningham virus [progressive multifocal leukoencephalopathy], Herpes simplex virus (HSV), and *Cryptococcus*, etc. can occur.

Gastrointestinal and Hepatic Manifestations

Candidiasis, periodontal disease, salivary gland disease, oral hairy leukoplakia, and oral ulcerations can occur. Chronic or recurrent diarrhea with malabsorption, abdominal pain, dysphagia, and failure to thrive are common symptoms of gastrointestinal (GI) disease. GI disease can be caused by bacteria [*Salmonella, Campylobacter, Mycobacterium avium complex* (MAC), MTB], protozoa (*Giardia, Cryptosporidium, Isospora*, microsporidia), viruses (CMV, HSV, rotavirus), or fungi (*Candida*). Infections may be localized or disseminated. HIV or AIDS enteropathy is the syndrome of malabsorption with partial villous atrophy which is not associated with a specific pathogen and has been postulated to be a result of direct HIV infection of the gut. Disaccharide intolerance is common in those with chronic diarrhea. Maintaining proper nutrition is important in children with failure to thrive. Hepatomegaly is common (viral replication in reticuloendothelial system). Fluctuating serum levels of transaminases with or without cholestasis is common. ARV drugs [PIs or nucleoside reverse transcriptase inhibitors (NRTIs)] or other drugs used for the treatment of OIs (such as antitubercular therapy) can also cause elevation of liver transaminases. Chronic hepatitis can be caused by CMV, hepatitis B or C, or MAC and may lead to portal hypertension or hepatic failure. Pancreatitis may occur due to drug therapy [pentamidine, didanosine (ddI), or lamivudine] or OIs (MAC or CMV).

Cardiovascular System

The reasons for cardiac involvement can be prolonged immunosuppression due to HIV, intercurrent infections, nutritional deficiencies, OIs, immune-mediated reactions, and adverse effects of drug therapy (ZDV). Usually, the cardiac involvement is clinically silent. Dilated cardiomyopathy, coronary artery disease, left ventricular hypertrophy, pulmonary hypertension, and congestive cardiac failure can occur. Resting sinus tachycardia or sinus arrhythmia, pericardial effusion, cardiac tamponade, conduction disturbances, nonbacterial thrombotic endocarditis, and sudden death may be seen. Electrocardiography and

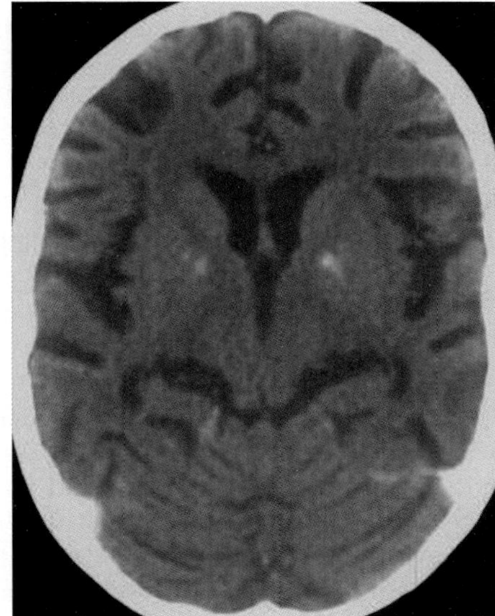

Fig. 5.23.3: *Computed tomographic scan of brain.* Note the bilateral basal ganglia calcification, generalized cerebral atrophy, and dilatation of ventricles in a child with HIV-encephalopathy.
(HIV: human immunodeficiency virus).

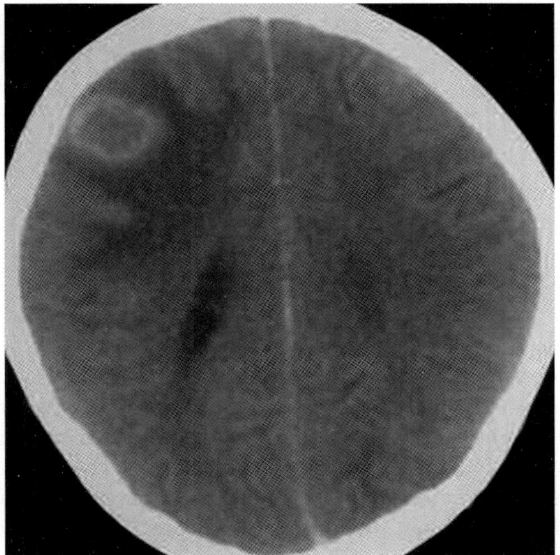

Fig. 5.23.4: *Computed tomographic scan of brain.* Note the ring-enhancing lesion in the right frontal cortex with perilesional edema (tuberculoma) in an HIV-infected child.
(HIV: human immunodeficiency virus).

echocardiography are helpful in assessing cardiac function. Supportive treatment is required (diuretics, vasodilators, and inotropes). Recent evaluation of HIV-infected children on long-term ART has revealed echocardiographic findings closer to normal, suggesting probable cardioprotective effect of ART.

Renal Disease

Nephropathy is an unusual presenting symptom of HIV infection. Renal disease can occur due to HIV infection of epithelial cells, immune-complex mediated, OIs, hyperviscosity (hyperglobulinemia), or use of nephrotoxic drugs (indinavir). Focal glomerulosclerosis (80%) progressing to renal failure in 6–9 months, mesangial hyperplasia (10–15%), segmental necrotizing glomerulonephritis, and minimal change disease may be seen. Polyuria, oliguria, hematuria, and acute renal failure have also been seen. Treatment consists of HAART and angiotensin-converting enzyme inhibitors. Nephrotic syndrome is the most common manifestation of pediatric renal HIV disease. Cases resistant to steroid therapy can be candidates for cyclosporine therapy.

Dermatological Disorders

Cutaneous manifestations seen in HIV-infected children are inflammatory or infectious disorders, which are not necessarily unique to HIV infection. The disorders tend to be more disseminated and respond less consistently to conventional therapy. Seborrheic dermatitis, severe eczema, recurrent or chronic episodes of HSV, herpes zoster, molluscum contagiosum, anogenital warts, candidial infections, tinea, onychomycosis, impetigo, and scabies are common. HIV-related characteristic conditions include oral hairy leukoplakia, bacillary angiomatosis, and Kaposi's sarcoma.

Hematologic Disorders

Anemia is frequent (20–70%) and can be due to chronic infection, inadequate nutrition (folic acid, vitamin B_{12}, or micronutrient deficiency), autoimmune factors, virus-associated conditions (hemophagocytic syndrome or parvovirus B19 red cell aplasia), and bone marrow suppression or due to adverse effect of drugs (ZDV). In those with low erythropoietin levels, subcutaneous recombinant erythropoietin may be useful. Leukopenia occurs in almost one-third of untreated cases (and neutropenia often occurs). If antineutrophil antibodies are the cause, then treatment with intravenous immunoglobulin (IVIG) is useful. Many drugs used for treatment or OI prophylaxis or ARV drugs (ZDV) may also cause leukopenia or neutropenia. Treatment with subcutaneous granulocyte colony-stimulating factor can be used. Thrombocytopenia may occur in up to 20% of patients. It may be immunologic (i.e. circulating immune complexes or antiplatelet antibodies), or due to drug toxicity or idiopathic. Treatment with IVIG or anti-D offers some improvement. If ineffective, a 2–3-day course of high-dose steroids is an alternative. ART can also reverse the thrombocytopenia. Patients are predisposed for thrombosis due to hyperviscosity (due to hypergammaglobulinemia) as well as protein C and protein S deficiency; however, clinical disease (due to venous or arterial thrombosis) is rare. Vitamin K may be used to correct coagulopathy due to deficient clotting factors (II, VII, and IX).

Malignancies

As compared to adults, malignant diseases are uncommon in children. Non-Hodgkin lymphoma and primary CNS lymphoma are known to occur. Epstein–Barr virus is associated with most lymphomas. Kaposi's sarcoma (caused by human herpes virus 8) is very rare in HIV-infected children.

Growth, Nutrition, and Endocrine System

Delay in growth and puberty may be seen due to infections, abnormalities in GI and metabolic functions, drugs, ART medications, and malnutrition. Thus, it is essential to assess nutrition and growth in all patients and counsel them on the same. The vitamin and mineral requirements are often up to five times normal and oral supplements/enteral tube feeds/parental feeding may be required. Other metabolic abnormalities include HIV-associated lipodystrophy, lipoatrophy, hyperlipidemia, insulin resistance, hyperinsulinemia, and hyperglycemia.

Other Organ Involvement

Other organ involvement such as HIV-arthropathy, myopathy, rheumatologic manifestations, etc. may also be seen.

DIAGNOSIS OF HUMAN IMMUNODEFICIENCY VIRUS INFECTION

Human Immunodeficiency Virus Antibody Detection

Since all infants born to HIV-infected mothers are antibody positive (IgG) at birth (passive transfer of maternal HIV antibody across the placenta), they cannot be used for the definitive diagnosis till 18 months of age (till maternally transmitted antibody is lost). Most uninfected infants lose the maternal antibody between 6 months and 12 months of age (seroreverters). Presence of IgA or IgM anti-HIV in the infant's circulation can indicate HIV infection (these immunoglobulins do not cross the placenta), but their assays are insensitive and nonspecific (not used clinically). In a child above 18 months of age, demonstration of IgG antibody to HIV by a repeatedly reactive enzyme immunoassay or enzyme-linked immunosorbent assay (ELISA) with a confirmatory test (immunoblot or immunofluorescence assay) establishes the diagnosis of HIV infection. Rapid HIV tests (single step with result within an hour) are also available.

Polymerase Chain Reaction, Culture and Human Immunodeficiency Virus p24 Antigen Assay

The HIV-DNA polymerase chain reaction (PCR) (qualitative test—test of choice) or HIV-RNA PCR (quantitative test—used to estimate viral load), HIV culture, or HIV p24 antigen immune-dissociated p24 are more useful in young infants for definitive diagnosis (by 1–6 months of age). At 4–6 months of age, the HIV culture or PCR can identify all infected infants. HIV-DNA PCR is preferred; about 40% of infected newborns have positive test results in the first 2 days of life, with more than 90% testing positive by 2 weeks of age.

Testing Protocols

Viral diagnostic testing should be performed within the first 48 hours of life. About 40% of HIV-infected infants can be identified at this time and many of these have a rapid progression of disease deserving aggressive therapy. In exposed children with negative virologic testing at 2 days of life, additional testing should be done at 1–2 months of age and at 4–6 months of age. A positive virological assay (detection of HIV by PCR or culture, or p24 antigen) suggests HIV infection and must be confirmed by a repeat test on second specimen as soon as possible. A diagnosis of HIV infection can be made with two positive virological test results obtained from different blood samples. HIV infection can be reasonably excluded, if an infant has had at least two negative virological test results with at least one test performed at or after 4–6 months of age.

In older infants, two or more negative HIV antibody tests performed at least 1 month apart after 6 months of age (in the absence of hypogammaglobulinemia or clinical evidence of HIV disease) can reasonably exclude HIV infection. For infants who are breastfeeding, a negative antibody test should be repeated 6–8 weeks after complete cessation of breastfeeding to confirm that the infant remains uninfected. In children above 18 months, ELISA antibody is reliable test (sensitivity and specificity above 99%). Positive ELISA should again be confirmed by Western blot test or repeat ELISA by using different kit. In developing countries, 2–3 ELISA tests (using different kits, one of which is a rapid ELISA test) can be used to confirm a positive report (same sample to be used).

Presumptive Diagnosis

Presumptive diagnosis is made in patients (below 18 months) who have symptoms and signs suggestive of HIV infection where virological testing is not available. Presumptive diagnosis is made when an infant is confirmed HIV antibody positive and diagnosis of any of the AIDS-indicator condition can be made (or if the infant is symptomatic with two or more of the following: oral thrush, severe pneumonia, or severe sepsis). Other factors supporting the diagnosis of severe HIV disease in an HIV-antibody-positive infant include recent HIV-related maternal death or advanced HIV disease in the mother and child's CD4 count below 20%. These infants can be started on ART.

Recent World Health Organization Guidelines (2016) on Diagnosis of Human Immunodeficiency Virus

The WHO recommends HIV virological testing at 4–6 weeks of age or at the earliest opportunity thereafter in all HIV-exposed infants. These include HIV-DNA on whole blood specimen or dried blood spots (DBSs), HIV-RNA on plasma or DBS, and ultrasensitive p24 antigen on plasma and DBS. HIV-exposed infants with nondetectable nucleic acid testing at 4–6 weeks should undergo HIV serological testing at around 9 months of age (or at the time of the last immunization visit) to rule out HIV infection. HIV-exposed infants who have reactive serological assay at 9 months of age should have a virological test to identify infected infants who need ART (repeat if negative or breastfeeding). Symptomatic infants should undergo serological testing and if positive, virological confirmation. Children above 18 months should be tested with serological methods as used in adults.

In all settings, children with a parent living with HIV should be routinely offered HIV testing and, if found to be either infected or at high risk of infection through breastfeeding, should be linked to services for treatment or prevention.

MANAGEMENT OF HUMAN IMMUNODEFICIENCY VIRUS INFECTION

Though there is no cure for HIV infection, goals of treatment are to achieve normal growth and development, prevent OIs and organ involvement, and maintain good health and an acceptable quality of life.

Antiretroviral Therapy

Antiretroviral therapy does not eradicate the virus but only suppresses the virus, thus changing course of the disease to a chronic illness. ART should be given in consultation with an expert in pediatric HIV disease.

Principles of Antiretroviral Therapy

It is necessary that the OIs are stabilized before initiating the ART. Suppression of HIV replication to an undetectable level restricts the selection of ARV-resistant mutants.

Sustainable suppression of HIV replication is best achieved by simultaneous initiation of combinations of ARV agents and adherence to complex drug regimens.

Drugs Used in Antiretroviral Therapy and Combination Therapy

Three main types of ART drugs include NRTIs, NNRTIs, and PIs. ARV agents are categorized by their mechanism of action (ability to inhibit the HIV reverse transcriptase or protease enzymes). Maximum viral suppression is possible by targeting different points in the viral life cycle and stages of cell activation, and delivering drug to all tissue sites. Thus, combination of three drugs, a thymidine analog NRTI [azidothymidine (AZT)/ZDV], a nonthymidine analog NRTI [2′,3′-dideoxy-3′-thiacytidine (3TC)-lamivudine] to suppress replication in both active and resting cells, and a PI [lopinavir/ritonavir (LPV/r) or nelfinavir] or an NNRTI (EFV or NVP), is effective. Doses and adverse effects of various commonly used agents are listed in **Table 5.23.3**. HAART refers to a three-drug combination (two NRTIs plus one NNRTI or PI). Most NNRTI and PI drugs are inducers or inhibitors of the cytochrome P450 system. There are syrup formulations of ZDV, 3TC, NVP, and EFV. Fixed drug combinations (which help in reducing the pill burden and improve compliance) are available through the national program. d4T and ddI are no longer recommended in first-line regimes of pediatric ART.

Adherence Issues

Adherence to treatment is a vital factor in deciding whether and when to initiate ART and whether the ART regimen will be successful. Compliance below 80–90% results in suboptimal suppression of viral load. Poor adherence to ART regimens results in subtherapeutic drug concentrations and enhances development of drug resistance (particularly with PIs and NNRTIs). It is mandatory for participation of the family or caretaker in the decision to initiate ART as ART regimens are often unpalatable and require extreme dedication on the part of the caretaker and the child. Education on drug administration, follow-up visits, relationship of drug adherence to viral suppression, and commitment of the family and the child are important in achieving success in ART treatment. Adherence support interventions recommended are peer-counselors, use of mobile phone text messages and reminder devices, cognitive-behavioral therapy as well as behavioral skills training/medication adherence training, use of once-daily and fixed-dose combinations.

Initiation of Antiretroviral Therapy and Regimens

Various guidelines are available to initiate appropriate ART regimen. Ideally, HIV-infected children with symptoms or with evidence of immune dysfunction should be treated with ART, regardless of age or viral load. Recent WHO guidelines (2016) have recommended initiating ART in all HIV-infected infants, children, and adolescents irrespective of CD4 count or WHO clinical staging with priority in all infected children below 2 years of age, in those children 2–5 years of age with CD4 count below or equal to 750 cells/mm^3 (or below 25%, whichever is less), in children equal or more than 5 years of age (and adolescents) with CD4 count below or equal to 350 cells/mm^3, and children with WHO clinical stages 3 and 4 (irrespective of CD4 counts). Also any child below 18 months of age with presumptive clinical diagnosis of HIV warrants ART initiation. WHO has emphasized on discontinuation of d4T in first-line regimens due to metabolic toxicities and encouraged use of fixed-dose combinations and once-daily regimens for ART. For infants less than 2 weeks, two NRTIs (AZT + 3TC) plus NVP should be started and changed at 2 weeks to abacavir (ABC) (or AZT) + 3TC + LPV/r. Children below 3 years of age (irrespective of NNRTI exposure) should be started on a LPV/r-based regimen with two NRTIs [ABC + 3TC OR AZT + 3TC] or NVP-based regimen [NVP or raltegravir (RAL)] if LPV/r is not feasible. In children between 3 years and 10 years, two NRTIs along with one NNRTI [EFV (or NVP alternative)] are recommended with preferred regimen being ABC + 3TC + EFV [others are ABC + 3TC + NVP, AZT + 3TC + EFV (or NVP) or tenofovir (TDF) + 3TC [or emtricitabine (FTC)] + EFV (or NVP)]. In adolescents (10–19 years of age) more than 35 kg, two NRTIs + one NNRTI or one integrase strand transfer inhibitor should be used. Preferred option is TDF + 3TC (or FTC) + EFV, alternatives being ABC (or AZT) + 3TC + EFV (or NVP), TDF + 3TC (or FTC) + NVP (or DTG or EFV at lower dose of 400 mg/day). Children with TB should be initiated as soon as possible on ART regardless of CD4 cell count or WHO clinical staging, within 8 weeks of starting ATT. While on ATT, for children less than 3 years of age, three NRTIs (AZT + 3TC + ABC) can be started and changed over to PI or NNRTI-based regimen once ATT is over. In children more than 3 years old, two NRTIs with EFV or three NRTIs may be started. In case the child is already on an ART while starting ATT, it may be modified to three NRTIs (AZT + 3TC + ABC) or continuation with LPV/r with high-dose RTV (if already on a LPV/r-based regimen) or continuation of NVP at 200 mg/m^2 (if already on NVP-based regimen) for children less than 3 years of age. For those more than 3 years already on ART, NVP, or LPV/r may be substituted with EFV or three NRTIs (AZT + 3TC + ABC) or continuation of LPV/r with high-dose RTV (if on LPV/r-based regimen). ART should also be initiated regardless of WHO clinical staging or CD4 cell counts in children and adolescents coinfected with HBV with evidence of severe chronic liver disease/cirrhosis, TDF + FTC (or 3TC) being recommended as NRTI backbone.

Table 5.23.3: Commonly used antiretroviral drugs.

Antiretroviral drug	*Class of drug*	*Daily dosage*	*Adverse effects*
AZT/ZDV	NRTI	8 mg/kg or 480 mg/m^2 (two divided doses)	Anemia, neutropenia, pancytopenia, gastrointestinal intolerance, headache, liver toxicity, myopathy, lactic acidosis, or severe hepatomegaly with steatosis, lipodystrophy, lipoatrophy
Lamivudine (3TC)	NRTI	8 mg/kg (two divided doses)	Gastrointestinal symptoms, rash, pancreatitis, peripheral neuropathy, lactic acidosis
d4T	NRTI	2 mg/kg (two divided doses)	Lipodystrophy, lactic acidosis, peripheral neuropathy, pancreatitis, headache, nausea, anemia, rash
ABC	NRTI	16 mg/kg (two divided doses)	Hypersensitivity, gastrointestinal symptoms, rash, pancreatitis, elevated triglycerides, lipodystrophy, lactic acidosis
ddI	NRTI	240 mg/m^2 (two divided doses)	Gastrointestinal symptoms, pancreatitis, peripheral neuropathy, lactic acidosis
TDF	NRTI	8 mg/kg once daily	Nausea, vomiting, diarrhea, lactic acidosis, or hepatomegaly with steatosis, chronic kidney disease, acute kidney injury, and Fanconi syndrome, decreased bone mineral intensity
FTC	NRTI	6 mg/kg (maximum 240 mg) once daily	Headache, insomnia, skin discoloration, nausea, diarrhea, lactic acidosis with hepatic steatosis, neutropenia
NVP	NNRTI	• 120–200 mg/m^2 once daily for first 2 weeks. • 240–400 mg/m^2 (two divided doses)	Hepatitis, rash, hypersensitivity, headache, fever, nausea
EFV	NNRTI	10–20 mg/kg (200–600 mg) depending on weight once a day BSA-directed dosing: Oral: 367 mg/m^2/dose once daily	Severe skin and hypersensitivity reactions, neurological and psychiatric symptoms, hepatotoxicity, potential teratogenicity
NFV	PI	90–110 mg/kg (two divided doses) for > 2 years of age	Gastrointestinal symptoms, lipid abnormalities, hepatitis
LPV/r	PI	600 mg/m^2 LPV with 150 mg/m^2 ritonavir (two divided doses)	Gastrointestinal symptoms, lipid abnormalities, pancreatitis, hepatotoxicity, ECG abnormalities (PR and QRS prolongation, Torsades de pointes)
RTV	PI	Not used individually, used to enhance other PIs, dose varies as per PI	Gastrointestinal symptoms, lipid abnormalities, pancreatitis, hepatitis
ATV/r	PI	Used in more than 6 years with 100 mg RTV in all groups and once daily; *15 kg to < 20 kg*: 150 mg; *20–40 kg*: 200 mg; *>40 kg*: 300 mg	Nephrolithiasis, indirect hyperbilirubinemia, ECG abnormalities (PR and QRS interval prolongation)
DRV/r	PI	Used in 3–10 years of age *10 kg to < 15 kg*: 20 mg/kg DRV + 3 mg/kg RTV; 15 kg to < 30 kg: 375 mg DRV + 50 mg RTV bid; *30 kg to < 40 kg*: 450 mg DRV + 100 mg RTV bid; *>40 kg*: 600 mg DRV + 100 mg RTV bid	Fatigue, headache, rashes, gastrointestinal manifestations, lipid abnormalities, elevated liver enzymes, hyperglycemia
DTG	INSTI	50 mg once daily (>12 years of age)	Severe skin and hypersensitivity reactions, hepatotoxicity
RAL	INSTI	12 mg/kg in two divided doses	Hepatotoxicity, hypersensitivity/rash, rhabdomyolysis, myopathy, myalgia

(ABC: abacavir; ATV/r: atazanavir; AZT: azidothymidine; BSA: body surface area; d4T: stavudine; ddI: didanosine; DRV/r: darunavir; DTG: dolutegravir; ECG: electrocardiogram; EFV: efavirenz; FTC: emtricitabine; INSTI: integrase strand transfer inhibitor; LPV/r: lopinavir/ritonavir; NFV: nelfinavir; NNRTI: non-nucleoside reverse transcriptase inhibitors; NRTI: nucleoside reverse transcriptase inhibitors; NVP: nevirapine; PI: protease inhibitor; RAL: raltegravir; RTV: ritonavir; TDF: tenofovir; ZDV: zidovudine)

Immune Reconstitution Inflammatory Syndrome

Immune reconstitution inflammatory syndrome (IRIS) is a collection of signs and symptoms resulting from ability to mount an immune response to antigens or organisms associated with immune recovery on ART. IRIS may present with *paradoxical* unexpected clinical deterioration in a HIV-infected patient with previously diagnosed and/or treated infection, or *unmasking* of disease clinically unapparent/subclinical infections prior to ART initiation as immune function is being restored with ART. It can occur in up to 10% of all patients initiated on ART. The incidence is up to 25% in those with CD4 count below 50 cells/mm^3. Most of these are associated with mycobacterial infections (MTB), *P. carinii*, *Toxoplasma*, *Cryptococcus*, hepatitis B and C viruses, CMV, herpes zoster, etc. It is characterized by fever and worsening of the clinical manifestations of OIs or new manifestations, typically within the first few weeks (2–12 weeks) after initiation of ART, but may also occur up to several months after initiation of ART. Deciding whether the symptoms represent worsening of a current infection or a new OI or an IRIS or drug toxicity is often difficult. IRIS is generally self-limiting and ART should be continued in those who can tolerate it with reassurance. The unmasked OI needs to be treated. Also, life-threatening reactions may require alleviation of exaggerated inflammatory reaction by short course of corticosteroids. The incidence of IRIS may be reduced by early diagnosis of HIV and initiation of ART (before CD4 falls below 200 cells/mm^3) and screening of OIs with optimal treatment prior to ART initiation.

Changing the Antiretroviral Therapy

Antiretroviral therapy should be changed when the existing regimen is failing in an adherent child (treatment failure) as seen by increase in plasma viral load (virological failure—persistent viral load above 1,000 RNA copies/mL seen in two consecutive viral load measurements 3 months apart after at least 6 months of initiation of ART with adherence support), deterioration of the CD4 cell count (immunological failure in patients on ART-persistent CD4 counts below 200 cells/mm^3 in children less than 5 years and persistent CD4 counts below 100 cells/mm^3 for child above 5 years), or clinical failure [appearance/reappearance of WHO clinical staging 3 or 4 events (except TB) after at least 6 months of effective ART]. Also, development of toxicity or intolerance to drugs is a reason to consider a change in therapy. Potential cross-resistance and adherence issues should be looked into. When a decision is made to change the ARV therapy, all drugs should ideally be changed. However, in many situations (previous ART experience, intolerance, or toxicity), this may not be possible and hence, at least two drugs should be changed based on the resistance mutation genotype (if available) or previous ART regimen used. After failure on a first-line NNRTI-based regimen, a boosted PI (LPV/r preferred with ATV/r being alternative if child > 3 months; however, there is no suitable formulation for children <6 years) plus two NRTIs are recommended for the second-line therapy. After failure of regimen containing AZT or d4T plus 3TC (or FTC), the preferred regimen is substitution with ABC or TDF + 3TC (or FTC). In case of failure of regimen containing ABC or TDF + 3TC (or FTC), the preferred regimen is substitution with AZT + 3TC. For those who have received a PI-based first-line regimen, two NRTIs + RAL is the preferred regimen for use below 3 years of age (alternative of continuing same till 3 years, then switching over to two NRTIs + EFV); while two NRTIs + EFV is the preferred regimen (alternative regimen is two NRTIs + RAL) for those above 3 years of age till 10 years. For adolescents more than 10 years of age, the preferred regimen is two NRTIs + ATV/r or LPV/r [alternative regimen is two NRTIs + darunavir (DRV/r)]. In case of failure of second-line ART, third-line ART needs to balance benefits versus risks using newer ARV medications that have minimum cross-reactions with previously used ARV drugs. Continue tolerated second-line ART, if third line not possible or provide symptomatic management with pain relief and OI prevention if ART is stopped. The possible third-line regimens are RAL (or DTG) + 2 NRTIs or DRV/r + 2 NRTIs or DRV/r + RAL (or DTG) + one to two NRTIs.

Monitoring the Antiretroviral Therapy

Clinical assessment and laboratory tests play a key role in the follow-up of HIV-positive individuals. Viral load (DBS specimens using venous or capillary blood) is now preferred to diagnose and confirm treatment failure. New WHO recommendations encourage routine viral load testing at 6 months and 12 months after starting ART and, if the patient is stable on ART, every 12 months thereafter and support stopping CD4 count tests where viral load tests are available. In the case of unavailability of viral loads, CD4 counts and clinical monitoring may be used to evaluate those at high risk of disease progression and mortality. Thus CD4 is still important to assess baseline risk of disease progression, decisions regarding initiation and stopping prophylaxis for OIs and initiating ART in settings where universal treatment is not possible.

Toxicities of Antiretroviral Therapy

Adverse reactions to ART drugs are many **(Table 5.23.3)** and should be based on report of the child on ART (or caregiver), history, clinical findings, or laboratory reports. Due to similarity in manifestations, it is necessary to rule out concurrent medications and diseases (OIs, IRIS, etc.) while considering adverse reaction to ART. Based on the seriousness of the adverse event, mild reaction (Grade 1) requires reassurance with no change in ART, moderate reaction (Grade 2) requires continuation of ART as long as possible with single drug substitution (if no improvement occurs). Stress should be given on need to adhere to ART despite some toxicity in both mild and moderated reactions. Severe reactions (Grade 3) require substitution of the offending drug with continuation of remaining regimen, while severe life-threatening reactions, such as Stevens-Johnson syndrome and lactic acidosis (Grade 4), require immediate discontinuation of all drugs while treating the event and reintroducing a modified regimen once the patient stabilizes **(Table 5.23.3)**.

Resistance to Antiretroviral Therapy

High mutation rate of HIV impairs the success of ART. Resistance to ART should be suspected in the case of multiple failed regimens or suboptimal viral load response to treatment. For some drugs (NNRTIs or 3TC), a single mutation is associated with resistance, while for other drugs (AZT, ABC, TDF, and most PIs) several mutations are needed for developing resistance. Testing for drug resistance is becoming the standard of care and should be done before initiating ART as well as changing ART due to failure. The phenotypic assay measures the virus susceptibility in various concentrations of the drug, and the genotypic assay predicts the virus susceptibility from mutations identified in the HIV genome isolated from the patient. Treatment success is noted to be higher in patients whose ART is guided by genotype or phenotype testing.

Drug Interactions

Rifampicin reduces levels of NNRTIs and PIs. Antifungals increase levels of NVP, LPV, and saquinavir. Drug interactions of ART can also occur with oral contraceptives, lipid-lowering agents, and anticonvulsants. Amongst ART drugs, EFV is not used with NVP, NVP should not be used with ATV/r, and LPV/r requires dose adjustments when used with NVP.

Monitoring

Monitoring is required in patients on ART and even those not on ART. In addition to clinical monitoring, investigations are required for monitoring the disease activity and response to treatment. Screening for HBV and HCV serology is recommended. Complete hemogram, liver functions, urine and stool examination, fundoscopy, echocardiography, and height should be done at least annually. HIV viral load testing should be done at 6 months and 12 months after initiating ART, and every 12 monthly thereafter. CD4 counts may be done every 6 months until the patients are stable on ART. Additional investigations may be required depending on the symptomatology, OIs suspected and organ involved. Checking the immunization status and looking for symptoms of OIs is required at each visit. It should be ensured that the child is on cotrimoxazole prophylaxis, and concomitant medications should be noted. Assess criteria for ART initiation at every visit and also assess the family situation.

Counseling

Disclosure of HIV-positive status of self or parents or caregivers should be done in children of school age (6–12 years old). Younger children should be gradually prepared for disclosure by incremental updating of their status adapting to their cognitive skills and emotional maturity. Counseling the parents or caretakers about the disease, course of illness and therapy is of utmost importance in treatment of patients. Decision for treatment should be taken after confirming issues of adherence in the light of understanding of the caretaker, the availability of medications, access to healthcare and socioeconomic condition. Starting ART is not an emergency and adherence should be ensured.

Prophylactic Regimens (Table 5.23.2)

Pneumocystis carinii pneumonia prophylaxis has already been discussed. Prophylaxis against MAC is required in children with severe immunosuppression (i.e. CD4 lymphocyte count less than 750 cells/mm^3 in children less than 1 year, less than 500 cells/mm^3 in 1–2 years age, less than 75 cells/mm^3 in 2–6 years age, and less than 50 cells/mm^3 in children greater than 6 years age OR in WHO clinical stage 4 irrespective of CD4 counts), and the drugs of choice are clarithromycin (7.5 mg/kg twice a day orally) or azithromycin (20 mg/kg once a week orally or 5 mg/kg daily orally). Lifelong secondary prophylaxis with clarithromycin (or azithromycin) and ethambutol is recommended in diagnosed cases of MAC. Prophylaxis may be discontinued in an asymptomatic child, if CD4% is more than 15% for 6 months where ART has been continued for more than 12 months or if child aged ≥ 2 years has received stable combination ART for ≥ 6 months and has sustained (>3 months) CD4 cell count recovery well above the age-specific target for initiation of prophylaxis. IVIG (dose 400 mg/kg every 4 weeks) has been recommended to prevent recurrent serious bacterial infections for symptomatic patients who have suffered from at least two documented serious bacterial infections within 1 year; have laboratory—documented inability to make antigen-specific antibodies; or in those who have hypogammaglobulinemia. For postexposure ARV prophylaxis, the preferred ARV regimen in children below 10 years of age (duration is for 28 days) consists of AZT + 3TC backbone [alternatives—ABC + 3TC or TDF + 3TC (or FTC)] with LPV/r as the preferred third drug (alternatives—ATV/r, RAL, DRV, EFV, and NVP as per age). For adolescents (10–19 years of age), TDF + 3TC (or FTC) is the preferred backbone with LPV/r or ATV/r as the third drug (alternative being RAL, DRV/r, or EFV).

Immunization, Nutrition, and Supportive Treatment

Immunization is an important mode of preventing infections. All routine vaccinations can be given if the child is asymptomatic or has mild symptoms. Live vaccines (varicella, measles-mumps-rubella) are contraindicated in symptomatic patients with severe immunosuppression (CD4% < 15%) or AIDS. Inactivated or killed vaccines should be preferred to live vaccines (e.g. inactivated polio vaccine instead of oral polio vaccine); however supplemental doses or revaccination may be needed after ART-induced immune reconstitution. Besides the national immunization schedule, additional vaccines such as varicella, MMR (measles-mumps-rubella), IPV (inactivated polio vaccine), pneumococcal and hepatitis A are recommended as per IAP schedule. However live vaccines should be avoided in symptomatic children, till there is improvement in CD4 counts subsequent to ART. However, immunizations may not always offer adequate protection in HIV-infected children. Counseling and psychosocial support is the cornerstone for management of HIV-infected children, whether or not they receive ART. The caretakers should be counseled about the importance of good handwashing, avoiding raw or undercooked food (prevent *Salmonella* infection), avoiding drinking or swimming in lake or river water or being in contact with young farm animals (to prevent Cryptosporidium infection), and the risk of playing with pets (to prevent *Toxoplasma gondii* from cats). Simple interventions, such as good general hygiene (including food and water), dental care, adequate nutrition (including nasogastric and parenteral nutrition, if required), balanced diet, timely immunizations, vitamin A supplementation, counseling about micro- or macronutrient deficiency, using locally available nutritious foods, plotting weight and height on growth charts, provision of safe and stimulating environment, developmental evaluation and interventions, such as occupation therapy or speech therapy, etc., can help a child with HIV to be free of infections and grow well. Early nutritional intervention is essential due to the interrelationship amongst nutrition, growth, and HIV, the nutritional needs depending on the severity and stage of disease and recent complications, such as persistent diarrhea or OIs. It is recommended that in asymptomatic patients, the energy intake should be increased by 10% of recommended dietary allowance, while in symptomatic patients, it needs to be increased by 25–30%. In severely malnourished patients, 50–100% additional energy is required.

PROGNOSIS

Better understanding of the pathogenesis with availability and access to healthcare and medications, including effective ART, has considerably changed the outcomes. In the developed countries, progression of HIV to AIDS and the mortality rate have decreased with improved quality of life. Even with partial decrease in the viral load, children have significant clinical and immunologic advantages. High viral load (greater than 100,000 copies/mL) or CD4 lymphocyte percentage of below 15% is associated with higher mortality and morbidity. In the developing countries where limitations exist, as regards availability of ART and diagnostic tests, clinical staging system can be used to predict progression of disease. Lymphadenopathy, splenomegaly, hepatomegaly, Lymphocytic interstitial pneumonia, and parotitis are the indicators of a comparatively better prognosis. Children with OIs (PCP or MAC), encephalopathy, or severe wasting syndrome have poor prognosis (75% die before 3 years of age). Persistent fever with or without oral thrush, serious bacterial infections (meningitis, pneumonia, and sepsis), hepatitis, persistent anemia (less than 8.0 g/dL) with or without thrombocytopenia (less than 100,000/mm^3) also suggest a poor prognosis.

PREVENTION

Prevention of Perinatal Transmission

Mother-to-child transmission (MTCT) of HIV (during pregnancy, labor or delivery, or after delivery through breastfeeding) is a significant contributor to the HIV pandemic, accounting for 9% of new infections globally. Prevention of perinatal transmission from mother to child has been achieved (to as low as 2%) by effective access to HIV testing and counseling, initiation of lifelong ART with support for adherence, retention, and viral suppression for mothers living with HIV, safe delivery practices, optimal infant feeding practices, and access to postnatal ARV prophylaxis for infants. In some situations, the mother may be counseled about the potential benefit of cesarean section to reduce the risk for vertical transmission. ART should be initiated urgently in all pregnant and breastfeeding women, even if they are identified late in pregnancy or postpartum, because the most effective way to prevent mother-to-child HIV transmission is to reduce maternal viral load. As the coverage of ARV medicines provided to pregnant HIV-infected women to prevent perinatal transmission has increased from 47% to 76% since 2010, so has the new infections in children declined by 47% during the same period.

The World Health Organization Recommendations for Prevention of Perinatal Transmission (2016)

The use of ARV drugs during pregnancy and breastfeeding is advocated for maternal health, prevention of infection in the exposed baby and reduction of sexual transmission. The WHO (2016) guidelines recommend lifelong ART to all pregnant and breastfeeding women irrespective of WHO clinical stage or CD4 counts. This has been implemented in order to accelerate scaling up on ART and prevention of MTCT (PMTCT) globally, ensure global access of pregnant women to ART and achieve global goals of eliminating new pediatric infections and keeping mothers alive. The preferred first-line therapy in mothers is TDF + 3TC (or FTC) + EFV. Infant prophylaxis is another component of the PMTCT, whereby WHO (2016) recommends that all infants born to mothers with HIV infection on ART should receive prophylaxis with NVP and/or AZT. In infants born to mothers at high risk for acquiring HIV (received ART for less than 4 weeks before delivery, viral load more than 1,000 copies/mL in the 4 weeks before delivery, diagnosed during pregnancy/postpartum/feeding), dual prophylaxis should be given with AZT (twice daily) and NVP (once daily) for first 6 weeks of life, irrespective of feeding practices (breastfed or formula fed). In breastfed infants who are at high risk of acquiring HIV, prophylaxis should be continued for an additional 6 weeks (total of 12 weeks of infant prophylaxis) using with AZT (twice daily) and NVP (once daily) or NVP alone. Infants of mothers on ART should receive 6 weeks of daily NVP (if breastfeeding) or 4–6 weeks of daily NVP (or twice daily AZT) if on replacement feeding.

Human Immunodeficiency Virus and Breastfeeding (The World Health Organization Recommendations)

Since HIV is known to be transmitted through breastfeeding, it is necessary to balance HIV prevention (by omission of breastfeeding) with protection from other causes of childhood mortality. Complete avoidance of breastfeeding may be ideal to prevent this transmission but needs to be weighed against the possibility of the child having infections (due to unhygienic practices and nonavailability of support systems for replacement feeding) and undernutrition (by the use of suboptimal replacement feeding), thus causing morbidity and mortality. The WHO has recommended setting of national or subnational recommendations for infant feeding in HIV-exposed children. Counseling and support should be given to the mothers known to be HIV infected to either breastfeed and receive ARV interventions or avoid breastfeeding completely to prevent transmission of HIV to the child. It is necessary to consider the socioeconomic and cultural context of the population, availability and quality of health services, local epidemiology, and main causes of infant and child mortality. Mothers who are HIV infected should be provided lifelong ART or ARV prophylaxis to reduce transmission to the infant. In countries recommending breastfeeding with ARV drugs, HIV-infected mothers should exclusively breastfeed for first 6 months, continue breastfeeding for at least first 12 months of life, and may extend breastfeeding till 24 months or longer with good ART adherence. Breastfeeding minimizes mortality due to pneumonia, diarrhea, and malnutrition in the first year of life, while presence of ARV drugs reduces risk of infant transmission. When ARV drugs are not available, breastfeeding may still provide infants a greater chance of survival, and mothers should be counseled to exclusively breastfeed for first 6 months of life and continue breastfeeding thereafter unless environmental and social circumstances are safe and supportive of replacement feeding. Mothers who decide to stop breastfeeding should do so gradually over a period of 1 month. In such cases, the infants should be provided with nutritionally appropriate and safe replacement feeds. For those on replacement feeding, it is necessary to ensure safe water and good sanitation, sufficient supply for normal growth and development, adequate hygiene (to prevent diarrhea and malnutrition), family support and access to comprehensive child healthcare.

Other Measures

Early identification of mothers with HIV (to provide ART drugs to both mother and newborn baby) can be ensured by recommended prenatal visits and pregnancy care. In addition, screening for sexually transmitted infections, nutritional support, and counseling about infant feeding and family planning should be provided. Rapid HIV testing should be provided to women in labor/immediate postpartum with unknown HIV status, to enable early ART/infant prophylaxis if tested positive. Deliveries should be conducted in facility with trained skill birth attendants avoiding unnecessary instrumentation or premature rupture of membranes. In HIV-exposed infants, at birth, the baby's mouth and nostrils should be wiped as soon as the head is delivered, infants should be handled with gloves till all blood and maternal secretions are washed off, and the cord should be clamped soon after birth (avoid milking). Postdelivery, appropriate follow-ups, linkages to treatment and postpartum care should be ensured. Infants should be provided with initial care during the first immunization visit at 4–6 weeks of age (reinforce safe feeding practices, early infant diagnosis, and ARV coverage), while mothers should be reviewed for postpartum checkup, family planning advice, and review of ARV therapy and adherence.

Indian Initiatives

The Government of India set up the National AIDS Control Program (NACP)-I in 1992 and the National AIDS Control Organization (NACO). The State AIDS Control Societies were set up in 25 societies and 7 union territories. In 1999, the second phase of the NACP-II was introduced; in 2007, the third phase of the NACP-III was initiated; and the fourth phase of the NACP-IV was in progress between 2012 and 2017. The main objectives for NACP-IV were the reduction of new infections, providing comprehensive care and support to all people living with HIV, and treatment facilities for all those requiring it. The National Pediatric HIV/AIDS initiative was launched in November 30, 2006, and till September 2016, nearly 80,634 children living with HIV/AIDS were in active care at ART centers, and 55,606 were receiving free ART. Having already succeeded in achieving the targets of the Millennium Development Goals by 2015 (over 50% reduction in annual new HIV infections and AIDS-related deaths), the NACO has developed a 7-year National Strategic Plan (NSP) on HIV/AIDS and sexually transmitted infections for India (NSP 2017-2024 with total estimated budget of Rs. 33,088.19 crores for the period), which envisions "An AIDS Free India by 2030."

BIBLIOGRAPHY

1. ACO (2017). National Strategic Plan for HIV/AIDS and STI 2017–2024. New Delhi: National AIDS Control Organization, Ministry of Health and Family Welfare, Government of India. [online]. Available from http://naco.gov.in/sites/default/files/Paving%20the%20Way%20for%20an%20AIDS%204.12.17.pdf. [Accessed October, 2018].
2. AIDSinfo (2013). Panel on opportunistic infections in HIV-exposed and HIV-infected children. In: Guidelines for the prevention and treatment of opportunistic infections in HIV-exposed and HIV-infected children. Department of Health and Human Services. [online]. Available from http://aidsinfo.nih.gov/contentfiles/lvguidelines/oi_guidelines_pediatrics.pdf [Accessed October, 2018].
3. Shah SR, Tullu MS, Kamat JR. Clinical profile of pediatric HIV infection from India. Arch Med Res. 2005;36:24-31.
4. Tullu MS, Kher A. Laboratory diagnosis of HIV infection. In: Shah I, Shah NK, Manglani M (Eds). IAP Speciality Series on Pediatric HIV. Mumbai: Indian Academy of Pediatrics; 2006. pp. 30-5.
5. Tullu MS, Thombare T. HIV and acquired immunodeficiency syndrome. In: Gupta P, PSN M, Ramji S, Lodha R (Eds). PG Textbook of Pediatrics, 2nd edition. New Delhi: Jaypee Brothers Medical Publishers; 2018. pp. 1428-45.
6. Udgirkar VS, Tullu MS, Bavdekar SB, et al. Neurological manifestations of HIV infection. Indian Pediatr. 2003;40: 230-4.
7. World Health Organization, United Nations Children's Fund (UNICEF). (2016). Guidelines: updates on HIV and infant feeding: the duration of breastfeeding and support from health services to improve feeding practices among mothers living with HIV. Geneva: World Health Organization. [online]. Available from http://apps.who.int/iris/bitstream/handle/10665/246260/9789241549707-eng.pdf?sequence=1 [Accessed October, 2018].
8. World health Organization. (2016). Consolidated guidelines on the use of antiretroviral drugs for treating and preventing HIV infection. Recommendations for a public health approach, 2nd edition. Geneva: World Health Organization. [online]. Available from http://apps.who.int/iris/bitstream/handle/10665/208825/9789241549684_eng.pdf;jsessionid=AA98EB5E5BA9F114762F0E6F0F193E21?sequence=1 [Accessed October, 2018].
9. World Health Organization (2014). Supplement guidelines—on post-exposure prophylaxis for HIV and the use of co-trimoxazole prophylaxis for HIV-related infections among adults, adolescents and children. Recommendations for a public health approach. December 2014 supplement to the 2013 consolidated guidelines on the use of antiretroviral drugs for treating and preventing HIV infection. [online]. Available from http://apps.who.int/iris/bitstream/10665/145719/1/9789241508193_eng. pdf? [Accessed October, 2018].
10. Yogev R, Chadwick EG. Acquired immunodeficiency syndrome (human immunodeficiency virus). In: Kliegman RM, Stanton BF, St Geme III JW, Schor NF, Behrman RE (Eds). Nelson Textbook of Pediatrics, 20th edition. Philadelphia, PA: Saunders (Elsevier); 2016. pp. 1645-66.

5.24 Leptospirosis

S Ramesh

INTRODUCTION

Leptospirosis is an acute febrile generalized disease whose manifestations can range from mild self-limiting disease to fatal multiorgan involvement. Leptospirosis, an infectious disease that affects humans and animals, is considered the most common zoonosis in the world. It is caused by pathogenic (spirochetes) bacteria that belong to the genus *Leptospira*. The genus *Leptospira* was originally thought to have two species—*Leptospira interrogans* which is pathogenic and *Leptospira biflexa* which is nonpathogenic. More recent research work has identified seven genomospecies of pathogenic *leptospira*, which have been divided into more than 250 serovars according to their antigenic composition.

EPIDEMIOLOGY

The rat is the principal source of infection. *Leptospira* exists as a commensal in the kidneys of rats. Other important reservoirs include wild mammals, and domestic and farm animals. The infected animals excrete spirochetes in urine for an extended period of time. Human infection occurs due to exposure to water or soil contaminated with rat urine.

Leptospirosis occurs as an epidemic in India during the monsoon and immediate postmonsoon period. It can also be endemic in areas due to exposure to leptospire contamination of stagnant water with sewerage. Recreational activities such as swimming, canoeing, and water skiing in contaminated water are other reasons for acquiring leptospirosis.

PATHOPHYSIOLOGY

Leptospira gains access to the human body through cuts and abrasions in the skin and intact mucous membranes. The primary lesion caused by the leptospire is damage to the endothelial lining of small blood vessels, leading to vasculitis with leakage and resultant ischemic damage to the liver, kidneys, meninges, and muscles.

CLINICAL FEATURES

The clinical spectrum of leptospirosis varies widely. It frequently presents with an abrupt onset of fever, associated with rigors, myalgia, and headache. Conjunctival suffusion, if present is considered an important finding in leptospirosis. According to the World Health Organization, the disease can present in one of the four ways:

1. As a nonspecific febrile illness
2. As Weil's syndrome with jaundice, renal failure, hemorrhage, and myocarditis
3. As meningitis or meningoencephalitis
4. As pulmonary hemorrhage with respiratory failure

According to The Indian Leptospirosis Society, this illness should be suspected when a child presents with history of abrupt onset fever with body ache or headache and with any one or more of the following features:

- Jaundice
- Oliguria
- Cough and breathlessness
- Hemorrhagic tendency
- Signs of meningeal irritation or altered sensorium or convulsions

Leptospirosis can occur more commonly as anicteric disease, with less severe manifestations or rarely as an icteric form which is more severe.

Anicteric Leptospirosis

It occurs as a biphasic illness with septicemic phase followed by the immune phase. Distinction between first and second phase may not always be clinically apparent.

Septicemic Phase

The septicemic phase is associated with the multiplication of *leptospira* in the bloodstream, cerebrospinal fluid (CSF), and other tissues. The child may present with fever of abrupt onset, associated with muscle pain, headache, nausea, vomiting, abdominal pain, etc. Less common findings include a transient skin rash, photophobia, and mild signs of meningism. The septicemic phase lasts for 4–7 days.

Immune Phase

The septicemic phase is followed by an immune phase characterized by the development of circulating antibodies to *leptospira* and disappearance of the organisms. There is brief asymptomatic interlude between the septicemic and immune phase. The important clinical features during the immune phase are as follows:

- Fever is less pronounced than in the early phase.
- Aseptic meningitis with abnormal CSF pleocytosis is seen occasionally among children.
- Hepatitis is characterized by enlargement of the liver, elevation of serum bilirubin with a modest increase in liver enzymes.
- Renal involvement is characterized by abnormal findings in the urinalysis (hematuria, proteinuria, and casts), azotemia with oliguria or anuria. Renal failure is the principal cause of death in fatal cases.

Icteric Leptospirosis (Weil's Syndrome)

Weil's syndrome is characterized by hepatic, renal, and vascular dysfunction in addition to the other symptoms of anicteric leptospirosis. Individuals with Weil's syndrome usually develop jaundice without hepatocyte destruction and azotemia by the third day to seventh day of illness. The liver may be enlarged, and there may be right upper quadrant tenderness. With increasing severity of jaundice, the individual is at greater risk of developing renal failure, hemorrhage, and cardiovascular collapse. Uremia, oliguria, and anuria may occur with the onset of kidney failure unless dialysis is provided. Fatalities due to icteric leptospirosis are typically due to renal failure, cardiopulmonary failure, and fatal hemorrhage.

LABORATORY DIAGNOSIS

Leptospira can be cultured from blood or CSF during the first 10 days of illness and from the urine several weeks beginning from second week. The following are the tests currently available for routine diagnosis.

Dark-Field Microscopy

Dark-field microscopy is used to detect leptospires in blood within the first 10 days of illness and from the urine from the second week onward. False-positive results are common due to extrusion of fibrillar material from red blood cells which mimics leptospirosis. Urine samples must be examined within half an hour of collection.

Detection of Antibodies to Leptospira

Antibodies against *leptospira* start appearing 5–10 days after the onset of fever. Therefore, timing of tests is important. Serologic tests form the mainstay in the diagnosis of leptospirosis.

Macroscopic Slide Agglutination Test

It is a genus-specific test and uses killed *Leptospira* as antigen.

Immunoglobulin M Enzyme-linked Immunosorbent Assay and Immunoglobulin M-Specific Dot Enzyme-Linked Immunosorbent Assay Tests

These tests detect genus-specific immunoglobulin M (IgM) antibodies which tend to become positive early in the disease starting from around fifth day of illness.

The sensitivity of the above-mentioned tests is about 80–90%, but they are not specific. They do not differentiate between pathogenic and saprophytic *Leptospira*, and the infecting serovar cannot be identified. These are the tests which are done in most commercial laboratories and are the source of confounding the diagnosis of a febrile illness.

Microscopic Agglutination Test

It is a serovar-specific test and is the gold standard in serological tests to detect *leptospira* due to its high specificity. It detects serovar-specific antibodies, both immunoglobulin G and IgM antibodies. Microscopic agglutination test is usually positive 10–12 days after the onset of symptoms and reaches a peak by the third week. It involves the use of a battery of live *leptospiral* cultures to be used as antigen and is done in specialized laboratories. Available antisera may not identify all known *leptospira* serotypes. Serotypes commonly seen in the community are usually identified including the virulent and serious types. An initial high titer of 1:800 or rising titers (four-fold increase from baseline) obtained at least 2 weeks apart is diagnostic.

Molecular Tests

Molecular techniques such as real-time polymerase chain reaction and loop-mediated isothermal amplification have been developed for diagnosis of leptospirosis. Next-generation sequencing is a technology for the sequencing of an exponentially greater number of genes than conventional deoxyribonucleic acid sequencing. Currently, these investigations are not readily commercially available.

TREATMENT

Initiation of treatment early in the disease before seventh day shortens the clinical course.

Hospitalized Children with Severe Leptospirosis

Intravenous (IV) crystalline penicillin is the drug of choice, and the dose is 250,000 U/kg/24 h given in four divided doses. Maximum dose is 6–12 million units per day. Alternative drugs include injections of ceftriaxone 75 mg to 100 mg/kg in a single dose or two divided doses, doxycycline 4 mg/kg/day IV in two divided doses, with the maximum dose of 200 mg/day. Doxycycline can be used in children above 8 years of age.

- For children less than 8 years with allergy to penicillin and B-lactam, azithromycin 10 mg/kg IV on day 1 followed by 5 mg/kg once daily is administered.
- The duration of treatment is for at least 7 days.

Children with Less Severe Illness and Outpatients

For children above 8 years who are not hospitalized, oral doxycycline 2 mg/kg in two divided doses not exceeding 200 mg/day for a total of 7 days is given. For children less than 8 years of age, oral azithromycin 10 mg/kg on day 1 followed by 5 mg/kg on subsequent days or oral amoxycillin 25–50 mg/kg in three divided doses is advised.

PREVENTION

Rodent control and avoidance of contact with contaminated water and soil help to prevent infection. Parents should instruct their children not to wade through flood waters or play in stagnant water.

BIBLIOGRAPHY

1. Azimi P. Leptospira. In: Kliegman RM, Behrman RE, Jenson HB, Stanton BF (Eds). Nelson Textbook of Pediatrics, 18th edition. Philadelphia: Saunders; 2009. pp. 1271-2.
2. Tullu MS, Karande S. Leptospirosis in children: a review for family physicians. Indian J Med Sci. 2009;63:368-78.
3. World Health Organization and International Leptospirosis Society. (2003). Human leptospirosis: guidance for diagnosis, surveillance and control. Geneva. [online] Available from http://www.who.int/iris/handle/10665/42667. [Accessed September, 2018].

5.25 Tuberculosis

Aparna Mukherjee, Anuj Singh, Rakesh Lodha

INTRODUCTION

Tuberculosis (TB) is one of the most common causes of mortality worldwide. An estimated 6.3 million new cases of TB were seen in 2016, of which 1.3 million died due to TB in 2016. Children represent about 11% of all TB cases. Approximately 67 million children are infected with TB (latent TB) and are therefore at risk of developing disease in the future. Despite the best of efforts, childhood TB is still underreported in most of the countries.

EPIDEMIOLOGY

Incidence of TB cases varies among different populations and regions from under 10 per 100,000 population in most high-income countries to 150–300 in most of the 30 high-burden countries. The World Health Organization (WHO) South-East Asia Region (WHO-SEAR) accounted for 45% of the incident cases. TB is the ninth leading cause of death worldwide; it is the main cause from a single infectious agent. About 82% of TB deaths among human immunodeficiency virus (HIV)-negative people occurred in the WHO African Region and the WHO-SEAR in 2016; these regions accounted for 85% of the combined total of TB deaths in HIV-negative and HIV-positive people. India accounted for 33% of global TB deaths among HIV-negative people, and for 26% of the combined total of TB deaths in HIV-negative and HIV-positive people. As per India TB report 2018, the incidence was 211 per 100,000 and mortality of 32 per 100,000 population.

The incidence of drug-resistant TB has increased over the past few years and is a challenge for the whole world due to diagnostic and therapeutic challenges. In 2016, worldwide estimates for multidrug-resistant (MDR)/rifampicin (RIF)-resistant TB in new, and previously treated cases were 4.1% and 19%, respectively.

PATHOGENESIS

Mycobacterium tuberculosis (MTB) bacilli are acid-fast, nonspore-forming, nonmotile, pleomorphic, weakly gram-positive curved rods 1–5 μm long, typically slender, and slightly bent. They may appear beaded or clumped under microscopy. They are obligate aerobes that grow in synthetic media containing glycerol as the carbon source and ammonium salts as the nitrogen source. Other closely related mycobacteria, such as *Mycobacterium bovis*, *Mycobacterium africanum*, and *Mycobacterium microti*, along with MTB form the MTB complex. The characteristic property is acid-fastness, which is imparted by the ability to form stable mycolate complexes with arylmethane dyes that resist discoloration with ethanol.

The spectrum of affliction by MTB includes exposure, infection, and disease.

- *Exposure* means that the child had significant contact with a person with infectious TB but lacks proof of infection.
- *Infection* occurs when an individual inhales droplets, which contain mycobacteria, which survive intracellularly in lung and lymphoid tissue. In this stage, child is *asymptomatic* and has a normal physical examination.
- *Disease* occurs when the signs or symptoms or radiographic manifestations become apparent.

Not all infected individuals have the same risk of developing disease. An immunocompetent adult with untreated TB infection has approximately a 5–10% lifetime risk of developing disease. In contrast, an infected infant has a 40% chance of developing disease within 9–12 months.

Lung is the portal of entry in majority of cases. Bacilli enter alveolar passage in an aerosol droplet and interact with macrophages or type II pneumocytes and are phagocytosed in a process initiated by bacterial contact with macrophage mannose and/or complement receptors. On entry into a host macrophage, MTB initially resides in an endocytic vacuole called the phagosome. If the normal phagosomal maturation cycle occurs, i.e. phagosome-lysosome fusion, these bacteria may encounter a hostile environment that includes acidic pH, reactive oxygen intermediates, lysosomal enzymes, and toxic peptides. Interferon-gamma (IFN-γ) plays a key role for a protective immune response. IFN-γ, produced mainly by CD4+ (cluster of differentiation), CD8+ T cells, and the natural killer cells, synergizes with tumor necrosis factor-α and activates macrophages to kill intracellular bacilli. Bacteria may evade destruction by preventing phagosome-lysosome fusion and cause macrophage necrosis. These bacilli, which survive within macrophage, are carried to regional lymph nodes. The *primary complex (Ghon complex)* of TB includes local infection at the portal of entry and the regional lymph nodes that drain the area.

There is tissue reaction at initial foci over next 2–12 weeks; and hypersensitivity develops, which heal by calcification or fibrosis. Occasionally, this portion may continue to enlarge and lead to focal pneumonitis and pleuritis, and if caseation is intense then may lead to cavitation. During the development of the primary complex, tubercle bacilli are carried to most tissues of the body through the blood and lymphatic vessels.

Disseminated TB occurs if host cellular immunity is inadequate. Bacterial replication is more likely to occur in organs with conditions that favor their growth, such as lung apices, brain, kidneys, and bones. The time between initial infection and apparent disease is variable. Pulmonary TB that occurs after 1 year of primary infection is due to endogenous growth of bacilli. This reactivation of TB is rare in children but common in adults and adolescents. Occasionally reinfection can occur in immunocompromised individuals or those living in highly endemic areas.

DIFFERENCES BETWEEN TUBERCULOSIS IN ADULTS AND CHILDREN

Childhood TB is not simply a reflection of the adult spectrum of disease. Characteristics of TB in children include the paucibacillary nature; preponderance of primary focus and lymph node disease; higher chance of dissemination into serious manifestations, such as miliary TB, TB meningitis (TBM), and spinal TB; higher burden of extrapulmonary TB (EPTB); challenges in diagnosis due to inability to expectorate sputum; and difference in pharmacokinetic or pharmacodynamics characteristics of antitubercular drugs.

PULMONARY TUBERCULOSIS

Intrathoracic involvement in children is varied and may include the following:

- *Primary focus:* Primary focus or Ghon focus that results from primary infection is usually a single focus of parenchymal involvement with or without pleural component. The primary focus along with the draining regional lymph node is called the primary or Ghon complex. This may get complicated and result in cavitation or intrabronchial spread.
- *Lymph node disease:* As a result of primary infection, parahilar and paratracheal nodes may be involved; complications may include airway involvement leading to alveolar collapse or pneumonia.
- *Pleural or pericardial effusion:* This represents a hypersensitivity reaction resulting in straw-colored fluid with high lymphocyte count. If mycobacterium bacilli grow in pleural space, localized empyema is formed. Pericardial effusion may lead to constrictive pericarditis.
- *Miliary disease:* This results from hematogenous dissemination of bacilli; < 2 mm nodules are seen on chest X-ray extending up to the periphery.
- *Adult-type cavitory lesion:* This is usually seen around 8–10 years of age and beyond.

Clinical Features

Pulmonary TB can present with cough and/or fever for more than 2 weeks, not responding to a course of antibiotic for 7–10 days; weight loss (more than 5% of the highest recorded weight in the past 3 months) or not gaining weight; poor appetite; lethargy or easy fatigability; and night sweats. There may be history of contact with an open case of TB within the last few years.

Diagnosis

Tuberculin Skin Test (Mantoux Test)

Tuberculin skin test (TST) is an intradermal skin test with 5 TU of purified protein derivative (PPD)-S or 2 TU of PPD RT 23 or equivalent, read after 48–72 hours. An induration of 10 mm or more is considered positive. In immunocompromised individuals, induration of 5 mm or more is considered positive. Positive TST merely indicates presence of tubercular infection and not disease; hence, it can only *aid in diagnosis* of TB disease and not *confirm* it.

Imaging

- *Chest X-ray:* Radiological features highly suggestive of TB include hilar or paratracheal lymph nodes with or without parenchymal involvement, miliary pattern, fibrocavitary lesion. Some examples are given in **Figures 5.25.1 to 5.25.4**. If left untreated, miliary nodules may coalesce and may reach 3–5 mm in size, radiologically, described as a "snow-storm" appearance.
- *Contrast-enhanced computed tomography (CECT) chest:* Computed tomography (CT) chest may be done in cases where the chest X-ray is not conclusive. CECT chest enables evaluation of parenchymal lesion; identification of necrosis in lymph nodes; description of pleural, airway, and diaphragmatic pathologies; and evaluating visualized bones. CECT features suggestive of TB include necrotic lymph node with a low-density center surrounded by rim enhancement (rim sign), 2–4 mm centrilobular nodules, and tree-in-bud appearances (sharply marginated linear branching opacities around terminal and respiratory bronchioles) indicating endobronchial spread, thick-walled cavity surrounded by parenchymal lesion indicating active disease. CT may also be useful in undertaking guided aspiration/biopsy from mediastinal nodes for cyto/histopathology and microbiological diagnosis.

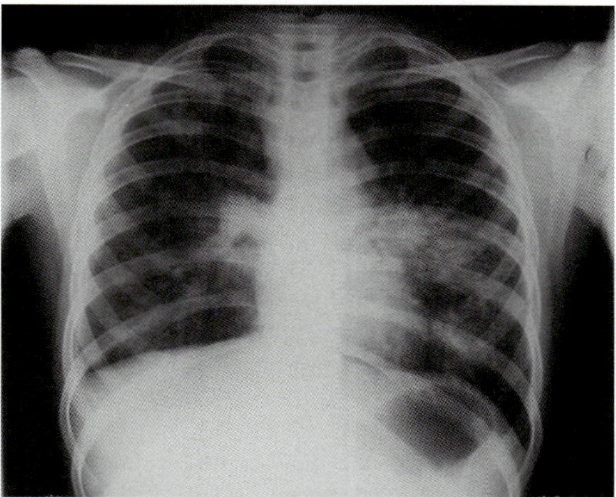

Fig. 5.25.1: Chest X-ray showing bilateral infiltrates.

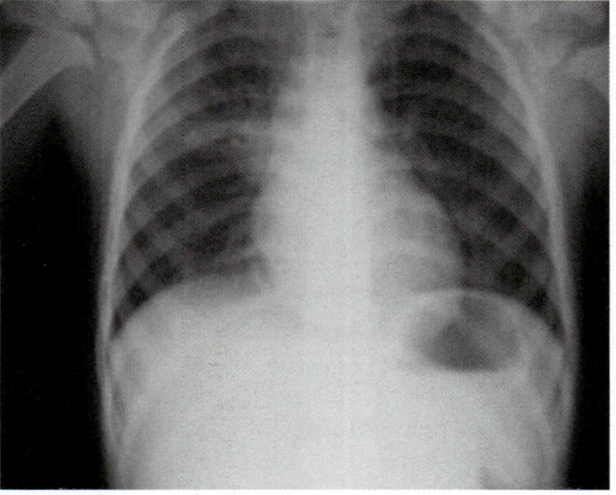

Fig. 5.25.2: Chest X-ray of a 5-year old with collapse consolidation of the right middle lobe.

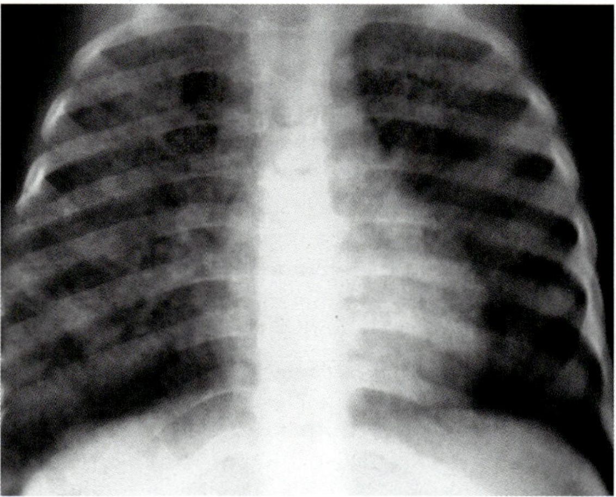

Fig. 5.25.3: Chest X-ray of a 2.5-year-old girl with miliary tuberculosis.

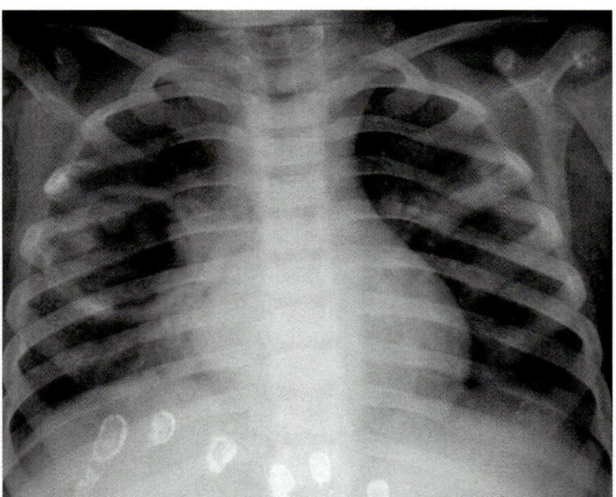

Fig. 5.25.4: Chest X-ray showing a cavitary lesion.

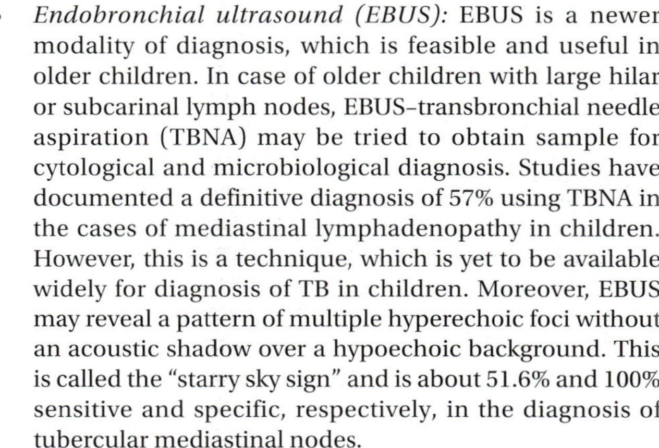

- *Endobronchial ultrasound (EBUS):* EBUS is a newer modality of diagnosis, which is feasible and useful in older children. In case of older children with large hilar or subcarinal lymph nodes, EBUS-transbronchial needle aspiration (TBNA) may be tried to obtain sample for cytological and microbiological diagnosis. Studies have documented a definitive diagnosis of 57% using TBNA in the cases of mediastinal lymphadenopathy in children. However, this is a technique, which is yet to be available widely for diagnosis of TB in children. Moreover, EBUS may reveal a pattern of multiple hyperechoic foci without an acoustic shadow over a hypoechoic background. This is called the "starry sky sign" and is about 51.6% and 100% sensitive and specific, respectively, in the diagnosis of tubercular mediastinal nodes.
- *Magnetic resonance imaging (MRI) chest:* This mode of diagnosis can be employed for follow-up of mediastinal nodal disease instead of CT chest to reduce radiation exposure. The presence of diffusion restriction in lymph nodes along with peripheral enhancement suggests active disease.

Microbiological Confirmation

In spite of the fact that approximately 50% of intrathoracic TB in children is diagnosed clinico-radiologically, every attempt should be made to document a microbiological confirmation in each case.

- *Sample collection:* A major challenge in microbiological diagnosis of childhood TB is the difficulty in obtaining appropriate sample, as children usually cannot expectorate sputum. Gastric aspirate/lavage and induced sputum are feasible options of collecting respiratory samples even in ambulatory, nonhospitalized children.

- *Examination of smear from respiratory samples under light microscopy after Ziehl-Neelsen (ZN) staining:* It is still the most widely accessible investigation in majority of high-burden areas. In spite of a high specificity, the sensitivity of smear examination remains variable (25–80%).
- *Culture:* Löwenstein-Jensen (LJ) culture media (LJ medium) is the most widely used solid media for the determination of characteristic features of colonial morphology, growth rate, and pigment production. The yield of culture varies from 30% to 50%. Excessively long period required for the isolation of MTB by conventional culture techniques has led to the development of other techniques for culture: BACTEC radiometric assay, Septi-Chek acid-fast bacilli (AFB) system, and mycobacterial growth indicator tube (MGIT) culture. BACTEC-MGIT 960 culture system uses a fluorescent compound embedded in silicone on the bottom of the tube containing modified 7H11 broth with an antibiotic mixture and growth supplements for mycobacteria. As this fluorescent compound is sensitive to oxygen, depletion of the latter by the growth of mycobacteria unmasks the fluorescence, which can be detected by observing the tube under long-wave ultraviolet light. Liquid systems are more sensitive for detecting mycobacteria and may increase the case yield by 10% over solid media as well as reduce time to result from weeks to days. Average time to detection in these systems is 8–14 days, culture being declared negative if no result till 42 days. For drug susceptibility testing, the delay may be reduced to as little as 10 days, compared with 28–42 days with conventional solid media.
- *Microscopic observation drug susceptibility (MODS) assay:* MODS assay is an inexpensive, rapid, and sensitive diagnostic method utilizing manual liquid culture method (Middlebrook 7H9 broth culture) and an inverted light microscope to detect the growth of MTB in the form of "tangles or cords." In a study from Peru, where the assay was developed, MODS detected 94% of 1,908 positive sputum cultures, whereas conventional LJ culture detected only 87%. This assay is not yet available widely and has some problems as it is operator dependent and labor intensive, and more studies in nonresearch settings are needed to validate its use.
- *Nucleic acid amplification test (NAAT):* Polymerase chain reaction (PCR), fully automated platform of real-time PCR, and loop-mediated isothermal amplification (TB-LAMP) platform are the available variations of NAAT. Automated cartridge-based NAAT (CBNAAT), such as Xpert MTB/RIF test, is fully automated real-time PCR-based assay, which not only detects MTB, but also rifampicin (RIF) resistance. WHO as of now strongly recommends that CBNAAT should be used in children, when there is strong suspicion of MDR TB or in the case of HIV-TB coinfection. It may also be used in any case where pulmonary TB is suspected, depending on the available resources. The main advantage of this assay is the rapid turnover time, less chance of human error, and ability to simultaneously detect *MTB* and resistance to RIF. In a meta-analysis published by WHO, the overall pooled sensitivity of Xpert MTB/RIF compared against culture as a reference standard in children presumed to have TB was 66%; the samples used were induced sputum, expectorated sputum, and gastric lavage. The pooled specificity of Xpert MTB/RIF compared against the gold standard, culture was at least 98%. The sensitivity of Xpert MTB/RIF to detect RIF resistance in specimens from children was 86%.
- *Molecular drug resistance testing-Line probe assays:* Line probe assays are strip tests that simultaneously detect MTB bacteria as well as genetic mutations that indicate isoniazid (INH) and/or RIF resistance.

T-cell Based Interferon-gamma Release Assays

Interferon-gamma release assays (IGRA) are in vitro tests of cell-mediated immune response, which are mostly helpful in detecting latent TB infection, not disease. The two commercially available IGRAs are the QuantiFERON-TB (QFT) Gold In-Tube (GIT) assay (Cellestis Ltd, Carnegie, Australia) and the T-SPOT.TB assay (Oxford Immunotec, Oxford, the United Kingdom). The QFT-GIT assay is an enzyme-linked immunosorbent assay (ELISA)-based whole-blood test that quantitates IFN-γ released in response to antigenic stimulation from three TB-specific peptides, namely, early secreted antigenic target of 6 kDa (ESAT-6), 10-kDa culture filtrate protein (CFP-10), and TB7.7 in a simple in-tube format. T-SPOT.TB is an enzyme-linked immunospot assay designed to measure the number of IFN-γ-producing T-cells in response to ESAT-6 and CFP-10 peptides. The advantage of these assays lies in the fact that they are not affected by previous bacille Calmette-Guérin (BCG) vaccination, do not cross-react with most of the nontubercular mycobacterium (except *Mycobacterium kansasii*, *Mycobacterium szulgai*, and *Mycobacterium marinum*), are not affected by observer bias, and require only one visit for testing. The sensitivity of QFT assay and T-SPOT.TB assay is 75–85% and 90–95%, respectively. The sensitivity is lower in high-incidence regions. The shortcoming of these assays includes the inability to distinguish between latent and active TB and high cost. The immune response leading to the release of IFN-γ is inconsistent in children below 4 years of age; and hence, interpretation of IGRA may be difficult in this age group. The sensitivity of QFT-GIT is variable in children below 4 years of age with higher number of indeterminate results.

Antigen Detection Tests

Lipoarabinomannans (LAMs) are phosphorylated lipopolysaccharides, which are a major cell wall component of bacteria of the genus *Mycobacterium*. Antigen detection assays based on capture ELISA format to detect LAM in urine hold promise as an easy, point-of-care, noninvasive tool for diagnosing active TB. However, the low sensitivity of urinary LAM (17–50%) as compared with the gold standard of culture offsets the advantages. The specificity is acceptable (88–95%). This diagnostic tool may be particularly helpful in the selected subset of patients with HIV/TB coinfection, where the sensitivity increases.

Antibody Detection Tests

There is no role of any serological diagnosis in the form of antibodies against tubercular antigens in the diagnosis of any type of TB—pulmonary or extrapulmonary. Such tests are currently banned by the Government of India.

Flowchart 5.25.1 depicts an algorithm that is used to diagnose intrathoracic TB in children.

Treatment

Category-based treatment is applicable for children with TB as well. Category 1 antitubercular therapy (ATT) is to be started for new cases, which includes 2 months of intensive phase with INH, RIF, pyrazinamide, and ethambutol (HRZE), followed by 4 months of maintenance phase with INH, RIF, and ethambutol (HRE). A 10-month maintenance phase is required for osteoarticular and central nervous system (CNS) TB. **Table 5.25.1** shows the category-based ATT for children.

The medications should preferably be given daily on mg/kg body weight basis. A meta-analysis conducted on

Flowchart 5.25.1: Diagnostic algorithm for childhood intrathoracic tuberculosis.

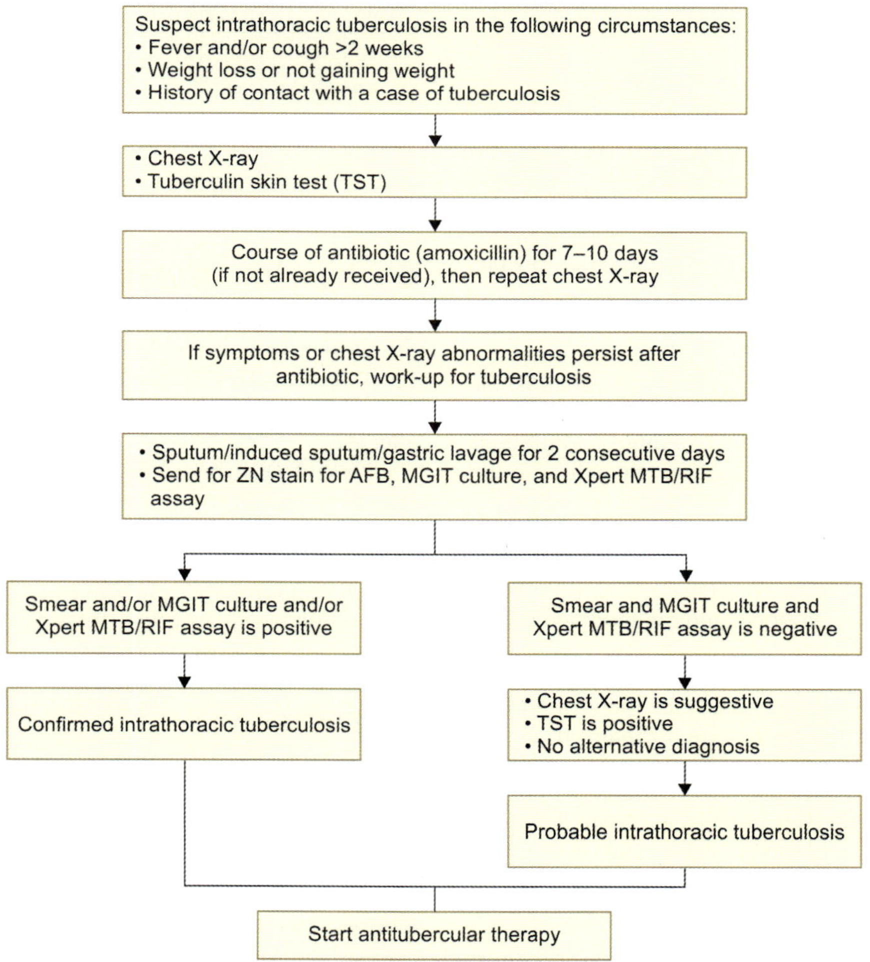

(AFB: acid-fast bacilli; MGIT: mycobacteria growth indicator tube; TST: tuberculin skin test; ZN stain: Ziehl–Neelsen staining)

Table 5.25.1: Category-based treatment for tuberculosis in children.

Category of treatment	*Inclusion criteria*	*Treatment regimen*	
		Intensive phase*	***Continuation phase***
New cases (Category 1)	• New smear-positive pulmonary tuberculosis • New smear-negative pulmonary tuberculosis • New extrapulmonary tuberculosis	2 HRZE	4 HRE[†]
Previously treated cases (Category 2)	• Relapse, failure to respond or treatment after default • Retreatment	2 HRZES + 1 HRZE	5 HRE

Note: The prefix number denotes the number of months.
*Intensive phase can be extended by 1 month in case of unsatisfactory response.
[†]Continuation phase to be extended for 10 months in cases of osteoarticular and central nervous system tuberculosis.
(H: isoniazid; R: rifampicin; Z: pyrazinamide; E: ethambutol; S: streptomycin)

studies in children showed that intermittent therapy of antitubercular drugs was less likely to cure than daily therapy. **Table 5.25.2** details the recommended daily doses of the four first-line antitubercular drugs according to the latest WHO guidelines. The dose of the antitubercular drugs should be adjusted according to the current weight of the child in each follow-up visit during therapy.

Table 5.25.2: Daily dose and maximum doses of isoniazid, rifampicin, ethambutol, and pyrazinamide in children.

Drug	*Dose (range) mg/kg body weight/day*	*Maximum dose mg/day*
Isoniazid	10 (7–15)	300
Rifampicin	15 (10–20)	600
Ethambutol	20–25	1,500
Pyrazinamide	30–35	2,000

Monitoring

Any child on ATT should be regularly monitored for the following:

- *Response to treatment:* Clinicoradiological improvement at 2 months and 6 months of ATT is assessed by weight gain, symptomatic improvement, and more than two-thirds resolution of radiological abnormalities. If AFB or MGIT is positive at baseline, gastric lavage and induced sputum should be repeated at 2 months for ZN staining and MGIT culture.
- *Adverse events:* Any feature suggestive of hepatitis, rash, and/or peripheral neuropathy should be promptly investigated. The antitubercular drugs should be modified if the child is symptomatic with abdominal pain, vomiting, or yellowish discoloration of sclera and urine; or if the liver enzymes are deranged (aspartate aminotransferase/alanine aminotransferase) more than five times the upper limit; or total bilirubin is raised. INH, RIF, and pyrazinamide should be stopped, and the modified regimen should contain ethambutol and a fluoroquinolone, such as levofloxacin. Injectable streptomycin may be added if the disease severity warrants. Once the symptoms are relieved and liver parameters are normalized, the first-line antitubercular drugs should be restarted sequentially, increasing every 5–7 days after checking the liver functions. Once the full dose of conventional antitubercular drugs is reached, the modified regimen may be stopped.

Role of Corticosteroids in Tuberculosis

Routinely there is no role of corticosteroids in the management of intrathoracic TB in children. However, in the case of superior mediastinal compression syndrome due to mediastinal nodes, oral corticosteroids may be used.

TUBERCULAR LYMPHADENITIS

Lymph node TB is the most common form of EPTB, especially in children. Approximately 35% of EPTB cases are lymph node TB. Deep-seated nodes of the mediastinum (mediastinal TB) or abdomen (abdominal lymph node TB) may also be affected.

A child with lymph node TB presents with matted, usually nontender lymph nodes >2 cm size at one or more sites, not responding to antibiotic treatment and persisting for > 1 month. The child may also have fever, poor appetite, and weight loss/inability to gain weight. The lymph node may become fluctuant and burst forming a sinus or ulcer with undermined edges **(Fig. 5.25.5)**.

Diagnosis

Tuberculin skin test: Positive TST ≥ 10 mm suggests tubercular infection but does not confirm disease. X-ray of chest should be done to evaluate pulmonary involvement.

Fine needle aspiration of the nodes: Antigravity Z technique should be applied for aspiration. Deep-seated nodes can be accessed by ultrasound guidance. Sample should be sent for cytopathology, AFB, MGIT culture, and CBNAAT assay. The cytopathological characteristics of tubercular lymphadenitis

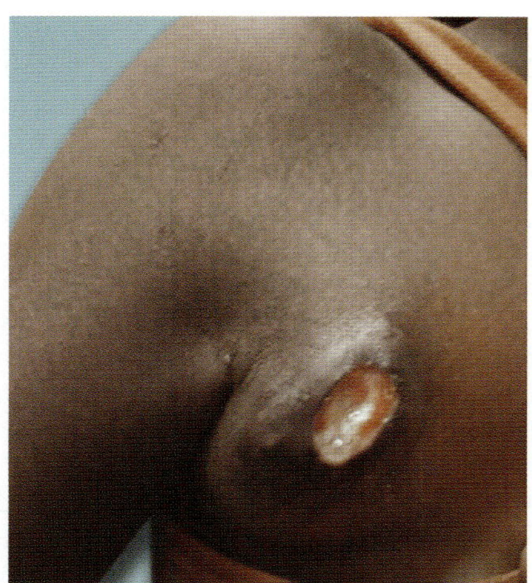

Fig. 5.25.5: Tubercular axillary lymph nodes with overlying ulcer formation.

include epithelioid cell granuloma with or without Langhans cell granuloma with or without necrosis. Staining for AFB is a must in all cases suspected to be lymph node TB.

Excision biopsy: It may be needed if cytopathology from aspiration is inconclusive, and there is high index of suspicion of malignancy.

Treatment

Treatment of tubercular lymphadenitis follows the same category-based principle of ATT, with category 1 regimen for new cases of lymph node TB being 2 months of HRZE, followed by 4 months of HRE. There is no role of surgery in treatment of tubercular lymphadenitis.

ABDOMINAL TUBERCULOSIS

Abdominal TB occurs in approximately 3.5 % of patients with EPTB. Approximately 30% of patients with intra-abdominal TB have evidence of pulmonary TB at the time of diagnosis. Miliary TB cases will have abdominal involvement in about one-third of cases.

Abdominal TB may involve the various regions of the gastrointestinal (GI) tract or the peritoneum, or both. The most common site of involvement in the GI tract is the ileocecal region, followed by ascending colon, jejunum, appendix, duodenum, stomach, esophagus, sigmoid colon, and rectum. In case of peritoneal involvement—it may be wet with development of ascites, dry type with adhesions, and fibrotic type along with pockets of ascites.

Abdominal TB is more common due to the ingestion of infected sputum rather than inhalation of the pathogen. Intra-abdominal TB may also arise from hematogenous spread or in some cases retrograde spread via fallopian tubes.

Abdominal TB may present acutely or insidiously. Clinical features of abdominal TB may be very nonspecific and include abdominal pain, fever, and weight loss. In the case of intestinal involvement, child may present with colicky pain, chronic diarrhea alternating with constipation and abdominal mass. Ascites is frequently present; subacute intestinal obstruction can also be the presenting complaint. Omental involvement may give rise to a characteristic doughy feel to the abdomen. Isolated involvement of the hepatobiliary system by MTB is rare; it usually is part of a more disseminated process. Hepatic involvement may be miliary with multiple miliary tubercles; granulomatous with tuberculomas; nodular with abscess formation; ductal; or nodal where nodes cause obstruction at the porta leading to jaundice.

Diagnosis

Diagnosis of abdominal requires the following:

- *Chest X-ray:* X-ray should be done in all the cases of presumptive abdominal TB to look for pulmonary involvement.
- *Ascitic fluid analysis:* Ascitic fluid is usually straw colored, exudative in nature, with majority of lymphocytes. Protein concentration is higher than 2.5 g/mL, serum-ascites-albumin gradient (SAAG) > 1.1.
- *Microbiological confirmation* should be attempted in all cases. Samples that can be sent for ZN staining, MGIT culture and CBNAAT assay include ascitic fluid, ultrasonography, or CT-guided fine needle aspirate or biopsy from the mesenteric/retroperitoneal nodes or peritoneum.

Treatment

- Category 1 ATT is advised for abdominal TB for a period of 6 months.
- Supportive treatment should be provided for ascites.
- Subacute intestinal obstruction is to be managed conservatively.

OSTEOARTICULAR TUBERCULOSIS

Bones and joints account for approximately 10% of EPTB. Spinal TB or Pott's spine is the most common type of bone TB, thoracic spine being the most common site. Spinal TB results from hematogenous spread from either a pulmonary site or extrapulmonary site, such as lymph node.

Tuberculosis of the spine may present with localized back pain for more than 6 weeks, fever, weight loss, or failure to gain weight. There may be localized tenderness with gibbus formation, with or without spinal cord involvement and neurological manifestations.

All suspected cases of spinal TB should undergo X-ray of spine, followed by MRI of spine. MRI spine demonstrates characteristic features of bone destruction earlier than X-ray and can also give important information regarding the spinal cord involvement. Chest X-ray should also be done in all cases to look for pulmonary involvement. Samples should be taken (guided by radiology) from any paravertebral collection and joint effusion for AFB, MGIT culture, and CBNAAT assay along with cytopathology.

The treatment option for bone TB is category 1 ATT for a total duration of 12 months (2 months HRZE, followed by 10 months of HRE). Development and progression of neurological deficit may need surgical intervention.

CENTRAL NERVOUS SYSTEM TUBERCULOSIS

Central nervous system TB includes an array of conditions—meningitis (TBM), cerebral and spinal tuberculoma, myelitis, and arachnoiditis. Approximately 1% of total TB cases are due to CNS TB. CNS TB can lead to considerable mortality and morbidity, especially, in younger children < 3 years of age.

Tuberculosis Meningitis

Tuberculosis meningitis may present as acute, subacute, or chronic meningitis. According to the Wallgren timeline, TBM develops within approximately 3 months of primary infection if not contained. TBM may initially present with nonspecific symptoms, such as fever, listlessness or apathy, poor appetite, failure to thrive, neck stiffness, and headache if the child is old enough to complain. Later it may progress to altered sensorium, seizures, and focal neurological deficits. Because of the nonspecific nature of the symptoms any meningitis such as presentation before one year of age should be investigated for TBM. Moreover, there is a close association of TBM with miliary TB and immunocompromised states.

The disease begins with the development of small tuberculous foci (Rich foci) in the brain, spinal cord, or meninges caseating into the subarachnoid space.

There are various clinical classifications of stages or severity of TBM. The British Medical Council Research criteria classify TBM into following stages:

- *Mild:* Fully conscious with no focal neurological deficit.
- *Moderate:* Conscious but with altered sensorium, confusion, lethargy, and moderate neurological signs, such as single nerve palsy, hemiparesis, and paraparesis.
- *Severe:* Comatose, multiple cranial nerve palsies, hemiplegia, and/or paraplegia.

Effort should be made for early diagnosis and treatment of TBM to avoid unfavorable outcome and lasting disability.

Diagnosis

- *Lumbar puncture and cerebrospinal fluid (CSF) analysis:* Clear appearance, pleocytosis with lymphocytic predominance, raised protein (0.5–2.5 g/L, and low CSF—plasma glucose ratio < 0.5). CSF should be sent for AFB, MGIT culture, and CBNAAT assay. Samples should also be sent for ruling out bacterial and fungal pathology.
- *Imaging:* Noncontrast CT brain shows basal hyperdense exudates; contrast studies may demonstrate basal meningeal enhancement, infarcts, or hydrocephalus. MRI brain is a better imaging option in determining the features of TBM, especially brainstem lesions and early infarcts. Contrast-enhanced MRI can help in visualization of leptomeningeal tubercles, vascular involvement (most commonly affecting the terminal portions of the internal carotid arteries and proximal parts of middle and anterior cerebral arteries).
- *Adenosine deaminase* does not have any role in diagnosing TBM.
- Like any other EPTB, a *chest X-ray* should always be done to look for pulmonary involvement.
- *Human immunodeficiency virus infection* should also be ruled out.

Main complications of TBM are hydrocephalus (communicating variety in 70–80% cases), vasculitis, stroke, and opticochiasmatic arachnoiditis leading to loss of vision.

Tuberculoma

Tuberculomas are granulomas in solid organs. CNS tuberculoma can occur anywhere in brain or spinal cord and may be present along with TBM. Clinical features of CNS tuberculoma are mainly seizures and/or focal neurological deficit; fever and headache may also be present.

Diagnosis

Important differential diagnosis includes neurocysticercosis, pyogenic abscess, and malignancy. The differentiating features between CNS tuberculoma and neurocysticercosis are outlined in **Table 5.25.3**. MRI brain is the main modality

Table 5.25.3: Differences between CNS tuberculoma and neurocysticercosis.

CNS tuberculoma	*Neurocysticercosis*
May present at any age	Rare before 3 years of age
Progressive neurological deficit	Usually no neurological deficit
Lesion size is usually >20 mm, irregular outline with marked cerebral edema, may be conglomerate	Usually smaller, regular rounded outline with less cerebral edema
May be supra- or infratentorial	Usually supratentorial
Likely to cause midline shift	Usually no midline shift
Magnetic resonance spectroscopy shows lipid peak	No lipid peak

(CNS: central nervous system)

of diagnosis of CNS tuberculomas. Tuberculomas may occasionally increase in size or number in the first 3 months after starting ATT; this is due to paradoxical reaction or immune reconstitution inflammatory syndrome.

Treatment of Central Nervous System Tuberculosis

Treatment of any form CNS TB entails 12 months of ATT (2 HRZE + 10 HRE) for new cases. Adjunctive steroid therapy in the form of prednisolone (4 mg/kg) or dexamethasone (0.6 mg/kg) for 4 weeks followed by tapering over next 2 weeks improves the outcome. Mannitol may be used for emergency management of cerebral edema. In more subacute cases and in hydrocephalus, acetazolamide or furosemide may be used. Surgical intervention may be needed for hydrocephalus in the form of ventriculoperitoneal shunting, if there is no response to medical management or if there is noncommunicating hydrocephalus. In the case of seizures, appropriate antiepileptic drug should be added.

TUBERCULOSIS AND HUMAN IMMUNODEFICIENCY VIRUS

With the spread of the HIV infection, there has been resurgence in TB. The two infections have significantly detrimental interactions. Coexistent TB and HIV infections accelerate the progression of both the diseases. HIV-infected children are more likely to have EPTB and disseminated TB; the course is also likely to be more rapid. An HIV-infected child with latent tubercular infection is more likely to develop the disease than a seronegative child.

Diagnosis

In the absence of significant immunosuppression due to HIV infection, the clinical manifestations of TB are not much different from that in seronegative children. Diagnosis of TB in HIV-infected children poses greater challenges than in other children. Even with the use of a lower cut off of 5 mm, the tuberculin test is often negative, particularly in children with severe immunosuppression. In extensive disease, the bacteriological confirmation rates are likely to be greater. All attempts should be made to isolate MTB. Other than providing definitive diagnosis, it offers the opportunity to do drug-sensitivity analysis. The incidence of MDR TB is higher in HIV-infected patients.

Management

Most current international guidelines recommend that TB in HIV-infected children should be treated according to the same category-based treatment as in non-HIV-infected children. A close follow-up is essential to diagnose nonresponse/drug resistance early. In a HIV-positive child, starting ATT takes precedence over antiretroviral therapy.

There is no clear-cut consensus for the *optimal timing of commencing antiretroviral therapy* when a child is on ATT, but all HIV-infected children who have developed TB have to be started on ART, irrespective of the CD4 count. The decision has to be taken weighing the possibilities of drug interaction, immune reconstitution syndrome, overlapping toxicities against the possibility of worsening immune status. However, it is advisable to start ART as soon as possible within 8 weeks of initiation of ATT. Earlier initiation of ART is more crucial in HIV-TB coinfected children with low CD4 values.

After timing, the next important concern in treatment of HIV-TB coinfected children is the *drug interaction between RIF and antiretroviral drugs,* particularly nevirapine (NVP) and efavirenz (EFV). RIF is known to be a potent inducer of hepatic microsomal cytochrome P450 (CYP 450) enzyme system. NVP and EFV are metabolized primarily by CYP3A4 and CYP2B6, respectively, both being induced by RIF. Some important studies in adults have shown that NVP and EFV levels are reduced by 20–40% when coadministered with RIF; changes in NVP levels are more than that of EFV. In children over 3 years of age or >10 kg body weight, a regimen of two nucleoside reverse transcriptase inhibitors (NRTIs) + EFV (the non-NRTI component) is suggested. Currently, in children under 3 years of age, regimen containing lopinavir with ritonavir boosting is the first choice. In the presence of coadministration of RIF, lopinavir needs to be superboosted with ritonavir (1:1 ratio). If superboosting is not possible, NVP can be used. When used along with RIF, no lead-in period should be given for NVP so that the child is not exposed to subtherapeutic levels. Moreover, NVP should be given at the highest possible dosage (200 mg/m^2/dose). Alternatively, rifabutin can be used instead of RIF as it is less affected by the induction of CYP3A4. All children diagnosed with TB-HIV coinfection should receive cotrimoxazole prophylaxis.

Please refer to Chapter 5.23, Pediatric Human Immunodeficiency Virus Infection or Acquired Immunodeficiency Syndrome, for more specific details.

MULTIDRUG RESISTANCE TUBERCULOSIS

Multidrug resistance TB is defined as a case of TB with MTB showing resistance to at least INH and RIF. In 2016, globally, an estimated 4.1% of new TB cases and 19% of previously treated cases have been diagnosed with MDR TB.

In the absence of a drug-sensitivity report, conventionally the second-line regimen is designed with at least 5–7 antitubercular drugs presumed to be still effective. Apart from ethambutol and pyrazinamide from the first-line drugs, an injectable aminoglycoside, such as kanamycin, a fluoroquinolone, such as levofloxacin, along with ethionamide and cycloserine are added. More drugs may be added in case-to-case basis. The usual duration of second-line ATT is 18–24 months. A child on this therapy should be very carefully monitored for clinical improvement and adverse events of the drugs prescribed.

PREVENTION

Prophylaxis

Isoniazid is prescribed for chemoprophylaxis at a dose of 10 mg/kg of body weight/day, for 6 months.

Tuberculosis preventive therapy or chemoprophylaxis should be provided in the following scenarios:

- All asymptomatic contacts, less than 6 years of age, of an open case of TB (smear positive), after ruling out active disease. Status of BCG vaccination or TST reading does not preclude one from receiving this chemoprophylaxis.
- All HIV-infected children with a known exposure to an infectious TB case, but with no active TB disease.
- All TST-positive children who are receiving immunosuppressive therapy.
- A child born to mother who was diagnosed to have TB in pregnancy, after ruling out congenital TB. BCG vaccination can be given at birth even if chemoprophylaxis is planned.

Vaccination

Bacille Calmette–Guérin is the only vaccine for TB disease used at present. The protection it provides against pulmonary TB is variable; however, it has 60–80% protective efficacy against more serious, disseminated diseases in children such as CNS TB.

BIBLIOGRAPHY

1. Marais BJ, Schaaf HS. Tuberculosis in children. Cold Spring Harb Perspect Med. 2014;4(9):a017855.
2. Thwaites GE, van Toorn R, Schoeman J. Tuberculous meningitis: more questions, still too few answers. Lancet Neurol. 2013;12:999-1010.
3. World Health Organization. Guidance for national tuberculosis programmes on the management of tuberculosis in children. Geneva, Switzerland: WHO; 2014.

5.26 Diphtheria

Monjori Mitra

INTRODUCTION

Diphtheria is a potentially acute disease caused by exotoxin-producing *Corynebacterium diphtheriae*, a gram-positive *Bacillus*. Morbidity and mortality result from the bacterial toxin that may cause obstructive pseudomembranes in the upper respiratory tract (croup) or damage myocardium and other tissues.

EPIDEMIOLOGY

Humans are the only natural reservoir of *C. diphtheriae*, although occasionally it has been isolated from a variety of domestic animals. Spread occurs in close-contact settings through respiratory droplets or direct contact with respiratory secretions or skin lesions. The majority of nasopharyngeal *C. diphtheriae* infections result in asymptomatic carriage, with clinical disease developing in only about one in seven individuals.

Diphtheria immunization protects against disease but does not prevent carriage. Vaccination with diphtheria toxoid (formalin-treated toxin) was introduced in the 1920s. Immunization of children in an era when the majority of older individuals had natural immunity resulted in a dramatic drop in the incidence of diphtheria and an even more rapid decline in the proportion of toxigenic strains isolated, presumably because the selective advantage of the *tox* gene promotion of greater replication and spread of the organism is lost in an immune host. In most Western countries, toxigenic *C. diphtheriae* has virtually been eliminated.

Vaccine-induced immunity to diphtheria wanes with time, and there is a growing cohort of individuals with no natural diphtheria immunity. Serosurveys indicate that 20–60% of adults in industrialized countries have diphtheria antitoxin levels below minimal protective levels. As long as a high proportion of the population remains susceptible, the danger of reintroduction or re-emergence of toxigenic strains exists. Since 1990, there has been a major resurgence of diphtheria in several countries of the former Soviet Union.

In 2005, India contributed 5,826 (71%) of the 8,229 diphtheria cases reported globally. New numbers released by the Central Bureau of Health Intelligence, under the Union Ministry of Health and Family Welfare in 2010, a total of 3,129 cases of diphtheria were reported out of which 731 were found to be from Delhi and a huge 90% of reported diphtheria deaths (163 out of 177) recorded in 2010 were also in Delhi. In the recent July 2015 update from World Health Organization global monitoring system data, India contributed 6,094 cases out of the total number of 7,382 reported cases.

PATHOGENESIS

Corynebacterium diphtheriae is a member of a group of aerobic, nonmotile, unencapsulated, nonsporulating, and pleomorphic organism. Both nontoxigenic and toxigenic *C. diphtheriae* strains exist. Toxigenicity is conferred when a nontoxigenic organism is infected with a beta-phage carrying the gene for the toxin (*tox*). *C. diphtheriae* has three biotypes: (1) gravis, (2) mitis, and (3) intermedius—that are distinguished by colonial morphology and varying biochemical and hemolytic reactions. Strains may be distinguished for epidemiologic purposes by molecular techniques. *Corynebacterium ulcerans* can also produce classic diphtheria, including local respiratory tract and distal toxic complications.

Corynebacterium diphtheriae colonizes the mucosal surface of the nasopharynx and multiplies locally without blood stream invasion. Released toxin causes local tissue necrosis with the formation of a tough, adherent pseudomembrane composed of a mixture of fibrin, dead cells, and bacteria. The membrane usually begins on the tonsils or posterior of the pharynx. In more severe cases, it spreads over the pharyngeal wall, fauces, and soft palate and into the larynx, resulting in respiratory obstruction. Toxin entering the blood stream causes tissue damage at distant sites, particularly the heart (myocarditis), nerves (demyelination), and kidney (tubular necrosis). Nontoxigenic strains may cause mild local respiratory disease, sometimes including a membrane.

CLINICAL MANIFESTATIONS

Anterior Nasal Diphtheria

Anterior nares colonization leads to chronic serosanguineous or seropurulent discharge and erosive rhinitis without fever or significant toxicity. A whitish membrane may be observed on the septum.

Pharyngeal and Tonsillar Diphtheria

The faucial (pharyngeal) form is most common. It is manifested with sore throat, malaise, and mild-to-moderate fever. Initially, there is mild pharyngeal erythema, usually followed by progressive formation of whitish tonsillar exudates, which over a period of 24–48 hours changes into a grayish membrane that is tightly adherent and bleeds on an attempted removal. Cervical adenopathy and soft tissue edema result in the typical bull neck appearance and stridor.

Laryngeal Diphtheria

Laryngeal involvement is manifested as hoarseness, stridor, and dyspnea.

Cutaneous Diphtheria

Classic cutaneous diphtheria is an indolent, nonprogressive infection characterized by a superficial, euthymic, nonhealing ulcer with a gray-brown membrane. Diphtheritic skin infections cannot always be differentiated from streptococcal or staphylococcal impetigo, and these conditions frequently coexist. In most cases, a primary process, such as dermatosis, laceration, burns, bite, or impetigo, becomes secondarily infected with *C. diphtheriae*. Extremities are more often affected than the trunk or head. Pain, tenderness, erythema, and exudate are typical. Local hyperesthesia or hypoesthesia is unusual.

COMPLICATIONS

Most complications of diphtheria, including death, are attributable to effects of the toxin. Myocarditis typically occurs in the first week or second week after the onset of respiratory symptoms and develops either suddenly or insidiously with signs of low cardiac output and congestive failure. Conduction disturbances, such as ST-T wave abnormalities, arrhythmias, and heart block, may occur without myocarditis.

Neurologic impairment is manifested as cranial nerve palsies and polyneuritis. Palatal or pharyngeal paralysis (or both) occurs during the acute phase; peripheral neuritis, symmetrical and predominantly motor, occurs 2–12 weeks after onset of the disease. Motor deficit may range from minor proximal weakness to complete paralysis. Complete recovery is the rule.

Other complications include otitis media and respiratory insufficiency due to airway obstruction, especially in infants.

DIAGNOSIS

The specimen should be collected immediately after clinical diagnosis with the swab from the inflamed tissue, and one is sent for staining and the other for the culture. It is obtained from the nose and throat and any other mucocutaneous lesion. A portion of membrane should be removed for culture. Evaluation of a direct smear using Gram stain is used to accurately identify the organism and subsequently with the special stain, such as Albert's stain, Ponder's stain; the metachromatic granular structure is identified.

Alert the laboratory to the suspicion of diphtheria because isolation of *C. diphtheriae* requires special culture media. *C. diphtheriae* may be grown on various selective media, including tellurite agar or specially enriched Loeffler, Hoyle, Mueller, or Tinsdale medium.

Culture isolates of coryneform organisms should be identified to the species level, and toxigenicity and antimicrobial susceptibility tests should be performed for *C. diphtheriae* isolates. Elek's test is used for toxigenicity to determine whether the organism is able to produce the diphtheria toxin or not.

DIFFERENTIAL DIAGNOSIS

The differential diagnosis includes streptococcal and viral tonsillopharyngitis, infectious mononucleosis, Vincent's angina, candidiasis, and acute epiglottitis.

MANAGEMENT

The goals of treatment are to neutralize the toxin rapidly, eliminate the infecting organism, provide supportive care, and prevent further transmission. The mainstay of therapy is equine diphtheria antitoxin and should be administered based on clinical grounds. A single dose ranging in quantity from 20,000 U for localized tonsillar diphtheria up to 100,000 U is given for extensive disease with severe toxicity. Antitoxin may be administered intramuscularly or intravenously; particularly for more severe cases, the intravenous route is preferred. Tests for sensitivity to antitoxin should be performed before administering it and desensitization carried out if necessary.

Antibiotic therapy should be started simultaneously. Parenteral penicillin (4–6 million units/day) or macrolides, such as erythromycin, clarithromycin, and azithromycin, are the drugs of choice. The antibiotic is given for 10–14 days.

General supportive care includes ensuring a secure airway, electrocardiographic monitoring for evidence of myocarditis, treating heart failure and arrhythmias, and preventing secondary complications of neurologic impairment, such as aspiration pneumonia. The patient should be in strict isolation until follow-up cultures are negative. Convalescing patients should receive diphtheria toxoid.

The local health department must be notified. Close contacts should have cultures performed and be administered prophylactic antibiotics. All contacts without full primary immunization and a booster within the preceding 5 years should receive diphtheria toxoid.

Antibiotic therapy is not a substitute for antitoxin therapy. Some patients with cutaneous diphtheria have been treated for 7–10 days. Elimination of the organism should be documented by negative results of at least two successive cultures of specimens from the nose and throat (or skin) obtained 24 hours apart after completion of therapy. Treatment with erythromycin is repeated if either culture yields *C. diphtheriae*.

PREVENTION

Immunization with diphtheria toxoid is the only effective means of primary prevention. The primary series is four doses of diphtheria toxoid (given with tetanus toxoid and pertussis vaccine) at 6 weeks, 10 weeks, 14 weeks, and 15–18 months, and a preschool booster dose is given at 4–6 years of age. Thereafter, boosters [tetanus and diphtheria (Td) or tetanus-diphtheria-acellular pertussis (Tdap)] should be given as part of the adolescent immunization visit (i.e. at 10 years and 16 years of age), followed by doses administered every 10 years. Since 2005, the Centers for Disease Control and Prevention (CDC) recommends the routine use of tetanus toxoid, reduced diphtheria toxoid, and acellular pertussis vaccine (Tdap) in adolescents 11–18 years of age in place of tetanus and diphtheria toxoid (Td) vaccines. In addition, the CDC recommends routine use of a single dose of Tdap for adults 19–64 years of age to replace the next booster dose of Td.

In countries that are rendered nonendemic through high immunization coverage, the primary vaccination series of the three doses should be extended by at least one booster dose. Revaccination of adults against diphtheria (and tetanus) every 10 years may be necessary to sustain immunity in some epidemiological settings. Particular attention should be given to revaccination of health-care workers. To further promote immunity against diphtheria, combined diphtheria toxoid and tetanus toxoid rather than tetanus toxoid alone should be used when tetanus prophylaxis is needed following injuries.

PROGNOSIS

Although most infections with *C. diphtheriae* are asymptomatic or run a relatively mild clinical course, high case-fatality rates (>10%) have been reported even in recent outbreaks. In prevaccination era, diphtheria had a very high case-fatality rate in the preschool children. With the widespread vaccination in both developed and developing countries, the incidence of diphtheria has decreased, but there is also a decrease in the circulating toxigenic *C. diphtheriae* organisms, resulting in less natural boosting of antibody levels. Hence, if adequate booster dose is not given, the chances of outbreaks will be there, leading to increase case-fatality rates.

Hence, the ideal public health policy should put efforts to reach at least 90% coverage with the three doses of diphtheria toxoid in children below 1 year of age. In countries where diphtheria has been successfully controlled, immunity levels should be maintained by booster doses.

BIBLIOGRAPHY

1. Bitragunta S, Murhekar MV, Hutin YJ, et al. Persistence of diphtheria, Hyderabad, India, 2003-2006. Emer Infec Dis. 2008;14(7):1144-7.
2. Buescher ES. *Corynebacterium diphtheria*. In: Kliegman RM, Stanton BF, Behrman RE (Eds). Nelson Textbook of Pediatrics, 18th edition. Philadelphia, PA: WB Saunders; 2009. pp. 1153-7.
3. Centers for Disease Control and Prevention. Respiratory diphtheria-like illness caused by toxigenic *Corynebacterium ulcerans*—Idaho, 2010. MMWR. 2011;60(3):77.
4. Clarridge JE, Popovic T, Inzana TJ. Diphtheria and other corynebacterial and coryneform infections. In: Hausler WJ, Sussman M (Eds). Topley and Wilson's Microbiology and Microbial Infections. New York, NY: Oxford University Press; 1998. p. 347.
5. Galazka AM, Robertson SE. Diphtheria: changing patterns in the developing world and the industrialized world. Eur J Epidemiol. 1995;11(1):107-17.
6. Philip AM. *Corynebacterium diphtheria*. In: Mandell GL, Bennette JE, Dolin R (Eds). Mandell, Douglas and Bennett's Principles and practice of infectious diseases, 7th edition. Philadelphia, PA: Churchill Livingstone; 2009. pp. 2678-93.
7. Sharma NC, Banavaliker JN, Ranjan R, et al. Bacteriological and epidemiological characteristics of diphtheria cases in and around Delhi—a retrospective study. Indian J Med Res. 2007;126(6):545-52.
8. World Health Organization. Diphtheria vaccine—WHO position paper. Wkly Epidemiol Rec. 2006;81:24-31.

5.27 Pertussis

Sailesh Gupta

INTRODUCTION

Pertussis or whooping cough is an infection of the respiratory tract characterized by a paroxysmal cough. Before the availability of a vaccine, pertussis was the major cause of morbidity and mortality among infants and children. In 1940s, vaccination reduced reported cases of pertussis by more than 99%. However, pertussis still remains a disease of public health concern.

EPIDEMIOLOGY

Bordetella pertussis and *Bordetella parapertussis* cause whooping cough. Bacteria spread via aerosolized droplets from coughing of infected individuals. Transmission can occur through direct face-to-face contact, sharing a confined space, or through contact with oral, nasal, or respiratory secretions from an infected source. The organism damages ciliated respiratory epithelium. Bronchopneumonia develops with desquamation of the epithelium of small bronchi, causing bronchiolar obstruction and atelectasis. Bronchiectasis may develop and persist.

The true global burden of pertussis is underestimated. The World Health Organization received reports of 136,036 confirmed cases of pertussis in 2013; however, worldwide it is estimated that there are actually 16 million pertussis cases every year, including approximately 195,000 childhood deaths. The case-fatality rate among infants in low-income countries may be as high as 4%. Neither natural infection, nor vaccination provides lifelong immunity. Protection against pertussis wanes 3–5 years after vaccination and is not detected after 12 years. Since the 1980s, incidence has cyclically increased, and peaks occur every 2–5 years. From 1980 to 2005, the reported incidence of pertussis in the United States dramatically increased across all age groups. Although the largest increase has been among adolescents and adults, the annual reported incidence remained highest among infants less than on 1 year old, at 55.2 cases per 100,000 populations. California experienced a pertussis epidemic in

2014. Pertussis is cyclical and peaks every 3–5 years as the numbers of susceptible persons in the population increases due to waning of immunity following both vaccination and disease. The last epidemic in California occurred in 2010; however, the overall incidence of pertussis has increased since the 1990s. One reason for the increase is the use of acellular pertussis vaccines, which cause fewer reactions than the whole-cell vaccines that preceded them, but do not protect as long. There is also a shift in the epidemiology of pertussis, with more cases being reported in older age groups, which is due to waning immunity to *B. pertussis*, a number of years after immunization. Adolescents and adults have been identified as the source of pertussis transmission to infants. Young infants are at greatest risk of hospitalization and death from pertussis; therefore, pregnant women are encouraged to receive tetanus-diphtheria-acellular pertussis (Tdap) vaccine during the third trimester of every pregnancy. Pertussis antibodies are transferred from vaccinated mothers to their infants and will help protect them until they are old enough to be vaccinated. Other options to prevent transmission to infants include vaccination of adolescents and adults in close contact with infants and vaccinating infants with pertussis vaccine at birth.

CLINICAL COURSE

It is observed that the frequency of pertussis cases in India is higher during the months of November to June. Typically, the incubation period of pertussis ranges from 3 days to 12 days. It is an illness lasting 6 weeks and goes through catarrhal, paroxysmal, and convalescent stages, each lasting from 1 week to 2 weeks. The catarrhal phase is similar to common upper respiratory infections with nasal congestion, rhinorrhea, sneezing, conjunctival injection, and discharge. While most infectious in the catarrhal phase, pertussis may remain communicable for 3 or more weeks after the onset of cough. Paroxysmal phase presents with paroxysms of intense coughing lasting up to several minutes. In older infants and toddlers, the paroxysms of coughing may be followed by a loud whoop as inspired air goes through a still partially closed airway. Infants younger than 6 months have apneic episodes and are at risk for exhaustion. Facial congestion with coughing and posttussive vomiting are common symptoms. Patients in the convalescent stage have a chronic cough, which may last for weeks. Uninterrupted coughing, feelings of suffocation or strangulation, and headaches may be seen in older children and adolescents, instead of the distinct stages.

Physical examination contributes little to the diagnosis in patients with uncomplicated pertussis. Fever is typically absent. Most patients do not have signs of lower respiratory tract disease. Conjunctival hemorrhages and facial petechiae result from intense coughing.

As per the guidelines from the Center for Disease Control, in 2015, a confirmed case of pertussis should have acute cough illness of any duration, with isolation of *B. pertussis* from a clinical specimen or cough illness lasting more than or equal to 2 weeks, with at least one of the following signs or symptoms—paroxysms of coughing, inspiratory "whoop," posttussive vomiting or apnea (with or without cyanosis) (for infants aged < 1 year only), and polymerase chain reaction (PCR) positive for pertussis or cough illness lasting more than or equal to 2 weeks, with at least one of the signs or symptoms mentioned earlier, and contact with a laboratory-confirmed case of pertussis.

Premature infants and patients with underlying cardiac, pulmonary, neuromuscular, or neurologic disease are at high risk for complications of pertussis (e.g. pneumonia, seizures, encephalopathy, and death). Older children, adolescents and adults often have mild or atypical illness. Approximately one-half of adolescents with pertussis cough for 10 weeks or longer. Complications among adolescents and adults include syncope, sleep disturbance, incontinence, rib fractures, and pneumonia. Infants less than 6 months old are more likely to have severe disease, to develop complications and to require hospitalization. Pneumonia occurs in approximately 13% of infants with pertussis either from *B. pertussis* infection or from secondary infection with other pathogens. Rarer, central nervous system complications such as seizures and encephalopathy are thought to result from severe paroxysm-induced cerebral hypoxia and apnea, hypoglycemia, and small intracranial hemorrhages. Reported deaths in young infants have increased considerably over last 20 years. From 1990 to 1999, the case-fatality rate was approximately 1% in infants younger than 2 months and less than 0.5% in infants aged 2–11 months. Males and females are equally affected.

The conditions that should be differentiated from pertussis include afebrile pneumonia syndrome, bronchiolitis, chlamydial infections, mycoplasma infections, and respiratory syncytial virus infection.

LABORATORY DIAGNOSIS

Laboratory confirmation of pertussis is difficult and delayed. Therefore typical symptoms along with history of incomplete or absent pertussis vaccination and lymphocytosis help in making a presumptive diagnosis of pertussis. Leukocytosis (15,000–50,000/μL) with absolute lymphocytosis occurs during the late catarrhal and paroxysmal phases and correlates with severity of the disease.

A confirmed case is defined as one with any cough illness in which *B. pertussis* is isolated and cultured, or a case with typical symptoms confirmed by PCR or epidemiologic linkage to a laboratory-confirmed case. Culture is considered the gold standard as it is the only 100% specific method for identification. Specimen for culture is obtained by deep nasopharyngeal (NP) aspiration, and inoculation in Bordet-Gengou agar, Regan-Lowe, or modified Stainer-Scholte media causes growth in 3–4 days. Recovery of organisms is highest during catarrhal and early paroxysmal stages. Previously immunized or antibiotic-treated patients may produce a negative culture; however, this does not exclude the diagnosis of pertussis.

Polymerase chain reaction assay and antigen detection are very sensitive, provide results rapidly, and can be used later in the disease course or after antimicrobial therapy, because the tests do not rely on the isolation of viable organisms. PCR should be tested from NP specimens taken at 0–3 weeks following cough onset but may provide accurate results for up to 4 weeks. Commercially, there are several different serologic tests used in the United States with unproven or unknown clinical accuracy. The optimal timing for specimen collection is 2–8 weeks following cough onset, when the antibody titers are at their highest; however, serology may be performed on specimens collected up to 12 weeks following cough onset.

Imaging studies typically add little to the diagnosis of pertussis. Chest roentgenogram may reveal perihilar infiltrates or edema with variable degrees of atelectasis. Consolidation is indicative of secondary bacterial infection or, rarely, pertussis pneumonia. Occasionally, pneumothorax, pneumomediastinum, or air in the soft tissues may be seen.

MANAGEMENT

Management aims at limiting the number of paroxysms, providing assistance when necessary and maximizing nutrition, rest, and recovery. The mainstay therapy in patients with active pertussis infections is supportive.

Antibiotics initiated during the second stage do not affect the duration and severity of illness but can hasten the eradication of *B. pertussis* and help reduce communicability. For patients aged 1 month or older, macrolides such as erythromycin (40–50 mg/kg/day in four divided doses for 14 days), clarithromycin (15–20 mg/kg/day in two divided doses for 5–7 days), and azithromycin (10–12 mg/kg/day once a day for 5 days) are the preferred agents. Azithromycin is the recommended agent in the youngest patients. Patients older than 2 months with hypersensitivity to macrolides may be treated with trimethoprim-sulfamethoxazole (8 mg/kg/day and 40 mg/kg/day in two divided doses for 5–7 days). Most patients older than 1 year can be treated on an outpatient basis. Frequent reviews are necessary based on patient's age, disease severity, and presence of comorbid conditions.

Hospitalization should be advised for patients at risk of severe disease and complications, including infants younger than 3 months; infants aged 3–6 months, unless observed paroxysms are not severe; premature infants; and infants or children with underlying pulmonary, cardiac, or neuromuscular disease. Vitals and oxygen saturation of hospitalized patients should be monitored continuously, especially in relation to coughing paroxysms. Attention should be paid the young infant's hydration and nutritional status. Patients who are severely ill may require treatment in an intensive care unit.

The use of corticosteroids and β2-adrenergic agents for the treatment of pertussis is not supported by current evidence.

PREVENTION

Administration of the vaccine containing cellular and acellular components stimulates the production of antibodies with specific protective properties. All children less than 7 years of age should receive the pertussis vaccine either diphtheria, tetanus whole-cell pertussis (DTwP) or diphtheria, tetanus, and acellular pertussis (DTaP). Adolescent 11 through 18 years of age should receive a single dose of Tdap. The preferred age of Tdap is 11 through 12 years of age. The Indian Academy of Pediatrics Immunization Schedule recommends vaccination with the whole-cell pertussis vaccine/combination for the primary series, reserving the acellular vaccine for special circumstances. However, there is no need to vaccinate a child additionally with DTwP if the primary immunization series is already completed with DTaP vaccine. The first and second pertussis vaccine boosters should preferably be DTwP, but DTaP may be used to avoid the high reactogenicity of DTwP.

BIBLIOGRAPHY

1. American Academy of Pediatric Committee on Infectious Diseases. Prevention of pertussis among adolescents: recommendations for use of tetanus toxoid, reduced diphtheria toxoid, and acellular pertussis (Tdap) vaccine. Pediatrics. 2006;117(3):965-78.
2. American Academy of Pediatrics. Pertussis. In: Pickering LK (Ed). Red book: 2006 report of the committee of infectious disease. Grove Village, IL: American Academy of Pediatrics; 2006. pp. 498-520.
3. Centers for Disease Control and Prevention. Preventing tetanus, diphtheria, and pertussis among adults: use of tetanus toxoid, reduced diphtheria toxoid and acellular pertussis vaccine. Morb Mortal Wkly Rep. 2006;55:1-33.
4. Centers for Disease Control and Prevention. Pertussis—United States, 1997–2000. Morb Mortal Wkly Rep. 2002;51(4):73-6.
5. Cherry JD, Heininger U. Pertussis and other *Bordetella* infections. In: Feigin RD, Demmler GJ, Cherry JD, Kaplan SL (Eds). Textbook of Pediatric Infectious Diseases, 5th edition. Philadelphia, PA: WB Saunders; 2004. pp. 1588-608.
6. Edwards K, Decker MD. Pertussis vaccine. In: Plotkin SA, Orenstein WA (Eds). Vaccines, 4th edition. Philadelphia, PA: Saunders; 2004. pp. 471-528.
7. Mikelova LK, Halperin SA, Scheifele D, et al. Predictors of death in infants hospitalized with pertussis: a case-control study of 16 pertussis deaths in Canada. J Pediatr. 2003;143(5):576-81.
8. Tiwari T, Murphy TV, Moran J. Recommended antimicrobial agents for the treatment and postexposure prophylaxis of pertussis: 2005 CDC guidelines. MMWR Recomm Rep. 2005;54:1-16.
9. Vitek CR, Pascual FB, Baughman AL, et al. Increase in deaths from pertussis among young infants in the United States in the 1990s. Pediatr Infect Dis. 2003;22(7):628-34.
10. Zhang L, Prietsch SO, Axelsson I, et al. Acellular vaccines for preventing whooping cough in children. Cochrane Database Syst Rev. 2011;3:CD001478.

5.28 Tetanus

Raju C Shah, Pratima R Shah

INTRODUCTION

Tetanus historically called *Lockjaw* is an acute often fatal, severe exotoxin-mediated infection caused by *Clostridium tetani*. Rosenbach in 1886 demonstrated for the first time these slender bacilli. The disease first described by Carlie and Rattone is characterized by severe muscular spasms or acute spastic paralysis and is caused by the action of a potent neurotoxin produced during the growth of the bacteria in dead tissues.

EPIDEMIOLOGY

Tetanus occurs worldwide and is an important cause of neonatal death in developing world. The causative organism *C. tetani* is part of the normal flora in human and animal intestines and is disseminated through the excreta and found in soil and dust. In spore form, they are hard and long lasting in soil and dust. As the spores of *C. tetani* are ubiquitous, wound contamination is unavoidable. The contamination of wound, unhygienic and improper handling of the umbilical cord in newborns, lack of hygienic habits, and aseptic care during and after delivery in women are the main risk factors for infection. Tetanus can occur in a child having chronic ear discharge.

It is the only vaccine-preventable disease that is infectious but not contagious from person to person. Among the burden of vaccine-preventable diseases world over, tetanus ranks fourth with 13% disease burden. The incidence is high in tropical countries with humid climate. According to WHO in 2009, global reported cases were 9,836 and estimated deaths in children less than 5 years were 61,000. The reported cases of tetanus in India in 2006 were 2,587, of which 600 cases were neonatal tetanus. More cases are reported from rural than urban areas.

In 2010, 4,797 neonatal tetanus cases were reported globally with 373 cases from India. According to the Child Health Epidemiology Reference Group (2008), an estimated 60,000 newborns die of the disease each year. In April 2015, WHO included India in the list of countries which has eliminated neonatal tetanus. It means that India has less than 1 case of neonatal tetanus per 1,000 live births in every district.

Worldwide, all countries are committed to "elimination" of maternal and neonatal tetanus (MNT), i.e. a reduction of neonatal tetanus incidence to below 1 case per 1,000 live births per year in every district. As of March 2018, 14 countries remain that have not eliminated MNT **(Box 5.28.1)**.

ETIOLOGY

The causative organism *C. tetani* is a gram-positive, anaerobic, spore forming organism. It forms terminal spores resembling drumsticks. The spores are resistant to boiling, usual antiseptics, and chemical agents like phenol. They can survive autoclaving at 121°C for 10–15 min.

Clostridium tetani usually enters the body through wound. The bacilli itself is noninvasive. The spores germinate in anaerobic conditions. They produce two types of toxins: tetanospasmin and tetanolysin. Of these, tetanospasmin is a neurotoxin and is responsible for the clinical signs and symptoms of the disease. Toxins act at several sites within the nervous system.

CLINICAL MANIFESTATIONS

The incubation period of tetanus is around 10 days (range 3–30 days). Based on clinical findings, three different forms of tetanus have been described:

1. The most common type (80%) is "generalized tetanus."
2. "Localized tetanus" produces pain and spasm of the muscles in proximity to the site of injury. Occasionally, this form of disease may precede generalized form.
3. "Cephalic tetanus" is a rare form of the disease seen in children with otitis media.

Generalized Tetanus

It is usually present with a descending pattern. The first sign most of the time is trismus or lockjaw due to spasm of masseter muscle. Headache, restlessness, and irritability may be the early symptoms followed by stiffness of the neck, difficulty in swallowing, and rigidity of abdominal muscles. The spasms can be precipitated by bright light, noise, and even touch. The

Box 5.28.1: Global magnitude of tetanus (2016).
• 13,778 reported cases
• 72,600 estimated deaths in <5 years (in 2011)

rigidity of facial muscles leads to the sardonic smile of tetanus or risus sardonicus, a typical grinning appearance. Rigidity and spasm of back and abdominal muscles cause arching (opisthotonos). Laryngeal and respiratory muscle spasm can lead to airway obstruction and asphyxia. Constipation and retention of urine may also occur. Hyperpyrexia, hypertension, excessive sweating, tachycardia, and cardiac arrhythmia can occur due to sympathetic nerve involvement. Paralysis is evident in the first week, stabilizes in second week, and ameliorates in the next 1–4 weeks.

Neonatal Tetanus

This typically occurs when the umbilical cord is cut with an unsterilized instrument or some unhygienic materials are applied to the stump of the cord. It manifests within 3–12 days of birth. It is generalized tetanus, a serious condition and often fatal. Progressive difficulty in feeding (sucking and swallowing) with associated hunger and crying are generally seen. Paralysis and diminished movement, stiffness to touch, spasms with or without opisthotonos are the clinical features. Opisthotonos may be extreme or sometimes absent.

Localized Tetanus

This is painful spasms to the site of infection precede generalized tetanus. Cephalic tetanus with bulbar muscle involvement is seen with wounds of the head, face, and nostrils or with chronic otitis media. Retracted eyelids, deviated gaze, trismus, risus sardonicus, spastic paralysis of the tongue, and pharyngeal muscles are the presenting features.

DIAGNOSIS

Diagnosis is mainly clinical. The typical setting is an injured unimmunized patient or baby born to an unimmunized mother presenting within 2 weeks with trismus, rigid muscles, and clear sensorium. The organism can be isolated from wound or ear discharge.

MANAGEMENT

It comprises wound debridement, immunoglobulin administration, antibiotics, and supportive care. The aim of therapy is to neutralize all toxins, eradication of *C. tetani*, and wound environment conducive to anaerobic multiplication and supportive care.

Human tetanus immunoglobulin (TIG) 3,000–6,000 U intramuscular (IM) is recommended to be given immediately. TIG has no effect on toxin, which is already fixed to the neural tissue and does not penetrate the blood-cerebrospinal fluid barrier. It can neutralize circulating tetanospasmin. If TIG is not available, human intravenous immunoglobulin can be used. Anti-tetanus serum is recommended only when TIG is not available. It can be given in a single dose of 50,000–100,000 U, half the dose IM and the rest intravenously after skin test.

Penicillin is the antibiotic of choice for *C. tetani.* Penicillin G 200,000 U/kg body weight can be given intravenously in four divided doses for 10–14 days. Local wound, discharging ears, and umbilical cord should be cleaned and debrided if needed.

All patients with generalized tetanus require muscle relaxant. Diazepam is preferred as it causes both muscle relaxation and seizure control. Initial dose is 0.1–0.2 mg/kg every 3–6 h given intravenously. Midazolam and baclofen can also be used. The best survival rates with generalized tetanus are achieved with neuromuscular blocking agents, such as vecuronium and pancuronium. These drugs produce general flaccid paralysis, which can be managed by mechanical ventilation.

Meticulous nursing care is imperative. The patient should be kept in a quiet, dark environment with minimum auditory or visual stimuli. Maintenance of nutrition, fluid and electrolyte balance, suctioning of secretions, and cardiorespiratory monitoring should be done. Provision for tracheostomy should be kept ready.

Wound Management

All wounds should be cleaned; necrotic tissue and foreign material should be removed. As shown in **Table 5.28.1**, wounds, which are not minor, require human TIG except those in fully immunized patients. In patients with a history of unknown or incomplete immunization, crush, puncture or bone projecting wounds, wounds contaminated with soil, saliva or feces, avulsion injuries, and compound fractures, 250 U of TIG should be given IM. In cases where the wound

Table 5.28.1: Wound management.

	Clean minor wounds		***All other wounds****	
History of tetanus toxoid doses	***TT/Td/ Tdap***	***TIG***	***TT/Td/ Tdap***	***TIG***†
Unknown, less than three doses, immunocompromised	Yes	No	Yes	Yes
More than three doses	No‡	No	No§	No

*Including, but not limited to, wounds contaminated with dirt, feces, soil, and saliva; puncture wounds; avulsions; and wounds resulting from missiles, crushing, burns, and frostbite.

† TIG: Tetanus immunoglobulin (250–500 U intramuscular).

‡ Yes, if more than 10 years since last dose.

§ Yes, if more than 5 years since last dose.

(Td: tetanus and diphtheria; TT: tetanus toxoid; Tdap: tetanus-diphtheria-acellular pertussis)

could not be properly debrided or wound more than 24 h old, 500 U of TIG should be given. Tetanus toxoid may be administered immediately depending on the immunization status of the child.

COMPLICATIONS

Aspiration of secretions leading to pneumonia is one of the major complications. Autonomic system irregularities in the form of cardiac arrhythmias, asystole, and labile blood pressure may be noted. Few children may get seizure-related injuries, rhabdomyolysis, myoglobinuria, bone fractures, and renal failure.

PROGNOSIS

The average mortality of tetanus is 45–55%. For neonatal tetanus, the mortality is 60–70%. The most important factor influencing outcome is the supportive care. Recovery from tetanus does not confer immunity; therefore, active immunization of the patients following recovery is imperative.

PREVENTION

Tetanus is an entirely preventable disease. Active immunization is the best method to prevent tetanus. WHO recommends a three-dose primary vaccination series with diphtheria containing vaccine followed by three booster doses. The three-dose primary series should begin as early as 6 weeks of age, with subsequent doses given with a minimum interval of 4 weeks between doses. The three booster doses should preferably be given during the second year of life (12–23 months), at 4–7 years, and at 9–15 years of age. Ideally, there should be at least 4 years between booster doses. After 7 years of age, Tdap (tetanus-diphtheria-acellular pertussis) (low-dose diphtheria and acellular pertussis) should be used as a booster dose.

Neonatal tetanus could be prevented by immunizing the pregnant women with two doses of tetanus toxoid or tetanus and diphtheria (Td) (preferably one-dose Tdap) between 16 weeks and 36 weeks of pregnancy, and with only one dose of Tdap or Td in the subsequent pregnancies.

BIBLIOGRAPHY

1. Arnon SS. Tetanus. In: Kliegman RM, Jenson HB, Behrman RE, Stanton BF (Eds). Nelson Textbook of Pediatrics, 18th edition. Philadelphia, PA: Elsevier; 2007. pp. 1228-30.
2. Centers for Disease Control and Prevention. Diphtheria, tetanus and pertussis: recommendations for vaccine use and other preventive measures. Recommendations of the Immunization Practices Advisory Committee (ACIP). MMWR Recomm Rep. 1991;40(RR-10):1-28.
3. Centers for Disease Control and Prevention. Epidemiology and prevention of vaccine-preventable diseases, 10th edition. Atlanta: Department of Health and Human Services, CDC; 2007.
4. World Health Organization. The "high risk" approach: the WHO—recommended strategy to accelerate elimination of neonatal tetanus. Wkly Epidemiol Rec. 1996;71:33-6.

5.29 Rickettsial Diseases

Narendra Rathi

INTRODUCTION

Family *Rickettsiae* comprises a group of microorganisms that phylogenetically occupy a position between bacteria and viruses. *Rickettsia* are small, nonflagellate, gram-negative pleomorphic coccobacilli adapted to obligate intracellular parasitism and transmitted by arthropod vectors, such as fleas, ticks, mites, and lice.

EPIDEMIOLOGY

Rickettsial diseases have a global distribution (except Antarctica) and recent reports suggest their continuing presence in India as well. The presence of rickettsial disease in India has been documented in Jammu and Kashmir, Himachal Pradesh, Uttaranchal, Rajasthan, Assam, West Bengal, Maharashtra, Kerala, and Tamil Nadu. Recent studies from western Maharashtra and central India have documented that rickettsial diseases are an important reemerging infections in India.

ETIOPATHOGENESIS

Family *Rickettsiae* comprises three genera, namely *Rickettsia, Orientia*, and *Ehrlichia*. Former members of this family, *Coxiella burnetii* which causes Q fever and *Rochalimaea quintana* causing trench fever, have been excluded because the former is not primarily arthropod-borne and the latter not an obligate intracellular parasite. Various members of this family can be grouped into four bio-groups as shown in **Table 5.29.1** based on the lipopolysaccharides group antigen.

Man is an accidental host except for louse-borne epidemic typhus caused by *Rickettsia prowazekii*. Transmission to humans occurs by infected arthropod vector or exposure to infected animal reservoir host. Vector-to-human transmission occurs as vector defecate while feeding (flea feeding reflex) so that feces contaminates pruritic bite wounds (seen with typhus fever group) or primarily by bite, where the regurgitation of infected saliva occurs during feeding (seen with spotted fever group and scrub typhus).

Vasculitis is the basic pathogenic mechanism and is responsible for skin rash, microvascular leakage, edema, and tissue hypoperfusion and end organ ischemic injury.

CLINICAL FEATURES

Early signs and symptoms of these infections are notoriously nonspecific, and hence, high index of suspicion is of paramount importance for their early diagnosis. Various clinical features of rickettsial infections are shown in the following sections.

Fever

Fever of undetermined origin is the most frequent presentation of rickettsial disease. Fever is usually abrupt onset, high grade, sometimes with chills, occasionally with morning remissions, and associated with headache and myalgia. In fact, the diagnosis of rickettsial disease should always be considered in patients with acute febrile illness accompanied with headache and myalgia, particularly in endemic areas with history of tick exposure or contact with dogs.

Headache and Myalgia

Severe frontal headache and generalized myalgia especially in muscles of the lumbar region, thigh, and calf are seen in variable proportion of cases.

Rash

Though rash is considered as hallmark of rickettsial disease, it is neither seen at presentation nor it is present in all the patients. Thus, it should be remembered that spotted fevers could be spotless too! Rash usually becomes apparent after 3–5 days of onset of symptoms. Initially, rash is in the form of pink, blanching, discrete macules which subsequently becomes maculopapular, petechial, or hemorrhagic. Sometimes palpable purpura (typical of vasculitis) is seen **(Fig. 5.29.1)**. Occasionally, petechiae enlarge to ecchymosis and gangrenous patches may develop. Rarely gangrene of digits **(Fig. 5.29.2)**, earlobes, scrotum, nose, or limbs may develop secondary to vasculitis and thrombosis. Distribution of rash is initially on the extremities near ankles, lower legs, and wrists. Thereafter, the rash spreads centripetally to involve the whole body. The presence of rash on palms and soles, considered so typical

Table 5.29.1: Bio-groups of rickettsia.

S. no.	Bio-group	Disease	Vector	Organism
1.	Spotted fever	RMSF	Tick	*Rickettsia rickettsii*
		Rickettsialpox	Mite	*Rickettsia akari*
		Indian tick typhus, boutonneuse fever, MSF	Tick	*Rickettsia conorii*
2.	Typhus	Epidemic louse-borne typhus	Louse	*Rickettsia prowazekii*
		Brill-Zinsser disease (recrudescent typhus)	Louse	*Rickettsia prowazekii*
		Endemic or murine flea-borne typhus	Flea	*Rickettsia typhi*
3.	Scrub typhus	Scrub typhus	Chigger	*Orientia tsutsugamushi*
4.	Miscellaneous	Ehrlichiosis and anaplasmosis	Tick	*Ehrlichia, Anaplasma*
		TIBOLA	Tick	*Rickettsia slovaca*
		DEBONEL	Tick	*Rickettsia slovaca*

(RMSF: Rocky mountain spotted fever; MSF: Mediterranean spotted fever; TIBOLA: tick-borne lymphadenopathy; DEBONEL: Dermacentor-borne necrosis-eschar-lymphadenopathy)

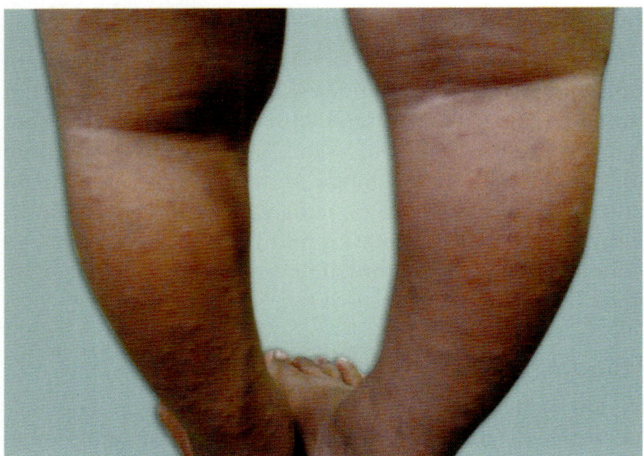

Fig. 5.29.1: Palpable purpuric rash.

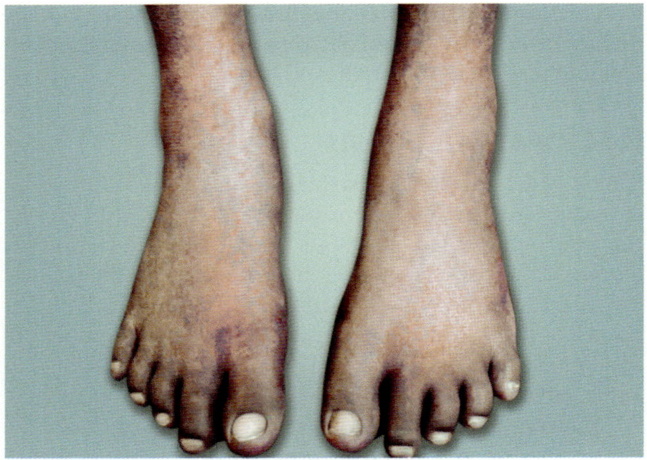

Fig. 5.29.2: Pedal edema with gangrenous changes in toes.

of rickettsial disease, can be seen in other diseases, such as infective endocarditis, syphilis, meningococcemia, enteroviral diseases, and adverse drug reactions. The rash of typhus group infections is quite atypical, initially appearing on trunk, spreading centrifugally, and usually sparing palms and soles.

Eschar

A necrotic eschar at the inoculating site is seen in variable proportion of Indian tick typhus, scrub typhus, and rickettsial pox cases. The site of initial tick bite is inapparent in other rickettsial infections. Eschar, a black necrotic area, resembles the skin burn of cigarette butt **(Fig. 5.29.3)**. A necrotic eschar usually has an erythematous rim and is associated with regional lymphadenopathy.

Generalized Lymphadenopathy and Hepatosplenomegaly

It is found in majority of scrub typhus patients.

Systemic Features

Clinical features referable to various systems are sometimes seen in rickettsial infections. Gastrointestinal symptoms, such as nausea, vomiting, abdominal pain, and diarrhea, are seen with varying frequency. Constipation is seen particularly in epidemic typhus. Respiratory symptoms, such as cough and distress, are sometimes seen. Neurological manifestations, such as dizziness, drowsiness, disorientation, tinnitus, photophobia, delirium, meningismus, and visual disturbances, are seen more commonly with typhus group infections.

Miscellaneous

Periorbital edema, conjunctival hyperemia, epistaxis, acute reversible hearing loss, and arthralgia are sometimes reported.

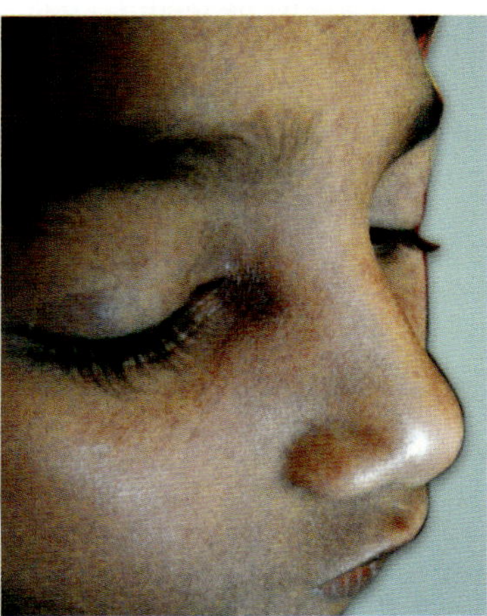

Fig. 5.29.3: Eschar near medial canthus of right eye.

MODALITIES OF DIAGNOSIS

Clinical laboratory findings include normal-to-low total leukocyte count, during early course of the disease with marked shift to left, low platelet counts, and high erythrocyte sedimentation rate. There may be hyponatremia, hypoalbuminemia, and raised hepatic transaminases.

Serological diagnosis is difficult during the acute stage of the disease as definite diagnosis usually requires examination of paired serum samples after convalescence. Most common serological test for confirmed diagnosis is indirect immunofluorescence assay, but not until the second week of the disease, diagnostic titer is detectable.

Blood or tissue samples can be tested for rickettsial nucleic acid by polymerase chain reaction, but it is relatively insensitive as the level of rickettsemia is very low.

Flowchart 5.29.1: IAP guidelines for diagnosis and management of rickettsial diseases.

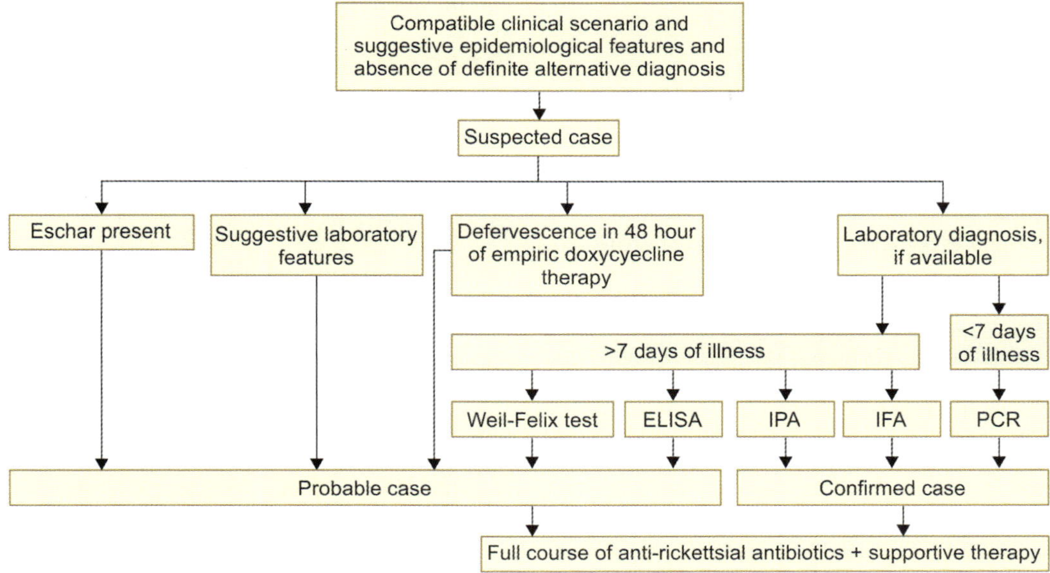

(IAP: Indian Academy of Pediatrics)

As no clinical or laboratory clues are specific for early diagnosis, diagnosis should be made with compatible clinical presentation, history of tick exposure, epidemiological data, suggestive laboratory parameters, and rapid defervescence with appropriate antibiotics.

Indian Academy of Pediatrics have formulated guidelines for rickettsial diseases in children and have elaborated an algorithm of case definitions **(Flowchart 5.29.1)**, various clinical scenarios in which rickettsial disease should be considered **(Box 5.29.1)**, epidemiological features which suggest these infections **(Box 5.29.2)**, differential diagnosis **(Box 5.29.3)**, and laboratory features which suggest diagnosis of these infections **(Box 5.29.4)**.

Box. 5.29.1: Compatible clinical scenario for rickettsial infection.

One or more of the following:
- Undifferentiated fever of more than 5 days.
- Sepsis of unclear etiology.
- Fever with rash.
- Fever with edema.
- Dengue-like disease.
- Fever with headache and myalgia.
- Fever with hepatosplenomegaly and/or lymphadenopathy.
- Aseptic meningitis/meningoencephalitis/acute encephalitic syndrome.
- Fever with cough and pulmonary infiltrates or community acquired pneumonia.
- Fever with acute kidney injury.
- Fever with acute gastrointestinal or hepatic involvement.

TREATMENT

Definitive treatment should be instituted based on clinical and epidemiological clues as early as possible to avoid severe disease and fatal outcome. Various antibiotics useful for treating different rickettsial diseases are tetracycline preferably doxycycline, chloramphenicol, macrolides (especially azithromycin, clarithromycin, and roxithromycin), and fluoroquinolones (especially ciprofloxacin, ofloxacin, pefloxacin, and levofloxacin).

Doxycycline is the drug of choice. Dose is 5 mg/kg/day in two divided doses for children below 45 kg and 200 mg/day in two divided doses for children above 45 kg. Duration of therapy should be minimum 5–7 days or at least 3 days after defervescence. It can be used for treatment of rickettsial diseases in children below 8 years of age as tooth discoloration is dose dependent.

Box. 5.29.2: Suggestive epidemiological features for rickettsial infections.

One or more of the following within 14 days of illness onset:
- Tick bite.
- Ticks seen on clothes or in and around homes or in areas where children play.
- Visit to areas which are common habitats of vectors like high uncut grass or weeds or bushes or rice fields or woodlands (where rodents share habitats with animals) or grassy lawns or river banks or poorly maintained kitchen gardens.
- Animal sheds in proximity of homes.
- Contact with pet or stray dog infested with ticks.
- Living in or travel to areas endemic for rickettsial diseases.
- Occurrence of similar clinical cases simultaneously or sequentially in family members, coworkers, neighborhood or pets.
- Exposure to rodents.

Box. 5.29.3: Differential diagnoses for rickettsial infections.

- *Viral diseases*: Enteroviral diseases, measles, dengue fever, chikungunya, and infectious mononucleosis.
- *Bacterial diseases*: Meningococcemia, leptospirosis, typhoid fever, scarlet fever, secondary syphilis, and infective endocarditis.
- *Protozoal diseases*: Malaria.
- *Vasculitis*: Kawasaki disease and thrombotic thrombocytopenic purpura.
- Adverse drug reactions.
- Differential diagnoses pertaining to each systemic presentation.

Box. 5.29.4: Suggestive laboratory features for rickettsial infections.

- Normal-to-low total leukocyte count with a shift to left in early stages and leukocytosis later.
- Thrombocytopenia
- Raised ESR and CRP
- Hyponatremia
- Hypoalbuminemia
- Elevated hepatic transaminases.

Chloramphenicol should be used in case of doxycycline allergy (50–100 mg/kg/day every 6 hours intravenously, maximum 3 g/day).

COMPLICATIONS

Respiratory (interstitial pneumonitis and *acute respiratory distress syndrome*), neurologic (meningoencephalitis), renal (acute renal failure), disseminated intravascular coagulation, hepatic failure, gangrene, and myocarditis are various complications seen in rickettsial infections.

PROGNOSIS

Untreated cases can have fatality rates as high as 30–35%, but when diagnosed early, they are often easily treated and carry extremely good prognosis.

PREVENTION

Avoiding tick bites, limiting exposure to tick habitats, inspecting the body carefully for ticks after being in a tick habitat, and removing attached ticks immediately by grasping with tweezers close to skin and pulling gently with steady pressure are various means of prevention. Antibiotic prophylaxis after tick bite is usually not beneficial.

BIBLIOGRAPHY

1. Edwards MS, Feigin RD. Rickettsial and ehrlichial diseases. In: Feigin RD, Cherry JD, Demmler-Harrison GJ, Kaplan SL, Steinbach WJ (Eds). Textbook of Pediatric Infectious Diseases, 6th edition. Philadelphia, PA: Saunders Elsevier; 2009. pp. 2669-83.
2. Rathi N, Rathi A. Rickettsial infections—Indian perspective. Indian Pediatr. 2010;47(2):157-64.
3. Rathi NB, Rathi AN, Goodman MH, et al. Rickettsial diseases in central India—proposed clinical scoring system for early detection of spotted fever. Indian Pediatr. 2011;48(11):867-72.
4. Rathi NB, Kulkarni A, Yewale V. IAP guidelines on rickettsial diseases in children. Indian Pediatr. 2017;54:223-9.

5.30 Leprosy

Rajeshwar Dayal

INTRODUCTION

Leprosy, also known as Hansen's disease, is a chronic granulomatous disease caused by *Mycobacterium leprae*. It particularly affects the skin and nerves along with affecting all the organs.

EPIDEMIOLOGY

According to World Health Organization (WHO), out of a total 214,783 new cases of leprosy in the world in 2016, 135,485 (63%) were residing in India. Of these, 8.94% were below 15 years of age. The global prevalence rate decreased from 0.31/10,000 population in 2014 to 0.23/10,000 population in 2016.

Leprosy is widely prevalent in India. In South East Asia Region also, India contributes the highest number of cases with a registered prevalence of 88,166 out of 115,180 cases. After the introduction of multidrug therapy (MDT) the total number of registered cases of leprosy in India came down to about 86,028 (prevalence rate of 0.66/10,000 population) in 2016 from 0.5 million (prevalence rate of 6.7/10,000 population) in 1997.

Pediatric leprosy constitutes about 9% of the total disease burden. The age group most commonly affected in the pediatric leprosy population is 5–14 years, though in very high-endemic countries, prevalence in age groups 0–4 years is also significant. Leprosy affects males more than females. It is not a hereditary disease, and it was found that infants born to leprous parents, if separated soon after birth and protected from the exposure, escaped from the disease. Human immunodeficiency virus infection has not been documented to alter the risk of leprosy in areas of high prevalence.

Achieving eradication of the disease from the elimination stage is a giant task. It requires the cases to be identified at an early stage and treated promptly so that deformity and spread of infection can be prevented. For the diagnosis of early and suspicious cases of leprosy, newer diagnostic concepts of molecular biological approaches, such as polymerase chain reaction (PCR), in situ PCR, and in situ hybridization, have evolved and are the need of the time.

ETIOLOGY

Leprosy is caused by *M. leprae*, which is an acid-fast, nonsporing bacillus, and occurs both intracellularly as well as extracellularly. In stained smear, it lies singly, as rods, or in clumps called globi. They have affinity for the Schwann cells and cells of reticuloendothelial system. Till date, it cannot be grown in any artificial media. *M. leprae* does not produce any toxin and is well adapted to reside within macrophages, yet it may survive outside the body for months.

Source of Infection and Mode of Transmission

The only source of infection is the infected human being. The capacity of multibacillary leprosy patients to infect is 4–11 times that of patients with paucibacillary leprosy.

Direct Transmission

For direct transmission, a prolonged and close contact is required. An "intrafamilial" contact with a patient is more risky than an "extrafamilial" one.

Untreated lepromatous patients discharge as many as 100 million bacilli from their nasal secretions every day. These bacilli remain viable outside the human body for several days. Inhalation of these bacilli, via droplets, is now regarded as the most common mode of entry of leprosy bacilli into the contact person. After inhalation, these inhaled leprosy bacilli enter the respiratory system from where they are disseminated by blood to skin and peripheral nerves where depending on the host immune response, the disease may manifest either as tuberculoid leprosy (where there is good cell-mediated immune response to *M. leprae*) or may manifest at lepromatous leprosy (LL) (where there is anergy to *M. leprae*).

Other portals of entry include scratched, abraded, or insect-bitten skin, which facilitates passage of organism via the droplets laden with leprosy bacilli through the epidermis into the dermis, and ingestion of infected breast milk.

Indirect Transmission

Mycobacterium leprae remains viable for several days outside the human body. Occasionally, leprosy may spread by fomites being used by a patient suffering from multibacillary leprosy. Localized infections via infected syringes and tattooing needles have been reported.

CLINICAL MANIFESTATIONS

Incubation Period

This varies from a few months to as long as 20 years with an average between 2 years and 5 years. Onset of this disease is usually gradual but may be sudden in highly susceptible people.

Early Signs of the Disease

- A hypopigmented patch in the skin, present for a long duration, nonirritating with loss of sensation to touch, pain, and temperature.
- Thickening of the skin, more red and shiny in appearance than the surrounding parts; this is more prominent on face and hands.
- Loss of sensation, numbness, feeling of "pins and needles" or "crawling of ants", tingling sensation in any part of the body, especially in hands and feet. There may be paresis in hands and feet or difficulty in fine movements of fingers.
- Appearance of spontaneous blisters and ulcers, especially in fingers.

CLASSIFICATION

According to the classification laid down by Indian Association of Leprologists, the cases have been divided into five broad groups, viz.

1. Indeterminate
2. Borderline
3. Tuberculoid
4. Lepromatous
5. Polyneuritic.

The borderline group is further subdivided into midborderline (BB), borderline lepromatous (BL), and borderline tuberculoid (BT) types.

Indeterminate Leprosy

This type of leprosy is seen in only 10–20% of infected individuals and is the earliest detectable form of leprosy.

This is characterized by the presence of a single hypopigmented macule measuring 2–4 cm in diameter, with a poorly defined border without any erythema or induration. Anesthesia may be minimal or even absent. Biopsy may show a granuloma but bacilli are rarely seen in the section. In 50–75% of patients, this lesion heals spontaneously, and in the remaining cases, it gradually progresses to one of the classic forms.

Tuberculoid Leprosy

It is characterized by the presence of single or few asymmetrical, well-defined, hypopigmented, erythematous, or copper-colored patches with sensory impairment. The entire patch or only its margins are raised above the level of the surrounding skin.

Initially, a single nerve trunk related to the lesions is affected. The nerve trunk becomes enlarged, hard, and tender and later may form a nerve abscess.

In this form of leprosy, the lepromin test is positive, and there is an absence of bacilli in the skin smear. On biopsy, foci of lymphocytes, epithelioid cells, and Langhan's giant cells are seen.

This form of leprosy is the most common, especially in children, and is relatively benign and stable with a good prognosis.

Borderline Leprosy

Borderline leprosy is further classified into three subtypes based on clinical and histological criteria.

1. *Borderline tuberculoid leprosy*: Here the lesions are greater in number but smaller in size than in tuberculoid leprosy. There may be small satellite lesions around older lesions, and the margins of the BT lesions are less distinct and the center is less atrophic and anesthetic. This form usually involves thickening of two or more superficial nerves.
2. *Midborderline leprosy*: In this subtype, the lesions are more numerous and heterogeneous. The lesions may become confluent or even plaques may be present. The borders are poorly defined and the erythematous rim fades into the surrounding skin. Hyperesthesia is more common than anesthesia.
3. *Borderline LL*: In BL leprosy, there are a large number of asymmetrically distributed lesions, which are heterogeneous in appearance. Macules, papules, plaques, and nodules may all coexist. Usually, the individual lesions are small unless confluent. Anesthesia is mild and superficial nerve trunks are spared.

Lepromatous Leprosy

Most cases of LL develop from borderline leprosy (BB or BL). This form of leprosy is relatively uncommon in the pediatric age group. There are two symptoms, which may precede the classical skin lesions by months or years, and serve to alert the physician to a possible early diagnosis. They are:

- Nasal symptoms
- Edema of legs.

The nasal symptoms chiefly constitute stuffiness, crust formation, and bloodstained discharge. Edema of legs and ankles is always bilateral, usually prominent late in the evening and disappears after overnight rest.

Skin lesions may take the form of macules, papules, nodules, and a combination of them. Numerous symmetrically distributed erythematous or coppery, shiny, macules with ill-defined margins are usually the first ones to appear. Patients may have a leonine facies due to the loss of eyebrows and eyelashes. There is no sensory impairment in these lesions, but as the disease progresses, many peripheral nerves get symmetrically affected. Due to enormous bacillary infiltration, nerves are initially softer and larger than normal and are tender. In advanced cases, nerves become thin and hard due to fibrosis and result in extreme anesthesia. The skin smear is almost always positive, and the lepromin test is negative.

This form of LL is the most infectious, prone to lepra reactions and if left untreated, the prognosis is poor.

The features of these varieties of leprosy are summarized in **Table 5.30.1**. As age advances, the disease moves from tuberculoid end of the spectrum toward the lepromatous end.

Neuritic Leprosy

These cases show nerve involvement but do not have any skin lesion. This may be of primary or secondary variety. In the former, the nerves are directly infected without any skin lesion, while in the latter, infection spreads up the nerves from leprous skin lesions. The affected nerves become thickened and tender, producing sensory motor and trophic changes in their areas of distribution. This dysfunction leads to deformities, neuropathic ulcers, and lagophthalmos, which may result in serious eye complications.

Neuritic leprosy most commonly involves the ulnar, median, lateral popliteal, tibial, great auricular and rarely radial nerves. It also affects the V and VII cranial nerves.

Reactions

Reactions are acute exacerbations due to changes in the host-parasite immune relationship. They are common during initial years of treatment. The types are noted in the following subsections.

Type 1

Reversal reaction: This is seen in borderline cases and consists of acute tenderness and swelling at the site of lesion. Irreversible nerve injury can occur if this reaction is not treated immediately.

Table 5.30.1: Clinical aspects of tuberculoid, borderline, and lepromatous leprosy.

Features	*Types of leprosy*				
	TT	*BT*	*BB*	*BL*	*LL*
Number of lesions	Single usually	Single or few	Several	Many	Very many
Size of lesions	Variable	Variable	Variable	Variable	Small
Surface of lesions	Very dry, sometimes scaly	Dry	Slightly shiny	Shiny	Shiny
Sensation in lesions	Absent	Markedly diminished	Moderately diminished	Slightly diminished	Not affected
Hair growth	Absent	Markedly diminished	Moderately diminished	Slightly diminished	Not affected
AFB in lesions	Nil	Nil or scanty	Moderate numbers	Many	Very many (plus globi)
AFB in nasal scrapings/in nose blows	Nil	Nil	Nil	Usually nil	Very many (plus globi)
Lepromin test	Strongly positive (+++)	Weakly positive (+ or ++)	Negative	Negative	Negative

(AFB: acid-fast bacilli; BB: midborderline; BL: borderline lepromatous; BT: borderline tuberculoid; LL: lepromatous leprosy; TT: tuberculoid)

Type 2

Erythema nodosum leprosum reactions: This occurs in lepromatous and BL cases as a systemic inflammatory response. There is high fever, migrating polyarthralgia, orchitis, iridocyclitis, and lymphadenitis. Tender red papules or nodules resembling erythema nodosum are seen characteristically.

DIAGNOSIS

Diagnosis of leprosy is based on the presence of any one of the following cardinal signs:

- Characteristic skin lesion with partial or total loss of sensation in the affected skin lesion or in the area of the skin supplied by the peripheral nerve involved with or without the presence of thickened nerves.
- Presence of acid-fast bacilli in the skin smear.

Smear Examination

Sites of bacteriological examination are usually from the most affected parts of the lesion. If no definite patches or areas of thickened skin are visible, smear should be taken from ear lobules and buttocks. Smears should be made by "slit and scrape" method and stained by Ziehl–Neelsen (ZN) staining. Smears are positive in LL, BL, and some BB and BT cases. It is of limited help in tuberculoid and indeterminate lesions and in patients with early atypical clinical presentation.

Histopathology

In some cases of indeterminate lesions, it becomes necessary to carry out a histological examination for the purpose of diagnosis and classification of the lesion.

Bacillary Index

It is a semiquantitative estimation of the density of bacilli present in the skin smears and biopsies and is measured on two scales, namely, (1) the Dharmendra scale and (2) Ridley scale. It measures the total acid-fast bacilli in microscopic field, which includes both live and dead bacilli.

Patients are labeled as having paucibacillary infection when there are less than or equal to five skin lesions and no bacilli on skin smears. They are labeled as having multibacillary infection when there are more than or equal to six skin lesions and bacilli are present on skin smears. The bacterial index can range from 0 (no bacilli in 100 oil immersion field) to 6 (>1,000 bacilli per field).

Footpad Culture

Inoculation of material into the mouse footpad is the only certain way to demonstrate multiplication of bacilli. This method is 10 times more sensitive at detecting *M. leprae* than slit skin smear examination.

Immunological Methods

Test for Cell-mediated Immunity

Lepromin test: This is a test using intradermal injection of 0.1 mL of lepromin (Dharmendra or Mitsuda antigen) into the inner aspect of forearm of the individual. The reaction is read at 48 hours (Fernandez reaction) and 21 days (Mitsuda reaction) to classify the stage of leprosy. Lepromin test is not a diagnostic test for leprosy but it has been found to be useful for classifying the disease. This test is positive in the cases of tuberculoid and BT; negative in LL, BL; and weakly positive and variable in BB leprosy. The lepromin-negative contacts have been found to be at much higher risk of developing disease than the lepromin-positive contacts. This test signifies cell-mediated immunity of a person. Two kinds of lepromin are commonly used:

1. Crude antigen of Mitsuda;
2. The refined antigen of Dharmendra.

Serological Assays

Specific serological tests can detect subclinical infection. The major serological assays include:

- *Fluorescent leprosy antibody absorption test*: This technique is highly sensitive in detecting the antibodies against *M. Leprae* antigen by immune-fluorescent technique and is useful in identifying healthy contacts of patients who are at risk of developing disease.
- *Radioimmunoassay*: It detects antibodies to the cell wall antigen of *M. Leprae.*
- *Enzyme-linked immunosorbent assay (ELISA)*: Phenolic glycolipid (PGL)-ELISA (PGL-ELISA) was found highly positive in multibacillary cases, but positivity in paucibacillary and subclinical cases was quite low. Further simplified dot ELISA and dipstick ELISA using a monoclonal antibody targeting PGL-1 have also been studied.

Serological testing is not useful for diagnosis as it does not detect most paucibacillary cases, and it remains positive even after treatment of multibacillary patients.

Molecular Biological Approaches

Identification of organisms can be done in a more rapid and specific way, both from culture and directly from clinical specimen, by recombinant deoxyribonucleic acid (DNA) technology. Based on the gene sequences of *M. Leprae*, several probes have been designed in recent years. During the recent years, several gene amplification techniques, such as PCR, for amplifying *M. Leprae*-specific sequences from variety of specimens have been published. These have been reported to be highly sensitive and specific.

In Situ Polymerase Chain Reaction

In situ PCR, also called slide PCR, is a method to run PCR directly on small tissue samples, tissue microarrays, or other small cell samples rather than extracting DNA or ribonucleic acid (RNA) first, and then performing PCR, real-time PCR or quantitative PCR from the extracted material. In our series, in situ PCR showed a positivity of 57.1% in early or localized form of leprosy [indeterminate (I)/BT] and 61.5% in BB or BL group. When compared to histopathological examination, a significant enhancement of 15% in diagnosis was seen. Hence, it can be concluded that in situ PCR, with added advantages of providing structural correlates and concomitant study of tissue pathology, improves diagnostic yield in early doubtful cases of leprosy and when histopathology in nonspecific.

In Situ Hybridization

In situ hybridization uses a labeled complementary DNA/RNA strand to localize specific DNA/RNA in a portion or section of tissue. In situ hybridization significantly enhances the diagnosis in early cases. In our series, it showed a positivity of about 42.8% in early I/BT and 46.7% in BB/BL group, thus enhancing the diagnosis by 18.1%.

In Situ Polymerase Chain Reaction on Slit Skin Smears

Another molecular biological approach is the utility of in situ PCR on the slit skin smears. It was found that with an average positivity of 72%, in situ PCR on slit skin smears was better than that on skin biopsies (60%). In addition, it has the added advantages of being minimally invasive and less cumbersome and can be performed even at sites from where skin biopsy is difficult.

Mycobacterium leprae-specific Repetitive Element Polymerase Chain Reaction

The *M. leprae*-specific repetitive element (RLEP) amplicon of *M. leprae* is specific for the organism and is a repetitive sequence in the chromosome. Our studies using the *RLEP PCR* techniques showed that it was significantly better than ZN staining. It is therefore a very valuable diagnostic tool.

MANAGEMENT

Leprosy patients should be treated with patience, perseverance, and understanding. Along with the medical treatment, the patients and their parents need moral support and reassurance. Parents should be explained hygienic measures, proper diet, and importance of taking treatment completely and regularly.

Multidrug Therapy

It is now a well-known fact that simultaneous administration of several different antibacterial agents may prevent the emergence of drug-resistant mutants.

The standard child (ages 10–14 years) treatment regimen for multibacillary leprosy is:

- *Rifampicin*: 450 mg once a month under supervision.
- *Clofazimine*: 150 mg once a month under supervision and 50 mg every other day.
- *Dapsone*: 50 mg daily.
- *Duration*: 12 months.

Table 5.30.2: World Health Organization (WHO) multidrug therapy regimens.

Type of leprosy	*Daily, self-administered*	*Alternate day, self-administered*	*Monthly, supervised*	*Months of treatment*
Paucibacillary	Dapsone (2 mg/kg)	–	Rifampicin (10 mg/kg)	6
Multibacillary	Dapsone (2 mg/kg)	Clofazimine (1 mg/kg)	Rifampicin (10 mg/kg) Clofazimine (6 mg/kg)	12

Courtesy: WHO. (2013). Leprosy elimination. [online] Available from <http://www.who.int/lep/mdt/en/> [Accessed October, 2018].

- The standard child (ages 10–14 years) treatment regimen for paucibacillary leprosy is:
- *Rifampicin*: 450 mg once a month under supervision.
- *Dapsone*: 50 mg daily.
- *Duration*: 6 months.

The dosage schedule for children below 10 years as recommended by WHO is shown in **Table 5.30.2**.

In the MDT, it is assumed that clofazimine is acceptable for children and, therefore, no child will require ethionamide or prothionamide which are potent hepatotoxic drugs. Parents should be advised to give rifampicin on empty stomach and clofazimine with meals or with a glass of milk. Red staining of skin and lesions are very common with clofazimine.

Treatment of Reactions

Drugs commonly used in these conditions are antimalarials, such as chloroquine (given orally), antimonials, e.g. potassium antimony tartrate IV and fantosin intramuscularly (IM), clofazimine, corticosteroids, and thalidomide (all the three given orally). Symptoms, such as iritis and neuritis, occurring during reactions (or occurring independently) should be properly treated in order to avoid irreversible sequelae, i.e. deformities and neuropathic ulcers.

PROPHYLAXIS

Leprosy Vaccine

The National Leprosy Eradication Programme (NLEP) has introduced the *Mycobacterium indicus pranii* (MIP) vaccine in a project mode in India from the year 2016. MIP vaccine has been shown to have both immunotherapeutic and immune-prophylactic effects in multibacillary leprosy patients and their contacts in both hospital and population-based trials. It also reduced the bacillary load, upgraded the lesions histopathologically, led to complete clearance of granuloma, reduced reactions, and neuritis and reduced the duration of MDT in leprosy patients. In the new field project undertaken under Indian Council of Medical Research and NLEP, the index leprosy patient will receive the MIP vaccine over and above the MDT. His family members and contacts would be immunized with MIP twice at an interval of 6 months with the expectation that their immunity is reinforced to evade leprosy on exposure to *M. leprae* from a patient. The utility of immunizing the index case is for rapid clearance of bacteria and clinical lesions. In contacts, MIP vaccination upgrades their immunity, thereby resisting the development of the clinical disease on exposure to *M. leprae* from those suffering from it.

Bacille de Calmette et Guérin Vaccine

The result of 5–9-year follow-up study conducted on 120,000 randomized individuals in South Africa indicates that the bacillus Calmette–Guérin (BCG) booster vaccination (two-dose BCG regimen given at 0 months and 3 months) provides 50–75% protection against leprosy. The combined BCG *M. leprae* vaccine offered no additional benefit.

In order to accelerate the elimination of leprosy as a public health problem in India, the following activities should receive high priority: 100% MDT coverage and accessibility, high treatment completion, and cure rates and inclusion of leprosy in the training curricula of the general health staff of all categories.

BIBLIOGRAPHY

1. Dayal R, Agarwal M, Natrajan M, et al. PCR and in-situ hybridization for diagnosis of leprosy. Indian J Paediatr. 2007;74:645-8.
2. Dayal R, Singh SP, Mathur PP, et al. Diagnostic value of in situ polymerase chain reaction in leprosy. Indian J Paediatr. 2005;72:1043-6.
3. Global leprosy update, 2016: accelerating reduction of disease burden. Wkly Epidemiol Rec. 2017;92:501-20.
4. Gupta P. Textbook of Preventive and Social Medicine, 4th edition. New Delhi: CBS Publishers and Distributors Private Limited; 2013.
5. Kamal R, Dayal R, Gaidhankar K, et al. RLEP PCR as a definitive diagnostic test for leprosy from skin smear samples in childhood and adolescent leprosy. Indian J Lepr. 2016;88:193-7.
6. Kamal R, Pathak V, Kumari A, et al. Addition of *Mycobacterium indicus pranii* vaccine as an immunotherapeutic to standard chemotherapy in borderline leprosy: a double-blind study

to assess clinical improvement (preliminary report). Br J Dermatol. 2017;176:1388-9.

7. Leprosy. In Park K (Ed). Textbook of Preventive and Social Medicine, 23rd edition. India: Bhanot Publishers; 2015. pp. 314-30.
8. Powell DA. Hansen disease (*Mycobacterium leprae*). In Kliegman B, Jenson S (Eds). Nelson Textbook of Pediatrics, 18th edition. Philadelphia, PA: Elsevier Saunders; 2008. pp. 1255-8.
9. Yan W, Xing Y, Yuan LC, et al. Application of RLEP real-time PCR for detection of *M. leprae* DNA in paraffin-embedded skin biopsy specimens for diagnosis of paucibacillary leprosy. Am J Trop Med Hyg. 2014;90:524-9.

5.31 Pandemic Influenza

Nitin Shah

EPIDEMIOLOGY

On March 18, 2009, Mexico reported cases of influenza-like illness (ILI) in children from whom a novel influenza type A virus was isolated. The disease then spread further in Mexico, USA and other parts of world. On June 11, 2009, the World Health Organization (WHO) declared phase 6 of the first influenza pandemic of the current century caused by novel H1N1 2009 type A strain.

In 2015, there was a resurgence of pH1N1 (p refers to pandemic status of the strain) influenza cases in India and some other parts of world. In the last week of February 2015, 652 out of 659 samples testing positive for influenza were due to pH1N1. As on March 31, 2015, the number of reported cases of pH1N1 influenza in India had crossed the figure of 30,000 and reported deaths caused had crossed figure of 2,000, which was very similar to the pandemic situation when it began in India. Rajasthan, Gujarat, and Andhra Pradesh were the worst affected states in 2015.

NOVEL H1N1 INFLUENZA STRAIN

Antigenic shift leading to point mutations in the H and or N antigens of the circulating influenza viruses occurs regularly, which results in outbreaks or epidemics in the community from time to time. When both the H and N antigens change such way that they are antigenically totally different from the past circulating strains, it is called antigenic shift and results in pandemic as the population has no immunity to the new virus.

The novel H1N1 2009 strain responsible for the recent pandemic in 2015 was a reassortant virus with gene segments from viruses of swine (European, North American, and Asian; five segments), birds (two segments), and humans (one segment). However, this novel virus was not infective in swine and was actually a misnomer. The novel H1N1 2009 virus was antigenically different from the earlier human H1N1 viruses. It was believed that this virus had no cross-protection from previous exposure to seasonal H1N1 virus. However, we now know that the novel H1N1 2009 virus infection was milder in elderly population, and hence, there seems to some cross-protection between this virus and the 1918–1919 H1N1 virus.

MODE OF INFECTION

The novel H1N1 virus is transmitted via nasopharyngeal route like any other influenza virus. Hence, virus spreads mainly via coughing, sneezing, hands, social contact, and from medical interventions, such as suctioning, nebulization, and open ventilation, which generates respiratory mist. It can spread by infected fomites such as shared napkins and handkerchiefs. Person is infective from 1 day before to 7 days after novel H1N1 infection. If illness persists beyond 7 days, person remains infective till resolution of symptoms.

CLINICAL MANIFESTATIONS

Pandemic H1N1 2009 infection, though milder than previous influenza pandemics and with less mortality, affected healthy young people more often than the elderly people. In India, 33% of cases were reported in 5–19 years of age group and 40% in 20–39 years of age group; seroepidemiology study done from Pune, India, during the peak transmission showed that the peak seroprevalence in general population was 7.7% in adults, 13.2% in children, 28.3% in 15–19 years old, and only 3.5% in more than 60 years old. Seroprevalence was higher in people exposed to children and sick patients and was 20% in hospital staff, 35.6% in general medical practitioners, 26% in school staff. Another study in the USA showed that 25–50% of cases who were hospitalized or died were young and healthy and had no comorbidities. Pregnancy, asthma, other lung diseases, diabetes, morbid obesity, autoimmune disorders and associated immunosuppressive therapies, neurological disorders, and cardiovascular disease are some of the risk factors for increased morbidity and mortality associated with pandemic influenza. A recent metaestimate of burden of influenza in developing countries compared to developed countries has shown that the incidence of influenza-like acute lower respiratory infections was 2.9-fold higher in children less than 5 years of age in developing countries compared to developed countries, proven influenza incidence was 2.8-fold higher and even mortality was significantly higher in children less than 5 years in developing countries.

Spectrum of illness can vary from nonfebrile upper respiratory tract infection to severe and often fatal pneumonia. Most develop typical ILI with cough, cold, fever, malaise, sore throat and headache, and recover spontaneously. Up to 40% can develop gastrointestinal (GI) symptoms such as diarrhea and vomiting. During peak transmission, 10–30% of patients presenting with ILI tested positive for novel H1N1 virus, 2–10% of these patients needed hospitalization, and 30% of hospitalized patients needed ventilation. Mortality due to pH1N1 2009 was estimated to be less than 0.5% (0.0004–1.47%), but it is difficult to estimate, as many cases are mild or subclinical giving an incorrect denominator.

The most commonly reported symptoms include cough, fever, sore throat, malaise, and headache. Fever is absent in some outpatients and in up to one in six surviving hospitalized patients. GI symptoms (nausea, vomiting, and/or diarrhea) occurred in up to 38% of outpatients in the USA. Approximately 2–5% of confirmed cases in the USA and Canada, as well as 6% in Mexico needed hospitalization. Among patients presenting with acute respiratory illness for care in Mexico, 13% tested positive for new influenza A (H1N1) virus infection (about one fifth have had seasonal influenza) of whom about 10% have been hospitalized and one third of those hospitalized required mechanical ventilation.

COMPLICATIONS

Most deaths occurred due to severe pneumonia, acute respiratory distress syndrome, or multiorgan failure with renal failure. Mean time from onset of disease to death is 10 days (2–22 days). A total of 30% of patients with fatal pandemic influenza had secondary bacterial infection mainly with *Pneumococcus* as proven by polymerase chain reaction (PCR) for *Pneumococcus* on postmortem lung specimens. Other complications known to occur though rare include rhabdomyolysis, renal failure, myocarditis, and hemophagocytic syndrome. There are patients who are at risk of developing complications following influenza infection because of underlying medical conditions that include those who have chronic pulmonary (including asthma), cardiovascular (except hypertension), renal, hepatic, neurologic, hematological, or metabolic (including diabetes mellitus) disorders; those who are immunosuppressed (including immunosuppression caused by medications or by human immunodeficiency virus), those who are or will be pregnant during the influenza season, those aged 6 months to 18 years and receiving long-term aspirin therapy and who therefore might be at risk for experiencing Reye syndrome after influenza virus infection, and residents of nursing homes and other chronic care facilities.

DIAGNOSIS

Definitive diagnosis of pH1N1 infection is made by real-time PCR test done on clinical specimens, such as nasopharyngeal swab, nasal swab, throat swab, wash or aspirate, or tracheal aspirate (in case of intubated child). The specimen should be collected by experienced clinician or microbiologist. The swab should be placed in transport medium-containing tube and stored and transported at 4°C within 24 hours of collection or else it should be stored at –70°C. Its sensitivity and specificity in a symptomatic patient is nearly 100%. Results normally take 24–48 hours. Serological testing is not recommended as it can only tell whether the strain is type A or type B and cannot differentiate between pH1N1 and other type A seasonal influenza strains.

The Government of India guidelines recommend to reserve PCR-based test only for severe hospitalized patients and not for outdoor patients who should be any way started on oseltamivir on clinical grounds. PCR-based test is also useful to monitor drug sensitivity to oseltamivir and genetic drift in the pH1N1 virus.

MANAGEMENT

Management includes supportive care in most and use of specific antimicrobial agent oseltamivir in select cases as per national guidelines.

National Guidelines

Once ILI is suspected one should follow the national guidelines in managing patients. Patients with some fever but no other features of ILI-like cough, cold, sore throat, vomiting, loose stools, etc. are classified as *group I* and are treated at home with paracetamol, adequate fluid intake, and asked to follow-up, if other symptoms of ILI develop.

Patients who have ILI but without dangers signs, such as respiratory distress, breathlessness, excessive vomiting, persistent high fever, somnolence, inability to take or retain adequate fluids, convulsion or cyanosis, etc., are classified as *group II* and are treated at home with oseltamivir as shown in **Table 5.31.1** along with paracetamol, adequate fluids, and asked to return for follow-up if any of the danger signs develop. Testing with nasopharyngeal swab for PCR is not recommended for *group II* patients. They are also counseled to take rest and measures of infection control at home as discussed later to prevent spread of infection to their contacts and in community.

Once any of the danger signs develop as mentioned before, these patients are classified as *group III* and are hospitalized in isolation wards created for treating pH1N1 patients. Their nasopharyngeal swab is sent for PCR at a government-approved laboratory. Pending the report, they are given oseltamivir. In addition, they are treated with intravenous or oral fluids, symptomatic treatment, oxygen therapy, and other respiratory support including ventilation as required. All measures of infection control are strictly undertaken as discussed later. Salicylates should be avoided in a child with ILI due to risk of Reye's encephalopathy.

Antiviral Therapy

The novel pH1N1 influenza A virus is susceptible to neuraminidase inhibitors (oseltamivir and zanamivir) but resistant to Matrix-2 ion-channel inhibitors (amantadine and rimantadine). Antiviral therapy should be started as early as possible, preferably within 48 hours of onset of illness to be maximally effective. However, it should be started, even if it is delayed at any stage of active disease when ongoing viral replication is anticipated or documented. It is especially recommended in individuals at high risk of complications, such as children less than 5 years of age, patients with progressive respiratory disease including pneumonia, and those with high-risk medical conditions.

Oseltamivir is preferred being oral agent and with minimum side effects and gives higher systemic level. Zanamivir is delivered by inhalation with low systemic absorption. Oseltamivir is the recommended treatment for lower respiratory tract complications. Rare neuropsychiatric symptoms such as confusion or abnormal behavior have occurred after beginning treatment for seasonal influenza with oseltamivir, particularly in children and adolescents, but the contribution of oseltamivir to these events is unknown.

Inhaled zanamivir has been temporally associated with bronchospasm, and patients with preexisting airway disease appear to be at increased risk for this severe adverse reaction. Recommended regimens of using antiviral therapy are shown in **Table 5.31.1**. There is no role of using preventive antiviral therapy due to risk of development of drug resistance. About 278 cases of oseltamivir-resistant novel H1N1 viruses have been reported to the WHO.

Table 5.31.1: Recommended antiviral treatment regimens.

Oseltamivir: For adolescents, 13–17 years of age and for adults the recommended oral dose is 75 mg oseltamivir twice daily for 5 days. For children, recommended doses are as follows:	
By weight:	
15 kg or less	30 mg orally twice a day for 5 days
15–23 kg	45 mg orally twice a day for 5 days
24–40 kg	60 mg orally twice a day for 5 days
>40 kg	75 mg orally twice a day for 5 days
For infants:	
<3 months	12 mg orally twice a day for 5 days
3–5 months	20 mg orally twice a day for 5 days
6–11 months	25 mg orally twice a day for 5 days
(Available as 75 mg per tablet and syrup containing 12 mg/mL)	
(Duration of treatment can be extended up to 10 days in a severe case)	
Zanamivir: Zanamivir is indicated for treatment of influenza in adults and children (>5 years). The recommended dose for treatment of adults and children from the age of 5 years is two inhalations (2 × 5 mg) twice daily for 5 days.	

Supportive Measures

Adequate hydration, proper nutrition, use of moist oxygen, early detection of respiratory failure and timely management with moist oxygen, and ventilatory support are some of the important general supportive measures. Antibiotics are not used routinely and are reserved for cases with suspected secondary bacterial infection. *Pneumococcus* and *Staphylococcus* are important organisms involved in secondary infection in pandemic influenza in children. Routine use of corticosteroids is best avoided. Infection control measures are of utmost importance in preventing spread of disease to close contacts.

PREVENTION

Novel H1N1 infection can be prevented by general measures as well as specific vaccination.

General Infection Control Measures

At Home

Hand hygiene and cough etiquette are important measures for a patient who is managed at home. Surgical mask is not as effective and tends to clog within 2–4 hours, making it ineffective and uncomfortable. Only N95 masks are highly effective in preventing spread of virus but are expensive, not easily available, and are best used in hospital set up. Hand sanitizers are useful in preventing spread of the virus to contacts. Isolation in home for 5–10 days also helps in preventing spread to contacts at workplaces.

At the Community Level

Availability of hand sanitizers at public places will help spread of virus for people touching things of common interest. Avoidance of mass gathering also will prevent spread of virus. Closure of schools, though practiced during peak transmission, is not found to be effective and is impractical. General awareness about how the virus spreads and messages regarding hand hygiene and cough etiquette help regulate personal behavior and spread of virus.

At the Healthcare Facility

Health-care personnel are at great risk of spread of virus from a suspected case of H1N1 influenza, especially, there is uncontrolled mist of respiratory tract secretions of the patient generated, such as with open nebulization, suctioning, or open ventilation systems. Use of protective gears, such as N95 mask (ideal) or surgical disposable mask, head cap and gowns, and strict hand hygiene before and after touching the patient are strongly recommended for those handling patients of H1N1 influenza which includes health-care workers and caretaker. Such patients also have to be isolated in a reserved area with separate entrance and exit where no or minimum human visitors are allowed.

Influenza Vaccines

First vaccine against novel H1N1 strain was a monovalent vaccine against novel H1N1 strain and was approved for manufacturing by US Food and Drug Administration on September 15, 2009, and was available for mass use in the United States on October 5, 2009. Now, novel H1N1 vaccines are available as a live-attenuated trivalent vaccine for intranasal administration and as trivalent inactivated split-virus or subunit vaccines (TIV) for injection which again are with or without adjuvant. Recently, quadrivalent inactivated vaccines containing one more type B strain are available in Western countries. There are several manufacturers of these vaccines. Most of the manufacturers use chicken eggs for producing these vaccines.

Vaccine Compositions

Before the current novel H1N1 pandemic, seasonal H1N1, H3N2, and type B influenza viruses were cocirculating since 1977. Accordingly, influenza vaccine was a trivalent vaccine containing circulating seasonal H1N1, H3N2, and type B strains. Manufacturing flu vaccines is literally a race against the time. Every year the circulating virus drifts and hence the vaccine strains change accordingly. The WHO reference laboratory collects samples isolated from patients with ILI from various sentinel sites in different countries throughout the year and decides on the strains to be used in the Northern vaccine (by February) and Southern vaccine (by August) and provides the seed vaccine virus to the manufactures. The manufacturers then prepare vaccine for commercial and public health use and come out with vaccine in next 6 months so as to be used before next flu season (by September for Northern vaccine and by March for Southern vaccine). Vaccines without adjuvant contain 7.5 μg of hemagglutinin (HA) of each of the three types (total 22.5 μg) per dose for children less than 3 years and 15 μg/dose of each of three types (total 45 μg) for more than 3 years of age. Vaccines with adjuvant usually contain half the dose of HA per virus type. Adjuvants used include ASO4, AFO3, etc.

In the year 2009, novel H1N1 strain replaced the circulating seasonal H1N1, H3N2, and B strains. Hence, monovalent vaccines (live as well as inactivated) containing novel H1N1 virus strain were manufactured and used. As the pandemic got over, gradually novel H1N1 strain became endemic and other strains circulating before the pandemic started cocirculating with the pandemic strain, and hence in 2010, like in past, trivalent flu vaccines (live as well as inactivated) were manufactured containing novel H1N1 strain [A/California/7/2009 (H1N1)-like], seasonal H3N2 strain [H3N2 (A/Perth/16/2009) (H3N2)-like], and type B strain (B/Brisbane/60/2008-like). The vaccine strains have remained the same even in 2011. The strains for 2014/2015 Northern influenza vaccines include A/California/7/2009 (H1N1)-like virus, A/Texas/50/2012 (H3N2)-like virus, B/Massachusetts/2/2012 (B)-like virus and for quadrivalent vaccine additional B type strain is B/Brisbane/60/2008 (B)-like virus. For 2015 Southern vaccines two strains are different and include A/California/7/2009 (H1N1)-like virus, A/Switzerland/9715293/2013 (H3N2)-like virus, B/Phuket/3073/2013 (B)-like virus and for quadrivalent vaccine additional B type strain is B/Brisbane/60/2008(B)-like virus. In 2015 cold adapted live trivalent nasal vaccine is available from on local manufacturer.

Schedule

Influenza vaccine is to be given annually as the vaccine changes every year as discussed before. Two doses are recommended at 4 weeks interval in the first year for children less than 9 years of age. Subsequently, one dose is given annually.

Inactivated Flu Vaccine

Inactivated flu vaccine can be used only for children more than 6 months of age; both for healthy subjects and population at risk of medical complications of influenza infection. Children from 6 months to 3 years of age receive 0.25 mL/dose and those above 3 years receive 0.5 mL/dose.

Live-attenuated Influenza Vaccine

Cold adapted live nasal flu vaccines are recommended only for healthy nonpregnant 2–60 years of age subjects.

Children aged 2–9 years require two doses given 1 month apart. Children above 9 years of age require one dose. Live-attenuated influenza vaccine (LAIV) should be used, if one has received another live vaccine within the last 4 weeks. Dose is split equally between two nostrils administered using a nasal sprayer. The Indian live nasal vaccine has been approved a single dose for all the ages where the vaccine is indicated.

Adverse Effects

These vaccines commonly cause local reactions in 30% of vaccine recipients such as soreness, swelling, and redness at the injection site, and less often fever, muscle- or joint-pains, or headache. These symptoms are generally mild; do not need medical attention, and last for 1–2 days. Fever, aches, and headaches can occur more frequently in children compared to elderly people. Rarely, such influenza vaccines can cause allergic reactions, such as hives, rapid swelling of deeper skin layers and tissues, asthma, or a severe multisystem allergic reaction due to hypersensitivity to certain vaccine components. Live vaccines are given via a nasal spray and can commonly cause runny nose, nasal congestion, cough, and can less frequently cause sore throat, low-grade fever, irritability and headache, and muscle aches. Wheezing and vomiting episodes have been described in children receiving live-influenza vaccines.

Immunogenicity

With experience of using seasonal flu vaccines in past, it has been shown that HA titers of more than 1:40 are considered as seroprotective and known to provide at least 50% protection against seasonal H1N1 disease. Monovalent novel H1N1 vaccines have shown that more than 90% of children achieve seroprotection rates with one or two doses. Two doses are better in children less than 3–9 years of age. In general, the geometric mean titer achieved after one or two doses are more than 1,000 U/mL. Adjuvant vaccines are better immunogenic, and hence need lesser antigen doses than non-adjuvant vaccines. The WHO recommends that children more than 6 months and less than 9 years need two doses.

Efficacy/Effectiveness

Randomized placebo-controlled vaccine efficacy trials using novel H1N1 vaccines are neither feasible nor ethical. Hence, case-controlled studies have looked at the effectiveness of the monovalent novel H1N1 vaccines in the UK, Germany, and Canada. The effectiveness has been found to be 96.8% (95.2–97.9) in 14–59 years old and 83.3% (71.0–90.5) in more than 60 years old in Germany. In Canada, the effectiveness was found to be 100% (79.5–100) in 6 months to 10 years old children. In the UK, the effectiveness was 77% (11–94) in children less than 10 years of age, 100% (80–100) in 10–24 years old, 22% (−153–76) in 25–49 years old, and 41% (−71–80) in 50+ years old.

Contraindications

Flu vaccine is not indicated in less than 6 months old children. TIV is contraindicated in patients with past history of anaphylactic reaction to egg or previous flu vaccine. Guillain-Barrè syndrome within 6 weeks of previous dose of flu vaccine is a precaution for subsequent use of TIV. Like with any vaccine, any severe acute illness is a temporary contraindication to use flu vaccine till the person recovers from the illness. LAIV is contraindicated in less than 2 years and more than 50 years old subjects. It is also contraindicated, if the child having moderate-to-severe febrile illness, receiving salicylates, has anaphylactic reaction to egg protein, have reactive airway disease, and patients at risk of medical complications following influenza infections, pregnant women, and contacts of immune-compromised conditions requiring protected environment such as stem-cell transplant recipients.

BIBLIOGRAPHY

1. Centers for Disease Control and Prevention. (2010). Prevention and control of influenza with vaccines—recommendations of the Advisory Committee on Immunization Practices (ACIP). CDC. [online]. Available from http://www.cdc.gov/mmwr/preview/mmwrhtml/rr5908a1.html [Accessed October, 2018].
2. John TJ, Moorthy M. 2009 Pandemic influenza in India. Indian Pediatr. 2010;47(1):25-31.
3. MOHFW. (2009). Guidelines on categorization of influenza a H1N1 cases during screening for home isolation, testing, treatment and hospitalization. [online]. Available from http://www.mohfwh1n1.nic.in [Accessed October, 2018].
4. Shah NK. H1N1 2009 pandemic: lessons learnt. Indian Pediatr. 2011;48(5):363-4.
5. Shah NK. H1N1 guidelines—reply. Indian Pediatr. 2010;47:102-3.
6. Shah N. Pertinent queries on swine flu (H1N1). Indian Pediatr. 2009;46:813-4.
7. World Health Organization. (2009). Guidelines for pharmacological management of pandemic (H1N1) influenza and other influenza viruses. [online]. Available from http://www.who.int/csr/resources/publications/swineflu/h1n1_guidelines_pharmaceutical_mngt.pdf [Accessed October, 2018].
8. World Health Organization. (2009). Antiviral drugs and pandemic (H1N1). [online]. Available from http://www.who.int/csr/disease/swineflu/fre quently_asked_questions/antivirals/en/ [Accessed October, 2018].

5.32 Typhoid Fever

Kakali Roy, Ritabrata Kundu

INTRODUCTION

Typhoid fever is a disease of the developing countries in the setting of poor public health, sanitation, and water supply as it spreads by fecal-oral route. In the developed country, it mainly occurs in travelers returning from the developing country.

ETIOLOGY

Typhoid fever classically caused by *Salmonella enterica* serotype Typhi, gram-negative rod-shaped bacilli in the family Enterobacteriaceae. All *Salmonella* organisms are closely related and are considered a single species, *S. enterica*. Similar but less severe clinical symptoms of paratyphoid fever produced by other *Salmonella*, namely *Salmonella paratyphi* A, B, and C; and *Salmonella choleraesuis*. Collectively they are known as typhoidal *Salmonella* serovars. Ratio of typhoid to paratyphoid fever is 10:1, and currently, paratyphoid fever is in rise. Enteric fever includes both typhoid and paratyphoid and cannot be differentiated clinically.

EPIDEMIOLOGY

There are about 50–60 million cases with 6 lakh deaths per year due to typhoid fever worldwide. The major brunt of the disease is in the developing countries including India which reports about 5 million cases annually. It is more common in children below 5 years of age.

Humans are the only reservoir and only known host to get infected. Carriers are asymptomatic who shed typhoid bacilli after disease. The bacilli are shed either from gallbladder through feces or in urine. Convalescent carrier and chronic carrier—the former sheds bacilli for about 3 months following the disease, whereas the later sheds for more than a year. Fortunately, carrier state is not common in children (<2%). It is more common with biliary abnormalities or concurrent schistosomiasis infection.

Transmission occurs by direct or indirect contact with food or water contaminated with feces or urine of infected person or carrier.

PATHOGENESIS

Infecting dose in typhoid fever is 10^3–10^6 bacilli. Those bacilli surviving the acidic environment of stomach will pass through the intestinal mucosa to invade the Peyer's patch, where macrophages engulf them but cannot kill. Subsequently, via mesenteric lymph node and lymphatics, they reach bloodstream. This primary viremia is usually asymptomatic. Then they multiply within the reticuloendothelial tissue of liver, spleen, bone marrow, lymph node, and Peyer's patch. After a critical density is reached, it induces macrophage apoptosis and gets released into bloodstream again. This results in secondary bacteremia which causes clinical symptoms. The gallbladder can get infected either via bacteremia or direct extension of infected bile. Organism via bile reenters the gut and is shed in stool. Gut epithelium overlying hyperplastic Peyer's patch may get sloughed out and result in ulceration which can bleed or progress to cause perforation. In neonate, the infection is transmitted vertically.

CLINICAL FEATURES

Incubation period is 7–21 days depending upon inoculum size and host's immunity status.

Most prominent feature is prolonged fever which persists for around 4 weeks if untreated. Fever typically rises in stepladder pattern but not seen these days with frequent use of antibiotics. It may present with nonspecific features, such as headache, chill, malaise, myalgia, cough, or arthralgia. At times, presents with gastrointestinal symptoms, such as anorexia, pain abdomen, nausea, vomiting, diarrhea (pea soup) followed by constipation. Physical finding of coated tongue, hepatosplenomegaly, abdominal tenderness, and jaundice may be present. Spleen is usually palpable at the end of first week.

In the second week, abdominal signs and symptoms progress and salmon-colored blanching and truncal maculopapular rose spot may develop, which is not appreciated in Indian complexion.

In third week or fourth week, central nervous system involvement, such as encephalopathy, neuritis, Guillain-Barré syndrome, and gastrointestinal bleed (<1%) may occur but rare in children.

DIAGNOSIS

Clinical presentation of enteric fever is nonspecific. No laboratory test is diagnostic other than positive culture.

- *Complete blood count:* Change in complete blood count (CBC) is nonspecific. Leukopenia is found in 20–25% cases, whereas leukocytosis makes the diagnosis less probable. White blood cell count remains normal mostly. In differential count, absolute eosinopenia and thrombocytopenia may be seen. Presence of severe anemia is unlikely, if present, points toward complications like perforation, hemolysis, or an alternative diagnosis like malaria.
- *Biochemical:* Mild elevation of bilirubin, serum glutamic oxaloacetic transaminase, and serum glutamic pyruvic transaminase may occur.
- *Culture:* Definitive diagnosis is by isolation of organism by culture of different specimen.
  - *Blood culture:* It is a gold standard investigation with overall sensitivity of 50% and specificity of 100%. Sensitivity is maximum in the first week and reduces with time. Factors for failure to obtain positive culture are shown in **Box 5.32.1**.

    BACTEC, an automated blood culture system, certainly increases the isolation rate. Blood culture should be done in all suspected cases as positive culture not only unequivocally establishes the diagnosis but also gives the sensitivity pattern which is important in this era of multidrug-resistant typhoid fever (MDRTF).
  - *Bone marrow culture:* Median bacteremia in bone marrow is high (9 CFU/mL) compared to blood. Bone marrow to peripheral blood ratio of organism is around 4.8 in the first week, which increases to 158 during third week because of decrease bacteria in peripheral blood. It is not preferred as being invasive but has sensitivity of 80–95% and good yield even in late disease treated with antibiotics.
  - *Stool, urine, and other culture:* These are not done routinely. Bacilli can be isolated in third week if untreated. Stool specimen of adequate amount should be processed within 2 hours or should be kept in 4°C. For the detection of carrier, several samples should be examined because of irregular shedding of organism. Sensitivity of urine culture is very poor. Duodenal string and skin snip culture of rose spots is of academic interest only.
- *Serological tests:* No tests are enough sensitive or specific to replace culture-based diagnosis.
- *Widal test:* It detects agglutinating antibodies against the somatic O and flagellar H antigen of *Salmonella typhi, S. paratyphi* A and B. "O" antigen is also shared by other *Salmonella* species and other members of Enterobacteriaceae family. Anti-O titer is mainly immunoglobulin M (IgM) type, rises and falls sharply early in the illness, whereas anti-H titer is both IgM and IgG type, rises late in the illness, and persists for a longer time.

Conventionally, positive Widal implies rising titer in paired samples done at a gap of weeks, but use of antibiotics dampens the immune response and may prevent rise in titer. In endemic area, baseline antibodies are present due to repeated subclinical infections with *Salmonella* and other Enterobacteriaceae. This antibody titer varies with age, socioeconomic condition, urban or rural area, and prior immunization status. In one study on 1,200 healthy blood donors from central India, anti-O and anti-H titer of more than 1:80 was seen in 14% and 8%, respectively. For optimal result, Widal test should be done by tube method after 5–7 days of fever, and single result of 1:160 against both O and H antigen should be taken as cutoff value for diagnosis.

It is most widely used diagnostic tool in India, but the sensitivity and specificity is suboptimal **(Box 5.32.2)**. It may be negative in up to 30% culture-positive enteric fever.

- *Enzyme immune assay test or typhidot test:* This is a simple, rapid test for early diagnosis and has high positive and negative predictive values. It detects IgM and IgG antibodies against a 50-kD outer membrane protein of *S. typhi* and is commercially available as typhidot. Detection of IgM indicates acute infection in early stage. As IgG antibodies can persist till 2 years following an infection, the test cannot distinguish between acute infection and convalescence phase. This test has been improved in modified typhidot M test, which detects only IgM antibodies.
- *Intermediate-density lipoprotein Tubex test:* Positive test detects only IgM antibodies against 09 antigens, specifically found in group D *Salmonella*. It is not positive with other groups of *Salmonella*-like paratyphoid.
- *Antigen detection tests:* To detect serum or urinary O, H, or Vi, antigens have suboptimal with variable sensitivity and specificity.

Box 5.32.1: Factors for failure to obtain positive culture.

- Inadequate laboratory media
- Too little volume of blood taken for culture (the median bacterial count in the peripheral blood is low, only 0.3 CFU/mL. At least 5 mL of blood should be collected for a ratio of 1:5 to 1:10 of blood to broth to neutralize the bactericidal effect of serum)
- Prior treatment with antibiotic
- Increased time gap between blood collection and inoculation

Box 5.32.2: Sensitivity and specificity of Widal test.

Causes of low sensitivity:
- Negativity in early infection
- Prior antibiotic therapy dampens antibody response
- Failure to mount an immune response in certain individuals

Causes of low specificity:
- Preexisting baseline antibodies in endemic areas
- Cross-reactivity with other gram-negative infections and nontyphoidal *Salmonella*
- Anamnestic reactions in unrelated infections such as malaria

Molecular methods, such as polymerase chain reaction, are still in experimental stage and not used in day-to-day practice. These tests are not evaluated extensively in the field condition. Still blood culture is taken as gold standard diagnostic tool.

MANAGEMENT

Appropriate antibiotic therapy in time considerably reduces mortality and morbidity. Along with general supportive measures, prompt recognition and treatment of complications are also important. Most cases can be managed at home with oral antibiotic and adequate care. Hospitalization is required for excessive vomiting, inability to take oral feed, severe diarrhea, abdominal distention, and other complications.

Antimicrobial Therapy

Multidrug-resistant *Salmonella* are resistant to first-line drugs, namely chloramphenicol, cotrimoxazole, and ampicillin are reported since 1990. Thereafter, fluoroquinolones, such as ciprofloxacin or ofloxacin, in a dose of 15–20 mg/kg/day were most effective drug, but minimum inhibitory concentration of ciprofloxacin has increased considerably during the past decade. Resistance to nalidixic acid is a surrogate marker of decreased susceptibility of fluoroquinolones. They have the advantage of lower stool carriage rate; however, Drug Controller General of India does not approve fluoroquinolones less than 18 years of age, except in cases of resistance to all other recommended antibiotics or in life-threatening infection.

Though there are reports that first-line antibiotics have again started to show efficacy in treating typhoid fever, they are not recommended as drugs for empirical treatment of enteric fever. They may be used if blood culture report shows sensitivity to them.

Third-generation cephalosporin (both oral and injectable) are recommended first-line treatment. They are also effective for MDRTF, including fluoroquinolone-resistant strains. For uncomplicated cases, among oral preparations, cefixime is used most widely in a dose of 20 mg/kg/day in two divided doses for 14 days and cefpodoxime is also used. Of these, two more studies with cefixime are there, and it is the drug of choice. For severe typhoid, among parenteral preparations, ceftriaxone, cefotaxime, cefoperazone are used, of which ceftriaxone is most convenient as used in once or twice daily dose (100 mg/kg/day). Once the child is afebrile and is able to tolerate orally, we can switch over to oral drug, i.e. oral third-generation cefixime to complete a 14-day course.

Recently, azithromycin in a dose of 10–20 mg/kg is being used as second-line alternative for uncomplicated typhoid fever, when there is no clinical improvement by day 5 with inconclusive culture report. As typhoid bacilli are intracellular organism, azithromycin has good efficacy, especially during relapse. Aztreonam (in three divided doses) and imipenem are potential second-line drug for complicated cases. Full treatment regimen is shown in **Tables 5.32.1 and 5.32.2**.

Table 5.32.1: Treatment of uncomplicated typhoid fever.

	First-line oral drug		*Second-line oral drug*	
Susceptibility	***Antibiotic***	***Daily dose (mg/kg)***	***Antibiotic***	***Daily dose (mg/kg)***
Fully sensitive	Third-generation cephalosporin e.g. Cefixime	20	Chloramphenicol	50–75
			Amoxicillin	75–100
			TMP–SMX	8 TMP
				40 SMX
MDR	Cefixime	20	Azithromycin	10–20
	Cefpodoxime	10		

(MDR: multidrug resistant; SMX: sulfamethoxazole; TMP: trimethoprim)

Table 5.32.2: Treatment of severe typhoid.

	First-line oral drug		*Second-line oral drug*	
Susceptibility	***Antibiotic***	***Daily dose (mg/kg)***	***Antibiotic***	***Daily dose (mg/kg)***
Fully sensitive	Ceftriaxone or Cefotaxime	100	Chloramphenicol	50–75
			Amoxicillin	75–100
			TMP–SMX	8 TMP
				40 SMX
MDR	Ceftriaxone or Cefotaxime	100	Aztreonam	50–100

(MDR: multidrug resistant; SMX: sulfamethoxazole; TMP: trimethoprim)

Duration of Therapy

Therapy should be continued for at least 14 days or 7 days after defervescence.

Relapse

Relapse after 2–3 weeks of fever resolution occurs in 5–10% of apparently successfully treated cases. They are sensitive to the same antibiotic used initially and should be given for 5–7 days in proper dose.

Complications in the developing countries are around 30% and occur during second week or third week of illness. It is mostly seen in late diagnosed case, delayed initiation of antibiotic, inadequately or inappropriately treated, associated with other illness, such as sickle cell disease, human immunodeficiency virus, innate immune deficiency, or in MDRTF.

Severe typhoid fever is seen in 1% or less of patients with high mortality rate of about 50%. These cases are with marked mental confusion, delirious, obtundation, stupor, coma (cerebrospinal fluid study should be done immediately), or shock (when systolic blood pressure is less than 80 mmHg with evidence of decreased skin, cerebral, or renal perfusion).

In severe typhoid fever, high-dose corticosteroid in the form of dexamethasone should be given as an initial dose of 3 mg/kg intravenous over 30 minutes, followed by 1 mg/kg every 6 hourly for 48 hours, which reduces mortality by 80–90%. Low dose hydrocortisone is not effective.

"Intestinal perforation," if confirmed, surgical repair should not be delayed. Antibiotic should be broadened to cover polymicrobial peritonitis.

Intestinal hemorrhage needs intensive care monitoring, surgical consultation, and sometimes blood transfusion.

Other complications include renal failure, pneumonia, respiratory failure, toxic myocarditis, arrhythmias, cardiac failure, shock, meningitis, localized abscess, arthritis, osteomyelitis, hemolytic anemia, cholecystitis, and very rarely disseminated intravascular coagulation and hemophagocytic lymphohistiocytosis. They are all occasionally encountered and should be managed accordingly. Biliary sludge due to ceftriaxone should be considered in cholecystitis.

PROGNOSIS

Poor prognostic factors are those responsible for complication are mentioned above. Recovery of neurological deficit is slow but complete. Immunity following enteric fever is partial. Mortality in the developed countries is 1%, whereas in the developing countries, it is 10%.

PREVENTION

Proper improvement of hygiene standard with supply of potable water will go in a long way to prevent this disease, but it is a distant dream in the developing countries. As chronic carriers are asymptomatic, they remain undiagnosed and should be picked up and treated, especially if they are food handlers.

Vaccine is the very important measure for prevention. Both polysaccharide and conjugated typhoid vaccine are available for this dreaded disease.

BIBLIOGRAPHY

1. Bhutta ZA. Enteric fever (typhoid fever). In: Stanton BF, Schor NF, St Geme JW (Eds). Nelson Textbook of Pediatrics, 20th edition. Philadelphia, PA: Elsevier; 2015. pp. 1388-93.
2. IAP recommendations and guidelines on diagnosis of enteric fever. In: Kundu R, Ganguly N, Ghosh TK (Eds). IAP Protocol on Infectious Diseases in Children, 1st edition. Kolkata: IAP Infectious Diseases Chapter; 2008. pp. 25-41.
3. Kalra A. Salmonella infections. In: Parthasarathy A, Kundu R, Agarwal R (Eds). Textbook of Pediatric Infectious Disease, 1st edition. New Delhi: Jaypee Brothers Medical Publishers; 2013. pp. 217-22.

5.33 Healthcare-associated Infections

Digant D Shastri

INTRODUCTION

Healthcare-associated infections (HAIs) (previously known nosocomial infections) refer to infections which were not present in a patient at the time of admission to healthcare setting; also, there were no evidence of incubation of such infections at the time of hospitalization. These occur worldwide and affect both the developed and resource-poor countries. Hospital-acquired infections increase the use of antibiotics, increase cost of treatment, extend hospitalization duration, and result in elevated morbidity and mortality. They are a significant burden both for the patient and for public health. Increased incidence of HAIs reflects a poor quality of health service delivery.

EPIDEMIOLOGY

Magnitude

The prevalence of HAIs at a given time in the developed countries varies between 3.5% and 12%. The European Centre for Disease Prevention and Control reports an average prevalence of 7.1% in European countries. The estimated incidence in the USA was 4.5% in 2002, corresponding to 9.3 infections per 1,000 patient-days and 1.7 million affected patients. The prevalence of HAI varies between 5.7% and 19.1% in low- and middle-income countries. The proportion of patients with intensive care unit (ICU)-acquired infection ranged from 4.4% to 88.9% with a frequency of overall infections as high as 42.7 episodes per 1,000 patient-days [World Health Organization (WHO)].

Sources

Source of infectious agents for causing HAI may be endogenous or exogenous:

- *Endogenous sources:* Normal flora present in one site can cause infection in any other site when antibiotics are given inappropriately or if there is a breach in the skin or mucosa, e.g. wounds and catheter, which allows the overgrowth of *Clostridium difficile*, *Candida*; gram-negative organisms in the gastrointestinal tract can invade the surgical site or the urinary tract.
- *Exogenous sources:* Bacteria are transmitted between the patients through direct contact, e.g. hands, saliva, droplets, or by staff via contaminated hands or by contaminated equipment, visitors by water or food.

Risk Factors for Healthcare-associated Infection

Hospitalized patient is usually in a "poor state of health," impairing his/her defense. Advanced age or premature birth, malnutrition, immunodeficiency (congenital or acquired) present a general risk, while other diseases can present specific risks; for instance, chronic obstructive pulmonary disease can increase the chances of respiratory tract infection. Invasive devices, such as intubation tubes, catheters, surgical drains, and tracheostomy tubes, all bypass the body's natural lines of defense against pathogens and provide an easy route for infection. Patients already colonized at the time of admission are instantly put at greater risk when they undergo invasive procedures. Treatment modality in patient may leave him/her vulnerable to infections: Immunosuppression and antacid treatment undermine the body's defenses, while antimicrobial therapy (removing competitive flora and only leaving resistant organisms) and recurrent blood transfusions have also been identified as risk factors **(Box 5.33.1)**.

Contributory Factors

- *Reuse of disposable material*: Lack of affordability due to financial constraints in private healthcare facilities or inadequate supply of disposable material in public sector hospitals.

Box 5.33.1: Risk factors for healthcare-associated infections.

- Prior antibiotic therapy
- Immunodeficiency
- Immunosuppression
- H_2 blocker administration
- Prior intralipid use (in newborn babies causing *Candida* infection)
- Parenteral nutrition, central venous line placement (in newborn babies causing candida infection)
- *Extremes of age*: Gestational age of less than 32-week-old people
- Hospital stay longer than 7 days
- Cerebral palsy (urinary tract infections in pediatric patients)
- Reintubation (ventilator-associated pneumonia)

- *Inadequate infrastructure* leading to overcrowding of patients and sharing of equipment (due to insufficient equipment).
- *Inadequate staff* leading to increase workload and increase chances of cross infections.
- *Lack of knowledge and application of basic infection control measures.*
- *Lack of well-written protocols.*
- *Lack of local and national guidelines and policies.*

CAUSATIVE AGENTS FOR HEALTHCARE-ASSOCIATED INFECTION

Healthcare-associated infections are caused by bacteria, fungi, viruses, and protozoa. About 90% of nosocomial infections are due to bacteria, whereas protozoans, viruses, and fungi account for the rest of 10%. The agents that are usually involved in hospital-acquired infections include *Streptococcus* spp., *Acinetobacter* spp., enterococci, *Pseudomonas aeruginosa* (*P. aeruginosa*), coagulase-negative staphylococci (CoNS), *Staphylococcus aureus* (*S. aureus*), *Bacillus cereus* (*B. cereus*), *Legionella*, and Enterobacteriaceae family members including *Proteus mirabilis*, *Klebsiella pneumoniae* (*K. pneumoniae*), *Escherichia coli* (*E. coli*), and *Serratia marcescens*. Out of these enterococci, *P. aeruginosa*, *S. aureus*, and *E. coli* have a major role. Urinary tract infections (UTIs) usually contain *E. coli*, while it is uncommon in other infection sites. Contrarily, *S. aureus* is frequent at other body sites and rarely causes UTI. In blood-borne infections, coagulase-negative *S. aureus* is the main causative agent. Surgical-site infections (SSIs) contain *Enterococcus* spp., which is less prevalent at respiratory tract. One tenth of all infections are caused by *P. aeruginosa*, which is evenly distributed to the entire body sites.

The distribution of bacteria in nosocomial infections is changing over time. For example *Proteus* spp., *Klebsiella* spp., and *Escherichia* spp. were responsible for HAI in the 1960s, but from 1975 to the 1980s, *Acinetobacter* spp. with *P. aeruginosa* created clinical difficulties. During the recent years, streptococci along with CoNS and coagulase-positive staphylococci reemerged and incidence level of *K. pneumoniae* and *E. coli* declined from 7% to 5% and 23% to 16%, respectively.

TYPES OF HEALTHCARE-ASSOCIATED INFECTIONS

National Healthcare Safety Network with Center for Disease Control (CDC) for surveillance has classified HAI sites into 13 types, with 50 infection sites, which are specific and based on biological and clinical criteria. The most common types are:

- Bloodstream infection (BSI)
- Pneumonia [e.g. ventilator-associated pneumonia (VAP)]
- Urinary tract infection
- Surgical-site infection

Catheter-related Bloodstream Infections

In ICUs longline insertions, vascular accesses are the important factors for catheter-related BSIs (CRBSIs), which are due to local colonization of commensals, such as CoNS leading to bacteremia and septicemia. Infections are due to skin colonization, hub contamination, infusion of contaminated fluids, and hematogenous seeding. The incidence of CRBSI varies widely among different healthcare institutions, ranging from 1.12 to 4.2 per 1,000 catheter days, the risk being higher in central lines than peripheral lines in the pediatric ICUs (PICUs).

Risk Factors

- Settings such as PICUs
- Site of catheterization
- Type of catheter
- Frequency of dressing
- Duration
- Length of hospital stay
- Type of antiseptic solutions
- Local and systemic antibiotics.

Common Organisms

The likely organisms are *Staph.* group 10–50%, *Enterococcus* 15–20%, methicillin-resistant *S. aureus* (MRSA) 20–25%, extended-spectrum beta-lactamase producing bacteria 15–20%.

Management

Empirical antibiotics with coverage against gram-positive and gram-negative organisms, including *Pseudomonas*, should be started and then should be modified based on the susceptibility pattern of isolated organisms. Antifungal therapy is added to empiric antibiotic coverage in some cases particularly those who are immunocompromised patients, those who have prolonged ICU stay as well as those who had exposure to antibiotics in the last 90 days. In case where disseminated viral infection is suspected, antiviral therapy (e.g. ganciclovir and acyclovir) may be added. The duration of therapy depends on isolated pathogen, retention of catheter, or presence of complications, such as endocarditis and sepsis. For most bacterial organisms, the duration of therapy is 10–14 days after blood cultures become negative. The removal of central line should be considered, if

- The line is no longer needed.
- The infection is caused by *S. aureus*, *Candida* species, or mycobacteria.
- The patient is critically ill.
- The patient fails to clear bacteremia in 48–72 hours.
- The symptoms of BSI persist beyond 48–72 hours.

Catheter-associated Urinary Tract Infections

Urinary tract infection is the most common HAIs associated with least morbidity. Occasionally it can lead to bacteremia, septicemia and rarely death. Majority of the time it is due to indwelling catheter. WHO defines positive culture, of more than 1 lakh count with a maximum of two isolated organisms.

Common Organisms

The bacteria responsible are *E. coli* and multiresistant *Klebsiella.*

Management

To avoid persistence and recurrence of infection, as far as possible, the indwelling catheters should be removed. On some instances, the removal of catheter may result in spontaneous resolution of bacteriuria or asymptomatic cystitis. Consider empiric antibiotic and antifungal therapy (immunocompromised individual) to avoid complications, such as pyelonephritis, renal scarring, and generalized septicemia. For children with sepsis, pyelonephritis, or urinary tract abnormalities, antibiotics of 10–14 days have been recommended by most of the experts.

Ventilator-associated Pneumonia

Ventilator-associated pneumonia occurs in ICU settings associated with high morbidity and mortality and enormous cost to the health care. Microorganisms colonize the stomach, upper airway, and bronchi and cause infection in the lungs (pneumonia): they are often endogenous (digestive system or nose and throat), but may be exogenous, often from contaminated respiratory equipment.

World Health Organization definitions of pneumonia include clinical and radiological criteria which are readily available but nonspecific: recent and progressive radiological opacities of the pulmonary parenchyma, purulent sputum, and recent onset of fever.

Diagnosis is more specific when quantitative microbiological samples are obtained using specialized protected bronchoscopy methods.

Risk Factors

Known risk factors for infection include:

- The type and duration of ventilation
- The quality of respiratory care
- Severity of the patient's condition (organ failure)
- Previous use of antibiotics.

Management

For management of VAP, one should initially start with broad-spectrum empirical antibiotic therapy, and the regime should be modified based on the culture results of sputum/endotracheal suction material/bronchial lavage wash. The choice of empiric antibiotic coverage should take into consideration the risk for multidrug-resistant (MDR) pathogens. The duration of antibiotics ranges from 14 days to 21 days.

Surgical-site Infections

World Health Organization defines SSI clinically as: "a purulent discharge around the wound or the insertion site of the drain, or spreading cellulitis from the wound." CDC classifies SSI as being either incisional or organ/space, occurred within 30 days after the operation, may be deep involving the organs or superficial involving the shin and soft tissues which are manipulated during the procedure.

The incidence depends on the place, hospitals, invasive procedures, elective or emergency surgery, persons, and quality of care, immune status of the individuals, age, and surgical site. Incidence varies from 1% to 20%.

Risk Factors

- Type of surgery—more in cardiothoracic orthopedic, GI surgeries
- In implanted surgeries and less in pinhole surgeries
- Wound type clean or contaminated
- Experience of the surgical team
- Duration of stay in the hospital
- Immune status of the child
- Emergency or elective surgery
- Duration of surgery and age
- Infection control policy of the hospital contributes greatly.

Common Organisms

Organisms involved in SSI depend upon the site of surgery, i.e. if surgery is close to perineum and hollow viscous organs, the organisms may be endogenous, such as fecal flora, e.g. *E. coli*, and sometimes anaerobes, such as *Bacillus fragilis.*

Staphylococcus aureus continues to be top in the list of pathogens isolated from SSI, followed by CoNS, *Enterococcus* spp., *E. coli, P. aeruginosa,* and *Enterobacter* spp. Other pathogens involved include *P. mirabilis, K. pneumoniae, Candida albicans,* and other *Streptococcus* spp.

Management

Management of SSIs must be dual prong approach—combination of surgical care and antibiotic therapy. After starting empirical antibiotic therapy the regime should be modified based on the culture results. Aggressive surgical interventions are needed for severe infections, such as streptococcal gangrene and extensive tissue necrosis, as antibiotics alone may not work.

PREVENTION OF HEALTHCARE-ASSOCIATED INFECTIONS

Standard precautions are to be applied to the care of all patients in all healthcare settings regardless of the suspected or confirmed presence of an infectious agent. This is the primary strategy in preventing transmission of infectious agents among patients and healthcare personnel. Transmission-based precautions are used in addition to standard precautions when caring for patients who are infected or colonized with pathogens transmitted by airborne, droplet, or contact routes.

- Preventive precautions to prevent transmission of airborne droplet infections include the use of single-patient rooms, negative air-pressure ventilation, and N95 respirator masks.
- Preventive precautions to prevent transmission of microorganisms via direct or indirect contact with infected or colonized persons include the use of single-patient room (if not feasible, cohort patients infected with the same organism), use of gowns and gloves, and hand hygiene after glove removal.
- Preventive precautions to prevent intravascular catheter-associated infections include avoidance of unnecessary catheter placement, removal of catheter as soon as possible, aseptic technique during catheter insertion, and minimal manipulation of catheter. Scrubbing the catheter hub with devices containing isopropyl alcohol has been found to reduce lumen contamination, organism density, and catheter-related and ultimately to reduce BSIs.
- Preventive precautions to prevent healthcare-associated bacterial pneumonia include education of healthcare workers (HCWs) about infection control procedures, thorough cleaning of devices for sterilization or disinfection, changing the breathing circuit only when it is visibly soiled, hand hygiene, and change of soiled gloves.

Other General Measures

Handwashing

Poor hand hygiene is responsible for 40% of infections transmitted in hospitals. Surveys have shown that the improvement in compliance with handwashing reduces HAIs. Accessibility of the handwashing stations and the use of alcohol gels improves compliance with handwashing. It is recommended to use a hand scrub after examination of each patient either by handwashing or use of alcohol-based hand rub. Hands should also be washed before and after aseptic procedures and after the removal of gloves. When washing hands with soap and water, wet hands first with water, apply an amount of product recommended by the manufacturer to hands, and rub hands together vigorously for at least 15 seconds, covering all surfaces of the hands and fingers then rinse hands with water and dry thoroughly with a disposable towel. While using an alcohol-based hand rub, apply recommended quantity of product to palm of one hand and rub hands together, covering all surfaces of hands and fingers, until the hands are dry. It is advisable to use a handwash formulation containing 60–95% alcohol alone or 50–95% alcohol in combination with a quaternary ammonium compound or 50–95% alcohol in combination with a hexachlorophene or 50–95% alcohol in combination with chlorhexidine gluconate **(Fig. 5.33.1)**.

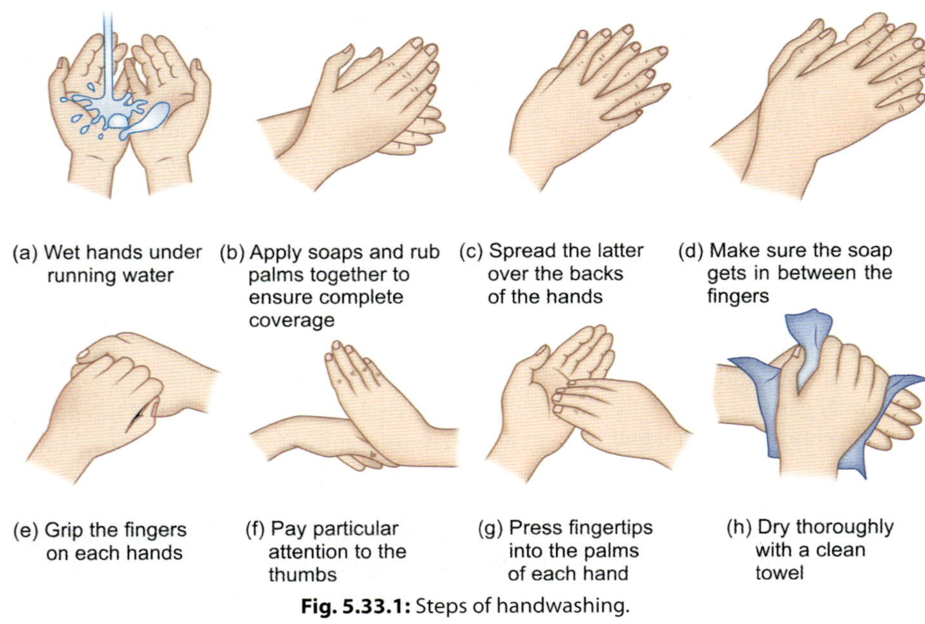

Fig. 5.33.1: Steps of handwashing.

Environmental Sanitation

Environmental surfaces could potentially contribute to cross-transmission through hand contact with contaminated surfaces, medical equipment, or patients. Daily wet mopping of floors and surfaces close to patient care is a must. Particular attention is to be paid for surfaces, such as door-knobs, which are most commonly handled by patients in the clinic. It is preferable to use a disinfectant over plain soap and water with a contact time of at least 30–60 seconds. Spills of blood on surfaces should be promptly cleaned with detergent, followed by bleach (1:100) using gloves.

Disinfection of Hospital Rooms

Disinfection of hospital rooms with hydrogen peroxide vapor in addition to standard cleaning reduces environmental contamination and the risk of infection with MDR organisms.

Safe Practices during Procedures

The use of invasive procedures increases the risk of nosocomial infections. For insertion of intravascular catheters and other invasive procedures and for obtaining blood cultures, 2% chlorhexidine, chlorhexidine in 70% alcohol, 10% povidone-iodine or alcoholic tincture of iodine should be used. Povidone-iodine should be left to dry for 2 minutes. Tunneling the catheter reduces the risk of nosocomial infection. Antimicrobial impregnated catheters can reduce catheter-related infections. The use of a strict, aseptic technique is paramount in the insertion of intravascular catheters. By using isolation rooms for patients with MRSA, *C. difficile*, vancomycin-resistant enterococci (VRE) and resistant gram-negative infections, the spread of infection can be reduced owing to improved awareness of the implementation of appropriate infection control precautions.

Biowaste Management

As per the Infection Management and Environment plan Policy framework, March 2007, by the Indian Ministry of Health, it is the duty of every occupier of a clinic, dispensary, nursing home, or hospital to take all steps to ensure handling and disposal of biowaste generated without any adverse effect to man health and the environment. Waste should be segregated as per the color coding provided by the Bio-Medical Waste Management Rules 1998 and disposed-off through biowaste management protocols **(Flowchart 5.33.1)**.

INFECTION CONTROL PROGRAM

The important components of the infection control program are:

- Basic measures for infection control, i.e. standard and additional precautions
- Education and training of HCWs
- Protection of HCWs, e.g. immunization
- Identification of hazards and minimizing risks
- Routine practices essential to infection control, such as aseptic techniques, use of single-use devices, reprocessing of instruments and equipment, antibiotic usage, management of blood/body fluid exposure, handling and use of blood and blood products, sound management of medical waste
- Effective work practices and procedures, such as environmental management practices including management of hospital/clinical waste, support services (e.g. food, linen), use of therapeutic devices
- Surveillance
- Incident monitoring
- Outbreak investigation.

Recommendations for Infection Control in Waiting Area

- The waiting room should be adequately ventilated. Ideally, it should provide at least 6 air exchanges/hour. A facility of handwash or alcoholic hand rub should be available.
- In office practice, the waiting time may be minimized by consultation on appointment and thereby minimizing the risk of exposure.
- The healthcare professionals should try for early pick up and triage of patients with obvious communicable diseases such as chickenpox, measles, and conjunctivitis while they are waiting in the waiting area and they should provide then consultation on priority. These will minimize exposure to other patients waiting for their turn.
- Prioritize the consultation for immunocompromised patients so as to minimize the chances of exposure to patients with communicable diseases.
- Regular cleaning of floors and surfaces in the waiting area through wet mopping is recommended as they can easily get contaminated with settling of droplets or contact with shoes. Any visible soiling by vomitus/urine/feces is to be promptly cleaned followed by disinfection.
- Toys are easily mouthed by children and can act as fomites. Toys should be washed with soap and water daily or when soiled by secretions. The risks of sharing toys/books should not outweigh the advantage of entertaining children, and toys should be removed, if supervised and regular cleaning is not feasible.
- Educational posters for respiratory etiquettes and emphasis about hand hygiene displayed in the waiting area can help in dissemination of information.

Maintenance of Reusable Medical Equipment

- The bell and diaphragm of stethoscope, ear curettes of otoscope, infantometer, and blood pressure cuffs are

Flowchart 5.33.1: Treatment of hazardous and nonhazardous waste.

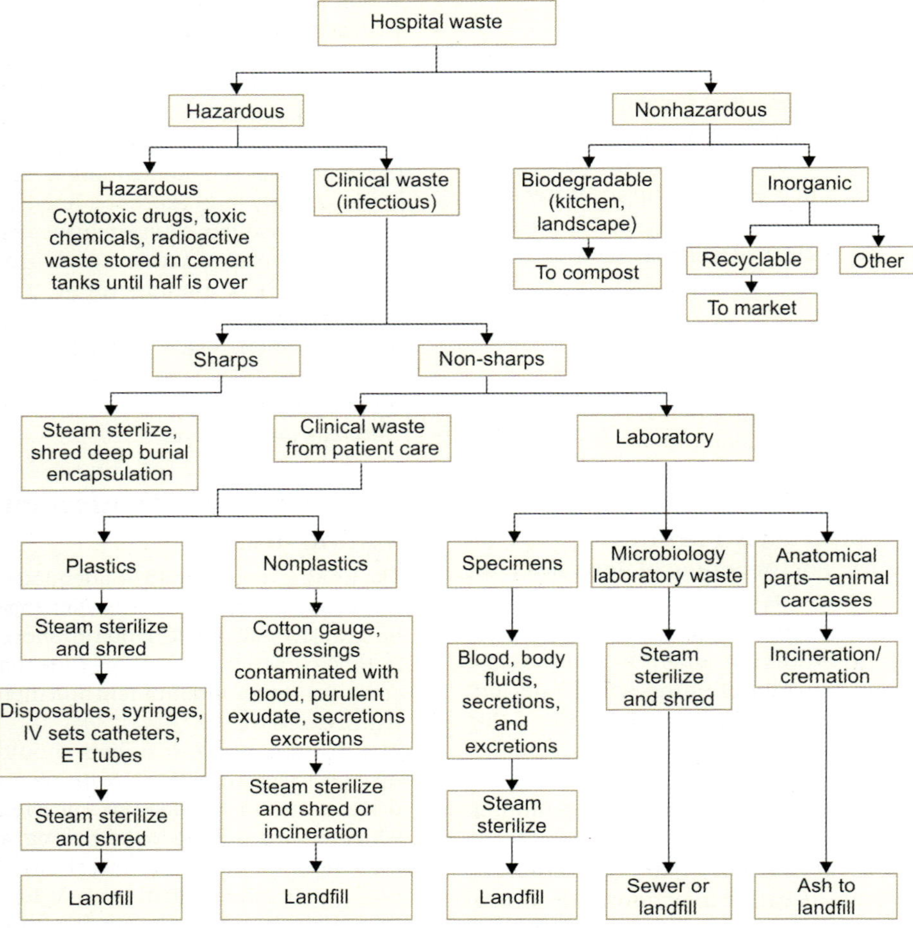

noncritical equipment which encounter intact skin, and therefore, they are at low risk of infection transmission and require low disinfection, such as washing with plain water and soap.

- Infant weighing scales can be washed with soap and water. Separate clean paper (clean newspaper, if sterile paper is not economically feasible) should be used for every baby to prevent risk of hypothermia and cross-contamination.
- Clinical thermometer should preferably be used in contact with intact skin, such as in axillary fold rather than mucous membrane, such as rectal mucosa. It can be washed with soap water or wiped with 70–90% ethyl or isopropyl alcohol with a contact time of at least 30 seconds and air dried.
- Metallic tongue depressors come in contact with mucous membrane and saliva and required sterilization after washing by either boiling or autoclave. Disposable sterile tongue depressors are recommended but are expensive.
- Nebulizer machine should be maintained as per manufacturer's instructions. In general, the mask and T-shaped part of the nebulizer machine should be washed with mild soap and water and air dried on clean cloth.
- Instruments required for suturing should be placed inside a clean-folded cloth, and the tray should be autoclaved.

Prevention of Occupational Infections of the Healthcare Workers

- *Equipment for personal safety*:
  - Gloves should be worn by the HCW just before any invasive procedure, or contact with sterile sites and nonintact skin or mucous membrane, or where there is risk of exposure to body fluids or blood, or while handling sharps and contaminated devices. The gloves should be removed soon after the procedure and disposed appropriately. Hands should be washed after removal of gloves.

    - A surgical mask should be worn, if there is high risk of the procedure to expose to respiratory secretions, splash of blood, and body fluids. For example—for procedures, such as nebulization-induced sputum collection for acid-fast bacilli. Mask should be appropriately disposed soon after use. Also it should be used only once and changed, if wet or soiled. For severe acute respiratory syndrome, coronavirus or avian influenza, current recommendations are for personnel to wear a N95 mask for pandemic influenza, a N95 mask is recommended only for personnel performing certain aerosol-generating procedures.
    - Gloves and facemask should be worn when handling biowaste.
- *Immunization*: All HCWs should be vaccinated against hepatitis B. It is recommended to be immunized against vaccine preventable diseases, such as measles, mumps, varicella, influenza, diphtheria, and tetanus.
- *Education and training of staff:* Rationale behind infection control practices should be taught to the staff. The correct methods of disinfection should be explained and supervised. Repeated discussions and training can help in maintaining high standards of compliance.
- *Personal hygiene*: The staff should maintain high standards of hand hygiene, keep nails short and free of false nails, and wear short sleeves.
- *Postexposure prophylaxis* should be promptly undertaken on exposure to needle-stick injury or exposure to contagious material.

BIBLIOGRAPHY

1. Canadian Pediatric Society. Infection control in paediatric office settings. Paediatr Child Health. 2008;13(5):408-19.
2. Coffin SE, Zaoutis TE. Healthcare-associated infections. In: Long SS, Pickering LK, Prober CG (Eds). Principles and Practice of Pediatric Infectious Diseases, 3rd edition. Philadelphia, PA: Churchill Livingstone; 2008. Chapter 101.
3. Healthcare Infection Control Practices Advisory Committee (HICPAC); Rutala WA, Weber DJ. (2008). Guideline for disinfection and sterilization in healthcare facilities. [online] Available from: http://www.cdc.gov/hicpac/Disinfection_Sterilization/3_4surfaceDisinfection.html [Accessed October, 2018].
4. Horan TC, Andrus M, Dudeck MA. CDC/NHSN surveillance definition of health care-associated infection and criteria for specific types of infections in the acute care setting. Am J Infect Control. 2008;36(5):309-32.
5. Mehta A, Rosenthal VD, Mehta Y, et al. Device-associated nosocomial infection rates in intensive care units of seven Indian cities: Findings of the International Nosocomial Infection Control Consortium (INICC). J Hosp Infect. 2007;67(2):168-74.
6. Patwardhan N, Kelkar U. Disinfection, sterilization and operation theater guidelines for dermatosurgical practitioners in India. Indian J Dermatol Venereol Leprol. 2011;77(1):83-93.
7. World Health Organization (2002). Prevention of hospital-acquired infections: A practical guide, 2nd edition. WHO/CDS/CSR/EPH/2002. [online] Available from: http://apps.who.int/medicinedocs/documents/s16355e/s16355e.pdf [Accessed October, 2018].
8. Rosenthal VD, Richtmann R, Singh S, et al. Surgical site infections, International Nosocomial Infection Control Consortium (INICC) report, data summary of 30 countries, 2005-2010. Infect Control Hosp Epidemiol. 2013;34(6):597-604.
9. Rosenthal VD. Central line-associated bloodstream infections in limited-resource countries: a review of the literature. Clin Infect Dis. 2009;49(12):1899-907.
10. Zaoutis TE, Coffin SE. Clinical syndromes of device-associated infections. In: Long SS, Pickering LK, Prober CG (Eds). Principles and Practice of Pediatric Infectious Diseases, 3rd edition. Philadelphia, PA: Churchill Livingstone; 2008. Chapter 102.

Section 6

Diseases of Central Nervous System

6.1 Neuroanatomic Localization in Children

Vrajesh Udani

INTRODUCTION

Pediatric neurological disorders are more diffuse than focal, and hence, accurate localization to discrete neurologic regions is difficult and probably not critical. As an example, children who have cerebral palsy do not really need the rigorous exercise of neuroanatomical localization in most instances. This chapter cannot cover the whole of neurologic localization and has highlighted this exercise in conditions, such as motor paralysis (hemiplegia, paraplegia, etc.), ophthalmoplegia, and visual loss.

LOCALIZATION IN THE MOTOR PATHWAYS

Lower Motor Neuron

Anatomy

The final common pathway of motor pathway is the lower motor neuron (LMN), i.e. alpha-motor neuron in the ventral horn of the spinal cord and the motor nuclei of the cranial nerves in the brainstem. Axons then exit as motor roots traverse in the peripheral nerve, which innervates the muscle extrafusal fibers via the neuromuscular junction and affects contraction **(Fig. 6.1.1)**. A "motor unit" comprises of the motor neuron, the axons from it, and the muscle fibers it innervates. These could be few, for example in extraocular muscles or several hundred in larger truncal muscles.

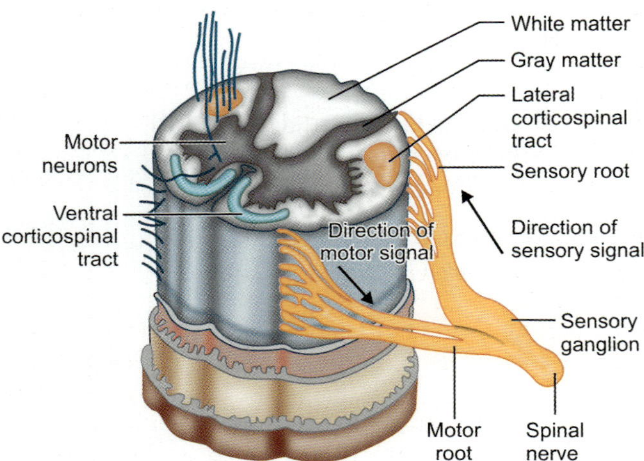

Fig. 6.1.1: Organization of a spinal segment.

Localization

The LMN disorders cause varying degrees of weakness, hypotonia, and areflexia. Motor neuron disorders (poliomyelitis or spinal muscular atrophies) cause muscle wasting, proximal more than distal weakness, and early areflexia. Radiculopathies are usually painful and can be symmetric [Guillain-Barré syndrome (GBS)] or less commonly asymmetric (intervertebral disk prolapse, tumors) with weakness or sensory loss or reflex change in a segmental distribution. Peripheral neuropathies (hereditary sensorimotor neuropathies) generally cause more distal weakness and sensory loss with early areflexia. GBS affects roots and peripheral nerves. Neuromuscular junction disorders (myasthenia, botulism, snake bite) often involve ocular and pharyngeal muscles early and have retained reflexes; often the weakness fluctuates. Muscle disease usually involves proximal more than distal muscles, and reflex loss is seen primarily in weak muscles.

Upper Motor Neuron

Anatomy

The corticospinal tract (CST) and corticobulbar tracts (CBT) exert direct supraspinal, mostly inhibitory influences on the alpha-motor neuron and cranial nerve motor nuclei **(Fig. 6.1.2)**. The CST arises not only from the primary motor cortex, lateral premotor cortex, and the medial supplementary motor cortex, but also receives input from the post-central sensory cortex and other areas. The motor cortex has somatotopic organization with maximum representation for the lips, jaw, thumb, and fingers. Anterior to the motor areas is the frontal eye field, which controls contralateral horizontal gaze. The CST descends into the corona radiate, posterior limb of the internal capsule where it is adjacent to ascending sensory fibers, the optic radiations, and the thalamus or caudate and putamen; from there it winds down into the cerebral peduncle in the anterior midbrain where it lies close to the oculomotor nerve and red nucleus. It then traverses the anterior pons

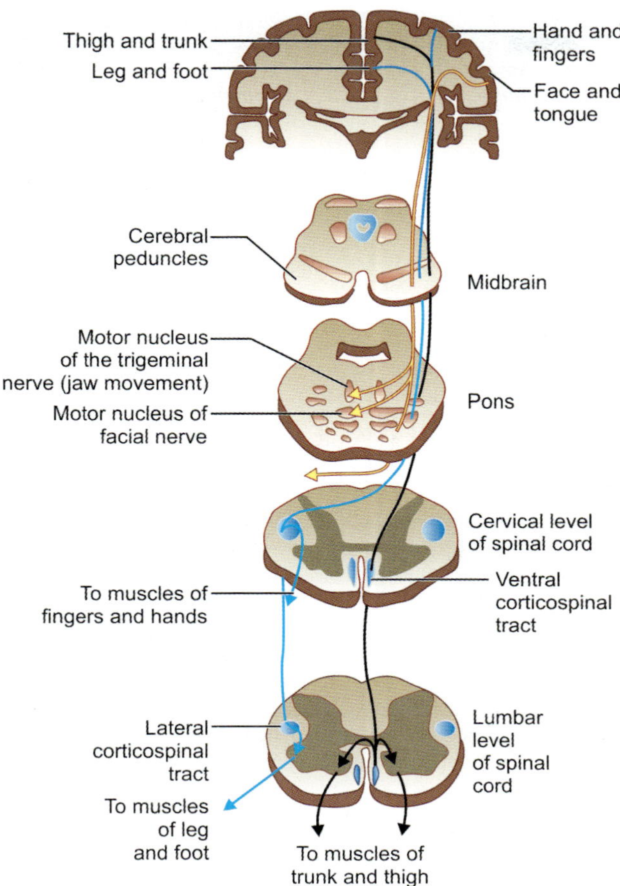

Fig. 6.1.2: The corticospinal and corticobulbar tracts.

where the VIth and VIIth nerve nuclei are situated and finally forms the medullary pyramid anterior to the lower cranial nerve nuclei; 90% of the CST fibers decussate and then descend in the spinal cord as the lateral CST. Brainstem cerebellar peduncles—superior, middle, and inferior—are close by and serve ipsilateral cerebellar functions.

The CBT has a similar origin and descends in the genu of the internal capsule, medial cerebral peduncle, and the pons; it provides bilateral input to the motor cranial nerve nuclei, i.e. the Vth, VIIth innervating the upper facial muscles, IXth, Xth, and XIIth; the VIIth nerve nuclei innervating the lower facial muscles and that part of the XII nucleus supplying the genioglossus receive contralateral corticobulbar input.

The CST lies in the lateral funiculus of the spinal cord, ventrolateral to the uncrossed ascending posterior columns, and posterior to the crossed lateral spinothalamic tract. A smaller ventral CST descends ipsilaterally.

Localization

The upper motor neuron (UMN) syndrome typically has weakness, spasticity, hyperreflexia, and extensor plantar, though in acute lesions, initial hypotonia and hyporeflexia may predominate. Distribution of weakness could be hemiplegia, quadriplegia [upper limb (UL) = lower limb (LL)], diplegia (LL > UL), double hemiplegia (UL > LL), paraplegia, and monoplegia. The lesions causing these various syndromes could be in the cortical motor or premotor cortices, subcortical white matter in the corona radiata, internal capsule, brainstem, and spinal cord. Generally, cortical or subcortical lesion cause incomplete deficits with less spasticity, while spinal cord and sometimes brainstem lesions cause more complete deficits and more spasticity. If there is an upper motor neuron (UMN) facial paresis on the same side as the paresis, the lesion is necessarily above the pons. **Table 6.1.1** outlines the clinical localization of lesions in the motor pathway.

LOCALIZATION OF LESIONS IN THE OCULAR MOTOR SYSTEM

Paralysis of the external ocular muscles can be caused by lesions in the brainstem ocular motor nuclei, the nerves, the neuromuscular junction, or the muscles. The ocular motor system is responsible for volitional and reflex vertical and horizontal conjugate eye movements whose primary goal is to keep a binocular image on the fovea at all times.

Anatomy

Six muscles, the recti and the obliques, control eye movements. The lateral rectus is innervated by the abducens (VI) nerve, and the superior oblique (SO) is innervated by the trochlear nerve (IV), while the other four muscles—the medial rectus, superior rectus, inferior rectus, and inferior oblique—are innervated by the oculomotor (III) nerve. **Figure 6.1.3** outlines the action of the different muscles. The levators of the eyelid are innervated primarily by the III nerve and also receive some sympathetic supply. Dilators of the pupils are mediated by the sympathetic supply, while the constrictors receive parasympathetic innervations.

Oculomotor (III) nerve ***(Fig. 6.1.4)***: The III nerve nucleus lies in the upper midbrain, fibers for the superior rectus cross to the opposite side, while the levators get bilateral innervations; all other muscles get ipsilateral innervations, including the parasympathetic pupilloconstrictor fibers.

After exit the III nerve traverses the subarachnoid space (SAS) and is close to the posterior communicating and the carotid arteries.

After the SAS, the nerve lies in the lateral wall of the cavernous sinus with the IV, VI, and the ophthalmic branch of the V nerve (V1) close to the intracavernous carotid artery. It then enters the orbital apex via the superior orbital fissure along with the aforementioned nerves, and here is also close to the optic nerve.

Table 6.1.1: The clinical localization of lesions in the motor pathway.

Site	*Motor syndrome*	*Characteristics*	*Associated symptoms/ signs*	*Common etiologies*
Cortical or subcortical white matter	• Hemiplegia • Diplegia • Quadriplegia • Monoplegia • Double hemiplegia	• Distal weakness > proximal • *Lateral lesions*: UL/ face > leg • Medial lesions • Leg > UL/face • Deficits rarely complete	• Seizures • Cortical sensory loss • Aphasia/Apraxia • CN gaze palsy (transient) • Bilateral lesions • Pseudobulbar palsy (drooling, dysphagia)	• Mono or hemiplegia • Stroke • Granulomas • Demyelination (ADEM) • Encephalitis (HSV) • Quad or diplegia • Brain injury (HIE, PVL, TBI) • Leukodystrophies
Internal capsule	Hemiplegia	Complete deficits (UL = LL = face)	• Hemisensory deficits • Hemianopia • Dystonia	• Stroke • TBM (granulomas/infarcts) • Encephalitis
Brainstem	• Hemiplegia • Quadriplegia	Complete deficits	• Ipsilateral CN deficits • Ipsilateral ataxia	• Glioma • Encephalitis/ADEM • Leigh's disease
Spinal cord	• Paraplegia • Quadriplegia • Hemiplegia • Hemicord syndrome	• Complete deficits • Severe spasticity • Flexor spasms • LMN signs at level of lesion; UMN signs below	• Bladder or bowel involved (earlier in intramedullary) • *Sensory level (Hemicord syndromes)*: Ipsilateral position or vibration loss, CN pain/ temperature	• Myelitis/ADEM • Trauma • Meningomyelocele • Neoplasm • Hereditary spastic • Paraparesis

(ADEM: acute disseminated encephalomyelitis; CN: contralateral; HIE: hypoxic-ischemic encephalopathy; HSV: herpes simplex virus; LL: lower limb; LMN: lower motor neuron; PVL: periventricular leukomalacia; TBI: traumatic brain injury; TBM: tuberculous meningitis; UL: upper limb; UMN: upper motor neuron)

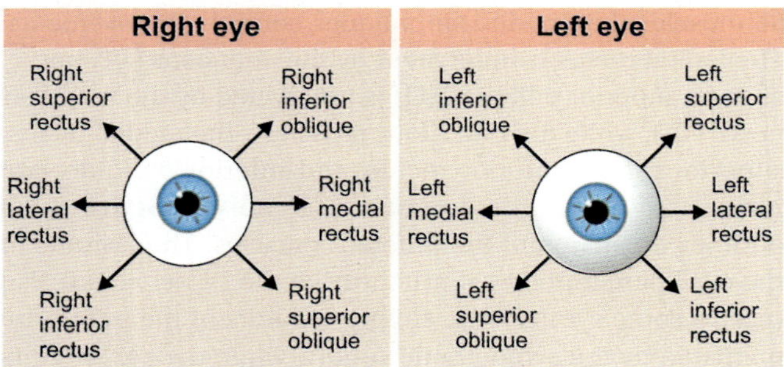

Fig. 6.1.3: Actions of the extraocular muscles.

Trochlear (IV) nerve **(*Fig. 6.1.4*)**: The nucleus lies in the lower midbrain after which it exits dorsally and decussates immediately and then has the longest intracranial course in the SAS making it vulnerable to traumatic injury.

The nerve then has a similar course in the cavernous sinus and the orbital apex before it innervates the SO.

Abducens (VI) nerve **(*Fig. 6.1.4*)**: The nucleus is in the pontomedullary junction near the facial nerve colliculus. The nerve then exits anteriorly after connecting to the contralateral III nerve via the medial longitudinal fasciculus (MLF).

In the SAS, the nerve ascends the brainstem and is close to the petrous apex and then courses over the tentorial edge.

The further course through the cavernous sinus and orbital apex before it innervates the lateral rectus is similar to the other ocular motor nerves.

Localization

Oculomotor nerve: Third nerve palsy would have ptosis, exotropia in primary gaze (due to unopposed action of the lateral rectus), absent adduction, elevation and weakened depression in the abducted eye. The pupil would be dilated and unreactive though partial palsies can spare the pupil.

Nuclear lesions cause ipsilateral weakness in adduction and ipsilateral depression in the abducted eye along with bilateral ptosis and bilateral deficit in elevation in abduction. Fascicular lesions in the brainstem often involve adjacent CST or substantia nigra or red nucleus to give crossed hemiplegia or tremor. Brainstem encephalitis, Leigh's disease, and late stages of herniation syndromes with bilateral midbrain lesions are some common causes in childhood.

In the SAS, isolated III nerve palsies are the rule, and the causes include uncal herniation, meningitis, tumors, parainfectious neuritis, and possibly recurrent ophthalmoplegic migraine. As the pupillomotor fibers are at the nerve periphery, extrinsic compressive lesions involve the pupil, while intrinsic lesions, such as in Miller-Fisher syndrome/GBS, usually spare it.

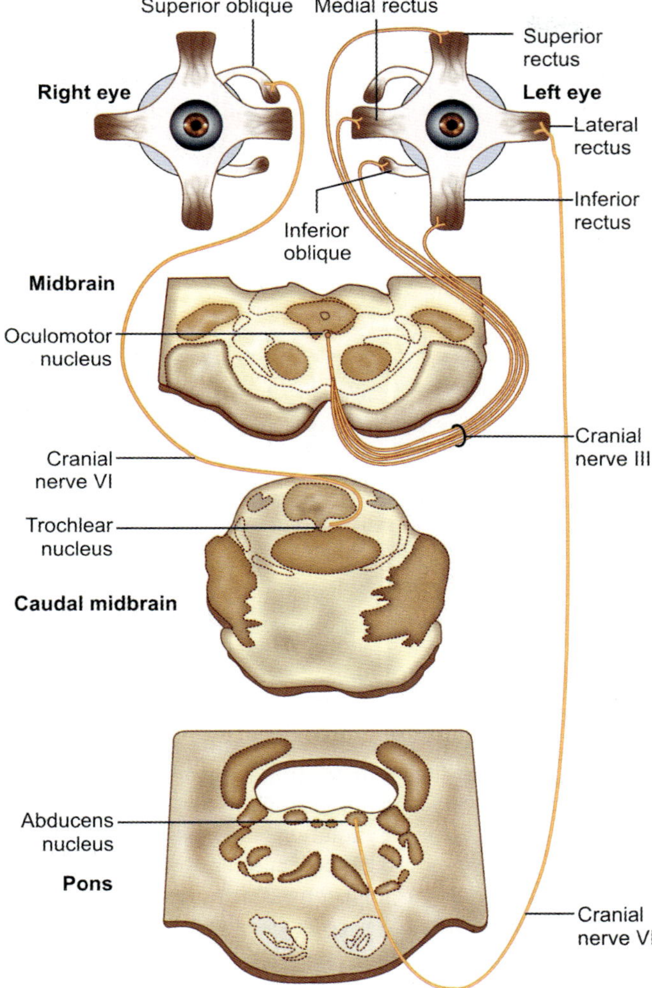

Fig. 6.1.4: The ocular motor nerves.

When pupils are spared, always consider ocular myasthenia (often unilateral, asymmetric); Miller Fisher syndrome often has bilateral involvement.

Trochlear nerve: The fourth nerve palsy causes paresis of depression in the adducted position with mild elevation of the eyeball in primary gaze. There is often a compensatory head tilt.

Isolated IV nerve palsy is seen after trauma and is also often congenital.

Abducens nerve: The sixth nerve palsy would have the paresis of ipsilateral abduction with esotropia in primary gaze.

Nuclear lesions often cause a combined VI and VII nerve palsy. Ipsilateral horizontal conjugate gaze is also affected. Contralateral hemiplegia may also occur. Common lesions include pontine glioma and congenital agenesis, such as in Moebius syndrome.

In the SAS, the nerve is susceptible to raised intracranial pressure (ICP) or even low ICP, and hence, one may get a "false localizing" sign. Meningitis, apical petrositis, and parainfectious neuritis are the other causes.

Convergence spasm with either unilateral or bilateral esotropia is a common mimic.

Multiple Ocular Muscle Weakness

Lesions at the cavernous sinus (such as thrombosis) and orbital apex (such as orbital cellulitis) cause proptosis, pain, multiple ocular motor palsies, and sensory loss in the area of the face innervated by the ophthalmic branch of the trigeminal nerve (V1); cavernous sinus lesions can have an associated Horner's syndrome due to involvement of the nearby ocular sympathetic fibers, while lesions at the orbital apex may have visual loss due to involvement of the adjacent optic nerve.

Other locations include the brainstem (glioma) where associated long tract signs are often seen, SAS (e.g. meningitis) and part of peripheral conditions such as GBS or the Miller–Fisher syndrome.

Ocular muscle involvement in myasthenia can mimic any pupil sparing ocular motor neuropathy. It is often diffuse or bilateral but can be remarkably asymmetric. Ptosis is almost invariable.

Chronic progressive external ophthalmoplegia can be isolated or part of many myopathies, most commonly mitochondrial. Ptosis with bilateral diffuse ophthalmoplegia and pupillary sparing is characteristic and is typically confused with ocular myasthenia.

SUPRANUCLEAR OR INTERNUCLEAR CONTROL OF EYE MOVEMENTS

Horizontal Gaze

Saccades (fast conjugate movements to a fixed target) are initiated in the frontal or parietal eye fields; fibers then descend and cross to innervate the prepontine reticular formation (PPRF) which projects to the adjacent abducens nerve nucleus. This then connects with the contralateral oculomotor nerve nucleus through the MLF. Pursuit movements are generated in the parietal-temporal-occipital junction with ipsilateral projections to the abducens nucleus.

Localization

Destructive lesions (e.g. infarcts) of the frontal eye field will paralyze (usually transiently) contralateral horizontal conjugate gaze so that the unopposed ipsilateral gaze will turn the eyes toward the lesion. Irritative lesions (focal seizures) will result in gaze to the opposite side.

Destructive lesions of the PPRF (e.g. glioma) will cause ipsilateral conjugate gaze paresis, and hence, the eye will look away from the lesion.

Congenital ocular motor apraxia is a disorder with defective or absent horizontal saccades; the children use head thrusts to fixate on an object. It is also seen with Joubert syndrome and ataxia telangiectasia.

Vertical Gaze

A cluster of nuclei in the upper dorsal midbrain (the pretectal area) controls vertical gaze. These centers then connect to the relevant oculomotor and trochlear nerve nuclei through the MLF to control upgaze and downgaze.

Localization

Lesions posterior to the pretectum, such as enlarged III ventricle in hydrocephalus, pineal tumors, etc., cause the Parinaud syndrome with upgaze palsy, upper lid retraction (these cause the "sunset sign" in hydrocephalus), and convergence retraction nystagmus. Lysosomal storage disorders, such as Gaucher and Niemann-Pick syndromes, are other important causes.

Localization in the Visual System

Localization of visual loss to different parts of the visual pathway is difficult in children and even more in infants because of the difficulties in testing visual acuity and visual fields accurately. Much of the following discussion is, therefore, more relevant in the older child and teenager.

Anatomy

The visual field and the retina have an inverted and reversed relationship; the upper visual field falls on the inferior retina and vice versa, and the nasal field falls on the temporal retina and vice versa **(Fig. 6.1.5)**.

The optic nerves receive their axons from the retinal ganglion cells (first-order neurons) and proceed through the optic canal in the posterior orbit where they lie close to the III, IV, V, and VI nerves entering the orbit.

A little more than half of the optic nerve fibers from the nasal retina (serving the temporal field) cross to the opposite side in the optic chiasm, while the uncrossed temporal retinal fibers (serving the nasal field) continue on the same side. Below the optic chiasm lies the pituitary gland, while above it is the hypothalamus.

The optic tract with contralateral nasal fibers and ipsilateral temporal fibers then synapses with the lateral geniculate body neurons, which then proceed to the primary visual cortex in the occipital calcarine cortex via the optic radiations. Fibers in the optic tract leave to reach the midbrain III nerve nucleus, which forms the efferent arc of the pupillary light reflex and causes ipsilateral and consensual pupillary constriction.

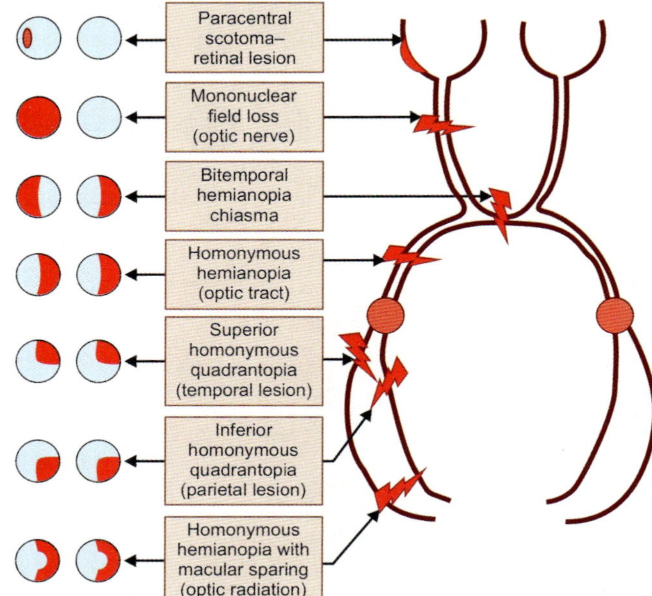

Fig. 6.1.5: The visual pathway: effects of lesions.

The inferior optic radiation courses through the temporal lobe and contains fibers for the upper visual field, while the superior parietal optic radiation has fibers for the inferior nasal field. Anteriorly the optic radiations are close to the internal capsule, which contains the motor and sensory long tracts.

The optic radiations then converge onto the visual cortex. The tip of the occipital lobe receives bilateral input from the macular region.

Localization

Monocular visual loss is due to lesions in the eye or the optic nerve. Binocular visual loss is due to the involvement of both eyes, both optic nerves, the optic chiasm, or posterior retrochiasmal lesions.

Optic neuropathies (ON) cause central visual loss, impaired color vision, abnormal visual fields, initially swollen (papillitis) or normal (retrobulbar) optic disks, which may become pale over 4–6 weeks. The relative afferent pupillary defect (RAPD) is seen in unilateral or asymmetric ON. With unilateral or asymmetric visual loss, there is reduced or no signal reaching the brainstem parasympathetic nuclei leading to less or no pupillary constriction bilaterally when light is flashed in the affected eye. This difference in pupillary constriction between the affected and the normal eye is the basis of the RAPD **(Fig. 6.1.6)**.

The most common acquired disorder is optic neuritis, which can be clinically isolated or associated with other demyelinating conditions, such as acute disseminated encephalomyelitis,

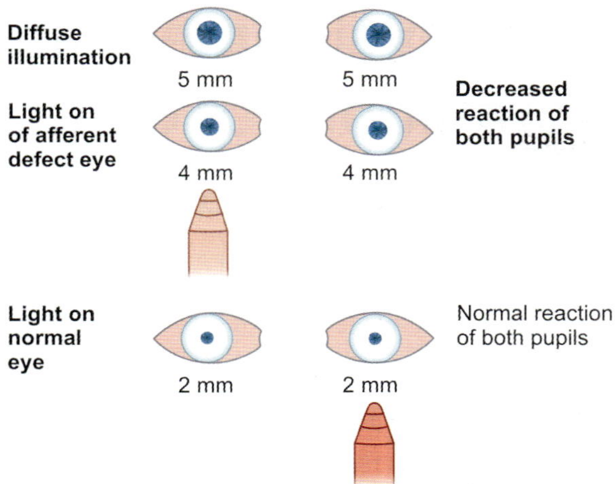

Fig. 6.1.6: Swinging flashlight test for relative afferent pupillary defect (RAPD).
Note: Pupils appear equal in ambiant light unless the defect is brought out by the swinging flashlight test.

neuromyelitis optica, or multiple sclerosis. Hereditary ON, such as Leber ON, are rarer causes of painless acute monocular visual loss, which can involve the other side as well.

When acute visual loss is associated with pain, diplopia, ptosis, ophthalmoplegia, and/or proptosis, an orbital process, such as cellulitis, should be considered. Though tumors, such as optic glioma, are slow growing and produce progressive visual loss, they are often noticed suddenly and may be mistaken as an acute optic neuritis.

Disk edema can be caused by an anterior optic nerve process, such as optic neuritis, or by raised ICP, i.e. papilledema. Early visual loss is typical of optic neuritis, while papilledema causes enlargement of the blind spot and visual loss as secondary optic atrophy occurs later.

Chiasmatic lesions, such as craniopharyngioma or glioma, characteristically produce mono or binocular visual loss, and as they involve crossing nasal fibers, they produce a bitemporal hemianopia. They may extend laterally and cause ocular motor neuropathies, if the cavernous sinus area is invaded or extend superiorly causing hydrocephalus.

Retrochiasmal lesions produce a homonymous hemianopia (HH). There is ipsilateral nasal and contralateral temporal field defects, congruent or incongruent, but which respect the vertical meridian. Lesions in the parietal optic radiations cause inferior quadrantic HH, and temporal optic radiations cause a superior quadrantic HH. Lesions in the occipital lobe produce a complete HH but the occipital tip, which represents macular (central) vision, is often spared, and hence, visual acuity may be unaffected. In bilateral occipital lesions, bilateral, often asymmetric HH and decreased visual acuity are usual. Pupils characteristically remain unaffected.

The causes of transient binocular visual loss include migrainous visual aura and occipital lobe seizures. More prolonged loss can be seen with posterior reversible edema syndrome; hypoxic, ischemic encephalopathy; traumatic brain injury, posterior circulation strokes, etc. Perinatal brain injuries, such as hypoglycemic brain injury and periventricular leukomalacia, are the most frequent causes as both have a predilection for the posterior areas.

BIBLIOGRAPHY

1. Biousse V, Newman N. Neuro-ophthalmology Illustrated. New York, NY: Thieme Medical Publishers; 2009.
2. Brazis P, Masdeu J, Biller J. Localization in Clinical Neurology, 6th edition. Philadelphia, PA: Wolters Kluwer/Lippincott Williams and Wilkins; 2011.
3. Campbell W. Dejong's the Neurologic Examination, 6th edition. Philadelphia, PA: Lippincott Williams and Wilkins; 2005.
4. Fenichel G. Clinical Pediatric Neurology: a Signs and Symptoms Approach, 5th edition. Philadelphia, PA: Saunders; 2005.
5. Swaiman K. Neurologic examination after the newborn period until 2 years of age. In: Swaiman K, Ashwal S, Farriero D (Eds). Pediatric Neurology Principles and Practice, 4th edition. Philadelphia, PA: Mosby Elsevier; 2006. p. 3746.
6. Swaiman K. Neurologic examination of the older child. In: Swaiman K, Ashwal S, Farriero D (Eds). Pediatric Neurology Principles and Practice, 4th edition. Philadelphia, PA: Mosby Elsevier; 2006. p. 1735.

6.2 Prenatal Development and Malformations of Central Nervous System

PA Mohammed Kunju

INTRODUCTION

With the widespread availability of imaging tools, such as magnetic resonance imaging (MRI) and ultrasound (US) scan, the diagnosis of congenital nervous system malformations has become common, and therefore, practicing pediatricians will often be asked to give opinion on outcome, possible management, and chance of recurrence. So an up-to-date knowledge of embryology and imaging features is necessary.

Current concept of neuroembryology has changed a lot from the classic descriptive morphogenesis to the integration of molecular genetic programming that direct cellular and regional differentiation. This approach has provided precise spatial and temporal sequences of the anatomic malformations, both macroscopic and functional.

Molecular genetic programming ranges from early processes that establish the axes of the neural tube and gradients of genetic expression to late processes that establish identity of specific types of neurons, the type of neurotransmitter they synthesize, and the synaptic connections they make. The variations in these stages may explain the unpredictable clinical manifestation of malformations. For example, the two cases of corpus callosum agenesis with nearly identical imaging findings may differ in that one may have epilepsy refractory to pharmacological control, whereas the other may have no clinical seizures at all.

NORMAL EMBRYONIC DEVELOPMENT AND OVERVIEW OF PATHOGENESIS

The events of neural maturation after initial induction and formation of the neural tube are:

- Neurulation or formation of the neural tube
- Proliferation of neuroblasts
- Programmed death (apoptosis) of excess neuroblasts
- Neuroblast migration
- Axonal growth
- Electrical polarity of the cell membrane
- Synaptogenesis
- Biosynthesis of neurotransmitters
- Myelination of axons.

Primary Neurulation

Neural plate is formed (18th day of gestation) as a thickening of the primitive ectoderm that overlies the notochord. Invagination of it, forms the neural groove (20th day), and neural tube is formed by separation from the overlying surface ectoderm. Initial closure (22nd day) of the neural tube is accomplished in the area corresponding to the junction of the cervical spinal cord and medulla and moves rapidly both caudally and rostrally. The rostral end of the neural tube closes (24th day) first, and the caudal neuropore closes (26th day) last between T11 and S2 vertebral level. Brain and upper spine is formed by this primary neurulation [for the timing of events **(Figs. 6.2.1A to C)**]. It can be understood that all these developments occur before the time women realize they are pregnant.

Secondary Neurulation

At 4–5 weeks of gestation, distal spine and the most caudal part of the spinal cord (i.e. conus medullaris and filum terminale) develop from the neuroepithelium caudal to the site of posterior neuropore closure by a process of secondary neurulation. This part of the spinal cord forms not as a tube, but rather as a solid cord of neural cells in which ependymal cells differentiate in its core and canalize the cord. Because of the differential growth between the vertebral column and the spinal cord, the conus becomes more rostral during the later development.

Brain Formation

The cells along with the caudal end of the neural tube form the hindbrain and spinal cord, and cells on the rostral end of the neural tube form the brain. The rostral end of neural tube expand and constrict to form the three primary brain vesicles. Craniocaudally, these are prosencephalon, mesencephalon, and rhombencephalon (mnemonic polymyalgia rheumatica). Prosencephalon becomes telencephalon [cerebral cortex and striatum (caudate and putamen)] and diencephalon (thalamus, hypothalamus, and globus pallidus). Mesencephalon is the midbrain. Rhombencephalon also becomes subdivided into

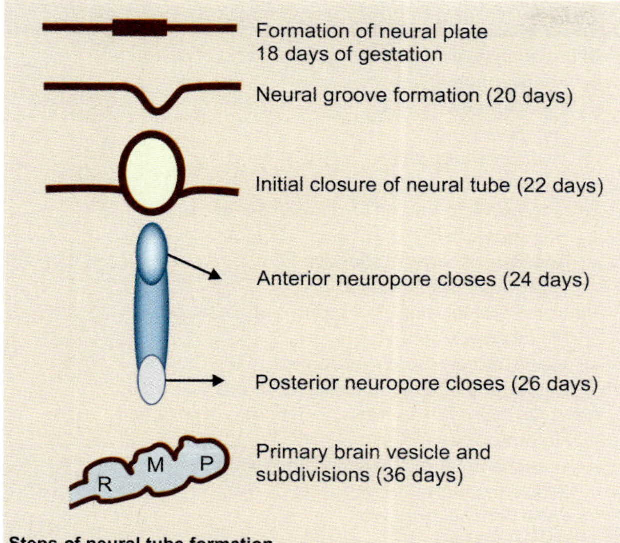

Steps of neural tube formation
Dates of events can be remembered as neural plate, neural groove, neural tube, anterior neuropore closure and posterior neuropore closure—18, 20, 22, 24 and 26 days respectively
(P: prosencephalon; M: mesencephalon; R: rhombencephalon)

A

Figs. 6.2.1A to C: (A) Steps of neural tube formation; (B) Cranial part of neural tube evolving as three primary vesicles; (C) Three primary brain vesicles and five secondary vesicles and the derived brain parts.

metencephalon (pons and cerebellum) and myelencephalon (medulla) **(Figs. 6.2.1B and C)**. The cavities of the brain vesicles are later designated as lateral ventricle (cavity of telencephalon), the third ventricle (cavity of diencephalon), aqueduct (cavity of mesencephalon), and the fourth ventricle (cavity of rhombencephalon).

The failure of primary neurulation leads to open neural tube defects (NTDs), and a defect in secondary neurulation leads to closed NTDs.

Neural Crest

During the rapid growth of cells within the neural plate and invagination of the neural groove to form neural tube, the differentiation of a conglomerate of cells occurs at the two fusing lips of the closing neural tube. These are the neural crest cells, which migrate distally along the predetermined pathways to form the peripheral/cranial sensory root ganglia, sympathetic and parasympathetic ganglia, chromaffin tissue, adrenal medulla, melanocytes, leptomeninges, and Schwann cells.

The failure of correct migration or differentiation of neural crest cells can lead to a number of abnormalities, such as Hirschsprung disease, neuroblastoma, DiGeorge syndrome, neurofibromatosis type 1, intestinal aganglionosis, melanoma, and albinism.

Neuronal Proliferation

The embryonic neural tube consists of three zones: (1) ventricular, (2) mantle, and (3) marginal. The proliferation of neuroepithelial cells in the ventricular zone generates neurons and glial cells by gestation week 6; active mitoses cease well before the time of birth (the end of the 15th week.) in most parts of the human nervous system, except few sites. A population of "stem cells" with mitotic potential in the subventricular zone and hippocampal dentate gyrus has generated considerable interest because of a potential for regeneration of the damaged brain.

Disorders of neuronal proliferation include hypoplasia of the brain (e.g. cerebellar hypoplasia), microcephaly, and megalencephaly.

Neuronal Migration

Neurons after mitotic proliferation at the subependymal germinal matrix (subventricular zone) migrate to their final site to establish the synaptic connections. This begins at 6 weeks of gestation (42 days). During the early phases of neuron production, neurons migrate via *somal translocation* as cells have to travel only short distance. Then migration proceeds along the radial glial fibers that span the entire cerebral mantle to pial membrane at the surface of the brain (*radial migration*). In the cortex, this occurs in an "inside-out" manner—layers 6–2 migrate in the reverse order. However, layer 1 migrates first.

Tangential migration: It does not require glial fibers and occurs parallel to the brain surface. This migration mode allows the passage of neurons from one brain compartment to another and occurs at the later stages of the development. Interneurons (GABAergic neurons) and neurons of basal ganglia migrate tangentially.

After the above steps, development further proceeds with axonal growth and dendritic arborization, establishment of electrical polarity of the cell membrane, synaptogenesis, biosynthesis of neurotransmitters (inhibitory and excitatory), and myelination of axons.

Defects in these steps are seen in various chromosomal, metabolic, and hypoxic encephalopathies and can lead to mental retardation and epilepsy.

MALFORMATIONS OF THE CENTRAL NERVOUS SYSTEM

The majority of malformations that occur early in gestation have a genetic basis, whereas those that begin late in gestation are more likely to be secondary to destructive lesions. Factors, such as radiation, drugs, malnutrition, chemicals, and infections, may induce malformations by a teratogenic influence that acts at a particular time of ontogenesis.

CLASSIFICATION OF CENTRAL NERVOUS SYSTEM MALFORMATIONS

The classification of central nervous system (CNS) malformations is provided in **Box 6.2.1**.

Box 6.2.1: Classification of central nervous system malformations.

- *Neurulation (neural tube defect) (3–4 weeks of gestation):*
  - Anencephaly
  - Iniencephaly
  - Encephalocele
  - Myelomeningocele
  - Chiari malformation
- *Prosencephalic formation (2–3 months of gestation):*
  - Holoprosencephaly
  - Agenesis of corpus callosum
  - Septooptic dysplasia
- Neuronal proliferation (3–4 months of gestation):
  - Microcephaly vera
  - Macrocephaly (Soto syndrome)
  - Neurocutaneous syndromes (tuberous sclerosis)
- *Neuronal migration disorders (3–5 months of gestation):*
  - Heterotopias
  - Lissencephaly/pachygyria complex
  - Schizencephaly
  - Focal cortical dysplasia
  - Polymicrogyria
- *Disorders of cerebellar development (32 days to 1 year gestation):*
  - Hypoplasia of the vermis, e.g. Joubert syndrome
  - Dandy–Walker malformation
- *Destructive brain lesions:*
  - Hydranencephaly
  - Porencephaly

DISORDERS OF NEURAL TUBE CLOSURE

Anencephaly

Anencephaly (Greek *an*, "without"; *enkephalin*, "brain"; with open cranium) is failure of the closing of anterior neuropore at 24 days of gestation. As a result, forebrain is exposed or extrudes from the skull, a condition known as exencephaly. Two types are recognized. In holoanencephaly, there is a complete absence of brain. In meroanencephaly, rudiments of the basal ganglia, brainstem, and cranial vault are replaced by an amorphous vascular neural mass (area cerebrovasculosa). Death in utero occurs in approximately 7% of anencephalic pregnancies; 34% of such babies are born prematurely and 53% at term.

The prenatal diagnosis is done by amniotic fluid examination for elevated α-fetoprotein and ultrasonographic finding of the absence of calvaria and brain above orbit as early as 12 weeks of gestation.

Spina Bifida and Cranium Bifidum

The failure of bony fusion in the posterior midline of the skull (cranium bifidum) or the vertebral column (spina bifida) results in a bony cleft through which the meninges and varying quantities of brain or spinal cord may protrude. The term dysraphism is used to indicate the persistent continuity between posterior neuroectoderm and cutaneous ectoderm. In spina bifida, the herniation is called meningocele or meningomyelocele, depending on whether the meninges herniate alone or together with spinal cord parenchyma and nerve roots. Spina bifida can be "aperta" with open NTD and "occulta" with closed NTD. Open NTD frequently involves the entire CNS with associated hydrocephalus and Chiari II malformation. Closed NTD is localized and confined to the spine and brain rarely affected.

In cranium bifidum, the term *encephalocele* refers to the herniation of brain tissue and meninges and meningocele when herniation only of meninges.

Encephalocele

Encephalocele is classified according to the anatomic site of cranial defect:

- Occipital encephalocele **(Figs. 6.2.2A and B)** lies between lambda and foramen magnum.
- Parietal encephalocele lies between bregma and lambda.

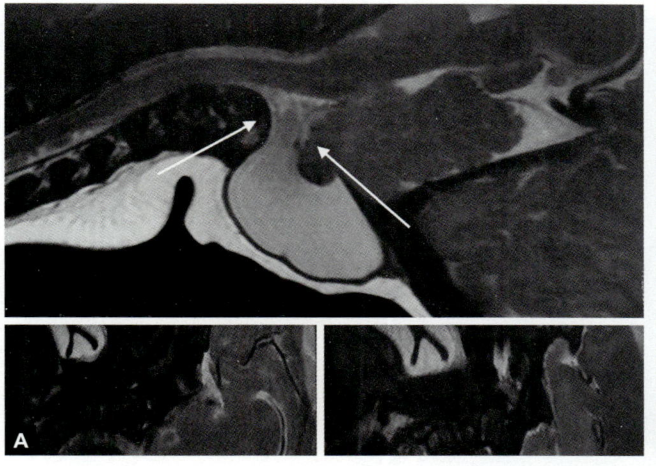

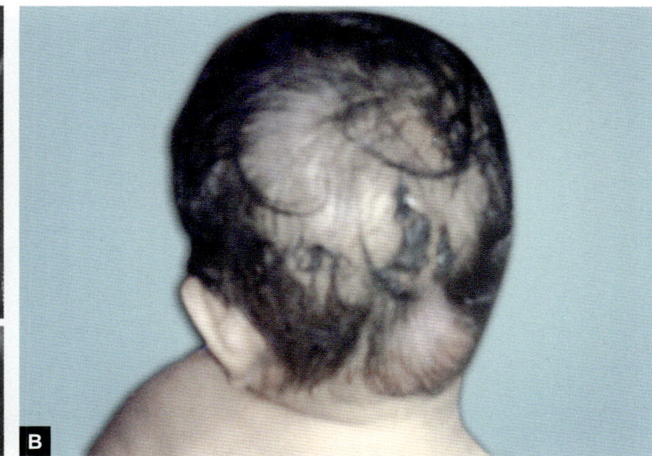

Figs. 6.2.2A and B: Occipital encephalocele.

- Sincipital (frontoethmoidal) encephalocele lies between bregma and anterior margin of ethmoid bone.
- Basal encephalocele herniates through ethmoid or sphenoid bone into nasal pharynx.

The treatment of choice of small encephaloceles is surgical excision and closure of overlying cutaneous defects. Seizures and hydrocephalus are common but treatable complications. Nasopharyngeal encephaloceles may be a cause of recurrent meningitis from cerebrospinal fluid (CSF) rhinorrhea.

Spina Bifida Occulta

In spina bifida occulta, no herniation of the meninges is present, and the skin of the back is completely epithelialized. Suspect in children with recurrent meningitis of occult origin:

- Examine for a small sinus tract in the posterior midline region, including the back of the head. Patches of hair, a lipoma, discoloration of the skin, or a dermal sinus **(Figs. 6.2.3A to C)** in the midline of the low back signifies an underlying malformation of the spinal cord, L5 and S1 spinal cord, including syringomyelia, diastematomyelia, and a tethered cord.
- Surgical referral mandatory.
- Clear indications for surgery include the finding of progressive neurologic defects, the presence of an associated tumor or a dermal sinus that carries the risk of meningitis or deep abscess, or a history of meningitis.

Myelomeningocele

Most lesions are lumbosacral in location, but myelomeningocele may also occur in the thoracic or even the cervical region, usually as an extension rostrally of lumbosacral lesions. In its full expression, the following features are present:

- The presence of unfused or excessively separated vertebral arches of the bony spine (spina bifida).
- Cystic dilation of the meninges that surround the spinal cord (meningocele).
- Cystic dilation of the spinal cord itself (myelocele).
- Type II Chiari malformation is commonly present and aqueductal stenosis coexists in 50% of the cases. Hydrocephalus is a common complication, which will require an early treatment **(Figs. 6.2.4A to C)**.
- The level of involvement determines much of the clinical deficit. Infants with myelomeningocele typically have an increasing neurologic deficit as the myelomeningocele extends higher into the thoracic region.
- A lesion in the low sacral region causes bowel and bladder incontinence associated with anesthesia in the perineal area but with no impairment of motor function.
- A myelomeningocele in the midlumbar region tends to produce lower motor neuron signs due to abnormalities and disruption of the conus medullaris.
- Infant with upper lumbar lesion shows a flaccid paralysis of the lower limb, an absence of deep tendon reflexes, poor response to touch and pain, and a high incidence of clubfeet and subluxation of the hips.

Treatment

The treatment of myelomeningocele is the surgical closure of small defects in the neonatal period itself. Large defects associated with complete paraplegia and flaccid neurogenic bladder, often accompanied by hydronephrosis, severe hydrocephalus, and other cerebral malformations, are dealt appropriately. A decision not to treat such infants or not to prolong survival poses a moral question addressed by the physicians in consultation with parents, hospital ethics committees, and other individuals whom the parents may identify. Aggressive treatment is the current strategy.

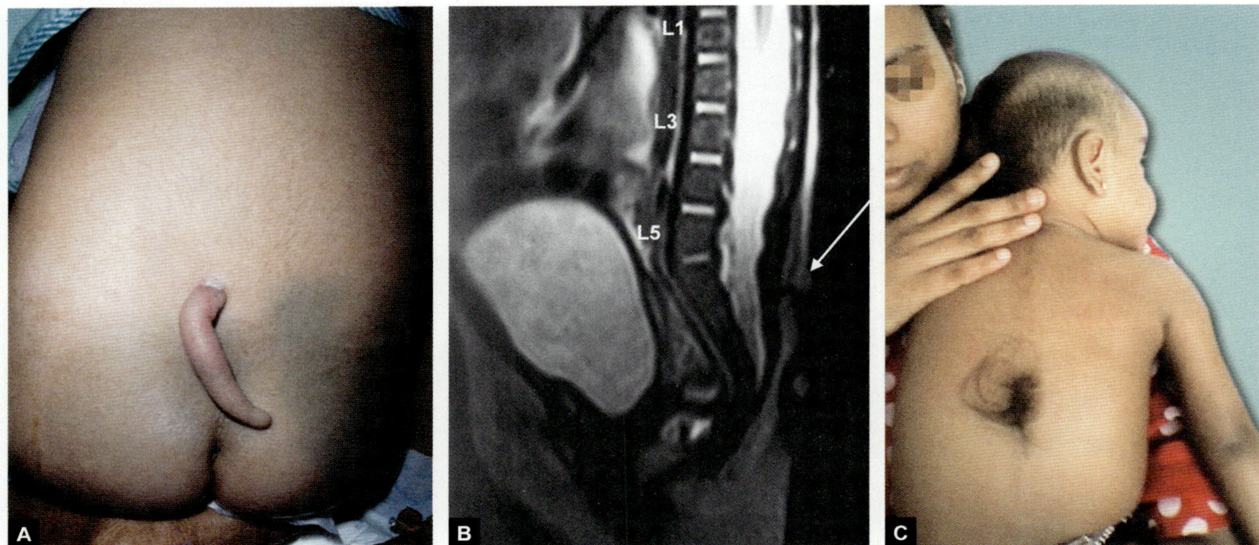

Figs. 6.2.3A to C: (A and C) Spina bifida occulta two clinical forms; (B) MRI with tethering and dermal sinus. (MRI: magnetic resonance imaging)

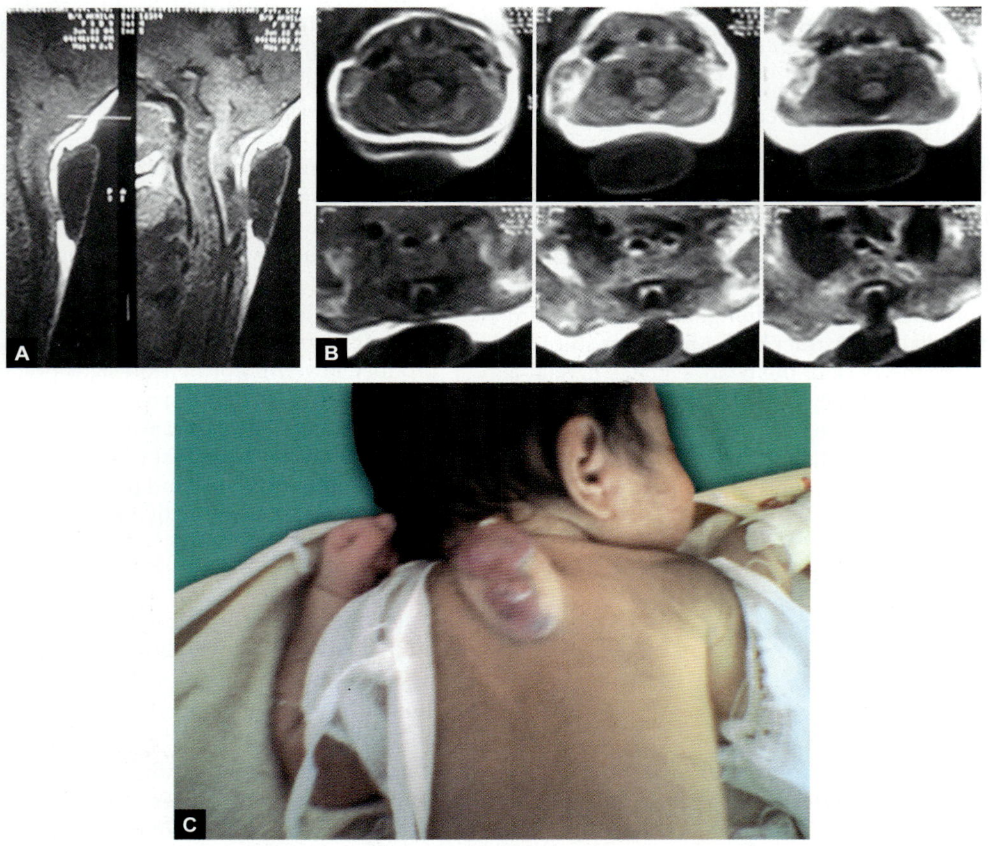

Figs. 6.2.4A to C: Cervical meningomyelocele with Arnold–Chiari malformation II. (A) Sagittal MRI of cervical spine and neck; (B) Axial sections—note the descend of cerebellum and brainstem to the spinal canal; and (C) Baby with cervical meningomyelocele.

These include the repair of myelomeningocele, a shunting procedure for hydrocephalus, early surgical decompression of the medulla, and cervical cord, if hindbrain dysfunction appears. Clubfeet and dislocated hips may require casting and operative procedures.

Neurogenic bladder: About 80% of the patients have this, which most commonly manifests as a small, poorly compliant bladder, and an open and fixed sphincter. Options of management include the following:

- Clean intermittent catheterization by parents and ultimately the patient prevents urinary tract infections and reflux leading to pyelonephritis and hydronephrosis.
- Periodic urine cultures and assessment of renal function.
- Artificial urinary sphincter to increase outlet resistance.
- Surgical urinary diversion (e.g. suprapubic vesicostomy).
- Augmentation cystoplasty to increase bladder capacity in combination with the use of oxybutynin.

Long-term ambulation potential: It is determined by the level of lesion.

- *Sacral:* As the patient is able to plantar flex the ankles and move the toes, nearly all children and adolescents will ambulate, with minimal assistive devices.
- *Low lumbar:* The patient is able to flex the knee and dorsiflex the ankle. Nearly half of the younger children and nearly all adolescents will ambulate, with varying degrees of braces or crutches.
- *Midlumbar:* The patient is able to flex the hips and extend the knee. The percentage of those able to ambulate is the midway between those with high and low lumbar lesions.
- *High lumbar:* The patient is able to flex the hips, but there is no knee extension. About one-third of the children and adolescents will ambulate, but only with extensive assistive devices.
- *Thoracic:* As no hip flexion, no young child will ambulate and one-third of the adolescents can be ambulated with the aid of extensive braces and crutches.

Prenatal Diagnosis and Prevention

Neural tube defects can be detected prenatally by ultrasonography, the α-fetoprotein level in amniotic fluid or maternal serum and amniotic fluid acetyl cholinesterase. Sonological diagnosis of a myelomeningocele is usually prompted by the recognition of the associated Chiari II malformation in the second trimester. Diagnostic signs are "lemon" and "banana" signs. Lemon sign is due to the abnormal cranial vault that is narrowed rostrally, and the banana sign represents the cerebellum surrounding the brainstem in a small posterior fossa.

The risk of recurrence of NTDs after one affected child increases to 3–4% and to 10% with two previous abnormal pregnancies. There is strong evidence that maternal periconceptional folic acid supplementation reduces the incidence of NTDs in pregnancies at risk by at least 50%. The US Public Health Service has recommended that all women of childbearing age and who are capable of becoming pregnant take 0.4 mg of folic acid daily, and that women who have previously had a pregnancy, resulting in an NTD, be treated with 4 mg of folic acid daily, beginning 1 month (preferably 3 months) before the time pregnancy is planned.

Chiari Malformations

Type I Malformation

The Chiari I malformation consists of the displacement of cerebellar tonsils at least 3–5 mm through the foramen magnum into the upper cervical canal. Type I is clinically the least severe and generally asymptomatic during childhood. The presentation may be insidious, and it is associated with mental retardation and epilepsy in a small minority. There may be paroxysmal vertigo, drop attacks, vague dizziness, and headache, which may be increased by the Valsalva maneuver. Occipital headache precipitated by exertion may progress to torticollis, downgaze nystagmus, periodic nystagmus, and oscillopsia. Magnetic resonance imaging findings in patients with Chiari I malformations include malformations of the base of the skull and of the upper cervical spine, including hydromyelia, syringomyelia, and syrinx.

Type II Malformation (Arnold–Chiari Malformation)

The vermis, pons, medulla, and an elongated fourth ventricle are displaced into the cervical canal. Type II is the most common of those diagnosed during childhood. A variety of cerebellar brainstem and cortical defects can occur. It is associated with encephalocele, noncommunicating hydrocephalus, and myelomeningocele in almost 100% of the cases.

Type III

Type III involves an occipitocervical bony defect with the herniation of cerebellum into the encephalocele. Type III comprises the features of types I and II, but the entire cerebellum is herniated throughout the foramen magnum, with a cervical spina bifida cystica. Hydrocephalus is a common feature.

Type IV

Type IV is cerebellar hypoplasia without a connection with the other malformations.

Syringomyelia and Hydromyelia

Syringomyelia is the development of a fluid-filled cavity or syrinx within the spinal cord. Hydromyelia is a dilatation of the central canal by CSF. This can occur as a developmental anomaly, associated with Chiari malformations, or can be an acquired lesion of the spinal cord secondary to trauma, infarction, or intramedullary tumors. Syringomyelia usually involves the cervical area. Symptomatic presentation depends primarily on the location of the lesion within the neuraxis. Common manifestations are dissociated sensory loss, muscle atrophy that begins in the hands, and spasticity of lower limbs. The identification and treatment of associated dysraphism have the greatest impact on arresting progression of syringomyelia. Surgery includes suboccipital and cervical decompression with laminectomy and syringotomy (dorsolateral myelotomy).

DISORDERS OF PROSENCEPHALIC FORMATION

Holoprosencephaly

Holoprosencephaly (HPE) is a malformation in which the two cerebral hemispheres appear fused in the midline due to a failure of cleavage in the midsagittal plane of the embryonic cerebral vesicle at 33 days of gestation. Four variant forms are described: (1) alobar, (2) semilobar, (3) lobar, and (4) the middle interhemispheric variant. The most common associations of HPE are chromosomal defects (trisomy 13 and deletions) and maternal diabetes mellitus. Facial abnormalities, including cyclopia, cebocephaly, and premaxillary agenesis, are common. Endocrine dysfunction may be present, associated with hypothalamic or pituitary involvement. The most severe form, alobar HPE, is characterized by a single ventricle, an absent falx, and fused basal ganglia. Mortality and morbidity are variable, and care must be taken before prognostication.

Treatment

The treatment of HPE depends on the complications, such as seizures, hydrocephalus, and hormonal disturbances. Educational potential and need for supports depend on the degree of mental retardation, speech, and visual impairment.

Agenesis of the Corpus Callosum

Agenesis of the corpus callosum (ACC) is an anomaly (2.3% prevalence) that may occur in isolation or in association with other CNS malformations. Agenesis of the corpus callosum may be complete, partial, or atypical. Secondary destruction of corpus callosum occurs with hypoxic ischemic encephalopathy (HIE), surgery, or infarcts. Other cerebral malformations may coexist with callosal dysgenesis, e.g. interhemispheric cysts, intracranial lipomas, and neuronal migration disorders (NMDs). Various genetic syndromes are associated with ACC, e.g. trisomy 8, 11, and 13; Aicardi syndrome consists of ACC, chorioretinal lacunae, vertebral anomalies, mental retardation, and infantile spasm in girls.

Clinical Symptoms

Clinical symptoms of ACC may be minimal in children of normal intelligence. Detailed neurological examination discloses deficits in the interhemispheric transfer of perceptual information for verbal expression. Mental retardation or learning disabilities occur in some cases. Epilepsy is common and may relate more to minor focal cortical dysplasia than to the callosal agenesis itself. Similarly, interhemispheric lipoma replacing part of the corpus callosum is associated with a high incidence of epilepsy. Hypertelorism is present in many and often is associated with divergent squint.

Diagnosis

Diagnosis of callosal agenesis depends on neuroimaging. In the newborn, before the closure of anterior fontanels occurs, ultrasonography will show the absence of the corpus callosum; it may also show parallel lateral ventricles, interhemispheric cysts, hydrocephalus, and other related anomalies. The electroencephalogram characteristically shows interhemispheric asynchrony (checkerboard pattern), with or without multifocal spikes. Computed tomography scan findings include widely separated, parallel lateral ventricles with straight medial border, colpocephaly (enlarged posterior horns), and extension of the third ventricle into the interhemispheric fissure (devil's horn appearance). Magnetic resonance imaging is the imaging procedure of choice.

Prenatal Diagnosis of Agenesis of the Corpus Callosum

Prenatal diagnosis is possible from 20 weeks of gestation.

DISORDERS OF NEURONAL PROLIFERATION

Microcephaly

Microcephaly is defined by a head circumference, as measured around the forehead and the occipital protuberance that is more than three standard deviations below the mean for age, gender, and race. Head circumference should also be compared with previous measurements of the same child, ideally from birth, to determine whether microcephaly is congenital or acquired. An abnormally small brain results either from anomalous development during the first 7 months of gestation (primary microcephaly—genetic) or from an insult incurred during the last 2 months of gestation or during the perinatal period (secondary microcephaly—nongenetic).

Primary Microcephaly

Primary microcephaly results from a variety of insults that cause anomalies of induction and migration. Microencephaly denotes a small brain or cerebral hypoplasia determined by imaging or neuropathologic examination. It can be transmitted as an autosomal recessive or as an autosomal dominant disorder. Numerous migrational anomalies are seen, including schizencephaly, lissencephaly, pachygyria, polymicrogyria, and ACC.

- *Autosomal recessive:* Characteristic facies with slanted forehead, prominent nose, and ears.
- *Autosomal dominant:* Milder phenotype.
- *Syndromes with microcephaly:* Down, Edward, Cri-du-chat, Cornelia de Lange, Rubinstein–Taybi, and Smith Lemli Opitz.

Secondary Microcephaly

Secondary microcephaly can be due to radiation during pregnancy; congenital TORCH infections [Toxoplasmosis; Other (syphilis, varicella zoster, parvovirus B19, etc.); Rubella; Cytomegalovirus and herpes simplex] drugs, such as phenytoin (fetal hydantoin syndrome); maternal alcoholism (fetal alcohol syndrome); maternal diabetes mellitus and maternal hyperphenylalaninemia; postnatal intracranial infections, hyperthermia; malnutrition; and hypoxic ischemic encephalopathy (HIE). Postnatally acquired progressive microcephaly can be due to Rett syndrome and human immunodeficiency virus encephalopathy.

- Investigations and management depend on the possible etiology and associated manifestations.
- The recurrence of microcephaly is relatively high; the exact frequency depends on the incidence among the kindred.
- Prenatal diagnosis by US has been attempted by serial biparietal diameter measurements. However, it discriminates poorly between affected and unaffected fetuses until late pregnancy.

Macrocephaly

Large head can be due to various causes other than hydrocephalus. The common causes starting from skull inward are provided in **Box 6.2.2**.

Box 6.2.2: Causes of macrocephaly.

- *Conditions with a thickened skull causing large head:*
  - Hemolytic anemia
  - Rickets
  - Cleidocranial dysostosis
- *Subdural:*
  - Hematoma
  - Hygroma
  - Empyema
- *Brain parenchyma:*
  - *Anatomical megalencephaly*: Genetic megalencephaly and Sotos syndrome
  - *Metabolic megalencephaly*: Alexander disease and Tay–Sachs disease
- *Brain and ventricle:*
  - Hydranencephaly
  - Porencephaly
- *Ventricle:*
  - Hydrocephalus
  - Holoprosencephaly

NEURONAL MIGRATION DISORDERS

Disorders of Neuronal Migration

Disorders of neuronal migration include heterotopia, focal cortical dysplasia, lissencephaly, and pachygyria. Three types of following aberrations can occur:

1. Neuroblasts never having begun migration from the periventricular region produce periventricular nodular heterotopia.
2. Neuroblasts after beginning migration arrested in the subcortical white matter and produce subcortical laminar heterotopia.
3. Neuroblasts reach the cortical plate but fails to form the normal cortical layers and lead to abnormalities of gyration, such as lissencephaly and pachygyria.

Recently with MRI, it is clear that the incidence of NMD is much greater than had been estimated. The conditions associated with NMD include the phakomatoses, a variety of metabolic, genetic, and chromosomal syndromes, and maternal and environmental causes. Migratory disorders develop when neuroblasts of the subependymal germinal matrix fail to reach their intended destination in the cerebral cortex.

Heterotopia

When gray matter lies in the white matter area, it is called heterotopia. They include subcortical laminar (band heterotopia) and bilateral periventricular nodular heterotopia.

In the first one, a band of gray matter heterotopia lies within the subcortical white matter parallel to the overlying cerebral cortex but separates from it by white matter **(Figs. 6.2.5A to D)**. In bilateral periventricular nodular heterotopia, islands of neurons and glial cells occur in the subependymal regions around the lateral ventricles. Intractable seizure is the common manifestation.

Lissencephaly (Agyria, Pachygyria, Macrogyria)

Lissencephaly means smooth brain. It is characterized by the absence of cerebral convolutions and a horizontally placed sylvian fissure giving a "Figure of 8" appearance on axial MRI. In pachygyria (macrogyria), the pathology is less severe

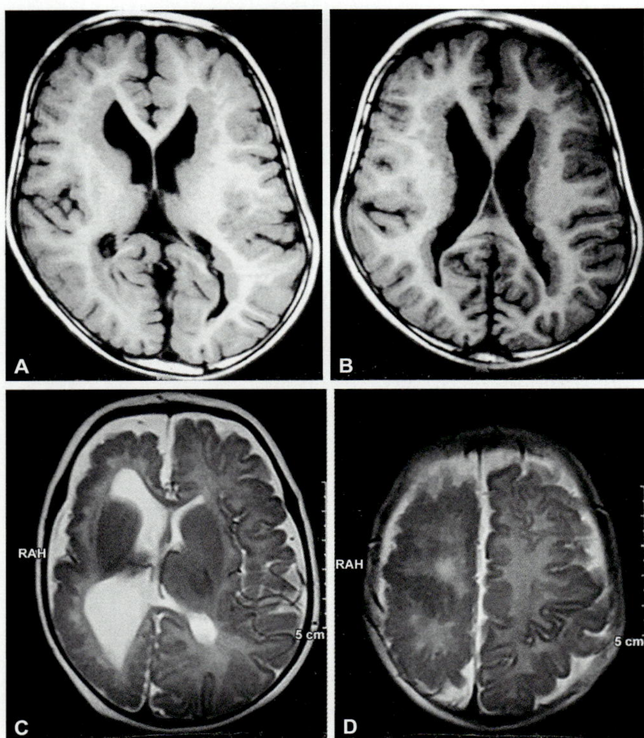

Figs. 6.2.5A to D: (A and B) Band heterotopias (nodular appearance along the outer border of lateral ventricle); (C and D) T2 MRI showing polymicrogyria and heterotopia on right side.
(MRI: magnetic resonance imaging)

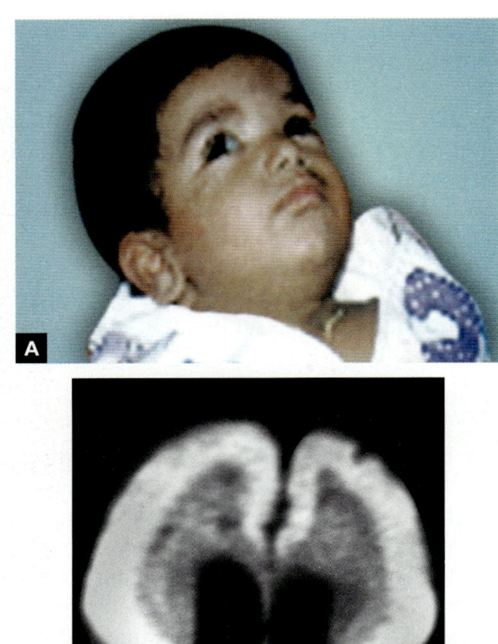

Figs. 6.2.6A and B: Lissencephaly: Miller–Dieker syndrome. (Note the facial features)

than that in lissencephaly, and the areas of normal laminar organization are seen.

Clinically, these infants present with severe infantile spasms, failure to thrive, microcephaly, and gross developmental delay. Eye abnormalities, such as hypoplasia of the optic nerve and microphthalmia, are seen. Two types of lissencephaly are described here:

1. Miller–Dieker syndrome, classical or type I lissencephaly with four-layered cortex. Children with Miller–Dieker syndrome have characteristic facies, including a prominent forehead and bitemporal hollowing.
2. Anteverted nostrils, a prominent upper lip, and micrognathia **(Figs. 6.2.6A and B)**.
3. Walker-Warburg syndrome and Fukuyama congenital muscular dystrophy, characterized by an almost complete absence of cortical layering.

Schizencephaly

Schizencephaly is characterized by clefts placed symmetrically within the cerebral hemispheres and extending from the cortical surface to the underlying ventricular cavity **(Fig. 6.2.7)**. It should be distinguished from porencephaly caused by a vascular insult to the brain. Porencephalic cysts communicate with the ventricular system or may extend to the cerebral cortical surface but do not destroy the thin pial membrane. Banks of schizencephaly will be lined by heterotopic gray matter.

The clinical picture of schizencephaly includes seizures, hypotonia, and hemiparesis or spastic. Imaging quadriparesis studies usually show bilateral, symmetric, or asymmetric clefts.

Polymicrogyria

Polymicrogyria results from an insult to the brain sustained before the fifth month of gestation. Brain will resemble a chestnut kernel and is characterized by gyri that are too small and too numerous. The clinically polymicrogyric children present as hypotonic cerebral palsy (mental retardation and hypotonia with active deep tendon reflexes). Another specific syndrome of opercular polymicrogyria or congenital bilateral perisylvian syndrome has been delineated

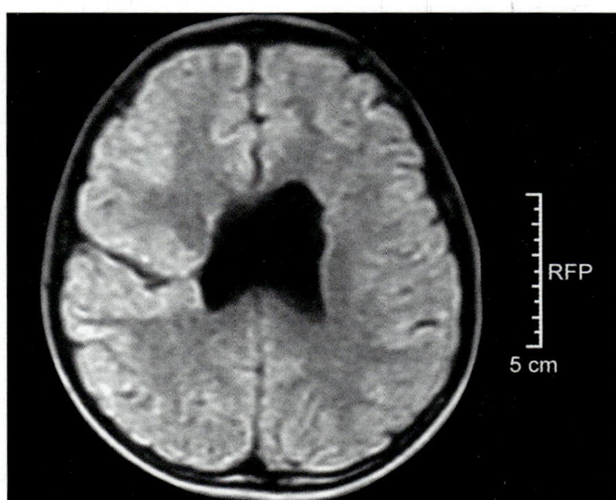

Fig. 6.2.7: Schizencephaly.
(Note the cleft on the right hemisphere with band of grey matter on both the banks)

(Figs. 6.2.5C and D). They have seizures, mental retardation, and pseudobulbar manifestation (dysarthria, abnormal tongue movements, and dysphagia).

DISORDERS OF CEREBELLAR DEVELOPMENT

Dandy–Walker Malformation

The Dandy–Walker malformation consists of posterior fossa cyst due to ballooning of the posterior half of the fourth ventricle. The failure of the foramen of Magendie to open is the primary pathology. Aplasia of the posterior cerebellar vermis, heterotopia of the inferior olivary nuclei, pachygyria of the cerebral cortex, and other cerebral and visceral anomalies are usually present. Infants present with a rapid increase in head size and a prominent occiput. Most children have evidence of long tract signs, cerebellar ataxia, and delayed motor and cognitive milestones, probably due to the associated structural anomalies. Management is like that of hydrocephalus.

DESTRUCTIVE BRAIN LESIONS

Hydranencephaly

The cerebral hemispheres are absent or represented by membranous sacs with remnants of frontal, temporal, or occipital cortex dispersed over the membrane. As it is presumed to be due to bilateral occlusion of the internal carotid arteries, posterior circulation structures, such as midbrain and brainstem, are relatively intact.

HYDROCEPHALUS

Hydrocephalus, an excessive volume of CSF in the skull, results from an imbalance between the formation of CSF and its absorption. The increased pressure and the ventricular enlargement follow account for the clinical findings. Any block in the CSF pathway from the site of formation to that of absorption results in increased CSF pressure.

By convention, hydrocephalus is divided into noncommunicating (obstructive) and communicating (nonobstructive) forms.

- In noncommunicating hydrocephalus, the obstructive site is within the ventricular system, including the outlet foramina of the fourth ventricle.
- Communicating hydrocephalus occurs when full communication occurs between the ventricles and subarachnoid space. It is caused by overproduction of CSF: choroid plexus papilloma, defective absorption of CSF (subarachnoid hemorrhage, meningitis, leukemic infiltrates, and intrauterine infections), or venous drainage insufficiency (achondroplasia or venous thrombosis).

The term congenital hydrocephalus applies to the ventriculomegaly that develops in the fetal and infancy periods, often associated with macrocephaly. The most common causes of congenital hydrocephalus are stenosis of the aqueduct of Sylvius, Arnold–Chiari malformation, and Dandy–Walker malformation. These patients may stabilize in the later years due to compensatory mechanisms but may decompensate, especially, following minor head injuries.

The incidence of congenital hydrocephalus is 3 per 1,000 live births.

Clinical Features

Clinical features of hydrocephalus are influenced by the patient's age, etiology, location of obstruction and duration are provided in **Box 6.2.3**.

Investigations

- MRI is the investigation of choice blockage clearly. Associated abnormalities such as Chiari malformation, cerebellar or periaqueductal tumors can also be seen. It is useful in differentiating hydrocephalus due to CSF block from "hydrocephalus ex vacuo" (enlargement of ventricular size due to cortical atrophy). Periventricular hyperintensiy seen in MRI is due to CSF driven transependymally into the periventricular white matter (interstitial edema) and is a relatively definite indication for surgery.
- Computed tomography scan is useful for identifying calcification in intrauterine infection **(Fig. 6.2.8)**.
- Ultrasound through the anterior fontanel in infants is useful for evaluating subependymal and intraventricular hemorrhage, and in following infants for possible development of progressive hydrocephalus.
- Genetic testing and counseling is recommended when X-linked hydrocephalus is suspected.

Box 6.2.3: Clinical features of hydrocephalus.

Signs and symptoms in infants:
- Poor feeding
- Head enlargement
- Irritability
- Sutural separation
- Reduced activity
- Dilated scalp veins
- Vomiting
- Tense anterior fontanel
- Open posterior fontanel
- Setting-sun sign
- Transillumination
- *Due to the underlying etiology:*
  - Features of spinal dysraphism
  - Cranial bruit in the cases of vein of Galen arteriovenous malformation
  - *Chorioretinitis*: Intrauterine infection, such as toxoplasmosis

Symptoms in children:
- Slowing of mental capacity
- Headaches (initially in the morning)
- Neck pain and head tilt suggesting tonsillar herniation
- Vomiting, more significant in the morning
- *Blurred vision*: Due to optic atrophy
- *Double vision*: Due to the sixth nerve palsy
- Failure of upgaze and of accommodation indicating pressure on the tectal plate
- *Macewen sign*: A "cracked pot" sound is noted on percussion of the head
- *Stunted growth and sexual maturation from the third ventricle dilatation*: obesity, precocious, or delayed puberty
- *Difficulty in walking secondary to spasticity*: Because the periventricular lower limb UMN fibers are stretched by the hydrocephalus

(UMN: upper motor neuron)

- Evaluate CSF in posthemorrhagic and postmeningitic hydrocephalus for protein concentration and to exclude residual.
- Infection.

Medical Management

Medical treatment is used to delay surgical intervention. It may be tried in premature infants with posthemorrhagic hydrocephalus (in the absence of acute hydrocephalus). Normal CSF absorption may resume spontaneously during this interim period.

- *Decreasing CSF secretion by the choroid plexus*:
  - Acetazolamide
  - Furosemide
- *Increasing CSF reabsorption*:
  - Isosorbide (effectiveness is questionable)

Surgical Care

Repeat Lumbar Punctures

Repeat lumbar punctures for hydrocephalus after intraventricular hemorrhage, since this condition can resolve spontaneously. If reabsorption does not resume when the protein content of CSF is less than 100 mg/dL, spontaneous resorption is unlikely to occur. Surgical treatment is the preferred therapeutic option.

Do monthly head circumference measurement, and if it exceeds more than 2.5 cm/month, surgical options to be considered.

Shunts

Only about 25% of the patients with hydrocephalus are treated successfully without shunt placement.

- Establish a communication between the CSF (ventricular or lumbar) and a drainage cavity (peritoneum, right atrium, or pleura).
- Remember that shunts are not perfect and that all alternatives to shunting should be considered first.
- A *ventriculoperitoneal* shunt is used most commonly.
- *A ventriculoatrial shunt (vascular shunt):* It shunts the cerebral ventricles through the jugular vein and superior vena cava into the right cardiac atrium. It is used when the patient has abdominal abnormalities (e.g. peritonitis, morbid obesity or after extensive abdominal surgery).
- *A lumboperitoneal* shunt is used for communicating hydrocephalus, CSF fistula, or pseudotumor cerebri.

Rapid-onset Hydrocephalus with Increased Intracranial Pressure

Rapid-onset hydrocephalus with increased intracranial pressure is an emergency. The following can be done, depending on each specific case:

- Ventricular tap in infants
- Open ventricular drainage in children and adults
- *Lumbar punctures* in posthemorrhagic and postmeningitic hydrocephalus
- Ventriculoperitoneal or ventriculoatrial shunt.

Endoscopic Third Ventriculostomy for Obstructive Hydrocephalus

Instead of the installation of a shunt hardware in the body, CSF pathway is diverted away from blockage by endoscopic third ventriculostomy. This allows the CSF to flow directly to the basal cisterns, thereby shortcutting any obstruction.

Prognosis

It depends on the etiology. Hydrocephalic children are at increased risk for various developmental disabilities.

Though gross mental retardation is absent, the mean intelligence quotient is reduced compared with the general

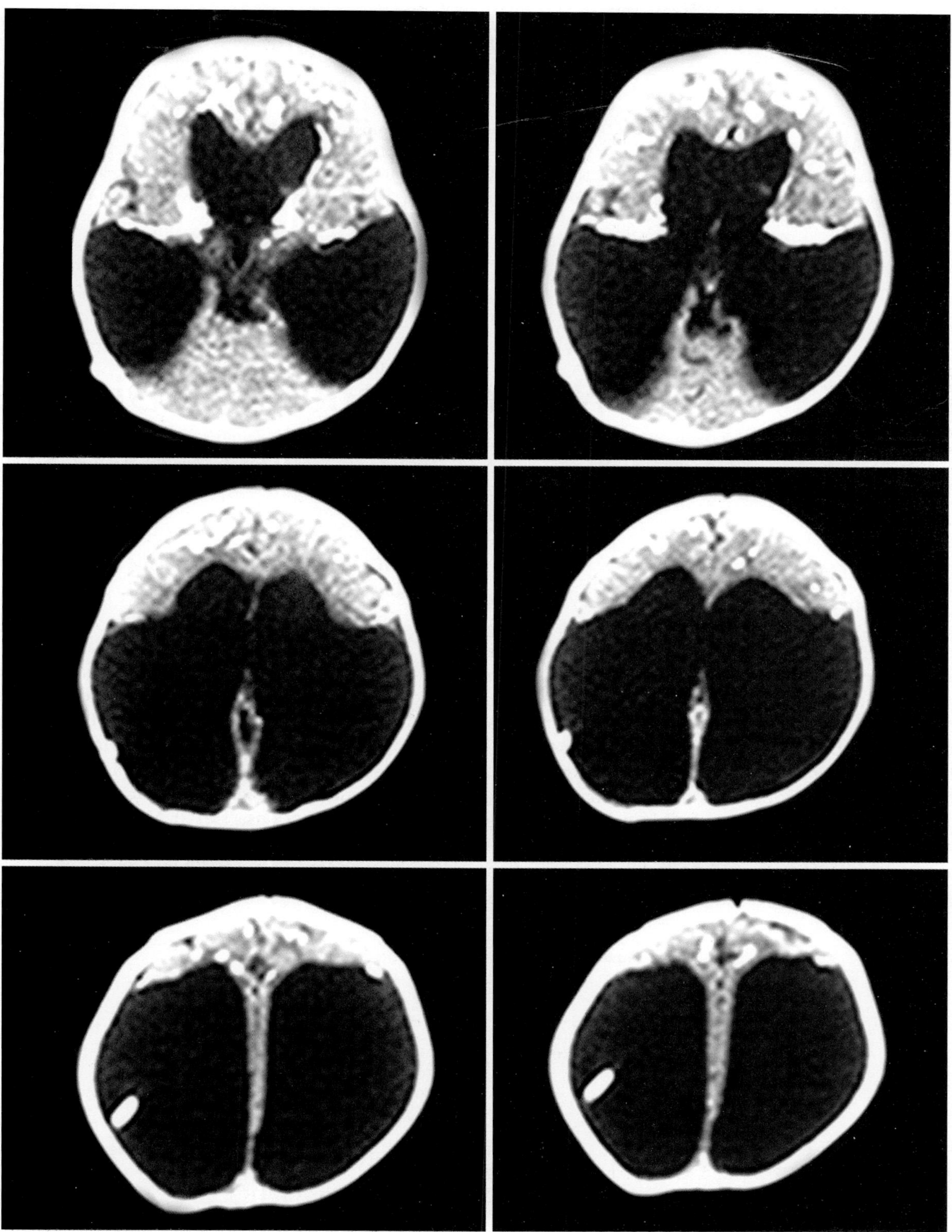

Fig. 6.2.8: CT scan brain showing hydrocephalus with calcification in a case of toxoplasmosis. (Note the tip of shunt tube in the right lateral ventricle.)

population. Long-term follow-up for the possible shunt complication, such as infection, block, and associated neurological deficits, must be done in a multidisciplinary setting.

BIBLIOGRAPHY

1. Eric Piña-Garza J. Fenichel's Clinical Pediatric Neurology: A Signs and Symptoms Approach, 7th edition. Philadelphia, PA: Elsevier Saunders; 2013.
2. Johnston MV, Kinsman S. Congenital anomalies of the central nervous system. In: Kliegman RM, Stanton B, St. Geme J, Schor N (Eds). Nelson Textbook of Pediatrics, 20th edition. Philadelphia, PA: Elsevier Saunders; 2016. pp. 2802-18.
3. Stiles J, Jernigan TL. The basics of brain development. Neuropsychol Rev. 2010;20(4):327-48.
4. ten Donkelaar HJ, Lammens M, Hori A. Clinical Neuro-embryology—Development and Developmental Disorders of the Human Central Nervous System. New York, NY: Springer; 2006.

6.3 Neurodegenerative Disorders

Naveen Sankhyan, Arushi G Saini

INTRODUCTION

Neurodegenerative disorders (NDDs) are characterized by neuroregression. They are genetic disorders causing progressive intellectual and neurological deterioration, which results from a progressive loss of neurons. Neuroregression in children is associated with loss of memory, ability to think, understand, and recognize along with personality changes or distressing behavior. Vision loss, hearing loss, tone abnormalities, and epilepsy are other common symptoms. This neurological deterioration is not explainable by any other concurrent systemic illness. Although most of the childhood NDDs are fatal, an accurate diagnosis is crucial for genetic counseling, prognostication, initiating prevention strategies, and prenatal diagnosis. Neuroregression may result from NDD, neurometabolic problems or may be acquired (**Flowchart 6.3.1**).

EPIDEMIOLOGY

The true burden of NDD in India remains unknown. However, most of the common NDDs have been reported from India. A recent single-center laboratory-based study of 464 patients from Hyderabad reported 23 different lysosomal storage disorders. Sphingolipidosis was the most frequent lysosomal storage disorder in this report followed by mucopolysaccharidosis (MPS). Neurometabolic diseases likely contribute to a significant proportion of neuroregression secondary to a genetic cause, although exact estimates are not available from India. Among the white-matter degenerations,

Flowchart 6.3.1: Causes of neuroregression.

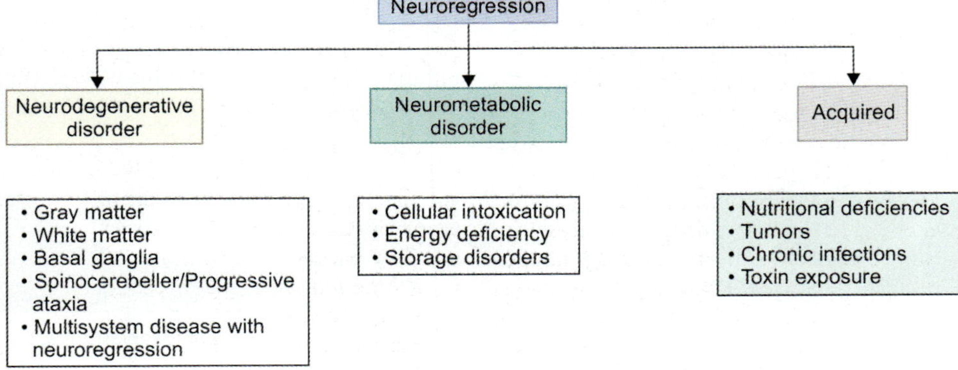

megalencephalic leukodystrophy with subcortical cysts is particularly common in India especially in the Agarwal community.

PATHOGENESIS

Both intrinsic and extrinsic factors are involved in pathogenesis. The underlying gene defect may affect the whole population of neurons or functionally related group of neurons. The nerve cells may be affected as a whole, or certain components may be preferentially involved, e.g. axon, myelin, etc. Some disease processes may affect synaptic connections, neurotransmitter synthesis or action, or neuromodulators. In some diseases, certain cellular proteins become structurally abnormal, accumulate and disrupt functions in the nervous system (proteopathies). Further, a dysfunction of the elimination pathways for damaged cellular components, such as uniquitin/proteasome system (UPS), lysosomal-autophagy and apoptosis pathways, contributes to the pathogenesis of NDDs. For most disorders, the precise process by which the abnormal enzyme activity or abnormal metabolite accumulation causes brain damage is being extensively studied but is yet to be defined. In some disorders, the culprit metabolite has been identified, e.g. psychosine in Krabbe leukodystrophy, polyglutamine in Huntington disease, and abnormal sterol in defects of cholesterol synthesis. Extrinsic factors, such as fasting, high protein load, fever, hypoglycemia, etc., may contribute to worsen the underlying condition, especially metabolic and mitochondrial disorders. Although central nervous system (CNS) has been considered as an immune-privileged organ, increasing evidence supports the role of chronic inflammation in various neurodegenerative diseases, such as Aicardi-Goutieres syndrome, neuronal ceroid lipofuscinoses, and several leukodystrophies and gangliosidoses. Metals, such as iron, copper, and manganese, have an important role in NDD and alterations in their homeostasis in the body can result in metal accumulation, free radical damage, and progressive illness.

APPROACH TO DIAGNOSIS

The first question we need to ask is "whether the development is delayed but improving or regressing?" **(Fig. 6.3.1)**. There are certain red-flag signs in children with a diagnosis of static encephalopathy **(Box 6.3.1)**, which should make us think about an underlying NDD. Once a NDD is suspected, the objective of a careful initial evaluation is to ascertain the age of onset, extent, and evolution of the disease [white matter, gray matter, cerebellum, etc. **(Table 6.3.1)**].

As a first step to clinical evaluation, pseudoregression should be excluded in all children with neuroregression. Regression can occur without an underlying neurodegenerative process due to poorly controlled seizures, overmedication with anticonvulsants, intercurrent systemic illness, raised intracranial pressure caused by brain tumor, hydrocephalus, chronic CNS infections, vitamin B_{12} deficiency, chronic lead poisoning, hypothyroidism, autistic regression, recurrent strokes, and secondary neurological problems in a child with static encephalopathy, e.g. loss of mobility due to development of joint contractures, seizures, movement disorder, etc. or depression or other emotional problems especially in older children.

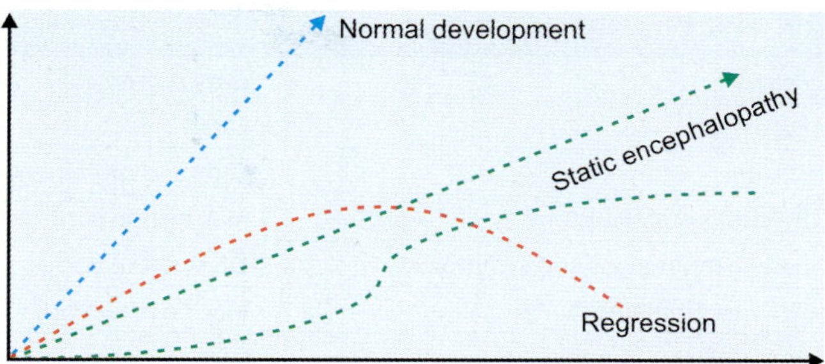

Fig. 6.3.1: Developmental trajectory in static encephalopathy versus neuroregression.

Box 6.3.1: Red-flag signs in children with encephalopathy suggestive of NDD.

- Excessive delay or arrest in psychomotor development
- No definite history of a preceding injury
- Family history of neurological symptoms
- Parental consanguinity
- Inadequately explained oculomotor abnormalities, involuntary movements, ataxia, muscle atrophy, or sensory loss
- Recurrent episodic altered mentation, vomiting, or abnormal movements (IEM)
- Progressive difficulty in walking
- Unsteady gait, ataxia, or involuntary movements
- Intentional myoclonus (polymyoclonus)
- Skeletal and visceral abnormalities

(IEM: inborn errors of metabolism; NDD: neurodegenerative disorder)

History and Examination

A detailed history is aimed at ascertaining the age of onset, and the spheres of development affected motor, cognitive, vision, and hearing. Family history of three generations obtained by pedigree charting is important to identify the possible modes of transmission. There are certain specific clues in general physical and systemic examinations, which give an indication to the nature of disorder **(Table 6.3.2)**. After a careful history and examination, one is generally able to decide about the range of pathology within the nervous system and whether other organ systems are involved or not. Broadly, if one can assign the patient into one of the following groups, the further evaluation is easier:

- *Gray-matter degenerations*: Poliodystrophies
- *White-matter degeneration*: Leukodystrophies
- Progressive ataxias
- Basal ganglia disorders
- Multisystem disorders with neuroregression.

Table 6.3.1: Clinical features of gray- and white-matter diseases.

Features	*Gray matter*	*White matter*
Dementia	Early	Late
Seizures	Early and prominent	Late
Psychological symptoms	May be present	Uncommon
Basal ganglia signs and symptoms	Often present	Absent
Retinitis pigmentosa	May be present	Absent
Primary optic atrophy	Rare	May be seen
Primary neuropathy	Rare	May be seen
MRI	Cortical atrophy, abnormalities in basal ganglia, cerebellum	Clearly identifies abnormalities in white matter
ERG	May be abnormal	Normal
Visual-evoked response	May be abnormal	Normal
Brainstem auditory-evoked responses	Usually normal	Abnormal

(ERG: electroretinogram; MRI: magnetic resonance imaging)

Table 6.3.2: Some clinical pointers in hereditary neurodegenerative disorders.

Organs or features	*Abnormality*	*Disorders*
Head	Microcephaly	NCL, Krabbe disease, Rett syndrome
	Macrocephaly	MPS, Alexander disease, Canavan disease, GM1 gangliosidosis, Tay-Sachs disease, MLSC
Hair	Alopecia	Biotinidase deficiency
	Pigmentary changes	PKU, Menkes disease
	Wooly, kinky hair	Menkes disease **(Fig. 6.3.2)**
Skin	Rash	Biotinidase, holocarboxylase deficiency
	Subcutaneous nodules	Farber disease
	Angiokeratomas	Fabry disease
	Fat pads, focal atrophy	Congenital disorders of glycosylation
	Hyperpigmentation	Adrenoleukodystrophy
Eyes	Cataract	Galactosemia, Zellweger disease, Wilson disease
	Retinitis pigmentosa	Peroxisomal disorders, NCL, mitochondrial encephalomyopathies, MPS, PKAN, ABLP
	Cherry red spot	Tay–Sachs disease, Niemann–Pick disease, GM1 gangliosidosis, Sialidosis
	Optic atrophy	NCL, MLD, Krabbe disease, Canavan disease, GM2 gangliosidosis
	Chorioretinitis	MPS, SSPE, Lowe syndrome
	Dislocated lens	Homocystinuria, sulfite oxidase deficiency
Ears	Deafness	MPS, ALD, mitochondrial disorders, peroxisomal disorders
	Hyperacusis	Krabbe, Tay-Sachs disease
Abdomen	Hepatosplenomegaly	MPS, GM1 gangliosidosis, Gaucher disease, Niemann-Pick disease
	Hernia	GM1 gangliosidosis, MPS
Nervous system	Peripheral neuropathy	MLD, Krabbe disease, mitochondrial disorders
	Hydrocephalus or raised intracranial pressure	MPS, infantile Alexander disease
Cardiac	Cardiomyopathy	FAOD, mitochondrial disorders, Friedreich ataxia, AVED, Pompe disease
	Valvular defects	MPS, Zellweger syndrome, Fabry disease

(ABLP: abetalipoproteinemia; ALD: adrenoleukodystrophy; AVED: ataxia with vitamin E deficiency; FAOD: fatty acid oxidation defects; MLD: metachromatic leukodystrophy; MLSC: megalencephalic leukodystrophy with subcortical cysts; MPS: mucopolysaccharidosis; NCL: neuronal ceroid lipofuscinosis; PKAN: pantothenate kinase-associated neurodegeneration; PKU: phenylketonuria; SSPE: subacute sclerosing panencephalitis)

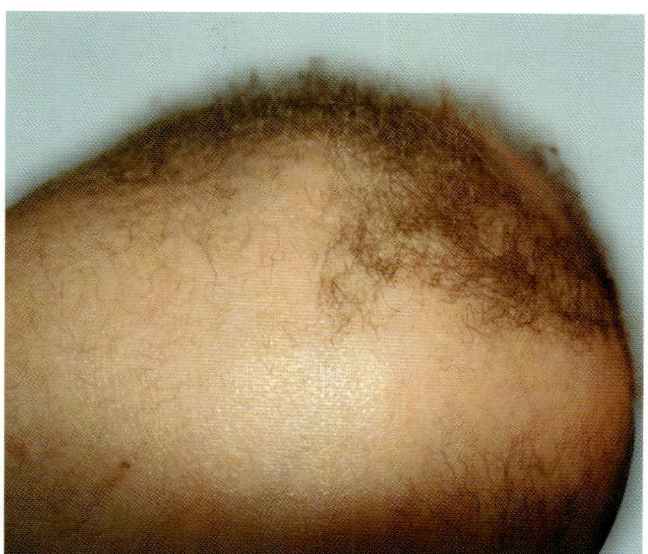

Fig. 6.3.2: Note the sparse, hypopigmented curly, stubby hair in a child with Menkes disease.

Flowchart 6.3.2: A simplified approach to a child less than 2 years with suspected degenerative brain disorder.

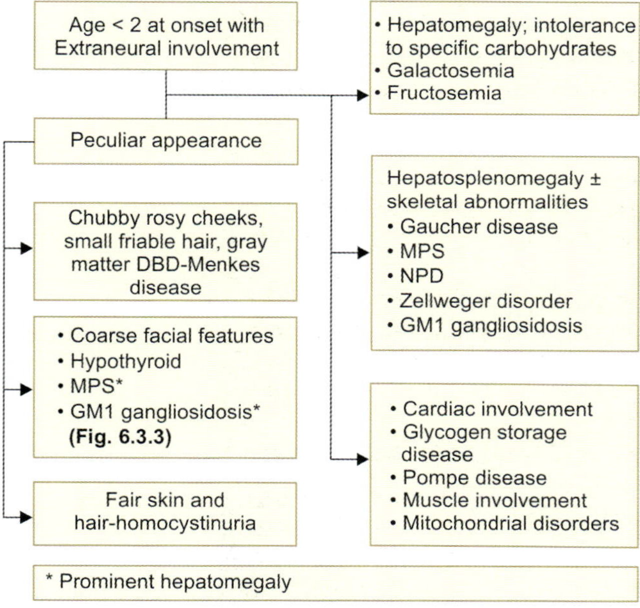

(DBD: degenerative brain disorder; MPS: mucopolysaccharidosis; NPD: Niemann–Pick disease)

Regression in a Child Below 2 Years (Flowcharts 6.3.2 and 6.3.3)

During infancy, delayed milestones are a common manifestation of neuroregressive disorders. Since the child has not gained many distinctive abilities, the loss of abilities is

Flowchart 6.3.3: A simplified approach to a child less than 2 years with suspected degenerative brain disorder with no extraneural abnormalities.

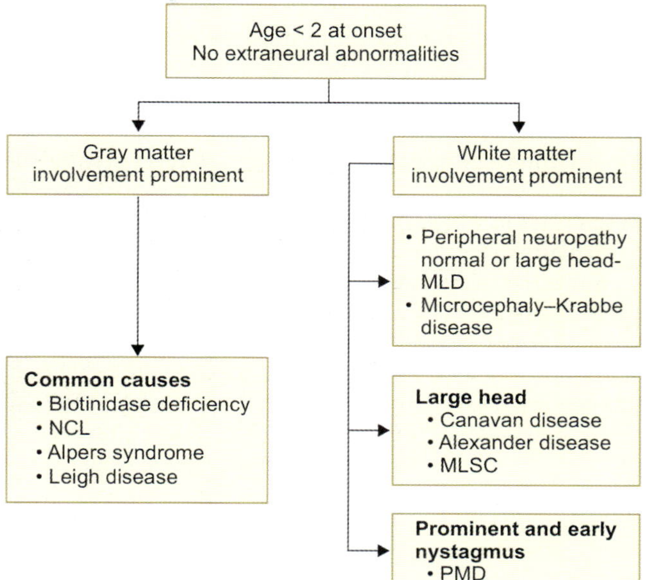

(MLD: metachromatic leukodystrophy; MLSC: megalencephalic leukodystrophy with subcortical cysts; NCL: neuronal ceroid lipofuscinosis; PMD: Pelizaeus–Merzbacher disease)

difficult to quantify or localize. Commonly, the affected infant lacks visual interest or socialization and has poor head control and inability to use hands. Other common symptoms are developmental retardation with severe hypotonia, especially with feeding difficulties and/or vomiting and failure to thrive.

Many disorders that present in the second year of life are frequently recognizable by the obvious loss of motor abilities. This may result from corticospinal, cerebellar, extrapyramidal, or peripheral nerve involvement. The second year of life is also the age for disorders with gradually increasing dysmorphism, skeletal abnormalities, and cognitive decline (MPS and mucolipidosis) to manifest. Some children may present with progressive mental deterioration, seizures, and vision loss. Yet another group of children presents with recurrent neurological deterioration interspersed with apparent recovery (organic aciduria, mitochondrial disorders, urea cycle disorders, etc.).

- In girls with regression in cognitive spheres starting in infancy and microcephaly and associated with loss of purposeful hand movements, Rett syndrome should be considered.
- In addition, a possibility of human immunodeficiency virus (HIV) encephalopathy should always be kept in mind and a systematic evaluation for risk factors should be undertaken.

Neuroregression in Later Childhood and Adolescence (Flowcharts 6.3.4 and 6.3.5)

In older children, the presentation of neuroregression begins after a considerable period of normal development. The onset and course of the disorder can also be more accurately determined.

It is now much easier to view individual patients as having the predominant involvement of a particular area of the nervous system. The major clinical problem one faces is the varied ways in which the same disorder can present. This is particularly so for autosomal dominant disorders.

Subacute sclerosing panencephalitis (SSPE), though not a hereditary NDD, is a common cause of neuroregression in our country. It should be considered in all children with behavioral changes, cognitive deterioration with or without myoclonic jerks.

In addition to extrapyramidal syndrome, severe self-mutilation behavior resulting in chewing of lips is shown in **Figure 6.3.4**.

Investigations

They are guided by history and examination.

Imaging

A high-resolution magnetic resonance (MR) imaging with spectroscopy would be the best to pick up abnormalities. Magnetic resonance imaging in certain patients may provide a diagnostic clue, e.g. pantothenate kinase-associated neurodegeneration with "Eye of Tiger" sign in globus pallidi **(Fig. 6.3.5)**, megalencephalic leukodystrophy with subcortical cysts **(Figs. 6.3.6A and B)**, SSPE **(Fig. 6.3.7)**, metachromatic leukodystrophy (MLD) **(Fig. 6.3.8)**,

Flowchart 6.3.4: Approach to progressive neurological deterioration in 2–5 years age group.

Primary involved area of CNS on history and examination

- Gray matter and coarseness → • MPS • Mucolipidosis
- Ataxia → • Ataxia • Telangiectasia • Mitochondrial disorders
- Progressive myoclonic epilepsy/gray matter degeneration → • NCL • MERRF
- Extrapyramidal syndrome → • PKAN • Lesch-Nyhan disease • Glutaric acidurial
- White matter disorder **(Figs. 6.3.2 and 6.3.3)** → • MLD • ALD

(ALD: adrenoleukodystrophy; CNS: central nervous system; MERRF: myoclonic epilepsy with ragged red fibers; MLD: metachromatic leukodystrophy; MPS: mucopolysaccharidosis; NCL: neuronal ceroid lipofuscinosis; PKAN: pantothenate kinase-associated neurodegeneration)

Flowchart 6.3.5: Approach to progressive neurological deterioration in 5–15 years age group.

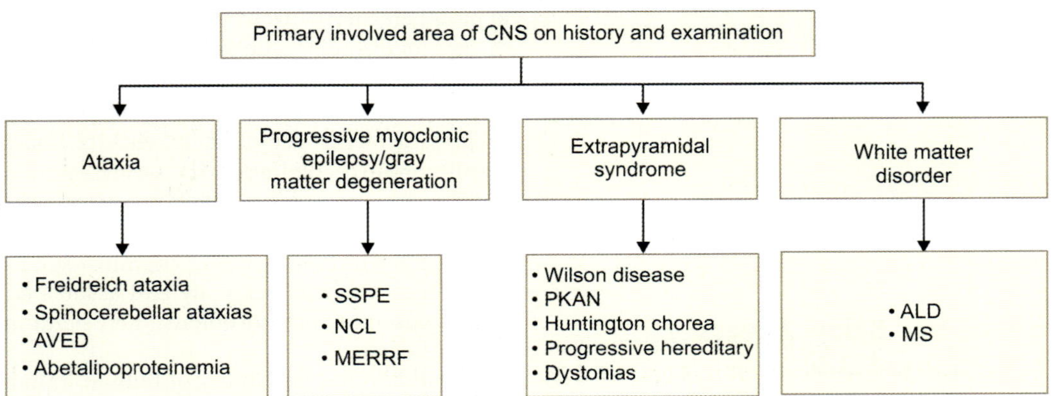

(ALD: adrenoleukodystrophy; AVED: ataxia with vitamin E deficiency; CNS: central nervous system; MERRF: myoclonic epilepsy with ragged red fibers; MS: multiple sclerosis; NCL: neuronal ceroid lipofuscinosis; PKAN: pantothenate kinase-associated neurodegeneration; SSPE: subacute sclerosing panencephalitis)

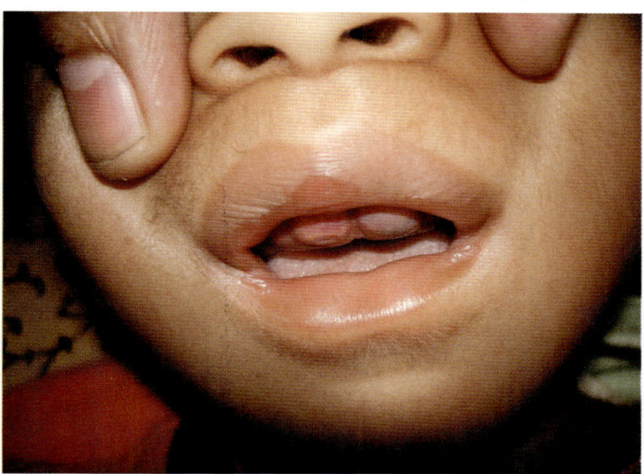

Fig. 6.3.3: Gum hypertrophy and coarsening in an 18-month-old child with infantile GM1 gangliosidosis.

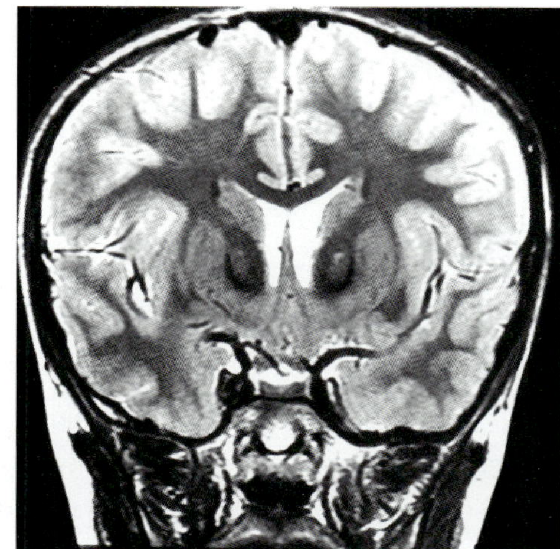

Fig. 6.3.5: Coronal T2W MRI in a child with pantothenate kinase-associated neurodegeneration showing the bilaterally hypointense globus pallidi with an area of central hyperintensity
(MRI: magnetic resonance imaging; T2W: T2 weight)

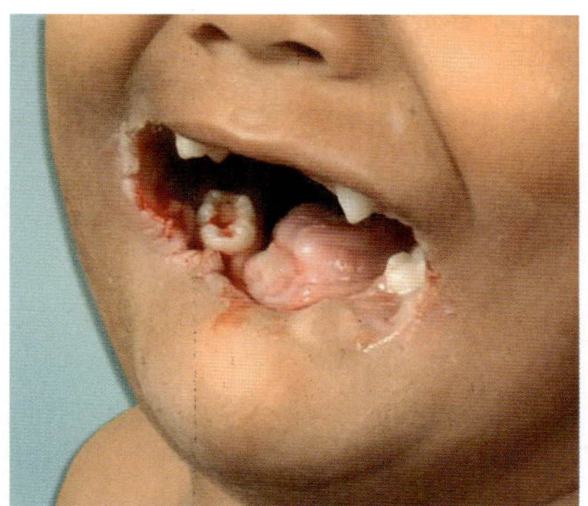

Fig. 6.3.4: Severe self-mutilation in a 3-year-old boy with Lesch–Nyhan disease.

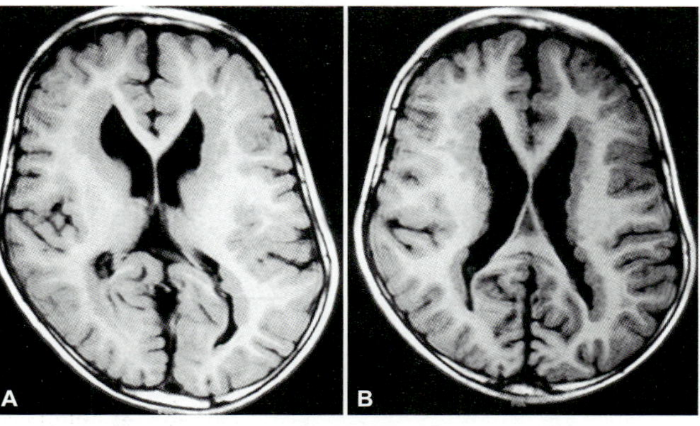

Figs. 6.3.6A and B: (A) Axial T2W MRI of brain showing abnormal diffusely hyperintense white matter in a 3-year-old child with "megalencephalic leukodystrophy with subcortical cysts"; (B) note the temporal cysts on the FLAIR image.
(FLAIR: fluid-attenuated inversion recovery; MRI: magnetic resonance imaging; T2W: T2-weighted)

adrenoleukodystrophy (ALD) **(Fig. 6.3.9)**, Wilson disease **(Fig. 6.3.10)**, mitochondrial encephalopathies, and creatine-deficiency disorders. Magnetic resonance imaging with spectroscopy helps in diagnosis of certain disorders, such as Canavan disease **(Figs. 6.3.11A and B)**.

Radiographs

A skeletal survey would be important to look for abnormalities in certain storage disorders, such as MPS **(Figs. 6.3.12A and B)** with infantile GM1 gangliosidosis, showing mild changes of dysostosis multiplex with breaking of the lumbar vertebra.

Urine and Blood Assay for Plasma Ammonia, Blood Lactate and Pyruvate, Plasma Amino Acids

These tests guide the course of further investigations in a suspected neurometabolic disorder to arrive at the diagnosis.

Electrophysiological Tests

These include "visual evoked potentials," brainstem auditory-evoked responses, "nerve conduction studies," electroencephalography, electromyography, and somatosensory-evoked potentials. These help to delineate the extent

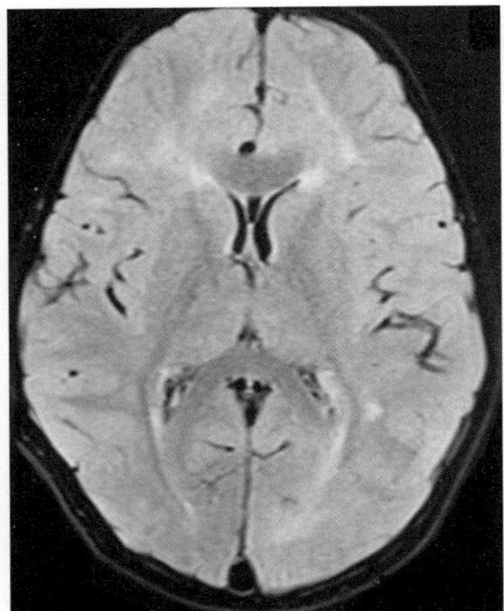

Fig. 6.3.7: Axial FLAIR-MRI of brain showing ill-defined, bilateral, asymmetrical, patchy hyperintensities in the periventricular and subcortical white matter of frontal and parieto-occipital regions in a child with SSPE.
(FLAIR-MRI: fluid-attenuated inversion recovery-magnetic resonance imaging; SSPE: subacute sclerosing panencephalitis)

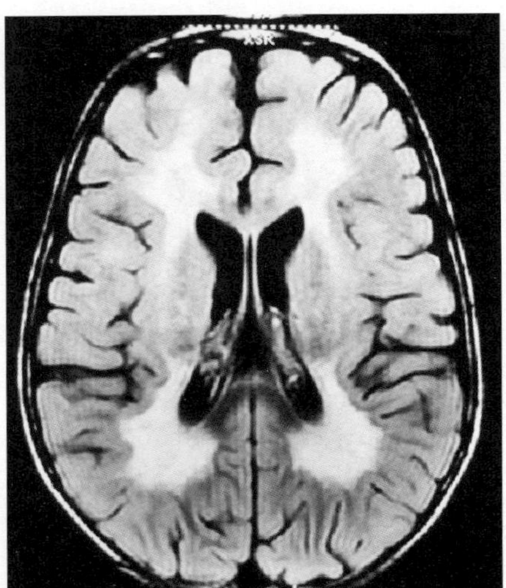

Fig. 6.3.8: Axial FLAIR-MRI of brain showing bilateral periventricular abnormal hyperintense white matter in a child with metachromatic leukodystrophy.
(FLAIR-MRI: fluid-attenuated inversion recovery-magnetic resonance imaging)

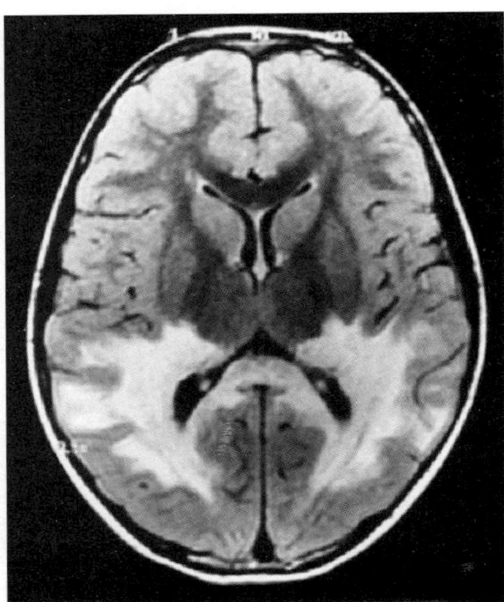

Fig. 6.3.9: Axial FLAIR-MRI of brain showing posterior dominant abnormal hyperintense white matter in a child with adrenoleukodystrophy. The splenium of corpus callosum also prominently involved.
(FLAIR-MRI: fluid-attenuated inversion recovery-magnetic resonance imaging)

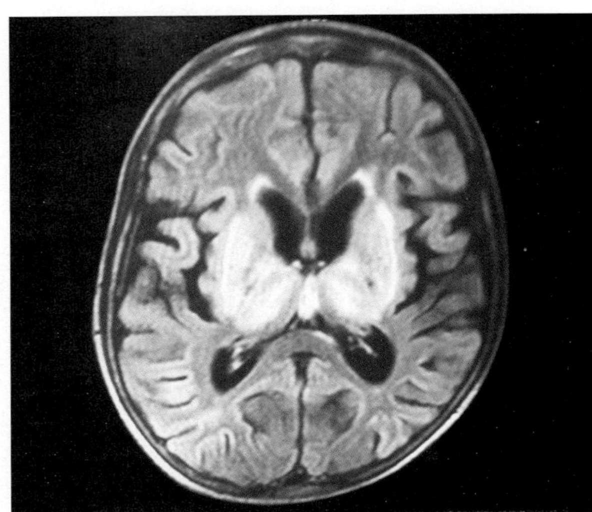

Fig. 6.3.10: MRI in a child with Wilson disease showing the involvement of bilateral basal ganglia.
(MRI: magnetic resonance imaging)

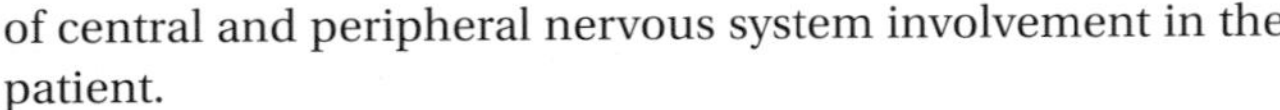

of central and peripheral nervous system involvement in the patient.

Other Tests

- *Histopathological and ultrastructural information from selected biopsies.*
- *Bone marrow*: Storage cells are seen in Niemann–Pick disease, Gaucher disease.
- *Conjunctival, skin, rectal biopsy*: Neuronal ceroid lipofuscinosis.
- *Muscle*: Mitochondrial disorders.
- *Hair microscopy*: Menkes disease.

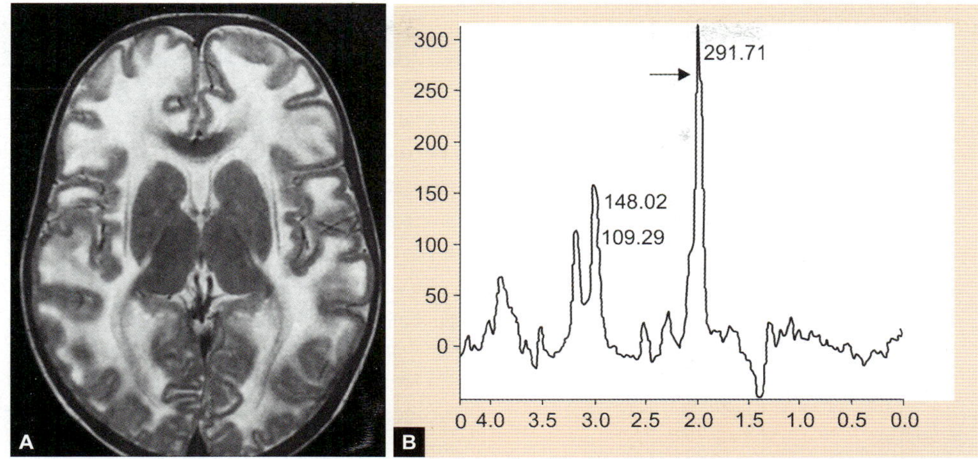

Figs. 6.3.11A and B: T2-weighted MRI image showing (A) diffuse, symmetrical white-matter hyperintensities involving the periventricular and subcortical white matter and (B) NAA peak on MR spectroscopy in a 2-year-old boy with progressively increasing head size and developmental delay suggestive of Canavan disease.
(MR: magnetic resonance; NAA: N-acetylaspartate)

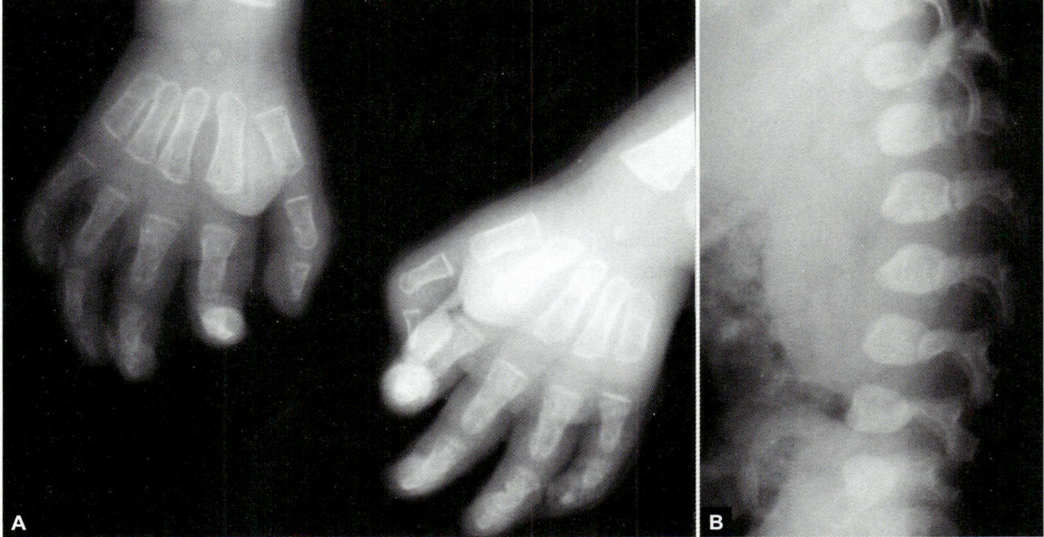

Figs. 6.3.12A and B: (A) X-ray of hands of a child with infantile GM1 gangliosidosis showing mild changes of dysostosis multiplex with early conical shape of proximal bases of 2–5 metacarpals with tapering of the proximal phalanges; (B) lateral radiograph of the spine in child.

Specific investigations are done based on clues obtained from preceding investigations:

- *Serology*: HIV, SSPE.
- *Urine copper, serum ceruloplasmin*: Wilson disease.
- *Urine MPS*: Mucopolysaccharidosis.
- *Enzyme analysis*: Lysosomal storage disorders, biotinidase deficiency.
- *Urine organic acids*: Organic acidemias.
- *Very long-chain fatty acids (VLCFA) and plasmalogen levels*: Peroxisomal disorders.
- *Mutation testing*: This can be undertaken, if the diagnosis is quite certain and the test is available.

MANAGEMENT

First, never miss out a treatable cause of neuroregression, such as hydrocephalus, HIV infection, hypothyroidism

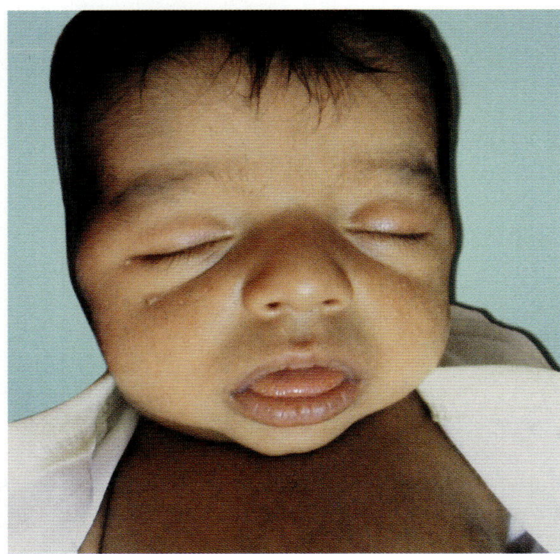

Fig. 6.3.13: Note the coarsening of facial features, large tongue in an infant with hypothyroidism.

(Fig. 6.3.13), lead toxicity, etc. It must be remembered that many NDD are amenable to treatment **(Table 6.3.3)**. Therapies under research include mitochondrial genome manipulation of heteroplasmic mitochondrial deoxyribonucleic acid mutations; defective mitochondrial replacement by genome editing, gene-editing tools, such as zinc finger nucleases, meganucleases, and transcription activator-like effector nucleases; CRISPR (clustered regulatory interspaced short palindromic repeats)-Cas9 (CRISPR-associated); and antiapoptotic drugs, such as minocycline, rasagiline, melatonin, resveratrol, and lithium.

Table 6.3.3: Few examples of treatment in neurodegenerative disorders.

Disease	*Therapeutic agent*
Gaucher disease	Enzyme replacement, miglustat
Fabry disease	Enzyme replacement
Attenuated variants of MPS I	Enzyme replacement
Pompe disease	Enzyme replacement
Ataxia (Co-Q deficiency)	Coenzyme Q10
Ataxia with vitamin E deficiency	Vitamin E
Minimally symptomatic X-linked adrenoleukodystrophy, Krabbe	Bone marrow transplant
MPS 1H-Hurler disease	Bone marrow transplant
Glycogen storage disease	Liver transplant
Glutaric aciduria-II, biotinidase deficiency	Cofactor replacement
Wilson disease	D-Penicillamine, trietine, zinc acetate, liver transplantation
Menkes disease	Copper sulfate
Creatine-deficiency disorders	Creatine supplements
Hypermanganesemia	Chelation
Glucose transporter disorder, Pyruvate dehydrogenase deficiency, Refsum disease	Special diet
Neurotransmitter disorder	Specific cofactors or drugs
Lesch-Nyhan disease	Allopurinol

(Co-Q: coenzyme Q10; MPS 1: mucopolysaccharidosis type 1)

Supportive Measures

It is never wise or correct to say that the disease is "untreatable." Such statements only result in the parents feeling a profound sense of anguish, abandonment, and loneliness. Something can almost always be done to help the child. Supportive treatment may add significantly to the quality of life of a child with NDD. Measures to reduce spasticity, dystonia, drooling, swallowing problems, control seizures, control pain, improve nutrition, prevent constipation, prevent bed sores, and to enhance mobility, all contribute to the quality of life of the patient and indirectly to the quality of life of the parents and any unaffected siblings. The use of mitochondrial cocktail, a mixture of oral vitamins and supplements, such as L-carnitine, coenzyme Q, riboflavin, thiamine, vitamin C and E, in disorders with impaired mitochondrial function, has been shown to produce modest improvements in broad patient outcomes in small-scale clinical trials. Formulating a chronic care and follow-up plan and communicating this to all professionals involved is of immense benefit to the child and the family.

PREVENTION

One of the very important aspects of management of a child with NDD is to accurately establish the diagnosis. This becomes important not only for proper care and prognostication but also for accurate prenatal diagnosis to prevent further children being affected by the same disease. The diagnosis may also help identify pauci- or presymptomatic siblings or other family members who may benefit from early therapy, e.g. zinc therapy in Wilson disease. It would be wise to refer the parents for prenatal diagnosis to an equipped center before they plan any future pregnancies.

PROGNOSIS

It is sensible to first confirm the diagnosis and then prognosticate. The prognosis in NDD depends on the underlying disorder. In general, an earlier onset of disease predicts a poorer outcome. However, several late onset diseases can also rapidly progress, e.g. adrenoleukodystrophy.

KEY MESSAGES

- A thorough clinical evaluation that includes a detailed history, family history, general physical and systemic evaluation forms an important starting point for further evaluation. If the history and examination are strongly indicative, more specific diagnostic testing can be undertaken, e.g. HIV testing, urine MPS, VLCFA, etc.
- Based on the clinical presentation, always keep the treatable causes in mind and exclude them systematically.
- Second-line investigations are undertaken best at research and referral centers with expertise in handling these children.
- While managing these children, always focus on issues, which make the child's and caregiver's life comfortable, e.g. control seizures, spasticity, adequate nutrition and skin care, etc.

BIBLIOGRAPHY

1. Fenichel GM. Clinical Pediatric Neurology: A Signs and Symptoms Approach, 5th edition. Philadelphia, PA: Elsevier; 2005.
2. Lyon G, Kolodny EH, Pastores GM. Neurology of Hereditary Metabolic Diseases in Children, 3rd edition. New York, NY: McGraw Hill Companies; 2006.
3. Michelson DJ, Shu SK. Cognitive and Motor Regression. In: Swaiman KF, Ashwal S, Ferriero DM (Eds). Pediatric Neurology, 4th edition. Philadelphia, PA: Elsevier; 2006. p. 82144.
4. Neurologic syndrome. In: Clarke JTR (Ed). A Clinical Guide to Inherited Metabolic Diseases, 3rd edition. Cambridge: Cambridge University Press; 2006. p. 2889.

6.4 Neurocutaneous Disorders

Devendra Mishra

INTRODUCTION

Neurocutaneous disorders are disorders, which frequently involve the skin in addition to the nervous system. Many of these may initially present with the cutaneous findings, and recognition of the characteristic features helps in identifying the disorder and anticipating the neurological problems. **Table 6.4.1** lists and summarizes the clinical features of these disorders. The more common ones would be discussed in detail.

TUBEROUS SCLEROSIS COMPLEX

It is a multisystem disorder with an incidence of nearly 1 in 5,800 live births (prevalence 1:10,000). It is transmitted as an autosomal dominant trait with variable penetrance. Two genes *tuberous sclerosis complex 1* [*TSC1* (located on 9q34, gene product hamartin) and *TSC2* (located on 16p13, gene product tuberin)] have been identified. The lesions are caused by hamartomas and hamartias, and there is a wide variation in clinical expression of the disease. Seizures occur in about 85%, mental retardation in around 50%, skin lesions in more than 95%, and autism in up to half of the patients. More importantly, diagnosis can be made even in the presence of only skin or neuroimaging findings; less than one-third fulfill the classic Vogt triad (epilepsy, low intelligence quotient, and adenoma sebaceum, also shortened as epiloia).

The neurological affection is the most important clinically. The major brain abnormalities include cortical tubers **(Fig. 6.4.1)**, and subependymal nodules (which may develop into subependymal giant cell tumors in 5–10% patients). Epilepsy is the commonest presenting feature and almost all types of seizures are reported. Majority have seizure onset during infancy with infantile spasms developing in up to one-third of children with tuberous sclerosis complex (TSC).

Skin manifestations include angiofibromas (erroneously called as adenoma sebaceum), which appear in the preschool age and are progressive. These are present as pinkish papules in patches around the nose, cheek, and chin **(Fig. 6.4.2)**. Hypopigmented macules over trunk and limbs (ash leaf macules) are apparent at birth and may increase in size with age. These are better seen with Wood's light. Connective tissue hamartomas (shagreen patch) are usually found in the lumbosacral region.

After the neurological involvement, renal involvement causes the most morbidity and consists of angiomyolipomas and renal cysts. The former is seen in up to 80% patients, may appear in childhood, and are occasionally symptomatic, causing pain, obstruction, or hemorrhage. More important from the pediatric perspective is the cardiac rhabdomyoma, which is seen in up to 60% and is maximal at birth or early childhood, regressing spontaneously later. They may even be detected prenatally. Depending on the location, these

Table 6.4.1: Characteristic features of various neurocutaneous disorders.

Disorder	Features
Tuberous sclerosis complex	• Hypopigmented macules (ash leaf macules) • Seizures (including infantile spasms) • Cortical tubers • Angiofibroma (adenoma sebaceum) • Connective tissue nevus (shagreen patch)
Neurofibromatosis	• *NF1*: Multiple *café-au-lait* spots, neurofibromas, Lisch nodules (iris hamartomas), axillary or inguinal freckling, optic glioma, learning difficulties • *NF2*: Vestibular schwannomas
Sturge–Weber syndrome	• Facial hemangioma (port-wine stain) • Leptomeningeal angioma • Seizures • Developmental delay
Ataxia-telangiectasia	• Progressive ataxia • Recurrent sinopulmonary infections • Ocular telangiectasia • Increased preponderance for lymphoreticular malignancies
Incontinentia pigmenti	• Hyperpigmented skin lesions • CNS abnormalities • Hypopigmented lesions in hypomelanosis of Ito
Klippel–Trenaunay–Weber syndrome	• Unilateral limb hypertrophy • Subcutaneous hemangioma • Macrocephaly • Hydrocephalus
von Hippel–Lindau disease	• Cerebellar hemangioblastoma • Retinal angiomas presenting in young adults
PHACE syndrome	• Posterior fossa malformations • Hemangiomas • Arterial abnormalities • Coarctation of aorta and other cardiac abnormalities, eye abnormalities

(CNS: central nervous system; PHACE: posterior fossa anomalies, hemangioma, arterial anomalies, cardiac anomalies, and eye anomalies)

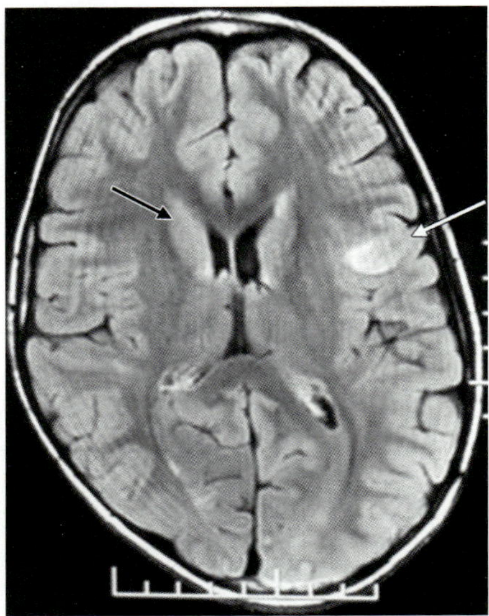

Fig. 6.4.1: MRI brain T1-weighted image showing cortical tubers (white arrow) and subependymal tubers (black arrow) in tuberous sclerosis. (MRI: magnetic resonance imaging)

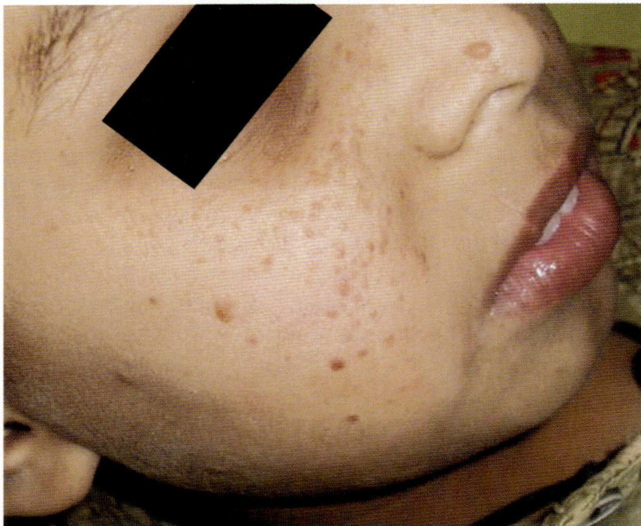

Fig. 6.4.2: Facial angiofibroma (adenoma sebaceum) in a child with tuberous sclerosis complex and autism.

can cause obstruction, conduction defects, and valvular dysfunction. Nearly half of the patients have retinal hamartomas and others have ocular problems. Hamartomas of other organ systems are also reported, and females may exclusively have pulmonary involvement.

Evaluation

Specific diagnostic criteria, which include major and minor features, have been provided. Neuroimaging, developmental assessment, and eye, cardiac, and renal evaluation are recommended at the time of diagnosis for all patients, and then as indicated by manifestations. Follow-up for neuroimaging is suggested every 1–3 years, as there is a possibility of development of subependymal giant cell tumor.

Management

Management includes medical management of epilepsy, and interventions for developmental and behavioral problems. Drug-resistant patients may be helped by epilepsy surgery, if a single tuber is responsible for majority of the seizures. Infantile spasms in TSC respond well to vigabatrin. Some associations between autism spectrum disorders and tuber load have been reported. Everolimus, a mammalian target of rapamycin inhibitor, reduces the volume of renal angiomyolipomas and has also been shown to reduce the seizure frequency.

NEUROFIBROMATOSIS

Two major types of neurofibromatosis have been delineated.

Neurofibromatosis 1

Neurofibromatosis 1 (*NF1*) is transmitted in autosomal dominant manner (gene *NF1* located on 17q11.2 chromosome, product is neurofibromin) with a prevalence of 1:4,000 and most commonly involves the nervous system and the skin. As opposed to TSC, the most common presentation in neurofibromatosis is the skin features, of which the most important are the *café au-lait* spots **(Fig. 6.4.3)**. These are present at birth and may increase in infancy. In prepubertal children, they need to be more than 5 mm in size and at least six in number to suspect neurofibromatosis. Inguinal freckling (starting in the preschool age) and later in the axillae and base of neck is also seen. Cutaneous neurofibromas are discrete, soft, or firm papules, which can occur at any age and at any location. Plexiform neuroma is a tumor involving a longitudinal section of a nerve and its branches.

Hamartomas of the iris (Lisch nodules) appear after 5 years of age and are seen in more than 90% adults with NF1. Optic gliomas and astrocytomas of the intracranial structures may occur. Magnetic resonance imaging (MRI) in under-five children may show unidentified bright objects. Congenital glaucoma may occur occasionally. Spontaneous limb fractures (with pseudoarthrosis), macrocephaly, short stature, and scoliosis are also reported. Approximately 50% patients have developmental disabilities including attention-deficit hyperactivity disorder.

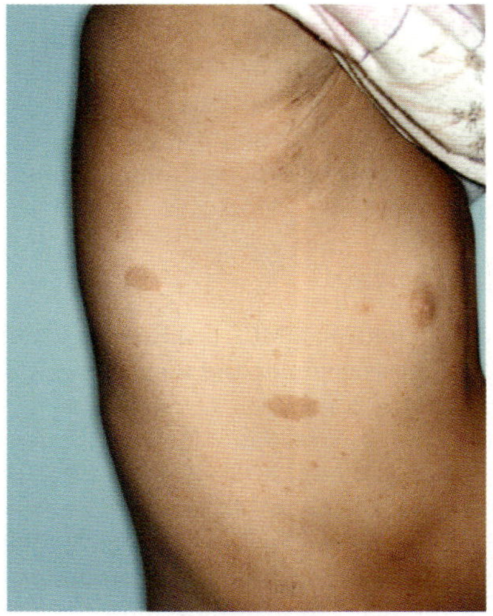

Fig. 6.4.3: *Café-au-lait* macules in neurofibromatosis 1.

Neurofibromatosis 2

It is the central form of neurofibromatosis. The hallmark is bilateral vestibular schwannomas, which may appear at any age and usually present with tinnitus with or without hearing loss. Juvenile lens opacities (present in approximately 80%) and retinal hamartomas are also seen in children. Magnetic resonance imaging evaluation is the investigation of choice, though brainstem auditory evoked responses may be helpful, especially for follow-up.

Management

No specific management is required for NF1 other than regular evaluation for complications, e.g. hypertension, focal neurological deficit, abnormal puberty, optic pathway tumor, and scoliosis. Almost 50% of the cases occur sporadically, and thus unaffected parents have a low recurrence risk. Schwannomas in neurofibromatosis 2 (NF2) are managed surgically. Genetic testing for diagnosis and prenatal testing are available for both NF1 and NF2.

STURGE–WEBER SYNDROME

This disorder, also called as encephalotrigeminal angiomatosis, is one of the most easily identifiable among the neurocutaneous disorders due to the characteristic facial features. The disease occurs sporadically with a prevalence of 1:50,000 and is due to the presence of residual embryonic blood vessels. The essential features are the angiomas of the face (port-wine stain) and ipsilateral leptomeningeal angiomas. It is referred to as complete when both central nervous system (CNS) and facial angiomas are present and incomplete when only the face or CNS is affected (Roach scale). The usual facial involvement is in the upper face and eyelids, although lips, intraoral structures, and pharynx may also be involved. Trunk and extremities of either side are occasionally affected. Ipsilateral parietal and occipital regions are the most commonly affected by the leptomeningeal angiomas, which occasionally may be bilateral. The majority (75–90%) of the patients are present with seizures that are frequently refractory to medical management. Approximately one-third of the patients develop contralateral hemiparesis, and nearly half may have mental retardation and developmental problems. Around 60% patients have recurrent headaches. Ocular problems include glaucoma (in 25% patients due to choroidal involvement), heterochromia iris, and strabismus; fundus may be of a tomato-ketchup color.

Evaluation

Evaluation includes cranial MRI (preferably gadolinium enhanced) and/or computed tomography, which are diagnostic **(Fig. 6.4.4)**. By the age of 20 years, almost 90% have typical linear, parallel intracranial calcification evident

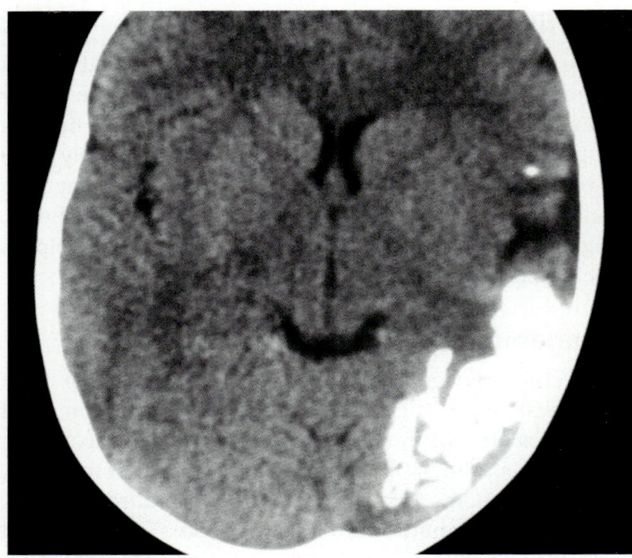

Fig. 6.4.4: Linear intracranial calcification on noncontrast CT of the head in an 8-year-old child with Sturge–Weber syndrome.

on skull radiograph (tram track sign) in parietal or parieto-occipital region. Ophthalmological assessment for ocular manifestations is essential.

Management

Management of seizures is like that due to any other cause. Epilepsy surgery is a viable option for drug-resistant seizures. Dermatological manifestations should be treated at the earliest (even in infancy), usually by pulsed dye laser therapy. Glaucoma should be managed medically or surgically depending on the underlying abnormality and response. Symptomatic and prophylactic therapy for headaches, as needed, should be offered.

ATAXIA-TELANGIECTASIA

It is a degenerative disease of the nervous system that is transmitted autosomal recessively [mutation in ataxia telangiectasia-mutated (ATM) gene on chromosome 11q22q23] and is characterized by progressive ataxia, recurrent sinopulmonary infections, ocular telangiectasia, and increased preponderance for lymphoreticular malignancies. Ataxia starts at around 2 years of age and gradually increases leading to loss of ambulation by 12 years. Telangiectasia, characteristically present on the bulbar conjunctiva **(Fig. 6.4.5)**, appears by the age of 3–6 years and may also be seen on the face or extremities. There may be presence of nystagmus, strabismus, and ocular motility abnormalities. Immunologic functions are deranged (commonly decreased secretory immunoglobulin A in 70% and elevated immunoglobulin M in around 60% patients), and there may be a loss of skin elasticity. Elevated α-fetoprotein levels help in diagnosis in early childhood. Patients have a greatly increased risk of developing tumors (lymphoma, leukemia, Hodgkin disease, brain tumors, etc.). Death usually occurs by adolescence or young adulthood and is due to infection or malignancy.

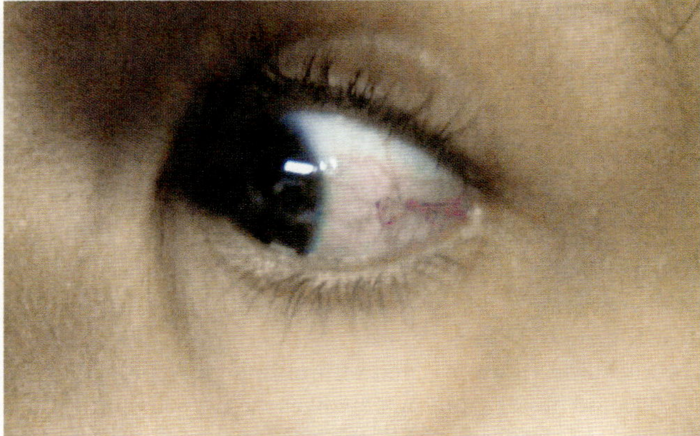

Fig. 6.4.5: Corneal telangiectasia in a girl with ataxia-telangiectasia.

Management

Ataxia is frequently resistant to treatment. Use of regular immunoglobulin infusion is useful in preventing infections. Ataxia telangiectasia-mutated heterozygosity is also a risk factor for malignancy, and regular surveillance of family members should be advised. Affected individuals are very sensitive to the effects of radiation exposure, including medical X-rays. Desferrioxamine has shown some promise in early clinical trials.

KEY MESSAGES

- The skin should be specifically examined in every patient with epilepsy or neurological problems.
- Recognition of suggestive dermatological findings helps in identifying a neurocutaneous disorder.
- Early diagnosis of neurocutaneous disorders helps in anticipating complications, optimizing management, and providing prognosis.

BIBLIOGRAPHY

1. Cardis MA, DeKlotz CMC. Cutaneous manifestations of tuberous sclerosis complex and the paediatrician's role. Arch Dis Child. 2017;102(9):858-63.
2. Little H, Kamat D, Sivaswamy L. Common neurocutaneous syndromes. Pediatr Ann. 2015;44(11):496-504.
3. Ruggieri M, Praticò AD. Mosaic neurocutaneous disorders and their causes. Semin Pediatr Neurol. 2015;22(4):207-33.
4. Rust RS. What the child neurologist should know about neurocutaneous conditions. Semin Pediatr Neurol. 2011;18(2):112-3.

6.5 Seizures, Epilepsy, and Nonepileptic Events

Rekha Mittal

INTRODUCTION

Seizures are the commonest pediatric neurological problem, by themselves or as manifestations of many underlying disorders. They may be easy to manage but often present a diagnostic or therapeutic dilemma. Correct diagnosis of seizures, identification of seizure types, documentation of epilepsy imitators (EIs), and correct classification into epilepsy syndromes, as far as possible, are essential for appropriate treatment and counseling.

TERMINOLOGY

Seizure

A seizure is the clinical manifestation (i.e. signs and symptoms) of an abnormal excessive paroxysmal synchronous neuronal activity in the brain. This abnormal neuronal activity is conducted to the body and produces a seizure. It could manifest in many ways **(Box 6.5.1)**. Having a seizure does not necessarily mean that the patient has epilepsy.

The type of seizure depends on:

- The area of the brain producing the discharge
- The type of discharge
- The age of the patient.

Thus there are many kinds of seizures.

Acute symptomatic seizures are seizures occurring during the course of an acute illness, e.g. meningitis or head injury are called provoked or acute symptomatic seizures.

Epilepsy: Epilepsy is defined neurophysiologically as a disease of the brain characterized by an enduring predisposition to generate epileptic seizures, and by the neurobiologic, cognitive, psychological, and social consequences of this condition. The definition of epilepsy requires the occurrence of at least one epileptic seizure.

Epileptogenesis is the sequence of events that converts normal neuronal networks into hyperexcitable networks.

Practically, epilepsy is a disease of the brain defined by any of the following conditions:

- At least two unprovoked (or reflex) seizures occurring greater than 24 hours apart
- One unprovoked (or reflex) seizure and a probability of further seizures, such as the general recurrence risk (at least 60%), after two unprovoked seizures, occurring over the next 10 years
- Diagnosis of an epilepsy syndrome

Epilepsy is taken as "resolved" for individuals:

- Who had an age-dependent epilepsy syndrome but are now past the applicable age
- Those who have remained seizure free for the last 10 years, with no seizure medicines for the last 5 years.

Symptomatic epilepsies are epilepsies where the cause is known, e.g. structural malformations or old brain insult, such as postmeningitis sequelae, posthypoxic ischemic encephalopathy, or stroke. Cryptogenic epilepsies are epilepsies, which are expected to have a cause, but despite investigations, no cause is found. These terms are not used anymore.

Epileptic Syndrome

This is a syndrome where epilepsy is a prominent feature and is defined by a cluster of features occurring together **(Box 6.5.2)**. It may have associated etiologic, prognostic, and treatment implications. There are many well-recognized syndromes, such as childhood absence epilepsy, West syndrome, and Dravet syndrome, etc.

Box 6.5.1: Clinical manifestations during seizures.

- Abnormal motor activity, which may be a tonic contraction or single or repetitive jerks
- Impairment or loss of consciousness or awareness
- Abnormal behavior
- Abnormal sensory phenomena, e.g. abnormal sensation in one part of the body, visual phenomena, smell, and/or taste
- Abnormal experience, e.g. fear, anger, illusions, or hallucination. Children often run to the parent when this occurs
- Autonomic symptoms

Box 6.5.2: Information required for identifying an epileptic syndrome.

- Seizure type(s) (seizure semiology plus EEG pattern)
- Age of onset and remission
- Developmental status and comorbidities
- Etiology
- Anatomy and imaging features
- Precipitating factors
- Prognosis (occasionally)

(EEG: electroencephalogram)

CLASSIFICATION OF SEIZURES, EPILEPSIES, AND EPILEPSY SYNDROMES

It is very important to classify seizures and epilepsy type and identify the epilepsy syndrome wherever possible, as this is important for starting correct treatment and prognostication, and it may also help to identify etiology and genetics.

In the past, there existed confusion regarding the epilepsies and seizure types. Many of the epilepsies were classified and described by the names of the persons who first described them. There was no uniformity in the classification and descriptions used in the different parts of the world varied.

The International League Against Epilepsy (ILAE) is an organization whose primary goal is to advance and disseminate knowledge about epilepsy. They described a classification of *seizures* in 1981, and *epilepsies* and *epileptic syndromes* in 1989. This was modified by the ILAE, in 2010, but this could not be adopted for the universal use. In September 2017, ILAE has published a new classification of seizures as well as epilepsies, and a brief account of this is presented below. **Figure 6.5.1** shows the current classification of seizures and epilepsies.

Steps in Classification

The main steps in the classification of epilepsies include the following:

- Classify seizure type
- Classify epilepsy type
- Identify epilepsy syndrome.

At every step (1) look for etiology and classify into one of the etiology groups and (2) identify comorbidities. *Attempts to classify the seizure and epilepsy types must be made after EIs have been ruled out.*

In some settings, classification according to seizure type may be maximum level of diagnosis possible. In other cases, there is simply too little information to be able to make a higher level diagnosis, e.g. when a patient has only had a single event.

Classification of Seizure Type (Fig. 6.5.2)

On the basis of the onset, seizures are of three main types:

1. *Generalized seizures*: They originate at some point within the cortex and rapidly engage bilaterally distributed networks and can include cortical and subcortical structures but not necessarily the entire cortex.
2. *Focal seizures*: They originate within the networks limited to one hemisphere. They may be discretely localized or more widely distributed.
3. *Focal to bilateral tonic-clonic seizures*: If focal seizures propagate to both hemispheres, the term focal to bilateral tonic-clonic seizure is used. The term "secondarily generalized seizures" is abandoned; "generalized" is used *only* for seizures that apparently originate simultaneously in both the hemispheres.
4. *Unknown onset:* If the seizure description or observation is unable to determine whether the seizure is focal or generalized.
5. *Unclassified:* If the seizures cannot be placed in any of the other types for any reason (e.g. insufficient information, poor description).

Steps in Seizure Classification

Step 1: Decide onset, whether "focal" or "generalized," if not sure the onset may be stated as "*unknown onset.*"

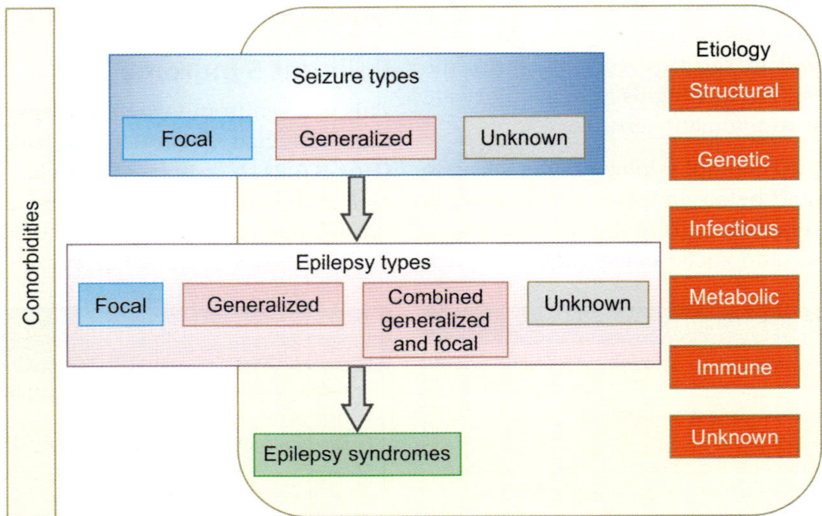

Fig. 6.5.1: Current classification of seizures and epilepsies.
Source: ILAE. https://doi.org/10.1111/epi.13709 here.

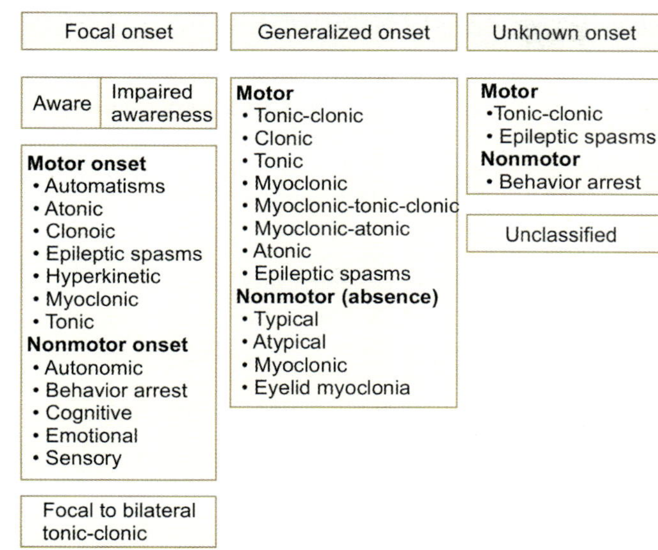

Fig. 6.5.2: ILAE 2017 classification of seizures—expanded version 1. (ILAE: International League Against Epilepsy)
Source: ILAE. https://doi.org/10.1111/epi.13670 here.

Step 2: Decide awareness: This is applicable to the focal or unknown onset seizures only and is *not* a parameter for generalized onset seizures. If awareness is impaired at any point during the seizure, it is classified as a focal or unknown onset *impaired awareness seizure*. If awareness is retained throughout, it is called a *focal aware seizure*. If unsure of the level awareness, one can omit awareness as a classifier.

Step 3: Decide motor or nonmotor: The types of motor and nonmotor seizures are given in **Figure 6.5.2** and the description in **Boxes 6.5.3A and 6.5.3B**. This can be done even without specifying level of awareness, e.g. a *focal tonic seizure*. A behavior arrest seizure shows the arrest of behavior as the prominent feature of the entire seizure. A transient behavior arrest at onset of a seizure is not behavior arrest seizure.

Step 4: *Add additional descriptors*: It is encouraged to add descriptions of other signs and symptoms, suggested descriptors, or free text. These do not alter the seizure type. Example: *focal emotional seizure* with tonic right arm activity and hyperventilation. A standard list of descriptors can be obtained from ILAE website.

Classification of Epilepsy Type

Before attempting classification, it is assumed that the patient has a diagnosis of epilepsy based on the 2014 definition as above. Not all epilepsies can be placed into a syndrome, and the epilepsy classification type is important where one is unable to make an epilepsy syndrome diagnosis or a diagnosis of etiology.

- *Generalized epilepsies*: There are only generalized seizures, e.g. absence, myoclonic, atonic, tonic, or tonic-clonic seizures, and the electroencephalogram (EEG) should show generalized spike-wave discharges. For a patient with generalized tonic-clonic seizures (GTCS) and a normal EEG, supportive evidence is needed, e.g. characteristic seizures, such as myoclonic jerks or a relevant family history.
- *Focal epilepsies*: There are only focal, multifocal, or hemispheric seizures. Many seizure types may be seen e.g. focal aware/impaired awareness seizures, focal motor/nonmotor seizures, and focal to bilateral

Box 6.5.3A: Brief clinical description of seizure types—focal.
Focal motor
Automatisms: A coordinated, purposeless, repetitive motor activity, which might appear normal in other circumstances
Atonic: Focal loss of tone
Clonic: Focal rhythmic jerking or epileptic spasms
Epileptic Spasm: Focal flexion or extension of arms and flexion of trunk
Hyperkinetic: Pedaling or thrashing motor activity
Myoclonic: Irregular, brief focal jerking
Tonic: Sustained focal stiffening or tightness
Focal nonmotor
Autonomic: Gastrointestinal sensations, a sense of heat or cold, flushing, piloerection (goose bumps), palpitations, sexual arousal, respiratory changes, or other autonomic effects
Behavior arrest: Cessation of all movement and unresponsiveness, which should be present for the *entire* seizure
Cognitive: Deficits in language, thinking, or associated higher cortical functions, e.g. déjà vu, jamais vu, hallucinations, or illusions
Emotional: Feeling of emotions, such as fear, anxiety, agitation, anger, paranoia, pleasure, joy, ecstasy, laughing (gelastic), or crying (dacrystic)
Sensory: Abnormal sensations, which may be somatosensory, olfactory, visual, auditory, gustatory, hot-cold sense, or vestibular

Box 6.5.3B: Brief clinical description of seizure types—generalized seizures.

Generalized motor

Generalized tonic-clonic seizures (*earlier known as grand mal seizures*): It starts with a tonic phase characterized by a generalized stiffening of the whole body, followed by rhythmic to and fro contractions of extremities. There may be a tongue bite in the tonic phase, with urinary or stool incontinence, and frothing during the clonic phase

Clonic seizures: These begin, progress, and end with sustained rhythmic jerking of limbs on both sides of the body and often head, neck, face, and trunk. Generalized clonic seizures are much less common than tonic-clonic seizures, but usually occur in infants

Tonic seizures: Bilateral limb stiffening or elevation, often with neck stiffening, and is not followed by clonic movements. The tonic activity can be a sustained abnormal posture, either in extension or flexion, sometimes accompanied by tremor of the extremities

Myoclonic seizures: Sudden contraction of a muscle or muscle group. They can be single or occur in clusters. They may be simply myoclonic, or myoclonic-atonic or myoclonic-tonic. Myoclonus differs from clonus by being briefer and not regularly repetitive. Myoclonus as a symptom may also have a nonepileptic etiology

Myoclonic-tonic-clonic: Seizures begin with a few myoclonic jerks followed by tonic-clonic activity. These seizures are commonly seen in patients with juvenile myoclonic epilepsy

Myoclonic-atonic: Brief jerking of limbs or trunk, followed by limpness. These seizures, previously called myoclonic-astatic seizures, are most commonly seen in Doose syndrome, but it can also be encountered in Lennox–Gastaut and other syndromes

Atonic seizures: Sudden generalized loss of muscle tone. Drop attack may result, with the patient falling on the buttocks or sometimes forward onto the knees and face. These are also often associated with underlying other neurological abnormalities, and other types of seizure may occur

Epileptic spasm: It presents as a sudden flexion, extension, or mixed extension-flexion of predominantly proximal and truncal muscles. They commonly occur in clusters and most often during infancy

Generalized nonmotor seizures: absence seizures

Typical absence: It starts and ends abruptly. There is no fall, and after the brief period of alteration consciousness (few seconds only), the child resumes activity as if nothing has happened

Atypical absence: Onset is gradual, the patient has alteration of consciousness for a variable duration (may be minutes), and ending is also gradual. Postural changes can occur, and they are often associated with other seizure types and neurological abnormalities and mental retardation

Myoclonic absence: An absence seizure with rhythmic 3 per second myoclonic movements, associated with 3 per second generalized spike-wave discharges. Duration is typically 10–60 seconds

Eyelid myoclonia with absence: Myoclonic jerks of the eyelids and upward deviation of the eyes, associated with the absence

tonic-clonic seizures. The interictal EEG typically shows focal epileptiform discharges, but the diagnosis is made on clinical grounds, supported by EEG findings.

- *Combined generalized and focal epilepsies*: Both types of seizures occur, and the interictal EEG may show both generalized spike-wave and focal epileptiform discharges, but epileptiform activity is not required for the diagnosis. Examples are Dravet syndrome and Lennox–Gastaut syndrome.
- *Unknown*: Where the onset of seizures is not clear.

IDENTIFICATION OF EPILEPTIC SYNDROMES

The ILAE also proposed a classification of epilepsies and epileptic syndromes in 1989, and an organization of epileptic syndromes in 2010, based on age of onset. However, in the 2017 position paper of the ILAE Commission for Classification and Terminology, *there are no "ILAE-approved" syndromes.* A list of syndromes with their complete description is given on their website *epilepsydiagnosis.org*.

Practically, an age-wise organization of the syndromes can still be useful and is given in **Table 6.5.1**.

Idiopathic generalized epilepsy: These are now referred to as genetic generalized epilepsies. These are epilepsies, which have no underlying cause except perhaps a genetic predisposition to epilepsy. It does not necessarily mean inherited, because de novo mutations can occur. The term "idiopathic generalized epilepsy" is permitted for only four syndromes: childhood absence epilepsy, juvenile absence epilepsy, juvenile myoclonic epilepsy (JME), and epilepsy with GTCS alone. The diagnosis of any of these syndromes does not require confirmation by genetic testing.

Self-limited focal epilepsies: There are several self-limited focal epilepsies, typically beginning in childhood, but may begin in later life as well. The earlier term "benign" is replaced with "self-limited" or "pharmacoresponsive;" e.g. epilepsy with centrotemporal spikes, formerly called "benign epilepsy with centrotemporal spikes" is now called "self-limited epilepsy with centrotemporal spikes."

Table 6.5.1: Epilepsy syndromes (according to ILAE).	
By the age of onset	***By etiology***
• *Neonatal period*: • Benign neonatal seizures • BFNS • EME • Early infantile epileptic encephalopathy (Ohtahara syndrome)	*Genetic:* Genetic defect directly contributes to the epilepsy, and seizures are the core symptom of the disorder
Infancy: • Migrating partial seizures of infancy • West syndrome • MEI • Benign infantile epilepsy • Benign familial infantile epilepsy • Dravet syndrome • Myoclonic epilepsy in nonprogressive disorders • Epilepsy of infancy with migrating focal seizures	*Structural:* Caused by a structural disorder of the brain, e.g. cortical malformations, tuberous sclerosis, lissencephaly
Childhood: • Early onset benign childhood occipital epilepsy (Panayiotopoulos type) • Epilepsy with myoclonic-atonic seizures • Benign childhood epilepsy with centrotemporal spikes • Autosomal dominant nocturnal frontal lobe epilepsy • Late onset childhood occipital epilepsy (Gastaut type) • Epilepsy with myoclonic absences • Lennox–Gastaut syndrome • Epileptic encephalopathy with CSWS including Landau–Kleffner syndrome • Childhood absence epilepsy	*Metabolic:* Caused by a metabolic disorder of the brain, e.g. pyridoxine deficiency, nonketotic hyperglycinemia
Adolescence: • JAE • JME • Epilepsy with GTCA • ADEAF • Other familial temporal lobe epilepsies • PME	*Infectious:* • Tuberculosis • Neurocysticercosis
Relation with age less specific: • Generalized epilepsies with FS+ • Familial focal epilepsy with variable foci • Reflex epilepsies – Idiopathic photosensitive occipital lobe – Visual-sensitive epilepsies – Primary reading epilepsy • Startle epilepsy	*Immune:* • Autoimmune encephalitis • Rasmussen encephalitis
	Unknown

Note: The word benign is recommended to be replaced with "self-limited."

(ADEAF: autosomal dominant epilepsy with auditory features; BFNS: benign familial neonatal seizures; CSWS: continuous spikes and waves during sleep; EME: early myoclonic encephalopathy; FS+: febrile seizures plus; GTCA: generalized tonic-clonic seizures alone; ILAE: International League Against Epilepsy; JAE: juvenile absence epilepsy; JME: juvenile myoclonic epilepsy; MEI: myoclonic epilepsy of infancy; PME: progressive myoclonus epilepsies)

EPIDEMIOLOGY

In India the prevalence of epilepsy is 5.59–10 per 1000 population in various studies. Males and females are equally affected, and these rates are the same in different geographical areas.

ETIOLOGY

Etiology is multifactorial, and almost any insult to the brain can result in seizures. Epilepsy can result from sequelae of prolonged seizures, as well as malformation of the central

Table 6.5.2: Etiology of seizures and epilepsy.

Causes of seizures	*Causes of epilepsy*
• *Infections*: Viral encephalitis, pyogenic meningitis, tubercular meningitis, neurocysticercosis • *Metabolic events*: Hypoglycemia, hypocalcemia, hypomagnesemia, dyselectrolytemia (hypernatremia/hyponatremia) • *Vascular events—cerebrovascular accidents* (thrombosis/embolism/hemorrhage): • Drug intoxication/side effects • Neoplasms • Hypoxia/anoxia, especially during delivery • Head trauma • Febrile seizures	*Sequelae of any of the acute causes of seizures:* • Cerebral malformations • Metabolic diseases • Degenerative brain disease • Neoplasms • Genetic

nervous system (CNS), genetic and metabolic causes **(Table 6.5.2)**.

PATHOPHYSIOLOGY

The pathophysiology of seizures is still not well understood. However, we do know that seizures are produced when there is an abnormality in the

- Neurotransmitters levels
- Ion channels
- Receptors.

In many of the genetic epilepsies, there is abnormality of the ion channels or the receptors due to mutations, resulting in epilepsies. These abnormalities can result in hyperexcitability of neurons, which thus lead to seizures.

The other epilepsies result from neuronal damage because of various insults, such as infections, trauma, and vascular events.

INVESTIGATIONS

Investigation of Seizures

The plan of investigations depends on suspected cause [see management of acute seizures and status epilepticus (SE)].

Investigation of Epilepsy

Electroencephalogram

An EEG is the most important test for investigating epilepsy. It is a graphic recording of the electric activity of the brain. An EEG is normal *not* due to normal patterns but *because* it has no abnormal patterns.

It is important to remember that EEG can be normal in the cases of epilepsy, while abnormal EEG does not necessarily mean an epileptic disorder. About 15% of the cases of epilepsy have a normal EEG, while 10% of the normal population has an abnormal EEG. Thus the EEG must be interpreted in the clinical context **(Box 6.5.4)**.

Box 6.5.4: EEG: information and limitations.

Information:
- Epileptic versus nonepileptic attacks
- Seizure type and epilepsy syndrome **(Figs. 6.5.1 to 6.5.4)**
- Photosensitivity
- Focal seizures—to identify focus **(Figs. 6.5.5 and 6.5.6)**
- Identify etiology e.g. SSPE **(Fig. 6.5.7)**
- Monitor progress—only in some epilepsies, e.g. typical absence seizures, West syndrome. In most cases, clinical response should be the criterion for judging response to treatment. Routine EEGs during treatment are *not* required

Limitations:
- Normal EEG does not exclude epilepsy
- Must always be interpreted in the clinical context
- With the exception of 3 Hz spike-wave discharges and hypsarrhythmia, EEG is a poor guide to seizure control
- Withdrawal of drugs: EEG is not required. Only clinical seizure control should decide whether drug is to be stopped

(EEG: electroencephalogram; SSPE: subacute sclerosing panencephalitis)

Ictal recordings are preferable over interictal ones. Special provocation procedures, such as sleep deprivation, hyperventilation, and photic stimulation, can be used to increase the yield of EEG.

Video EEG is an EEG recording where the EEG and video recording of the child are done at the same time. It may help to differentiate nonepileptic events (NEEs) from seizures and also help in identification of the type of seizure **(Fig. 6.5.8)**.

Neuroimaging

Neuroimaging gives important information about the etiology in the cases of symptomatic epilepsies **(Figs. 6.5.9 and 6.5.10)**.

Magnetic resonance imaging (MRI) is preferred since small lesions, such as cortical dysplasia, cannot be picked up on computed tomography (CT) scan. Generally neuroimaging should be done in all cases except where clinical features and EEG are suggestive of idiopathic epilepsy.

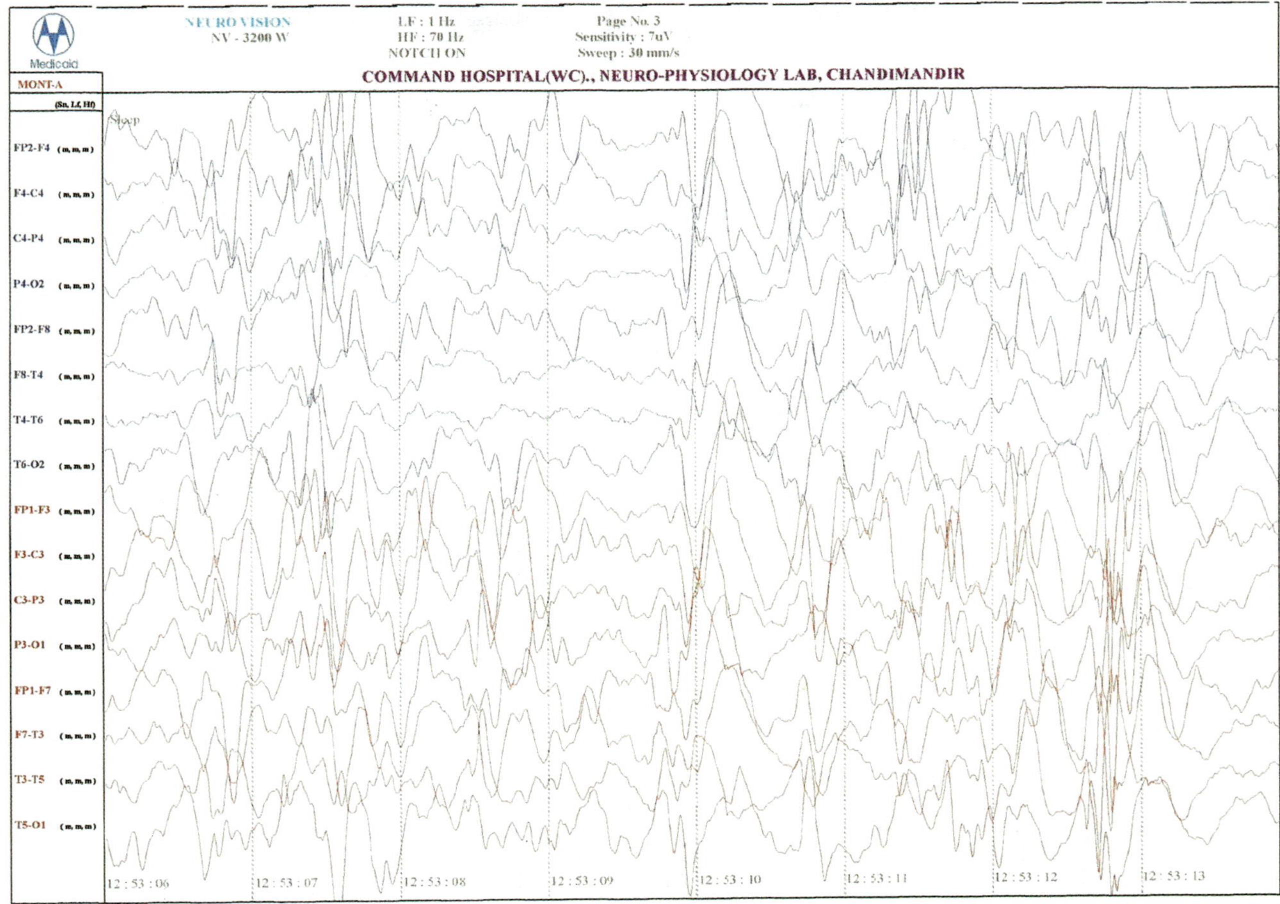

Fig. 6.5.3: Hypsarrhythmia, a high-voltage, chaotic EEG pattern, which changes, characteristic of infantile spasms here. (EEG: electroencephalogram)

Positron emission tomography and single photon emission CT (SPECT), done as pre-epilepsy surgery workup in refractory epilepsy, are functional scans and help in identifying epileptic foci.

Other Investigations

Other investigations depend on suspected etiology in the case of symptomatic epilepsies. They include metabolic and genetic tests.

NATURAL HISTORY

In any given population with epilepsy, it may undergo remission without treatment in 30% of the cases, as estimated by the studies of epilepsy in poor countries where no treatment has been given for epilepsy because of financial constraints. Of those who are treated, 60–70% undergo remission, while the remaining have intractable seizures.

DIFFERENTIAL DIAGNOSIS OF SEIZURES AND EPILEPSIES: THE EPILEPSY IMITATORS

Epilepsy imitators are the recurrent paroxysmal events which resemble seizures but are *not* the result of abnormal electrical discharges from the neurons. They are also known as nonepileptic attack disorder, NEEs, epilepsy mimickers, and pseudoseizures. These can also produce recurrent episodes of motor movement or apparent changes of consciousness or behavior that are also seen in children with epilepsy. Moreover, disorders that mimic seizures are more likely to occur in children who have epilepsy, associated with abnormal EEG or to be relieved by antiepileptic drugs (AEDs) making their diagnosis more difficult.

Incidence

Twenty to thirty percent of all patients reporting to epilepsy clinics are found to have EIs. As many as 30% of the patients

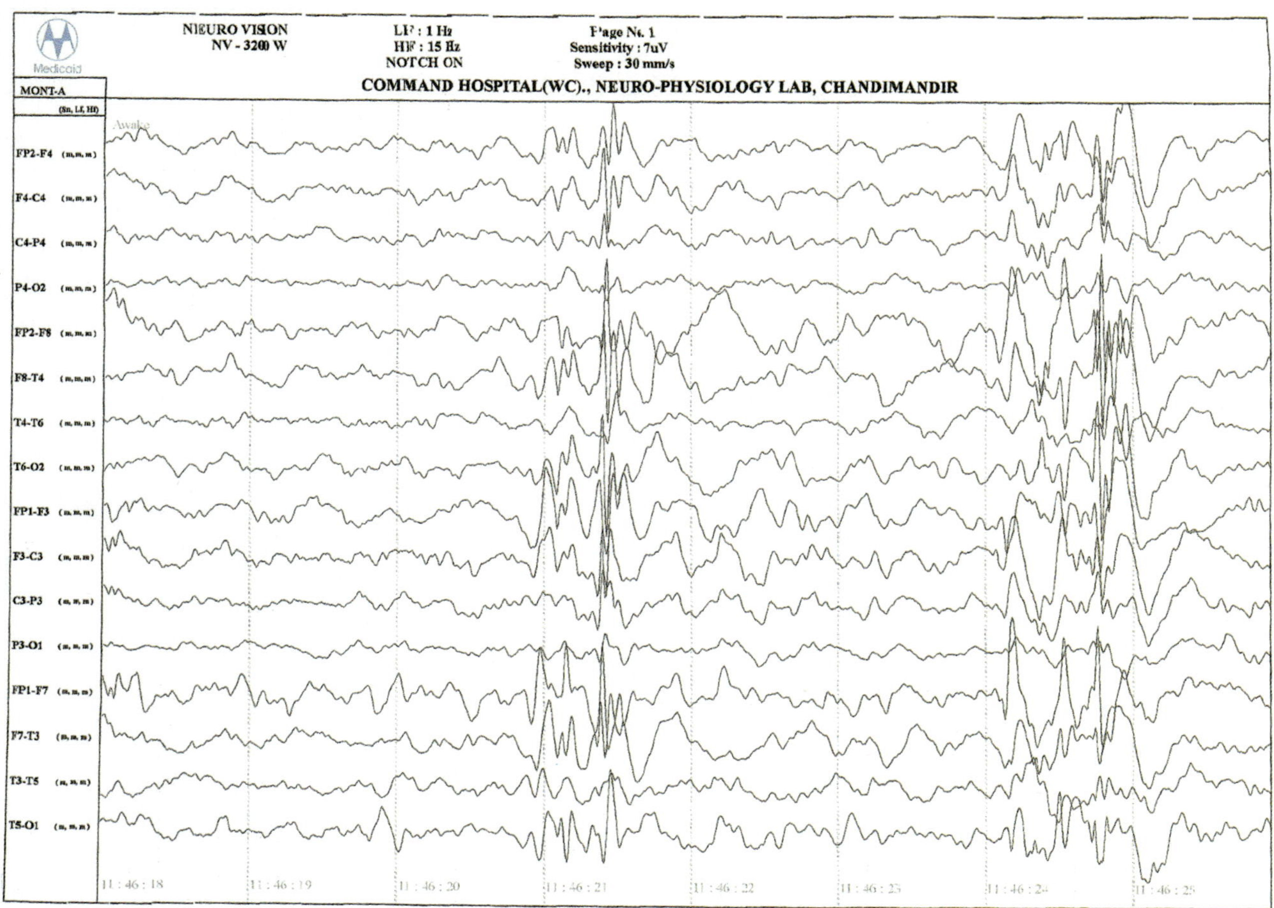

Fig. 6.5.4: Polyspike-wave discharges suggestive of myoclonic seizures here.

with EIs have real seizures as well. Epilepsy imitator and epilepsies both present at all ages and in many different forms. Therefore, many conditions can mimic epilepsy at different stages of a child's life.

Nonepileptic events can be divided into two groups:

1. *Physiological EIs*: These are various physiological phenomena which resemble seizures on observation or when described by parents.
2. *Psychogenic EIs*: These are seen mostly in children more than 5 years and are either conversion reactions or malingering.

Approach to Differentiation from Seizures

History and clinical examination can give clues to the correct diagnosis. A description of event, especially an eyewitness account, is very important in obtaining a correct diagnosis. The event should typically be suggestive of some type of seizure. A video recording by the parents may suggest the diagnosis. Developmental delay and neurological deficits are more likely to be associated with true seizures but may also be associated with EIs.

Age-based approach: Consider the types of seizures in an age-group, and if the event does not match the type of seizures occurring in that age-group, then one should review the EIs in that age-group **(Table 6.5.3)**, e.g. myoclonic jerks during sleep in a neonate may be confused with myoclonic seizures, daydreaming in a school-going child may be confused with focal impaired awareness seizures.

Attempts to observe the event: If possible, attempt to observe the event. This is possible, if the event occurs at a particular time or is precipitated by something, e.g. breath-holding spells—try to make the child cry. If *psychogenic seizures* are suspected, then the event may be induced by saline injections and suggestion to the patient that the injection will precipitate seizures.

Ancillary testing—EEG/video EEG: This is done when there is a doubt about the diagnosis of EI despite history and clinical observation of the patient.

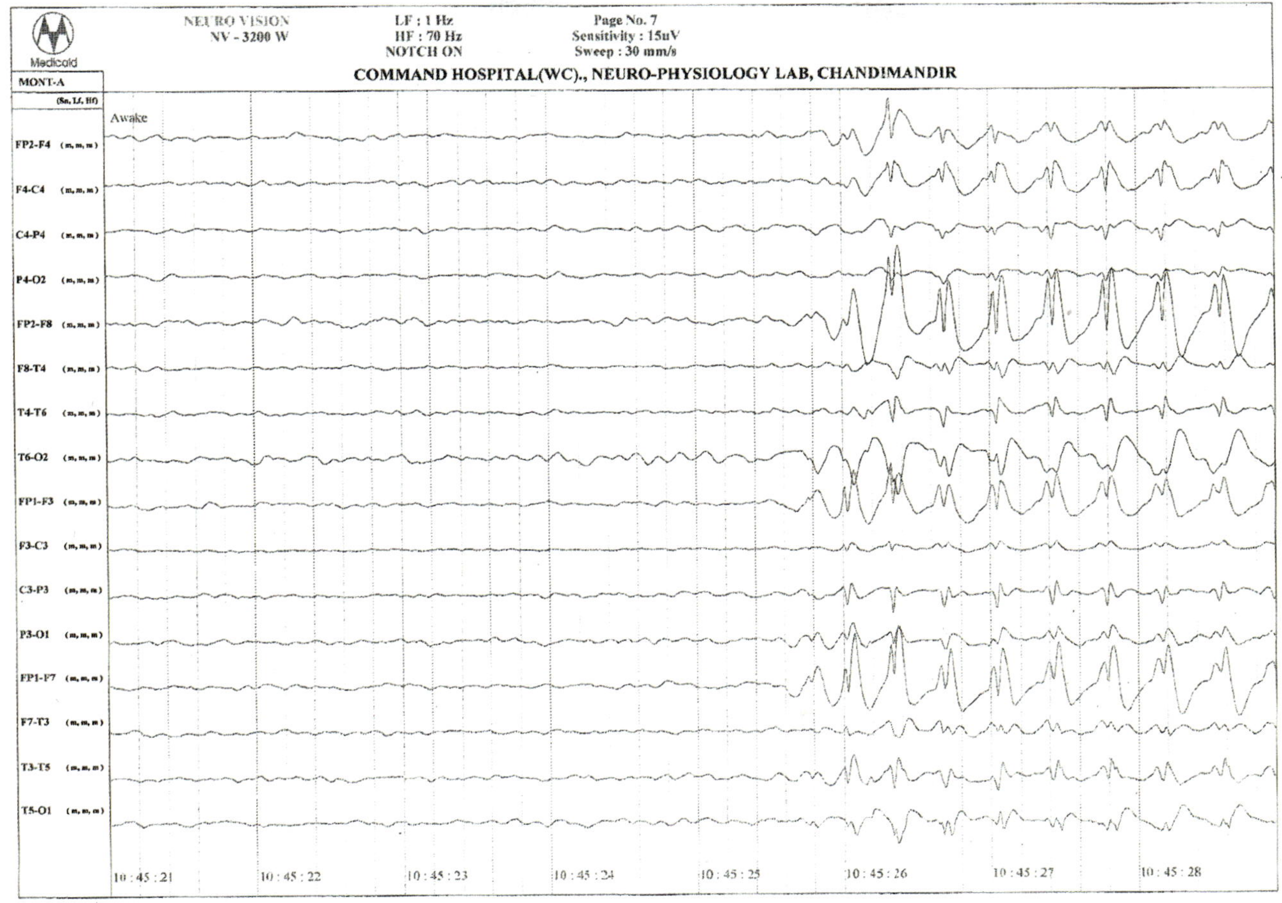

Fig. 6.5.5: Three/second spike-wave discharges suggestive of typical absence seizures here.

Sometimes true seizures and NEEs may coexist making differentiation between the two very difficult.

COMMON EPILEPSY IMITATORS

Breath-holding Spells

Breath-holding spells are stereotypic events that occur in response to a painful stimulus or an adverse emotional event leading to forceful crying. They occur in children 6 months to 2 years and disappear by 6 years of age. Males are more commonly affected than females in a ratio of 3:1. Family history may be present in the one-fourth of the cases.

Pathophysiology

The spell is actually a reflex, rather than a behavior problem as was thought earlier. They are of two types:

1. *Cyanotic* (*more common*): There is forceful expiration during crying, a respiratory pause (breath holding), resulting in hypoxia and cyanosis.
2. *Pallid*: Vagal stimulation, following a painful stimulus or during pause in respiration during expiration, results in cardiac asystole, hypoxia, and pallor.

Clinical Presentation

The child holds his/her breath following a sudden painful stimulus and becomes pale or after a prolonged expiration while crying and becomes cyanosed. He/she then loses consciousness for a brief period, usually less than a minute. There may be stiffening of the whole body, followed by a few clonic jerks, which may make the event appear like a seizure. He/she gradually regains consciousness with the return of normal color and may remain drowsy or sleep for some time. The attack may occur many times in a day.

Differential Diagnosis

These include epilepsy, syncope, and cardiac arrhythmias.

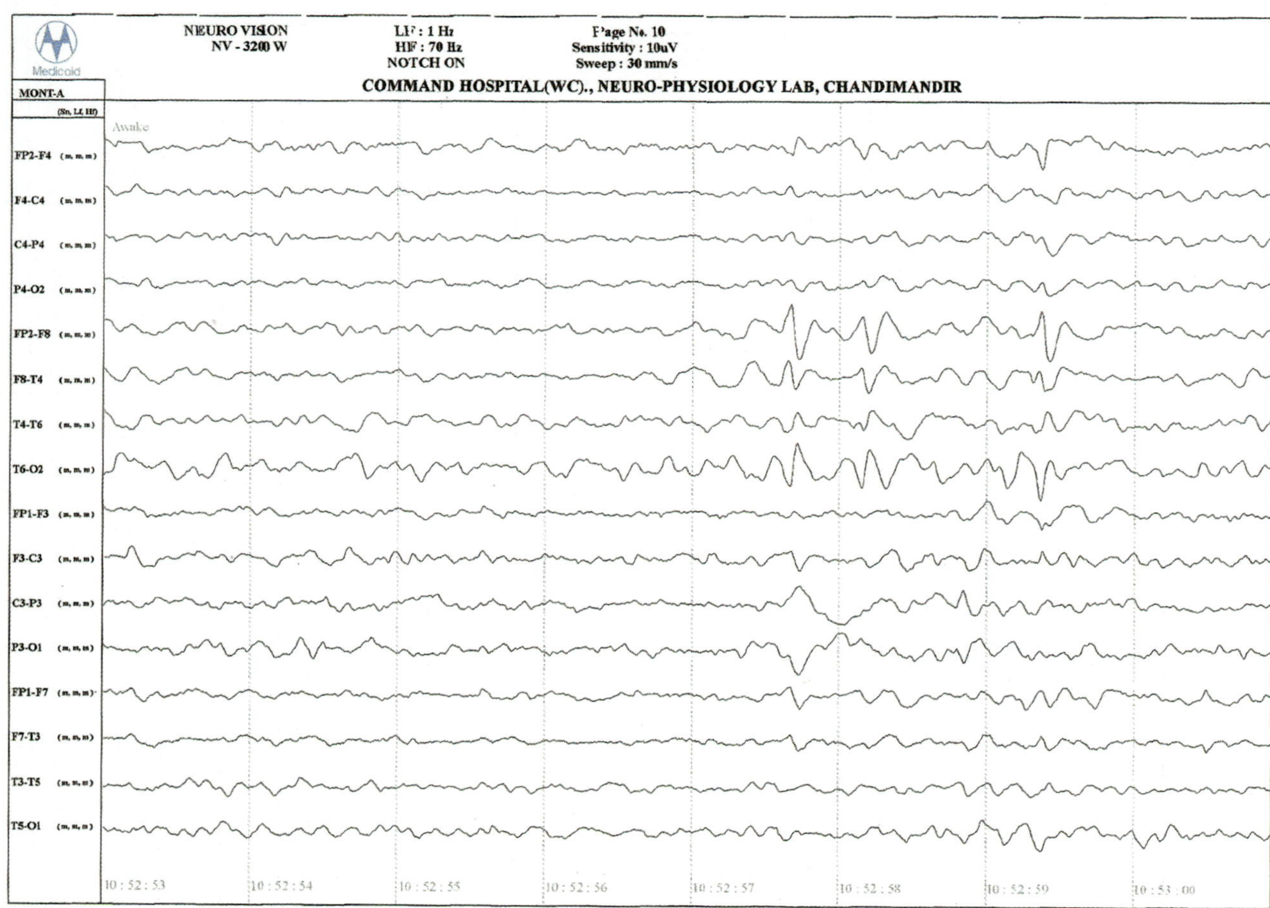

Fig. 6.5.6: Epileptic focus—right frontal region here.

Investigation

In the case of doubt, video EEG may be done. Work up for cardiac arrhythmias or anomaly in case that is suspected.

Management

- Counseling regarding the benign nature of the condition is a must to alleviate anxiety.
- Diverting the child's attention at the onset of crying can abort an attack.
- Some children have low hemoglobin levels; therefore, iron therapy may help in decreasing the frequency of attacks.
- In the case of severe multiple attacks, piracetam, in doses of 50 mg/kg/day in three divided doses, may be given and can significantly decrease the frequency of attacks.

Benign Neonatal Sleep Myoclonus

This is a myoclonus that is sometimes seen in neonates at the age of 1–2 weeks, up to 6 months of age. It comprises repetitive jerking or myoclonic movements of the different body parts and occurs only during sleep. Awakening the baby terminates the attacks. The baby remains neurologically normal. They may be mistaken for seizures and put on AEDs, to which there is no response. Electroencephalogram and video EEG are normal. Treatment is not required. Parents should be counseled about the benign nature of the condition.

Syncope

Syncope is a transient loss of consciousness, resulting in loss of tone and a fall, from which the patient makes a spontaneous recovery. Presyncope is the period just before consciousness is lost. It consists of a lightheaded feeling, weakness, and unsteadiness. It may result in a drop attack. About 20% of the children suffer from one or more attacks of syncope before the age of 15 years, but most of the syncopal attacks are benign in children.

Syncope can be differentiated from seizures by taking a detailed history. If there is a doubt, then the *tilt table test* can

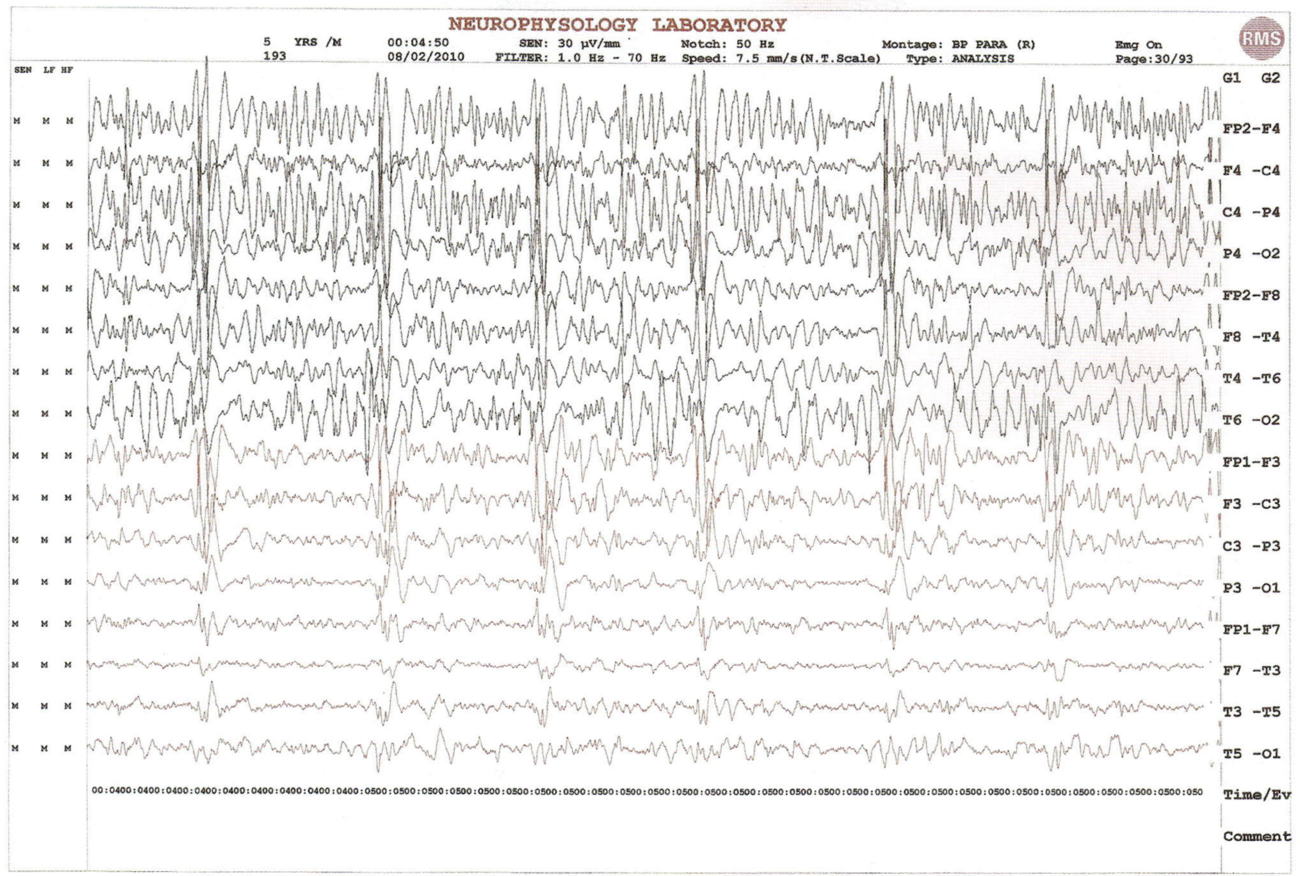

Fig. 6.5.7: Periodic complexes seen in SSPE here.
(SSPE: subacute sclerosing panencephalitis)

be done, which involves putting the patient in 70° position after strapping to a table and checking vital parameters and symptoms of syncope in that position. Cardiac syncope should be suspected if the syncope occurs during exercise or when lying down.

If the child has vasovagal syncope the child should avoid situations that precipitate the attack. During an attack the clothes should be loosened, and the patient made to lie down for some time. No attempt should be made to give mouth-to-mouth respiration.

Psychogenic Seizures

Psychogenic seizures are events that resemble seizures and occur due to emotional or psychological reasons. There is no accompanying epileptiform discharge in the brain. They are usually a conversion reaction, but may be a form of malingering as well. About 20–30% of the children attending epilepsy units may have psychogenic seizures. They are seen only after the age of 5 years.

Psychogenic seizures are mainly of two types:

1. Unresponsiveness with no motor activity
2. Unresponsiveness with varying degrees of motor activity, ranging from just shivering to thrashing around violently.

Both forms may be difficult to differentiate from true epilepsy, just based on history alone. It is important to try to observe an episode to discern whether it is a true seizure or a psychogenic one. A video EEG is must if any doubt remains about the reality of seizures.

Some clues to psychogenic seizures are given in **Box 6.5.5**. Once diagnosed, children should undergo neuropsychological testing and counseling. Most children/parents would opt for discontinuing the drugs. A trial of placebo may be given.

Sometimes, true seizures coexist with psychogenic seizures, when it becomes extremely difficult to differentiate true from psychogenic seizures, leading to either undertreatment or overtreatment.

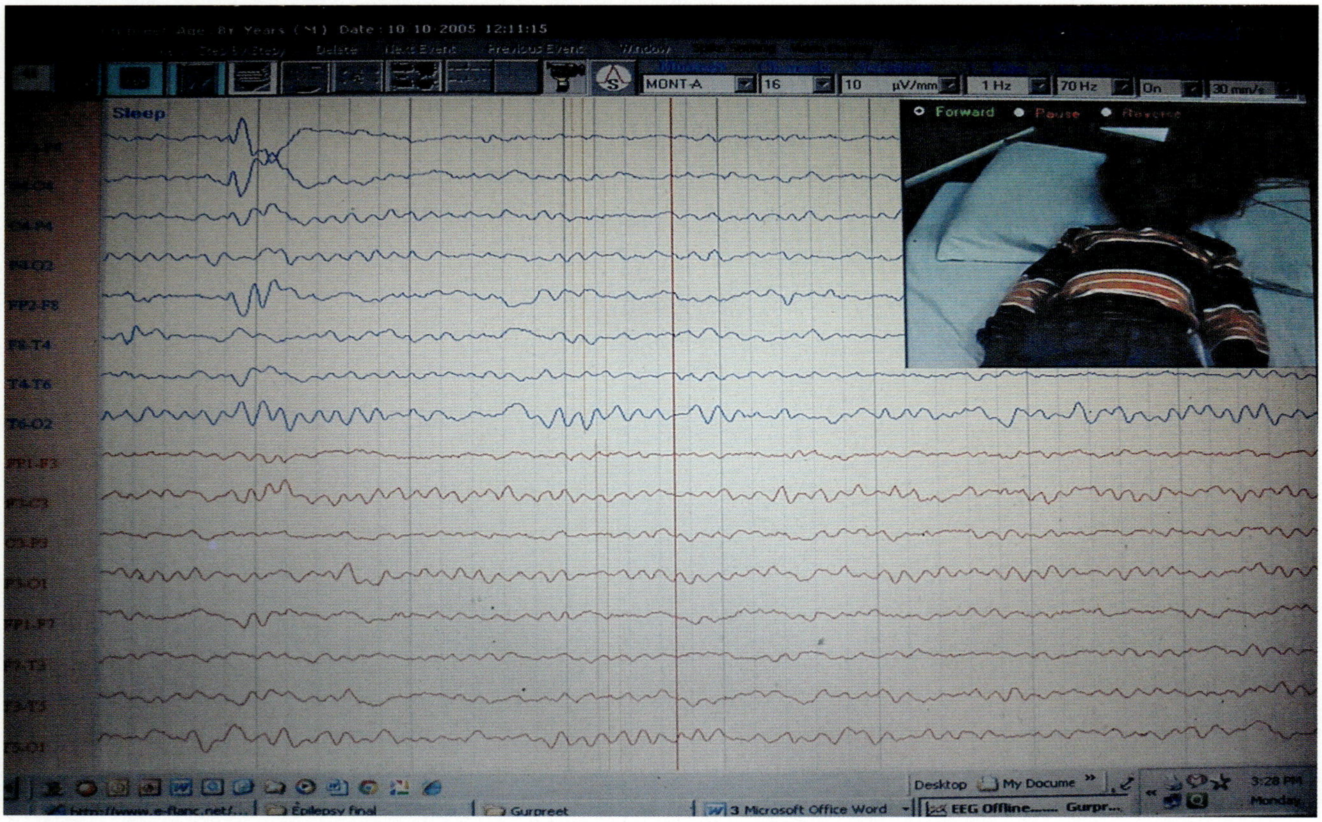

Fig. 6.5.8: Video EEG. Simultaneous EEG and video recording here
(EEG: electroencephalogram)

SELECTED TYPES OF SEIZURES AND EPILEPTIC SYNDROMES

Acute Seizures and Status Epilepticus

Most seizures terminate spontaneously without treatment, and if brought to medical attention, after administration of a fast-acting anticonvulsant drug. Status epilepticus means that seizures continue for a prolonged period. Physiologically, SE results from either the failure of the mechanisms responsible for seizure termination or from the initiation of mechanisms, which lead to abnormally, prolonged seizures. Two timings are important.

1. *T1-5 minutes of seizures*: After this time the seizure is unlikely to stop on its own. At this time the active treatment to abort seizures must be started.
2. *T2-30 minutes of seizures*: This can have long-term sequelae, including neuronal death, neuronal injury, and alteration of neuronal networks, depending on the type and duration of seizures.

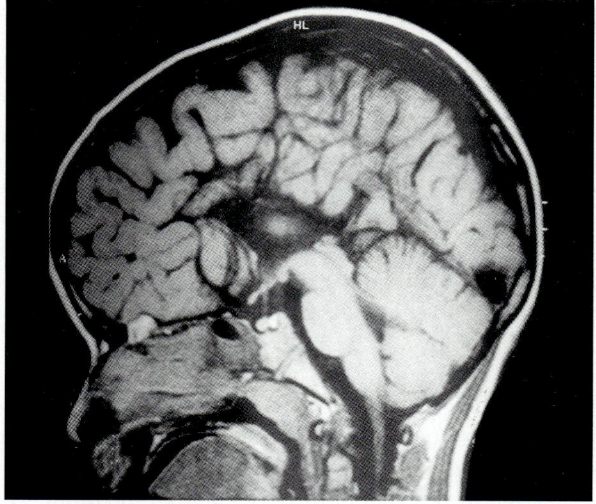

Fig. 6.5.9: Structural malformation of CNS—agenesis of corpus callosum here.
(CNS: central nervous system)

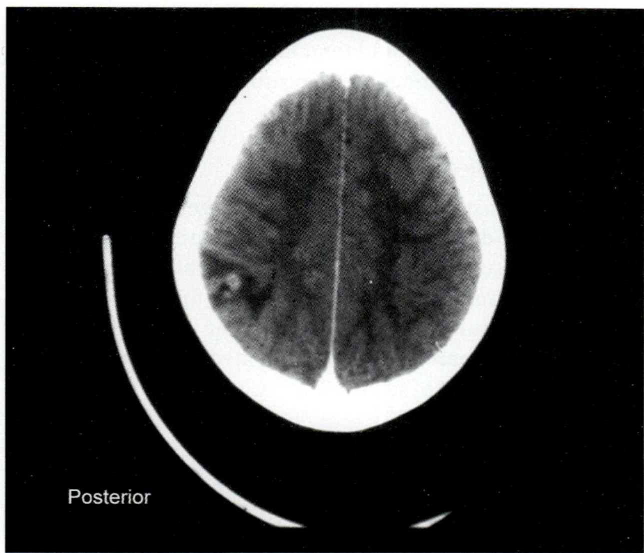

Fig. 6.5.10: Neurocysticercosis here.

Definition of Status Epilepticus

- *Status epilepticus*: ILAE defines SE as seizures that continue for more than 30 minutes or recurrent seizures for more than 30 minutes without the recovery of consciousness in between the attacks.
- *Practical definition*: If seizure duration is more than twice the duration of the usual seizures.
- *Refractory SE*: If seizures fail to respond to appropriate first- and second-line drug treatment and persists for more than 60 minutes.
- *Superrefractory SE*: If seizures continue for more than 24 hours after appropriate anticonvulsant treatment.

Incidence

Overall incidence is about 50 patients per 100,000 population per year. In children, SE is most likely in those less than 3 years. Almost 70% of the children less than 1 year with epilepsy may have SE.

Classification of Status Epilepticus

- *According to seizure type:* For example, generalized tonic-clonic, partial, and absence
- *According to the clinical presentation*:
    - *Convulsive status*: When the seizures have a predominant motor component. For example, GTCS, clonic, tonic, myoclonic, epilepsia partialis continua, and seizures in one half of the body
    - *Nonconvulsive status*: Absence, complex partial SE, and continuous spike waves during slow-wave sleep
- *According to EEG findings*

Pathophysiology

Convulsive SE can be life-threatening and causes permanent neuronal damage after 30 minutes of seizure activity due to excessive glutamate production leading to excessive neuronal depolarization, rise in intracellular sodium and calcium, cerebral edema and finally cell damage and death. Systemic changes include hypoxia, hypotension, and hyperpyrexia. Metabolic derangements, such as acidosis, hypoglycemia, and hyperkalemia, may result in cardiac, respiratory, and renal failure.

Table 6.5.3: Common epilepsy imitators at different ages.

Neonates—2 years	*Early childhood*	*Late childhood and adolescence*
Abnormal movements *During sleep:* • Benign neonatal sleep myoclonus • Sleep myoclonus *When awake:* • Self-gratification behavior • Jitteriness • Stereotypies • Myoclonic movements—benign myoclonus of early infancy • Paroxysmal tonic upgaze • Spasmus nutans • Opsoclonus myoclonus **Abnormal breathing phenomena** • Recurrent apneic attacks • Breath-holding spells	**Abnormal movements** *During sleep:* • Sleep myoclonus *When awake:* • Chorea • Tics • Paroxysmal choreoathetosis **Abnormal behavior** *During sleep:* • Sleepwalking • Night terrors • Nightmares • Confusional arousals *When awake:* • Panic/rage attacks • Delirium • Loss of consciousness/awareness • Daydreaming **Others** • Benign paroxysmal vertigo • Migraine	**Abnormal movements** • Psychogenic "seizures" • Loss of consciousness/awareness/tone • Psychogenic "seizures" • Syncope • Narcolepsy/cataplexy **Others** Fears and phobia

Etiology

Etiology of status is essentially the same as that of seizures and epilepsy **(Box 6.5.1)**. However, certain factors can precipitate seizures and SE in a person with epilepsy **(Box 6.5.6)**.

Management

The success of treatment of SE depends on how quickly the seizure is brought under control. The principles of management are well defined, but the protocols vary from institute to institute; what is important is that every medical care facility must have a very clear protocol or drill in the management of SE.

One does not have to wait for 30 minutes to set into motion, the treatment protocol for SE. Any patient who is brought with seizures to the hospital or whose seizures last for more than 5 minutes is to be treated as for SE.

The goals of management are to stop the seizure activity as soon as possible and prevent brain damage and systemic complications, and at the same time, to support airway-breathing-circulation, carry out a diagnostic evaluation **(Box 6.5.7)**, and treat the underlying condition.

A suggested management protocol is shown in **Table 6.5.4**.

Box 6.5.5: Features of psychogenic nonepileptic events.

- May be precipitated by an emotional event
- All episodes may not be similar
- No history of injury despite fall
- Memory of events during the episode may be present sometimes
- Thrashing movements are side to side rather than flexion extension and appear to vary with time
- Waxing and waning of movements
- Screwing up the eyes when attempts are made to examine then, and uprolling of eyes on attempts to passively open the eyes
- When hand is raised up, it falls on the side rather than on the face
- There is usually no frothing, but saliva may trickle out from the mouth. Voluntary tongue bite may occur
- No urinary incontinence—but may occur occasionally
- Patient appears to periodically be focused and interact with surroundings
- Attack terminates with an action, e.g. sprinkling water on the face, holding legs together, or rubbing hands
- Duration—variable but is often prolonged
- Patient may start crying before, during, or after the attack. Sometimes, tears may just flow

Box 6.5.6: Precipitating factors of seizures/status epilepticus in chronic neurological disorders.

- Febrile illness
- AED (substandard brands/different compositions)
- Sudden discontinuation of AED
- Sleep deprivation/fatigue/emotional upset
- CNS stimulants, such as theophylline

(AED: antiepileptic drugs; CNS: central nervous system)

Follow-up Advice

All parents must be taught home management of seizures with a benzodiazepine (nasal/buccal midazolam, rectal diazepam, or sublingual lorazepam). The child should be put on long-term anticonvulsants if he/she is found to have EEG abnormality, abnormal neuroimaging or he/she is far from medical facility, parents are not educated or confident about home management of seizures.

Prognosis

Mortality is 1–2% in the developed countries. Improvement in the prognosis of convulsive SE is due to more effective and prompter treatment.

Morbidity: Long-term complications include epilepsy, focal neurological deficit, post-status encephalopathy, and mental retardation. The recurrence of SE can occur in up to 13% of the cases.

Febrile Seizures

Definition

These are seizures, which occur between 3 months and 5 years of age, associated with fever, but without evidence of intracranial infection or defined cause for the seizure, and without any history of seizures earlier.

Epidemiology

About 2–4% of all children below the age of 5 years suffer from febrile seizures (FS). Incidence is equal in both sexes. About 25–40% children with FS have a family history of FS. Any

Box 6.5.7: Diagnostic evaluation of status epilepticus.

All cases:
- Blood biochemistry—glucose and electrolytes, and other metabolic parameters
- Ionized and total calcium, especially in children < 2 years
- Blood gases assessment

Associated fever:
- Blood counts
- CSF examination
- Urine examination
- Necessary cultures

Studies on case-to-case basis:
- EEG
- Neuroimaging
- Drug levels

(CSF: cerebrospinal fluid; EEG: electroencephalogram)

Table 6.5.4: Suggested protocol for the management of SE or any patient presenting with acute seizures.

Time	***Action***	
0–5 minutes *Initial observation and management*	*Observe:* • Seizure activity—diagnose SE, assess patient's condition *Airway:* • Suction of secretions • Maintain airway • Administer oxygen *Breathing:* • Bag and mask ventilation; intubate and provide ventilatory support if required (This may be done at any time throughout the management process) *Circulation:* • Start IV line; draw samples for blood glucose and biochemistry. Glucose may be estimated by a glucometer. Start two lines if possible • If hypoglycemic or glycemic status is unknown—IV 25% glucose 2 mL/kg in > 6 months; < 6 months 10% glucose *Monitoring:* • Vital signs monitoring, especially pulse oximetry	
5–15 minutes or *If brought seizing to hospital* *Stabilization, monitoring, and ABC support* *Drug administration* *Start first-line drug:* *Any benzodiazepine* *(Rapid onset of action but short acting)*	*Stabilization and monitoring:* • Continue maintaining airway, breathing, circulation (ABC), and monitoring *Drug administration* *IV line established:* • *Lorazepam* 0.1 mg/kg (maximum 5 mg) at 2 mg/min OR • *Midazolam* at 2 mg/min 0.1–0.2 mg/kg OR • *Diazepam* 0.2 mg/kg (maximum 10 mg) at 5 mg/min • Dose can be repeated once if seizures do not stop after 5 minutes	*No IV access:* • Diazepam rectally 0.5 mg/kg OR • Midazolam intranasally/buccal 0.2–0.4 mg/kg, intramuscular 0.1–0.2 mg/kg OR • Lorazepam sublingual 0.1 mg/kg • Repeat once if seizures do not stop in 5 minutes
15–35 minutes *Monitoring and ABC support* *Drug administration* *Second-line drug* *Phenytoin/fosphenytoin* *(Slower onset of action but longer acting)*	*No response, seizures recur, or initial seizures >10 minutes:* • *PHT* 20 mg/kg @ 1 mg/kg min IV infusion (solution only in saline as PHT is incompatible with dextrose or calcium) OR • *FOS* 20 mg/kg of PE @ 3 mg/kg/min (150 mg/min) (Solution in dextrose or saline) (1.5 mg of FOS = 1 mg of PHT)	• *FOS* IM 20 mg/kg PE. Divide in half and give two separate injections for more rapid action
35–60 minutes *(Established SE)* *Monitoring and ABC support* *Shift to ICU* *Drug administration* *Repeat second-line drug in smaller dose* *Start third-line drug*	*Monitoring and ABC support:* • Continue maintaining ABC, monitoring *Drug administration:* • Repeat *PHT/FOS* 5 mg/kg two doses to maximum dose of 30 mg/kg • Start third-line agent *If ICU available:* • *Midazolam drip* 0.2 mg/kg IV bolus, followed by infusion of 0.2–2 mg/kg/h *If ICU is not available:* (At this point, every institute needs to decide its protocol depending on the facilities available) • Injection Valproate 20 mg/kg bolus over 5 minutes, then maintain at 5 mg/kg/h for 6 hours seizure free; or maintenance dose of 10 mg/kg 6 hourly OR/followed by • Injection Phenobarbitone 20 mg/kg @ 2 mg/kg/min IV OR/followed by • Injection Levetiracetam 20–30 mg/kg @ 5 mg/kg/min infusion IV • At any point when ICU becomes available, midazolam infusion should be started if seizures are continuing PLUS • Give mannitol 0.25 mg/kg/3% saline, if there are features of raised intracranial pressure to reduce cerebral edema	

Contd...

Contd...

Time	*Action*
After 60 minutes (refractory stage) *Monitoring and ABC support* *ICU care* *EEG monitoring* *Drug administration: Induce coma*	• Continue maintaining ABC, monitoring (ventilatory support is required at this stage) • Continuous EEG monitoring if available *Drug administration:* • Continuous infusion of *midazolam* in increasing doses till seizure control OR • *Pentobarbital*: Loading dose: 20 mg/kg over 1 hour, followed by a maintenance infusion of 0.25–5 mg/kg/h OR • *Thiopentone*: Loading dose: 5–10 mg/kg over 2–5 minutes, maintenance 2–10 mg/kg/h OR • *Propofol*: Loading dose 1–3 mg/kg, maintenance 2–10 mg/kg/h

Remember:
- In children, most SE is symptomatic, hence, investigate thoroughly to find etiology
- LP should not be done in a convulsing patient
- There is no place of oral administration of drugs in acute seizures; where IV access is a problem, rectal/buccal/nasal routes should be used
- Most children can be managed successfully with BZP or PHT
- FOS is preferred if cost is not an issue (cost of FOS is three times cost of PHT; 10 kg child—cost of PHT loading approximately ₹ 25 and cost of FOS ₹ 75)
- Start the next drugs only after full loading doses of PHT/PB have been given
- Give the full loading dose in one dose as this is more effective, rather than suboptimal doses many times
- If the child is on AEDs, give half the loading dose of the drug
- For hypotension, inotropes may be required
- Choice of drug depends on cost and availability, as well as the ICU and monitoring facilities. It is better to give valproate rather than phenobarbitone and midazolam rather than pentobarbitone if ventilation facility is not available
- *After seizure control*: Discontinue drug infusion at 12 hours. If seizures recur reinstate drug and try weaning off at 12 hourly intervals
- Continue maintenance doses of PHT and phenobarbitone 12–24 hours after loading dose administration
- End point of treatment: on EEG—no electrographic seizures or burst suppression pattern; if no EEG monitoring is available: clinical seizure control
- Prognosis depends on how fast the seizures are controlled

(AEDs: antiepileptic drugs; BZP: benzodiazepines; EEG: electroencephalogram; ICU: intensive care unit; IM: intramuscular; IV: intravenous; LP: lumbar puncture; SE: status epilepticus; FOS: fosphenytoin; PB: phenobarbital; PE: phenytoin equivalent; PHT: phenytoin)

infection that causes fever can cause FS. In view of the high incidence of family history, children with FS are said to have a genetic predisposition to FS.

Type of Seizures in Febrile Seizures

Febrile seizures are generalized tonic, clonic, or tonic-clonic seizures, occasionally hypotonic, but never myoclonic. If focal seizures occur, they may be unilateral and may be followed by Todd paralysis, suggesting a focal origin of the seizures.

Febrile seizures are of two types—(1) simple and (2) complex **(Table 6.5.5)**.

Table 6.5.5: Types of febrile seizures.

Simple	*Complex*
• <15 minute duration • No focal features s/o focal origin of seizure • Only one attack in one febrile episode	• >15 minutes duration • Focal features present including Todd paralysis • More than one attack in one febrile episode

Investigations

Electroencephalogram is not required for the diagnosis or management of FS, whether simple or complex, even when they are recurrent. An abnormal EEG does not change the management of FS and is therefore not recommended as part of the assessment of a child with FS. Neuroimaging is not required in simple FS but may be done in
- Micro/macrocephaly, a neurocutaneous syndrome or preexisting neurological deficit
- Persistent postictal neurological deficit after the FS
- Recurrent complex FS.

Management

The management of attack of the first FS and subsequent long-term management of FS is shown in **Flowchart 6.5.1**.

Prognosis

- *Risks following FS*: About 35% of all children will have recurrence after the first FS. Management/prevention of recurrences is shown in **Flowchart 6.5.1**.
- *Risk of epilepsy*: Overall risk of epilepsy following FS is 2–5%. Preventing FS does not decrease the risk of epilepsy.
- *Risk of mesial temporal sclerosis (MTS)*: There is a strong association between the development of refractory temporal lobe epilepsy/MTS and complex FS (especially prolonged or focal). However, it remains unclear whether the prolonged FS was the cause of MTS, or whether a

Flowchart 6.5.1: Algorithm for the management of febrile seizures.

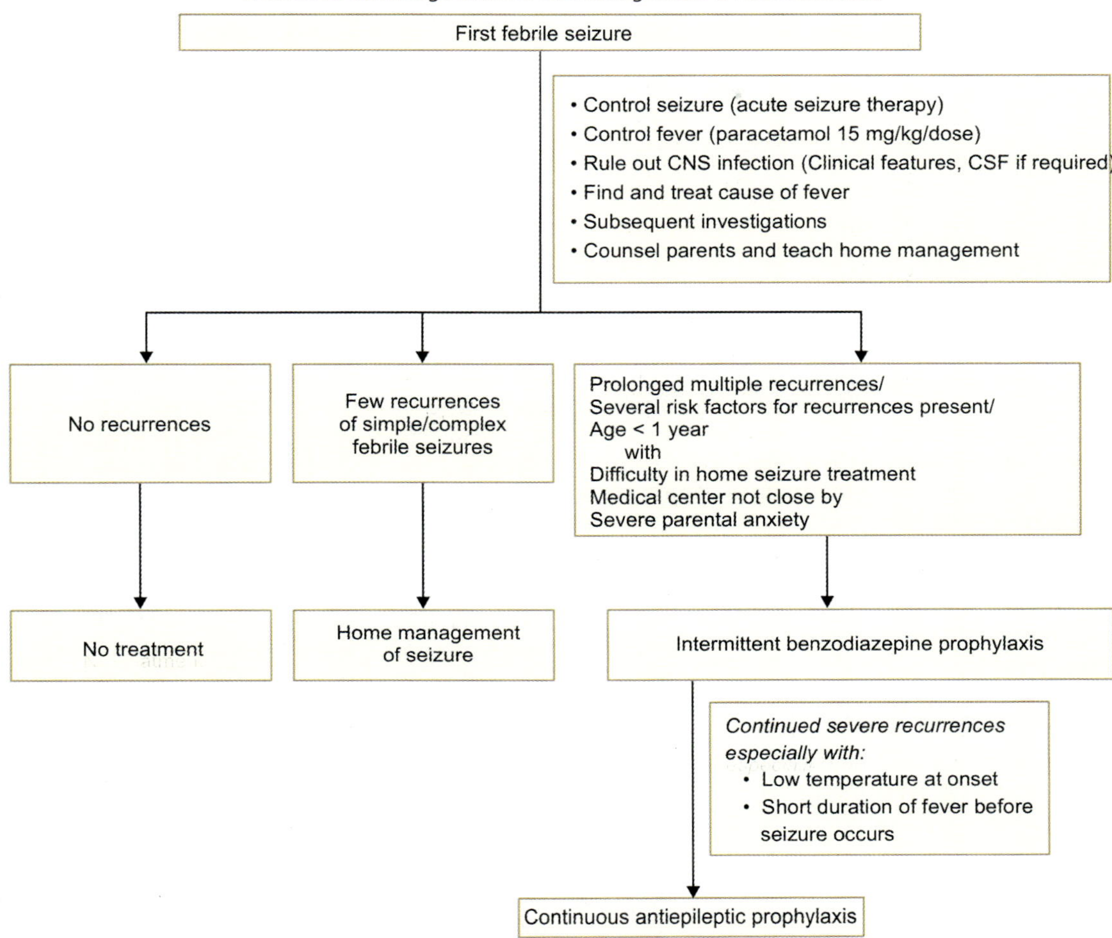

Source: Reproduced with permission from Indian Journal of Pediatrics; 2014.

pre-existing MTS predisposes the child to have prolonged FS.

- *Mental and neurological development* remains normal if it was normal before the onset of FS.
- *Mortality* is not increased in children with FS as compared to the normal population.

West Syndrome

This is an epileptic syndrome with three essential features:

1. Characteristic seizures called *infantile spasms*. The child has a sudden spasm of the body, in which the head, neck, or trunk undergoes a contraction, resulting in either flexion (flexor spasms), but sometimes extension (extensor spasms), or flexion of one part and extension of the other (mixed spasms). The severity of the spasms can be very mild when parents may notice only a mild vibration, to severe resulting in complete folding over of the body. They occur in clusters, and each cluster has many jerks. They are maximum on getting up from sleep or when falling asleep. (Infantile spasms may be used synonymously with West syndrome by many people).
2. *Electroencephalogram findings of hypsarrhythmia*, which is a high voltage completely chaotic EEG, which changes every second, with spikes from multiple foci.
3. *Developmental regression* with the onset of seizures. In many cases, developmental delay pre-exists.

The onset is around 3–4 months of age, and they may remit with treatment or spontaneously by around 2 years age, or they may remain uncontrolled and evolve into other syndromes (Lennox-Gastaut syndrome) or seizure types (tonic, atonic, atypical absences, or myoclonic).

Etiology

Almost any CNS insult can result in infantile spasms **(Table 6.5.2)**. Tuberous sclerosis is often associated with infantile spasms.

Pathophysiology

It is postulated that the hypsarrhythmia and spasms originate from the brainstem.

Investigations

Electroencephalogram is a must to diagnose the syndrome. Magnetic resonance imaging is the imaging modality of choice. It may show CNS malformation, or evidence of an earlier CNS insult. Biochemical investigations are necessary to rule out inborn errors of metabolism.

Treatment

Following options are available:
- *Steroids*: Adrenocorticotrophic hormone or prednisolone.
- *Vigabatrin*: Especially in infantile spasms due to tuberous sclerosis or symptomatic infantile spasms.
- *Other AEDs*: Valproate, benzodiazepines, lamotrigine, topiramate, levetiracetam.
- *Pyridoxine* may be tried in refractory cases, especially when no cause for spasms has been identified.
- *Epilepsy surgery*: Focal cortical lesions should be considered if the child has not shown a response to three trials of different AEDs.

Childhood Absence Epilepsy

This is idiopathic generalized epilepsy with a genetic basis. The onset is at 4–8 years; girls are more affected than boys.

Seizures

Typical absence seizures are seen with the sudden loss of consciousness, associated with automatisms in the form of lip smacking, eye blinking, and hand picking. The seizure terminates suddenly as child resumes activity as if nothing happened. Many attacks occur every day. The attacks can be precipitated by hyperventilation. Child is neurologically normal.

Electroencephalogram

It shows 3-Hz spike-wave discharges on a normal background. Hyperventilation precipitates 3 Hz discharges on EEG and the seizure clinically.

Treatment

Valproate and ethosuximide.

Prognosis

The response to treatment is very good. Seizures remit by 10–12 years of age. However, many children may develop GTCS which are infrequent. Others may develop myoclonic jerks and would then be labeled JME, another epilepsy syndrome of adolescence.

Benign Epilepsy with Centrotemporal Spikes

This is a common childhood focal epilepsy syndrome, of genetic basis. It accounts for 8–20% of pediatric patients with epilepsy. It has a characteristic age of onset, seizure pattern, neurodevelopmental profile, imaging, and electroencephalographic pattern.

Seizures

Age of onset: Mostly around 7–8 years, with a range of 1–14 years.

Seizures occur during nonrapid eye movement sleep, mainly at sleep onset or just before awakening, but in occasional children during waking hours as well. The seizures are infrequent, and a child may have just one or two seizures in a year. The seizures are brief (1–3 minutes), unilateral abnormal sensation and/or motor activity, speech arrest, and drooling, with sometimes retained awareness. The child remains neurodevelopmentally normal.

Electroencephalogram

The EEG shows unilateral or bilateral centrotemporal spikes which are markedly increased during sleep. Neuroimaging is normal.

Treatment

Seizures remit in most children by the age of 15 years, and the EEG normalizes. Many children may not be given treatment, in consultation with the parents, as the seizures are nocturnal and infrequent. If daytime seizures occur or seizures are frequent, or atypical features are seen, then carbamazepine or oxcarbazepine is the drug of choice; or if side effects develop, then levetiracetam or valproate may be used.

MANAGEMENT OF EPILEPSY

Drug Therapy

Decision-making: Should Antiepileptic Drug be Started?

The most important consideration in the management of epilepsy is the possibility of recurrence of the seizure, and drug treatment is considered only once recurrent seizures are confirmed. The decision should be taken after counseling the parents, especially after a first seizure.

Generalized tonic-clonic seizures: They recur in only around 40% of the cases; hence, the first episode of GTCS does not require treatment with long-term AEDs. Exceptions to this rule include situations wherein the first episode of GTCS was SE, where the patient resides in a place, which is far off from medical facility, or parents are overanxious and unable to administer home treatment of acute seizures.

Partial, absence, atonic, and myoclonic seizures: Because of the high rates of recurrence of seizures, treatment is indicated in these cases. Most of the time, the patient will have had multiple seizures when they report.

Choice of Antiepileptic Drugs (Table 6.5.6)

The efficacy of the four first-line AEDs (phenytoin, phenobarbital, carbamazepine, and valproate) in the

Table 6.5.6: Drugs used in treating epilepsy.

Conventional AEDs					
AED	***Indications***	***Preparation***	***Dose***	***Side effects/toxicity***	***Remarks***
PHT	• Focal seizures • GTCS	• *Suspension:* 30 mg/5 mL 125 mg/5 mL • Tablet 100 mg	*5–8 mg/kg/day* In two divided doses	• Gum hypertrophy • Rash • Steven–Johnson syndrome • Toxicity • Ataxia • Nystagmus • Blurring of vision	Younger children require higher doses Since it has a long half-life, the drug may be started with the target dose Make sure about which preparation the patient is using, because of wide variation in the concentration in different preparations Avoid PHT in children if cost is not a factor
Phenobarbitone	• Neonatal seizures • Status epilepticus • Tonic-clonic • Focal seizures • Clonic febrile	• Tablets 30 mg • Syrup 30/5 mL	3–5 mg/kg/day Single dose or two divided doses	• Sedation • Hyperkinetic behavior • Dependence	Younger children require higher doses Since it has a long half-life, the drug may be started with the target dose
Valproate	• Broad-spectrum, effective against any seizure type • Idiopathic generalized epilepsies—childhood absence epilepsy, juvenile myoclonic epilepsy, infantile spasms • Lennox–Gastaut syndrome	• Tablets 200 mg, 400 mg • Syrup 200 mg/5 mL	*20–40 mg/kg/day* Doses up to 80 mg/kg/day may be used provided there are no side effects Three divided doses Sustained release preparation—two divided doses	• Hepatotoxicity • Drowsiness • Lethargy • Weight gain • Hyperammonemia • Teratogenicity	Precaution in children < 1 year
Carbamazepine	• Focal seizures • GTCS	• *Suspension:* 100 mg/5 mL • Tablets 200 mg, 400 mg, 600 mg • Sustained release tablets are also available 200 mg, 500 mg	*10–40 mg/kg/day* Three divided doses	• Rash • Bone marrow depression • Steven–Johnson syndrome	*Start with low dose* *Not* to be used in absence and myoclonic, atonic, and atypical absence seizures The suspension is thick and settles at the bottom; it needs to be shaken thoroughly
Nitrazepam	Myoclonic seizures	Tablets 5 mg, 10 mg	0.5 mg/kg/day two divided doses	• Drowsiness • Hypotonia • Ataxia	

Contd...

Contd...

AED	***Indications***	***Preparation***	***Dose***	***Side effects/toxicity***	***Remarks***
Clonazepam	Myoclonic seizures, atonic, tonic, atypical absence	Tablets 0.5 mg, 2 mg	*0.03–0.1 mg/kg/day* two to three divided doses	• Drowsiness • Hypotonia • Ataxia	
Clobazam	Add-on drug for any seizure type Intermittent use in febrile seizures, or seizures due to known precipitating causes	Tablets 5 mg, 10 mg, 20 mg	*0.5 mg/kg/day* one to two divided doses	*Drowsiness* Hypotonia Ataxia less than other benzodiazepines	
Newer AEDs					
Oxcarbazepine	Same as carbamazepine	• Tablet • 150 mg, 300 mg, 600 mg • Suspension	*8–10 mg/kg/day in two divided doses* Target maintenance—30 mg/kg/day Maximum 50 mg/kg/day	Fewer side effects, such as allergies and bone marrow suppression	Drug level monitoring is not required
Vigabatrin	• *Monotherapy:* Infantile spasms especially those due to tuberous sclerosis • Add-on: Refractory focal seizures	Tablet 500 mg	• *Start with 40 mg/kg/day* • Target maintenance dose 80–100 mg/kg/day • Maximum 120–150 mg/kg/day	• Visual field defects • Blindness	*Not easily available/ manufactured in India* Perimetry/fundoscopy regularly to check for visual complications
Lamotrigine	• Broad-spectrum add-on drug. Multiple seizure types • Monotherapy—refractory focal seizures in children > 12 years • Add-on focal/ generalized epilepsy West syndrome, Broad-spectrum add-on drug for epilepsy with multiple types of seizures, e.g. Lennox–Gastaut syndrome	Tablets 25 mg, 50 mg, 100 mg	• *With valproate: start with 0.15 mg/kg/day* Increase by 0.3 mg/kg/day every 2 weeks till maintenance dose of 1–5 mg/kg/day • *Monotherapy*: 0.3 mg/kg/day Increase by 0.6 mg/kg/day every 2 weeks till maintenance dose of 4.5–7.5 mg/kg/day With enzyme inducing drug start with 0.6 mg/kg/day increase by 1.2 mg/kg/day every 2 weeks till dose of 5–15 mg/kg/day. All doses divided into BID doses	Rash, headache drowsiness	*Use with care with valproate* Level is affected by other AEDs May aggravate myoclonic seizures sometimes
Topiramate	• *Monotherapy: Focal or generalized epilepsy* • Add-on focal/ generalized epilepsy West syndrome, Broad-spectrum add-on drug for epilepsy with multiple types of seizures, e.g. Lennox–Gastaut syndrome	Tablets 25 mg, 50 mg, 100 mg, 200 mg	• Start with 0.5 mg/kg/day • Increase to 5 mg/kg/day • *Maximum dose*: 8 mg/kg/day	• Drowsiness • Ataxia • Metabolic acidosis • Hyperammonemia especially with valproate	Good drug with few drug interactions

Contd...

Contd...

AED	Indications	Preparation	Dose	Side effects/toxicity	Remarks
Levetiracetam	• Add-on for myoclonic seizures • Focal seizures or generalized seizures	Tablets 250 mg, 500 mg, 750 mg	*Start with 10 mg/kg/day* 20 mg/kg/day increase weekly Increase to 60 mg/kg/day In two divided doses	• Headache • Anorexia • Drowsiness • Behavior problems	• Safe drug for children • No drug interactions with other AEDs
Gabapentin	• Add-on for refractory focal epilepsy without generalization • Neuralgias	Tablets 10 mg, 300 mg, 400 mg, 600 mg	*Start with 10–15 mg/kg/day* Target dose < 5 years 40 mg/kg/day >5 years 30 mg/kg/day Three divided doses	• Headache • Anorexia • Drowsiness • Behavior problems	Worsens myoclonus and absences
Rufinamide	Add-on for Lennox–Gastaut syndrome and refractory focal seizures in children > 4 years	• Tablets 200 mg, 400 mg • Suspension 40 mg/mL	Start with 5–10 mg/kg/day in two divided doses with meals, increase weekly by 5–10 mg/kg/day to maximum dose of 45 mg/kg/day	• Drowsiness • Headache • Vomiting • Behavior changes	*Precaution:* In severe hepatic dysfunction, drugs affecting QT interval

(AEDs: antiepileptic drugs; GTCS: generalized tonic-clonic seizures: PHT: phenytoin)

management of common epileptic disorders including generalized tonic-clonic as well as focal seizures is nearly similar.

The decision regarding specific drug depends upon:
- The type of seizures and epileptic syndrome
- Side effects
- Cost
- Lifestyle of the patient.

Monotherapy should be the rule. Polytherapy should be avoided because of drug interactions, and subsequent alteration of drug efficacy.

Starting Antiepileptic Drug

Start an AED in a small dose and build up gradually to an optimal dose. It is best to calculate a target dose, and start with one-third of that and increase by one-third every week till target dose is reached in the case of drugs with short half-lives, such as carbamazepine and valproate. Phenytoin and phenobarbitone may be started with the full optimum dose at starting. If seizures continue, increase gradually till maximum tolerated dose is reached or seizure is controlled.

Treating a Relapse

Restart the same drug in the same dose as it was effective in controlling seizures earlier.

Changing Antiepileptic Drug

Start the second drug in a small dose and build it up to a dose effective in controlling seizures.

Taper off the second drug as above.

Principles of Combination Therapy

- Use drugs with different mechanisms of action.
- Drugs should have large therapeutic index.
- Few side effects.
- Keep in mind drug interactions: Combination may cause increased toxicity or decreased efficacy.

Drug Level Monitoring

Drug levels may be estimated in certain specific situations **(Box 6.5.8)**, but this is not usually required. Drug dosage

Box 6.5.8: Indications of drug level monitoring.

- Uncontrolled seizures despite adequate doses of the correct AED (trough levels)
- Breakthrough seizures
- AED toxicity (peak levels)
- In polytherapy
- Change in AED dose or regimen
- Other systemic disease altering drug metabolism or excretion
- To check compliance

(AED: antiepileptic drug)

Seizure Diary

Name of Child ____________ Age ____________ Sex ____________

Month ____________ Year ____________

Types of seizure (in case the child has multiple types of seizures)

Type 1 Type 2 Type 3 Type 4

AEDs

Name Dose Timing

Date	Type of seizure	Time of onset	Time of control	Precipitating factor (in case any identified)	Routine AED given Yes/No	Any AED given to control acute seizure	Remarks

Instructions:
A separate page has to be made every month
Any skipping of doses/alteration of AED is to be recorded
In case of multiple types of seizures, each seizure type should be assigned a number, and the number noted
Remarks: Anything unusual to be brought to the doctor's notice.

(This diary should preferably be made in the language used locally)

Fig. 6.5.11: A sample seizure diary.

should be decided by clinical control of seizure or appearance of side effects. Drugs whose levels are useful include phenytoin, carbamazepine, phenobarbitone, and valproate.

Follow-up

Parents should be instructed to maintain a seizure diary **(Fig. 6.5.11)** containing the details of seizure type, duration, and frequency. Initial follow-up should be

- After 4 weeks
- If breakthrough seizures occur
- If side effects occur.

Subsequent follow-up should be, if seizures are controlled 3 monthly.

Indications for Hospitalization

- Status epilepticus
- To observe the seizure type
- To distinguish between seizure and NEE
- Serious adverse reactions
- To check compliance.

Duration of Treatment

Treatment is usually from 18 months to 24 months seizure-free period. Increasing duration AED therapy beyond 2 years does not decrease the risk of relapse. Certain other epilepsies may warrant earlier stopping, e.g. benign centrotemporal epilepsy, acute symptomatic epilepsy due to inflammatory granulomas.

Stopping Antiepileptic Drug

Before tapering, the parents must be counseled about the risk of relapse after tapering

- The drug must never be stopped abruptly, it must be tapered gradually over 4–12 weeks.
- If patient is on multiple drugs, taper only one drug first.
- Wait for 1 month after tapering the first drug.
- Taper the next drug.

Referral to Pediatric Neurologist

- Children less than 2 years
- Uncontrolled seizures
- Suspected syndromes.

Counseling

Explain disease: Parents should be informed about the nature of the disease and chances of recurrence, with and without treatment. Some epilepsies are inherently refractory to treatment, and the poor outcome in such cases should be explained to the parents at the outset.

Lifestyle: Patients should be advised to allow the child to continue a normal lifestyle. School teachers should be informed about the nature of disease and should be specifically told not to be biased against these children. Some caution is advocated in possibly dangerous circumstances, such as cycling, swimming, and activities near fire, particularly in the first year of remission.

REFRACTORY EPILEPSY

The child is said to have refractory epilepsy if he continues to have one or more seizures per month, despite a trial of the correct AEDs in adequate doses for 2 years. However, for young infants and children with developing brains, 2 years is too long a period to wait before labeling as refractory, therefore, the time period is now defined as 6 months.

A child with refractory epilepsy needs to be reworked up to:

- Confirm true seizures
- Confirm correct seizure type and epileptic syndrome
- Confirm adequate correct and doses of AED.

Investigations: EEG, MRI, and SPECT are repeated.

Management options include:

- Newer AEDs
- Epilepsy surgery—to remove epileptogenic foci.
- Ketogenic diet—the diet induces ketosis by high-fat and low-carbohydrate diet. Ketosis has an anticonvulsant effect in certain types of epilepsies.
- Vagal nerve stimulation—a device (the impulse generator) is implanted under the skin in the chest with a coil around the vagal nerve. It is activated in the case of an impending seizure by passing a magnet across it. The impulses generated stimulate the vagus nerve and control the seizure.

KEY MESSAGES

- Seizures are the clinical manifestation of abnormal excessive paroxysmal discharges in the brain.
- Epilepsy is at least two unprovoked (or reflex) seizures occurring greater than 24 hours apart, or one unprovoked (or reflex) seizure and a probability of further seizures, such as the general recurrence risk (at least 60%) after two unprovoked seizures, occurring over the next 10 years or the diagnosis of an epilepsy syndrome.
- There are many different types of seizures, depending on the part of the brain involved.
- Investigation of seizures, especially after the first attack, is carried out to find the etiology of the seizure.
- Investigation for epilepsy is carried out to find out the etiology of epilepsy as well as to identify and classify the type of seizures, epilepsy, or epileptic syndrome.
- Attempts must be made to classify the seizure and epilepsy type, as well the epileptic syndrome.
- Though EEG can help in diagnosis as well as classification of epilepsy, it must always be interpreted in the clinical context.
- All attempts must be made to rule out NEEs before starting treatment, as well as when there is poor response to first-line AEDs.
- Cost factor must be considered before deciding on the AED to be started.
- Drug preparations/brands must not be changed in a well-controlled patient.
- Parents and older children must be counseled about all the aspects of epilepsy and its management before starting treatment.
- Caregivers must be taught prehospital management of seizures with a benzodiazepine (rectal diazepam/nasal or buccal midazolam). The procedure must be demonstrated with normal saline before sending the patient home.

BIBLIOGRAPHY

1. Berg AT, Berkovic SF, Brodie MJ, et al. Revised terminology and concepts for organization of seizures and epilepsies: report of the ILAE Commission on Classification and Terminology, 2005-2009. Epilepsia. 2010;51:676-85.
2. Fisher RS, Cross JH, French JA, et al. Operational classification of seizure types by the International League against Epilepsy: position paper of the ILAE Commission for Classification and Terminology. Epilepsia. 2017;58:522-30. France
3. Hausler M, Kluger G. To treat or not to treat (pediatric perspective). In: Auvin S, Sankar R (Eds). Acute Seizures in Children in the Emergency Setting. United Kingdom: John Libbey Eurotext; 2013. pp. 139-46.
4. Ma L, Yung A, Yau E, et al. Clinical guidelines on management of prolonged seizures, serial seizures, and convulsive status epilepticus in children. HK J Pediatr. 2010;15:52-63.
5. Mittal R. Recent advances in febrile seizures. Indian J Pediatr. 2014;81:909-16.
6. National Clinical Guideline Centre. The epilepsies: the diagnosis and management of the epilepsies in adults and children in primary and secondary care. In: Pharmacological Update of the Clinical Guideline 20. London, UK: Royal College of Physicians; National Institute for Health and Clinical Excellence: Guidance; 2012.
7. Passi G (Ed). Epilepsy in children. New Delhi: Jaypee Brother Medical Publishers (P) Ltd.; 2014.
8. Scheffer IE, Berkovic SE, Capovilla G, et al. (2014). The organization of the epilepsies: report of the ILAE Commission on Classification and Terminology. [online] Available from: <http://www.ilae.org/visitors/centre/Documents/OrganizationEpilepsy.pdf> [Accessed October, 2018].
9. Scheffer IE, Berkovic S, Capovilla G, et al. ILAE classification of the epilepsies: position paper of the ILAE Commission For Classification and Terminology. Epilepsia. 2017;58:512-21.
10. Shinnar S, O'Dell C. Treatment decisions in childhood seizures. In: Pellock JM, Bourgeois BFD, Dodson WE, Nordli DR, Jr., Sankar R (Eds). Pediatric Epilepsy—Diagnosis and Therapy. 3rd edition. New York, NY: Demos Medical Publishing; 2008. pp. 403-12.

6.6 Headache and Migraine

Munni Ray

INRODUCTION

Headaches in children and adolescents are common, and a steady alarming increase in their incidence has been attributed to the rapidly changing untoward lifestyle habits.

EPIDEMIOLOGY

This common neurological disorder has both a high incidence and prevalence, and the burden of this disease impacts not only the child but also the family including school performance, social life, mental health, and quality of life.

Bille reported that 75% of children complain of a significant headache by the age of 15 years. Migraine was reported in 3.9% of the children aged 7–15 years, which increased from 1.7% in 7-year old to 5.3% in 15-year old. It was more common in boys aged less than 7 years, whereas in adolescents, girls had a higher prevalence.

ETIOPATHOGENESIS

Headaches in children can either be primary such as migraine or tension-type headaches (TTH) or secondary. Secondary headaches have a cause and effect association with a specific etiology, whereas primary headaches are intrinsic to the nervous system.

The etiopathogenesis of the different types of headaches in children is dependent upon the five different temporal patterns of headaches. The primary headaches are of generally the acute recurrent variety such as migraine, whereas the chronic nonprogressive types are TTH and chronic daily headaches. The acute and the chronic progressive types of headaches occur generally due to secondary causes, and they are primarily present in the emergency. The list of etiologies, which present as secondary headaches, is provided in **Table 6.6.1**. The major pathophysiologic basis of life-threatening causes of acute or chronic progressive headaches is raised intracranial pressure.

The biological basis of the primary headaches at a molecular level is yet uncertain and different etiopathogenetic theories such as neurovascular theory, release of neuropeptides, and channelopathies have been cited.

Table 6.6.1: Secondary causes of acute headache.

Causes	*Proportion of disease contribution to acute headache in emergency room (%)*
Viral illness	40–70
Sinusitis	1–6
Post-traumatic headache	5–7
Meningitis or encephalitis	2–9
Streptococcal pharyngitis	5–10
Brain tumor	2–3
Postictal headache	1–4
Intracranial hemorrhage	1
Sinus venous thrombosis	<<1
Ischemic stroke	<<1
Intracranial cyst rupture	<<1
Ventriculoperitoneal shunt malfunction	<<1

CLINICAL FEATURES

The diagnosis of pediatric headaches is challenging as children have limitations in describing their symptoms. Moreover, one individual may have more than one disorder. An orderly approach is required for the proper diagnosis. Crucial elements include a thorough history (based on the information given by the child primarily and then by the parents) supplemented by general, neurological, and psychological evaluation, as well as laboratory testing and neuroimaging in selected patients.

The headache history is crucial, and the questions enquired are highlighted in **Box 6.6.1**. The "red flags," which suggest the possibility of secondary headache, are first or worst headache ever in life, recent headache onset, increasing severity or frequency, occipital location, headache awakening from sleep associated with severe vomiting, and that associated with straining. Once these features are identified, the pediatrician must conduct the work-up indicated and thereby diagnose any secondary headache disorder that is present.

In the absence of secondary headache, the clinician proceeds to diagnosing a primary headache disorder. If the headache is atypical or difficult to classify, the possibility of secondary headache should be reconsidered.

Box 6.6.1: Helpful questions for obtaining headache history.

- When did the headache begin?
- How did the headache begin?
- What is the temporal pattern of the headache?
- What is the headache frequency?
- How long does the headache typically last?
- Do the headaches happen at any time or circumstance?
- Is there an aura or prodrome?
- Where is the pain?
- What is the pain like?
- Are there any associated symptoms?
- What do you do during the headache?
- Would I know you had a headache if I saw you?
- What makes the headache better or worse?
- Are there any symptoms between headaches?
- Are there any other health problems?
- Are you taking medications?
- Is there a family history of headaches?
- What do you think is causing the headaches?

Useful strategies to help improve headache diagnosis in children might be the following:

- Take history with enough time and patience, and with age-appropriate terminology.
- Ask the patient (assisted by parents) to keep an appropriate headache diary (e.g. depicting headache characteristics, associated symptoms, and triggers) over a period of weeks and the degree of disability as well as medication usage.

The assessment of headache severity in children should be done using combination of pain rating scale and visual analog scale according to age and cognitive levels of subjects.

PHYSICAL EXAMINATION

The general examination should include vital signs, growth parameters, head circumference, skin examination, and ophthalmological assessment. Although a frequent parental concern, headaches caused by poor visual acuity are easily identified by most patients. In most patients, serious medical and neurologic disorders can be excluded by a detailed history and examination. Children with headaches related to serious pathology have demonstrable neurologic signs, and the three important features are: (1) Papilledema, (2) Sensorial alteration, (3) Paralysis.

Headache Examination

This includes examination of:

- Cervical spine
- Vascular evaluation for skull bruits
- Ears
- Temporomandibular joint
- Nerves including supraorbital nerves, occipital nerves, and examination of nerves IX through XII
- Eyes
- Sinuses
- Teeth

Psychological Examination

Assessment of psychosocial background is of immense importance. The evaluation process should be completed with scales for depression, anxiety, etc., and family interview. The impact of the headache on a child's life must be part of the evaluation using Pediatric Quality of Life 4.0 and Pediatric Migraine Disability Assessment (PedMIDAS).

MODALITIES OF DIAGNOSIS

Diagnostic studies are seldom required unless risk factors are identified. Nonetheless, many families and physicians feel compelled to embark on investigations for children with headaches, but unwarranted investigations may be counterproductive as it can undermine ones attempts at reassurance. Routine laboratory studies and performance of lumbar puncture are not recommended. If the history or physical examination raises concern about meningitis or encephalitis, a lumbar puncture will be necessary. In headaches caused by pseudotumor cerebri, the lumbar puncture may be both diagnostic and therapeutic. Electroencephalography is not indicated as it is unlikely to determine an etiology or distinguish migraine from other types of headaches. Neuroimaging on a routine basis is not indicated in children with recurrent headaches and a normal neurologic examination. Physicians should consider imaging in children with an abnormal neurologic examination or in whom red flag alerts such as associated seizures, a recent onset of severe headaches, a change in headache type, or associated features to suggest neurologic dysfunction are present. The routine use of neuroimaging may lead to the discovery of incidental benign abnormalities, which may cause undue alarm, and headaches may wrongfully be attributed to these incidental findings. In the emergency, setting a computed tomography of the head is preferred and a plain scan is highly sensitive in acute hemorrhage, whereas magnetic resonance imaging is the investigation of choice otherwise.

Once the secondary headache disorders are ruled out, the primary headaches, such as migraine, TTH, etc. are diagnosed as per criteria laid down by the International Classification of Headache Disorders (ICHD) in 2004 **(Box 6.6.2)**.

TREATMENT

The mainstay of treatment of secondary headaches is to manage the underlying cause. The priority of a pediatrician managing a child with primary headaches is to reassure confidently that the headaches are not caused by a life-threatening etiology. Management of pediatric primary headaches is complex, and nonpharmacological therapy is the first line of treatment **(Flowchart 6.6.1)**. Maintaining a headache diary may be remarkably therapeutic. Noting

Box 6.6.2: International Classification of Headache Disorders II criteria for pediatric migraine without aura and episodic tension-type headaches.

Criteria for Pediatric Migraine without Aura

A. At least five attacks fulfilling criteria B–D below
B. Headache attacks lasting 1–72 hours
C. *Headache has at least two of the following characteristics*:
   - Unilateral location may be bilateral, frontotemporal (not occipital)
   - Pulsing quality
   - Moderate or severe pain intensity
   - Aggravation by or causing avoidance of routine physical activity (e.g. walking and climbing stairs)
D. *During the headache, at least one of the following*:
   - Nausea, vomiting, or both
   - Photophobia and phonophobia, which may be inferred from behavior
E. Not attributed to another disorder

Criteria for Episodic Tension-type Headaches

1. At least 10 episodes fulfilling 2–4
2. Headache lasting 30 minutes to 7 days
3. *Two or more of the following*:
   a. Pressing or tightening quality
   b. Mild-to-moderate severity
   c. Bilateral
   d. Not aggravated by routine activity
4. *Both of the following:*
   a. No nausea or vomiting
   b. Phonophobia or photophobia is absent

triggers in the diary and their careful avoidance is important. Other approaches include appropriate sleep hygiene, regular physical activity, and limiting caffeine. Behavioral therapies such as relaxation techniques and biofeedback have shown good efficacy. Psychological interventions aim to reduce psychosocial stressors, provide more social support for families, and help the patient to improve his coping abilities. These techniques are useful in children with both migraine and TTH.

Pharmacologic approaches to migraine include rescue and prophylactic medications. Both ibuprofen (10 mg/kg) and acetaminophen (15 mg/kg) are safe and efficacious as rescue medications in managing acute attacks when given early and in appropriate doses. Parents should be cautioned to limit the use of these drugs to a maximum of 2-3 times per week to avoid medication overuse headaches. Nasal sumatriptan is the only serotonin receptor antagonist, which has been useful in managing acute headaches in adolescents. For prophylaxis of migraine in children, the recommended drugs are propranolol (2–4 mg/kg/day), flunarizine (5 mg/day), valproate (20–40 mg/kg/day) and topiramate (1–10 mg/kg/day), cyproheptadine (0.25–1.5 mg/kg/day), and amitriptyline (10–25 mg/day). These drugs are to be used in those who have frequent attacks (1-2 attacks per week) or disabling headaches (PedMIDAS score > 30) with the aim to lower the frequency to 1-2 attacks per month and disability for at least 4–6 months.

PROGNOSIS

Almost half of childhood headaches persist into adulthood, and long-term follow-up studies have indicated that there is a tendency to transform from one subtype of headache to the other.

PREVENTION

As migraine is a disorder with genetic basis, prevention of development is unlikely, although use of biobehavioral techniques as well as prophylactic medications may help in reducing attacks.

RECENT ADVANCES

International Classification of Headache Disorders II has improved the identification of childhood migraines. Recent studies have highlighted the presence of osmophobia as an important associated feature in children with migraines and presence of cutaneous allodynia is under evaluation. Use of headache drawings in evaluation of children has greatly improved the diagnostic aspect. Identification of comorbidities in childhood headaches, such as obesity, epilepsy, allergy, emotional and sleep disorders, etc. influences management choices, overall outcome, and response. Almotriptan has been recently recommended for treatment of headaches in adolescents.

Flowchart 6.6.1: Practice guidelines for evaluation and management of a child with headaches.

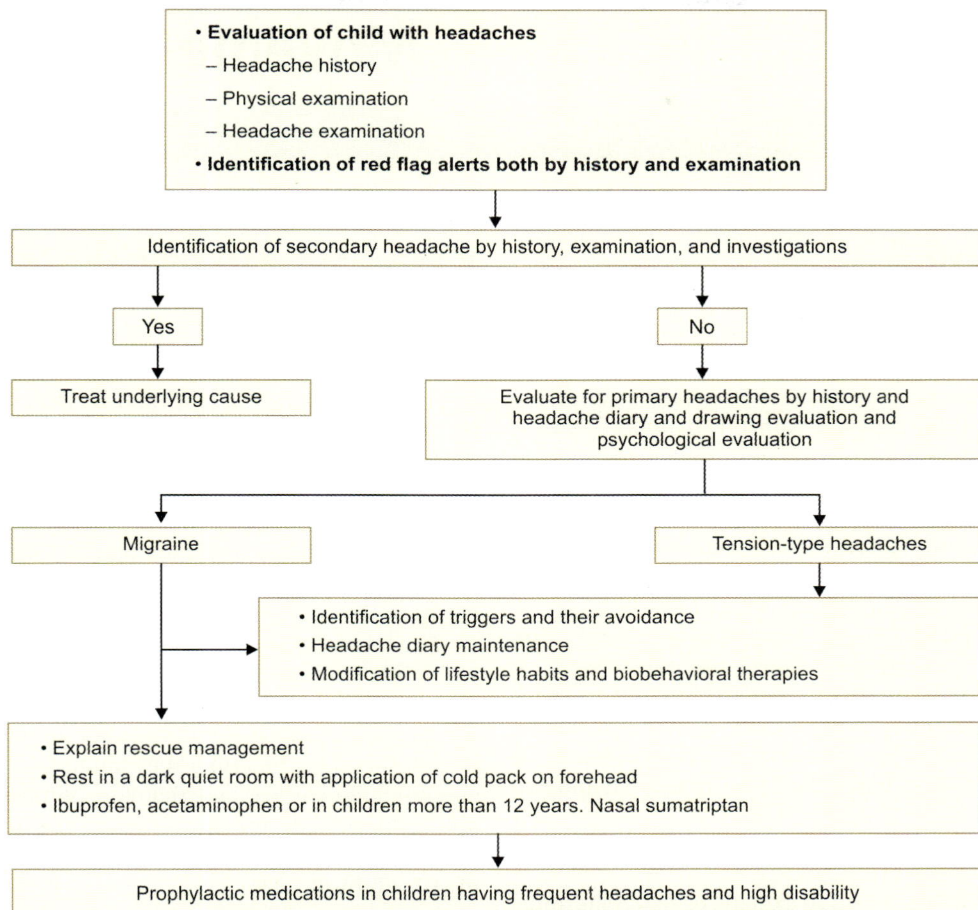

KEY MESSAGES

- Pediatric headaches are common.
- Secondary headaches are usually present in emergency, and they should be promptly diagnosed and managed.
- Majority of recurrent headaches are primary in nature.
- Appropriate identification by using headache history, clinical examination, and headache diary analysis helps in appropriate diagnosis using ICHDII.
- Biobehavioral therapy along with pharmacological managements is to be used to reduce school absenteeism, headache-induced disability, and improve quality of life.

BIBLIOGRAPHY

1. Bille BS. Migraine in school children. A study of the incidence and short-term prognosis, and a clinical psychological and electroencephalographic comparison between children with migraine and matched controls. Acta Paediatr. 1962;51: 16-151.
2. Brenner M, Oakley C, Lewis D. The evaluation of children and adolescents with headache. Curr Pain Headache Rep. 2008;12:361-6.
3. Headache Classification Subcommittee of the International Headache Society. The International classification of headache disorders, 2nd edition. Cephalalgia. 2004;24:9-160.
4. Hershey AD. Recent developments in pediatric headache. Curr Opin Neurol. 2010;23:249-53.
5. Kienbacher C, Wöber C, Zesch HE, et al. Clinical features, classification and prognosis of migraine and tension type headache in children and adolescents: a long term follow-up study. Cephalalgia. 2006;26:820-30.
6. Lewis DW, Ashwal S, Dahl G, et al. Practice parameter: evaluation of children and adolescents with recurrent headache: report of the Quality Standards Subcommittee of the American Academy of Neurology and the Practice Committee of the Child Neurology Society. Neurology. 2002;59:490-8.
7. Termine C, Ozge A, Antonaci F, et al. Overview of diagnosis and management of paediatric headache. Part II: therapeutic management. J Headache Pain. 2011;12:25-34.

6.7 Movement Disorders

Anoop Verma

INTRODUCTION

Pediatric movement disorders (MDs) are commonly encountered clinical entities day-to-day practice. These disorders may represent an underlying genetic disorder, a metabolic disorder, or a hypoxic-ischemic insult during the perinatal period. There is growing concern for both consensus definitions and ongoing research into the causes, clinical spectrum, and management of the pediatric MDs. Treating these cases is largely based on the experience rather than evidence because of the paucity of literature. Hope in near future we can provide better diagnosis and care for children with MDs.

A MD is typically defined as dysfunction in the implementation of appropriate targeting and velocity of intended movements, dysfunction of posture, the presence of abnormal involuntary movement, or the performance of normal appearing movements at inappropriate or unintended times. Movement disorders are divided into two major categories:

1. "*Hyperkinetic MD*", e.g. tics, chorea, ballismus, dystonia, myoclonus, stereotypies, and tremors.
2. "*Hypokinetic MD*" referred as akinetic or rigid syndrome, e.g. parkinsonism. These are rare in children.

When faced with an MD, some key questions need to be asked:

- Is the pattern of movements normal or abnormal?
- Are the movements hyperkinetic or hypokinetic?
- Are the movements paroxysmal or continuous?
- Has the MD changed over time?
- Can the movements be suppressed voluntarily? (e.g. tics)
- Is the abnormal movement heralded by a premonitory sensation or urge?
- Is there any clinical clue of focal neurological deficit or systemic disease?
- Is there any family history of similar disorder? (e.g. dominant or recessive)
- Is there any history of hypoxic-ischemic encephalopathy or neonatal hyperbilirubinemia? (e.g. athetosis and dystonia)
- Is there any history of precipitating factors? (e.g. drugs, infections, or muscular exercise)
- Does the MD abate with sleep?

TYPES AND PATHOPHYSIOLOGY OF MOVEMENT DISORDERS

A qualitative appreciation is required to diagnose MDs. Various types of MDs and their brief descriptions of pathophysiology are given in **Table 6.7.1**.

Most MDs have their origin in the basal ganglia dysfunction, which is based on their organization and function within the complex information circuits of the brain, although virtually the entire nervous system is engaged in motor control, e.g. upper motor neuron, lower motor neuron, cerebellar circuitry, basal ganglia circuitry, motor association cortex, and sensory system.

The basal ganglia consist of five large subcortical nuclei, e.g. caudate nucleus, putamen, globus pallidus, substantia nigra, and subthalamic nuclei. They participate in controlling the movement but do not have either direct input or output with the spinal cord; rather they interact with the prefrontal and premotor cortices and, therefore, influence the planning and initiation of the movement. The disease process selectively involves these structures resulting in various types of MDs **(Table 6.7.1)**.

APPROACH TO DIAGNOSIS

- The first step is to categorize the abnormal movement into one of the common types **(Table 6.7.1)**. Examine whether the abnormal movements interfere with voluntary movements.
- Tics and stereotypies are distinct motor behaviors, e.g. limb chorea, facial tics, other oral movements of lip and tongue biting can be present in neuroacanthocytosis. Tics and obsessive-compulsive disorders can be associated with pediatric autoimmune neuropsychiatric disorders associated with streptococcal infections. Repetitive stereotyped hand movements, such as wringing and/or repeatedly putting hands into the mouth, occur in Rett syndrome.
- Fixed muscle contractures, jerks, and spasms seen after peripheral trauma need to be distinguished from dystonia and myoclonus.
- The neurological examination needs to be tailored to the clinical history.

Table 6.7.1: Types of movement disorders, phenomenology, and anatomical correlate.		
Movement disorder	***Brief description***	***Anatomical correlate***
Chorea	Abrupt, large amplitude involuntary movements of proximal more than distal muscles	Contralateral caudate nucleus, putamen, striatum
Athetosis	Slower writhing irregular movements predominantly distal	Striatum, subthalamic nucleus
Dystonia	Co-contraction of agonist and antagonist, which cause twisting and repetitive movements or abnormal postures	Contralateral striatum, putamen, thalamus
Ballismus	Violent flinging movements of entire limb	Contralateral subthalamic nucleus, thalamus
Myoclonus	An extremely brief contraction of a muscle group leading to involuntary purposeless jerk of affected limb	Cerebral or cerebellar cortex and dentate nucleus
Ataxia	Inability to control movements and typically is caused by cerebellar dysfunction	Cerebellum
Tics	Rapid, involuntary, briefly suppressible, repetitive, nonrhythmic, and stereotyped movements. Simple motor tic involves only one group of muscles, such as eye blinking, head jerking, or shoulder shrugging. Complex motor tics are typically more purposeful appearing and of a longer nature. They may involve a cluster of movements and appear coordinated	Unknown
Tremor	Rhythmic oscillation about a certain point or position involving one or more body part	Brainstem, cerebellum, spinal cord
Stereotypies	Repetitive, patterned involuntary movements that have no apparent function	Unknown

- For MDs that are situation specific, home videos can provide useful information.
- The most common MDs seen are tics, dystonia, and chorea. Myoclonus is commonly associated with epilepsy syndromes.

Differences from Epilepsy

- Movement disorders disappear during sleep, seizures persist or may worsen.
- Movement disorders have more stereotyped appearance and are more persistent than seizures.
- Seizures are often characterized by the loss of consciousness or awareness whereas MD is not.
- Seizures are accompanied by epileptiform activity in electroencephalography whereas MD is not.

Disorders with Chorea as the Predominant Manifestation

Sydenham's Chorea (Chorea Minor or Saint Vitus Dance)

This is a disease characterized by rapid, uncoordinated jerking movements affecting primarily the face, feet, and hands. It results from childhood infection with Group A beta hemolytic *Streptococcus* and is reported to occur in 20–30% of patients with acute rheumatic fever.

The other causes of chorea in childhood are cerebral palsy, drug-induced chorea, systemic lupus erythematosus, and antiphospholipid antibody syndrome.

Sydenham's chorea is treated with penicillin prophylaxis up to the age of 21 years to prevent a recurrence, even if the patients lack the signs and symptoms of rheumatic fever. Valproic acid is the first drug of choice. Carbamazepine can also be used. Dopamine-receptor-blocking drugs, such as tetrabenazine and antipsychotics, are indicated only if other medications fail.

Disorders with Tremor as the Predominant Manifestation

Metabolic Causes

Tremors may be the most prominent manifestation of various metabolic causes (Wilson disease and phenylketonuria, hypoglycemia, hyperthyroidism, deficiencies of magnesium and thiamine). It is a feature of many neurodegenerative disorders or cerebellar disease.

Familial Essential Tremor

It is a slowly progressive neurological disorder characterized by a tremor of the arms or hands that is apparent during voluntary movements, such as eating and writing.

Drugs and Toxins

It may also manifest as toxicity to drugs and toxins (amphetamines, caffeine, corticosteroids, and alcoholism and tobacco withdrawal).

The therapy for tremors is based primarily on the etiology. Children with essential tremor often do not require treatment, since their disability is minimal. The usual options are topiramate and beta-blockers.

Disorders with Dystonia as the Predominant Manifestation

Primary Dystonia

Early-onset dystonia can be broadly divided into two major categories: (1) Dystonia-1 (DYT1) early onset generalized dystonia and (2) Non-DYT1 early-onset dystonia. The distinction is that DYT1 generalized dystonia is known to be caused by a specific mutation in the *DYT1* gene. However, not all primary generalized dystonia that begin in childhood are caused by this specific mutation. These forms are simply referred to as non-DYT1 generalized dystonia.

DYT1 dystonia is primary. Non-DYT1 dystonia may be primary or secondary.

Other names to describe DYT1 generalized dystonia include Oppenheim's dystonia, primary torsion dystonia, early-onset dystonia, childhood-onset dystonia, and idiopathic torsion dystonia. Lesser used terms include dystonia musculorum deformans.

Other names to describe non-DYT1 generalized dystonia include primary torsion dystonia, early-onset dystonia, childhood-onset dystonia, and idiopathic torsion dystonia. Lesser used terms include dystonia musculorum deformans.

Historically, early-onset generalized dystonia has also been referred to as idiopathic torsion dystonia and dystonia musculorum deformans.

Idiopathic torsion dystonia (DYT1 dystonia): It is the most common form of primary dystonia and is inherited as an autosomal dominant trait. The typical phenotype consists of childhood onset limb dystonia, which gradually progresses over subsequent years to become generalized, affecting trunk and limb muscles. The diagnosis rests on clinical presentation with normal perinatal history, normal intelligence, and no biochemical abnormalities. Confirmation is usually by genetic analysis.

Dopa-responsive dystonia (DRD): This is also known as DYT5 dystonia, Segawa syndrome. The most important type is DYT5. Segawa disease has a characteristic diurnal variation. Symptoms improve on awakening and are worse later in the day. Although uncommon, the importance of DRD lies in its dramatic and sustained response to levodopa. The clinical presentation is like DYT1 dystonia, with childhood limb onset dystonia and gradual progression to generalized dystonia, with mild parkinsonism in some patients. Confirmation is by mutation analysis.

Secondary Dystonia

There are several causes of secondary dystonia particularly infections, trauma, metabolic disorders, and degenerative disorders; these must be considered in appropriate settings.

Tic Disorders

Simple Motor Tics

Tics are possibly the most common primary MDs in childhood. About 5% and 24% of school children have a single transient tic that may last from several weeks to a few months and then disappear spontaneously. Simple motor tics are typically sudden, brief, and meaningless movements that usually involve only one group of muscles, such as eye blinking, head jerking, or shoulder shrugging.

Tourette Syndrome

It is an inherited neuropsychiatric disorder with onset in childhood. It is characterized by multiple physical (motor) tics and at least one vocal (phonic) tic. These tics characteristically wax and wane, can be suppressed temporarily, and are preceded by a premonitory urge.

Parents are to be educated and reassured. Treatment of tics is needed only when they cause any functional impairment. Clonidine is considered as the first-line medication. Other drugs that can be used are olanzapine, risperidone, and metoclopramide. The current strategy in the treatment of Tourette syndrome is behavior modification therapy.

Miscellaneous Disorders

Stereotypies and Self-injurious Behavior

Some stereotypies are simple rhythmic movements, e.g. body rocking, waving, flapping the hands, staring, and touching, whereas others, such as head banging, can be self-injurious.

Lesch–Nyhan Syndrome

Lesch–Nyhan syndrome, an X-linked recessive disorder of purine metabolism, is characterized by mental retardation, spasticity, extrapyramidal symptoms, and intense self-mutilation (e.g. lip biting) with intact pain sensation. These patients have elevated uric acid levels. The self-mutilating behavior improves with carbidopa-levodopa, naltrexone, and serotonin reuptake inhibitors.

Drug-induced Movement Disorders

Acute Dystonic Reactions (Figs. 6.7.1A and B)

Acute dystonic reactions can be induced by dopamine depleting drugs, e.g. antihistamines, antipsychotics, antiemetics (domperidone, metoclopramide, or prochlorperazine) tetrabenazine, and antimalarials. The dystonia usually occurs on the first day of drug exposure and affects the head, neck, and trunk muscles with neck retraction, tongue protrusion, trismus, and oculogyric crisis. It is treated with anticholinergics (benztropine) or benzodiazepines.

Akathisia

Akathisia (restlessness) is induced by antidepressants, antipsychotics, antihistamines, calcium channel blockers, carbamazepine, or metoclopramide. If the offending drug cannot be stopped, propranolol or benzodiazepines may alleviate the symptoms.

Chorea

Chorea can result from the use of phenytoin, lamotrigine, amphetamines, antihistamines, antipsychotics, and metoclopramide.

Tardive Syndromes

Tardive syndromes are a group of delayed onset abnormal involuntary MDs induced by drugs. Tardive dyskinesia has a slow onset and characterized by rhythmic involuntary movements of tongue, face, and jaw usually after long antipsychotic drug use. Tardive dystonia (usually of the face and neck), akathisia (during neuroleptic or even afterward), tics (tardive tourettism), myoclonus (of the neck or upper arms), and tremor can also result from chronic antipsychotic use.

Tremor

Tremor may be caused by many drugs such as amphetamine, albuterol, terbutaline, caffeine, carbamazepine, valproic acid, ephedrine, and pseudoephedrine. It is reversible once the cause has been removed.

MANAGEMENT (TABLE 6.7.2)

Chorea: For symptomatic treatment, tetrabenazine, pimozide, benzodiazepines, haloperidol, or valproate can be used. All children with Sydenham's chorea are to be treated as if they had acute rheumatic fever with penicillin for 10 days to eradicate active streptococcal infection and prophylactic long-acting penicillin therapy until a minimum age of 21. Steroid treatment has also been shown to be of benefit. In lupus-associated chorea, the control of the underlying disease with high-dose steroids is recommended.

Idiopathic torsion dystonia: Management is usually ineffective. High-dose anticholinergic drug therapy (trihexyphenidyl, 30 mg/day) may be useful. Other drugs used are baclofen, benzhexol, carbamazepine, and benzodiazepines. All juvenile onset dystonic patients deserve a trial of L-dopa. Botulinum toxin may be used in focal dystonia.

Dopa-responsive dystonia: It is managed by small doses of levodopa, which rapidly and completely relieve the symptoms.

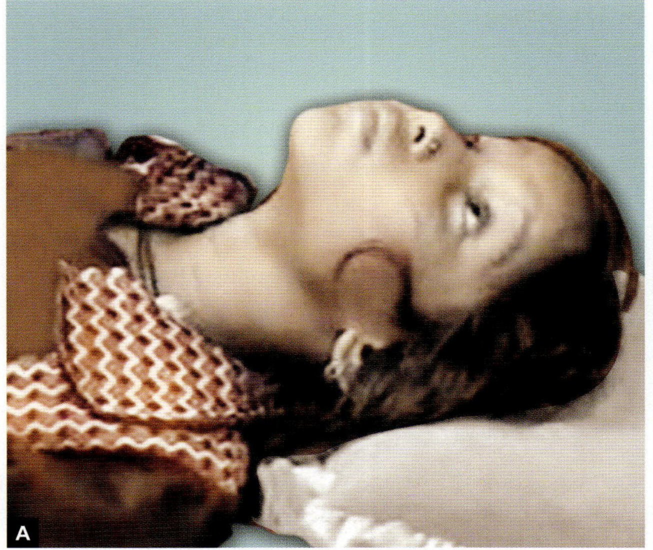

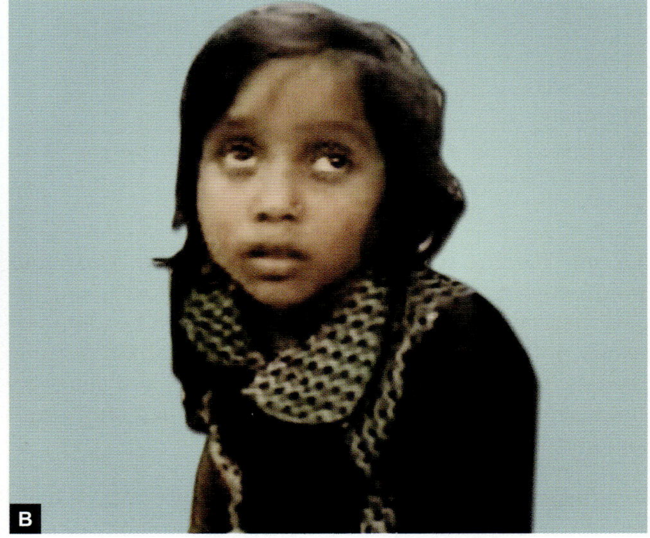

Figs. 6.7.1A and B: Acute dystonic reaction: (A) Neck retraction (B) Oculogyric crisis caused by metoclopramide.

Table 6.7.2: Summary of drugs used in movement disorders.

Drug	*Dosage*	*Precautions*	*Indications*
Pimozide	• 0.05 mg/kg/day • Increase gradually up to 0.2 mg/kg/day, maximum 10 mg/day	• Prolonged QT interval • Cardiac arrhythmia	Gilles de Tourette syndrome
Haloperidol	• *Initial*: 0.25–0.5 mg/day • Increase by 0.25–0.5 mg weekly • Maximum 0.15 mg/kg/day	Liver, kidney disease	• Choreiform movement • Epilepsy • Rheumatic chorea • Thyrotoxicosis • Hemiballismus • Gilles de Tourette syndrome
Tetrabenazine	• Dosage for children not established • Suggested half of adult dosage • Adult dosage 12.5 mg bid • Increment of 12.5 mg every 5–7 days • Maximum 3 mg/kg/day	• Pregnancy • Lactation • Depression • Patient on levodopa, reserpine	• Chorea • Hemiballismus • Myoclonus • Buccolingual dyskinesia • Certain dystonia
Trihexyphenidyl	• Begin with 0.5 mg/day < 4 years, 1 mg/day > 4 years • Increase 1 mg every 5 days till benefit or side effect	• Glaucoma • Sick sinus syndrome • Cardiac failure • Tachycardia	• ITD • Myoclonus • Drug-induced MD • Torticollis
L-Dopa, carbidopa	Start 1 mg/kg/day; up to 5 mg/kg/day	• Hypersensitivity • The use of monoamine oxidase inhibitors • Narrow angle glaucoma	• DRD • Dystonia • Parkinson state
Carbamazepine	• *Less than 6 years of age*: 5 mg/kg/day oral; may increase every 5–7 days by 5 mg/kg/day • *6–12 years*: Initially 10 mg/kg/day; increase by 5 mg/day at weekly intervals • *Usual dose*: 10–30 mg/kg/day	• Porphyria • Hepatic failure • MAOs	• Chorea • Athetosis • Ballismus • Paroxysmal kinesigenic dyskinesia
Sodium valproate	• Start 5–10 mg/kg/day, up to 15–30 mg/kg/day • Above 20 kg–400 mg/day	• Liver disease • SLE • Porphyria	• Chorea • Athetosis • Ballismus
Clonazepam	• *Initial*: 0.01–0.03 mg/kg/day in 2–3 to divided doses • Increase 0.25–0.5 mg/day every 3–5 days • Maximum dose 0.2 mg/kg/day	Hypersensitivity to benzodiazepine	• ITD • Torticollis • Myoclonus • Startle syndrome
Propranolol	1–2 mg/kg/day	Avoid in cardiac failure, asthma	Tremors

(DRD: dopa-responsive dystonia; ITD: idiopathic torsion dystonia; MAOs: monoamine oxidase inhibitors; MD: movement disorders; SLE: systemic lupus erythematosus)

Tics and Tourette syndrome: Tics and Tourette syndrome do not require treatment as their natural history is one of exacerbation and remission. The parents must be told that tics are not a sign of progressive neurological illness and are made worse by stress and will diminish when ignored. The drug treatment in selected cases includes pimozide, clonidine, fluphenazine, and haloperidol.

Drug-induced movement disorders: Drug-induced MD is best managed by stopping the offending drug and supportive care. The acute drug-induced dystonia are usually self-limiting or respond to treatment with benztropine. **Table 6.7.2** shows a summary of dugs commonly used in the management of MDs.

KEY MESSAGES

- Establishing phenomenology is the key to diagnosis to MD.
- Every type of MD has its own characteristic, and combinations of them are also not rare, try to find the dominant one and existence of others also.

- Presence of neurological and non-neurological causes of abnormal movement, epilepsy, and epilepsy mimic also must be considered.
- After having reached to clinical-based MD type, proceed for diagnostic work-up to locate the cause behind and accordingly plan for treatment.
- Home videos can aid diagnosis in paroxysmal MDs.

BIBLIOGRAPHY

1. Fenichel GM. Movement disorders, Chapter 14. In: Clinical Pediatric Neurology, 4th edition. Philadelphia: WB Saunders Company; 2001. p. 281
2. Fernandez-Alvarez E. Movement disorders in children: recent advances in management. Indian J Pediatr. 2009;76:531-6.
3. Grosset KA, Grosset DG. Prescribed drugs and neurological complications. J Neurol Neurosurg Psychiatry. 2004;75(Suppl. 3):iii2-8.
4. Jarman PR, Wood NW. Genetics of movement disorders and ataxia. J Neurol Neurosurg Psychiatry. 2002;73 (suppl 2):II22-6.
5. Nygaard TG, Wooten GF. Dopa-responsive dystonia: some pieces of puzzle are still missing. Neurology. 1998;50:853-5.
6. Rojahn J. Self injurious and stereotypic behavior of non-institutionalized mentally retarded people: prevalence and classification. Am J Ment Defic. 1986;91(3):268-76.

6.8 Encephalitis and Encephalopathies

Rashmi Kumar

INTRODUCTION

The term "encephalitis" means the inflammation of the brain parenchyma, part or all the "encephalon." It is an important cause of death and permanent neurologic disability in both children and adults.

Commonly, encephalitis has an infectious cause. Actual invasion by a viral agent causing direct neuronal injury is the most common cause of encephalitis, when it is called "viral encephalitis" (VE). Nonviral agents can also cause inflammation of the brain parenchyma. Encephalitis and meningitis are overlapping syndromes. Pathologically, some degree of both meningeal and parenchymal inflammation is found in most patients with viral and nonviral invasion of the brain. Therefore, the term "meningoencephalitis" is often used.

Direct injury by invasion may result in acute, subacute, or chronic manifestations. Sometimes the inflammation is not due to invasion but is an indirect immunologically mediated injury.

Noninflammatory diffuse cerebral dysfunction is termed as "encephalopathy"; common causes include metabolic, toxic, or ischemic. Encephalopathy can be acute or chronic. The term encephalopathy is also used for altered mentation due to any cause. The World Health Organization coined the term acute encephalitis syndrome (AES) in 2006 for the surveillance of Japanese encephalitis (JE). This is defined as "an illness in a person of any age and at any time of the year characterized by acute onset of fever with alteration of consciousness, stupor, coma and/or new onset of convulsions excluding simple febrile convulsions." Basically, this means acute illness with fever and altered sensorium with or without convulsions. It may have infectious (including VE) and noninfectious causes.

VIRAL ENCEPHALITIS

Several groups of viruses can invade the brain to cause encephalitis. Some of these, such as arboviruses, *herpes simplex*, rabies, etc. are "neurotropic"; i.e. they have a predilection for the brain, while others, such as measles, mumps, and influenza, only occasionally invade the brain.

- *Arbo or "Arthropod-borne" viruses*: Western equine, Eastern equine, Venezuelan equine, Japanese, St Louis, West Nile, and Murray valley encephalitis viruses: These viruses are naturally transmitted between the insects and the vertebrate animals that decide the geographical habitat and seasonal occurrence of the infection.
- *Herpesviruses*: Herpes simplex 1 and 2, *Varicella-zoster-virus*, Epstein–Barr, *Cytomegalovirus*, human herpesvirus-6, and herpes simian B virus.
- *Enteroviruses*: Polioviruses, coxsackievirus, echo, *Enteroviruses* 70 and 71.
- *Orthomyxoviruses*: Influenza viruses.
- *Paramyxoviruses*: Measles, mumps, parainfluenza, Nipah virus.
- *Adenoviruses*
- *Rhabdovirus*
- *Parvoviruses*.

Epidemiology

Japanese encephalitis is the most common VE in Asia and causes the maximum number of cases worldwide. Arboviruses have their own specific geographical distribution depending on the activity of their insect vectors and tend to cause epidemics or outbreaks. For example, JE transmission occurs between the mosquito, *Culex tritaeniorrhynchus*—a rice field breeding mosquito—and the pig. Man is an incidental "dead-end" host. In the recent years, incidence of JE has come down in many regions of India probably due to vaccination. Rabies is prevalent in most countries of the world. Herpes simplex encephalitis (HSE) is the most common form of sporadic encephalitis in Western countries. Mumps, measles, and rabies encephalitis have been largely eradicated from many developed countries due to effective vaccination program. Japanese encephalitis and rabies are public health problems in India.

Pathogenesis

The illness begins with the entry of the infecting agent and replication at an extraneural site. Most viruses reach the nervous system hematogenously, and the probability of an encephalitis depends on the degree of viral amplification at the extraneural site and the ensuing viremia. Other viruses gain access to the brain by the neuronal route. For example, the rabies virus replicates locally at the site of animal bite then enters nerve endings and travels retrograde via axons to the brain. Upon reaching the brain, the virus replicates in neurons and may lead to cell death. There are varying degrees of parenchymal and meningeal inflammation, edema, and necrosis. Some viruses may have a predisposition to involve specific areas of the brain, such as temporal lobe in *Herpes simplex* and hippocampus in rabies.

Clinical Features

Clinical manifestations depend on whether the brain parenchyma or meninges are predominantly involved producing an encephalitic or meningitic syndrome, respectively. The same virus may produce a meningitic picture in one and encephalitic picture in another patient. The severity of manifestations may vary widely either as a mild febrile illness associated with headache to a severe disorder with convulsions, coma, neurological deficits, and death. Usually, the onset is abrupt with fever and declining mental status. There may be irritability, agitation, screaming spells, confusion, delirium, drowsiness, stupor, or coma. Headache may be complained of in older children. Typical features include an initial stage of fever, headache, and vomiting lasting for less than a week, followed by convulsions, coma, and neurological deficits with or without signs of meningeal irritation. Severe cases may be associated with life-threatening rise in intracranial tension, decerebration, or flaccid coma. Typically, this stage lasts for 7–10 days after which there is a gradual recovery with or without sequelae. Some patients may have a biphasic course. Occasionally, VE can be subacute in the onset or present as stroke, a movement disorder, or a behavioral disturbance (as seen with HSE). Chronic encephalitis can present like a degenerative brain disorder.

Examination should include a search for the skin rashes often seen with enteroviral encephalitis, measles, dengue, and varicella zoster. Parotitis often occurs with mumps. Concurrent upper respiratory infection is a characteristic of influenza. Patients with rabies may have the characteristic hydrophobia or aerophobia. A constellation of frontotemporal signs with aphasia, personality change, and focal deficits or focal seizures is a characteristic of HSE. Rabies initially presents with nonspecific symptoms, such as fever, discomfort, and headache, soon followed by specific symptoms, such as insomnia, anxiety, confusion, excitation, hallucinations, agitation, hypersalivation (increase in saliva), difficulty in swallowing, hydrophobia (fear of water), and aerophobia (fear of drafts of fresh air). Death usually occurs within days of the onset of these symptoms. Rarely, rabies may present as an ascending paralysis simulating Guillain–Barré syndrome. Japanese encephalitis is associated with prominent extrapyramidal signs in the form of rigidity and abnormal movements, especially in the convalescent stage.

Even when the diagnosis of VE is made, identification of the etiologic agent is a daunting task. Neurological signs do not reliably identify the underlying etiology despite the propensity of certain neurotropic viruses to affect specific focal areas of the brain. Geographic and seasonal factors, history of recent travel, contact with animals, animal bite, occupation, and immune status of the patient need to be considered.

Investigations

- *Blood counts:* In the acute stage, blood counts usually reveal a polymorphonuclear leukocytosis. Low platelets count and high packed cell volume in the patients from endemic areas may point toward dengue infection.
- *Cerebrospinal fluid examination:* This is an essential investigation but should be done when considered safe. Cerebrospinal fluid (CSF) in VE typically shows a pleocytosis of up to 300 cells/mm^3, which can be either predominantly lymphocytic or polymorphonuclear, with normal to slightly raised protein and normal sugar level. Cerebrospinal fluid pleocytosis (>5 cells/mm^3) is present in more than 95% cases of acute VE and exceeds 500 cells/mm^3 in 10% cases of average variance extracted. The CSF in the acute VE is indistinguishable from aseptic or viral meningitis.

- *Samples for viral culture* from respiratory secretions, throat swab, CSF, blood, urine, and stool should be taken as early as possible, collected in appropriate transport media, and sent to the reference laboratory.
- *Serological investigations in acute serum for specific IgM antibody level*: JE is commonly diagnosed by the antibody capture ELISA for IgM antibody in acute phase serum and CSF.
- *Polymerase chain reaction (PCR)* is being developed to provide a rapid and accurate diagnostic tool for a host of pathogens and is the mainstay of diagnosis. This is widely used for the diagnosis of HSE with high sensitivity (>90%) and specificity (100%).
- *Tests for rabies:* No single test is enough for antemortem diagnosis of human rabies. Saliva can be tested by virus isolation or reverse transcription, followed by polymerase chain reaction. Skin biopsy specimens are examined for rabies antigen in the cutaneous nerves at the base of hair follicles. Immunofluorescent staining of corneal smears and skin biopsy specimen does not have a high yield. Serological assays are not suitable for the diagnosis of rabies, as virus-specific antibodies in serum tend to appear on an average 8 days after the onset of clinical symptoms. The fluorescent antibody test is considered the gold standard for the diagnosis in animals postmortem.
- *Neuroimaging of brain:* This is now a standard investigation in the patients with suspected VE. Neuroimaging is often normal, may reveal cerebral edema, diffuse low attenuation, patchy hypodensities, or specific abnormalities as in HSE. Cranial neuroimaging may also be useful in ruling out other treatable intracranial disorders and acute disseminated encephalomyelitis (ADEM). Magnetic resonance imaging (MRI) is the procedure of choice. Characteristic abnormalities are found in HSE which shows early changes of focal edema in the medial aspects of the temporal lobes, orbital surfaces of the frontal lobes, insular cortex, and cingulate gyrus **(Fig. 6.8.1)**. In infants and young children, however, more widespread changes may be seen. In JE, neuroimaging shows distinct hypointensity in the thalamus, basal ganglia, and brain stem.
- *Electroencephalography (EEG)* shows diffuse slow waves as a nonspecific finding in VE. In HSE, characteristic changes of 2–3 Hz periodic lateralized epileptiform discharges originating from the temporal lobes are seen in less than half of the cases, in later stages.

In practice, the diagnosis of VE is presumptive, based on clinical assessment and exclusion of other possibilities. Specific virologic investigations are complex, time consuming, and expensive, even in advanced centers; etiological diagnosis is possible in only a small proportion of clinically suspected cases.

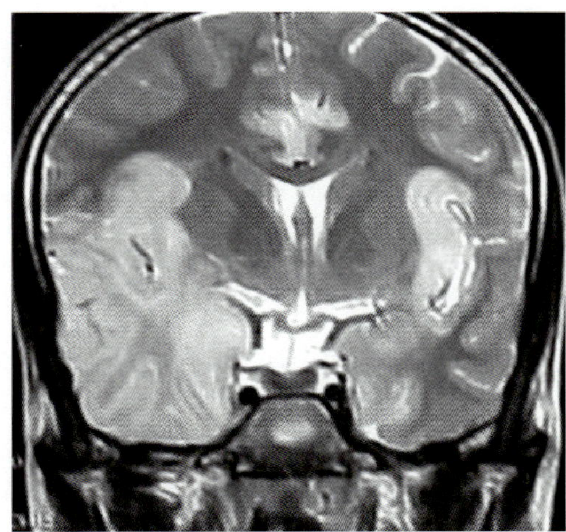

Fig. 6.8.1: MRI brain in Herpes simplex encephalitis showing temporal lobe change.

Treatment

Supportive treatment is the mainstay of therapy for a child with presumed VE. A severe case should be managed in an intensive care unit.

The measures include maintenance of airways, breathing and circulation, hydration, electrolyte status, and control of pyrexia and convulsions. It is prudent to use the appropriate parenteral antibiotics to cover for meningitis. Raised intracranial tension should be controlled with mannitol infusion (0.25–1.0 g/kg every 4–6 hours), hypertonic saline, intravenous furosemide, or intermittent positive pressure ventilation to keep the arterial CO_2 tension between 25 mm Hg and 30 mm Hg. Proper nursing care must be given. The role of steroids in acute VE is debatable.

Specific therapy is recommended in encephalitis due to Herpes group of viruses. Acyclovir in a dose of 10 mg/kg administered as an intravenous infusion over 1 hour every 8 hours for 14–21 days (21 days in immunocompromised) is indicated in HSE. Success of antiviral therapy depends on early institution of therapy. Acyclovir is also recommended for varicella zoster encephalitis. Oseltamivir can be considered for influenza encephalitis.

NONVIRAL INFECTIOUS ENCEPHALITIS

Nonviral agents which can cause encephalitis include:

- *Bacteria*:
  - Pyogenic and tuberculous meningitis
  - *Mycoplasma pneumoniae*
  - *Listeria monocytogenes*
  - *Spirochetes*: Syphilis, leptospirosis, lyme disease
  - Brucellosis

- *Legionella*
- *Salmonella typhi*
- Cat scratch disease (Bartonellosis)

- *Rickettsia*: In recent years, scrub typhus, caused by *Orientia tsutsugamushi*, has emerged as an important cause of AES in India. IgM against this organism is found in up to 60% of AES in the Gorakhpur area. Multisystem involvement with liver, kidney, pulmonary dysfunction, and low platelets is found along with features of meningoencephalitis.
- *Fungi*: *Cryptococcus*, *Histoplasma*, *Aspergillus*, mucormycosis, *Candida*, and coccidioidomycosis, especially in immunocompromised children
- *Protozoa*: *Plasmodium*, *Trypanosoma*, *Naegleria*, *Acanthamoeba*, *Toxoplasma gondii*, schistosomiasis, *Echinococcus granulosus*.
- *Metazoa*: Trichinosis, *Echinococcus*, *Cysticercus*, *Schistosoma*.
- *Human slow viral infections*: Subacute sclerosing panencephalitis (SSPE), progressive rubella panencephalitis, Creutzfeldt–Jakob disease, Kuru, and progressive multifocal leukoencephalopathy. Human immunodeficiency virus (HIV)-acquired immune deficiency syndrome (AIDS) itself causes a subacute or chronic encephalitis but the associated immunosuppression may predispose to encephalitis by other pathogens.

Postinfectious or Postvaccine Acute Disseminated Encephalomyelitis

This is a postinfectious immune inflammation, common postinfectious causes being measles, rubella, mumps, varicella zoster, influenza A and B, rickettsia, and *M. pneumoniae*, while vaccines associated with this syndrome include rabies, measles, and yellow fever. The illness is monophasic with altered consciousness, convulsions, and multifocal neurological signs affecting cerebellum, optic nerves, long tracts, spinal cord, and peripheral nerve roots. Fever may be absent at the onset of symptoms. A history of a viral exanthem or vaccine in the recent past is often available. Cerebrospinal fluid may reveal a mild pleocytosis. Characteristic plaque-like lesions are seen scattered in white matter, at times in deep gray matter and other areas of the neuraxis in MRI **(Fig. 6.8.2)**. Treatment options include high-dose pulse steroids, intravenous immunoglobulins, and plasmapheresis. The initial presentation of multiple sclerosis can be indistinguishable from ADEM.

Autoimmune Encephalitis

This entity of neurological syndromes associated with serum and/or CSF antibodies against ion channels, receptors, and associated proteins is well recognized in adults. The illness may be part of a paraneoplastic neurological disorder; the clinical picture can localize specific areas of the central nervous system. In large US and UK cohorts, 23–40% of the patients were under the age of 18 years. Neuropsychiatric manifestations, mutism, movement disorder, seizures, and cognitive decline are the important symptoms.

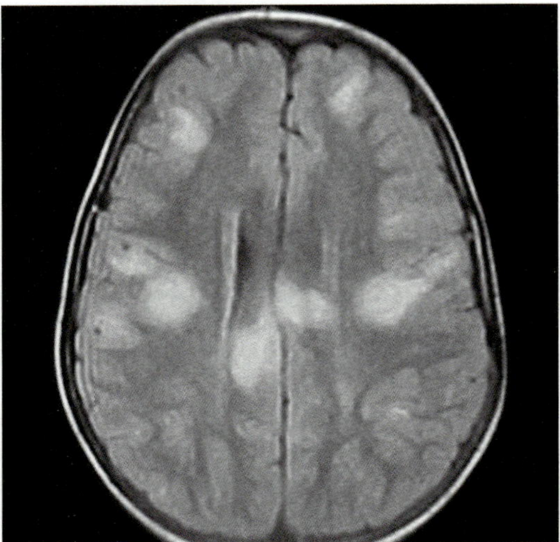

Fig. 6.8.2: MRI brain in acute disseminated encephalomyelitis showing plaque-like lesions in deep white matter.

ENCEPHALOPATHIES

Clues must be sought to differentiate encephalopathy from encephalitis, but the distinction is not always possible on clinical grounds. General features of encephalopathies are:

- Absence of fever or meningeal signs
- Absence of focal neurologic signs or focal seizures
- No peripheral leukocytosis
- Normal CSF
- Diffuse slowing on electroencephalography
- Normal imaging studies.

Other Causes of Acute Encephalitis Syndrome

The presence of fever is not enough to make a diagnosis of infective or inflammatory encephalitis, since encephalopathy may be precipitated by systemic infection, or sepsis without cerebral inflammation or some other cause of fever may coexist.

- *Infectious encephalopathies*: These include infectious disorders associated with encephalopathy without actual invasion of the brain parenchyma. Important causes include cerebral malaria, enteric encephalopathy, dengue encephalopathy, shigellosis, and sepsis syndrome.
- *Fever from any cause associated with metabolic or toxic encephalopathy* can produce a picture of AES. Examples of such metabolic/toxic causes include Reye syndrome, dyselectrolytemia, diabetic, uremic or hepatic coma, poisoning, and heat stroke. Recent outbreaks of AES in

Saharanpur and Muzaffarpur, Bihar, are examples of toxin-related AES.

- *Fever from any cause associated with a structural lesion* in the brain, such as tumor or vascular insult.

Dengue Encephalopathy

The occurrence of neurological manifestations in dengue infections has been recognized for long. Dengue infection may produce a picture of acute febrile encephalopathy with/without rash, swelling (nonpitting edema on face and body), bleeding manifestations, low platelet count, and deranged liver function without frank jaundice. The cause of encephalopathy in dengue was believed to be vasculitis with fluid exudation, cerebral edema, hypoperfusion, and hyponatremia. Over the last two decades, neurotropic potential of dengue virus with virus invasion of the brain producing "encephalitis" has been well documented primarily from studies in the Southeast Asia.

Reye Syndrome

This syndrome of acute encephalopathy with fatty infiltration of the liver usually presents with a history of a preceding viral infection (upper respiratory infection in 90%; varicella in 5–7%). A strong association exists with preceding intake of salicylates. Abrupt onset of protracted vomiting is followed by delirium, combative behavior, and stupor. Most children have a mild course but rapid progression to seizures, coma, and death may occur. Mild hepatomegaly and hypoglycemia are common. Hepatic dysfunction is suggested by raised liver enzymes (>3-fold), raised serum ammonia, and abnormal coagulogram, but serum bilirubin is usually normal. Liver is yellow to white because of high triglyceride content, and biopsy reveals diffuse microvesicular fatty infiltration without any evidence of inflammation or necrosis. Reye syndrome has been reported from different parts of India.

Prognosis and Outcome

Even when meningoencephalitis are not fatal, they have the potential to cause permanent neurological handicap in the child. Therefore, the treatable infections must be identified early and energetically treated. The outlook is somewhat better with the noninflammatory encephalopathies.

CHRONIC ENCEPHALITIS AND ENCEPHALOPATHIES

Some viral encephalitides are chronic and may present like a neurodegenerative disorder. These include SSPE, progressive rubella panencephalitis, HIV, toxoplasma, and human slow virus infections—Kuru, progressive multifocal leukoencephalopathy, and Jacob-Creutzfeldt disease.

Diffuse cerebral dysfunction can follow asphyxia, trauma, vascular insult, CNS infection, and metabolic disorders (hypoglycemia, hyponatremia, and inborn errors of metabolism). Degenerative brain disorders and epileptic encephalopathies are also present as chronic encephalopathy.

KEY MESSAGES

- Encephalitis and encephalopathies are important causes of hospital admissions among children in India.
- Encephalitis refers to inflammation of brain parenchyma and can be caused by a large variety of infections. Japanese encephalitis and scrub typhus are major causes in India.
- Encephalopathy or noninflammatory diffuse cerebral dysfunction can be caused by several toxic and metabolic causes.
- These conditions have the potential of permanent neurologic handicap in the survivors.
- Specific treatment is available for many nonviral infections and HSE.

BIBLIOGRAPHY

1. Chaudhuri A, Kennedy PGE. Diagnosis and treatment of viral encephalitis. Postgrad Med J. 2002;78:575-83.
2. Glaser CA, Honarmand S, Anderson LJ, et al. Beyond viruses: clinical profiles and etiologies associated with encephalitis. Clin Infect Dis. 2006;43:1565-77.
3. Hacohen Y, Wright S, Waters P, et al. Paediatric autoimmune encephalopathies: clinical features, laboratory investigations and outcomes in patients with or without antibodies to known central nervous system autoantigens. J Neurol Neurosurg Psychiatry. 2013;84(7):748-55.
4. Kumar R. Encephalitis and encephalopathy. In: Singh M (Ed). Medical Emergencies in Children, 5th edition. New Delhi: Sagar Publications; 2011.
5. Prober CG. Central nervous system infections. In: Behrman RE, Kleigman RM, JensonHB, Stanton BF (Eds). Nelson Textbook of Pediatrics, 18th edition. Pennsylvania, PA: WB Saunders Co.; 2008. pp. 2512-23.

6.9 Infections of the Central Nervous System

Pratibha Singhi

INTRODUCTION

Infections of the central nervous system (CNS) are serious diseases that are associated with high mortality and morbidity. Early diagnosis and appropriate management are extremely important. The presentation of various CNS infections is often nonspecific and includes fever, headache, and altered sensorium, at times seizures and focal neurological deficits. Clues from a detailed history, epidemiology, examination, and appropriate investigations are required for a precise diagnosis. Central nervous system infections can broadly be categorized into:

- *Meningitis*: Acute, subacute, or chronic
- *Acute encephalitis*: Diffuse or focal
- Encephalopathy with systemic infections
- Postinfectious syndromes.

Several organisms including bacteria, viruses, parasites, and fungi can cause CNS infections. In this chapter, bacterial meningitis, brain abscess, and neurocysticercosis (NCC) are discussed.

ACUTE BACTERIAL MENINGITIS

Etiology

The causative organisms for acute bacterial meningitis depend on the age, nutritional and immune status of the child, and associated clinical conditions **(Table 6.9.1)**.

The three major causative organisms in children are *Haemophilus influenzae, Neisseria meningitidis*, and *Streptococcus pneumoniae*, and in neonates, gram-negative bacilli, group B streptococci, and *Listeria monocytogenes*.

Epidemiology

Bacterial meningitis may be sporadic or epidemic, it commonly occurs in infants and children although it can occur at any age. In the developed countries, a substantial reduction of *H. influenzae* type B (Hib) and pneumococcal meningitis has occurred because of widespread immunization. However, these organisms continue to cause meningitis in many developing countries. Poor socioeconomic conditions, overcrowding, malnutrition, and human immunodeficiency virus (HIV) further contribute to the high incidence of meningitis in the developing countries.

Haemophilus influenzae type B meningitis occurs usually in children between 3 months and 3 years of age. Pneumococcal meningitis occurs throughout childhood and is particularly seen in children with pneumonia, otitis media, sinusitis, cerebrospinal fluid (CSF) leaks, head injury, sickle cell disease, and thalassemia major. Meningococcal meningitis occurs mainly in school-age children and young adults. Meningitis caused by Hib, *Pneumococcus*, and *Meningococcus* is rare in the first 3 months of life because of the transplacental transfer of protective maternal antibodies.

Table 6.9.1: Common causative organisms for bacterial meningitis in various age-groups.

Age	*Causative organisms*	*Initial antibiotics and doses (mg/kg/day)*
<1 month	Gram-negative bacilli (*Escherichia coli, Pseudomonas*) Group B streptococci, *Listeria monocytogenes*	*Cefotaxime 100; q8 hour or Ampicillin 50–100; q6–8 hour plus Gentamicin 2–2.5; q8 hour
1–3 months	*Haemophilus influenzae* type B *Streptococcus pneumoniae* *Neisseria meningitides* Gram-negative bacilli Group B streptococci *Listeria monocytogenes*	Ceftriaxone 100; q24 hour or Cefotaxime 100; q8 hour plus Ampicillin
>3 months	*Haemophilus influenzae* type B *Streptococcus pneumoniae* *Neisseria meningitidis*	Ceftriaxone or cefotaxime plus †Vancomycin 15; q6 hour or ‡Ampicillin and Chloramphenicol

*In places with aminoglycoside-resistant gram-negative organisms.
†In places with ceftriaxone-resistant pneumococci.
‡If ceftriaxone not affordable.

Pathogenesis

Bacterial meningitis occurs through the hematogenous route in most cases. Inhaled bacteria adhere to the nasopharyngeal mucosa, evade mucosal host defense mechanisms, and enter the blood stream, and then the CSF by penetrating the blood–brain barrier (BBB). This is facilitated by various neurotropic and virulence factors. Nonhematogenous spread of bacteria into the CSF can also occur from contiguous sites of infection, such as otitis media, sinusitis, and mastoiditis or through direct communication of the subarachnoid space (SAS) with the skin or mucosa as in head trauma, dermal sinuses, and through infected CSF shunts.

Bacterial multiplication and autolysis in the SAS lead to the release of bacterial components that trigger a strong inflammatory response. Several inflammatory cytokines and chemokines, including interleukins and tumor necrosis factor (TNF), are produced that in turn lead to the release of other inflammatory mediators, including platelet-activating factor, matrix metalloproteinases (MMP), nitric oxide, and free oxygen radicals that lead to the disruption of the BBB. Leukocytes pass from the blood into the CSF leading to CSF pleocytosis, and further release of various toxic mediators that adversely affect the cerebral blood flow and cerebral metabolism and contribute to the development of cerebral edema.

Neuropathology

The inflammatory exudates cover the brain and cerebral blood vessels and cause vasculitis and thrombosis; ischemia may lead to cerebral infarction. Cerebral edema may be marked and may lead to cerebral herniation. Neuronal damage occurs due to these multitudes of factors.

Clinical Presentation

Typically, meningitis presents acutely with fever, headache, vomiting, altered sensorium, stiff neck, and in some cases, seizures and photophobia. The child may have a preceding upper respiratory infection, pneumonia, or otitis media. Fever may be absent in very small infants, in severely malnourished or immune-compromised children, and in children on previous antibiotic therapy. Younger children may not be able to complain of headache but may be irritable. Seizures may be the presenting feature in almost one-third of children with meningitis; they may be recurrent and prolonged. Impairment of sensorium at presentation may be minimal but worsens gradually with progression of the disease. In some cases of meningococcal meningitis, a fulminant course with sepsis, shock (Waterhouse–Frederiksen syndrome), rapidly progressive cerebral edema, and raised intracranial pressure (ICP), evolving over a few hours may occur.

On examination, neck rigidly and other signs of meningeal irritation are seen. These include:

- *Kernig's sign:* With thighs flexed on abdomen, passive extension of knee produces pain in the back.
- *Brudzinski's sign:* Passive flexion of neck produces flexion of both lower limbs.
- *Tripod sign:* In the sitting position, the child supports himself with both arms extended behind the back, which is kept straight.
- *Knee-kiss sign:* The child cannot bend forward to kiss his knees.

Meningeal signs may be minimal or absent in neonates and young infants, and in malnourished and deeply comatose children. In infants, a bulging fontanel is an important sign of meningitis.

Symptoms and signs of raised ICP (headache, vomiting, and respiratory abnormalities) may appear within 24–28 hours. Papilledema at presentation is uncommon, and if present, a computed tomography (CT) scan must be done to exclude a mass lesion or a complication. Focal signs may be due to subdural collection, cortical infarction, or cerebritis. Associated findings such as a maculopapular or petechial rash in meningococcal infections, otitis media or pneumonia in pneumococcal infections, and pustular skin lesions in staphylococcal infections may be seen.

In neonates, meningitis may be present with nonspecific symptoms of sepsis with poor feeding, lethargy, fever, vomiting, irritability, high-pitched cry, and at times seizures. The anterior fontanel may be level or full and, in some cases, there may be enlargement of head with separation of sutures.

Diagnosis

As early diagnosis of meningitis is extremely important, it should be suspected in any child with lethargy, unconsciousness, inability to feed, stiff neck, and seizures. It is important to note that the absence of fever or meningeal signs does not exclude the diagnosis of bacterial meningitis.

Differential Diagnosis

The differential diagnoses according to presentation include:

- *Acute onset fever and meningismus*: Aseptic meningitis, pneumonia with right upper lobe involvement, retropharyngeal abscess, and cervical lymphadenitis.
- *Coma*: Encephalitis, Reye's syndrome, metabolic problems, hepatic encephalopathy, intoxications, and other causes of nontraumatic coma. Cerebral malaria is an important differential diagnosis in endemic regions. Blood films for malarial parasites should be taken in children with splenomegaly and anemia.
- *Focal signs*: Cerebral abscess, stroke, herpes encephalitis, intracranial bleeds, and other space-occupying lesions; get urgent neuroimaging.

- *Subacute presentation*: Tubercular, fungal, and parasitic meningitis.

Laboratory Diagnosis

Cerebrospinal fluid examination: It is essential for the diagnosis of meningitis. Lumbar puncture (LP) should be done as early as possible in all cases of suspected meningitis and in the following:

- Neonates and very young infants who present as nonspecific sepsis;
- *Children with febrile seizures*: Up to 18 months of age, or if the child looks ill or is on previous antibiotics.

Contraindications of LP include:

- Raised ICP
- Focal neurological symptoms or signs
- Shock/cardiorespiratory instability
- Thrombocytopenia (platelet count < 50,000/mm^3)/ coagulation disorder
- Local infection at LP site.

Appropriate antibiotics should be given early in all cases of suspected meningitis even if the LP is delayed. Early antibiotic administration for 24 hours does not significantly alter the CSF cellular response but may decrease the yield on culture and on Gram stain.

Computed tomography scan before the LP is not routinely needed; it is indicated in children with focal neurological symptoms or signs, papilledema, critically raised ICP, or suspicion of a mass lesion. Computed tomography is normal in most cases of bacterial meningitis, including those with subsequent herniation; a normal CT does not rule out raised ICP.

Typically, the CSF pressure is raised; there is polymorphonuclear leukocytosis, decreased glucose, and increased protein concentration. The cell count may vary from a few to hundreds to over a thousand leukocytes; almost 90% cases have a CSF cell count over 100/mm^3. In the developing countries, the reported CSF cell counts are not very high in most cases. A cloudy CSF under pressure is almost diagnostic of bacterial meningitis. Cell count should be done within half an hour of CSF collection. In normal children, the CSF has 0–5 mononuclear cells/mm^3; polymorphonuclear cells are very rarely seen. The presence of a single polymorphonuclear cell in the clinical setting of meningitis should be considered significant. In neonates, the upper limit of normal extends to 20–30 WBCs (white blood cells)/mm^3; however, the mean CSF cell count is generally 5–10 WBCs/mm^3.

The CSF glucose levels are less than 40 mg/dL in more than half the cases; a CSF to serum glucose ratio of 0.4 or less is 80% sensitive and 98% specific in children above 2 months of age. In neonates, a CSF to serum glucose of less than or equal to 0.6 is abnormal. The blood glucose should be collected before the LP.

At times, the CSF can be completely normal in early stages of bacterial meningitis, particularly in neonatal meningitis; a repeat LP after few hours may show abnormalities; antibiotic therapy must therefore be started in all cases with a strong suspicion of bacterial meningitis. **Table 6.9.2** shows the CSF characteristics helpful in differentiation of acute bacterial meningitis from aseptic and tubercular meningitis.

Occasionally, an initial polymorphonuclear response can be seen in viral meningitis and an initial lymphocytic response in bacterial meningitis. The CSF sugar is normal in most cases of viral meningitis but may be low in some cases; however, it is rarely below 20 mg/dL.

Organism Identification

- *Cerebrospinal fluid Gram stain:* It is quick, reliable, and inexpensive, positivity depends on the number of organisms in the CSF—at least 10^5 CFU/mL of CSF is required. The yield is markedly increased by examining fresh centrifuged sediment of the CSF.
- *Acridine orange*: It stains the nucleic acid of some bacteria so that they appear bright red orange under a fluorescent microscope. It stains the intracellular bacteria better than the Gram stain and may be positive even when the Gram stain is negative.
- *Cerebrospinal fluid culture*: A positive CSF culture is the gold standard for organism identification. High positivity

Table 6.9.2: Cerebrospinal fluid characteristics in various types of meningitis.

Types of meningitis	*Cerebrospinal fluid appearance*	*Cell count*	*Polymorphonuclear cells*	*Lymphocytes*	*Protein (mg/dL)*	*Glucose*
Bacterial	Cloudy	Few 100 to >1,000	+++	+	Raised 100 to >500	↓↓
Partially treated	Clear	5 to few 100	++	+	Raised 100–500	↓
Tubercular	Clear	<500	–	+++	Raised 100–500	↓↓
Viral	Clear	10–500	+	++	N (<50) or raised up to 100	N

(≈75%) reported from the developed countries is not seen in the developing countries because of prehospital antibiotic therapy, delayed plating, inadequate storage, and transport of CSF.

- *Rapid diagnostic tests*: Rapid diagnostic tests detect bacterial antigen by countercurrent immune-electrophoresis, enzyme-linked immunosorbent assay (ELISA), and latex agglutination tests. They are helpful in providing early diagnosis and in differentiating viral from bacterial meningitis. A negative test does not exclude bacterial meningitis. These tests are expensive and are not routinely used.
- *Multiplex polymerase chain reaction (PCR) assays*: PCR can rapidly detect many organisms; however, they are not available in most developing countries.
- *Samples from other sites of infection*: Samples from other sites of infection, such as pleural fluid, cellulitis, otitis, aspiration of petechiae in suspected meningococcemia, and urine in young infants, should also be collected for organism identification.
- *Other nonspecific tests*: Nonspecific tests, such as raised peripheral white blood count, C-reactive protein, CSF lactate and procalcitonin, have limited specificity.

Cerebrospinal fluid presepsin (biomarker of bacterial infection in CSF) has been found to be superior to CSF leukocytes and proteins in diagnosing bacterial infections; however, this is still experimental.

Course and Complications

If treated properly, children improve within 48–72 hours, and the fever comes down within 4–5 days. Persistent fever (>10 days) may be due to thrombophlebitis, subdural effusions, spread of infection (such as pneumonia, arthritis, or osteomyelitis), drug fever, and rarely resistant organisms. The common complications of bacterial meningitis are listed in **Box 6.9.1**.

A neuroimaging in the form of CT scan/magnetic resonance imaging (MRI) is indicated in the following situations—in a child who does not show clinical improvement and has sudden unexplained deterioration, new onset seizures or focal neurologic signs, signs of raised ICP, persistent fever, or enlarging head. Subdural effusions, infarct, hydrocephalus, cerebritis, or cerebral abscess may be detected. Magnetic resonance imaging detects parenchymal complications earlier than CT. Ultrasound of the head is helpful in neonates and in infants with open fontanel.

Box 6.9.1: Complications of bacterial meningitis.

- Late onset seizures
- Subdural empyema
- Infarcts, cerebritis, and brain abscess ventriculitis
- Hydrocephalus
- Cranial nerve involvement
- Sensorineural deafness
- Diabetes insipidus
- Spread of infections to distant sites (pneumonia, pericarditis, arthritis, and osteomyelitis)

Systemic complications

- Septic shock DIC, ARDS, and septic or reactive arthritis

(ARDS: acute respiratory distress syndrome; DIC: disseminated intravascular coagulation)

Management

Appropriate intravenous (IV) antibiotics and supportive therapy should be started as soon as possible. Delay in initiation of antibiotics is an independent strong risk factor for mortality. Close monitoring is essential to detect and manage any acute life-threatening complications, such as shock or raised ICP. Ideally this is done in a pediatric intensive care unit (PICU) until the child is stable. In resource-poor countries, at least the severely ill children should receive intensive care.

Antibiotic Therapy

This should be broad enough to cover all the likely pathogens according to the age of the child and the prevalent epidemiology and resistance patterns of organisms. Once the organism is isolated on culture, and its susceptibility is determined, antibiotic therapy is targeted accordingly. If no organisms are isolated, the initial antibiotics should be continued for at least 7–10 days.

The standard recommendation for the duration of antibiotics is 10–14 days for *S. pneumoniae* and *H. influenzae*, and 7 days for *N. meningitides*. Shorter durations of antibiotic therapy (5 days) have also been found effective. A minimum of 3 weeks of antibiotics is required for gram-negative, staphylococcal, and neonatal meningitis.

With proper treatment, the CSF culture and Gram stain become negative within 24–48 hours, and the CSF glucose normalizes over 72 hours. The increase in cells and proteins may persist for several days. A repeat LP either during treatment or at the end of therapy is not routinely needed unless there is the appearance of new symptoms or signs.

Supportive Treatment

Airway, breathing, and circulation must be maintained. Shock, raised ICP, seizures, and status epilepticus must be urgently and appropriately managed. Enough fluids should be given to maintain normovolemia, normal blood pressure, and thereby adequate cerebral perfusion. Cerebral perfusion pressure targeted therapy in neurocritical care units is associated with better outcome. Electrolyte imbalances should be promptly corrected.

- *Corticosteroid therapy*: Early dexamethasone therapy (0.15 mg/kg/6 hourly × 4 days) has been recommended in the developed countries as it reduces mortality, severe hearing loss, and neurological sequelae in the cases of Hib and pneumococcal meningitis. However, no beneficial effect of corticosteroids has been found in children from low-income countries and thus they are not recommended.

- *Oral glycerol*: Oral glycerol for the first 48 hours (6 g/kg/day q6 hour) may reduce neurological sequelae. The use of glycerol reduces the risk of subsequent deafness; however, it has not been found to have any effect on death/seizures.
- *Other therapies for modulation of inflammatory pathways*: Other therapies for modulation of inflammatory pathways, such as isoform of nitric oxide synthase, inhibition, endothelin agonists, antioxidants, neurotrophin, glutamate antagonist, TNF neutralization, MMP inhibition, and caspase inhibition, are still experimental.
- *The role of IV immunoglobulin*: The role is limited to children with immune-deficient states and in some cases of neonatal meningitis.

Prognosis

Coma, raised ICP, status epilepticus, shock, and respiratory depression are important predictors of mortality and morbidity. Neurologic sequelae including hearing loss, hydrocephalus, epilepsy, spasticity, visual and cognitive deficits, and developmental delay are common.

Prevention

To prevent secondary meningitis, children with Hib or meningococcal meningitis should be isolated for 24 hours.

Chemoprophylaxis

- *Haemophilus influenzae* type B *meningitis*: Rifampicin (20 mg/kg/day twice daily for 4 days) for all household contacts if there is at least one unvaccinated contact less than 4 years old. Rifampicin for the index case before discharge if ampicillin and/or chloramphenicol were used, as they do not eradicate *H. influenzae*; it is not needed if ceftriaxone was used.
- *Meningococcal disease*: Rifampicin (10 mg/kg 12 hourly for 2 days) for household and day care contacts. Ceftriaxone single intramuscular dose (125 mg for children < 12 years and 250 mg for older children and adults). Ciprofloxacin 500 mg or azithromycin 500 mg single dose in adults.
- *Primary prevention*: It is possible by immunization against the common pathogens causing meningitis.

BRAIN ABSCESS

Brain abscess is a focal infection of the brain parenchyma, which may be bacterial, tubercular, fungal, or parasitic.

Bacterial Brain Abscess

Epidemiology

It is rare in the developed countries (0.3–1.3 per 100,000 people per year), but not uncommon in the developing countries.

Etiology

Streptococci, staphylococci, gram-negative organisms, anaerobic bacteria, and several unusual organisms may cause brain abscess. In neonates' gram-negative organisms particularly *Klebsiella*, *Citrobacter diversus*, and *Proteus mirabilis* are common. The causative organisms of the abscess are determined mainly by the underlying/predisposing condition. In about one-third of cases, polymicrobial sepsis is seen.

Pathogenesis

Brain parenchyma gets infected by the hematogenous route, contiguous spread from an adjacent infection, trauma, or a neurosurgical procedure. The predisposing conditions and likely organisms are shown in **Table 6.9.3**.

Following hematogenous infection, the pathogens localize in the poorly vascularized areas of the brain, such as the gray-white junction, and cause cerebritis. The inflammation and edema progress through four stages in 4–6 weeks:

1. Early cerebritis (1–3 days).
2. Late cerebritis (4–9 days).
3. Early fibroblastic capsule formation (10–14 days).
4. Late capsule formation (>14 days) when a dense fibrous capsule is formed.

Most brain abscesses occur in the cerebral hemispheres, some in the cerebellum and brainstem, depending on the etiology. Multiple scattered abscesses are common with hematogenous infections; those secondary to direct spread are usually single and occur in contiguous brain parenchyma.

Clinical Presentation

Clinical presentation is variable; usually it is subacute with fever, headache, vomiting, altered sensorium, seizures, neck rigidity, and focal neurological deficits depending on the site of the abscess. Occasionally, the presentation may be acute if the abscess ruptures in the ventricles. Papilledema, the sixth nerve palsy, and occasionally cerebral herniation syndromes may occur secondary to raised ICP. Neonates and young infants present with nonspecific features of irritability, lethargy, poor feeding, seizures, bulging fontanels, and an enlarging head; focal signs are rare.

Differential diagnosis includes tumors, focal encephalitis, such as herpes, and other focal suppuration.

Table 6.9.3: Predisposing conditions for brain abscess and likely organisms.

Predisposing conditions for brain abscess	*Likely organisms*
Hematogenous spread	
Cyanotic congenital heart disease particularly tetralogy of Fallot	*Streptococcus viridans* *Staphylococcus aureus* Microaerophilic streptococci *Haemophilus* species
Subacute bacterial endocarditis	*Streptococcus viridans* Microaerophilic streptococci *Staphylococcus aureus* *Haemophilus* species
Chronic pulmonary infection	Streptococci Staphylococci Anaerobic bacteria
Orofacial infections	Anaerobic bacteria Streptococci (aerobic and anaerobic) *Staphylococcus aureus*
Sinus infections	Streptococci (aerobic and anaerobic) *Staphylococcus aureus* *Haemophilus* species Anaerobic bacteria *Pseudomonas*
Malnutrition and immunocompromised status	*Staphylococcus aureus* Gram-negative organisms Anaerobic organisms Unusual organisms
Direct spread	
Chronic otitis, mastoiditis	Streptococci (aerobic and anaerobic) *Staphylococcus aureus* *Haemophilus* species *Proteus* Anaerobic bacteria *Pseudomonas*
Infected dermal sinuses; epidermoid cysts and encephalocele; neurosurgical procedures, such as ventriculoperitoneal shunts, penetrating skull injury, and fracture of the skull base	*Staphylococcus aureus* *Staphylococcus epidermidis* Streptococci *Enterobacteriaceae*
Complication of meningitis	Organisms causing the underlying meningitis particularly Gram-negative staphylococci

Diagnosis

Neuroimaging: Typically brain abscess appears as a characteristic ring-enhancing lesion with central hypodensity and surrounding edema on CT **(Fig. 6.9.1)**. In early cerebritis, the ring enhancement may be incomplete, and a double contrast CT may be helpful in defining the capsule. The MRI is more sensitive than CT in the diagnosis of cerebritis. Magnetic resonance imaging with magnetic resonance spectroscopy (MRS) and diffusion-weighted imaging helps in differentiating bacterial abscess from tubercular/fungal abscesses.

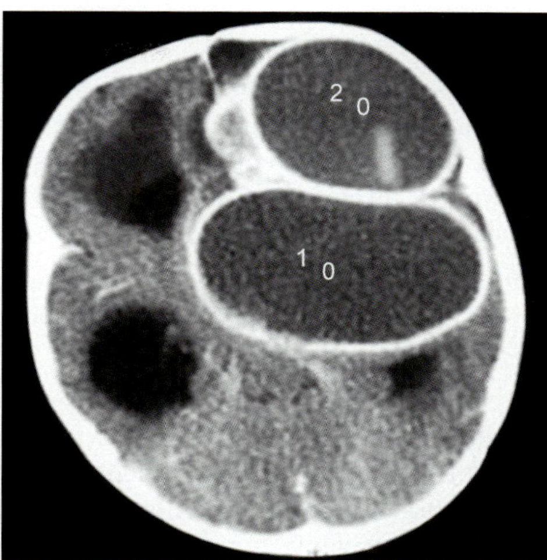

Fig. 6.9.1: CT showing large abscesses.

Thallium single-photon-emission CT and fluorine-18 fluorodeoxyglucose positron emission tomography are effective in differentiating brain abscess from tumor in doubtful cases.

Organism identification: It is done by Gram stain and culture of the aspirate. Blood cultures are positive in less than 25% cases with hematogenous infections.

Electroencephalogram: It may show focal slowing, spikes, or periodic lateralizing discharges.

The underlying source of infection: It should be identified by a detailed history, examination, and appropriate investigations.

Management

Management involves appropriate antibiotics and surgical drainage or excision of the abscess. Urgent decompression is required in the cases with critically raised ICP. Stereotactic aspiration guided by precision mapping of the lesion's location with CT or MRI may be used to drain inoperable sites. Magnetic resonance (MR) fluoroscopy may also be used to guide aspiration instead of stereotactic aspiration.

Antibiotics: Antibiotics alone are used in early cerebritis, very small abscesses (<2 cm), or abscesses in deep-seated/critical areas of the brain. A broad-spectrum combination to cover anaerobic, gram-negative, gram-positive, and staphylococcal species is used until a specific organism is identified. Ceftriaxone/cefotaxime, metronidazole, and vancomycin are generally used. Penicillin and chloramphenicol can be used, if cephalosporins are not affordable. Subsequent antibiotics are tailored to the organism identified. Antibiotics in highest doses are given IV for at least 6 weeks. Patients with HIV infection may require therapy for toxoplasmosis.

Steroids: In children with marked cerebral edema, IV corticosteroids are used for a short period to reduce cerebral edema and raised ICP.

Supportive management: Supportive management for raised ICP, seizures, and general PICU care is the same as for any critically ill child. There is no scientific evidence to recommend the use of prophylactic anticonvulsants. Proper treatment of the source of infection should be done.

Prognosis

Early adequate management is associated with 90% cure rate. Poor prognostic factors include multiple large abscesses, underlying cyanotic heart disease, rupture of abscess into the ventricular system, and low Glasgow Coma Scale at presentation. Delayed treatment is associated with significant neuromorbidity.

Prevention

Early treatment of orofacial and dental infections and antibiotic prophylaxis for children with cyanotic congenital heart disease undergoing procedures associated with bacteremia and after penetrating skull injury or craniotomy are some helpful measures.

NEUROCYSTICERCOSIS

Neurocysticercosis caused by the infection of the CNS with encysted larvae of *Taenia solium* is a common cause of acquired epilepsy in many developing countries.

Pathogenesis

Neurocysticercosis is acquired through the feco-oral route, by eating the food contaminated with *T. solium* eggs that are passed in feces of persons with intestinal teniasis (which occurs by eating undercooked pork infected with cysticerci). In the human intestine the eggs hatch to release larvae that penetrate the intestinal mucosa and migrate throughout the body to produce human cysticercosis. Most mature cysts are found in the CNS, skeletal muscle, subcutaneous tissue, and the eyes. Cysticerci often live asymptomatically within host tissues for years (vesicular cysts), evading host response after which they degenerate (colloidal or granular nodular stage) and cause symptoms.

Clinical Manifestations

Neurocysticercosis is classified into parenchymal and extraparenchymal (ventricular, cisternal, ophthalmic, or spinal). The latter is uncommon in children. Most children present with single degenerating parenchymal cysts, some with multiple cysts.

Parenchymal Neurocysticercosis

Parenchymal NCC usually presents after 5 years of age; some cases are seen in preschoolers and even in infants.

- Seizures occur in 70–90% of cases; usually they are partial (84–87%) and of short duration. Status epilepticus occurs in 2–32% cases.
- Almost one-third of children have headache and vomiting. Papilledema and focal neurological deficits are uncommon.
- Cysticercal encephalitis with severe acute raised ICP may rarely occur in children with innumerable cysts and extensive cerebral edema.

Extraparenchymal Neurocysticercosis

Extraparenchymal NCC is rare in children as compared to adults and may present as arachnoiditis, obstructive hydrocephalus, or chronic meningitis. Spinal cysticercosis may present as transverse myelitis or other spinal cord syndromes. Ophthalmic cysticercosis can cause visual deficits and limitation of eye movements.

Diagnosis

Diagnosis is with neuroimaging. On CT the most common finding is a "single", small (<20 mm) ring, or disk-enhancing lesion with surrounding edema [single small enhancing CT lesion (SSECTL)] **(Fig. 6.9.2)**. The scolex appears as a

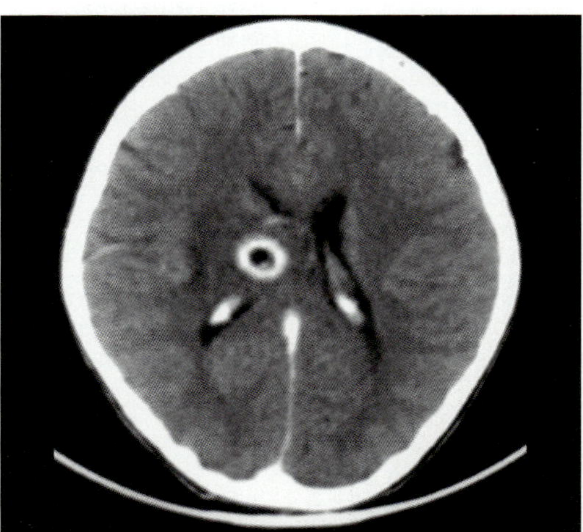

Fig. 6.9.2: CT scan of the head in a child with neurocysticercosis showing a cyst with a scolex.

bright, high-density eccentric nodule in these cysts and is pathognomonic of NCC. It represents the degenerating stage (colloidal) of the cyst. Some children may have 2–3 lesions or multiple lesions; disseminated NCC with numerous cysts—"starry sky" appearance is typical of NCC **(Fig. 6.9.2)**. Calcified cysts are few millimeters in size, single or multiple, and generally without any surrounding edema.

Extraparenchymal NCC: Hydrocephalus, enhancement of tentorium and basal cisterns due to arachnoiditis, and occasionally infarcts may be seen.

Magnetic resonance imaging is better for identification of scolex and visualization of extraparenchymal cysts.

Laboratory Tests

Serologic tests have a low positivity (17–25%) particularly for single lesions. Both ELISA and the enzyme-linked immunoelectrotransfer blot assay are more sensitive in the cases with multiple brain lesions than in those with single lesions.

Stool examination for tapeworms, blood counts, and X-rays of skeletal muscles are not useful. Biopsy of subcutaneous nodules can corroborate the diagnosis. CSF is normal in most cases but may show increased cells and proteins and hypoglycorrhachia in NCC meningitis.

Differential Diagnoses

In the cases where the scolex is not well seen, the differential diagnosis mainly includes tuberculoma. The presence of raised ICP, progressive focal neurological deficit, CT lesion more than 20 mm, lobulated irregular shape, and marked edema causing midline shift favor the diagnosis of tuberculoma.

Tuberculomas are more often seen in the base of the brain, whereas NCC lesions are more common near the gray-white junction of the cortex. Sophisticated imaging techniques, such as proton MRS and three-dimensional constructive interference in steady state, are being tried to distinguish NCC from tuberculoma. Mantoux test, chest X-ray, and other tests should be done for the exclusion of tuberculosis.

Other differential diagnoses include microabscess, low-grade astrocytoma, cystic cerebral metastasis, toxoplasmosis, and fungal lesions.

Since NCC is pleomorphic, it should be considered in the differential diagnosis of seizures and other neurological disorders.

Treatment

Carbamazepine or phenytoin is used for seizure control, usually for a period of 1 year seizure-free interval if the lesion has disappeared on follow-up CT and longer if the lesion is persistent or calcified. Prednisolone 1–2 mg/kg orally or IV dexamethasone for 3–5 days are used if there is edema or features of raised ICP.

Cysticidal Therapy

Albendazole (15 mg/kg/day, 4 weeks) or praziquantel (50 mg/kg/day for 15 days) has been found effective for the destruction of vesicular cysts. It is also associated with higher and faster resolution of SSECTL. However, whether cysticidal therapy improves long-term seizure control is debatable. Albendazole is the drug of choice as it is more effective than praziquantel, less expensive, and better tolerated. Cysticidal therapy is contraindicated in the cases with

- Markedly raised ICP, particularly in disseminated NCC.
- In ophthalmic NCC, as the host inflammatory response may cause sudden elevations of ICP/damage to the eye.
- Such cases should be treated with corticosteroids alone.

Cysticidal therapy is not indicated for calcified lesion(s) as the parasite is already dead.

Shunt placement may rarely be required for hydrocephalus. Ventricular cysts can be removed endoscopically. As NCC is a polymorphic disease, treatment needs to be individualized.

Follow-up

A repeat CT is generally done after 3–6 months to determine whether the lesions have resolved.

Outcome

Outcome depends on the type of NCC, cyst location, and numbers. Single lesions disappear within 6 months in over 60% cases, and risk of seizure recurrence is low. Cases with multiple lesions and calcifications have frequent seizure recurrences.

Prevention

Prevention is possible by ensuring proper hygiene and sanitation, and animal husbandry.

KEY MESSAGES

- Early diagnosis and administration of appropriate antibiotics are essential to reduce morbidity and mortality of bacterial meningitis.
- Infants and neonates usually do not have typical signs and symptoms of meningitis.
- Lumbar puncture should be done in all cases of suspected meningitis (unless contraindicated) and in all neonates with sepsis.
- Supportive management for raised ICP and seizures along with adequate fluid and electrolyte therapy are extremely important.

- Clinical presentation of brain abscess is often atypical in children; neuroimaging must be done in suggestive settings.

BIBLIOGRAPHY

1. Bonfield CM, Sharma J, Dobson S. Pediatric intracranial abscesses. J Infect. 2015;71(1):S42-6.
2. Brouwer MC, McIntyre P, de Gans J, et al. Corticosteroids for acute bacterial meningitis. Cochrane Database Syst Rev. 2010;(9):CD004405.
3. Kocherry XG, Hegde T, Sastry KV, et al. Efficacy of stereotactic aspiration in deep-seated and eloquent-region intracranial pyogenic abscesses. Neurosurg Focus. 2008;24(6):E13.
4. Kumar R, Singhi S, Singhi P, et al. Randomized controlled trial comparing cerebral perfusion pressure-targeted therapy versus intracranial pressure-targeted therapy for raised intracranial pressure due to acute CNS infections in children. Crit Care Med. 2014;42(8):1775-87.
5. Peltola H, Roine I. Improving the outcomes in children with bacterial meningitis. Curr Opin Infect Dis. 2009;22:250-5.
6. Prasad K, Kumar A, Gupta PK, et al. Third generation cephalosporins versus conventional antibiotics for treating acute bacterial meningitis. Cochrane Database Syst Rev. 2007;(4):CD001832.
7. Salinas R, Prasad K. Drugs for treating neurocysticercosis (tapeworm infection of the brain). Cochrane Database Syst Rev. 2010;(1):CD000215.
8. Singhi P, Singhi S. Acute bacterial meningitis. In: Singhi P, Griffin DE, Newton CR (Eds). Central Nervous System Infection in Childhood. London: Mac Keith Press; 2014. pp. 160-81.
9. Singhi P, Suthar R. Neurocysticercosis. Indian J Pediatr. 2015;82(2):166-71.
10. Wall EC, Ajdukiewicz KM, Heyderman RS, et al. Osmotic therapies added to antibiotics for acute bacterial meningitis. Cochrane Database Syst Rev. 2013;3:CD008806.

6.10 Coma

Arun Bansal

INTRODUCTION

Coma is a common childhood neurological emergency that can have a devastating outcome. It can occur from trauma or a wide range of nontraumatic causes. The incidence of nontraumatic coma is 30/100,000 children per year and that of traumatic coma is 670/100,000.

DEFINITIONS

Clouding of Consciousness

Clouding of consciousness describes states of reduced wakefulness characterized by impaired attention and memory. Patients may be distractible, hyperexcitable, and irritable with slow thought processes.

Stupor

Stupor is a condition of unresponsiveness, similar to deep sleep, from which the patient can be aroused only by vigorous and repeated stimuli. Even when aroused, communication is by monosyllabic sounds and simple behaviors and as soon as the stimulus ceases the stuporous subject lapses back into the unresponsive state.

Coma

Coma is a state of unconsciousness in which the eyes are closed and sleep-wake cycles are absent. There is no understandable response to external stimuli or inner need, and the patient neither utters understandable responses nor accurately localizes noxious stimuli.

It is differentiated from:

- Lethargy, drowsiness caused by a condition other than sleep.
- Stupor, a state of somnolence in which a patient can be transiently aroused.
- Delirium, a state of confusion in which attention, concentration, and memory can be impaired.

Vegetative State

Vegetative state (VS) consists of:

- No evidence of sustained, reproducible, purposeful or voluntary behavioral responses to visual, auditory, tactile, or noxious stimuli.
- No evidence of language comprehension or expression.
- Intermittent wakefulness manifested by the presence of sleep-wake cycles (i.e. periodic eye-opening).

Vegetative state may be a transient, persistent, or permanent condition. Transient VS lasts less than 4 weeks and is often associated with a favorable outcome. The term persistent is applied when VS lasts longer than 4 weeks, regardless of etiology. The VS is considered permanent (i.e. irreversible) after 3 months following nontraumatic brain injury and after 12 months following traumatic injuries.

Minimally Conscious State

Minimally conscious state is defined as a condition of severely altered consciousness in which the patient demonstrates minimal but definite behavioral evidence of self or environmental awareness.

Brain Death

Brain death is defined as the permanent absence of all brain functions including those of the brainstem. Brain-dead patients are irreversibly comatose and apneic with absent brainstem reflexes.

ETIOLOGY

Coma is caused by wide variety of causes **(Box 6.10.1)**. They are broadly classified into traumatic or nontraumatic. In nontraumatic coma, infections are the most common cause of coma. In the experience from the authors' center, out of 100 children with nontraumatic coma, 60% were due to infections, 19% had toxic-metabolic causes, 10% had status epilepticus, and 7% had intracranial bleed.

Box 6.10.1: Causes of coma.

- *Focal lesions*:
  - Intracranial bleed; arteriovenous malformation
  - Stroke
  - Accidental/nonaccidental head injury
  - Brain abscess
  - Focal encephalitis (herpes)
- *Diffuse lesions*:
  - Accidental/nonaccidental head injury
  - *Infections*: Bacterial, malaria, enteric, *Shigella*, rickettsia
  - *Postinfectious*: Acute necrotizing encephalopathy
  - *Vascular*: Venous thrombosis
  - *Diffuse hypoxic injury*: Postcardiac arrest, shock
  - *Metabolic causes*:
    - *Electrolyte disturbances*: Sodium
    - Acid-base abnormality
    - *Endocrine*: Hypoglycemia, diabetic ketoacidosis
    - Inborn error of metabolism
- Hepatic failure
- Renal failure
- Hydrocephalus
- Hypertensive encephalopathy
- Nonconvulsive status
- Postictal
- Drugs, toxins, and poisoning

Clinical Tips to Differentiate Coma by Etiology

Detailed and clear history is important to approach a case of coma. History of accidental or nonaccidental trauma differentiates between traumatic and nontraumatic coma. Presence of fever points toward an infective cause of coma though fever may precipitate a metabolic cause of coma too. Infants with systemic infection and coma can present with hypothermia. History of drowning, choking, aspiration, drug/toxin exposure, or dog bite should be elicited. Coma due to inborn error of metabolism can occur at any age, but symptoms of failure to thrive, neurodevelopmental delay, and seizures with history of consanguinity may precede encephalopathy. A child with history of seizures may be having nonconvulsive status.

EVALUATION OF A CHILD WITH COMA

Coma is a medical emergency and requires multidisciplinary approach. It includes simultaneous assessment, evaluation, and treatment.

Stabilization of any child with coma is a priority. Patency of the airway and adequate breathing should be ensured, as a comatose child is more prone to aspiration because of loss of protective reflexes. Any child having Glasgow Coma Scale (GCS) less than eight should preferably be intubated. If breathing is not adequate, mechanical ventilation should be initiated. Hemodynamic status should be monitored and fluid bolus be (20 mL/kg) given on evidence of shock. Hypoglycemia, if present, should be treated, and hematological, biochemical, and acid-base status should be assessed and derangements corrected. Evidence of internal and external injuries must be sought and any temperature instability must be treated. If seizures are present, anticonvulsants must be given and treated accordingly.

Examination

Vitals

All vitals should be recorded as they can give a vital clue. Hypertension can cause hypertensive encephalopathy or may be a Cushing's response to raised intracranial pressure (ICP). Seizures, retinal hemorrhage, and pulmonary edema can occur secondary to hypertension. Hypotension may be seen in shock, myocardial dysfunction, or adrenal insufficiency and can lead to decreased cerebral perfusion. Fever may indicate infection. Tachycardia may be because of early shock, sepsis, or fever. Bradycardia may be in response to raised ICP. Tachypnea with lung findings may indicate respiratory focus. Silent tachypnea may be metabolic because of acidosis due to diabetic ketoacidosis, drug/toxin, uremia, etc.

General Examination

Skin/mucosal membranes should be examined for anemia, icterus, rash, skin bleeds, purpura, and neurocutaneous markers. Look for any evidence of trauma in the form of hematoma, fracture, or bruises. Measure head size for microcephaly, palpate fontanels, look for sutural separation, and auscultate head for any bruise. Height and weight must be measured to rule out failure to thrive.

Systemic Examination

Cardiac examination is important to look for any evidence of heart lesion, which may lead to stroke, palpate abdomen for hepatosplenomegaly, which may be present in various infections or metabolic disorders, and respiratory examination is helpful to detect underlying pneumonia or empyema.

Neurological Examination

Careful neurological examination is important to localize the cause and the lesion. Prior administration of neuromuscular drugs or anticonvulsants may hamper the examination.

Grading of Coma

Level of consciousness need to be recorded objectively, and the most common scale used is GCS, but it cannot be used in younger children, especially in children less than 3 years of age. Modified GCS has been recommended for these young children and has been endorsed by the British Paediatric Neurology Association. Each component of the score should be reported separately (e.g. E3, M3, and V2) as compared to summed up score (e.g. GCS 5, 7, or 12) as it has been shown that summed up scores cannot be equated with clinical assessment.

Eye Findings

Examine pupillary reaction to light, direct, and consensual. Pupillary reaction correlates with the severity of coma. Preserved pupillary reaction, despite other brainstem abnormal signs, indicates toxic/metabolic cause. Unilaterally fixed and dilated pupil is evident of transtentorial herniation, provided topical administration of mydriatics has been ruled out. Corneal reflex gets diminished/absent in children with deep coma. Presence of nystagmus may be because of ongoing status, barbiturate, or phenytoin poisoning. Persistent ocular deviation also indicates ongoing nonconvulsive seizures. Ophthalmoplegia, ocular bobbing, convergent or divergent spasms, episodes of lid retraction, and spontaneous blinking usually suggest brainstem dysfunction. Extraocular movements should be tested with the doll's eye maneuver. Papilledema and retinal hemorrhages can be ruled out on fundus examination.

Motor Examination

Examine bulk, tone, posture, asymmetry, and reflexes in motor system. Decerebration is usually a reflection of raised ICP and central herniation. Decortication and decerebration can result from metabolic, toxic, and structural "causes" of coma. Flaccidity and areflexia are grave signs in a comatose child. Focal seizures, if present, may help in localization. Myoclonic jerks are seen with anoxic and hepatic encephalopathy. Dystonia or dyskinesia in a comatose child without antecedent history of a neurometabolic disease may be present in Japanese B encephalitis, tubercular meningitis, and inborn errors of metabolism or phenothiazine, phenytoin, or metoclopramide toxicity.

Pattern of Respiration

Abnormal respiratory patterns help in localization of the disease. The different patterns are:

- Normal
- *Cheyne–Stokes*: Cerebral hemispheres, rarely, upper pons
- *Central neurogenic hyperventilation*: Brainstem *tegmentum*
- *Apneustic*: Mid or low pontine dysfunction
- *Ataxic*: Medulla
- *Apnea*: Medullary dysfunction.

Other Neurological Signs

Neck rigidity is present in meningitis, herniation, or trauma. Meningeal irritation can also be assessed by Brudzinski's and Kernig's sign. Raised ICP can lead to various herniation syndromes, which can be subfalcine, transtentorial, or transforaminal.

INVESTIGATIONS

Comatose child may need a variety of investigations. The list is exhaustive, and some may be needed in all and some may be tailored according to the differential diagnosis **(Table 6.10.1)**. If lumbar puncture is contraindicated, the most appropriate therapeutic agents should be started. Computed tomography (CT) scan is the most common neuroimaging available and is the first-line investigation. The CT and magnetic resonance imaging (MRI) complement each other in *traumatic brain injury (TBI)*. While CT helps in diagnosing conditions, which require urgent surgical treatment such as bleed, MRI helps in diagnosing acute axonal injury. Always discuss with neuroradiologist to plan the investigation, which is best for the patient and is cost-effective.

MANAGEMENT

Management of the comatose child starts as soon as the child presents to the physician **(Table 6.10.2)**. Maintain the airway, breathing, and circulation as discussed earlier.

Table 6.10.1: List of investigations.

Sample	*Patients*	*Indications*
Blood		
Complete blood count	All	Infection
Blood glucose	All	Hypoglycemia/hyperglycemia
Serum electrolytes	All	Metabolic disturbances
Calcium, phosphate	All	Metabolic disturbances
Liver function tests	All	Hepatic encephalopathy, metabolic, toxic, infections
Renal function tests	All	Uremic encephalopathy, infections, metabolic, toxic
Arterial blood gas	All	Acidosis
Ammonia	All	Metabolic, toxic, infections
Lactate	All	Infections, metabolic, toxic
Culture	Specific	Infections
Peripheral blood film for malaria	Specific	Cerebral malaria
Viral markers	Specific	Viral encephalitis
Leptospira serology	Specific	Leptospirosis
Weil–Felix test	Specific	Rickettsial infections
Widal test	Specific	Enteric encephalopathy
Toxicology screen	Specific	Poisoning
Enzyme studies	Specific	Metabolic, neurodegenerative, syndromic
Urine		
Culture	Specific	Infections
Reducing substances	Specific	Metabolic disorders
Toxicology screen	Specific	Poisoning
Ketones	Specific	Metabolic, diabetic ketoacidosis
Cerebrospinal fluid		
Cell count, protein, sugar, culture	Specific	Infections
Viral markers	Specific	Viral encephalitis
Tuberculosis work-up	Specific	Tubercular meningitis
Fungal culture, serology, galactomannan enzyme immunoassay	Specific	Infections
Neuroimaging		
CT head (contrast/plain)	All; except documented uncomplicated metabolic causes, such as diabetic ketoacidosis, hypoglycemia	Trauma, infections, bleed, tumor, vascular cause
CT angiography	Specific	Vascular cause
MRI	Specific	Infections, acute disseminated encephalomyelitis, acute necrotizing encephalopathy of childhood, neurometabolic disorders
Electrophysiological studies		
Conventional electroencephalogram	Specific	Seizure, nonconvulsive status, infections
Continuous electroencephalogram	Specific	Seizures, comatose children on paralysis

(CT: computed tomography; MRI: magnetic resonance imaging)

Table 6.10.2: Management of coma.

General management	
Raised ICP	• Head in midline, normothermia, 30° head end elevation, euvolemia and adequate sedation, and analgesia • In impending herniation, hyperventilation, and mannitol (0.25–1 g/kg)/3% hypertonic saline (0.1–1.0 mL/kg/h) • Target ICP < 20 mm Hg or CPP > 50 mm Hg
Seizures	• Benzodiazepines (IV diazepam/ lorazepam at 0.1 mg/kg) followed by IV phenytoin loading dose at 20 mg/kg over 30 minutes • Nonconvulsive status may be present and should be looked through subtle clinical signs or continuous EEG
Specific management	
Hypoglycemia/ Hyperglycemia	• Correct hypoglycemia with IV 25% dextrose 2–4 mL/kg bolus followed by slow infusion of 5% dextrose containing fluid to prevent recurrence. Close monitoring of blood sugar is essential as hyperglycemia may also be detrimental • The underlying cause of hyperglycemia, such as DKA is treated
Infections	• *Bacterial*: Broad-spectrum antibiotics • *Herpes*: Acyclovir • *Cerebral malaria*: Antimalarials (quinine/artesunate derivatives) • *Rickettsia*: Oral doxycycline or IV azithromycin • *TBM*: Antitubercular treatment
Drug poisoning	• Specific antidote

(CPP: cerebral perfusion pressure; DKA: diabetic ketoacidosis; EEG: electroencephalogram; ICP: intracranial pressure; IV: intravenous; TBM: tuberculous meningitis)

Steroids have no role in TBI. But they are useful in acute disseminated encephalomyelitis, tubercular meningitis, and enteric encephalopathy. Decompressive craniectomy should be considered in cases of severe TBI or refractory raised ICP. Adequate nutrition should be provided in all cases of coma, and some cases may need to be fed through nasogastric tube.

PROGNOSIS AND OUTCOME

Nontraumatic Coma

The outcome of coma depends on the etiology, depth, and duration of impaired consciousness. Mortality in these children has varied between 25% and 35%. Factors, which predict increasing mortality, are usually infants or small children (<3 years), poor pulse volume, abnormal respiratory pattern and apnea, abnormal pupillary size and reaction, abnormal extraocular movements, absent corneal reflex, abnormal motor muscle tone, and motor-GCS less than eight. All children with nontraumatic coma should be given aggressive multidisciplinary rehabilitation program till 12 months before giving any outcome.

Traumatic Coma

Children with trauma show much better outcome than their initial evaluation suggests. Severity of trauma and poor socioeconomic status are predictors of poor outcome. Refractory raised ICP also predict poor outcome.

KEY MESSAGES

- Coma is a medical and neurological emergency.
- Broadly, it can be divided into traumatic or nontraumatic coma.
- Causes of nontraumatic coma are quite varied.
- The basic principles of management include rapid assessment and stabilization, detailed history and clinical examination to assess depth of coma, localization of lesion in the central nervous system and possible clues to etiology, and treatment includes general and specific measures.
- Because coma has a high rate of mortality and morbidity in children, and the clinician may be unsure of the outcome very early in the course, it is important to have strategies to define prognosis.

BIBLIOGRAPHY

1. Bansal A, Singhi SC, Singhi PD, et al. Nontraumatic coma. Indian J Pediatr. 2005;72:467-73.
2. Kirkham FJ. Non-traumatic coma in children. Arch Dis Child. 2001;85:303-12.
3. Kochanek PM, Carney N, Adelson PD, et al. Guidelines for the acute medical management of severe traumatic brain injury in infants, children, and adolescents. Pediatr Crit Care Med. 2003;4:S1-75.
4. Seshia SS, Bingham WT, Griebel RW. Coma in childhood. Handbook Clin Neurol. 2008;90:329-50.
5. Sharma S, Kochar GS, Sankhyan N, et al. Approach to the child with coma. Indian J Pediatr. 2010;7:1279-87.
6. Singhi PD, Bansal A, Ramesh S, et al. Predictive value of electroencephalography and computed tomography in childhood non-traumatic coma. Indian J Pediatr. 2005;72:475-9.
7. Singhi S, Singhi P, Baranwal AK. Bacterial meningitis in children: critical care needs. Indian J Pediatr. 2001;68:737-47.
8. Stevens RD, Bhardwaj A. Approach to the comatose patient. Crit Care Med. 2006;34:31-41.
9. Wong CP, Forsyth RJ, Kelly TP, et al. Incidence, aetiology, and outcome of non-traumatic coma: a population based study. Arch Dis Child. 2001;84:193-9.

6.11 Primary Brain Tumors

Kamer Singh Rana, JN Goswami

INTRODUCTION

Primary brain tumors are one of the most devastating diseases encountered today. It is the second most common childhood malignancy, next to leukemias, accounting for almost one quarter of the total childhood neoplasms. Age-adjusted incidence varies among countries from 1.12 to 5.14 cases per 100,000/year for children and adolescents less than 19 years of age. Incidence is more common in boys.

Childhood brain neoplasms differ from those of adulthood brain tumors regarding their site of origin, clinical presentations, tendency to disseminate, histological features, and their biological behaviors. Astrocytoma and embryonic tumors are more common in children, whereas metastases, glioma, and meningioma are seen predominantly in adults. Incidence of infratentorial tumors and tumors with malignant behavior (medulloblastoma and ependymoma) decreases with increasing age, whereas the occurrence of supratentorial tumors and tumors with benign nature (pilocytic astrocytoma/glioma) increases with age. Local dissemination is faster in young children. Manifestations and outcomes depend upon the location, behavior of the tumor, degree of surgical resection, and response to adjuvant therapy.

Though significant advances in the field of diagnosis and treatment have occured over the years, overall survival rate remains modest. The survivors face considerable morbidity throughout their lives due to long-term sequelae of the surgical or adjuvant radio and chemotherapy. Introduction of molecular diagnostics has helped in understanding the behavior of these neoplasms and response to treatment. World Health Organization (WHO) has changed the classification and grading of childhood neoplasms due to fast evolving molecular diagnostics. Aggressive surgery is the undisputable primary modality of treatment, but long-term postsurgical sequelae are still very high. Distressing cognitive/endocrinal and growth-related issues are intolerable after adjuvant therapy. There is a great hope that innovative treatment modalities, such as immunotherapy and gene therapy, will improve the overall survival and quality of life of these children in coming times.

ETIOLOGY

Etiology of childhood brain neoplasms remains unknown. Two strong risk factors are associated with childhood brain neoplasms namely, genetic syndromes and exposure to therapeutic ionized radiotherapy. The common genetic syndromes associated with increased risk of brain neoplasms are shown in **Table 6.11.1**. Inheritance pattern in all of these familial disorders is autosomal dominant.

Primitive embryonic tissue can also be a potential risk for the development of primitive neuroectodermal tumors. Craniopharyngioma, a common midline supratentorial tumor in children, arises from persistent remnants of craniopharyngeal pouch. Intracranial germ cell tumors with the exception of mature teratoma are seen commonly during adolescence. This is probably due to hormonal drive to gonadal development, which interacts with potential tumor cells within brain. Another potent risk factor is therapeutic ionizing radiation exposure. The common neoplasms reoccurring after radiations are malignant glioma and meningioma and can be as late as 5–15 years. Other possible risk factors are higher birth weight, nervous system anomalies, diagnostic ionizing radiations, advanced parental age, folic acid deficiency, exposure to electromagnetic radiations (cell phones), immunosuppression, and residual pesticides. Etiology in majority of the brain tumors is probably multifactorial, where genetic instabilities and environmental factors play a role in the pathogenesis. The common genetic mutations associated with childhood brain

Table 6.11.1: Common genetic syndromes associated with primary brain tumors.

Genetic syndrome and mutations	***Brain tumors***
NF1 and NF2	Pilocytic astrocytoma of visual pathways
TSC1 and TSC2	Giant cell astrocytoma
VHL	Hemangioblastoma of cerebellum
Li-Fraumeni (Germ cell line TP53)	Glioma Medulloblastoma
Atypical teratoid/rhabdoid tumor syndrome (SMARCB1, SMARCA4)	Atypical teratoid/rhabdoid tumor
Gorlin syndrome (Germ line PTCHED-1)	Medulloblastoma

(NF: neurofibromatosis; TP53: tumor protein p53; TSC: tuberous sclerosis complex; VHL: Von-Hippel-Lindau)

Table 6.11.2: Common childhood neoplasms with genetic mutations.

Tumor	*Genetic mutations*
Astrocytoma (diffuse and anaplastic) grades II and III	*IDH* (>80%), *TP53* (94%), *ATRX* (86%)
Glioblastoma mutant grade IV Glioblastoma wild-type grade IV	*IDH1* (>95%), *ATRX* (90–95%), *TP53* (62–65%), *IDH2* (2–5%) *TP53* (25–35%) *TERT* promoter (>80%) *EGFR* amplification, *CDKN2A* homogeneous deletion (35–50%)
Oligodendroglioma grades II and III	*IDH* (98%), 1p/19q codeletion (100%), *TERT* promoter (96%), *MG MT* methylation (85%)
Subependymal giant cell astrocytoma grade I	*TSC1* and *TSC2* (100%)
Pilocytic astrocytoma grade I	*BRAF-KIAA* 1549 fusion (70%), *BRAF-V600E* (15%)
Diffuse midline glioma grade IV	Histone *K27M* (100%), *ATRX* (50%), *TP53* (50%)
Craniopharyngioma	*BRAF V 600E* and *CTNNB1* (100%)
AT/RT grade IV	*SMARCB1* (95%), *SMARCA4* (2%)
Medulloblastoma grade IV	*TERT* promoter (21%)
Meningioma	*TRAF7/KLF4* (100%)

(AT/RT: atypical teratoid/rhabdoid tumor)

tumors are depicted in **Table 6.11.2**. These mutations help in establishing the correct diagnosis and prognostication. Some of them are useful markers for tumor prediction.

CLASSIFICATION

Brain tumors can be classified according to their location **(Table 6.11.3)**, immunohistochemical or molecular markers, and behavior of the neoplasm. WHO has revised the classification of childhood brain neoplasms based on their molecular behaviors in 2016. In brain tumors, the terms "benign" and "malignant" often are misleading. Malignant tumors, such as medulloblastoma, may be curable in up to 80%, if it occurs in older children or when well localized and completely surgically resectable. On the contrary, some benign tumors, such as low-grade astrocytoma and glioma, can disseminate to surrounding normal brain and may be quite difficult to remove completely and behave like a malignant mass.

Supratentorial tumors peak during the first year of life and after 10 years of age, whereas infratentorial tumors are more common in 1–10 year age-group children. In India, the most common childhood brain tumors are astrocytoma, medulloblastoma, and craniopharyngioma.

STAGING AND GRADING OF PRIMARY BRAIN TUMORS

Staging of the central nervous system (CNS) tumors depends upon the degree of surgical resectability, the residual tumor mass left after the surgery, and the extent of the spread beyond the primary location of the tumor. Staging of the CNS tumors is usually performed based on magnetic resonance imaging (MRI) images of the brain and the spinal cord and/or by cerebrospinal fluid (CSF) analysis for tumor cells. Scans taken after surgery are used to determine left out tumor mass. CNS tumors, those have the tendency to spread, are exposed to both the scan images and CSF studies. Patients with medulloblastoma, for example will often have their CSF examined for the presence of tumor cells. These patients also require spinal cord scans because of the tumor's tendency to spread to the spinal cord. Since embryonal and glial neoplasms rarely spread to non-neuronal sites, evaluation for disease spread outside nervous system is not recommended.

Immunohistology and molecular diagnostics have been incorporated to determine treatment response and risk stratifications. Same neoplasm at different location and at different age of presentation can have different underlying mutations and different behaviors, for example the underlying genetic mutations and behavior of the midline and cortical gliomas are different.

Grading helps in deciding the benign or malignant nature of the tumor, treatment response, and outcome. The higher the grade, the more malignant is the tumor. Based on the WHO grading system, there are four tumor grades—I, II, III, and IV **(Table 6.11.4)**.

Clinical Features

Clinical features depend on location, size, evolutional behavior of the tumor, and the age of the child. Aggressively growing

Table 6.11.3: Classification of brain tumors based on their anatomical localization and common ages of occurence.

Infratentorial (43.2%)	*Supratentorial (40.9%)*	*Multiple sites and spinal cord (15.9%)*
• *Astrocytoma (40%)*: 5–15 years • *Medulloblastoma (40%)*: 1–4, 7–10 years • *Brainstem glioma (10–20%)*: 5–15 years • *Ependymoma (10–20%)*: 1–4 years • *Atypical teratoid/rhabdoid (3%)*: 1–3 years	• Cortical glioma • Low grade (50%): 1–15 years • High grade (20%): 10–19 years • Diencephalic (10%): 0–3 years • Craniopharyngioma (10%): 5–15 years • Choroid plexus papilloma (<1%): 0–12 years	• Astrocytoma • Glioma • Ependymoma

Table 6.11.4: World Health Organization grading of primary brain tumors.

Grade of the tumor	***Characteristics***	***Examples***
Grade I (Benign)	• The least malignant tumors associated with long-term survival • Their growth is slow, and the appearance under microscope is almost normal • Surgery alone may be an effective treatment	• Pilocytic astrocytoma • Subependymal giant cell astrocytoma • Craniopharyngioma • Neurofibroma • Choroid plexus papilloma • Meningioma
Grade II (Semibenign)	• These tumors are slow growing and look slightly abnormal under a microscope • Some can spread into nearby normal tissue and recur • Surgery with additional adjuvant therapy is required	• Ependymoma • Diffuse astrocytoma IDH mutant • Neurocytoma • Atypical choroid plexus papilloma • Atypical meningioma
Grade III (Semimalignant)	• By definition, these tumors are malignant • The cells of a grade III tumor are actively reproducing abnormal cells, which grow into nearby normal brain tissue • These tumors tend to recur, often as a grade IV	• Anaplastic astrocytoma IDH mutant • Anaplastic ependymoma • Anaplastic ganglioglioma • Anaplastic meningioma
Grade IV (Malignant)	• The most malignant tumors • These reproduce rapidly, look bizarre when viewed under the microscope, and easily invade into nearby normal brain tissue • They form new blood vessels, so they can maintain their rapid growth • They also have areas of dead cells in their centers	• Glioblastoma IDH mutant and wild type • Pineoblastoma • Medulloblastoma (all subtypes) • Atypical teratoid/rhabdoid tumors

(IDH: isocitrate dehydrogenase)

tumors manifest early with severe symptoms, whereas initial signs and symptoms of slow-growing tumors are subtle.

Subtentorial tumors become symptomatic in the beginning because of the compact space. Extra-axial subtentorial tumors obstruct CSF pathways and present with early features of raised information and communication technology, such as early morning headache, vomiting, bradycardia, hypertension, visual disturbances, papilledema, mental changes, and gait disturbances. Intra-axial masses in the subtentorial region, such as pontine glioma, present with the features of multiple cranial nerves palsy and long tracts signs. Supratentorial tumors present with seizures and focal neurological deficit.

In infants and young children, presentations can be nonspecific, and there are difficulties in detection and evaluation. Before closure of skull sutures and fontanels, the only manifestations can be progressively enlarging head size without features of raised intracranial pressure and focal neurological symptoms and signs. Slowly growing neoplasms may present with developmental delay in the beginning and regression of developmental milestones in the later part of progression. There may be disk pallor instead of papilledema, particularly in suprasellar masses. Sun setting sign is a common feature of raised intracranial tension, manifested by impaired upward gaze with persistent downward gaze due to dilated third ventricle with pressure on tectum due to obstructive hydrocephalus.

Hypothalamic neoplasms in children may present with diencephalic syndrome, characterized by the failure to thrive and emaciation in an otherwise normal child. These children may present with gelastic seizures, particularly in hypothalamic hamartoma. Such children are usually irritable with significant developmental delay but some of them are happy and euphoric also.

Expanding neoplasms also cause secondary brain dysfunction because of herniation due to pressure gradient in different compartments. Herniation causes overcrowding of brain matter, stretching and rupturing of blood vessels, edema, and pressure over vital structures, notably cranial nerves and vital centers in the brainstem.

Diagnosis

Key features while assessing the primary brain neoplasms are the site, size, type of brain tissue involved, surgical resectability, and spread within the brain and spinal cord. Neuroimaging, histopathology, immunology, and molecular diagnostics are the primary tools used in diagnostic assessment of the brain tumors.

- Magnetic resonance imaging with Gadolinium-diethylenetriaminepentaacetic acid (GD-DTPA) is a generally preferred diagnostic mean **(Figs. 6.11.1 to 6.11.4)**. Most tumors enhance with contrast. MRI is better

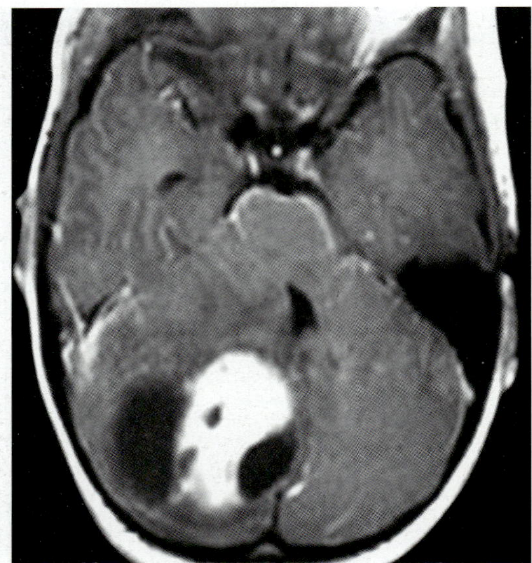

Fig. 6.11.1: Postgadolinium T1-weighted transverse MRI image of brain showing a well-defined heterogeneously enhancing mass lesion in the right cerebellar hemisphere. Biopsy proven case of cerebellar astrocytoma. (MRI: magnetic resonance imaging; T1: transverse 1)

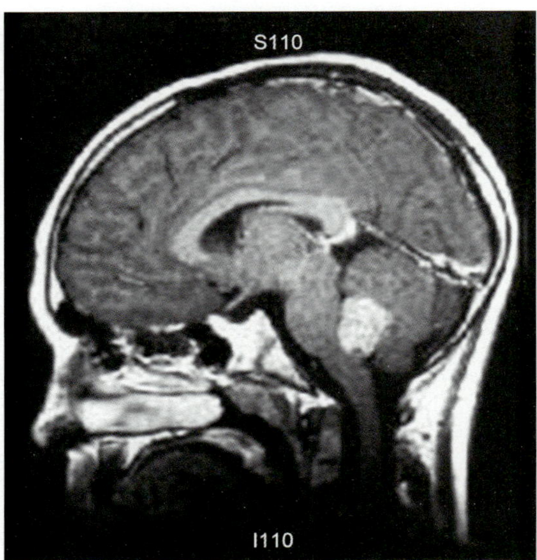

Fig. 6.11.2: Postgadolinium T1-weighted sagittal MRI image of brain showing a well-defined intensely enhancing mass lesion expanding the fourth ventricle and displacing the brainstem anteriorly. Biopsy proven case of medulloblastoma. (MRI: magnetic resonance imaging; T1: transverse 1)

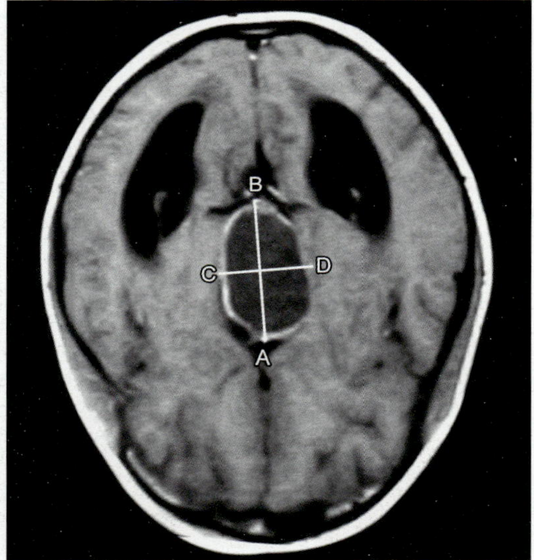

Fig. 6.11.3: Postgadolinium T1-weighted coronal MRI image of brain showing a well-defined rim-enhancing lesion in the third ventricle. Biopsy proven case of the third ventricle ependymoma. (MRI: magnetic resonance imaging; T1: transverse 1)

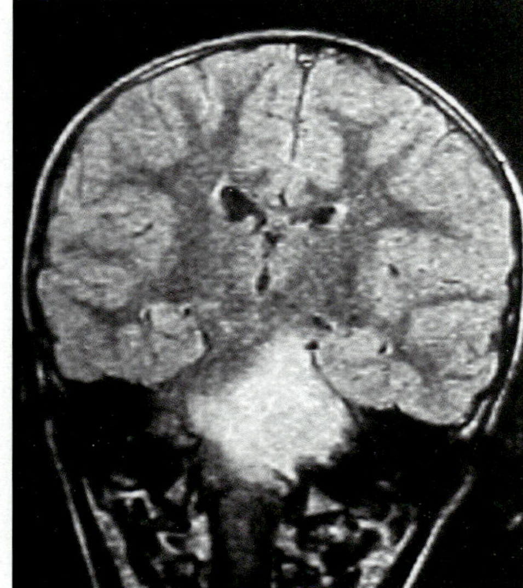

Fig. 6.11.4: FLAIR coronal MRI images of brain showing an ill-defined mass lesion expanding the pons. Biopsy proven case of pontine glioma. (FLAIR: fluid-attenuated inversion recovery; MRI: magnetic resonance imaging)

in delineating benign masses from malignant growths, inflammatory and infectious conditions, and normal brain tissue. Tumors in the posterior fossa, temporal lobe, sellar and chiasmatic regions are also best visualized with MRI.

- Positron emission tomography and MR spectroscopy have a role in characterization of brain tumors, in follow-up and in differentiation from other nonmalignant conditions.
- Computed tomography is the imaging modality of choice in an emergency.

Cerebrospinal fluid studies for malignant cells are advised in tumors, having tendency to spread.

Immunohistopathology of the resected tumor and molecular testing have improved diagnostic accuracy, better targeted therapy, and prognostication.

TREATMENT

Surgery remains the mainstay and the initial step in the treatment of brain tumors. Total resection may not be possible in many cases, but partial resection is useful to reduce the bulk of tumor thus permitting destruction of the remaining malignant cells by the irradiation or chemotherapy. Partial resection provides tissue for immunohistology that is essential for the specific diagnosis and characterization of tumor's behavior. Significant postsurgical sequelae are unavoidable in many situations. Hypothalamic and pituitary abnormalities are common in supratentorial midline tumors, such as craniopharyngioma. Cerebellar mutism syndrome, characterized by postoperative mutism, emotional liabilities, irritability, hypotonia, and other cerebellar deficits, is seen primarily but not exclusively after medulloblastomas resection. This is thought to be secondary to disruption of cerebellar dentate nuclei or pathways between dentate nuclei and cortex. It can be permanent in 50% of cases.

Radiotherapy can be used either as an adjuvant to surgery or definitive therapy. Many pediatric brain tumors are radiosensitive. Newer radiotherapy techniques are more precisely targeted to the tumor with less radiation doses and minimal or no collateral damage to surrounding brain tissue. Newer modalities include brachytherapy, three-dimensional conformal radiation therapy, confronted proton beam radiation therapy, intensity modulated radiation therapy, and stereotactic radiotherapy. Radiotherapy is the pillar of palliative care in most malignant and aggressive neoplasms or infiltrative benign masses not amenable to surgery. The overall survival has improved with radiotherapy, but long-term sequelae are a concern. Common long-term effects are endocrinal, growth/development, and cognition. Long-term sequelae depend upon the age of the child, dose and type of radiation, and pre-existing brain injury. Secondary neoplasms after radiation exposure are another long-term concern.

Addition of chemotherapy has increased median survival rates for high-risk neoplasms. The common chemotherapeutic agents used are deoxyribonucleic acid alkylators and alkaloids. Overall success remains unchanged, reasons are impairments to drug delivery across blood-brain barrier and resistant to drugs. Newer strategies have been designed to concentrate chemotherapy agents directly into the tumor with least effect on the body stem cells and regional delivery systems, such as intrathecal or intraventricular.

Recent advances in biological therapy include primarily supportive care measures, such as the use of hematopoietic growth factors and autologous stem cell harvesting and reinfusion. Identification of major targets, such as the *epidermal growth factor receptor, platelet-derived growth factor receptor, vascular endothelial growth factor*, and key signaling pathways, such as the *mitogen-activated protein kinase* and *phosphatidylinositol 3-kinase* (*PI3K*)/AKT/*mammalian target of rapamycin (mTOR) pathway*, has enhanced the knowledge of physicians in understanding the tumor behavior and design-tailored therapy.

Immunotherapy, a novel modality to treat deadly or incurable brain neoplasms, has a supportive role in prolonging survival and improving the quality of life of such children. Adverse effects and toxicity related to conventional treatment of brain tumors significantly reduces the quality of patient's life. Although most immunotherapy approaches are not successful in solid tumors, several early phase clinical trials are beginning to reveal a potential role of immunotherapy in the treatment of brain neoplasms. Promising immunotherapy includes de novo activation of T cells through cancer vaccines, oncolytic viral therapy, or *ex vivo* engineered cell therapy. Monoclonal antibodies are also showing promising role; however, the main concern is how to deliver across the blood-brain barrier.

In gene therapy, genetic material is transferred to cancer cells to either stop or slow the growth and multiplication of these cells. Genetic material in the cells also increases the susceptibility to other treatment modalities. Gene transfer technology has used many viruses as delivery agents.

Endocrine dysfunctions are common before and after surgery and after craniospinal radiation or chemotherapy for supratentorial midline neoplasms. Complete endocrine workup before surgery for midline tumors is essential for better outcome. Children with tumors near hypothalamic-pituitary axis are prone for fluid and electrolytes abnormalities during perioperative period. All children (except those having Cushing disease) with midline tumors near pituitary hypothalamic axis are administered hydrocortisone 100 mg every 6–8 hourly during surgery and postoperative period for 3 days. Hydrocortisone is continued, if serum cortisol levels are low. Endocrinal follow-up is recommended after the resection of a craniopharyngioma and other midline masses and cranial irradiation for a long time.

Prophylactic antiepileptic drugs, such as intravenous phenytoin 10 mg/kg as slow loading followed by 4–8 mg/kg/day, are recommended during perioperative period. Psychological assessment is critical as these children are more prone for cognitive and behavioral problems (**Table 6.11.5**).

Table 6.11.5: Common childhood brain tumors.

Type of tumor	Salient features
Glioma	• Gliomas arise from glial precursors and are differentiated along astrocytic and oligodendroglial lineage. Occurs through all ages and throughout neuraxis. Histologically these are either low-grade (WHO grade I or II) or high-grade gliomas (WHO grade III or IV) • Low-grade gliomas are the most common brain tumors in childhood constituting more than 20% of all childhood primary brain tumors. The common sites are cerebellum, visual pathways, and diencephalon. According to WHO grading system, gliomas are either grade I or grade II. Common tumors in grade I are pilocytic astrocytoma, subependymal giant cell astrocytoma, and astrocytic astrocytoma. Grade II examples are oligodendroglioma, oligoastrocytoma, neurocytoma, and diffuse astrocytoma • Common genetic abnormalities in low-grade astrocytoma are gain in chromosome 7, 4, 5, 6, 8, and 11 and deletion of 17p and 1q. In DIPG, the genetic aberrations are gain of chromosome 1q, 2p, 2q, 8q, and 9q and common deletions of 16q, 14q, 17p, and 20p. High-grade gliomas have more association with familial genetic syndromes, such as Li-Fraumeni, Turcot type-1, and CMMR-D syndrome. Common tumors in this group according to WHO grading are: glioblastoma (IV), anaplastic oligodendroglioma (III), and anaplastic oligoastrocytoma (III) • Clinical presentations depend upon the location, age of the child, and behavior of the tumor. High-grade gliomas present with recent history of symptoms and progress very fast. Low-grade tumors present slowly, and presentations can be atypical. In DIPG the median duration of symptoms is about 1 month. Signs include cranial nerves palsy, cerebellar and long tract signs. Rarely pathological laughter can also be the presenting symptom • Modalities of investigations are MRI brain with contrast and MRS. Treatment options are radical surgical resection, radiotherapy, and chemotherapy. In DIPG, radiotherapy is the mainstay of treatment; chemotherapy and surgery have poor role. In glioblastoma, management is radical surgery, followed by radiations. In adults, temozolomide is considered the standard care, but in pediatric glioblastoma, its role is limited
Medulloblastoma	• Embryonal tumor of the cerebellum believed to arise from the stem cells and neuronal progenitor cells in and around the cerebellum. Accounts for 20% of primary brain neoplasms and 40% of all posterior fossa tumors • It has bimodal incidence peak between 3 years and 4 years and 7 years to 10 years of age. Commonly associated with familial syndromes, such as Gorlin (germline mutation of *PATCHED*-1 gene on chromosome 9), Turcot's type-1 (mutations of the adenomatous polyposis gene), and Li-Fraumeni syndrome (germline mutation TP53). Rarely medulloblastoma has association with Rubinstein–Taybi and Fanconi syndrome. Therapeutic radiation exposure is another risk factor. • Age of onset, sex predilection, and outcome depend upon the molecular subgrouping. Commonly present with the features of raised intracranial pressure. Macroscopic bleed and rapid progression can lead to sudden altered sensorium and coma. Classical sun setting sign is seen rarely • Medulloblastoma can spread along neuraxis but there are no signs and symptoms of dissemination. Lesion is well-defined, homogenous; hypointense on T1-weighted images and hyperintense on T2. Majority of them enhance with contrast. • Treatment is surgical excision, followed by radiotherapy and chemotherapy. Posterior fossa mutism syndrome is the most common complication following surgery seen in almost 20–30% children. With current means of treatment, most of the children are expected to survive more than 5 years after the diagnosis. Majority of the survivors are left with neurocognitive delay, endocrinal problems (commonest growth hormone deficiency). High-grade gliomas are the common recurring neoplasms after adjuvant therapy and are very resistant to treatment.
Craniopharyngioma	• Craniopharyngioma is a benign tumor histologically, but its unique relationship with vital structures, such as optic pathways and hypothalamic-pituitary axis and its high recurrence rate, makes the management very challenging. It arises from the embryonic remnants of the Rathke's pouch in the parasellar region. Tumor is partially calcified and heterogeneous having solid and cystic components • Histologically, it has three variants: adamantinomatous, papillary, and rarely mixed variety. Often infiltrates the surrounding critical structures. • Tumor has a bimodal age distribution with peaks at age 5 years and 15 years and another peak in adults between 50 years and 75 years of age. The diagnosis is delayed because of the slow growth. Headache due to raised intracranial pressure is the presenting complaint in about 75%. Visual complaints due to pressure on visual pathways are observed in more than 50%. Hypothalamic and pituitary dysfunctions as presenting complaints are seen in 25–50% cases. Growth hormone deficiency is seen in 75% of children with craniopharyngioma, followed by deficiency of gonadotropins (93%). Diabetes insipidus develops in the two-thirds of cases • Preoperative endocrinal workup is essential. MRI contrast shows enhancing cystic capsule and solid tumor. • Presently, there is no consensus on optimal management strategies. Treatment can be radical surgery, subtotal resection with radiation, and intracystic irradiation/bleomycin/interferon. Frequent follow-up with neuroimaging is essential to detect early recurrence. Hypothalamic-pituitary dysfunction is common and includes obesity, hyperphagia, memory deficit, thermoregulation instability, labile behavior, and sleep-awake cycle abnormalities.

Contd...

Contd...

Type of tumor	*Salient features*
Ependymoma	• Second most common primary malignant neoplasm of the central nervous system, accounting for about 10% of all childhood primary brain tumors. More than 50% of the intracranial ependymomas arise in children less than 5 years of age. In adults, spinal origin predominates. Prevalence is slightly more in males. During childhood, 75% of them originate in the fourth ventricle. • Most common presentation is features of raised intracranial pressure. Some of the children may present with cerebellar or lower cranial nerves features. Very young child is brought with excessive irritability or lethargy. • Probable location of origin is ependymal lining of ventricles and central canal; however, these may arise anywhere along neuraxis not related to ependymal lining. Dissemination via cerebrospinal fluid is reported in 10–20%. In adults, the most common spinal site is filum terminale. • MRI typically displays iso- to hypointensities on T1W and hyperintensities on T2W images. Contrast enhancement is heterogeneous. There is genetic and epigenetic heterogeneity between different spinal cord and intracranial locations. In intracranial ependymomas, there is upregulation of *RAF-1* gene and, in spinal cord, there is upregulation of PLA2GS-ITIH2 and HOX family of genes. In supratentorial neoplasms, EPHB–EPHRIN is overexpressed, while there is a loss of chromosomes 22q, 6q, and 17q in infratentorial tumors. • Treatment is primarily surgical excision, followed by chemo- and radiotherapy. Recurrence is common, and outcome becomes poor with subsequent recurrences. Prognostic features are degree of surgical resection, age (older children better outcome), and location (supratentorial, the outcome is better).
AT/RT	• Highly malignant tumor that occurs predominantly in children younger than 3 years of age. It accounts for 3% of total childhood primary central nervous system neoplasms. About 15% of children less than 3 years of age with primary brain tumors have AT/RT. • Due to aggressive nature of the disease, children present with very brief onset of symptoms. Clinical presentations depend upon the location of the tumor and the age of the child. Infratentorial neoplasm presents with the features of raised intracranial pressure, and presentation of supratentorial masses is seizures and focal neurodeficits. Other nonspecific features can be progressively enlarging head, neuroregression, and lethargy. AT/RT can arise in the spinal cord also, and manifestations are those of spinal cord compression. • MRI shows heterogeneous intensities on T1W and T2W images because of intralesion bleed. Contrast enhancement is also heterogeneous because of bleed in the mass lesion. MRS typically shows high choline peak and absent or reduced *N*-acetyl-aspartate peak. Histological picture is mixed of rhabdoid cells, primitive neuroectodermal cells, epithelial and mesenchymal cells. Genetically, there is complete or partial loss of chromosome 22 (mutated genes—*SMARKB1*, *SMARKA4*). • Treatment is radical surgical excision. Chemotherapy is the mainstay of adjuvant therapy. Radiotherapy can also be given. Outcome is poor due to high toxicity related to adjuvant treatment.

(AT/RT: atypical teratoid/rhabdoid tumor; CMMR-D: constitutional mismatch repair deficiency; DIPG: diffuse intrinsic pontine glioma; MRI: magnetic resonance imaging; MRS: magnetic resonance spectroscopy; T1: transverse 1; T2: transverse 2; T1W: transverse 1 weight; T2W: transverse 2 weight; TP53: tumor protein p53; WHO: World Health Organization)

BIBLIOGRAPHY

1. Canabas R, Saurez G, Alert J, et al. Prolonged use of nimotuzumab in children with central nervous system tumors: safety and feasibility. Cancer Biother Radiopharm. 2014;29:173-8.
2. Jain A, Sharma MC, Suri V, et al. Spectrum of brain tumors in India: a multi-institutional study. Neurol India. 2011;59:208-11.
3. Kim KE, Kim KU, Kim DC, et al. Cytogenetic characterization of central nervous system tumors: the first comprehensive report for a single institute in Korea. J Korean Med Sci. 2009;24:453-60.
4. Kimbly JJ, Jennifer C, Jill SBS, et al. Childhood brain tumors epidemiology: a brain tumors epidemiology consortium review. Cancer Epidemiol Biomarkers Prev. 2014;23:2716-36.
5. Lieberman NAP, Vitanza NA, Crane CA. Immunotherapy for brain tumors: understanding early success and limitations. Expert Rev Neurother. 2018;18:251-9.
6. Louis DN, Perry A, Reifenberger G, et al. The 2016 WHO classification of the tumors of the central nervous system: a summary. Acta Neuropathol. 2016;131:803-20.
7. Packer RJ. Pediatric neuro-oncology: an overview. In: Swaiman KF, Stephen A, Donna MF, Nima FS, Richard SF, Adrea LG, Phillip LP, Michel IS (Eds). Swaiman's Pediatric Neurology: Principles and Practice, 6th edition. Edinburgh: Elsevier. pp. 957-62.
8. Sung HP, Jaekyung W, Seong IK, et al. Molecular testing of brain tumors. J Pathol Transl Med. 2017;51:205-23.
9. Veeravagu A, Lee M, Jiang B, et al. The role of radiosurgery in the treatment of craniopharyngiomas. Neurosurg Focus. 2010;28:E11.
10. Wibroe M, Cappelen J, Caster C, et al. Cerebellar mutism syndrome in children with brain tumors of posterior fossa. BMC Cancer. 2017;17:439.

6.12 Raised Intracranial Pressure

Sunit Singhi

INTRODUCTION

Raised intracranial pressure (ICP) is a life-threatening condition that is commonly seen in emergency with both traumatic and nontraumatic neurological illnesses. Unless recognized and treated early, it may cause secondary brain injury due to reduced cerebral perfusion pressure (CPP) and progress into herniation syndrome and death.

PATHOPHYSIOLOGY

Monro-Kellie doctrine states that in a noncompliant skull vault, ICP is the sum of pressure exerted by the brain (≈80%), blood (≈10%), and cerebrospinal fluid [CSF (≈10%)]. The volume of brain tissue increases without a significant change in ICP only if there is an adaptive reduction in CSF and cerebral blood volume, but when these adaptations have been exhausted, ICP increases exponentially.

Normal Values

The normal range for ICP varies with age. The usual normal range is considered as 5–15 mm Hg. In newborn term infants, it is 1.5–6 mm Hg; in young children, 3–7 mm Hg; and in older children, 10–15 mm Hg. ICP more than 20 mm Hg is considered as intracranial hypertension requiring treatment. For all practical purposes, if symptoms and signs of raised ICP are present, one should consider that ICP is more than 20 mm Hg and treat accordingly. Sustained ICP values more than 40 mm Hg indicate severe life-threatening raised ICP.

Cerebral Perfusion Pressure

Cerebral perfusion pressure is the pressure at which brain is perfused. It provides an indirect measure of adequacy of cerebral blood flow (CBF). It is calculated as the difference between mean arterial pressure (MAP) and ICP (CPP = MAP – ICP). Generally, accepted minimal CPP values necessary to prevent ischemia are as follows: infants or toddlers: more than 40–50 mm Hg; children: more than 50–60 mm Hg. CPP less than 40 mm Hg is a significant predictor of mortality in children with traumatic brain injury.

Autoregulation maintains a steady CBF within a CPP range of 50–150 mm Hg. It is lost at CPP values less than 50 mm Hg. Once autoregulation is lost, CBF and cerebral blood volume become dependent on changes in systemic blood pressure.

Box 6.12.1: Common causes of raised intracranial pressure.

- *Increase in brain volume:*
  - *Cytotoxic edema:* Encephalitis, meningitis, head injury, Reye's syndrome
  - *Vasogenic edema*: Hypoxic ischemic injury (hypoventilation, shock), ischemic stroke or infract
  - *Metabolic encephalopathy*: Hyperpyrexia, hepatic failure, lead intoxication
  - *Space-occupying lesions*: Hematomas, tumors, abscesses
- *Increases in blood volume*:
  - *Venous obstruction*: Cerebral venous thrombosis
  - *Vasodilatation*: Due to hypoxia, drugs, or hypercapnia
  - Status epilepticus
- *Increases in cerebrospinal fluid volume*:
  - Obstructive hydrocephalus, communicating hydrocephalus
  - *Impaired reabsorption*: Subarachnoid hemorrhage
  - *Increased production*: Tumors
- Idiopathic or benign intracranial hypertension

ETIOLOGY

Common causes of raised ICP with respect to pathophysiology are shown in **Box 6.12.1**.

CLINICAL FEATURES

Clinical symptoms and signs of raised ICP are highly variable and depend on the nature and location of the primary brain insult, and the rate of increase in ICP.

In awake patients, irritability, headache, vomiting, confusion and decreased alertness, neck retraction, and tense fontanel on palpation may be presenting features. Papilledema, though a reliable sign of raised ICP, is usually absent in acute conditions.

In unconscious or comatose patients, raised ICP should be suspected in all patients with head injury, meningitis encephalitis, liver disease, and diabetes mellitus. The clinical features strongly favoring raised ICP are abnormal posturing (decerebration or decortication), abnormal pupillary dilatation, hypertension, bradycardia, irregular breathing, sixth nerve palsy, and papilledema.

Computed tomography (CT) scan signs of brain swelling are predictive of increased ICP, but the CT scan may be normal even in the presence of documented raised ICP.

MANAGEMENT

Goals and Principles of Therapy

The immediate goal is to prevent progression to herniation or to reverse the herniation if present, and then to maintain adequate CPP.

The principle therapeutic measures include maintaining normoxia and normocarbia, avoiding factors that aggravate or precipitate raised ICP, namely fever, hypoxia, hypoglycemia, hypotension, and any noxious stimulation, treatment of underlying cause whether intracranial or extracranial, maintain adequate MAP (more than 50th centile for given age and gender) with help of fluid and, if needed, vasoactive therapy and bringing ICP down with hyperosmolar therapy and other measures.

Therapeutic modalities to treat raised ICP are shown in **Box 6.12.2** and an overall approach in **Flowchart 6.12.1**.

AIRWAY, BREATHING, AND CIRCULATION

Airway

In unconscious patients, airway patency should be ensured by positioning the patient on the side and suctioning of the oral secretion. Oro- or nasopharyngeal airways can be used. Endotracheal intubation and assisted ventilation are needed in patients with a modified Glasgow Coma Scale less than or equal to eight, signs of respiratory distress, declining O_2 saturation, irregular respiratory efforts, inadequate chest movements, or central cyanosis.

Box 6.12.2: Therapeutic modalities to reduce raised intracranial pressure.

- *General measures and first-tier therapy:*
  - Head in neutral position, 30° elevation
  - *Ensure oxygenation*: Normoxia and normocarbia ($PaCO_2$ = 35 mm Hg)
  - *Ensure adequate circulating volume*: Normovolemia
  - Maintain normal BP
  - Ventilation to achieve $PaCO_2$ = 35 mm Hg
  - Osmotic diuretic; mannitol 0.25–0.50/kg IV over 20 minutes, repeat SOS or hypertonic (3%) saline infusion: 10 mL bolus, 0.1–1.0 mL/kg/h infusion
  - *Dexamethasone*: 1–2 mg/kg IV q6 hourly cytotoxic cerebral edema (brain abscess, granuloma, and tumor)
  - *Cerebrospinal fluid drainage*: Obstructive hydrocephalus
  - Prevent all events that increase intracranial pressure

Fever: Hypothermia; *Pain*: Adequate sedation, analgesia; *Seizures*: Anticonvulsant, loud noise, invasive stimuli

- *Second-tier therapy:*
  - Profound hyperventilation ($PaCO_2$ 30–35 mm Hg)
  - *Barbiturates coma*: Thiopental or pentobarbital
  - Moderate hypothermia (32–34°C)
- *Third-tier therapy:*
  - Decompressive craniectomy or temporal lobectomy
  - Hyperventilation to $PaCO_2$ < 30 mm Hg (use transiently)

(BP: blood pressure, IV: intravenous)

Breathing

Start 100% oxygen with nonrebreathing mask and if needed use bag valve mask ventilation to ensure adequate oxygenation. Short-term hyperventilation is required in patients with signs of impending herniation (unequal pupils, posturing).

Circulation

Maintain euvolemia and use isotonic fluids. If there are signs of poor perfusion, give a bolus of normal saline 20 mL/kg. Maintain good blood pressure to achieve desired CPP, if needed, by using fluid and vasoactive agents (dopamine, norepinephrine). Colloids are not recommended.

GENERAL MANAGEMENT

Head position: Elevate head end of bed by 30° and keep head in neutral position to promote venous drainage.

Temperature: Keep below 38°C. If child is febrile, use paracetamol 15 mg/kg/dose and surface cooling.

Sedation and analgesia: Use midazolam 1–3 μg/kg/min, morphine 0.1 mg/kg/dose q6 hourly, and titrate to achieve a level that the patient responds to commands only and is asleep.

Glucose control: Keep random blood sugar around 150 mg/dL. Hypoglycemia (<60 mg/dL) and hyperglycemia (>180 mg/dL) should be avoided.

Seizure prophylaxis: Use phenytoin 20 mg/kg intravenous (IV) loading, followed by 5–8 mg/kg/day for the first 7 days for seizure prophylaxis in patients with severe head injury, focal symptoms and signs, and central nervous system infections.

Use lidocaine 1 mg/kg/dose 5 minutes before endotracheal suctioning and procedure. Do not repeat within 2 hours.

Gastrointestinal (GI) bleed prophylaxis: Use antacid 1 mL/kg/dose q8 hourly or pantoprazole 1 mg/kg/dose q12 hourly (if GI bleed is present use pantoprazole).

Anemia: Maintain Hb concentration around 10 g/dL to help cerebral oxygen delivery.

Hypertension: Characteristically increase in systolic pressure is common in response to raised ICP. Generally, it is left untouched in acute raised ICP unless underlying cause is

Flowchart 6.12.1: Approach to management of raised intracranial pressure.

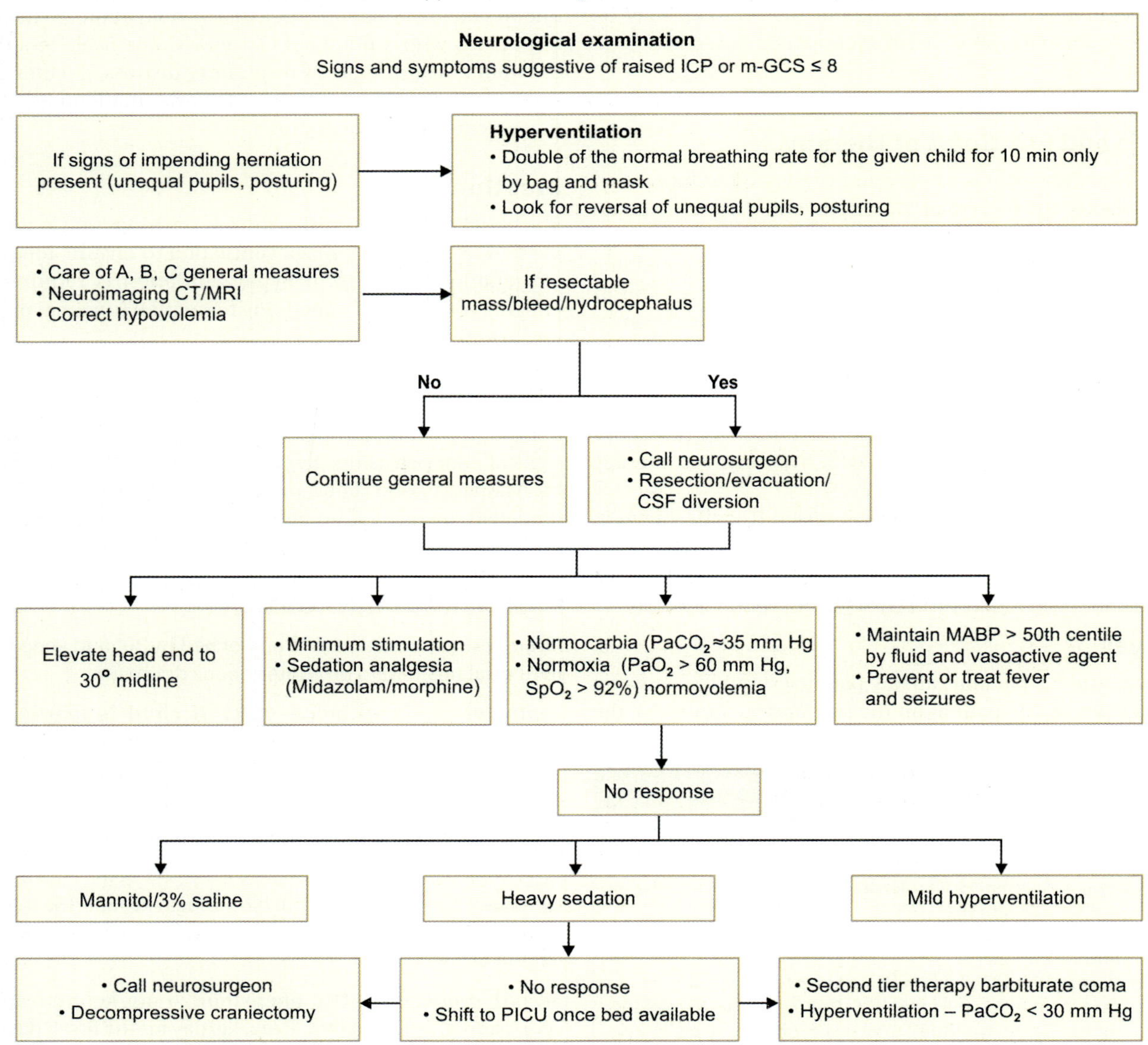

(CSF: cerebrospinal fluid; CT: computed tomography; ICP: intracranial pressure; MABP: mean arterial blood pressure; m-GCS: motor-Glasgow Coma Scale; MRI: magnetic resonance imaging; PICU: pediatric intensive care unit)

hypertensive encephalopathy. Treatment is reasonable in patients with evidence of rapidly worsening brain edema on CT scan, and those with a persistent extreme surge in blood pressure. If it is decided to treat hypertension, vasodilating drugs, such as nitroprusside, nitroglycerin, and nifedipine, should be avoided; these could increase ICP. Sympathomimetic-blocking drugs (esmolol, labetalol) or centrally acting alpha-receptor agonists (clonidine) are preferred, because they reduce blood pressure without affecting ICP.

First-tier Treatment

After initial general measures, if signs of raised ICP persist, use first-tier therapy.

Mild Short-term Ventilation

Mild short-term ventilation should be undertaken, if danger of impending herniation is present (see above under breathing). Monitor for reversal of unequal pupils, posturing, and improvement in mentation, after that target a $PaCO_2 \approx 35$ mm Hg. There is no role for prophylactic hyperventilation.

Heavy Sedation

Use morphine and midazolam and titrate the dose to achieve a state where child is asleep and has sluggish response to glabellar tap.

Osmotherapy (Mannitol, Hypertonic Saline)

Mannitol: An amount of 2.5 mL/kg of 20% mannitol given as a rapid infusion reduces blood viscosity and improves microvascular CBF, cerebral oxygenation, and CPP with reduction in cerebral blood volume initially. Within 15–30 minutes, it reduces ICP through direct osmotic effect on neural cells with reduction in total brain water and reduced CSF production. If further dose is required, use 1.25–2.5 mL/kg/dose. Do not repeat mannitol in less than 4 hours. Monitor the urine output and take care of hypovolemia. Mannitol is contraindicated in decompensated shock, oliguria, anuria, and heart failure.

Hypertonic saline (3% HS): HS creates an osmotic force to draw water from the interstitial space of the brain parenchyma into the intravascular space. It promotes rapid CSF absorption, increases cardiac output, and expands intravascular volume, thereby augmenting the CPP with a positive inotropic effect. Usual loading dose is 10 mL/kg followed by 0.1–1 mL/kg/h. In cerebral edema, the initial serum sodium goal is commonly set at 145–155 mEq/L and is intensified up to 160 mEq/L, if clinically indicated. Monitor serum sodium and creatinine every 6 hours. It is contraindicated, if serum sodium is more than 150 mEq/L, and/or osmolality is more than 320 mOsmol/L. Therapy must be tapered after 24 hours of continued infusion to prevent rebound raise of ICP.

Mannitol versus HS: It is unclear which of these two therapies is superior for reduction of ICP. A recent systematic review found that HS appears to achieve a greater reduction in ICP than other osmotic agents in head injury patients. In a study of nontraumatic encephalopathies, there was less mortality with use of HS as compared to mannitol.

Other Therapeutic Measures

Corticosteroids

Corticosteroids are commonly used for primary and secondary brain tumors to decrease vasogenic edema. The most commonly used regimen is IV dexamethasone 0.15 mg/kg/dose every 6 hours (maximum 16 mg/day). Routine use in head injury is not recommended.

Antibiotics or Antiviral Agents

A febrile child with raised ICP should receive empiric ceftriaxone (50 mg/kg IV q12 hourly), acyclovir 30 mg/kg IV in three divided doses 8 hourly as infusion over 1–2 hours for herpes encephalitis, and IV quinine if child is a resident of *Plasmodium falciparum* endemic area and has hypoglycemia and anemia.

INVESTIGATIONS

Random blood sugar, iCa^{2+}, serum electrolytes, hemogram, blood culture, and febrile encephalopathy work up.

Neuroimaging

Obtain neuroimaging (CT/magnetic resonance imaging) in all patients with raised ICP soon after stabilization. CT will readily identify intracranial bleed, hydrocephalus, cerebral edema, compartmental shifts, infarct, abscess, or intracranial space-occupying lesions. Initial normal CT does not rule out an evolving lesion of an infection or raised ICP. In herpes simplex encephalitis, CT head is abnormal in approximately 50% of cases but may be normal in the first 4–5 days.

Monitoring

Monitor continuously for all vital parameters (temperature, heart rate, respiratory rate, and blood pressure) and level of consciousness (hourly), neurological status, brainstem signs, oxygenation (SpO_2), $EtCO_2$, ICP, and CPP. Also assess adequacy of sedation and analgesia, input and output, and bowel sounds. After a dose of mannitol, monitor the urine output hourly. Random blood sugar should be monitored at least every 6 hours, and if hypoglycemia or hyperglycemia is present, monitor blood sugar every 1–2 hours. Serum sodium should be monitored every 4–6 hours, if 3% saline is used. Electroencephalogram should be monitored to look for nonconvulsive seizure, if child is comatose.

KEY POINTS

- Raised ICP is a life-threatening condition; unless recognized and treated early, it may progress into herniation syndrome and death.
- Symptoms and signs are neither sufficiently sensitive nor specific; hence, a high index of suspicion and vigilance is needed for early recognition.
- Immediate goal of management is to prevent or reverse herniation and to maintain good CPP.
- The therapeutic measures include stabilization of airway, breathing, and circulation, along with neutral neck position, head end elevation by 30°, adequate sedation

and analgesia, minimal stimulation, and hyperosmolar therapy (mannitol or 3% saline).

- Short-term hyperventilation (to achieve $PCO_2 \approx 30$ mm Hg) using bag ventilation can be resorted to if signs of impending herniation are present.

BIBLIOGRAPHY

1. Bansal A, Singhi SC, Singhi PD, et al. Non traumatic coma. Indian J Pediatr. 2005;72:467-73.
2. Gwer S, Gatakaa H, Mwai L, et al. The role for osmotic agents in children with acute encephalopathies: a systematic review. BMC Pediatr. 2010;10:23-30.
3. Knapp JM. Hyperosmolar therapy in the treatment of severe head injury in children: mannitol and hypertonic saline. AACN Clin Issues. 2005;16:199-211.
4. Mayer MJ, Megyesi J, Meythaler J, et al. Acute management of acquired brain injury part II: an evidence-based review of pharmacological interventions. Brain Inj. 2010;24:706-21.
5. Singhi P, Singhi S, Baranwal AK. Bacterial meningitis in children: critical care needs. Indian J Pediatr. 2001;68:737-47.
6. Singhi SC, Tiwari L. Management of intracranial hypertension. Indian J Pediatr. 2009;76:519-29.
7. Thompson AE, Salonia R. Airway management. In: Fuhrman BP, Zimmerman JJ (Eds). Pediatric Critical Care, 4th edition. Philadelphia, PA: Elsevier Saunders; 2011.

6.13 Stroke

Satinder Aneja

INTRODUCTION

Stroke is defined by the World Health Organization as a clinical syndrome of rapidly developing focal or global disturbance of brain function lasting more than 24 hours or leading to death with no obvious nonvascular cause. Stroke can result from rupture of a vessel (hemorrhagic stroke), occlusion of artery (arterial ischemic), or a vein/venous sinus (sinovenous thrombosis). An acute onset of focal neurological deficit may not always be due to vascular derangement but may result from metabolic derangements—also referred to as "stroke-like syndrome." Neuroradiological diagnosis based on newer imaging techniques has contributed to the increased recognition of cerebrovascular disease that was overlooked in previous years. Cerebrovascular disease in children is most frequently associated with several conditions, many of which are genetic. In addition, the brain of a child is immature and has more plasticity than adult brain, so recovery and final outcome is better in younger patients than adults.

EPIDEMIOLOGY

The reported incidence ranges from 3 to 8 per 100,000 children per year. Arterial ischemic strokes (AIS) constituted 80% of cases. Neonates are at significantly increased risk for stroke compared with older infants and children. At all ages, there is an unexplained male predominance for ischemic stroke. Ethnic and geographic variations in stroke incidence and mortality have been reported.

ETIOLOGY

Stroke is broadly classified into ischemic stroke due to interruption of blood flow to a part of brain, and hemorrhagic stroke due to rupture of blood vessels with bleeding into the cerebral parenchyma.

The common causes of ischemic and hemorrhagic strokes are summarized in **Table 6.13.1**. The most frequently reported risk factors for stroke in children include cardiac disorders, coagulation disorders, sickle cell disease, vasculopathies, arterial dissection, and genetic disorders. Risk factors in children with AIS are definable in approximately 80% of cases, are age-related, and differ significantly from adults. Embolic stroke secondary to congenital heart disease is a frequent cause of stroke during childhood. Several cardiac disorders are associated with stroke in children, including congenital heart disease, cardiac procedures, and acquired heart disease.

Infections of central nervous system (CNS), e.g. acute bacterial meningitis, tuberculous meningitis, are common causes of stroke in children in tropical countries. Occlusion of blood vessels by perivascular exudates and endarteritis is the underlying cause of stroke in infections of CNS. Varicella has been identified as an important risk factor for childhood stroke and is reported to account for a significant proportion of ischemic strokes. The stroke may occur a week to months after varicella infection. The exact mechanism is not known but vascular changes with irregular stenosis and beading has been observed. A wide variety of infections are known to trigger stroke.

Table 6.13.1: Risk factors of stroke in children.

Ischemic stroke	*Hemorrhagic stroke*
• *Heart disease*: – Congenital heart disease – Rheumatic heart disease – Infective endocarditis – Complication of cardiac surgery • *Hematologic disorders*: – Sickle cell anemia – Leukemia – Polycythemia • *Prothrombotic states*: – Protein C, protein S deficiency – AT III deficiency – Antiphospholipid antibodies • *Vasculopathies*: – *Infective* ▪ Pyogenic ▪ Tuberculosis ▪ Fungal ▪ AIDS ▪ Postvaricella vasculopathy – *Noninfective* ▪ Moyamoya disease ▪ SLE ▪ Polyarteritis nodosa ▪ Takayasu arteritis • *Hereditary/metabolic:* – Homocystinuria – Raised lipoprotein(a) • *Trauma:* – Blunt cervical arterial trauma – Arterial dissection – Oral foreign bodies injuring carotid artery • *Miscellaneous*: – Hypotension – Iron deficiency anemia	• *Vascular malformation:* – Arteriovenous malformations – Aneurysm – Angiomas • *Hematological:* – Leukemia – Thrombocytopenia – Hemophilia – Disseminated intravascular coagulation • *Trauma:* – Falls – Shaken body syndrome – Birth trauma

(AIDS: acquired immune deficiency syndrome; AT: antithrombin; SLE: systemic lupus erythematosus)

Cervicocerebral arterial dissections have been increasingly recognized as a cause of stroke. Arterial dissections may occur in internal carotid artery or vertebral artery. In each arterial system, the segment of the artery involved can be extracranial or intracranial. Cervicocerebral dissections are often preceded by some form of trauma to the neck.

Iron deficiency anemia is a risk factor for stroke in children. The possible underlying mechanism includes thrombocytosis leading to hypercoagulable state and anemic hypoxia.

Moyamoya disease is characterized by progressive stenosis and occlusion of the cerebral arteries at the circle of Willis. In response to the stenosis, an abnormal network of small collateral vessels develops, creating the characteristic "puff of smoke" appearance on angiograms. Children with Moyamoya disease present with recurrent transient ischemic attacks as well as AIS. In general, there is a progressive neurologic deterioration that is characterized by significant impairment of motor and cognitive function.

Risk factors for cerebrovascular disease are outlined in **Table 6.13.1**.

CLINICAL FEATURES

The clinical features at presentation vary with age of the patient, the type of stroke, and extent of involvement. Older children usually present like adults with hemiplegia, hemisensory loss, aphasia, and other neurological deficits appropriate to the vascular territory affected. The age at which the hemiplegia appears may vary with the specific cause. Trauma and bacterial infections are most common during the preschool years. Cerebral occlusive vascular disease associated with cyanotic congenital heart disease is most frequently observed during first 2 years of life.

The clinical picture is partly dependent upon the primary disease responsible for the hemiparesis. Neurological manifestations both in the otherwise healthy child and in the child with a precipitating condition vary according to the rapidity of development and the site and extent of damage. Embolism produces a rapidly evolving clinical picture, with maximum involvement within a few minutes. Thrombosis is slower in development and may progress either intermittently or progressively during a period of hours or days. There may be a prodromal period of days to weeks, consisting of febrile upper respiratory infections or frontal headache contralateral to the hemiparesis.

There are three clinical distinct syndromes of stroke, i.e. AIS, cerebral sinovenous thrombosis (CSVT), and hemorrhage.

Arterial Ischemic Stroke

It is the most common clinical type of stroke seen accounting for nearly two-thirds of children with stroke. Anterior circulation is affected in more than 80% of patients, and middle cerebral artery is the most common vessel involved. It typically presents with acute onset of neurological deficit, such as hemiparesis with upper limb involved with or without seizures. Seizures at the onset of stroke are relatively frequent in children and indicate cortical involvement. In older children with involvement of dominant hemisphere, aphasia is prominent feature. In patients with lesions at internal capsule, there is dense hemiplegia with facial nerve palsy of upper motor neuron type. Infarcts in posterior circulation and large infarcts involving middle cerebral artery may present with alteration of sensorium. Focal signs may be absent in neonates or young infants, in whom seizures may be the only manifestation of clinical stroke.

Cerebral Sinovenous Thrombosis

Cerebral sinovenous thrombosis commonly occurs in the setting of acute illnesses, e.g. sepsis or dehydration and head and neck infections. The presentation is influenced by age, extent and location of thrombus, and presence of associated venous infarction. It is more common in neonates. The main neurologic manifestations of sinovenous thrombosis in the children are a decreased level of consciousness, headache, and focal neurologic signs such as hemiparesis, and cranial nerve palsies. Signs of raised intracranial pressure (ICP) typically develop gradually over hours and days. Diffuse neurologic signs and symptoms, such as headaches and papilledema are commonly seen. The primary neurologic manifestations of CSVT in the neonates comprise seizures and diffuse neurologic signs. Underlying risk factors, including prothrombotic states, may "predispose" the patient to thrombosis, while acute illnesses often act as triggering factors.

Hemorrhagic Stroke

The hemorrhage can be parenchymal or extracerebral. Onset is apoplectic in hemorrhagic stroke with loss of consciousness and seizures. Signs of raised ICP and mass effect are usual. There may be meningismus (signs of meningeal irritation) if there is subarachnoid hemorrhage.

DIAGNOSTIC EVALUATION

Any child presenting with sudden onset of one or more of the following symptoms should arouse suspicion of stroke and should undergo immediate neurological evaluation. These are:

- Focal weakness
- Speech disturbances
- Ataxia
- Altered mental status
- Headache
- Signs of raised ICP
- Seizures with additional neurological symptoms.

The diagnostic evaluation in a patient with stroke is aimed at confirming the diagnosis of cerebrovascular disease, define extent, type of stroke (ischemic or hemorrhagic), and to determine the vascular territory (large vessel versus small vessel) and, if possible, to identify the underlying etiology of stroke. The stroke-like picture can be seen in variety of conditions **(Box 6.13.1)** and the diagnosis of cerebrovascular disease must be confirmed by neuroimaging. The causes of stroke in children are varied and it is important to identify the underlying cause as it has implications on the management, future recurrences, prognosis, and even genetic counseling of the family.

Box 6.13.1: Differential diagnosis of stroke.

- Inflammatory granuloma
- ADEM
- Migraine
- Intracranial infections
- Cerebral tumors
- Neonatal seizures
- Posterior leukoencephalopathy syndrome
- MELAS

(ADEM: acute disseminated encephalomyelitis; MELAS: mitochondrial encephalomyopathy, lactic acidosis, and stroke-like episodes)

The evaluation requires accurate history, thorough clinical examination, investigations, and neuroimaging. A patient presenting with stroke should be investigated in a systematic fashion. All patients coming with acute onset neurological deficit should first undergo neuroimaging. Magnetic resonance imaging (MRI) is the investigation of choice since computed tomography (CT) cannot pick up an infarct in early stage. In case MRI cannot be done, a plain CT scan is mandatory. This will help to differentiate between infarction and hemorrhage and rule out other diagnosis. A combination of noncontrast-enhanced CT and CT angiography may be done if MRI is not available as it has good correlation with diffusion-weighted stroke MRI.

Magnetic resonance imaging is a valuable tool for evaluation of stroke and should be used as a first-line investigation, but it is more expensive, less readily available, and more time consuming. Diffusion-weighted MRI is even more sensitive than conventional MRI. The other advantage of MRI is that magnetic resonance angiography and magnetic resonance venography can be done at the same time if necessary. This helps to elucidate noninvasively the vascular anatomy of cerebral vessels and demonstrates stenosis or occlusion in ischemia and vascular malformation in cases with hemorrhage. Hence, it helps to obviate the need for invasive cerebral angiography in majority of patients. Imaging of the cervical and proximal intracranial arterial vasculature should be performed in all children with AIS.

After confirming the existence of infarct or hemorrhage, one should investigate further to determine the etiology of stroke. All patients should have a thorough cardiac examination, chest X-ray, electrocardiogram, and echocardiogram as underlying heart disease is a very common cause of stroke in the pediatric population. If transthoracic echocardiography is noncontributory and the suspicion of cardiac source of embolism is high, the patient should be subjected to transesophageal echocardiography.

Cerebrospinal fluid analysis is mandatory in a stroke patient with unexplained fever or signs of central nervous infections.

Patients with cryptogenic stroke should be screened for prothrombotic states and metabolic causes. This should include evaluation for protein C, protein S deficiency, activated protein C resistance, increased lipoprotein-A, increased plasma homocysteine, factor V Leiden, and *MTHFR TT677* mutations and antiphospholipid antibody.

TREATMENT

Management of Acute Phase

Children with stroke should be preferably managed in tertiary care centers with facilities for diagnosis and intensive care. Currently, there is a lot of delay in recognizing childhood stroke by families and health professionals, which may account for increased mortality and sequelae.

In acute stage, maintaining perfusion and homeostasis is the priority. Raised ICP should be looked for and appropriately managed. Large volume infarct and posterior circulation stroke is more likely to develop raised ICP. Initial supportive care includes admission to an intensive care setting, 30° elevation of the head of the bed, maintenance of euvolemia and normal temperature, prevention of hypotension, and control of seizures. The most important indicators for raised ICP are deteriorating level of consciousness and the worsening of neurologic dysfunction. Decompressive craniectomy may be lifesaving and considered in such patients.

On presentation, it is essential to make the distinction between hemorrhagic and ischemic stroke, since the former require neurosurgical intervention. Tissue plasminogen activator (TPA) is the standard treatment for acute ischemic stroke for adults. The use of TPA in pediatric age has been reported from several pediatric centers. Similarly, endovascular therapy has been used in children with large vessel occlusion who presented early, and treatment could be initiated within 6 hours. Because of lack of high-quality evidence, TPA and endovascular therapy are currently not recommended for routine use in children.

Anticoagulation is recommended in certain situations to limit the propagation of thrombosis. Provided there is no significant hemorrhage on brain imaging, anticoagulation with low molecular weight heparin and oral anticoagulants is recommended in children with:

- Confirmed extracranial arterial dissection associated with AIS
- Cerebral venous sinus thrombosis
- Cardioembolic stroke.

The treatment for hemorrhagic stroke in children depends on the cause and the condition of the patient. The proper characterization of these lesions is essential to determine the best therapy. Treatments for vascular malformations include surgery, endovascular embolization, and radiosurgery.

Other therapy in acute phase of stroke depends upon the underlying cause. Patients with sickle cell disease benefit from blood transfusion or exchange transfusion. Antibiotics are required if there is suspicion or evidence of infection such as septic CSVT.

After stabilizing the patient, a thorough search should be made for the underlying cause responsible for the event and specific treatment should be instituted for the underlying etiology.

Revascularization surgery should be considered in patient with Moyamoya disease to prevent recurrences. Patients with underlying cardiac disease may require definitive treatment.

Prevention of Recurrence

Antiplatelet agents are prescribed for the secondary prevention of ischemic stroke in children. Aspirin is the most common antiplatelet agent used for this purpose. All patients with ischemic stroke should be started on aspirin (1–5 mg/kg) to prevent recurrence. This is given for a period of 1–2 years.

Prognosis

The reported mortality for AIS ranges from 7% to 28% and from 6% to 54% for hemorrhagic stroke. The functional outcome in cases of ischemic infarct depends upon the size and location of infarct as well as the age of child. Most children improve over time. However, as the brain is developing, some problems such as epilepsy and learning difficulty become evident as the child grows. Clinically detectable neurologic deficits may be seen in nearly 60% of patients on long-term follow-up.

Rehabilitation

Early rehabilitation of children with stroke is usually undertaken from the time of diagnosis in the setting of the acute ward. Early therapy of the hemiplegia is essential, as its proper application may well determine ultimate motor function. As soon as possible after admission, a child with stroke should have an evaluation of:

- Ability to feed safely
- Communication
- Positioning requirements
- Risk of pressure sores.

All children affected by stroke should have a multidisciplinary assessment after stabilization. A comprehensive assessment of speech and language should be made and where speech and language therapist indicated should be involved in the rehabilitation program.

BIBLIOGRAPHY

1. Amlie-Lefond C, Sébire G, Fullerton HJ. Recent developments in childhood arterial ischaemic stroke. Lancet Neurol. 2008;7:425-35.
2. Australian Childhood Stroke Advisory Committee. Guidelines for diagnosis and management of childhood stroke. Australian Childhood Stroke Advisory Committee; 2017.
3. Dlamini N, Billinghurst L, Kirkham FJ. Cerebral venous sinus (sinovenous) thrombosis in children. Neurosurg Clin N Am. 2010;21:511-27.
4. Greenham M, Gordon A, Anderson V, et al. Outcome in childhood stroke. Stroke. 2016;47:1159-64.
5. Lopez-Vicente M, Ortega-Gutierrez S, Amlie-Lefond C, et al. Diagnosis and management of pediatric arterial ischemic stroke. J Stroke Cerebrovasc Dis. 2010;19:175-83.

6.14 Floppy Infant: Clinical Approach

Bibek Talukdar

INTRODUCTION

The term floppy infant literally means an infant who is extremely hypotonic. Clinically, the condition refers to an infant with generalized hypotonia with onset at birth or in early life. The onset of floppiness in these infants is usually subacute to chronic that continues to persist. Floppy infant, often termed floppy infant syndrome, is not a disease but a clinical condition associated with many diseases and disorders. They usually present with floppiness, diminished motor activity, and/or certain complications, such as feeding difficulty, aspiration, pneumonia, and respiratory failure. Even if they present with complications, floppiness remains the predominant feature.

Presentation can be acute and stormy with marked hypotonia and floppiness in some disorders, such as perinatal insult following hypoxic ischemic encephalopathy and certain inborn errors of metabolism (IEM). However, the course is usually prolonged and hypotonia continues to remain as a predominant feature.

Many acute systemic disorders can have significant floppiness at presentation that can be severe at times; however, these cases are usually not labeled as floppy infants but are diagnosed according to the primary cause and they reverse with recovery from primary condition. Examples of such disorders are septicemia, meningitis, encephalitis, acute severe malnutrition, hypokalemia, Guillain–Barré syndrome, bulbar poliomyelitis, acute transverse myelitis, neonatal myasthenia, and infant botulism.

ETIOLOGY

Many conditions or diseases can be associated with floppiness. A list of such disorders based on published data is shown in **Table 6.14.1**. They can be grouped into central nervous system (CNS) disorders, neuromuscular disorders (NMDs), genetic disorders, metabolic disorders (mostly IEM), and miscellaneous disorders. The proportions of cases in different areas differ in different reports, due to variation in methodology and diagnostic approach. Central hypotonia accounts for 60–80% of cases and peripheral hypotonia 15–30% of cases. The most common CNS disorder seen commonly is perinatal asphyxia and its sequel, the most common NMD is spinal muscular atrophy (SMA), and the most common genetic disorders are Down and Prader–Willi syndromes. Metabolic and other disorders as causes of floppy infant are relatively uncommon.

APPROACH TO DIAGNOSIS

The workup of floppy infants is aimed at finding the causes that are quite diverse. A systematic approach through good history, examination, and etiology-oriented diagnostic investigation is necessary. In history, emphasis should be given on bad obstetrical history, prenatal-intranatal-neonatal problems, postneonatal problems, development, and past and family histories.

Neurological Examination

Neurological examination needs to be thorough with special emphasis on tone, power, reflexes, sensation, and neurodevelopment. The most important areas in examination of a floppy infant are tone and power of muscles.

Muscle tone in floppy infant is examined by:

- Observing the posture that is lying flabby with diminished movement of the extremities.
- Observing the resistance to passive movements at different joints that is reduced to variable extent.

Table 6.14.1: Diseases associated with or causing hypotonia in floppy infants.

• ***Central nervous system disorders*** – *Malformations:* ▪ Pontocerebellar hypoplasia ▪ Holoprosencephaly – *Perinatal problems:* ▪ Birth anoxia and hypoxic ischemic encephalopathy ▪ Birth trauma ▪ Intracranial hemorrhage ▪ Hypotonic CP • ***Neuromuscular disorders*** – *Anterior horn cell disease*: ▪ Spinal muscular atrophy types I and II – *Polyneuropathy:* ▪ Guillain–Barré syndrome ▪ Bulbar poliomyelitis • ***HMSN type III (Dejerine–Sottas)*** ***Congenital hypomyelinating neuropathy*** – *Neuromuscular junction disorders*: ▪ Myasthenia-transient neonatal and congenital forms ▪ Infant botulism – *Developmental disorder of muscle*: ▪ Myotubular myopathy ▪ Nemaline rod myopathy ▪ Central core disease ▪ Minicore and multicore disease ▪ CMFTD ▪ Benign congenital hypotonia – *Muscular dystrophy*: ▪ Myotonic muscular dystrophy ▪ CMD ▪ Fukuyama disease ▪ Walker–Warburg syndrome ▪ Muscle-Eye-Brain disease – *Metabolic myopathy*: ▪ Pompe disease (glycogenosis type II)	• ***Genetic disorders (syndromes)*** – Down syndrome – Prader–Willi syndrome – Trisomies • ***Metabolic disorders (mostly inborn errors of metabolism)*** – *Aminoacidopathy*: ▪ Hyperphenylalaninemia from deficiency of the cofactor BH4 ▪ Homocystinuria due to defects in methylcobalamin formation ▪ Maple syrup urine disease due to deficiency of E3 subunit ▪ Multiple carboxylase deficiency—infantile form ▪ Isolated 3-methylcrotonyl cocarboxylase deficiency ▪ Methylmalonic acidemia ▪ Nonketotic hyperglycinemia, neonatal form ▪ Mevalonic aciduria ▪ Propionic acidemia ▪ Methylmalonic acidemia ▪ Glutaric aciduria type I ▪ Canavan disease – *Lipid metabolism disorders:* ▪ Infantile Refsum disease ▪ Zellweger syndrome ▪ Leigh disease ▪ Late-onset metachromatic leukodystrophy – *Miscellaneous disorders:* ▪ Hypothyroidism ▪ *Congenital laxity of ligaments* - Ehler–Danlos syndrome - Marfan syndrome

(CMD: congenital muscular dystrophy; CMFTD: congenital muscle fiber-type disproportion; CP: cerebral palsy; HMSN: hereditary motor and sensory neuropathy)

Box 6.14.1: Few classic signs in floppy infants.

Some classic signs in a floppy infant:
- *Hypotonic posture*: Infant assuming a frog-leg posture with hands and legs everted and externally rotated **(Fig. 6.14.1)**
- Sparse or diminished motor movement of the extremities
- Very little resistance on passive movement of joints
- Head lag
- Body assuming the posture of inverted "U" on ventral suspension **(Fig. 6.14.2)**
- More severe the hypotonia more prominent are these signs

Significant hypotonia in floppy infants is often associated with a few characteristic signs as shown in **Box 6.14.1**. Hypotonia in floppy infants is usually accompanied by varying degrees of motor weakness that needs careful assessment to rule out NMDs.

Muscle power in floppy infant is examined by:
- Observation of movement, spontaneous and on stimulation
- Using the standard pull-push technique at joints giving varying resistance (kinetic power)
- By trying to move a limb held static by the infant and feeling the resistance (static power).

Many cases of floppy infant do have associated muscle weakness. Basically, hypotonia is reduced resistance to passive motion at joints and weakness is reduction in maximum muscle power that can be generated. It is useful to try to look at carefully whether muscle tone is affected more or muscle power. Muscle power is usually more severely affected in NMDs, whereas it is usually less severely affected in CNS, genetic, and metabolic disorders. Attempt should also be made to find whether weakness is proximal or distal. Proximal weakness is more common in myopathies and muscular dystrophies, and distal weakness is more common in peripheral neuropathies.

Tendon reflexes, if found to be good to exaggerated, suggests CNS disorder. Plantar reflex if found to be extensor, again suggests CNS disorder. Findings of sensory abnormality will suggest hereditary sensory neuropathy.

Detailed *neurodevelopmental assessment* is essential in all cases. Varying degree of neurodevelopmental delay is common in many cases of floppy infant especially those with genetic, metabolic, endocrine, and CNS etiology.

Clinical Pointers

Certain features in history and examination can give valuable clues to etiology and should be looked for in all cases of floppy infant. Some such features are given in **Table 6.14.2**. At the end of the examination, efforts should be made to find as to which etiological group a particular case belongs to, i.e. CNS, neuromuscular, genetic, metabolic, or miscellaneous disorders **(Table 6.14.1)**. These will help in proper planning of investigations.

- A *CNS cause* should be suspected in the presence of:
  - History of prenatal, intranatal, neonatal, and postneonatal problem
  - Weakness relatively less severe compared to the degree of hypotonia
  - Tendon reflexes that are well-preserved to brisk
  - History of seizures
  - Cognitive dysfunction with or without hearing and visual deficits.

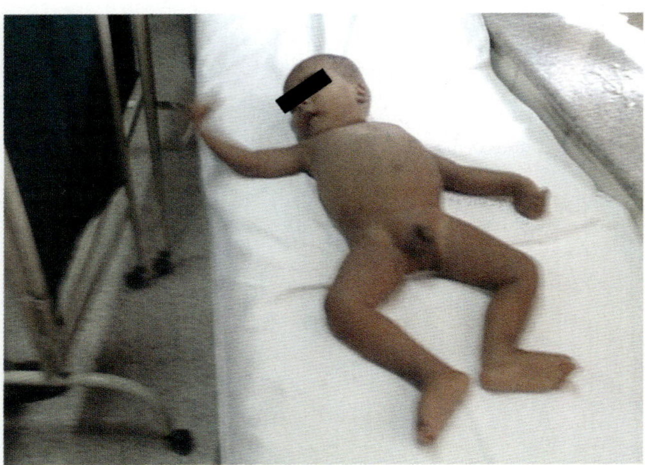

Fig. 6.14.1: Typical frog-leg posture in SMA. (SMA: spinal muscular atrophy)

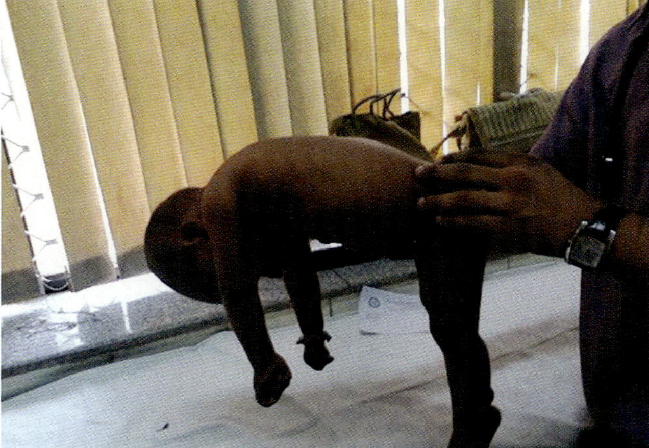

Fig. 6.14.2: Inverted U on ventral suspension in SMA child. (SMA: spinal muscular atrophy)

Table 6.14.2: Clinical clues to possible diagnosis in floppy infants.

Historical findings	***Diagnostic clues***
Miscarriage, consanguinity	Genetic and metabolic disorders
Decreased fetal movement	Myotubular myopathy, nemaline rod myopathy
Polyhydramnios	Myotubular myopathy
Maternal myasthenia	Myasthenia gravis
Maternal myotonia	Myotonic muscular dystrophy
Constipation	Botulism
General examination findings	
Dysmorphism	Genetic disorders and syndromes, some IEMs
Dolichocephaly	CMFTD, nemaline rod myopathy
Macrocephaly	Canavan disease
Inverted V-shaped upper lip	Myotonic muscular dystrophy
Tented upper lip	Fukuyama muscular dystrophy
Upslanting palpebral fissure	Zellweger syndrome

Contd...

Contd...

High-arched palate	Myotubular myopathy, CMFTD, nemaline rod myopathy, myotonic muscular dystrophy
Cleft palate	Nemaline rod myopathy
Joint contracture	CMFTD, CMD, central core disease, Ulrich anomaly
Scoliosis and kyphosis	SMA, central core disease, minicore disease, multicore disease
Arthrogryposis	Nemaline rod myopathy, CMD, congenital hypomyelinating neuropathy
Pes cavus	Central core disease
Subluxation of hip	CMFTD
Undescended testes	Myotubular myopathy
Neurologic examination findings	
Visual impairment	Muscle-eye-brain disease, Walker–Warburg syndrome
Ocular anomalies	Muscle-eye-brain disease, Walker–Warburg syndrome
Impaired corneal reflex	Botulism
Third nerve palsy	Botulism
Ptosis	Myasthenia gravis, myotubular myopathy
Facial nerve palsy	Botulism, some CNS disorders
Bulbar palsy	Bulbar poliomyelitis, GBS, botulism, nemaline rod myopathy, some CNS disorders
Hypotonia disproportionate to weakness	Benign congenital hypotonia, CMFTD, myofibrillar myopathy
Fasciculation	SMA
Insensitivity to pain	HMSN III, congenital hypomyelinating neuropathy
Other systemic examination findings	
Cardiomyopathy	Pompe disease, myofibrillar myopathy, some IEMs
Cardiac anomaly	Central core disease, minicore disease, some IEMs
Hepatomegaly	Pompe disease, some IEMs

(CMD: congenital muscular dystrophy; CMFTD: congenital muscle fiber-type disproportion; CNS: central nervous system; GBS: Guillain–Barré syndrome; HMSN: hereditary motor sensory neuropathy; IEM: inborn errors of metabolism; SMA: spinal muscular atrophy)

- A *NMD* should be suspected in the presence of:
  - Profound motor weakness proportional to the severity of hypotonia
  - Decreased or absent tendon reflexes
  - Relatively preserved cognitive function
  - No history of seizure
  - Fatigable weakness.
- A *genetic or metabolic cause* should be suspected in the presence of:
  - History of bad obstetric history (previous abortions, still births)
  - Consanguinity
  - Positive family history
  - Dysmorphism
  - Neurodevelopmental delay.

Neurodevelopmental delay probably due to a metabolic cause should be suspected in the presence of certain additional features characteristic of IEM, such as vomiting, feeding difficulty, lethargy, recurrent dehydration, acidosis, seizures, coma, respiratory abnormality, organomegaly, rash, and failure to thrive.

INVESTIGATIONS

Etiology of floppy infant is diverse, and there cannot be a set of routine investigation for the condition. Investigations must be guided by clinical suspicion based on history and clinical examination. A useful approach to investigation is to try to clinically categorize the possible cause, i.e. CNS, neuromuscular, genetic, metabolic, or miscellaneous disorder and then proceed accordingly. Such planning should help in avoiding many investigations which are quite costly and ultimately do not help in diagnosis. However, it may not always be possible to pinpoint the etiology on clinical grounds alone as several signs and symptoms are shared by many diseases, especially NMDs. Thus, a balanced approach is needed in investigating cases of floppy infant.

If a CNS cause is suspected, there is hardly any need for extensive investigation as diagnosis in most cases can be arrived at based on the history and examinations, i.e. sequel of birth anoxia. Imaging is often done to confirm any brain pathology if clinically suspected. Imaging specially magnetic resonance imaging (MRI), however, appears to give valuable clues to the etiology quite often and probably should be done in all floppy infants belonging to the category of CNS disorder. Many a times an unexpected diagnosis also comes up. Finding an etiology may at times may be useful in parental counseling for future, i.e. in developmental and metabolic disorders.

If NMD is suspected, certain investigations are needed to establish the etiology. These are serum muscle enzymes [commonly creatine phosphokinase (CPK)], nerve conduction velocity studies, electromyography, muscle biopsy, and genetic studies. The CPK is usually raised in muscular dystrophies. Nerve conduction velocity is useful in differentiating whether the weakness is neurogenic or myopathic. Nerve conduction velocity is essential for diagnosis of Guillain-Barré syndrome and useful in botulism. Electromyography is essential when myopathy is suspected. Electromyography also has special utility in diagnosis of myasthenia, myotonic dystrophy, and botulism. Imaging of the muscles (i.e. ultrasound and MRI) has also been used to diagnose dystrophic muscles. A muscle biopsy with special staining is needed to arrive at the definitive diagnosis of myopathies.

Molecular genetic studies are now becoming almost essential for most of the NMDs as several diseases are confirmed with certainty using this technique, since muscle biopsy findings on many occasions are overlapping. Deoxyribonucleic acid (DNA) markers are commonly studied. Genetic studies are relatively easy and less invasive; its value has been clearly established in SMA, i.e. survival motor neuron (*SMN*) gene mutation. In conditions where genetic abnormalities have been clearly defined, as in SMA, genetic studies are preferred first. Spinal muscular atrophy is the most common cause of floppy infant. The current recommendation is that when NMD is suspected, *SMN* gene mutation should be studied first. If positive, there is no need of muscle biopsy. If negative, muscle biopsy is undertaken. Genetic studies thus have obviated muscle biopsy, which is difficult in infant.

Whenever genetic or metabolic causes are suspected, appropriate genetic or metabolic studies are undertaken. For dysmorphism and suspected syndromes, karyotyping and DNA-based molecular diagnostic studies are usually undertaken. Workup for metabolic causes is usually started with screening tests in blood and urine followed by confirmatory tests, such as amino acidogram, analysis of enzymes and metabolites. Investigations for disorders in the *miscellaneous category* are based on clinical suspicion.

BIBLIOGRAPHY

1. Bassam BA. Floppy infant. In: Katirji B, Kaminiski HJ, Preston DC, Ruff RL, Shaprio BE (Eds). Neuromuscular Disorders in Clinical Practice. Boston, MA: Butterworth-Heinemann; 2002. pp. 1311-8.
2. Bodensteiner JB, Riggs JE, Schocher Jr. SS. Congenital myopathies. In: Katirji B, Kaminiski HJ, Preston DC, Ruff RL, Shaprio BE (Eds). Neuromuscular Disorders in Clinical Practice. Boston, MA: Butterworth-Heinemann; 2002. pp. 1114-27.
3. Connolly AM, Iannaccone ST. Anterior horn cell and cranial motor neuron disease. In: Swaiman KF, Ashwal S, Ferriero DM (Eds). Pediatric Neurology, 4th edition. Philadelphia: Mosby Elsevier; 2006. pp. 1859-85.
4. Dua T, Das M, Kabra M, et al. Spectrum of floppy children in Indian scenario. Indian Pediatr. 2001;38:1236-43.
5. Paro-Panjan D, Neubauer D. Congenital hypotonia: is there an algorithm? J Child Neurol. 2004;19:439-42.
6. Peredo DE, Hannibal MC. The floppy infant: evaluation of hypotonia. Pediatr Rev. 2009;30:e66-76.
7. Prasad AN, Prasad C. Genetic evaluation of the floppy infant. Semin Fetal Neonatal Med. 2011;16:99-108.
8. Prasad AN, Prasad C. The floppy infant: contribution of genetic and metabolic disorders. Brain Dev. 2003;25:457-76.

6.15 Neuromuscular Disorders

Sheffali Gulati, Shruthi NM

INTRODUCTION

Neuromuscular disorders (NMDs) are a heterogeneous group of disorders, which result from pathology anywhere in the motor unit. The motor unit comprises a single anterior horn cell and all the muscle fibers that are innervated by it. NMDs comprise neuronopathy (primary disorder of anterior horn cell), neuropathy (primary disorder of axon or its myelin), neuromuscular junction disorders, and myopathy (primary disorder of muscle). NMDs may be hereditary [e.g. spinal muscular atrophy (SMA), congenital myopathies] or acquired [e.g. inflammatory myopathies, myasthenia gravis (MG)]. Many NMDs are multisystem disorders affecting multiple organ systems, e.g. myotonic muscular dystrophy (affects brain and eye) and mitochondrial cytopathies.

In recent times, inherited NMDs have witnessed a paradigm shift in their recognition from histopathology to genetic identity. Detailed history and careful physical examination are the fundamental tools in the evaluation of a child with NMD. **Table 6.15.1** enumerates key features to differentiate between various NMDs.

CLINICAL APPROACH

Weakness and hypotonia are the cardinal features of NMDs. The maintenance of normal tone requires intact central and peripheral nervous system. Dysfunction of either or both leads to hypotonia. Cerebral (central) hypotonia differs from peripheral hypotonia (due to motor unit disorders) by having preserved muscle stretch reflexes, extensor plantar, preserved power (hypotonia is out of proportion to weakness and predominance of axial weakness), persistence of neonatal reflexes, associated seizures, dysmorphic features, and malformations of brain or other organs. Mixed hypotonia occurs in both the central and peripheral nervous system involvement with relatively preserved power and areflexia/hyporeflexia. **Table 6.15.2** shows common etiologies of peripheral and central hypotonia.

Weakness is a common feature of motor unit dysfunction. Different patterns of weakness such as limb-girdle, scapuloperoneal, distal upper limbs and proximal lower limbs, facial, oculopharyngeal, and axial weakness exist. In general, muscle involvement results in proximal weakness (except myotonic dystrophy and Miyoshi myopathy), and nerve involvement leads to distal weakness. Anterior horn cell involvement leads to generalized weakness. Neuromuscular junction disorders lead to fatigable weakness with predilection to facial/ocular muscles and limb-girdle muscles. Key features to differentiate and localize motor unit disorders have been enumerated in **Table 6.15.1**.

History: Key points in history should include three-generation pedigree, consanguinity, drug or teratogen exposure (alcohol, solvents, and drugs), reduced fetal movements, history of polyhydramnios, detailed birth and perinatal history (details of resuscitation and feeding history), family history of recurrent infantile deaths, and developmental history. Detailed history of neuromuscular symptoms such as age at onset, progression, extent of involvement, pattern of involvement, positive and negative symptoms, fluctuations, precipitating factors, associated features of central nervous system, and other system involvement should be taken.

Evaluation: One should perform focused general, musculoskeletal and neurologic, and systemic examinations to direct further diagnostic workup. Electrodiagnostic studies, including nerve conduction studies and electromyography, are considered extensions of physical examination and help to guide further tests, such as muscle/nerve biopsy or genetic testing. With this approach and skilled synthesis of all available information, one can make an accurate diagnosis and also anticipate complications, provide prognostic information, and guide for specific molecular therapies if available.

MUSCLE DISORDERS

Congenital Myopathy

Congenital myopathies are heterogeneous group of muscle diseases, and they typically present with hypotonia, motor delay, and muscle weakness with variable age of onset. Majority of the patients present from birth to early infancy or childhood. Usually, they have a benign course with nonprogressive hypotonia and weakness leading to predominant motor delay. Sometimes the severe forms present with early-onset respiratory distress and feeding difficulties. Children may have myopathic facies (long facies, temporal hallowing, dolichocephaly, high-arched palate, tented upper lip, and open mouth). There may be variable

Table 6.15.1: Key features to differentiate between motor unit disorders.

Site of involvement	*Proximal (P) vs distal (D) involvement*	*Facial involvement*	*Atrophy*	*Muscle stretch reflexes*	*Sensations*	*Electrophysiological studies*	*Muscle biopsy*
Anterior horn cell	P ≥ D	Absent	Yes	Absent	Normal	Evidence of denervation and fasciculation	Type grouping
Nerve	D > P	Absent	Yes	Depressed/ Absent	Decreased	Abnormal nerve conduction studies and denervation potentials on EMG	Denervation pattern
Neuromuscular junction	Variable, fatigable	Present (ptosis and ophthalmoparesis)	No	Normal	Normal	Repetitive nerve stimulation—abnormal decrement/ increment	Normal
Muscle	P > D	Present variably (ptosis in congenital myopathies)	Late stages	Depressed	Normal	Low-amplitude short-duration polyphasic motor unit action potential on EMG	Usually characteristic

(EMG: electromyogram)

Table 6.15.2: Differential diagnosis of hypotonia.

Central hypotonia (floppy strong)	*Peripheral hypotonia (floppy weak)*	*Mixed hypotonia*
Chromosomal disorders: • Prader–Willi syndrome • Trisomy *Static encephalopathies:* • Cerebral malformations • Cerebellar disorders • Hydrocephalus • Perinatal insult *Neurometabolic:* • Acid maltase deficiency • Biotinidase deficiency • GM1/GM2 gangliosidoses • Peroxisomal disorders • Congenital disorders of glycosylation *Infections:* • Sepsis/meningitis • Intrauterine infections *Benign congenital hypotonia* *Genetic defects:* • Lowe syndrome • Familial dysautonomia	*Anterior horn cell:* • Spinal muscular atrophy • Poliomyelitis • Enteroviral infections *Neuropathies:* • Giant axonal neuropathy • Hereditary sensory autonomic neuropathies • Congenital hypomyelinating neuropathy • Charcot–Marie–Tooth disease • Guillain–Barré syndrome • *Infections*: Diphtheria, human immunodeficiency virus • Traumatic neuropathies • *Toxic neuropathies*: Lead, porphyria *Neuromuscular junction disorders:* • Myasthenia gravis • Congenital myasthenic syndromes • Botulism *Myopathies:* • Central core disease • Myotubular myopathy • Nemaline rod myopathy • Congenital fiber-type disproportion myopathy • Metabolic myopathies • Inflammatory myopathies *Muscular dystrophy:* • Dystrophinopathies • Myotonic dystrophy • Facioscapulohumeral dystrophy • Congenital muscular dystrophy • Emery–Dreifuss muscular dystrophy	• Hypothyroidism • Acid maltase deficiency • Hypoxic ischemic encephalomyelopathy • Familial dysautonomia • Infantile neuronal degeneration • Motor unit disease with superimposed asphyxia • Mitochondrial disorders • Lysosomal storage disorders • Peroxisomal disorders

(GM1: ganglioside M1; GM2: ganglioside M2)

involvement of facial, extraocular, bulbar, and respiratory muscles. Intellectual function is usually preserved, and primary cardiac involvement is rare.

There are four broad pathological variants:

1. *Protein inclusion myopathies*, such as nemaline rod and myosine storage myopathies;
2. *Core myopathies*, such as central core and multiminicore myopathies;
3. *Myopathies with internalized nuclei*, such as myotubular myopathy (MTM) and centronuclear myopathy; and
4. *Myopathies associated with abnormal fiber size*, such as congenital fiber-type disproportion myopathy.

Histopathological review at All India Institute of Medical Sciences, New Delhi, has found core myopathies to be the most common variant.

Diagnosis is based on history, clinical findings, electrophysiology, muscle biopsy, and genetic testing. In muscle biopsy the presence of morphological and ultrastructural sarcolemmal skeletal changes and the absence of histological features of dystrophies, such as fiber necrosis, fibrosis, fatty, and inflammatory infiltration, are the defining features of congenital myopathy. Creatine phosphokinase (CPK) is usually normal. Popularly they have been classified based on the major characteristic features seen on muscle biopsy, e.g. rods (nemaline myopathy), cores (central core disease and multiminicore disease), central nuclei (centronuclear/MTM), and selective atrophy/hypotrophy of type 1 fibers (congenital fiber-type disproportion). Genetic diagnosis is gaining importance in view of the prognostic implications and for genetic counseling.

At present, *treatment* is mainly supportive with focus on rehabilitative measures. There are no curative therapies. Therapies, such as L-tyrosine for nemaline myopathy, salbutamol in core myopathies, pyridostigmine in centronuclear myopathy and MTM, *N*-acetyl cysteine in selenoprotein N1 (SEPN1) and ryanodine receptor 1 (RYR1)-related myopathies, gene and enzyme replacement therapies in MTM, microribonucleic acids and histone deacetylases in RYR1 myopathies, are under investigation.

Table 6.15.3 depicts common congenital myopathy subtypes with their clinical, muscle biopsy and muscle magnetic resonance imaging features.

Congenital Muscular Dystrophies

The congenital muscular dystrophies (CMDs) are early-onset muscle disorders (onset within 2 years of age) that are usually progressive. Affected infants typically present as floppy infants, skeletal abnormalities, and other organ involvement, such as eye and brain, to variable extents. Early joint contractures and spinal deformities are particularly prominent. The muscle biopsy is consistent with dystrophic process (even if not fully developed, with variation in fiber size, necrosis, increased endomysial fibrosis, and regenerative changes) without histological evidence of another neuromuscular disease. CPK levels are usually elevated but can be normal.

However, now it is known that there is overlap between the CMDs and the congenital myopathies on the clinical, morphological, and genetic level. Recently, classification of CMDs has underwent major revision with emerging knowledge of genes causing CMDs. **Table 6.15.4** gives an outline of classification of CMDs.

Laminin alpha 2-related CMDs are the most common variants with variable spectrum. Abnormalities on neuroimaging are found in laminin alpha 2 deficiency (white matter changes) and dystroglycanopathies (structural brain abnormalities). Normal cognitive abilities and neuroimaging are found in collagen VI deficiencies and SEPN1-related CMDs. Dystroglycanopathies have severe presentations with eye and brain involvement (Walker–Warburg syndrome, Fukuyama CMD, and muscle-eye-brain disease). Collagen VI-deficient CMDs (Ullrich and Bethlem myopathy) have prominent skeletal manifestations with early proximal joint contractures and distal joint laxity **(Fig. 6.15.1)**. Serum CPK levels are normal or mildly increased in collagen VI-deficient CMD, SEPN1-related CMD, and lamin A/C-related CMD, whereas those with primary merosin deficiency (laminin alpha 2 deficiency) or secondary merosin deficiency (dystroglycanopathies) have raised levels (>4 times normal).

No specific therapy is available for any of the variants, and treatment is mainly focused on supportive respiratory, cardiac, orthopedic, and general care.

Muscular Dystrophies

Muscular dystrophies are heterogeneous, inherited disorders characterized by progressive muscle degeneration and loss of strength defined by the presence of variable dystrophic changes on muscle biopsy. They are caused by various defects of the cytoskeletal proteins or enzymes leading to the degeneration of the muscle fibers and replacement by fibrous tissue. Classically, there is involvement of facial, axial, and limb-girdle muscles, with the involvement of cardiac and smooth muscles in some subtypes. They may be X-linked (dystrophinopathies), autosomal dominant [limb-girdle muscular dystrophy (LGMD) type 1], or recessively inherited (LGMD type 2). Dystrophinopathy (Duchenne and Becker) is the most common muscular dystrophy having a prevalence of 1 in 3,500 live male births. It accounts for approximately 60% of all the muscular dystrophy cases.

Dystrophinopathies

Dystrophinopathies are a group of disorders resulting from mutations in the dystrophin gene (located on the short arm of X chromosome in the Xp21 region). Dystrophin is expressed

Table 6.15.3: Clinical features and genetics of subtypes of congenital myopathy.

Subtype (with genes and inheritance)	*Clinical features and muscle biopsy*	*Muscle MRI features*
NM		
ACTA1, NEB, TPM2, TPM3, TNNT1, CFL2, KBTBD13, KLHL40	• NEB mutation is the most common cause of NM (>50%), autosomal recessive inheritance • Most common presentation is congenital • Severity may vary from mild to lethal. Significant bulbar involvement, facial weakness, neck weakness, foot drop, variable extremity weakness, chest deformity, and scoliosis are common • Ophthalmoparesis is infrequently observed except in some specific genetic variants, such as *LMOD3* • *Muscle biopsy* shows rods in Gomori Trichrome staining as dark red/purple dense bodies in the cytoplasm or as intranuclear inclusions	Relative sparing of thigh with early involvement of lower leg with sparing of tibialis anterior and gastrocnemius
Core myopathies (central core disease and multiminicore disease)		
RYR1, SEPN1, ACTA1, TTN, MYH7, KBTBD13	• *RYR1* is the most common cause of both central (autosomal dominant *RYR1*) and multiminicore (autosomal recessive *RYR1*) myopathies • Risk of malignant hyperthermia is high in patients having *RYR1* mutations • *SEPN1* (multiminicore disease) mutation-related myopathy presents with congenital axial weakness (head drop) and thin built with reduced muscle mass • Spinal rigidity may be marked. Scoliosis and congenital dislocation of hip may be present • The presence of ptosis, ophthalmoparesis, and facial weakness is more common with *SEPN1* than *RYR1*-related disorders • *Muscle biopsy* shows regions with lack of staining on oxidative stains. Central core disease shows single central cores with well-defined borders, best appreciated on longitudinal sections – Multiminicore disease shows multiple smaller cores with less-defined boundaries	• Marked involvement of sartorius, vasti, adductor magnus, and sparing of RF, AL, and hamstrings • Calf level-lateral head of gastrocnemius, soleus with sparing of peroneal, medial head of gastrocnemius, and anterior compartment
Centronuclear myopathies		
MTM1, DNM2, BIN1, RYR1, TTN, SPEG	• *MTM1* (X-linked) and *DNM2* (autosomal dominant) are the common mutations associated • It may present with varying severity from newborn to adulthood. Diagnostic clues are facial weakness, neck flexors weakness, ptosis and external ophthalmoplegia, swallowing, and respiratory weakness along with distal predominant extremity weakness • *Muscle biopsy* shows increased fibers with internalized nuclei (>25%) in H/E staining and radial sarcoplasmic strands and central aggregates of staining material on NADH stain. Myofiber hypotrophy and type 1 fiber predominance is seen	Predominant and progressive distal lower leg involvement (soleus, peroneal, TA) and in thigh recti and hamstrings involved with sparing of sartorius and gracilis

Contd...

Contd...

Subtype (with genes and inheritance)	*Clinical features and muscle biopsy*	*Muscle MRI features*
CFTD		
ACTA1, TPM3, TPM2, RYR1, SEPN1	• Most common is due to *TPM3* mutations (autosomal dominant). Majority has less severe phenotype and many of them can walk into adulthood • *Muscle biopsy* shows variation in fiber sizes (type 1 fibers consistently smaller than type 2 by >25%, type 1 fiber predominance of >75%) or ratios, with no cores, rods, or central nuclei	No characteristic findings

(AL: adductor longus; CFTD: congenital fiber-type disproportion; HE: hematoxylin/eosin; *LMOD3*: leicin 3; MRI: magnetic resonance imaging; NADH: nicotinamide adenine dinucleotide; NEB: nebulin; NM: nemaline myopathy; RF: rectus femoris; RYR1: ryanodine receptor 1; SEPN1: selenoprotein N1; TA: tibialis anterior)

Table 6.15.4: Classification of CMDs.

Subtypes of CMDs and associated genes	*Clinical phenotypic spectrum*
COL6-RD • *COL6A1, COL6A2, COL6A3*	• UCMD, autosomal recessive • BM, milder disease course, ambulatory, autosomal dominant
Laminin alpha 2 related dystrophy (LAMA2-RD, includes MDC1A and merosin deficient (MD) • *Gene: LAMA2*	• Nonambulant LAMA2-RD (complete merosin deficiency in muscle biopsy) • Ambulant LAMA2-RD (partial merosin deficiency)
Alpha Dystroglycan related dystrophy (aDG-RD, also alpha dystroglycanopathy) • *Common genes: FKRP, FKTN, POMT1, POMT2, POMGnT1*	• Walker–Warburg syndrome • Muscle-eye-brain disease; Fukuyama CMD; Fukuyama-like CMD • CMD with cerebellar involvement; cerebellar abnormalities may include cysts, hypoplasia, and dysplasia • CMD with mental retardation and normal brain on imaging • CMD with no mental retardation; no evidence of abnormal cognitive development • LGMD with mental retardation or without mental retardation (milder weakness, may be later onset) and a structurally normal brain on imaging
LMNA-related dystrophy (LMNA-RD, includes LMNA-CMD, and Emery–Dreifuss) • *LMNA*	• *CMD presentation*: Dropped head syndrome, axial and scapula-peroneal involvement, and absent or early loss of ambulation • Milder presentations fuse with early-onset Emery-Dreifuss muscular dystrophy
SEPN1-related myopathy (SEPN1-RM, also rigid spine CMD) • *SEPN1*	• *CMD presentation:* Present with cervicoaxial weakness, scapular winging, facial and bulbar involvement, progressively developing joint contractures, spinal rigidity, and scoliosis; secondary respiratory insufficiency and cardiac involvement common

(aDG-RD: alpha-dystroglycan-related dystrophy; BM: Bethlem myopathy; CMD: congenital muscular dystrophy; COL6-RD: collagen VI-related dystrophies; LAMA2-RD: laminina-2-related dystrophy; LGMD: limb-girdle muscular dystrophy; LMNA: lamin A/C; MDC1A: congenital muscular dystrophy type 1A; SEPN1: selenoprotein N1; UCMD: Ullrich congenital muscular dystrophy)

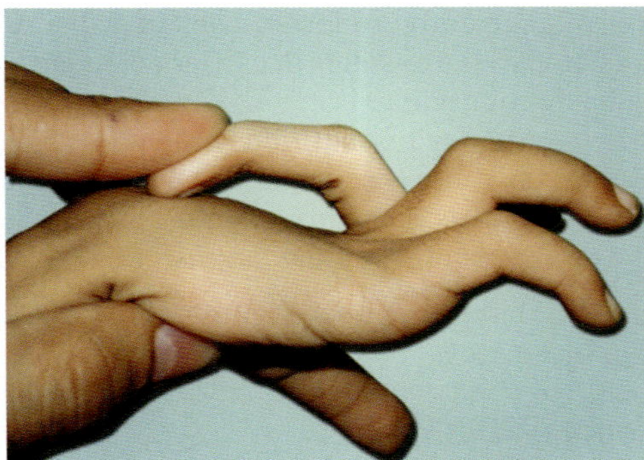

Fig. 6.15.1: Ullrich muscular dystrophy-distal hyperextensible joints.

in skeletal, cardiac, smooth muscles and brain. These may be affected variably in dystrophinopathies. Dystrophin is located underneath the sarcolemma and is responsible for the cytoskeletal stability. Decreased dystrophin will lead to membrane instability and susceptibility to mechanical stress and calcium-mediated cell injury, resulting in degeneration of the muscle fibers.

Duchenne Muscular Dystrophy and Becker Muscular Dystrophy

- *Duchenne muscular dystrophy (DMD):* It is the most common dystrophinopathy with an incidence of 1 in 3,500 live male births.

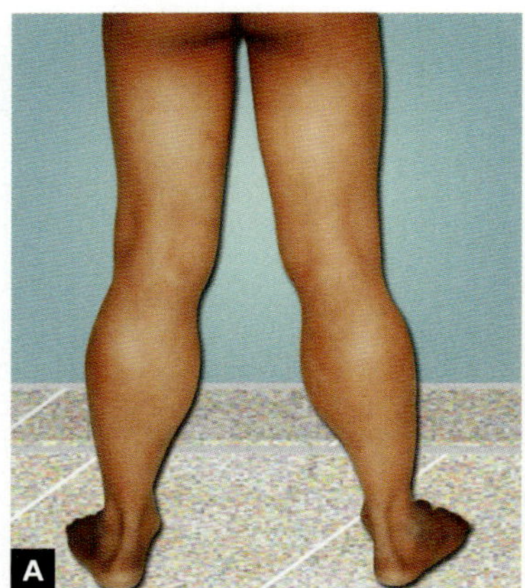

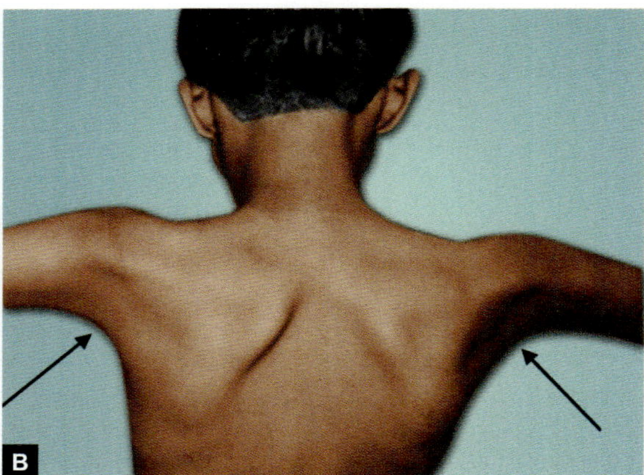

Figs. 6.15.2A and B: Duchenne muscular dystrophy: (A) Calf hypertrophy; and (B) Valley sign.

- *Becker muscular dystrophy (BMD):* Its rarer allelic variant, differs from DMD by its later age of onset (usually greater than 6 years of age), more prolonged unaided ambulation (greater than 15 years), more incidence of myalgias, occasional rhabdomyolysis following exercise, and cardiac findings, which are "out of proportion" to limb weakness. Symptomatic cardiac involvement is more common in BMD. Cognitive impairment is not prominent, but these patients may have behavioral issues, such as impaired attention and learning difficulties. Both form the two ends of a spectrum.

Clinical features: Children with DMD often have delayed motor milestones. Gait disturbances often become apparent at 3–4 years of age. Waddling gait, Gower sign, and calf muscle hypertrophy **(Figs. 6.15.2A and B)** are classical findings at this stage. Neck flexor muscle weakness is seen early. Other muscles may also show hypertrophy (extensor digitorum brevis, calf and tongue muscles). The progression of weakness may plateau between 3 years and 6 years of age. Subsequently, there is increasing gait difficulty, contractures, and increased lumbar lordosis. Natural history studies have shown that the age of loss of independent ambulation in untreated DMD is between 8.8 years and 10.5 years. After the loss of ambulation, there is worsening kyphoscoliosis, increasing upper limb weakness, and bulbar dysfunction.

Weakness of intercostal and diaphragmatic muscles with spinal deformity compromises respiratory function. Cardiomyopathy and arrhythmias are the major cardiac manifestations in DMD. The cause of death in DMD patients is usually the combination of respiratory insufficiency and cardiomyopathy. Other clinical features of DMD may include variable degree of intellectual disability and impaired gastric motility and smooth muscle dysfunction.

More than 90% of the female carriers are asymptomatic. However, few may have variable degree of weakness with elevated creatine kinase levels. Full DMD phenotype may be present in the case of complete inactivation of normal X chromosome. Increased risk of cardiomyopathy may be seen in female carriers.

Diagnosis

- *The serum creatine kinase* levels are greatly elevated (>10 times). It has no correlation with severity of the disease or response to treatment. Other muscle enzymes are also elevated. The levels decrease as the muscle mass is lost with the progression of the disease.
- *Genetics:* Multiplex polymerase chain reaction (PCR) can detect intragenic deletions (65% cases), Southern blotting and quantitative PCR detects duplications (5% cases), and multiplex ligation-dependent probe amplification detects the rest 30–35% (small insertion or deletion, single base changes, or splicing). In around 90% of the boys with DMD, the "out-of-frame" mutation disrupts the normal dystrophin transcription, resulting in almost undetectable dystrophin. The "in-frame" mutations result in the production of some abnormal molecular weight dystrophin leading to BMD phenotype. This "reading frame rule" was proposed by Koenig and has a sensitivity of 93–96% in predicting DMD. Mutation analysis is currently preferred over invasive methods, such as biopsy. It also helps in carrier detection, prenatal and genetic counseling.
- *Muscle biopsy* may be required in deletion of negative cases and to differentiate between DMD and BMD. Genetic diagnosis is mandatory in biopsy confirmed cases as per recent recommendations.

Management: Management of a child with DMD is briefly outlined in **Box 6.15.1**.

Other Common Dystrophies

Other common dystrophies apart from dystrophinopathies are summarized in **Table 6.15.5**.

Metabolic Myopathies

The metabolic myopathies are a group of muscle disorders resulting from failed energy production related to defects in glycogen, lipid, or mitochondrial metabolism. Fatty acid oxidation is the chief source of energy for resting muscle with glucose utilization accounting for 10–15% of total oxygen consumption. During exercise, for the initial 5-10 minutes, high-energy phosphates are used, followed by glycogenolysis. At around 90 minutes of exercise, glucose and free fatty acids are the major sources. During prolonged exercise, free fatty acids and triglycerides are the major fuel sources.

Affected older children and adults present primarily with exercise intolerance, weakness, and myoglobinuria; newborns and infants present with severe multisystem disorders. In patients with glycolytic/glycogenolytic defects, symptoms are induced by either brief isometric exercise, such as lifting heavy weights, or by less intense but sustained dynamic exercise. With disorders of lipid metabolism, the abnormalities are usually induced by prolonged exercise and prolonged fasting. Investigations include serum CPK, urine myoglobin, serum ammonia, tandem mass spectrometry, gas chromatography-mass spectrometry, electrophysiological studies, forearm ischemia exercise test, muscle biopsy, and molecular studies.

Box 6.15.1: Management of a child with Duchenne muscular dystrophy.

Physical therapy:
- Effective stretching and appropriate positioning at various joints, assistive devices to prevent contractures, avoid high-resistance strength training

Surgery:
- Persistent contractures and spinal fusion

Steroids:
- Standard of care
- Usually started in children more than 2 years of age with static or declining functions; in less than 2-year-old steroids are not started in presymptomatic or plateau phase
- Most effective dose 0.75 mg/kg/day of prednisolone (increased till the child reaches 40 kg weight with a cap at 30–40 mg/day of prednisolone); daily schedule more effective than alternate day dosing
- Deflazacort (0.9 mg/kg/day; maximum 36–39 mg/day) may be preferred in children with excessive weight gain with prednisolone or with pre-existing behavioral problems but has increased incidence of cataracts
- *Nonambulatory DMD children:* Low-dose (0.3–0.6 mg/kg/day) prednisolone may be started with the aim of preserving upper limb strength, reducing the progression of scoliosis and delaying the decline in respiratory and cardiac function
- *Before starting steroids:* Adequate immunization (pneumococcal/influenza/varicella); screening with chest X-ray and Mantoux test
- *Monitoring of children on steroid therapy:* Screening for side effects of steroids (cushingoid features, obesity, cataracts, hypertension, glucose intolerance, infections, growth, hirsutism, acne, behavioral changes, polyuria/polydipsia, GERD/PUD, fractures, and color of urine after exercise)
- *In the case of side effects*: Reduce steroid dose by 25–33%, reassess monthly, up to a minimum effective daily dose of steroid is reached (3 mg/kg/day); switch to alternative regimen (intermittent day regimen: 10 days on and 10 days off/10 days in a month; alternate day regimen: 0.75–1.25 mg/kg on alternate days or high-dose weekend regimen) if side effects still persist

Follow-up:
- *At each visit*: Monitor weight/height/body mass index, blood pressure, and blood sugar
- Annual SMR staging
- Annual ophthalmologic evaluation
- Pulmonary function tests (6 monthly in nonambulatory; annually in ambulatory patients)
- Echocardiography (once in 2 years < 10 years of age; annually > 10 years of age)
- Serum calcium, phosphate, 25(OH) vitamin D (biannually)
- DEXA scan annually
- Respiratory and cardiac care
- *Orthopedic management*: Surveillance for scoliosis after 5 years of age (surgery if > 25% scoliosis or reduction in vital capacity > 30%)
- Management of gastrointestinal problems
- Psychosocial management

Newer therapies:
- Antisense oligonucleotide and exon skipping (for out-of-frame deletions): Eteplirsen (Exondys 51; FDA approved in 2016), Drisapersen
- Read through stop codon strategies (for nonsense mutations): PTC124 (Ataluren)
- *Utrophin upregulation*: SMT C1100 (phase 1B trials on go)
- Stem cell therapy and gene transfer therapies—used in research settings only
- *Drugs under trial*: Givinostat (histone deacetylase inhibitor, phase II trials); isosorbide dinitrate with ibuprofen
- Drugs, such as oxandrolone, azathioprine, creatine monohydrate, nifedipine, leucine, selenium, vitamin e, methysergide, pizotifen, sildenafil, tadalafil, inhibitors of myostatin and idebenone, have been tried in research without much benefits and evidence for use

[DEXA: dual energy X-ray absorptiometry; DMD: Duchenne muscular dystrophy; FDA: Food and Drug Administration; GERD: gastroesophageal reflux disease; PUD: peptic ulcer disease; SMR: sexual maturity rating (Tanner staging)]

Box 6.15.2: Presentation of juvenile myasthenia gravis.

Clues from history:
- Slowly progressive course with relapsing-remitting tendency with variable or fatigable weakness
- *Perinatal:* Reduced fetal movements, polyhydramnios, arthrogryposis
- *Infancy*: Hypotonia, weakness, weak cry, feeding difficulties, and recurrent apneic episodes
- *Childhood*: Difficulty in chewing or swallowing, fatigability or hoarse voice, diplopia especially on sustained gaze or continuous activity, such as reading, weakness of jaw, orthopnea secondary to diaphragmatic weakness; limb-girdle weakness; ocular symptoms are the most common

Clues on neurological examination:
- *Eye signs:* Ptosis (may be asymmetric); peep sign (on attempting to tightly close eyes, after few minutes the cornea gets exposed due to inability to sustain contraction of orbicularis oculi), ophthalmoparesis, curtain sign (when examiner lifts the more affected eyelid, contralateral less affected eyelid ptosis worsens)
- *Facial weakness:* Compensatory wrinkling of forehead (due to hypercontracted frontalis to maintain eye opening), expressionless facies, snarl on trying to smile, inability to close the jaw
- *Other cranial musculature*: Bulbar weakness, tongue may show triple longitudinal furrowing
- *Skeletal musculature*: Proximal limb weakness and tachypnea/shallow respiration

Box 6.15.3: Diagnosis of myasthenia gravis.

- *Edrophonium testing:* A rapid acting, short duration cholinesterase inhibitor. Effects are seen within 10 seconds and persist till 120 seconds; positive: transient resolution of the clinical signs (ptosis/ophthalmoplegia/dysarthria); diagnostic dose is 0.1–0.2 mg/kg [may be repeated every minute to a total maximum dose of 5 mg (weight < 34 kg) or 10 mg (weight > 34 kg)]; should be done in a monitored setting with available atropine and cardiorespiratory resuscitation kit
- *Infants*: Edrophonium is not recommended for use in infants due to high risk of arrhythmias and short duration of action, which precludes objective assessment. Neostigmine (Prostigmine methylsulfate) by intramuscular injection slower in action, response anticipated in 10–15 min and maximum in 30 minutes, a more objective assessment of response can be made; dose used is 0.125 mg/kg in an infant and 0.04 mg/kg in an older child. If the result is equivocal or negative, the dose may be repeated in 4 hours. **Figures 6.15.4A and B** demonstrate a positive response to neostigmine challenge test
- *Ice pack test:* It may be helpful for the diagnosis of ocular myasthenia; should only be interpreted as positive when there is clear and unequivocal improvement in ptosis following a 2-minute application of an ice pack to the affected eyelid
- *Electrophysiological testing:* RNST—The fatigability of neuromuscular transmission is demonstrated by a decrement of more than 10% in compound muscle action potential after repetitive nerve stimulation (2–5 Hz). SFEMG may show increased jitter or variation in contraction time in muscle fibers. RNST is positive in 80% of the generalized MG with 50–100% sensitivity and in 50% of the ocular MG with 10–20% sensitivity. SFEMG is virtually always abnormal and is the most sensitive test
- *Serum antibodies:* Acetylcholine receptor antibodies may be positive (up to 80% in the generalized MG and in up to 50% of the ocular MG patients); positivity rates are lower in peri and prepubertal children (50–60%). Specificity is up to 98%. Anti-MuSK antibodies may be demonstrable in 40% of the seronegative myasthenia gravis patients and is 80–90% specific
- *Muscle biopsy:* It is not indicated routinely
- X-ray chest or CT of anterior mediastinum may show thymoma/thymic hyperplasia
- Thyroid profile should always be done in suspected juvenile myasthenia gravis patients

(CT: computed tomography; MG: myasthenia gravis; MuSK: muscle-specific kinase; RNST: repetitive nerve stimulation test; SFEMG: single fiber electromyography)

Management

- *Chronic treatment*: The aims of treatment for MG patients should be to induce and maintain complete clinical or pharmacological remission with minimal adverse effects.
- *Nonimmune modulatory:* Pyridostigmine
- *Immune modulatory:* Steroids, steroid-sparing agents, and thymectomy **(Table 6.15.6)**.

Spontaneous remission is seen in 20% of the patients. Drugs are withdrawn if the patient remains asymptomatic up to 1 year.

Treatment of Acute Exacerbations/Crisis

Causes: Disease progression, stressor/illness, withdrawal of chronic treatment, use of contraindicated medication **(Box 6.15.4)**. A close differential diagnosis is cholinergic crisis due to overdosage of acetylcholinesterase (AChE) inhibitors.

Short-term immunotherapy: Intravenous immunoglobulin 2 g/kg over 2–5 days and plasmapheresis.

Supportive care: Temporary nil per os or nasogastric tube feeding to prevent aspiration. Close respiratory monitoring and provide ventilatory support if necessary.

Cholinergic crisis: Cholinergic symptoms and signs may include diarrhea, urinary incontinence, miosis, bronchospasm, salivation, and lacrimation. If patient is in crisis, withhold AChE inhibitor.

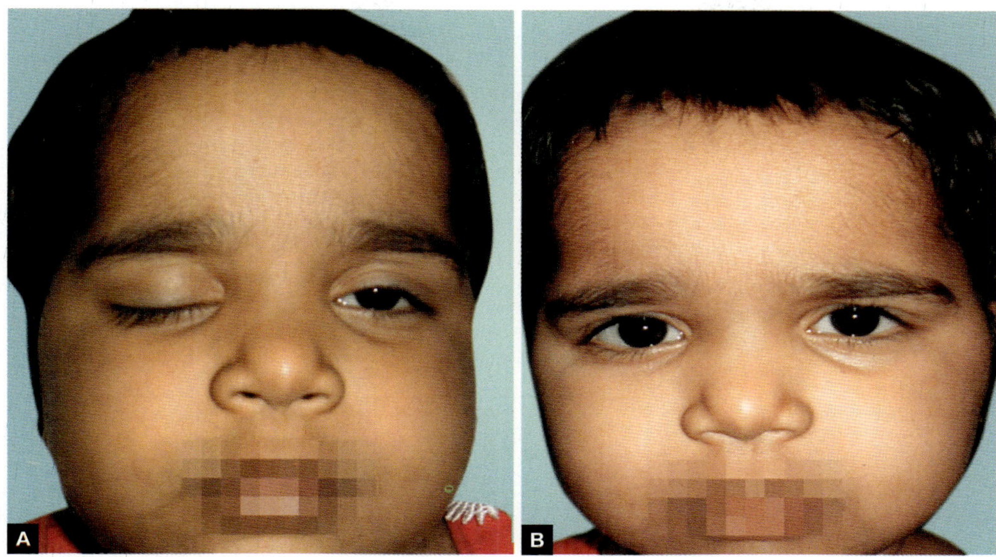

Figs. 6.15.4A and B: Juvenile myasthenia gravis; neostigmine challenge test: (A) Pre- and (B) Post-test; also note the asymmetric ptosis.

Table 6.15.6: Management of juvenile myasthenia gravis.

Drugs	***Mechanism of action***	***Dose***	***Indications***	***Monitoring/precautions***
Pyridostigmine	AChE inhibitor	• 1–7 mg/kg in 5 or 6 divided doses 30 minutes before meals • *Maximum dose*: 300 mg • Dose of IV pyridostigmine is 1/30th of oral dose	First line for all JMG patients	May use glycopyrrolate/atropine for muscarinic side effects
Corticosteroids	Exact mechanism unknown; immunosuppressive; reduces anti-AChR antibody level	• *In nonacute setting:* Start at low dose (@ 0.5 mg/kg/day); dose can be gradually increased as tolerated; once in remission, decrease dose gradually; effect starts within 2–3 weeks, full improvement is seen in 3 months; occasionally steroids can worsen the symptoms • *Acute setting*: Intravenous pulse steroids at 30 mg/kg/day for 3–5 days	*Cases:* Unresponsive to pyridostigmine and acute settings	Monitor for side effects
Azathioprine	Purine antimetabolite—inhibits T-cell proliferation	1–3 mg/kg/day as single dose; may be increased by 0.5–1 mg/kg/day every 4–8 weeks; takes a longer duration for the effects to appear, maximal effect is observed by 18–20 months	May be used as steroid-sparing drug; may be used alone also	• CBC, hepatic function monthly • Withhold treatment if counts • <3,000; reduce if < 4,000 percubic millimeter
Mycophenolate mofetil	Selectively blocks purine synthesis in T and B cells by inhibiting the action of inosine-5-monoposphate dehydrogenase	1,000–1,500 mg every 12 hourly; slow onset of action with maximum benefit seen by 9–10 months	May be used as steroid-sparing drug	Monthly CBC for 1 year, then 3 monthly

Contd...

Contd...

Drugs	*Mechanism of action*	*Dose*	*Indications*	*Monitoring/precautions*
IVIG	Blocks Fc receptor of antibodies	• *Acute setting:* 2 g/kg/day IV over 2 days or 5 days • *Maintenance:* 1 g/kg/day × 2 days every 4–8 weeks • Maximal benefit observed over 1–2 weeks; effect persists up to 1 month	May be used in myasthenic crises or as maintenance therapy if child unresponsive to other immune-modulatory therapy	Monitor for side effects
Plasmapheresis	Removes AChR antibodies from circulation	• *Acute setting:* 3–5 exchanges every other day; number may depend on the severity • *Maintenance:* 3–5 exchanges/month	May be considered in children who failed to respond to anti-AChE; and in crises	Monitor for side effects
Thymectomy	Immunomodulator	–	Necessary in thymoma; may be considered in nonthymomatous hyperplasia; thymectomy within 2 years of diagnosis results in a higher rate of remission; benefit may be delayed for years; timing of surgery is debatable	Undertaken with caution in very young children due to the occurrence of immunological abnormalities

(AChE: acetylcholinesterase; CBC; complete blood count; IVIG: intravenous immunoglobulin; JMG: juvenile myasthenia gravis)

Box 6.15.4: Medications exacerbating myasthenia gravis.

- *Absolutely contraindicated: Curare, penicillamine, Botox, and IFN-α*
- Relatively contraindicated
  - *Antibiotics:* Fluoroquinolones (ciprofloxacin, levofloxacin, etc.)
  - Macrolides (erythromycin, azithromycin, etc.)
  - Aminoglycosides (gentamicin, tobramycin, etc.)
  - Quinine
  - Class IA antiarrhythmic (procainamide, quinidine, lidocaine, etc.)
  - Magnesium
- *Use with caution:* Calcium channel blockers, lithium, statins, and steroids

Congenital Myasthenia Syndromes

Congenital myasthenia syndromes (CMS) are a genetically determined heterogeneous group of neuromuscular junction disorders. Age of onset is variable ranging from neonatal period to adulthood. Patients may present with ptosis, external ophthalmoparesis, facial weakness, general hypotonia, proximal greater than distal muscle weakness, and variable degrees of functional impairment. More than 20 CMS disease gene have been identified till date; amongst them, the most common cause of CMS is the gene, responsible for defects in AChR. **Table 6.15.7** gives outline of classification and therapeutics for common subtypes of CMS.

PERIPHERAL NEUROPATHIES IN CHILDHOOD

Peripheral neuropathy is a heterogeneous group of disorders affecting peripheral nerves which can be acquired or genetic in origin. Hereditary neuropathy is represented by Charcot-Marie-Tooth disease (CMT), a heterogeneous entity, the most common inherited NMD with estimated prevalence of 40 per 100,000. Acquired neuropathies are usually due to vitamin deficiencies, drugs/toxins, immune dysfunction, and focal mononeuropathies. Among the acquired causes, Guillain-Barré syndrome (GBS) is the most common with annual incidence of 1.2–2.3 per 100,000. Outline of diagnostic approach to peripheral neuropathy is depicted in **Flowchart 6.15.1**.

Charcot–Marie–Tooth Disease and Hereditary Motor Sensory Neuropathy

It is the common hereditary neuropathy and comprises a heterogeneous group of inherited, nonmetabolic neuropathies. Salient features include positive family history, long slowly progressive course, and foot deformities. Individuals with CMT1 have a hypertrophic demyelinating neuropathy (onion bulbs in histopathology) and reduced nerve conduction velocities, whereas CMT2 denotes individuals with an axonal neuropathy and normal or slightly reduced nerve conduction velocities. CMT3 (Dejerine-Sottas disease) refers to individuals with a demyelinating peripheral neuropathy having a more severe phenotype presenting in infancy. CMT4 refers to autosomal recessive CMT, whereas CMT 1, 2, and 3 are historically considered autosomal dominant conditions.

Distal weakness, impaired sensation, and diminished or absent reflexes are the salient features. Individuals present

Table 6.15.7: Outline of classification and therapeutics of common subtypes of congenital myasthenia syndromes.

Subtypes	*Treatment*	*Caveats*
Presynaptic defects		
Choline acetyltransferase deficiency	Pyridostigmine parenteral neostigmine for acute apneic episodes	Recurrent apneas are common. They are floppy and weak with respiratory and bulbar muscle involvement. Severely affected patients may not respond to any cholinergic drugs and may require permanent respiratory support
SNAP25B deficiency	Amifampridine	
Synaptic defects		
Acetylcholinesterase deficiency	Salbutamol or ephedrine	Avoid pyridostigmine and amifampridine
Laminin-β2 deficiency	Ephedrine	Avoid pyridostigmine
Postsynaptic defects		
Primary acetylcholine receptor deficiency	Pyridostigmine; amifampridine also helps; salbutamol may be given in refractory cases	Most common variant of CMS
Slow-channel syndrome	Quinine, quinidine, or fluoxetine	Avoid pyridostigmine and amifampridine
Fast-channel syndrome	Pyridostigmine and amifampridine	Avoid quinine, quinidine, or fluoxetine
Dok-7 deficiency	Salbutamol or ephedrine	Presents as limb-girdle myasthenia. Avoid pyridostigmine
End-plate rapsyn deficiency	Pyridostigmine, amifampridine, and salbutamol	—

(CMS: congenital myasthenia syndromes; SNAP25B: synaptosomal-associated protein 25)

with complaints of clumsiness; slippage of slippers; difficulty in running or climbing stairs; or impaired fine motor skills, such as writing, buttoning clothes, or tying shoelaces. High arches, hammertoes, pes cavus, and claw hands are useful clinical indicators for hereditary neuropathy. Sensory symptoms may include numbness, dysesthesias, or ataxia. Autonomic symptoms, such as abnormal sweating, cardiac arrhythmias, hypotension, or bowel and bladder dysfunction, may accompany peripheral neuropathy.

One should keep in mind that in large families with known hereditary neuropathies, only 20% of the affected family members seek medical attention because of symptoms. One should inquire in detail before arriving at a conclusion regarding family history—difficulty with running; sports or military activities; high-arched feet or flat feet; hammer or curled-up toes; claw hands; wasting of muscles; foot troubles; foot ulcers; use of orthosis, arthritis, or poliomyelitis (incorrect diagnosis); and difficulty in walking on heels and toes.

There are various gene locations and known protein abnormalities associated with various forms of CMT (hereditary motor sensory neuropathy) and the clinical subtypes.

Guillain–Barré Syndrome

It is a common cause of acute flaccid paralysis in children. Many subtypes have been described and include acute inflammatory demyelinating polyradiculoneuropathy (AIDP), acute motor axonal neuropathy (AMAN), acute motor and sensory axonal neuropathy, and the Miller-Fisher syndrome (MFS). There are many variants of GBS, such as acute pandysautonomia, acute sensory neuropathy, Bickerstaff brainstem encephalitis, acute paraplegic variant, acute ophthalmoparesis variant, pharyngo-cervico-brachial variant, and polyneuritis cranialis.

About the two-thirds of GBS cases have an antecedent infection 1–6 weeks prior to symptom onset, generally an upper respiratory tract infection or gastroenteritis. The clinical manifestations include an acute-onset symmetrical ascending weakness (both proximal and distal) with frequent facial weakness and respiratory weakness in the one-fourth of the cases. Dysautonomia is also common. Pain and refusal to walk may be the initial manifestations. The axonal forms of GBS exhibit is more common in Asian population, including India compared to western population, and is usually associated with *Campylobacter* infection. Weakness reaches its nadir by 2–4 weeks, with AMAN variants having a severe and faster progression. Areflexia is commonly seen, though AMAN variants may have preserved reflexes.

The diagnosis depends on classical clinical picture, electrophysiological findings, and cerebrospinal fluid

Flowchart 6.15.1: Diagnostic approach.

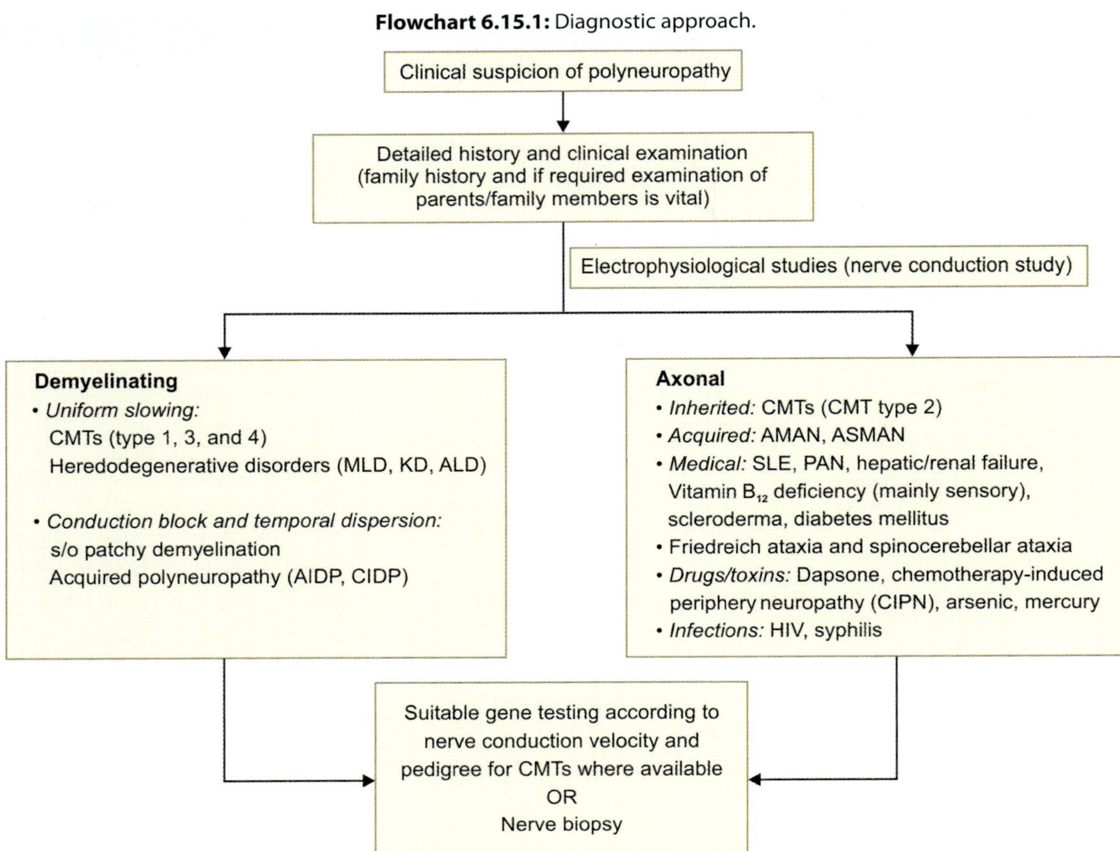

[A(C)IDP: acute (chronic) inflammatory demyelinating polyneuropathy; ALD: adrenoleukodystrophy; AMAN: acute motor axonal neuropathy; ASMAN: acute sensory motor axonal neuropathy; CMT: Charcot–Marie–Tooth disease; KD: Krabbe disease; MLD: metachromatic leukodystrophy; PAN: polyarteritis nodosa; SLE: systemic lupus erythematosus]

(CSF) examination. Electrophysiology may reveal absent F-responses or H-reflexes, reduced compound muscle action potentials or sensory nerve action potentials (in axonal forms), prolonged distal latencies, reduced conduction velocities, abnormal temporal dispersion, and conduction blocks (in demyelinating types). CSF analysis may reveal raised CSF protein concentration (80%) with the mononuclear cell count being either normal (albuminocytologic dissociation) or less than 50 cells/mm^3. Both electrophysiological studies and CSF analysis may be normal in the first week of the illness. Certain antibodies may also be detected in some subtypes, such as anti-ganglioside M1 and anti-ganglioside D1a antibodies in AMAN variant, anti-ganglioside Q1b in MFS variant, but are not helpful in early establishment of diagnosis. Antigen involved in AIDP is unknown. **Boxes 6.15.5 and 6.15.6** give clinical diagnostic criteria and management principles for the patients suffering from GBS, whereas **Table 6.15.8** gives differential diagnosis of GBS.

ANTERIOR HORN CELL DISORDERS

Spinal muscular atrophy is the most common anterior horn cell disorder encountered in children. It will be discussed briefly below. Other disorders affecting the anterior horn cells are infective (polio, nonpolio enteroviruses, human immunodeficiency virus, West Nile virus, human T-lymphotropic virus, Lyme disease and Japanese encephalitis); inflammatory (para/postinfectious/ autoimmune, such as multifocal motor neuropathy and sarcoidosis); hereditary (amyotrophic lateral sclerosis or other motor neuron disorders that commonly manifest in adults), toxic; paraneoplastic; and vascular causes.

Spinal Muscular Atrophy

Spinal muscular atrophy (SMA) is an autosomal recessive NMD characterized by the degeneration of motor neurons of the spinal cord which results in progressive muscle

Box 6.15.5: Clinical diagnostic features for Guillain–Barré syndrome.

Features required for diagnosis:
- Progressive symmetrical weakness in more than one limb (might start with weakness only in the legs)
- Areflexia (or decreased tendon reflexes)

Features that strongly support diagnosis:
- Progression of symptoms over days to 4 weeks
- Minimal sensory symptoms
- Pain (often present) and autonomic dysfunction
- Cranial nerve involvement (may involve bilateral 7th cranial nerves)
- High concentration of protein in CSF and albumin cytological dissociation
- Typical electrodiagnostic features

Features that should raise doubt about the diagnosis:
- High-grade fever at the onset of illness
- Severe pulmonary dysfunction with limited limb weakness at onset
- Severe sensory signs with limited weakness at onset and sharp sensory level
- Persistent and significant bowel bladder involvement
- Slow and staggered course of weakness progression (may consider subacute or chronic inflammatory demyelination)
- Marked persistent asymmetry of symptoms
- Increased CSF cell count (>50 × 10^6/L) suggesting other infections, such as HIV

(CSF: cerebrospinal fluid; HIV: human immunodeficiency virus)

Box 6.15.6: Management of a patient with Guillain–Barré syndrome.

Give good general care:
- Regularly monitor pulmonary function (initially every 2–4 h, in stable phase every 6–12 h)
- Regularly check for autonomic dysfunction (blood pressure, heart rate, pupils, and ileus)
- Check for swallowing dysfunction
- Recognize and treat pain and prevent decubitus ulcers and contractures
- Prevent and treat infections and pulmonary embolism
- Prevent corneal ulceration due to facial weakness

Consider specific treatment with IVIg or PE
- *Indications to start IVIg or PE*
- Severely affected patients (inability to walk unaided)
- *Start IVIg preferably within first 2 weeks from onset*: 2 g/kg over 2–5 days or 5 × PE with total exchange volume of five plasma volumes in 2 weeks (can be given up to 4 weeks from the onset of illness)

Indications for retreatment with IVIg:
- *Secondary deterioration after initial improvement or stabilization (treatment-related fluctuation)*: Treat with 2 g/kg over 2–5 days
- No proven effect of retreatment with IVIg in patients who continue to worsen

Is there an indication for admission to an intensive care unit?
- Rapid progressive severe weakness often with impaired respiration (vital capacity < 20 mL/kg)
- Respiratory failure
- Insufficient swallowing with high chance of pulmonary infection/aspiration
- Severe autonomic dysfunction

Fluctuations during the course of disease or continued slow progression:
- *Consider treatment-related fluctuation*: Repeat treatment
- Consider acute-onset CIDP (A-CIDP) and treat accordingly (intravenous steroids)

(A-CIDP: acute-onset chronic inflammatory demyelinating polyneuropathy; IVIg: intravenous immunoglobulin; PE: plasma exchange)

weakness and paralysis. SMA is one of the most common fatal autosomal recessive disorders, with an estimated incidence of 1 in 10,000 live births. SMA is caused by mutations in the survival motor neuron (*SMN*) gene present on 5q13. The homozygous absence of the SMN1exon 7 is most commonly observed in the majority of patients and is being utilized as a reliable and sensitive SMA diagnostic test. SMN2 produces less full-length transcript than SMN1; the number of SMN2 copies has been shown to modulate the clinical phenotype, more the number of copies less severe the phenotype. SMA is conventionally classified according to the age of onset and highest motor function achieved, including SMA type 0 to describe the severe forms of prenatal onset SMA **(Table 6.15.9)**. A very summary of recent advances in management of SMA is given in **Box 6.15.7**.

Table 6.15.8: Common differential diagnosis of Guillain–Barré syndrome.

Muscle disorders	*Neuromuscular junction disorders*	*Neuropathies*	*Central nervous system disorders*	*Others*
• Inflammatory myopathy • Periodic paralysis • Hypokalemia • Infections	• Myasthenia gravis • Eaton–Lambert syndrome • Botulism	• Diphtheritic neuropathy • Acute intermittent porphyria • Traumatic neuritis • Vasculitic neuropathy	• Acute myelopathy • Acute anterior poliomyelitis • Acute transverse myelitis • Brainstem stroke • Brainstem encephalitis • Acute cerebellar ataxia	*Antalgic conditions:* • Fracture • Trauma • Bone pain • Joint synovitis • Discitis • Scurvy • Leukemia

Table 6.15.9: Subtypes of spinal muscular atrophy.

Subtypes	*Age of onset*	*Maximum function achieved*	*SMN copy number*
Type 0 (very severe)	Neonatal with prenatal signs	Never sits	
Type 1 (severe) (Werdnig–Hoffman disease)	0–6 months	Never sits	SMN2 $\leq$ 2 copies
Type 2 (intermediate)	7–18 months	Sits but never stands	SMN2: 3 copies
Type 3 (mild) (Kugelberg–Welander disease)	>18 months	Stands and walks	SMN2: 3–4 copies
Type 4 (adult)	10–30 years	Stands and walks	SMN2: 4 or more copies

(SMN: survival motor neuron)

Box 6.15.7: Therapeutic approaches in spinal muscular atrophy.

- *SMN1 gene replacement*: Gene therapy (under research only)
- *SMN2 activation*: Histone deacetylase inhibitors (valproate, phenylbutyrate, and sodium butyrate have been found to be not useful) and hydroxyurea
- *Promotion of exon 7 inclusion*: Antisense oligonucleotides (Spinraza, first disease modifying therapy approved, requires repeated intrathecal administrations)
- *Stabilization of SMN protein*: Aminoglycosides
- *Cell replacement*: Cell therapy (under research only)
- *Neuroprotection*: Riluzole, gabapentin, creatine, albuterol, olexosime

(SMN: survival motor neuron)

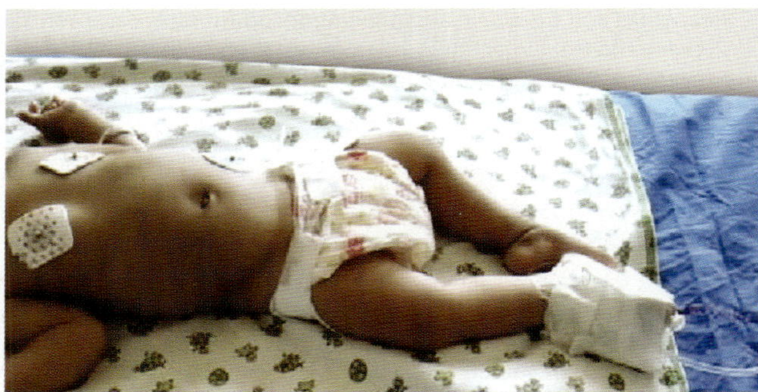

Fig. 6 15.5: Frog-like posture in a child with spinal muscular atrophy type 1.

Type 1 disease presents with profound hypotonia and flaccid weakness. Weak sucking, poor swallowing, labored breathing during feeding, frequent aspiration of food or secretions, and weak cry are commonly seen. Aspiration pneumonia is an important cause of morbidity and mortality. In the supine position, the lower extremities may be abducted and externally rotated in a "frog-leg" position, and the thorax is flattened anteroposteriorly, hence is bell shaped because of intercostal weakness **(Fig. 6.15.5)**. Children with type 2 disease are usually able to sit unaided. They may develop kyphoscoliosis, tremors (polyminimyoclonus), poor swallowing, and respiratory insufficiency. Types 3 and 4 patients are usually able to walk. They may mimic LGMD or myopathy.

KEY MESSAGES

- Detailed history and examination, in a child with suspected neuromuscular disease, is essential to localize the lesion in the motor unit.
- Family history with pedigree drawing is imperative to reach appropriate diagnosis.
- Investigations must be planned judiciously while managing children with NMD.
- Never miss potentially treatable conditions, such as neuromuscular junction disorders, which may mimic common muscle disorders. They may also have potentially fatal complications, if unrecognized.
- Genetic counseling and prenatal diagnosis are important in selected clinical scenarios. When we come across

families with multiple sibs affected with common conditions, such as SMA and DMD, the medical fraternity carries the blame for not offering appropriate genetic counseling and prenatal diagnosis.

- Early diagnosis is supported by the knowledge of the common initial clinical presentations of specific NMDs, and in many cases, the early diagnosis has potential implications for treatment and prevention of secondary conditions.

BIBLIOGRAPHY

1. Berardo A, DiMauro S, Hirano M. A diagnostic algorithm for metabolic myopathies. Curr Neural Neurosci Rep. 2010;10(2):118-26.
2. Bonnemann GC, Wang HC, Quijano-Roy S, et al. Diagnostic approach to the congenital muscular dystrophies. Neuromuscul Disord. 2014;24(4):289-311.
3. Bushby K, Finkel R, Birnkrant DJ, et al. Diagnosis and management of Duchenne muscular dystrophy, part 1: Diagnosis and pharmacological and psychosocial management. Lancet Neurol. 2010;9(1):77-93.
4. Engel AG, Shen XM, Selcen D, et al. Congenital myasthenic syndromes: pathogenesis, diagnosis and treatment. Lancet Neurol. 2015;14(4):420-34.
5. England JD, Gronseth GS, Franklin G, et al. Evaluation of distal symmetric polyneuropathy: the role of laboratory and genetic testing (an evidence-based review). Muscle Nerve. 2009;39(1):116-25.
6. Joint Task Force of the EFNS and the PNS. European Federation of Neurological Societies/Peripheral Nerve Society Guideline on management of chronic inflammatory demyelinating polyradiculoneuropathy. Report of a joint task force of the European Federation of Neurological Societies and the Peripheral Nerve Society. J Peripher Nerv Syst. 2010;15(3):185-95.
7. Jungbluth H, Ochala J, Treves S, et al. Current and future therapeutic approaches to the congenital myopathies. Semin Cell Dev Biol. 2017;64:191-200.
8. Lilleker JB, Keh YS, Roncaroli F, et al. Metabolic myopathies: a practical approach. Pract Neurol. 2018;18(1):14-26.
9. McDonald MC. Clinical approach to the diagnostic evaluation of hereditary and acquired neuromuscular diseases. Phys Med Rehabil Clin N Am. 2012;23(3):495-563.
10. North KN, Wang CH, Clarke N, et al. Approach to the diagnosis of congenital myopathies. Neuromuscul Disord. 2014;24(2):97-116.

6.16 Cerebral Palsy, Intellectual Disability, and Autism Spectrum Disorder

MS Mahadeviah

CEREBRAL PALSY

Cerebral palsy (CP) as it is commonly known is the most common cause of physical disability in children. It encompasses a group of nonprogressive disorders causing physical disability mainly in the various areas of body movement. Despite all the progresses in newborn care, its prevalence remains at 2–2.5 per 1,000. The prevalence in India is not definitively established. Although CP is described as a static encephalopathy, the neurological features may change over the time.

Definition

Cerebral palsy describes a group of permanent disorders of movement and posture causing activity limitation. It is also attributed to nonprogressive disturbances that occurred in the developing fetal or infant brain. The motor disorders of CP are often accompanied by the disturbances of sensation, perception, cognition, communication and behavior, epilepsy, and secondary musculoskeletal problems. CP excludes motor disorders of spinal, peripheral nerve, muscular or mechanical origin. Although it is stated that there is no explicit upper age limit, CP usually refers to the first 2–5 years when there is active growth of the brain.

Etiology

At present, 75–80% of causes of CP point to prenatal factors, which are responsible for abnormal development of brain. Main etiological factors in 10–20% of children with CP are intrapartum asphyxia and exposure to maternal infections, such as chorioamnionitis, sepsis, urinary tract infections, and fever with elevated levels of cytokines. Prematurity, especially infants weighing less than 1,000 g, is a major risk factor resulting in intraventricular hemorrhage and periventricular leukomalacia.

Perinatal and neonatal causes, such as sepsis, neonatal seizures, cerebral ischemia, and low Apgar scores, are present in substantial number of children with CP.

Clinical Features

The most common presentation of CP is delay in motor development, such as head control, sitting, standing, and walking. All types of CP are characterized by abnormal muscle tone, reflexes, or motor development and coordination. Other features include asymmetrical reaching for objects, abnormal movements and postures. Associated manifestations include delay in speech, visual difficulties, intellectual disability (ID), and seizures.

Classification

Cerebral palsy at present is broadly classified into spastic, dyskinetic, hypotonic, ataxic, and mixed.

Spastic Cerebral Palsy

Spastic type of CP accounts for 70–75% of the cases with CP. Spastic CP is further classified into spastic diplegia, spastic hemiplegia, spastic quadriplegia, spastic monoplegia, and spastic triplegia, as described here:

- *Spastic diplegia:* It refers to the spasticity predominantly of the lower extremities with minimal or no involvement of upper extremities. The major causes include prematurity, ischemia, and infections leading to periventricular leukomalacia. These children have relatively better cognitive functioning.
- *Spastic hemiplegia:* It refers to involvement of left or right side of the extremities; upper usually greater than lower. Spastic hemiplegia has the best prognosis for ambulation but is more prone to develop seizures. In 20–30% the pathology is contralateral cerebral infarcts.
- *Spastic quadriplegia:* It refers to equal involvement of all the four extremities with generalized spasticity. They have considerable clinical manifestations of drooling, difficulties in feeding, seizures along with speech disability, hearing disability, visual disability, and ID. The most common pathologies are periventricular leukomalacia and multicystic cortical encephalomalacia. The prognosis for independent ambulation is poor.
- *Spastic monoplegia and triplegia:* These are rare.

Dyskinetic Cerebral Palsy

This includes children with athetoid or choreoathetoid movements along with head lag, variable tone, drooling, tongue thrust, rigidity, and dystonia. In the past, dyskinetic CP was common with neonatal hyperbilirubinemia secondary to Rh incompatibility, which may still be a cause in the developing countries. Other factors include severe birth asphyxia, lesions in basal ganglia, and mitochondrial disorders.

Differential Diagnosis

It is important to rule out disorders of motor disability. Detailed history and examination should be directed to rule out progressive neurological disorders (degenerative), muscular disorders (myopathies and muscular dystrophies), spinal cord tumors, and genetic syndromes.

Investigations

At the present state-of-the-art of medical practice, a magnetic resonance imaging (MRI) scan of the brain is necessary. Ophthalmic evaluation, hearing tests, speech and language evaluation, psychological and educational evaluation, electroencephalogram (EEG), and other investigations should be done depending on the clinical profile.

Management

Management of children with CP involves a multidisciplinary team, which should include a developmental pediatrician, physiotherapist, occupational therapist, orthotic specialist, orthopedic surgeon, psychologist, educational specialist, speech pathologist, and social worker along with consultants in neurology, psychiatry, ophthalmology, assistive technology, and otolaryngology as necessary.

Counseling the Parents

Counseling the parents is the greatest challenge the professional faces. It is important to teach the parents regarding the activities of daily living, such as feeding, bathing, dressing, and follow-up of therapy that is being done by the physiotherapist and occupational therapist. Frequent follow-up, addressing the special needs of children and parents, should be the most important service.

Drugs

Some of the common drugs used are muscle relaxants, such as baclofen, dantrolene sodium, and benzodiazepines. One of the most popular drugs that is used to relieve spasticity is Botox (botulinum toxin), which when injected to specific muscle groups is effective in reducing spasticity. However, it is important to have specific evaluations for such therapies because of the cost involved. Levodopa and carbamazepine are recommended in children with dystonia and rigidity.

Physiotherapy

Management includes prevention of contractures, which is the main goal of physiotherapist and orthopedic surgeon.

Surgical Procedures

Surgical procedures such as tendo-Achilles lengthening, adductor tenotomy, psoas transfer, and soft tissue release to prevent dislocation of hip. Posterior rhizotomies are useful in selected cases with spastic diplegia.

Prognosis

Cerebral palsy is a lifelong disorder, and hence parents and adolescents require constant counseling. Independent ambulation is the dream of every parent. Children with hemiplegia and diplegia have better prognosis than children with quadriplegia. Anticipatory guidance should be provided regarding ambulation and education for future planning. A gross motor function classification system provides the best guidance to clinician for prognosis.

INTELLECTUAL DISABILITY

Definition

The term ID has now replaced the earlier term "mental retardation" (MR) as per Federal Statute in the United States (Public Law III—256 Rosa's Law) as the term, MR, was considered offensive.

Intellectual disability is defined as "significantly subaverage general intellectual functioning, existing concurrently with deficits in adaptive behavior and manifested during the developmental period that adversely affects a child's educational performance," according to the US Special Educational Plan, the Individuals with Disabilities Education Act.

Prevalence

Intellectual disability affects the population in varying proportions; however, 75% of these cases fall under mild ID. Severe ID accounts for less than 5% of the population of affected children.

Pathogenesis

There are no specific pathological correlates for ID. The more severe the ID, greater are the chances of finding abnormalities in the brain. These include reduction in brain volume (microcephaly), disorders of cell migration, heterotopias, polymicrogyria, pachygyria, and dendritic changes.

Classification

At present, various levels of severity are defined based on adaptive functioning and not on intelligence quotient (IQ). It is the level of adaptive functioning that determines the level of support required.

- *Mild ID:* IQ level 50–70
- *Moderate ID:* IQ level 35–50/50–55
- *Severe ID:* IQ level 25–35/35–40
- *Profound ID:* IQ level below 20–25.

Severity levels for ID and functioning are described in three domains: conceptual, social, and practical domains.

Etiology

Intellectual disability is multifactorial in etiology. The causes include socioeconomic to genetic, metabolic, endocrine and infectious disorders, and induced by toxins and trauma. Mild forms, which are the most common one, occur four times greater in children of women with poor education and socioeconomic status. A list of common causes of IDs is given in **Box 6.16.1**.

Clinical Features

Essential features of ID are deficits in general mental abilities (criterion A), impairment in everyday adaptive functioning, in comparison to an individual age, gender, and socioculturally matched peers (criterion B), and onset during developmental period (criterion C).

Any dysmorphic feature, such as microcephaly, macrocephaly, and facial features, as present in Down syndrome and Turner syndrome should raise suspicion of ID. Developmental delay involving milestones, such as head control, sitting, standing, walking, and talking, are the earliest presentations. Special attention should be paid to speech and language development. Children with mild ID may later present with scholastic backwardness with global difficulties in learning.

Diagnosis

The diagnosis of ID is based on both clinical assessment and standardized testing of intellectual and adaptive functions.

According to the Diagnostic and Statistical Manual of Mental Disorders-4, three criteria must be met for the diagnosis of ID:

Box 6.16.1: Common causes of intellectual disability.

- *Parental causes*:
  - Consanguinity
  - Maternal age and nutrition
  - Infections
  - Toxemias
  - *Metabolic diseases*: Diabetes mellitus
  - *Drugs*: Alcohol (fetal alcohol syndrome)
- *Perinatal and neonatal*:
  - Prematurity
  - Low birth weight
  - Fetal distress and asphyxia
  - Difficult labor
  - Multiple births
  - Sepsis
  - Seizures
  - Hyperbilirubinemia
- *Postnatal*:
  - Malnutrition
  - *Infections*: Viral and bacterial (TORCH, HIV)
  - Trauma resulting in head injury
  - Child abuse and neglect
- *Genetic, chromosomal, and dysmorphic syndromes*:
  - Down syndrome
  - Klinefelter syndrome
  - Turner syndrome
  - Fragile X syndrome
  - X-linked mental retardation
  - Williams syndrome
  - Cornelia De-Lange syndrome
  - Neurocutaneous syndromes (tuberous sclerosis)
  - Neurofibromatosis
- *Inborn errors of metabolism*:
  - Phenylketonuria
  - Galactosemia
  - Mucopolysaccharidosis
- *Endocrine*:
  - Hypothyroidism and iodine deficiency

The list is endless. To make a broad statement, any adverse effect on the developing brain from conception to 18 years can cause intellectual disability

(HIV: human immunodeficiency virus; TORCH: toxoplasmosis, other (syphilis, varicella-zoster, parvovirus B19), rubella, cytomegalovirus, and herpes infections).

1. An IQ below 70
2. Significant limitations in two or more areas of adaptive behavior (as measured by an adaptive behavior rating scale, i.e. communication, self-help skills, interpersonal skills, and more) and
3. Evidence that the limitations became apparent before the age of 18 years.

An accurate medical history is the most important part of the diagnosis. The history should include prenatal, perinatal, postnatal, developmental, dental and visual, general health, school performance and behavior. Detailed history about family should include parental education, family income, socioeconomic status, history of the ID, epilepsy, genetic disorders, and mental health.

A detailed physical examination should note general physical appearance, dysmorphic features, neurocutaneous markers, eye contact, detailed developmental and neurological examination should be done.

Investigations

Ideally newborn screening for thyroid function and metabolic disorders should be done depending on the clinical diagnosis and age of the child. Further investigations, such as cranial computed tomography scans; MRI of brain; EEG; hearing, speech, and language studies; ophthalmic, psychological, and psychoeducational evaluations, should be performed.

Management

Since ID is a lifelong condition, management requires a multidisciplinary team that consists of a pediatrician, psychologist, education specialists, speech pathologist, social worker, and occupational therapist. Consultants should include pediatric neurologists, psychiatrist, and ophthalmologist. The key to the success of management depends on the inclusion of parents as equal partners in management.

Early diagnosis in infancy is important. Medical professionals should pay attention to parents' concerns regarding child's development. A definitive diagnosis of developmental delay, if not the definitive cause can easily be done in most cases by 2 years. Delay in neck control by 6 months, sitting by 12 months, walking by 18 months, and talking by 2 years should alert every pediatrician of the possibility of ID.

Drugs

There is no scientific evidence for the use of medications to improve brain functions. Perhaps the only drug that successfully cures ID is thyroxine for hypothyroidism if initiated in the newborn period. Antiepileptic drugs, such as phenobarbitone, phenytoin, carbamazepine, and valproate, are used to treat various seizure disorders, which are present in children with ID.

Prevention

- *Primary prevention:* These include counseling regarding proper maternal and infant nutrition, healthcare, prenatal immunization with rubella vaccine, folic acid supplements, genetic counseling, and if indicated prenatal screening for malformations. The specific measures for children include proper nutrition, health education in school, and universal immunization.

- *Secondary prevention:* Early diagnosis and rehabilitation; frequent developmental screening.
- *Tertiary prevention:* Research and liaisons with governmental agencies for proper funding and support to the families.

Prognosis

Since 75–80% of children with ID have mild degree of ID, attaining independent living and fair educational skills are good.

Mild Intellectual Disability

Given excellent rehabilitation, these children with ID who have minimal impairment in sensory motor area can hardly be differentiated from normal population. They develop good social and communication skills. Academic skills up to the fifth to sixth standard can be achieved by teenage years. As adults, they can be self-supportive and can lead independent lives. They however need to be supervised and assisted during social and economic stress.

Moderate Intellectual Disability

They constitute 10% of children. Most of them can acquire communicative skills, which can be provided by vocational training. They however have limited academic skills. They face considerable difficulties in adolescent period because of the lack of social skills and peer relationships. As adults they will require sheltered workshops and need supervision.

Severe Intellectual Disability

They constitute 3–5% of children. Some of the children can profit to a limited extent by academic input. Concentration should be on acquiring self-care skills. Adult years must be spent at home or community homes.

Profound Intellectual Disability

They constitute only 1–2%. These children have identifiable neurological and genetic diagnosis. With intense training, they can develop some communication skills. However, they will require home care with individual supervision and treatment of associated conditions.

AUTISM SPECTRUM DISORDER

Essential features of autism spectrum disorder (ASD) include permanent impairment of reciprocal social communication and social interaction (criterion A), restrictive repetitive patterns of behavior, interest, or activities (criterion B). These symptoms are present from early childhood and limit or impair everyday functioning (criterion C and D). Manifestations of the disorder vary greatly depending on the severity of autistic condition, development level, and chronological age, hence the term "spectrum." The ASD now encompasses disorders previously referred to as early infantile autism, childhood autism, Kenner's autism, high-functioning autism, atypical autism, pervasive development disorder, not otherwise specified, childhood disintegrative disorder, and Asperger disorder. Readers are advised to refer to Chapter 6.19 for a detailed description on *childhood autism*. Asperger syndrome and Rett syndrome are described in brief here.

Asperger Syndrome

Asperger syndrome differs from autistic disorder in that there are no delays in language. Single words are spoken at 2 years and phrases at 3 years, and no delays are noted in cognitive development. These children have appropriate self-help skills and adaptive behaviors. However, there is impairment in social interaction, restricted, repetitive behavior, interest, and activities. Asperger syndrome may manifest later than autistic disorder. Social interaction becomes more noticeable in school age. Major milestones may be delayed and children with Asperger syndrome exhibit clumsiness. Asperger syndrome is a lifelong disorder and is more common among males.

Rett Syndrome

The Rett syndrome is a disorder of early development of brain. Rett syndrome is caused by mutations in the gene *MECP2*. Infants have normal head size till 6 months of age and then decrease is noted in brain growth. Major clinical features are the hand-wringing movements and loss of purposeful use of hands. Autistic behavior is noted at 2–3 years of age. Children with Rett syndrome develop seizures. Death occurs usually in the third decade from cardiac arrhythmias.

BIBLIOGRAPHY

1. American Psychiatric Association (2010). DSM-5 development. [online] Available from: http://www.dsm5.org/Pages/Default.aspx [Accessed October, 2015].
2. Denckla MB, James LS. An update on autism: a developmental disorder. Pediatrics. 1991;87:751-96.
3. Francis K. Autism Interventions: a critical update. Dev Med Child Neurol. 2005;47:493-9.
4. Morris C. Definition and classification of cerebral palsy. Dev Med Child Neurol. 2007;109;3-7.
5. Nelson KB. The epidemiology of cerebral palsy in term infants. Ment Retard Dev Disabil Res Rev. 2002;8:146-50.
6. Palisano R, Rosenbaum P, Walter S, et al. Development and reliability of a system to classify gross motor function in children with cerebral palsy. Dev Med Child Neurol. 1997;39:214-23.
7. Rutter M, Scopler E. Autism and pervasive developmental disorders. Concepts and diagnostic issues. J Autism Dev Disord. 1987;17:159-86.
8. Stromme P, Hagberg G. Etiology in severe and mild mental retardation: a population based study of Norwegian children. Dev Med Child Neurol. 2000;42:76-86.

6.17 Learning Disabilities and Attention-Deficit Hyperactivity Disorder

Sunil Karande

INTRODUCTION

Learning disabilities (LDs) and attention-deficit hyperactivity disorder (ADHD) are two common neurodevelopmental disorders that occur in up to 5–10% of children.

LEARNING DISABILITY

Definition

Learning disability is a group of neurodevelopmental disorders, which manifest in childhood as persistent difficulties in learning to efficiently read (dyslexia), write (dysgraphia), or do mathematical calculations (dyscalculia) despite normal intelligence, conventional schooling, intact hearing and vision, adequate motivation, and sociocultural opportunities.

Etiopathogenesis

Learning disability is believed to be a result of functional disruption in neural systems and is genetically inherited. Dyslexia or "specific-reading disability" is the most common and most carefully studied, affecting 80% of all those identified as learning-disabled. Children with dyslexia have deficits in "phonologic awareness," viz. they have difficulty developing an awareness that words, both written and spoken, can be broken down into smaller units of sound and that, in fact, the letters constituting the printed word represent the sounds heard in the spoken word.

Clinical Features

A history of language delay, or of not attending to the sounds of words (trouble playing rhyming games with words or confusing words that sound alike), along with a family history, are important red flags for dyslexia. Children with LD present with persistent "academic problems" such as reading slowly and incorrectly, skipping lines while reading aloud, making repeated spelling mistakes, untidy/illegible handwriting with poor sequencing, and inability to perform even simple additions and subtractions. These children invariably fail to achieve school grades that are commensurate with their intelligence.

Diagnosis

A conclusive diagnosis of LD cannot be made until the child is about 7–8 years old. Unlike children having LD, some of the children are "normal late developers" who by the age of 7–8 years on their own outgrow their learning problems.

An evaluation for LD should be considered for all children presenting with learning problems in preschool/school. A multidisciplinary team comprising of pediatric neurologist, counselor, clinical psychologist, and special educator is needed to assess each child referred for poor school performance. The sequence of evaluations done is as follows:

- Audiometric and ophthalmic examinations are done to rule-out hearing and visual deficits, as they are common causes of poor school performance. Also, children with uncorrectable hearing and visual deficits (of >40% disability) do not qualify for a diagnosis of LD but are diagnosed as having "hearing impairment" and "visual impairment," respectively.
- The pediatric neurologist then takes a detailed clinical history and does a detailed clinical examination to exclude medical causes, e.g. hypothyroidism and chronic lead poisoning, and neurological causes, e.g. cerebral palsy and Wilson disease, and to identify behavioral causes, e.g. ADHD, depression, conduct disorder (CD), or oppositional defiant disorder (ODD), of poor school performance.
- The counselor takes a detailed interview of the parents/family members to rule out that emotional problem due to stress at home/school is not primarily responsible for the child's poor school performance.
- The clinical psychologist conducts the standard Wechsler Intelligence Scale for Children test to determine that the child's global intelligence quotient (IQ) score is average or above average (≥85). This helps to exclude children having "borderline intellectual functioning" IQ score (71–84) also known as "slow learners" who also present with poor school performance.
- The fifth edition of Diagnostic and Statistical Manual of Mental Disorders (DSM-V) has recommended adopting intellectual disability as a rule-out criterion rather than using average IQ as a rule-in criterion for diagnosing LD. The DSM-V recommendation effectively eliminates the slow learners' category. However, this recommendation

has raised a controversy and till date in India has not been accepted.

- The special educator assesses the child's academic achievement by administering a standard educational test (e.g. Curriculum-Based Test, Woodcock-Johnson Test of Achievement) to assess the child's performance in areas such as reading, spelling, written language, and mathematics. An academic achievement of up to 2 years below the child's actual school grade placement or chronological age is considered diagnostic of LD.
- The child psychiatrist plays an important role in confirming the diagnosis of ADHD, a comorbid condition found in 12–24% of children with LD.

Treatment

The cornerstone of treatment of LD is remedial education, and it should begin early when the child is in primary school. Using specific teaching strategies and teaching materials, the special educator formulates an *Individual Educational Program* to reduce or eliminate the child's deficiencies in specific learning areas of reading, writing, and mathematics identified during the child's educational assessment. The child has to undergo remedial education sessions twice or thrice weekly for a few years to achieve academic competence. However, even after adequate remedial education, subtle deficiencies in reading, writing, and mathematical abilities persist.

The management of LD in the more time-demanding setting of secondary school is based more on providing provisions (accommodations). These provisions, e.g. exemption from spelling mistakes, availing extra time for all written tests, dropping a language and substituting it with work experience, dropping algebra and geometry and substituting them with lower grade of mathematics and work experience, are meant to help the child cope up in a regular mainstream school.

Complications

The "academic problems" of children with LD also have an adverse impact on their self-image, peer and family relationships, and social interactions.

Prognosis

It is well known that favorable outcome of LD is dependent on early diagnosis, regular remedial education for a few years, availing the necessary provisions, and a supportive home and school environment.

Practice Guidelines

Every pediatrician can facilitate early detection of LD by enquiring about every child's school performance during a consultation and guiding the parents for getting their child's psychoeducational assessment done, when LD is suspected.

ATTENTION-DEFICIT HYPERACTIVITY DISORDER

Definition

Attention-deficit hyperactivity disorder is a neurodevelopmental disorder characterized by persistent hyperactivity, impulsivity, and inattention that significantly impairs educational achievement and/or social functioning.

Epidemiology

There is no data available from India of the prevalence rates of ADHD. Data from Western countries indicate that 8–12% of school-going children have ADHD.

Etiopathogenesis

Recent functional magnetic resonance imaging brain studies indicate that the disorder may be caused by atypical functioning in the frontal lobes, basal ganglia, corpus callosum, and cerebellar vermis. Pharmacological studies have also implicated dysregulation of frontal-subcortical-cerebellar catecholaminergic circuits (dopamine and norepinephrine neurotransmitter systems) in the pathophysiology of the disorder. Family studies have provided strong evidence that genetics plays a major role in conferring susceptibility to ADHD. Studies have indicated that low birth weight and psychosocial adversity (for example severe parental discord, low-social class, and foster placement) are predisposing risk factors for ADHD.

Clinical Features

A history of being asked to leave preschool for disruptive behavior, or of being avoided by peers for play activities, along with a family history, are important red flags for ADHD.

Diagnosis

The diagnosis is made by ascertaining whether the child's specific behaviors meet the DSM-V criteria **(Table 6.17.1)**. These criteria define three presentations of ADHD:

1. Attention-deficit hyperactivity disorder primarily of the inattentive type
2. Attention-deficit hyperactivity disorder primarily of the hyperactive-impulsive type
3. Attention-deficit hyperactivity disorder, combined type

A child meets the diagnostic criteria for ADHD by documentation of:

- A persistent pattern of inattention and/or hyperactivity-impulsivity that interferes with functioning or development. Six or more of the symptoms have persisted

Table 6.17.1: Diagnostic and Statistical Manual of Mental Disorders-V criteria for diagnosing attention-deficit hyperactivity disorder.

Behavior domains	
Inattention (9 criteria)	***Hyperactivity-impulsivity (9 criteria)***
• Careless with details • Fails to sustain attention in tasks • Appears not to listen • Does not finish instructed tasks • Poor in organizing tasks • Avoids tasks that require sustained mental effort • Loses things • Easily distracted by extraneous stimuli • Forgetful in daily activities	*Hyperactivity (6 criteria):* • Fidgets with hands or feet or squirms in seat • Leaves seat when should be seated • Runs about or climbs excessively and inappropriately • Cannot play or engage in leisure activities quietly • Always "on the go" or "driven by a motor" • Talks excessively *Impulsivity (3 criteria):* • Blurts out answer before question is completed • Has difficulty awaiting turn • Interrupts or intrudes others' conversations or games

Note: Criteria for presentations are 6/9 on either list, or for combined presentation, 6/9 on both lists together with certain prerequisites (see text)

for at least 6 months to a degree that is inconsistent with developmental level and which has negatively impacted social and academic activities. The symptoms are not solely a manifestation of oppositional behavior, defiance, hostility, or failure to understand tasks or instructions.

- Several inattentive or hyperactive-impulsive symptoms are present in two or more settings (for example at home and at school) for at least past 6 months.
- Several inattentive or hyperactive-impulsive symptoms were presented prior to age 12 years.
- Clear evidence of clinically significant impairment in academic or social functioning, or in both.
- These symptoms not occurring exclusively during the course of schizophrenia or another psychotic disorder and are not better explained by another mental disorder (e.g. mood disorder, anxiety disorder, dissociative disorder, personality disorder, substance intoxication, or withdrawal).

For older adolescents and adults (age 17 years and older), five or more symptoms are required.

Treatment

Optimal treatment of ADHD requires integrated behavioral and medical (combined) treatment.

Behavioral Therapy

Parents are taught how to:

- Reinforce positive behaviors by praise or by using daily contingency charts (star or "happy face" charts).
- Extinguish negative behaviors by active ignoring.
- Effectively punish for intolerable behaviors.

Simple psychoeducational interventions at school such as seating the child near the teacher to minimize classroom distractions, or assigning a specific teacher to review daily assignments with the child are effective in improving the behavior and academic performance of affected children.

Medications

Medications are not recommended for use in children who are below 6 years of age. Methylphenidate (MPH) and atomoxetine are the two drugs, which are being currently prescribed. Most children with ADHD improve on the stimulant MPH and maintain their improvement without intolerable adverse events. Short-acting MPH is now available in our country. Its behavioral effects begin within 30 minutes of oral administration and last for 3–5 hours. The daily dose should be individualized by titration and careful monitoring and it ranges from 5 mg to 20 mg twice daily to three times daily. Side effects include anorexia, stomachache, headache, irritable mood, tics, and sleep difficulties. These side effects are usually mild and responsive to dose adjustment and often abate with continuous use. Continuous use has been associated in some children with slowing of physical growth (approximately 1 cm/year during the first 1–3 years of treatment), which is transient and of unclear cause. In Western countries, long-acting MPH is available and it permits once-daily administration (18–54 mg) and its behavioral effects last for 10–12 hours. It is used to ensure compliance in children who feel embarrassed to take medication in school.

Atomoxetine, a nonstimulant highly selective noradrenalin reuptake inhibitor, is a relatively new drug with efficacy comparable to MPH. The starting once-daily dose is 0.5 mg/kg/day and increased after 4 days to 1.2–1.4 mg/kg/day. Its most commonly reported adverse effects are transient and include dyspepsia, nausea, vomiting, decreased appetite, and weight loss.

In general, medication is best titrated against desirable effects such as behavioral control, improved educational achievement and peer group relations, and development of intolerable adverse effects. Medication can be discontinued on Sundays and school holidays. Also, periodic (yearly) discontinuation for a brief period during summer vacations is often used to reaffirm the need for continuing medication.

Complications

Between 18% and 35% of children with ADHD have one or more associated psychiatric disorders such as anxiety disorder, depression, ODD, and CD. Also, up to 15–20% of children with ADHD have associated LD. It is known that children with combined LD and ADHD have more severe learning problems than children who have LD but no ADHD, and also more severe attention problems than children who have ADHD but no LD.

Prognosis

It is well known that favorable outcome of ADHD is dependent on early diagnosis and treatment and a supportive home and school environment. If ADHD remains undetected the child may experience academic failure, rejection by peers, and develop low self-esteem. Recent studies suggest that 30–60% of affected children continue to show significant symptoms of ADHD into adolescence and young adulthood. Adolescence may bring about a reduction in the overactivity but inattention, impulsiveness, and inner restlessness remain. DSM-V has suggested that ADHD is not limited to childhood and may extend across the whole life span causing impairment even later in life.

It is now well recognized that the presence of a child with ADHD results in increased likelihood of disturbances to family and marital functioning, disrupted parent-child relationships, and increased levels of parent stress, particularly when ADHD is comorbid with ODD or CD.

Practice Guidelines

Pediatricians should initiate an evaluation for ADHD when a child presents with symptoms that include academic underachievement and failure, disruptive classroom behavior, inattentiveness, poor self-esteem, or problems with establishing or maintaining social relationships. Those familiar with its management can even initiate the medication management but will need to liaise with a child psychiatrist/developmental pediatrician when intolerable side effects or treatment failures occur or if comorbid conditions are suspected.

KEY MESSAGES

- With appropriate remedial education and provisions, children with LD achieve academic competence in regular mainstream schools.
- Optimal treatment of ADHD requires integrated behavioral and medical treatment.

BIBLIOGRAPHY

1. Al-Yagon M, Cavendish W, Cornoldi C, et al. The proposed changes for DSM-5 for SLD and ADHD: international perspectives—Australia, Germany, Greece, India, Israel, Italy, Spain, Taiwan, United Kingdom, and United States. J Learn Disabil. 2013;46:58-72.
2. Biederman J, Faraone SV. Attention-deficit hyperactivity disorder. Lancet. 2005;366:237-48.
3. Demonet JF, Taylor MJ, Chaix Y. Developmental dyslexia. Lancet. 2004;363:1451-60.
4. Sharma N, Mishra R, Mishra D. The fifth edition of Diagnostic and Statistical Manual of Mental Disorders (DSM-5): what is new for the pediatrician? Indian Pediatr. 2015;52:141-3.

6.18 Global Developmental Delay and Early Intervention

Sunanda K Reddy

INTRODUCTION

Global developmental delay (GDD) constitutes a subset of developmental disabilities, currently gaining ground as a diagnostic entity. Some prefer to use it as an umbrella term to denote developmental lag in various domains along with significant intellectual impairment.

The diagnostic and statistical manual of mental disorders, fifth edition, defines GDD as "the failure of an individual under age 5 years to meet expected developmental milestones across multiple areas of intellectual functioning."

DEFINITION

Global developmental delay is defined as "a significant delay in two or more of the following developmental domains: gross/fine motor, speech or language, cognition, social/personal-adaptive and activities of daily living (ADLs)". Significant delay implies a discrepancy of 25% or more from the expected rate, or 1.5–2 standard deviation (SD) from the norm.

In practice, however, the term GDD is usually reserved for children younger than 5 years of age, showing the symptom complex with a yet undefined profile that includes poor cognitive and psychomotor functions, whereas the term "mental retardation (MR)" or "intellectual deficit disorder" is applied to older children when intelligence quotient testing is more reliable and valid.

EPIDEMIOLOGY

There is a paucity of studies related to GDD in the population. The relatively new concepts and the prevailing controversies regarding terminology, coupled with the difficulties in ascertaining diagnosis in young children whose capacities are evolving, pose challenges to epidemiological studies.

The exact incidence and prevalence in India are not known. Studies in India, mostly in resource-poor settlements, have found a prevalence of 1.5–2.15% of developmental delay in children less than 2 years of age. The double burden of infectious diseases along with poverty correlates, such as malnutrition and risks associated with urbanization, exposure of mothers and infants to toxic substances, may contribute to the growing numbers of children with GDD in the developing countries.

ETIOPATHOGENESIS

Evidence from several studies during this decade points to the heterogeneous nature of the underlying diseases and suggest that the predominant categories of cerebral dysgenesis, chromosomal disorders, multiple malformation syndromes, hypoxic-ischemic encephalopathy, and antenatal toxin exposures account for global functional delays in nearly two thirds of children.

At present time, our knowledge of the prime movers for observed etiology (e.g. gene responsible for a particular cerebral dysgenesis) may not be sufficient, and one may be describing in pathogenic terms (e.g. periventricular leukomalacia and cerebral dysgenesis). The more recent developments in genomics have suggested a high association with chromosomal aberrations, especially when delay is also associated with autistic traits. An approach of conceptualizing etiology as a diagnostic aid that can translate into useful clinical information for prognosis and management is gaining momentum, consistent with practice parameters and guidelines proposed by the Child Neurology Society and the American Academy of Neurology.

CLINICAL PICTURE

There is no definitive clinical picture as GDD is a symptom complex associated with a variety of conditions. Child invariably presents with significant delay in two or more major developmental domains. Expected features include microcephaly or occipitofrontal circumference 2 SD below the mean, dysmorphic features, and identifiable neurological deficits. Global developmental delay from prenatal causes may be associated with growth retardation and multisystem involvement (congenital heart disease, hepatosplenomegaly, seizures, etc.). Associated sensory problems in hearing, vision, and/or disequilibrium reactions may be seen with a specific etiological yield. Adaptive problems and behavioral alterations are common in both prenatal and postnatal insults.

A family history of miscarriages or difficulties in learning in family members and a history of intrapartum complications may be elicited in some children. A history of birth asphyxia, seizures, and abnormal neurological findings in the newborn period and infancy are often predictors of GDD, especially in the presence of dysmorphism. Clinically identifiable features emerge as the child grows, and follow-up evaluation of babies often points to an underlying condition.

Clinical evaluation of the growing child with GDD must include a follow-up for global mental functions, particularly looking at the evolving capacities. These include the degree/quality of awareness and alertness, orientation, intellectual functions including cognitive development, global psychosocial functions, or interpersonal skills to establish reciprocal social interactions, temperament, attention, energy, and drive functions. Abnormalities in these areas constitute soft neurological findings for GDD, and the developmental variability must alert the pediatrician to look for developmental deviations.

DIAGNOSTIC EVALUATION AND INVESTIGATIONS

Establishing an accurate etiologic diagnosis is not always possible; nevertheless the diagnostic process is necessary for accurate genetic counseling and rehabilitative planning. Clinical assessment remains vital for guiding investigations.

Early diagnosis of GDD is possible by regular newborn follow-up and periodic evaluation for developmental lag in the first 2 years of life. Every static abnormality or failure to acquire new skills must be alarm symptoms when applying the *developmental surveillance* approach for identifying developmental and behavioral disorders.

A developmental assessment based on in-depth history and clinical examination is paramount. Quite often, a detailed developmental history including prenatal, perinatal, neonatal history and developmental patterns in infancy may suggest diagnosis or the framework needed for early identification of delays. Evidence for poor capacity for self-help/ADLs expected for the age calls for a detailed diagnostic evaluation. Tests for adaptive functioning and psychomotor development using standard developmental scales appropriate for the age must be undertaken. The Bayley Scales of Infant Development, Wechsler Scales (Wechsler Preschool and Primary Scale of Intelligence-III), Vineland Adaptive Behavior Scale are some tests administered for the purpose in children less than 5 years of age. A diagnostic formulation in terms of maturation and development can also form the basis for the early intervention (EI) and identification of special education needs. Repeated developmental assessments over time are more informative than one-off assessment.

The basic investigations may include thyroid profile testing, TORCH (toxoplasmosis, rubella, cytomegalovirus, herpes simplex, and HIV) screen, and magnetic resonance imaging/computed tomography scans of brain. One should consider referring children to care settings with good diagnostic facilities whenever etiological diagnosis is important to prognosticate and provide appropriate intervention. The subcommittee of the American Academy of Neurology and Practice committee of Child Neurology Society had made evidence-based recommendations concerning the evaluation of the child with a nonprogressive GDD.

Neuroimaging and karyotyping may be done for all with dysmorphism and congenital anomalies. Metabolic testing (e.g. serum amino acids) and biochemical analysis are additionally undertaken in tertiary settings for specific management.

A case for genetic evaluation is strong in current practice because of the increased evidence of clinical syndromes associated with chromosomal aberration.

A suggested approach as a diagnostic strategy linked to intervention for children with GDD is described in **Flowchart 6.18.1**.

The contemporary approach to diagnostic assessment of children with developmental disorders is based on the guiding principle that diagnostic assessment is a "dead end" unless it generates a focus/plan for intervention.

MANAGEMENT AND EARLY INTERVENTION PRACTICE GUIDELINES

Early intervention is a term traditionally associated with the services managed by professionals with a transdisciplinary approach for a child with developmental disability during the preschool years to help overcome the developmental lag.

In the resource-poor settings, EI or help in the early years starts as a high-risk follow-up clinic linked to primary care and extends to become a cost-effective family-centered model. Drawing from the fundamental neurodevelopment perspectives, the caregiver, who is often a developmental therapist or a pediatrician, works to create a developmental setting in which the key to a child's progress is mother-child participation.

The basis for EI is that there are critical periods of development and interventions, to be most effective, should happen before those periods. The second reason is that the central nervous system (CNS) has the feature of neuroplasticity or intrinsic ability of neural structure to form functional neuronal networks for new learning.

Helping the child with GDD during the early years is critical for later development. Developmental gains may not always be measurable in quotients, but some benefits are obvious.

Early intervention prevents developmental decline and deviant patterns of development that are seen in GDD. Professional intervention is particularly effective in addressing the motor and sensory impairments and seizures that are often seen as comorbidities.

Even in a child with severe impairment, providing sensory inputs and appropriate experiences early in life contributes to information gains (early infant stimulation). Guidance to parents is a crucial component of EI. An early acceptance of the problem and early efforts to help the child overcome the biological disadvantage helps parents understand their child better and cope with the difficult situations.

The components for EI depend on the primary impairment and can vary with the child's needs. Developmental therapy focuses on mobility, manipulation, and communication. In the presence of GDD without significant motor impairment, activities promoting sensory integration, balance, and communication become important. Evidence of visual and auditory impairments in this group is high and management should address this after appropriate visual and audiometric assessment at the time of diagnostic.

In children with special learning needs from GDD, EI brings down inappropriate behaviors and improves social competence.

Challenging behaviors (aggression, oppositional defiant behaviors) may require behavior management techniques as well as environment engineering. Medication is of little use, except for short-term psychopharmacological management in select cases. Family counseling and respite care should be integral part of EI and management plan. Support care instituted early with interdisciplinary management should be multimodal to address the diverse needs of the child: health, education, recreation, social activities, and direct efforts to ameliorate the effects of associated impairments and behaviors to improve functional outcomes and participation.

A program for "early infant stimulation" is facilitated by early identification of problems at birth or at discharge from nursery. Early and intensive support through home visits by health workers, and multicomponent stimulation programs that are culture-sensitive and context-specific can promote developmental outcomes. The key care provider and the team of professionals (developmental therapist, speech therapist, pediatrician, clinical psychologist, and other members) in a transdisciplinary/interdisciplinary mode of EI look to addressing risks and enhancing promotion of health and abilities as well as to prevent secondary problems through direct support to the child and the family.

Flowchart 6.18.1: Diagnostic strategy linked to intervention for children with global developmental delay—Algorithm for the evaluation of the child with developmental delay.

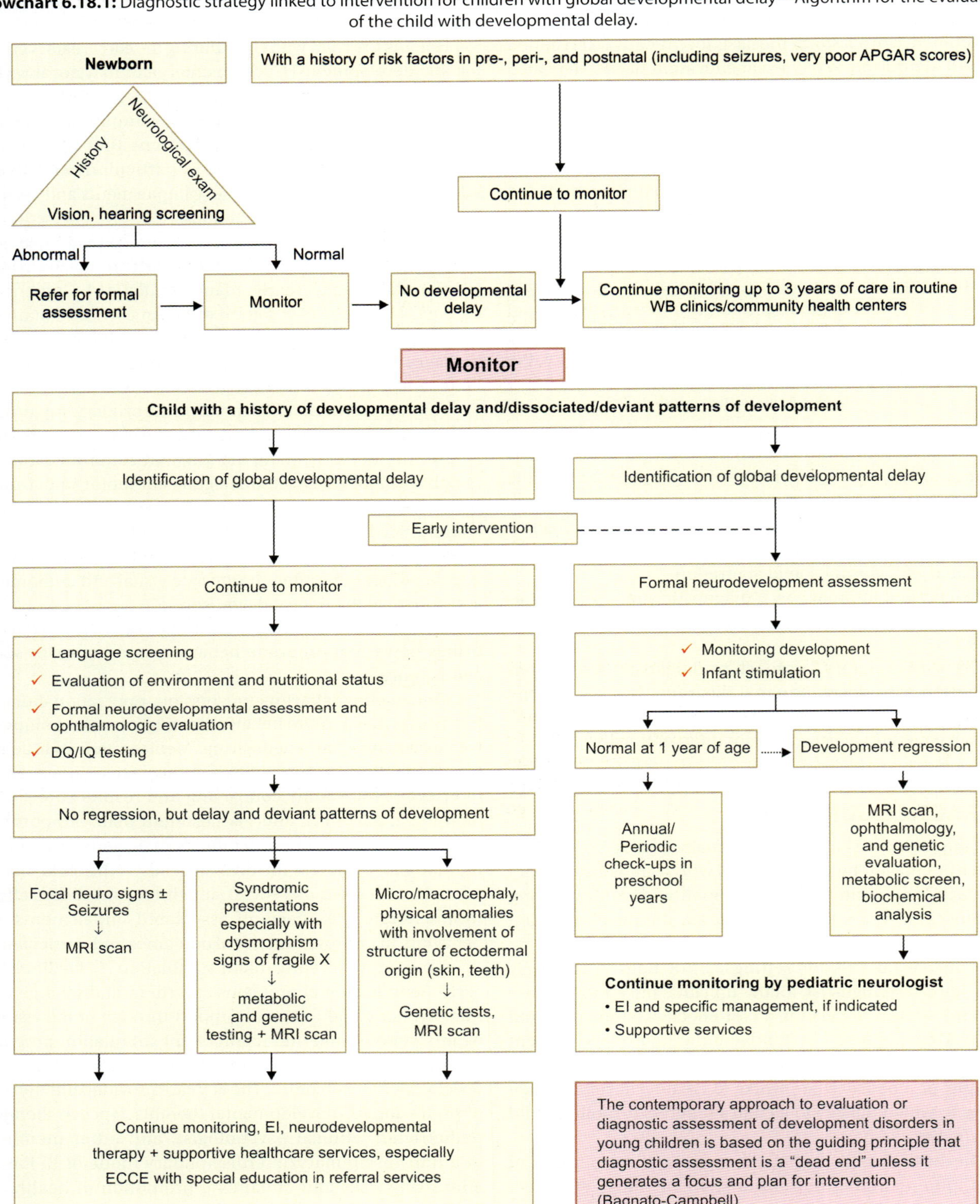

(DQ: developmental quotient; ECCE: early childhood care and education; EI: early intervention; IQ: intelligence quotient; MRI: magnetic resonance imaging)

Severe chronic multiple special needs due to associated systemic problems should consider the functional limitation, family needs, and resources in creating a framework for care based on the International Classification of Functioning, Disability and Health.

PROGNOSIS

Global developmental delay often evolves into a more specific developmental disorder, the most common being intellectual disability (MR).

The ultimate impact of GDD is shaped by the nature and extent of the impairments, the developmental patterns and cadence of change, services available for EI, family supports, and other environmental factors. Some infants with mild delay may do well in terms of functioning in later years due to neuroplasticity and effect of CNS maturation coupled with EI. However, the majority may be diagnosed in late childhood as having communication disorders, autism, specific syndromes, such as Rett syndrome. Those with limitations in ADLs and poor adaptive abilities may grow into adults requiring extensive supports. Appropriate management with a lifespan approach and social support is essential.

PREVENTION

In the field of developmental impairments, prevention includes prospective interventions to avert progression to disabilities.

Prevention at the primary level is possible by efforts to reduce the contributory illness and determinants of GDD and/or MR. Good prenatal services and obstetric care, good nutrition and administering measles-mumps-rubella vaccine to all girls, fortification of food with iodine, iron, folic acid, and general awareness campaigns for promoting health-seeking behaviors, as well as screening for early identification, can go a long way in decreasing the magnitude of GDD.

Primary prevention strategies remain the best for developing countries. Recent literature pointing to increased genetic associations in GDD makes a case for comanagement among families, the clinical unit, and clinical genetics specialty unit for both prevention and family centric services.

BIBLIOGRAPHY

1. American Academy of Pediatrics; Council on Children with Disabilities, Section on Developmental Behavioural Pediatrics, Bright Futures Steering Committee, Medical Home Initiatives for Children with Special needs, Project Advisory Committee. Identifying infants and young children with developmental disorders in the medical home: an algorithm for developmental surveillance and screening. Pediatrics. 2006;118:405-20.
2. American Psychiatric Association. Diagnostic and Statistical Manual of Mental Disorders, 5th edition. Arlington, VA: American Psychiatric Publishing; 2013.
3. Glader L, Plews-Ogan J, Agarwal R. Children with medical complexity: creating a framework for care based on the International Classification of Functioning, Disability and Health. Dev Med Child Neurol. 2016;58:1116-23.
4. Glascoe FP. Developmental screening and surveillance. In: Kliegman B, Jenson S (Eds). Nelson Textbook of Pediatrics, 18th edition. Philadelphia, PA: Elsevier; 2007. pp. 74-81.
5. McDonald L, Rennie A, Tolmie J, et al. Investigation of global developmental delay. Arch Dis Child. 2006;91:701-5.
6. Mithyantha R, Kneen R, McCann E, et al. Current evidence-based recommendations on investigating children with global developmental delay. Arch Dis Child. 2017;102:1071-6.
7. Shevell MI, Ashwal S, Donley D, et al. Practice parameter, evaluation of the child with global developmental delay: report of the quality standards subcommittee of the American Academy of Neurology and the Practice Committee of the Child Neurology Society. Neurology. 2003;60:367-80.
8. Shinawi M, Liu P, Kang SH, et al. Recurrent reciprocal 16p11.2 rearrangements associated with global developmental delay, behavioural problems, dysmorphism, epilepsy, and abnormal head size. J Med Genet. 2010;47(5):332-41.
9. Srour M, Mazer B, Shevell MI. Analysis of clinical features predicting etiologic yield in the assessment of global developmental delay. Pediatrics. 2006;118:139.
10. Tikaria A, Kabra M, Gupta N, et al. Aetiology of global developmental delay in young children: experience from a tertiary care centre in India. Nat Med J India. 2010;23:324-8.

6.19 Autism Spectrum Disorder

Jaya Shankar Kaushik

INTRODUCTION

Autism is a neurodevelopmental disorder characterized by impairment in social communication along with presence of restricted, repetitive pattern of behavior, interest, and activities. The current diagnostic criteria of autism spectrum disorder (ASD) based on Diagnostic and Statistical Manual of Mental Disorders (DSM)-5 clubs all pervasive developmental disorders (Asperger syndrome, Rett syndrome, and pervasive developmental disorder not otherwise specified) into a single umbrella diagnosis of "ASD."

BURDEN

Autism and developmental disability monitoring cohort (2010) estimated that 1 in every 68 children is identified with ASD. In an Indian study representing rural, urban, and tribal population, a prevalence rate of 0.15% was estimated. All the epidemiological studies show a significantly greater number of boys than girls with autism. Male-to-female ratios vary from 4:1 to 5:1. Few studies have demonstrated higher prevalence among those with higher socioeconomic status.

There has been a recent surge in number of cases diagnosed with ASD. This could be attributed to increasing awareness about the entity or probably secondary to broadened diagnostic criteria of ASD. Average age at diagnosis is around 3–4 years and children with better cognitive skills are often diagnosed only when social demands exceed their limited capacity. There is growing emphasis on early diagnosis and early intervention. Although children can be diagnosed as early as 18 months, reliability of diagnosis is often established by 3 years. Children with ASD were diagnosed earlier as intellectual disability (ID). Nearly 60–70% of children with ASD may have low intelligence quotient scores (<70). Children with ASD and ID are more likely to have seizures, microcephaly, and syndromic or metabolic etiology.

RISK FACTORS

There is no single factor that is believed to be causative for ASD. A combination of genetic, environmental, and epigenetic factors has been implicated. Sibling studies have shown that risk of developing autism is 10–18% if one child is affected and 25% if two siblings are affected with ASD. There are large numbers of metabolic, genetic, and monogenic disorders associated with ASD **(Box 6.19.1)**.

Few maternal risk factors implicated in ASD include maternal drug intake (thalidomide and sodium valproate), gestational diabetes mellitus, prenatal stress, oral contraceptive consumption, and advanced maternal and paternal age. Other perinatal complications including pre-eclampsia, intracranial hemorrhage, and perinatal asphyxia have also been linked to ASD. Few environmental chemicals such as mercury, cadmium, nickel, vinyl chloride, and other air pollutants have been postulated to increased risk for developing ASD. There is no causative link between measles mumps rubella vaccine with ASD.

PATHOGENESIS

Pathogenesis of ASD is challenging considering the genetic complexity and heterogeneity in evidence from

Box 6.19.1: Box outlining diseases associated with autism spectrum disorder.

Diseases associated with autism spectrum disorder

Metabolic disorders:
- Phenylketonuria
- Adenylosuccinate lyase deficiency (disorder of purine metabolism)
- Adenosine deaminase deficiency
- SSADH
- Disorder of creatine transport and metabolism (arginine: glycine amidinotransferase deficiency and guanidinoacetate methyltransferase deficiency)
- Cerebral folate deficiency
- Smith–Lemli–Opitz syndrome
- Mitochondrial disorders

Chromosomal disorders:
- Dup 7q11.23
- Dup or Del 16p 11.2
- Del 17q 12
- Del or Dup 15q13
- Del 22q 13

Monogenic disorders:
- Neurofibromatosis
- Tuberous sclerosis
- Fragile X syndrome

(SSADH: succinic semialdehyde dehydrogenase deficiency)

Flowchart 6.19.1: Approach to diagnosis and management of children with Autism spectrum disorder.

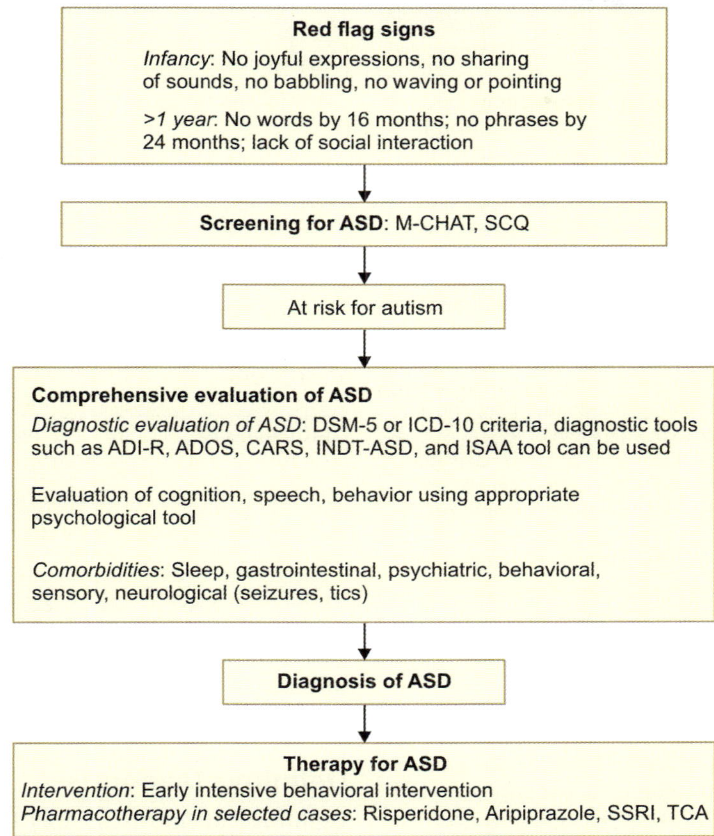

(ADI-R: Autism Diagnostic Interview Revised; ADOS: Autism Diagnostic Observation Schedule; ASD: autism spectrum disorder; CARS: childhood autism rating scale; DSM-5: Diagnostic and Statistical Manual for Mental Disorder; ICD: International Classification of Diseases; INDT-ASD: INCLEN Diagnostic Tool for Autism Spectrum Disorder; ISAA: Indian Scale for Assessment of Autism; M-CHAT: modified checklist for autism; SCQ: Social Communication Questionnaire; SSRI: selective serotonin reuptake inhibitor; TCA: tricyclic antidepressant)

neuropathology, neurotransmitter, and animal models. It is considered a "developmental disconnection syndrome" with impairment in long-range neural connections between normally cooperative brain in frontal and anterior temporal lobe region. Neuropathology studies in ASD have revealed cortical dysgenesis, migration defects, abnormal lamination, increased synaptic spine density, and increased cortical minicolumns. Functional magnetic resonance imaging has shown deranged connectivity along frontoparietal, frontotemporal, and frontostriatal circuits. At molecular level, mutations in genes for synaptic activity, synaptic adhesion, and scaffolding have been implicated in pathogenesis of ASD.

DIAGNOSIS

Approach to diagnosis and management has been summarized in **Flowchart 6.19.1**. Clinical diagnosis of ASD is often based on criteria described in the DSM. DSM-5 includes two domain levels:

1. Impairment in social interaction and social communication (three items).
2. Restrictive, repetitive patterns of behavior, activity, and interest (four items).

Diagnosis of ASD requires all three of three items in first domain and at least two of four items in second domain. In addition, these symptoms must be present in the early childhood. In many occasions when the symptoms are mild, they get manifest only when the child grows up and is not able to cope up to the expectations of his age or in other words, symptoms manifest when social demands exceed limited capacity. These symptoms must cause significant impairment in social, occupational functioning. DSM-5 criteria for diagnosis of ASD have been outlined in **Box 6.19.2**.

Box 6.19.2: Diagnostic and Statistical Manual for Mental Disorder-5: Diagnostic criteria for autism spectrum disorder.

- Persistent deficits in social communication and social interaction across multiple contexts as manifest by following:
  1. *Deficits in social-emotional reciprocity*: Ranging from abnormal social approach, failure to normal back to forth conversation, to reduced sharing of interests, emotions or affect, failure to initiate or respond to social interaction
     - Deficits in nonverbal communicative behavior used for social interaction ranging from poorly integrated verbal and nonverbal communication, abnormal eye contact and body language, deficits in understanding and use of gestures, to total lack of facial expression, and nonverbal communication.
     - *Deficits in developing and maintaining relationships:* Ranging from difficulties adjusting behavior to suit social contexts, difficulties in sharing imaginative play, and in making friends to absence of interest in others.
- Restricted, repetitive patterns of behavior, interests, or activities as manifested by at least two out of four following symptoms:
  1. Stereotyped or repetitive speech, motor movements, or use of objects or speech
  2. Insistence on sameness, inflexible adherence to routines, or ritualized patterns of verbal or nonverbal behavior
  3. Highly restricted, fixated interests that are abnormal in intensity or focus
  4. Hyper- or hyporeactivity to sensory input or unusual interest in sensory aspects of environment
- Symptoms must be present in early childhood (but may not manifest until social demands exceed limited capacities)
- The symptoms cause clinically significant impairment in social, occupational, or other important areas of functioning
- These disturbances are not better explained by GDD or intellectual disability

(GDD: global developmental delay)

Comorbid conditions include psychiatric conditions, behavioral disturbance, sensory disturbance, neurological disturbance, gastrointestinal, and sleep-related issues **(Table 6.19.1)**. Conditions that are commonly associated with ASD include attention-deficit hyperactivity disorders (ADHDs), anxiety, depression, and conduct disorder. *Diagnostic overshadowing* occurs when salient features of one disorder, for example ID, overshadow the consideration of another disorder say ASD. In such a case, when symptoms of ASD can be explained solely by ID, diagnosis of ASD alone is not made. DSM-5 allows comorbid diagnosis. Hence one can make a diagnosis of ASD-ID, ASD-ADHD, ASD-global developmental delay, and so on.

SCREENING

Screening tool (age of administration) for autism includes Modified Checklist for Autism in Toddlers, Revised with Follow-up (M-CHAT R/F) (16–30 months), Early Screening for Autistic Trait (14–15 months), Infant Toddler Checklist (6–24 months), Social Communication Questionnaire (SCQ) (more than 4 years), Social Responsiveness Scale (more than 2.5 years), and Gilliam Autism Rating Scale (GARS) (3–22 years). Most commonly used screening tool for ASD includes M-CHAT R/F for children below 3 years of age and SCQ in children above 3 years.

Table 6.19.1: Comorbid conditions of autism spectrum disorder.

Broad category	*Comorbid condition*
Psychiatric	• Anxiety (43–84%) • Depression (2–30%) • Obsessive-compulsive disorder (37%) • Oppositional defiant disorder (7%) • Behavioral problems
Behavioral	• Disruptive • Irritable • Aggressive behavior (8–32%) • Self-injurious behavior (34%)
Sensory disturbances	• Tactile (80–90%) • Auditory sensitivity (5–47%)
Neurological	• Seizures and epilepsy (5–49%) • Tics (8–10%)
Gastrointestinal	• GERD (8–59%) • Constipation (8–59%)
Sleep disturbances	Sleep disruptions (52–73%)

(GERD: gastroesophageal reflux disease)

Definitive Diagnosis

Definitive diagnosis of ASD is based on DSM-5 criteria or International Classification of Diseases-10 criteria. Differential diagnosis and comorbidities of ASD must be considered before reaching a final diagnosis. The diagnostic tools could be parental interview based or observation based. Interview-based diagnostic tools include Autism Diagnostic Interview-Revised, parent interview for autism, GARS, and Pervasive Developmental Disorder Screening Test. Observation-based diagnostic tools include Childhood Autism Rating Scale, Autism Diagnostic Observation Schedule, INCLEN Diagnostic Tool for ASD, and Indian Scale for Assessment of Autism.

Differential Diagnosis

The most common differential diagnosis of ASD includes ID, ADHD, and social communication disorder. Children with isolated impairment of social interaction and communication without restrictive repetitive behavior are often labeled under social communication disorder. Clinical features of ASD and ID tend to overlap, leading to ambiguity of comorbid diagnosis of ASD and ID versus ID alone explaining the autistic features. DSM-5 allows comorbid diagnosis of ID, ADHD, and other genetic diagnosis unlike DSM-IV. Hence, diagnosis of ASD with ID is possible under DSM-5.

TREATMENT

Behavioral Intervention

Early intensive behavioral intervention is based on early delivery (before 5 years) and intensively (25–40 hours a week). Objective is to train and teach children, how to learn and to equip them to be able to benefit from school-based services. Parent-mediated intervention include their training in structured behavioral method which can be applied at home, thus reducing the time at therapy centre, making the intervention more enjoyable and natural.

Pharmacological Treatment

Existing drugs are not effective for core symptoms of ASD. These drugs often act on comorbid symptoms: methylphenidate is useful for hyperactivity, risperidone for aggressive and irritable behavior, aripiprazole for abnormal motor stereotypies, and aggressive behavior. Other medications targeting irritable, aggressive, and impulsive behaviors include selective serotonin reuptake inhibitor, tricyclic antidepressant, gabapentin, clonidine, guanfacine, memantine (*N*-methyl-D-aspartate receptor antagonist). Melatonin can be useful for sleep disturbances.

Support to Family

Autism is a lifelong condition with a wide range of fluctuation in the clinical course. Access to appropriate medical services, educational materials, and social support is required for families. There is a delay between symptom recognition by parents and final diagnosis of autism. There is emerging need for infrastructure, trained therapist, and medical insurance to care for children with ASD in India. Prohibitive cost of intensive behavioral intervention in private sector is a major limiting factor in care of Indian children with ASD.

NATIONAL EFFORTS

Right for Person with Disability Act Bill was notified by Government of India in its official gazette in 2016, which covers ASD as 1 of 21 disabilities. National trust for welfare of persons with autism, cerebral palsy, mental retardation, and multiple disabilities is a statutory body of Ministry of Social Justice and Empowerment has been set up to enable and empower persons with disability including ASD. There are large numbers of government schemes for benefit of children with ASD in India along with legal provisions and educational services available. There is a website of National Trust which can be accessed for details of available government schemes [URL: http://thenationaltrust.gov.in/content/innerpage/schemes.php].

BIBLIOGRAPHY

1. American Psychiatric Association. Autism spectrum disorder. In: Diagnostic and Statistical Manual of Mental Disorders DSM-5, 5th edition (revised). Washington, DC: American Psychiatric Association Publishing; 2013. pp. 50-9.
2. Barua M, Kaushik JS, Gulati S. Legal provisions, educational services and health care across the lifespan for autism spectrum disorders in India. Indian J Pediatr. 2017;84:76-82.
3. Chen JA, Peñagarikano O, Belgard TG, et al. The emerging picture of autism spectrum disorder: genetics and pathology. Annu Rev Pathol. 2015;10:111-44.
4. Filipek PA, Accardo PJ, Ashwal S, et al. Practice parameter: screening and diagnosis of autism: report of the Quality Standards Subcommittee of the American Academy of Neurology and the Child Neurology Society. Neurology. 2000;55:468-79.
5. Levy SE, Mandell DS, Schultz RT. Autism. Lancet. 2009;374:1627-38.
6. Mukherjee SB. Autism spectrum disorders—diagnosis and management. Indian J Pediatr. 2017;84:307-14.
7. Nickel RE, Huang-Storms L. Early identification of young children with autism spectrum disorder. Indian J Pediatr. 2017;84:53-60.
8. Toriello HV. Approach to the genetic evaluation of the child with autism. Pediatr Clin North Am. 2012;59:113-28.
9. Warren Z, McPheeters ML, Sathe N, et al. A systematic review of early intensive intervention for autism spectrum disorders. Pediatrics. 2011;127:1303-11.

Section 7

Diseases of Cardiovascular System

7.1 Clinical Approach to Pediatric Cardiology

S Srinivasan

INTRODUCTION

The objectives of clinical examination of the cardiovascular system in newborns, young infants, and older children are as follows:

- To ascertain without delay the presence of any life-threatening critical congenital heart disease (CHD) in neonates or other CHD associated life-threatening complications, such as cardiogenic shock, pulmonary edema, tachyarrhythmias or bradyarrhythmias, endocarditis, cardiac tamponade.
- To institute appropriate, immediate, and urgent resuscitative measures before resorting to detailed history taking and physical examination.
- To carry out proper history taking and clinical examination to ascertain the presence of a cardiovascular problem and identify the nature of underlying cardiac conditions in terms of structural involvement.
- To ascertain its etiology congenital/acquired, genetic (chromosomal/dysmorphogenetic).
- To assess the severity of the condition and the functional restriction.
- To identify the presence or absence of other related and associated complications and its impact on child's nutritional, growth and developmental status of the child.

HISTORY TAKING

The mother must be allowed to give her own account of the presenting symptoms, which necessitated her to bring the child to medical attention and narrate the evolution of these symptoms from the time of their onset. Only open-ended questions must be used. The historical points of interest, of course, will vary considerably, depending upon the age of the patient, the presenting signs, symptoms, and complaints. If the child is brought in a state of breathlessness, cyanosis, or shock, precious time must not be wasted in taking elaborate history. Neonates with marked shortness of breath, cyanosis, and pallor with lethargy need immediate attention with regard to adequacy of breathing, circulation (perfusion) and airway patency, quick clinical and investigative assessment (pulse oximetry and echocardiography) to rule out life-threatening, acute cardiac emergency states, e.g. ductus-dependent congenital cardiac lesions that restrict pulmonary or systemic blood flow. Other relevant and important details in history taking that have bearing on the diagnosis of the cardiac condition, its severity, and in planning treatment and counseling have been summarized in **Table 7.1.1**.

Moreover, while taking the history, one should take note of the evolution of symptoms according to chronology

Table 7.1.1: Important documentation of history relating to causative or precipitating factors.

History of abnormal facial features or minor or major congenital malformations	Many chromosomal disorders, such as Down syndrome; Turner syndrome; other trisomies; and other genetic, metabolic, and isolated malformations, may indicate the presence of associated congenital heart diseases (CHD)
Past history	Any physical symptoms, health problems, hospital visits or admissions in the past for recurrent chest infections, bacterial endocarditis, symptoms suggestive of rheumatic fever, such as arthritis, abnormal movements, tuberculosis, and delayed motor development, rashes, skin peeling in palms, soles, tips of fingers and toes, sore throat preceding onset of joint pains
Prenatal history	• History of acute or chronic infections in various trimesters—fever, rashes • Other maternal illness—metabolic disorders, such as gestational diabetes, autoimmune disorders, such as SLE • Drugs—phenytoin, lithium, other anticonvulsants • Substance abuse; alcohol, addictive drugs, etc. • Exposure to irradiation, pollutants, others

Contd...

Contd...

Birth history, immediate postnatal and neonatal history*	Delayed crying and breath initiation, bluishness, sucking and feeding difficulty, lethargy, importance of finding out the gestational age, birth weight, need for resuscitation, need for breathing and oxygen support, prolonged stay in neonatal unit, need for tube feeding or intravenous fluids, type of medications given during neonatal stay in the hospital and subsequent to discharge
Nutritional history	Children with cardiac conditions with frequent heart failure or recurrent infections will have loss of appetite, and their nutritional intake will be greatly compromised
History of growth and developmental impairment	• Growth impairment and failure to thrive in the first few years of life is commonly noted in moderate-to-severe cardiac structural lesions. Tall stature or short stature, delayed gross motor milestones have a bearing on underlying cardiac disease • In a child with tall stature, the possibility of Marfan syndrome must be considered. In a female child with short stature, Turner syndrome and associated coarctation of aorta must be ruled out • Moderate-to-severe CHD will be associated with delay in gross motor milestones in relation to other areas of development. Chromosomal and dysmorphogenetic syndromes with associated heart diseases may exhibit global developmental delay
Family history	• Record any of the following present in the family members: sudden death, SIDS, rheumatic fever, structural or congenital cardiac abnormalities in siblings, genetic or dysmorphogenic syndromes in the family • The estimated recurrence risk of CHD is 2–6% when a previous sibling is affected, nearly 30% with two siblings affected and 3%, if one of the parents is affected
History of functional limitations	School attendance and absenteeism, academic performance, inability to participate in games and sports activities
Treatment history	Past and present treatment (medical and surgical) details
Personal/socioeconomic history	In a developing country with the majority of the population being below the poverty line, long-term treatment facilities including surgical corrections at appropriate age may not be possible. Hence, children and adults at all ages may have CHD with or without advanced complications, such as PAH

(PAH: pulmonary arterial hypertension; PDA: patent ductus arteriosus; SIDS: sudden infant death syndrome; SLE: systemic lupus erythematosus)
*Preterms have higher incidence of PDA. These preterms also go into heart failure early in their first week with even moderate-sized defects with left to right shunts.

and mode of presentation, duration, progression, severity, relieving factors, aggravating factors, associated symptoms, and functional impairment.

Cardiac Symptoms

Symptoms of CHD can be very varied and subtle at times and may manifest anytime from fetal period to adulthood **(Box 7.1.1)**. Many of these symptoms may not be the presenting problem, and therefore, it has to be elicited by asking pertinent questions.

GENERAL PHYSICAL EXAMINATION

Examination of an infant and young child needs a lot of tact, and the general principles of examining a child should be applied. Although it is a usual routine to follow a definitive order in clinical examination, in a young child, such an orderly examination may not be always possible because of their apprehensive and anxious nature. In a sleeping child, it is better to perform auscultation of the precordium for the nature of cardiac sounds and presence of murmurs and other sounds. Infants and young children must be comfortably seated in

Box 7.1.1: Presentation of cardiac problems.

Fetus (diagnosed by fetal echocardiography):
Hydrops, arrhythmias, cardiomegaly

Neonate and infant:
- Heart failure (tachypnea with feeding or activities, labored breathing/dyspnea, feeding difficulties, sweating on head), failure to thrive
- Cyanosis, circulatory failure, collapse, abnormal heart rate/rhythm, murmur, weak femoral pulses
- Noticeable excessive precordial activity or pulsations observed by mother, sleep disturbances, recurrent lower respiratory infections
- Dysmorphism, noncardiac congenital abnormalities

Older child:
- Heart failure (exercise intolerance, shortness of breath with activities), palpitation
- Increased precordial pulsations or prominence, dizzy or fainting spells, syncope
- Chest pain on activity, recurrent lower respiratory infections, failure to thrive, murmur
- Hypertension, as a part of multisystem disease (rheumatic fever, Kawasaki disease), seizures (presenting as a complication of cyanotic heart disease), cyanotic spells, squatting

the mother's lap with their dresses removed earlier before sitting in front of the examiner. The standard format of general physical examination has been summarized in **Table 7.1.2**.

Table 7.1.2: Proforma for general examination in a cardiac patient.

General appearance	Comfortable, consolable, state of distress
Posture/decubitus	
General health	
Body build and proportion	
Nutritional and growth status	Anthropometry
Features of chromosomal/ genetic/dysmorphogenic syndromes	Down syndrome, Turner syndrome, other trisomies, William's syndrome, Noonan syndrome, etc.
External isolated/multiple congenital external malformations	Short neck, webbing, polydactyly, syndactyly, camptomelia
Oral cavity, teeth, and pharynx	Sore throat, caries
Skin	Rashes, erythema marginatum, nodules, desquamation
Joints	Rheumatic fever, rheumatoid arthritis
Abnormal movements	Chorea
Dependent edema	Sites—feet, legs, back, eyelids
Lymph nodes	Kawasaki disease, tuberculosis
Clubbing of fingers and toes	Cyanotic heart defects, bacterial endocarditis
Central cyanosis, differential cyanosis	

It is important to remember that vital signs should be examined first before undertaking detailed cardiac examination. The pertinent points to note are airway, breathing (rate, type, and sign of distress), circulation (capillary filling time, details of pulse, and blood pressure), and temperature.

CARDIAC EXAMINATION

Precordium

The objectives of inspection of the chest is to identify chest wall asymmetry if present, in the form of precordial prominence, pectus excavatum, carinatum, kyphosis, scoliosis, and Harrison's sulcus; abnormal pulsations in the neck, suprasternal notch, parasternal region, epigastric region, and over the back; the location of apical impulse—left side or right side; and scars of previous operative procedures.

Jugular Venous Pulse and Pressure

The jugular venous pulse waveform consists of three positive upstrokes—a, c, and v—and two negative waves—*x* descent after a and c waves, and *y* descent after v wave. The abnormalities of various waveforms have been summarized in **Table 7.1.3**.

Arterial Pulse

Pulse is the peripherally transmitted waveform of propagated arterial blood from the aortic root along the arterial tree generated by systolic contraction of the left ventricle. The travel speed of the arterial pulse wave is 10 times faster than that of the blood column. The importance of palpating the arterial pulse at various sites, e.g. both radials, femoral,

Table 7.1.3: Abnormal jugular venous pulse and its clinical interpretation.

"A" wave abnormalities		
Large "a" waves	Forcible contraction of right atrium against obstruction at AV valve area	Tricuspid stenosis, RA myxoma
	Increased resistance offered by noncompliant right ventricle	Severe PAH, PS (moderate-to-severe), RV cardiomyopathy, acute pulmonary embolism
Cannon or very large giant "a" waves	Contraction of right atrium against a closed tricuspid valve	Tricuspid atresia, AV dissociation, complete heart block
	Regular cannon waves	Junctional rhythm, isorhythmic AV dissociation
	Irregular cannon waves	Complete heart block, classic AV dissociation, ventricular pacing, ventricular ectopics
Absent "a" waves	Ineffective atrial contraction	Atrial fibrillation, marked sinus tachycardia
"V" wave abnormalities		
Large "v" waves	Rapid and excessive RA filling	TR, TAPVD, ASD with MR

(ASD: atrial septal defect; AV: atrioventricular; MR: mitral regurgitation; PAH: pulmonary arterial hypertension; PS: pulmonary stenosis; RA: right atrial; RV: right ventricular; TAPVD: total anomalous pulmonary venous drainage; TR: tricuspid regurgitation)

brachialis, popliteal, posterior tibials, dorsalis pedis, carotids, and superficial temporal arteries, should be kept in mind at the beginning of each clinical posting and perhaps throughout life so as to ensure that one does not miss coarctation of aorta, and thromboembolic phenomena need to be repeatedly emphasized to the students at every posting of theirs. The various types of abnormal pulses have been depicted in **Table 7.1.4**.

Precordial Palpation

The learning objectives of palpation of the precordium are (1) to identify the site and type of apical impulse whether

Table 7.1.4: Abnormal pulses.

Pulsus parvus	Low-volume pulse with slow rise; its presence suggests the possibility of severe AS or severe low-output states, such as severe heart failure
Pulsus tardus	Slow-rising pulse with a late peaking closer to the second sound and is reported in fixed LV obstructive lesions
Hypokinetic pulse	Weakly felt, small-volume pulse felt with difficulty in the cases of low-cardiac-output states, such as shock, severe heart failure, myocarditis, cardiac tamponade, constrictive pericarditis, severe left heart obstructive lesions, such as MS and AS, and aortic outflow obstructions, such as aortic arch syndromes and coarctation of aorta
Hyperkinetic (bounding) pulse	High amplitude, large-volume pulse with rapidly rising ascending wave felt in augmented high-cardiac-output states with decreased peripheral arterial resistance and wide pulse pressure, e.g. anxiety, exercise, fever, anemia, thyrotoxicosis, arteriovenous fistulas, beriberi, moderate MR, moderate-sized ventricular septal defects, AR, PDA
Water hammer/ collapsing pulse	The pulse is elicited by suddenly and gently elevating the child's arm above his/her shoulder, while the radial pulse is continuously felt by the palmar surface of the examiner's hand instead of the usual three fingertips. It is a large-volume pulse with sudden and rapid upstroke with equally rapid downstroke. The term "water hammer" refers to a famous Victorian era English toy. Collapsing pulse indicates rapid and reverse diastolic run off into the left ventricle in AR and rapid run off to the peripheral vessels due to decreased systemic peripheral vascular resistance. AR, PDA, AP window, and RSOV into the right ventricle and arteriovenous fistulas. Collapsing pulse in a cyanotic child suggests truncus arteriosus with truncal regurgitation, pulmonary atresia with AP collaterals, TOF with AP collaterals or PDA. Collapsing pulse is also felt in hyperkinetic states, such as anemia, fever, thyrotoxicosis, pregnancy, and beriberi
Bisferiens pulse	Pulse with two beats in a single systolic wave upstroke; when the examiner's palpating finger feels two positive upward peaks during systole, it is termed pulsus bisferiens, better appreciated over the carotids than radials. They indicate the presence of severe AR or AR with AS or HOCM
Corrigan's pulse	Prominently visible dancing pulsation over the carotids in AR
Brisk/jerky pulse	Pulse with a sharp, tapping upstroke with normal volume, and downstroke is characteristic of HCM
Anacrotic pulse	It is felt in severe AS, is a small-volume (low amplitude), slow-rising (ana = up, and crotos = beat) upstroke wave with late peaking. The anacrotic notch occurs during the early half of the ascent; earlier it is felt, severe is the AS. In severe MS, the notch is felt in the latter half of the ascending limb
Dicrotic pulse	It refers to pulse waveforms with two peaks in each wave, one in systolic ascending limb and the second prominent one in the descending limb of the wave during diastole. This is seen in cardiac conditions with low stroke volume and decreased peripheral arterial resistance—typhoid fever, LV failure, dilated cardiomyopathies, and cardiac tamponade
Pulsus paradoxus	It occurs when there is an exaggerated decrease in pulse volume and blood pressure more than 10 mm Hg recorded during inspiration. In normal individuals, there is usually a normal physiological drop of systolic blood pressure during inspiratory phase ranging from 5 mm Hg to a maximum of 10 mm Hg, which may be appreciated by experienced clinicians on feeling the arterial pulse in the absence of tachycardia. Hence, the term paradox used as adjective is not true. It is seen in cardiac tamponade, pericardial effusion, constrictive pericarditis, acute severe asthma, and in conditions that obstruct superior vena cava return to right atrium as noted in anterior and superior mediastinal tumors
Pulsus alternans	It refers to occurrence of alternating pulse of high and low amplitudes or volumes in the presence of normal rhythm and is indicative of moderate-to-severe LV failure
Pulsus bigeminy, pulsus trigeminy	It refers to coupling of two or three beats, followed by a pause with a stronger beat after the pause. It occurs in AV block and sinoatrial block with ventricular escape

(AP: aortopulmonary; AR: aortic regurgitation; AS: aortic stenosis; AV: atrioventricular; HCM: hypertrophic cardiomyopathy; HOCM: hypertrophic obstructive cardiomyopathy; LV: left ventricular; MR: mitral regurgitation; MS: mitral stenosis; PDA: patent ductus arteriosus; RSOV: ruptured sinus of Valsalva; TOF: tetralogy of Fallot) normal or abnormal; (2) to identify the presence of abnormal pulsations, heaves, and thrills in specified precordial sites—left parasternal and epigastric regions, suprasternal notch, second left intercostal space (LICS); and (3) to ascertain enlargement of right ventricle, left ventricle or both, or dilatation of great arteries—aorta and pulmonary arteries.

Apical Impulse

Apical impulse refers to the outermost and lowermost definitive palpable outward thrust of cardiac impulse in the lower precordium imparted by the anterior movement of left ventricular (LV) apex during early systolic contraction of the left ventricle. Its location, amplitude, duration, size, character, or contour must be recorded.

In the first, 3–4 years of life after birth, the normal location of the apical impulse is in the fourth LICS 1–2 cm lateral to the midclavicular line (MCL). Between 4 years and 8 years, the location is in the fifth LICS on the MCL. Beyond 8 years, it lies in the fifth LICS 1–2 cm or half an inch medial to the MCL. The apex beat is shifted to the left in cardiomegaly, scoliosis, pectus excavatum, and right-sided pneumothorax or effusion. It is shifted to the right side in the cases of congenital dextrocardia, acquired dextroposition (heart pushed or pulled to the right side as in left-sided pleural effusion or pneumothorax), and diaphragmatic hernia. **Table 7.1.5** summarizes different types of apical impulse.

Other Palpable Sounds and Pulsations

The second heart sound (S2) may be palpable in pulmonary hypertension. The third heart sound (S3) may be rarely palpable in severe mitral regurgitation (MR) or dilated cardiomyopathy. The fourth heart sound (S4) is more often palpable in adults than in children in the following conditions: hypertrophic cardiomyopathy, severe aortic stenosis (AS), acute MR, and long-standing hypertension. Suprasternal pulsations are seen and palpable in patent ductus arteriosus, AS, aortic regurgitation, coarctation of aorta, and aortic aneurysm. Pulsations in the parasternal area without a perceptible or palpable left parasternal lift is characteristic of right ventricular (RV) volume-overload conditions, such as atrial septal defect, tricuspid regurgitation, moderate-to-large ventricular septal defect without pulmonary arterial hypertension in addition to hyperdynamic high-output states. Epigastric pulsations are seen and the impulse is felt in RV volume-overload states. Apart from these sounds, murmurs are also palpable in various areas.

Parasternal Heave

Parasternal heave is both seen and felt by the ulnar border of the examiner's hand over the left parasternal region of the precordium overlying the heart. It indicates RV enlargement.

Heart Sounds

The first heart sound (S1) is produced by the closure of mitral and tricuspid valves marking the beginning of systole. It is best heard over the apex and in mitral area. The S2 is produced by the closure of semilunar valves of aorta and pulmonary arteries. The normal variable split of S2 is because the pulmonary component (P2) is normally heard 30 ms after the aortic component(A2) during inspiration (increased RV ejection time and pulmonary artery hangout interval) and within 20 ms during expiration. The S3 is low

Table 7.1.5: Characteristics of apical impulse.

Tapping apical impulse	Palpable S1 noted in MS; it represents a hypokinetic, underfilled left ventricle. Tapping apical impulse is also felt in ASD
Hyperdynamic apex	Suggests LV dilatation seen in high-cardiac-output states, and ventricular volume overloads seen in MR and AR, VSD, or PDA. In hyperdynamic apex, the apical impulse, in addition to being shifted outward and downward, has increased amplitude with brisk upstroke, is felt in more than one ICS, usually over two or three ICSs exceeding 3 cm. It is ill sustained with the duration of impact between the one third and half of systole
Heaving apex	It is said to be present when the systolic thrust is sustained and increased in duration almost like a wave felt for more than the two thirds of systole with increased amplitude and is confined to one ICS. It is indicative of pressure overload and LVH seen in AS, systemic arterial hypertension, or coarctation of aorta
Retractile apical impulse	Indicative of constrictive pericarditis where there is systolic retraction away from the chest wall, and forward or positive diastolic thrust
Double apical impulse	It suggests AS with AR, HOCM, LBBB, and in adults, LV aneurysm. Triple or quadruple impulse may be felt in HOCM
Absence of apical impulse	Dextrocardia, pericardial effusion, obesity, apex under the rib, emphysema, or large pleural effusion on the left side

(AR: aortic regurgitation; AS: aortic stenosis; ASD: atrial septal defect; HOCM: hypertrophic obstructive cardiomyopathy; ICS: intercostal space; LBBB: left bundle branch block; LV: left ventricular; LVH: left ventricular hypertrophy; MR: mitral regurgitation; MS: mitral stenosis; PDA: patent ductus arteriosus; S1: first heart sound; VSD: ventricular septal defect) pitched, may be normally heard in early diastole, and is caused by rapid ventricular filling. It may also be heard in athletes and pregnant women. If S3 occurs in a child with cardiac symptoms, one should suspect diastolic overload conditions or LV dysfunction (dilated left ventricle, decreased ejection fraction, constrictive pericarditis) or LV failure. The S3 gallop refers to an exaggerated sound with a cadence heard when significant tachycardia occurs with the above conditions. The S4 is often an abnormal sound, and it is low pitched, late diastolic sound produced by forceful atrial contraction against certain degree of resistance and decreased ventricular compliance during late ventricular filling. The characteristics of various heart sounds have been summarized in **Table 7.1.6**.

Table 7.1.6: Characteristics of different heart sounds.

Intensity of S1	***Cardiac conditions***
Loud	Exercise, sinus tachycardia, short PR interval states, such as WPW syndrome, MS, tricuspid stenosis, atrial myxoma
Soft	Long PR interval, pericardial effusion, MR, TR, calcific MS, myocarditis and cardiomyopathy, proximal LBBB
Split S1	Ebstein anomaly, RBBB, large ASD
Intensity of S2	
Loud S2	*Soft S2*
Increased A2: Systemic hypertension, aortic root dilatation, L-TGA, TOF	*Decreased A2*: Severe AS, AR, calcific aortic valve
Increased P2: Pulmonary hypertension, ASD	*Decreased P2*: PS, TOF, TGA
Splitting of S2	*Cardiac conditions*
Wide (both A2 and P2 audible in inspiration and expiration)	*Due to early A2 closure*: VSD, MR
	Due to late P2 closure: PAH, PS, RBBB, pulmonary embolism, LV ectopic beat
	Increased hangout interval due to decreased impedance to pulmonary artery: ASD, PS, TAPVC, Ebstein, idiopathic dilatation of pulmonary artery
Wide and fixed split	ASD, severe RV failure
Paradoxical or reverse split	Delayed A2
P2, then A2 (split audible in expiration but not in inspiration)	*Mechanical*: AS, hypertension, CAD *Electrical*: Proximal LBBB; RV ectopics
	Decreased impedance to aorta: PDA, poststenotic dilatation in AS
Single S2	*Absent A2*: HLHS, aortic atresia
	Absent P2: Pulmonary atresia, truncus arteriosus, absent pulmonary valve
	Very soft/masked P2: TOF, TGA, severe PS
	Synchronous A2 and P2: Severe PAH, PPH, Eisenmenger VSD
Intensity of S3	
LV overload states	MR, VSD, PDA
RV overload states	TR, ASD
LA S4 gallop	Aortic valvular stenosis, systemic arterial hypertension
Right atrial S4 gallop	PAH, PS, Ebstein anomaly, ASD, prolonged PR interval

(A2: aortic component of S2; AR: aortic regurgitation; AS: aortic stenosis; ASD: atrial septal defect; CAD: coronary artery disease; HLHS: hypoplastic left heart syndrome; LA: left atrial; LBBB: left bundle branch block; LV: left ventricular; L-TGA: levo-transposition of great arteries; MR: mitral regurgitation; MS: mitral stenosis; P2: pulmonary component of S2; PAH: pulmonary arterial hypertension; PDA: patent ductus arteriosus; PPH: primary pulmonary hypertension; PR: pulmonary regurgitation; PS: pulmonary stenosis; RBBB: right bundle branch block; RV: right ventricular; S1: first heart sound; S2: second heart sound; S3: third heart sound; S4: fourth heart sound; TAPVC: total anomalous pulmonary venous connection; TGA: transposition of great arteries; TR: tricuspid regurgitation; TOF: tetralogy of Fallot; VSD: ventricular septal defect; WPW: Wolff–Parkinson–White)

Other Abnormal Sounds

Clicks, opening snap, and pericardial friction rub are the other added sounds one should try to detect during auscultation.

Heart Murmurs

Heart murmurs are audible sound waves in the range of 20–2,000 Hz that occur as a result of turbulent blood flow due to functional or structural hemodynamic alterations in the pattern of blood flow in the heart chambers across the valves or the atrial or ventricular septum or in the vessels as in coarctation of aorta, renal artery stenosis or pulmonary arteriovenous collaterals or malformations.

When the presence of murmur over the precordium is appreciated by the student, it becomes essential to make a clinical decision whether the murmur is functional/innocent or organic/pathological due to an underlying cardiac disorder. When one or more of the following are present, the murmur is likely to be pathologic and requires further evaluation: symptoms, cyanosis, systolic murmur that is loud (grade 3/6, harsh, and long in duration), diastolic murmur, abnormal heart sounds, presence of a click, and abnormally strong or weak pulses. The characteristics of organic heart murmurs have been summarized in **Table 7.1.7**.

Innocent Murmurs

A murmur heard in a child without structural heart disease is termed innocent murmur. The child has no cardiac-related symptoms or other signs on careful history and physical examination, and basic investigations, such as chest X-ray, electrocardiogram, and echocardiogram, are normal. A significantly large proportion of children have innocent murmurs beginning at 3–4 years of age.

The characteristics of innocent or functional murmurs are usually the following: they are localized to specific areas, short, often early or midsystolic, grade 1/6 or 2/6 (not

Table 7.1.7: Characteristics of organic heart murmurs.

<table>
<tr><th colspan="4">Organic systolic murmurs</th></tr>
<tr><td>Pansystolic</td><td>Ejection</td><td colspan="2">Mid/late systolic</td></tr>
<tr><td>MR
TR
VSD</td><td>AS
PS
ASD
VSD</td><td colspan="2">MVP</td></tr>
<tr><th colspan="4">Organic diastolic murmurs</th></tr>
<tr><td>Early diastolic</td><td>Mid-diastolic</td><td colspan="2">Presystolic</td></tr>
<tr><td rowspan="2">AR
PR</td><td>• MS
• TS
• Carey Coomb's murmur of mitral valvulitis
• Austin flint murmur in AR</td><td colspan="2">Severe MS</td></tr>
<tr><td>Secondary flow murmurs (ASD, VSD, PDA, MR, TR)</td><td colspan="2"></td></tr>
<tr><th colspan="4">Organic continuous murmurs</th></tr>
<tr><td colspan="2">Acyanotic
• PDA
• Aortopulmonary window, rupture of sinus of Valsalva into right ventricle or pulmonary artery
• Coronary arteriovenous fistulas
• Systemic arteriovenous fistulas
• Peripheral pulmonary artery branch stenosis
• ALCAPA
Cyanotic
• Pulmonary arteriovenous fistulas
• Truncus arteriosus
Blalock-Taussig shunt</td><td>Secondary collaterals in
• TOF
• Aortic coarctation
• Aberrant LCA with RCA collaterals</td><td>Combination of defects
• VSD + AR
• AR + AS
• MR + AR/TR + MR + AR</td></tr>
</table>

(ALCAPA: anomalous left coronary artery from the pulmonary artery; AR: aortic regurgitation; AS: aortic stenosis; ASD: atrial septal defect; LCA: left coronary artery; MR: mitral regurgitation; MS: mitral stenosis; MVP: mitral valve prolapse; PDA: patent ductus arteriosus; PR: pulmonary regurgitation; PS: pulmonary stenosis; RCA: right coronary artery; TOF: tetralogy of Fallot; TR: tricuspid regurgitation; TS: tricuspid stenosis; VSD: ventricular septal defect) associated with thrill), and vary in intensity with change in posture; decreasing in intensity when the child stands, sits up, or strains during a Valsalva maneuver.

BIBLIOGRAPHY

1. Allen HD, Philips JR, Chan DP. History and physical examination. In: Moss AJ, Allen HD (Eds). Moss and Adams' Heart Disease in Infants, Children and Adolescents, 7th edition. Philadelphia, PA: Lippincott; 2008. pp. 66-80.
2. Fyler DC, Nadas AS. History, physical examination, and laboratory test. In: Keane J, Fyler DC, Lock J (Eds). Nadas' Pediatric Cardiology. Philadelphia, PA: Saunders; 2006. pp. 101-6.
3. Geggel RL, Fyler DC. History, growth, nutrition, physical examination, and routine laboratory tests. Nadas' Pediatric Cardiology, 2nd edition. Philadelphia, PA: WB Saunders; 2008.
4. Park MK. Basic tools in routine evaluation of cardiac patients. In: Park MK (Ed). Pediatric Cardiology for Practitioners, 5th edition. Philadelphia, PA: Mosby Elsevier; 2008. pp. 3-39.
5. Roy DL. Cardiovascular assessment of infants and children. In. Goldbloom RB (Ed). Pediatric Clinical Skills, 3rd edition. Philadelphia, PA: Saunders; 2003. pp. 169-89.
6. Tandon R. Bedside diagnosis of congenital heart disease. In: Bahl VK (Ed). Cardiology Update 2008. New Delhi: Cardiological Society of India; 2008. pp. 484-90.
7. Thompson WR, Mehrotra SM. Approach to heart diseases in children: cardiac history and physical examination. In: Raid A (Ed). Heart Diseases in Children: a Pediatrician's Guide. New York, NY: Springer; 2011. pp. 3-16.

7.2 Congenital Heart Disease

R Krishna Kumar

INTRODUCTION

Congenital heart disease (CHD) encompasses a broad and extremely diverse range of conditions that can manifest anytime from fetal life to late adulthood. In common parlance, CHD refers to structural heart defects that are present at birth. Conditions, such as hypertrophic cardiomyopathy and mitral valve prolapse, may have a congenital basis, but these are often discussed separately. Similarly, electrical and conduction disorders, such as prolonged "QT" syndrome, Brugada syndrome, arrhythmogenic right ventricular dysplasia, and congenital complete heart block, are not usually categorized as CHD even though in the strictest terms they should perhaps be. In this chapter, we will be discussing common structural defects that are present at birth.

The bewildering array of CHD is intimidating to the uninitiated pediatrician. Many defects are quite complex, and a very large number of combinations often defy predictable patterns. The most significant challenge that a student faces is striking the right balance between acquiring an in-depth understanding of individual conditions and acquiring a broad overall understanding of most "commonly encountered" CHDs.

A practical approach lies in remembering the following:

- The most important role of the pediatrician today is to ensure that, as far as possible, serious CHD should not be missed; this is especially true for the neonatal period and during infancy where maximal attrition from CHD occurs.
- History, physical examination, chest X-ray, and electrocardiogram (ECG) are the traditional tools available to the pediatrician. With this, it is usually possible to identify whether CHD is present except perhaps in the early newborn period where CHD diagnosis can be challenging.
- Despite numerous anatomic possibilities, the physiologic categories of CHD are limited and can be understood. Understanding the basic hemodynamic and physiologic concepts are important because they have an important bearing on clinical picture, interpretation of echocardiographic reports, natural history and decision-making on the timing of surgical or catheter intervention.
- The traditional diagnostic tools allow classification of physiologic categories in a significant proportion of babies. The limitations of the traditional tools in identifying the precise anatomy are substantial, and this is exposed by the widespread use of echocardiography.
- Numerous recent advances have dramatically changed the outlook of children with CHD. As a result, some form of palliation or correction is feasible for most CHD provided this is undertaken in a timely fashion.
- The improved understanding of CHD today suggests that management needs to be individualized or

tailored to each patient. Today, it is possible to identify and determine the severity of all the specific lesions through echocardiography. Recognizing the numerous combinations and specific features with each lesion, each patient needs to be approached according to the specifics of the lesion(s).

- It is increasingly evident that a substantial proportion of children with CHD have significant problems in other organ systems. A growing proportion of children with CHD are being identified to have specific chromosomal (such as CATCH 22) and single-gene disorders. The pediatrician has an important role in identifying them because they have significant bearing on eventual outcomes and counseling of the family.
- Despite significant recent advances, long-term concerns after palliation and many forms of "correction" of CHD are significant, and many of these children need lifelong follow-up.

This chapter will expand on the above-mentioned points. A detailed description of individual congenital heart defects is beyond the scope of this chapter, and the reader should refer to standard textbooks of pediatric cardiology. Brief descriptions of "common" CHDs are included in a section at the end of the chapter.

EPIDEMIOLOGY OF CORONARY HEART DISEASE

Congenital heart disease account for about 10% of infant deaths and nearly half of all deaths due to congenital malformations in the developed countries. The prevalence of CHD diagnosed in the first 12 months is estimated at 6–8 per 1,000 live births. Of these, at least 25% are life-threatening CHDs that require very early intervention. A large recent prospective study was recently undertaken from Cochin, and 5,487 consecutive newborns were screened. Of these, 425 had CHD (prevalence: 7.75%) and 17 (0.31%) had major CHD (lesions that are likely to require early intervention). The rest (408 patients, 7.44%) were minor CHD [such as small muscular ventricular septal defects (VSDs), closing patent ducts, and small atrial septal defects (ASDs)/patent foramen], most of which were normalized by 6 weeks. In a larger and more recent study from Delhi, involving nearly 20,000 consecutive newborns, CHD was identified in 159 (prevalence 8.36 per 1,000 live births). Of these, 70 had a major CHD (3.68 per 1,000 live births), of whom 44 had serious CHDs (requiring surgical or catheter intervention in the first year of life), and 26 had critical CHDs (requiring intervention in the first month of life).

Extrapolating this data on a national scale suggests that the absolute burden of CHD in India is substantial. For a population of 1.2 billion, it can be expected that there would perhaps be approximately 100,000 newborns born each year with CHD requiring some form of intervention early in life. In relative terms, CHD is of importance in those parts of the country that are showing improved human development indices (such as Kerala, Tamil Nadu, Himachal Pradesh, and Goa). In these regions' infant mortality form readily, preventable conditions (such as diarrhea and respiratory infections) has declined substantially.

It is estimated that only 6–10% of newborns and infants with CHD are receiving timely surgery in India. Most newborns with CHD escape timely detection. Even after diagnosis is made, the economic and logistic barriers to reach a center and successfully undergo surgery are substantial in our country. As a result, CHD has a unique profile in India (such as in other low- and middle-income countries). This is characterized by remarkable early attrition, late survival selected by natural history and significant numbers of older children with complications, such as pulmonary hypertension, overt (brain abscess and stroke) and covert (neurodevelopmental abnormalities) neurological damage.

ETIOPATHOGENESIS

The link between etiology and embryogenesis of CHD is often very complex. A lot of recent research has focused on the chain of events in early embryogenesis of the heart and great vessels. As a result, there have been dramatic conceptual upheavals. The details are beyond the scope of this chapter. In simplified terms, the pediatrician should recognize today that a growing proportion of patients with CHD have an identifiable genetic basis. **Table 7.2.1** summarizes common genetic conditions that are associated with CHD. The association with acquired conditions and teratogens and occurrence of CHD is summarized in **Table 7.2.2**.

PHYSIOLOGY AND PHYSIOLOGIC CLASSIFICATION OF CONGENITAL HEART DISEASE

Once the basic physiologic concepts are understood, it is relatively easy to understand clinical manifestations (history and physical examination). These concepts enable better interpretation of chest X-ray, ECG, and echocardiographic findings and allow correct management decisions (timing of surgical or catheter interventions).

For many years, CHD has been broadly classified as cyanotic and acyanotic with certain specific subtypes in each category **(Table 7.2.3)**. While broad classifications based on physiology works for many situations, there are several patients who cannot be classified into common physiologic categories. In addition, there are often specific issues, such as valve regurgitation that dictate the clinical presentation. The broad categories of CHD in **Table 7.2.3** have limitations, and some patients may have a combination of lesions belonging to more than one category. For example, a child may have a

Table 7.2.1: Common genetic conditions that are linked to the occurrence of congenital heart disease.

Specific condition	*Genetic basis*	*Cardiac lesions*	*Other manifestations*
CATCH 22 syndrome	Microdeletion on long arm of chromosome 22, 22q11 deletion; autosomal dominant inheritance	Interrupted aortic arch, tetralogy of Fallot (TOF), ventricular septal defect (VSD), persistent truncus arteriosus, double outlet right ventricle	Cleft palate, hypocalcemia, thymic hypoplasia, nasal regurgitation of feeds, feeding disorders, failure to thrive, gastroesophageal reflux, facial dysmorphism, delayed speech, hypernasal speech, learning disabilities, behavioral disorders (ADHD), older children may have psychiatric disorders
Williams–Beuren syndrome	Microdeletion at chromosome 7q11.23 (elastin gene located in this segment); autosomal dominant inheritance	Supravalvar aortic stenosis, pulmonary arterial stenosis, aortic and mitral valve abnormalities, adult systemic hypertension	Distinctive facies (periorbital fullness, stellate iris pattern, full lips-wide mouth, elfin appearance) strabismus, mental retardation, cognitive disability, hyperacusis, hypersocial personality, failure to thrive, short stature, hypercalcemia, hypothyroidism, chronic urinary tract infections, nephron-calcinosis
Down syndrome	Chromosomal trisomy for chromosome 21 (rarely Robertsonian translocation or mosaicism), sporadic mutation	AV canal defect, perimembranous VSD, TOF, PDA	Characteristic facies, clinodactyly, single palmar crease mental handicap; hypotonia, hearing and vision loss, early-onset dementia
Turner syndrome	Chromosomal (45, X karyotype and variants mosaicism, structurally abnormal X chromosome)	Predominantly left-sided lesions (i.e. bicuspid aortic valve (BAV), coarctation); risk for aortic root dilatation	Variable phenotype; short stature, gonadal dysgenesis, lymphedema, renal anomalies, normal intelligence but can have learning disability
Noonan syndrome	Protein tyrosine phosphatase, non-receptor type (PTPN11) mutations in 50%; half of cases are de novo autosomal dominant inheritance in the next generation	Pulmonic stenosis (20–50%) hypertrophic cardiomyopathy (20–30%) atrial septal defect (ASD)	Variable phenotype, short stature, webbed neck, dysmorphic facies, varying developmental delay; cryptorchidism; coagulation defects
VATER association	No specific recurring etiology, sporadic; very small risk to offspring	VSD, TOF	Vertebral defects, anal atresia, TEF, renal and limb anomalies, normal intelligence
Holt-Oram syndrome	TBX5 mutation (70%); 15% familial, autosomal dominant inheritance	Ostium secundum ASD, VSD, conduction defects	Upper limb anomalies of varying degrees (especially radial ray) in 100%
Charge	CHD7 mutation (60%) or deletion; most cases are de novo autosomal dominant inheritance	Commonly right-sided lesions branch pulmonary artery stenosis and conotruncal lesions (TOF, VSD)	Colobomas, growth failure, developmental delay, choanal atresia, genital hypoplasia, ear anomalies, and hearing loss
Alagille syndrome	Pulmonary valve, artery, and branch PA most commonly affected; TOF in 7–15%	JAG1 mutation (90%) or deletion (7%); 50–70% of cases are de novo; autosomal dominant inheritance	Hepatic disease, dysmorphic facies, butterfly vertebrae, renal anomalies, neurovascular anomalies

(ADHD: attention deficit hyperactivity disorder; CHD7: chromodomain-helicase-DNA-binding protein 7; JAG1: jagged1; PA: pulmonary atresia; TBX5: T-box transcription factor 5; TEF: tracheoesophageal fistula; VATER: vertebrae, anus, trachea, esophagus, renal)

Table 7.2.2: Etiology of congenital heart disease (CHD)—prenatal exposure to acquired factors.

Acquired condition	***Association with CHD***
Diabetes	A variety of forms of CHDs are now linked with maternal gestational and pregestational diabetes. The list includes transposition, atrioventricular septal defects, ventricular septal defect (VSD), hypoplastic left heart syndrome, cardiomyopathy, and patent ductus arteriosus (PDA)
Febrile illnesses in the first trimester	Any febrile illness during the first trimester of pregnancy may have a twofold increase in the risk of CHD
Maternal rubella	Specific cardiac manifestations of rubella embryopathy include: PDA, pulmonary valve abnormalities, peripheral pulmonary stenosis, and VSD
Epilepsy	The association is perhaps because of the risk of CHD from anticonvulsant medications
Lupus (apart from typical symptoms of SLE, it may be useful to ask for history of previous abortions)	Maternal systemic lupus erythematosus (SLE) is associated with the risk of complete heart block in the offspring
Phenylketonuria	Phenylketonuria is associated with a >six-fold increase in the risk of CHD (specifically VSD, TOF, PDA, and single ventricle)
Vitamin deficiency	Multivitamin supplements including folic acid derivatives have been shown to protect against the occurrence of CHD in two studies. Multivitamins may also reduce the risk of CHD associated with febrile illnesses in the first trimester
Prenatal exposure to medications in the first trimester	The list of medications known to be associated with a risk of CHD in the offspring includes: anticonvulsants, non-steroidal anti-inflammatory drugs (NSAIDs), trimethoprim–sulfonamide, thalidomide, and vitamin A congeners
Occupational exposure	Exposure to organic solvents, herbicides, pesticides, ionizing radiation may increase the risk of CHD in the offspring

(TOF: tetralogy of Fallot)

large VSD with moderate pulmonary stenosis (PS) and mild pulmonary hypertension.

Another way of understanding the physiology of CHD is to list the various physiological perturbations **(Table 7.2.4)** that are commonly associated with CHD. Here again it is evident that many defects have more than one physiological perturbation. The table is, however, useful in that it illustrates various mechanisms by which CHD produces clinical manifestations. The reader is encouraged to study this table carefully. A thorough understanding of physiology of individual forms of CHD can be acquired through detailed study of individual lesions. This is clearly beyond the scope of this chapter.

Here, the focus will be on illustrating selected key physiological concepts that are important to understand many lesions. These include

- Pretricuspid versus post-tricuspid shunts
- The VSD-PS physiology
- Single-ventricle physiology
- Duct-dependent lesions
- Unfavorable streaming and parallel circulation.

Pretricuspid versus Post-tricuspid Shunts

Acyanotic heart disease with left-to-right shunts is traditionally classified as pretricuspid and post-tricuspid shunts. There are important differences in physiology that have an important bearing on clinical manifestations and natural history.

Left-to-right shunts at the level of the atria are known as pretricuspid shunts. They include ASDs and partial anomalous pulmonary venous connection. The left-to-right shunt and the consequent excessive pulmonary blood flow are dictated by relative stiffness of the two ventricles. Since the right ventricle (RV) is relatively stiff (noncompliant) at birth and during early infancy, the shunt is small. Over the years the RV progressively enlarges to accommodate the excessive pulmonary blood flow. The pulmonary vasculature also becomes more capacious to gradually accommodate the excessive blood flow. This explains why ASDs typically do not manifest with the symptoms of pulmonary overcirculation during infancy and childhood. The clinical signs are also easily explained by the physiology of pretricuspid shunts. The diastolic flow murmur of ASD is across the much larger tricuspid valve and is, therefore, subtle or even inaudible. The second heart sound split is wide and fixed largely because of the prolonged "hang-out" interval resulting from increased capacitance of the pulmonary circulation. In addition, the large communication at atrial level minimizes any differences in the impact of respiration on the right versus left heart. Pulmonary arterial hypertension (PAH) is typically absent or at most mild. The presence of moderate or severe PAH in

Table 7.2.3: Broad physiologic categories of congenital heart disease.

Physiologic category	***Examples***
Acyanotic congenital heart disease	
Simple left-to-right shunts	
Pretricuspid	Partial anomalous pulmonary venous drainage, atrial septal defect
Post-tricuspid	
Ventricular	Ventricular septal defects (VSDs)
Great artery	Aortopulmonary window, patent arterial duct, coronary cameral fistula, ruptured sinus of Valsalva
Combination of pre- and post-tricuspid	Atrioventricular septal defect, left ventricle to right atrial communications
Obstructive lesions Inflow: Left sided	Cor triatriatum, obstructive lesions of the mitral valve apparatus
Outflow	
Right ventricle	Infundibular stenosis, pulmonary valve stenosis, branch pulmonary artery stenosis
Left ventricle	Subaortic membrane, valvar aortic stenosis, supravalvar aortic stenosis, coarctation of aorta
Miscellaneous lesions	Coronary artery abnormalities, congenital mitral and tricuspid valve regurgitation
Cyanotic heart disease Reduced pulmonary blood flow	Pulmonary atresia (PA) with intact ventricular septum, critical pulmonic stenosis (PS) with R-L shunt at atrial level, Ebstein anomaly, isolated RV hypoplasia
Intact interventricular septum	
Unrestrictive ventricular communication	All conditions listed under VSD with PS or PA physiology*
Miscellaneous conditions	Pulmonary arteriovenous malformation, anomalous drainage of systemic veins to LA
Increased pulmonary blood flow	
Pretricuspid	Total anomalous pulmonary venous communication common atrium
Post-tricuspid	All single-ventricle physiology lesions† without PS, persistent truncus arteriosus
Pulmonary hypertension	Shunt reversal after the development of pulmonary vascular obstructive disease in any of the conditions associated with increased pulmonary blood flow (Eisenmenger physiology)

(LA: left atrium; R-L: right-to-left; RV: right ventricle)
**VSD with PS or PA physiology*: This includes all conditions with an unrestrictive interventricular communication and pulmonary stenosis or pulmonary atresia. *Included in this list are the following*: Tetralogy of Fallot, double outlet right ventricle, single ventricle, transposition with VSD, corrected transposition with VSD, atrioventricular septal defect and tricuspid atresia.
†Admixture lesions are all conditions with a single-ventricle physiology.

Table 7.2.4: Physiological perturbations in congenital heart disease.

Physiological derangement	***Hemodynamic consequences***	***Clinical consequences***	***Examples***
Increased pulmonary blood flow	Inefficient circulation, pulmonary congestion, pulmonary hypertension	Failure to thrive, heart failure symptoms, tachypnea, frequent respiratory infections	All post-tricuspid shunts, some large pretricuspid shunts
Reduced pulmonary blood flow	Hypoxia in the presence of an atrial or ventricular septal defect; reduced cardiac output, if both septa are intact	Cyanosis, fatigue	All congenital heart defects that are associated with pulmonary stenosis
Mixing of systemic and pulmonary venous return (single-ventricle physiology)	Some hypoxia will result, but the exact oxygen saturation will be dictated by pulmonary blood flow. If pulmonary blood flow is increased (shunt ratio of 2:1 or more) saturations are usually above 85%	Cyanosis of varying severity depending on pulmonary blood flow	All forms of univentricular hearts; double-inlet left ventricle (LV) or right ventricle (RV), tricuspid atresia, primitive hearts associated with asplenia, and polysplenia

Contd...

Contd...

Physiological derangement	*Hemodynamic consequences*	*Clinical consequences*	*Examples*
Unfavorable streaming and parallel circulation	Hypoxia tends to be severe unless pulmonary blood flow is significantly elevated	Severe cyanosis in the face of excessive pulmonary blood flow	All variations of transposition of the great arteries; double outlet RV with subpulmonic ventricular septal defect (VSD) (Taussig-Bing)
Pulmonary venous hypertension	Pulmonary venous congestion with pulmonary arteriolar vasoconstriction and resultant elevation in pulmonary vascular resistance	Tachypnea from pulmonary edema, severe elevation in pulmonary vascular resistance translates into reduced pulmonary blood flow and increased cyanosis	Obstructed total anomalous pulmonary venous connection, cor triatriatum, congenital mitral stenosis, mitral atresia with restrictive atrial septal defect (ASD), pulmonary venous stenosis
Elevated pulmonary vascular resistance	Inability to increase cardiac output during exercise or stress, increased right-to-left shunting across associated defects	Fatigue on effort, patients with defects in the atrial or ventricular septum will have increasing cyanosis	All conditions associated with increased pulmonary blood flow increase the risk for the development of increased pulmonary vascular resistance
Left-sided atrioventricular valve regurgitation	Left ventricular volume overload, elevation in left atrial pressures, pulmonary venous congestion	Tachypnea, fatigue on effort	Atrioventricular septal defects, corrected transposition, ASDs (5–10% have associated mitral valve prolapse and MR), congenital MR, anomalous coronary artery from pulmonary artery
Right-sided atrioventricular valve regurgitation	Right ventricular volume overload elevated right atrial pressures, systemic venous congestion	Fatigue, right heart failure	Ebstein anomaly, congenital anomalies of tricuspid valve
Left ventricular hypertrophy	Elevated filling pressures with resulting in left heart failure	Tachypnea from pulmonary venous congestion	All forms of left ventricular outflow tract obstruction, hypertrophic cardiomyopathy
Right ventricular hypertrophy	Elevated right-sided filling pressures with systemic venous congestion	Right heart failure: liver enlargement, fluid accumulation (edema and ascites)	Advanced forms of right ventricular outflow obstruction: critical pulmonary stenosis, advanced pulmonary hypertension
Reduced coronary perfusion	Left ventricular dysfunction	Tachypnea, fatigue	Anomalous left coronary artery from pulmonary artery
Pulmonary valve regurgitation	Dilation of branch pulmonary arteries with airway compression, right ventricular dilation	Respiratory symptoms in infants with tetralogy of Fallot (TOF) and absent pulmonary valve, fatigue on effort in patients with long-standing pulmonary valve incompetence	TOF with absent pulmonary valve, because of pulmonary hypertension (usually mild)
Aortic valve regurgitation	Left ventricular dilation	Fatigue and palpitation	Bicommissural aortic valve, in association with subpulmonic and some perimembranous defects

(MR: mitral regurgitation)

ASD is worrisome and may suggest the onset of irreversible changes in the pulmonary vasculature.

Post-tricuspid shunts are different in that there is direct transmission of pressure from the systemic to the pulmonary circuit at the ventricular level (VSD) or great arteries [patent ductus arteriosus (PDA) and aortopulmonary (AP) window]. For patients with large posttricuspid shunts, symptoms begin in early infancy, typically after some regression of elevated pulmonary vasoconstriction in the newborn period together with progressive development of the pulmonary vascular tree. The excessive pulmonary blood flow returns to the left atrium (LA) and flows through the mitral valve, resulting in the apical diastolic flow murmur that is a consistent marker of large posttricuspid shunts. The LA and ventricle are dilated because of this extra volume. Elevation in pulmonary artery (PA) pressures is an inevitable consequence of large (or unrestrictive) posttricuspid shunts and is labeled as hyperkinetic PAH. This needs to be distinguished from the elevation of pulmonary vascular resistance that results from sustained exposure to increased pulmonary blood flow.

Ventricular Septal Defect: Pulmonary Stenosis Physiology

This situation is characterized by a large communication at the ventricular level together with varying degrees of obstruction to pulmonary blood flow. Typically, this is in the form of subvalvar (infundibular), valvar, annular (small valve annulus), and occasionally supravalvar stenosis. The free communication between the two ventricles results in the equalization of pressures. Severity of PS dictates the volume of blood flowing through PAs and, therefore, amount of oxygenated blood returning via pulmonary veins. Severe PS results in right-to-left shunt across the VSD with varying degrees of hypoxia and, consequently, cyanosis. Cyanosis is directly proportionate to the severity of PS. Since the RV is readily decompressed by the large VSD, heart failure is unusual. The best example of VSD-PS physiology is tetralogy of Fallot (TOF). In its least severe form, TOF is often not associated with cyanosis (pink TOF). Here, PS is significant enough to result in a large pressure gradient across the right ventricular outflow tract (RVOT), but not severe enough to result in a reduction in pulmonary blood flow. Pink TOF is typically associated with a loud ejection systolic murmur (ESM) because of a reasonable volume of blood flowing across the RVOT. As the severity of PS increases, pulmonary blood flow declines and the intensity of murmur declines progressively. Other examples of VSD–PS physiology include double outlet RV (DORV) with subaortic VSD and PS, corrected transposition with PS, and atrioventricular (AV) septal defect with PS. These conditions are often indistinguishable from TOF at the bedside.

Single-ventricle Physiology

This refers to a group of conditions where there is complete mixing of pulmonary and systemic venous returns. In addition to single ventricle (double-inlet ventricle), a variety of conditions come under the category of single ventricular physiology. Atresia of one of the AV valves, severe hypoplasia of one of the ventricles, and severe straddling of one of the AV valves over a large VSD are all examples of situations where there is mixing of pulmonary and systemic venous returns. The clinical manifestations are dictated by whether there is PS. In the absence of PS, there is excessive pulmonary blood flow especially in infants because of the relatively lower pulmonary vascular resistance. As a result, the proportion of oxygenated blood from pulmonary veins that mixes with the systemic venous return is high. As a result, cyanosis is minimal and measured oxygen saturation may be in the 90s. However, the price for this preserved oxygenation is heart failure and development of permanent elevation of pulmonary vascular resistance pulmonary vascular obstructive disease (PVOD). Over time, if the child survives infancy, pulmonary vascular resistance progressively increases with increasing cyanosis.

Single ventricle and its physiologic variants can be associated with varying degrees of PS. Here, the situation is quite like VSD-PS physiology except for relatively severe hypoxia because of free mixing systemic and pulmonary venous return.

Duct-dependent Lesions

An infant or a newborn with CHD that is dependent on the patency of the ductus arteriosus for survival can be termed as suffering from duct-dependent lesion. Typically, these are newborns in which either the systemic blood supply is critically dependent on an open PDA duct-dependent systemic circulation (DDSC) or pulmonary blood flow is duct-dependent pulmonary circulation (DDPC).

Closure of the PDA in DDSC results in systemic hypoperfusion (often mislabeled as neonatal sepsis). Examples of DDSC include hypoplastic left heart syndrome where the entire systemic circulation is supported by the RV through the PDA and interrupted aortic arch where the descending aortic flow is entirely through the PDA. Severe coarctation and critical aortic stenosis (AS) are also the examples of DDSC.

Closure of PDA in DDPC results in severe hypoxia and cyanosis in the affected newborn. Examples of DDPC include all forms of pulmonary atresia (irrespective of underlying heart defect) where the PDA is the predominant source of pulmonary blood flow. There are examples of pulmonary atresia where pulmonary blood supply is from major AP collaterals. These children may survive even after the PDA closes. Critical pulmonic stenosis ("nearly atretic" pulmonary valve) can present as duct-dependent pulmonary blood flow.

Neonates with duct-dependent physiology require prostaglandin E1 (PGE1) for survival. Early recognition of a duct-dependent situation allows early initiation of PGE1 and stabilization until definitive procedure can be accomplished.

Unfavorable Streaming and Parallel Circulation

Unfavorable streaming refers to a situation where oxygen-rich pulmonary blood flow is directed toward the pulmonary valve and poorly oxygenated blood toward the aortic valve. An extreme form of unfavorable streaming is the parallel circulation in transposition of the great arteries (TGA) with intact ventricular septum. Here survival is dependent of the presence of a communication (ideally at atrial level) that allows mixing of pulmonary and systemic venous return. The presence of a VSD may improve the situation in TGA but significant cyanosis is usually present unless the pulmonary blood flow is torrential.

RECOGNITION OF CONGENITAL HEART DISEASE

The manifestations of CHD are different in a neonate, an infant or a child. It is often easy to recognize the presence of CHD in older children. In infants, and particularly in newborns, manifestations of heart disease can often be subtle. Further, several conditions that do not involve the cardiovascular system can result in clinical manifestations that overlap with those resulting from heart disease. Notwithstanding these difficulties, it is possible to identify the presence of heart disease in most infants and newborns after careful clinical evaluation. The following clinical features should alert the pediatrician regarding the presence of CHD.

Cyanosis

Cyanosis may be peripheral or central. Peripheral cyanosis almost exclusively involves lips and extremities. Normal neonates may have bluish extremities that respond to warming or moving the extremities. Saturations of 90% or lower while breathing room air beyond the first 20 minutes are considered abnormal. Similarly, some infants may have peripheral cyanosis following exposure to cold. Central cyanosis involving the mucous membranes and trunk along with the lips and extremities strongly suggests the likelihood of CHD. Unfortunately, however, cyanosis often remains unnoticed. This is particularly true in the Indian context, where it is difficult to detect cyanosis is the presence of a dark skin complexion. Further, cyanosis is often masked by anemia. When central cyanosis is suspected, its presence should be confirmed, and severity quantified by measuring oxygen saturation using a skin oximeter probe. Unfortunately, however, the availability of this instrument is limited to a few selected institutions.

Difficult Feeding and Poor Growth

The parent of an infant with CHD may complain that the child has difficulty with feeds. This is usually a feature of an infant with congestive heart failure resulting from CHD. The history may be of slow feeding, small volumes consumed during each feed, tiring easily following feeds and requirement of periods of rest during feeds. Not infrequently, no history of feeding difficulty may be obtained, but examination of the growth charts will reveal that the child's growth rate is not appropriate for age. A recent decline in growth rate (falling off the growth curve) or weight that is inappropriate for age (<5th percentile) may result from a large left-to-right shunt. Characteristically, growth retardation affects weight more than height.

Difficult Breathing

Tachypnea (respiratory rates consistently more than 60/min in infants < 2 months; > 50/min in older infants; >40/min after 1 year), is a characteristic manifestation of heart failure in newborns (preterm newborns may normally have respiratory rates of up to 60/min). For infants, subcostal or intercostal retractions together with flaring of nostrils (alae nasi) are frequently associated with tachypnea.

Frequent Respiratory Infections

Respiratory infections that are frequent, severe, and difficult to treat are common in infants with CHD associated with large left-to-right shunts, resulting in increased lung blood flow. Not infrequently, heart disease may be detected for the first time during an episode of respiratory tract infection.

Clinical Stigmata of Specific Syndromes

Evidence of the presence of chromosomal anomalies or other syndromes that are known to be associated with CHD should alert the clinician to the presence of specific cardiac defects that are known to be associated with these conditions. The list of such conditions is a long one. Trisomy 21 is the most common chromosomal anomaly that is associated with heart disease. Other common examples include trisomy 13, trisomy 18, Turner syndrome, Noonan syndrome, velocardiofacial and the DiGeorge syndrome **(Table 7.2.1)**.

CARDIOVASCULAR EXAMINATION

A thorough and systematic cardiovascular examination provides valuable clues to the presence of heart disease. With practice such an examination can be accomplished in a short time. For the pediatrician, a thorough familiarization with what is normal is a useful initial step. It is useful to answer the following questions that can serve as a checklist for a preliminary cardiac examination. This checklist is, not at all, comprehensive and is designed primarily for answering the question: Does the patient have heart disease? It can also help identify the broad physiologic category of heart defect.

- *Are the arterial pulsations normal?*
  Is the pulse volume normal or increased?

Is there a discrepancy of pulsation in any of the four extremities?

A careful evaluation of pulsations in all extremities should always be a part of physical examination. Coarctation is readily diagnosed when weak femoral artery pulsations are detected in comparison to brachial or radial artery. When a discrepancy in pulses is suspected, four-extremity blood pressure measurements should be obtained. An automated noninvasive blood pressure instrument is preferred over manual recording for four-extremity blood pressure measurement.

- *Does the precordium feel normal?*
  Are there visible precordial pulsations?
  Is the apex beat displaced, hyperdynamic or heaving? Is there a thrill palpable?
- *Are the heart sounds normal?*
  Can the two components of the second heart sound be separated?
  Is there an additional heart sound in diastole (such as S3)?
  Are there any additional systolic sounds (ejection clicks)?
- *Is (or are) there a murmur (or murmurs)? If so:*
  Is it systolic or diastolic or both systolic and diastolic (diastolic murmurs always have a structural basis)?
  Is it loud (grade 3 or louder murmurs are seldom innocent)?

DIAGNOSIS

Electrocardiogram and Chest X-ray

If there is a suspicion of heart disease on the basis of the history or physical examination, an ECG and a chest X-ray should be obtained. The ECG should be interpreted keeping the age of the child in mind. Interpretation of the chest X-ray should involve evaluation of the cardiac silhouette and lung vasculature. The X-ray also provides information about the location of abdominal organs (for determination of the situs) and the aortic arch. Beyond the neonatal period, a normal ECG and chest X-ray make the diagnosis of a hemodynamically significant heart defect unlikely. In the newborn, however, ECG and chest X-ray change and may take a few days to evolve. For the newborn, particularly in the first few days, a "normal" ECG and a normal X-ray do not rule out serious heart disease.

Echocardiography

Echocardiography has revolutionized the diagnosis of CHD, and its high diagnostic yield makes this investigation very cost effective in most situations. This statement is, however, only true if it is performed by an experienced individual who understands anatomy and physiology of CHD. In many children with CHD, a very thorough evaluation is possible, and all the questions addressed in the checklist (below) can be answered. This is particularly true for infants and newborns in which excellent images are readily obtained. Such patients can undergo a definitive procedure based on the information provided by the echocardiogram. Transesophageal echocardiography can supplement transthoracic studies. This is particularly true for patients with poor echocardiography windows that do not permit adequate imaging. Unlike adults, children undergoing transesophageal echocardiography often require general anesthesia. Echocardiography has a few inherent limitations; however, it consistently fails to define certain structures, such as the PA branches beyond the hila of the lungs. Here cardiac computed tomography (CT) or cardiac magnetic resonance (CMR) imaging work well. Newer modalities, such as three-dimensional echocardiography, are in the evolving phase and at present do not add significance to two-dimensional echocardiography.

Checklist of Diagnosis of Congenital Heart Disease through Echocardiography

- What is the visceral and atrial situs (solitus, inversus, or ambiguous)?
- What are the systemic venous connections like? Is the inferior vena cava (IVC) intact? Is there a separate left superior vena cava? If so, how does it drain?
- What is the relationship of the abdominal aorta to the IVC?
- What is the appearance of the atria like? Is the atrial septum intact? Is there an ASD or a patent foramen ovale? If so, what direction does blood flow?
- How do the atria connect to the ventricles (concordant or discordant)?
- Is it possible to identify two separate AV valves?
- How are the AV valves in their appearance and function?
- The ventricles, their size, shape, and function?
- Are the various components of the interventricular septum intact?
- Is there any outflow tract obstruction?
- How do the ventricles connect to the great arteries?
- What is the appearance and function of the semilunar valves?
- What is the great artery relationship?
  - Are the branch PAs in continuity? Is there any branch PA stenosis?
  - What side is the aortic arch? What is its branching pattern? Is there a PDA or a coarctation?
  - What is the coronary artery anatomy?
  - How is the hemodynamics and physiology altered?

Cardiac Magnetic Resonance Imaging

Cardiac magnetic resonance imaging (MRI), a useful noninvasive imaging modality, has established itself as an important modality for the evaluation of CHD. It is especially useful in older patients and postoperative patients where imaging from echo is limited. In addition, CMR has tremendous value in defining extracardiac structures, such as branch PAs, pulmonary veins, and AP collaterals. Very useful physiologic data (especially blood flow calculations at several locations) is also obtained through MRI. It is likely to replace cardiac catheterization in most situations. Limitations with CMR include limited expertise for interpretation and requirement of general anesthesia to enable breath holding.

Computed Tomography

Anatomic information from CT is like that of MRI. Computed tomography overcomes some of the key limitations in MRI because it has a much lower image acquisition time. However, exposure to ionizing radiation is a major concern. In addition, unlike in adults, children have faster resting heart rates that come in the way of satisfactory imaging of coronary arteries.

Diagnostic Cardiac Catheterization

The role of diagnostic cardiac catheterization for patients with CHD has declined considerably with the availability of high-quality echocardiography, MRI, and CT. Since cardiac catheterization is an invasive procedure, its performance requires careful planning, so that the information desired may be obtained with the minimum risk to the patient. Simply stated, a diagnostic cardiac catheterization may be performed whenever noninvasive investigations do not provide crucial information that is required for operation. Accurate estimation of filling pressures and PA pressures, determination of blood flows and vascular resistance, definition of coronary arteries are often best performed through cardiac catheterization.

NEWBORN SCREENING FOR CONGENITAL HEART DISEASE

Notwithstanding its significant limitations, pulse oximetry offers the best prospect of detecting CHD among all the available tools in the newborn period. Clinical examination alone has very poor sensitivity and specificity. Systematic efforts to examine the utility of pulse oximetry for screening for newborn heart disease in Indian settings have yielded mixed results. Among the 19,009 newborns screened in the recent study from Delhi, pulse oximetry detected 39 major (sensitivity 55.7%, specificity 68.3%) and 22 critical CHDs (sensitivity 84.6%, specificity 68.3%). Addition of pulse oximetry to clinical examination significantly improved sensitivity for major CHDs (35.7–75.7%) and critical CHDs (11.5–84.6%). There are important challenges in applying screening for newborn CHD on a national scale. The existing numbers of centers are simply not capable of dealing with existing volume of cases that are incidentally identified. With the introduction of widespread systematic screening, there is likely to be a substantial increase in the numbers of children that will completely overwhelm the existing programs. A nationwide screening program can only be introduced after downstream consequences of identifying large numbers of children with CHD are fully considered.

DEFINITIVE TREATMENT AND PALLIATION FOR CONGENITAL HEART DISEASE

To ensure the best possible results of management of CHD, it is necessary to assemble a team of especially qualified individuals who should ideally be a part of a comprehensive pediatric heart program. The details are shown in **Flowchart 7.2.1.** Definitive treatment for CHD requires the collaborative (and not competitive) use of surgery and catheter-based interventions.

Surgery

Surgery is still the best option for definitive treatment or palliation of most forms of CHD. A simple scheme of classification of surgery for CHD is shown in **Flowchart 7.2.2**. This classification is a practical one and is from the point of view of follow-up issues. A detailed description of all congenital heart operations is clearly beyond the scope of the chapter. Congenital heart operations are also broadly classified as open heart [requiring the use of cardiopulmonary bypass (CPB)] and closed heart (not requiring CPB). Most corrective operations and many palliative operations fall under the category of open-heart operations. These procedures are generally a more significant and expensive undertaking because of the use of the CPB circuit and a substantially larger number of disposable items. The morbidity of open-heart operations is proportionate to the duration of exposure to CPB and the cross-clamp time (the period when heart beating is deliberately brought to a standstill using cardioplegia).

Catheter Interventions for Congenital Heart Disease

The scope of catheter interventions has grown by leaps and bounds in the last two to three decades, and this treatment option has transformed the care of many children with CHD. Many simple defects, such as secundum ASD, PDA, selected muscular VSD, can now be closed in the catheterization laboratory. In addition, balloon valvotomy is now the first line of treatment for congenital stenosis of the pulmonary and aortic valves. Additional details of catheter intervention procedures are shown in **Table 7.2.5**. The advantages of catheter-based interventions are obvious, and this has become an increasingly appealing option for many children. The procedures are far less traumatic than surgery, accomplished with greater ease, allow rapid recovery, and leave behind no scars.

Flowchart 7.2.1: The constituents of a comprehensive pediatric heart program for optimal care of children with congenital heart disease. For the best and consistently reproducible results in newborn and infant heart surgery the presence of such a team is vital.

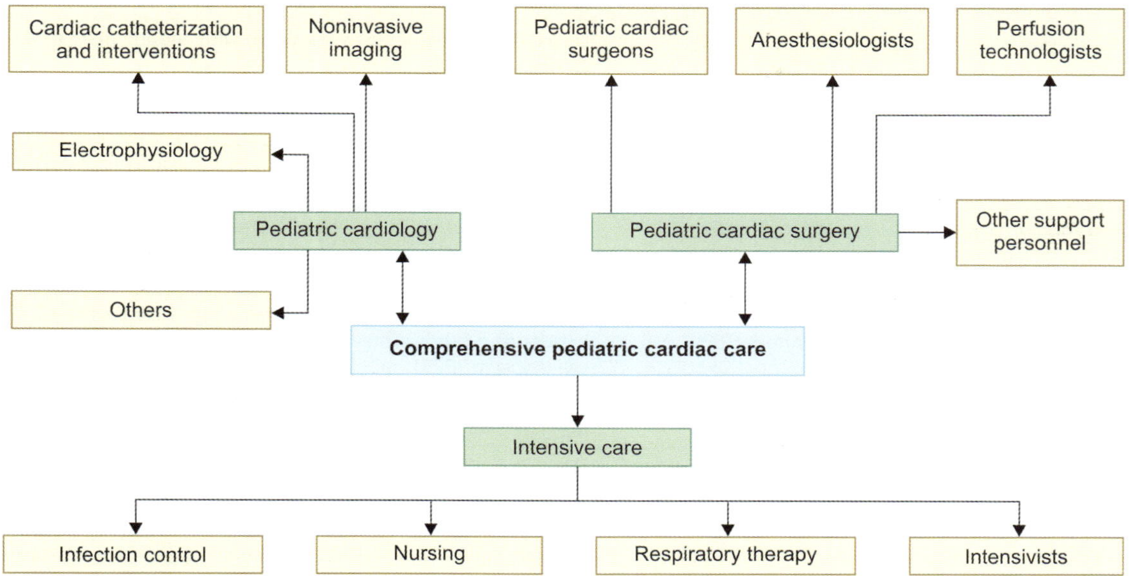

Flowchart 7.2.2: Classification of common congenital heart operations.

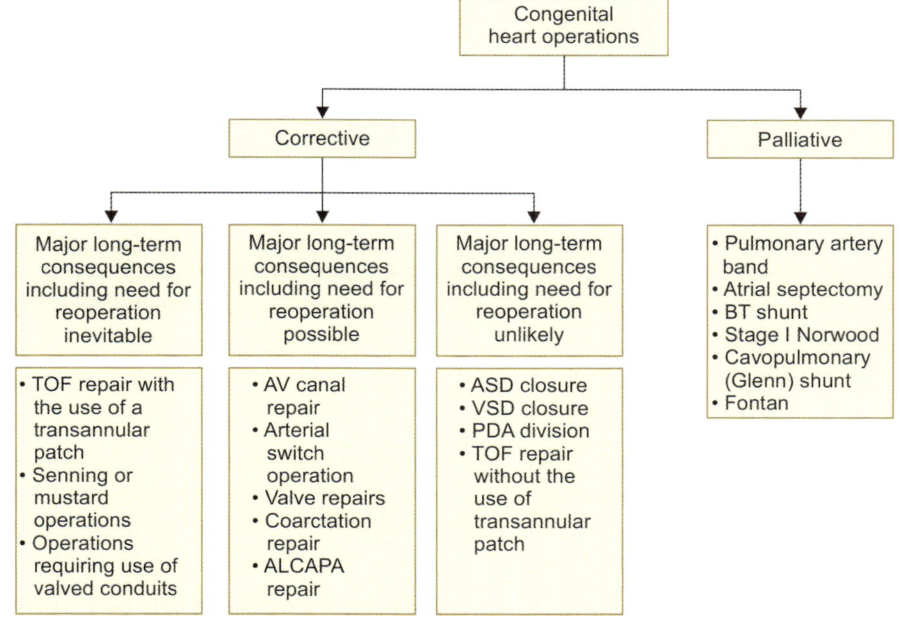

(ALCAPA: anomalous left coronary artery arising from the pulmonary artery; ASD: atrial septal defect; BT shunt: Blalock–Taussig shunt; PDA: patent ductus arteriosus; TOF: tetralogy of Fallot; VSD: ventricular septal defect)

COMPLICATIONS OF CONGENITAL HEART DISEASE

Several adverse complications occur because of CHD **(Table 7.2.6)**. For the sake of simplicity, we will focus on the selected common complications.

Pulmonary Arterial Hypertension

Pulmonary arterial hypertension occurs commonly in the context of CHD. With increasing emphasis on early correction, the magnitude of the problem is on the decline in most developed nations. Unfortunately, because most

Table 7.2.5: Congenital heart defects amenable to catheter-based interventions.

Lesion	*Procedure*	*Remarks*
Atrial septal defect	Device closure	Only defects in the fossa ovalis region with enough margins are suited for device closure
Patent ductus arteriosus (PDA)	Coil or device closure	Most PDAs can be closed in the Cath lab with the exception of large PDA in small infants
Muscular ventricular septal defect (VSD)	Device closure	Device closure is an option for relatively older infants and children (>8 kg)
Membranous VSD	Device closure	This is controversial because of the small but definite possibility of heart block. However, an increasing number of children with membranous defects are being offered closure
Pulmonary valve stenosis	Balloon pulmonary valvotomy (BPV)	Treatment of choice for most forms at all ages. Dysplastic valves in Noonan syndrome may not respond well to balloon pulmonary valvuloplasty (BPV)
Aortic valve stenosis	Balloon aortic valvotomy	Initial treatment of choice at all ages; eventually the dilated aortic valves may need surgical management
Branch pulmonary artery stenosis	Balloon dilation with stenting	Stenting is often preferred to surgery in branch PA stenosis
Coarctation of aorta	Balloon dilation with or without stenting	Surgery is the preferred option in the newborn period because recurrence after balloon is very common. For older infants, balloon is a reasonable alternative. Older children and adolescents (>10 years) may be offered stenting for a more complete relief. Neither balloon or stenting has a proven advantage over surgery
Coronary artery fistula	Coil or device closure	Treatment of choice
Pulmonary arteriovenous malformations	Coil or device closure	Treatment of choice when discrete. For diffuse malformations coil or device, closure is not an option
Duct-dependent pulmonary circulation	Stenting of the PDA	Stenting can be offered in carefully selected cases as an alternative to the Blalock–Taussig shunt
Pulmonary atresia with intact ventricular septum	Perforation of the valve followed by balloon dilation	Emerging as the procedure of choice in selected institutions with the facility and expertise
Ruptured sinus of Valsalva aneurysm	Device closure	A reasonable option in carefully selected cases
Transposition of the great arteries	Balloon atrial septostomy	Short-term palliation before definitive surgery (arterial switch operation)

(Cath lab: catheterization laboratory; PA: pulmonary atresia)

children with CHD do not receive timely attention, this is still a problem of considerable magnitude in low- and middle-income countries.

The lesions that have the greatest likelihood include cyanotic heart disease with increased pulmonary blood flow. Here irreversible changes in pulmonary vasculature develops rapidly often during infancy itself. Therefore it is particularly important to correct or appropriately palliate these lesions early (ideally within the first few months of life). Large acyanotic post-tricuspid shunts are also prone to early development of PAH and should be ideally corrected early, preferably within the first year. In pretricuspid shunts, PAH develops slowly and unpredictably. Most patients with ASD will have mild or no PAH throughout their lives. A small proportion develops accelerated changes in the pulmonary vasculature. Some of the key features responsible for the development of PAH are summarized in **Figure 7.2.1**.

Infective Endocarditis or Endarteritis

Endocarditis can complicate CHD with a suitable substrate. This includes the presence of a region of significant turbulence created by high-pressure gradients. Examples include restrictive VSD and PDA, TOF (pulmonary valve) and other VSD-PS situations, and left ventricular outflow tract obstruction. Some surgical operations [such as the Blalock–Taussig (BT) shunt] are also associated with increased risk of infective endocarditis or endarteritis. Lesions with little

Table 7.2.6: Common adverse consequences of congenital heart disease (CHD).

Lesion category	***Adverse consequences***
Duct-dependent systemic blood flow in the newborn: • Hypoplastic left heart syndrome • Critical coarctation • Interrupted aortic arch • Critical aortic stenosis	Systemic hypoperfusion and death with closure of the duct
Duct-dependent pulmonary blood flow in the newborn: • Pulmonary atresia intact ventricular septum • Pulmonary atresia with other CHD conditions • Critical pulmonary stenosis • Severe Ebstein anomaly	Fetal hypoxia and death with the closure of the ductus
• Conditions associated with increased pulmonary blood flow: Left-to-right shunts • Admixture lesions with increased pulmonary blood flow: Transposition with ventricular septal defect (VSD), persistent truncus arteriosus, double outlet right ventricle, tricuspid atresia with unrestricted pulmonary blood flow, single ventricle, etc.	*Early:* • Heart failure • Lower respiratory infections that are frequent prolonged and difficult to treat growth retardation *Late:* • Pulmonary vascular obstructive disease and Eisenmenger syndrome *Development of valve dysfunction:* • Aortic regurgitation in VSD • Mitral regurgitation in atrial septal defect (ASD)
• Conditions with reduced pulmonary blood flow and right-to-left *shunting in the heart* Tetralogy of Fallot (TOF) Other conditions with TOF (VSD with pulmonic stenosis) physiology	• Cyanotic spells • Brain infarction • Brain abscess • Seizure disorder • A variety of adverse long-term neurodevelopmental consequences • Cognitive impairment • Lower intelligence quotient (IQ) • Learning disturbance • Problems associated with polycythemia
Obstructive lesions: • Aortic and pulmonary valve stenosis • Subaortic obstruction • Supravalvar aortic stenosis • Isolated infundibular stenosis • Coarctation • Peripheral pulmonic stenosis	• Heart failure • Sudden death • Dysrhythmias
Congenital valve regurgitation	• Heart failure • Ventricular dysfunction • Dysrhythmia

or no turbulent flows, such as ASD, are not associated with increased risk. Typically, the risk of endocarditis increases after dentition begins. Current guidelines do not routinely recommend antibiotic prophylaxis for many conditions (including some of the above lesions). However, the importance of maintaining good dental hygiene in all children with CHD cannot be overemphasized.

Growth and Nutrition

This is affected in all forms of CHD and is particularly striking in large left-to-right shunts. Children with CHD show a high prevalence (59% in recent Indian studies) of significant malnutrition (weight is more affected than height), and this tends to improve after correction, irrespective of the underlying lesion. However, catch-up growth is slow, especially if CHD is corrected late.

Myocardial Dysfunction and Myocardial Damage

Chronic volume overload results in ventricular enlargement and ventricular dysfunction that is typically reversed after correction. A small proportion of patients with severe hypoxia

Contd...

Management of cyanotic spells
• *Start vasopressor infusion*: Methoxamine given IV at dose of 0.1–0.2 mg/kg/dose or IM (0.1–0.4 mg/kg/dose). *Phenylephrine:* 5 µg/kg as bolus and then 1–4 µg/kg/min as infusion • If spells are persistent, consider paralyzing the child, elective intubation and ventilation and plan for surgery, which can be corrective or palliative (BT shunt) • If convulsions occur—consider IV diazepam 0.2 mg/kg or IV midazolam 0.1–0.2 mg/kg/dose, as slow push *After a spell:* • After a spell is successfully managed, a careful neurological examination is mandatory. In the case of suspicion of neurologic insult during a spell, a CT scan is to be done to assess the presence and extent of cerebral infarcts • Initiate maximally tolerated beta-blockade (propranolol 0.5–1.5 mg/kg/dose 8 hourly or 6 hourly). The dose can be titrated by the heart rate response. Beta-blockade may help improve resting saturation and can decrease frequency of spells • Do a detailed segmental analysis by 2-D echo for complete diagnosis • Plan toward early corrective or palliative operation (depending on the age and anatomy) • Continue therapeutic (if anemic) or prophylactic iron therapy (if not anemic) *Prevention:* • Parents of patients diagnosed to have a cyanotic congenital heart defect should be counseled, if the possibility of occurrence of a spell is anticipated: • Explain to them the circumstances when a spell may occur • Avoid dehydration • Rapid control of temperature whenever fever occurs • Encourage early surgical repair Obtaining IV access in a cyanotic child can precipitate spells. This can be avoided by sedating child with IM ketamine (3–5 mg/kg) and/or by using local anesthetic skin ointment (Emlap) before attempting for venous access or blood sampling

(2D echo: two-dimensional echocardiography; BT: Blalock–Taussig; CT: computed tomography)

Table 7.2.8: Spontaneous closure of heart defects.

Variable	***Effect of likelihood of spontaneous closure***
Age at evaluation	Younger patients have a higher likelihood of spontaneous closure of defects. Most ASDs and most VSDs that are destined to close or become very small do so before the age of 3 years. PDAs have a tendency to close in the first 2–4 weeks after which they seldom close, particularly in a preterm infant
Size of the defect	Larger defects have little likelihood of spontaneous closure. ASDs > 8 mm is unlikely to close spontaneously. Similarly, large unrestrictive VSDs are also unlikely to close
Location of the defect	Only fossa ovalis ASDs tend to close. Primum and sinus venosus type of ASDs do not close muscular VSDs have the highest likelihood of spontaneous closure. Perimembranous VSDs can also close spontaneously. Outlet (subpulmonic) VSDs may close by prolapse of the aortic valve with the risk of aortic regurgitation. Inlet VSDs and misalignment type of VSDs (such as those occurring in TOF) do not close spontaneously

(ASD: atrial septal defect; PDA: patent ductus arteriosus; TOF: tetralogy of Fallot; VSD: ventricular septal defect)

PDA (during the first few months of life). The variables that influence likelihood of spontaneous closure include age at evaluation (the likelihood of spontaneous closure declines with age, and most ASDs and many VSDs are unlikely to close after the first 3 years of age), size of the defect (smaller defects are more likely to close), and location of the defects (fossa ovalis ASDs, perimembranous and muscular VSDs can close on their own). **Table 7.2.8** summarizes the variables that influence spontaneous closure. It is important to recognize the possibility of spontaneous closure while interpreting echocardiogram reports in infancy.

SURVIVAL OF PATIENTS WITH CONGENITAL HEART DISEASE

The natural history of common forms of CHD is shown in **Figure 7.2.1**. This figure is an approximation but serves to illustrate the fact that, without correction, many children with CHD (especially those with cyanotic CHD) will not survive beyond infancy or early childhood. This is dramatically altered by correction through surgery and in some situations through catheter interventions.

Following surgical correction, the natural history of many CHDs is dramatically improved. With accumulating follow-up data, however, it is becoming increasingly apparent that many "curative" operations have important long-term sequelae. The best example is surgery for TOF. For many years, it was thought that TOF repair was curative. A transannular patch that sacrifices the pulmonary valve and leaves behind severe pulmonary regurgitation was not thought to be of major importance. However, after 25–30 years of experience, most patients will develop progressive RV dilation with increased risk of late heart failure and sudden cardiac death.

Similarly, there are growing long-term concerns after the arterial switch operation (aortic root dilation, silent coronary occlusion), AV canal repair (AV valve regurgitation), and coarctation (residual hypertension, aortic aneurysm). In addition, there are operations that involve placement of conduits (pulmonary atresia, Rastelli operations for TGA-VSD-PS). These require replacement with growth.

The Fontan operation, a final solution for all univentricular hearts (single-ventricle physiology), is best described as palliative with several significant long-term concerns.

PREVENTION OF CONGENITAL HEART DISEASE

Education of the lay public on the dangers of consanguinity, drugs, and teratogens in the first trimester of pregnancy, widespread immunization against Rubella can prevent CHDs to limited extent. However, since most CHDs do not yet have an identifiable etiology, there is no effective strategy available for their prevention in the periconceptional period. Fetal echocardiography is emerging as a modality for CHD prevention after 14–16 weeks of gestation. Fetal echo is best suited to diagnose relatively severe forms of CHD. Conditions that are involving major chamber discrepancy (such as hypoplastic left heart syndrome), single ventricles and common AV canal can be identified in a simple screening protocol (the four-chamber view). With some refinement (outflow tract and three vessel views), additional conditions, such as TOF, large VSD, TGA, persistent truncus arteriosus, can be picked up as well.

The most significant challenge of fetal echocardiography lies in identifying the population at risk. The low incidence of CHD together with relatively small proportion of CHD that occur in "high-risk" pregnancies makes fetal screening of CHD and inefficient exercise. Further, the expertise and equipment required for accurate fetal echocardiography is scarce in regions with poorly developed facilities for pediatric heart care.

Once a serious CHD is identified, it is vital to counsel the families carefully and thoroughly about the postnatal manifestations, natural history, surgical options, and their long-term outlook. Before 20 weeks of gestation, medical termination of pregnancy (MTP) is an option. After legal period of MTP, fetal echocardiography enables directed delivery at a center with a comprehensive pediatric heart program. This overcomes the logistic challenges of transporting a newborn with CHD and allows prompt institution of treatment in the newborn period (such as PGE1 for duct-dependent lesions).

It is a common practice to recommend fetal echocardiography for future pregnancies after the diagnosis of serious CHD in a child. This practice is likely to have a low yield because only 2–8% of CHD tend to recur. The highest chance of recurrence is with obstructive lesions of the left heart.

The detection of certain specific chromosomal anomalies in a child should prompt an evaluation of parents to identify a carrier state. The examples of these conditions include partial deletion of chromosome 22 (22q11 or the CATCH 22 syndrome), translocation variants of trisomy 21 through fluorescence in situ hybridization or Karyotyping. The growing list of single-gene mutations that are known to be associated with CHD that can be detected through laboratory tests may enable precise counseling for a larger proportion of families where a child is affected with CHD.

SELECTED INDIVIDUAL CONGENITAL HEART DEFECTS

The following section has a brief description of selected individual heart defects. This is an incomplete list of conditions. It is important to recognize that many patients have one or more defects. It is, therefore, important to individualize the approach depending on the exact combination of lesion and the overall clinical situation.

ATRIAL SEPTAL DEFECT

Incidence: Atrial septal defects occur as an isolated anomaly in 5–10% of all CHDs.

Anatomy: Based on anatomy, ASDs are classified as follows:

Fossa ovalis ASD: They are in the central portion of atrial septum, in the position of foramen ovale. Only these defects are amenable to closure in the catheterization laboratory.

Sinus venosus ASD: In the region of superior vena cava (SVC)—right atrium junction. These defects do not have a superior margin because the SVC straddles the defect.

Ostium primum ASD: These defects are created by failure to seal the septum primum. They are in the lower part of the atrial septum, and the inferior margin of the defect is formed by the AV valve.

Coronary sinus ASD: An unroofed coronary sinus is a rare communication between the coronary sinus and the LA, which produces a clinical picture like other types of ASD.

Physiology: The physiology of ASD is that of a pretricuspid shunt [*see* Section on "Physiology and Physiologic Classification of Congenital Heart Disease" (page 494)]. The heart murmur in ASD originates from the pulmonary valve because of the increased blood flow through this normal sized valve; therefore, the murmur is systolic in timing. An increased flow through the tricuspid valve may result in a diastolic rumble at the lower left sternal border. The dilated RV cavity prolongs the time required for the depolarization of RV, resulting in delayed P2. This delay also results from the prolonged "hang-out" interval because of the very low resistance in the pulmonary circulation.

In addition, the large ASD tends to abolish respiration-related fluctuations in systemic venous return to the right side of the heart; thereby the fixed S2.

Natural history and complications: Heart failure is exceptional in infancy. Pulmonary hypertension is also relatively rare. A small proportion of patients develops PAH. It appears that those who are destined to develop PAH do so relatively early (often in the second or third decade). Atrial septal defect closure is primarily recommended to prevent complications in late adulthood. These include atrial arrhythmias and heart failure.

Treatment: Fossa ovalis defects with good margins can be closed percutaneously in the catheterization laboratory with occlusive devices. Others require surgical closure. Closure is recommended before school entry to prevent late complications. Small defects (<8 mm) can be observed. Spontaneous closure is well recognized in small defects that are diagnosed in infancy or early childhood.

VENTRICULAR SEPTAL DEFECT

Incidence: Ventricular septal defect accounts for 15–20% of all CHDs. It is the most common heart defect.

Anatomy: The ventricular septum may be divided into a small membranous portion and a large muscular portion **(Fig. 7.2.2)**. The muscular septum has three components: the inlet, the trabecular, and the outlet septum. The trabecular septum is further divided into central, marginal and apical portions. A VSD may be classified into perimembranous, inlet, outlet, central muscular, marginal muscular, and apical muscular defects.

Pathophysiology: The physiology is that of a posttricuspid left–right shunt. The magnitude of the shunt is determined by the size of the VSD and the level of pulmonary vascular resistance (PVR). The lower the PVR, the greater the magnitude of left-to-right shunts. In VSD, the LV starts contracting before RV, and

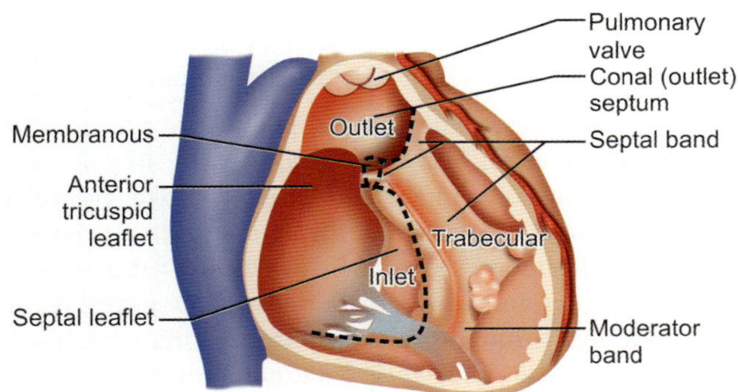

Fig. 7.2.2: En-face view of the right ventricular septal surface to show various landmarks that are used to classify ventricular septal defects.

high-pressure gradient is maintained between two ventricles throughout systole. Hence, the murmur is pansystolic. Passing through a normal mitral valve, the relatively larger volume of blood results in a middiastolic murmur at the apex. This is a very useful clue indicating a large flow and operability of the lesion.

Since the LV has two outlets, it empties relatively early; this results in early A2. Since ejection into RV and PA is increased, P2 is delayed. Therefore, the S2 is widely split but varies with respiration. In a large VSD with increasing pulmonary vascular resistance, S2 splitting becomes less and less obvious. It is single once PVR is significantly elevated because of the reduced "hang-out" interval.

Treatment: Decisions to close a VSD is dictated by many considerations that include anatomic subtype, number and size of the defects, age at diagnosis, symptom status, comorbidity and logistics of follow-up. Infants with large defects should be referred to a center for infant heart surgery early. The consequences of delaying surgery in the hope that the defect will close spontaneously are, sometimes, quite devastating. They include pneumonia that is severe and refractory to treatment, severe malnourishment, and premature pulmonary vascular disease. Catheter closure is usually unrealistic in early infancy because of technical challenges. The long-term results of surgical closure in infancy are excellent.

PATENT DUCTUS ARTERIOSUS

It is the persistence of normal fetal channel connecting the aorta and PA and accounts for 5–10% of all CHDs. Functional closure of the ductus occurs within 12–24 hours after birth due contraction of the medial smooth muscle. Anatomic closure occurs between 2 weeks and 3 weeks and is produced by fibrosis of the ductal tissue. Prematurity is associated with delay in process of closure of the PDA.

Anatomical and Physiological Considerations

The PDA needs to be understood in two circumstances: as a source of pulmonary blood flow in cyanotic heart disease with reduced pulmonary blood flow and as a cause of left-to-right shunts. In the former situation, the PDA tends to be vertical, often from the undersurface of the aorta, while in the latter, it connects the roof of the main PA with the proximal descending thoracic aorta. In this section, we will focus on the latter only. The PDA is programmed to close early in life. In the cases where the ductus fails to close normally, blood will shunt from left to right into PA and lungs. This occurs increasingly as the PVR drops and the pressure in the aorta exceeds that of PA. The volume of shunted blood will increase pulmonary blood flow, increase venous return to LA, and cause LA/LV volume overload. The flow in the PDA occurs throughout the cardiac cycle. This results in a murmur which starts in systole after S1, peaks at S2, and continues in diastole. This is continuous murmur. The passage of increased blood across the mitral valve produces a mid-diastolic murmur as in any other posttricuspid shunt. The prolonged LV systole results in delayed closure of the aortic valve and a late A2. With large PDA, S2 may be paradoxically split. The excessive diastolic back flow from the aorta results in a low diastolic pressure and bounding pulses.

Clinical Circumstances

Preterm Infants

Persistent patency of ductus arteriosus in preterm infants is well recognized in the era of modern preterm care. The prevalence of PDA in babies less than 1750 g is 45%, and it increases closer to 80% in very-low-birth-weight babies less than 1200 g weight. Patent ductus arteriosus with significant left-to-right shunt is associated with varied complications, such as necrotizing enterocolitis, intraventricular hemorrhage, and chronic lung disease in preterm babies. Effective and timely treatment of PDA enhances preterm survival and reduces the risk of complications. Studies showed that closure of hemodynamically significant PDA is beneficial but the timing and the best method of closure is not clear.

A hemodynamically significant duct is identified clinically by features of heart failure, bounding pulses, evidence of pulmonary overcirculation (tachypnea, tachycardia, and continued requirement of mechanical ventilation). An easily audible murmur often accompanies the hemodynamically significant duct, but this is typically absent if the duct is large and unrestrictive. Echocardiography aids considerably in determining the hemodynamic significance of a PDA. A size of greater than 1 mm/kg body weight is considered the minimum for the PDA to be of significance. Additional findings that suggest an important PDA include flow reversal in descending aorta and LA and LV enlargement.

Older Infants

Older infants with PDA present like any other posttricuspid shunts (such as VSD).

Treatment

Three modalities of definitive treatment are available for the PDA, and they need to be tailored to anatomy and clinical circumstances. For the preterm infant, indomethacin or ibuprofen should ideally be the first line of treatment. The younger the gestational age of the infant, the lesser is the likelihood of a response to indomethacin or ibuprofen. Beyond 10-day postnatal age, the ductus rarely responds to indomethacin.

In these circumstances, surgery should be considered.

Catheter closure has emerged as a very promising option for all forms of PDA. Two methods are available. They include coil occlusion and closure with occlusive devices. Today, surgery is reserved for large ducts in small infants.

AORTOPULMONARY WINDOW

This uncommon malformation consists of communication usually nonrestrictive between the adjacent walls of the ascending aorta and pulmonary trunk. The pathophysiology of aortopulmonary (AP) window is like that of a large PDA. In 80% of the patients the murmur is systolic rather than continuous and is punctuated by eddy sounds. A moderately restrictive AP window (rare) can generate a continuous murmur. Apical mid-diastolic murmur represents increased flow across the mitral valve. Aortopulmonary window requires early surgical correction.

OBSTRUCTIVE LESIONS

These lesions can be divided into two groups:

1. *Ventricular outflow obstructive lesions:*
    - Aortic stenosis
    - Pulmonary stenosis
    - Coarctation of aorta
2. *Stenosis of AV valves/ventricular inflow tract:*
    - Congenital mitral stenosis (MS)
    - Supramitral ring
    - Cor triatrium
    - Tricuspid stenosis.

Features common in ventricular outflow obstruction are concentric hypertrophy of the chamber proximal to obstruction due to pressure overload and an ESM due turbulent flow of blood through the obstruction.

Congenital Aortic Stenosis

The most common cause of congenital aortic stenosis (AS) is bicommissural aortic valve. The partial or complete fusion of commissures between right-left or right-noncoronary commissures results in variable degrees of severity of AS. Very severe stenosis presents early in newborn period with left ventricular dysfunction and heart failure; less sever forms present later.

Other forms of LV outflow tract obstruction are less common and include subaortic membrane and supravalvar AS. The latter is seen in association with the Williams-Beuren syndrome.

The symptoms of AS are related to LV outflow obstruction and include effort angina, dyspnea, syncope, and fatigue on effort. There is a significant risk of sudden death with severe AS, especially in adolescent and young adults.

The murmur of AS is loudest over the ascending aorta (i.e. upper right sternal border or aortic valve area) and characteristically radiates to the carotid arteries. Constant systolic ejections click just after the first heart sound is a consistent physical finding in bicommissural aortic valve. This is highly sensitive and specific in children and often better heard at the apex. The ECG is characterized by evidence of LV hypertrophy (voltage with strain in severe cases). Severe aortic valve stenosis can be relieved by balloon dilation in the catheterization laboratory. Many of these patients require aortic valve surgery to deal with progressive aortic regurgitation. Other forms of AS require surgical relief.

Congenital Pulmonary Stenosis

Like in AS, pulmonic stenosis may involve the valve or occur above or below the valve. Subvalvar or infundibular PS (double-chambered RV) results from hypertrophied muscle bundles within the RV cavity. In the common form of pulmonary valve stenosis, the valve is thickened, with fused or absent commissures. This valve characteristically domes in systole; the resultant click is best heard during expiration when the excursion of the valve is exaggerated by a relatively under-filled RV cavity. Another form of pulmonary valve stenosis is the dysplastic valve (frequent in Noonan syndrome) that is characterized by tethering of the leaflets to the adjacent main PA with narrowing of the main PA at the sinotubular junction.

Supravalvular PS often refers to the narrowing of branch PAs.

Most patients are acyanotic and well developed. Newborns with critical PS are cyanotic and tachypneic. The majority of patients are asymptomatic in infancy and childhood. Dyspnea and fatigue are mild, if the RV maintains normal stroke volume at rest and augments its stroke volume with exercise. The murmur of PS is loudest over main PA (i.e. second left intercostal space) and is associated with systolic thrill. The intensity and length of ESM is directly proportional to the severity of PS.

Wide spitting of S2 due to delayed closure of pulmonary valve. The pulmonary component of S2 is soft. An inconstant ejection click louder in expiration is also audible at the site of the murmur the interval between S1 and click varies inversely with the degree of PS. The ECG shows right ventricular hypertrophy (RVH). Neonates with critical PS may show predominant LV forces because of associated hypoplasia of RV.

Balloon valvotomy is a relatively simple intervention is now accepted as the standard treatment for valvar PS. While dysplastic valves have a characteristically suboptimal response, balloon is still attempted in them.

Coarctation of Aorta

Isolated coarctation is more common in males (3:1) and characterized by narrowing of aorta typically located near aortic attachment of ligamentum arteriosum or PDA.

It can be a localized or discrete narrowing or associated with long segment tubular hypoplasia of the segment proximal to the coarctation (isthmus). There are two types of presentations described: (1) symptomatic newborns or infants with heart failure and (2) relatively asymptomatic adolescent or young adults who may have "minor" symptoms in the form of headache, epistaxis, and leg fatigue.

Depending on the severity of obstruction, the femoral pulses are both weak and delayed (due to delayed upstroke of arterial pulse in lower extremity sites) or absent. This is a valuable physical sign and an excellent screening test in newborns as well.

In older children a systolic murmur is present over descending aorta, distal to obstruction (in left interscapular region). Sometimes, a continuous murmur of collaterals between vessels arising from pre- and postcoarctation segment is present over the back of the chest.

Hypertension with significant difference in upper and lower limb systolic blood pressure (>20 mm Hg) exaggerates on exercise. Is an inevitable consequence in older children and this accounts for most of the late morbidity? In addition, vascular complications, such as aortic dilation with aneurysm formation, and berry aneurysms in cerebral vasculature are commonly seen. The ECG in symptomatic infant shows RVH, while LVH is present in older children and adult.

Newborns with severe coarctation require surgery for lasting relief. In older children, balloon dilation is a less invasive option, and in adolescents and adults, stenting of the coarctation segment can yield maximum reduction in gradient. Irrespective of the treatment modality chosen, all patients with coarctation should ideally be followed lifelong for hypertension and vascular complications that may occur despite relief of the obstruction.

Congenital Mitral Stenosis

Congenital MS results from a variety of mechanisms that include a membrane at the level of the annulus (supramitral ring), thickening of chordal apparatus and reduction of leaflet motion, single papillary muscle (parachute mitral valve). The onset and severity of symptoms are related to the severity of MS. Congenital MS is often associated with other forms of left heart obstruction (LV outflow obstruction at various levels), coarctation (as a part of the Shones complex), and other CHD (such as VSD, DORV). Clinical examination is characterized by the typical mid-diastolic murmur with presystolic accentuation. However, unlike in rheumatic MS, the opening snap is unusual. Management is challenging. Surgical relief is often the only option (balloon mitral valvotomy seldom works for congenital MS). However, this too is unsatisfactory in most situations.

Cor Triatriatum

This is a rare anomaly in which LA is divided into two compartments by an abnormal fibromuscular septum with small opening, producing pulmonary venous return obstruction. Embryologically, this results from the failure of incorporation of embryonic common pulmonary vein into LA. Therefore the upper compartment is a dilated common pulmonary vein, and the lower compartment is the true LA. It produces pulmonary venous and PAH as in MS. This condition is easily amenable to surgery.

Tetralogy of Fallot

Among the cyanotic CHDs, TOF has a relatively favorable natural history that allows survival beyond infancy in about 75% of cases. As a result, it is the most common CHD encountered beyond the age of 1 year. The disease has been a subject of intense study over several decades.

The physiology is that of VSD with PS and has been described earlier in this chapter.

Anatomically, it is characterized by the classic tetrad: severe RV outflow obstruction, large VSD, aortic that overrides the VSD and RVH. Within this classic tetrad, there are numerous anatomical variations, most of which have an important bearing on treatment strategies **(Table 7.2.9)**.

Corrective operation for TOF involves closure of the VSD and relief of the RVOT obstruction. There is growing emphasis on retaining the pulmonary valve during initial repair to prevent pulmonary regurgitation and its major late consequences (RV dilation, arrhythmia, heart failure, and sudden death). However, this is not often possible, if the component(s) of the RVOT are small.

Although corrective operation is feasible in very young infants, many centers opt for palliative options initially. Palliation is possible in the very young through the BT shunt, balloon dilation of the pulmonary vale, or stenting of the patent arterial duct (if present). Cyanotic spells are a major concern in severe TOF, and its management and prevention has been elaborated upon in the section on complications.

Ebstein Anomaly

There is downward displacement of septal and the posterior leaflets of the tricuspid valve into the RV cavity. A portion of RV is incorporated in RA (atrialized RV). This contracts asynchronously with the RV, resulting either in right-to-left shunting via a patent foramen ovale (majority) or heart

Table 7.2.9: Anatomic variations in tetralogy of Fallot and their significance.

Structure	***Common variation***	***Implications***
RVOT	Degree of stenosis at various levels: infundibulum, valve, pulmonary annulus, main PA	Severe stenosis manifests early; annular narrowing requires correction with a transannular patch with significant late sequelae; predominant stenosis of the valve may allow palliation with a balloon valvotomy in selected cases
Branch PAs	Stenosis of LPA, absence of either branch PA, hypoplastic PAs	Small branch PA may not allow correction at an early age, sever stenosis of LPA origin will need to be addressed at the time of surgery, absence of one branch PA may require the placement of a conduit
Pulmonary valve	Absent pulmonary valve with aneurysmal branch PAs	This results in a dramatically different manifestation. There is severe airway compression in the worst affected and the manifestations are essentially related to respiratory consequences
VSD	Extension of the VSD to the inlet or outlet septum, restrictive VSD with sever right ventricular hypertrophy and strain, additional muscular VSD	Surgical approach needs to be tailored accordingly
Coronary arteries	Origin of left anterior descending artery from right coronary artery. This abnormal vessel may cross the RVOT	The abnormal vessel comes in the way of corrective surgery. If it is running along the pulmonary annulus, a transannular patch is not feasible, and this may require a conduit
Atrial communication	ASDs, PFO	While it is necessary to close and ASD, a PFO is often helpful in the early postoperative period. Many surgeons chose to leave it behind because it helps with early postoperative recovery
Aortopulmonary collaterals	Large major aortopulmonary collaterals	These collaterals will need to be clearly defined. They will need to be closed if their supply overlaps with the native PA supply

(ASD: atrial septal defect; LPA: left pulmonary artery; PAs: pulmonary arteries; PFO: patent foramen ovale; RVOT: right ventricular outflow tract; VSD: ventricular septal defect)

Table 7.2.10: Cardiac emergencies in the newborn.

Physiologic category	*Conditions*	*Manifestation*
Duct-dependent systemic blood flow*	Hypoplastic left heart syndrome, critical coarctation, interruption of aortic arch, critical aortic stenosis	Heart failure, shock, circulatory failure, acidosis
Duct-dependent pulmonary blood flow*	Pulmonary atresia, critical pulmonary stenosis, Ebstein anomaly	Cyanosis, hypoxia
Obstruction of pulmonary venous return	Obstructed total anomalous pulmonary venous return, mitral atresia with a restrictive patent foramen ovale	Cyanosis, hypoxia, heart failure
Parallel circulation with poor mixing	Dextro-transposition with intact ventricular septum	Cyanosis, hypoxia
Valve regurgitation	Congenital mitral valve regurgitation	Heart failure
High-output state	Atrioventricular (AV) malformations (usually intracranial)	Heart failure
Myocardial dysfunction	Myocardial diseases (inflammatory and metabolic)	Heart failure
Tachyarrhythmia	Atrial flutter, neonatal atrioventricular reentrant tachycardias, ectopic trial tachycardia	Tachycardia, heart failure
Bradyarrhythmia	Complete heart block	Bradycardia, heart failure

*Some of the duct-dependent conditions (critical PS, AS, coarctation) manifest with varying severity. The most severe forms manifest early (in the first few days) with absolute dependence on the duct for survival. Others may manifest later in the neonatal period (first few weeks) with heart failure or cyanosis and may not be strictly "duct dependent."

failure (rare). In addition, there is also an additional leak through the severely deformed tricuspid valve. Presentation is variable and dependent on the severity of the involvement. Severe disease may manifest in the newborn period. Mild disease may resent for the first time in adulthood. Reentrant arrhythmias are a frequent accompaniment, and this may result from accessory (bypass) tracts in the region of the displaced leaflets.

NEONATAL HEART DISEASE

Because of the fact that many heart diseases that present in the newborn period are potentially fatal and need to be recognized early, it is important to be familiar with them. **Table 7.2.10** describes the most common CHD that present in the newborn period. For a detailed description on the individual conditions, the reader should refer to standard textbooks included in the reference.

SELECTED HEART DISEASE THAT PRESENT IN THE NEWBORN PERIOD

Dextro-transposition of the Great Arteries

This condition is characterized by parallel circulation resulting from aorta arising from RV and PA arising from LV. Hypoxia is inevitable, and survival is dependent upon communications at the atrial, ventricular, or great vessel level that allows mixing between the two parallel circulations. Such a communication is created at the atrial level by a balloon atrial septostomy procedure or by PGE1 that opens the closing ductus arteriosus. The neonatal arterial switch operation has dramatically transformed the outlook of transposition. This operation needs to be done early. The operation is ideally performed within 2–4 weeks for dextro-TGA (D-TGA) with intact ventricular septum because of the regression of the LV that is connected to the low resistance pulmonary circuit. In D-TGA with a large VSD the concern relates to rapid development of PVOD, and these babies often need surgery before 3 months of age.

Total Anomalous Pulmonary Venous Connection

This condition, as the name suggests, involves all pulmonary veins that typically come together in a confluence or a common chamber, which then drains into the right atrium often via one of the systemic venous channels draining into the heart.

The critical determinant of physiology is whether pulmonary venous drainage is obstructed or not. Obstructed total anomalous pulmonary venous connection (TAPVC) presents early, often in the newborn period with heart failure and hypoxia. Severe pulmonary hypertension is invariably present. Emergency surgery often offers the only prospect for survival. Unobstructed TAPVC presents variably, often a little later in infancy. A small fraction of unobstructed TAPVC (~10%) remains relatively symptom free and present late like an ASD.

BIBLIOGRAPHY

1. Allen HD, Shaddy RE, Driscoll DJ, et al. Moss Adams' Heart Disease in Infants, Children and Adolescents, 7th edition. Philadelphia, PA: Kluwer/Lippincott William and Wilkins; 2008.
2. Kumar RK, Shrivastava S. Pediatric heart care in India. Heart. 2008;94:984-90.
3. Kumar RK, Prabhu SS, Ahamed Z. IAP Specialty Textbook of Pediatric Cardiology. New Delhi: Jaypee Brothers Medical Publishers (P) Ltd.; 2008.
4. Saxena A, Mehta A, Ramakrishnan S, et al. Pulse oximetry as a screening tool for detecting major congenital heart defects in Indian newborns. Arch Dis Child Fetal Neonatal Ed. 2015;100(5):F416-21.
5. Vaidyanathan B, Sathish G, Mohanan S, et al. Clinical screening for congenital heart disease at birth: a prospective study in a community hospital in Kerala. Indian Pediatr. 2011;48:25-30.
6. Vaidyanathan B, Radhakrishnan R, Aravindakshan DS, et al. What determines nutritional recovery in malnourished children undergoing correction of congenital heart defects? A prospective study. Pediatrics. 2009;124:e294-9.
7. Viswanathan S, Kumar RK. Assessment of operability in congenital cardiac shunts with increased pulmonary vascular resistance. Catheter Cardiovasc Interv. 2008;71:665-70.

7.3 Rheumatic Fever and Rheumatic Heart Disease

Savitri Shrivastava

INTRODUCTION

In early 20th century, there has been a marked decline in the prevalence of rheumatic fever (RF) in developed world. The earlier decline is related to the improved standards of living hygiene, health, literacy (particularly of females), medical facilities, etc. Further decline occurred with easy availability of penicillin to treat streptococcal throat infection. The reported incidence of RF in Indian series varies from 0.42 to 10.9 per 1,000, and the prevalence of rheumatic heart disease (RHD) using clinical criteria as reported varies from 0.56 to 11 per 1,000. Studies from some parts of India (Kerala/Chandigarh) suggest that there is a decline in the prevalence. Recent studies in India using echocardiography show a prevalence of RHD from 0.12 to 0.67 per 1,000.

ETIOPATHOGENESIS

Several studies have suggested that RF follows group A beta hemolytic streptococcal pharyngitis. Outbreaks of RF usually occur with epidemics of pharyngitis due to rheumatogenic strains of streptococci. Rheumatic fever and recurrences can be prevented with specific antimicrobial treatment. The most accepted postulation is that M proteins from the rheumatogenic strains share certain epitomes with cardiac myocytes and sarcolemmal membrane protein. Antibodies produced in the host by these epitomes cross-react with cardiac tissues and produce pancarditis (i.e. involving pericardium, myocardium, and endocardium). The data is not clear if this host response is related to genetic programming, acquired alterations in host defense or immunological mechanisms.

Pathologically, acute RF results in diffuse exudative and proliferative reaction resulting in infiltration with lymphocytes, polymorphonuclear leukocytes, histiocytes, and eosinophils. In some areas, typical Aschoff nodules are formed with aggregation of multinucleated giant cells. These inflammatory changes are diffuse affecting heart, large joints, brain, and subcutaneous tissue. Long-term sequelae occur as a result of involvement of endocardium of valvular and subvalvular regions resulting in valvular heart disease. The most common involvement is of mitral valve [most common being mitral regurgitation (MR)], followed by aortic [aortic regurgitation (AR) is more common], tricuspid, and very rarely pulmonary valves. Microscopically, there is edema, inflammatory cell infiltration, and capillary proliferation. Inflammatory infiltrates are also frequently seen in myocardium with scanty injury and loss of myocardial fibers. Pericardial involvement results in fibrinous pericarditis, which may result in pericardial effusion which is serosanguinous. It usually resolves completely, never causing constrictive pericarditis. Small pericardial effusion is common but cardiac tamponade rarely occurs.

Acute RF with carditis results in valvular regurgitation most commonly of the mitral valve of variable severity. This is due to plastering and thickening of posterior leaflet, thickening and retraction of anterior leaflet, and lack of normal coaptation. With aortic involvement, AR is the most common abnormality. Rarely, the tricuspid valve is involved; pulmonary valve is usually not involved in the acute attack.

CLINICAL FEATURES

The classical clinical picture of RF consists of streptococcal sore throat followed 10 days to few weeks later by various manifestations of RF, although the history of acute streptococcal sore throat is available only in 50% of patients. The guidelines for the diagnosis of acute RF were originally suggested by T Duckett Jones in 1944, subsequently revised by the American Heart Association in 1965, updated in 1992 and later revised and updated **(Table 7.3.1)** by World Health Organization in 2003. The criteria have been revised in 2015. The guidelines consist of major, minor, and essential criteria. Two major or one major and two minor criteria are required in the presence of essential criteria to diagnose acute RF. It is important to emphasize that these guidelines are meant to help a physician in making a firm diagnosis of RF and do not mean that a physician should not use his/her clinical judgment in diagnosing acute RF in the absence of these criteria.

Table 7.3.1: Revised Jones criteria for the diagnosis of acute rheumatic fever.

Major criteria	***Minor criteria***
Carditis	Arthralgia
Chorea	Previous rheumatic fever or rheumatic heart disease (RHD)
Erythema marginatum	
Polyarthritis	Fever
Subcutaneous nodules	• Elevated erythrocyte sedimentation rate (ESR) or C-reactive protein or leukocytosis • Prolonged PR interval on electrocardiogram (ECG)
Essential criteria	
Evidence for recent streptococcal infection as indicated by: • Increased levels of antibodies against streptococci • Positive throat culture for group "A" *Streptococcus* • Recent scarlet fever	

Major Criteria

Carditis

The rheumatic carditis is a pancarditis involving pericardium, myocardium, and endocardium. Carditis occurs in 34–90% of patients with acute RF. It is an early manifestation of RF so that by the time a patient seeks help, the patient already has evidence of carditis. Almost 80% of those patients who develop carditis do so within the first 2 weeks of the onset of RF.

- *Pericarditis:* Pericarditis results in precordial pain, which may be quite severe. On auscultation, a pericardial friction rub is present. Clinical pericarditis is seen in approximately 15% of those who have carditis. The electrocardiogram (ECG) may show ST and T changes consistent with pericarditis. As a rule, rheumatic pericarditis is associated with only small pericardial effusion and does not result in either tamponade or constrictive pericarditis. A patient of rheumatic pericarditis always has additional MR or AR murmurs or both. If after the disappearance of the pericardial friction rub, there are no murmurs, it is unlikely to be due to RF.
- *Myocarditis:* The features diagnostic of myocarditis are (1) cardiac enlargement, (2) soft S1, (3) protodiastolic (S3) gallop, (4) congestive cardiac failure, and (5) Carey Coombs murmur. Carey Coombs murmur is a low-pitched delayed diastolic mitral murmur heard during the course of acute RF. It tends to disappear after the myocarditis subsides. Most likely it is due to increased diastolic flow secondary to MR across inflamed rigid mitral valve. The disappearance can be explained by the decrease in the left ventricular (LV) size following subsidence of myocarditis and better function of mitral valve—papillary muscle complex resulting in decrease in MR and subsidence of inflammation causing decrease in turbulent flow.
- *Endocarditis:* Endocardial lesions are most important and tend to leave permanent scarring in most cases. The endocardial inflammation is most severe and common in the mitral and aortic valves, less common in the tricuspid valve, and least in the pulmonary valve. The inflammation results in regurgitation murmurs. The most common finding of carditis is apical pansystolic murmur of MR occurring in 92–95% of patients. Aortic valve involvement results in early diastolic murmur of AR. Aortic valve is involved in 20–25% of cases; it is an isolated finding in only 5–8% of cases. Pathologically, tricuspid valve involvement is seen in 30–50% of cases. Clinical involvement of tricuspid valve in the first attack of RF is extremely uncommon. Pulmonary valve involvement alone is almost never seen in acute RF.

Noncardiac Manifestations of Rheumatic Fever

- *Arthritis*: Rheumatic arthritis is a fleeting polyarthritis involving large joints, such as knees, ankles, and elbows. Uncommonly smaller joints can be involved. The arthritis is typically migratory. The affected joints have redness, warmth, swelling, pain, and limitation of movements. It is an early manifestation and occurs in 30–50% of cases in our country; there is no residual damage of the joints.

- *Subcutaneous nodules*: Subcutaneous nodules appear as nontender, nodules varying in size from pin head to almond on bony prominences, such as shin, wrist, elbow, knee, ankle, spine, and occiput. They are late manifestations occurring around 6 weeks after the onset of RF, rarely as early as 3 weeks after the onset. In Indian series, their incidence is 5–20%. Usually they disappear in a few days to a few weeks rarely lasting even up to 1 year. Patients who have nodules always have carditis. Persistence of nodules is associated with chronic carditis.
- *Chorea*: Chorea is characterized by purposeless jerky movements resulting in abnormal speech, muscular incoordination, dropping of articles, awkward gait, and weakness. There is also emotional instability. Chorea is three to four times more common in females. It is a late manifestation occurring about 3 months after the onset of acute RF. It is reported to occur in 5–36% of cases. It is usually self-limiting.
- *Erythema marginatum*: The rash is reddish, not raised above the skin and nonitching, with serpiginous margins. It starts as a red spot with a pale center, increasing in size to coalesce with adjacent lesions to form serpiginous margin. It increases by applying heat. Though specific but seen extremely rarely in India, probably due to dark complexion.

Minor Criteria

They are divided into clinical and laboratory examinations.

Clinical

- *Fever*: Usually present in 90% of patients, the temperature usually goes up to 39.5°C.
- *Arthralgia*: Subjective joint pains without physical signs are labeled as arthralgias. Many Indian authors take it as major criteria.
- History of previous RF or RHD.

Laboratory

- Acute phase reactants consists of polymorphonuclear leukocytosis, increased erythrocyte sedimentation rate (ESR), and presence of C-reactive protein (CRP). The leukocyte count usually is between 10,000/mm^3 and 15,000/mm^3. The ESR is almost always elevated during acute RF and remains so for 4–10 weeks in almost 80% of patients. In a small proportion of patients, it may remain elevated even beyond 12 weeks. C-reactive protein is a beta globulin, which is increased uniformly in all patients of acute RF. Absence of raised CRP goes strongly against the diagnosis of acute RF. Presence of increased CRP, however, is not diagnostic since it becomes positive in many infections.
- *Electrocardiogram*: Prolonged PR interval is a nondiagnostic criterion since it can occur in many infections. Higher grades of block, such as second-degree atrioventricular (AV) block, especially of the Wenckebach type, may also be seen. Complete AV block is extremely rare as a manifestation of acute RF. Prolongation of QTc (corrected QT interval) is suggestive of myocarditis.

Essential Criteria

The essential criteria include evidence of recent streptococcal infection.

- The best out of these is the presence of antibodies against streptococci. The most common in use is the antistreptolysin "O" titer. Considerable confusion exists regarding the levels, which should be considered significant as the normal values differ significantly in different areas. Elevated levels of antistreptolysin "O" only indicate previous streptococcal infection, and not RF. The higher the level, more the likelihood of a recent streptococcal infection; lower level considered "normal" do not necessarily exclude a recent streptococcal infection. Rising titers of antistreptolysin "O" is a strong evidence of a recent streptococcal infection. To increase the sensitivity, other antibodies can also be tested. Antideoxyribonuclease B, antihyaluronidase, and streptozyme are used by many centers. Single antibody sensitivity is 70%. With two antibodies tested, it rises to 90%, and with three antibodies tested, it rises to 95%. With paired sera testing of single antibody, the sensitivity is 80% rising to 99% if paired sera of two antibodies are tested.
- Positive throat culture for streptococci is relatively uncommon when a patient presents with acute RF. Positive throat culture cannot be equated with the diagnosis of RF. Positive throat culture means that streptococci are present in the throat. The patient may or may not have RF.
- The third feature suggestive of the diagnosis of recent streptococcal infection is the history of recent scarlet fever. The desquamation of skin of palms and soles indicates that the patient has had scarlet fever within the previous 2 weeks. Scarlet fever is rare in India.

TREATMENT

There is no specific treatment. Management is symptomatic combined with suppressive therapy **(Table 7.3.2)**. In suppressive therapy, either aspirin or steroids can be used. The total duration of aspirin or steroid therapy is generally 12 weeks. With aspirin, the full doses are given for 10 weeks and then tapered off in the next 2 weeks. The dose of aspirin is 90–120 mg/kg/day in four divided doses (if facilities for blood salicylate level estimation are available, the dose is modified to maintain a blood salicylate level of 20–25 mg/dL for 10 weeks and later tapered off over 2 weeks).

Table 7.3.2: Treatment of acute rheumatic fever.

Bed rest
• It is advised in all patients with carditis till activity subsides • Total bed rest may have to be continued for 2–3 months, especially in the presence of congestive failure
Diet
• Salt restriction is not necessary unless congestive cardiac failure is present • Easily digestible nutritious diet with vitamin supplements should be given
Antimicrobial therapy
• *Penicillin*: After testing skin sensitivity, procaine penicillin 400,000 U, intramuscularly (IM), twice daily for 10 days or a single dose of benzathine penicillin or oral penicillin for 10 days, followed by prophylactic injection of benzathine penicillin • 1.2 mega units every 21 days above 10 years of age • 0.6 mega units 1 M every 15 days, if the age is less than 10 years • Alternatively oral penicillin V in a dose of 250 BID daily • Patients sensitive to penicillin should be advised to take erythromycin 20–40 mg/kg in two divided doses
Suppressive therapy
• Aspirin or steroids are given as suppressive therapy • For patients having carditis with congestive cardiac failure, use of steroids is generally mandatory • For carditis without congestive cardiac failure, one may use either steroids or aspirin, but most use steroids • For patients without carditis, it is preferable to use aspirin
Management of chorea
• Usually self-limiting • Complete physical and mental rest • In resistant cases, phenobarbitone, 3–5 mg/kg/day • Chlorpromazine, diazepam, diphenhydramine, haloperidol, or promethazine can also be used

Full doses of steroids are given as prednisolone 2 mg/kg/day for 3–4 weeks and then tapered gradually to cover a total period of 10–12 weeks.

PREVENTION

It would be ideal to provide primary prevention of RF. Primary prevention requires identification of streptococcal sore throat and its treatment with penicillin in the population. The treatment modalities have been summarized in **Table 7.3.3**. Its success depends on the awareness of parents regarding dangers of sore throat. Therefore, for primary prevention, it is necessary to educate the community regarding the consequences of streptococcal sore throat. Logistically, it is difficult in our country since it requires (1) identification of sore throat, which is dependent on education of parents; (2) rapid laboratory confirmation of streptococcal infection of the throat; and (3) medical help and availability of penicillin.

Table 7.3.3: Drugs for primary prophylaxis of acute rheumatic fever (treatment of streptococcal sore throat).

Drugs	***Dose***	***Sore throat treatment (duration)***
Benzathine penicillin G (deep IM injection) after sensitivity test (AST)	1.2 million unit (>27 kg) 0.6 million unit (<27 kg)	Single dose
Penicillin V (oral)	*Children*: 250 mg qid *Adult*: 500 mg tid	10 days
Azithromycin (oral)	12.5 mg/kg/day once daily	5 days
Cephalexin (oral)	15–20 mg/kg/dose bid	10 days

Secondary prevention consists in giving long-acting benzathine penicillin intramuscularly. The dose is 1.2 mega units once every 3 weeks in patients above the age of 10 years or 0.6 mega units every 2 weeks below the age of 10 years. The injection is painful, and some patients get fever for 24–36 hours following the injection. As such, it is preferable to give the injection on a Saturday afternoon to avoid loss of studies for the child.

In the presence of carditis, ideally penicillin prophylaxis should continue lifelong. Less than ideal would be to continue it till the age of 35 years. If there is only polyarthritis but no carditis, usually the penicillin prophylaxis should be given for 5 years after the attack, and subsequently, all clinical attacks of streptococcal sore throat should be treated with penicillin. If there is allergy to penicillin (which is very rare in children), erythromycin can be used but this is not ideal.

CHRONIC RHEUMATIC HEART DISEASE

In pediatric cardiac practice, roughly 20–25% of cases have RHD, with crippling valvular heart disease in many of them. Mitral valve is the most common valve involved in RHD. It may be regurgitant, stenotic, or may have combined regurgitation and stenosis, combined mitral and aortic valve disease in the next common subset. Isolated aortic valve involvement is seen only in 2–8% of cases. Isolated rheumatic tricuspid valve disease does not occur. Tricuspid stenosis occurs rarely and mostly with mitral stenosis (MS).

MITRAL REGURGITATION

Clinical Features

Exertional fatigue and palpitation are common features. Exertional dyspnea and features of right-sided cardiac failure are late manifestations of severe grades of MR and LV failure.

There is no tachycardia, tachypnea, or basal rales unless significant LV overload/failure occurs. The pulse pressure is wide with significant MR. The cardiac size increases with increasing severity of MR resulting in LV hyperdynamic impulse downward and outward. There may be a palpable LVS3. The S1 may be soft, normal, or loud. It may be masked by the murmur. The S2 is normal with mild MR; with severe grades of MR, it becomes wide variable split due to early A2 as LV systole is shortened due to part of stroke volume regurgitating in the left atrium. With severe MR and congestive heart failure (CHF), P2 becomes loud due to high pulmonary arterial pressures. Left ventricular S3 is generally audible with significant MR due to increase in early diastolic filling. Moderate-to-severe degree of MR results in a low-pitched delayed diastolic murmur at the apex, which may be palpable as a diastolic thrill. A diastolic thrill is more commonly felt with MR than a systolic thrill. Systolic thrill is uncommonly felt at apex in MR as the blood is regurgitating in the left atrium, which is posteriorly placed. The diagnostic feature of MR is a pansystolic murmur best heard at the apex and radiating to the axilla. With significant MR, a low-frequency delayed diastolic murmur is audible at the apex; the duration of murmur increases with increasing severity of MR. If MR is severe, the diastolic rumble is audible throughout diastole but has no presystolic accentuation in the absence of MS. In patients with severe MR, there are also features of CHF, such as raised jugular venous pressure (JVP) and hepatomegaly.

Differential Diagnosis

In a child with MR, one should keep in mind other causes, such as mitral valve prolapse, cleft mitral valve, levo-transposition with regurgitant left AV valve, and connective tissue disorders.

Investigations

- *Electrocardiogram*: It reveals sinus rhythm and may be normal with mild MR. With increasing degree of MR, left atrial (LA) overload and LV volume overload are seen. Left atrial enlargement results in bifid "P" wave (P-mitrale). LV enlargement results in tall R waves in left-sided leads (I, augmented vector left, V5, V6) with deep "Q" waves indicating volume overload of left ventricle. In the cases of severe MR, right ventricular (RV) hypertrophy may be seen due to the development of pulmonary hypertension.
- *Chest X-ray*: Significant MR results in LA and LV enlargement with the changes of pulmonary venous hypertension.
- *Echocardiogram*: It clearly shows the altered valve pathology, degree of LA and LV enlargement and function, and quantum of regurgitation.

Management

Symptomatic patients with moderate-to-severe MR will need decongestive therapy [including angiotensin-converting enzyme (ACE) inhibitors]. The patients should be carefully evaluated if the mitral valve could be repaired surgically. Patients with severe MR with decreasing LV ejection fraction need early surgical intervention. If the valve cannot be repaired, they will need mitral valve replacement.

RHEUMATIC MITRAL STENOSIS

Clinical Features

In pediatric age group, male patients commonly have MS. The patient complains of shortness of breath on exertion initially. With increasing severity, this becomes more severe, and the child becomes breathless on walking short distances. Subsequently, the child starts getting paroxysmal nocturnal dyspnea and breathlessness at rest. In the later stages, with the development of severe pulmonary hypertension and tricuspid regurgitation (TR), features of CHF develop. The patient can also have hemoptysis or pulmonary edema due to severe pulmonary venous hypertension. On examination, there may be tachycardia and low pulse volume. Jugular venous pressure is normal with mild MS. With severe MS and TR, elevated JVP with prominent "V" wave (due to regurgitation of blood into right atrium) and rapid "Y" descent is seen (in the presence of TR without tricuspid stenosis). Enlarged and tender hepatomegaly, which may be pulsatile, is seen with severe TR. Respiratory rate with mild MS is normal; tachypnea develops with significant MS. Basal crepitations are also heard with significant MS. If the patient develops pulmonary edema, severe respiratory distress, extensive rales, and cyanosis are seen.

Precordial examination reveals normal heart size in most cases. Cardiac enlargement is seen in the presence of CHF and TR. The apex beat is tapping; parasternal heave is present with the development of pulmonary hypertension. At this stage, P2 many also be palpable. Mild TR does not result in RV dilatation. Therefore, there is no parasternal pulsation. Significant TR results in RV dilatation resulting in parasternal lift. If the pressure in the right ventricle is elevated, parasternal pulsations can be seen, and on palpation, parasternal heave is felt. A systolic thrill is rarely felt along left or right sternal border. A diastolic thrill could be felt at the apex. On auscultation, the S1 is loud; S2 is normally split with loud pulmonary component, loudness depending on the degree of pulmonary hypertension. An opening snap—hallmark for the diagnosis of MS—is audible at the apex at the beginning of diastole. The closer the opening snap is to the A2, the severe is the MS. A low-pitched delayed diastolic rumble is audible at the apex with presystolic accentuation immediately after the opening snap. In the presence of significant TR, systolic pulsations can be felt over the liver, which enlarges with the development of CHF. A systolic murmur along the left sternal border increasing with inspiration or leg raising is the hallmark for the diagnosis of TR. With significant regurgitation, S3 can be heard in the tricuspid area; if the quantum of regurgitation is significant, a delayed diastolic murmur across tricuspid valve is heard. Rarely, an opening snap and presystolic accentuation of the diastolic murmur is heard, if tricuspid stenosis is present.

Investigations

- *Electrocardiogram*: The rhythm is usually sinus. With increasing pulmonary hypertension, increasing degree of right axis deviation, RV hypertrophy (tall R wave in right-sided leads), and right atrial (RA) overload (tall peaked "P" wave) are seen.
- *Chest X-ray*: Heart size is usually normal, with the development of TR and CHF. Cardiomegaly develops due to RA and RV enlargement. The left atrium is enlarged. Features of varying grades of pulmonary venous and arterial hypertensions are also seen.
- Two-dimensional echocardiogram with color flow mapping clearly shows the stenotic mitral valve; the mitral valve area can be calculated. The gradient across the mitral valve is calculated by taking the velocity of the mitral inflow on Doppler. The peak velocity of TR gives the estimate of pulmonary arterial pressures.

Differential Diagnosis

Cor triatriatum, supramitral ring, congenital MS, and LA myxoma are rare entities that can sometimes mimic MS.

Management

Salt-restricted diet and diuretics are useful to reduce the pulmonary venous congestion. If there is evidence of cardiomegaly and CHF, digoxin is useful. Basically, the mitral obstruction has to be relieved. Presently, balloon dilatation of mitral valve percutaneously is the method of choice. If it is not feasible, surgical closed mitral valvotomy is done. Both procedures have identical results. Both these procedures relieve the commissural fusion, and to some extent, the subvalvular fusion but chordae shortening and fusion are not relieved. If there is marked fibrosis of the valve and subvalvular apparatus, open surgical commissurotomy may be needed.

AORTIC REGURGITATION

Clinical Features

Aortic regurgitation is common in male patients. The presenting symptom is usually palpitation and increased neck pulsations due to high stroke volume. Exertional fatigue and dyspnea develop in patients with significant AR, which become more prominent with the development of CHF. The pulse pressure is the best clinical parameter to assess the degree of AR. The wider the pulse pressure, severe is the regurgitation. The wide pulse pressure results in several signs **(Table 7.3.4)**. It also results in prominent neck, suprasternal, peripheral, and abdominal pulsations. The pulse shows a sharp rise and fall the so-called water hammer pulse that becomes more evident on elevating the arm. Nodding of the head with cardiac cycle may be seen (de Musset's sign). The increased pressure difference between the systolic pressure of upper and lower limbs is called Hill's sign. Normally, this difference is less than 20 mm Hg. With mild, moderate, and severe regurgitation, it is 20–40, 40–60, and greater than 60 mm Hg, respectively. Pistol-shot sounds can be heard over large arteries with significant regurgitation. If slight pressure is applied over these arteries, a systolic murmur can be heard, and if pressure is applied distally, a diastolic murmur is heard. This is called Duroziez sign. Palpation of the precordium may be unremarkable with mild AR; with significant regurgitation, the cardiac apex is displaced down and out and is of LV hyperdynamic type. The greater the amount of regurgitation, the bigger is the heart size. Rarely with severe regurgitation, the whole of the precordium is pulsatile. The S3 may be felt over the LV apex. In some cases, a systolic thrill may be felt in second left intercostal space. The S1 is soft, the S2 is normally split with mild-to-moderate regurgitation; it may be paradoxical with severe regurgitation, particularly with LV failure. The murmur of AR is high-pitched decrescendo

Table 7.3.4: Peripheral signs of aortic regurgitation (AR).

Sign	Description
Corrigan's pulse	Dancing carotids
De Musset's sign	Head nodding
Quincke's sign	Capillary pulsations over nail bed
Traube's sign	Pistol-shot sounds over femorals
Hill's sign	Lower extremity blood pressure > upper extremity blood pressure >20 mm Hg—mild AR >40 mm Hg—moderate AR >60 mm Hg—severe AR
Muller's sign	Systolic pulsation of uvula
Rosenbach's sign	Pulsatile liver
Gerhardt's sign	Enlarged pulsatile spleen
Light house sign	Blanching and flushing of forehead
Landolfi's sign	Alternating constriction and dilatation of pupil
Becker sign	Visible pulsations of retinal arteries seen through ophthalmoscope

diastolic starting with A2. A systolic ejection murmur is commonly heard in the aortic area conducted to the neck in the cases with significant AR. Delayed diastolic rumble is heard in some cases of AR (Austin Flint murmur). Some of the other signs have been listed in **Table 7.3.4**.

Investigations

- *Electrocardiogram:* The ECG may be normal with mild AR. If significant regurgitation is present, the ECG shows evidence volume overload of left ventricles—increased LV voltage with prominent "Q" waves and tall "T" waves. In patients with severe AR, particularly in the presence of CHF, LA overload may also be seen.
- *X-ray chest:* In the cases of mild AR, there is no cardiomegaly, and aorta may be prominent. With increasing AR, heart size enlarges due to enlarged left ventricle. Changes of pulmonary venous hypertension develop with severe regurgitation and LV failure.
- *Echocardiography:* Two-dimensional and color Doppler echocardiography can confirm the diagnosis and also estimate the severity of AR, degree of LV enlargement and function.

Differential Diagnosis

In the case of isolated AR, one should look for Marfan syndrome, Hurler syndrome, and nonspecific aortoarteritis. The other causes of AR, such as congenital aortic valve disease, rupture sinus of Valsalva, or ventricular septal defect with AR, should be kept in mind.

Management

Mild AR is well tolerated. Significant AR causing LV dilatation may benefit with ACE inhibitors. If the left ventricle is progressively dilating and the patient is symptomatic or there is evidence of CHF, decongestive therapy along with ACE inhibitor should be started and patient planned for surgery, aortic valve repair, or replacement. In most of these patients, the aortic valve repair is not possible, and they end up with valve replacement. The improvement with surgery is remarkable, but with prosthetic valve, the child has to take lifelong anticoagulant therapy with its own inherent hazards.

TRICUSPID REGURGITATION

Tricuspid regurgitation is commonly seen in patients of rheumatic mitral valve disease (20–50%). It can be functional or organic. If TR is present in the absence of severe pulmonary arterial hypertension (PAH), it is likely to be organic, but if PAH is present, it can be either functional, organic, or both.

Clinical Features

There are no specific symptoms of TR except pain in right hypochondria and fatigue due to low cardiac output. The symptoms will depend on the lesion with which TR is associated. The signs diagnostic of TR are prominent "V" wave with rapid "Y" descent in JVP, systolic pulsations over liver, systolic murmur at lower left or right sternal border, increasing in severity with inspiration. It may sometimes be associated with a systolic thrill, enlarged right ventricle, S3, and delayed diastolic rumble over tricuspid area. Tricuspid stenosis results in slow Y descent in JVP, diastolic rumble with presystolic accentuation in the tricuspid area, and rarely an opening snap before the diastolic rumble. The other physical finding will be of the associated lesion; isolated tricuspid valve diseases of rheumatic etiology do not occur.

Investigations

Electrocardiogram may reveal evidence of RA and RV overload pattern in addition to other changes due to the associated lesions. Significant TR results in cardiac enlargement due to the dilatation of right atrium and right ventricle. Two-dimensional and color Doppler evaluation easily confirms tricuspid valve disease. The degree of regurgitation is estimated by color flow mapping.

Management

The presence of significant TR results in cardiomegaly and CHF, and the patients need decongestive therapy. The complete management will depend on the associated valvular lesions. Severe grades of TR results in dilatation of tricuspid annulus. If the tricuspid annulus is greater than 21 mm/m^2, then it has to be repaired by annuloplasty in addition to the other valvular lesions at surgery.

BIBLIOGRAPHY

1. Gewitz MH, Baltimore RS, Tani LY, et al. Revision of the Jones criteria for the diagnosis of acute rheumatic fever in the era of Doppler echocardiography: a scientific statement from the American Heart Association. Circulation. 2015;131(20):1806-18.
2. Jones TD. The diagnosis of rheumatic fever. JAMA. 1994;126:481-4.
3. Kumar PK, Paul M, Francis TP. RHD in Indian: are we ready to shift from secondary prophylaxis to vaccinating high-risk children? Curr Sci. 2009;97:397-404.
4. Misra M, Mittal M, Singh R, et al. Prevalence of rheumatic heart disease in school-going children of Eastern Uttar Pradesh. Indian Heart J. 2007;59:42-3.
5. Padmawati S. Rheumatic fever and rheumatic heart disease in India at the turn of the century. Indian Heart J. 2001;53:35-7.

7.4 Congestive Heart Failure

Anita Saxena

INTRODUCTION

Congestive heart failure (HF) is a complex syndrome resulting from multiple causes, which are different in children as compared to adults. This term is increasingly being replaced by HF, since peripheral congestion may not be present in all cases. Several definitions have been proposed for HF, which again reflects our less than complete understanding of this enigma. A commonly used definition is "it is a pathophysiological state in which an abnormality of cardiac function is responsible for the failure of the heart to pump blood at a rate commensurate with the requirements of the metabolizing tissues, or does so only at elevated filling pressures." In the case of children, this requirement includes growth and development.

Heart failure in infants and children is commonly secondary to congenital heart defects (shunts or obstructive lesions). Less common causes include cardiomyocyte dysfunction secondary to myocarditis/cardiomyopathies. Heart failure in children is often a transient state that is secondary to an underlying condition. Palliated congenital heart disease (CHD) leading to HF is increasingly being recognized.

CAUSES OF HEART FAILURE IN INFANTS AND CHILDREN

Children can have diverse causes of HF depending on the age, geographical location, and many other factors. The prominent causes of HF or ventricular dysfunction in children have been provided in **Table 7.4.1. Table 7.4.2** enumerates the likely causes of HF by age at presentation. This is important as the symptoms and signs of HF can be confusing or nonspecific in children.

Table 7.4.1: Causes of heart failure in children by underlying pathology.

Cause	*Comment*
Volume overload (relative or absolute)	CHD with increased pulmonary blood flow (VSD, PDA, AVSD, TGA, truncus, TAPVC, etc.)* arteriovenous fistula or malformations, anemia, thyrotoxicosis†
Obstructive lesions/atretic valves or great vessels	AS, PS, mitral valve atresia or stenosis, coarctation of aorta, aortic interruption‡
Regurgitant lesions (MR/TR)	Congenital (e.g. as part of AVSD, Ebstein anomaly), acquired (e.g. RF/RHD), postoperative*
Myocyte dysfunction (pump failure)	
Primary	Inborn errors of metabolism, muscular dystrophies, DCM, drug induced, hemoglobinopathies†
Inflammatory	Myocarditis, Chagas, HIV*
Hemodynamic	Obstructive or regurgitant lesions, HT‡
Abnormal rate/rhythms	Tachycardiomyopathy, bradycardia, AV dyssynchrony†
Abnormal morphology	SV physiology‡, ALCAPA
Ischemic	CAD (including premature CAD)†
Postoperative	Post-bypass, SV surgeries, post-TGA repair‡
Abnormal homeostasis	Hypothermia, hypoxia, hypocalcemia, hypoglycemia, sepsis† (peculiar to neonatal period)

(ALCAPA: anomalous left coronary artery from the pulmonary artery; AS: aortic stenosis; AV: atrioventricular; AVSD: atrioventricular septal defect; CAD: coronary artery disease; CHD: congenital heart disease; DCM: dilated cardiomyopathy; HIV: human immunodeficiency virus; HT: hypertension; MR: mitral regurgitation; PDA: patent ductus arteriosus; PS: pulmonary stenosis; RF: rheumatic fever; RHD: rheumatic heart disease; SV: single ventricle; TAPVC: total anomalous pulmonary venous connection; TGA: transposition of the great arteries; TR: tricuspid regurgitation; VSD: ventricular septal defect)

*Common.

†Rare (may be common in specific age group/settings).

‡Uncommon.

Table 7.4.2: Common causes of heart failure by age at presentation.

Day 1 of life/fetal	*1–2 months*
• Asphyxia • Metabolic • Systemic arteriovenous fistula • Myocarditis • Hematological • SVT, CHB, severe TR (Ebstein anomaly), severe MR	• VSD • PDA • AVSD • Aortopulmonary window • Unobstructed TAPVC • TGA and malposition complexes • ALCAPA • DCM
First week of life	***2–6 months***
• Critical AS/PS • Obstructive TAPVC • Hypoplastic left heart • Coarctation of aorta • Adrenalin sufficiency • TGA with intact septum • Day 1 causes	• Causes at 1–2 months • Coarctation of aorta • Aortic stenosis
Second week of life	***Older children***
• Large VSD • Large PDA • AVSD • Persistent truncus arteriosus • Unobstructive TAPVC	• RF/RHD • CHD with complications • Cardiomyopathies • Severe PS with TR • Palliated/postoperative CHD • Tachycardiomyopathies • Severe hypertension

(ALCAPA: anomalous left coronary artery from the pulmonary artery; AS: aortic stenosis; AVSD: atrioventricular septal defect; CHB: complete heart block; CHD: congenital heart disease; MR: mitral regurgitation; PDA: patent ductus arteriosus; PS: pulmonary stenosis; RF: rheumatic fever; RHD: rheumatic heart disease; SVT: supraventricular tachycardia; TAPVC: total anomalous pulmonary venous connection; TGA: transposition of the great arteries; TR: tricuspid regurgitation; VSD: ventricular septal defect)

Heart failure presenting on the first day of life is commonly due to metabolic abnormalities and not CHD. Conditions producing fetal HF, such as Ebstein anomaly or abnormal heart rate/rhythm, are also causes of HF on day 1 of life.

Obstructive and duct-dependent lesions can present with HF or acute circulatory shock soon after birth. Heart failure due to left-to-right shunts occurs later (4–6 weeks) as the pulmonary vascular resistance falls, though large ventricular septal defect (VSD), patent ductus arteriosus (PDA), atrioventricular septal defect (AVSD) may present earlier. Children with isolated atrial septal defect (ASD) are mostly asymptomatic; if an infant is diagnosed to have ASD and is in failure, the likely diagnosis is the much more malignant CHD, total anomalous pulmonary venous connection (TAPVC).

Heart failure secondary to CHD is unusual after the first year of life unless complicated by infective endocarditis (IE), anemia, infections, or arrhythmias. Thus older children (usually beyond 2 years) are likely to have other causes for HF, such as acute/chronic rheumatic heart disease (RHD), myocarditis, cardiomyopathies, and postoperative CHD.

EPIDEMIOLOGY OF HEART FAILURE IN CHILDREN

Epidemiology of HF in children is a difficult science given the fact that symptoms, etiology, diagnostic criteria, and outcomes are quite heterogeneous. The incidence of CHD is about 8 per 1,000 (0.8%) of live births, of which one-third to one-fourth are severe enough to warrant attention. Half of these result in HF.

Rheumatic fever (RF)/RHD is an important cause of HF in children in the developing countries, such as India. While the incidence and prevalence of RF and RHD are well documented, there are no data on presentation with HF in this group, although a significant majority of acute rheumatic carditis and established juvenile multiple sclerosis will present with the features of HF.

CLINICAL FEATURES

The clinical features of HF in children vary according to the cause and age of the child. An important point to remember is that raised jugular venous pressure, peripheral edema, effusions, and chest crepitations are not seen in neonates and are unlikely in young children as a sign of HF. Chest crepitations, in fact, suggest the possibility of underlying chest infection, which so often accompanies HF in children, especially, in high pulmonary flow situations.

Common clinical features of HF in children have been given in **Table 7.4.3**. These features are quite nonspecific in neonates and may resemble features of septicemia. Thus a high index of suspicion is required. Routine examination for lower limb pulses is very important; otherwise, coarctation of aorta will be missed. Coarctation of aorta is not a cause of HF beyond infancy, and hence in such cases, other diagnoses, such as nonspecific aortoarteritis, should be sought. One must also remember that neonates with coarctation of aorta or even interruption of aortic arch may have normal lower limb pulses due to PDA. Closure of PDA could be disastrous in these babies. Some of the other important clinical considerations are as follows:

Central cyanosis with HF should always be taken seriously in a neonate, especially, if associated with soft or no murmur.

- An ASD or VSD does not cause HF in the first 2 weeks of life; prompt evaluation should be done for TAPVC or associated coarctation of aorta, respectively.
- A premature newborn with respiratory distress and a murmur is likely to have a PDA causing HF.
- Rule out tachyarrhythmia as a cause of HF, if heart rate is above 220 beats/min.
- Associated extracardiac and chromosomal abnormalities may provide clues for the diagnosis of CHD.

Table 7.4.3: Clinical features of heart failure by age and associated findings.

Newborn/neonates	
• Tachypnea • Tachycardia • Hepatomegaly • Cardiomegaly • Feeding difficulties • Excessive sweating • Subcostal recession • Cyanosis and wheeze • Shock	• Bounding pulses in arteriovenous malformations, PDA, truncus • Asymmetric upper and lower limb blood pressure in aortic arch anomalies • Central cyanosis in TGA, TAPVC, truncus, tricuspid atresia with no PS • Differential cyanosis in PPHN and R-L shunt through patent ductus • Multiple heart sounds in Ebstein anomaly • Ejection systolic murmur in AS/PS • Syndromic anomalies (Down and Noonan syndromes) HLHS, coarctation of aorta, interrupted aortic arch, critical AS, tachyarrhythmias, myocarditis
Infants	
• Poor feeding • Lethargy • Excessive sweating • Tachypnea, tachycardia • Slow weight gain • Hepatomegaly	• Precordial bulge, signs of pulmonary hypertension and less impressive systolic murmurs suggest larger L-R shunts • Crepitations should alert to the possibility of chest infection • Cyanosis in TAPVC, TGA with VSD, AVSD, truncus • Findings of CHF and cyanosis in suspected ASD suggest TAPVC • Later onset of HF in infancy can be due to certain forms of TAPVC and ALCAPA
Older children	
• Poor weight gain • Effort intolerance, orthopnea • Cardiomegaly • Gallop rhythm, murmurs • Peripheral edema • Basilar crepitations • Fatigue • Hepatomegaly • Raised JVP	• Diastolic murmur in a child with known VSD suggests associated AR • Pericardial rub in appropriate settings suggests acute RF • Hypertension and unequal pulses or bruits suggest nonspecific aortoarteritis • Findings of raised JVP, ascites, and anasarca should lead to the suspicion of constrictive pericarditis or restrictive cardiomyopathy

(ALCAPA: anomalous left coronary artery from the pulmonary artery; AR: aortic regurgitation; AS: aortic stenosis; ASD: atrial septal defect; AVSD: atrioventricular septal defect; CHF: congestive heart failure; HF: heart failure; HLHS: hypoplastic left heart syndrome; JVP: jugular venous pulse; L-R: left-to-right; PDA: patent ductus arteriosus; PPHN: persistent pulmonary hypertension of the newborn; PS: pulmonary stenosis; RF: rheumatic fever; TAPVC: total anomalous pulmonary venous connection; TGA: transposition of the great arteries; VSD: ventricular septal defect)

- Older children with tetralogy of Fallot (TOF) or TOF physiology may develop HF due to complications, such as anemia, IE, aortic regurgitation, large aortopulmonary collaterals.

The established New York Heart Association HF classification is not applicable in children. Functional classification for children has been proposed by many authors, the most acceptable is modified Ross classification, given in **Table 7.4.4**.

Table 7.4.4: Ross classification of heart failure.

Class I	Asymptomatic
Class II	• Mild tachypnea or diaphoresis with feeding in infants • Dyspnea on exertion in older children
Class III	• Marked tachypnea or diaphoresis with feeding in infants • Marked dyspnea on exertion • Prolonged feeding times with growth failure
Class IV	Symptoms, such as tachypnea, retractions, grunting, or diaphoresis at rest

INVESTIGATIONS

The cornerstones for rapid clinical diagnosis of HF in children are chest radiograph and an electrocardiogram (ECG).

Chest Radiograph

Chest radiograph should be done in all patients with suspected HF; an echocardiogram is not a substitute for radiograph. It enables the diagnosis of cardiomegaly, quantification of pulmonary blood flow, presence of associated chest infection, pleural effusion, etc. as well as showing pathognomonic cardiac silhouette in certain disease states. A cardiothoracic ratio of greater than 60% in neonates and greater than 55% in older children suggests that cardiomegaly though expiratory films should be interpreted with caution. A large thymus can also give false impression of cardiomegaly in neonates and infants **(Fig. 7.4.1)**. Cardiomegaly with increased pulmonary blood flow (pulmonary plethora), prominent main and branch pulmonary arteries are the features of significant left-to-right shunts **(Fig. 7.4.2)**. Typical radiographs are rare but if present are diagnostic of certain CHD, e.g. egg-on-side appearance in transposition of the great arteries (TGA) **(Fig. 7.4.3)**, normal heart size with ground glass lungs in obstructed TAPVC **(Fig. 7.4.4)**, figure-of-eight appearance in unobstructed supracardiac TAPVC **(Fig. 7.4.5)**, and so on digitalization is not performed. One can start directly with oral maintenance dose at 10 µg/kg/day (the available digoxin elixir has 50 µg/mL; hence, the dose is 0.1 mL/kg twice daily).

- Continuous infusion of diuretics is recommended in the cases of acute decompensated HF. Monitoring and supplementation of K^+ is necessary at higher doses, as hypokalemia is associated with increased arrhythmic deaths.

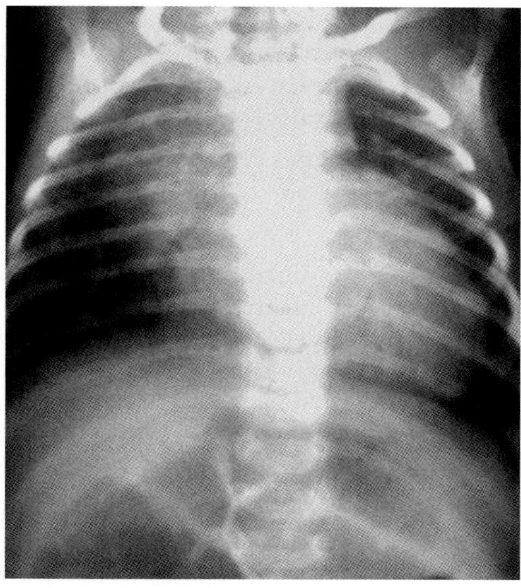

Fig. 7.4.1: A large thymus may give false impression of cardiomegaly in neonates and infants.

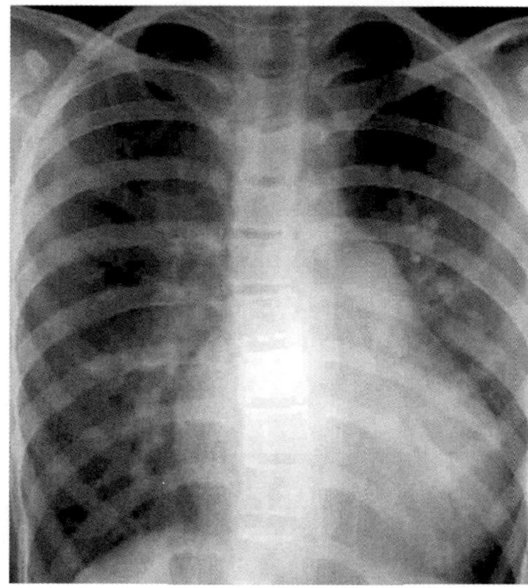

Fig. 7.4.2: Features of significant left-to-right shunts: cardiomegaly with increased pulmonary blood flow (pulmonary plethora), prominent main and branch pulmonary arteries.

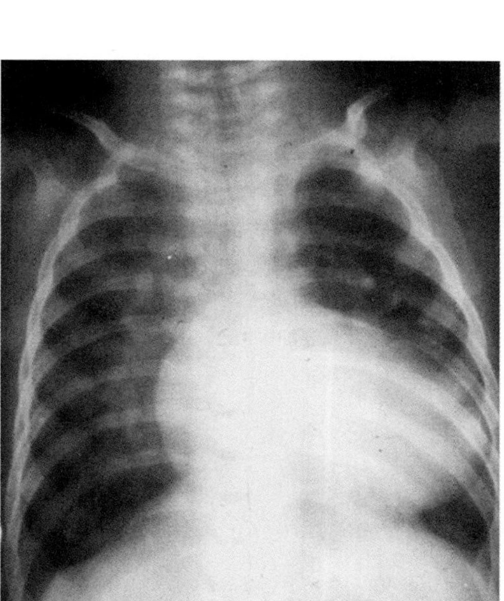

Fig. 7.4.3: Egg-on-side appearance in transposition of great arteries (TGA).

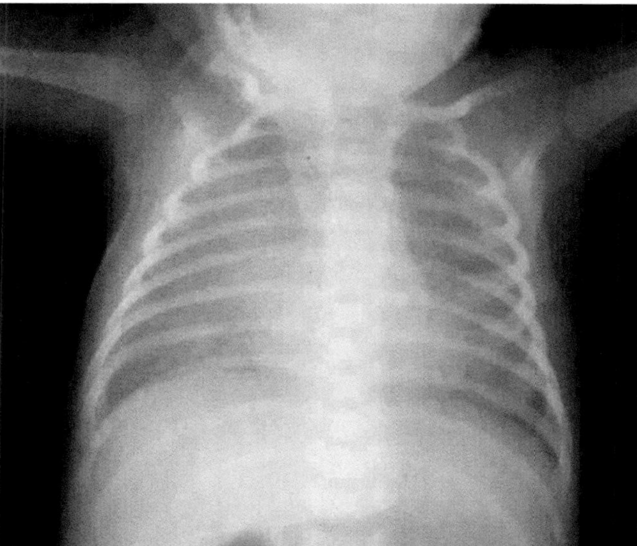

Fig. 7.4.4: Normal heart size with ground glass lungs in obstructed total anomalous pulmonary venous connection (TAPVC).

Electrocardiogram

An ECG is a much underutilized investigation in children. It is often useful for diagnosing type of CHD and in tachyarrhythmia. Biventricular hypertrophy **(Fig. 7.4.6)** with volume overload of the left ventricle is seen in large VSD, the most common cause of HF in infants. Tachycardiomyopathy, a potentially reversible cause of HF, due to incessant supraventricular tachycardia (such as ectopic atrial tachycardia) can only be picked up by ECG. Similarly, bradyarrhythmias due to congenital complete heart block are detected on ECG **(Fig. 7.4.7)**. Anomalous left coronary artery from pulmonary artery produces a very specific pattern, pathologic "q" waves in anterolateral leads **(Fig. 7.4.8)**. Left axis deviation in a child with large shunt lesion suggests AVSD as a cause of HF **(Fig. 7.4.9)**. Rarely, hypocalcemia may cause left ventricular dysfunction; ECG shows prolonged QTc interval with terminal "T" wave inversion **(Fig. 7.4.10)**.

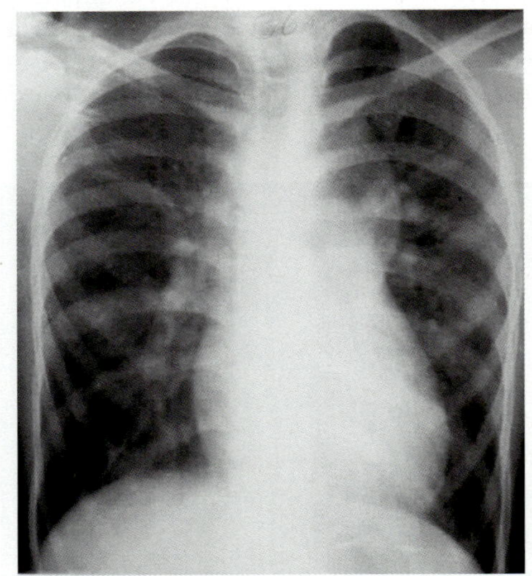

Fig. 7.4.5: Figure-of-eight appearance in unobstructed total anomalous pulmonary venous connection (TAPVC).

Echocardiogram

An echocardiogram is invaluable in the diagnosis of HF. It confirms the presence of structural heart disease and aids in the management strategy. Echocardiogram is an operator-dependent test, and to avoid wrong diagnosis, it should always be interpreted in an integrated fashion with clinical, radiographic, and ECG findings.

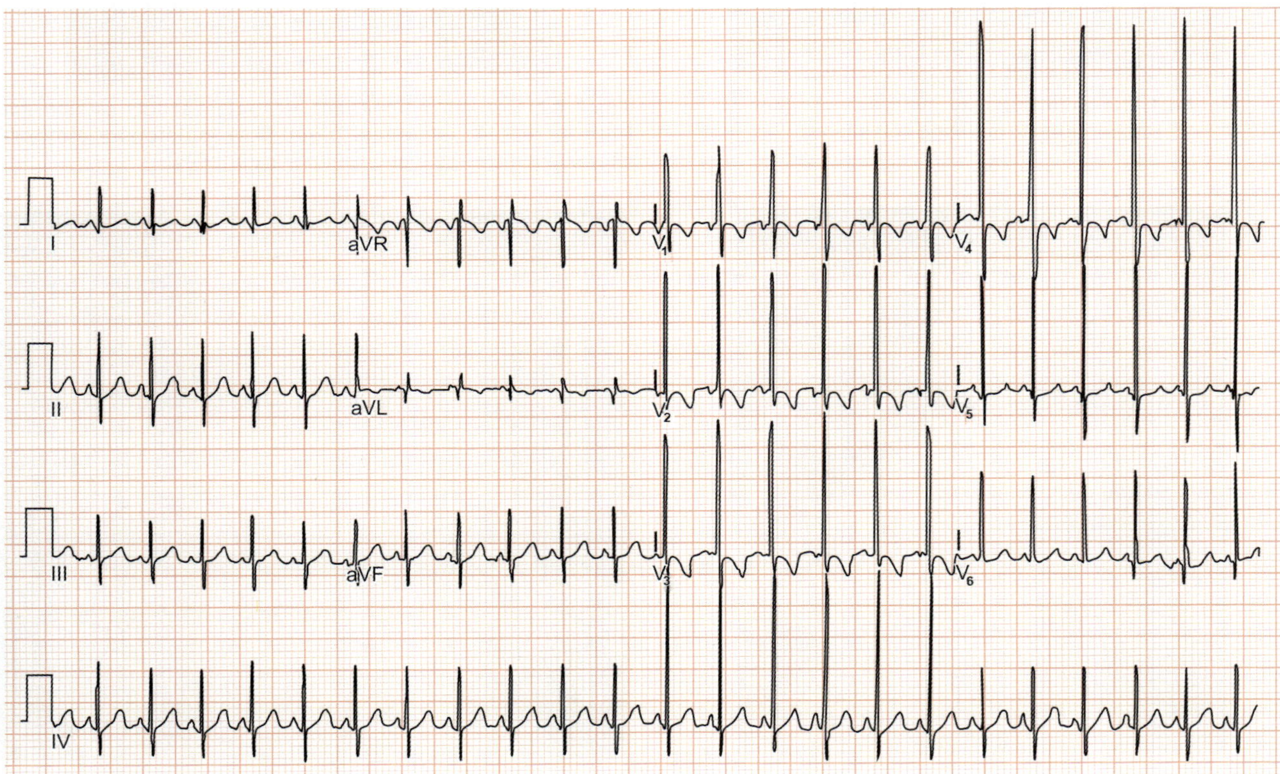

Fig. 7.4.6: Biventricular hypertrophy with volume overload of the left ventricle seen in large ventricular septal defect (VSD).

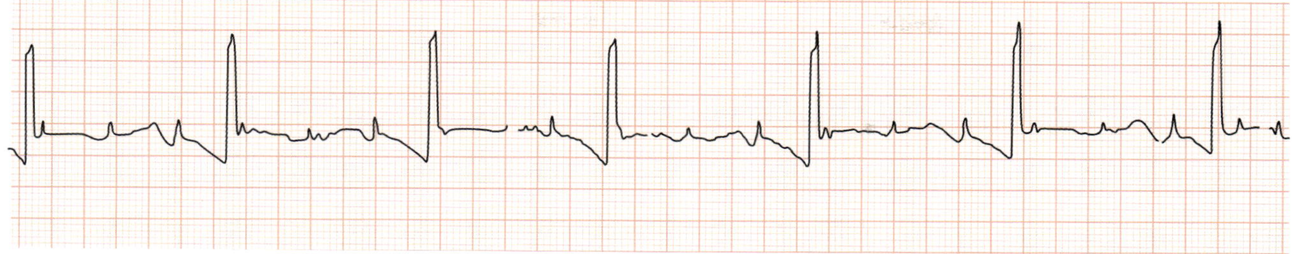

Fig. 7.4.7: Electrocardiogram detecting bradyarrhythmias due to congenital complete heart block.

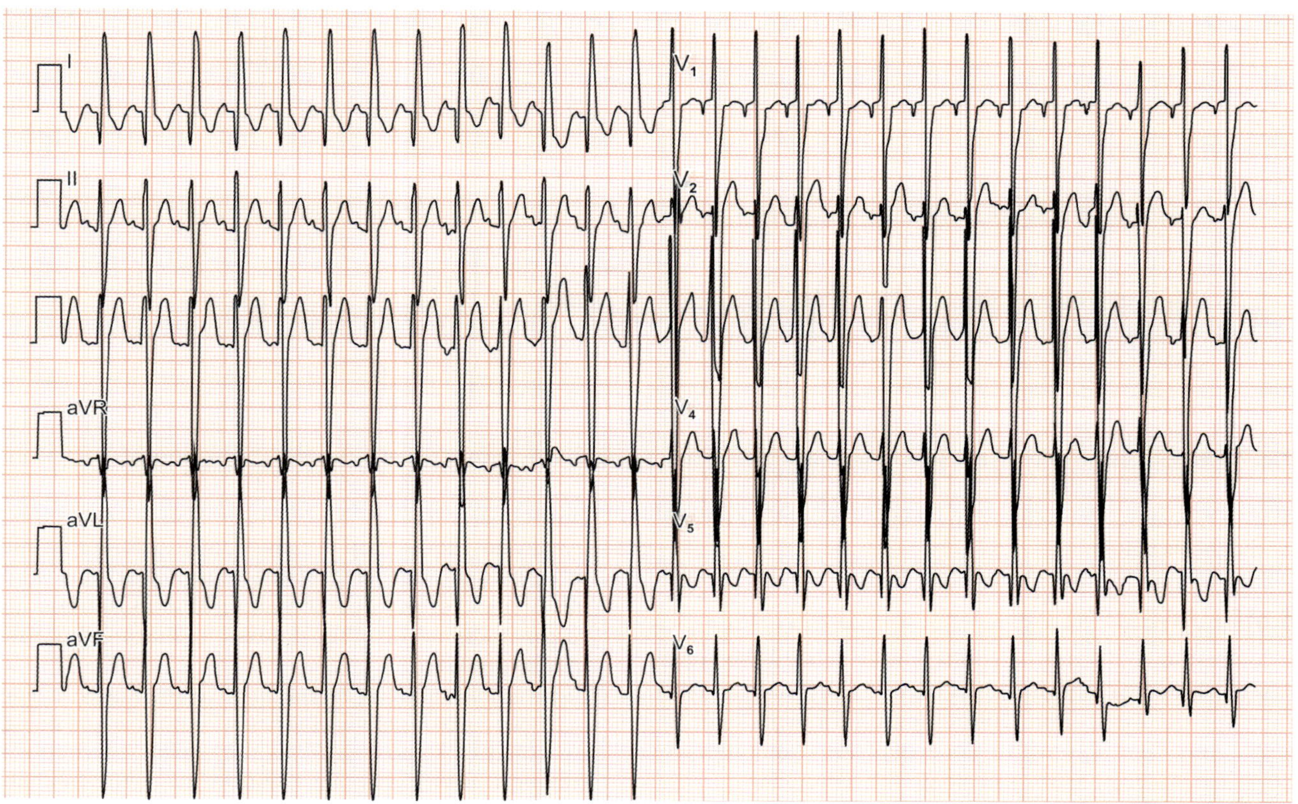

Fig. 7.4.8: Anomalous left coronary artery from pulmonary artery (ALCAPA) producing a very specific pattern, pathologic "q" waves in anterolateral leads.

Other Investigations

- *B-type natriuretic peptide*, a cardiac natriuretic hormone, secreted in escalating fashion in ventricular dysfunction and progressive HF, is increasingly used in acute settings for differentiation of HF from pulmonary causes of respiratory distress. B-type natriuretic peptide is significantly elevated in HF, and its trend over time can have important predictive value. A failure to decrease on follow-up may indicate increased risk of death or needing a heart transplantation.
- *Hemoglobin* estimation is important as anemia can cause decompensation in children with underlying heart disease but no HF.
- *Electrolytes*, such as serum calcium, phosphorus, and blood glucose, should be routinely measured in all children with HF, especially neonates, where their abnormalities are an uncommon but reversible cause of ventricular dysfunction.
- *Tests to screen for hypoxia and sepsis* also constitute the evaluation of HF in a newborn. Antistreptolysin O

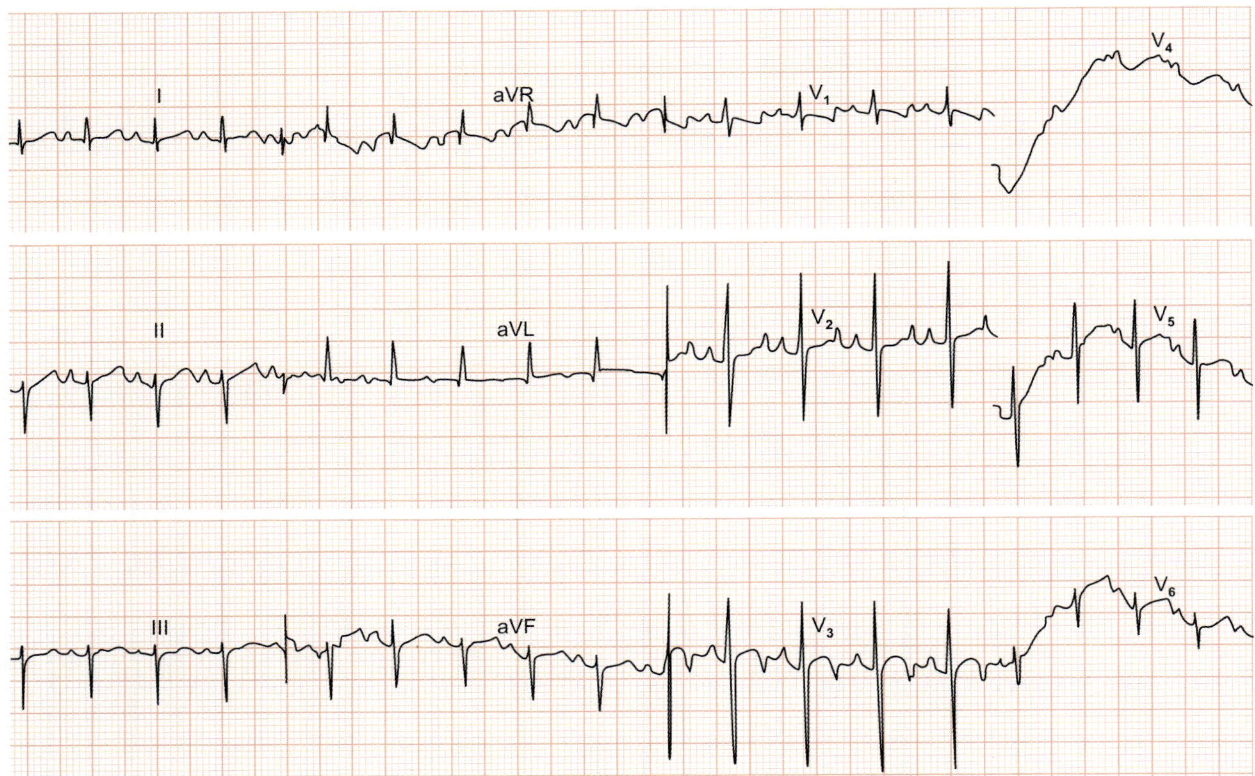

Fig. 7.4.9: Left axis deviation in a child with large shunt lesion suggesting atrioventricular septal defect (AVSD) as a cause of heart failure.

and C-reactive protein are invaluable in workup for the diagnosis of RF.

MANAGEMENT

In contrast to HF therapy in adults, few evidence-based data exist to guide the management of HF in children. Most of the drugs for HF are used in children based on experience in adults. Angiotensin-converting enzyme (ACE) inhibitors are the preferred drugs, to be used along with a diuretic.

- Treatment of HF in children, such as in adults, should consist of treatment of the cause, precipitating factors (anemia, IE, infections, acute RF, electrolyte imbalance, noncompliance with drug or diet, arrhythmias) and treatment of the congested state.
- *Digoxin* has a very narrow safety window in children and adults alike. It should be avoided in premature babies, those with renal compromised state and the cases with acute myocarditis. Electrolytes (K^+, Ca^{++}, and Mg^{++}) should be carefully monitored to avoid potentiation of toxicity and development of arrhythmias (which are more often bradyarrhythmias in children). Generally initial total digitalization is not performed. One can start directly to oral maintenance dose at 10 µg/kg/day (the available digoxin elixir has 50 µg/mL, hence the dose is 0.1 mL/kg twice daily).
- During early infancy, *supplementation of potassium* is usually not required up to 2 mg/kg of dose for furosemide or equivalent. In the cases requiring higher doses and in older children, a combination of loop diuretic and spironolactone (or other potassium-sparing diuretics) may be preferred.
- *Angiotensin-converting enzyme inhibitors* should be avoided in HF caused by lesions having pressure overload physiology, e.g. in aortic stenosis (AS), as they might interfere with compensatory hypertrophy. The incidence of ACE-inhibitor-induced cough is much less in children as compared to adults. One should avoid combining ACE inhibitors with spironolactone as there is a risk of hyperkalemia.
- *Beta-blockers* therapy has been shown to be beneficial in adults with HF. Some studies in children have also shown improvement in ventricular function on beta-blockers in patients of dilated cardiomyopathy. These drugs are underutilized in children with HF, partly due to the fear of aggravation of HF symptoms. One should start with a low dose and gradually uptitrate it. Beta-blockers should not be administered in acute decompensated HF.
- In neonates and infants, active *fluid restriction* is not recommended. Calorie supplementation, either by increasing the density of milk or giving commercially available high-calorie formulas, is recommended. In older children, fluid and salt restrictions are generally required.

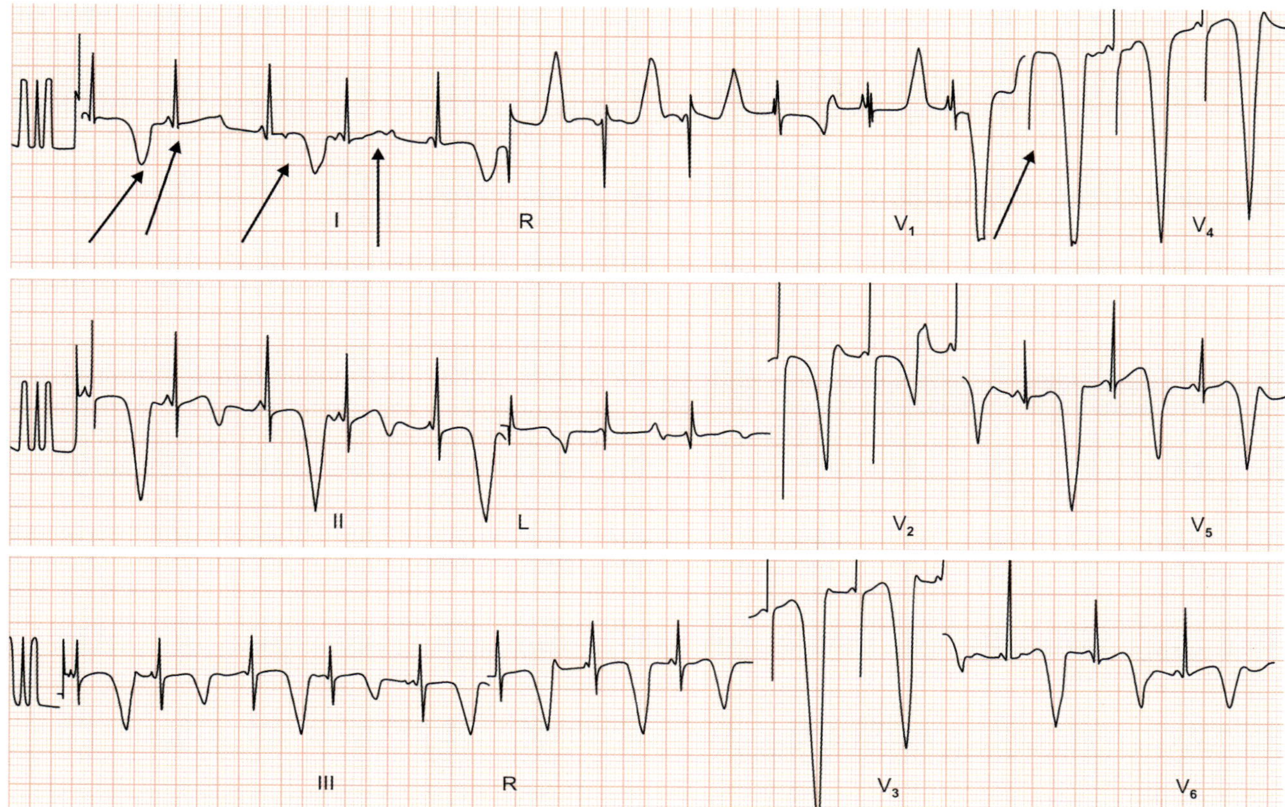

Fig. 7.4.10: Electrocardiogram showing prolonged QTc interval with terminal "T" wave inversion in hypocalcemia.

Children should be asked to avoid extra salt as is present in fries, chips, pizzas, and other similar food items.

Key concepts in the management of HF in children are listed below.

Management of Heart Failure in Subgroups

Neonates

They may present with HF and circulatory collapse due to ductus-dependent CHD, such as tight coarctation of the aorta, interruption of the aortic arch, critical AS, and TGA with intact septum and restrictive interatrial communication. These disorders require maintenance of duct patency with prostaglandin infusion till the time more definitive treatment can be employed. Because these children are very sick, they should be transferred to tertiary centers with expertise in their care after initial resuscitation and prostaglandin infusion (if required).

Infants with Congenital Heart Disease Awaiting Surgery

Short-term medical treatment is required for stabilization and alleviation of symptoms. This is a very common group because most of CHDs causing HF require surgical intervention. These children present with HF and frequently have comorbidities, such as sepsis or chest infection.

Children Requiring Long-term Medical Therapy

Several causes of HF in children require prolonged medical therapy. Examples include moderate-sized VSDs, PDA, myocarditis/cardiomyopathy, etc. Therapy is also required for long-term in residual defects following surgery and in valvular diseases where the risk-benefit ratio is not in favor of surgery.

Drugs for the Treatment of Heart Failure

The advances in medical science have ensured a wide variety of evidence-based and emerging therapies for the treatment or palliation of HF **(Table 7.4.5)**. There are several newer agents, the roles of which are still investigational, in adults and in children. These include natriuretic peptides (e.g. nesiritide), calcium sensitizers (e.g. levosimendan), vasopressin antagonists (e.g. tolvaptan), renin inhibitors (e.g. aliskiren), endothelin antagonists (e.g. sitaxentan), etc. Some, such as oral phosphodiesterase inhibitors, antiinflammatory molecules, nitric oxide agonists, and neuropeptidase antagonists, have not proven useful or found to have excess side effects.

Tables 7.4.6 to 7.4.8 outline the treatment of HF in children and dosages of common drugs used for the treatment in acute and chronic settings.

Mechanical Circulatory Support

Last decade has seen increasing utilization of ventricular assist devices (VAD) in children with end-stage HF. Ventricular assist devices has the advantage over extracorporeal membrane oxygenation that it can be used for long-term support for HF while waiting for heart transplantation. The Berlin Heart Excor was the first VAD used in children, and a number of trials have proved its efficacy. Ventricular assist devices are associated with high rates of side effects, including stroke. Postoperated patients of CHD generally do not do well on VAD.

Table 7.4.5: Treatment options for chronic heart failure.

Established	***Investigational***
Pharmacotherapy • Angiotensin-converting enzyme (ACE) inhibitors • Beta-blockers • Digoxin • Diuretics • Aldosterone antagonists • Anticoagulants (with severe ventricular dysfunction) *Cardiac transplantation:* • *Surgery:* – Definite (for structural diseases) – Ventricular assist devices – Extracorporeal membrane oxygenation – Intermittent inotrope infusion (weekend pulsed dobutamine)	*Pharmacotherapy* • Angiotensin receptor blocker • Nesiritide • Levosimendan Ventricular remodeling Cardiac resynchronization therapy Implantable cardiac defibrillator Stem-cell therapy

Cardiac Transplantation

The heart transplantation has been used for the treatment of end-stage heart disease in children for nearly five decades with the first infant transplant done in the late 1960s. Around 350 pediatric cardiac transplantations are done annually, representing about 10% of total cardiac transplantations. The majority of the transplantations are carried out for end-stage heart disease due to cardiomyopathies. Other causes include CHDs, such as hypoplastic heart syndrome, and other complex CHDs, single ventricle, palliated heart disease. The 1-year survival has approached 90%. However, given the fact that the surgery is done in few centers globally and the available donor hearts have remained static over last many years to few hundreds, it is clear that heart transplantation can be a solution for a minority only.

Stem-cell Therapy

A heightened interest has developed in stem-cell therapy for HF. Several trials have been completed, or are ongoing in adults with HF, predominantly due to ischemic heart disease. Stem-cell therapy is being investigated worldwide under experimental settings for the children with refractory HF.

Table 7.4.6: Treatment algorithm for acute heart failure in neonates.

Supportive measures	
Avoid hypothermia and hypoglycemia; check for hypocalcemia	
Maintenance of adequate oxygenation	Monitoring of blood gases if perfusion is poor ventilate, if required, with modest PEEP to achieve PaO_2 of 50–60 mm Hg and SaO_2 of 75–85% to avoid pulmonary congestion
Adequate hydration	Stop oral feeds if severe tachypnea
IV access	IV and CVP lines (umbilical vein cannula)
IV inotropes for shock	Isoproterenol 0.5–2 µg/kg/min Dopamine 5–20 µg/kg/min Dobutamine 5–20 µg/kg/min Avoid digoxin or use cautiously
Milrinone	Inotrope and vasodilator load with 25–50 µg/kg/min; maintain at 0.25–1 µg/kg/min
Diuretics	Furosemide 2–4 µg/kg PO/IV
Vasodilators	Captopril 0.1–1 mg/kg/day PO q 8 hourly Sodium nitroprusside 0.5–4 µg/kg/min IV Careful monitoring of blood pressure is necessary
Prostaglandin infusion for ductus-dependent lesions	Start at 0.1 µg/kg/min (up to 0.4 µg/kg/min if no response), taper to the lowest dose possible (0.005 µg/kg/min) monitor for apnea; keep minimum required dose

(CVP: central venous pressure; IV: intravenous; PEEP: positive end-expiratory pressure; PO: per oral)

Table 7.4.7: Oral dosages of common drugs used to treat chronic heart failure.

Digoxin	10 µg/kg/day (in two divided doses for children < 5 years)
Furosemide	1–4 mg/kg/day (1–2 doses)
Spironolactone	2–4 mg/kg/day (two doses)
Captopril	*Neonates*: 0.4–1.6 mg/kg/day in three divided doses *Infants and children*: 0.5–4 mg/kg/day in three divided doses
Enalapril	0.1–0.5 mg/kg/day (two doses); avoid in neonates
Losartan	0.5 mg/kg/day once daily
Metoprolol	0.1–0.2 mg/kg/dose (two doses) and increase to 1 mg/kg/dose or maximally tolerated dose over weeks or months
Carvedilol	0.05 mg/kg/dose (twice daily) and increase to 0.4–0.5 mg/kg/dose (twice daily) or maximally tolerated dose

Table 7.4.8: Stepwise guide to the management of heart failure.

Step 1	*In acute decompensation*: Bed rest, propped-up position, humidified oxygen sodium and, if required, volume restriction
Step 2	Start digoxin (not in myocarditis) Assess reversible and precipitating causes Assess the need for surgery/interventional procedure in the case of structural heart disease
Step 3	Add ACE inhibitor. In the case of ACE-inhibitor-induced cough, switch to ARB like losartan Switch to nitrates if ACE inhibitor/ARB is not tolerated
Step 4	Add carvedilol in compensated HF, especially, in the cases with tachycardia
Step 5	Once or twice weekly dobutamine therapy Consider stem-cell coronary infusion
Step 6	Cardiac transplantation Ventricular assist device as bridge in the case of delays or even destination therapy

(ACE: angiotensin-converting enzyme; ARB: angiotensin receptor blocker; HF: heart failure)

CONCLUSION

Heart failure in children is a complex syndrome with heterogeneous etiology and presentation. Unlike adults, HF in children is commonly due to structural heart disease and reversible conditions, thus lending it amenable to definitive therapy or short-term aggressive therapy. Thus the overall outcome with HF is better in children than that in adults. Clinical presentation of HF in younger children can be nonspecific requiring heightened degree of suspicion. In particular, some conditions that can present with acute shock are important to recognize, as they can be effectively treated or palliated on an urgent basis. While the general principles of management are similar to those in adults, there is a dearth of evidence base in pediatric HF. It would require a judicious balance of extrapolation from adult medicine (thus avoiding generation of redundant evidence) and the development of children-specific treatments (thus recognizing the inherent differences in HF of children and adults) to optimize the outcomes in this challenging field.

BIBLIOGRAPHY

1. Burch M. Heart failure in the young. Heart. 2002;88:198-202.
2. Gazit AZ, Oren PP. Pharmaceutical management of decompensated heart failure syndrome in children: current state of the art and a new approach. Curr Treat Options Cardiovasc Med. 2009;11:403-9.
3. Kay JD, Colan SD, Graham TP. Congestive heart failure in pediatric patients. Am Heart J. 2001;42:923-8.
4. Moffett E, Chang AC. Future pharmacologic agents for treatment of heart failure in children. Pediatr Cardiol. 2006;27:533-51.
5. Ramakrishnan S, Kothari SS, Bahl VK. Heart failure—definition and diagnosis. Indian Heart J. 2005;57:13-20.
6. Saxena A, Anil OM, Juneja R. Clinical and echocardiographic outcome in patients receiving carvedilol for treatment of dilated cardiomyopathy. Indian J Pediatr. 2013;80:549-54.
7. Shaddy RE, Boucek MM, Hsu DT, et al. Carvedilol for children and adolescents with heart failure: a randomized controlled trial. JAMA. 2007;298:1171-9.
8. Wong DT, George K, Wilson J, et al. Effectiveness of serial increases in amino-terminal pro-B-type natriuretic peptide levels to indicate the need for mechanical circulatory support in children with acute decompensated heart failure. Am J Cardiol. 2011;107:573-8.
9. Working Group on Management of Congenital Heart Diseases in India. Consensus on timing of intervention for common congenital heart disease (Saxena A, Ramakrishnan S, Tandon R, et al.). Indian Pediatr. 2008;45:117-26.

7.5 Diseases of Endocardium, Myocardium, and Pericardium

Srikanta Basu

INFECTIVE ENDOCARDITIS

Infective endocarditis (IE) is defined as the "endovascular microbial infection of cardiovascular structures," involves infection of the endocardium or of the endothelium of the great vessels. This condition usually occurs as a complication of congenital heart disease (CHD) or rheumatic heart disease (RHD) but rarely develops without preexisting heart disease. It is associated with 16–25% of mortality, and 20% of the patients require emergency surgery.

EPIDEMIOLOGY

Infective endocarditis is more common in adults as compared to the children and accounts for 0.8–3.3 cases for each 1,000 admissions to hospital with a cumulative risk of 6.1 per 1,000 children up to 18 years. The incidence in children and neonates may be rising due to increasing use of newer devices, indwelling catheters, increasing sophistication of resuscitative techniques, especially, in sick babies, and due to overall improved survival. In India or in the other developing countries, RHD still forms a significant proportion of cases with IE.

In general, cardiac lesions with steep pressure gradients (ventricular septal defect, patent ductus arteriosus, left-sided valvular regurgitation) are associated with increased risk of IE. It is extremely rare in patients with atrial septal defects. Tetralogy of Fallot, bicuspid aortic valve, and children who had undergone repair or palliation for cyanotic CHD are also at higher risk of IE. In newborn, endocarditis often involves right-sided structures, and the diagnosis may be difficult with a very high mortality rate.

ETIOPATHOGENESIS

Gram-positive cocci are the most likely organisms, although gram-negative rods and fungi can cause IE. *Streptococcus viridans* is the most common causative agent, followed by *Staphylococcus aureus* in children beyond the age of 1 year. This has been reported in Indian studies as well. However, *S. aureus* and fungus are more common in children where vascular indwelling catheter or prosthetic valve is used and in immunocompromised patients.

The cardiac lesions consist of vegetations of fibrin, leukocytes, platelets, and bacteria. Many clinical manifestations are related to destructive aspects of the infection or to embolization of portions of the vegetation. Endocarditis, particularly from *Staphylococcus*, may cause valvular damage, such as perforation of the aortic cusps or ruptured chordae tendineae of the mitral valve. Embolization may occur into the pulmonary or the systemic circulations and cause infarction, abscess, or inflammation of various tissues. Emboli to the lungs, kidneys, spleen, or brain are reported most frequently because in each location there are major clinical or laboratory findings of the phenomenon.

CLINICAL FEATURES

The clinical presentation is insidious with prolonged fever, malaise, myalgia, anorexia, weight loss, pallor, arthralgia, and headache. The classical signs, such as Janeway lesions, Osler's node, and Roth spot, are rarely seen in children. The diagnosis should be suspected in any child with a significant cardiac murmur and a prolonged fever. Congestive cardiac failure may develop, especially if aortic or mitral valve regurgitation is created by the infection. Signs and symptoms of embolic phenomenon should be sought. Signs of recurrent pneumonia or a pleuritic type of pain may indicate embolization of infected material to the lungs. Signs of systemic embolization, such as splenomegaly, hematuria, splinter hemorrhages, and central nervous system signs, should be sought in any febrile patient with a cardiac anomaly, and rarely the children may present with these signs acutely. Acute IE has a fulminant course often requiring emergency intervention. It presents with high-grade fever, rapidly changing signs and symptoms, and shock; and *S. aureus* is the most common causative organism.

DIAGNOSIS

The diagnosis can be confirmed by obtaining the organisms from a blood culture. Usually three blood cultures should be taken aseptically within the first 12 or 24 hours, and 2–3 mL of blood may be enough. Blood culture may be negative in nearly 7% of the cases, although studies from India have shown that the percentage is much higher, which may be due to prior use of antibiotics, and insufficient sample of blood for culture specially in our setup. Nonspecific acute-phase reactants, such as erythrocyte sedimentation rate, C-reactive protein, and rheumatoid factor, are usually elevated; the tests may also be useful in following the progress of therapy. Echocardiography has become an important modality for the diagnosis of IE and is taken as major criteria in the modified Duke's classification **(Tables 7.5.1 and Box 7.5.1)**. It is important to remember that diagnostic yield of echocardiography is influenced by the image quality, size of vegetation [vegetation less than 2–3 mm may not be well seen by transthoracic echocardiography (TTE)], location of vegetation, and the experience of echocardiographer. The absence of valve changes or vegetations does not exclude endocarditis. Transthoracic echocardiography is very sensitive in children due to better acoustic window, but occasionally, transesophageal echocardiography is advised in situation when window is poor, in patients with prosthetic valve, grafts, or conduits, rarely in aortic valve endocarditis or aortic root abscess.

Table 7.5.1: Modified Duke's criteria.

Major criteria
A. Positive blood culture for IE
• Typical microorganism consistent with IE from two separate blood cultures as noted below: – *Streptococcus viridans, Streptococcus bovis* or HACEK group or *Staphylococcus aureus* – Community-acquired enterococci in the absence of a primary focus • Microorganisms consistent with IE from persistently positive blood cultures defined as: – Two positive cultures of blood samples drawn > 12 hours apart, or – All of three or a majority of four separate cultures of blood (with first and last sample drawn 1 hour apart) – Single positive blood culture for *Coxiella burnetii* or antiphase 1 IgG antibody titer > 1:800
B. Evidence of endocardial involvement
Echocardiogram positive for IE (TEE recommended for patients with prosthetic valves rated at least "possible IE" by clinical criteria, or complicated IE paravalvular abscess; TTE as first test in other patients)
• Positive echocardiogram for IE is defined as: – Oscillating intracardiac mass on valve or supporting structures, in the path of regurgitant jets, or omni-planted material in the absence of an alternative anatomic explanation, or – Abscess, or – New partial dehiscence of prosthetic valve • New valvular regurgitation (worsening or changing of preexisting murmur not sufficient)
Minor criteria
• *Predisposition*: Predisposing heart condition or intravenous drug use • *Fever*: Temperature > 38.0°C (100.4°F) • *Vascular phenomena*: Major arterial emboli, septic pulmonary infarcts, mycotic aneurysm, intracranial hemorrhage, conjunctival hemorrhages, and Janeway lesions • *Immunologic phenomena*: Glomerulonephritis, Osler's nodes, Roth spots, and rheumatoid factor • *Microbiological evidence*: Positive blood culture but does not meet a major criterion as noted above* or serological evidence of active infection with organism consistent with IE • Echocardiographic minor criteria eliminated

(HACEK: *Haemophilus* species, *Actinobacillus actinomycetemcomitans*, *Cardiobacterium hominis*, *Eikenella corrodens*, *Kingella* species; IE: infective endocarditis; TEE: transesophageal echocardiography; TTE: transthoracic echocardiography)

*Excludes single positive cultures for coagulase-negative staphylococci and organisms that do not cause endocarditis.

Box 7.5.1: Diagnosis of infective endocarditis (IE) according to the modified Duke's criteria.

Definite IE:
- *Pathologic criteria*: Microorganism demonstrated by culture or histologic examination of vegetation, emboli, intracardiac abscess; or active endocardial lesions on pathology examination
- *Clinical criteria*: Two major criteria, or one major criterion and three minor criteria, or five minor criteria

Possible IE: One major criterion and one minor criterion, or three minor criteria

Rejected:
- Firm alternative diagnosis explaining evidence of IE; or
- "IE syndrome" resolved within 4 days of antibiotic therapy; or
- No pathological evidence of IE at surgery or autopsy within 4 days of antibiotic therapy; or
- Does not meet criteria for "possible IE" as above

MANAGEMENT

The aim of the management is to treat infection with antibiotics, manage complications, and surgical intervention in selected cases. If the patient is very ill, antibiotic treatment can be initiated empirically after the cultures are taken. However, in all the other cases, initiation of therapy should await the results of blood cultures. Exact treatment depends upon the organism isolated and its antibiotic sensitivities. Usually, penicillin (or vancomycin if sensitive to penicillin) and gentamicin are the preferred antibiotics that are administered parenterally. The total duration of therapy for native valve endocarditis varies from 2 weeks to 6 weeks. Duration of therapy depends on the type of etiological agent, site of valvar infection, and complications. Following completion of therapy, blood cultures should be obtained to verify eradication of the infection. The American Heart Association has listed various regimens for IE in adults, and the same can be followed in children with dose modification. Fungal endocarditis may be difficult to treat and may require surgery along with antifungals, such as amphotericin B, for a duration of 6–8 weeks followed by oral antifungals, such as fluconazole, for prolonged duration of time (may take up to a year). The

Box 7.5.2: Indications for surgery in acute phase of infective endocarditis.

- Myocardial or periannular abscess
- Continued bacteremia after 2 weeks of antibiotic therapy
- Worsening of heart failure due to valvular regurgitation
- Embolic events
- Fungal endocarditis
- Prosthetic valve dysfunction

Box 7.5.3: Complications of infective endocarditis.

- *Embolic events*: Cerebral, pulmonary, renal, coronary
- Congestive heart failure
- Persistent bacteremia or fungemia
- Periannular extension of abscess
- Metastatic infection
- Glomerulonephritis/renal failure
- Mycotic aneurysm
- Arrhythmia or development of new heart block

indications of surgery in the acute phase have been listed in **Box 7.5.2**. The aims of the surgery are to repair the cardiac defects, eradicate infection, and to prevent complications. Despite the availability of antimicrobials, endocarditis can lead to major complications **(Box 7.5.3)**. Complications are more likely to occur in patients with prosthetic valve, age less than 2 years, left-sided IE, fungal and staphylococcal IE, symptom continuing for more than 3 months, and cyanotic CHDs.

PROPHYLAXIS

Antibiotics are recommended for the prevention of IE prior to certain medical and dental procedures. The guidelines by the American Heart Association have undergone changes in 2007. The cardiac conditions for which prophylaxis is recommended have been listed in **Box 7.5.4**. Presently, it is recommended for all dental procedures that involve treatment of gingival tissue or periapical region of the teeth or oral mucosal perforation, for invasive procedures that involve incision or biopsy of respiratory mucosa, such as tonsillectomy and adenoidectomy. It is no longer recommended for genitourinary or gastrointestinal tract procedures solely for bacterial endocarditis prophylaxis. The application of these guidelines in the Indian context is debated by various pediatric cardiologists. The drugs recommended are oral amoxicillin (50 mg/kg), intravenous ampicillin, and those allergic to penicillin can take cefazolin, ceftriaxone, clindamycin, cephalexin, azithromycin, or clarithromycin. The antibiotic should be given before the procedure and up to 2 hours after the procedure in those who did not take it earlier.

Box 7.5.4: Cardiac conditions for which antibiotic prophylaxis is recommended for dental, respiratory tract, infected skin, skin structures, or musculoskeletal tissue procedures.

- Prosthetic cardiac valve or prosthetic material used for cardiac valve repair
- Previous IE
- Unrepaired cyanotic CHD, including palliative shunts and conduits
- Completely repaired congenital heart defect with prosthetic material or device, whether placed by surgery or by catheter intervention during the first 6 months after the procedure
- Repaired CHD with residual defects at the site or adjacent to the site of a prosthetic patch or prosthetic device (which inhibits endothelialization)
- Cardiac transplantation recipients who develop cardiac valvulopathy

(CHD: congenital heart disease; IE: infective endocarditis)

MYOCARDIAL DISEASES

CARDIOMYOPATHY

Cardiomyopathy refers to a group of diseases of heart muscle that is not secondary to structural heart disease, hypertension, or pulmonary vascular disease. These are categorized by the World Health Organization as dilated, hypertrophic, restrictive, and arrhythmogenic right ventricular dysplasia—cardiomyopathy. One more form of cardiomyopathy, i.e. left ventricular (LV) noncompaction (spongy myocardium or fetal myocardium) is also recognized as a distinct form of cardiomyopathy by the American Heart Association. This entity is not so rare as was previously believed as the incidence in various studies in children varies between 8% and 9% and mimics dilated cardiomyopathy (DCM) as far as clinical features and outcome are concerned. Cardiomyopathy is characterized by the abnormality of systolic and/or diastolic function. Factors identified as causes of myocardial damage have been shown in **Table 7.5.2**.

Dilated Cardiomyopathy

Dilated cardiomyopathy is the most common type of heart muscle disease in children where both the ventricles are dilated with reduced contractility. Most cases of DCM are idiopathic.

Etiopathogenesis

Three major factors, viz. preceding viral myocarditis, autoimmunity, and underlying genetic predisposition, have been implicated in the pathogenesis of myocardial damage in DCM. Injury to the myocardial cells is the initiating factor that leads to cell death. If considerable cell loss occurs, the myocardium fails to generate enough contractile force to produce adequate cardiac output and leads to chronic

Table 7.5.2: Etiology of myocardial damage.

Infections	***Metabolic, endocrinal, nutritional***
Viral infections (myocarditis): • Coxsackievirus B • Adenovirus • Parvovirus • Human immunodeficiency virus • Echovirus • Rubella • Varicella • Mumps • Epstein-Barr virus • Cytomegalovirus • Measles • Polio *Others*: • Diphtheria • *Mycoplasma* • Tuberculosis • Lyme disease • Psittacosis • Rocky mountain spotted fever • *Toxoplasma* • *Toxocara* • *Cysticercus* • *Histoplasma* • *Coccidioidomycosis* • *Actinomycosis*	• Pompe disease • Carnitine deficiency syndrome • Hyperthyroidism • Carcinoid syndrome • Infant of diabetic mother • Kwashiorkor • Pellagra • Thiamine deficiency • Selenium deficiency
Familial—hereditary	***Coronary arteries***
• Mitochondrial myopathy syndrome • Hypertrophic cardiomyopathy • Duchenne or Becker muscular dystrophies • Friedreich ataxia • Kearns-Sayre syndrome • Other muscular dystrophies	• Kawasaki disease • Anomalous left coronary artery *Drugs—toxins:* • Doxorubicin • Cyclophosphamide • Chloroquine • Hemosiderosis
Connective tissue—granulomatous—infiltrative: • Systemic lupus erythematosus • Scleroderma • Rheumatoid arthritis • Sarcoidosis • Amyloidosis • Dermatomyositis • Leukemia	*Others* • Anemia • Sickle cell disease • Endomyocardial fibroelastosis • Histiocytosis

heart failure (CHF). Overstretching of the ventricles causes myocardial thinning, cavity dilatation, secondary valvular regurgitation, and compromised myocardial perfusion. The resulting subendocardial ischemia perpetuates myocyte damage.

Myocardial remodeling is an important contributor to worsening heart failure (HF). Lost myocyte cells are replaced with fibrous tissue, thereby decreasing the compliance of one or more ventricles and adversely affecting performance. Aldosterone, angiotensin II, catecholamines, endothelins, and mechanical factors, such as excessive myocardial stretch and ischemia, have been identified as mediators of remodeling.

Altered gene expressions resulting in calcium-handling abnormalities, downregulation of myosin or conversion to the less active beta isoform, and abnormal beta-receptor signal transduction have all been identified at the molecular level in the chronically failing heart.

Clinical Features

Children with DCM usually present typically after HF. Cough, poor feeding, irritability, and difficulty in breathing are usually the initial presenting symptoms. Older children complain of easy fatigability, dyspnea, and palpitation and rarely may present with pulmonary edema. Clinical examination may reveal displaced apical impulse, muffled heart sound with a prominent S3 or S4. Murmurs are usually not audible but rarely the murmur of mitral regurgitation (MR) or tricuspid regurgitation (TR) may be heard. The liver may be enlarged, and in older children, other signs of venous congestion, such as neck vein congestion and peripheral edema, may be observed. A short duration of symptoms (2–4 weeks) may suggest myocarditis. The infant or young child with the disease is often tachypneic, tachycardic with weak peripheral pulses and has cool extremities and hepatomegaly. Blood pressure is low with a decreased pulse pressure, accentuated P2, murmurs of MR and TR; murmurs may be inconspicuous initially if the patient presents with acute HF and cardiomegaly.

Cardiomyopathy should always be suspected in cases of acute decompensated HF in emergency and primary-care settings, especially if the infant presents with lethargy, weakness, abdominal pain, and unexplained tachypnea or disproportionate tachycardia. Even in the absence of cardiomegaly in chest X-ray, myocarditis should always be considered in the differential diagnosis in cases presenting with a viral prodrome and nonspecific respiratory or abdominal symptoms associated with tachycardia, hypotension, or cardiac rhythm abnormalities. One should rule out three important correctable causes of DCMs, i.e. anomalous left coronary artery from the pulmonary artery, tachycardiomyopathy, and hypocalcemia in newborn and young infants.

Diagnosis

The main aim for diagnostic evaluation for a patient with DCM is to identify the underlying etiology so that an etiology-specific therapy can be planned. Even in best of centers the cause is usually identified in only 34% of children. An additional purpose is to determine the extent of myocardial dysfunction and its complication, such as clot formation in the heart (**Fig. 7.5.1**). **Table 7.5.3** provides a list of useful diagnostic tests.

Screening of Family Members

Recent reports suggest a genetic cause for more than 50% of patients with DCM. With the advancement of molecular genetics techniques, prospective controlled studies on screening of family members have revealed a genetic transmission up to 20–30% cases with DCM and a prevalent autosomal trait. Due to limited awareness about the genetic predisposition, screening and echo of family members are not performed, but it is advisable in view of above findings.

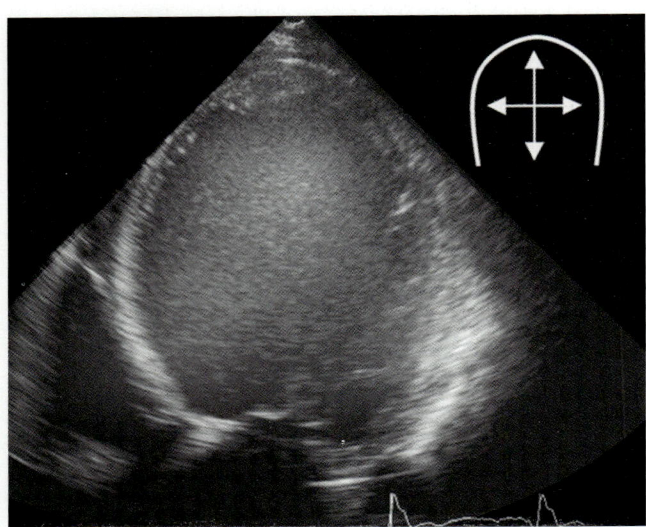

Fig. 7.5.1: Transthoracic echocardiogram of patient with dilated cardiomyopathy (apical four-chamber view shows dilated left ventricle).

Treatment

Treatment involves supportive management of CHF (discussed in detail in Chapter 7.4, Congestive Heart Failure). Ideally, etiology-specific treatment is recommended, but it requires clear proof of association of etiology, which is not possible always, other various treatment modalities (immunoglobulins or carnitine) are administered without good evidence. These treatment modalities have been enlisted in **Table 7.5.4**.

Immunoglobulins and immunosuppression: Intravenous immunoglobulin (IVIG) has been used as an immune modulator, which neutralizes pathogenic antibodies and suppresses the ongoing process and is used in cases of myocarditis. Pediatric Cardiac Society of India in a consensus review (2009) has recommended IVIG in cases where symptoms are preceded by viral illness, or when history is short (<3 months) or cardiac enzymes are elevated. The role of immunosuppressive agents (prednisolone, azathioprine, or cyclosporine) is debatable and is not recommended routinely due to lack of convincing evidence.

Table 7.5.3: List of investigations in dilated cardiomyopathy.

Investigations	***Findings and comments***
Chest X-ray	Cardiomegaly and features of pulmonary venous congestion
Electrocardiogram	Low-voltage waves, "ST" segment depressions with "T" wave inversion in the anterolateral precordial leads, prominent "Q" wave, changes suggestive of arrhythmias
Echocardiogram **(Fig. 7.5.1)**	EF and FS. LV systolic dysfunction in children is currently defined by a fractional shortening < 25% and/or an ejection fraction < 55%. Quantification of MR, clots, thrombus, and coronaries; rule out any structural heart lesion
Basic laboratory tests	Hemogram, ESR, glucose, urea, creatinine, LFT, electrolytes, calcium, phosphorous, ABGs
Metabolic screening	Blood lactate, serum ammonia, urinary ketones
Muscle enzymes	CPK, CPK-MB, cardiac troponin T
Biomarkers: BNP/NT-proBNP	Differentiates symptoms due to lung disease or heart failure, can be used as a confirmatory test in the acute evaluation of pediatric HF
Screening and echocardiogram of family members	Screening of first-degree relatives of the case
Endomyocardial biopsy and viral culture	Not advised routinely and should only be performed if confirming the clinical diagnosis of myocarditis will have a clear effect on the patient treatment plan
CMRI with gadolinium contrast	Can detect patchy myocardial involvement and provide additional information by tissue and scar characterization

(ABGs: arterial blood gases; BNP: B-type natriuretic peptide; CMRI: cardiac magnetic resonance imaging; CPK: creatine phosphokinase; CPK-MB: creatine phosphokinase-muscle/brain; EF: ejection fraction; ESR: erythrocyte sedimentation rate; FS: fractional shortening; HF: heart failure; LFT: liver function test; LV: left ventricular; MR: mitral regurgitation; NT-proBNP: N-terminal pro-b-type natriuretic peptide)

Table 7.5.4: Treatment options for dilated cardiomyopathy.

Treatment options	***Comments***
Digoxin	Can be given in myocarditis but loading dose is to be avoided
Furosemide + spironolactone	Helps in reducing systemic and pulmonary venous congestion
Intravenous inotropes and vasodilators (dobutamine, dopamine, amrinone, milrinone)	• Dobutamine is the first choice in the stage of decompensation • Milrinone is becoming the first-line treatment as it causes less mechanical stress as compared to other cardiotonics • To be used cautiously in cases of hypotension
ACE inhibitors (captopril, enalapril)	• Benefits by reducing systemic vascular resistance • Initiate treatment with captopril and can be changed to enalapril • Avoid during acute decompensated state
Beta-blockers and carvedilol	Carvedilol is the most widely used and improves symptoms and LV failure. It should be considered in the absence of overt heart failure, particularly in the presence of tachycardia
Anticoagulation and aspirin	All children with DCM and severe LV dysfunction (EF < 30%) should ideally be anticoagulated and in the absence of monitoring INR, aspirin can be tried. Presence of LV thrombus is a strong indication for oral anticoagulation
Carnitine	If metabolic screening suggests carnitine deficiency (elevated ammonia levels, high blood lactate, or presence of urinary ketones), carnitine can be given

(ACE: Angiotensin converting enzyme; DCM: Dilated cardiomyopathy; EF: Ejection fraction; INR: International normalized ratio; LV: Left ventricular)

Surgical and other interventions: Reduction cardiomyoplasty or Batista operation, assist devices, extracorporeal membrane oxygenation, and artificial heart are some procedures, which are often used as option to "bridge to transplantation procedure" and are very expensive. Cardiac transplantation is the final treatment for DCM with severe LV dysfunction and reported survival benefit of 1 year being 90%, 5 years 75%, and 20 years 40%.

Stem-cell therapy: This is other promising option and several researches are going in adult and pediatric population.

Prognosis

In a small proportion of pediatric patients, DCM may resolve completely. In few pediatric case series the mortality from DCM at 5 years after presentation varied from 33% to 66%. In a large case series from All India Institutes of Medical Sciences on 128 children, it was reported that 54% improved on medication and of these 24% became symptom free without medication. Around 35% deteriorated despite therapy, and 19% died. Female sex was only multivariate predictor of death. Overall, the prognosis of DCM will improve only if various etiologies are understood and etiology-specific therapy is instituted.

Hypertrophic Cardiomyopathy

Hypertrophic cardiomyopathy (HCM) is a condition in which myocardial thickness is increased. In contrast to DCM the LV cavity has a normal or decreased size. During systole, the hypertrophied myocardium bulges into the LV outflow tract and may result in subaortic obstruction.

Etiology and Genetics

The disease may be caused by one of many possible mutations of genes coding for various contractile proteins. This condition frequently occurs as an autosomal dominant with a variable penetrance. Multiple generations may be involved. Manifestations can begin at any age. Siblings of the proband may not be affected as children but may show evidence of the disease as they reach adolescence and adulthood. The natural history and prognosis are variable; sudden death is not uncommon even in patients who have no important obstruction or sentinel arrhythmia.

Clinical Features

Patients with HCM usually come to medical attention in one or more of the following ways:

1. Detection of a murmur
2. An angina kind of chest pain
3. An abnormal electrocardiogram (ECG)
4. From family screening or a positive family history or
5. From evaluation of syncope, palpitations, or out of hospital cardiac arrest

The physical findings can be variable. The peripheral pulse may be of bisferiens character with rapid upstroke, and palpation of the apex may reveal a double impulse. A long systolic ejection murmur is present along the left sternal border and faintly radiates to the base. The murmur varies in intensity with change in position; it is usually the loudest with the patient standing in contrast to functional flow murmurs. Third and fourth sounds may be present.

Investigations

Chest X-ray is not diagnostic, and ECG shows the evidence of left and frequently biventricular hypertrophy with or without ischemic changes. Septal changes are evidenced by abnormal "q" waves in V5 and V6. The echocardiogram may reveal asymmetric septal hypertrophy. Left ventricular thickness more than or equal to 2 standard deviation above the mean (*Z* score >) for age, sex, or body size is diagnostic of HCM in children, the interventricular septum may be 2–3 cm thick compared with the normal, which is less than or equal to 1 cm. Systolic anterior motion of the mitral valve anterior leaflet is a classic two-dimensional echocardiographic finding. It results from the high-velocity flow occurring in the LV outflow tract. This creates low pressure, which "pulls" the valve leaflet toward the interventricular septum during systole. Cardiac catheterization and angiography are rarely required.

Treatment

The greatest risk with HCM is sudden death despite medical and surgical treatment. For symptomatic patients, beta-blockers or verapamil can be tried, and for the control of arrhythmias, disopyramide and amiodarone are the drugs of choice. Digitalis, other inotropic drugs, and afterload reducing agents, which increase the gradient, are contraindicated. It is necessary that patients with HCM should undergo a 24-hour Holter to document for arrhythmias and should be restrained from strenuous games and exercises. Implantable automatic cardioverter/defibrillator devices may abort potentially lethal arrhythmia in some patients.

For patients with significant LV outflow tract obstruction, surgical myomectomy or alcohol ablation can be done. There is increasing evidence that elimination of the obstruction prolongs life and relieves symptoms.

Prognosis

Although ultimately fatal in majority, interval between discovery and death often goes in decades. The risk of sudden death in recent population-based studies has shown to be nearly 1% per year. Following features may be associated with higher risk for sudden death: diagnosis in childhood, septal thickness exceeding 3 cm, nonsustained ventricular tachycardia, failure of normal increase of systolic blood pressure during exercise, family history of premature death associated with HCM, significant LV outflow tract obstruction, and prior cardiac arrest.

Restrictive Cardiomyopathy

This is the rarest form of cardiomyopathy characterized by poor ventricular compliance and limited filling. It may be idiopathic or may be associated with a systemic disease, such as scleroderma, amyloidosis, sarcoidosis, or inborn error of metabolism (mucopolysaccharidoses).

The two common types are endocardial fibroelastosis with normal or less than normal left ventricle and endomyocardial fibrosis. Endomyocardial fibrosis is endemic in Kerala, but rare in North India.

Symptoms are nonspecific and like those of CHF seen with DCM. In contrast to DCM the left ventricle is of normal size and may have normal systolic function. This condition alters diastolic ventricular function, so the clinical manifestations are those of elevated left and right atrial pressures.

Examination reveals hepatic and splenic enlargement and jugular venous distension. Electrocardiographic abnormalities are usually limited to atrial enlargement. Chest X-ray shows pulmonary vascular congestion with a relatively normal cardiac silhouette. The echocardiogram reveals striking dilatation of the atria and great veins but normal or small ventricles. Physiologically, the condition is like constrictive pericarditis, and differentiating the two can be difficult. Overall, the prognosis is poor in infants and children, and cardiac transplantation is advised once the diagnosis is made.

A comparison of the three variants of cardiomyopathy has been summarized in **Table 7.5.5**.

PERICARDIAL DISEASE

Pericarditis is the inflammation of the visceral and parietal layer of pericardium. The causes are variable and are listed in **Table 7.5.6**. Pericardial effusion is the accumulation of excess fluid in pericardial sac. The symptoms that result from pericardial fluid depend upon the status of the myocardium and the volume and the speed at which the fluid accumulates. It may be exudative due to bacterial infections, serous to increased capillary pressures (e.g. CHF) or decreased plasma oncotic pressure (e.g. hypoproteinemia). Cardiac tamponade is a life threatening, slow or rapid compression of the heart due to accumulation of fluid, blood, clots, or gas in the pericardial space leading to significant impairment of ventricular filling with reduction in stroke volume and cardiac output. It is most commonly associated with viral infections, neoplasm, uremia, and acute hemorrhage. Constrictive pericarditis is due to adherent thick noncompliant pericardium that restricts ventricular filling. In children, tuberculosis is the most common cause in India.

Table 7.5.5: Overview of myopathy.

	Dilated	***Hypertrophic***	***Restrictive***
Prevalence	50/100,000	1/500	Unknown
Inheritance	25–50% AD, AR, X-L, MT	50% AD	Unknown
Ventricular function	Systolic and diastolic dysfunction	Diastolic dysfunction	Severely reduced diastolic function
Arrhythmias	Atrial, ventricular, and conduction disturbances	Atrial and ventricular dynamic systolic outflow obstruction	Atrial fibrillation normal to reduced systolic function
Echocardiographic findings	Dilated LV cavity with normal to thin wall thickness	Asymmetric, concentric or apical LV hypertrophy	Normal or small ventricular cavity size, marked biatrial enlargement
Medical management	ACE inhibitors diuretics (furosemide, spironolactone) digitalis β2-blocking agents	Propranolol pacemaker calcium antagonists (digitalis/catechols and nitrates contraindicated, and diuretics may worsen symptoms)	Antiarrhythmic agents careful use of diuretics, milrinone
Surgical/interventional	ICD, resynchronization biventricular pacing transplantation	ICD, septal myomectomy transplantation	ICD transplantation
Sudden death	Yes	Depends on gene 0.7–11% per year, associated with exercise	1.5% per year

(ACE: angiotensin converting enzyme; AD: autosomal dominant; AR: autosomal recessive; ICD: implantable cardioverter defibrillator; LV: left ventricular; MT: mitochondrial; X-L: X-linked)

Table 7.5.6: Causes of pericardial diseases.

Congenital:
- Absence of pericardium
- Pericardial cyst

Infectious:
- Viral (*coxsackievirus A and B, Epstein-Barr virus, hepatitis, HIV, adenovirus*)
- Bacterial (*Staphylococcus, Haemophilus influenzae type B Streptococcus, Pneumococcus*)
- Tuberculosis
- Fungal (*histoplasmosis, actinomycosis*)
- Parasitic (*Toxoplasmosis, Echinococcosis*)

Connective tissue diseases:
- Rheumatic fever
- Rheumatoid arthritis
- Systemic lupus erythematosus
- Systemic sclerosis
- Kawasaki disease
- Wegener granulomatosis

Hematology-oncology:
- Bleeding diathesis
- Malignancy (primary, metastatic)
- Radiotherapy induced

Postprocedural:
- Postcardiac catheterization
- Cardiac surgery
- Central line placement

Drugs:
- Anticoagulants
- Antithrombolytics
- Hydralazine
- Phenytoin
- INH
- Rifampicin

Others:
- Renal failure
- Hypothyroidism
- Chylopericardium

(HIV: human immunodeficiency virus; INH: isonicotinylhydrazide)

Clinical Features

The clinical manifestations of pericarditis, which may vary from a simple inflammatory response with no cardiovascular compromise to cardiac tamponade and constrictive pericarditis, are noted in **Table 7.5.7**. The differentiation of the constrictive pericarditis and restrictive myocarditis can be challenging.

Table 7.5.7: Manifestations and management of pericarditis.

	Nonconstrictive pericarditis	*Pericardial effusion*	*Cardiac tamponade*	*Constrictive pericarditis*
Symptoms	• Retrosternal chest pain (occasionally radiating to back) • Aggravated by supine position • Relieved by leaning forward, dyspnea	• May be asymptomatic • Dull ache • Other features of cardiac tamponade	• Dyspnea • Fatigue • Anorexia • Cough • Cold extremities	• Exercise intolerance • Syncope with exertion • Dyspnea • Fatigue • Anorexia
Signs	• Fever • Tachypnea • Pericardial rub • Distant heart sound	• Muffled heart sound • Ewart sign (dullness of posterior left chest wall) • Tachycardia	• Raised JVP • Hypotension • Tachycardia • Pulsus paradoxus (decrease in systolic blood pressure > 10 mm Hg with each inspiration) • Decreased capillary refill time • Silent precordium • Distant heart sound • Hepatomegaly	• Tachycardia • Pedal edema • Raised JVP • Hepatomegaly • Ascites • Pericardial knock • Signs of low cardiac output
ECG	• "ST" segment elevation in all leads • PR segment depression	• Decreased voltage "QRS" complex • Electrical alternans	• Electrical alternans • Sinus tachycardia • Low-voltage waves • Electrical alternans	• Low-voltage waves • Intraventricular conduction delay
Chest X-ray	Normal	Globular, symmetrical cardiomegaly	Globular, symmetrical cardiomegaly	• Normal • Pericardial calcification or effusion
Echocardiography	Usually normal	An echo-free space (suggesting fluid) around the heart	• Global fluid collection • Compressed and collapsing chambers with hyperdynamic cardiac function	• Flattening of the left ventricular posterior wall endocardium • Abnormal septal motion • Dilated SVC, IVC, atria
Treatment	• Treat the cause; symptomatic treatment with rest • Analgesic and rarely antibiotics	• Treat the underlying condition • Pericardiocentesis if sudden accumulation of fluid • NSAIDs or steroids are required occasionally	• Needle pericardiocentesis or surgical drainage, pericardial stripping or window in recurrent condition	• Analgesic, corticosteroids, and antibiotics • Pericardiectomy is definitive treatment but mostly unwarranted as many cases, including TB, resolve spontaneously

(ECG: electrocardiogram; IVC: inferior vena cava; JVP: jugular venous pressure; NSAIDs: nonsteroidal anti-inflammatory drugs; SVC: superior vena cava; TB: tuberculosis)

Management

The management of these conditions will depend on the cause and they are listed in **Table 7.5.7**.

BIBLIOGRAPHY

1. Baddour LM, Wilson WR, Bayer AS, et al. Infective endocarditis: diagnosis, antimicrobial therapy, and management of complications: a statement for healthcare professionals from the Committee on Rheumatic Fever, Endocarditis, and Kawasaki Disease, Council on Cardiovascular Disease in the Young, and the Councils on Clinical Cardiology, Stroke, and Cardiovascular Surgery and Anesthesia, American Heart Association: endorsed by the Infectious Diseases Society of America. Circulation. 2005;111(23):e394-433.
2. Jefferies JL, Towbin JA. Dilated cardiomyopathy. Lancet. 2010;375:752-62.

3. Kantor PF, Lougheed J, Dancea A, et al. Presentation, diagnosis, and medical management of heart failure in children: Canadian Cardiovascular Society guidelines. Can J Cardiol. 2013;29:1535-52.
4. Wilson W, Taubert KA, Gewitz M, et al. Prevention of infective endocarditis guidelines from the American Heart Association: a guideline from the American Heart Association Rheumatic Fever, Endocarditis, and Kawasaki Disease Committee, Council on Cardiovascular Disease in the Young, and the Council on Clinical Cardiology, Council on Cardiovascular Surgery and Anesthesia, and the Quality of Care and Outcomes Research Interdisciplinary Working Group. Circulation. 2007;116:1745-54.
5. Working Group on Management of Congenital Heart Diseases in India. Consensus on timing of intervention for common congenital heart disease. Indian Pediatr. 2008;45:117-26.
6. Working Group on Management of Congenital Heart Diseases in India. Drug therapy of cardiac diseases in children (Saxena A, Ramakrishnan S, Tandon R, et al.). Indian Pediatr. 2009;46(4):310-38.

7.6 Cardiac Arrhythmias

S Srinivasan

INTRODUCTION

Cardiac arrhythmias refer to occurrence of *irregularities in rate or rhythm or both of the heartbeats* due to disturbances or alterations or dysfunction in cardiac electrical impulse generation, conduction or excitability. Arrhythmias are more often seen in hearts with abnormal conduction pathway structures or altered cardiac structural or pathological states than seen in normal hearts during certain physiological states. They may occur in periodic or paroxysmal episodes or have continuous runs unless terminated by appropriate therapeutic interventions. When heart rate slows down to less than 60 per minute, it is termed as *bradycardia*, and when the same is more than 120 per minute, it is called *tachycardia*.

The myocardial contraction is initiated by electrical impulses (action potentials due to phasic alteration in electrical voltage of membrane potential by the influx of ionic Na^+ and Ca^{++} causing depolarization and efflux of K^+ resulting in repolarization) generated in the sinoatrial node (SA node) located at the junction of superior vena cava and right atrium by a well-regulated sequence of electrically charged transmembrane ion exchanges through highly specialized channels. The SA node acts as an electrical impulse generator or pacemaker with its own intrinsic rate depending upon the age of the child, controlled by the autonomic nervous system. The impulses thus generated by the SA node pass through the internodal pathways in atrium to the atrioventricular (AV) node and bundle of His, and then its right and left branches having specialized fibers for rapid transmission of electrical impulses on either side of the interventricular septum to depolarize the atria and ventricles in sequence determined by the slower conductivity of AV node. The right and left bundle branches terminate in millions of small Purkinje fibers projecting through the myocardium. The action potentials passing through the specialized internodal pathways in the atria depolarize the atrial myocytes. The respective right and left branches depolarize the myocytes of the corresponding right and left ventricles with the interventricular septum. The cardiomyocytes contract by a process termed "excitation-contraction coupling".

If the sinus rate generated by master pacemaker SA node slows down considerably, shift in pacemaker activity occurs, and the AV node (nodal rhythm) or the myocytes of the ventricle (idioventricular rhythm) takes over the function of impulse generation and propagation **(Table 7.6.1)**.

The SA node, consisting of specialized electrical impulse generating cardiac fibers with few contractile myofibril elements and nerve terminals from the autonomic nervous system, has inherent automatic rhythmicity to generate regular electrical impulses to be conducted to AV node, thus

Table 7.6.1: Cardiac cell types, their location, and their inherent electrical pacemaker potentials.

Pacemaker	*Location*	*Inherent rate (beats/min)*
Sinoatrial node	RA at SVC junction	60–100
Atrioventricular node	RA at posteroinferior area of interatrial septum	40–60
Purkinje fibers	Throughout the ventricles	2–40
Ventricular cardiomyocytes	Throughout the ventricles	2–40

(RA: right atrium; SVC: superior vena cava)

setting the pace for cardiac contractility to occur at a regular rate. Hence, it is also known as the primary pacemaker or generator of the heart.

The AV node is stimulated by the transmission of impulses at a specific rate per minute from SA node and transmits them to the contractile elements, e.g. the myocardial fibers of the ventricles. AV node is thus directed by the SA node to intensify and transmit or relay the electrical signals to the ventricular myocardium to contract at a specific rate. AV node functions mostly as a receiver and a pace transmitter or relay station and occasionally takes over as a pacesetter. AV node is not influenced directly by the autonomic nervous system unlike SA node. It is governed by the SA node automaticity, rhythmicity, and conductivity.

If the SA nodal generated rate slows down considerably, shift in pacemaker activity occurs, and the AV node (nodal rhythm) or the ventricle (idioventricular rhythm) takes over the function of impulse generation and propagation.

On the standard surface electrocardiogram (ECG) recording, the "P" wave in the PQRST represents the depolarization wave spreading from SA node throughout the atrial musculature causing atrial contraction ahead of ventricular depolarization and contraction. Its duration is usually 0.08–0.1 second. The atrial rate is calculated by determining the time interval between P waves. The brief isoelectric period after the P wave and before the inscription of QRS represents the travel time of electrical impulse within the AV node with decreased conduction velocity and the bundle of His.

The *PR interval* duration, the distance between the onset of P wave to the beginning of QRS complex (normal duration: 0.12–0.20 second), is the time duration between the onset of atrial and ventricular depolarizations. A prolonged PR interval beyond the upper range of the normal for that age (more than 0.2 second) indicates delay between SA node and AV node, termed AV block.

The *QRS complex* represents ventricular depolarization. The distance between two successive QRS complexes in a child with regular rhythm helps in arriving at the ventricular rate. When this time gets prolonged beyond the upper range of normal for that age (range: 0.06–0.1 second), it indicates slowed and impaired conduction within the ventricles occurring in bundle branch blocks or in situations where an abnormal ventricular focus acts as an abnormal ectopic pacemaker directing the rate of ventricular contractions.

The *ST segment*, the isoelectric segment that follows the QRS, is the time taken for ventricular depolarization. An elevated or depressed ST segment from isoelectric line is of diagnostic importance in ischemic, hypoxic, or inflammatory insults to the ventricular myocardium and pericardium.

The *T wave* representing ventricular repolarization is longer in duration than its depolarization. It may be sometimes followed by a "U wave" representing the late phase of repolarization. When present, its prominence or inversion indicates abnormal physiological or pathological states affecting repolarization.

The *QT interval* is the average ventricular electrical action potential representing the total duration of ventricular depolarization and repolarization time (heart-rate-dependent range 0.2–0.4 second). Prolonged QT interval indicates increased risk for the development of tachyarrhythmias; and hence, it is vital to accurately determine and interpret the duration of QT interval as normal, prolonged, or short. It is often expressed as "corrected QT interval (QTc)." Thus heart rate independent "QTc" is calculated by dividing the QT interval by the square root of the RR interval (interval between two successive ventricular depolarizations). Prolonged QTc interval is beyond 0.44 second.

SINUS RHYTHMS

Sinus Bradycardia and Sinus Tachycardia

Sinus bradycardia (heart rate less than what is mentioned in **Table 7.6.2** for that age) occurs in older children who are athletic. It also occurs following therapy with drugs, such as parasympathomimetic drugs or poisons, antisympathomimetic drugs, such as beta-blockers, digitalis, and verapamil; and pathological conditions, such as hypothyroidism, hypothermia, and raised intracranial pressure.

Sinus tachycardia (heart rate more than what is mentioned in **Table 7.6.2** for that age) occurs with sympathetic

Table 7.6.2: Approximate range of normal heart rate variability in neonates, infants, and children.

Age range	*Heart rate*	*Age range (years)*	*Heart rate*
Neonates	100–160	3–5	80–120
1–5 months	90–150	6–10	70–110
6–12 months	80–140	11–14	60–105
1–3 years	80–130	15–20	60–100

stimulation after exercise, fever, anxiety, anemia, pregnancy, heart failure, thyrotoxicosis, and administration of drugs, which stimulate sympathetic nervous system.

Sinus arrhythmia is a manifestation of normal automatic nervous activity with increase in sinus heart rate during inspiration and a decrease during expiration. This is seen in young children.

TACHYARRHYTHMIAS

Supraventricular Tachycardia (Supraventricular Tachyarrhythmia, Paroxysmal Atrial Tachycardia, Atrioventricular Nodal Reentrant Tachycardia)

Supraventricular tachyarrhythmia is the most common of the rapid rhythm abnormalities encountered in children, the greatest frequency being recorded in infancy. It is known to occur in fetus as early as in the middle fetal life.

The two basic mechanisms of initiation of supraventricular tachycardia (SVT) are:

1. Impulse generation abnormalities, e.g. increased automaticity resulting in ectopic impulse formation.
2. Propagation abnormalities in ectopic impulse generated (reentry loop or closed circuit propagation), termed "reentrant tachycardia".

The sites, in which these mechanisms operate, determine the type of SVT:

- Reentry of the electrical impulse back into the conducting system either through an accessory pathway (Wolff-Parkinson-White syndrome) or accessory pathway reentry
- Atrioventricular nodal reentry
- Atrioventricular junctional focus
- Ectopic localized atrial focus of enhanced automaticity.

In AV reentrant tachycardia, retrograde conduction occurs from the ventricles back to the atrium by a concealed bypass tract.

In the absence of antegrade conduction by the bypass accessory pathway, reentry through the AV node or through a concealed bypass tract is responsible for more than 90% of all SVTs. AV nodal reentrant tachycardia, being the most common of all SVTs, has no specific predisposing factors. It most often occurs in children who are otherwise normal. In infancy, it is more common in children below 6 months of age.

Symptoms

These children are often asymptomatic. In infants, if it persists for more than 24 hours, symptoms and signs of congestive heart failure occur along with pallor, fatigue, and tachypnea. An older child may sense palpitation with sudden onset. Syncope and hypotension may be the presenting symptoms. Acute pulmonary edema can ensue.

Supraventricular tachyarrhythmia occurring in the fetus, when prolonged, results in heart failure and nonimmune hydrops fetalis.

Diagnosis

The heart rate is regular and often ranges between 200 per minute and 320 per minute, and all impulses are conducted to the ventricles. The onset of the paroxysm is as sudden and abrupt as its termination.

Whenever the heart rate in an infant is more than 200 beats/min (ranging up to 320 beats/min) and in a child more than 180 beats/min and often regular and in the absence of possible causes for sinus tachycardia, SVT is strongly suspected and confirmed by immediate electrocardiographic examination. There may be symptoms or history suggestive of SVT either now or in the past.

Electrocardiogram shows marked tachycardia (>200 per minute) with regular narrow QRS complexes, and the P waves may be normal, absent, buried in the QRS complex, or appear as distortions at the terminal part of the QRS complexes. When QRS complexes become wider in presence of associated bundle branch block, it becomes difficult to differentiate from ventricular tachycardia (VT).

Treatment

Stable children with abrupt, brief episode without symptoms:

First step: Simple vagal stimulation techniques or maneuvers, such as carotid sinus massage, placement of ice water bags over the face, and then child blowing through a closed straw, can effectively terminate SVT in the majority of cases. The progress must be however monitored by concurrent ECG recording.

Second step: Medical management—with unsuccessful vagal stimulation tactics, in a stable child with normal perfusion and with normal QRS less than 0.08 second, immediate vascular access is established. Adenosine, with its short half-life, is the drug of choice for all ages. Intravenous rapid bolus administration of 0.1 mg/kg of adenosine (maximum first dose of 6 mg and second dose of 12 mg) is resorted to. Verapamil is the next drug of choice and may be given in children above 1 year of age if adenosine is not readily available. Beta-blockers, disopyramide, and digitalis are less preferred alternatives, and digoxin is not helpful in acute case.

Third step: Electroconversion or direct-current (DC) cardioversion—if administration of adenosine (two blouses) is not terminating the normal or narrow QRS complex SVT, electrical DC cardioversion (first dose: 0.5–1 J/kg, and second dose, if first dose is ineffective: 2 J/kg) is performed with trained pediatric team in advanced life support system and resuscitation. Sedation before cardioversion is given to a conscious child.

Fourth step: Prevention of recurrences—further recurrences of SVT due to AV nodal reentry is achieved by the use of drugs, such as digitalis, beta-blockers, or calcium channel blockers, which act primarily on the antegrade slow pathway.

- Temporary percutaneous venous, atrial or ventricular pacing terminates the attack when drugs fail to do so or in recurrent cases.
- Catheter radiofrequency ablation of the reentrant circuit is frequently being resorted to in refractory cases.
- Cryoablation using cold energy is another recent, potentially safe, faster, and more effective method which is being increasingly employed and being evaluated.
- Surgical ablation is rarely resorted to.

Wolff–Parkinson–White Syndrome (Preexcitation Syndrome)

An abnormal band of specialized electrically conductible atrial tissue acts as an accessory pathway bypassing the junctional tissue. This occurs in association with some congenital heart diseases, and most commonly with Ebstein anomaly.

Wolff-Parkinson-White syndrome refers to antegrade conduction by AV bypass tract resulting in a short PR interval, a slurred upstroke of the QRS complex termed delta wave and a wide QRS complex. Differential conducting speeds of accessory and normal pathways with differing refractory periods cause reentry phenomenon to occur resulting in paroxysmal SVT. Atrial flutter and atrial fibrillation also occur commonly in this condition. This, in turn, may lead to very rapid ventricular rates, even resulting in VT and ventricular fibrillation (VF) because of the lack of decremental conducting properties in the bypass tract as in AV node.

Supraventricular tachyarrhythmia is treated as mentioned earlier. Class 1A drug (quinidine, procainamide, disopyramide) or Class 1C (flecainide) may be used to slow conduction and increase refractoriness primarily in the bypass tract. Flecainide is to be limited to be used in otherwise normal heart. Digitalis and verapamil can precipitate VF by shortening the refractory period of the bypass tract.

Radiofrequency ablation of an accessory pathway is another treatment option commonly used in patients with reentrant rhythm or atrial ectopic tachycardia. It is often used electively in children and teenagers, as well as in patients who require multiple agents or find drug side effects intolerable or for whom arrhythmia control is poor. The overall initial success rate ranges approximately from 80% to 95%, depending on the location of bypass tract. Surgical ablation of bypass tract may also be successful in related patients **(Table 7.6.3)**.

ATRIAL TACHYARRHYTHMIAS

Atrial Ectopic Beats or Extrasystoles

Premature atrial beats are recognized by abnormally shaped premature "P" waves, followed by near normal PR interval with normal QRS complex. Rarely, QRS complex may be aberrant. They may occur in normal newborns and disappear with age and do not cause symptoms. Multiple atrial premature beats may sometimes result in transient atrial fibrillation.

Atrial Flutter and Atrial Fibrillation

These two types of atrial arrhythmias are less common in children than in adults.

Atrial Flutter

Atrial flutter is uncommon in children. In atrial flutter, the characteristic feature is a very rapid atrial activity (250–400 beats/min) with the ventricles responding to every second to fourth atrial beat, resulting in a regular or regularly irregular tachycardia.

Causes: Being rare in children, it may however be seen rarely in congenital heart diseases, resulting in a grossly enlarged atria, e.g. mitral or tricuspid insufficiency, atrial septal defects (ASDs), tricuspid atresia, Ebstein anomaly, acquired rheumatic mitral valvular heart disease, acute viral myocarditis, cardiomyopathy, pericarditis, hypertension, and intra-atrial surgery.

Pathophysiology: An electrically active (irritable), abnormal focus in atria produces abnormal impulse, which gets

Table 7.6.3: Intravenous antiarrhythmic agents commonly employed in SVT, atrial, and ventricular tachyarrhythmias.

Drug (types of arrhythmia)	***Dosage***	***Comments***	***Monitoring***
Adenosine (SVT)	0.05 mg/kg through a central line; double the dose until effect is seen to a maximum of 0.4 mg/kg	Caution in asthmatics, contraindicated in preexisting types 2 and 3 AV block without pacemaker	
Verapamil (SVT)	0.05–0.2 mg/kg IV (maximum 5 mg) over 5–10 minutes	Contraindicated in children < 12 months of age	For hypotension
Propranolol	0.05–0.15 mg/kg IV slowly every 5 minutes (maximum 0.3 mg/kg, 5 mg)	Contraindicated in children with asthma, congestive heart failure. Not to be given with verapamil	Pulse, BP
Esmolol (SVT, VT)	0.5 mg/kg bolus over 1 minute; maintenance: 50–300 µg/kg/min	Contraindicated in children with asthma, congestive heart failure, hypersensitivity, sick sinus syndrome, second- and third-degree heart blocks	Pulse, BP
Procainamide (AF, AVN, and VT tachyarrhythmias)	10–20 mg/kg IV over 30–45 months maintenance 20–60 µg/kg/min	Continuous monitoring	Dizziness, hypotension
Lidocaine (VAs)	1–2 mg/kg IV over 15 months by continuous infusion: 30–50 µg/kg/min maintenance	Causes respiratory depression, hypotension	BP
Lignocaine (VAs)	1 mg/kg IV bolus 20–50 µg/kg/min IV		
Amiodarone (SVT, AAs and VAs)	Ventricular fibrillation: 5 mg/kg IV load over 20 minutes, then 5–15 µg/kg/min (maximum 15 mg/kg/day) SVT: 5 mg/kg over 10 min × 5 doses	Safety and efficacy in pediatric patients have not been well established	
Phenytoin (VAs)	20 mg/kg over 30 min IV LD		

(AAs: atrial arrhythmias; AF: atrial fibrillation; AVN: atrioventricular node; BP: blood pressure; IV: intravenous; LD: loading dose; SVT: supraventricular tachycardia; VAs: ventricular arrhythmias; VT: ventricular tachycardia)

repeatedly propagated by a circus rhythm, resulting in extremely rapid atrial rate. All of these rapid atrial beats cannot get transmitted through AV node. Varying degrees of AV block result in anywhere from 2:1 to 8:1 atrial ventricular rate ratios.

Symptoms: Symptoms depend upon the ventricular rate. No symptoms occur in atrial flutter with reasonable ventricular rate.

Prolonged episodes of atrial flutter with very rapid ventricular rate precipitate left ventricular (LV) dysfunction characterized by syncope, dyspnea, and other features of LV failure.

Electrocardiogram is characteristic showing the rapid and regular atrial saw-toothed flutter "F" waves.

Treatment: Direct-current cardioversion is the most effective method of reverting back to sinus rhythm.

Drugs: If the clinical status is stable, the ventricular rate is first slowed by the administration of AV node blocking drugs, such as beta-blockers, calcium channel antagonist (verapamil) or digitalis.

Once the ventricular rate is slowed, attempt is made to convert the flutter into normal sinus rhythm by the use of Class 1A drugs (quinidine, procainamide, or disopyramide), Class 1C drugs (flecainide), or amiodarone. The same drugs also prevent recurrences of atrial flutter and fibrillation.

Atrial Fibrillation

Atrial fibrillation is characterized by totally distorted, chaotic, rapid, and ineffective atrial contractions with irregular and erratic ventricular response resulting in the diagnostic "irregularly irregular" radial arterial pulse with pulse deficit. It may be paroxysmal or persistent. Atrial fibrillation is extremely uncommon in neonates, infants, and young children.

Causes: The causes mentioned above in atrial flutter may also lead to atrial fibrillation. Chronic rheumatic heart disease with mitral valve disease with significant atrial dilatation in adolescents in tropical countries and chronic unoperated moderate-to-severe ASDs in older children may develop atrial fibrillation. In sick sinus syndrome, atrial fibrillation may occur in the tachycardiac phase.

Symptoms: Symptoms occur with rapid ventricular rate—fatigue, palpitation, giddiness or syncope, symptoms of heart failure, and symptoms of systemic embolization in children with mitral valvular disease.

The ECG is characteristic with no organized discernible "P" waves, except for irregular, fibrillatory "F" waves in the baseline with irregular but normal QRS complexes.

Treatment: The therapeutic goal is to immediately slow down the ventricular rate by using either beta-blockers (propranolol) or calcium channel antagonists (verapamil). Quinidine or other Class 1A drugs as mentioned above or Class 1C drugs, such as flecainide, may then correct the condition to sinus rhythm. If no response occurs within 24 hours, electrical DC conversion is resorted to. The causative factors have to be immediately attended. Anticoagulation 2 weeks prior and 2 weeks after any attempt at cardioversion is indicated to prevent the dreaded thromboembolic complications in situations where atrial fibrillation has been persistent for more than 48–72 hours.

In exceptional circumstances of refractory atrial fibrillation, surgical or transvenous catheter radiofrequency ablation may be resorted to deliberately induce complete heart block (CHB) with simultaneous permanent pacemaker implantation.

VENTRICULAR TACHYARRHYTHMIAS

Ventricular Tachycardia

Ventricular tachycardia is defined as a tachycardia arising below the bundle of His with at least three or more ectopic ventricular beats in sequence. Sustained VT means a run of ventricular premature contractions in succession for a period of 30 seconds or more. Nonsustained VT represents episodes less than 30 seconds.

Monomorphic VT has regular rate and rhythm with the same QRS complex morphology.

Polymorphic VT has variable rate and variable QRS morphology.

The mechanisms involved in VT are the same as mentioned above for generation of SVT, e.g. ectopic automaticity of impulse generation, reentry and altered propagation in the ventricular myocardium.

Ventricular tachycardia, a potentially life-threatening arrhythmic condition in all age-groups, is thankfully less common in children. It accounts for 6% of all childhood tachyarrhythmias. When it occurs, it indicates the presence of a serious underlying structural or functional cardiac problem. VT with pulses may cause high variability in heart rate, varying from normal to even 200 beats/min. It compromises stroke volume and hence the cardiac output. The prognosis is poor and carries a great risk of mortality unless corrected immediately.

Causes

Electrolyte disturbances, such as hypokalemia, hypomagnesemia, severe acidosis, hypoxia, proarrhythmogenic drugs, myocarditis, ischemic myocardial damage, anomalous origin of the coronary artery, cardiomyopathy, mitral valve prolapse, prolonged QT interval (congenital or acquired), Wolff-Parkinson-White syndrome, cardiac tumors, and drug abuse with cocaine or amphetamine, are all known predisposing factors. In a significant number of children with VT, an underlying cause may not be found.

Symptoms

Symptoms vary depending upon the duration, type, and the underlying cause initiating the VT, and they include dizziness, syncope, chest pain, palpitations, breathlessness, and cardiac arrest.

Diagnosis

Electrocardiography: VT must be differentiated from SVT, and the golden rule is that all wide QRS tachycardia should be considered and treated as VT until proved otherwise. The helpful electrocardiographic features in the diagnosis of VT are the wide or broad QRS complexes (prolonged QRS duration), usually unidentifiable P waves, regular and fast ventricular beats usually around 120 beats/min. T waves with opposite polarity to QRS, ventricular arrhythmias dissociation, capture fusion beats, extreme left axis deviation, no response to carotid sinus massage, or intravenous administration of adenosine. The features that differentiate VT from SVT with wide QRS are the variation in RR intervals and the presence of fusion complexes.

Treatment

- *Acute management of VT*:
  - In "unstable" VT child, instantaneous synchronized cardioversion with 2 J/kg is the treatment of choice. The dose may be increased, if needed. It is mandatory to have electric defibrillator in every emergency room and intensive care areas and in all wards or in each floor of the hospital.
  - In "stable" VT child, drug treatment with 5 mg/kg of amiodarone is administered intravenously over 30–60 minutes. The other drug that is employed is intravenous procainamide at a dose of 15 mg/kg over the same period.
- *Drugs*:
  - *Lignocaine*: If defibrillator to deliver DC shock is not available or if VT is relatively well tolerated, bolus dose of lignocaine (1 mg/kg) is intravenously administered with continuing intravenous infusion at a rate of 10–50 mg/kg/min.

- Bretylium is an alternative drug in lignocaine refractory cases. Mexilitine, flecainide, disopyramide, and amiodarone are suitable alternatives.
- Phenytoin is effective in VT, especially when it occurs following the digitalis toxicity.

- *Treatment or elimination of the precipitating factors and prevention of recurrences*:
  - Whatever underlying precipitating factor must be identified and effectively treated or eliminated. Electrolyte disturbances, such as hypokalemia, hypomagnesemia, and others, such as drugs, have to be identified and immediately corrected or stopped. Myocardial tumor, anomalous origin of the coronary artery, and similar surgical problems are appropriately tackled.
- *Alternative treatment strategies*:
  - When the drug therapy fails in control or prevention of recurrences, other modalities of treatment are contemplated and executed as mandated by the causative factors.
  - Implantation of automatic cardioverter, implantable defibrillator, or surgical resection of the diseased myocardial area.

Ventricular Fibrillation

Ventricular fibrillation is a chaotic ventricular tachyarrhythmia with no effective ventricular contraction. The ECG record shows a wavy line without any discernible QRS complexes; P waves may be discernible.

Ventricular fibrillation may be a preterminal event in many conditions, disturbances, or diseases. Hypokalemia, digitalis or quinidine toxicity, myocardial inflammation or damage, catecholamines, aminophylline, anesthetic drugs, and plant toxins may precipitate VF. Uncontrolled VT or multifocal ventricular ectopic beats or long QT interval syndromes may result in VF. If not terminated instantaneously, death ensues.

A thump in the chest may restore sinus rhythm. External cardiac massage with artificial ventilation and DC defibrillation are immediate measures to be undertaken. The precipitating factors are corrected without delay. After defibrillatory conversion to VT, VT is treated with drugs as mentioned above. Refractory cases are treated by implantable automatic cardioverter–defibrillator.

BRADYARRHYTHMIAS

Sinus Arrest and Sinoatrial Block

Sinus arrest is failure of impulse formation within the SA node.

Sinoatrial arrest refers to blockade of the generated sinus impulse from reaching the atrium.

Though rare in children, these disturbances may occur secondary to digitalis toxicity and extensive atrial surgery.

Atrioventricular Block

Atrioventricular block occurs when interference occurs in normal conduction of the electrical impulses from the atria to the ventricles through the AV node.

First-degree Atrioventricular Block

Prolongation of *PR interval* beyond the *stipulated normal range for that age and heart rate* without conduction blockade of any of the atrial impulses to the ventricles is defined as *first-degree heart block*. No evidence of heart disease is seen in the majority of such cases. However, it may be seen in children with coronary heart disease, such as ASD, corrected transposition of the great vessels, Ebstein anomaly, primary myocardial disease, rheumatic carditis, diphtheria, and in children receiving drugs, such as digitalis and quinidine. Children with first-degree block are asymptomatic and need no treatment except for the treatment of primary cause.

Second-degree Atrioventricular Block

Some of the atrial impulses are blocked, and hence, not conducted to the ventricles.

In *Mobitz type I (Wenckebach phenomenon)*, while PP interval remains constant, progressive increase in PR interval occurs with successive beats until an atrial impulse seen as P wave is not conducted to the ventricle (absent QRS complex). The PR interval is again shorter in the cycle following the dropped ventricular complex. It will then progressively increase to result in another blocked ventricular impulse.

In *Mobitz type II*, atrial conduction is blocked at constant intervals, e.g. once every three, four or five beats with no change in the PR interval.

It is less often noticed in individuals with normal hearts. The same predisposing factors mentioned in first-degree AV block also play a role. No treatment is necessary. If Stokes–Adams syndrome occurs, although rare, pacemaker insertion is undertaken.

Complete or Type 3 (Third-degree) Atrioventricular Heart Block

Complete AV block refers to complete non-propagation of SA nodal generated electrical impulses to the AV nodes. There is total dissociation between the SA node and AV node, and the AV node starts generating its own electrical impulse at its inherent slow-paced rhythmicity with a rate ranging between 50 per minute and 100 per minute in neonates and infants, and between 50 per minute and 60 per minute in older children and adults.

Idioventricular rhythm: Rarely when AV node stops generating impulses or there is a failure of conduction in the bundle of His, the ventricular myocytes intrinsically generate their own action potential to be propagated to adjacent ones causing the heart to beat at a rate of 20–40 per minute.

Congenital or Acquired Complete Atrioventricular Heart Block

Congenital CHB is a rare entity with a reported incidence of 1 in 20,000 live births.

Causes: Autoimmune injury of the fetal conduction tissue by immunoglobulin G antibodies transferred from mother with active or inactive systemic lupus erythematosus is one of the well-known causes of this condition. The reported incidence of fetal CHB in women with anti-Ro/SSA (Sjögren's-syndrome-related antigen A) *antibodies* is 1–5%, and in the cases of a previously affected child, it rises 6–25%. In neonates with lupus rash, the incidence of CHB may be as high as 20%. It is seein association with congenitally corrected transposition of the great arteries.

Other autoimmune diseases, such as rheumatoid arthritis, are reported to cause congenital heart block. Myocarditis and postsurgical repair involving ventricles are other known causes of acquired CHB. In utero, it may result in hydrops fetalis. It may also result in fetal wastage. In some children, it may occur at 3–6 months of age.

Symptoms: Older children are asymptomatic. Syncope, fatigue, irritability, and night terrors may be some of the symptoms.

Diagnosis: Slow, bounding pulse less than 60 per minute not increasing by more than 10–20 beats/min after exercise or atropine administration; cannon A waves; and varying intensity of the S1 are clinically diagnostic of this condition. ECG strip is diagnostic with regular P waves with same PP interval but with varying PR intervals.

Prognosis and treatment: The prognosis of this condition is usually good. In symptomatic children with Stokes-Adams syndrome, insertion of artificial pacemaker is imperative to prevent sudden death. All cardiac depressants should be avoided.

Drug treatment: Isoproterenol, atropine, or epinephrine is temporarily employed.

Temporary transvenous ventricular pacing is often employed to increase the heart rate temporarily until pacemaker placement can be arranged.

Transthoracic epicardial pacemakers: Permanent measure is to go for permanent implantable epicardial pacemakers.

Indications for cardiac pacing:
- Neonates with extremely low ventricular rate below 50/min
- Associated with congenital cardiac malformations, such as cyanotic heart disease, single-ventricle physiology, complete AV septal defect or significant AV valve disease
- The onset or the presence of symptoms and signs of low cardiac output or heart failure
- Life-threatening wide complex rhythms, such as prolonged QT interval or ventricular arrhythmia, unstable escape rhythm.

BIBLIOGRAPHY

1. Losek JD, Endom E, Dietrich A, et al. Adenosine and pediatric supraventricular tachycardia in the emergency department: multicenter study and review. Ann Emerg Med. 1999;33:185-91.
2. Sacchetti A, Moyer V, Baricella R, et al. Primary cardiac arrhythmias in children. Pediatr Emerg Care. 1999;15:95-7.
3. Walsh EP, Saul JP, Triedman JK (Eds). Cardiac arrhythmias in the pediatric patient. Philadelphia, PA: Lippincott Williams and Wilkins; 2001.
4. Wolff G, Gelband H, Deal BJ. Arrhythmias in infants and children: current concepts in diagnosis and management of atrial arrhythmias in infants and children. New York, NY: Futura Publishing Inc.; 1998.
5. Ziegler VL, Gillette PC (Eds). Practical management of pediatric cardiac arrhythmias. New York, NY: Futura Publishing Inc.; 2001.

Section 8

Diseases of Respiratory System

8.1 Examination of the Respiratory System

TU Sukumaran

INTRODUCTION

Respiratory disorders are as common in children as it is in adults. A systematic history taking coupled with a physical examination is necessary for arriving at a diagnosis. In this chapter, author has discussed the practical aspects of the examination of the respiratory system.

Physical examination consists of general assessment of the patient, vital signs, and examination of upper and lower respiratory tract.

GENERAL ASSESSMENT

Look for Danger Signs

These include abnormal breathing patterns, altered sensorium, convulsions, cyanosis, inability to drink, sweating, hypotonia, repeated vomiting, dehydration, and paralysis. Altered sensorium and convulsions indicate hypoxemia.

Vital Signs

Tachypnea (Fast Breathing)

This usually occurs in pneumonia but can also occur in anxiety, asthma, collapsed lung cardiac failure, pulmonary edema, pneumothorax, and pleural effusion. The rate of breathing should be assessed by counting it for 1 minute; it should be repeated in case of any doubt. Rapid, shallow breathing denotes respiratory muscle paralysis. Metabolic acidosis of any etiology is characterized by an increased rate and depth of breathing.

Tachycardia

Sinus tachycardia may be a manifestation of respiratory tract infection. Anxiety, cardiac failure, respiratory failure, and simultaneous intake of sympathomimetic drugs should also be considered.

Temperature

Fever indicates upper (sinusitis, otitis media, tonsillopharyngitis, and mastoiditis) as well as lower respiratory tract infection. Common causes for high fever in lower respiratory illness are pneumonia, empyema, lung abscess, and bronchiectasis. Low-grade fever occurs in mycoplasma infections.

Blood Pressure

Blood pressure should always be recorded. Hypertension and pulsus paradoxus indicate serious respiratory impairment.

Examination of the Respiratory System

- Apnea, which is cessation of breathing for more than 20 seconds, is associated with bradycardia or neurologic impairment. A duration of less than 20 seconds, which is associated with pallor, limpness, cyanosis, or convulsions, should be a cause for alarm.
- Cheyne-Stokes breathing is characterized by rhythmic waxing and waning of the depth of respiration, with regularly recurring periods of apnea. It is seen in congestive heart failure and raised intracranial pressure with cerebral cortical impairment.
- Biot's breathing also called ataxic respiration is characterized by irregular periods of apnea, alternating with periods of four or five breaths of identical depth, and indicates severe brain stem damage.
- Kussmaul breathing is rapid deep breathing of metabolic acidosis.
- Gasping or jaw breathing is of slow rate with rapid inspiration, prominent jaw movement, and slow expiration. It indicates severe hypoxia due to any cause.

Work of Breathing

This includes flaring of alae nasi, head nodding (sternomastoids and scalene overactivity), and chest retractions (intercostals, subcostal, suprasternal, and infrasternal).

Chest and Abdominal Movements

Observe the chest movements from the side in supine and standing positions to confirm that both sides are moving equally and to assess the relative contributions of chest and abdomen. In normal inspirations, the lower chest flares out and the abdomen moves forward by the actions of the lower intercostal muscles and diaphragm, respectively. When the intercostals are paralyzed, as in spinal muscular atrophy, inspiration causes the lower chest to be drawn inward by the diaphragm, and the outward movement of the abdominal wall is prominent. Such movements can occur also in upper airway occlusion and are caused by the violent action of the diaphragm. The reverse movement is seen in diaphragm weakness, in which the abdomen is drawn inward during inspiration (paradoxical breathing). In unilateral phrenic nerve paralysis, the abdomen is drawn in on the paralyzed side during inspiration but is normal (i.e. moves out) on the nonparalyzed side.

Cyanosis in respiratory diseases indicates a serious degree of hypoxia and can be identified by the hyperoxia test. Associated circulatory failure or underlying cardiac lesions should be ruled out.

Clubbing in respiratory diseases is seen early in cystic fibrosis, bronchiectasis (of at least 1 year duration) lung abscess, empyema, and malignancies.

Indicators of Serious Chronic Respiratory Illness

These include persistent fever, limitation of physical activity, chronic purulent sputum, cyanosis, clubbing, persistent tachypnea, labored breathing, growth retardation, persistent chest hyperinflation, and a family history of heritable lung diseases.

Examination of the Upper Respiratory Tract

Use a bright torch to examine the nose, ears, and throat.

Signs of Allergic Problems

People with allergic rhinitis frequently develop a transverse nasal crease resulting from repeated rubbing of the nose to relieve the itching (Darier's line). Another feature of nasobronchial allergy is dark circles under the eyes (allergic shiners).

Changes in the Anatomical Structures

The nasal passages may be narrow, as in midface hypoplasia associated with various syndromes. Congenital abnormalities, such as a deviated nasal septum, should be looked for. Extensive nasal polyps cause widening of the nasal bridge. Signs, such as the presence of ulceration, crusting, purulent or a blood-stained discharge, presence of foreign bodies, trauma, and tumors (vascular and nonvascular) should be noted.

Examination of Sinuses

Sinus tenderness can be elicited over the affected sinus.

Examination of the Ears

The ears should be examined for congenital anomalies, infections, foreign bodies, and impacted wax. Gently move the pinna and tragus; tragal pain suggests otitis externa. Examine the mastoids and retroauricular areas for eczema, tenderness, and lymph node enlargement. For better visualization of the external ear canal and tympanic membrane, pull the pinna up and posteriorly with the thumb and index finger.

Otoscopic evaluation is a must for patients with fever of unknown or known origin, as well as those with ear symptoms. In the latter situation, the healthy side should be evaluated first. The otoscope should have a strong light and the speculum should be of the largest size that can fit comfortably into the ear canal. Gently place the otoscope over the external auditory meatus and inspect the external ear canal. Carefully advance it to observe the tympanic membrane. Absence of the normal light reflex, dull appearance, bulging, retraction, perforation, and so on should be noted.

Examination of the Throat

The tonsils should be examined for size (hypoplastic in X-linked agammaglobulinemia, enlarged in infections and tumors), congestion, follicles, or membranes. Other symptoms of pharyngeal infection are redness and mottling over the soft palate and uvula. In a retropharyngeal abscess, the neck is hyperextended, and respiration becomes noisy with gurgling sounds and pooling of secretions. In lateral pharyngeal abscess, the features are torticollis toward the same side, trismus, and bulging in of the lateral pharyngeal wall. Peritonsillar abscess also is characterized by trismus and torticollis. Adenoidal tissue hypertrophy on the posterior pharyngeal wall may reveal cobble stoning.

The integrity of the palate should be investigated by palpation to exclude a submucous cleft. A bifid uvula is a clue to an occult submucous cleft palate.

Examination of the Lower Respiratory Tract

Neck

The important aspects to be assessed in relation to the respiratory tract are the trachea, neck vein, and the presence of surgical emphysema.

Trachea

This is inspected and palpated for deviation (in the standing or sitting position), with the examiner facing the patient. Tracheal deviation causes the clavicular head of the sternomastoid muscle on that side to appear prominent (*Trail sign*). In severe respiratory distress, "tracheal tug" (i.e. pulling in of the trachea) occurs because of the vigorous contraction of the diaphragm pulling down the mediastinum. Gently palpate the trachea with the middle finger at the suprasternal notch. Should there be massive pleural effusion, pneumothorax, and large intrathoracic cysts and tumors, the trachea will shift to the opposite side. It is pulled to the same side in upper lobe collapse, fibrosis, and pleural adhesions.

Signs of Superior Mediastinal Obstruction

Signs of superior mediastinal obstruction are edema of the head and neck, cyanosis, proptosis, Horner syndrome, and distended nonpulsatile neck veins. The common cause is mediastinal mass, notably because of a lymphoma.

Examination of the Chest

Inspection

This should be performed with the chest as maximally exposed as the custom permits, with the eyes at the level of the chest, from head and foot ends, and from front and lateral aspects. Evaluate the overall shape and appearance of the chest. Assess the shoulders for drooping (indicates painful conditions of the chest wall on the same side, pleurisy, pneumonia, collapse, and fibrosis), position of the cardiac apical impulse, and precordial shape. The anteroposterior diameter of the chest is increased in hyperinflation. A localized bulge indicates parietal wall inflammatory swellings, hematoma, or tumors. In pleural effusion or pneumothorax, intercostal spaces (ICS) appear bulging. Look for chest movements. Localized paucity of movements occurs in trauma and in painful conditions of the chest wall and pleura, pleural effusion, pneumothorax, pneumonia, collapse, and tumors of the lung.

Palpation

This includes measurement of the expansion of the chest at the level of the nipples after deep inspiration and expiration. Expansion of identical sides of the chest should be assessed. Chest movements are assessed over supraclavicular, upper interscapular and lower interscapular areas from the back, and infraclavicular and inframammary areas from the front. To do this, encircle the chest from both sides with four fingers and palm, with the thumbs meeting in the midline but not touching the chest wall. On inspiration, if one thumb remains closer to the midline, it indicates reduced chest movements on that side. Tactile vocal fremitus is compared for spoken words over identical areas on both sides of the chest with the medial margin of the right palm.

Percussion

The examiner should master the technique of percussion to feel, rather than hear, the normal and abnormal lung resonance. The patient should be in a comfortable position, i.e. sitting or lying down. The left middle finger (the pleximeter) is placed parallel to the long axis over the area to be percussed; back of the middle phalanx of the pleximeter finger is struck, as a tapping movement arising from the wrist. The plexor finger should immediately be raised after the tap. The terminal phalanx of the plexor finger should be at right angles to the metacarpal bone and the pleximeter finger while the blow is delivered. Proceed down the ICS in mammary line, with each blow being compared with that on the other side. The upper border of liver dullness reaches the fifth ICS on the right side in the mammary line and will shift to one space lower down on deep inspiration (tidal percussion). On the left side, the normal resonance is replaced by the tympanitic note of the stomach at the same level. The cardiac dullness should be verified on the left side and will be more resonant in emphysema. To percuss the lateral side of chest, patients' limbs should be raised above the shoulders with the hands resting over the vertex—one over the other. Each ICS is percussed and compared with the opposite side, with the examiner standing or sitting on the side to be percussed. The normal resonance on the right side is replaced by liver dullness in the seventh space in the midaxillary line and on the left side by the tympanitic note of the stomach almost at the same level.

Percussion of the back should start from the supraclavicular area, i.e. from the medial to the lateral side, the pleximeter finger being placed across the area with the tip directed forward. A band of lung resonance that normally presents in the central area (Kronig isthmus) will be replaced by a dull note in massive pleural effusion, consolidation, neoplasia, or collapse of the apical part of lung. Subsequently, the upper and lower interscapular and the infrascapular spaces should be percussed. The normal resonance is replaced by the dullness at the 9th and 10th ICS in the infrascapular area on the right (liver) and left side (spleen), respectively.

Resonance is the normal feel and sound caused by air being set into vibration. Lung resonance is increased in airway obstruction and pneumothorax; in the latter situation, it reaches up to a tympanitic note. Localized obstruction occurs in congenital lobar emphysema or in partial obstruction by a foreign body in the bronchus (check valve or ball valve). Overall, hyperinflation occurs in obstructive airway disease, as in asthma pushing down the liver dullness. Percussion note is impaired or dull when the lung becomes more solid (pneumonia, consolidation, collapse, fibrosis, sequestration, abscess, infarction), or the pleura becomes thickened or contains fluid (pleural effusion, empyema, hemothorax) or solid (mesothelioma). A feel of resistance below the pleximeter finger is perceived in pleural effusion, as if percussed against a wall, and is described as a "stony dullness."

In hydropneumothorax, a *shifting dullness* can be identified by percussing the chest (from anterior to posterior) in the supine, lying position of the patient. As the fluid shifts to the posterior part of the chest in the lying position, the dull lower chest (in the sitting position) becomes resonant anteriorly and a definite level below which there is complete dullness can be demonstrated.

Auscultatory Percussion

It is helpful to detect mediastinal masses. The patient sits with arms resting on both thighs while the examiner sits facing the patient. With the tip of the terminal phalanx of the middle finger of the dominant side, light percussion is directly applied over the sternum from the center to either side, while the note is auscultated from behind over the corresponding areas. The area of impaired resonance reveals the size of the mediastinal mass.

Auscultation

Developing an expertise in interpreting auscultatory findings is an experimental process and, as such, there is no substitute for the experience of having listened to a large number of patients, both with and without lung disease. Follow a consistent pattern for auscultation to avoid missing any area. Start from the infraclavicular area and proceed to mammary, inframammary, axillary, and infra-axillary areas, each time comparing with the opposite side. Segmental auscultation is the technique of comparing breath sounds of homologous segments. The examiner should sit facing the patient when auscultating the anterior aspect of the chest. The lateral side of the chest can be auscultated from front as well as from behind the patient. Posteriorly, auscultation is performed in the same way as in the order of percussion, with the examiner sitting behind the child.

The parameters to be assessed are the breath sounds, added sounds, and vocal resonance. Assess the intensity and quality of the breath sounds. Intensity may be normal (when the lung tissue is inflating normally), reduced, or increased. It is reduced in airway obstruction, lung damage, pleural thickness, effusion, and pneumothorax. The normal breath sounds are vesicular. The inspiration is loud and high-pitched followed by harsh low-pitched expiration (without a pause in between), which is of short duration, i.e. almost up to half of inspiration. The cycle is followed by a pause. In bronchovesicular breathing, the expiration is prolonged up to or more than the inspiration, and there is no pause in between. This is typical of asthma.

Bronchial breathing is louder in intensity. Expiration is high-pitched, loud, and prolonged (equal to or more than the duration of inspiration). There is a pause in between. The normal vesicular breathing is replaced by bronchial breathing when the lung becomes more solid (as in consolidation, collapse consolidation, fibrosis, abscess lung, massive pleural effusion, and neoplastic growth) or contains a cavity. In these situations, the sounds generated in large airways are transmitted more efficiently and resemble those obtained by listening over the trachea. Adventitious sounds are wheezes, crackles, pleural rub, mediastinal crunch, peristaltic sounds, and crepitus.

Wheezes arise from narrowed intrathoracic airways. Monophonic wheeze is due to localized narrowing of a single bronchus, as in foreign body aspiration or bronchial adenoma. Widespread polyphonic wheezes (of differing intensity), usually heard in expiration, indicate diffuse airway obstruction as in asthma.

Crackles or crepitations are short bubbling or crackling noises arising from large airways with secretions (coarse), or from small airways (fine), and from alveoli containing exudates (fine). These sounds are produced by sudden changes in gas pressure from the rapid opening of previously closed small airways or alveoli. Crackles are heard in obstructive airway disease, pneumonia, and pulmonary edema. Localized loud and coarse crackles may indicate bronchiectasis.

The added sounds should be differentiated from conducted sounds from the throat and pharynx. Conducted sounds disappear after suction and changes in position and are heard with equal intensity over equidistant parts of the chest and better by auscultation in front of the mouth and neck.

Pleural rub has a rubbing, superficial, leathery character and is heard during an identical phase of inspiration and expiration; unlike crackles, it does not change after coughing. The intensity increases as the chest piece is pressed firmly, it can be felt also with the palpating hand.

Mediastinal crunch (Hamman's sign) is heard in emphysema and left-sided pneumothorax. A crunching sound will be heard over the left sternal border during a systole.

Peristaltic sounds are gurgling sounds occasionally heard over the lower part of the left side. Frequent peristaltic sounds with other clinical evidences indicate diaphragmatic hernia.

In addition to peristaltic and diaphragmatic sounds, crepitus sounds may occur over the region of a broken rib or surgical emphysema. Additional false sounds arise by the movement of the stethoscope on the patient's skin and should be differentiated from the symptomatic sounds.

Vocal resonance is the sound perceived by the chest piece, as the voice is transmitted through the lungs. The child is auscultated while saying one or his name in the same order of auscultation, and both sides are compared. The intensity of resonance will be decreased in airway obstruction, collapse, pleural effusion, or pneumothorax (except when bronchial breathing is present). Intensity is increased over consolidation, cavity, infraction, and collapse consolidation. If the patient is asked to whisper the same words, they will be heard clearly in the examiners ears (*whispering pectoriloquy*) in massive consolidation and bronchopleural fistula **(Table 8.1.1)**.

Table 8.1.1: Salient features of common lower respiratory diseases in children.

Parameter	*Acute asthma*	*Consolidation*	*Collapse*	*Pleural effusion*	*Pneumothorax*
Respiratory rate	↑	↑↑	↑↑	↑↑↑	↑↑↑
Chest in-drawing	+++ Overall	++ Spares affected region	++ Spares affected region	++ Spares affected region	++ Spares affected region
Chest expansion	Overall reduction	Reduced over affected area	Reduced over affected area	Reduced over affected area	Reduced over affected area
Tracheal and mediastinal shift	Nil	Nil	Toward the affected side	Toward the opposite side	Toward the opposite side
Lung resonance	Hyperresonant, liver dullness pushed down	Dull over affected area	Dull over affected area	Stony dullness over affected area	Tympanitic over affected area
Breath sound intensity	N/↓	↑	↓/– over affected area	↓/– over affected area	↓/– over affected area
Breath sound quality	Bronchovesicular	Bronchial	Vesicular/Bronchial	Vesicular	Vesicular
Vocal resonance	Normal	↑↑	↓↓	Imperceptible	Imperceptible

BIBLIOGRAPHY

1. Empey D. The respiratory system. In: Swash M (Ed). Hutchison's Clinical Methods, 10th edition. London: WB Saunders and Company Ltd; 1995. pp. 60-8.
2. Kuruvilla VJ, Thulasi Prasad K. Clinical Evaluation of Newborns, Infants and Children, 2nd edition. New Delhi: Jaypee Brothers Medical Publishers; 2009. pp. 112-20.
3. Silverman M, Callaghan CL. Practical Pediatric Respiratory Medicine, 1st edition. New Delhi: Viva Books (P) Ltd.; 2005.

8.2 Diagnostic Procedures and Investigations in Respiratory Diseases

D Vijayasekaran

Taking and methodical clinical examination help to arrive at provisional diagnosis and to confirm investigations are required. Children with chronic lung problems require many investigations where the judicious approach is important **(Table 8.2.1)**.

HEMATOLOGICAL TESTS

Complete blood count may give information about the current infection. Estimation of hemoglobin, differential leukocyte count, and peripheral blood smear is helpful to arrive at a diagnosis. Leukocytosis [white blood cell (WBC) above 16,000/μL] and leucopenia (WBC below 4,000/μL) may suggest infection. The presence of lymphocytosis suggests pertussis and increased atypical lymphocytes suggest infectious mononucleosis. C-reactive protein increases with infections both viral and bacterial. It is useful in monitoring the disease. Raised erythrocyte sedimentation rate suggests chronic infection and inflammatory disorders.

TUBERCULIN SKIN TEST (MANTOUX TEST)

One tuberculin unit purified protein derivative with Tween 80 is injected intradermally and the reaction read between 48 hours and 72 hours. Mantoux test is considered positive if the induration is 10 mm or more. Similar to Mantoux test, Interferon Gamma Release Assays also detect tuberculosis (TB) infection; however, like Mantoux test, it does not distinguish between the latent and active infection. Since

Table 8.2.1: Investigations and procedures in respiratory diseases.

Common	*Optional*
Hematology • Complete blood counts • ESR • CRP	*Pulmonary function tests* • Spirometry • Peak expiratory flow rate
Imaging studies • Chest X-ray • Ultrasound • CT and MRI • Contrast radiography • Fluoroscopy • Radionuclide lung scan	*Endoscopy* • Fiberoptic bronchoscopy • Bronchoalveolar lavage • Rigid bronchoscopy • Laryngoscopy
Microbiology Gastric lavage/Induced sputum/ Sputum/Blood culture	*Monitoring* • Pulse oximetry • Capnography • Polysomnography
• Immunoglobulin assay • Radioallergosorbent assay • Tuberculin skin test • Allergic skin tests	*Others* • Thoracentesis • Intercostal drainage • Video-assisted thoracoscopy • Sweat chloride

(CRP: C-reactive protein; ESR: erythrocyte sedimentation rate; CT: computed tomography; MRI: magnetic resonance imaging)

it uses selective antigens, namely early secretory antigenic target and culture filtrate protein 10, it is not affected by prior bacillus Calmette-Guérin and infection due to nontuberculous mycobacterium.

IMAGING

Chest Radiography

X-ray chest is considered as an extension of clinical examination. The standard chest radiograph is the posteroanterior but in younger children, the anteroposterior view is taken for convenience. Chest X-ray delineates four densities, namely air, fluid, soft tissue, and bone density **(Figs. 8.2.1A to D)**.

Before viewing the chest radiograph, it is assumed that technical qualities (projection, orientation, rotation, and penetration) are fulfilled. Chest radiograph is useful in the diagnosis of pneumonia. In chest radiograph, the right margin of the mediastinum is formed by superior vena cava and right atrium from above downward and left margin by aorta, pulmonary artery, left atrial appendage, and left ventricle. Mediastinal shift occurs in lung problems, such as collapse (same side of lesion), obstructive emphysema, pneumothorax, and pleural effusion (opposite side).

Contrast Radiograph

Barium swallow gives information about the upper gastrointestinal tract especially in the evaluation of gastroesophageal reflux, achalasia, and hiatus hernia. Barium meal study helps in the evaluation of malabsorption syndromes, abdominal TB, and ileocecal problems.

Computed Tomography Scan

Computed tomography (CT) provides more information than the plain chest radiograph because of its higher resolution, cross-sectional perspective, and studying bone-related problems. Technological advancements have enabled the modern multidetector CT. It renders images in coronal and sagittal sections and also three-dimensional reconstruction.

Magnetic Resonance Imaging

Magnetic resonance imaging (MRI) uses magnetic properties of atoms and radio waves. MRI does not depend on ionizing radiation, so it is safer than CT. MRI is more useful in differentiating the soft tissue shadows particularly in studying the vessels.

Fluoroscopy

The combination of fluoroscopy along with barium swallow forms a useful investigation in the evaluation of children with gastroesophageal reflux disease. For the study of the diaphragmatic movements and suspected foreign body, fluoroscopy plays a significant role.

Ultrasound Chest

Ultrasound is an imaging study that uses high-frequency sound waves to look at the organs. In the chest, it helps in the evaluation of diaphragm, eventration, and pleural diseases.

MICROBIOLOGY

Microbiological tests in children pose many disadvantages, such as sputum collection (children less than 7 years do not expectorate), contamination from upper airway flora, and difficulty in differentiating infection from colonization. The preferred specimens in the diagnosis of TB are gastric lavage (GL) and induced sputum.

GeneXpert Tuberculosis

Since Löwenstein-Jensen medium takes longer duration (6–8 weeks) to culture TB bacilli, newer diagnostic tests are used which include Mycobacterium Growth Indicator System and GeneXpert TB (Xpert *Mycobacterium tuberculosis*/ rifampicin). The latter is a cartridge-based nucleic acid amplification test and identifies both tubercle bacilli and rifampicin resistance (multidrug-resistant TB). It is an excellent tool for the diagnosis of TB from the body fluid specimens.

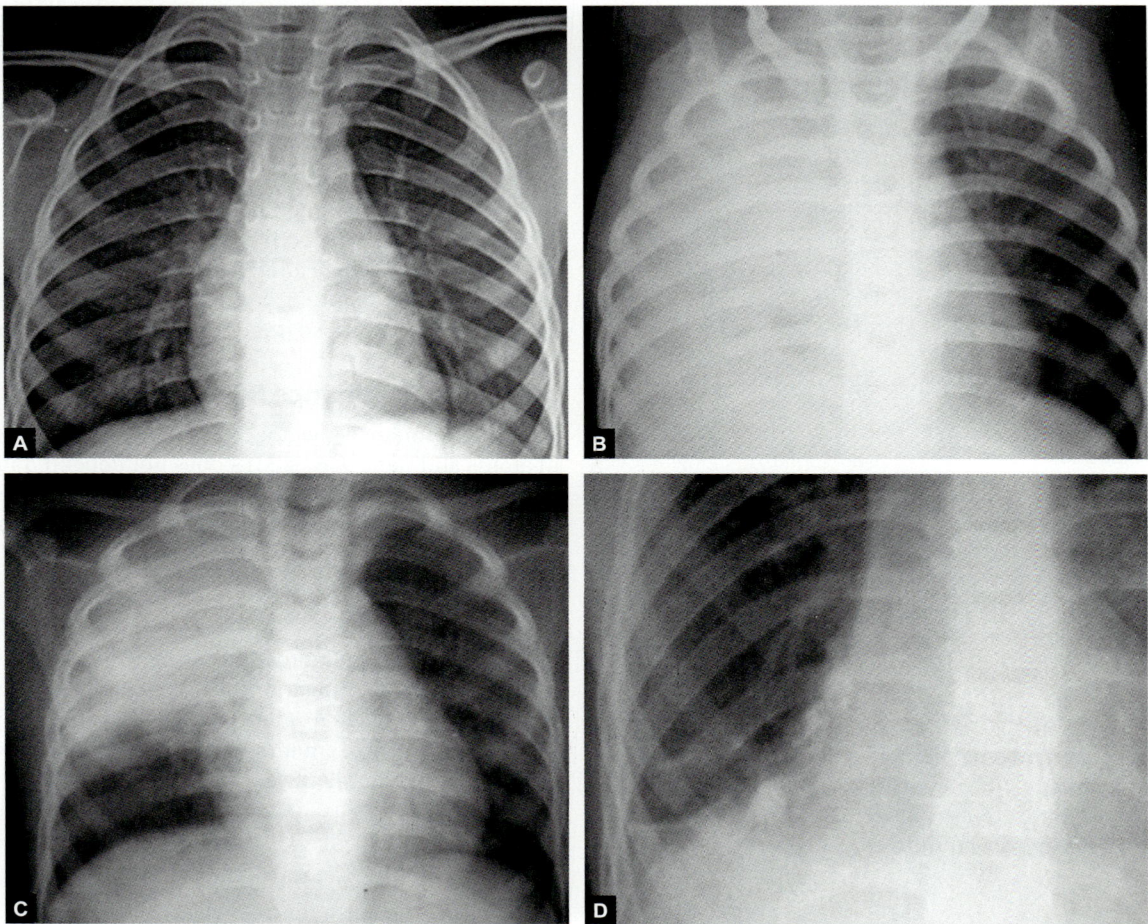

Figs. 8.2.1A to D: X-ray chest showing four densities, namely, air, fluid, soft tissue, and bone density.

GASTRIC LAVAGE AND INDUCED SPUTUM

Pediatric TB is a paucibacillary disease. GL is done in the early morning to isolate the acid-fast bacilli. GL can also be done as an ambulatory procedure after 4–6 hours of fasting. While doing induced sputum collection, the child is nebulized with 3% hypertonic saline to induce sputum. Secretions are then collected from the throat or nasopharynx. Recent studies report that induced sputum yields higher results than GL.

ALLERGY TESTING

Allergy testing can be done by allergy immunoassays and allergy skin prick test. Immunoassays are blood tests (in vitro test) which measure the specific immunoglobulin E to a suspected allergen. The advantages claimed by allergy immunoassays are safety aspect (no systemic reaction), and not affected by the drugs (antihistamines or steroids). Skin prick test is a manual test (in vivo test) considered as more sensitive with a greater selection of antigens.

PULMONARY FUNCTION TESTS

Spirometry

Spirometry differentiates lung diseases (functionally) into obstructive and restrictive diseases but does not give any information about the etiology.

Spirometry measures the forced vital capacity (FVC) and not the individual lung volumes. The other indices, such as forced expiratory volume in 1 second (FEV_1), the ratio of FEV_1 with FVC (FEV_1/FVC), and forced expiratory flow 25–75% of FVC, are derived from FVC by the machine **(Figs. 8.2.2A and B)**.

Achieving a good FVC curve is the most important aspect of spirometry. For this, a child (after appropriate coaching) should take a deep breath to full inhalation followed by a brief hold and then a sustained exhalation (at least 3 seconds) with maximum effort to produce a good curve (flow volume curve or loop).

Spirometry helps to differentiate obstructive and restrictive lung diseases. FVC is diminished in both

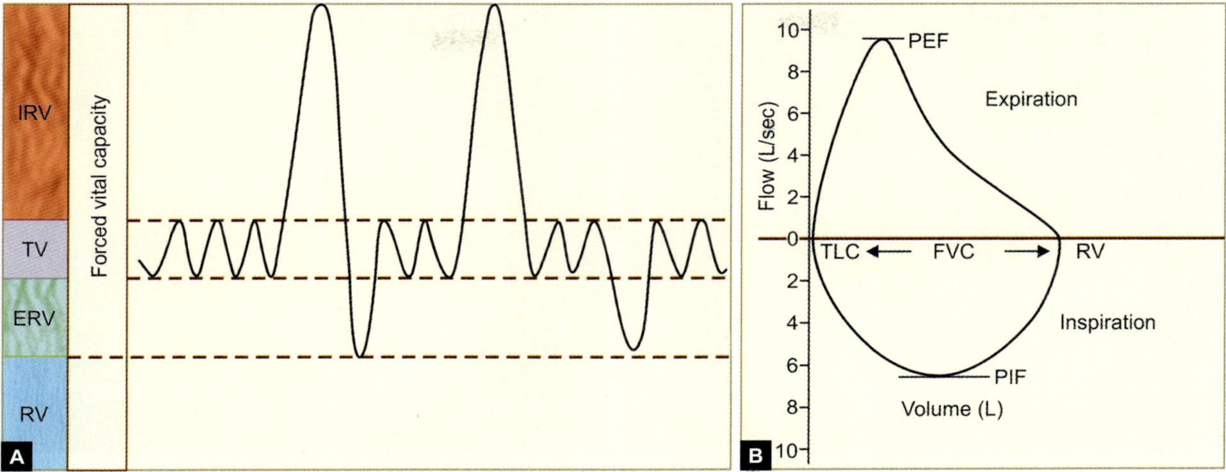

Figs. 8.2.2A and B: Spirometry recordings of lung volumes and flow volume loop.

obstructive and restrictive diseases. FEV_1 is decreased in obstructive diseases. FEV_1/FVC ratio may be normal or even increased in restrictive diseases.

Peak Expiratory Flow Rate

Peak flow meter records peak expiratory flow rate (PEFR), the greatest flow obtained on forced expiration after full inspiration. PEFR is effort dependent and measures mostly large airway function. It plays a major role in monitoring asthma therapy (correlates with FEV_1) and sudden fall may be an indicator of an impending asthma attack.

ARTERIAL BLOOD GAS ANALYSIS

Arterial blood gas (ABG) analysis reveals oxygenation status, adequacy of ventilation, and acid-base balance. Many serious acid-base disturbances can coexist without significant clinical manifestations.

The radial artery at the wrist is the most preferred site of ABG specimen collection as it has adequate collaterals. Heparinized syringe with 22-gauge needle should be held like a pen with a 45° angle (with the beveled edge of the tip facing downward) and the artery should be punctured just 2 cm above the wrist crease; the sample should be analyzed immediately.

The normal power of hydrogen of our body is 7.4 (range 7.36–7.44), depending upon the levels of $PaCO_2$ and HCO_3. The disturbances blood gases result in four simple acid-base disorders, namely metabolic acidosis (↓ HCO_3), metabolic alkalosis (↑ HCO_3), respiratory acidosis (↑ $PaCO_2$), and respiratory alkalosis (↓ $PaCO_2$).

Metabolic acidosis results due to loss of HCO_3 from the body (diarrhea) or due to the addition of acids (lactic acid, ketoacids). Anion gap calculation is used to differentiate the above two. Metabolic alkalosis results due to loss of acids (H^+ ions) from the GI tract (vomiting) or through renal mechanisms (Bartter syndrome). Mild respiratory disorders cause hypoxemia resulting in respiratory alkalosis due to CO_2 washout (↓ $PaCO_2$). Advanced respiratory diseases and neuromuscular dysfunction lead to carbon dioxide retention ($PaCO_2$ > 45 mm Hg) resulting in respiratory acidosis.

Table 8.2.2: Fiberoptic bronchoscopy—indications.

Diagnostic	*Therapeutic*
• Persistent pneumonia, atelectasis • Prolonged stridor and wheezing • Suspected foreign body, endobronchial TB • Suspected airway anomaly • Evaluation of hemoptysis and hemosiderosis • Bronchoalveolar lavage	• Removal of mucous plug/ bronchial cast • Removal of retained secretions • Drug instillation • Bronchoscopy-guided ET intubation • Tracheostomy evaluation • Endobronchial biopsy

(ET: endotracheal; TB: tuberculosis)

FIBEROPTIC BRONCHOSCOPY

Fiberoptic bronchoscopy (FBS) is an important diagnostic technique, done under local anesthesia. The diagnostic indications and therapeutic utility are increasing **(Table 8.2.2)**. After lignocaine gel is applied into the nostril, lignocaine solution is instilled through the suction channel of bronchoscope as "spray and proceed technique." Dynamic problems with vocal cord pathology, laryngomalacia, tracheomalacia, and foreign body are better identified with FBS **(Figs. 8.2.3A to D)**.

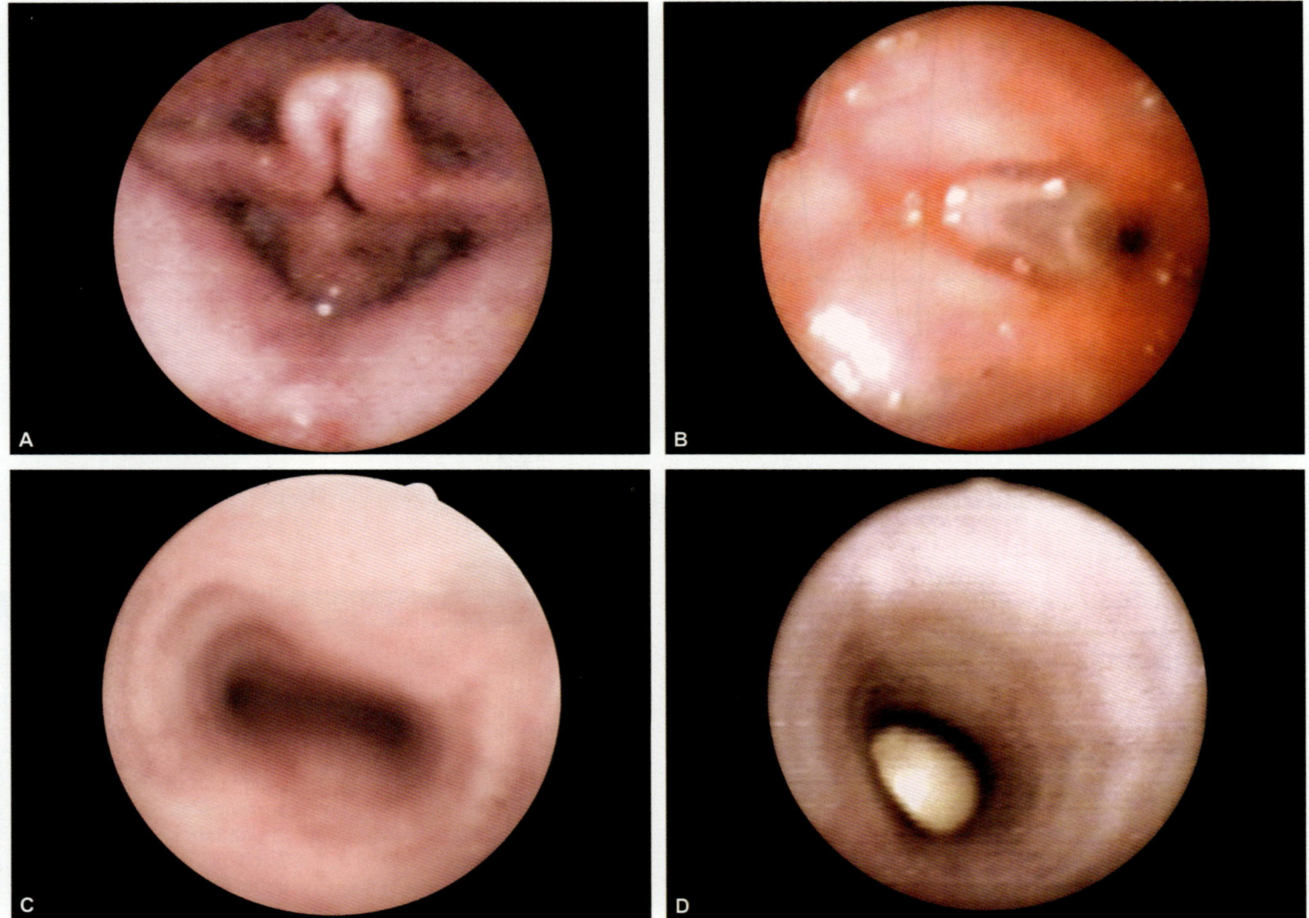

Figs. 8.2.3A to D: Bronchoscopic view of laryngomalacia, laryngeal web, tracheomalacia, and central foreign body.

BRONCHOALVEOLAR LAVAGE

Bronchoalveolar lavage (BAL) is a diagnostic procedure and allows the recovery of both cellular and noncellular components from the epithelial surface of the lower respiratory tract. BAL is rightly called as the "liquid biopsy of the lung." After wedging the scope into the desired subsegmental bronchus, BAL is performed by instilling 2 mL/kg of sterile, normal saline. BAL is helpful in diagnosing opportunistic infections, such as *Pneumocystis jirovecii*, *Cytomegalovirus*, *Aspergillus fumigatus*, and *Mycobacterium tuberculosis*.

THORACENTESIS

Thoracentesis or pleural tap is done to diagnose pleural fluid (preferably after ultrasonographic confirmation). Nature of the fluid and biochemistry may be useful to differentiate transudate versus exudates **(Table 8.2.3)**.

Table 8.2.3: Comparison of transudate and exudate.

	Transudate	***Exudate***
Pathophysiology	↑ Hydrostatic and ↓ oncotic pressure	Inflammation Infiltration of pleura
Appearance	Clear	Turbid pus, straw color
Protein (g/dL)	<3	>3
LDH (IU/L)	<200	>200
pH	>7.2	<7.2
Glucose	<40 mg/dL	>40 mg/dL
Pleural fluid/serum protein	<0.5	>0.5
Pleural fluid/serum LDH	<0.6	>0.6
Cause	Congestive cardiac failure, nephrotic syndrome, cirrhosis, hypoproteinemia	Complicated parapneumonic effusion, empyema

(LDH: lactic dehydrogenase; pH: power of hydrogen)

Intercostal Drainage

Intercostal drainage is the procedure to remove pus from the pleural cavity by inserting a chest tube. Fifth intercostal space at the midaxillary line is the ideal site.

SWEAT CHLORIDE

Sweat is collected by pilocarpine-induced iontophoresis. Electric current (3 mA) is passed for 30 minutes and about 100 mg of sweat is collected. Chloride estimation is done by titration. Sweat chloride more than 60 mEq/L on two occasions suggests cystic fibrosis.

BIBLIOGRAPHY

1. Dheda K, Udwadia ZF, Hugget JF. Utility of antigen-specific interferon gamma assay for the management of tuberculosis. Curr Opin Pulm Med. 2005;11:195-202.
2. Shulman ST, Bisno AL, Clegg HW, et al. Clinical practice guideline for the diagnosis and management of group A streptococcal pharyngitis: 2012 update by the Infectious Diseases Society of America. Clin Infect Dis. 2012;55:e86-e102.

8.3 Respiratory Distress

Madhumati Otiv

INTRODUCTION

Respiratory distress and respiratory failure together account for nearly 50% of the pediatric emergency services or intensive care units. Children with respiratory distress primarily may be having respiratory or nonrespiratory cause of respiratory distress. With supportive care for respiratory distress along with aggressive treatment of the underlying cause, most children recover uneventfully. Delayed recognition and intervention of the respiratory distress develops into cardiopulmonary compromise and hence poor outcome. Infants and young children become fatigued and/or decompensate more quickly than older children and adolescents due to smaller airways, increased metabolic demands, decreased respiratory reserves, horizontal ribs with poor mechanical advantage, easy fatigability of intercostal muscles leading to inadequate compensatory mechanisms. This chapter describes definitions of respiratory distress and failure, diagnosis, pathophysiology, clinical features with emphasis of early diagnosis of respiratory failure, and some lifesaving maneuvers. Management of individual causes of respiratory distress is discussed elsewhere in this book.

DEFINITIONS

Tachypnea is *increase in the respiratory rate beyond the physiological limit* ***(Table 8.3.1)*** while dyspnea or respiratory distress is characterized by signs of *increased work of breathing (characterized by stridor, wheeze, tachypnea or hyperpnea, use of accessory muscles, and/or retractions).* A patient with inadequate respiratory effort may be too sick to exhibit signs of increased work of breathing such as retractions but may have an abnormal pattern of respiration, e.g. agonal, gasping, irregular, paradoxical, or a respiratory rate that may be *inappropriately slow for the clinical condition.*

Respiratory failure is defined as inability of the respiratory system to fulfill the gas exchange needs of the patient. Most of the times, physical examination alone is sufficient to realize if the cardiopulmonary compromise is present or imminent. Blood gas estimation or any other investigation such as chest X-ray should never delay the institution of life supporting measures and initiation of treatment of probable underlying disease. Respiratory failure when seen through the prism of

Table 8.3.1: World Health Organization definition of tachypnea in children.

Age	*Breaths/min*
<2 months	>60
2–12 months	>50
1–5 years	>40
>5 years	>20

pediatric assessment triangle (Consciousness, Breathing, Circulation), it is clinically characterized by *features such as "altered sensorium, dusky color, poor tone, weak or absent cry, poor pulses, or capillary refill time (CRT) (normal CRT = less than 2 seconds)".*

ETIOLOGY AND PATHOGENESIS

Of all the functions of respiratory system, oxygenation, and ventilation (CO_2 removal) are the prime functions, which depend upon matching of ventilation to perfusion. Ideally almost all the right ventricular output (Q) must return to the left heart only after taking part in gas (V) exchange. This may not happen if the lung volume is lost (e.g. pneumonia, acute respiratory distress syndrome, atelectasis), resulting in poor ventilation [low V/Q (ventilation-perfusion)] or due to shunt (cyanotic heart, severe acute asthma alveolar overinflation—high V/Q).

Respiratory rate or work of breathing (tachypnea or dyspnea) is sensitive to hypoxemia (e.g. low cardiac output, respiratory disease), metabolic acidosis (e.g. low HCO_3 of sepsis, diabetic ketoacidosis), respiratory acidosis (e.g. high $PaCO_2$ of severe asthma, cyanotic spell), or even high metabolic demands (sepsis, fever, exercise). Deterioration of sensorium also results in abnormal pattern of respiration, such as periodic or irregular respiration and respiratory failure.

Thus, respiratory distress can be the result of number of diseases, which may be respiratory or nonrespiratory. Cause of respiratory distress can usually be found out after a very careful and detailed history and physical examination. **Table 8.3.2** shows etiological classification of respiratory distress. Of these, life-threatening conditions such as epiglottitis, anaphylaxis, foreign body, tension pneumothorax, chest trauma (flail chest), cardiac tamponade must be identified rapidly for urgent intervention.

CLINICAL FEATURES AND EVALUATION

Goals of Clinical Examination

- To identify respiratory failure.
- To localize the origin of respiratory distress/respiratory failure.

As mentioned earlier in this chapter, identification of respiratory failure can be done by simple clinical examination. If child is in respiratory failure, urgent resuscitation as per Pediatric Advanced Life Support (PALS) guidelines is the priority. Once respiratory failure is excluded, localization of respiratory distress by physical signs should be done which will help in designing treatment to prevent the child from going into respiratory failure **(Table 8.3.3)**. While examining, it is important to provide oxygen in a comfortable way that the child can tolerate as far as possible in mother's lap as crying narrows the airway diameter and worsens the respiratory distress. At times, a child in distress finds his own comfortable posture that gives maximum advantage such as head extension in case of upper airway obstruction.

Initial and ongoing identification, evaluation, and intervention are always a priority, while important and relevant part of history taking can be done simultaneously.

Table 8.3.2: Etiological classification of acute respiratory distress in children.

Respiratory causes of respiratory distress	*Nonrespiratory causes of respiratory distress*
• *Respiratory tract infection:* - Epiglottitis* - Retropharyngeal abscess - Peritonsillar abscess - Croup - Tracheitis - Bronchiolitis - Pneumonia • Asthma • Anaphylaxis* • *Foreign body**: - Upper airway - Lower airway - Esophageal • Biologic or chemical weapons • *Chest wall/thoracic:* - Air leak (e.g. tension pneumothorax*) - Chest wall deformity (e.g. thoracic dystrophy, flail chest*) - Mass lesion (e.g. pulmonary sequestration, malignancy)	• *Cardiovascular:* - Heart failure - Cyanotic heart disease - Pericarditis - Cardiac tamponade* - Myocarditis • *Trauma*: - Blunt or penetrating (e.g. pneumothorax, lung contusion) - Inhalational injury (e.g. airway burn, smoke inhalation) • *Nervous system*: - Depressed ventilation (from ingestion, injury, or infection) - Hypotonia (poor pharyngeal tone, ineffective respiratory effort) - Loss of airway protective reflexes • *Metabolic/Endocrine*: - Acidosis (e.g. diabetic ketoacidosis, severe dehydration, sepsis) - Hyperthyroidism/hypothyroidism • *Hematologic*: - Decreased oxygen carrying capacity (e.g. severe anemia, methemoglobinemia) • *Gastrointestinal:* - Splinting from abdominal pain, abdominal distension, aspiration as a gastroesophageal reflux

*Life-threatening.

Table 8.3.3: Localization of source of respiratory distress by physical findings.

Upper airway obstruction • *Sniffing position*: Neck flexed, head extended to open airway • *Nasal flaring*: Also seen with lower airway disease • Prolonged inspiration • *Retractions*: Supraclavicular, suprasternal • *Abnormal voice*: Hoarseness, stridor, barking cough • Transmitted upper airway sounds (stridor)	***Lower airway disease*** • *Retractions*: Intercostal, subcostal • *Nasal flaring*: Also seen with upper airway obstruction • *Prolonged expiration*: Lower airway obstruction • *Wheezing*: Intrathoracic airway obstruction • *Grunting*: Expiratory sound heard in young children with severe hypoxia or severe pain from an intra-abdominal process • Crackles (rales), pleural rub, bronchophony • *Pulsus paradoxus*: Caused by lower airway obstruction
Cardiac disease • Gallop or other murmur • Jugular venous distention • Hepatomegaly • *Pulsus paradoxus*: Cardiac tamponade	***Metabolic disease*** • Acidotic breathing in DKA • Findings suggestive of chronic/acute renal disease
CNS disease • CNS involvement (altered sensorium, seizures, posturing)	***Others*** • Acute abdomen • Trauma • Poisoning

(CNS: central nervous system; DKA: diabetic ketoacidosis)

Table 8.3.4: Indications for investigations in respiratory distress.

Test	*Indications*
• *Bedside*: Pulse oximetry • Electrocardiogram	• All children with respiratory distress • Suspected cardiac disease
• Arterial blood gas • Electrolytes, glucose, and ammonia	Gas exchange evaluation in respiratory failure, a rapidly deteriorating patient
• Toxicology screen (e.g. organophosphate poisoning, salicylate, paracetamol) • Carbon monoxide/methemoglobin	• Only when suspected based on history • Carbon monoxide poisoning patients may be pink, and methemoglobin may be cyanosed
Lateral neck radiograph	Useful for evaluation of upper airway obstruction
Chest radiograph	Should be performed for all children with persistent asymmetric breath sounds and for most children with significant respiratory distress
Expiratory or bilateral decubitus chest radiograph	May help in foreign body aspiration
Unilateral decubitus chest radiograph	This study can distinguish a pulmonary infiltrate from an effusion
Abdominal radiographs (supine and upright, or cross-table lateral)	May demonstrate signs of abdominal obstruction or perforation
Computed tomography of the head	May demonstrate mass, injury, or hydrocephalus
Computed tomography pulmonary angiography	May indicate a pulmonary embolism
Abdominal computed tomography	May be useful to evaluate abdominal causes of respiratory distress
V/Q scan	Indicated for possible pulmonary embolism

(V/Q scan: ventilation–perfusion scan)

Clues in history are generally tale-telling such as infective cause in a febrile child, a cardiac cause when disproportionate tachycardia with hepatomegaly, a foreign body in a healthy child with sudden chocking event, acute asthma exacerbation in a known asthmatic, anaphylaxis on exposure to some allergen, drug or bite, or central nervous system cause when sensorium altered before marked respiratory distress. Child with trauma requires a very close observation, especially the chest and abdominal injuries may not be very obvious initially and can decompensate in a subject who could be conscious and compensated hemodynamics at the time of admission.

INVESTIGATIONS

After initial clinical evaluation based on the suspected cause further investigation should be done **(Table 8.3.4)**.

Table 8.3.5: Lifesaving maneuvers to relieve acute respiratory distress.

Condition	***Maneuver***	***Comments***
Complete upper airway obstruction	Needle cricothyrotomy	Temporary measure, can provide oxygenation, not ventilation
Foreign body	Back blows/chest thrusts (<1 year of age)	Maneuvers should only be used for patients who are unable to phonate
	Abdominal thrusts (≥1 year of age)	
	Manual removal with finger sweep	Perform this maneuver only when foreign body is visible in the oropharynx
	Laryngoscopy and removal with Magill forceps	
Laryngospasm	Positive pressure with a ventilation bag and tight fitting mask	
Soft tissue upper airway obstruction	Head tilt/chin lift	
	Jaw thrust	Use for patients who may have cervical spine injury
	Nasopharyngeal airway	May be tolerated by a conscious patient
	Oropharyngeal airway	Use only in an unconscious patient
Respiratory failure	Bag-mask ventilation	Consider upper airway obstruction if unable to ventilate with proper size equipment and technique
	Endotracheal intubation	Use for patient who requires more than a few minutes of assisted ventilation. Consider for patient with complete subglottic upper airway obstruction
Tension pneumothorax	Needle thoracocentesis	Most patients will require chest tube placement following emergent decompression
Cardiac tamponade	Pericardiocentesis	

Table 8.3.6: Equipment for tackling respiratory distress/failure.

Essential for office practice and indoor facility	Optional for office/desirable indoor pediatric hospital/essential for level one PICU
• Stethoscope, manual BP apparatus, pulse oximeter • Glucometer • IV access material, IV sets, IV fluid • Oxygen tank (two) preferably with heated humidifier • Oxygen delivery devices (O_2 box, simple mask, nonrebreathing mask, nasal prongs) • Suction catheters and machine • Intubation equipment • Needle thoracocentesis facility • Lifesaving drugs (adrenaline, atropine, $NaHCO_3$, calcium gluconate, 10% and 25% dextrose, NS/RL, lorazepam, phenytoin Na, phenobarbitone, midazolam, ketamine, vecuronium/Atracurium, frusemide, adenosine)	• Multipara monitor with NIBP • Chest X-ray • Bedside USG • Facility to do blood gas analysis • Syringe pump • Defibrillator • Central line insertion • Intercostal drain • Access to 24 hour pharmacy • Access to 24 hour brain imaging • Access to 24 hour blood bank • Facility for pediatric bronchoscopy • Humidified high-flow nasal cannula/noninvasive ventilation facility • Short-term ventilation

(BP: blood pressure; IV: intravenous; NIBP: noninvasive blood pressure; NS: normal saline; PICU: pediatric intensive care unit; RL: Ringer's lactate; USG: ultrasonography)

LIFESAVING MANEUVERS TO RELIEVE ACUTE RESPIRATORY DISTRESS

Familiarity with some lifesaving maneuvers is useful in emergency **(Table 8.3.5)**. Some of the essential skills are opening of airway, bag and mask ventilation, clearing of airway, and endotracheal intubation. A child with suspected nasal or airway foreign body may be handed over to a center where anesthesia backup is, unless it is extremely urgent, because back blows of abdominal thrust may dislodge from a bronchus and block airway at the carina.

MANAGEMENT PRINCIPLES

Golden hour management is as per PALS guidelines. After initial assessment of consciousness, breathing, and circulation, a quick distinction needs to be done between respiratory failure and distress, where former may need endotracheal intubation while latter may need oxygen through a nonrebreathing mask. Judicious fluid administration based of circulation status is needed. Remaining treatment is depending upon underlying cause of the respiratory distress, which is discussed elsewhere in this book.

However, the office/indoor facility needs to be prepared for dealing with such emergent situation in terms of equipment **(Table 8.3.6)**.

8.4 Upper Respiratory Tract Infections

Sushil K Kabra

INTRODUCTION

Acute respiratory infections are the major causes of morbidity and mortality in children and of particular significance in the developing countries, such as India. Outpatient attendance attributed to acute respiratory infections is as high as 20–40% of all out patients and 12–35% of inpatients. The overall incidence of acute respiratory infection in the children under the age of 5 years may be between 3 and 8 episodes/child/year. Majority of these are due to upper respiratory tract infections (URTI).

Upper respiratory tract infection is a vague term, which includes infection of nasal cavity, throat, nasopharynx, ears, and sinuses. URTIs are common causes of morbidity in children.

ACUTE NASOPHARYNGITIS

Infection of nasopharynx is also called common cold. It is probably the most common infection in children. In young children, 3–8 episodes of common cold may occur in a year.

Etiology

Acute nasopharyngitis is caused by viruses. The common viruses include rhinovirus and corona viruses. The other viruses include adenoviruses, influenza, parainfluenza, or respiratory syncytial viruses. These are spread by droplet infection. Predisposing factors include chilling, sudden exposure to cold air, and overcrowding. Rhinitis could also be due to allergy.

Clinical Features

Clinical features of common cold are due to congestion, swelling, and increased secretion of nasopharyngeal mucosa. Clinical manifestations are more distressing in infants and young children. The common manifestations include nasal discharge (initially watery followed by thick white to yellowish), nasal block, cough, and conjunctival congestion. Nasal block causes difficulty in feeding, irritability, excessive crying, and mouth breathing. Occasionally it may be complicated by secondary bacterial sinusitis and otitis media. Otitis media should be suspected in a child with no relief in crying, even after treatment for nasal block. If a course of common cold is prolonged beyond 7–10 days, sinusitis should be considered in a school-going child.

Treatment

Acute nasopharyngitis is usually caused by virus, is self-limiting, and requires no specific treatment. For fever, paracetamol can be given every 4–6 hours. For nasal block, normal saline can be instilled in nostrils every 4–6 hours, especially before feeds. The child may be given plenty of warm liquids to drink. There is no role of antibiotics, antihistamines, local decongestive drops, or steroids. Home remedies for cough and cold, such as *tulsi*, ginger, or honey, may be beneficial in common cold. However, the mother should be told to bring the child to hospital immediately, if there is rapid respiration, lower chest in drawing, poor feeding, or persistent vomiting.

ACUTE PHARYNGITIS

Acute pharyngitis includes infection of pharynx and tonsils. This is also called acute tonsillopharyngitis. Most of the times, it is associated with rhinitis, sinusitis, and occasionally laryngitis.

Etiology

This is commonly caused by viruses, such as rhinovirus, coronavirus, influenza, parainfluenza, and adenoviruses.

About 10–20% of sore throats are caused by bacteria. The most important bacterial pathogen is group A beta-hemolytic *Streptococcus*. Rarely, *Corynebacterium diphtheriae* may present with acute pharyngitis.

Clinical Features

Children with acute pharyngitis may have fever, sore throat, pain during deglutition, nasal discharge, conjunctival congestion, and discomfort in throat. There may be enlargement of tonsils and soreness in throat. Sore throat may lead to dysphagia and drooling of saliva. Cervical lymph nodes may be enlarged and tender. Examination may reveal grayish-white pseudomembrane specifically in infection with *diphtheria* and Epstein–Barr virus. Infection due to group "A" *Streptococcus* may show pus points over tonsillar surface, palate, or pharyngeal wall.

Viral pharyngitis is self-limiting and recovers in 5–7 days. Pharyngitis caused by group "A" beta-hemolytic *Streptococcus* may lead to suppurative complications, such as retropharyngeal and peritonsillar abscesses. Presence of these complications may be indicated by high-grade fever, severe dysphagia, and bulge in the posterior wall of pharynx or around tonsils. The nonsuppurative complications due to streptococcal pharyngitis include acute rheumatic fever and acute glomerulonephritis. These complications can be prevented by administration of antibiotics.

It is very difficult to differentiate viral from bacterial pharyngitis. Presence of exudates/pus points on pharynx with enlarged tender cervical nodes and absence of nasal discharge suggests bacterial pharyngitis.

Diagnosis

Acute pharyngitis is a clinical diagnosis. At times, it is very difficult to differentiate nasopharyngitis from pharyngitis. Diagnosis of streptococcal pharyngitis can be made with presence of exudates, enlarged tonsils, and absence of nasal discharge. The diagnosis can be confirmed by throat swab culture. Now, a rapid diagnostic test based on latex agglutination is also available for diagnosis of streptococcal pharyngitis and can be carried out in office practice.

Treatment

The major consideration in treatment of acute pharyngitis is to prevent acute rheumatic fever. If a clinical diagnosis of streptococcal pharyngitis is made, a throat swab should be taken, or rapid diagnostic test performed to demonstrate streptococci, and penicillin should be administered.

Penicillin can be given orally or by intramuscular route. The duration of oral penicillin is for 10–14 days. If compliance is a problem, a single injection of long-acting (benzathine) penicillin can be given. The other alternative antibiotics are ampicillin, amoxicillin, or oral cephalosporins. If an individual is sensitive to penicillin, he/she may be treated with one of the macrolide antibiotics, such as erythromycin, roxithromycin, clarithromycin, or azithromycin.

ACUTE SUPPURATIVE OTITIS MEDIA

Acute suppurative otitis media (ASOM) is a common cause of morbidity in children specifically infants and young children. It is defined as inflammation of mucoperiosteal lining of the middle ear. If the duration of illness is more than 2 weeks, it is termed as *chronic suppurative otitis media*. Children are more prone for ASOM because the eustachian tubes communicating throat with ears are straight and short. Acute suppurative otitis media may be one of the complications of other respiratory infections.

Etiology

Acute suppurative otitis media in children is commonly caused by *Streptococcus pneumoniae, Haemophilus influenzae*, and *Moraxella catarrhalis*. Very rarely, it may be caused by *Staphylococcus* and gram-negative organisms. The latter is more common in immunocompromised hosts.

Clinical Features

Acute suppurative otitis media presents with fever, ear pain, ear discharge, and restlessness. In young children, this is a common cause of excessive crying. Once the tympanic membrane perforates, the child may get relief in pain but could develop pus discharge from ear. Acute suppurative otitis media may cause infection of mastoids in older children. The intracranial extension may lead to pyogenic brain abscess. Sometimes, ASOM may cause lower motor neuron facial palsy. Children may develop middle-ear effusion even after treatment with antibiotics; it is self-limiting and resolve in majority in a 12-week time. If it persists, these children should be sent to otolaryngologists for consideration of grommet insertion. Chronic middle-ear effusion may lead to hearing impairment.

Diagnosis

In a setting of URTI, if a child is crying excessively, his/her ears should be examined by otoscope. Eardrum may be inflamed and bulging with loss of normal anatomy with fluid in middle ear. Otoscopic examination should be part of routine examination in young children, presenting with fever without localization.

Treatment

Acute suppurative otitis media is a bacterial infection and should be treated with antibiotics. The antibacterial useful in

ASOM includes ampicillin, amoxicillin, oral cephalosporins, or macrolide. Children below 2 years of age may be treated with antibiotics from the time of diagnosis. However, children above 2 years of age with mild disease may be treated with analgesics and for 2–3 days for improvement in clinical symptoms without antibiotics. In severe disease as indicated by presence of high fever (explosive onset, severe otalgia, and toxic appearance and high-grade fever more than 102°F) and children with mild disease in beginning but deterioration in 48–72 hours, one should consider starting antibiotics. The antibiotic of choice is amoxicillin. The antibiotics continued for 10 days to prevent recurrence and development of chronicity. If the child is not improving by 3–4 days, an alternative antibiotic, such as injectable third-generation cephalosporin or amoxicillin-clavulanic acid combination, may be started. In severe cases, injectable third-generation cephalosporin (cefotaxime or ceftriaxone) may be started.

For relief from pain, paracetamol or one of the nonsteroidal anti-inflammatory drugs, i.e. ibuprofen, may be given round the clock. Occasionally, tympanocentesis may be required to relieve pain. There is no role of local antibiotic drugs in ASOM.

For treatment of chronic otitis media, it is recommended to keep the ears dry by cotton wick. A course of oral antibiotics sometimes may be useful.

ACUTE SINUSITIS

In children, ethmoid and maxillary sinuses are present in infancy. Sphenoid sinuses are well developed by 3–5 years, and frontal sinus develops between 6 years and 11 years of age. Infection of sinuses is common and associated with nasopharyngitis and pharyngitis.

Etiology

Commonly, the viruses causing pharyngitis and nasopharyngitis are responsible for sinusitis. Sometimes, they may be invaded by bacterial pathogens. The common bacterial pathogens include *S. pneumoniae, H. influenzae,* and *M. catarrhalis*. Gram-negative bacteria and fungi may invade paranasal sinuses in immunocompromised patients.

Clinical Features

Common presentation of sinusitis includes nonresolving rhinitis or common cold even after 7 days, thick purulent nasal discharge, fever, and tenderness over sinuses. In young infants, there may be swelling around the eyes. There may be headache—unilateral, bilateral, temporal, or occipital depending on sinus involvement.

Diagnosis

Usually prolonged course of nasopharyngitis in the form of persistence of fever and nasal discharge could be due to sinusitis. If tenderness over sinuses can be demonstrated or periorbital puffiness is present in young children, a clinical diagnosis of sinusitis can be made. It can be confirmed by demonstrating opacity or mucosal thickening or fluid level in paranasal sinuses on X-ray films. Other imaging modalities, such as computed tomography or magnetic resonance imaging scan of sinuses, may be done in immunocompromised host or complicated cases.

Treatment

The clinical significance of sinusitis is due to bacterial invasion. A course of amoxicillin, ampicillin, or oral cephalosporin should be given to the child. The supportive care includes normal saline in nostrils and paracetamol for fever and pain relief. There is no role of routine administration of antihistamines.

BIBLIOGRAPHY

1. Arroll B. Antibiotics for upper respiratory tract infections: an overview of Cochrane reviews. Respir Med. 2005;99:255-61.
2. Banerjee S, Bharaj P, Sullender W, et al. Human metapneumovirus infections among children with acute respiratory infections seen in a large referral hospital in India. J Clin Virol. 2007;38:70-2.
3. Bharaj P, Sullender WM, Kabra SK, et al. Respiratory viral infections detected by multiplex PCR among pediatric patients with lower respiratory tract infections seen at an urban hospital in Delhi from 2005 to 2007. Virol J. 2009;6:89.
4. Kumar P, Medigeshi GR, Mishra VS, et al. Etiology of acute respiratory infections in infants: a prospective birth cohort study. Pediatr Infect Dis J. 2017;36:25-30.
5. Mirza A, Wludyka P, Chiu TT, et al. Throat culture is necessary after negative rapid antigen detection tests. Clin Pediatr (Phila). 2007;46:241-6.
6. Simasek M, Blandino DA. Treatment of the common cold. Am Fam Physician. 2007;75:515-20.
7. Tiewsoh K, Kaur J, Lodha R. Management of upper respiratory tract infection. Indian J Pediatr. 2008;75:S28-32.

Nebulized Adrenaline

It should be given immediately to children with severe croup. The doses are 0.5 mL/kg of body weight of 1:1,000 dilutions to a maximum of 5 mL. The onset of action is seen within 30 minutes and the effect lasts for about 2 hours. In case of persistent stridor, the dose can be repeated every 2–4 hours.

Intubation

Children with signs of impending respiratory failure should be intubated for a better control on airway. An endotracheal tube of 0.5 mm smaller than expected for the child's size is selected. Intubation is maintained till an air leak develops to a maximum of 5 days.

Discharge from the Hospital

The child who is given adrenaline nebulization can be discharged if he is stridor free at rest 4 hours after the dose, and the one who is given oral steroids is stridor free at rest post half an hour after the dose.

Reporting Back to the Hospital

Parents should be instructed to report back to the hospital in case stridor at rest reappears, irrespective of what treatment was given to the child.

OUTCOME

Croup is a common infectious condition amongst small children. Most children have mild symptoms and are treated at home and the illness resolves in 3–4 days. It is observed that if the child's symptoms are minimal at discharge, return within 24 hours is unlikely. Only about 5% of children discharged from the emergency department after corticosteroid therapy need to return because of worsening of symptoms. Intubation is rarely required. In Canada, of all children with croup, about 4% have been estimated to require hospitalization, and intubation was required for only 1 of the 170 hospitalized children or 1 in 4,500 of all children with croup.

BIBLIOGRAPHY

1. Bjornson CL, Johnson DW. Croup in children. CMAJ. 2013;185:1317-23.
2. Bjornson C, Russell K, Vandermeer B, et al. Nebulized epinephrine for croup in children. Cochrane Database Syst Rev. 2013;(10):CD006619. doi: 10.1002/14651858.CD006619.pub3.
3. Mandell GL. Douglas and Bennett's Principles and Practice of Infectious Disease, 5th edition. Philadelphia, PA: Churchill Livingstone; 2009.
4. Ortiz-Alvarez O. Acute management of croup in the emergency department. Paediatr Child Health. 2017;22:166-73.
5. Rankin I, Wang SM, Waters A, et al. The management of recurrent croup in children. J Laryngol Otol. 2013;127(5):494-500.
6. Smith DK, McDermott AJ, Sullivan JF. Croup: diagnosis and management. Am Fam Physician. 2018;97(9): 575-80.

8.6 Pneumonia

Rohit C Agrawal

INTRODUCTION

Pneumonia probably is one of the oldest diseases, as old as antiquity known to humankind and has always remained a subject of challenge to medical science, despite extensive research. Pneumonia is number one cause of under-five childhood mortality across the globe, particularly in developing countries. Unfortunately, over the years the mortality remained almost the same, and hence, it is also been called as "forgotten killer" or "silent killer".

EPIDEMIOLOGY

Approximately 150 million episodes of childhood pneumonia are reported every year from the world, out of which 95% are from developing countries. A total of 15 countries account for nearly 75%, and 6 countries including India account for 50% cases. India alone bears the brunt of 25% disease burden.

According to Million Death Study, out of the 7.6 million under-five childhood mortality world over is 16%, i.e. 1.2 million deaths are due to pneumonia. More than 90% of the deaths due to pneumonia among young children occur in 68 poor nations, mostly from Africa and Asia.

In India, the disease burden is huge. The 45 million episodes are estimated annually with 6.6 million hospitalizations, which contribute to 24% national disease burden and 0.37 million deaths annually.

DEFINITION

Pneumonia is defined as an inflammatory process involving lung parenchyma usually due to microorganisms. It is referred as "pneumonitis" when the cause is noninfective. Pneumonia is mainly classified as:

- *Community acquired:* Pneumonia acquired outside the hospital environment in a previously healthy immune-competent subject. The patient should not have been hospitalized within 14 days prior to the onset of symptoms.
- *Nosocomial pneumonia*: Pneumonia acquired within hospital setting more than 48 hours after hospitalization (hospital-acquired pneumonia) or more than 48–72 hours after endotracheal intubation (ventilator-associated pneumonia).

This classification does not include "recurrent pneumonia" which is defined as two episodes of pneumonia in 1 year or 3 episodes in any timeframe, with clearing of pneumonia in between, "persistent pneumonia", where there is no clinic-radiological resolution after 3–4 weeks of appropriate and adequate antibiotic therapy, and "aspiration pneumonia" which occurs due to aspiration of foreign materials in the lower airways.

ETIOLOGY

It depends on various factors, such as age, immune status, underlying comorbidity, and various risk factors, as shown in **Flowchart 8.6.1**.

The causative agents may be viral, bacterial, or atypical pathogens. They are usually age specific as shown in **Table 8.6.1**.

Most common bacterial pathogens are *Streptococcus pneumoniae* and *Haemophilus influenzae*, which together are responsible for 60–70% of total pneumonia cases, followed by viruses, which account for 30–35% of pneumonia cases.

Mycoplasma pneumoniae and *chlamydia* are most common causes of "atypical pneumonia" in school-going children older than 5 years of age accounting for 11–30% cases. *Legionella* is infrequent but serious cause of atypical pneumonia. Significant proportion of pneumonia is due to mixed infection (8–40%), and in 20–60% of cases, pathogens are not identified.

Table 8.6.1: Etiology of pneumonia—relation to age.

Age group	*Etiology*
0–3 months	• Gram-negative *Enterobacteriaceae* • Enterococci • *Chlamydia trachomatis* • Group B streptococci • *Haemophilus influenzae* • *Streptococcus pneumoniae* • *Listeria monocytogenes*
3 months–5 years	• *Streptococcus pneumoniae* • Viruses • *Haemophilus influenzae* • *Staphylococcus* • *Mycoplasma pneumoniae*
>5 years	• *Streptococcus pneumoniae* • *Mycoplasma pneumoniae* • Viruses • *Staphylococcus* • *Streptococcus pyogenes*

Flowchart 8.6.1: Predisposing factors for CAP.

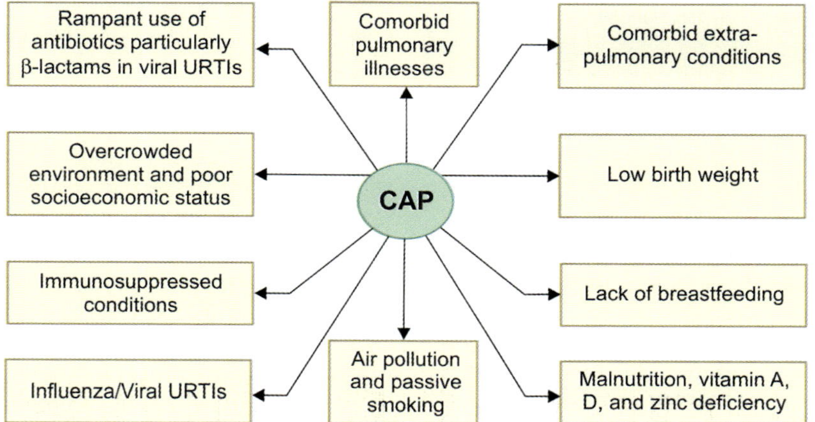

(CAP: community-acquired pneumonia; URTI: upper respiratory tract infections)

Source: Berman S. Epidemiology of acute respiratory infections in children of developing countries. Rev Infect Dis. 1991;13(6):S454-62.

PATHOGENESIS

Pneumonia is usually preceded by respiratory viral infection, which disturbs the defense mechanism of the lungs and disrupts the normal epithelial layer of respiratory tract and as a result there is dysfunction of ciliary brush border clearing mechanism. There is inhibition of phagocytosis by alveolar macrophages. Thus, bacteria and other organisms invade the lung parenchyma and produce a pneumonic lesion. The invasion could be either direct spread from nasopharyngeal tract by respiratory droplet infection or could be by invasion through hematogenous dissemination within the lung parenchyma. When the spread is hematogenous, it is called *invasive or bacteremic pneumonia* and when the spread is direct, it is called mucosal or *nonbacteremic pneumonia.* However, the pathogenesis is still ill understood.

CLINICAL FEATURES

Constellation of symptom-triad of fever, cough, rapid breathing, and/or difficult breathing is classical clinical manifestation of pneumonia. Diagnosis of pneumonia is essentially clinical. Tachypnea is single most sensitive and specific sign to diagnose pneumonia, as sensitive as 66–88% of auscultation (*see* Table 8.3.1, Chapter 8.3 for grading of tachypnea).

Clinical features may differ from neonate to older child. In the neonate, there could be absence of cough and fever, and common presenting features are excessive irritability or lethargy, difficulty in feeding, intermittent apneic spells, cyanosis ±, progressive air hunger, and rapid clinical deterioration with or without evidence of sepsis. In severely malnourished children, the breathing efforts will be poor. The World Health Organization has graded pneumonia as given in **Table 8.6.2** based on symptoms.

Assessment and grading of severity is most important for successful management.

Table 8.6.2: The World Health Organization grading of pneumonia.

Pneumonia	Fever less than 38.5°C, cough and tachypnea, no feeding difficulties, no dehydration
Severe pneumonia	High-grade fever more than 39°C, difficulty in feeding, tachypnea, respiratory distress with ICR or SCR, dehydration, grunt, bronchial breath sounds on auscultation with or without crackles, $SpO_2 \geq 92$ at room air, radiological opacity on chest X-ray +/–
Severe to very severe pneumonia	Inability to feed, altered sensorium, intermittent apneic spells, cyanosis, excessive diaphoresis, narrow pulse pressure, acidemia, and $SpO_2 < 92$ at room air

(ICR: intercostal retraction; SCR: subcostal retraction; SpO_2: peripheral capillary oxygen saturation)

DIAGNOSIS

Diagnosis of pneumonia is essentially clinical and seldom requires laboratory support. Absence of past history of recurrent cough and presence of fever with fast breathing is a hallmark presentation in clinical diagnosis of pneumonia. It should always be remembered that there are no definite differentiating markers between viral, bacterial, and atypical pneumonia. However, there are certain clinical clues, which can help to nail down on etiological diagnosis **(Table 8.6.3)**.

Characteristics of Viral Pneumonia

- Acute—sudden onset
- Younger age
- Preceding upper respiratory catarrh
- Wheeze with crackles
- Clinical evidence of hyperinflation with scattered exudates on radiology due to segmental atelectasis.

For optimum antimicrobial management of pneumonia, it is prudent to differentiate between bacterial, viral, and atypical pneumonia clinically, as it is often very difficult to isolate the offending pathogen **(Table 8.6.4)**.

LABORATORY DIAGNOSIS

- *Acute phase reactants*, such as complete blood cell, C-reactive protein, erythrocyte sedimentation rate, have poor sensitivity and specificity. They do not distinguish between viral and bacterial etiology, nor they help in making decision of antibiotic choice; however, they may be useful tools for monitoring the course of the disease.

Table 8.6.3: Clinical clues which help in diagnosis of etiological diagnosis of pneumonia.

Predisposing factors	*Organisms (apart from usual ones)*
Pyoderma, measles, pneumatoceles	*Staphylococcus*
HIV	*Pneumocystis carinii*
Neutropenia	Gram-negative, *Aspergillus*
Cystic fibrosis	*Pseudomonas, Staphylococcus*
Severe PEM	Gram-negative, *Staphylococcus*
Preceding coryza, wheeze	Viral
Young afebrile infant with neonatal conjunctivitis	*Chlamydia*
Multisystem involvement (rash, anemia, hepatitis, encephalitis)	*Mycoplasma*
Marked leukocytosis	Bacteria
Acute otitis media	*Streptococcus pneumoniae/ Haemophilus influenzae*

(HIV: human immunodeficiency virus; PEM: protein-energy malnutrition)

Table 8.6.4: Differential diagnosis between typical and atypical pneumonia.

Features	***Typical pneumonia***	***Atypical pneumonia***
Age	More common in young infants, children, and in older children	School-going children, adolescents, and adults
Onset	Acute/sudden	Gradual/insidious
Facies	Toxic	Well
Rigors	Shaking chills	Chilliness
Wheeze	Rare or nil	Common
Cough	Productive	Nonproductive/ paroxysmal
Sputum	Purulent/bloody	Mucoid
Temperature	High 102–104°F	Mild-moderate < 102°F
Pleurisy	Frequent	Rare
Consolidation	Frequent	Rare
Extrapulmonary manifestations	Uncommon	Common
Gram staining (sputum)	Neutrophils	Mononuclear cells
Sputum culture	Occasional growth of microbe	Rarely any growth
WBC count	>15,000/mm^3; shift to left	>15,000/mm^3; no shift
Chest radiography	Defined density	Nondefined infiltrates

(WBC: white blood cell)

- *Radiology* is not routinely required in nonsevere pneumonia to confirm the diagnosis. At times, it may not correlate with the clinical signs; there is also wide variation in the interpretation by radiologists. Moreover, reliability in predicting the etiology is poor. However, chest X-ray may be indicated in very severe disease, ambiguous picture, no improvement/worsening more than 48–72 hours of therapy, suspected complications, and known immune-compromised child **(Figs. 8.6.1A to C)**.
- *Microbiology*—sputum culture or blood culture though more specific, but the yield is very poor (10–15%). There is also a risk of growing normal nasopharyngeal flora.
- *Serology*—Serology, latex agglutination, urinary antigens for pneumococcus and *Haemophilus influenzae* b (Hib), rapid antigen detection test, and cold agglutinins for mycoplasma are not easily available, expensive with time lagging, and have poor sensitivity.
- *Invasive procedures*, such as bronchoscopy, bronchoalveolar lavage, and lung aspiration, have high sensitivity and specificity; however, they are too invasive and unethical to be advised in office practice.
- *Pulse oximetry* is a mandatory tool for monitoring the course of the disease in all the hospitalized children.

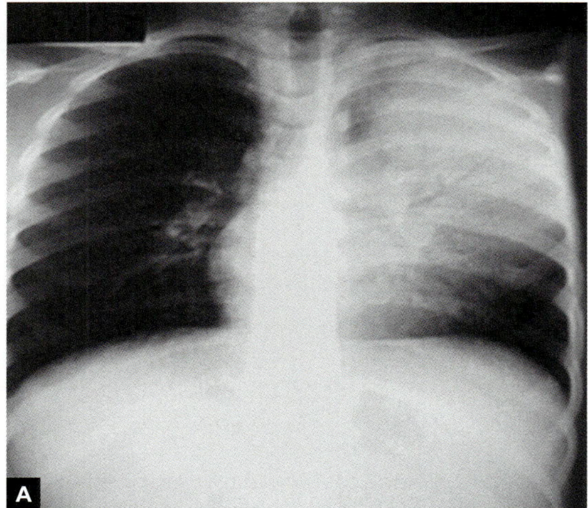

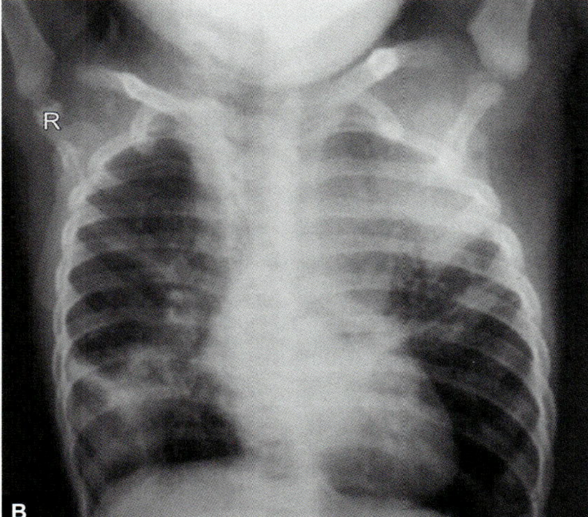

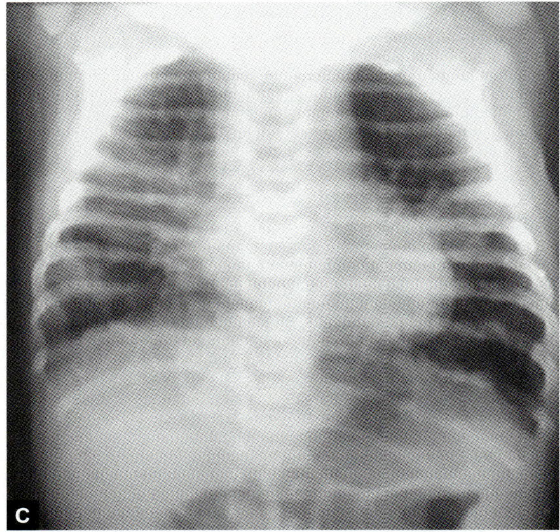

Figs. 8.6.1A to C: Radiologic findings in: (A) Bacterial lobar consolidation; (B) Bronchopneumonia; and (C) Interstitial pneumonia.

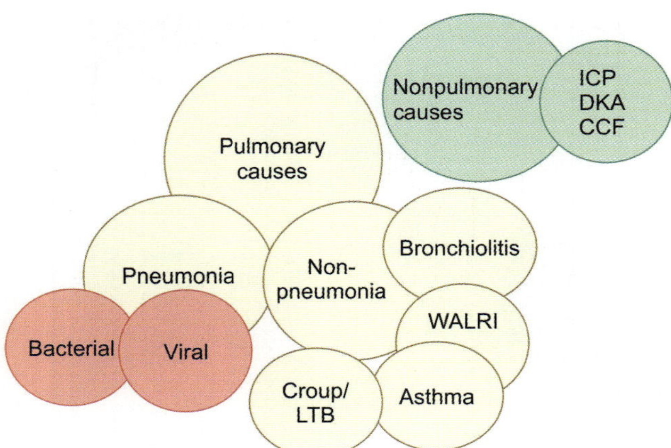

Fig. 8.6.2: Triad of fever + cough + tachypnea is symbolic of LRTI; but all LRTIs are not pneumonias.

(CCF: congestive cardiac failure; DKA: diabetic ketoacidosis; ICP: intracranial pressure; LRTI: lower respiratory tract infection; LTB: laryngotracheobronchitis; WALRI: wheeze-associated lower respiratory infection)

Differential Diagnosis

Though symptom complex of fever, cough, and rapid/difficult breathing is classical presentation of pneumonia; it should be differentiated from other masqueraders, which may mimic with same symptomatology. One should remember all cases of fever, cough, and breathlessness need not be pneumonia **(Fig. 8.6.2)**.

MANAGEMENT

The mainstays of management are antibiotics and supportive treatment. It is imperative to understand that all pneumonias deserve antibiotics for two reasons, one because pneumonia is number one cause of childhood mortality, particularly in developing world where children die due to either need of antibiotics or delayed initiation of antibiotic therapy and two, as differentiation between viral and bacterial is difficult. Empirical antibiotics are rational in pneumonia.

Nonsevere pneumonia above the age of 3 months can be managed at domiciliary level with oral antibiotics. However, any pneumonia below the age of 3 months should be hospitalized and treated with parenteral antibiotics. The choice of antibiotics though empirical should be determined by age, severity, predisposing conditions if any, and local epidemiology and drug resistance pattern.

Outpatient Management

All nonsevere pneumonias more than 3 months of age, when the child is not toxic, accepting oral feeds, not dehydrated, maintaining normal saturation, and fever less than 38.5°C can be managed at domiciliary level with supportive care, such as maintenance of hydration, nutrition, and antipyretics and adjuvants, if needed. The choice of oral antibiotic is as shown in **Table 8.6.5**.

Table 8.6.5: Choice of antibiotics.

Age	*First-line*	*Second-line*
3 months–5 years	Amoxicillin*	Co-amoxiclav/Cefuroxime/ Chloramphenicol
>5 years	Amoxicillin*	Macrolide†/Co-amoxiclav/ Cefuroxime

**Standard doses*: 40–45 mg/kg/day in two or three divided doses.
†*Erythromycin*: 30–40 mg/kg/day in three divided doses; *Clarithromycin*: 15 mg/kg/day in two divided doses; *Azithromycin*: 10 mg/kg/day in once a day dose.

Box 8.6.1: Indications for hospitalization.

- Infants less than 3 months
- Severe malnutrition
- More than two risk factors
- Comorbidities
- Associated complications
- Respiratory rate more than 70 per minute in infants and more than 50 per minute in older children
- Respiratory distress—grunting, alae nasi flare, ICR, or SCR
- Cyanosis or SpO_2 less than 92% in room air
- Poor oral intake/dehydration
- Inappropriate observation or supervision at home

(ICR: intercostal retraction; SCR: subcostal retraction; SpO_2: oxygen saturation)

First-line oral antibiotics should be given minimum for 5 days and second line for 7 days. Child should be followed-up after 48 hours, and if there is clinical improvement, the child should be continued with the same management. If the condition clinically deteriorates after 48 hours, one should revise the diagnosis, look for associated complication and comorbidities, changing the antibiotic to second line, and if be the need, the child should be hospitalized **(Box 8.6.1)**.

Inpatient Management

Management comprises specific antimicrobial along with supportive care of nutrition, hydration, oxygen if needed, antipyretics (paracetamol), and bronchodilators along with chest physiotherapy if needed **(Table 8.6.6)**.

In case of methicillin-sensitive *Staphylococcus aureus*, the duration should be for 2 weeks, and in case of methicillin-resistant *S. aureus*, it should be 4–6 weeks.

The duration for intravenous antibiotics should be for 5–7 days in uncomplicated cases; however, switchover to oral antibiotics may be considered if accepted orally.

Table 8.6.6: Specific antimicrobial therapy in pneumonia.

Age	*First-line*	*Second-line*
<3 months	Cefotaxime‡/Ceftriaxone† ± Aminoglycosides‖	
3 months–5 years	Ampicillin/Co-amoxiclav* or Ampicillin + Chloramphenicol	Ceftriaxone†/ Cefotaxime‡
>5 years	• Ampicillin/Penicillin G • Co-amoxiclav/ Macrolide (if mycoplasma suspected)	Ceftriaxone†/ Cefotaxime‡ and Macrolides
Suspected staphylococcal infection	Cefuroxime§ or Co-amoxiclav or IV 3rd generation Cephalosporins + Cloxacillin	Ceftriaxone†/ Cefotaxime‡ and Vancomycin/ Teicoplanin/Linezolid

**Co-amoxiclav*: 30–40 mg/kg/day.
†*Ceftriaxone*: 50–100 mg/kg/day.
‡*Cefotaxime*: 100–200 mg/kg/day.
§*Cefuroxime*: 20–30 mg/kg/day.
‖*Aminoglycosides*: 15 mg/kg/day in single or two divided doses.

The switchover therapy for injectable third-generation cephalosporins should be either cefpodoxime (10 mg/kg/day in two divided doses) or cefdinir (15 mg/kg/day in two divided doses) and should never be cefixime as it has no activity against *Pneumococcus* and poor activity against community pathogens responsible for pneumonia.

Despite rational choice of antibiotics in right dose and for optimal duration, if there is failure in clinical improvement, one needs to:

- Check the diagnosis and rule out foreign body, aspiration pneumonia, and interstitial lung disease.
- Look for underlying comorbidity, such as lung abscess, empyema, bronchiectasis, left-to-right shunts, gastroesophageal reflux disease, asthma, cystic fibrosis, and ciliary dyskinesia.
- Evaluate immune suppression in the host, such as human immunodeficiency virus and hypogammaglobulinemia.
- Test phagocytic dysfunctions for chronic granulomatous disease.
- Look for drug resistance, particularly if child is from day-care center has received multiple courses of beta-lactams and corticosteroids.
- Search for the possibility of polymicrobial etiology.
- There is no need to chase for follow-up X-rays since total radiological resolution may take 4–8 weeks' time depending on offending organisms.

COMPLICATIONS

These include empyema, pneumothorax, persistent bacterial bronchitis bronchogenic dissemination, septicemia, osteomyelitis, multiple systemic abscesses, septic arthritis, and meningitis.

PROGNOSIS

Prognosis is good provided there is appropriate recognition and proper referral by the healthcare provider and early initiation of antibiotics. Unfortunately, only 15–20% cases of pneumonia receive proper and adequate antibiotics, which is the main reason for high infant mortality due to pneumonias particularly in developing countries.

PREVENTION

A multifaceted approach is needed to prevent and control childhood pneumonia. These include:

- Exclusive breastfeeding for first 6 months of life
- Weaning to solid foods after 6 months of age, preferably with homemade foods
- Avoidance of risk factors, such as overcrowded environment, biofuels, exposure to pollution, and bottle-feeding
- Protection from malnutrition and supplementation of vitamin A and D
- Optimum immunization with diphtheria-pertussis-tetanus, measles, Hib, pneumococcal vaccines at appropriate ages.

8.7 Bronchiolitis

A Balachandran

INTRODUCTION

Bronchiolitis is a common viral respiratory illness in children. It accounts for a substantial portion of the pediatric burden of illness all over the world; it is the most common and serious lower respiratory tract syndrome that results in hospital admission among infants and is associated with considerable morbidity. It is generally a self-limiting condition and is most commonly due to respiratory syncytial virus (RSV) infection. Babies with chronic lung disease are at risk for more severe RSV-associated illness. Bronchiolitis occurs most frequently among children younger than 12 months of age. Most cases occur between late autumn and early spring, with sporadic cases throughout the year.

DEFINITION

Bronchiolitis is a clinical syndrome characterized by the acute onset of respiratory symptoms in a child younger than 2 years of age. Typically the initial symptoms of upper respiratory tract viral infection, such as fever and coryza, progress within 4–6 days to include evidence of lower respiratory tract involvement with the onset of cough and wheezing.

RISK FACTORS

In bronchiolitis, an increased risk for hospitalization is seen among infants attending day care, those exposed to passive smoking and overcrowding in the household. Environmental and genetic factors may also contribute to the severity of disease. High-risk factors include age less than 3 months, premature delivery, low birth weight, congenital heart disease, chronic lung disease (e.g. cystic fibrosis), recurrent aspiration pneumonitis, bronchopulmonary dysplasia (BPD), congenital lung malformations, tracheoesophageal fistula, neurogenic disorders (interfering with pulmonary toilet), immunodeficiency, and malnutrition.

The high-risk groups are vulnerable for rapid deterioration and more severe disease. Children with a pulmonary patch (consolidation or atelectasis) on radiograph, hypoxia, repeat episodes of apnea and extreme tachypnea at admission are at higher risk of admission to the intensive care unit and may need mechanical ventilation.

ETIOLOGY

Bronchiolitis is usually a result of a viral respiratory tract infection. Respiratory syncytial virus is the most common underlying infecting agent. Other viral pathogens, such as influenza, parainfluenza, adenovirus, coronavirus, and rhinovirus, can also cause bronchiolitis. *Mycoplasma* is also implicated occasionally in children with lower respiratory tract infection and wheezing.

PATHOLOGY

Respiratory syncytial virus infection results in the loss of epithelial cilia and sloughing of epithelial cells in the airways. This leads to the collection of desquamated airway epithelial cells, polymorphonuclear cells, and lymphocytes within the airway. There may also be cellular infiltration and airway mucosal edema with very little or no alveolar infiltration. In acute bronchiolitis, sloughed epithelial cells, neutrophils, and lymphocytes appear to be the major contributors to airway obstruction. The complete plugging of some airways and partial plugging of others may lead to localized atelectasis of some units of lung parenchyma and overdistention of other units. These results in ventilation–perfusion mismatch causing hypoxemia, which is generally relieved by the administration of oxygen (O_2).

CLINICAL FEATURES

Clinical features are quite variable. Initially, they present like any other viral upper respiratory tract infection with cough or cold with or without fever. Later, disturbing cough, tachypnea, respiratory distress, and poor feeding may develop depending on the severity of illness. Fever is present in almost 50% of the infants. In patients with adenovirus or influenza-associated bronchiolitis, fever is often higher than 39°C. On examination, infants typically may have tachypnea, respiratory distress, audible wheezing, rales or rhonchi, crackles, poor air movement, and the expiratory phase is usually prolonged. Other concomitant findings, such as conjunctivitis, rhinitis, and otitis media, may be present. Once hypoxia sets in, there can be lethargy, seizure, and death.

GRADING OF BRONCHIOLITIS

Based on the ability to feed, the respiratory effort, and O_2 saturation (SaO_2) observed at admission, each infant's condition can be clinically graded as mild, moderate, and severe bronchiolitis **(Table 8.7.1)**.

INVESTIGATIONS

Bronchiolitis is a clinical diagnosis. The specific and supportive investigations, which can be done in bronchiolitis, are discussed further.

- Nasopharyngeal aspirate for RSV and viral culture.
- Full blood counts.
- Serum electrolytes, to look for evidence of syndrome of inappropriate antidiuretic hormone secretion, especially when intravenous (IV) fluids, are needed.
- Blood culture if temperature more than 38.5°C.
- Arterial blood gas (ABG) analysis to look for carbon dioxide (CO_2) retention when there is evidence of respiratory failure.
- The chest X-ray need not be done routinely and is indicated only in children with severe respiratory distress or when there is diagnostic dilemma. The radiographic findings of bronchiolitis include hyperinflation, patchy infiltrates that are typically migratory and attributable to postobstructive atelectasis, and peribronchial cuffing. Because bronchiolitis is not a disease of the alveolar spaces, a secondary bacterial pneumonitis should be suspected if a true alveolar infiltrate is seen on chest radiograph.

Table 8.7.1: Grading of bronchiolitis.

	Mild	*Moderate*	*Severe*
Ability to feed	Ability to feed normally	Appear short of breath during feeds	May be reluctant or unable to feed
Respiratory effort	Little or no respiratory distress	Moderate distress with some chest wall retractions and nasal flaring	Severe distress with marked chest wall retractions, nasal flaring, and grunting May have frequent or prolonged apneic episodes
Oxygen saturation	*Saturations*: SaO_2 more than 92%	Saturations less than 92%, correctable with oxygen	Saturations less than 92%, may or may not be correctable with oxygen

DIFFERENTIAL DIAGNOSIS

Congenital anomalies, such as vascular ring, congenital heart disease, gastroesophageal reflux, aspiration pneumonia, or foreign body aspiration can mimic the symptoms of bronchiolitis.

MANAGEMENT

Supportive care is the mainstay of therapy for infants with bronchiolitis. Children with mild bronchiolitis can be managed on outpatient basis. They need to be followed and reviewed earlier if there is clinical worsening. Infants in high-risk group are better hospitalized and managed even if they are graded as mild in view of their propensity to deteriorate rapidly, whereas moderate and severe cases have to be definitely admitted and monitored. Considerable unexplained variation exists in the inpatient management of bronchiolitis **(Flowchart 8.7.1)**.

NONCONTROVERSIAL ISSUES

Oxygen

The drug of choice in bronchiolitis is O_2. Oxygen is used when the SaO_2 is less than 94% or in a combination of clinically significant respiratory distress, a respiratory rate above 60/min, and difficulty in feeding. The aim of humidified O_2 supplementation is to maintain SaO_2 above 95% using suitable device, preferably in a nonthreatening fashion. Noninvasive strategies that may be effective in reducing work of breathing, improving gas exchange, and avoiding the need for endotracheal intubation include heated humidified high-flow nasal cannula (HFNC) therapy and continuous positive airway pressure (CPAP) ventilation. During recovery, SaO_2 of 90–92% in room air is acceptable if baby is feeding well and not distressed except in children with chronic lung disease.

Fluid Therapy

If the infant tolerates well, oral feeds are continued, as is the case with mild-to-moderate severity. Intravenous fluids are needed to maintain hydration in moderate-to-severe or severe respiratory distress (marked retractions, nasal flaring), marked tachypnea (>60/min), coughing and choking with feeds, vomiting, decreased intake, apneic episodes, and tiring during feeds. Normal general maintenance fluids with normal maintenance volumes are used with N/2 or N/4 dextrose saline.

Nasogastric Feeding

Nasogastric (NG) feeding is avoided during acute phase and is reserved for recovery phase. During acute phase, the NG tube blocks one nostril and increases upper airway resistance, which in turn further increases the work of breathing.

Flowchart 8.7.1: Management algorithm.

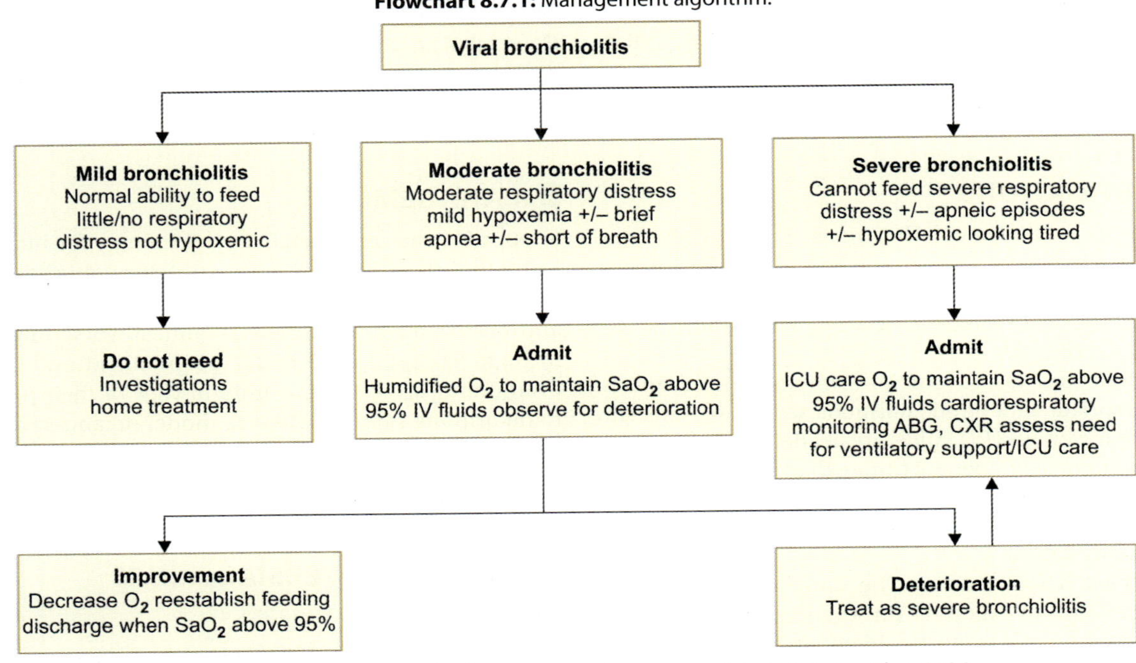

Source: Respiratory tract infection—group education module, IAP Action Plan; 2006.

Symptomatic Management

Symptomatic management, such as antipyretics, is needed to relieve fever.

CONTROVERSIAL ISSUES

Bronchodilators

The role of bronchodilators (salbutamol and epinephrine) in acute bronchiolitis is controversial. Though there is no absolute contraindication, bronchodilators neither treats hypoxemia nor affects the duration or progress of bronchiolitis. Inhaled beta-agonist therapy when used should be on a case-by-case basis, by critically evaluating its effectiveness in the individual patient. They might be of benefit in intermediate conditions, such as early wheezers or children with atopy.

Since mucosal edema is an important component of airway obstruction in infants with bronchiolitis, a logical approach to therapy might be to use a combined (alpha-adrenergic and beta-adrenergic agonist), such as epinephrine (0.3 mL/kg of 1:1,000 solution). Till date there is no definitive evidence to support the use of nebulized epinephrine in all children with moderate or severe bronchiolitis. When the effect of epinephrine was compared with placebo, the improvement in respiratory symptoms across studies has been in consistent and potentially short lived. It may therefore be appropriate, for clinicians to use nebulized epinephrine as a potential rescue medication for patients who are to be admitted.

There is no role for ipratropium bromide in the management of bronchiolitis.

Hypertonic Saline

Hypertonic saline has the potential to reduce airway edema and mucus plugging, the predominant feature of acute bronchiolitis. Several trials have indicated the potential benefit of hypertonic saline (3% NaCl) in acute bronchiolitis with conflicting results.

Sedation

Sedation should be avoided in an irritable child as this may be a sign of hypoxia and sedation further compromises the respiratory drive of the child.

Antibiotics

There is no role for routine or prophylactic antibiotics in bronchiolitis. Since secondary bacterial infections of the lower respiratory tract are unusual in children with bronchiolitis.

Aerosolized Ribavirin

Respiratory syncytial virus is the most common cause of bronchiolitis but specific antiviral therapy for symptomatic infants has been of limited value. Aerosolized ribavirin, used to treat mild to moderately ill infants with laboratory confirmed RSV bronchiolitis neither prevents the need for mechanical ventilation nor reduces the length of hospital stay. It is not recommended at present for treatment of bronchiolitis.

Noninvasive Ventilation

Humidified HFNC or CPAP may potentially benefit infants with bronchiolitis, by tenting to open the smaller airways during all phases of respiration, preventing air trapping and obstructive disease, and by serving as a constant ipratropium stimulus in infants with a propensity to experience apnea.

Role of Steroids

There is no role of systemic (parenteral/oral) or inhaled steroids in the management of bronchiolitis.

Intensive Care Unit Management

It will be needed if there is:

- Progression to severe respiratory distress, especially in high-risk group.
- Any significant apneic episodes (more than 15 seconds or associated with desaturation) or frequent recurrent brief apneic episodes.
- Persistent desaturation despite O_2; where ABG shows the evidence of respiratory failure, i.e. partial pressure of O_2 less than 80 mm Hg; partial pressure of CO_2 more than 50 mm Hg; pH less than 7.25.

Other Nonstandard Therapies

Antirespiratory Syncytial Virus Preparation

The use of immunoglobulin with a neutralizing activity against RSV [RSV-immune globulin intravenous (IGIV)] or RSV-specific humanized monoclonal antibody (palivizumab) have failed to improve outcomes in infants with or without risk factors, hospitalized with RSV infection.

Heliox

It is a mixture of helium and O_2 (80:20%). It can flow through airways with less turbulence and resistance than O_2. Only very small benefit is observed in a limited group of children who were administered heliox; hence, it is not recommended for routine use.

DISCHARGE CRITERIA

The infant is considered fit for discharge if the child did not require supplemental O_2 for more than10 hours, had minimal or no chest recession, and is feeding adequately, without the need for IV fluids.

COMPLICATIONS

Complication rates are higher in prematurely born infants with congenital heart disease and infants with other congenital abnormalities compared to infants without risk factors. Serious respiratory complications include respiratory failure, apnea, and pneumothorax. Others include secondary infection, cardiovascular involvement, and electrolyte imbalance.

PROGNOSIS

The need for supplemental O_2 (based on SaO_2 in room air) at admission is highly predictive of the length of the hospital stay. The case fatality rate for bronchiolitis is highest among infants less than 3-month age.

PREVENTION

Respiratory syncytial virus is highly contagious and spreads via inhalation of small particle aerosols or direct transfer via hand-to-hand contact. Respiratory syncytial virus cross infection is common but is largely preventable by:

- Simple hand washing by nursing, medical, other staff, and parents.
- Isolation of RSV-infected cases will minimize this problem.
- Palivizumab (RSV Ig) prophylaxis in BPD may be beneficial and has to be decided on case-by-case basis.

BIBLIOGRAPHY

1. Balachandran A, Gowrishankar NC. Bronchiolitis. In: Subramanyam L, Shivabalan S, Gowrishankar NC, Vijayasekaran D, Balachandran A (Eds). Essentials of Pediatric Pulmonology, 3rd edition. New Delhi: Jaypee Brothers Medical Publishers (P) Ltd.; 2008. pp. 91-5.
2. Christakis DA, Cowan CA, Garrison MM, et al. Variation in inpatient diagnostic testing and management of bronchiolitis. Pediatrics. 2005;115(4):878-84.
3. Coffin SE. Bronchiolitis: inpatient focus. Pediatr Clin North Am. 2005;52(4):1047-57.
4. Dayan SP, Roskind GC, Levine AD, et al. Controversies in the management of children with bronchiolitis. Clin Pediatr Emerg Med. 2004;5:41-53.
5. Grimaldi M, Gouyon B, Michaut F, et al. Severe respiratory syncytial virus bronchiolitis: epidemiologic variations associated with the initiation of palivizumab in severely premature infants with bronchopulmonary dysplasia. Pediatr Infect Dis J. 2004;23(12):1081-5.
6. King VJ, Viswanathan M, Bordley WC, et al. Pharmacologic treatment of bronchiolitis in infants and children: a systematic review. Arch Pediatr Adolesc Med. 2004;158(2):127-37.
7. Respiratory tract infection-group education module. IAP consensus protocol for the management of respiratory tract infection for children. IAP Action Plan; 2006.
8. Wainwright C, Altamirano L, Cheney M, et al. A multicenter randomized double-blind controlled trial of nebulized epinephrine in infants with acute bronchiolitis. N Engl J Med. 2003;349(1):27-35.

8.8 Empyema

Varinder Singh

INTRODUCTION

Involvement of the pleural space with pulmonary infections has been recognized since the ancient times. Bacterial pneumonia with associated pleural empyema is the most common cause of pleural effusion found in the pediatric population. They need to be understood differently from parapneumonic effusions, which are exudative thin effusions which can be seen in a significant proportion of those admitted with a severe and complicated pneumonia. Parapneumonic effusion and empyema lie on a continuum: the stage of the effusion is best assessed using chest ultrasound. While the simple effusions have free-flowing pleural fluid, more complex effusions have fibrin strands and loculations, whereas an empyema has multiple loculations and often a thick pleural rind. Importantly, a clinician must know that while most of the parapneumonic effusions resolve with an adequate and appropriate antimicrobial therapy, but antibiotics alone are almost never sufficient to treat empyema (frank pus in the pleural cavity).

DISEASE BURDEN

The reported global incidence of parapneumonic effusion and empyema is 3.3 per 10,000 children, but this varies with different populace and economic level. Some of the developed nations are showing an increased prevalence lately. It is more common in infants and young children under 5 years of age.

ETIOPATHOGENESIS

Staphylococcus aureus, *Streptococcus pneumoniae*, and *Streptococcus pyogenes* are the organisms most commonly implicated in empyema thoracis. While *S. pneumoniae* is the most common organism implicated in the most Western and developed countries, the prevalence of *Haemophilus influenzae* pneumonia with empyema has decreased following *H. influenzae* type b vaccination. In India, *S. aureus* continues to be the most common organism. *S. pneumoniae, H. influenzae,* and gram-negative bacilli form rest of the burden. Frank tuberculous empyema is very uncommon.

CLINICAL FEATURES

Clinical signs vary depending on the age of the patient, stage of the effusion, and type of prior antibiotic therapy. A high index of suspicion and appreciation of factors that predispose to development of empyema facilitates its recognition. Children usually present with a severe pneumonia, or a pneumonia that does not respond well to initial therapy. Lack of response to the antibiotics after 48 hours of treatment should raise the suspicion of an effusion. However, some may also present with a fever without clear focus, or with chest or abdominal pain.

Usual features of pneumonia, such as fever, tachypnea, hypoxia, and respiratory distress, may be present. Few children may also be septicemic, dehydrated, and/or in respiratory failure. Fever may not be present in the immunocompromised or debilitated patients. On physical examination, decreased chest expansion, decreased or bronchial breath sounds, dullness to percussion, and mediastinal shift are common signs. Few may also have pleural friction rub, bronchophony or egophony above pleural effusion, swelling/splinting of the chest, or a preference to lie on the affected side. Oxygen saturation ($SpaO_2$) levels below 92% may indicate severe disease.

Some children may have other stigmata of staphylococcal infection, such as skin pustules or boils, infected scabies, pyomyositis, septic arthritis, and pyopericardium.

DIAGNOSIS

Chest Skiagram: Frontal Views

Frontal views form the most important and primary investigation for patients with pleural disease. There is no role for a routine lateral or decubitus views. The earliest sign to be seen is the obliteration of the costophrenic angle. White opacity of the lateral part or whole of hemithorax is usually seen. Skiagrams, however, cannot differentiate empyema from a parapneumonic effusion. Scoliosis may also be seen.

Sonography of Chest

It is a very useful tool for the diagnosis, guidance of thoracocentesis, or pleural catheter placement. It is especially helpful when the radiograph shows a white out. Sonography can distinguish solid from liquid pleural abnormalities with much higher accuracy compared to skiagrams. Sonography gives valuable information regarding size of the effusion, the presence of adhesions or loculations, and the echogenicity of the pleural fluid. Sonographic appearance of pleural fluid varies according to the stage of effusion, ranging from an anechoic completely echo-free or sonolucent parapneumonic effusion to very echogenic fluid with septa as seen in frank empyema. Ultrasonography shows limiting membranes, suggesting the presence of loculated collections even when they are not so well seen on computed tomography (CT) scan.

Computed Tomography Scan

Empyema appears well-defined, smooth, round or elliptical on CT scan. The parietal and visceral layers are separated by interposed empyema fluid, giving rise to the "split pleura sign" of empyema. The CT scans should not be performed routinely as it exposes the child to a very high radiation dose while most information for diagnosis and for guiding treatment decisions can be received from a good sonogram. It may have a limited role in the cases which do not respond to the initial medical management or before a surgery to delineate the anatomy and to rule out a lung abscess.

Pus/Aspirate

The next most important investigation is the aspiration of the fluid and to confirm that it is pus. Fluid/pus aspirated should be sent for Gram stain and culture to guide the therapy. In case nonpus fluid is aspirated, it should also be subjected to cytological and biochemical examination to differentiate between the transudative and exudative effusions.

MANAGEMENT

The treatment options for management of empyema thoracis are antibiotics, with any of the following:

- Insertion of chest drain alone
- Intercostal drainage with addition of fibrinolytics
- Open decortication
- Video-assisted thoracic surgery
- Rib resection/thoracoplasty/lobectomy.

All children with empyema should be admitted to a hospital and given intravenous antibiotics, and tube thoracostomy should be done. Small collections (<10 mm in a child below 2 years and < 20 mm in a child above 2 years) with no significant symptoms or distress may respond to antibiotic therapy alone; otherwise all symptomatic cases need drainage. Repeated thoracocentesis is not recommended except in a few with very thin pus. If the aspirate is in the form of thick pus, a chest tube must be inserted at the outset.

Drainage

The chest tube can be placed following marking done by an ultrasound. If the initial aspiration fails, the drainage may be done under the ultrasound. Conscious sedation can be used for the chest tube insertion with all the personnel and equipment necessary for resuscitation.

The chest tube is connected to an underwater seal bottle which must always be kept below the level of the patient's chest. The drain should be clamped for 1 hour once 10 mL/kg is initially removed. In older children and adolescents, not more than 1.5 L should be drained at one time. A chest radiograph is repeated after the chest drain insertion to check the placement of tube and lung expansion.

The chest tube can be removed when the drainage decreases to less than 30–50 mL/day, and there is no air leak from any accompanying bronchopleural fistula and the lung has expanded. A nonfunctional drain (no air column movement) should also be removed, and the need for replacement must be assessed by repeat imaging. Loculation should be ruled out. The chest tube should be removed during expiration or a Valsalva maneuver. The chest X-ray is repeated after 24 hours to check for any recollection.

The agents, such as urokinase, streptokinase, and alteplase, have been used to facilitate the drainage. Their use is recommended for complicated parapneumonic effusion (thick fluid with loculations) or empyema (frank pus), as it increases the drainage and obviates the need for more invasive procedures, shortens hospital stay. The treatment, however, is expensive and has side effects which can be serious.

Supportive Management

Oxygen

Oxygen (in cases with peripheral $SpaO_2 < 92\%$) and fluid therapy, if child is dehydrated or unable to drink, should be provided. Adequate analgesia should be given, especially if the child has a chest tube. It helps to prevent scoliosis and aids mobilization.

Antipyretics

Antipyretics should be judiciously used as fever is one of the parameters used to assess response.

Antimicrobial Therapy

The choice of empirical antibiotics is based on the likeliest causative organisms. Antistaphylococcal penicillin (cloxacillin 100–200 mg/kg/day), along with third-generation cephalosporin, such as ceftriaxone, may be used as a first-line drug. Aminoglycoside may be used instead of ceftriaxone. Co-amoxiclav is another good alternative drug. The preferred route of therapy is intravenous for initial 2 weeks or so, and it can then be replaced by oral therapy. The total duration of therapy is 4–6 weeks.

Response to Therapy

Children may continue to be febrile for 5–7 days after starting antibiotic therapy in the case of *S. pneumoniae* and *H. influenzae* and a little longer in the case of *S. aureus* infection. The clinical response to therapy should be assessed with parameters, such as decrease in fever, normalization of laboratory parameters, such as white blood cell count, C-reactive protein, decrease in drain volume, clearing in chest X-ray, improvement in the overall condition of the patient.

In case of nonresponse after 96 hours of treatment, high spiking fever, and persistent drainage, second-line treatment may be instituted. A combination of vancomycin with ceftazidime is suggested.

Parenteral therapy is continued till the child becomes afebrile or at least till the chest tube is removed and subsequently can be started on oral antibiotics to finish 4–6 weeks of therapy.

Failure of medical therapy, persisting sepsis, and large pleural collection beyond 10 days should prompt surgical referral. Cases of chronic empyema in a symptomatic child should be referred for open thoracostomy and decortication. Cases with persistent bronchopleural fistula will also benefit from surgical intervention. A persistent radiological abnormality in a symptom-free child is not an indication for surgery.

KEY MESSAGES

- There is no "one size fits all" treatment for the parapneumonic effusions and empyema.
- *The pathology of empyema is a dynamic process*: It is not feasible to manage all stages of it with a single-therapeutic strategy.
- Management, therefore, needs to be tailor-made, using the broad principals described above on a case-by-case basis and requires clinical experience.
- The outcome is usually good.
- Key steps in treatment are diagnostic thoracocentesis, preference for percutaneous drain.
- The use of fibrinolysis in the early empyema stage may be guided by the user's experience, affordability, and cost versus benefit expected.
- Nonresolving cases may benefit from surgical intervention. However, efforts to achieve complete radiological clearance are largely nonproductive and inconsequential.
- In the long-term, most children will eventually show a complete expansion of the lung, if appropriately treated in the early phase.

8.9 Suppurative Lung Disease

L Subramanyam

INTRODUCTION

Suppurative disease of the lung includes bronchiectasis, lung abscess, and empyema. Bronchiectasis and lung abscess will be presented here. Empyema has been discussed separately in this section.

BRONCHIECTASIS

Bronchiectasis is a structural abnormality characterized by abnormal, dilation, and distortion of the bronchial tree, resulting in chronic obstructive lung disease. This condition is typically the end result of a variety of pathophysiologic processes that render the bronchial walls weakened, easily collapsible, chronically inflamed, and plugged with mucus secretions.

The prevalence of bronchiectasis in the developed nations has gradually declined in recent years, probably because of improvements in sanitation and housing, immunizations against respiratory illnesses (e.g. measles and pertussis).

Pathophysiology

The continued cycle of infection, inflammation, and airway injury with impaired mucociliary clearance results in loss of the airway muscular and elastic components with dilation and distortion of the airways and increased mucus production. The airways become collapsible, limiting airflow, especially with forced expiration. The lung parenchyma is often involved, the developing areas of atelectasis, emphysema, and fibrosis. In addition, there is marked hypertrophy of the bronchial vasculature, which is prone to rupture.

Morphologically, bronchiectasis is classified as cylindrical, varicose, and saccular (cystic). Cylindrical is mildly enlarged bronchi that fails to taper distally; this is an early feature after an infection and can be reversed on appropriate management. Varicose type has a beaded appearance due to areas of constriction and dilation. Saccular is the most severe form, i.e. irreversible ballooning of airways.

Causes

Etiological factors in bronchiectasis are traditionally classified as congenital and acquired. Congenital causes of bronchiectasis, such as Williams–Campbell syndrome, associated with annular cartilage deficiency, and Marnier-Kuhn syndrome associated with tracheobronchomegaly, are uncommon. Acquired bronchiectasis is always due to two mechanisms, obstruction and infection. It is usually the net result of the classic triad of bronchial obstruction, infection, and inflammation causing progressive irreversible airway damage, resulting in bronchiectasis.

The types of disorders that cause bronchiectasis vary among populations and age-groups. As examples, infections and acquired causes of bronchiectasis predominate in the developing nations, whereas cystic fibrosis (CF), congenital anomalies of the airways, or immunodeficiency are more prominent in children of the developed nations.

The conditions that predispose to bronchiectasis can be classified into the following categories **(Box 8.9.1)**:

- Congenital anatomic defects
- Immunodeficiency states
- Abnormal secretion clearance
- Acquired bronchial obstruction
- Infections
- Miscellaneous disorders.

Box 8.9.1: Causes of bronchiectasis in children.

Congenital anatomic defects:
- Tracheobronchomalacia, tracheal/bronchial stenosis,
- Tracheal bronchus, bronchogenic cyst, vascular ring
- Pulmonary sequestration, congenital pulmonary airway malformation (CPAM)

Immunodeficiency states:
- *Primary abnormality*:
  - Congenital (Bruton's type) agammaglobulinemia
  - Selective IgA, IgG subclass deficiency
  - Severe combined T and B cell immunodeficiency
  - Chronic granulomatous disease
- *Secondary abnormality*:
  - HIV infection, malnutrition
  - Immunosuppressive therapy

Abnormal secretion clearance:
- Cystic fibrosis, PCD
- Kartagener's syndrome, Young syndrome
- Impaired cough (e.g. neuromuscular weakness condition)

Acquired bronchial obstruction:
- Intraluminal obstruction (foreign body, granuloma)
- *Extraluminal compression*: Lymphadenopathy (tuberculosis)
- Right middle lobe syndrome (usually seen in asthmatics)

Infections:
- Childhood infection (pertussis, measles)
- Persistent bacterial bronchitis
- Severe bacterial pneumonia
- Viral (adenovirus)
- Recurrent aspiration (tracheoesophageal fistula, vocal cord paralysis, and neurodevelopmental disorders)
- Other infections (*Mycobacterium tuberculosis*, fungal, mycoplasma)

Miscellaneous disorders:
- ABPA
- Alpha-1 antitrypsin deficiency
- Bronchiolitis obliterans, interstitial lung disease
- Genetic disorders (yellow nail syndrome)
- Autoimmune/connective tissue disorders (rheumatoid arthritis, scleroderma)
- Inhalation of toxic fumes (smoke, irritant gases)

(ABPA: allergic bronchopulmonary aspergillosis; HIV: human immunodeficiency virus; IgA: immunoglobulin A; IgG: immunoglobulin G; PCD: primary ciliary dyskinesia)

Clinical Manifestations

The most common symptom in children with bronchiectasis is persistent cough, which is present in 80–90% of children with bronchiectasis, and is typically "wet" or productive. About 50–70% of children also produce purulent sputum. The absence of sputum production does not exclude bronchiectasis, because children younger than 6 or 7 years old may not be able to expectorate sputum.

Some patients present with episodic exacerbations of infection, characterized by increased cough and sputum production that may be associated with change in color of sputum, fever, pleuritic chest pain, and dyspnea. These exacerbations typically respond to antibiotic therapy. Hemoptysis is caused by the erosion of inflamed airway tissue adjacent to pulmonary vessels. The amount of bleeding can range from mild, with blood-streaked sputum, to profuse amounts of fresh bleeding if larger pulmonary vessels rupture.

Dyspnea and exercise intolerance are uncommon at presentation but may develop as the disease progresses or may occur during an acute exacerbation of the disease due to intercurrent infection. Children with severe bronchiectatic lung disease may have clubbing, indicating severe hypoxemia due to mismatched pulmonary ventilation and perfusion. If the hypoxemia is prolonged and profound, it may lead to pulmonary hypertension and cor pulmonale.

The underlying disorder responsible for the bronchiectasis may also cause other symptoms at presentation and provide clues to the diagnosis. As for example, failure to thrive is frequently seen in diseases, such as CF and immunodeficiency disorders. Chronic sinusitis is common among children with CF, ciliary dysfunction disorders, and immunodeficiencies. The presence of congenital anomalies should alert the clinician to the possibility of associated anomalies that predispose to bronchiectasis (e.g. congenital heart disease and anomalies of the tracheobronchial tree).

Evaluation

The aims of evaluating children with suspected bronchiectasis are to:

- Confirm the diagnosis
- Define the distribution and severity of airway involvement
- Look for other system involvement associated with bronchiectasis (e.g. cor pulmonale)
- Identify familial and treatable underlying causes of bronchiectasis.

The evaluation includes a complete medical history, physical examination, radiographic imaging, as well as laboratory testing and pulmonary function test.

A complete medical history, including past medical, family, travel, and environmental history, is a crucial part of the evaluation and can be helpful in identifying the underlying cause for bronchiectasis. Certain features of the history should raise concern for specific underlying disorders; for example the history of choking suggests foreign body aspiration; chronic aspiration should be considered in patients with recurrent pneumonia, particularly those with neurologic dysfunction.

Pulmonary examination may reveal the following features: crackles and rhonchi, which are often heard over the area of bronchiectasis, wheezing, which is less common; clubbing of the nail bed, which is a basic clinical sign of bronchiectasis. Chest wall deformity can be seen in obstructive lung diseases (e.g. CF); in which, hyperinflation of the lungs results in increased anterior to posterior chest diameter.

On chest radiograph, findings, such as persistent/recurrent infiltrates or atelectasis in the same lobe/segment, should create suspicion of bronchiectasis. Multiple cystic changes/honeycomb pattern is characteristic of bronchiectasis **(Fig. 8.9.1)**. High-resolution computed tomography (HRCT) is the most sensitive imaging method to detect bronchiectasis. Features in HRCT which are suggestive of bronchiectasis include linear atelectasis, dilated and thickened airways (i.e. tram-tracking or parallel lines on longitudinal view or ring shadows on cross section)**(Fig. 8.9.2)**.

For patients with diffusely distributed bronchiectasis the minimum evaluation includes testing for CF [sweat chloride and deoxyribonucleic acid (DNA) testing] and immunodeficiency (including complete blood count with differential, immunoglobulins, and immunoglobulin G subclasses). Ciliary dyskinesia should be considered in patients with recurrent sinus and ear infections and evaluated with a nasal mucosal biopsy. Potential mechanisms of aspiration should be assessed using videofluoroscopy, esophageal pH monitoring, and/or nuclear scintigraphy. Direct laryngoscopy and bronchoscopy should be performed if laryngeal clefts or tracheoesophageal fistula are suspected and for patients with focal bronchiectasis to evaluate for airway obstruction (e.g. airway foreign body or congenital pulmonary anomalies).

Pulmonary function tests can be helpful to evaluate the severity of lung disease and should be performed in older children. Most patients with bronchiectasis have the features of obstructive lung disease, indicated by low forced expiratory volume in 1 second (FEV1) and FEV1/FVC (forced vital capacity) ratio.

Management

The initial therapy for patients with bronchiectasis is medical and aims at decreasing airway obstruction and controlling infection. Chest physiotherapy (postural drainage), antibiotics, and bronchodilators are essential. About 2–4 weeks of parenteral antibiotics are often necessary to manage acute

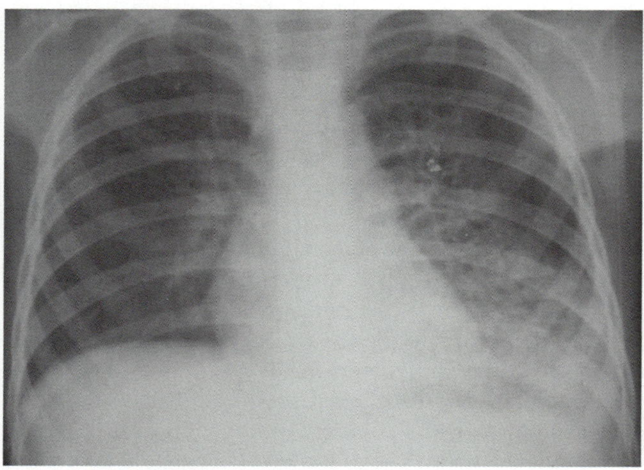

Fig. 8.9.1: Bronchiectasis left lower lobe.

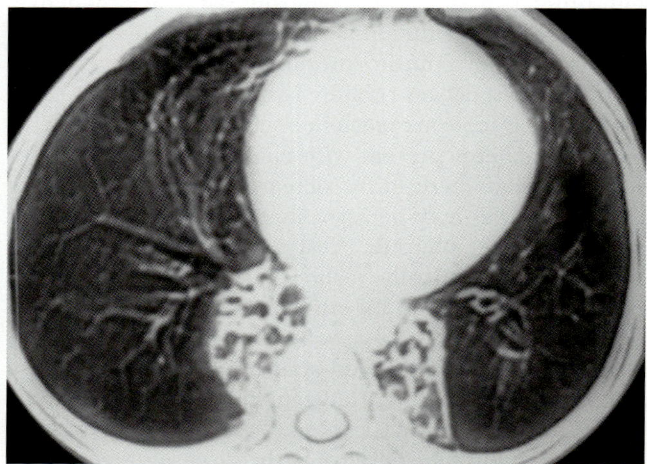

Fig. 8.9.2: Bilateral bronchiectasis lower lobes.

exacerbations adequately. Choice of antibiotic is dictated by the identification and sensitivity of organisms isolated from sputum (induced or spontaneous), or bronchoalveolar lavage fluid cultures. Low-dose, long-term macrolide therapy is found to be beneficial in idiopathic bronchiectasis. Nutritional support is important in these children. They should be routinely advised on adequate calories and good protein diet. Any underlying disorder (immunodeficiency, aspiration) that may be contributing to bronchiectasis must be addressed. When localized bronchiectasis becomes more severe or resistant to medical management, segmental or lobar resection may be warranted.

Prognosis

Overall the prognosis for patients with bronchiectasis has improved considerably in the past few decades. Early recognition of pneumonia, prompt treatment with appropriate antibiotics, prevention of predisposing conditions, and improved surgical outcomes are the likely reasons.

Prevention

Appropriate management of aspiration (gastroesophageal reflux, foreign body) and aggressive management of lower respiratory infections to prevent postinfectious bronchiectasis and routine immunization against respiratory pathogens (measles, pertussis, *Haemophilus influenzae*, viral influenza, pneumococcal) are helpful in preventing bronchiectasis.

LUNG ABSCESS

A lung abscess is an accumulation of inflammatory cells, accompanied by tissue destruction or necrosis that produces one or more cavities in the lung. A primary lung abscess occurs in a previously healthy patient with no underlying disorders. A secondary lung abscess occurs in a patient with underlying or predisposing condition. Abscess formation may result from inadequate or delayed treatment of lobar pneumonia. Aspiration is the most important predisposing factor for lung abscess, which may develop 1–2 weeks after the aspiration; other predisposing factors include airway obstruction and congenitally abnormal lung.

Etiology

Both anaerobic and aerobic organisms can cause lung abscesses. Common anaerobic bacteria that can cause a pulmonary abscess include *Bacteroides* spp., *Fusobacterium* spp., and *Peptostreptococcus* spp. Abscesses can be caused by aerobic organisms, such as *Streptococcus* spp., *Staphylococcus aureus*, *Escherichia coli*, *Klebsiella pneumonia*, and *Pseudomonas aeruginosa*. *S. aureus* is the organism most frequently involved.

Clinical Features

Clinical manifestations of lung abscess are nonspecific and similar to those of pneumonia. They include fever, cough, dyspnea, chest pain, anorexia, hemoptysis, and putrid breath. The course may be indolent. Physical examination typically reveals tachypnea, dyspnea, retractions with accessory muscle use, decreased breath sounds, and dullness on percussion in the affected area. Crackles may be heard on auscultation.

Diagnosis

The diagnosis is suggested by a chest radiograph demonstrating a thick-walled cavity with an air-fluid level **(Fig. 8.9.3)**, and it should be distinguished from pneumatocele, which is characterized by localized air collections with thin and smooth walls. Lung abscess should be suspected when consolidation is unusually persistent, when pneumonia remains persistently round or mass-like, and when the volume of the involved lobe is increased (as suggested by a bulging fissure). Lung abscess is confirmed by computed tomography. Interventional radiology may be helpful in obtaining a specimen from the abscess cavity for diagnostic studies.

Management

Treatment of lung abscess requires a prolonged course of antibiotic therapy usually initiated parenterally. Antibiotic choice should be guided by Gram stain and culture but initially should include aerobic and anaerobic coverage. Treatment regimens should include agent active against a penicillinase-resistant *S. aureus* and anaerobes. If gram-negative bacteria are suspected or isolated, an aminoglycoside should be added. The duration is determined by the clinical response but is usually a total of 4 weeks or 2 weeks after the patient is afebrile. The average duration for fever to subside is 3–4 days. About 80–90% of lung abscesses in children resolve

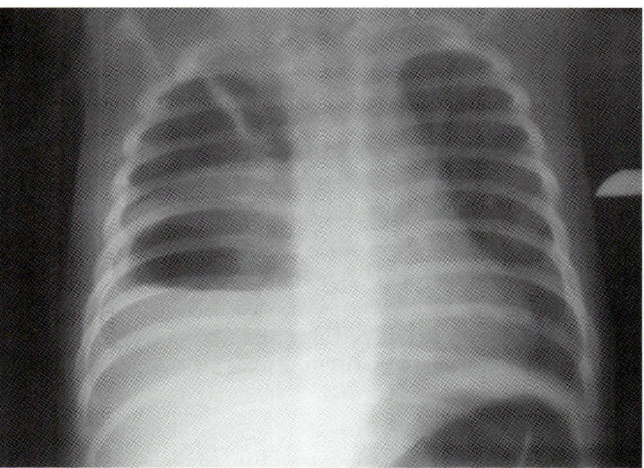

Fig. 8.9.3: Lung abscess right lower lobe with air-fluid level.

with antibiotic therapy alone and spontaneous drainage through the tracheobronchial tree, provided that bronchial obstruction is removed.

In the cases that fail to improve or worsen after 72 hours of the antibiotic therapy, needle aspiration or percutaneous catheter drainage may provide diagnostic information and therapeutic benefit without the increased risk of complications as occurs in children with necrotizing pneumonia. At least 3 weeks of intravenous antibiotic therapy should be delivered before lobectomy is considered for treatment failure.

Complications

The most common complication of lung abscess is intracavitary hemorrhage. This can cause hemoptysis or spillage of the abscess contents with the spread of infection to other areas of the lung. Other complications of lung abscess include empyema, bronchopleural fistula, septicemia, and cerebral abscess.

Prognosis

Overall, prognosis for children with primary pulmonary abscesses is excellent. Most children become asymptomatic within 7–10 days. Radiologic abnormalities usually resolve in 1–3 months.

BIBLIOGRAPHY

1. Chang AB, Redding GJ. Bronchiectasis. In: Kendig's disorders of the respiratory tract in children. Philadelphia: Saunders Elsevier; 2006. pp. 463-77.
2. Fakhoury K, et al. Causes, clinical manifestations, evaluation and management of bronchiectasis in children. UptoDate. 2018.
3. Lakser O. Bronchiectasis, lung abscess. Nelson Textbook of Pediatrics. Philadelphia, PA: Elsevier/Saunders; 2016. pp. 2094-7.
4. Redding GJ. Bronchiectasis in children. Pediatr Clin North Am; 2009;56(1):157-71.
5. UptoDate (2018). Causes, evaluation and management of bronchiectasis children; clinical features, diagnosis. [online]. Available from https://www.uptodate.com/contents/causes-clinical manifestations- and- management-of-bronchiectasis-in-children [Accessed November, 2018].
6. UptoDate (2018). Community-acquired pneumonia in children; clinical features, diagnosis. [online]. Available from https://www.uptodate.com/contents/community-acquired-pneumonia-in-children-clinical-features-and-diagnosis [Accessed November, 2018].
7. Vijayasekaran D, Shivbalan SO. Bronchiectasis. In: Subramanyam L, Shivabalan S, Gowrishankar NC, Vijayasekaran D, Balachandran A (Eds). Essentials of Pediatric Pulmonology, 3rd edition. New Delhi: Jaypee Brothers Medical Publishers (P) Ltd; 2008. pp. 196-200.

8.10 Bronchial Asthma

H Paramesh

INTRODUCTION

Asthma is an early onset environmental noncommunicable chronic lung disease, having significant psycho-socio-economic burden on family and the society. The disease is characterized by the following:

- Airway inflammation
- Airway obstruction mainly due to muscle spasm, associated with mucosal edema and accumulation of the mucus
- Airway hyperreactivity to aerobiologicals and irritants
- Airway remodeling in uncontrolled asthma.

EPIDEMIOLOGY

The incidence of asthma has steadily increased in both the developed and developing countries from 1970 to 2000. There is a marginal decrease in the incidence in Australia, Hong Kong, the United Kingdom, Italy, and Mexico after 2000, most probably due to saturation of the genetically predisposed population. However, the prevalence of persistent asthma needing constant medications is increasing.

A hospital-based study in Bengaluru showed that the prevalence of asthma steadily increased from 9% in 1979 to 29.5% in 1999. It decreased by 3% in 2004 and further by 1% in 2009. However, persistent asthma increased from 20% to 72% and persistent severe asthma from 4% to 11% from 1999 to 2009. The increased prevalence of asthma is noticed in the following situations:

- Urban children
- Rapid urbanization increasing prevalence in the semirural areas compared to rural.

- Children attending schools in heavy traffic areas, especially from the lower socioeconomic population.
- Children living in poorly ventilated homes and single room dwelling huts.
- Children living in houses with smokers.
- Children living in houses where cow dung cakes, agricultural waste, and firewood are used as cooking fuel.
- During Diwali and similar festivals, there is a 100% increase in emergency room visits for acute asthma episodes due to increase in sulfur dioxide (SO_2) in the air from bursting of the fire crackers.
- The prevalence in children less than 5 years is about 75%; above 5 years of age around 25%.
- *Male predominance*: The male-to-female ratio is 2:1 owing to the relatively small airways with which boys are born and inherited as an autosomal dominant trait.
- Positive family history of asthma either in parents, siblings, or grandparents.
- Air pollution not only triggers asthma but also changes genetic pattern.
- Nonatopic changing to atopic.

ETIOPATHOGENESIS

The etiological factors can be classified as biologicals and irritants as shown in **Table 8.10.1**.

Aerobiologicals

Children develop sensitivity to indoor allergens, as they grow older in the atmosphere they are reared. The predominant indoor allergen is the house dust mite. It takes 100 dust mites/g of dust to get sensitized and 500 dust mites/g of dust to produce wheezing. About 50% of the perennial asthma is due to dust mites. The pollen and mold sensitivity is observed less frequently, whereas cockroach sensitivity is fairly common.

Viral Infection

The precipitating factor for an asthma attack in 40% of the children is viral upper respiratory tract infections. Most children develop rhinitis with or without fever, followed by cough. In these children, chest congestion persists over 10 days, often with wheeze. The incidence varies from 29% to 54% in both atopic and nonatopic individuals. Respiratory syncytial virus and rhinoviruses are the predominant viruses triggering asthma.

Table 8.10.1: Etiological factors in asthma.

Biologicals	***Irritants***
Dust mites	Tobacco smoke
Cockroaches	Cooking fuel smoke
Pollens	Mosquito coil smoke
Fungi	Sprays
Pets—saliva, urine	Perfumes
Viral infections	Formaldehyde and volatile organic compounds from compressed wood and panel board furniture, etc.
Food	—

Season

Seasonal variation of asthma attacks is experienced by 35% of the children. The incidence is higher during monsoon, followed by winter, and is less common in summer. An increase of asthma attacks in summer from 2% to 28.5% in 17-year period has been noted, which is attributed to an increase in automobile emission from slow traffic and the bright sun converting the oxides of nitrogen to ozone (O_3), which aggravates the asthma sensitivity; in addition, O_3 has the cumulative effect.

Food

Diet plays a multifaceted role in shaping the observed worldwide trends of childhood allergies. Sensitivity can occur by ingestion, inhalation of cooking fumes, and from skin contact. Both early and late-phase reactions are observed. Only 10% of the asthmatics react to food and drinks. Eight foods—groundnut, egg, crustaceans, milk, fish, tree nuts, wheat, and soybean—account for 90% of the food allergies globally. In our country, we can add lentils, black gram, and many legumes. The incidence of food allergy is 4–8% in children globally. A community survey done in Mysuru and Bengaluru showed an incidence of only 1.88%. However, many parents of asthmatic children have misconceptions and perceptions about food allergy, especially fruits, such as guava, banana, citrus fruits, grapes, and tomato.

Pets

Pets are not the major factor for the asthma in India. Cats are more allergic than dogs. The saliva, urine, and dander are the causes for allergy sensitization. Specific immunotherapy for cat's allergy is beneficial, but dogs are not established equally. Dogs are stress busters, and in some asthmatic children, pet therapy (dog) has been recommended.

Air Pollution

Air pollution is both outdoor and indoor. The important outdoor pollutants are black smoke, respirable suspended particulates, SO_2, nitric oxide (NO), carbon monoxide (CO), O_3 produced by the combustion of fossil fuels, factories, mines, paper pulp mills, and automobile exhaust. Nitrogen oxide triggers asthma in 65% of the patients and also sensitizes to dust mites allergy. Ozone triggers asthma in 43% of the patients, and SO_2 sensitizes the asthmatics by tenfold.

PATHOPHYSIOLOGY

Asthma is a complex condition where interaction of genetics and environment occurs involving many inflammatory cells which release a wide range of mediators. These mediators act on the cells of the airway leading to smooth muscle contraction, mucus hypersecretion, plasma leakage, edema, activation of cholinergic reflexes, and activation of sensory nerves, which lead to amplification of the continuing inflammatory response. The chronic inflammation leads to the structural changes, including subepithelial fibrosis and smooth muscle hypertrophy and hyperplasia. This late process is less easily reversed than the acute changes and might end up with airway remodeling.

To mount an allergic response, one has to be sensitized to an allergen. When an allergen enters the epithelial cell, the dendritic cells below the epithelial cell act like a custom officer—catch the allergen by their long arms and break the allergen into small pieces called epitopes. These are handed over to the T-lymphocytes, the orchestrator of the immune system, which give the instruction to various cells for appropriate action. The B-lymphocytes are instructed to handle pollens, which produce interleukins (IL4 and IL13) to make immunoglobulin E (IgE) antibodies. The IgE arms the mast cell, the muscle man of immune system. The mast cell binds very large number of IgE molecules of various allergens. The activation of mast cell (mast cell degranulation) releases histamine. The continued exposure to allergen brings eosinophils (dreaded cell for parasites) into action. The eosinophilic granules release toxic chemicals, such as eosinophil cationic protein, eosinophil-derived neurotoxin, and major basic protein, which damage the epithelium and sensory nerves causing hyperresponsiveness to nonallergic stimuli. The mast cells are responsible for the early-phase reaction and eosinophils for the late-phase reaction in general.

CLINICAL FEATURES

All that wheezes is not asthma but most asthmatics do not wheeze. The common clinical features include the following:

- *Recurrent cough*: The majority of children present with recurrent cough 90% of the time. The cough is more at night or early morning; induced by physical or emotional stress (crying, laughing, and shouting).
- *Recurrent wheeze* is a prominent feature of the lower airway obstruction. Many people mistake rattling in the chest as wheeze. Wheezing is not felt on palpation of the chest.
- *Retractions* are a common feature for airway obstruction, depending on the severity of asthma; they may be present over subcostal, intercostal, or suprasternal areas, with flaring of nostrils.
- *Posttussive vomiting* (vomiting after a bout of coughing) occurs in 5% of the cases.
- Abdominal pain rarely occurs due to the overworking of expiratory abdominal muscles in 3% of the children.
- Chest pain is present rarely in 1% of the children.
- Other comorbid conditions, such as allergic rhinitis, sinusitis, serous otitis media, eczema, and conjunctivitis, may be present.

DIAGNOSIS

Diagnosis of asthma is mainly by the history and physical examination. The diagnosis of asthma in infants and preschoolers is often difficult due to poor cooperation for diagnostic procedures, hesitation by pediatricians, time-consuming and practicality, and ethical issues. However, an early diagnosis is essential for timely treatment to improve the quality of life, physical and psychological development; to prevent chronic pulmonary disease due to "airway remodeling;" to educate on the preventive measures; to cut the healthcare cost; and to prognosticate.

Preschool Children

The diagnosis of asthma is made based on clinical features only with following features:

a. *Variable respiratory symptoms of:*
   - Wheeze
   - Shortness of breath
   - Chest tightness
   - Cough persisting more than 2 weeks at night
b. *Associated with other features:*
   - Having wheeze, cough with emotional stress, (crying laughing shouting) or physical stress (running, jumping playing) in the absence of any respiratory infections
   - Having eczema, allergic rhinitis, family history of atopy
   - Improvement with controller medicines during 2–3 months treatment and relapse after cessation.
c. However one has to document the variable expiratory airflow limitation at least once preferably before starting controllers.

The phenotype classification of asthma in children over 2 years of age helps the clinician to distinguish the types of asthma and provide appropriate management and prognostication as shown in **Flowchart 8.10.1**.

School-going Children

- *Peak expiratory flow (PEF)* measurement before and after salbutamol nebulization with improvement (12–15%) is highly suggestive of reversible airway obstruction in asthma. This simple and less expensive procedure can be used to monitor the therapeutic response. Early asthma attack can be recognized by measuring diurnal variation in PEF. It measures the air coming out of larger and medium-sized airways.

Flowchart 8.10.1: Identification of asthma phenotypes.

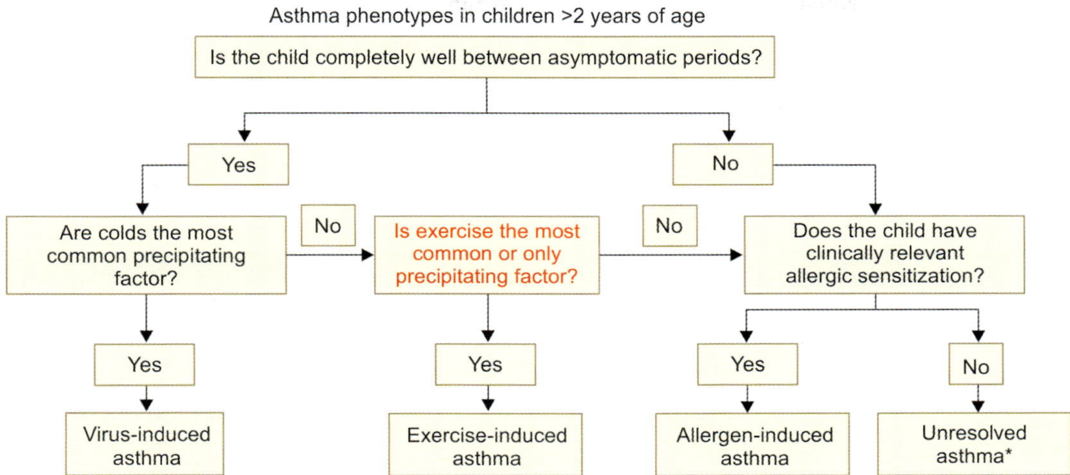

*Children may also be atopic. Different etiologies, including irritant exposure and as yet not evident allergies, may be involved here.
Source: Bacharier LB, Boner A, Carlsen KH, Eigenmann PA, Frischer T, Götz M, et al. Diagnosis and treatment of asthma in childhood: a PRACTALL consensus report. Allergy. 2008;63(1):5-34.

- *Spirometry* is the central tool for defining the obstructive airway disease. In asthma, there is decreased forced expiratory volume in 1 second (FEV_1), FEV_1/FVC_1 ratio (forced vital capacity/forced expiratory flow 25–75%).
- *Eosinophil count*: The increased eosinophil count in the blood is suggestive of an allergic phenomenon.
- *Total IgE level*: It is beneficial only to recognize the atopic background of asthma. It helps to predict a response to steroids, the prognosis, and the possibility of development of persistent as well as strongly advocated environment control.
- *Specific IgE level*: It is needed for specific immunotherapy and before the use of anti-IgE antibody treatment.
- *Chest X-ray* is not routinely needed to diagnose asthma. It is needed only when the diagnosis is not clear, or any complications are suspected. Children below 5 years do not have lung collaterals, and as a result, one may see subsegmental, segmental, or lobar atelectasis quite often in radiographs, which might be misdiagnosed and treated as recurrent pneumonia.
- *Breath nitric oxide* is used in some pulmonary centers for monitoring the eosinophilic airway inflammation. It is not used much in children for various reasons.
- *Breath volatile organic compound (VOC) analysis* offers the possibility of a rapid straightforward and noninvasive method to measure the control of asthma in future.
- *Skin testing with allergens* is the gold standard to identify the specific allergens and used before immunotherapy for aeroallergens.
- Bronchial challenge tests and other physiological tests do not have a major role in the diagnosis of asthma in children.

MANAGEMENT

The management of asthma includes:
- Education
- Environment control
- Pharmacotherapy
- Regular follow-up.

Education

The pediatrician must spend time to clear the misconceptions about the disease, sexual bias, noncommunicability of the disease, fear of inhalers, steroids, etc. In India, doctors should always include the grandparents in counseling. Individual counseling is preferred in adolescents.

Environment Control

It is the most important factor in the control of asthma. The aim should be to avoid allergens and irritants:
- *Dust mites*: Avoid carpets, upholstered furniture, use plastic covers to pillows and mattresses for easy washability and expose them to sunlight once a week, wash soft toys periodically and wet mop the floorings.
- *Cockroach*: Cover garbage and unused food containers.
- *Fungus*: Attend to damp walls, have good ventilation, and clean the shower curtains weekly.
- *Pets*: Keep them away from sleeping area, if possible outside the house.
- Avoid strong odors, smoke, mosquito coil burning, and especially tobacco smoke.
- Have indoor plants to absorb formaldehyde and VOCs from modern furniture, etc. and expose to sunlight once

a week and remove the water from trays once a week. The recommended plants in our country are bamboo, anthurium, money plant, fern, and chrysanthemum.

Pharmacotherapy

The drugs used in the management of asthma include quick relievers, controllers, and long-term symptoms relievers as listed in **Table 8.10.2** and dosages in **Table 8.10.3**. The choice of the drugs depends on the age and severity of the wheezing episodes **(Fig. 8.10.1 and Table 8.10.3)**. It should be ideally carried out in a stepwise manner:

- Always use a quick reliever as a rescue treatment in acute exacerbation of persistent asthmatics on preventers. Inhalation method is the best way to administer medication to avoid adverse reactions and for quick actions.

Table 8.10.2: Classification of drugs used for the management of asthma.

Quick relievers	***Controller***	***Long-term symptoms relievers***
• Used for acute attacks to relieve bronchospasm as and when needed • *Short-acting beta-2-agonists:* – Salbutamol – Terbutaline • Adrenaline • Aminophylline	• Used for long-term to control the inflammation and to prevent further attacks • Leukotriene receptor antagonists • *Steroids:* – Oral – ICS • Theophylline	• Used to relieve bronchospasm for longer hours • *Long-acting beta-2-agonists:* – Salmeterol – Formoterol – Bambuterol • Always use with inhaled steroids

(ICS: inhaled corticosteroids)

Table 8.10.3: Dosage of Drugs.

Drugs	***Dosage***
Salbutamol	• *<1 year:* Nebulizer: 0.05–0.15 mg/kg/dose every 4–6 hours with subsequent doses titrated based on clinical response • *1–4 years:* Nebulizer: 1.25–2.5 mg every 4–6 hours with subsequent doses titrated based on clinical response • *5 years or more:* MDI: 2 puffs (216 µg) every 4–6 hours as needed; DPI: 200 µg inhaled every 4–6 hours. May increase to 400 µg inhaled every 4–6 hours, if necessary • *5–11 years:* Nebulizer: 2.5 mg every 4–6 hours with subsequent doses titrated based on clinical response • *12 years or more:* Nebulizer: 2.5–5 mg every 6 hours as needed; MDI: 2 puffs (180 µg) every 4–6 hours
Levosalbutamol	Half dose of salbutamol
Terbutaline	• *<12 years*: Nebulization: 0.01–0.03 mg/kg/dose with the minimum dose of 0.1 mg; maximum dose is 2.5 mg diluted with 1–2 mL of normal saline every 4–6 hours • *>12 years:* Inhalation aerosol: 2 inhalations separated by 60 second every 4–6 hours. Do not repeat more often 4–6 hours
Salmeterol	• 1 puff (50 µg) every 12 hours in > 4 years • Combination with fluticasone propionate. 50 µg, 125 µg, 250 µg
Formoterol	12 µg (1 inhalation) every 12 hours (2 puffs—6 µg/puff) in children 5 years or more. Total daily dose should not exceed 24 µg. Combination available with Budesonide or Mometasone furoate as 100 µg, 200 µg, and 400 µg
Montelukast Sodium	• *6 months to 5 years:* 4 mg OD • *6–14 years*: 5 mg OD • *15 years and above*: 10 mg OD
Theophylline	• *Age < 1 year*: [0.2 × (age in weeks)] + 5 = mg/kg/day • *Age ≥ 1 year*: 16 mg/kg/day
Tiotropium bromide	Age 12 years or > –2.5 µg/day (2 inhalations orally of 1.25 µg OD)
Beclomethasone	100 µg
Budesonide	100 µg
Budesonide nebulized	250 µg
Fluticasone propionate	100 µg
Mometasone	100 µg
Ciclesonide	Low dose—100 µg, medium dose—double (200 µg), high dose—quadruple (400 µg)

(DPI: dry powder inhaler; MDI: metered dose inhaler)

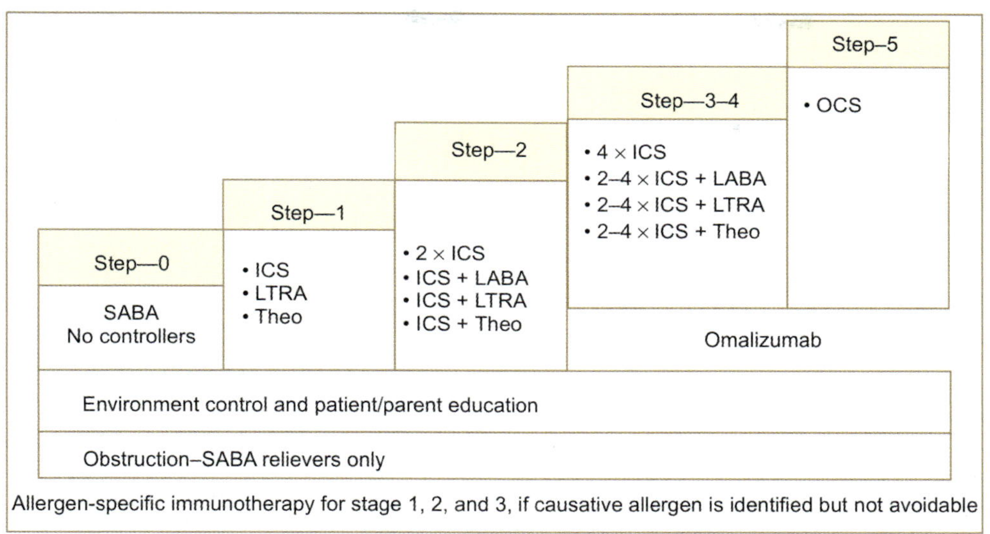

Fig. 8.10.1: Pharmacotherapy in bronchial asthma (ICON on Pediatric Asthma).
(EIB: exercise-induced bronchoconstriction; ICON: International Consensus; ICS: inhaled corticosteroid; LABA: long-acting beta-2 agonist; LTRA: leukotriene receptors antagonist; SABA: short-acting beta-2 agonist; OCS: oral corticosteroid)

Note:
- The stepwise approach is meant to assist not to replace the clinical decision-making and required to meet individual patient needs.
- If alternative treatment is used and response is inadequate, discontinue it and use the preferred treatment before stepping up.

Quick-relief medication for all patients:
- Short-acting beta-2 agonist as needed for symptoms. Intensity of treatment depends on the severity of symptoms: up to three treatments at 20-min intervals as needed. Short course of oral systemic corticosteroids may be needed.
- Use of SABA more than 2 days a week for symptom relief (not prevention of EIB) generally indicates inadequate control and the need to step-up treatment.

Source: Adapted from ICON.

Table 8.10.4: Level of control of asthma.

Parameters	*Controlled*	*Partly controlled*	*Poorly controlled*
Daytime symptoms	Less than 2 times/week	More than 2 times/week	Three or more features of partly controlled asthma in any week
Limitations of activities	None	Any	
Nocturnal symptoms of disturbed sleep	None	Any	
Need for relievers or rescue treatment	Less than 2 times/week	More than 2 times/week	
Lung functions PEF or FEV1	Normal	Less than 80% of predicted or personal best	
Exacerbation	None	One or more per year	One in any week

(FEV1: forced expiratory volume in 1 second; PEF: peak expiratory flow)

- It is always preferable to use spacer for inhalation therapy by which one can expect quick results using 1/10th dose of oral medications with less adverse reaction.
- In children, less than 5 years of age, static treated spacer and mask or a mouthpiece can be used whenever the child is capable of using the spacer; above 5 years, spacer with mouthpiece, dry powder inhaler (DPI), or breath-activated pressurized meter dose in inhaler are used.
- Nebulizer usage is a second choice; and 500 mL plastic bottle spacer is an effective spacer in all ages; and one should consider the child's ability to use the device, preference, and cost. Always rinse or gargle after the use of inhaled steroids in DPI.

Follow-up

Regular follow-up is needed to assess the level of controlling of asthma by using the parameters as listed in **Table 8.10.4**. Always give hope, confidence, and encourage sports activities. The pneumonic for the follow-up would be:

- ILL—What makes you ill?
- HELL—When do you feel worst?
- PILL—Medication used dosage
- SKILL—Technique of inhalation and nasal spray
- WELL: Follow instruction of your physician, environment control, lifestyle, yoga exercise, and regular follow-up.

COMORBIDITIES

The most common comorbid conditions are as follows:

- *Allergic rhinitis*: Nearly the three-fourths of asthmatic children develop allergic rhinitis, which complicates and worsens asthma. Nasal breathing is protective to asthma. Always evaluate as a unified airway disease, and a successful treatment of allergic rhinitis can control asthma.
- *Sinusitis*: Nearly 9% of the asthmatics have sinusitis, and the incidence in uncontrolled asthma is nearly 35%. The sinusitis is a result of blockage of osteomeatuses of sinuses due to edematous nasal mucosa and compromise in the mucociliary function of sinus.
- *Otitis media*: Nearly 25% of the children have serous otitis media due to the blockage of eustachian tube from edema of nasal mucosa.
- *Gastroesophageal reflux disease (GERD)*: GERD is quite common in infants, which we need not be worried about, but GERD as a cause for worsening of asthma is seen only in the few cases of refractory asthma. It should be suspected in children with prominent asthma symptoms while eating or sleeping or who prop up in bed by themselves to relieve nocturnal symptoms. The gold standard for diagnosis is esophageal pH monitoring.
- *Acute severe asthma*: Asthma attacks can be very severe in untreated or improperly treated cases needing hospitalization for intensive treatment. This occurs when the early signs of severity are missed or ignored by the patients, parents, and physicians.

Management of Acute Severe Asthma in Hospitalized Patient

To cover all aspects in acute severe attack of asthma and to prioritize the treatment, please remember six "M"s in aiming the therapy as shown in **Table 8.10.5**.

NUTRITIONAL MANAGEMENT OF ASTHMA CHILDREN

- Suggest smaller frequent meals for better diaphragmatic work and also to help to decrease the chances of gastroesophageal reflux.
- Always prefer homemade traditional food.
- Encourage fresh fruit, vegetables, butter, curd, pickles fish, and food with omega-3 fatty acids. Traditional food habits.
- Avoid salty snacks, carbonated water.

Table 8.10.5: Six "M"s in the management of acute severe asthma in children.

Principle of management	*Pathogenetic mechanism*	*Management*
Metabolic correction	Hypoxemia, metabolic acidosis	Humidified oxygen by mask, nasal prongs
Muscle spasm to be relieved	Airway obstruction	Beta-2-agonists + ipratropium bromide in O_2-driven nebulizers
Mucosal edema	Inflammation, airway obstruction	• Systemic or oral prednisolone or methylprednisolone • IV or inhaled fluticasone 1,500 µg
Mucus secretions	Excess mucus secretion and airway obstruction	Appropriate hydration, staccato type of coughing
Monitor for infection	Pneumonia, otitis media, sinusitis	Antibiotics
Mechanical ventilation	Respiratory acidosis, apnea ventilation failure	Ventilatory care as last resort

(IV: intravenous)

PROGNOSIS

Children with viral infection-triggered asthma tend to outgrow the disease by 5 years of age when the immune system attains adult levels. Some more outgrow the disease by 8 years when the airway caliber reaches adult levels, more so in boys. During adolescent period, the majority tends to outgrow the attacks. However, those with atopic asthma (high IgE level) and children with low lung capacities and girls have the tendency for asthma remaining for an indefinite period.

PREVENTION

The *primary prevention* is to prevent sensitization to allergens. Avoid unnecessary use of spectrum antibiotics.

Children born prematurely, small for date children and infants who gain weight more are prone for airflow limitation and a prelude for airway remodeling one has to guide them properly.

The *secondary prevention* is to prevent the occurrence of symptoms in sensitized child which is to avoid environmental triggers predominantly the tobacco smoke and indoor pollutants, such as dust mites, cockroach, fungi, pollens, and other smokes.

The *tertiary prevention* is to control the symptoms by environment control and long-term use of anti-inflammatory drugs and quick relievers as rescue medicines in any exacerbations.

RECENT ADVANCES

- Recognition of unified airway disease and chronic inflammatory disease concept.
- The asthma phenotypes based on inflammatory cells and mediators released by eosinophils, neutrophils, T-lymphocytes, and vascular endothelial cells.
- The importance of environment control.
- The use of breathing exercise or yoga to avoid chest and spinal deformity which increase morbidity and mortality.
- Use of anti-IgE antibody treatment in the difficult cases.
- The use of immunotherapy preferably by sublingual route.
- Obesity is recognized as a major risk factor for the development of asthma, especially in girls. A decrease in lung function is proportionately related to obesity.

PRACTICE GUIDELINES

Use quick reliever as and when necessary and use preventers in steps 2–5 as described in **Figure 8.10.1**.

Depending on the response either step-up or step-down the dose of preventers, some studies recommend starting with high dose and then reducing the dose earlier.

PRACTICAL TIPS

- Aim at good control of asthma with good education and bonding with patient, parents, and grandparents for better compliance.
- Avoid prolonged use of systemic steroids or high dose of inhaled steroids.
- Always use spacer preferably clear, valved one for better delivery. For metered dose inhaler, slow inhalation, and for powder inhaler, faster inhalation is needed.
- Always assess the compliance and technique of inhalation during follow-up while infusing trust, hope, and confidence.
- Counsel the adolescent separately and stress on ill effect of tobacco smoke.
- Stress on good environment control and to have indoor plants which needs to be exposed to sunlight and to remove water from the tray once a week.

KEY MESSAGES

- Please keep it in mind that while dealing with a biological system based on expert opinion, there should be enough room for individualization.
- Always look for availability, accessibility, and affordability in managing our children with asthma.
- Do realize that different forms of asthma respond differently to drugs.
- Phenotype-based treatments are likely to be more effective and safer than standard uniform treatment that we currently offer to all asthma phenotypes.
- Be optimistic as newer research needs a link between clinicians, researchers, and pharmacological companies for better, cost-effective individual treatment of patients.

BIBLIOGRAPHY

1. Bisgaard H, Bonnelykke K. Long-term studies of the natural history of asthma in childhood. J Allergy Clin Immunol. 2010;126(2):187-97.
2. Global Initiative for Asthma. (GINA) Global strategy for asthma management and prevention, 2018: www.ginasthma.org.
3. Gregori D, Gulati A, Paramesh H, et al. Children obesity from global determinants to local consequences: the Indian perspective. Indian J Pediatr. 2014;81:S-24.
4. Papadopoulos NG, Arakawa H, Carlsen KH, et al. International consensus on (ICON) pediatric asthma. Allergy. 2012;67: 976-97.
5. Paramesh H, Mohanty NC, Kumar R, et al. Airway Disease Education & Expertise (ADEX) NEXT Working Group Recommendations—Persistent (Chronic) Cough in Pediatric Practice. NIJP Index Copernicus Int. 2017;6(4); 230-43.
6. Paramesh H, Nagaraju K, Sukumaran TU, et al. Airway disease education and expertise (ADEX) in pediatrics: adaptation for clinical practice in India. Indian Pediatr. 2016;53:154-8.
7. Paramesh H. Air pollution and allergic diseases: social determinants and sustainability in the control and prevention. Indian J Pediatr. 2018;85(4):284-94.
8. Paramesh H. Textbook of Practical Pediatric Pulmonology. New Delhi: Jaypee Brothers Medical Publishers (P) Ltd.; 2009. pp. 192-7.
9. Petsky HL, Cates CJ, Lasserson TJ, et al. A systemic review and meta-analysis: tailoring asthma treatment on eosinophilic markers (exhaled nitric oxide or sputum eosinophils). Thorax. 2012;67:199-208.
10. Saadeh D Salameh P, Baldi I, et al. Diet and allergic diseases among population aged 0 to years: myth or reality? Nutrients. 2013;5(3):399-423.

8.11 Aerosol Therapy

Jagdish Prasad Goyal, Prawin Kumar

INTRODUCTION

Aerosol therapy is the delivery of aerosolized medication directly into the airways. It has been used as a part of the treatment for a variety of respiratory diseases in children. The first evidence of the use of aerosol therapy has been found in Hippocrates era where hot vapors were used for the management of respiratory diseases. In the modern era, use of aerosol therapy began with the introduction of Medihaler-Epi in 1956.

The aerosol forms used are bronchodilators, steroids, and antibiotics. Aerosol therapy has revolutionized the care of asthma and other chronic respiratory diseases, viz. cystic fibrosis, primary ciliary dyskinesia. The newer bronchodilator and anti-inflammatory drugs are becoming available to use as aerosol therapy.

BASICS OF AEROSOL THERAPY

The aerosol therapy delivers the drug directly into the lung and has several significant advantages over systemic drug delivery.

- Smaller medication dose to achieve the desired therapeutic effect with lesser side effect as compared to oral or the parenteral route.
- Faster onset action for the reversal of acute episode of bronchospasm.
- Easy and convenient to administer by patient, parents, and healthcare providers.
- Aerosol therapy is painless as compared to parenteral route of drug administration.

FACTORS AFFECTING AEROSOL THERAPY

Aerosol particle characteristics, including the size (diameter), density, electrical charge, hygroscopy, shape, and the velocity of the aerosol, determine the efficacy of aerosol therapy. Any particle size larger than 5 µm is likely to be filtered out in the upper airways and fail to reach the larger airways. Aerosol particles less than 5 µm in size readily reach the periphery of the lung. Chemical and physical properties of the aerosolized drug also play an important role in drug delivery. Furthermore, the hygroscopic property of aerosolized drug may have unfavorable effects on the drug delivery. The shape and velocity of particles eventually may affect drug deposition in airways. A high velocity of aerosolized drug particles may lead to drug deposition in upper airway, while slow velocity enhances drug deposition in the lower airways.

The host factors also play an important role in drug deposition in the lower airways. Patient's disease state and severity, breathing pattern, preference for device and technique are important factors which affect drug delivery. It has also been observed that increased breath-holding time is associated with better drug deposition in the lung.

INDICATIONS OF AEROSOL THERAPY

Aerosol therapy is indicated in a variety of respiratory conditions. In children the most common indication for use of aerosol therapy is in the long-term management of bronchial asthma in which both the inhaled corticosteroid and long-acting β2-agonist are used. Short-acting β2-agonist is used in the management of acute asthma. The use of inhaled tobramycin is now well established in cystic fibrosis. Other antibiotics (pentamidine, colistin, etc.) and antifungal agents (amphotericin B) have also been used as inhaled form. Hypertonic saline in aerosolized form is used in cystic fibrosis patients before chest physiotherapy and for inducing sputum in tuberculosis patients.

AEROSOL DEVICES

Aerosol devices can broadly be divided into two categories: nebulizer and inhaler. Three types of nebulizers, namely jet nebulizer, ultrasonic nebulizer, and mesh nebulizer, are available for use in the aerosol therapy. The pressurized metered-dose inhaler (pMDI) and dry powder inhaler (DPI) are two inhaler devices.

NEBULIZERS

Nebulizers have been used widely to deliver aerosol therapy in children in a variety of respiratory condition. A wide variety of nebulizers are available to use for home and hospital with varying drug delivery. The pediatrician must be aware of various nebulizers available and consider a specific nebulizer for a specific drug to be delivered to the child.

Box 8.11.1: Steps for the correct use of nebulizer.

1. Hands should be washed prior to preparing each nebulizer treatment
2. Assemble tubing, nebulizer cup, and mouthpiece/mask
3. Place medicine into nebulizer cup (If using a multidose bottle of medicine, use correct amount of medication into the chamber along with saline solution)
4. Sit in upright position and hold the nebulizer vertically
5. Connect the nebulizer to power source
6. As the mist starts, encourage the child to take normal tidal breath with open mouth
7. Continue until the medicine is finished in the chamber. This may take 5–10 minutes

Indications

Nebulizer is indicated when a child is in respiratory distress and not able to take inhaled medication by other aerosol devices. It is also required for some medications, which are not available in a form suitable for other devices, including pentamidine, ribavirin, deoxyribonuclease, hypertonic saline, and tobramycin. The steps for correct use of nebulizer are shown in **Box 8.11.1**.

Advantages and Disadvantages

The major advantage of a nebulizer is that it needs only minimal patient coordination. The nebulizer may be used in acute exacerbation of asthma in emergency and intensive care setting. However, a nebulizer is large and a cumbersome device. It requires a power supply, and there is also a potential risk of drug delivery to the eye with a facemask. Drug delivery is variable among different types, brands, and models. Treatment time is long and may range from 5 minutes to 25 minutes. Assembly and cleaning are required.

Types of Nebulizers

Three types of nebulizers are available: (1) jet nebulizers, (2) ultrasonic nebulizer, and (3) mesh nebulizer. These three types of nebulizers work on different principals but have many common features.

Jet Nebulizer

A jet nebulizer works on the Bernoulli's principle and uses compressed gas source (oxygen or air) to generate aerosol that breaks up into small particles by hitting the inner surface of the chamber **(Fig. 8.11.1)**. The smaller particles move through the outlet to patient, whereas larger particles hold on to nebulizer chamber and get reaerosolized. The size of the nozzle and compressed gas flow determine the size of aerosol particles. The commonly used nebulizers deliver aerosol continuously, and only 10–20% of the aerosol drug reaches the airways. Jet nebulizers have been modified to overcome this problem in several ways including a one-way valve for inhalation and exhalation and breath-actuated nebulizer where the aerosol is generated only during inspiration.

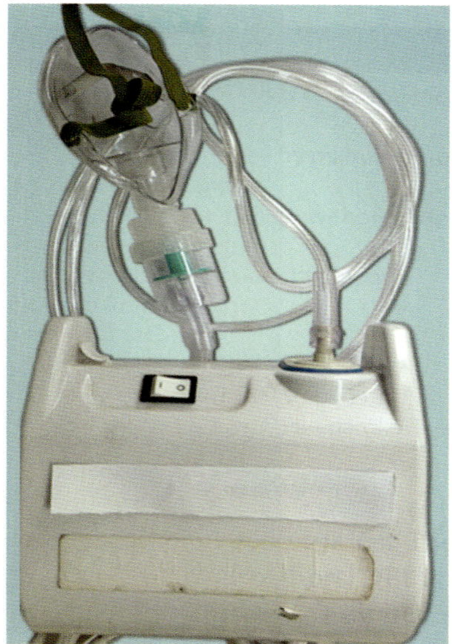

Fig. 8.11.1: Nebulizer with nebulization tubing and mask.

Ultrasonic Nebulizer

An ultrasonic nebulizer produces aerosol by means of electricity powered piezoelectric crystal to generate high-frequency vibration. The size of aerosol particles in ultrasonic nebulizer depends upon the frequency of vibration. It has been shown from studies that size of the aerosol particles generated from ultrasonic nebulizer is larger than jet nebulizer. Therefore, drug deposition in the upper airway is more as compared to the jet nebulizer.

Mesh Nebulizer

A mesh nebulizer is an aerosol device that uses a mesh with multiple, tiny openings to produce a liquid aerosol. In this aerosol device, liquid solution is passed through a fine mesh to produce aerosol. Mesh nebulizer generates aerosol with very small particle size. Research has shown that mesh nebulizer is superior to jet nebulizer in drug delivery due to small residual volume and particle size. Because of effective drug delivery of mesh nebulizer, it is sometimes necessary to adjust the dose of inhaled medication in view of possible adverse effect due to high dose. Both ultrasonic and mesh nebulizers are costlier than jet nebulizers.

Table 8.11.1: Age guidelines for preferred aerosol therapy in children.

Age of child	*Aerosol device*
Birth to 3 years	pMDI with spacer with mask or nebulizer with mask
4–5 years	pMDI with spacer, nebulizer with mask, DPI, breath-actuated pMDI (at the age of 5 years)
6–12 years	pMDI with spacer, nebulizer with mouthpiece, DPI, breath-actuated pMDI
>12 years	All devices

(DPI: dry powder inhaler; pMDI: pressurized metered-dose inhaler)

device-related, as well as environmental and clinical factors. The preferred device according to patient's age has been shown in **Table 8.11.1**.

Patient-related Factors

The selection of appropriate device depends upon the diagnosis. It should also be decided by patient's age, physical and cognitive ability. Patient's preference is also important in the selection of correct device as patients tend to use the device more regularly which they prefer.

Drug-related Factors

Some medications, especially hypertonic saline, antibiotics, are available only in liquid form and can be delivered only through nebulizers.

Device-related Factors

Easy to use, portability, and low maintenance cost are taken into account.

Environmental and Clinical Factors

It is very important to know the setting in which a device is to be used. There may be a different requirement of a device in the hospital and home setting. Depending upon the condition of the patient and frequency of requirement of aerosol therapy, device may be selected.

PATIENT EDUCATION FOR CORRECT USE OF THE DEVICE

It is important for healthcare provider to explain the advantages of aerosol therapy and dispel the myths and fears of patient and family. The healthcare provider should provide a demonstration for correct use and cleaning. Technique and compliance should be checked on every visit. The response to therapy and any adverse effect should be monitored.

BIBLIOGRAPHY

1. Ari A, Fink JB. Aerosol therapy in children: challenges and solutions. Expert Rev Respir Med. 2013;7:665-72.
2. Ari A, Fink JB. Guidelines for aerosol devices in infants, children and adults: which to choose, why and how to achieve effective aerosol therapy. Expert Rev Respir Med. 2011;5(4):561-72.
3. Atkins PJ. Dry powder inhalers: an overview. Respir Care. 2015;50:1304-12.
4. Berlinski A. Pediatric aerosol therapy. Respir Care. 2017;62(6):662-77.
5. Cheng YS. Mechanisms of pharmaceutical aerosol deposition in the respiratory tract. AAPS PharmSciTech. 2014;15(3): 630-40.
6. Ibrahim M, Verma R, Garcia-Contreras L. Inhalation drug delivery devices: technology update. Med Devices (Auckl). 2015;8:131-9.
7. Martin AR, Finlay WH. Nebulizers for drug delivery to the lungs. Expert Opin Drug Deliv. 2015;12:889-900.
8. Myrdal PB, Sheth P, Stein SW. Advances in metered dose inhaler technology: formulation development. AAPS PharmSciTech. 2014;15:434-55.
9. O'Malley CA. Device cleaning and infection control in aerosol therapy. Respir Care. 2015;60:917-27.
10. Rubin BK, Williams RW. Emerging aerosol drug delivery strategies: from bench to clinic. Adv Drug Deliv Rev. 2014;75:141-8.

Section 9

Diseases of Gastrointestinal System and Liver

9.1 Acute Diarrhea

Ashok K Patwari

INTRODUCTION

Worldwide, particularly in developing countries, diarrheal diseases still constitute significant causes of mortality and morbidity. There is considerable reduction in the mortality among infants suffering from acute diarrhea which is attributed to the proven efficacy of treatment with reduced osmolar oral rehydration solutions (ORS), oral zinc, proper diet monitoring, continuation of breastfeeds in young infants, and avoiding unnecessary medications. It is essential to understand various types of diarrhea based on duration and etiology as the approach and management differ.

DEFINITION

Diarrhea is usually defined as passage of three or more loose or watery stools in a 24-hour period, a loose stool being one that would take the shape of a container. However, for practical purposes, it is the recent change in consistency and character of stool and its water content rather than the number of stools that is important. Infants who are exclusively breastfed normally pass several soft or semiliquid stools each day; for them, it is practical to define diarrhea as an increase in stool frequency or liquidity that is considered abnormal by mother.

Acute Watery Diarrhea

It refers to diarrhea that begins acutely, lasts for less than 14 days, with passage of frequent loose or watery stools without visible blood. Vomiting may occur, and fever may be present. Loss of large volume of water and electrolytes can result in dehydration and dyselectrolytemia.

Dysentery

It is the term used for diarrhea with visible blood and mucus. It is often associated with fever and tenesmus. Common clinical features of dysentery include anorexia, rapid weight loss, and complications like renal failure and encephalopathy.

Persistent Diarrhea

It represents diarrhea, presumed to be caused by infectious agents that begins acutely, but is of usually long duration (more than 14 days). The episode may begin either as acute watery diarrhea (AWD) or as dysentery. Marked weight loss is common. Diarrheal stool volume may also be great, with a risk of dehydration. Persistent diarrhea should not be confused with "chronic diarrhea" which is recurrent or long-lasting diarrhea due to noninfectious causes such as sensitivity to gluten or inherited metabolic disorder.

EPIDEMIOLOGY

Acute diarrhea constitutes a leading cause of morbidity and mortality among children below 5 years of age in developing countries. In India, diarrhea is the third leading cause of childhood mortality attributed to 13% of all deaths per year in children under 5 years of age. About 80% of these deaths occur in the first 2 years of life, main causes being dehydration, complications associated with dysentery, malnutrition, and serious infections such as pneumonia.

Most of the diarrheal episodes occur during the first 2 years of life (highest incidence 6–11 months), in low socioeconomic status, in nonbreastfed infants, and in association with measles, severe malnutrition, and immunodeficiency.

ETIOPATHOGENESIS

In developing countries, the organisms most frequently associated with AWD include enterotoxigenic *Escherichia coli* (ETEC), enteropathogenic *Escherichia coli* (EPEC), *Shigella dysenteriae,* and *Campylobacter jejuni.* Rotavirus is a common cause of severe diarrhea, vomiting, and fever leading to rapid dehydration. *Vibrio cholerae* is an important organism in endemic areas and during epidemics. Nontyphoidal *Salmonella* is a common organism in areas where commercially processed foods are widely used and in hospital outbreaks. Most of these organisms produce watery diarrhea. The main cause of acute dysentery is *S. dysenteriae, C. jejuni* and infrequently enteroinvasive *Escherichia coli* (EIEC) or *Salmonella*. Epidemics of dysentery are usually caused by *S. dysenteriae* type 1. *Entamoeba histolytica* can cause dysentery in adults but is a less common cause in young children.

Diarrhea may also be caused by several antibacterial agents like ampicillin, cotrimoxazole, chloramphenicol, amoxicillin, clindamycin, etc. Pseudomembranous colitis is the most severe form of antibiotic-associated diarrhea.

CLINICAL FEATURES

Most enteropathogens can cause diarrhea by more than one mechanism. Hence, the clinical presentation depends upon the underlying pathophysiological changes taking place in the gastrointestinal tract. Three clinical types of diarrhea have been defined, each reflecting a different pathogenesis and requiring different approach to treatment.

Secretory Diarrhea

It is characterized by AWD with profound losses of water and electrolytes due to sodium pump failure as a result of the action of identified toxins. This group is at risk for rapid development of dehydration and electrolyte imbalance. Common causes are ETEC and *Vibrio cholerae*.

Invasive Diarrhea (Dysentery)

Intestinal mucosal cells are invaded by the microorganisms which set-up an inflammatory reaction clinically presenting with blood and mucus in the stools. This group is prone to develop other complications like intestinal perforation, toxic megacolon, rectal prolapse, convulsions, septicemia, and hemolytic uremic syndrome (HUS).

Osmotic Diarrhea

Injury to enterocytes may result in brush border damage and epithelial destruction leading to decreased mucosal disaccharidase activity. Clinical presentation is characterized by passage of large, frothy, explosive, and acidic stools. High osmolar solutions given orally (e.g. carbonated soft drinks and ORS with high sugar content) can also result in osmotic diarrhea. Besides worsening in the hydration status of the child, there is a danger of developing hypernatremia.

DIAGNOSIS

Diagnosis of acute diarrhea is based on clinical history of passing frequent, loose or watery stools, with or without vomiting, fever, pain in abdomen or blood in the stools. Many children may have symptoms and signs of other associated illnesses like cough, skin rashes/measles, or urinary symptoms. The clinical triad of rotaviral diarrhea is fever, vomiting, and profuse watery stools with tendency for dehydration.

Dehydration is the most common and life-threatening consequence of diarrhea. Loss of water and electrolytes in the diarrheal stool results in depletion of the ECF volume, electrolyte imbalance, and clinical manifestation of dehydration. The first symptom of dehydration appears after fluid loss of 5% of body weight. When fluid loss reaches 10%, shock often sets in, and the cascade of events that follows can culminate in death unless there is immediate intervention to rehydrate.

Routine stool examination is not recommended except in situations such as young infants with fever, suspected protozoan *Giardia* or *Entamoeba histolytica* as a cause, extra-gut infections or persistent colitis or disaccharide intolerance and prolonged/persistent diarrhea with malnutrition. Stool culture is invariably noncontributory.

Diarrhea when prolonged or recurrent, is a major cause of malnutrition in children, owing to use of bottle feeds, stoppage of breastfeeds, and lack of energy dense feeds and hygiene like hand washing, low food intake during the illness (poor appetite, vomiting, oral thrush or stomatitis, diluting/withholding of food, etc.), reduced nutrient absorption in the intestines, and increased requirements as a result of infection. Repeated and prolonged episodes of diarrhea have even more deleterious effects and may eventually result in growth failure, intercurrent infections, and problems associated with severe malnutrition and even death.

MANAGEMENT

Principles of Treatment

- General assessment of the child.
- Assessment of hydration status. Several clinical signs and symptoms can help in detecting dehydration. However, a simple assessment chart based on a few reliable clinical signs can be referred for quick assessment of dehydration **(Table 9.1.1)** and administration of appropriate fluids for prevention and treatment of dehydration.

Table 9.1.1: Assessment of hydration status in a patient with diarrhea.

Clinical signs	*No dehydration*	*Some dehydration*	*Severe dehydration*
General condition	Well, alert	Restless, irritable	Lethargic or unconscious
Eyes	Normal	Sunken	Sunken
Thirst*	Drinks normally, not thirsty	Drinks eagerly, thirsty	Drinks poorly, not able to drink
Skin pinch	Goes back quickly	Goes back slowly	Goes back very slowly
Decide hydration status	The patient has "no signs of dehydration"	If the patient has two or more signs, there is "some dehydration"	If the patient has two or more signs, there is "severe dehydration"
Treatment plan	*Plan A*	*Plan B*	*Plan C*

*In a young infant less than 2 months of age, thirst is not assessed and decision regarding "some" or "severe dehydration" is made if "two" of the three signs are present.

- Correction of electrolyte and acid-base imbalance.
- Proper feeding to provide normal nutritional requirements
- Zinc supplementation.
- Treatment of associated problems like dysentery and persistent diarrhea.
- Nutritional rehabilitation.
- Health education for prevention of diarrhea.

ORAL REHYDRATION THERAPY

Concept of oral rehydration therapy (ORT) has revolutionized the management of diarrhea with the discovery of coupled active transport of glucose and sodium in the small bowel, resulting in the passive absorption of water, and other electrolytes even during copious diarrhea. Oral rehydration therapy includes:

- ORS solution of recommended composition
- Solution made from sugar and salt (if prepared correctly)
- Food-based solutions with appropriate concentration of salt, like lentil soup, rice, *kanji,* butter milk, etc.
- Plain water given along with continued feeding.

Low Osmolarity Oral Rehydration Salts Solution

The standard WHO-ORS, used for over three decades, has saved millions of lives but did not decrease diarrheal duration or stool output. More effective low osmolarity ORS **(Table 9.1.2)** is now recommended as the universal solution for treatment and prevention of dehydration for all causes of diarrhea and at all ages.

Table 9.1.2: Low osmolarity ORS formulation recommended by WHO/UNICEF.

Reduced osmolarity ORS	*g/L*	*Reduced osmolarity ORS*	*mmol/L*
Sodium chloride	2.6	Sodium	75
Glucose, anhydrous	13.5	Chloride	65
Potassium chloride	1.5	Glucose, anhydrous	75
Trisodium citrate, dihydrate	2.9	Potassium	20
		Citrate	10
		Total osmolarity	245

(ORS: oral rehydration solutions; UNICEF: United Nations International Children's Emergency Fund; WHO: World Health Organization)

Prevention and Treatment of Dehydration

Management of "No Dehydration"

The objective of treatment is prevention of dehydration and malnutrition (Plan A). The management can be successfully carried out at home, by the mother/caretaker who is advised to:

- Give more fluids than normal **(Table 9.1.3)**
- Continue feeding
- Bring the child back after 2 days, or earlier if he has any of the danger signs (thirsty, irritable/restless, fever, high purge rate, repeated vomiting, and blood in the stool, eating or drinking poorly, and lethargic).

Table 9.1.3: Guidelines for replacement of fluid and electrolytes in children with "no dehydration" (Plan A).

Age	*After each loose stool, offer**
<6 months	Quarter glass or cup (50 mL)
7 months to 2 years	Quarter to half glass or cup (50–100 mL)
2–5 years	Half to one glass or cup (100–200 mL)
Older children	As much as the child can take

* Fluids which can be offered include ORS, lemon water, buttermilk, rice *kanji*, lentil soup, light tea, etc.

Management of "Some Dehydration"

The objective of treatment is to treat dehydration and electrolyte imbalance, and to continue feeding. These children should be rehydrated with ORS under supervision in a health facility (Plan B).

Correction of dehydration:

- For correction of fluid and electrolyte deficit on account of dehydration, 50–100 mL/kg body weight (75 mL/kg) of ORS must be administered, over a period of 4 hours. If the child wants more, more ORS should be given. Breastfeeding should be continued.
- Older children should have free access to plain water.
- Acceptance of ORS, purge rate, and vomiting should be closely monitored.

Reassess after 4 hours:

- If still dehydrated, deficit therapy should be repeated (Plan B) and milk/food should also be offered.
- If rehydrated, it is treated as "no dehydration" with maintenance therapy with ORS as in plan A.
- If ORT is not successful, it is treated as "severe dehydration" with intravenous (IV) fluids as in plan C.

Management of "Severe Dehydration"

The primary objective is to quickly rehydrate the child in a hospital with facilities for IV fluid therapy. Ringer's lactate is the preferred solution for rehydration and is given as 100 mL/kg over 6 hours in infants less than 1 year and over 3 hours in older children **(Table 9.1.4)**. If Ringer's lactate is not available, other alternatives like normal saline may be used.

Rehydration of Severely Malnourished Children

Rehydration of severely malnourished children deserves special attention owing to certain pathophysiological

Table 9.1.4: Deficit fluid therapy for "severe dehydration" (Plan C).

	Infants (<1 year)	*Older child (>1 year)*
Volume of Ringer's lactate	30 mL/kg body weight within first 1 hour, followed by 70 mL/kg body weight over next 5 hours	30 mL/kg body weight within half an hour, followed by 70 mL/kg body weight over next 2.5 hours
Monitoring	*Assess for improvement every 1–2 hours:* • If not improving, give IV infusion more rapidly • Encourage oral feeding by giving ORS 5 mL/kg/hr, along with IV fluids, as soon as the child is able to drink *Reassess hydration status:* • After 6 hours (infants) and 3 hours (older children) assess hydration status and choose appropriate plan for hydration (Plan A, B or C)	

changes in water and electrolyte balance peculiar to protein energy malnutrition (PEM). Dehydration may be over or underestimated in the presence of marasmus or edema, respectively. These children are at risk to develop hypoglycemia and electrolyte imbalance. Rehydration with ORS solution should be preferred because IV fluids can easily cause overhydration and heart failure. Therefore, it is recommended that severely malnourished children are slowly rehydrated, carefully monitored, and feeding is started early.

Feeding during Acute Diarrhea and Dysentery

Nutritional management of acute diarrhea and dysentery takes optimal advantage of intestinal absorption capacity, which is affected to some extent during diarrhea, by feeding small, frequent, energy dense food taking into consideration the age, pre-illness feeding pattern, and state of hydration of the child **(Table 9.1.5)**. Feeding is continued in children with no dehydration, and resumed as early as possible in some dehydration.

Zinc Supplementation for Treatment of Diarrhea

Zinc deficiency is common in children from developing countries because of intake of predominant vegetarian diets and the high content of dietary phytates. Increased fecal losses during many episodes of diarrhea aggravate preexisting zinc deficiency. WHO and Indian Academy of Pediatrics (IAP) recommend zinc supplementation as an adjunct to ORS in the treatment of diarrhea. The National IAP Task Force recommends that all children older than 6 months suffering from diarrhea should receive a uniform dose of 20 mg of elemental zinc as soon as diarrhea starts and continue for a total period of 14 days. Children aged 2–6 months should

Table 9.1.5: Feeding during diarrhea.

Stage of hydration	*Recommended schedule of feeding*
During rehydration phase	
• Breastfed infants	• Continue breastfeeding and resume normal feeding after rehydration is completed
• Nonbreastfed infants	• Should be preferable given only ORS till they are rehydrated • Animal milk/food should be offered, if rehydration takes longer than 4 hours
• Severely malnourished children	• Offer some food as soon as possible
After rehydration phase	
• Breastfed infants	• Breastfeed more frequently
• Nonbreastfed infants	• Offer undiluted milk as before
• Infants 6–12 months	• Give easily digestible energy rich complementary foods in addition to breast/animal milk
• For older children	• Give thick preparation of staple food with extra vegetable oil or animal fats, rich in potassium (Legumes, banana), carotene (dark green leafy vegetables, red palm oil, carrot, pumpkin) • Encourage to eat at least six times a day

be advised 10 mg/day of elemental zinc for a total period of 14 days.

Use of Antimicrobial Agents

Antibiotic therapy should be reserved only for cases of dysentery and suspected cholera **(Table 9.1.6)**. Every case of diarrhea needs to be carefully evaluated for the presence of blood in the stools which indicates dysentery and to identify cases of suspected cholera (high purge rate with severe dehydration in a child above 2 years in an area where cholera is known to be present). In view of widespread resistance to trimethoprim-sulfamethoxazole (TMP-SMX) and reported resistance to nalidixic acid, IAP Task Force recommends ciprofloxacin as first-line drug in areas where resistance rates to TMP-SMX exceeds 30%. No chemoprophylaxis is needed for contacts.

Associated nongastrointestinal infections, such as pneumonia, meningitis, urinary tract infection, etc. should also be carefully looked for and appropriately treated. In severe malnutrition, the usual signs of infection such as fever are often absent, yet multiple infections are common in these children. Therefore, it is assumed that all severely malnourished children may have an underlying infection

Table 9.1.6: Antimicrobials used to treat specific causes of diarrhea in children.

Cause	*Drug of choice*	*Dose*
Cholera	*First-line* Doxycycline *Second-line* Ciprofloxacin*	 Single dose of 6 mg/kg PO Single dose 15 mg/kg
Dysentery	*First-line* Ciprofloxacin** *Second-line* Pivmecillinam Ceftriaxone	 15 mg/kg two times a day orally 3 days 20 mg/kg four times a day PO × 5 days; 50–100 mg/kg once a day IM × 2–5 days
Amebic dysentery	Metronidazole	30 mg/kg/day in three divided doses PO × 5–10 days
Acute giardiasis	Metronidazole or Tinidazole	15 mg/kg/day in three divided doses PO × 5 days 15 mg/kg/day in three divided doses PO × 5 days

*Can be used if there is resistance to doxycycline or no clinical response.
**In view of widespread resistance to trimethoprim-sulfamethoxazole (TMP-SMX) and reported resistance to nalidixic acid, Indian Academy of Pediatrics Task Force recommends ciprofloxacin as first-line drug in areas where resistance rates to TMP-SMX exceeds 30%

which should be treated with broad-spectrum parenteral antibiotics.

Nutritional Rehabilitation

Nutritional support to a child following an episode of acute or persistent diarrhea is of immense importance in view of the known adverse impact of diarrheal diseases on the nutrition of a young child. The need for proper feeding after an episode of diarrhea has even greater importance particularly because the efforts made by the mother/caretaker to feed during convalescence are more rewarding when these children tend to have better appetite. Therefore, one extra meal, at least for 2 weeks after an episode of acute diarrhea and for at least 1 month after persistent diarrhea, stressing the need for "catch up growth", is likely to help in nutritional rehabilitation of these children.

COMPLICATIONS

Electrolyte Imbalance

With appropriate use of ORT, access to plain water and continued feeding, the risk of electrolyte disturbances is minimized. However, following electrolyte disturbances may be encountered in some cases.

Hypernatremia

Some children with diarrhea, especially young infants, develop hypernatremic dehydration which usually follows use of hypertonic drinks (canned fruit juices, carbonated cold drink, and incorrectly prepared salt and sugar solutions, ORS with high glucose content). Children with hypernatremic dehydration (serum sodium > 150 mEq/L osmolality > 295 mOsm/kg) are extremely thirsty, out of proportion to their other signs of dehydration and sometimes have convulsions. These children can be successfully treated with low-osmolarity ORS. However, if the child is unable to drink orally, Ringer's lactate can be initially given to treat shock and later switch over to ORT with low osmolarity ORS.

Hyponatremia

Patients who ingest only large amount of water or watery drinks that contain very little salt, may present with hyponatremia (serum sodium < 130 mEq/L, osmolality < 275 mOsm/kg), which may be clinically associated with lethargy and seizures. ORS is safe and effective therapy for hyponatremia as well. For children who are unable to drink orally, IV infusion of Ringer's lactate can effectively treat hyponatremia.

Hypokalemia

Inadequate replacement of potassium losses during diarrhea can lead to potassium depletion and hypokalemia (serum potassium < 3 mEq/L), which may result in muscle weakness, paralytic ileus, renal impairment, and cardiac arrhythmias. Severe potassium depletion particularly in malnourished children may lead to acute onset flaccid paralysis ranging from neck flop to quadriparesis and even respiratory paralysis. The potassium deficit can be corrected by using ORS solution for rehydration therapy and by feeding potassium rich foods (e.g. banana, fresh fruit juices) during and after diarrhea. Oral potassium supplementation (2 mEq/kg/day) is indicated in malnourished children. In transient flaccid paralysis due to hypokalemia, potassium can be administered parenterally by using 15% solution of potassium chloride (1 mL = 2 mEq of potassium), but not exceeding 40 mEq/L of IV fluids after ensuring adequate renal functions.

Hypoglycemia

Continued feeding during an episode of diarrhea minimizes the risk of getting hypoglycemia. However, some children, particularly those severely malnourished, are at a risk of getting hypoglycemia. Early feeding can prevent hypoglycemia in these cases. Sick young infants (less than 2 months) who are not able to breastfeed or have low weight for age and a child with symptoms of hypoglycemia should be given 20–50 mL (10 mL/kg) expressed breast milk or locally appropriate animal milk (with added sugar). If neither of these is available, give 20–50 mL (10 mL/kg) sugar water.

Metabolic Acidosis

During acute diarrhea, large amounts of bicarbonate may be lost in the stool. If the kidneys continue to function normally, most of the lost bicarbonate is replaced and a serious base deficit does not develop. Metabolic acidosis tends to correct spontaneously in most of the cases as the child is properly rehydrated. ORS solution contains adequate bicarbonate/citrate to counter acidosis in less severe cases. However, in severe dehydration, compromised renal function leads to rapid development of base deficit and metabolic acidosis. Hypovolemic shock occurs because of rapid loss of water and electrolytes in severe diarrhea. This results in excessive production of lactic acid, which may further contribute to metabolic acidosis. Rapid IV infusion of Ringer's lactate, containing 28 mEq/L of lactate (metabolized to bicarbonate), is recommended in severe dehydration. However, in the presence of circulatory failure, bicarbonate precursors (e.g. citrate, lactate) may not be readily metabolized in the body. If the patient presents with severe metabolic acidosis, (pH < 7.20, serum $HCO_3^- < 8$ mEq/L) sodium bicarbonate in a bolus dose of 2–3 mEq/kg can be given to correct acidosis. Attention should be paid to serum potassium concentration as correction of acidosis in a patient with low potassium can lead to life-threatening severe hypokalemia.

Acute Renal Failure

Severe dehydration and shock lead to decrease in renal blood flow resulting in prerenal type of acute renal failure. Immediate replacement of fluids is generally helpful to revive kidney functions unless renal failure is irreversible. In case fluid challenge, after rehydration fails to reverse the process, the child needs to be hospitalized and managed as per acute renal failure protocol.

Hemolytic Uremic Syndrome

Some children with invasive diarrhea due to *S. dysenteriae* or enteroinvasive *E. coli* may have hemolytic uremic syndrome (HUS) due to nephrotoxin liberated by these organisms. These children develop intravascular hemolysis with acute renal failure. This is a serious condition and needs to be managed in a hospital setting.

PROGNOSIS

Acute diarrhea is a self-limiting disorder. Early administration of ORS or home available fluids prevents onset of dehydration. Appropriate use of low osmolarity ORS in some dehydration and Ringer's lactate in severe dehydration can prevent all diarrheal deaths.

PREVENTION

Diarrheal diseases can be prevented to a great extent by improving infant feeding practices and personal, and domestic hygiene. Some of the interventions, which are feasible and cost effective include:

- Promotion of exclusive breastfeeding up to 6 months of age
- Improved complementary feeding practices
- Use of clean drinking water and sufficient water for personal hygiene
- Hand washing
- Use of sanitary toilets
- Safe disposal of the stool of young children
- Measles vaccination.

Rotavirus Vaccines

Recent studies have demonstrated safety and efficacy of two new live, oral, attenuated rotavirus vaccines in middle- and high-income countries, thereby suggesting a combined preventive and treatment strategy (vaccine, low osmolarity ORS, and zinc supplementation) to significantly reduce child mortality. However, the diversity of rotavirus strains and high prevalence of mixed infections are unique features of rotavirus epidemiology in India. Currently an Indian made Rota virus vaccine is included under National Immunization Program.

KEY MESSAGES

- Diarrhea is a self-limiting disorder and does not need any antibiotic for treatment.
- Oral rehydration with low osmolarity ORS, continued feeding and zinc supplementation is the key to treatment of diarrhea in children.
- Intravenous fluids are indicated in a few cases who have severe dehydration or unable to drink orally. Ringer's lactate is the most suitable solution for IV therapy.
- A child with diarrhea should be thoroughly examined for associated illnesses.
- Exclusive breastfeeding up to 6 months of age and hand washing significantly reduce incidence of diarrhea.

BIBLIOGRAPHY

1. Bhatnagar S, Bhandari N, Mouli UC, et al. Consensus Statement of IAP National Task Force: Status Report on Management of Acute Diarrhea. Indian Pediatr. 2004;41:335-48.
2. Integrated Management of Neonatal and Childhood Illness. Physician Chart Booklet. Ministry of Health and Family Welfare, Govt. of India; 2009.

9.2 Persistent and Chronic Diarrhea

Gadadhar Sarangi

PERSISTENT DIARRHEA

Less than 10% of infants are likely to suffer from persistent diarrhea and the risk factors broadly include host factors, disease characteristics, contributed by caregiver or attending physician. The severity may vary from mild to severe type and whatever the type of presentation, the basic defect is small intestinal mucosal damage, infection including small intestinal bacterial overgrowth (SIBO), malnutrition, and growth failure with significant morbidity and mortality depending on the severity.

Definition

The World Health Organization (WHO) has defined persistent diarrhea (PD) as a diarrheal illness with passage of three or more loose stools of presumed infectious etiology, which starts acutely but lasts for more than 14 days. It is a continuum of acute diarrhea. Intractable diarrhea of infancy often begins before the age of 3 months with more than three liquid stools lasting for more than 2 weeks less than 1 year of age accompanied by either weight loss or no weight gain during this period.

Etiology

Common causes of PD include persistent infection with one or more enteric pathogens, secondary malabsorption of carbohydrates and fat, intestinal parasitosis and infrequently dietary protein allergy/intolerance.

Pathology

Prolonged cell-mediated immune (CMI) damage to the small intestinal mucosa is probably the final common pathway by which a variety of noxious influences like nutritional, infective, and possibly allergic stimuli perpetuate the syndrome of persistent diarrhea in children in developing countries. There is impairment and considerable delay in the repair of damaged epithelium of the gut. Carbohydrate, fat, and protein malabsorption ensues as a result of the damage to the upper small intestinal mucosal absorptive surface. The loss of brush border enzymes and direct absorption of macromolecular foreign proteins result in food into lance and allergy (Cow's milk or wheat protein allergy). Overgrowth of bacteria in small bowel and altered intestinal flora are also marked as a consequence. Infection culminates in injury to the small intestinal absorptive mucosa and malabsorption of both macro- and micronutrients are the untoward events in the patients.

Clinical Presentation

Three clinical types of persistent diarrhea are recognized:

1. Mild form is characterized by several motions/day without significant weight loss and dehydration and can be managed successfully as outpatients with good follow-up.
2. Moderate form is characterized by several motions/day with marginal weight loss, without dehydration and nontolerance to milk and milk products and need frequent admissions due to acute exacerbations with complications, improper treatment, and no follow-up.
3. Severe form of persistent diarrhea is often life-threatening and is heralded by dehydration, weight loss, and nontolerance to milk and cereals. Secondary infection often coexists with this category **(Figs. 9.2.1A and B)** and these infants need to stay in the tertiary care hospitals for indefinite period till they recover, needing intestinal biopsy, total care including total/partial parenteral, and enteral nutrition support with elemental diets. The mortality is still high in most of the centers in developing countries.

Diagnosis

The emergency risk factors arising out of dehydration, malnutrition, and infection should be assessed. Stool examination for culture and reducing sugar with pH will help in management. The effect of previous treatment modalities and diet regimen should be evaluated. The attitude and cooperation of the parents remains the cornerstone in therapy.

Management

The management of persistent diarrhea is given in **Tables 9.2.1 and 9.2.2**.

Antimicrobials in Persistent Diarrhea

These are useful in the presence of gross blood in the stool or more than 10 pus cells/HPF (quinolones/oral third-generation

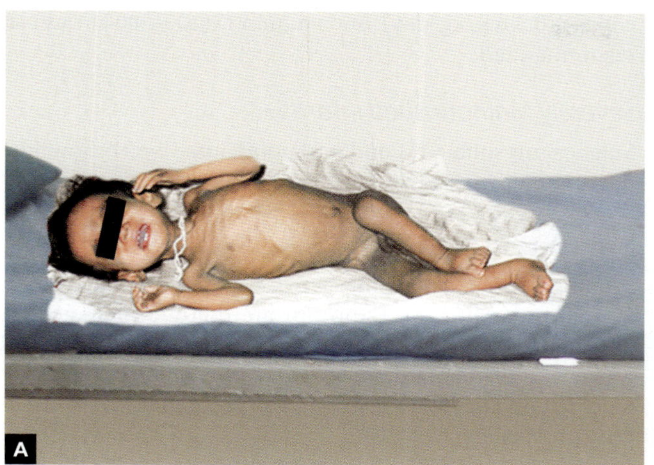

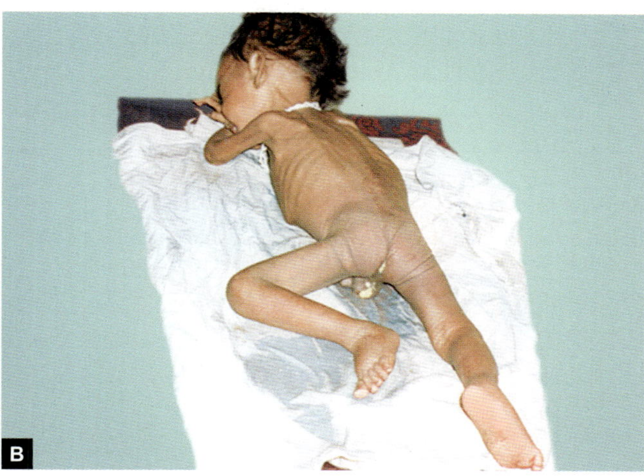

Figs. 9.2.1A and B: Persistent diarrhea with marasmic kwashiorkor as a result of infection and malnutrition.

Table 9.2.1: Management guidelines for persistent diarrhea.

Mild persistent diarrhea	
Try low milk formula feeds (rice, milk, sugar, and oil—diet of plan A) *Moderate persistent diarrhea* Do not try milk. Permit cereal-based feeds (rice/wheat/Bengal gram/ragi, sugar, and oil—diet of plan B)	
Severe persistent diarrhea	
Phase-I	Resuscitation < 24 hours
Phase-II	Partial control of diarrhea, sustained maintenance of vital signs Electrolyte, metabolic, and hemodynamic balance by partial parenteral nutrition (PPN), intravenous fluids, colloids, parenteral antimicrobials (1–4 days)
Phase-III	5 days onward (nutritional rehabilitation) Monitor weight Hypoosmolar, hypoallergenic, home available caloridense nonoffending (lactose free) feeds (plan B) in gradual increments depending upon tolerance. If it fails, diet of plan C (chicken/egg white, glucose and oil) along with partial parenteral nutrition (PPN) to be given. If no response, total parenteral nutrition (TPN) will be life saving.
Criteria for changing over from Plan A to B to C: • Purge volume and rate more than 7 stools/day at the end of 7 days. • Tendency for dehydration • No weight gain/weight loss despite oral intake of 100 cal/kg/day × 3 days	

cephalosporins), systemic sepsis (parenteral ampicillin and aminoglycosides), severe malnutrition, very young infants (<3 months of age) associated extra-gut infections [e.g. urinary tract infection (UTI), lower respiratory tract infection (LRTI)], and HIV (ampicillin and aminoglycosides).

Table 9.2.2: Diets for persistent diarrhea.

Plan A (milk rice diet for persistent diarrhea)	
Ingredient	***Amount (g)***
Puffed rice	12.5
Milk	40.0
Sugar	2.25
Oil	2.0
Water to make	100.0
The above will yield the following:	
Energy density	96 kcal/100 mL
Protein	10.0%
Carbohydrate	55.87%
Lactose	1.73%
Fat	33.9%
Amino acid score	1.0%
Note: Puffed rice is ground and appropriate quantities are mixed with sugar and oil. Boiled water is then added to make a thick gruel. This feed has a shelf life of around 3 hours.	
Plan B (egg-based milk-free diet for persistent diarrhea)	
Ingredient	***Amount (g)***
Puffed rice	13.5
Egg	11.0
Sugar/glucose	3.5
Oil	3.5
Water to make	100.0
The above will yield the following:	
Energy density	92.2 kcal/100 mL

Contd...

Contd...

Ingredient	***Amount (g)***
Protein	9.5%
Carbohydrate	56.9%
Fat	33.29%
Amino acid score	1.0%
Note: Egg white is added to the mixture of weighed rice, sugar, and oil. Boiled water is added to make a thick gruel weighing 100 g.	
Plan C (chicken-based diet for persistent diarrhea)	
Ingredient	***Amount/L***
Chicken	100 g
Glucose	20–40 g
Coconut oil	40–50 g
KCL (15%)	7.5 mL
$NaHCO_3$ (7.5%)	20–30 mL
Water to make	1,000 mL
The above will yield energy 720 kcal and protein 26 g	

Note:
- It is prepared by grinding the precooked boneless chicken stuff in a mixer. Glucose, oil, and some water are added to it and the feed is brought to a boil. Additional water is added to make a final volume of 1 L. Finally, KCl, and $NaHCO_3$ are added to safeguard against spoilage. It is stored in a refrigerator.
- Glucose is initially added in 2% concentration and then built up to 4% by increasing 1% every alternate day. To reduce osmolar load a mixture of glucose and sugar may be employed.
- Any vegetable oil may be employed in place of coconut oil.

Antiprotozoal Drugs

For *Giardia* or *Entamoeba histolytica* trophozoites in the stool (metronidazole).

Lactobacilli and Saccharomyces boulardii

These are only adjuncts with little benefit.

Indications for Total Parenteral Nutrition in Persistent Diarrhea

- Protracted diarrhea with recurrent dehydration
- Intolerance to plan C treatment
- Weight loss or no weight gain even after plan C treatment.

Supplemental Vitamins and Minerals

About twice recommended daily allowance of supplemental multivitamins and minerals are to be given for at least 2–4 weeks. Special attention to be given for vitamin A 200,000 units for children above 12 months or 100,000 IU for infants to be given. Zinc, 20 mg/day for 14 days to be given to children above 6 months and below 6 months it is to be given 10 mg/day for 14 days. Folic acid (1 mg/day), elemental copper (0.3 mg/kg/day), and vitamin D (200–400 U/day) are recommended.

Severely Malnourished Infants

Magnesium sulfate IM and oral potassium in recommended doses should be given for at least 2 weeks.

Prevention

Promotion of breastfeeding, active and prompt management of acute diarrhea, and appropriate dietetic management during diarrhea with judicious administration of drugs will prevent PD of infancy. Rotavirus and other enteric vaccines do help in reducing PD. Role of zinc and probiotics in prevention is controversial.

Predisposing Factors

Prevention factors during the management of AWD such as bottle feeding and stopping breast milk, in advertent and empiric use of banned drugs, malnutrition, extra-gut infections especially nonbreastfed infant of less than 4 months of age, immune deficiency, infections like adenovirus, enteroaggregative *Escherichia coli* (EAggEC), EPEC, *Salmonella*, *Clostridium difficile*, *Candida*, HIV, etc. Small bowel overgrowth with significant mucosal atrophy should be focused.

CHRONIC DIARRHEA

Definition

Chronic diarrhea is characterized by increased stool frequency of more than three times a day, stool weight/volume of more than 10 g/kg/day in infants, and 200 g/day in toddlers with a duration of 4 weeks as the cutoff point. Most children have insidious onset and noninfective diarrhea for more than 14 days.

Pathophysiology

Reduced net water absorption, as low as 1% can cause diarrhea.

Osmotic Diarrhea

Failure to absorb luminal solutes and consequently osmotic retention of water in the gut: Example, disaccharidase deficiency primary or secondary to gut mucosal injury; excessive consumption of sugar where the absorptive capacity is overwhelmed, e.g. fructose and sorbitol, fruit juices. The diarrhea usually sees when the offending nutrient is removed from diet or after fasting within 24 hours.

Osmotic diarrhea can result from:

- Intestinal damage as in enteric infections
- Reduced absorptive surface area—active celiac disease.
- Defective digestive enzyme or nutrient carrier—lactase deficiency
- Decrease intestinal transit time—functional diarrhea
- Nutrient overload exceeding the digestive capacity—sorbitol in fruit juice or over feeding.

The undigested or excess nutrients get fragmented to organic acids and increase the intraluminal osmotic load in the colon.

Secretory Diarrhea

Increased net secretion of electrolytes and fluid from the intestine: Electrogenic secretion is induced by increase in intracellular concentration of cyclic adenosine monophosphate (AMP), cyclic guanosine monophosphate (GMP) or calcium in response to microbial enterotoxins or endogenous endocrine or nonendocrine moieties. The electrolyte water flux to the lumen overtaking absorption results in loading the colon with diarrhea. It can result from:

- Inhibition of NaCl absorption in villous enterocytes.
- Increase in electrogenic chloride secretion from the crypt cells.
- Extensive resection of the gut as in operations for necrotizing enterocolitis or intestinal atresia results in reduction of anatomic surface area resulting in diarrhea.
- Inflammatory processes like regional enteritis and ulcerative colitis involving a significant portion of the gut causes chronic diarrhea.

The differences between osmotic and secretory diarrhea are given in **Table 9.2.3**.

Causes

The common causes of chronic diarrhea are given in **Table 9.2.4**.

Table 9.2.3: Difference between osmotic and secretory diarrhea.

Character	*Osmotic diarrhea*	*Secretory diarrhea*
Stool volume	Moderately increased	Very large
Response to fasting	Diarrhea stops	Diarrhea continues
Reducing substance	Positive	Negative
Stool osmolality	Increased	Normal
Stool osmotic gap [Stool osmolality: 2 (Stool $Na^+ + K^+$)]	>100 mOsm/kg	<100 mOsm/kg
Stool Na^+	<70 mEq/L	>70 mEq/L
Stool pH	<5	>6

Table 9.2.4: Common causes of chronic diarrhea.

Infancy
• Postgastroenteritis malabsorption syndrome • Protein energy malnutrition • Cow's milk/soy protein intolerance • Secondary/primary disaccharidase deficiencies • Cystic fibrosis • Chronic nonspecific diarrhea of infancy (Toddler's diarrhea)
Childhood
• Excessive consumption of carbonated fluids (Chronic nonspecific diarrhea) • Secondary disaccharidase deficiency • *Intestinal parasites: Giardia, Entamoeba histolytica, Cryptosporidium* • *Postgastroenteritis*: Malabsorption syndrome • Celiac disease • Cystic fibrosis • Intestinal infection: Enteropathogens, *Mycobacterium tuberculosis* • Tropical sprue
Adolescence
• Irritable bowel syndrome • Inflammatory bowel disease: Crohn disease, ulcerative colitis • Giardiasis • Lactose intolerance

Evaluation

The evaluation should be done in a stepwise manner in order to avoid confusion in diagnosis **(Table 9.2.5)**.

Treatment

Treatment depends upon the cause.

- Restriction of carbonated drinks or excess fruit juice will reduce stool frequency in chronic nonspecific diarrhea. In diarrhea, due to secondary carbohydrate intolerance, reduction of lactose or sucrose in the diet will help. Lactase can be used to aid indigestion of lactose. If diarrhea persists, elimination of lactose/sucrose depending upon the situation is indicated.
- If stool examination reveals more fat, malabsorption syndrome (MAS) remains a distinct possibility. Postgastroenteritis MAS needs predigested formula to which a great proportion responds favorably.
- Infants presenting with secretory diarrhea in the first month of life need nutritional support as the likely cause is congenital defect in transport proteins.
- In instances, where chronic diarrhea is a manifestation of a disease, the etiology should be established and specific treatment instituted.

Table 9.2.5: Evaluation of patients with chronic diarrhea.

Phase-I	*Clinical history:* *Characteristics of the stool:* Small bowel diarrhea is with large volume foul smelling stool with undigested food particle. Large bowel diarrhea has blood, mucus, urgency, and tenismus and sometimes associated with explosive passage of motion with bloating. Toddler's diarrhea has loose stool with undigested food particles. *Carbohydrate intolerance*: Frequent explosive loose watery stools and bloating *Fat malabsorption*: Pasty, loose, and foul smelling stool. Extraintestinal symptoms of IBD should be looked for. Specific amounts of fluids ingested per day will indicate the overloading of gut with osmotically active substances. History of repeated infections seen in cystic fibrosis or immune deficiency syndromes. *Physical examination including nutritional assessment.* Assessment of dehydration. Nutritional assessment for growth failure. Extraintestinal manifestations of IBD like joint pain, swelling and erythema. Signs of nutrient deficiency like perianal dermatitis of zinc deficiency, rickets of vitamin D deficiency, night blindness and keratomalacia of vitamin A deficiency, bruising of vitamin K deficiency, and other deficiency signs of B complex vitamins should be looked for. Per rectal examination is important for Hirschsprung disease and IBD. *Stool examination* for pH, reducing substance, and smear for white and red blood cell count, stool fat globules, ova, cyst, and parasites should be performed. *Stool for culture* and stool for *Clostridium difficile* toxin. *Blood studies* include complete blood cell count, erythrocyte sedimentation rate, serum electrolytes, blood urea nitrogen, and creatinine.
Phase-II	Sweat chloride test for cystic fibrosis IgA anti-endomyseal antibody, tissue transglutaminase antibody for celiac disease 72 hours stool fat estimation in fatty diarrhea Stool electrolytes, stool osmolarity (stool osmotic gap) Fecal alpha-1-antitrypsin for protein-losing enteropathy. Stool pH, reducing substance, stool electrolytes, stool osmotic gap, and breath hydrogen test to determine osmotic versus secretory diarrhea Fecal elastase/chymotrypsin, secretin tests for pancreatic insufficiency Stool magnesium sulfate Phosphates
Phase-III	Endoscopic studies Small bowel biopsy Sigmoidoscopy or colonoscopy with biopsies. Barium studies Imaging: Ultrasound, MRI, and scintigraphy
Phase-IV	Hormonal studies Vasoactive intestinal polypeptides 5-hydroxy indole acetic acid Gastrin Secretin assay

(IBD: inflammatory bowel disease)

- Nitazoxanide therapy can be instituted where *Giardia lamblia* or *Cryptosporidium parvum* are suspected or found.

CONCLUSION

Chronic diarrhea may occur in many diseases including a variety of infectious and immunological conditions. Rare diseases with intracatable and chronic diarrhea have provided important insights into the gut physiology and immunology. All the informations have opened the way to more efficient management for both common and rare conditions of chronic diarrhea.

BIBLIOGRAPHY

1. Bavdekar A, Matthai J, Sathiyasekaran M, et al. IAP Speciality series on Pediatric Gastroenterology, Vol. 5 and 6. New Delhi: Jaypee Brothers Medical Publishers (P) Ltd; 2008. pp. 42-76.
2. Bhutta ZA, Ghishan F, Lindley K, et al. Persistent and chronic diarrhea and malabsorption: Working group report of the second world congress of pediatric gastroenterology, hepatology, and nutrition. J Pediatr Gastroenterol Nutr. 2004;39(Suppl 2):S711-6.
3. Bhutta ZA, Hendricks KM. Nutritional management of persistent diarrhea in childhood: A perspective from the developing world. J Pediatr Gastroenterol Nutr. 1996;22:17-37.
4. Cohen SA. Use of nitazoxanide as a new therapeutic option for persistent diarrhea: A pediatric perspective. Curr Med Res Opin. 2005;21(7):999-1004.
5. Grimwood K, Forbes DA. Acute and persistent diarrhea. Pediatr Clin North Am. 2009;56(6):1343-61.

6. Guearino A, Branski D, Winter HS. Chronic diarrhea. In: Kliegman, Stanton, St Geme, Schor (Eds). Nelson Textbook of Pediatrics, 1st South Asian Edition. India: Elsevier; 2015. pp. 1875-82.
7. Lima AA, Guerrant RL. Persistent diarrhea in children: Epidemiology, risk factors, pathophysiology, nutritional impact, and management. Epidemiol Rev. 1992;14:222-42.
8. Mathai J, Raju B, Bavdekar A. Pediatric gastroenterology chapter, Indian Academy of Pediatrics. Chronic and persistent diarrhea in infants and young children: Status statement. India Pediatr. 2011;48(1):37-42.
9. Schiller LR, Pardi DS, Sellin JH. Chronic diarrhea: Diagnosis and management. Clin Gastroenterol Hepatol. 2017;15(2):182-93.
10. Schiller LR. Chronic diarrhea. Gastroenterology. 2004;127:287-93.

9.3 Malabsorption Syndrome

Ujjal Poddar

INTRODUCTION

Malabsorption syndrome (MAS) is defined as the failure of absorption of one or more nutrients. Over the years, the spectrum of MAS in India has changed. Initial studies of 1960s and 1970s were mainly on young (<5 years) malnourished children and the focus was on stool examination to isolate infections and infestations. Almost half of those cases were due to gastrointestinal infestations like *Giardia*. Nevertheless, with improvement of nutritional status, personal hygiene, and appropriate use of antimicrobials, the prevalence of gastrointestinal infestations (especially *Giardia*) as a primary cause of MAS has decreased tremendously. Due to increasing awareness, easy availability of diagnostic tools such as serology and endoscopic biopsy, the focus has now shifted from infestation to celiac disease. Recent studies have shown that celiac disease is the most common cause of MAS in the West as well as in India (especially in North India) both in children as well as in adults.

PATHOGENESIS

Malabsorption syndrome is grossly divided into two categories:

1. Impaired breakdown of nutrients (*maldigestion*).
2. Defective mucosal uptake and transport of adequately digested nutrients (*true malabsorption*).

The latter one may be specific malabsorption of a nutrient or a group of nutrients or generalized malabsorption or panmalabsorption (malabsorption of broad range of nutrients).

Maldigestion

The luminal phase of digestion requires pancreatic enzymes, bile salts, and the absence of either of them give rises to failure of digestion of carbohydrate (lack of pancreatic amylase), fat (pancreatic lipase and bile salts), and proteins (pancreatic trypsin and chymotrypsin). Similarly, small intestinal bacterial overgrowth (SIBO) due to surgical causes (stricture, fistulae, blind loop, diverticula, etc.) or due to reduced motility of gut (pseudo-obstruction) can cause maldigestion by breaking down bile salts (deconjugation of conjugated bile salts) in the proximal small intestine by bacteria and thereby rendering them (conjugated bile salts) unavailable for mixed micelle formation for fat digestion. Even carbohydrate and protein malabsorption can happen in SIBO, primarily due to bacterial degradation of carbohydrate and mucosal injury by bacterial overgrowth, leading to brush-border enzyme deficiency. Other prominent feature of SIBO is vitamin B_{12} deficiency, as bacteria utilize vitamin B_{12}.

Malabsorption

Diseases that cause small intestinal mucosal damage like celiac disease, tropical sprue, food protein allergy [like cow's milk protein allergy (CMPA)], etc. give rise to panmalabsorption of carbohydrate, proteins, and fat due to deficiency of brush-border enzymes and lack of transport system located on the apical surface of enterocytes. The important brush-border enzymes for carbohydrate digestion are lactase (lactose malabsorption), maltase (maltose: up to nine residue oligosaccharides), and sucrase (sucrose malabsorption). For proteins, these are oligopeptidases (cleave amino acids from 3 to 8 residue peptides), dipeptidases, and tripeptidases. In malabsorption, the unabsorbed carbohydrate (oligosaccharides, disaccharides like lactose, sucrose) and proteins (oligopeptides, dipeptides, and tripeptides) reach colon, where colonic bacteria ferment carbohydrate and produce short chain fatty acids (propionic acid, acetoacetic acid, and butyric acid), and gas (hydrogen, methane and carbon dioxide). Short chain fatty acids (2–4 carbon length) in colon produce osmotic effect and draw

Flowchart 9.3.1: Approach to suspected malabsorption syndrome.

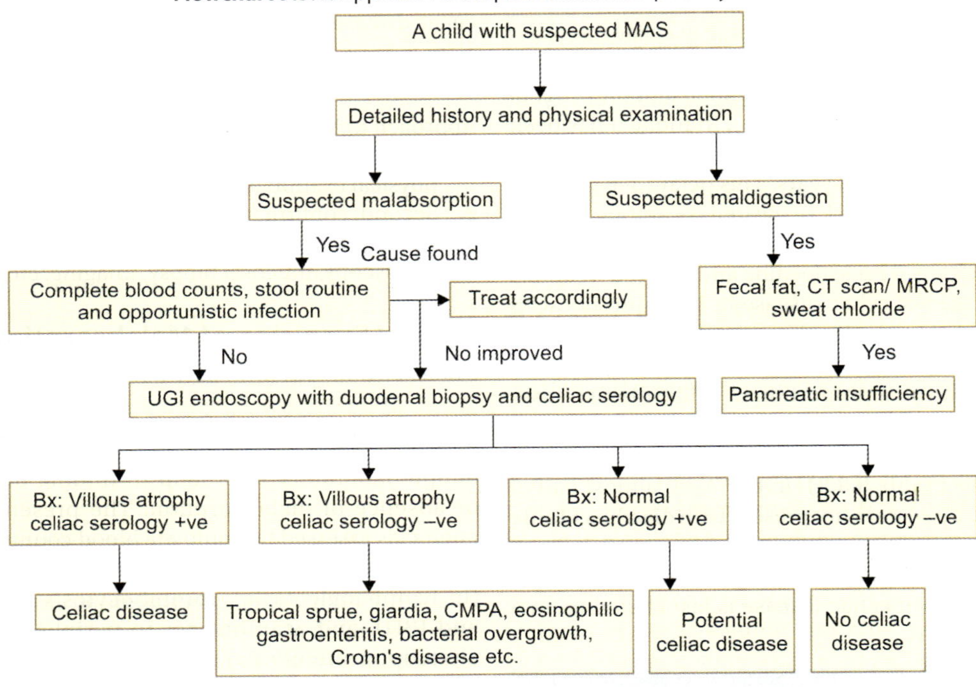

(Bx: biopsy; CMPA: cow's milk protein allergy; MAS: malabsorption syndrome; MRCP: magnetic resonance cholangiopancreatography; UGI: upper gastrointestinal tract)

eosinophilic gastroenteritis, Crohn's disease, etc. However, in most cases of MAS, the mucosal biopsies are abnormal (show villous atrophy) but not diagnostic of a condition such as celiac disease, tropical sprue, CMPA, severe protein energy malnutrition (PEM), prolonged iron, and folate deficiencies, etc. Approach to MAS is given in **Flowchart 9.3.1**. In a suspected case of CMPA, rectal biopsy plays a pivotal role (eosinophilic proctitis: >6 eosinophils per high power field). In this era of sophisticated investigations, simple stool examination (consecutive 3 days) cannot be ignored especially in young malnourished children to document parasitic infestations.

Diagnosis of Celiac Disease

Celiac disease is diagnosed by modified European Society of Pediatric Gastroenterology and Nutrition (ESPGAN) criteria. According to these criteria, small intestinal biopsy should be suggestive of celiac disease showing villous atrophy and the patient should show unequivocal clinical response to gluten-free diet (GFD) in weeks. However, there are many conditions other than celiac disease, which can give rise to villous atrophy, especially in India. Hence, if these criteria are applied in our population then celiac disease will be overdiagnosed. To overcome this problem, additional criteria, over and above ESPGAN criteria are needed. The best option to confirm the diagnosis is gluten challenge but it is cumbersome and requires repeated endoscopic biopsies and needs parents and child's cooperation. On the contrary, celiac serology is simple, effective, and if positive at the time of diagnosis and becomes negative on follow-up on "GFD", it confirms the diagnosis.

The best antibody test is anti-endomysial antibody (EMA) with a sensitivity and specificity of 97%, but it is a technically demanding test (done by indirect immunofluorescent technique). On the other hand, antitissue transglutaminase (tTG) is almost as good as EMA and it is done by enzyme-linked immunosorbent assay (ELISA) technique. The sensitivity and specificity of tTG is around 95%. In a prospective study in 180 children with celiac disease, it was shown that the tTG has got 95% concordance with EMA and its sensitivity and specificity were 94% and 97%, respectively. Hence, in Indian setting tTG is the best antibody to diagnose celiac disease. Nevertheless, in first 2 years of life when IgA antibody titers against tTG and EMA may not be adequate to be detected by these tests, and in IgA deficiency state (which is 10 times more common in celiac disease than that in general population), IgA plus IgG deamidated gliadin peptide (anti-DGP) antibody is shown to be superior to IgA-tTG and IgA-EMA tests.

Recently, ESPGHAN has modified its criteria to diagnose celiac disease and as per these new criteria, duodenal biopsy is not essential in all cases. In a symptomatic case, if tTG is more than 10 times upper limit of normal then second-line of investigations should be EMA and HLA testing, if both (EMA, HLA-DQ2/8) are positive then a patient can be labeled as celiac disease without a biopsy. However, this approach is not suitable in Indian setting as both EMA and HLA tests are scarcely available and prohibitively expensive. Hence, we should stick to biopsy-based criteria.

Proposed Criteria to Diagnose Celiac Disease in India

- Small intestinal biopsy should show villous atrophy.
- Celiac serology (EMA or tTG) should be positive.
- There should be unequivocal clinical response to GFDs in weeks along with disappearance of celiac serology on follow-up.

MANAGEMENT

Besides managing the underlying cause of MAS, these patients need supplements with iron, folic acid, multivitamins, and calcium. Severely malnourished children should be supplemented with extra calories and proteins. Caution should be maintained to avoid being too aggressive in restarting feeding in a severely malnourished MAS patient as they are at risk of developing "refeeding or nutritional recovery syndrome". In such situation the dictum is "start low, go slow". All such patients should be supplemented with thiamine, calcium, phosphate, magnesium, potassium, and feeding should be started with half of the daily requirements and to be increased gradually over a week.

Parasitic infestations are quite common in MAS patients but many of them are associated with another cause for MAS. Hence, just treatment of isolated parasites (like metronidazole for *Giardia*, nitazoxanide for *Cryptosporidium*) may not cure the condition. All such children should be followed-up and if their symptoms persist despite antiparasitic treatment they should be investigated for underlying diseases like celiac disease or CMPA.

In CMPA, besides stopping cow's milk the attention should be paid to foods containing milk-proteins such as biscuits, dairy products, butter, ghee, etc. as even a minute quantity of milk proteins can cause persistence or flare of the disease. All such children should be supplemented with calcium as milk is the richest source of calcium. Fortunately, CMPA is a self-limiting condition and most children (>90%) grow out of this condition by 3–5 years of age.

On the contrary, celiac disease is a lifelong condition and the patient (and parents) should be given a clear understanding that the gluten cannot be introduced at any stage of life.

KEY MESSAGES

- The etiology of MAS depends on age and geographic location.
- Protracted diarrhea due to CMPA and parasitic infestations are common causes in first 2 years of life.
- Celiac disease is the most common cause of MAS in more than 2 years of age in North India.
- Consecutive 3 days stool examination needs to be done in all cases before embarking on sophisticated investigations.
- Endoscopy and mucosal biopsy play important role in the diagnosis.
- Nondiarrheal manifestations of celiac disease are not uncommon in India and a high index of suspicion is required to diagnose atypical/non-classical celiac disease.
- Parasitic infestations are common in patients with MAS and many a times they are not the primary cause of malabsorption.
- Adequate supplements with minerals, vitamins, and gradual introduction of feed are the key to prevent nutritional recovery syndrome in severely malnourished MAS patients.

BIBLIOGRAPHY

1. Behera B, Mirdha BR, Makharia GK, et al. Parasites in patients with malabsorption syndrome: A clinical study in children and adults. Dig Dis Sci. 2008;53:672-9.
2. Husby S, Koletzko S, Korponay-Szabó IR, et al. European Society of Pediatric Gastroenterology, Hepatology and Nutrition guidelines for the diagnosis of celiac disease. J Pediatr Gastroenterol Nutr. 2012;54:136-60.
3. Mohindra S, Yachha SK, Srivastava A, et al. Celiac disease in Indian children: Assessment of clinical, nutritional, and pathologic characteristics. J Health Popul Nutr. 2001;19:204-8.
4. Poddar U, Thapa BR, Nain CK, et al. Celiac disease in India: Are they true cases of celiac disease? J Pediatr Gastroenterol Nutr. 2002;35:508-12.
5. Poddar U, Thapa BR, Nain CK, et al. Is tissue transglutaminase autoantibody the best for diagnosing celiac disease in children of developing countries? J Clin Gastroenterol. 2008;42:147-51.
6. Poddar U, Thapa BR, Singh K. Clinical features of celiac disease in Indian children: Are they different from the West? J Pediatr Gastroenterol Nutr. 2006;43:313-7.
7. Poddar U, Yachha SK, Krishnani N, et al. Cow's milk protein allergy (CMPA): An entity for recognition in developing countries. J Gastroenterol Hepatol. 2010;25:178-82.
8. Rastogi A, Malhotra V, Uppal B, et al. Etiology of chronic diarrhea in tropical children. Trop Gastroenterol.1999;20:45-9.
9. Sharma A, Poddar U, Yachha SK. Time to recognize atypical celiac disease in India. Indian J Gastroenterol. 2007;26:269-73.
10. Yachha SK, Misra S, Malik AK, et al. Spectrum of malabsorption syndrome in North Indian children. Indian J Gastroenterol. 1993;12:120-5.

9.4 Vomiting and Gastroesophageal Reflux Disease

Shashidhararao Nagabhushana

INTRODUCTION

Vomiting is a very common symptom in pediatric practice associated with not only a gastrointestinal but also other system involvement like central nervous system (CNS), renal, psychological, etc. Red flags like persistent/severe vomiting, copious bilious vomiting with colic/visible peristalsis, presence of other signs of raised intracranial pressure and failure to thrive warrants specific evaluation for its cause.

DEFINITION

Vomiting is forceful expulsion of the stomach contents. It occurs in three phases, i.e. (1) nausea, (2) retching, and (3) emesis. In very young children and in those with raised intracranial pressure, vomiting is induced without nausea.

Regurgitation (posseting) is effortless expulsion of gastric contents through the mouth. It is common in neonates and infants, is often a developmental process and does not need therapy; symptoms resolve with age and the child thrives well. In contrast, gastroesophageal reflux disease (GERD) is abnormal as in addition to vomiting it is usually associated with complications like aspiration, pneumonia, and esophagitis and the child may not thrive well. It therefore needs early recognition and prompt therapy.

PATHOPHYSIOLOGY AND ETIOLOGY

The causative mechanisms can be depicted as shown in **Flowchart 9.4.1**. The common causes of vomiting in children and at different age groups are provided in **Tables 9.4.1 and 9.4.2**, respectively.

Flowchart 9.4.1: Mechanism of vomiting in children.

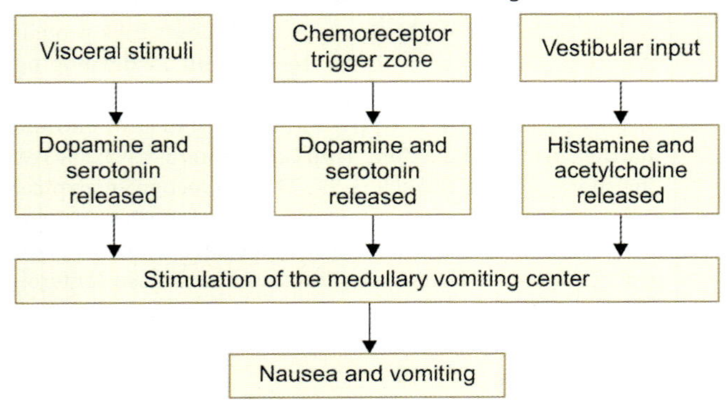

APPROACH TO MANAGEMENT

An accurate history and thorough physical examination helps in proper diagnosis. The child's age and the clinical profile dictate the most probable etiology **(Table 9.4.2)**.

- Enquire about the duration, frequency, and presence of blood or bile in the vomitus.
- Ask about associated abdominal pain, recent changes in feeding pattern, changes in urine color, drug consumption, and presence of associated fever or altered sensorium.
- Look out for symptoms and signs attributable to the respiratory, gastrointestinal, urinary, and CNS in that order.
- Assess the child for signs of dehydration.
- In neonates and infants with acute vomiting, the possibility of serious infections like sepsis, meningitis or urinary tract infection needs to be considered and ruled out, i.e. the cause of vomiting may be outside the gastrointestinal tract.
- In a neonate, vomiting may be the first sign of intestinal obstruction.

Table 9.4.1: Etiology of vomiting.

Common	*Less common*	*Rare*
Gastroenteritis/ gastritis	Surgical abdomen	Inborn errors of metabolism
Motion sickness	Gastroesophageal reflux	Migraine variant
Acute hepatitis	• Pyelonephritis	• Cyclic vomiting syndrome
	• Cholecystitis	• Chronic renal failure
	• Raised intracranial pressure	• Endocrine causes
	• Brain tumor, increased intracranial infection	• Diabetic ketoacidosis
	• Pseudotumor	• Addison's disease
	• Vestibular dysfunction	• Psychogenic

Table 9.4.2: Common causes of vomiting by age of presentation.

Etiology	*Newborn*	*Infant and child*
Infections	• Sepsis • Meningitis	• Gastroenteritis • Meningitis • Respiratory tract infections
Anatomic	• Atresia and webs • Duplications • Malrotation/ volvulus	• Pyloric stenosis • Intussusception
Gastrointestinal	• Overfeeding/ posseting Gastroesophageal reflux • Gastritis-swallowed meconium	• Gastroesophageal reflux • Gastritis • Hepatitis • Appendicitis
Renal	Urinary tract infection	Urinary tract infection
Neurologic	• Birth trauma	• Subdural hematoma • Increased intracranial tension • Migraine
Metabolic		Uremia
Endocrine		• Congenital adrenal hyperplasia • Diabetes mellitus • Acute intermittent porphyria
Others		• Cyclical vomiting • Toxin ingestion

Box 9.4.1: Features indicating organic causes.

- Persistent forceful vomiting
- Abdominal distension
- Palpable mass/abdomen or visible peristalsis
- Failure to gain weight/loss of weight
- Altered sensorium/failure to accept/demand feeds
- Bulging fontanels/persistent headache
- Sudden onset in a well-child/vomiting in an ill child with fever
- Persistent irritability in an infant with vomiting
- Persistent copious bilious vomiting

- Vomiting due to benign nonorganic causes does not lead to significant dehydration or weight loss.
- If a behavioral element is present, nonorganic causes can be considered.
- Remember that parental perception of how sick their child is in between episodes of vomiting helps us to determine the seriousness of the illness and the measures to be adopted.

The clinical features that indicate common organic causes of vomiting are given in **Box 9.4.1**.

INVESTIGATIONS

The history, age of the child, and the clinical features on presentation most often guide the appropriate investigations to be done. These include:

- Urine for evidence of infection (pus cells, granular casts, bacteria, Gram stain, culture, and sensitivity), proteinuria, and abnormal metabolites.
- Blood for evidence of systemic infection [leukocytosis, toxic granules, band forms, C-reactive protein (CRP), appropriate cultures, etc.].
- Liver function tests.
- Renal function tests, electrolyte studies, and metabolic screening tests (e.g. lactate, organic acids, ammonia, etc.).
- Stool for blood, pus cells, evidence of parasitic infestations.
- Radiological studies: Plain and contrast X-rays of abdomen, ultrasound or endoscopy.
- Lumbar puncture and CSF analysis in children with clinically suspected intracranial infection.
- CT or MRI scans of skull and/or sinuses or abdomen as and when indicated.

MANAGEMENT

The steps of management include recognition and treatment of the primary causes of vomiting in addition to symptomatic therapy and correction of dehydration **(Flowchart 9.4.2)**. Symptomatic treatment includes stomach wash in neonates and infants, with holding oral fluids for a few hours and gradually restarting in sips. If a child is persistently vomiting, dehydrated or has electrolyte imbalances, IV fluids are indicated. The preferred fluid is normal saline.

Vomiting due to simple gastroenteritis is relieved by a single dose of antiemetic. It is always prudent to remember that organic causes of vomiting do not satisfactorily respond despite adequate doses of antiemetics. In clinical practice, hasty use of an antiemetic without definite diagnosis of the cause has to be avoided. Antiemetics like metoclopramide or domperidone hasten stomach emptying and are useful if used judiciously. Ondansetron, a serotonin antagonist, is effective in the treatment of chemotherapy-induced as well as in managing refractory causes of vomiting.

CYCLIC VOMITING SYNDROME

Typically cyclic vomiting syndrome (CVS) is seen in schoolgoing children (4–18 years of age) presenting with severe, periodic, discrete, stereotypical, short term, early morning or nocturnal, self-limiting episodes with abdominal pain with high intense retch and apprehension. In 70–80%, a uniform symptom-free interval of 4 weeks in children and 3 months in adults is noted. Associated headache, sometimes with family history of migraine gives a clue for diagnosis.

Alarm features are absent except dehydration needing IV fluids.

Flowchart 9.4.2: Management of vomiting in children.

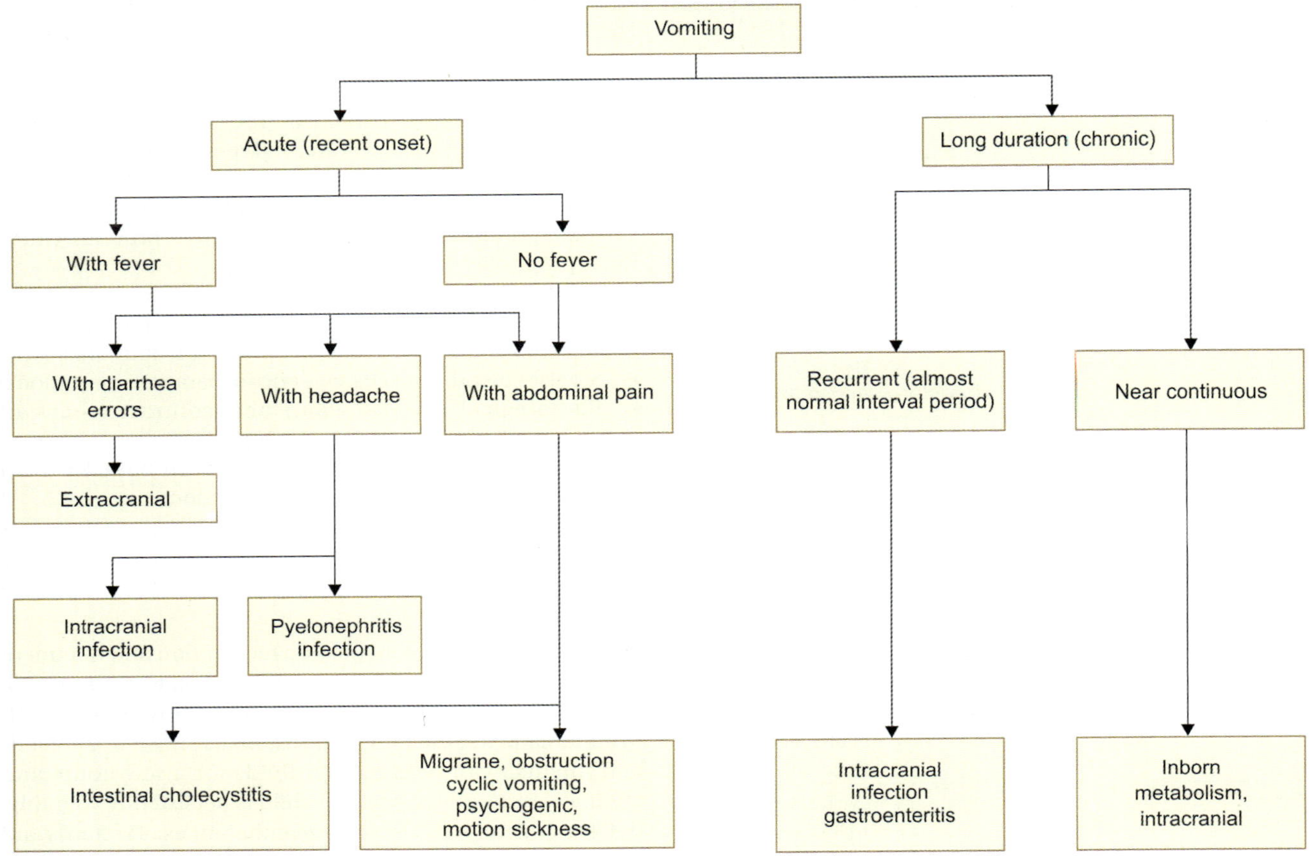

Diagnosis

It is mainly clinical with high degree of suspicion especially when there are no positive findings in physical examination and by exclusion. CVS needs to be differentiated from chronic vomiting **(Table 9.4.3)**, gastroparesis and intestinal pseudo-obstruction.

Management

Cyclic vomiting syndrome was previously thought to be a migraine variant (because of positive family history and response to antimigraine treatment), but the current view is that both are separate clinical entities. Treatment of CVS consists of rest, IV rehydration with dextrose saline administration and ondansetron, and preventers such as amitriptyline and cyproheptadine.

RECURRENT VOMITING

Common causes of recurrent vomiting in children include gastroesophageal reflux (GER) or GERD and functional vomiting due to CVS. Other causes include following chemotherapy, intracranial space occupying lesions (SOL), anatomic obstruction, metabolic causes, psychogenic, and organic causes especially of pancreatic and renal etiology. In adolescence GERD, functional causes especially migraine, CVS, intracranial SOL, and psychogenic vomiting are the leading causes.

Management depends upon the cause. It is important first to assess the hydration status and attend to life-threatening complications before going in for specific investigations for etiology. Always ascertain whether the vomitus is bilious, especially copious as in GI obstruction, bloody or contaminated with blood.

GASTROESOPHAGEAL REFLUX

Gastroesophageal reflux is one of the common causes of chronic abdominal pain in children with increasing incidence (1–8%). Children often suffer from involuntary passage of gastric contents into esophagus.

Pathological GER is GERD characterized by alarm symptoms like irritability, abdominal colic, epigastric or retrosternal burning pain, failure to thrive, GI bleed, dysphagia

Table 9.4.3: Differential diagnosis of cyclic vomiting and chronic.

Cyclic vomiting syndrome	***Chronic vomiting***
High intensity	Low intensity
Low frequency	High frequency
Very high need for IVF and rehydration	Not often required
Family history of migraine +ve (5 fold)	Low
Migraine symptoms +ve with triggers	Nil
Evaluation of lesions outside gut	Gut-peptic esophagitis

(IVF: intravenous fluid)

or odynophagia, belching, apnea, satiation, extraesophageal manifestations such as globus, throat clearing, recurrent aspirations, nocturnal cough or wheeze, dental erosions, and caries of teeth.

Regurgitation with abnormal posturing in neonates and very young infants is Sandifer syndrome.

The high-risk group includes children with neurological abnormalities, obesity, transient lower esophageal sphincter (LES) relaxations (TLESR), asthma, and those with nocturnal refluxing.

Clinically regurgitation of milk lasts up to 3–4 months of life and many get over it by 12–24 months. Chronic untreated esophagitis is rare and can result in strictures, Barret's esophagus, and adenocarcinoma in adults.

Diagnostic modalities include barium swallow, which has low sensitivity and specificity, 24-hour ambulatory esophageal pH monitoring (which however cannot detect nonacid reflux), and nuclear scintigraphy (99mTc milk scan). These are especially useful in children with GERD-associated asthma or pneumonia. Upper GI endoscopy grading and biopsy are useful for Barret's esophagus. Other special tests such as esophageal manometry and impedance for bolus nonacid reflux are done depending on specific situations.

Management Outlines of Gastroesophageal Reflux and Gastroesophageal Reflux Disease

- Physiological GER in infants, being a benign condition, needs often lifestyle modifications (LSM) like positioning (head up prone position at 45° angle), small, frequent, thick feeds; and in severe cases nasogastric drip feeds, addition of rice cereal and prokinetics (e.g. domperidone).
- Acid inhibitors like ranitidine 3–5 mg/kg/dose twice or thrice daily along with LSM for nonerosive reflux.
- Proton pump inhibitors (PPI) 1 mg/kg/day 1 hour before breakfast along with LSM for relief of symptoms of erosive esophagitis and healing are recommended.
- Barrier agents like sucralfate and alginates may give symptomatic relief.
- Antacids are outdated in view of better and effective drugs being available.
- Prokinetic drugs like levosulpiride, cinitapride are useful in adolescents and adults only.
- Extraesophageal manifestations of GERD need specific tests to confirm the etiology and more aggressive treatment with twice daily long-term PPI (for at least 3 months) and follow-up.
- Indications for surgery include refractoriness to adequate medical treatment, life-threatening complications like aspiration pneumonia, failure to thrive, dysphagia, odynophagia, hematemesis, anemia, and rarely Barrett's ulcer especially in adolescents. In impaired neurodevelopmental children, Nissen fundoplication laparoscopic or endoscopic techniques are popular modalities of treatment.

BIBLIOGRAPHY

1. Anderson CM, Burke V, Gracey M. Pediatric Gastroenterology, 2nd edition. Oxford: Blackwell Scientific Publication; 1987. p. 86.
2. Flake ZA, Scalley RD, Bailey AG. Practical selection of antiemetics. Am Fam Physician. 2004;69:1169-74, 1176.
3. Graef JW. Manual of Pediatric Therapeutics, 4th edition. Boston: Little Brown Company; 1988. pp. 33-34.
4. Illingworth RS (Ed). Common Symptoms of Disease in Children, 9th edition. Oxford: Blackwell Scientific Publication; 1998. pp. 69-82.
5. Indian Academy of Pediatrics. Vomiting: In: Rapid Approach to Common Symptoms-Standardization of Pediatric Office Practice; 2005. pp. 51-53.
6. Kliegman RM, Behrman RE, Jenson HB, et al. (Eds). Nelson's Textbook of Pediatrics, 19th edition. Philadelphia: Saunders Elsevier; 2004. pp. 1199-200.
7. McIntosh N, Helms P, Symth R, et al. (Eds). Forfar and Arneil's Textbook of Pediatrics, 7th edition. Edinburgh: Churchill Livingstone; 2008. pp. 658-63.
8. Rudolph AM, Hoffmann JIE, Rudolph CD (Eds). Approach to a child with acute, chronic or cyclic vomiting. In: Rudolph's Pediatrics, 20th edition. USA: Prentice Hall International Inc; 1991;(2):1523-24.

9.5 Parasitic Bowel Disease

BD Gupta

DEFINITION

A parasite is an organism that grows, feeds and is sheltered by or within a different organism while contributing nothing to survival of its host. The only possible exception is that the intestinal parasites may have some protective role on inflammatory bowel disease in human host. Unlike protozoa, most helminths do not multiply within the human body, except *Strongyloides stercoralis.*

EPIDEMIOLOGY

Intestinal parasitic infestation is more common in developing countries, though worldwide the vulnerable groups are children of both urban poor and rural population. Parasitic infestation is seen in both asymptomatic and symptomatic children in a hospital-based study. A study on rural and urban school children showed parasitic infestation rate of 91% and 33%, respectively. In one study, a single intestinal parasitic infestation was present in 65.7% out of which 48% were helminthic and 19.3% were protozoan. Multiple intestinal parasitic infestations were observed in 34.2% among which protozoa were 4.2%, helminths 8.5%, and both were present in 25.9% of children. Among the helminths, hookworm was present in 28%, *Ascaris lumbricoides* in 20.1%, *Enterobius vermicularis* in 16.1%, *Trichuris trichiura* in 6.3%, and *Taenia* in 3.3% of children while among the protozoa, *Entamoeba histolytica* was present in 14.8%, *Giardia* in 6.3%, and others in 2.8% of children.

Most often the larva or ova of intestinal parasites are passed intermittently in stools and hence repeated examination of fresh stool is recommended for better yield rate especially in immune-deficient children when we screen them for parasites causing diarrhea such as *Giardia lamblia, Cryptosporidium, S. stercoralis* and so on.

CLASSIFICATION

Parasitic bowel diseases are a group of infectious diseases due to protozoa and helminths and are a major cause of morbidity in infants and children in many parts of the world.

Parasitic bowel diseases may be classified according to their etiological agents as follows:

- *Protozoan diseases:* Due to *E. histolytica, G. lamblia, Balantidium coli, Cryptosporidium parvum, Blastocystis hominis, Isospora belli, Cyclospora cayetanensis,* and Microsporidia.
- *Helminthic diseases:* Due to
  - *Nematodes: Ascaris lumbricoides, E. vermicularis,* hookworms, i.e. *Ancylostoma duodenale* and *Necator americanus, Trichinella spiralis,* and *T. trichiura.*
  - *Trematodes: Fasciolopsis buski, Nanophyetus salmincola,* and *Heterophyes heterophyes.*
  - *Cestodes: Taenia solium, Taenia saginata, Diphyllobothrium latum, Hymenolepis nana,* and *Echinococcus granulosus.*

ETIOPATHOGENESIS

Parasitic bowel diseases are endemic in areas of world with poor levels of sanitation and low socioeconomic standards. Two distinct modes of transmission are known, namely feco-oral route and cutaneous route.

1. Protozoa like *E. histolytica, G. lamblia, and B. coli* infect humans by ingestion of cysts while nematodes like *A. lumbricoides, T. trichiura, E. vermicularis,* and cestodes like *T. saginata, T. solium,* and *D. latum* spread by ingestion of contaminated food and water with eggs of respective parasites.
2. Hookworms like *A. duodenale* and *N. americanus* enter the human body through skin penetration by their larvae. These larvae undergo extraintestinal migration through the venous circulation and lungs before they are swallowed to reach intestines.

Various parasites localize themselves at various sites in small as well as large intestine as per their suitable environment, e.g. *E. histolytica* dwell in colon, *G. lamblia* colonize in the lumen of duodenum and proximal jejunum, *B. coli* infests the large intestine, *A. lumbricoides* in small intestine, *T. trichiura* in cecum and ascending colon, and *E. vermicularis* typically inhabits cecum, appendix, and adjacent areas of ileum and ascending colon.

Various parasites cause symptoms due to invasion (*E. histolytica*), obstruction (*A. lumbricoides*), reduced absorptive surface (*G. lamblia*), and blood loss (hookworms).

It has been observed that parasitic bowel diseases have a role in prevention of inflammatory bowel diseases (IBD) like Crohn's disease, which are most prevalent in highly industrialized countries with temperate climate and occur rarely in tropical third world countries with poor environmental sanitation. Many helminths live within and migrate through human gut and interact with the mucosal immune system. The host mounts a mucosal response including Th2 cytokine production limiting helminthic colonization, as helminths and their eggs are probably most potent stimulus of mucosal Th2 response. This may modulate immune reaction to parasitic, bacterial, and viral infections. Perhaps, failure to acquire these parasites and experience mucosal Th2 conditioning predisposes to Crohn's disease and celiac disease, which is an overtly active Th1 inflammation. In some countries, the patient intensely infects them with worms like *N. americanus* and this is considered as a possible treatment for inflammatory bowel disease such as celiac disease. On the other hand, celiac disease may be aggravated by coexistent *G. lamblia* infestation and the disease may improve after treatment of giardiasis.

CLINICAL FEATURES

Parasitic bowel disease is associated with wide variety of clinical manifestations ranging from asymptomatic carrier stage to various intestinal and extraintestinal manifestations. The clinical features depend largely on the parasite, site of involvement, mechanical factors, and interference with host's nutrition.

General Symptoms

Most of parasites present with pain abdomen and diarrhea, which can be acute, chronic or recurrent; bloody or nonbloody; with or without tenesmus, abdominal cramps, bloating, and flatulence. Other symptoms include nausea, vomiting, anorexia, weight loss, fever, abdominal distension, malaise, myalgia, and headache.

Various other clinical features caused by different parasites are summarized in **Table 9.5.1**.

Table 9.5.1: Clinical manifestations.

Clinical manifestation	*Parasitic bowel disease(s)*
Nutritional deficiency (Vitamin A deficiency)	Ascariasis, giardiasis, and infection by intestinal flukes
Anemia	
Iron deficiency	Hookworm disease
B_{12} or folic acid deficiency	*Diphyllobothrium latum* (Diphyllobothriasis), trichuriasis
Malabsorption syndrome	Giardiasis, ascariasis, hookworm disease, and infestation by intestinal flukes
Weight loss	Giardiasis, hookworm disease, diphyllobothriasis, and spore-forming protozoa like cryptosporidiasis, isosporiasis, and cyclosporiasis
Intestinal obstruction	Ascariasis, teniasis
Rectal prolapse	Giardiasis, trichuriasis
Extraintestinal involvement	
Liver	Amebiasis, intestinal flukes
Muscles	Trichinosis, flukes, spore-forming protozoa, e.g. microsporidia
Skin	Cutaneous larva migrans—hookworm, *Strongyloides stercoralis*
Brain	Amebiasis, trichinosis, microsporidiosis, teniasis—neurocysticercosis
Lungs	Amebiasis, ascariasis, hookworm disease *S. stercoralis*
Immunodeficiency states	*Associated parasites: Cryptosporidium parvum, Isospora belli, Cyclospora cayetanensis*, microsporidium (AIDS), giardiasis, amebiasis

LABORATORY DIAGNOSIS

Parasitic bowel diseases can be diagnosed by examination of stool samples under direct microscopy. Repeated fresh samples (3 times) may be required to reach diagnosis of clinically suspected organisms. The stool examination may be supported by blood examination for evidence of eosinophilia and various serological tests specifically designed for the organism under consideration. Stool examination along with endoscopically obtained smears and tissue biopsy helps a lot in diagnosis of specific parasitic infestation. Ideally fresh stools should be examined within 30 minutes of passage for evidence of trophozoites/cysts in case of *E. histolytica* or *G. lamblia*. Stool samples preserved in polyvinyl alcohol helps in diagnosis of these organisms. Serological tests like indirect hemagglutination are available for *E. histolytica*. *Enterotest* on duodenal fluid for giardiasis is another alternative. Blood enzyme immunoassay (EIA) or direct fluorescent antibody test for *Giardia* antigen are now the tests of choice for giardiasis in most situations.

Stool examination and demonstration of oocysts helps in diagnosis of spore forming intestinal protozoa like *Cryptosporidium, Isospora, Cyclospora*, etc. Other tests for these parasites are EIA, indirect immunofluorescence and polymerase chain reaction (PCR). Multiplex PCR testing for multiple parasitic pathogens may become a viable option for testing in future.

Demonstration of eggs of helminths in stool is the mainstay of diagnosis of most of parasites. For ascariasis, Kato's thick smear examination of stool is easy and sensitive method. Fertilized eggs signify infection with both male and female worms, while unfertilized eggs show infection with female worm only. Enterobiasis can be diagnosed by examining cellophane tape imprint from perianal area. For trichinosis, serologic tests like bentonite flocculation test, muscle biopsy, and levels of muscle enzymes like creatine kinase and lactic dehydrogenase (LDH) help in diagnosis.

MANAGEMENT

Treatment of various parasitic infestations is summarized in **Table 9.5.2**.

PREVENTION AND CONTROL

Parasitic bowel diseases essentially are much more prevalent in areas of poor sanitation and environmental conditions. Hence, these diseases can be prevented by following certain measures, viz. safe disposal of human excreta, safe water supply, proper food hygiene, personal and community

Table 9.5.2: Common parasitic infections and their treatment.

Etiological agent	*Major clinical features*	*Treatment*	*Alternative Drug(s)*
Entamoeba histolytica	• Diarrhea • Dysentery • Liver abscess	• Metronidazole 35–50 mg/kg/day orally in 3 doses for 10 days • Diloxanide furoate 20 mg/kg/day orally in 3 doses for 10 days Either is followed by: • Idoquinon 30–40 mg/kg/day PO in 3 doses for 20 days • Paromomycin 25–35 mg/kg/day PO in 3 doses for 7 days	• Ornidazole 30–50 mg/kg/day orally in two doses for 5 days • Nitazoxanide 7.5 mg/kg twice daily for 3 days
Giardia lamblia	• Diarrhea • Malabsorption	• Metronidazole 5–10 mg/kg tid orally for 5 days • Nitazoxanide 7.5 mg/kg twice daily for 3 days	• Quinacrine 2 mg/kg tid orally for 5 days • Albendazole 400 mg OD for 5 days • Tinidazole 50 mg/kg (maximum two gram) once • Furazolidone 6 mg/kg/day Q 6hrs for 10 days • Paromomycin 25–30 mg/kg/day PO in 3 doses for 7 days
Balantidium coli	• Diarrhea • Dysentery • Painful abdomen	Metronidazole 45 mg/kg/day q 8 hours orally for 5 days	• Tetracycline 40 mg/kg (maximum 2 g) q 6 hours for 10 days (>8 years) • Iodoquinol 40 mg/kg/day q 8 hours PO (20 days)
Cryptosporidium	• Severe diarrhea with malabsorption in AIDS patients	Nitazoxanide 100 mg bid orally for 3 days (1–3 years); 200 mg bid for three days (4–11 years)	• Paromomycin 25–35 mg/kg/day in 3 doses for 7 days • Azithromycin 10–15 mg/kg/day orally for 4 weeks followed by Paromomycin 25–35 mg/kg/day in two doses orally for 8 weeks
Isospora belli	• Severe diarrhea with malabsorption in AIDS patients	Trimethoprim 5 mg/kg/dose + sulfamethoxazole 25 mg/kg/dose 8 hourly for 10 days; then bid for 3 weeks	• Ciprofloxacin or pyrimethamine ± folinic acid in sulfa-intolerant patients
Cyclospora	• Severe diarrhea with malabsorption in AIDS patients	Trimethoprim 5 mg/kg/dose + sulfamethoxazole 25 mg/kg/dose bid orally for 7 days	Ciprofloxacin (adults)
Microsporidium	• Severe diarrhea with malabsorption in AIDS patients	Albendazole 400 mg bid for 3 weeks	Nitazoxanide 7.5 mg/kg bid for 3 days Atovaquone
Ascaris lumbricoides	• Abdominal pain • Cough • Nausea	• Albendazole 400 mg orally once • Mebendazole 100 mg bid orally for 3 days or 500 mg once • Pyrantel pamoate 11 mg/kg once	• Piperazine citrate 75 mg/kg per day for two days, 65 mg/kg/dose 12 hourly for six doses • Ivermectin 200 μg/kg/day od orally for 1–2 days
Strongyloides stercoralis	• Loeffler like syndrome • Abdominal pain • Diarrhea • Malabsorption	Ivermectin 200 μg/kg/day once orally for 1–2 days	• Thiabendazole 50 mg/kg bid orally for 2 days • Albendazole 400 mg bid for 7 days

Contd...

Contd...

Etiological agent	*Major clinical features*	*Treatment*	*Alternative Drug(s)*
Enterobius vermicularis	• Pruritus ani • Sleeplessness	• Pyrantel pamoate 11 mg/kg once (max 1 g) • Mebendazole 100 mg bid PO for 3 days • Albendazole 400 mg once (Therapy to be repeated after 2 weeks)	Ivermectin 200 μg/kg/day orally for 1–2 days
Trichuris trichiura	• Chronic dysentery • Rectal prolapse • Anemia	Mebendazole 100 mg bid orally for 3 days or 500 mg once	• Albendazole 400 mg once for 3 days • Ivermectin 200 μg per kg daily for 3 days
Hookworm infection (Ancylostoma duodenale, Necator americanus)	• Chronic dysentery • Rectal prolapse • Anemia	• Albendazole 400 mg/day orally once • Mebendazole 100 mg bid for 3 days	Pyrantel pamoate 11 mg/kg/day (maximum 1 g) once for 3 days
Hymenolepis nana	• Abdominal pain • Loss of appetite • Diarrhea • Anemia • Hypoalbuminemia	• Praziquantel 25 mg/kg orally once (if available) • Nitazoxanide 7.5 mg/kg bid orally for 3 days	Albendazole 400 mg/day for 3 days Niclosamide 11–34 kg–1 g PO on day 1 then 500 mg PO for 6 days >34 kg–1.5 g PO on day 1 and then 1 g/day PO for 6 days
Trichinella spiralis	• Abdominal pain • Discomfort	• Mebendazole 200–400 mg tid orally for 3 days, then 400–500 mg tid for 10 days • Steroids to be given for severe symptoms	Albendazole 400 mg bid orally for 8–14 days
Diphyllobothrium latum	• Diarrhea • Fever • Periorbital edema • Myalgia • Megaloblastic anemia • Leukopenia • Thrombocytopenia	Praziquantel 5–10 mg/kg orally once	Niclosamide 50 mg/kg once

hygiene, health education, and early diagnosis and treatment of symptomatic and asymptomatic cases.

BIBLIOGRAPHY

1. Chen XM, Keithly JS, Paya CV, et al. Cryptosporidiasis. N Engl J Med. 2002;346:1723-31.
2. Conteas CN, Berlin OG, Ash LR, et al. Therapy for human gastrointestinal microsporidiasis. Am J Trop Med Hyg. 2000;63:121-7.
3. Cresese J, Gaze ST, Loukas A. Changed gluten immunity in celiac disease by *Necator americanus* provides new insights into autoimmunity. Int J Parasitol. 2013;43:275-82.
4. Elliott DE, Urban JF JR, Argo CK, et al. Does the failure to acquire helminthic parasites predispose to Crohn's disease. FASEB J. 2000;14:1848-55.
5. Kliegman RM, Stanton BF, Geme III JW, et al. (Eds). Infectious diseases. In: Nelson Textbook of Pediatrics, 19th edition. New Delhi: Reeds Elsevier First Asian Edition; 2016. pp. 1673-756.
6. Mitch L. (2016). Parasitic worms may prevent Crohn's disease by altering bacterial balance. [online] Available from: www.sciencemag.org/news/2016/04/parasitic-worms-may-prevent-crohn-s-disease-altering-bacterial-balance. [Accessed November, 2018].
7. Mohammadi R, Hosseini-Safa A, Ehsani Ardakani MJ, et al. The relationship between intestinal parasites and some immune-mediated intestinal conditions. Gastroenterol Hepatol Bed Bench. 2015;8(2):123-31.
8. Park K. Intestinal infections. In: Park K (Ed). Park's Textbook of Preventive and Social Medicine, 21st edition. Jabalpur: Banarsidas Bhanot; 2015. pp. 202-45.
9. Tripathi KD. Antiamoebic and other antiprotozoal drugs and anthelmintic drugs. In: Tripathi KD (Ed). Essentials of Medical Pharmacology, 6th edition. New Delhi: Jaypee Brothers Medical Publishers (P) Ltd; 2010. pp. 797-816.
10. Vohra P. Intestinal parasites in children. In: Bavdekar A, Mathai J, Sathiyasekaran M, Yachha SK, (Eds). IAP Specialty Series on Pediatric Gastroenterology, Vol. 9. New Delhi: Jaypee Brothers Medical Publishers (P) Ltd; 2008. pp. 107-24.

9.6 Gastrointestinal Bleeding

Neelam Mohan

INTRODUCTION

Gastrointestinal (GI) bleeding could result from bleeding from esophagus to anus. It has been divided into upper, middle, and lower depending on the site of bleeding. GI bleeding may be overt or obscure. Overt bleeding may present as hematemesis, melenemesis, melena, or hematochezia. Obscure GI bleed is defined as bleeding from GIT that persists or recurs without any obvious etiology after a diagnostic endoscopy. It accounts for around 5% of all GI bleeds. Occult bleeding may present as positive fecal occult blood test (e.g. guaiac testing), laboratory evidence of anemia, and iron deficiency, or symptoms of anemia or blood loss (e.g. fatigue, light headedness, syncope, dyspnea, and angina).

DEFINITIONS

- *Upper GI bleeding* is defined as bleeding from a source in the esophagus, stomach, or duodenum proximal to the duodenojejunal junction (ligament of Treitz).
- *Mid-GI bleeding*: GI bleeding occurs between ampulla of Vater and terminal ileum.
- *Lower GI bleeding*: Refers to colonic GI bleeds.
- *Obscure GI bleeding* is overt GI bleeding from remote sites where both upper GI endoscopy and ileocolonoscopy do not reveal the cause for GI bleeding.
- *Spurious hematemesis* can present as swallowed blood in a neonate or the source can be from oral cavity or as part of malingering/attention seeking ill health behavior.
- *Major GI bleeding is* alarming with overt clots of blood, tarry stools (melena) with over 100 mL of bleeding, and postural hypotension/shock.
- *Hematemesis*: Vomiting of fresh blood.
- *Melenemesis*: Vomiting of altered blood.
- *Melena*: Passage of black, tarry, sticky, offensive, and loose stools.
- *Hematochezia*: Passage of fresh blood in stool. It is most commonly associated with a colonic source of bleeding. If hematochezia is from an upper GI site, it reflects major bleeding with rapid transit which present with hemodynamic instability and increased mortality.

EPIDEMIOLOGY

Upper GI bleed is an indication for upper GI endoscopy in 5% of children and 5% of total GI bleeding may present as obscure GI bleeding. Need for hospitalization in patients with LGI bleed is only one-third of upper GI bleeding patients. Etiological spectrum varies in neonates, infants, and older children **(Table 9.6.1)**. A meticulous history, physical examination, and step-by-step evaluation is necessary in a tertiary care center preferably by trained pediatric gastroenterologist along with team of imaging, nuclear medicine, intervention specialists, and sometimes surgeons.

ETIOLOGY

Tables 9.6.1 to 9.6.3 list the causes of GI bleeding from upper and lower GI tract in children.

Table 9.6.1: Causes of upper gastrointestinal bleed.

Newborn	*Infant*	*Children*
• Swallowed maternal blood • Hemorrhagic disease of newborn • Stress gastritis • Cow's milk protein allergy • Acid peptic disease • Vascular anomaly • Coagulopathy	• Stress ulcer/gastritis • Acid-peptic disease • Mallory-Weiss tear • Vascular anomaly • Duplication cyst • Varices • Webs • Intestinal obstruction	• Mallory-Weiss tear • GERD/acid-peptic disease • Varices • Stress ulcer/erosive gastritis • Caustic injury • Foreign body • Vasculitis—HSP • Crohn's disease • Intestinal obstruction • Dieulafoy lesion • Hemobilia • Pancreatic pseudoaneurysm

(GERD: gastroesophageal reflux disease; HSP: Henoch-Schönlein purpura)

Table 9.6.2: Common causes of rectal bleeding in children.

Infant	*Older child*
• Anal fissure • Milk protein intolerance • Necrotizing enterocolitis • Swallowed maternal blood • Vitamin K deficiency	• Anal fissure • Intussusception • Infectious enterocolitis* • Amebiasis • Meckel diverticulum • Juvenile polyp

*Shigella; *E. coli*; *Cl. difficile*; Salmonellosis.

Table 9.6.3: Less common causes of rectal bleeding in children.

Infant	*Older child*
• Vascular lesions • Bleeding diathesis • Hirschsprung enterocolitis • Meckel diverticulum • Malrotation with volvulus • Intestinal duplication • Intussusception	• Inflammatory bowel disease • Ischemic/collagenous colitis • Vascular malformations • Intestinal duplication • Bleeding diathesis • Henoch-Schönlein purpura • Hemolytic uremic syndrome • Hemorrhoids, rectal varices • Perianal cellulitis • Rectal prolapse • Solitary rectal ulcer • Hereditary polyposis syndrome • Sexual abuse and anorectal trauma • Eosinophilic proctocolitis • Nodular lymphoid hyperplasia

Mallory-Weiss Tears

It occurs at the gastroesophageal (GE) junction primarily on the gastric side, resulting, from retching or coughing followed by hematemesis. It is less frequently seen with children.

Hemorrhagic and Erosive Gastropathy

It refers to subepithelial hemorrhage and erosions. These are restricted to the mucosa, where no large blood vessels are present and therefore do not cause major bleeding. Erosions are reported in around 2–10% of patients with upper GI bleeding. The most common causes are nonsteroidal anti-inflammatory drug (NSAID) use and stress. Prevalence in neonatal intensive care unit (NICU) is around 44% but only 5% are clinically significant.

Peptic Ulcer

Incidence of bleeding due to NSAID-induced erosive gastritis is common but bleeding ulcers appears to be rare compared to adults. Approximately one-third of patients found to have an ulcer with active bleeding or a nonbleeding visible vessel will have further bleeding requiring surgery if treated expectantly. These patients should receive endoscopic therapy and IV infusion of proton pump inhibitor (PPI). In less than 10 years of age, around 77% of the peptic ulcer disease (PUD) is in duodenum. Hematemesis and perforation are more in secondary PUD. Factors associated with PUD include:

- *Primary*: Related to *Helicobacter pylori*, bile reflux
- *Secondary*: Related to
  - NSAID intake
  - *Stress:* Shock, ischemia
  - Drugs
  - Corrosives
  - Ménétrier disease
  - Zollinger-Ellison syndrome.

Variceal Bleeding

In India, portal hypertension in children is caused more often by extrahepatic portal vein obstruction [EHPVO (68–76%)], cirrhosis (24–28%); and infrequently due to congenital hepatic fibrosis (3%), noncirrhotic portal fibrosis, and Budd-Chiari syndrome. In portal hypertension, there are several sites where natural porto-systemic shunts appear **(Table 9.6.4)**, the most common sites are esophagus, stomach, and rectum. EHPVO is also the most common cause of GI bleeding in children (70%). Predictors of variceal bleed include large varices and presence of red color signs (red wale marking, diffuse redness, and hematocystic malformation).

Gastric varices are found most commonly with splenic vein thrombosis or after endoscopic sclerotherapy (EST) of esophageal varices.

Extrahepatic Portal Vein Obstruction and Portal Hypertension

The mean age of presentation is 5–6 years. In India, 83% of patients with EHPVO present with upper GI bleeding before

Table 9.6.4: Conn's classification of esophageal varices.

Grade 1	On inspiration only	Can be effaced	Straight	Red
Grade 2	Both on inspiration and expiration	Cannot be effaced	Straight	Red
Grade 3	Projecting into lumen <50%, wavy	Cannot be effaced	Straight	Blue
Grade 4	Projecting into lumen more than 50% and coiled	Tense	Tortuous	Blue

the age of 20 years. Hematemesis with or without melena is the most common presentation; only 8–10% patients may not bleed. Upper GI bleeding is massive and recurrent, but risk of rebleeding after major episode is less than in cirrhosis; though fairly uniform and occurs once in every 2 years. The average number of bleed is 2.5–5 episodes per patient.

Firm splenomegaly is almost universal in patient with EHPVO. It can be present as early as 1 month of age and is usually seen before 3 years of age. Splenomegaly is mild (<6 cm) in 42%, moderate (6–10 cm) in 40%, and massive (>10 cm) in 18%. Children with EHPVO do not grow as much as their healthysiblings.

Variceal bleeding in EHPVO is well tolerated with reference to the liver function, viz. following the GI variceal bleeding, they usually do not develop encephalopathy even with massive GI bleed and they have normal liver functions. They may develop transient ascites following major bleeding episode. Persistent or massive ascites in children with EHPVO should make one doubt about the diagnosis or suggest the possibility of presence of coexistent cirrhosis. Recurrent GI bleeding in EHPVO decreases with age. Abdominal ultrasonography and Doppler study are diagnostic.

In portal hypertension occurring secondary to chronic liver disease (CLD) the presentation is usually dominated by manifestations of primary disease. The major causes in children are viral hepatitis, neonatal cholestasis, autoimmune liver disease, metabolic liver disease like Wilson's disease, glycogen storage disease, etc.

Children with EHPVO when compared to CLD, have more chances of UGI bleed, more previous bleeding episodes, long duration of symptoms and absence of jaundice, preservation of liver function, and less Hb value.

Esophageal varices can be classified as small (<5 mm), medium (5–10 mm), or large (>10 mm) according to size or graded by endoscopy according to Conn's classification **(Table 9.6.4)**.

Gastric varices are found most commonly with splenic vein thrombosis or after EST of esophageal varices. It can be further classified **(Fig. 9.6.1)** endoscopically according to location (Sarin Classification).

- *Gastroesophageal varices (GOV)*: Gastric varices continuing with esophageal varices
  - *GOV1*: Extending towards lesser curvature
  - *GOV2*: Extending towards fundus
- Isolated gastric varices (IGV): Gastric varices discontinuous with esophageal varices or present in absence of esophageal varices
  - *IGV1*: Fundal varices, tortuous, nodular
  - *IGV2*: Ectopic varices (body, antrum, and pylorus).

Ectopic varices account for 5% of all variceal bleed. Duodenum is a common site.

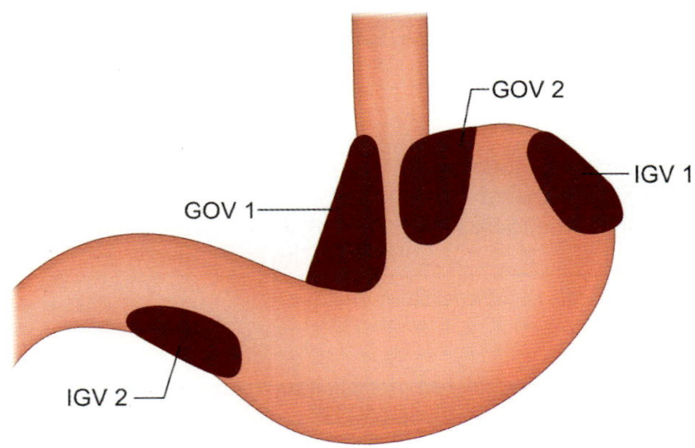

Fig. 9.6.1: Gastric varices (Sarin classification). (GOV: gastroesophageal varices; IGV: isolated gastric varices)

Table 9.6.5: Clinical clues to etiology in a gastrointestinal bleed patient.

Bleeding etiology	*Clinical clues*
Mallory-Weiss tear	Emesis before hematemesis, pain +
Esophageal ulcer	Odynophagia, GERD, H/O pill ingestion
Stress gastritis/PUD	Sick patient in ICU, respiratory failure/NSAID ingestion/pain
Angiodysplasia	Renal failure, hereditary hemorrhagic telangiectasia
Aortoenteric fistula	H/O aortic aneurysm or surgery
CLD	Variceal bleed significant, painless, splenomegaly, jaundice, stigmata of CLD, ascites

(CLD: chronic liver disease; GERD: gastroesophageal reflux disease; NSAID: nonsteroidal anti-inflammatory drug; PUD: peptic ulcer disease)

EVALUATION OF GASTROINTESTINAL BLEEDING

Vital signs include the pulse rate and the blood pressure in lying, sitting and if possible, in standing position for postural hypotension. It is essential to monitor urine output and fluid intake and respiratory rate throughout fluid resuscitation of patients in shock and altered sensorium/coma. Hyperventilation is an early sign of developing acidosis.

Physical examination to evaluate capillary perfusion, skin color for the presence of cyanosis, pulse, blood pressure, respiratory pattern, and level of consciousness should continue on an ongoing basis during active bleeding. Nasogastric aspirations that are grossly blood confirm upper GI sources while a negative aspiration does not rule out.

Some clinical clues to etiology in a GI bleed patient are given in **Table 9.6.5**. Presence of melena followed by any

Flowchart 9.6.1: Approach to etiology for upper gastrointestinal bleed (UGI).

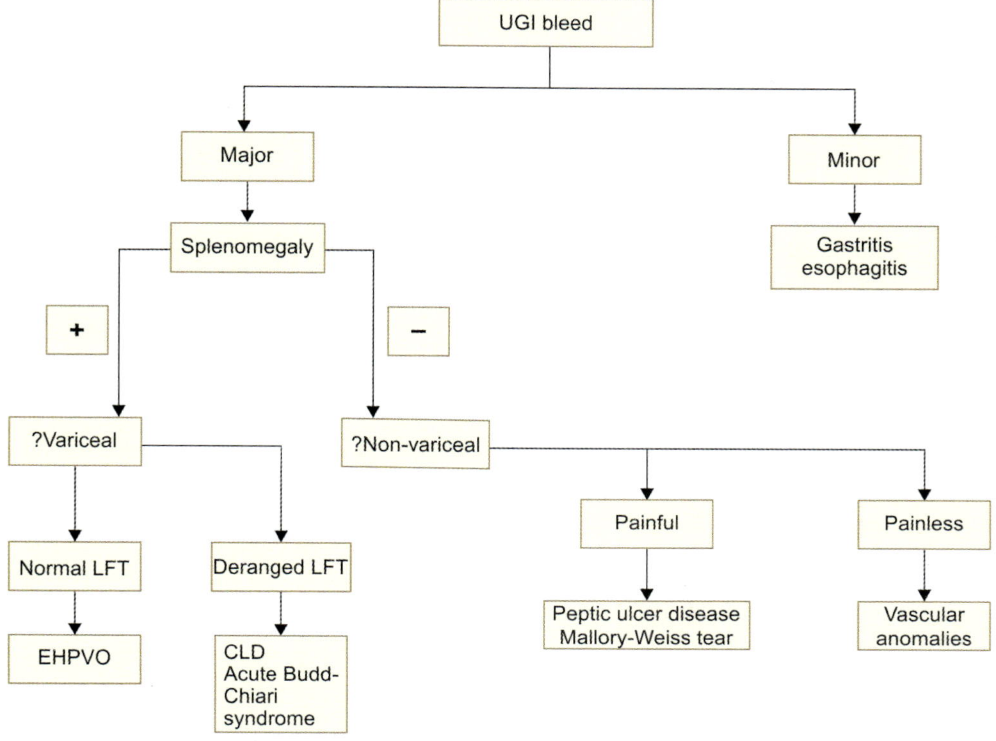

(CLD: chronic liver disease; EHPVO: extrahepatic portal vein obstruction; LFT: liver function test)

bright colored blood in stool indicates rebleed and these patients with melena should be monitored and managed in the pediatric intensive care unit. In patients with smaller amount of doubtful bleed, it is important to first confirm whether it is blood or something else by guaiac test **(Table 9.6.6)**.

Flowchart 9.6.1 provides a schematic approach to the diagnosis of etiology of upper gastrointestinal bleeding (UGIB).

MANAGEMENT

Management includes resuscitation, identification of the cause of bleed, control of bleed, and its prevention **(Box 9.6.1)**.

Box 9.6.1: Treatment goals.

- Immediate assessment of severity and causes
- Establish and maintain the intravascular volume.
- Packed red blood cell transfusion: Maintain Hb > 8–10 g%
- FFP transfusion with INR > 1.5–2 , platelets transfusion if platelet < 50,000/mm^3.
- Labs: Hemogram, LFT, BUN, Creatinine, PT, APTT, USG abdomen—Doppler, Endoscopy.
- Determine source and site of blood loss
- Stop gastrointestinal bleeding
- Prevention of further bleed.

(APTT: activated partial thromboplastin time; BUN: blood urea nitrogen; FFP: fresh frozen plasma; INR: international normalized ratio; LFT: liver function test; PT: prothrombin time; USG: ultrasonography)

Resuscitation

This includes achieving hemodynamic stability and treatment of hypovolemic shock. Adequate IV access should be established and carefully monitor pulse, blood pressure, and central venous pressure. Oxygen is given to counter hypoxia due to acute blood loss. An increase in the pulse rate of more than 20 beats per minute or a decrease in diastolic blood pressure of more than 10 mm Hg or a decrease in systolic of more than 20 mm Hg within 3 minutes of standing, indicates a greater than 20% loss of intravascular volume. As blood loss increases to 20–25%, the pulse rate increases more than 150 beats per minute. When the intravascular volume deficit exceeds 25%, the capillary refill is prolonged as blood is shunted from the skin to the brain and kidneys. Urine output decreases with further compromise and metabolic acidosis result; in short, all features of hypovolemic shock develop. Urine output and fluid intake must be carefully monitored throughout fluid resuscitation in patients with shock. Urine output in children is normally 2–3 mL per kg per hour, and urine output less than

1 mL per kg per hour is indicative of renal hypoperfusion. As blood loss exceeds 40%, compensation fails, pulses are lost, cerebral perfusion decreases, and the patient passes from lethargy to coma. The respiratory rate should also be carefully monitored. Hyperventilation is an early sign of a developing acidosis induced by a decrease in central nervous systems pH.

Physical examination by an experienced observer to evaluate capillary perfusion, skin color for the presence of cyanosis, pulse, blood pressure, respiratory pattern, and level of consciousness should continue on an ongoing basis throughout the hemorrhage to enable rapid recognition of shock. To enhance the ability to anticipate shock, it is helpful if the rate of bleeding is assessed periodically. In UGIB this is best accomplished through lavage of the stomach by means of a nasogastric tube placed in the stomach. Nasogastric aspiration that are grossly bleeding confirm upper GI sources but a negative aspiration does not rule out. Up to 15–18% of patients with UGIB have nonbloody nasogastric aspirate. The amount of blood lost in the stool should also be monitored, estimated, and recorded and any change in color from melena to bright red blood should be noted as a possible sign of increased blood loss and hypovolemic shock. It is prudent that all patients with significant gastrointestinal bleeding be monitored in a pediatric intensive care unit for changes in vital signs and urine output until they are stable and bleeding has ceased. For Calculating Transfusion Requirement - Quantity of Packed red blood cells - [(70 mL/kg × weight in kg) (desired hemoglobin–present hemoglobin)]/23 g hemoglobin per 100 dL of packed red blood cells; rough guideline - 5 mL of packed RBC/kg will raise the Hct. 3 points and Hb. 1g/dL (5:3:1).

Control of Acute Variceal Bleeding

It can be by the following modalities:

Pharmacotherapy

The most widely used agents to stop variceal bleeds are given in **Table 9.6.6**.

Balloon Tamponade

Sengstaken–Blackemore tube (three lumen and two balloons for esophageal and gastric variceal bleeds), Linton-Nachlas tube (three lumen and single balloon more effective for gastric variceal than esophageal bleed), and the Minnesota tube (four lumen and two balloons) are handled by experienced specialists as a lifesaver in active variceal bleeding if emergency sclerotherapy or banding is unavailable or not technically possible because visibility is obscured. In patients with active bleeding, an endotracheal tube should be inserted to protect the airway before attempting to place the esophageal balloon tube. Continued bleeding during balloon tamponade indicates an incorrectly positioned tube and bleeding from another source. After resuscitation, and within 12 hours, the tube is removed and endoscopic treatment repeated.

Endotherapy (Endoscopic Variceal Ligation or Sclerotherapy)

- *Endoscopic variceal ligation*: Using multiband ligator banding has less complications and is more effective than sclerotherapy. However, it is not possible in small children between 2 years and 3 years of age **(Table 9.6.7)**.

Table 9.6.6: Drugs used to stop variceal bleeding.

Drug	*Mechanism of action*	*Dose*	*Comments*
Vasopressin	Potent non-selective vasoconstrictor. Lowers the portal pressure by causing splanchnic arterial vasoconstriction and reducing the splanchnic blood flow to the varices	Given in a bolus of 0.33 U/kg of body weight diluted with 2 mL/kg of 5% dextrose given over a period of 15–20 minutes	Nitroglycerine, a vasodilator, may reduce the cardiac side effects of vasopressin by increasing local concentration of NO and reducing cardiac output
Terlipressin	Synthetic analog of vasopressin acts by immediate vasoconstriction. Its use in children requires further evaluation It is more effective in controlling bleeding (up to 79%) than vasopressin without any adverse side effects	Given as IV injections (2 mg) every 4 hours till bleeding free interval of 24–48 hours is achieved	
Somatostatin	Acts by inhibiting release of several vasodilatory hormones such as glucagon It induces selective splanchnic vasoconstriction	Recommended dosage is 1–3 bolus injections (250 µg/bolus) during first hour of therapy followed by infusion of 250 µg/hour of continuous infusion for 2–5 days	There is lower failure rate and complications in comparison to vasopressin Disadvantage is its short half-life
Octreotide	A synthetic analog of somatostatin with half-life of 90 minutes	1–2 µg/kg over 2–5 min, then 1–2 µg/kg per hour for 5 days	Side-effects are uncommon

Table 9.6.7: Comparison of endoscopic variceal ligation (EVL) and endoscopic sclerotherapy (EST).

	EVL	***EST***
Indications	Large varices, difficult in small children	Any size
Complications	Less (4%)	More (25%)
Rebleeding rate	Low (4%)	More (25%)
Sessions needed	More (17%)	Less (10%)
Recurrence of varices	Increase	IGV and GOV
Gastric varices	Increase	Increase

(GOV: gastroesophageal varices; IGV: isolated gastric varices)

- *Endoscopic sclerotherapy*: Injection of sclerosant into (intravariceal) or around (perivariceal) the varices. Various sclerosants used in esophageal varices are polidocanol, sodium tetradecyl sulfate, absolute alcohol, sodium morrhuate and in bleeding gastric varices, injection of glue (N-butyl-2-cyanoacrylate) is done.
- *Complications of endotherapy:* Fever, chest pain, dysphagia, superficial mucosal ulcerations (6–70%), esophageal perforation, pulmonary complications, and esophageal stricture.

Transjugular Intrahepatic Portosystemic Shunt

Transjugular intrahepatic portosystemic shunt (TIPS) is ideal for patients whose bleeding is not controlled by endoscopy. It is effective only in portal hypertension of hepatic origin and contraindicated in portal vein thrombosis, biliary block, septicemia, and severe hepatic encephalopathy. Complications include thrombosis of stent and encephalopathy.

Indications for Surgery

Failure of medical treatment, hypersplenism, isolated splenic vein thrombosis, patients from remote and underprivileged places, and of rare blood group. Emergency devascularization and esophageal transection (modified Tanner) or elective Warren distal splenorenal shunt or rarely Rex shunt (superior mesenteric vein to left portal vein branch with venous graft) or liver transplantation are useful.

Prophylaxis

For secondary prophylaxis, beta-blockers (propranolol) may be used in a dose of 1–2 mg/kg lowers venous flow, and the portal pressure by decreasing the heart rate by 25% and the blood pressure by 15 mm Hg and causing splanchnic vasoconstriction and decreasing portal venous flow.

Control of Nonvariceal Bleeding

Treatment depends on the cause of the bleeding. Various treatment modalities are H_2 receptor antagonists/PPIs, vasoactive agents, endotherapy including electrothermal agents such as endoclips and argon plasma coagulation **(Table 9.6.8)**.

Identifying the Other Sources of Gastrointestinal Hemorrhage

The other sources can be identified by esophagogastroduodenoscopy, colonoscopy, Meckel's scans (99m-Tc-pertechnetate scan) bleeding isotope scan, angiography, capsule endoscopy, double balloon enteroscopy, imaging, upper GI radiography, and barium enema, and preoperative endoscopy.

- *Endoscopy*: Esophago-gastroduodenoscopy or colonoscopy is very useful to detect esophagitis, Mallory-Weiss tears, varices, gastritis, ulcer, vascular malformations, etc. Bleeding from an ulcer is controlled using injection with adrenaline and recently hemoclips are also available for clipping at the site of vessel bleed at the base of the ulcer.
  Similarly, colonoscopy helps diagnosis and therapy of common causes like polyps and the less common vascular malformations and diagnosis of colitis, inflammatory bowel disease (IBD), solitary rectal ulcer, vascular malformations, etc.
- *Angiography*: It is indicated in active GI bleeding and the rate of bleeding must be at least 0.5 mL/minute. The diagnostic yield of emergency arteriography is low.

Table 9.6.8: Pharmacotherapy.

Drug	***Mechanism of action***	***Dose***	***Comments***
Ranitidine	H_2 receptor antagonist	20–40 mg/kg/day in 2–3 divided doses	
Famotidine	H_2 receptor antagonist	1–2 mg/kg/day in 2 divided doses	
Omeprazole	Proton pump inhibitor	1–3.3 mg/kg/day (<20 kg) 10 mg/day (>20 kg)	Approved for > 2 years old
Esomeprazole	Proton pump inhibitor	0.2–1 mg/kg/day	Approved for > 1 years old
Lansoprazole	Proton pump inhibitor	0.8–4 mg/kg/day (<30 kg) 15 mg/day (>30 kg)	Approved for > 1 years old
Pantoprazole	Proton pump inhibitor	Adult dose—40 mg/day	
Sucralfate	Cytoprotective agent	40–80 mg/kg/day	

Nowadays computed tomography (CT) angiography is preferred and conventional angiography is hardly used.

- *UGI radiology*: Radiographic studies are particularly useful in the diagnosis of esophageal strictures, malrotation of the bowel, or deep ulcerations.
- *Meckels's scan*: Because technetium (Tc) 99m pertechnetate is actively accumulated by cells in gastric mucosa, it can be used to identify the presence of ectopic gastric mucosa in a Meckel's diverticulum or intestinal duplications. More than 90% of bleeding Meckel's diverticula do contain gastric mucosa. A Meckel's scan should be considered whenever significant lower GI has occurred.
- *Bleeding scan*: It is a noninvasive study with a low radiation exposure. Tc sulfur or Tc-pertechnetate-labeled red blood cell scan are used. Tc sulfur red cell scan can detect site of bleeding even when the rate of bleeding is as low as 0.1 mL/minute. However, its half-life is only 2 minutes. Tc-pertechnetate-labeled red blood cell scan can visualize the site of bleeding when the bleeding rate is 0.5 mL/mt or higher. However, the longer half-life of the labeled red blood cells enables the images of the gastrointestinal system to continue for up to 24 hours. The Tc-pertechnetate-labeled blood cell scan should be considered when a small intestinal source of bleeding is suspected. In most institutions, the Tc-pertechnetate-labeled red blood cell scan is used to direct subsequent localized angiography. The nuclear scan can be readily repeated in patients with intermittent bleeding.
- *Barium enema*: Barium enema is useful in neonates and infants presenting with malrotation with secondary intestinal volvulus, intussusception which can be diagnosed and in many cases treated by barium enema. The barium enema is also effective in identifying the presence of polyps.

Specific Management of Common Conditions Presenting as Lower Gastrointestinal Bleeding

- *Anal fissure*: Treatment of constipation, laxatives, Sitz bath, topical 0.2% glyceryl nitrate twice daily.
- *Solitary rectal ulcer syndrome*: Sucralfate enema, twice daily, for 3–6 weeks with training on "not to strain during defecation" and yttrium-aluminum garnet (YAG) laser treatment for severe bleeds.
- *Hemorrhagic infective colitis*: Antimicrobials.
- *Polyps*: Colonoscopic snare polypectomy.
- *Inflammatory bowel disease and ulcerative colitis*: 5-aminosalicylic acid, steroids, cyclosporine, and total colectomy.
- *Crohn's disease*: Steroids, azathioprine, infliximab, metronidazole, and ciprofloxacin.
- *Vascular lesions*: Therapeutic endoscopy.
- *Portal colopathy and variceal bleed*: Octreotide, transjugular intrahepatic portosystemic stent shunt, and shunt surgery.

Flowchart 9.6.2: Approach to a case of upper gastrointestinal bleed.

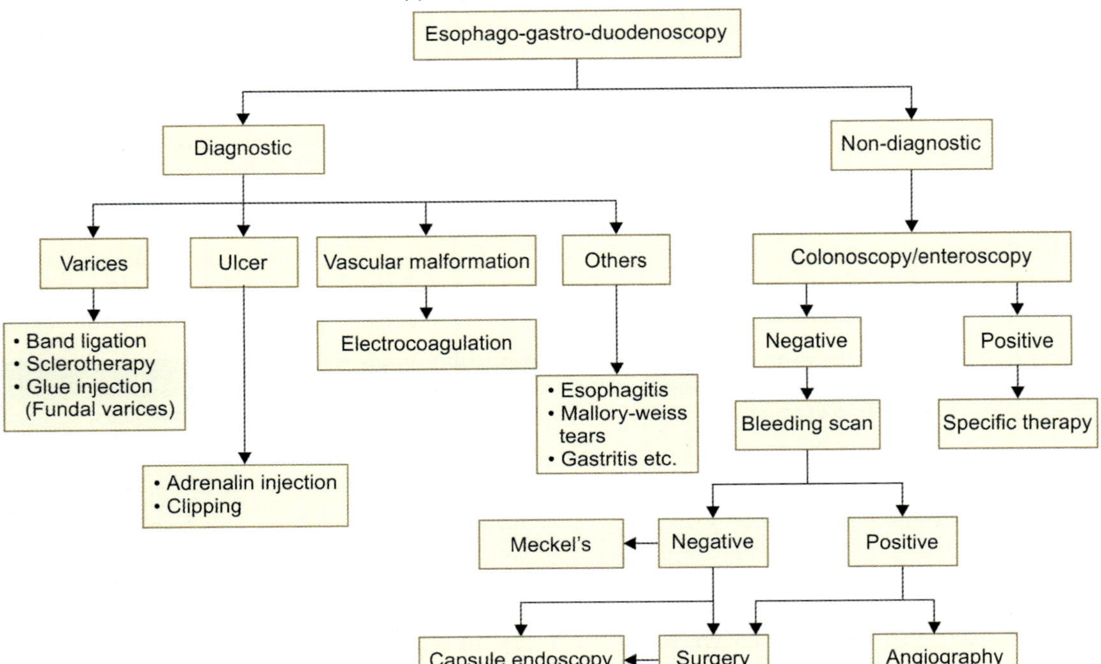

Flowchart 9.6.3: Approach to a case of lower gastrointestinal bleed.

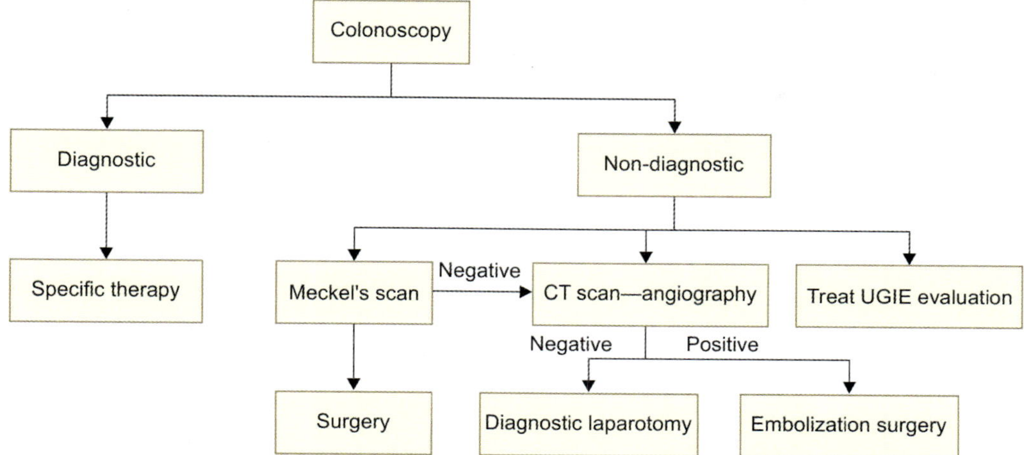

(CT: computed tomography; UGIE: upper gastrointestinal endoscopy)

Flowchart 9.6.4: Management of obscure bleeding

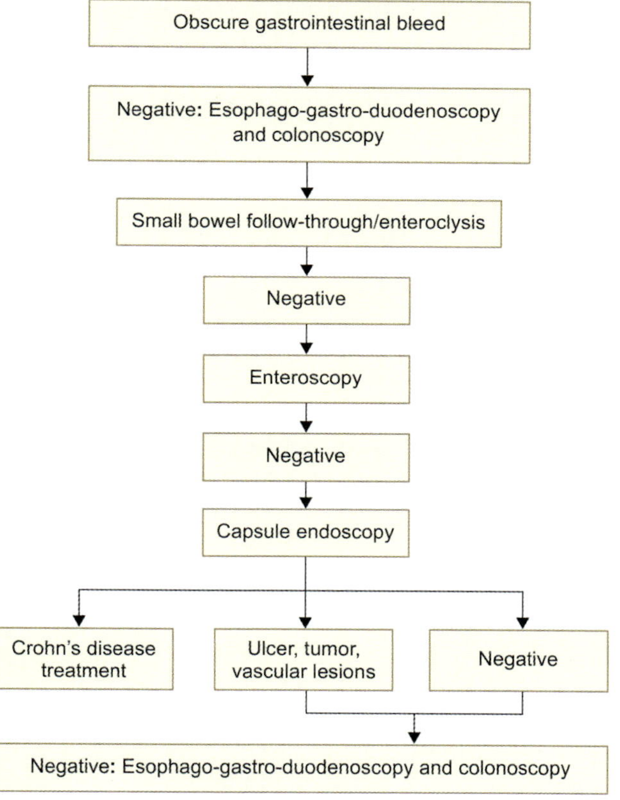

Indications for Surgery in Lower Gastrointestinal Bleeding

Intraoperative enteroscopy using pediatric colonoscpe or enteroscope may be useful to identify small bowel lesions.

- Surgery of Meckel's diverticulum, duplication of small bowel, and Hirschsprung disease (HD).
- Portosystemic shunt, esophageal transection, and TIPS.
- Liver transplantation may be necessary in the upper GI hemorrhage refractory to medical, endoscopic, and radiologic interventions.
- In lower GI hemorrhage, hemicolectomy or subtotal colectomy is occasionally required.
- Complications due to endotherapy such as perforation

Flowcharts 9.6.2 and 9.6.3 summarize the approach to a case of upper GI and lower GI bleed, respectively.

Obscure Gastrointestinal Bleed

It may occur as overt or occult bleed often in small bowel such as Crohn's, anastomotic, cytomegalovirus (CMV)/viral, or other infections like vascular (angiodysplasia, Dieulafoy's lesion, varices, or lymphangioma) or tumors (polyps, carcinoid, or lymphoma), and others like Meckel's diverticulum, diverticulosis, etc.

Various diagnostic modalities include small bowel follow through, enteroclysis, push enteroscopy, and capsule endoscopy. Rarely, surgery with intraoperative endoscopy may be required **(Flowchart 9.6.4)**.

BIBLIOGRAPHY

1. D'Amico G, Pagliaro L, Bosch J. Pharmacological treatment of portal hypertension. An evidence based approach. Semin Liver Dis.1999;19:475.
2. Garcia-Tsao G, Sanyal AJ, Grace ND, et al. Prevention and management of gastroesophageal varices and variceal hemorrhage in cirrhosis. Hepatology. 2007;46(3):923-38.
3. Gottumukkala SR, Lauren G, Das A, et al. American Gastroenterological Association (AGA) Institute medical position statement on obscure gastrointestinal bleeding. Gastroenterology. 2007;133(5):1694-6.
4. Poddar U, Borkar V. Management of extrahepatic portal venous obstruction (EHPO): Current strategies. Trop Gastroenterol. 2011;32(2):94-102.

9.7 Constipation

VR Ravikumar, VS Sankaranarayanan

INTRODUCTION

Constipation is a symptom of an underlying disorder seen in approximately 10–25% of all patients presenting in a pediatric gastroenterology clinic. A normal bowel pattern is considered as a sign of good health. Constipation in children is common, often chronic (persisting for more than 2 weeks) associated with consequences such as chronic abdominal pain, fecal soiling, voiding dysfunction, psychosocial stress, and behavioral problems resulting in poor quality of life.

DEFINITIONS

For practical clinical purposes, constipation is defined as infrequent defecation, painful defecation, or both. In most cases stools are too large, too hard, not frequent enough, and/or painful to pass.

The North American Society for Pediatric Gastroenterology Hepatology and Nutrition (NASPGHAN) defines constipation as "a delay or difficulty in defecation, present for 2 weeks or more, and sufficient to cause significant distress to the patient".

According to Rome III definition of chronic constipation, symptoms must include at least two of the following for the past 2 months:

- Two or fewer defecations per week
- At least one episode of fecal incontinence per week in a toilet-trained child
- History of excessive stool retention or retentive posturing
- History of painful or hard bowel movements
- Presence of large fecal mass in the rectum
- History of large diameter stools that may obstruct the toilet.

Consequences

Hard stools are difficult and painful to push leading to "pooping is pain" and stool withholding resulting in fecal retention. With rectal distension, excessive absorption of fluid and decreased sensory perception follow with hard stools. This leads to fissure in ano, painful defecation with partial evacuation. The vicious cycle results in "toilet-o-phobia", further impaction with fecaloma formation. This affects toilet training.

Encopresis (Fecal incontinence): Defecation reflex is normal. Chronic fecal retention leads to megarectum and megacolon with involuntary overflow and fecal soiling or encopresis.

Obstipation is the absence of passage of both feces and flatus and indicates underlying organic obstruction or pseudo-obstruction.

Functional constipation: Nearly 90% of children with constipation have functional constipation (c.f. for organic cause) at the school entry age. The contributing factors include stool-withholding habits after experience of passing painful bowel movement, denying natural calls in the school or teachers not giving permission to defecate and retentive defecation posturing. Characteristically the "red flags" (vide infra) are absent.

ETIOLOGY

The common causes of constipation are listed in **Table 9.7.1**. Neuronal intestinal dysplasia, visceral myopathy, Chagas disease, small left colon syndrome, and neurofibromatosis are some of the rare causes leading to pseudo-obstruction.

Table 9.7.1: Common causes of constipation.

Newborn	***Infants and children***
Prematurity	*Diet*: Poor dietary habits, lack of fiber
Underfeeding, formula feeds	Weaning formulas
Hypothyroidism	Hypothyroidism
Hirschsprung disease	Hirschsprung disease
Low anorectal anomalies (e.g. anteriorly placed anus)	Functional or psychogenic
Spinal abnormalities	Irritable bowel syndrome (constipating type)
Meconium plug syndrome	*Central nervous system (CNS)*: Hypoxic ischemic encephalopathy, cerebral palsy, mental retardation
Presacral/pelvic mass	*Drugs*: Antispasmodics, antimotility drugs, phenothiazines, codeine containing cough syrups, vincristine and vinblastine

CLINICAL FEATURES

Assessment of a Child with Constipation

A careful history and thorough physical examination including per rectal examination will suffice to diagnose functional constipation provided there are no "red flags".

"Red flags" suggesting organic cause of constipation are failure to thrive, abdominal distension, lack of lumbosacral curve, sacral agenesis, flat buttocks, patulous or anteriorly placed anus, tight empty rectum, gush of air and liquid stool on withdrawal of finger per rectal examination and absent anal wink or cremasteric reflex, and lower limb weakness.

Timing of constipation: At the time of initiating complementary feeds or toilet training (1–2 years); school entry or school age.

Hirschsprung disease and functional constipation: **Table 9.7.2** highlights the differences between Hirschsprung disease and functional constipation.

Table 9.7.2: Differences between Hirschsprung disease and functional constipation.

Functional constipation	***Hirschsprung disease***
More common	Less common
Meconium history—normal	Delayed passage
Onset beyond infancy	From birth
Fecal soiling	Spurious diarrhea
Abdominal distension—rare	Common
Loaded rectum	Empty rectum, grips finger, gush of air, and fluid on release
Failure to thrive or enterocolitis—rare	Common

INVESTIGATIONS

Good history and physical examination with rectal examination are essential.

- Less than 5% organic—tests rarely needed
- *X-ray abdomen* may show loaded colon **(Fig. 9.7.1A)**
- *Barium enema*: Dilatation from anal verge in habit constipation **(Fig. 9.7.1B)**; transition zone in Hirschsprung disease **(Fig. 9.7.1C)**; and rarely to look for strictures
- *Colonic manometry* may be helpful in refractory constipation
- *Rectal mucosal biopsy* in Hirschsprung disease, intestinal neuronal dysplasia, and solitary rectal ulcer.
- Do not forget to screen for hypothyroidism, diabetes mellitus, lead poisoning, celiac disease, and hypercalcemia.

MANAGEMENT

The main steps in the management of constipation are:

- Ensure there is no organic cause, treat if present
- Diet, fluids, exercise, and toilet training
- Pharmacotherapy
- Disimpaction
- Maintenance—prevention of reimpaction
- Behavioral therapy
- Education and re-education (counseling).

Consultation with a pediatric gastroenterologist or pediatric surgeon is appropriate if the child's history or examination findings suggest an underlying organic cause (e.g. Hirschsprung disease). Also seek consultation when the child fails routine therapy or when management is otherwise complex.

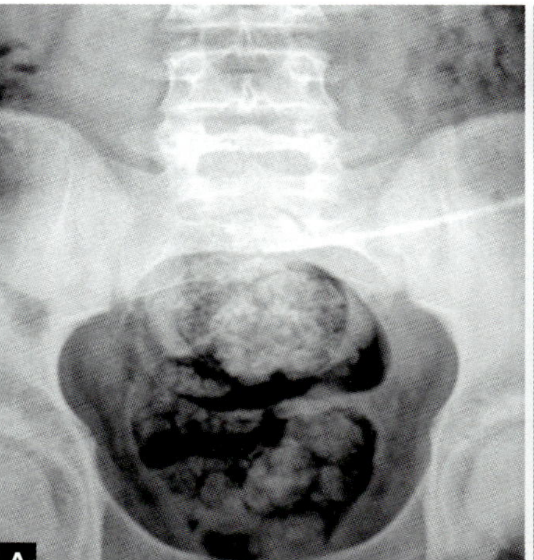

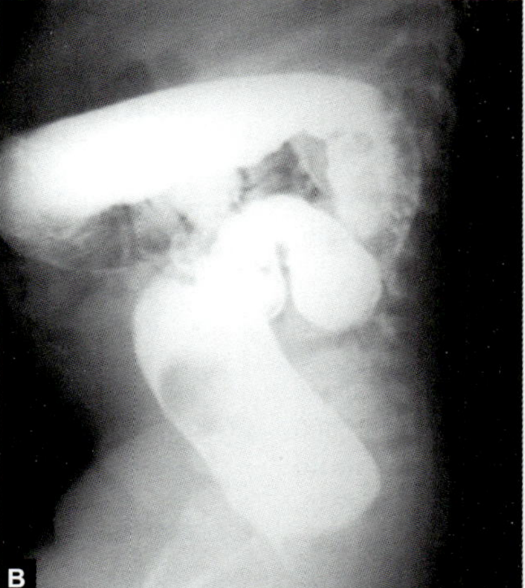

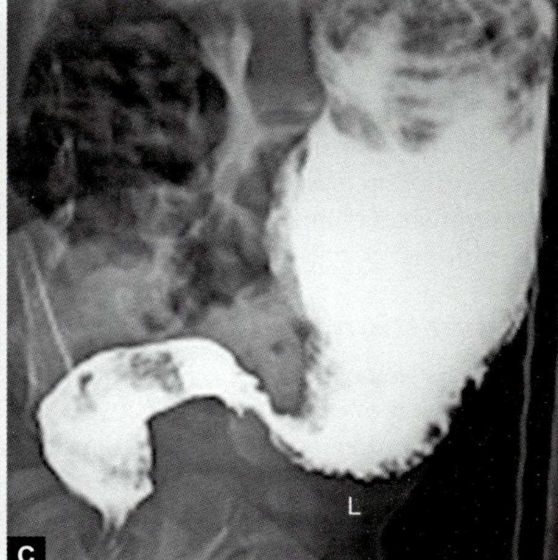

Figs. 9.7.1A to C: (A) Plain X-ray abdomen showing colon loaded with feces in a child with fecal impaction; (B) Habitual constipation with dilatation from anal verge; and (C) Hirschsprung disease showing transition zone.

Table 9.7.3: Laxatives dose and side effects.

Laxative	*Dose*	*Side effects*
Lubricant: Mineral oil	1–3 mL/kg/day once daily or in divided doses for a short period only	Do not give to infants Anal leakage, lipoid pneumonia
Osmotic: Lactulose, lactitol or sorbitol	1–3 mL/kg/day in two doses	Bloating, cramps and diarrhea
Polyethylene glycol (PEG)	5–10 mL/kg/day	Nausea, vomiting, cramps, diarrhea
Magnesium hydroxide	1–3 mL/kg/day in two doses	Hypermagnesemia, hypophosphatemia, hypocalcemia
Stimulant: Bisacodyl	*>2 years*: 5–10 mg daily orally; 5 mg per rectally	Cramps, diarrhea, anal irritation
Senna	• *>6 years*: 5–15 mL/day (8.8 mg/5 mL) • *2–6 years*: 2.5–7.5 mL/day	Melanosis coli, hepatitis

Diet

Diet in constipation includes fiber-containing items like sprouted whole grains, pulses, beans, and sorbitol-rich fruits (Apple with peel, guava, pomegranate, pear, and prune juice), green leafy vegetables, and water. Fiber intake is recommended over 2 years of age and the dose is calculated as age in years plus 5 g/day. Involvement of dietician is beneficial.

Laxatives

Laxatives such as lubricants, osmotic, and stimulants for maintenance are required for a longer period over years to regulate the bowel habits. These should be explained to the parents at the onset. Guidelines for maintenance dose of commonly used drugs are given in **Table 9.7.3**.

Mechanism of Action of Fiber in Chronic Constipation

Fiber is a bulk laxative available as psyllium (Isphagol), methylcellulose, and polycarbophil. *Dose*: Age in years + g/day (1–1.5 g/kg). Bloating is the side effect. Commercial fiber preparations are recommended above three years of age only. Combinations of fiber with lactulose or lactitol/PEG preparations are available in the pharmacy. Fiber and excess dietary carbohydrates have the mechanical effect of water holding and increase the bulk of the stool and osmotic effect respectively. The bulk of the stool is also increased by bacterial overgrowth, colonic bacterial fermentation, gas production and production of SCFA. Both mechanisms will stimulate the faster transit of colonic fecal mass and also reduce the colonic absorption.

Disimpaction

- *Polyethylene glycol (PEG)* is preferred as it is noninvasive. It is given orally in a dose of 20–25 mL/kg/hr (up to 1000 mL/hr) until clear colonic content is evacuated. It should be administered only under supervision in small children; Ryle's tube may be required for administration. Single dose of prokinetic and intravenous fluids may be needed in some children.
- *Mineral oil* is not recommended in infants.
- *Rectal suppositories* are useful in infants—glycerine suppository 1 g for pediatric size and 2–3 g for adolescents.
- *Rectal enema with* glycerine, sodium phosphate, saline or dioctyl sodium sulfosuccinate is invasive; not preferred by most children—but may be required in some cases.
- *Rectal digital disimpaction* is quick but invasive; painful, increases defecation phobia though it is effective especially in stubborn children withholding stools. If necessary, it may be done under anesthesia (cases refractory to all measures).
- *Topical applications*: Twice daily anal applications of petroleum jelly, zinc oxide cream, diltiazem, nitroglycerine or sucralfate with 2% xylocaine jelly using ear bud are effective for painful defecation due to anal cracks.

Maintenance Therapy

Maintenance therapy is aimed to avoid reimpaction and to ensure regular passage of stools with the help of diet modification, laxatives, and behavioral therapy. The caregivers are trained on a simplified use of stool diary and recording of daily stool and defecation details. These include:

- The parents are apprised about the need for long-term treatment and regular follow-up to make sure fecal impaction is not re-established
- Maintenance medication, diet, fluid intake, and exercise, toilet training to be continued for several weeks after regular bowel habits are established
- *Medication*: PEG 3350 with electrolytes if no fecal impaction.
  - *Dose*: Half the dose used for disimpaction regimen (1 g/kg/day). Dose can be adjusted depending on symptoms and response.
  - *Side effects*: Nausea, vomiting, and bloating (osmotic effects).
  - Add stimulant laxative (lactulose or lactitol for hard stools) if PEG is not effective.
  - No abrupt stoppage of treatment.
- Initial weekly review for 2–3 weeks with parents and stool diary helpful.

Behavioral Therapy

Behavioral therapy includes proper toilet training after feeds, three times daily for 5–10 minutes. One word, one person, one year, one stool/day, one sitting posture policy is ideal. Schoolteachers should be informed about the child's problem and management.

Education and Counseling

- Explain physiological basis of constipation and soiling. The National Institute of Clinical Excellence (NICE) guidelines recommend that the child should never be blamed for soiling
- Need to adhere to long-term medication and a regular toilet pattern
- Avoid antispasmodics and antidiarrheal drugs for pain and fluid fecal soiling (pseudodiarrhea)
- If needed, meeting with teacher in school
- As optimum dose is unpredictable for any child, initial weekly meeting for 2–3 weeks is suggested to help family titrate the dose.

Follow-up Schedule

- *Monthly follow-up* till regular bowel movement is achieved. Check diary, physical, and rectal examination. Laxative dose is to be adjusted
- *Follow-up of 3 months for next 2 years.* Continue same dose of laxative for at least 3 months (distended bowel to regain its function) and then slow tapering (early withdrawal of laxative is the most common cause of recurrence.)
- *Yearly follow-up.*

Refractory Constipation

Children with refractory constipation with recurrent impaction, not responding to routine use of laxatives, diet, and behavioral therapy need evaluation of organic diseases and timely referral for specific investigations such as rectal biopsy or to rule out anatomic defects by referral to pediatric surgeons or pediatric gastroenterologists for anorectal manometry, metabolic screen (hypothyroidism, cystic fibrosis, hypercalcemia, celiac disease, lead poisoning, mental retardation, etc.), colonic transit study, colonic manometry or ileo-colonoscopy, and magnetic resonance imaging (MRI) of lumbosacral spine for spinal dysraphism.

These patients, especially school-going children, may need to be diagnosed whether they are functional or organic, or have irritable bowel syndrome (IBS)-constipating type; or if functional whether they are of slow transit or normal transit type or pelvic floor dysfunction (rectoanal dyskinesia) which needs biofeedback training.

KEY MESSAGES

- Constipation is a common problem in children and often presents as chronic periumbilical pain with difficulty and delay in passing dry stools.
- Nearly 95% are functional and often does not need any investigation; diagnosis is invariably clinical including rectal examination and long-term follow-up is essential.
- Management includes drugs, diet modification, toilet training, and regular follow-up and behavioral therapy.
- Refractory cases need referral to the pediatric gastroenterologist for further work-up to know the cause and for management guidance.

BIBLIOGRAPHY

1. Medscape (2017). Pediatric Constipation. [online] Available from: https://emedicine.medscape.com/article/928185-overview [Accessed November, 2018].
2. North American Society for Pediatric Gastroenterology, Hepatology and Nutrition. Evaluation and treatment of constipation in children: Summary of updated recommendations of the North American Society for Pediatric Gastroenterology, Hepatology and Nutrition. J Pediatr Gastroenterol Nutr. 2006;43:405-7.
3. Srivastava A. Management of functional constipation. Indian J Pediatr. 2008;(Supp 75):519-25.
4. Tabbers MM, DiLorenzo C, Berger MY, et al. Evaluation and treatment of functional constipation in Infants and children: Evidence-based recommendations from ESPGHAN and NASPGHAN. J Pediatr Gastroenterol Nutr. 2014;58:258-74.
5. Thapa BR. Constipation in children. In: Bavdekar A, Matthai J, Sathiyasekaran M, et al. (Eds). IAP Speciality series on Pediatric Gastroenterology. New Delhi: Jaypee Brothers Medical Publishers (P) Ltd. 2008;10:125-44.

9.8 Hirschsprung Disease

Kanishka Das

DEFINITION AND EPIDEMIOLOGY

Hirschsprung disease (HD), after Harald Hirschsprung, a pediatrician, is a disorder of bowel motility characterized by uncoordinated peristalsis and functional bowel obstruction. With a worldwide incidence of 1 of 5,000 live births and an overall 4:1 male preponderance, 80–90% of HD occurs sporadically in full-term births and the rest account for the rare genetic/familial/syndromic forms.

EMBRYOLOGY, ETIOPATHOGENESIS AND PATHOPHYSIOLOGY

The ganglion cells originate in the neural crest and migrate aborally along the bowel till the proximal anal canal; further they migrate centripetally into the myenteric plexus and then the submucous plexus. These parasympathetic ganglion cells of the intrinsic enteric nervous system employ nitric oxide as the neurotransmitter and modulate smooth muscle excitatory/

inhibitory interactions in the bowel to effect a relaxation during rest and a coordinated antegrade peristalsis with a luminal bolus. HD results from a failure of such migration or destruction of the ganglion cells in a hostile local environment. Additionally, there is a deficiency of pacemaker cells of intestine-interstitial cells of Cajal (ICC). The resultant loss of receptive relaxation of the distal aganglionic bowel in response to the antegrade propulsive peristalsis of the proximal ganglionic bowel leads to uncoordinated peristalsis and functional bowel obstruction. The extrinsic nerves supplying the bowel respond by proliferation and elaboration of both cholinergic (excitatory) and adrenergic (inhibitory, excitatory) neurotransmitters; the excitatory effects of both predominate to render the aganglionic colon and internal anal sphincter spastic.

CLASSIFICATION

In the classic rectosigmoid form (85%) of HD, the aganglionosis commonly involves the anal canal and the rectum with a transition to normal ganglionic bowel at the sigmoid; rarely the aganglionosis extends proximally into the rest of the colon (long-segment, colonic), terminal ileum [total colonic aganglionosis (TCA)] or more proximally till the esophagus [total intestinal aganglionosis (TIA)]. Such "long-segment disease" is characterized by relative female preponderance and association with familial, syndromic, and genetic forms **(Fig. 9.8.1)**. Ultrashort segment HD (USSHD) refers to a localized spasm/achalasia of the internal anal sphincter identifiable at manometry. Indeed, TCA and USSHD are now considered as entities distinct from classical HD.

CLINICAL FEATURES

A clinical presentation of large bowel obstruction presenting at any time from the postnatal period to adulthood but dating back to infancy/early childhood is characteristic. Currently, nearly 90% is diagnosed in the neonatal period or early infancy. Failure to pass meconium within 48 hours of birth is a cardinal clinical feature seen in 80–90% infants with HD but also with 30–40% children without HD, and 30–35% healthy preterm babies. Symptoms of abdominal distension, poor feeding, nonbilious vomiting, and progressive constipation are characteristic. Infantile constipation often manifests at weaning, and the recurrent symptom complex of constipation-spurious diarrhea-abdominal distension culminates in failure to thrive during childhood.

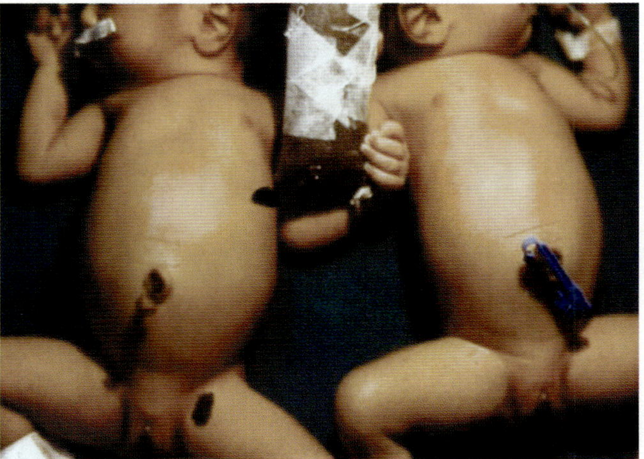

Fig. 9.8.1: Total colonic aganglionosis (TCA) in twin female neonates, the pigmented skin lesions suggest a neurocristopathy.

Hirschsprung enterocolitis is an immune-mediated toxic fulminant sepsis occurring at any age, even after definitive management is completed. It presents with fever, malaise, foul smelling, and often bloody diarrhea and abdominal distension; sometimes progressing to perforation of the cecum or appendix, particularly in the neonate.

Common-associated anomalies include trisomy 21 (5–15%), bowel atresias, and anorectal malformations. HD may be associated with neoplastic or non-neoplastic manifestations of aberrant migration of neural crest cells into the skin, retina, thyroid, adrenal, etc. the "neurocristopathies," e.g., multiple endocrine neoplasia (MEN) syndromes, neuroblastoma, and skin pigmentation.

The physical findings vary with the presentation; typical features in nonacute states are anemia, malnutrition, gaseous abdominal distension, visible/palpable bowel loops, a spastic tight anus at per rectal examination, and a rectal blast of stool and gas at withdrawal of the finger after per rectal examination.

DIFFERENTIAL DIAGNOSIS AND INVESTIGATIONS

Although HD is more common than several other conditions that may mimic it in the neonatal period, the differential diagnosis includes meconium plug syndrome, small left colon syndrome (diabetic mother), distal small bowel/colonic atresia, meconium ileus-cystic fibrosis complex, and other medical conditions like hypothyroidism and sepsis. Historical clues and clinical features direct the confirmatory investigations. Habitual constipation in the older child can be differentiated from HD by several factors that predominate in the former: a normal meconium history, secondary/recent onset of constipation, lack of significant abdominal distension, fecal loading of rectum, and perianal soiling, poor dietary fiber, evidence of associated voiding disturbances, and psychological overlay. The diagnosis of HD is based on an amalgamation of information from the following investigative modalities.

Anorectal Manometry

The principle of anorectal manometry (ARM) is an absence of the normal rectoanal inhibitory reflex (RAIR)—inhibition of the resting rhythmic activity of the internal anal sphincter with rectal distension in HD (including USSHD). This is preserved in the normal and the habitually constipated child. Though it is minimally invasive and has 75–95% accuracy, it is not widely available and difficult in the young uncooperative child. It may be performed under sedation/ anesthesia. Though the RAIR has been detected by 26 weeks of gestation, it is often poorly developed in the term neonate and inconsistent. However, histopathological confirmation of the diagnosis is required prior to surgical intervention.

Radiography

Plain abdominopelvic X-ray and contrast enema remain the basic diagnostic investigations that are easily performed and interpreted. An erect plain X-ray showing generalized dilatation of bowel; especially the peripherally placed colonic loop and an absence of the normal rectal gas shadow in the pelvis suggest the common rectosigmoid form of HD.

The contrast enema is diagnostic in the majority of rectosigmoid disease. A dilated sigmoid and a narrow rectum, a reversed rectosigmoid ratio and a conical transition zone between the two is characteristic of rectosigmoid HD **(Fig. 9.8.2)**. The mixed barium-stool picture in the delayed contrast enema film at 24 hours is also reliable. In associated colitis, a saw tooth mucosal contour due to irregular uncoordinated contractions of the aganglionic segment is seen. In distal small bowel obstruction, it clarifies the wide differential diagnosis; the "question mark microcolon" of TCA is typical **(Fig. 9.8.3)**. Despite precautionary measures and guarded interpretation, a significant false positive/negative rate is recognized in diagnosis of long-segment colonic disease and TCA; further the site and extent of the transition zone is unpredictable on radiology. In conclusion, the contrast enema is a good screening investigation prior to histological confirmation of HD by rectal biopsy.

HISTOPATHOLOGY

Histopathological evaluation is the gold standard for diagnosis with a 93–98% sensitivity and specificity. A rectal biopsy is essential to confirm the diagnosis of all forms of HD and further colonic, appendicular, or ileal biopsies are examined to determine the proximal extent of aganglionosis (leveling). The rectal biopsy may be full or partial (mucosubmucosal) thickness depending on the histological method employed and is taken at least 2 cm above the dentate line to avoid the physiological hypoganglionic anal zone. A suction apparatus for a rectal biopsy is available. At laparotomy/laparoscopy, the gross transition zone, where evident, guides the siting of more proximal leveling biopsies. Various histological methods are in use and include:

- Simple paraffin H and E staining on formalin fixed tissues
- Intraoperative evaluation with fresh frozen tissue—H and E, histochemical staining, e.g. acetylcholinesterase (AChE)
- Immunohistochemistry on formalin fixed tissues, e.g. Calretinin.

The histological features **(Fig. 9.8.4)** seen in the aganglionic (absence of ganglion cells, hypertrophic nerve bundles in described locations), ganglionic (regularly distributed normal morphology ganglion cells along the entire circumference, normal nerve fibers in the different plexi), and intervening transition segment (a variable mixture of both features) are well known; these are clearly visualized with AChE staining of the proliferating extrinsic cholinergic nerve fibers in characteristic patterns. The routine rectal biopsy is normal in USSHD.

Fig. 9.8.2: Contrast enema (lateral view) showing a narrow rectum and a dilated sigmoid diagnostic of rectosigmoid Hirschsprung disease (HD).

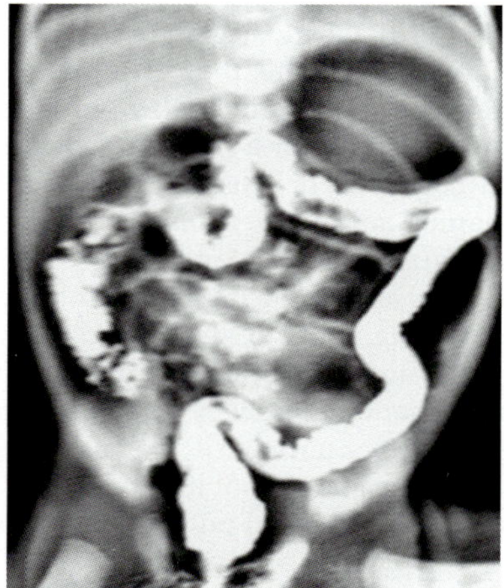

Fig. 9.8.3: Contrast enema (anteroposterior view) in total colonic aganglionosis (TCA). Note the question mark microcolon and the dilated small bowel.

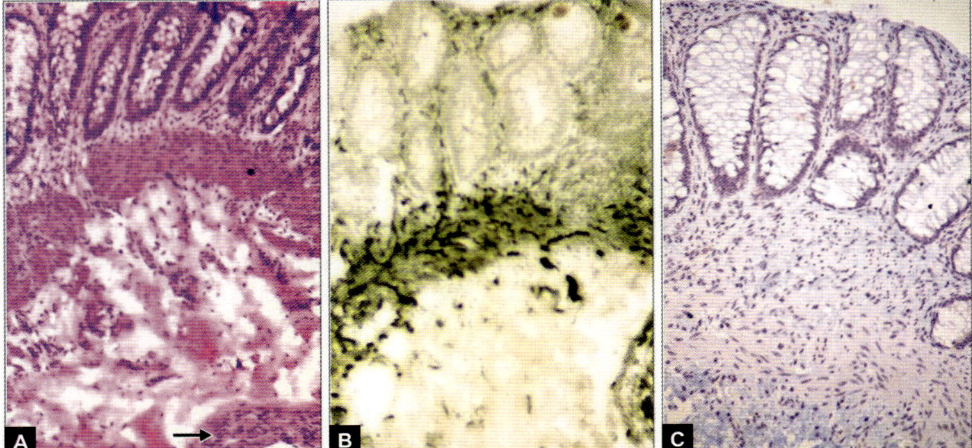

Figs. 9.8.4A to C: Histological confirmation of Hirschsprung disease on a rectal biopsy. At frozen section evaluation, the H&E section (A) shows rectal mucosa and submucosa with a hypertrophic nerve bundle in the submucosa (arrow) and absence of ganglion cells. Concurrent acetylcholinesterase stain (B) shows increased cholinergic activity in the mucosa in a typical pattern. Calretinin stain (C) on formalin-fixed tissue shows lack of the normal intrinsic nerve fiber distribution in the muscularis mucosa and lamina propria.
Courtesy: Suravi Mohanty, Pediatric Pathologist, St John's Medical College, Bengaluru, Karnataka, India.

GENETICS

Hirschsprung disease is multifactorial state with a sex-modified heterogeneous inheritance involving dominant, recessive, and polygenic forms in multiple pathways and more than 10 genes. The two major gene loci for diagnostic purposes are the long arm of chromosome 10 and the 13q22-*EDNRB* gene. However, variable expressivity and incomplete sex-dependent penetrance have limited attempts at prenatal diagnosis, pedigree analysis, and genetic counseling.

MANAGEMENT

The management of HD is based on the surgical principle of near total or total resection of the aganglionic bowel and apposition of the distal most ganglionic bowel within a centimeter of the dentate line, thus dividing the cranial half of the spastic internal anal sphincter. This may be achieved in a single stage pull through or a staged procedure with initial leveling stoma (colostomy or ileostomy) and a subsequent pull through (Duhamel, Soave, Swenson/or their modifications) by an abdominal/transanal, combined, or laparoscopic-assisted procedure at any age depending on the modalities of diagnosis, leveling, and surgical expertise available at a center. Generally, an initial stoma is preferred in poor risk malnourished patients, massively dilated proximal bowel, emergency settings (enterocolitis, bowel perforation, and peritonitis), or nonavailability of intraoperative histological leveling. In TCA, conventional pull-through procedures are generally modified to patch a longitudinal strip of aganglionic colon along the ganglionic ileum to facilitate optimal fluid reabsorption and avert troublesome diarrhea. USSHD is usually amenable to botulinum injections or a transanal longitudinal myotomy/myectomy of the internal anal sphincter.

In toxic acute states without bowel perforation, resuscitation with intravenous fluids, triple antibiotics (beta-lactam, aminoglycosides, and metronidazole), gentle rectal washes with warm saline, and other supportive critical care is vital prior to further surgical management.

PROGNOSIS AND OUTCOME

The majority of HD being sporadic rectosigmoid disease, early management with standard protocols outlined above yields an excellent outcome. Long-term complications or sequel like frequency of bowel movement, incontinence—perianal soiling, anastomotic strictures, recurrent constipation, residual/secondary aganglionosis, and variable somatic retardation occur in less than 10%, especially in long-segment disease and TCA and those managed without accurate histological leveling. Associated anomalies and neurocristopathies also influence the outcome.

BIBLIOGRAPHY

1. de Lorijn F, Boeckxstaens GE, Benninga MA. Symptomatology, pathophysiology, diagnostic work-up, and treatment of Hirschsprung disease in infancy and childhood. Curr Gastroenterol Rep. 2007;9(3):245-53.
2. Langer JC. Hirschsprung disease. In: Coran AG, et al. (Eds). Pediatric Surgery. Philadelphia: Saunders; 2014. pp. 474-91.
3. Swenson O. Hirschsprung's disease: A review. Pediatrics. 2002;109:914-8.
4. Szylberg L, Marszalek A. Diagnosis of Hirschsprung's disease with particular emphasis on histopathology. A systematic review of current literature. Prz Gastroenterol. 2014;9(5):264-9.
5. Tam PKH, Garcia-Barcelo M. Genetic basis of Hirschsprung's disease. Pediatr Surg Int. 2009;25:543-58.
6. Teitelbaum DH (Ed). Hirschsprung disease and related conditions. Semin Pediatr Surg. 2012;21(4):281-3.

9.9 Abdominal Pain

Srinivas Sankaranarayanan

INTRODUCTION

The evaluation of tummy ache can challenge both parents and the physician. Several disorders can cause abdominal pain; the most common medical causes being gastroenteritis and constipation, and the most common surgical cause being appendicitis.

DEFINITION

The traditional definition of recurrent abdominal pain (RAP) used over the last 40 years is based on Apley and Naish's criteria of at least three pain episodes over a 3-month period interfering with daily function. This has been replaced by the term chronic abdominal pain which refers to pain present continuously or occurring on and off for a minimum period of 2 months. It is a description, not a diagnosis, and can be due to organic disease or functional causes.

A child with chronic abdominal pain poses a formidable challenge as the parents may be terribly worried; child may be distressed, and the practitioner may be concerned about ordering multiple tests to avoid missing occult disease.

EPIDEMIOLOGY

The prevalence of chronic abdominal pain in community-based US studies is estimated to be up to 19%. Yet only in a small number of children is the pain caused by organic disease and in the majority the pain is functional or nonspecific, i.e., without demonstrable evidence of a pathologic condition. Functional or nonspecific abdominal pain is uncommon under 5 years of age.

The differential diagnosis of abdominal pain in children varies with age, gender, genetic, and environmental factors. Besides organic and functional components are not mutually exclusive, since psychological complications of organic disease are common in children. Hence, the diagnostic approach to abdominal pain in children relies heavily on the history provided by the parent and child to direct a stepwise approach to investigation rather than multiple "exclusionary" investigations.

ETIOLOGY

Table 9.9.1 lists some of the causes of chronic abdominal pain in children. It should be noted that organic causes account for only a small proportion of children with chronic abdominal pain as compared to nonorganic causes.

CLINICAL FEATURES

History

- The *location of the pain* is important, and the child may indicate the location of the pain by pointing with one finger or with the whole hand. Apley's observation that "the further the pain from the umbilicus, the greater the likelihood of organic disease" has held up reasonably well and most children with nonspecific abdominal pain present with mild intermittent pain around the region of the umbilicus. Epigastric pain raises the suspicion of gastroesophageal reflux disease (GERD)/acid peptic disease. Lower abdominal pain should make one suspect conditions like constipation or appendicitis.
- History of *recent medications* is important as antibiotics may predispose the patient to intestinal bacterial overgrowth, acne medications may induce pill esophagitis and tricyclic antidepressants may cause constipation.
- *Family history* of peptic disease, irritable or inflammatory bowel disease (IBD), pancreatitis, biliary disease, or migraine should be determined.
- Younger children often deny heartburn, but other features of peptic disease or GERD include nausea, epigastric pain, and early satiety. Older children and adolescents may complain of typical symptoms including heartburn/sour eructation and/or dysphagia.
- Pancreatic pain is often severe, upper abdominal and radiates to the back—often lasting for 1–2 hours. The child typically doubles up in pain and refuses food. The pain is severe enough to need narcotic agents for pain relief.
- The influence of pain on the child's daily activity is assessed through questions about school attendance, athletic endeavors and peer relationships.
- Whenever possible, a few minutes should be taken alone with adolescents to address concerns in the absence of parents and to elicit honest answers about sexual issues, psychological fears and the disruptions to lifestyle caused by the parents' interventions.
- The *"red flag"* symptoms that should trigger a search for organic disease include a history of abdominal distension, involuntary weight loss, deceleration of linear growth, prolonged fever, bile stained or persistent vomiting,

Table 9.9.1: Causes of chronic abdominal pain in children.

Gastrointestinal causes	*Liver, spleen, and biliary tract disorders*	*Genitourinary causes*
• Constipation • Reflux esophagitis • *Helicobacter pylori* gastritis • Peptic ulcer • Lactose intolerance • Giardiasis • Mesenteric adenitis syndrome • Inflammatory bowel disease	• Liver abscess • Cholelithiasis • Recurrent or chronic pancreatitis	• Urinary tract infection • Urinary calculi • Hydronephrosis • Dysmenorrhea • Pelvic inflammatory disease
Surgical causes • Malrotation with intermittent volvulus • Chronic appendicitis		
Miscellaneous • Lead poisoning • Vasculitis-like Henoch-Schönlein purpura • Familial Mediterranean fever • Angioneurotic edema • Acute intermittent porphyria		
Functional disorders (as classified by Rome III criteria) • Irritable bowel syndrome • Functional dyspepsia • Abdominal migraine • Childhood functional (nonspecific) abdominal pain • Childhood functional abdominal syndrome		

chronic diarrhea, dysphagia, nocturnal symptoms, family history of IBD, and pain persistently located away from the central abdominal area.

Examination

Anthropometric data of weight, height, and growth velocity are documented. Blood pressure is recorded, and the weight-for-height is plotted to assess malnutrition or obesity. The physician should percuss the liver span, document the spleen and kidney size, and determine the influence of leg movement (psoas sign). Examination for pain should be performed with gentle and deep pressure as well as with rebound.

Abdominal and rectal examinations will identify constipation, perianal inflammatory lesions of Crohn's disease, abdominal tumors such as neuroblastoma or Wilms tumor, hydronephrosis, and the presence of umbilical or abdominal wall hernias. The pelvic examination may suggest gynecologic problems, such as endometriosis, ectopic pregnancy, or ovarian cysts or torsion.

The red flag signs of organic disease include:
- Pallor/clubbing/pedal edema
- Growth faltering
- Localized tenderness
- Localized fullness or palpable mass
- Organomegaly
- Presence of perianal abnormalities.

DIAGNOSIS AND EVALUATION

Laboratory Testing

The common laboratory tests performed in the evaluation of abdominal pain in children include:
- Complete blood cell counts
- Erythrocyte sedimentation rate (ESR)/C-reactive protein (CRP)
- Urinalysis
- Stool testing for parasites or *Giardia* antigen
- Stool occult blood and stool calprotectin
- Serum albumin
- Liver enzymes, serum amylase, lipase
- Serology testing for celiac disease and *Helicobacter pylori*.
- Anemia, leukocytosis, thrombocytosis, elevated CRP, or ESR are frequently seen in inflammatory disease (IBD). Low serum albumin levels are seen in intestinal diseases with significant mucosal damage. An elevated stool calprotectin is an indirect marker of inflamed gastrointestinal mucosa—hence is often used as a screening test for IBD.

Hydrogen breath testing for lactose intolerance is indicated if empiric dietary interventions are inconclusive.

Imaging Investigations

Sonography of the Abdomen and Pelvis

This is usually *performed as the first investigation* in the evaluation of chronic abdominal pain to exclude nonintestinal origin of the pain, which includes gallstones, renal stones, and pancreatitis.

With the use of high-resolution ultrasonogram (USG) probes, there is increasing detection of mesenteric lymph nodes. Mesenteric lymph nodes should be considered as significant only when their transverse diameter is more than 10 mm in size or if there is matting/ascites/evidence of bowel thickening. The syndrome of mesenteric adenitis causes colicky pain in the right lower quadrant and can closely mimic appendicitis. Sonography of the pelvis is also indicated to look for visualization of the ileum for Crohn's disease, lymphadenopathy, or possible pelvic or ovarian disease in adolescent girls.

Barium Studies

A barium contrast of the upper GI tract may be useful to rule out malrotation especially if episodes of colicky abdominal pain are associated with bilious vomiting.

Abdominal Computed Tomographic Scan

Abdominal computed tomographic (CT) scan with contrast allows evaluation of the pancreas, extraintestinal mass lesions, abscess, retroperitoneal disease, and better imaging of the small bowel in IBD.

Endoscopy

Upper endoscopy is rarely indicated as a first-line investigation. The yield is maximal in patients with epigastric pain, symptoms of GER or positive celiac screen. Biopsies of the esophagus, gastric antrum and duodenum may be indicated even in the absence of macroscopic disease to identify microscopic diagnostic features of reflux esophagitis, *H. pylori* infection, eosinophilic gastritis, granuloma of Crohn's disease, and villous injury with enteropathy. Colonoscopy up to 10 cm of terminal ileum is mandatory in all children with suspected IBD as they may have Crohn's disease affecting the small bowel (ileum) and yet completely sparing the large bowel (colon) presenting as abdominal pain.

Empiric Intervention

The child's response to empiric intervention is also part of the diagnostic evaluation. This may include:

- Addition of laxatives to rule out constipation
- A trial of H_2 blocker in children with GERD or peptic ulcer disease prior to confirmatory investigations
- A trial of lactose elimination.
- Empiric trials of antispasmodic, anxiolytic or antidepressant medications are not indicated.

MANAGEMENT

If specific causes for the pain are discovered, then the management is specific and directed to treat them. Functional abdominal pain is discussed in detail below.

Functional Abdominal Pain

When RAP is not associated with a detectable organic issue or pathology, this medical condition can be renamed functional abdominal pain syndrome (FAPS) or, better, according to the recent European Society for Paediatric Gastroenterology Hepatology and Nutrition (ESPGHAN) Rome IV criteria, functional abdominal pain disorders (FAPDs). Yet, the affected children and their families can still experience anxiety and concerns that can interfere with school, sports, and regular daily activities and lead to frequent attendances at pediatric emergency departments or pediatric gastroenterology clinics. Children with FAPS frequently report significant limitations to life activities and may also manifest distinct psychopathologies, including depression, anxiety, and somatoform disorders.

According to the most recent criteria, FAP can generally be clinically diagnosed (i.e. without the requirement of additional diagnostic aids) when the physical examination of the child is overall normal and there are no alarming signs or symptoms.

The cornerstone of the diagnosis is a detailed history about the abdominal pain and any other associated symptoms, including onset, duration, frequency, site, characteristics, and triggering or relieving factors. Laboratory tests and radiological investigations are generally not mandatory for the diagnosis of FAP; they should be considered whenever concerns of an organic pathology must be ruled out or when, during the physical examination of the child, the physician recognizes some of the "red flag" signs.

Pathophysiology

The pathophysiology of "functional or nonspecific abdominal pain" is thought to involve abnormalities in the enteric nervous system leading to dysregulation of brain gut communications. Two factors are of primary importance in the perception of nonspecific abdominal pain:

1. Visceral hypersensitivity
2. Altered intestinal motility.

There is increasing evidence that visceral hyperalgesia (decreased threshold of pain to changes in intraluminal pressure) has been triggered by mucosal inflammation secondary to infection, allergies or IBD.

The pathophysiology of adult functional disorders such as IBD has been extensively studied. Immune, neuronal and genetic factors have been studied. Serotonin has been found to be decreased in the enterochromaffin cells of the rectal mucosa. Alterations in bowel flora can cause dysregulation and result in IBD.

Management of Functional Abdominal Pain

As a specific cure is not possible, children with FAP should be evaluated and treated in a manner that includes a biopsychosocial approach, thus engaging in a therapeutic patient-physician partnership. The management of nonspecific abdominal pain begins with the acknowledgment that the pain is real, that extensive investigations are not warranted. Education of the family in simple understandable language is an important part of treating a child with nonspecific abdominal pain such as likening the abdominal pain to a headache and giving examples of hyperalgesia like a healing scar. The primary goal of therapy is not eradication of pain but resumption of a normal lifestyle with regular school attendance, extracurricular activities and a normal sleep pattern. Parents must be discouraged from reinforcing the symptoms by allowing the child to miss school and paying too much positive attention to the pain.

It is important to identify, clarify and reverse possible physical and psychological stress factors that may exacerbate or maintain pain.

Nonpharmacological therapies include:

- Dietary modification
- Probiotic supplementation, and
- Biopsychosocial intervention.

Dietary intervention may involve excluding or reducing a specific ingredient or a group of foods from the diet, such as lactose; fructose; dairy products; fermentable oligosaccharides, disaccharides, monosaccharides, and polyols (FODMAPs); and gluten, or even increasing the daily intake of other foods, such as fiber-rich food and water.

Psychological approaches including cognitive behavioral therapy and gut-directed hypnotherapy have been tried with some success in children with nonspecific or functional abdominal pain but it is customary for such children to have been evaluated in more detail and undergone more investigations including an upper endoscopy and lower endoscopy to rule out IBD before such therapy is commenced.

Drug Therapy

Drug therapy for pain-related functional gastrointestinal disorders (FGIDs) has generally been directed at symptoms alleviation rather than at precise pathophysiological abnormalities. However, with increased understanding on the etiology of visceral hypersensitivity and dysmotility, newer strategies are being developed which include 5HT3 antagonists.

Since pain-related FGIDs tend to be chronic, waxing and waning, a quick cure is unlikely. As they have a high rate of spontaneous remission, a stepwise approach is necessary with the initial step being education, alleviation of stress factors, and diet modifications.

Children with chronic pain are a diagnostic and therapeutic challenge as they often have two or more different pain diagnoses (like tension type headache, migraine, and musculoskeletal pain) and they are prone to misuse of analgesics and are severely impaired. They are at increased risk for developmental stagnation. Adequate treatment and referral are essential to interrupt progression of the chronic pain process into adulthood.

KEY MESSAGES

- The two most common causes of chronic abdominal pain in children are constipation and nonspecific abdominal pain.
- Detailed history taking and physical examination will give us a clue to the cause of abdominal pain and helps us to rationalize investigations.
- Understanding and counseling about the pathophysiology of nonspecific or functional abdominal pain plays a pivotal role in the management.

BIBLIOGRAPHY

1. Abbott RA, Martin AE, Newlove-Delgado TV, et al. Psychosocial interventions for recurrent abdominal pain in childhood. Cochrane Database Syst Rev. 2017;1:CD010971.
2. Banz VM, Sperisen O, de Moya M, et al. A 5-year follow up of patients discharged with non-specific abdominal pain: Out of sight, out of mind? Intern Med J. 2012;42(4):395-401.
3. Brusaferro A, Farinelli E, Zenzeri L, et al. The management of paediatric functional abdominal pain disorders: Latest evidence. Paediatr Drugs. 2018;20(3):235-47.
4. Di Lorenzo C, Colletti RB, Lehmann HP, et al. Chronic abdominal pain in children: A clinical report of the American Academy of Pediatrics and the North American Society for Pediatric Gastroenterology, Hepatology and Nutrition. J Pediatr Gastroenterol Nutr. 2005;40:245-8.
5. Lake A. Chronic abdominal pain in childhood: Diagnosis and management. Am Fam Phys. 1999;59:1823-30.
6. Martin AE, Newlove-Delgado TV, Abbott RA, et al. Pharmacological interventions for recurrent abdominal pain in childhood. Cochrane Database Syst Rev. 2017;3:CD010973.
7. Newlove-Delgado TV, Martin AE, Abbott RA, et al. Dietary interventions for recurrent abdominal pain in childhood. Cochrane Database Syst Rev. 2017;3:CD010972.
8. Thornton GC, Goldacre MJ, Goldacre R, et al. Diagnostic outcomes following childhood non-specific abdominal pain: A record-linkage study. Arch Dis Child. 2016;101(4):305-9.
9. Zernikow B, Wager J, Hechler T, et al. Characteristics of highly impaired children with severe chronic pain: a 5-year retrospective study on 2249 pediatric pain patients. BMC Pediatr. 2012;16:12-54.

9.10 Inflammatory Bowel Disease

Moinak Sen Sarma

INTRODUCTION

Inflammatory bowel disease (IBD) is a chronic inflammatory disease of the GI tract and is of two main types: (1) Crohn's disease (CD) and (2) ulcerative colitis (UC). In about 10% cases the findings are labeled as unclassified IBD. Nearly 25% of all IBD patients present in the pediatric age group. Worldwide the incidence of IBD, more so CD is increasing in children. Large population-based studies have shown an incidence of 1.2–11.8 cases per 100,000 predominantly in the West. Higher latitude and northern hemisphere report higher incidences. There are population-based data available from India. The average age of presentation in children is 10–11 years. However, it is recently described in all the age groups including infancy.

PATHOPHYSIOLOGY

Being an immune-mediated disease, there is a complex interaction of innate and adaptive immunity, gut bacteria, genetic predisposition, and environmental factors **(Fig. 9.10.1)**. Genome-wide association studies have revealed more than 200 genetic loci responsible for the pathogenesis of IBD. These genes that code for proteins modify the body's immunity. A dysregulation in the gut barrier integrity and immune homeostasis may lead to alterations in biodiversity (proliferation and suppression of various gut bacterial species) triggering a chronic inflammation in the gut. The microbiome change in CD is better documented than the other IBDs. The older concept of hygiene hypothesis (people raised in sanitary conditions have higher risk of immune-mediated diseases) is gradually receding as IBD is now being reported frequently in lower socioeconomic strata too.

Genetics is a very important risk factor for IBD and up to 19–41% children in the West may have an affected family member with IBD. Having a first-degree relative with IBD increases the risk to about 30-fold. Susceptibility has been linked to some HLA subtypes, and linkage analysis has identified multiple other susceptibility loci on several chromosomes. Environmental factors (not yet identified) also seem to play a role because there is often nonconcordance among monozygotic twins. It is possible that viral infections can initiate the inflammatory process. Dietary triggers are unproven. CD causes transmural (mucosa, submucosa, muscular layers, and serosa) inflammation of various part of gastrointestinal tract (GIT) where as in UC the inflammation is limited to the colonic mucosa only. **Tables 9.10.1 and 9.10.2** summarize the disease distribution of UC and CD and classify the diseases based on their extent, respectively.

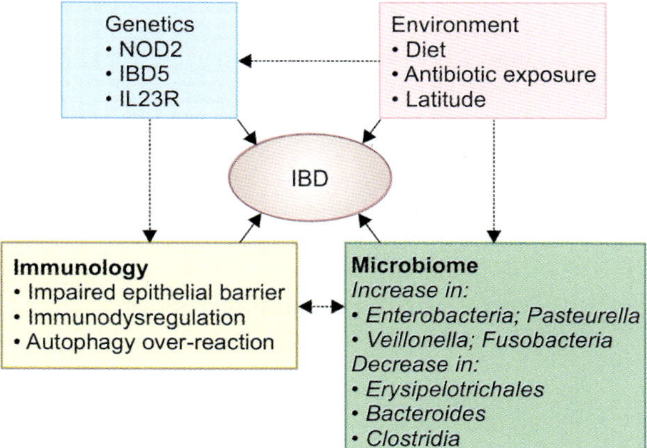

Fig. 9.10.1: Pathophysiology of inflammatory bowel disease (IBD): Complex interaction of diet, genetics, immunology, and gut microbiota.

CLINICAL FEATURES

Children with CD present with abdominal pain, diarrhea (with or without blood) and constitutional symptoms (fever and anorexia). The classical triad of diarrhea, abdominal pain and weight loss is seen in only 25% of children. In contrast children with UC present with bloody diarrhea. In Asia, children with

Table 9.10.1: Disease distribution in IBD.

Ulcerative colitis	*Crohn's disease*
Distal colitis (proctitis/ proctosigmoiditis): 5–20%	*Ileocolonic disease*: 50–70%
Left side colitis (up to splenic flexure): 10–40%	*Isolated colonic involvement*: 10–20%
Pancolitis: 50–90%	*Small bowel*: 10–15%
	Associated: • Upper gastrointestinal involvement: 30–40% • Perianal disease: 20–25%

Table 9.10.2: Paris classification for disease extent of IBD.

Crohn's disease	***Ulcerative colitis***
Age at diagnosis A1a: <10 years A1b: 10–17 years A2: 17–40 years A3: >40 years	*Extension* E1: Proctitis E2: Left-sided colitis (distal to splenic flexure) E3: Extensive (up to hepatic flexure) E4: Pancolitis
Location L1: Distal one-third ileum ± limited cecal disease L2: Colonic L3: Ileocolonic L4: Upper GI or rest of small bowel involvement	*Severity* S0: Never severe S1: Ever severe
Behavior B1: Non-stricturing B2: Stricturing B3: Penetrating B2B3: Both stricturing and penetrating P: Perianal	
Growth G0: No growth delay G1: Growth delay	

both UC as well as CD have growth failure or weight loss due to late referral. In the West, children with IBD present relatively early, and hence growth failure is more often encountered in CD than UC. **Table 9.10.3** summarizes the clinical, histologic and endoscopic differences between UC and CD.

Extraintestinal manifestations **(Table 9.10.4)** are seen in 25–30% children with IBD. They can precede, follow or occur concurrently with the intestinal disease and may be related or unrelated to activity of the intestinal disease. Of all the extraintestinal manifestations, arthralgia or arthritis are the most common manifestation (15%).

DIAGNOSIS

The initial evaluation of a child with suspected IBD includes a detailed clinical, family and treatment history. A complete examination includes growth charting, perianal and rectal examination for fistulae, tags and fissures. Laboratory tests may reveal anemia and thrombocytosis (67%), low albumin, high ESR and C-reactive protein (CRP) in 40–60% and these are reliable indicators of IBD.

Fecal inflammatory markers such as fecal calprotectin are popular in the West for screening of IBD. However, it has many fallacies especially in developing countries. Fecal calprotectin may not be sufficiently raised in early stage of disease, has poor specificity and elevated in intercurrent gastrointestinal infections (bacterial, parasitic, *H. pylori* infection and small bowel bacterial overgrowth). *Antineutrophil cytoplasmic antibody (ANCA)* is found in about 66% of UC patients and in only a few CD cases. *Anti-Saccharomyces cerevisiae antibody (ASCA)* is present in about 50% of CD patients and is uncommon in UC. Because there is overlap between CD and UC, none of these tests can discriminate absolutely between the two conditions. The use of antibodies is complementary and ancillary in the diagnosis of IBD. In fact, they may have a role in prognostication of the disease. ASCA positive CD patients are likely to have ileal involvement and greater need for surgery in future. ANCA positive CD has left colonic disease, sparing of terminal ileum and lesser need for surgery.

Table 9.10.3: Differentiation between Crohn's disease and ulcerative colitis.

Parameters	***Crohn's disease***	***Ulcerative colitis***
Distribution	• Entire GI tract • Transmural inflammation • Discontinuous lesions	• Colon only • Mucosal disease • Continuous involvement
Bloody diarrhea	• Less common	• Common
Abdominal pain	• Common	• Less common
Growth failure	• Common	• Less common
Perianal disease	• Present (abscess, fistulae, tags: **Fig. 9.10.2A**)	• Absent
Histopathology	• Noncaseating ill defined (<300 µm) granuloma (throughout GI tract) • No goblet cell dysplasia • Focal discontinuous crypt architectural distortion • Focal discontinuous chronic inflammation • Focally enhancing gastritis (biopsy of stomach) • Pyloric gland metaplasia (terminal ileum)	• No granuloma • Widespread crypt architectural distortion • Diffuse inflammatory infiltrate • Basal plasmacytosis • Goblet cell depletion • Crypt abscess • Paneth cell metaplasia
Endoscopy **(Figs. 9.10.2B to F)**	• Deep irregular serpiginous or aphthous ulcers • Normal intervening mucosa (skip lesion) • Ileal involvement, rectal sparing (60%) • Internal fistulae	• Diffuse superficial ulceration • Granularity, loss of vascular pattern, friability • Rectal involvement (80–90%) ileal sparing (unless back-wash ileitis) and cecal patch in left-sided colitis

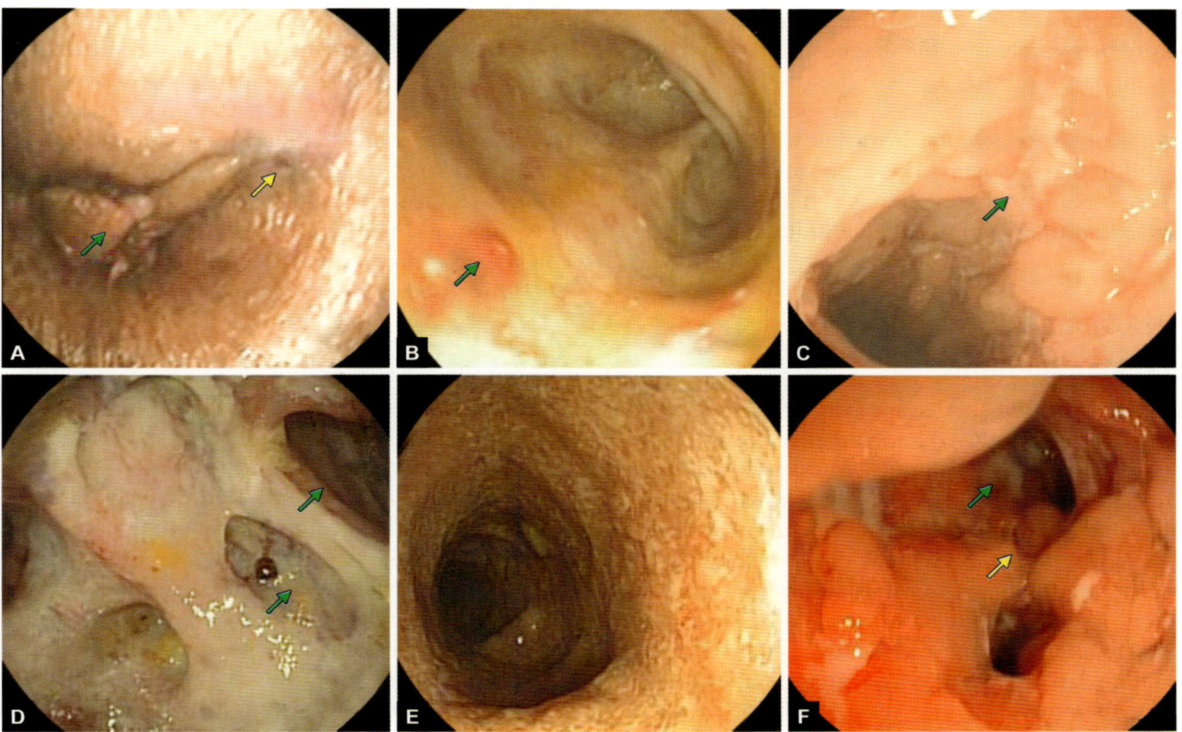

Figs. 9.10.2A to F: (A) Yellow arrow: mucocutaneous fistula; green arrow: perianal tag in CD; (B) Green arrow: aphthous ulcers in CD; (C): Green arrow: linear serpiginous ulcer in CD; (D) Green arrows: internal fistulae of colon to small bowel; (E) Superficial continuous ulcers in UC; and (F) Green arrow: ileal ulcer; yellow arrow: ileocecal valve destruction.

Table 9.10.4: Extraintestinal manifestations in IBD.

System	*Extraintestinal manifestation*
Joints	Nondeforming arthritis (large joints > small joints) and arthralgia Enthesitis Sacroiliitis Ankylosing spondylitis (HLA-B27 positive)
Skin/oral cavity	Oral ulcers Pyoderma gangrenosum Erythema nodosum Alopecia areata "Metastatic" Crohn's disease (ulcers and granulomatosis of penis, vulva, labia)
Eye	Uveitis Episcleritis
Liver/biliary tract	Primary or autoimmune sclerosing cholangitis Autoimmune hepatitis Pancreatitis Cholelithiasis Fatty liver Asymptomatic hyper-transaminasemia IgG4 cholangiopathy
Bones	Osteopenia and osteoporosis
Coagulation	Venous thrombosis (portal vein, hepatic vein, mesenteric veins)
Kidneys	Renal stones (oxalate)

Table 9.10.5: Diagnostic modalities available for IBD.

Diagnostic modality	*Importance*
Colonoscopy with ileal intubation Multiple biopsies from disease sites UGI endoscopy with biopsies	Most important to differentiate UC versus CD To look for granulomas
Small bowel imaging Barium enteroclysis, CT or MR enterocylsis	For small bowel strictures fistula Extramural complications may be seen in CT/MRI
MRI pelvis	Fistula, pelvic and genitourinary abscess
Capsule endoscopy	Ideal to evaluate small bowel involvement after excluding intestinal stricture that may result in retention of capsule. Disadvantage: biopsies cannot be taken
Enteroscopy	Limitation of not able to pass bigger diameter enteroscopes in younger children

Table 9.10.5 summarizes the diagnostic modalities available for IBD. UGI endoscopy, colonoscopy and small bowel imaging are mandatory for mapping of disease and confirmation of diagnosis. Biopsies from endoscopically involved and uninvolved sites at the onset are essential.

Basal plasmacytosis is the earliest diagnostic feature with the highest predictive value for the diagnosis of UC. Preserved crypt architecture does not rule out early UC. Therefore, repeat biopsies are recommended not sooner than 6 weeks after the initial assessment for the diagnosis of UC. At onset, CD in children is associated with more colitis and less ileitis. The frequency of granulomas is higher in the upper gastrointestinal tract is of assistance in differentiating CD from UC.

MANAGEMENT

General Management

Classification of severity of disease is by pediatric ulcerative colitis activity index (PUCAI) and pediatric Crohn's disease activity index (PCDAI). While PUCAI takes consideration of grading of clinical parameters (abdominal pain, rectal bleeding, stool number, consistency, nocturnal awakening, and daily activity), PCDAI is a much more elaborate grading that incorporates clinical as well as laboratory parameters (hematocrit, ESR, and albumin), examination (height, weight, abdominal tenderness, perirectal disease, and extraintestinal manifestations). Both the indices are important for assessing response to therapy.

The goals of treatment are to control inflammation, mucosal healing, improve growth, and ensure a good quality of life with the least toxic therapeutic regimen. Ensuring proper nutrition with caloric supplementation [120% of recommended daily allowance (RDA)] is a necessity for children with IBD. Calcium and vitamin D supplementation should be given as these children are at an increased risk of osteoporosis. As IBD is a chronic disease with remissions and exacerbations, proper counseling of both patient and family at diagnosis is essential. Exclusive enteral nutrition (EEN) with elemental, semielemental or polymeric formulae are popular in the West to induce remission in mild-moderate CD as compared to drug therapy. EEN may not be effective in severe pancolitis, fistulizing or perianal CD. Duration of EEN therapy should be 6–8 weeks. Drug therapy must be considered if there is no response by second week of EEN. EEN is not used as modality of therapy in UC.

Drugs

The main drugs used for IBD are listed in the **Tables 9.10.6 and 9.10.7**. There are two phases of therapy: induction and maintenance.

Steroids have a central role, as they are the most commonly used induction agents in moderate to severe UC and all severities of CD and IBD-U. Prednisolone is started as 2 mg/kg (maximum 40 mg/day and 60 mg/day in case of unsatisfactory response in older children) for 2–4 weeks followed by gradual tapering over 6–8 weeks by which time clinical remission is seen in majority. Toxicity of steroids must be monitored from time to time (every 2–3 weeks) with mandatory examination of blood pressure, intraocular pressure and cataract formation. Role of budesonide in place of prednisolone (for lesser steroid toxicity) in maintenance therapy in CD is not well established in children.

In cases of UC with steroid dependence, relapse or steroid refractory course and invariably in all cases of CD, *azathioprine* (1–2 mg/kg) is added on for maintenance. A

Table 9.10.6: Drugs used in IBD (first-line therapy).

Drug	*Dosage and route*	*Indication*	*Main side effects*
Sulfasalazine *Or* 5-aminosalicylic acid or mesalamine *(Active moiety of sulfasalazine)*	• 40–60 mg/kg/d oral • 50–100 mg/kg/d oral • Enema	• Anti-inflammatory (local action) in mild UC and maintenance • Enema in mild to moderate left sided colonic disease	• Folate deficiency • Pancreatitis • Steven-Johnson syndrome • Hepatotoxicity • Oligospermia (with sulfasalazine)
Prednisolone	• 1–2 mg/kg oral	• Induction therapy (first line) in all types of IBD	• Cushingoid facies • Hypertension • Glaucoma • Cataract • Fractures • Hyperglycemia • Growth impairment
Thiopurines: Azathioprine (AZA) 6-Mercaptopurine *(Active moiety of AZA)*	• 2–3 mg/kg/d oral • 1–2 mg/kg/d oral	• Frequent relapses* • Steroid dependence# • Steroid resistance% • Maintenance in moderate to severe disease	• Myelosuppression • Hepatotoxicity • Pancreatitis

**Frequent relapses: 2–3 relapses per year.*
#Steroid dependency: Initial remission but recurrence while tapering or inability to stop steroids in 14–16 weeks of initiation.
%Steroid resistance: Non-response to optimal doses of oral steroids within 7–14 days of initiation and good compliance.

Table 9.10.7: Drugs used in IBD (second-line therapy).

Drug	Dosage and route	Indication	Main side effects
Methotrexate	• 15 mg/m^2 IM weekly	• Steroid sparing • Refractory disease and/or intolerant to thiopurines	• Hepatotoxicity • Myelosuppression • Folate deficiency
Cyclosporine Tacrolimus	• 2–4 mg/kg/d IV infusion followed by 5–8 mg/kg/d oral • 0.1 mg/kg oral	• Rescue therapy for maximum 4 weeks in severe refractory UC	• Nephrotoxicity • Hypertrichosis • Gum hyperplasia • Hypertension • Paresthesia
Biological agents (infliximab, adalimumab)	• Infliximab 5 mg/kg IV at 0, 2, 6 weeks and thereafter 8–weekly • Adalimumab 2.4 mg/kg first dose followed by 1.2 mg/kg second dose followed by 0.6 mg/kg every 2 weekly	• Fistuling CD • Perianal disease • Severe disease not responding to immunomodulators	• Infusion reaction • Autoimmunity • Demyelination • Psychiatric problems • Flare infections • Hepatosplenic T-cell lymphoma
Thalidomide	• 1.5–2.5 mg/kg oral	• Refractory CD and intolerant to biological agents (very selective group)	• Irreversible peripheral neuropathy • Agitation • Hallucination

small dose of steroids may be additionally required in a minority along with azathioprine to maintain remission. Azathioprine is chosen as a steroid-sparing agent, which takes approximately 2–3 months for optimal action. On azathioprine, regular monitoring of blood counts for bone marrow suppression and liver enzymes for hepatotoxicity is required.

Second-line agents are used in select situations. Patients who are steroid-resistant and thiopurine-intolerant are invariably considered for *biologicals.* Infliximab and adalimumab have been used with response rates of 50–60% to achieve remission. Adalimumab has a better safety profile (infusion reactions) as compared to infliximab and can be used if antibodies to infliximab have developed leading to infliximab nonresponse. Biologicals may be combined with immunomodulators in severe disease. In developing countries, biologicals can only be started if tuberculosis is ruled out. Biologicals are anti-tumor necrosis factor (TNF) alpha agents that will uncover a tubercular granuloma and allow the mycobacteria to disseminate. Biologicals are also contraindicated in the presence of active suppurative infections.

Additionally, for perianal fistulizing CD, antibiotics (ciprofloxacin 20 mg/kg, metronidazole 10–20 mg/kg, or rifaximin 10–30 mg/kg) for 4–6 weeks have shown good short-term response. In mild-moderate non-fistulizing, non-stricturing CD, exclusive enteral nutrition with polymeric, semi-elemental or elemental formulations may be used for 6–8 weeks for induction of remission, followed by a maintenance first line immunomodulator. Oral 5-ASA has a role in induction of remission in mild UC and maintenance phase of mild-moderate UC. Topical 5-aminosalicylic acid (5-ASA) may be used in localized left sided UC. 5-ASA has limited role in CD. Combining oral 5-ASA with topical 5-ASA is more effective than oral alone in UC. Rectal 5-ASA is superior and should be preferred over rectal steroid therapy in UC.

Surgery

In IBD, cumulative risk of surgery increases with duration of disease (CD: 18%, 27%, and 32% at 1, 5, and 10 years, respectively and UC: 8% and 20% at 1 and 5 years, respectively). Surgery is indicated in UC patients with severe acute colitis refractory to medical disease. Uncontrolled hemorrhage, perforation, toxic megacolon, abscesses and obstruction are the other indications for surgery. Proctocolectomy is curative in UC but creating an ileal pouch for fecal continence is done with caution in a girl child due to reduced chances of fecundity later in adulthood. Since surgery is not curative in CD, its use must be limited, and the length of bowel resection must be minimized. Risk of adenocarcinoma colon is 8% after 20 years of disease in pediatric UC and should be suspected with new onset of symptoms after years of remission or features of large bowel obstruction and occult GI blood loss.

Acute Severe Ulcerative Colitis

Approximately 18–25% of UC may experience acute severe symptoms (PUCAI > 65) at any point of time during their disease course (>10 years) and will be transiently steroid refractory. In this scenario, associated infections such

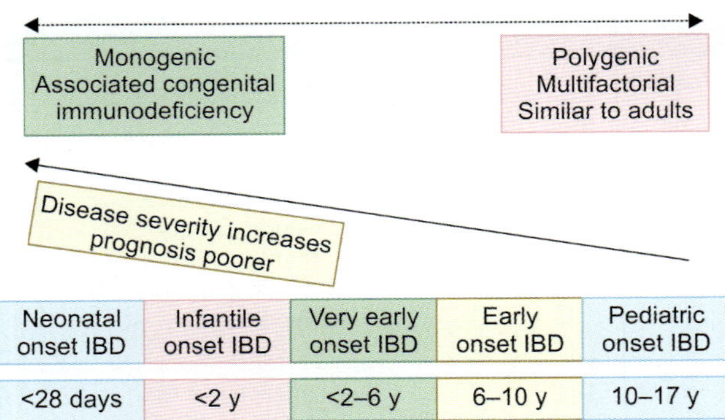

Fig. 9.10.3: New classification of pediatric inflammatory bowel disease (IBD).

as *Clostridium difficile* (stool toxin assay and passage of membranes per rectum), cytomegalovirus (deep colonic ulcers, immunohistochemistry and CMV inclusion bodies in colonic biopsies), concurrent fungal infections (stool for fungal hyphae) and infective colitis (stool culture for shigella, enterohemorrhagic *Escherichia coli,* etc.) must be considered and appropriately treated. Toxic megacolon (TMC, see below) should be looked for.

Considering the case as a steroid refractory state, intravenous (IV) methylprednisolone 1–1.5 mg/kg/d should be started. If there is failure of response to methylprednisolone by day 5, then second-line rescue therapy with IV cyclosporine/oral tacrolimus or infliximab must be considered. Both cyclosporine and infliximab are equally efficacious with similar response (75–80%) for remission. Cyclosporine is given for 3–4 months but therapy with infliximab is indefinite and hence infliximab has lower future colectomy rates. Failure of second-line therapy by day 14 is an indication for colectomy. Colectomy is also indicated if during the course the patient develops perforation or hemorrhage. Response and failure in acute UC is monitored by PUCAI.

Toxic Megacolon

Toxic megacolon is a complication seen in the setting of acute severe ulcerative colitis (ASUC). It is to be diagnosed if transverse colon diameter in an erect X-ray abdomen is more than 40 mm (<10 years age) and more than 56 mm (>10 years age) with evidence of systemic toxicity (fever, tachycardia, dehydration, dyselectrolytemia, altered sensorium, hypotension or shock). Intravenous antibiotics (such as ampicillin, gentamycin, and metronidazole), correction of electrolyte imbalance, food restriction, and preparation for surgery compose the mainstay of initial therapy for TMC. Rectal decompression tube and positional changes have limited benefits. Failure of medical management is an indication for emergency colectomy.

Table 9.10.8: Settings to suspect monogenic IBD (1 or more features).

Feature	*Comment*
Very early onset of symptoms	Most commonly < 2 years age
Family history	Consanguinity, sib death, affected sib or multiple family members, known immunodeficiency state in family
Atypical endoscopy or histology	Apoptotic enterocolitis, unusual, and coalescent pattern of ulcers
Resistance to conventional therapies	Failure of response to steroids, immunomodulators, and biological therapy
Ectodermal defects	Skin lesions (epidermolysis bullosa, eczema), nail dystrophy, hair abnormalities (wooly hair, trichorrhexis nodosa)
Early onset perianal disease	Deep fistula (mucocutaneous, rectogenitourinary), abscess
Reticuloendothelial abnormalities	Lymph node abscesses, splenomegaly, cyclical neutropenia
Recurrent infections or unexplained fever	Deep seated infections, atypical infections (intestinal or non-intestinal), multisystemic life-threatening infections
Hemophagocytic lymphohistiocytosis	Induced by Epstein Barr virus or cytomegalovirus
Associated autoimmunity	Arthritis, serositis, thyroiditis, type 1 diabetes
Early onset tumors	Non-Hodgkin lymphoma, hamartomas

Early Onset IBD

Recently pediatric IBD has been reclassified as shown in **Fig. 9.10.3**. IBD starting less than 2 years age comprises less than 5% of all pediatric IBD and requires detailed immunological workup for immunodeficiencies of monogenic inheritance. Some of the notable genetic defects associated with the infantile onset IBD are IL (interleukin)-10, IL-10 receptor A, IL-10 receptor B, ADAM-17, XIAP, TTC7A (apoptotic enterocolitis), IPEX syndrome, atypical severe combined immunodeficiency (Omenn syndrome), Wiskott-Aldrich syndrome, agammaglobulinemia, hyperIgM syndrome, common variable immunodeficiency (CVID) and chronic granulomatous disease. These diseases are primary immunodeficiencies, which manifest as recurrent infections and IBD.

Setting to suspect monogenic IBD is shown in **Table 9.10.8**. The very early onset, infantile and neonatal IBD have markedly poor prognosis. They have severe course, fistulizing disease, and resistance to biological therapy and often require colectomy or colonic diversion. Allogeneic hematopoietic stem cell transplants (HSCT) have shown to produce 80% remission in those who do not respond to standard therapy.

Due to the significant risk associated with HSCT, including graft-versus-host disease and severe infections, it is important to determine the genetic basis for each patient's VEOIBD before selecting HSCT as a treatment approach.

DIFFERENTIAL DIAGNOSIS OF IBD

Abdominal tuberculosis: In developing countries, tuberculous colitis is a very close differential diagnosis and possibly more common than IBD. Hence while working up for IBD, simultaneous evaluation for tuberculosis is mandatory. The discriminatory features are shown in **Table 9.10.9**. Basic work-up required are chest X-ray, Mantoux test and CT enterography. In select scenarios and high index of suspicion, HRCT chest is required. Circular transverse ulcers are commonly seen in tubercular colitis. Tissue biopsies should be also processed for TB-PCR, ZN stain, TB culture and GeneXpert/Line probe assay. Interferon gamma release assay is not recommended due to poor sensitivity. Occasionally it is very difficult to differentiate IBD versus abdominal TB despite thorough workup and hence a trial and response to at least 8–12 weeks of ATT is required. Paradoxically 20% of CD may report a transient clinical response to ATT which leads to further confusion in a case scenario of diagnostic dilemma. In this scenario, objective findings (resolution of imaging and mucosal changes) is considered response to ATT and suggestive of TB (Logan's criteria of TB).

Bovine milk allergy, multiple food protein allergy and eosinophilic colitis: This is to be considered in setting of infantile IBD. Temporal correlation with introduction of bovine milk or soy, colonic aphthous ulcers and eosinophilic infiltration of colonic biopsies are features.

Table 9.10.9: Discriminatory features favoring tuberculosis.

Clinical	Contact history, peripheral lymphadenopathy, disseminated disease (pulmonary, CNS), abdominal lymph nodal masses
Laboratory	Mantoux positivity, exudative ascites (lymphocyte predominant with high adenosine deaminase)
Imaging	Necrotic calcified or conglomerate abdominal lymph nodes, peritoneal thickening, pericardial effusion, lung involvement (military, bronchiectasis, mediastinal lymph nodes), and calcified space occupying lesions in brain
Histopathology	Caseating large well-defined granulomas (>300 μm size)
Microbiology	Acid-fast bacilli in Ziehl-Neelsen (ZN) stain, culture positivity or positive GeneXpert/line probe assay

Acquired immunodeficiency syndrome: Presentation may mimic IBD colitis. It is suspected in the presence of recurrent urinary, sinopulmonary or dermatological infections (extensive scabies, dermatophytoses), hepatosplenomegaly, generalized lymphadenopathy, thrombocytopenia, and hypergammaglobulinemia.

LONG-TERM ISSUES IN PEDIATRIC IBD

Bone density and linear growth (on steroids), nutrition (due to anorexia, recurrent pain abdomen, small bowel strictures, and malabsorption), immunizations (live vaccines contraindication due to immunosuppression), drug compliance (due to polytherapy, affordability of biologicals, adolescence), psychosocial issues (due to cosmetic stigmata of surgery, recurrent infections), school absenteeism (recurrent hospital admissions), fertility potential (due to drug toxicity, colectomy), and cumulative cancer risks are some of the long-term issues prevailing in IBD.

BIBLIOGRAPHY

1. Gower-Rousseau C, Dauchet L, Vernier-Massouille G, et al. The natural history of pediatric ulcerative colitis: a population-based cohort study. Am J Gastroenterol. 2009;104:2080-8.
2. Levine A, Koletzko S, Turner D, et al. ESPGHAN revised porto criteria for the diagnosis of inflammatory bowel disease in children and adolescents. J Pediatr Gastroenterol Nutr. 2014;58:795-806.
3. Oliveira SB, Monteiro IM. Diagnosis and management of inflammatory bowel disease in children. BMJ. 2017;357:j2083.
4. Ruemmele FM, Veres G, Kolho KL, et al. Consensus guidelines of ECCO/ESPGHAN on the medical management of pediatric Crohn's disease. J Crohns Colitis. 2014;8:1179-207.
5. Sawczenko A, Sandhu BK. Presenting features of inflammatory bowel disease in Great Britain and Ireland. Arch Dis Child. 2003;88:995-1000.
6. Turner D, Travis SP, Griffiths AM, et al. Consensus for managing acute severe ulcerative colitis in children: a systematic review and joint statement from ECCO, ESPGHAN, and the Porto IBD Working Group of ESPGHAN. Am J Gastroenterol. 2011;106:574-88.
7. Turner D, Levine A, Escher JC, et al. Management of pediatric ulcerative colitis: joint ECCO and ESPGHAN evidence-based consensus guidelines. J Pediatr Gastroenterol Nutr. 2012;55:340-61.
8. Uhlig HH, Schwerd T, Koletzko S, et al. COLORS in IBD Study Group and NEOPICS. The diagnostic approach to monogenic very early onset inflammatory bowel disease. Gastroenterology. 2014;147:990-1007.e3.
9. Vernier-Massouille G, Balde M, Salleron J, et al. Natural history of pediatric Crohn's disease: a population-based cohort study. Gastroenterology. 2008;135:1106-13.

9.11 Hepatomegaly: A Practical Diagnostic Approach

Sheila Bhave

INTRODUCTION

Hepatomegaly, often associated with enlargement of the spleen, is a common clinical problem in infants and children. Many disease processes, which may or may not be primarily hepatic, cause liver enlargement.

The pathophysiological mechanisms causing hepatomegaly are:

- Infection, inflammation (hepatitis, fibrosis)
- Kupffer cell hyperplasia
- Venous congestion
- Storage (glycogen, fat, and other metabolites)
- Infiltrations
- Tumors and neoplasia.

CLINICAL EVALUATION

Practical Clues

Is the Liver Really Enlarged?

The liver occupies most of the right upper quadrant of the abdomen attached to the lower surface of the diaphragm. The liver accounts for 1/20th of body weight in neonates and 1/50th of that of the adult.

In infancy and early childhood, the liver and spleen may be felt normally up to 3 cm below the costal margin. In chest diseases, such as pneumothorax, bronchiolitis, and emphysema and in chest deformities such as in rickets, the liver may be pushed down giving an "apparent" hepatomegaly. Hence, percussion for the upper border of the liver is important in the assessment of hepatomegaly especially to recognize "pushed down liver" which should be differentiated from true hepatomegaly.

Size, Margin, Contour, and Consistency of Liver

The liver is to be palpated like any routine palpation of abdomen from left iliac fossa in an anticlockwise manner. Sometimes right subcostal palpation by cupping method from above especially for shrunken firm to hard liver will be useful. Size of the liver is better assessed by "liver span", i.e., the height of the liver in right midclavicular line (superior border by percussion and inferior border by palpation as shown in **Fig. 9.11.1**). Normal liver span at various ages is:

- Less than 1 year: 4–5 cm
- 1–5 year: 5–7 cm
- 5–12 years: 7–9 cm
- More than 12 years: 9–12 cm.

Besides the size of the liver, the consistency and character of the surface and margin should be evaluated. Liver should be examined for tenderness and auscultated for any murmurs. The abdomen should also be palpated for other masses and for enlargement of the spleen. Epigastrium should always be palpated for the left lobe. Enlarged liver with firm to hard consistency and sharp margin usually implies cirrhosis or fibrosis. Soft, enlarged, and tender liver occurs in inflammatory and congestive processes such as viral hepatitis and congestive heart failure. An isolated mass felt in an otherwise normal liver or an asymmetric enlargement may suggest tumor or cyst.

The spleen is to be measured in its long axis, i.e. left upper quadrant to right iliac fossa. Although tip of the spleen is palpable in up to 5–10% of normal infants and children, it has to enlarge at least two to three times to be appreciably felt on physical examination.

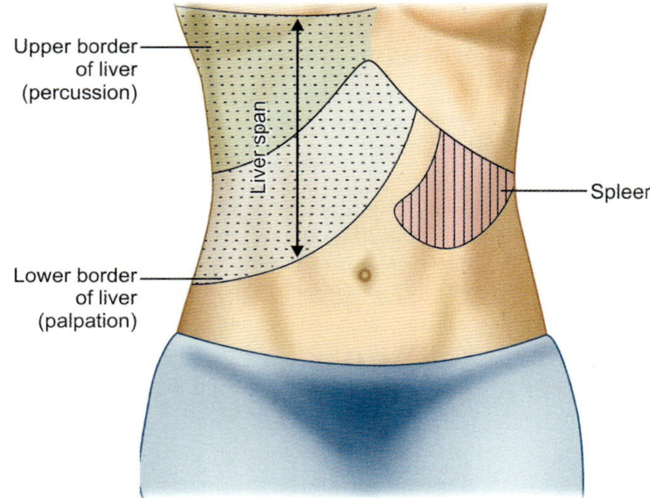

Fig. 9.11.1: Assessment of hepatosplenomegaly.

Is Hepatomegaly due to a Primary Liver Disorder or a Part of a Generalized Disease?

Common pediatric conditions such as protein energy malnutrition, anemia, and tuberculosis can cause significant hepatomegaly. History and general clinical examination can give important clues to these diseases. Primary liver disorders usually present with signs of liver cell failure (e.g. jaundice and ascites) and abnormal liver function tests.

Age of the Child

The age of onset is an important clue to the etiology of pediatric liver disease **(Table 9.11.1)**. Neonatal cholestasis syndrome presents in early infancy; Indian childhood cirrhosis occurs typically in preschool children whereas Wilson disease (WD) affects older children and adolescents.

Other Clues in History and General Physical Examination

Helpful clues are:
- *Onset*: Acute (viral hepatitis) or chronic (as in cirrhosis and chronic hepatitis).
- *Fever*: Typhoid, dengue, malaria, and tuberculosis.
- *Family history and consanguinity*: Wilson disease and thalassemia.
- *Hepatotoxic drugs*: Antitubercular, antiepileptic, and anticancer drugs.
- *Anemia*: Hemolytic anemia and leukemia.
- *Lymphadenopathy*: Disseminated tuberculosis and malignancy.

  Some other clinical clues to diagnosis are given in **Table 9.11.2**.

Important Associated Features in Differential Diagnosis of Hepatomegaly

- *Jaundice*: Obstructive, hemolytic, and hepatocellular types; each type is associated with different group of diseases.
- Splenomegaly is commonly associated with hepatomegaly because of common pathogenetic mechanisms. Causes of predominant and massive splenomegaly are seen in **Table 9.11.3**.
- Ascites, edema, and bleeding tendencies are signs of liver damage.
- Drowsiness (precoma and coma) and gastrointestinal hemorrhage (hematemesis, melena) are ominous signs of impending hepatic failure **(Box 9.11.1)**.

Table 9.11.1: Common causes of hepatosplenomegaly according to age.

Neonates and infants	*Children and adolescents*
Intrauterine infections	*Infections:* Acute viral hepatitis A–E, dengue, typhoid, and leptospirosis
Neonatal cholestasis syndrome Biliary atresia Neonatal hepatitis	*Infection*: Chronic tuberculosis, malaria, and kala-azar
Erythroblastosis (Rh, ABO incompatibility) Congestive heart failure Sepsis, systemic viral infections	*Liver cirrhosis* Indian childhood cirrhosis Budd-Chiari, Veno-occlusive disease Chronic active hepatitis
Metabolic liver disease Galactosemia Tyrosinemia, Alpha-1 antitrypsin deficiency Hemochromatosis	*Metabolic liver disease* Wilson disease Glycogen storage disease Gaucher disease Niemann-Pick disease Mucopolysaccharidosis Nonalcoholic fatty liver disease
Secondaries Wilms tumor Neuroblastoma	*Extrahepatic portal hypertension* Hepatic fibrosis Cystic fibrosis
	Hematological disorders Hemolytic anemia Leukemia, lymphoma
	Cysts (congenital, hydatid) Abscesses (amebic, pyogenic)

APPROACH TO HEPATOSPLENOMEGALY

Differential Diagnosis and Useful Investigations

Important aspects of the approach to diagnosis of hepatosplenomegaly are:
- Accurate clinical history and thorough clinical examination.

Table 9.11.2: Associated clinical manifestations which aid in the diagnosis of hepatomegaly.

Clinical features	*Suggestive of*
Microcephaly/ Hydrocephalus	Intrauterine infections (e.g. Rubella, toxoplasmosis, and CMV)
Cataracts	Galactosemia, Wilson disease
KF ring	Wilson disease
Tremors, dysarthria	Wilson disease
Mental retardation	Galactosemia, lipid storage disorder
Engorged neck veins	Congestive heart failure, constrictive pericarditis
Rickets	Wilson disease, tyrosinemia cystinosis
Cystic kidneys	Congenital hepatic fibrosis
Skin rashes	Histiocytosis Collagen vascular disorders

(CMV: cytomegalovirus; KF ring: Kayser–Fleischer ring).

Table 9.11.3: Causes of massive hepatosplenomegaly.

Predominant enlargement of	
Liver	***Spleen***
Glycogen storage disease (type 1)	Gaucher disease
Congenital hepatic fibrosis	Hemolytic anemia
Extrahepatic biliary atresia	Extrahepatic portal hypertension
Cyst (hydatid, abscess)	Chronic myeloid leukemia (juvenile)
Chronic extrahepatic cholestasis	Myelofibrosis
Tumors, primary or secondary, Acute Budd-Chiari syndrome	Chronic malaria, kala-azar, Hypersplenism, tropical splenomegaly

- Multidisciplinary approach.
- *Neonatal/infantile liver disease*: Usually presents with persistent jaundice (Jaundice beyond 15–21 days must always be investigated, even in the breastfed baby) **(Flowchart 9.11.1)**.
- Hepatomegaly (with or without splenomegaly) in preschool or older children **(Flowchart 9.11.2)**.
- *Assess severity:* Clinical signs of liver cell failure and laboratory tests **(Box 9.11.1)**. Most useful lab tests are:
  - Plasma albumin (low levels suggestive of chronicity)
  - Increased coagulation time (severity of hepatic dysfunction)
  - Low fasting blood sugar levels indicating poor hepatic function.

Box 9.11.1: Clinical signs of liver cell failure and chronic liver disease.

- Hepatomegaly (especially enlarged left lobe)
  - Alternately a "small" liver or a "hard" liver
- Firm splenomegaly
- Jaundice (usually prolonged/recurrent)
- Pruritus
- Ascites
- *Bleeding:*
  - Varices (Hematemesis, melena)
  - Epistaxis
  - Bruising/petechiae
- *Encephalopathy:*
  - Confusion, irritability, somnolence progressing to coma
  - Asterixis (flapping tremors)
- *Cutaneous features:*
  - Spider angiomata
  - Xanthomata
  - Papular acrodermatitis
  - Clubbing
  - Palmar erythema
- Rickets
- Clubbing
- Hypotonia
- Growth failure/malnutrition
- Malabsorption of fats and fat soluble vitamins
- Hepatorenal failure

The scheme of investigations should be directed judiciously at detecting the etiology and the mechanism of

Flowchart 9.11.1: Approach to diagnosis of hepatomegaly in neonatal period/infancy.

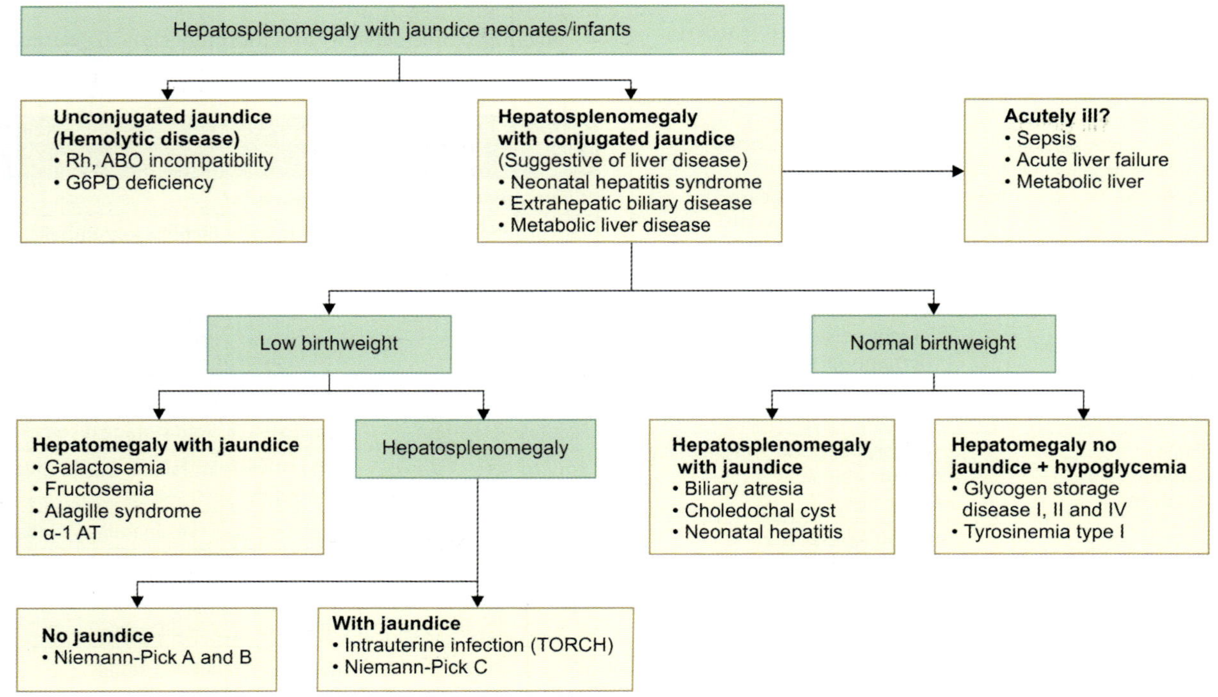

Flowchart 9.11.2: Approach to diagnosis of hepatosplenomegaly in the older child.

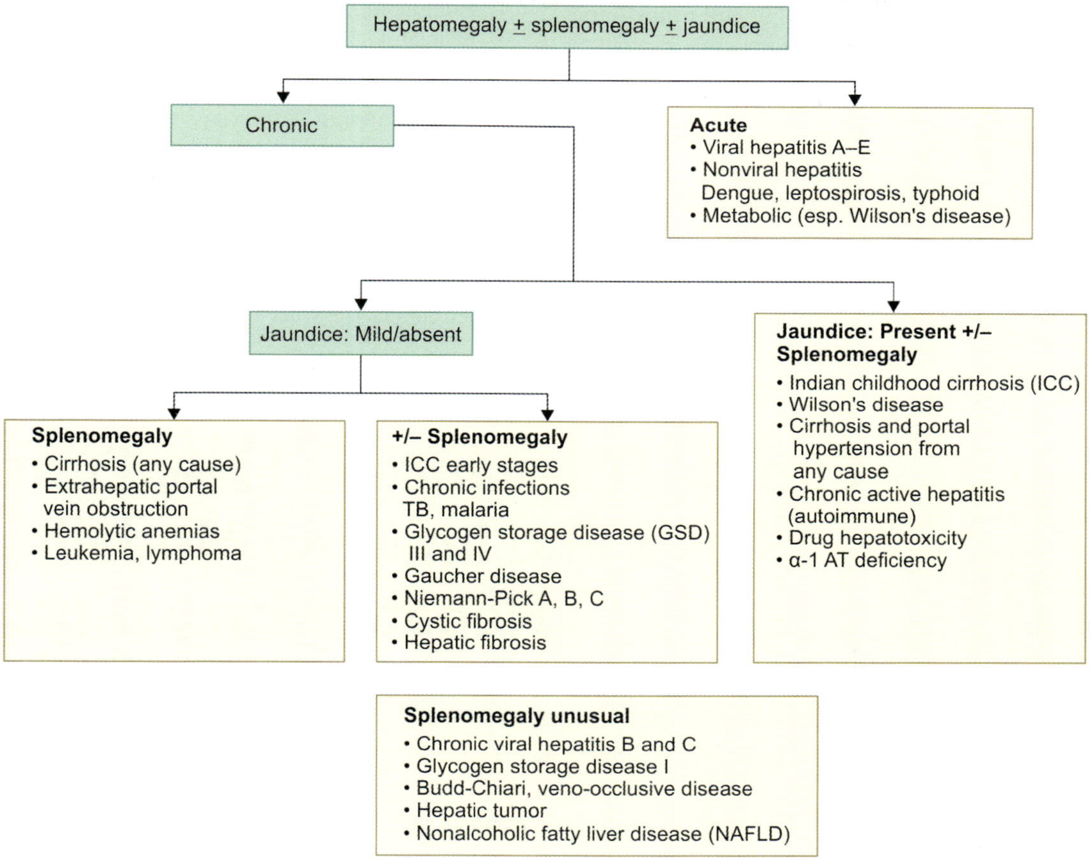

Hepatomegaly ± splenomegaly ± jaundice

- Chronic
  - Jaundice: Mild/absent
    - **Splenomegaly**
      - Cirrhosis (any cause)
      - Extrahepatic portal vein obstruction
      - Hemolytic anemias
      - Leukemia, lymphoma
    - **+/– Splenomegaly**
      - ICC early stages
      - Chronic infections TB, malaria
      - Glycogen storage disease (GSD) III and IV
      - Gaucher disease
      - Niemann-Pick A, B, C
      - Cystic fibrosis
      - Hepatic fibrosis
  - **Jaundice: Present +/– Splenomegaly**
    - Indian childhood cirrhosis (ICC)
    - Wilson's disease
    - Cirrhosis and portal hypertension from any cause
    - Chronic active hepatitis (autoimmune)
    - Drug hepatotoxicity
    - α-1 AT deficiency
- **Acute**
  - Viral hepatitis A–E
  - Nonviral hepatitis Dengue, leptospirosis, typhoid
  - Metabolic (esp. Wilson's disease)

Splenomegaly unusual
- Chronic viral hepatitis B and C
- Glycogen storage disease I
- Budd-Chiari, veno-occlusive disease
- Hepatic tumor
- Nonalcoholic fatty liver disease (NAFLD)

hepatomegaly as also the extent and severity of the disease. Base line and special additional tests are given in **Box 9.11.2**.

Progress of Liver Disease and Hepatomegaly

Important conclusions can be based on careful follow up of hepatomegaly. Benign hepatomegaly associated with common febrile illnesses of children usually recedes

Box 9.11.2: Laboratory tests in diagnosis of hepatosplenomegaly.

- *Hemogram*: Band cells, erythrocyte sedimentation rate (ESR), reticulocyte count, C-reactive protein (CRP)
- Urine routine, culture
- *Liver function tests*
  - Serum bilirubin (Conjugated/unconjugated)
  - Serum glutamic pyruvic transaminase (SGPT) or alanine transaminase (ALT)
  - Serum glutamic oxaloacetic transaminase (SGOT) or aspartate transaminase (APT)
  - Serum alkaline phosphatase (ALP)
  - Serum gamma glutamyl peptidase (GGT)
  - Serum albumin, globulin

Contd...

Contd...

- *Coagulation profile*: Prothrombin time (PT), partial thromboplastin time with kaolin (PTTK)
- Blood sugar levels
- Serum ammonia
- Liver biopsy
- *Imaging studies:*
  - Ultrasonography (USG) abdomen
  - Computed tomography/magnetic resonance imaging (CT/MRI) scan
  - Radionuclide scanning
- *Additional special tests:*
  - *Viral markers*: Hepatic A–E, dengue
  - *Autoimmune markers*: Autoimmune hepatitis
  - *TORCH titers*: Intrauterine infections
  - Metabolic studies
  - *Metabolic screen (urine) and confirmatory tests*: Metabolic liver disease
  - *Enzyme estimations*: Galactosemia, Gaucher disease, and Niemann-Pick disease
  - *Urine succinylacetone*: Tyrosinemia
  - *Copper studies*: Ceruloplasmin, urinary Cu, Cu stains on liver biopsy, hepatic Cu: ICC, Wilson disease
  - *Alpha-fetoprotein*: Hepatoblastoma, tyrosinemia
  - *Sweat chloride*: Cystic fibrosis

completely within a few weeks. Cases of acute viral hepatitis also usually resolve within 6 weeks. On the other hand, continued hepatomegaly with signs of progressive liver failure must be evaluated for chronic liver diseases and cirrhosis.

BIBLIOGRAPHY

1. Bhave SA. Chronic liver disorders in children. In: Bavdekar A, Mathai J, Sathiyasekaran M, Yachha SK (Eds). Pediatric Gastroenterology (IAP Specialty Series). New Delhi: Jaypee Brothers Medical Publishers (P) Ltd; 2008. pp. 188-96.
2. Bhave SA. Indian childhood cirrhosis (Update). In: Gupte S (Ed). Recent Advances in Pediatric Gastroenterology, Hepatology and Nutrition. New Delhi: Jaypee Brothers Medical Publishers (P) Ltd; 2000. pp. 322-31.
3. Boamah L, Ballistreri W. Manifestations of liver disease. In: Kliegman RM, Behrman RE, Jenson HB, Stanton BE (Eds). Nelson's Textbook of Pediatrics. New Delhi: Elsevier (India); 2008. pp. 1661-6.
4. Consensus Report on Neonatal Cholestasis Syndrome (NCS). Pediatric gastroenterology subspecialty Chapter of Indian Academy of Pediatrics. Indian Pediatr. 2000;37:845-51.
5. Kelly DA. The approach to the child with liver disease: Differential diagnosis and useful investigations. In: Kelly DA (Ed). Diseases of the Liver and the Biliary System in Children, 3rd edition. UK: Wiley-Blackwell Publishing; 2008. pp. 21-35.

9.12 Clinical Relevance of Liver Function Tests and Imaging Modalities in Hepatobiliary Disorders

Geetha M

LIVER FUNCTION TESTS

Liver function tests (LFTs) are a set of basic investigations done in all suspected hepatobiliary diseases. They should be interpreted with the background of the clinical history and physical findings to yield meaningful conclusions.

The frequently requested LFTs include serum bilirubin (total, direct and indirect), alanine aminotransferase (ALT) and aspartate aminotransferase (AST), serum alkaline phosphatase (SAP), gamma-glutamyltransferase (GGT), proteins (total, albumin and globulin) and prothrombin time (PT). In addition to the initial and basic urine tests, urine tests for bilirubin pigment, bile salt, and urobilinogen are also done. Blood glucose and serum ammonia are also relevant with useful clinical implications. The other blood tests requested sometimes in a clinical context are lactate dehydrogenase (LDH), bile acids, and 5'-nucleotidase (5'NT).

No single test alone is enough to provide complete estimate of the function of liver. LFTs reflect liver cell injury (AST, ALT, and LDH), indicate the synthetic function of liver (albumin, PT and blood glucose), cholestasis (SAP, GGT, and LDH), and organic ion transport or drug metabolism status (serum bilirubin, bile acids and urine bilirubin and urobilinogen).

Bilirubin

This is the most common LFT usually done. By itself, it gives a very little information. The normal value is less than 1 mg/dL of which 20% is conjugated. The type of jaundice can be categorized as direct, indirect or mixed hyperbilirubinemia.

- Hemolytic conditions have elevated indirect serum bilirubin with normal enzymes and PT.
- Benign conditions such as Gilbert syndrome have mildly increased indirect bilirubin level.
- Bilirubin levels more than 30 mg/dL would suggest:
  - Concomitant hemolysis + significant liver injury as in hepatitis A (HAV), hepatitis E (HEV), HAV + HEV, drugs or superadded sepsis
  - Acute viral hepatitis (AVH-HAV)/HEV/HAV + HEV on herbals
  - Sepsis and renal impairment can also increase bilirubin levels.

Aminotransferases

They consist of ALT and AST, earlier called serum glutamic pyruvic transaminase (SGPT) and serum glutamic oxaloacetic transaminase (SGOT), respectively. These enzymes are in the cytoplasm of the hepatocytes and are released when there is hepatocellular damage resulting in elevated serum levels. The normal adult values are less than 45 IU/L. The same values are extrapolated for children. The value may range from two times the upper limit of normal (ULN) to ten times ULN.

- In AVH, the level can increase up 10,000 IU/L or more.
- The three most common causes of very high ALT and AST (>2,000 IU/L) are AVH, toxic hepatitis (e.g. paracetamol poisoning and drug induced) and ischemic hepatitis.
- If in this scenario, the PT is also prolonged, the prognosis is poor. Conversely, if the PT is normal, irrespective of the bilirubin level, the child has a good prognosis.
- Conditions where transaminases are raised 5–50 times of the ULN range, are viral hepatitis, toxic hepatitis, autoimmune hepatitis, Wilson disease, storage diseases (e.g. glycogen storage disorders), and infections such as leptospirosis, dengue, and malaria.
- Conditions where transaminases are elevated up to 200–300 IU/L are same as earlier; and include sepsis like urinary tract infection (UTI) with bacteremia especially in younger children, non-alcoholic steatohepatitis (NASH), cholestasis, and extrahepatic causes such as cholecystitis with choledocholithiasis.
- In cirrhosis and obstructive jaundice, the levels are usually below 400 IU/L.
- In patients with choledocholithiasis with cholangitis the value can sometimes rise above 400 IU/L but rapidly declines within 2–3 days.
- Between the two transaminases, ALT is more liver-specific. AST can be raised in extrahepatic conditions such as myopathies, myositis, cardiac diseases, etc. since it is also found in muscle tissue.

Alkaline Phosphatase and Gamma-glutamyltransferase

In children, the alkaline phosphatase (ALP) levels are higher than in adults and this is contributed by the growing bones. The normal values in adults are up to 100 IU/L while in children it can rise up to 400–500 IU/L. Hence, it is not unusual to find an isolated raised ALP. Also, in conditions such as rickets and intestinal obstruction, the levels may be markedly raised.

To differentiate bone ALP from liver ALP, a GGT test can be done. If this is normal, the raised ALP is extrahepatic in origin.

A raised GGT or 5′NT along with raised ALP indicates a hepatic cause. The value may be raised four to ten-fold or greater in obstructive jaundice. Elevated ALP with low GGT is suggestive of progressive familial intrahepatic cholestasis [progressive familial intrahepatic cholestasis (PFIC) 1 and 2]; but elevated ALP with normal or above normal GGT is seen in PFIC 3, blood group B or O and bone disease associated with chronic renal failure.

Proteins

Serum albumin is also low in varieties of diseases other than liver diseases such as protein energy malnutrition (PEM) and nephrosis. In liver disease, its value is indicative of the synthetic function of liver. It is not very helpful in acute conditions but in cases of jaundice it helps to identify, if there is an underlying chronic liver disease. In acute conditions, albumin and total proteins may be transiently reduced but subsequently it normalizes.

Reversal of albumin: globulin ratio (A:G ratio) less than 1 (normal > 1.1) associated with low serum albumin (<3 g/dL), PT more than 3 seconds of control and AST:ALT of more than 1 are biochemical laboratory clues for chronic liver disease.

Prothrombin Time

Among all the LFTs, it is the PT, which carries the greatest importance, especially in acute liver disease. This test is done along with a control since the value can differ slightly from laboratory to laboratory. The normal value is 14 seconds. A prolongation of PT more than 2 seconds of ULN which is not corrected by vitamin K injection is generally considered a poor prognostic factor; if PT is more than 4 seconds, liver biopsy is not advisable and if persistently high, one should get liver transplant team's opinion.

International normalization ratio (INR) standardizes PT to different reagents. Normal INR value is 0.8–1.2.

- If INR value is more than 1.5, liver biopsy is not advisable.
- If INR is more than three in fulminant hepatic failure, it indicates poor prognosis and an important factor taken into consideration for liver transplantation.

In case of acute viral hepatitis, if the enzymes are very high but the PT continues to remain normal, the prognosis and outcome is good.

Caution in Interpretation of LFTs

Abnormal LFT need not always mean liver disease such as:

- Elevated bilirubin seen in Gilbert and Dubin-Johnson syndromes.
- Isolated elevation in serum ALP seen in growing children and rickets.
- Mild AST/ALT elevation in myopathies.
- Hypoalbuminemia can occur in other extrahepatic causes.
- Prolonged PT in vitamin K deficiency.
- Elevated ammonia in urea cycle disorders.
- Hypoglycemia in sepsis.

Normal LFT need not mean absence of liver disease:

- Serum transaminases and other synthetic liver functions could be transiently normal in chronic hepatitis, well-compensated cirrhosis, non-cirrhotic portal fibrosis (NCPF), methotrexate hepatotoxicity, etc.

    The terminology LFT is a misnomer: a conventional LFT tests the degree of liver injury or severity of cholestasis but not of liver synthetic function and most tests are not specific to the liver; hence, LFT is only a colloquial term.

IMAGING MODALITIES

Various imaging modalities are available for the hepatobiliary system, each with its unique indications and limitations. The common tests, which are performed, include ultrasonogram (USG) of abdomen, computed tomography (CT) scan of abdomen, magnetic resonance imaging (MRI) of abdomen, hepatobiliary scintigraphy, endoscopic retrograde cholangiopancreatography (ERCP), and endoscopic ultrasonography.

Ultrasonogram of Abdomen

This is the simplest and cheapest modality for imaging the liver and usually suffices in most cases. It provides information regarding organomegaly, any lesions, masses, portal flow, collaterals, presence of ascites, obstructive causes, etc. The presence of dilated intrahepatic radicals indicates that the source of obstruction is extrahepatic. The only notable exception to this is extrahepatic biliary atresia (EHBA). In case of doubtful masses in the liver, CT abdomen may be required for accurate delineation.

CT Abdomen

CT scan helps delineate masses of liver, causes of obstructive jaundice-like cholecystitis and choledocholithiasis, choledochal cyst, and ductal disease much more accurately. However, for diffuse, infiltrative lesions, such as storage disorders it is not very useful. The arterial and portal phases can help differentiate hemangiomas from other tumors.

Magnetic Resonance Imaging/Magnetic Resonance Cholangiopancreatography

This modality of imaging of the hepatobiliary system is helpful in identifying choledochal cyst, distal common bile duct stones (CBD) stones and microliths, strictures, etc.

Hepatobiliary Scintigraphy

This is a very useful test especially in early infancy to help diagnose cases of EHBA. Children with severe cholestatic jaundice are primed with phenobarbitone and imaging is done. Mebrofenin is the preferred agent used. The hepatocytes actively take up the dye and promptly secrete it into the biliary tree. In cases of EHBA, the uptake is prompt, but excretion is not seen even after 24 hours. In cases of neonatal hepatitis, the uptake itself is slow but excretion can be detected. However, in severe cases of neonatal hepatitis, it may not be possible to differentiate it from EHBA with this test and hence it is useful in only about 80% of the cases.

Tc-99m labeled hepatoiminodiacetic acid derivative (HIDA) scanning is also useful in conditions of suspected bile leak, e.g. trauma, postsurgical and even spontaneous perforation of bile duct.

Endoscopic Retrograde Cholangiopancreatography

This is an invasive test by which the biliary system and the pancreatic duct can be imaged by injecting dye through the ampulla of Vater. The image obtained is like percutaneous cholangiography (PTC). However, it has the advantage of offering therapeutic potential. CBD stones can be imaged and removed, strictures dilated, and obstructions stented. Biopsy can also be obtained by brush method. Earlier on, it was the diagnostic test for choledochal cyst but with the advent of magnetic resonance cholangiopancreatography (MRCP), it is no longer used for this indication.

Endoscopic Ultrasound

This is a relatively newer modality of investigation. The test involves the use of a specialized endoscope, which has an ultrasonic transducer at the tip and helps in imaging the organs from inside the bowel. Hence certain areas, which are not clearly delineated in CT scan, e.g. the lower CBD can be better imaged. In addition, it helps image the left lobe of liver, pancreas and any submucous bulges. It also offers the advantage of being able to biopsy any suspicious lesion as well as drainage of pseudocyst of pancreas up to 6 cm distance.

Though there are many tests available for investigating and imaging the hepatobiliary tree, a judicious combination of these tests in a logical manner will help clinch the diagnosis in most cases, rather than doing all the tests at once.

KEY MESSAGES

- Interpret LFTs in the clinical context.
- Careful history including drugs/sibling history of chronic liver disease (CLD) is a must for interpretation.
- Physical examination especially BMI (fatty liver), and stigmata of CLD should be done in all cases.
- Prothrombin time (PT) and serum albumin should be included in routine LFT.
- Include blood sugar and arterial ammonia in sick children.
- Ultrasonogram abdomen is a very useful investigation.
- Investigate for treatable causes and get hepatologist's opinion early when in doubt.

BIBLIOGRAPHY

1. Boyer TD, Manns MP, Sanyal AJ. Zakim and Boyer's hepatology. A Textbook of Liver Disease, 6th edition. Philadelphia: Saunders Elsevier. 2009;4:235-50.
2. Feldman M, Friedman LS, Brandt LJ. Sleisenger and Fordtran's Gastrointestinal and Liver Disease, 9th edition. Philadelphia: Saunders-Elsevier; 2010. pp. 1227-37.
3. Suchy FJ, Sokol RJ, Balistreri WF. Liver Disease in Children, 3rd edition. New York: Cambridge University Press. 2007;8:163-78.
4. Yamada T, Alpers DH, Kalloo AN, et al. Principles of Clinical Gastroenterology, 5th edition. Chichester: Wiley-Blackwell Publication; 2009. pp. 400-22.

9.13 Viral Hepatitis

Malathi Sathiyasekaran

INTRODUCTION

Hepatitis or inflammation of the hepatocytes may be acute or chronic in its presentation. Acute hepatitis is a self-limiting illness characterized by an abrupt onset of symptoms with the hepatocellular inflammation usually resolving completely within 4 weeks. When there is a continuing inflammation beyond 6 months (3 months in children), it is labeled as *chronic hepatitis*. Viruses are the most important causative agents of hepatitis and the term viral hepatitis refers to the illness caused by the major hepatotropic viruses—hepatitis A, B, C, D, E and rarely G (HAV, HBV, HCV, HDV, HEV and HGV), though several other viruses such as coxsackieviruses, Epstein-Barr virus (EBV), *Herpes simplex* and cytomegalovirus (CMV) can cause hepatitis. This chapter highlights the features of acute viral hepatitis (AVH) caused by the common hepatotropic viruses.

DEFINITION

Acute viral hepatitis is a systemic viral infection predominantly affecting the liver with a characteristic constellation of clinical (jaundice, nausea, vomiting and right hypochondrial pain), biochemical (elevated serum bilirubin and/or transaminases) and pathological features (hepatocellular inflammation and necrosis), which resolves spontaneously or progresses to acute liver failure or chronic hepatitis.

EPIDEMIOLOGY

In India sporadic AVH is caused mainly by the two enterally transmitted viruses namely hepatitis A (60–70%) and hepatitis E (10–20%). The two parenterally transmitted viruses namely HBV (10–15%) and HCV (<1%) are less common causes of acute sporadic hepatitis. Improvement in socioeconomic status has resulted in a shift in epidemiology of HAV with older children being susceptible to the infection. The prevalence of hepatitis B in India ranges from 2.4% to 16% and HCV is around 1–2.5%. HEV has been isolated in all the major epidemics in India and is more common in North India especially in regions around the river Ganges. Infections due to HAV and HEV are self-limiting and do not progress to chronicity, whereas HBV and HCV infections may progress to chronic hepatitis, cirrhosis and hepatocellular carcinoma.

ETIOPATHOGENESIS

- *Hepatitis A virus (HAV)* is a 27 nm picornavirus spread by the orofecal route with an incubation period of 15–50 days. The necroinflammatory reaction is believed to be an immune response of the host to the HAV.
- *Hepatitis E virus (HEV)* is a 30 nm RNA virus of the *Genus Hepevirus* with several genotypes. HEV is transmitted by the orofecal route with an incubation period of 15–40 days similar to HAV. The mechanism of hepatocyte injury is most likely due to an immune-mediated reaction.
- *Hepatitis B virus (HBV)* is a 42 nm of hepadnavirus family, which causes an immune-mediated injury. The severity of the illness depends on the degree of immune response by the host. HBV is a highly infective virus with an incubation period of 60–180 days and is transmitted by blood, blood products and body fluids. The three antigens hepatitis B surface antigen (HBsAg), envelope antigen (HBeAg) and core antigen (HBcAg)—the corresponding antibodies and the viral HBV DNA are useful biomarkers in diagnosis and monitoring therapy. HBsAg appears in the blood 6 weeks after infection and usually disappears within 6 months. Persistence of HBsAg beyond 6 months indicates chronicity. HBeAg appears soon after HBsAg and disappears within 6 weeks. Persistence of this antigen beyond 6 weeks indicates progression to chronicity. HBcAg is detected only in hepatocytes and not in the serum. The presence of anti-HBc IgM indicates recent infection, whereas presence of anti-HBc IgG indicates past infection. Anti-HBs is the protective antibody and may be present following immunization or natural infection. Quantification of HBV DNA is essential to determine the phase of chronic infection. Perinatal transmission of HBV is a unique problem seen in children and is more common in areas of high endemicity. The relaxed DNA of the hepatitis B virus on entering the hepatocyte becomes a closed circular covalent DNA (cccDNA) and integrates with the host DNA.
- *Hepatitis C virus (HCV)* is a 30–80 nm RNA virus of flaviviridae family and results in a complex immune response. HCV has an incubation period of 60–150 days and is less infective; but more sinister than HBV and is spread by blood and blood products. Perinatal transmission occurs when mothers have a high HCV viral load.

- *Hepatitis D virus (HDV)* is a defective virus with a small RNA molecule and an envelope constituted by HBsAg. This virus infects only those who are HBsAg positive and presents either as superinfection or co-infection depending on whether HDV infects a child with pre-existing chronic HBV infection or infects along with HBV.

CLINICAL FEATURES

In most young children with acute viral hepatitis, the presentation may be subclinical or anicteric whereas in older children the three stages of AVH, viz. the prodrome, icteric stage and convalescence may be more distinct. The clinical presentation is common to all the types of viral hepatitis with a prodrome, which usually lasts for 2–7 days characterized by nausea, vomiting, high-colored urine, fever and right hypochondrial pain followed by jaundice, pale stools and tender hepatomegaly. The icteric stage usually lasts for 7–14 days but may persist as long as 12 weeks in older children. The recovery is heralded by the disappearance of the constitutional symptoms, improvement in appetite and decrease in the size of liver.

HAV and HEV Hepatitis

Older children with HAV infection may present with atypical manifestations such as ascites, pleural effusion, firm hepatomegaly and disturbing pruritus. Extrahepatic manifestations due to circulating immune complexes are uncommon and include evanescent skin rash, transient arthralgia, pancreatitis, vasculitis, thrombocytopenia, triggering of autoimmune hepatitis, red cell aplasia, myocarditis, nephritis, cryoglobulinemia and Guillain-Barré syndrome. Acute liver failure occurs in less than 1% of children.

Infection due to HEV is similar to HAV. During HEV epidemics children usually have a milder or subclinical infection. Pregnant women present with acute liver failure associated with a high maternal mortality (1–20%) and stillbirths.

HBV and HCV Hepatitis

The majority of children with acute HBV infection are anicteric. Those with icteric hepatitis may be symptomatic for 1–2 months. Immune-mediated extrahepatic manifestations such as maculopapular or urticarial rash, migratory arthritis, nephritis and papular acrodermatitis of childhood (Gianotti-Crosti syndrome) may be present. Since the risk of chronicity is inversely proportional to the age of acquisition of the illness, a neonate born to a mother who is HBsAg and HBeAg positive has about 90% chance of acquiring the infection. This decreases to 30% if the age of acquisition is 1–5 years and 5–10% if acquired after the age of 5 years. The five stages in the natural history of HBV infection, viz. immune tolerant, immune-active HBeAg positive, immune-active HBeAg negative, inactive HBsAg carrier and viral clearance are categorized according to the transaminase and HBV DNA levels. These terminologies have been changed to chronic hepatitis B (CHB) HBeAg positive infection or disease and chronic hepatitis B (CHB) HBeAg negative infection or disease **(Table 9.13.1)**. In perinatal transmission the phase of immune tolerance characterized by high viral DNA, normal transaminases and minimal hepatic inflammation lasts for many years and is associated with a low annual HBeAg clearance.

Table 9.13.1: Interpretation of serologic markers in hepatitis B infection.

HBsAg	*HBeAg*	*Anti-HBe*	*Anti-HBc*	*Anti-HBs*	*HBV DNA*	*ALT*	*Significance*
+	+	–	IgM	–	>200,000 IU/L	>1,000 IU/L	Acute hepatitis
+	+	–	IgG	–	>200,000 IU/L	Normal	Immune tolerance No treatment (CHB HBeAg positive infection)
+	+	–	IgG	–	>20,000 IU/L	>2 UL/ N	Immune active HBeAg positive. TREAT (CHB HBeAg positive hepatitis)
+	–	+	IgG	–	>2,000 IU/L	>2 UL/ N	Immune active HBeAg negative TREAT (CHB HBeAg negative hepatitis)
+	–	+	IgG	–	<2,000 IU/L	Normal	Inactive carrier. No treatment (CHB HBeAg negative infection)
–	–	±	IgG	+	Not detected	Normal	Viral clearance
–	–	–	–	+	Not detected	Normal	Effective HBV vaccination

(CHB: chronic hepatitis B; HBV; hepatitis B virus)

Acute HCV hepatitis takes a milder course in children and acute liver failure occurs in lesser than 1%. The symptoms of malaise, fatigue and jaundice are mild but the transaminases are elevated for a longer period. Approximately 40–50% may progress to chronicity and later to cirrhosis and hepatocellular carcinoma. Sporadic hepatitis in children due to HCV is rare and is reported in children receiving multiple blood transfusions.

DIAGNOSIS OF ACUTE VIRAL HEPATITIS

Basic investigations, such as urine for bile salts, bile pigments, total bilirubin with fractionation, alanine transaminase (ALT) and aspartate transaminase (AST) will suffice in most children with AVH. Prothrombin time is a useful test for assessing prognosis. Complete blood counts, blood glucose, urea, creatinine, total protein and albumin are checked when the child is hospitalized. Hepatitis is diagnosed only if the transaminases are more than twice the upper limit of normal. In viral hepatitis, ALT is markedly increased more than 20 times the upper limit of normal and is higher than AST indicating cytoplasmic rather than mitochondrial injury. Investigations for etiology are not necessary unless there are atypical manifestations or the child is hospitalized. All children should be screened for HBsAg. The presence of anti-HAV IgM or anti-HEV IgM confirms the diagnosis of acute HAV and HEV hepatitis respectively. HBsAg positivity along with anti-HBc IgM indicates acute HBV hepatitis; whereas anti-HCV IgM positivity indicates acute HCV hepatitis.

Infection due to nonhepatotropic viruses, such as measles, parvovirus B19, *Herpes simplex* 1 and 2, dengue virus, cytomegalovirus (CMV), EBV and human immunodeficiency virus (HIV) may present with jaundice and moderate elevation of transaminases. The associated clinical features of the underlying illness and specific serologic tests will help in diagnosis. Other causes of hepatitis such as leptospirosis, typhoid fever, Wilson disease (WD) and autoimmune hepatitis should be excluded if there are atypical manifestations or features suggestive of nonviral hepatitis.

Ultrasound examination is done to exclude liver abscess or gallstones. Liver biopsy is not recommended in children with AVH, but is essential in those with suspected acute or chronic liver disease or chronic hepatitis.

MANAGEMENT

The majority of children with AVH will recover spontaneously and require only supportive treatment. A nutritious diet should be provided and undue physical exertion, hepatotoxic drugs and constipation should be avoided. Children with persistent vomiting, fever, fluid retention, altered sensorium or gastrointestinal bleed require hospitalization. Severe cholestasis can be managed with ursodeoxycholic acid (UDCA) in a dose of 20 mg/kg/day.

There is no role for antiviral agents in acute HAV and HEV hepatitis. There are few case reports of antiviral agents such as lamivudine and entecavir in children with acute severe HBV hepatitis. Patients with acute hepatitis C who have persistent viremia (i.e. HCV RNA positive for 12 weeks) following infection require treatment. The current recommendation is to initiate treatment with interferon (IFN)-alpha or pegylated interferon (PEG-IFN) as early as possible in asymptomatic patients infected with HCV genotype 1, while treatment may be delayed in icteric individuals with significant symptoms and those with genotype 2 and 3. The new direct acting antivirals (DAAs) have an excellent sustained viral response and are now recommended in children and adolescents.

COMPLICATIONS

Acute viral hepatitis is a self-limiting illness and most of the children recover without any sequel. Fever, hyperbilirubinemia, prolonged cholestasis, ascites and coagulopathy may be a presentation in older children. The most important complication is acute liver failure. Chronic hepatitis, cirrhosis and hepatocellular carcinoma are the complications seen in HBV and HCV infections.

PROGNOSIS

The majority of children with acute HAV and HEV hepatitis recover without any complications. Hepatotoxic drugs, indigenous medications and underlying metabolic liver disease may precipitate acute liver failure.

PREVENTION

General Measures

Infections due to HAV and HEV can be prevented by improving environmental sanitation and hygiene. Drinking clean water, washing hands and hygienic preparation of food are essential in preventing the transmission of HAV and HEV. Since, HBV and HCV are spread parenterally, proper screening of blood and blood products is necessary prior to transfusion. Disposable needles should be used and unnecessary needle pricks including tattooing should be avoided.

Immunization

Hepatitis A virus can be prevented by active immunization with two doses of hepatitis A vaccine given 6 months apart after the age of 18 months. Active immunization with three doses of hepatitis B vaccine given at 0, 1, and 6 months is recommended with the first dose preferably given soon after birth.

Table 9.14.1: Salient clinical differences between chronic hepatitis and cirrhosis liver.

Chronic hepatitis	*Cirrhosis*
3-6 months or longer	Complications often +
Signs/symptoms of CLD x 3–6 months	More prolonged
No variceal bleed	Variceal bleeds
Minimal or no splenomegaly	Firm splenomegaly
No epigastric veins	Tortuous and flow away from umbilicus
Ascites unusual	Ascites often present
Liver firm sharp edged and large	Nodular, hard and shrunken
Liver span increased	Decreased
Encephalopathy unusual	Often present
Growth failure late stage	Often present
SMR low late stage	Usual and early
Reversible with treatment	Irreversible
Prognosis better	Prognosis not good
Liver transplant—No	Recommended

(CLD: chronic liver disease; SMR: sexual maturity rating)

Cirrhosis is potentially a lethal, chronic and diffuse liver disease characterized by prolonged liver injury resulting in necro-fibro-inflammatory regeneration (nodule formation) response. When the chronic illness is silent, the child may have only firm hepatomegaly or hepatosplenomegaly with abnormal liver function tests (LFT), e.g. reversal of albumin to globulin (A:G) ratio and it is termed compensated (Child score A cirrhosis). When the patient develops jaundice, ascites, gastrointestinal variceal bleeding and/or hepatic encephalopathy, it is termed "decompensated (Child score B cirrhosis)". Advanced/end-stage (Child score C cirrhosis) denotes patients with poor prognosis invariably needing liver transplant.

A subset of children with CLD may decompensate following an acute insult. Superinfection with hepatotropic viruses on CLD in children manifests as ACLD, ACLF and non-ACLF. Hepatitis E virus is the most common superinfection in the population. The mortality in ACLF is five times higher than that in the non-ACLF group. Pediatric end-stage liver disease (PELD) score is useful in differentiating likely survivors and non-survivors. The salient differences between chronic hepatitis and cirrhosis are provided in **Table 9.14.1**.

Complications of Decompensated Cirrhosis and End-stage Chronic Liver Disease

This is characterized by ascites, coagulopathy, encephalopathy, gastrointestinal (GI) bleeds, hepatorenal syndrome, hepatopulmonary syndrome (cyanosis), spontaneous

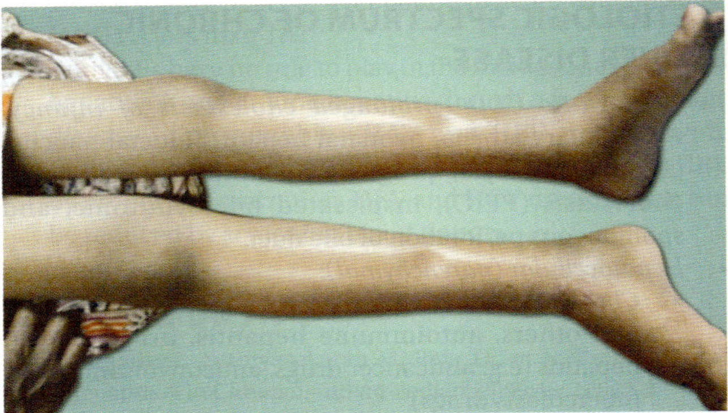

Fig. 9.14.3: Pitting pedal edema in decompensated cirrhosis.

bacterial peritonitis and hepatocellular carcinoma (especially following HBV, HCV, and HDV induced-cirrhosis). Growth failure, malabsorption and malnutrition are other prominent clinical features.

DIAGNOSTIC LABORATORY INVESTIGATIONS

The choice of laboratory tests requested is aimed to help early diagnosis and complications, status of liver function, etiology and prognosis of especially end-stage CLD.

Is there cirrhosis of liver? Clinical evidence of decompensation with liver cell failure as mentioned above with supportive evidence of defective synthetic function of liver such as hypoalbuminemia, reversal of albumin globulin ratio, raised prothrombin time (× two- to threefold) and raised international normlized ratio (INR) more than 3 are diagnostic of cirrhosis. Elevated liver transaminases with conjugated hyperbilirubinemia suggest active liver injury. Presence of pruritus and deep icterus and elevated cholestatic enzymes like serum alkaline phosphatase (SAP) and gamma-glutamyl transpeptidase (GGT) suggests evidence of cholestasis due to both intrahepatic and extrahepatic causes. Raised SAP and low or normal GGT is diagnostic of progressive familial intrahepatic cholestasis (PFIC) type 1 and 2, but raised SAP and high GGT is diagnostic of PFIC type 3.

Ultrasonogram (USG) of abdomen may reveal splenomegaly, tortuous and dilated splenic vein, portal vein collaterals, hyperechoic liver with dilated intrahepatic portal vein radicals, caudate lobe enlargement, minimal ascites and right-sided pleural effusion, leino-renal collaterals, etc. in cirrhotic patients. Choledochal cyst, extrahepatic biliary atresia, Budd-Chiari syndrome, etc. can also be recognized by USG abdomen.

USG color Doppler of spleno-porto-venous axis is useful in diagnosing the reversal of portal venous flow pattern and collateral circulation.

Upper GI endoscopy will reveal presence of esophageal and gastric fundic varices and frequently portal hypertensive congestive gastropathy and also indicate the need for endotherapy (endoscopic band ligation or sclerotherapy).

Complete hemogram may show pancytopenia indicating hypersplenism or persistent thrombocytopenia suggesting end-stage liver disease, which are poor prognostic markers whereas leukocytosis occurs in intercurrent infections.

Recurrent hypoglycemia and coagulopathy (high prothrombin time despite vitamin K and high INR) are poor prognostic markers.

Psychometry tests and serum ammonia may be needed in minimal hepatic encephalopathy and overt hepatic encephalopathy.

Brain proton MR spectroscopy for metabolites in children with suspected MHE show significant correlations with plasma ammonia and branched chain amino acids (BCAA) to aromatic amino acids (AAA) ratio. As in adults, brain MRS in children may be helpful in establishing a diagnosis of MHE.

Etiologic workup will depend on the clinical context, and includes infective causes (such as hepatitis B and C, TORCH, HIV), drugs depending on history, specific metabolic workup, bone marrow and liver biopsy for storage disorders specifically Wilson disease and liver copper-related disease workup, including ophthalmic referral for Kayser–Fleischer (KF) ring as well as cataract or cherry-red spots in lipid storage disorders.

Prognostic evaluation by Child scoring **(Table 9.14.2)** and model for end-stage liver disease (MELD) score is also necessary. In addition, chronic liver cell failure patients may need repeated laboratory tests pre-, peri-, and post-liver transplantation stage apart from donor screening tests. Fibroscan of liver is coming up in certain centers to assess degree of liver fibrosis.

Liver biopsy: Liver biopsy is the gold standard and confirmatory for chronic hepatitis and cirrhosis liver. Presence of periportal fibrosis and necrosis, nodular regeneration with loss of hepatic lobular architecture are the confirmatory findings for cirrhosis and the histopathological findings of portal and lobular inflammation (interface necro-fibro-chronic inflammation and ballooning degeneration) suggest chronic hepatitis. It helps in diagnosis, disease activity, classification, follow-up and identifying etiology like EHBA, Alagille syndrome with ductal paucity, HBV (ground-glass hepatocytes), PFIC, alpha-1 antitrypsin deficiency, hemochromatosis, Wilson disease, Caroli disease, fibropolycystic disease, etc.

Differential Diagnosis

- Extrahepatic portal hypertension (absent liver cell failure, abdominal wall veins)
- Chronic hepatitis (absence of nodular liver, abdominal wall veins and portal hypertension).

COURSE AND PROGNOSIS

It is variable, depending on Child scoring **(Table 9.14.2.)**.

Interpretation: Any two of the above will guide physician:

- *Child score A*: Patient with good liver dysfunction.
- *Child score C*: Patient with poor liver function and surgical/invasive procedures will carry increased mortality in 90% in non-bleeding cirrhosis patients.

Pediatric end-stage liver disease (PELD) is a disease severity scoring system for children under 12 years of age. It is calculated from the patient's albumin, bilirubin, and International Normalized Ratio (INR) together with the patient's age and degree of growth failure. This score is also used by the United Network for Organ Sharing (UNOS) for prioritizing allocation of liver transplants.

The PELD score is based on both laboratory data and growth data. These values are used together with the patient's degree of growth failure to determine the PELD score. The adult version of PELD is called MELD.

It is calculated according to the following formula:

$$\text{PELD} = 4.80\,[\text{Ln serum bilirubin (mg/dL)}] + 18.57\,[\text{Ln INR}] - 6.87\,[\text{Ln albumin (g/dL)}] + 4.36\,(<1 \text{ year old}) + 6.67\,(\text{growth failure})$$

MANAGEMENT

- Early detection and management of complications due to decompensated cirrhosis.
- There is no specific treatment of cirrhosis per se that will arrest or reverse the cirrhotic changes. Treatment of portal hypertension, ascites and hepatic encephalopathy has been discussed separately.

Table: 9.14.2: Child's prognostic grading of chronic liver disease (CLD) and cirrhosis (Modified Pughs).

Prognosis	***Compensated (A)***	***Guarded (B)***	***Decompensated (C)***
Jaundice (bilirubin)	Mild or nil < 2 mg/dL	Moderate 2–3 mg/dL	Intense > 3 mg/dL
Ascites	–	Mild and treatable	Severe/refractory
Albumin	>3.5 g/dL	3–3.5 g/dL	<3 g/dL
Encephalopathy	–	Past history	++
Prothrombin time	N or ×1 ↑	×2 ↑	Multiple times of normal ↑

- Treatment of specific cause if any, like Wilson disease, drug-induced hepatitis, and hepatitis B and C.
- Patients with compensated cirrhosis can lead to a normal life and no specific diet is helpful.
- Hepatic herbal supportive, antioxidants, liver cell membrane protectives and maintenance of adequate calories, fluid and electrolytes, vitamins especially fat-soluble vitamins are routinely recommended with variable outcome.
- Liver transplantation is the future hope in EHBA, tyrosinemia, glycogen storage disease, acetyl transferase deficiency and severe bile acid metabolic defects such as PFIC.

HEPATIC ENCEPHALOPATHY

Encephalopathy is characterized by:

- *Grade I*: Irritability, incoherent speech, mental confusion and violence
- *Grade II*: Drowsiness and somnolence, flapping tremor and fetor hepaticus
- *Grade III*: Exaggerated reflexes with upgoing plantar reflexes and stupor
- *Grade IV*: Coma.

Metabolic complications like hypoglycemia, dyselectrolytemia, renal failure, coagulopathy with bleeds, hyperammonemia, convulsions, etc. may supervene in Grade III and IV encephalopathy. Early detection of hepatic encephalopathy may be done by demonstrating constructional apraxia (inability to draw or copy a star).

Predisposing Causes

Gastrointestinal bleeds with excess protein in the bowel, rapid abdominal paracentesis, intercurrent infections (gram-negative septicemia), use of hepatotoxic drugs (morphine), major surgical procedures and electrolyte imbalance (diuretics) are the common precipitating factors.

Management Guidelines

Goal of therapy is to identify the complications of hepatic encephalopathy and decompensated cirrhosis and prevent by avoiding predisposing factors mentioned above.

Specific Treatment

These include:

1. *To identify any site of bleeding* by fiberscopy and treat appropriately, variceal bleed, gastric or duodenal erosions, etc.
2. *Maintenance of fluid and electrolyte balance:* Sodium restriction may be required despite hyponatremia which may be dilutional.
3. *Diuretics (spironolactone/loop diuretics):* Preferable to avoid loop diuretics which may induce hypokalemia; potassium preparations for hypokalemia.
4. *Parenteral IV glucose* for hypoglycemia.
5. *Infection:* Culture studies of ascitic fluid and if positive to treat infection as indicated. (Remember that liver disease may influence drug choice and dose). The role of rifampicin in hepatic encephalopathy in pediatric age group needs more study.
6. *Lactulose* to produce two liquid stools daily (15–30 mL twice or thrice daily). It produces osmotic diarrhea, prevents absorption of ammonia from colon and prevents proliferation of ammonia-producing organisms. Lactitol and ammonia-reducing drugs such as sodium benzoate are more beneficial.
7. *Selective intestinal decontamination* by administration of non-absorbable antibiotics (norfloxacin, neomycin).
8. *Sedation:* Short-acting benzodiazepines such as oxazepam, midazolam are preferred.
9. *Coagulation defects to be corrected* with fresh frozen plasma or clotting factors and vitamin K (single dose).
10. *Parenteral vitamins* (fat soluble and water soluble especially B complex vitamins).
11. *Variceal bleed* to be treated by somatostatin, octreotide, vasopressin or glypressin or endoscopic band ligation or sclero/glue therapy and Sengstaken tube.
12. *Specific causes of cirrhosis and management of treatable causes* like Wilson disease, autoimmune hepatitis, drug-induced, hepatitis B and C, etc. recommended.
13. *Liver transplantation* is life-saving for end-stage cirrhosis liver though cost prohibitive.

PORTAL HYPERTENSION

Clinical criteria include variceal upper GI bleed, splenomegaly, tortuous veins on anterior abdominal wall away from umbilicus especially in intrahepatic type and ascites getting localized in all end-stage cirrhosis in the presence of portal hypertension.

Cirrhotic portal hypertension will have history suggestive of CLD and clinical features of underlying cause for portal hypertension. Nodular and shrunken liver, abdominal veins and features of decompensation with extrahepatic manifestations of CLD will differentiate from patients of extrahepatic portal hypertension where the above features are absent until late stage. However, laboratory workup including ultrasound and Doppler abdomen will help to identify the pathology in the splenoportovenous (SPV) axis.

Diagnosis

- *Pressure criteria:* Portal venous pressure more than 10 mm Hg (normal < 10 mm Hg).
- *Hepatic venous pressure gradient:* If more than 12 mm it is a useful predictor of impending variceal bleed.

Abdominal ultrasound, esophago-gastroduodenoscopy, LFTs, and complete hemogram as mentioned earlier are relevant for diagnosis and management.

Management

Management of portal hypertension should include emergency resuscitation of patients with upper GI bleeding, control of bleeding with somatostatin and analogs or vasopressin and glypressin, emergency endoscopy therapy, and long-term prevention of variceal bleeds with propranolol (1 mg/kg/day) and isosorbide mononitrate. Proper counseling of close relatives for long-term follow-up and the natural course of the illness is mandatory.

Indications for Surgical Management

These include:

- Recurrent rebleeds even after 4–6 endotherapy sessions
- Hypersplenism
- Outstation patients (from remote places) where medical treatment is not available
- If patient is not fit for surgery or not willing for surgery TIPS (transjugular intrahepatic portosystemic shunt).

CHRONIC LIVER DISEASE

Clues for Etiology

- *Family or sibling history of liver disease*: Metabolic liver disease [Wilson disease, glycogen storage disease (GSD), tyrosinemia, galactosemia, Niemann-Pick disease, Gaucher disease, hemochromatosis, alpha-1 antitrypsin deficiency, urea cycle defects, PPD peripheral neuropathy, parotidomegaly and Dupuytren's contracture] or hepatomegaly in alcohol-induced liver disease
- *KF ring, sun flower cataract:* Wilson disease **(Table 9.14.3)**
- *Hyperpigmentation:* Hemochromatosis
- *History of blood transfusion or tattooing*: Hepatitis B/ hepatitis C
- *Scratch marks and xanthomas*: Chronic cholestasis
- *Drug history* in CLD and drug abuse in Hepatitis B infection
- *Dysmorphic facies*: Ductal paucity syndrome, e.g. Alagille syndrome
- *Early onset liver cell failure (LCF) and decompensation with neonatal cholestasis (NCS)* in tyrosinemia, galactosemia, hemochromatosis and alpha-1 antitrypsin deficiency
- *Severe itching/chronic diarrhea or malabsorption* in Byler's disease (PFIC 1)
- *Cataract* in congenital rubella syndrome, galactosemia and Wilson disease
- *Seborrheic dermatitis/otitis media/lumpy-bony swellings/ hepatosplenomegaly/cholestasis* in histiocytosis
- *Restricted growth/frequent eating habits/large liver/ cherubic face/tendency to be drowsy on fasting/acidosis* in GSD 1

Diagnostic Laboratory Investigations

- If ascites is present serum sodium, potassium, bicarbonate, chloride, urea and creatinine levels may help.

Table 9.14.3: Chronic liver disease (CLD) extrahepatic manifestations.

Clinical features	***Suggestive of***
Broad forehead, small chin, saddle nose, low set ears, posterior embryotoxon, cardiac and renal anomalies Developmental delay	Alagille syndrome
Cataracts	Galactosemia, Wilson disease, rubella syndrome
KF rings, tremors, dysarthria, extrapyramidal signs	Wilson disease
Progressive liver cell failure, renal tubular dysfunction, hypophosphatemic rickets	Tyrosinemia type I
Mental retardation	Galactosemia, lipid storage
Rickets	Wilson disease, tyrosinemia
Cystic kidneys	Congenital hepatic fibrosis
Skin rashes Blue berry muffin	Histiocytosis CMV infection
Pruritus	EHBO, PFIC, chronic hepatitis B/C infection with cholestasis, Alagille syndrome

(PFIC: progressive familial intrahepatic *cholestasis*; KF: Kayser-Fleischer)

- Serology for hepatitis B (HBsAg, HBeAg, anti-HBeAB, HBV DNA), anti-HCV (ELISA) and HCV RNA, CMV, EB virus, HIV, and TORCH group.
- Autoantibodies (ANA, anti-SMA, Anti-LKM, and p-ANCA)
- Serum ceruloplasmin, 24-hour urinary copper and slit-lamp examination for KF ring for Wilson disease
- Urine reducing sugars and for inherited metabolic liver disease screening tests, GALT assay (galactosemia)

Biochemical Clues for Chronic Liver Disease and Cirrhosis Liver

1. Persistently low serum albumin (<3 g/dL)
2. Persistently raised serum gammaglobulin and low albumin with reversal of A:G ratio (<1)
3. Prolonged PT (>3 times above normal limits)
4. AST:ALT ratio > 1.
5. Persistently elevated transaminases and SAP in chronic biliary disorders.

Differential Diagnosis

- Extrahepatic portal hypertension (absent liver cell failure, abdominal wall veins)
- Chronic hepatitis (absence of nodular liver, abdominal wall veins and portal hypertension)

Note: Chronic hepatitis or cirrhosis of liver is the end stage of CLD ultimately whatever may be the cause.

Management

- Early detection and management of complications due to decompensated cirrhosis
- Treatment of specific cause if any, like Wilson disease, drug-induced hepatitis, and hepatitis B and C.
- Patients with compensated cirrhosis can lead a normal life and no specific diet is helpful.
- Maintenance of adequate calories, fluid and electrolytes, vitamin especially fat-soluble vitamins
- Liver transplantation.

Complications of Chronic Liver Disease

These include portal hypertension with ascites, hypersplenism, variceal bleeding, synthetic dysfunction of liver, such as, hypoalbuminemia, coagulopathy, hypoglycemia, growth failure, reduced SMR and the end-stage complications like hepatic encephalopathy/minimal hepatic encephalopathy, hepatorenal/hepatopulmonary syndromes and in late stages hepatocellular carcinoma. **Table 9.14.4** summarizes the brief details about various disorders and the management principles.

Liver Transplantation: Common Indications

These include extrahepatic biliary atresia, fulminant hepatic failure (AVH, paracetamol toxicity), PFIC, tyrosinemia type 1, Wilson disease, Alagille syndrome, nonsyndromic HDP, cryptogenic, polycystic liver disease (Caroli), hepatitis B and C cirrhosis, GSD type IV, autoimmune end-stage liver disease, Budd-Chiari syndrome and hepatoblastoma.

Table 9.14.4: Chronic liver disease (CLD)—various disorders, clinical features and treatment.

Disease	*Defect*	*Clinical*	*Diagnosis*	*Treatment and Prevention*
Extrahepatic biliary atresia (EHBA)	Postinflammatory obstruction of biliary tract, chronic cholestasis, progressive fibrosis and secondary biliary cirrhosis	Full-term, normal birth weight and growth velocity, no dysmorphic facies, early dark urine with diaper stain and persistent pale stools, firm and moderate large liver	• *Rectal swab*—persistent pale stool • *Both SAP and GGTP* high • *USG abdomen:* Absent GB • *Hepatobiliary radioisotope study:* Uptake normal but excretion into intestine even after 24 hours—NIL • *Liver biopsy:* Ductular proliferation, widened portal tract, bile plugs and dense fibrosis cirrhosis • *Preoperative cholangiogram*: gold-standard-confirmation	• Medical conservative: EBF, MCT, vitamins UDCA (empiric) • Early Kasai portoenterostomy (<4–6 weeks ideal) • Liver transplant
Idiopathic (Giant cell) hepatitis	No cause detectable Sporadic/familial forms—of late, less common	• Normal birth weight • No dysmorphism • *Onset*: Neonatal, self-limiting • Neonatal conjugated hyperbilirubinemia in a normal infant. With no other clinical clue for cause • Recovery usually complete	• Raised transaminases and cholestatic enzymes • *USG abdomen:* Normal • *Liver biopsy:* Lobular disarray, ballooning and focal necrosis of hepatocytes and giant cell formation and extramedullary erythropoiesis	• Supportive—conservative
Alagille syndrome	Autosomal dominant *JAG-1* gene mutation on chromosome 20p12	• Chronic cholestasis • *Dysmorphism*: Triangular facies-broad forehead, pointed chin, saddle nose, bulbous tip, hypertelorism, low set ears, posterior embryotoxon • Renal anomalies • Cardiac abnormalities • X-ray—butterfly vertebra, curved phalanges, short ulna	• *Liver biopsy:* Ductal paucity—reduced ratio of interlobar bile ducts to portal tracts. (Normal = 0.9–1.8 In ductal paucity ≤ 0.5)	• Supportive UDCA, • Liver transplant

Contd...

Contd...

Disease	***Defect***	***Clinical***	***Diagnosis***	***Treatment and Prevention***
Tyrosinemia type-I	• Fumarylacetoacetate hydrolase deficiency, an enzyme for oxidative degradation pathway of phenyl-alanine and tyrosine • Gene mutation • Accumulation of succinyl acetone in liver and kidneys causing damage	• Progressive liver failure • Renal tubular dysfunction • Hypophosphatemic rickets and excretion of tyrosine metabolites. • Large liver with fibrosis-cirrhosis liver and after 2 years of age hepatocellular carcinoma • Acute form—early liver cell failure features and death by 8 months	• Abnormal LFT, very high alpha-fetoprotein (× 1–100 times) • Urine succinylacetone present urine aminoaciduria	• Restrict phenylalanine and tyrosine in diet • *Drug therapy:* Nitisinone (Orfadin) Prevents accumulation of succinyl acetone • *Dose:* 1 mg/kg/day PO, bid, 1 hour bf initially-step-up dose to 2 mg/kg/day
Galactosemia	• Autosomal recessive • Deficiency of galactose-1-phosphate uridyl transferase (GALT; EC2.7.712) • Accumulation of galactose and toxic metabolites and damage to liver and CNS	• Clinical spectrum varies according to type and number of *GALT* gene mutations • Onset in neonatal period, soon after breast milk and top milk with jaundice, hepato-splenomegaly, liver dysfunction, hypoglycemia, renal tubular dysfunction, hypotonia, cataract, and *E. coli* sepsis. • Untreated cases develop cirrhosis and die	*Measurement of GALT activity in RBC. Urine Benedict's test* for reducing substance +ve	Galactose –restricted diet (milk and milk products including breast milk) life long
PFIC (Progressive familial intrahepatic cholestasis) (3 types)	• Autosomal recessive • Gene mutation bile • Transport defects. • *Type 1 (Byler disease)*: *FIC1* gene encoding on P-type ATPase protein amino-phospholipid transport-chromo-some 18q21-22 • *Type 2:* SPGP (Sister of P-glycoprotein) gene encoding on BSEP (Bile salt export pump)-located on chromosome 2q 24 • *PFIC3: MDR3* gene mutations (multi-drug resistance-3) encoding on biliary phospholipid Transporter located on chromosome 7q21	• All types have pruritus, jaundice, fat soluble vitamin deficiency • *Type 1*: Systemic involvement—liver, pancreas, diarrhea. Cirrhosis in 1st decade of life. • Bad prognosis. • Onset delayed until adulthood. • History of cholestasis of pregnancy in the mother	• *Raised SAP* and *Normal/ low GGT.* • *Liver biopsy*—Paucity of intralobular bile ducts and granular bile in electron microscopy • SAP raised and Normal/ *low GGPT.* • *Liver biopsy:* Giant-cell hepatitis, canalicular/ hepatocellular cholestasis, amorphous bile • *Both SAP and GGTP are raised.* • *Liver biopsy* like EHBA	• UDCA • Liver transplant in 2nd decade • Supportive • Liver transplant in 1st decade • Supportive, UDCA • Liver transplant

Contd...

Contd...

Disease	*Defect*	*Clinical*	*Diagnosis*	*Treatment and Prevention*
ICC (Indian childhood cirrhosis)	Copper contaminated milk feeds	• Age—6 months to 5 years. • Boys predominance. • 20% sib history +ve. Not a disease of poverty. • Clinically early stage–nonspecific findings (irregular fever, altered appetite, mild abdominal distension, prolonged AVH like presentation) • Onset may be insidious or acute. • Jaundice may be present. • Liver initially leafy edge and firm • Later hard micronodular cirrhosis. • Decompensation in end stage.	*LFT*—abnormal but not diagnostic. *Liver biopsy:* intralobular pericellular creeping fibrosis, Mallory hyaline orcein + for Liver copper, no fatty changes no other histological clue	*D. penicillamine* Zinc Steroids? *Prevention:* Remove copper from diet
Neonatal hemochromatosis	• Congenital • Maternal factor • Iron deposition in liver and almost all organs except reticuloendothelial system	• Rare. • Early liver cell failure with congenital cirrhosis. Shrunken liver • If not treated—early death. • History of oligohydramnios, placental edema, IUGR/ stillbirth	• High degree of suspicion. • Complete saturation of iron binding capacity • Iron-staining buccal mucosa. • Minor salivary gland biopsy tissue. • Decreased intensity on T2-weighted MRI (pancreas, heart) characteristic of iron. Serum ferritin elevated.	• N-acetyl cysteine • Selenium • Desferrioxamine • Vitamin E, and Prostaglandin E_1 alpha. • Sepsis management • Liver transplant

(AVH: acute viral hepatitis; bf: before food; EBF: exclusive breastfeeding; EHBA: extrahepatic biliary atresia; IUGR: *intrauterine growth restriction;* MCT: medium chain triglyceride; PFIC: progressive familial intrahepatic cholestasis; PO: per oral; UDCA: ursodeoxycholic acid)

Table 9.14.5: Acute liver failure (ALF): Indicators of poor prognosis and immediate referral for liver transplantation.

Clinical	*Biochemical*
Increasing depth of jaundice	*Serum bilirubin > 300 mmol/L (>17.6 mg/dL)
Rapidly decreasing liver size	Decreasing transaminase levels
Recurrent/persist hypoglycemia	<4 mmol/L needing often dextrose infusions
Coagulopathy—bleeds	*Prothrombin time > 60 sec (INR > 3.5 and in paracetamol poisoning > 6.5)
Clinical acidosis	*Acid-base pH < 7.3 (acetaminophen poisoning)
Hepatic encephalopathy Grade 2/3	Raised serum ammonia levels
*Age < 10 years with jaundice > 7 days before encephalopathy	

Note: * King's College criteria

Clinical and biochemical indicators of poor prognosis and immediate referral for liver transplantation are defined **(Table 9.14.5)**.

KEY MESSAGES

- Chronic hepatitis, metabolic liver disorders and neonatal cholestasis are the leading causes of CLD.
- Minimal hepatic encephalopathy, a new entity, needs focus in the CLD workup
- Children with decompensated cirrhosis require both prevention and appropriate management of life-threatening complications and periodic counseling regarding liver transplant.

BIBLIOGRAPHY

1. Alam S, Khanna R. Chronic liver disease. In: Gupta P, Menon PSN, Ramji S, Lodha R (Eds). PG Textbook of Pediatrics. New Delhi: Jaypee Brothers Medical Publishers (P) Ltd.; 2015;2:Chapter 37.8, 1476-89.

2. Arora NK, Bhatia V. Chronic Liver Disease in India. Indian J Pediatr. 2008;75:S69-73.
3. Bacon BR, O'Grady JG, DiBisceglie AM, et al. Specific diseases of liver and biliary tree. In: Comprehensive Clinical Hepatology, 2nd Edition. Philadelphia: Mosby; 2010. pp. 14-36 and 205-56
4. Bavdekar A. Metabolic liver disease. In: Bavdekar A, Mathai J, Sathiyasekaran M Yachha SK (eds). IAP speciality series on Paediatric Gastroenterology. 2008;(16):217-27.
5. Foerster BR, Conklin LS, Petrou M, et al. Minimal Hepatic Encephalopathy in Children: Evaluation with Proton MR Spectroscopy. Am J Neuroradiol. 2009;30(8):1610-3.
6. Hardy S, Kleinman ER. Cirrhosis and chronic liver failure. In: Suchy FJ, Sokol RJ, Balistreri WF (Eds). Textbook of Liver Disease in Chidren, 2nd edition. Phildelphia: Lippincott Williams and Wilkins; 2001. pp. 89-127.
7. Jagadisan B, Srivastava A, Yachha SK, et al. Acute-on-chronic liver disease in children from the developing world: recognition and prognosis. J Pediatr Gastroenterol Nutr. 2012;54(1):77-82.
8. Sathiyasekaran M. Approach to a child with CLD. Indian J Pract Pediatrics, Hepatology 2002;4(4):362-9 and IAP speciality series on Paediatric Gastroenterology 2008;14:188-96.
9. Yacha SK. Portal hypertension in children. An Indian perspective. J Gastroenterol Hepatol. 2002;17:S228-31.

9.15 Neonatal Cholestasis Syndromes

A Riyaz

INTRODUCTION

Prolonged jaundice is frequent in the first 3 months of life, with most infants having unconjugated hyperbilirubinemia. Neonatal cholestasis syndromes (NCS) are characterized by prolonged conjugated jaundice beyond 2 weeks of life and high colored urine with or without pale stools. The presence of high level of conjugated bilirubin (>20% of total bilirubin if serum bilirubin > 5 mg/dL or > 1 mg/dL if total serum bilirubin < 5 mg/dL) is suggestive of NCS.

EPIDEMIOLOGY

Incidence: In 2–15% cases of neonatal jaundice, the jaundice lasts beyond 2 weeks of age and only 0.2–0.4% of these have conjugated hyperbilirubinemia. The estimated incidence of NCS is around 1 in 2,500 live births in the West and it constitutes about 30% of all hepatobiliary disorders in children in India.

CLASSIFICATION

Based on the primary site of pathology, NCS may be classified as intrahepatic (medical) or extrahepatic (surgical).

- *Intrahepatic cholestasis* is seen in TORCH infections (toxoplasmosis, other intrauterine infections, rubella, cytomegalovirus (CMV) and *Herpes simplex* virus 2), septicemia, during total parenteral nutrition (TPN), and various inborn errors of metabolism such as galactosemia, gestational alloimmune liver disease (GALD) and progressive familial intrahepatic cholestasis (PFIC).
- In the *extrahepatic* group, biliary atresia (BA) is the most important.

The spectrum of diseases causing NCS in India and the West is quite different as shown in **Table 9.15.1**.

It is also useful to classify NCS as babies who are sick and non-sick, as the sick babies require urgent workup for prompt therapy **(Flowchart 9.15.1)**.

Transient Cholestasis

Transient cholestasis may be seen in severe perinatal diseases causing hepatic ischemia like fetal arrhythmia, and neonatal lupus causing congenital heart block and in

Table 9.15.1: The spectrum of neonatal cholestasis syndromes: West versus India.

Disease	*West*	*India (Multicentric)*
Biliary atresia/choledochal cyst	25%	38%
Neonatal hepatitis (NH)	15%	37%
Metabolic diseases	20%	4%
PFIC/Alagille syndrome/bile acid synthesis disorders	25%	3%
Alpha-1 antitrypsin deficiency	10%	—
Viral infections	5%	10%
Others	—	2%
Unknown	—	6%

(PFIC: progressive familial intrahepatic cholestasis)

Flowchart 9.15.1: Classification of neonatal cholestasis syndromes.

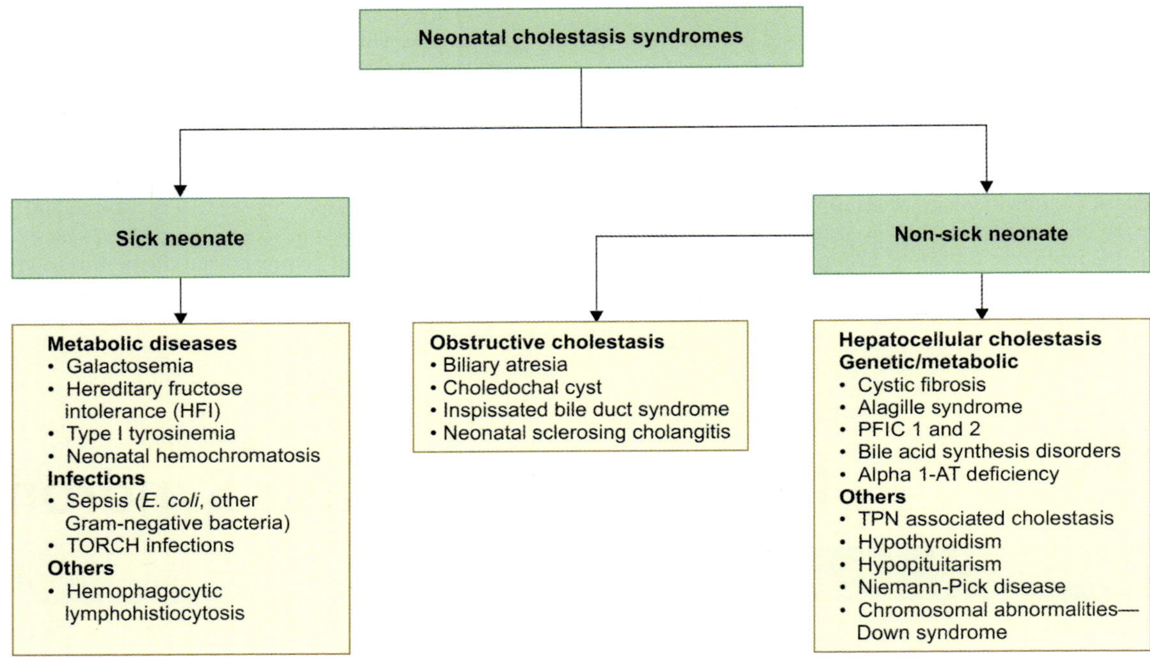

congenital hypothyroidism. Cholestasis rapidly reverses with appropriate therapy.

Physiologic Cholestasis

It is seen in preterm babies due to decreased expression of transport proteins of bile acids like NTCP (sodium taurocholate co-transporting protein) and BSEP (bile salt exporting pump).

TORCH Infections

TORCH infections are characterized by hepatosplenomegaly, failure to thrive, purpura, microcephaly, chorioretinitis and congenital heart disease in congenital rubella syndrome.

Idiopathic Neonatal Hepatitis

These infants tend to be small for gestational age (SGA) or premature. More than one child in a family may be affected. Liver biopsy shows extensive giant cell transformation, but bile ducts are relatively normal. It may be very difficult to differentiate idiopathic neonatal hepatitis (NH) from BA. The prognosis is much better than that of BA.

Gestational Alloimmune Liver Disease

This rare disease, previously called neonatal hemochromatosis, is a result of maternal alloimmune injury due to transplacental passage of specific reactive IgG that leads to fetal liver injury. The neonate presents with severe liver failure and is associated with marked iron deposition in the liver and extrahepatic tissues. The rate of recurrence of GALD in subsequent pregnancies is 90%. The combination of exchange transfusion and intravenous immunoglobulin (IVIG) is the current treatment of choice. High dose IVIG to mother dramatically reduces the risk for recurrence of disease.

Biliary Atresia

This is a fatal progressive fibroinflammatory cholangiopathy resulting in complete obliteration of the entire or portions of the extrahepatic and intrahepatic biliary tree within weeks of birth. The countries with the highest incidence of BA in the world are Japan and Taiwan.

The exact etiology of BA is not known. One prominent theory is that infections caused by Reovirus 3, Epstein–Barr virus, rotavirus and CMV and then perpetuated by an autoimmune disorder, may be responsible. Immunologic studies have further characterized roles of helper T-cells, B-cells, and natural killer cells in the immune dysregulation following viral replication and damage to biliary epithelium. Prominin-1-expressing portal fibroblasts may play an integral role in the biliary fibrosis associated with BA.

Recent studies have identified that common genetic variants in the *ADDUCIN-3* gene increased the risk of developing BA.

Biliary atresia is more common in term of female babies with normal birth weight. Stools are initially pale and then become completely acholic. Firm hepatomegaly is common. Splenomegaly is late and is a sign of hepatic fibrosis. Bleeding may occur due to uncorrected vitamin K deficiency, especially in breastfed babies.

Biliary atresia should be ruled out in any neonate with conjugated jaundice persisting beyond 14 days of life.

Choledochal Cyst

Choledochal cysts are a rare but important treatable cause of NCS. Ultrasonography, endoscopic retrograde cholangiopancreatography (ERCP) and percutaneous transhepatic cholangiography (PTC) are very useful in diagnosis. Treatment is by complete surgical excision with drainage of the biliary tract into the jejunum.

EVALUATION OF NEONATAL CHOLESTASIS SYNDROME

The workup should be done in a stepwise manner to establish the specific cause of cholestasis. Potentially life-threatening conditions like sepsis, galactosemia, tyrosinemia and endocrinopathies that need immediate intervention should be ruled out first and the next step is to rule out BA.

Clues in History and Examination

- *Intrauterine growth restriction*: TORCH infections
- *Gender*: BA and choledochal cyst are more common in girls
- *Consanguinity and similar illness in siblings*: Galactosemia, hereditary fructose intolerance (HFI), GALD, and PFIC
- *Escherichia coli sepsis*: Galactosemia
- *Recurrent abortions*: Gestational alloimmune liver disease
- *Precipitating factors*: Breastfeeds—galactosemia; ingestion of fruits—HFI
- *History of neonatal intensive care unit stay, severe ABO/Rh incompatibility, jaundice onset later than BA*: Inspissated bile duct syndrome
- *Seizures, vomiting*: Galactosemia, HFI, hypopituitarism, intracranial hemorrhage
- *History of lethargy, poor suck/latch* suggests neonatal sepsis or a possible metabolic decompensation which warrants urgent evaluation.
- *History of cholestasis in pregnancy* suggests a diagnosis of PFIC type 3 in the infant.
- *Abnormal urine odor*: Boiled cabbage/rancid butter urine in type I tyrosinemia
- *Dysmorphism*: Down syndrome, Zellweger syndrome, Alagille syndrome (triangular face), citrin deficiency (chubby face)
- *Microcephaly*: Congenital rubella, CMV, Smith-Lemli-Opitz syndrome
- *Deafness*: Zellweger syndrome, congenital rubella syndrome, CMV hepatitis
- *Post-axial polydactyly and syndactyly of toes II/III*: Smith-Lemli-Opitz syndrome
- *Early hepatosplenomegaly*: Neonatal hepatitis
- *Hard liver and ascites*: Ominous signs indicating that cirrhosis has already set in.
- *Bilious ascites and bile staining of scrotum (biliscrotum)*: Spontaneous perforation of bile duct
- *Exaggerated deep tendon reflexes and clonus* suggest cerebral irritation due to hepatic encephalopathy.
- *Lymph edema of extremities*: Aagenaes syndrome (Norwegian cholestasis)
- *Multiple joint contractures*: Arthrogryposis-renal dysfunction-cholestasis (ARC) syndrome
- *Congenital heart disease*: PDA and peripheral pulmonary stenosis in congenital rubella syndrome; peripheral pulmonary stenosis in Alagille syndrome; PDA and ASD in Smith-Lemli-Opitz syndrome.
- If the child has unusual craving for protein and fat rich food, and an aversion for carbohydrate-rich food, citrin deficiency should be considered.

Ophthalmologic Evaluation

- *Epicanthic folds:* Down syndrome and Zellweger syndrome
- *Cataract*: Galactosemia, HFI, congenital rubella syndrome, CMV hepatitis, Smith-Lemli-Opitz syndrome and Zellweger syndrome. In galactosemia and HFI, cataract may not be present at birth
- *Microphthalmia*: Rubella, CMV
- *Brushfield spots*: Down syndrome
- *Chorioretinitis*: NH due to CMV, toxoplasmosis, rubella
- *Posterior embryotoxon, Axenfeld anomaly*: Alagille syndrome **(Fig. 9.15.1)**
- *Cherry red spot*: Niemann–Pick disease type A
- *Glaucoma*: Zellweger syndrome
- *Retinitis pigmentosa*: Zellweger syndrome.

Neonatologists of Taiwan have introduced a novel screening program using an *infant stool card* **(Fig 9.15.2)** with different stool colors, which can be compared with the baby's stool color. This helps in the early suspicion of BA. Three colors (1–3) on this card are labeled abnormal (clay-colored, pale yellowish, and light yellowish), whereas the other 3 (4–6) are labeled normal (yellowish, brown, and greenish). It is an attractive idea to introduce this program to our country also to pick up BA early.

Investigations

- *Urine sugar*: Galactosemia, HFI
- *Urine microscopy*: Owl-eye bodies in CMV hepatitis
- *High serum/urinary succinyl acetone*: Type 1 tyrosinemia

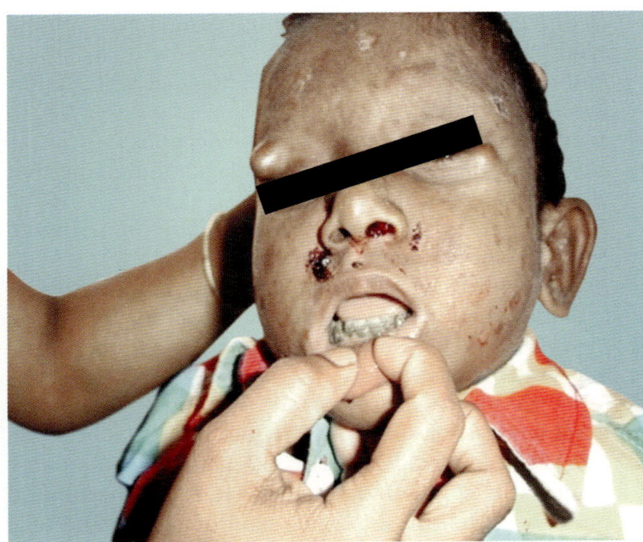

Fig. 9.15.1: Child with Alagille syndrome—note chlorodontia (greenish teeth).

- *Low/normal GGT*: PFIC I and II, Aagenaes syndrome, ARC syndrome, septo-optic dysplasia (De Morsier syndrome)
- TORCH screen
- Hepatitis B virus (HBV) serology
- Culture of blood, urine, and cerebrospinal fluid (CSF)
- *Buccal glandular biopsy*: For GALD.

Metabolic Workup

- *Hypoglycemia*: Galactosemia, HFI, and hypopituitarism
- *High sweat chloride*: Cystic fibrosis
- *Low RBC galactose-1-phosphate uridyltransferase*: Galactosemia
- *Alpha-fetoprotein levels*: Elevated in NH and normal in BA; extremely high in GALD and type I tyrosinemia
- *Abnormal genotype of protease inhibitor (PiZZ genotype) and low serum alpha-1 antitrypsin level*: Alpha-1 antitrypsin deficiency.

Radiological Workup

- *Diffuse cerebral calcification*: Congenital toxoplasmosis
- *Periventricular calcification*: Congenital CMV infection
- *Wimberger sign (erosion of the upper medial surface of tibia)*: Congenital syphilis
- *Celery stalk appearance of metaphysis*: Congenital rubella syndrome
- *Butterfly vertebrae, fused vertebrae, spina bifida occulta*: Alagille syndrome.

Ultrasonography

- *Non-imaged or small gallbladder in fasting state*: Suggestive of BA, but not diagnostic.
- *If normal gallbladder (GB) and bile ducts can be visualized*: BA is unlikely.
- *Triangular cord sign*: A cone-shaped fibrotic mass cranial to the bifurcation of the portal vein—highly suggestive of BA.
- In NH, GB is of normal size and contracts well after feeding.
- *Dilated intrahepatic biliary radicles* are not seen BA, as it is a progressive obliterative cholangiopathy.
- Gallbladder ghost triad in BA characterized by:
    - Small GB (length <1.9 cm)
    - An irregular or lobulated contour
    - A relatively indistinct lining and thin wall.

Radionuclide Hepatobiliary Scintigraphy

Technetium-99m-labeled derivatives of iminodiacetic acid are used to assess the continuity of the biliary tract with the small intestine.

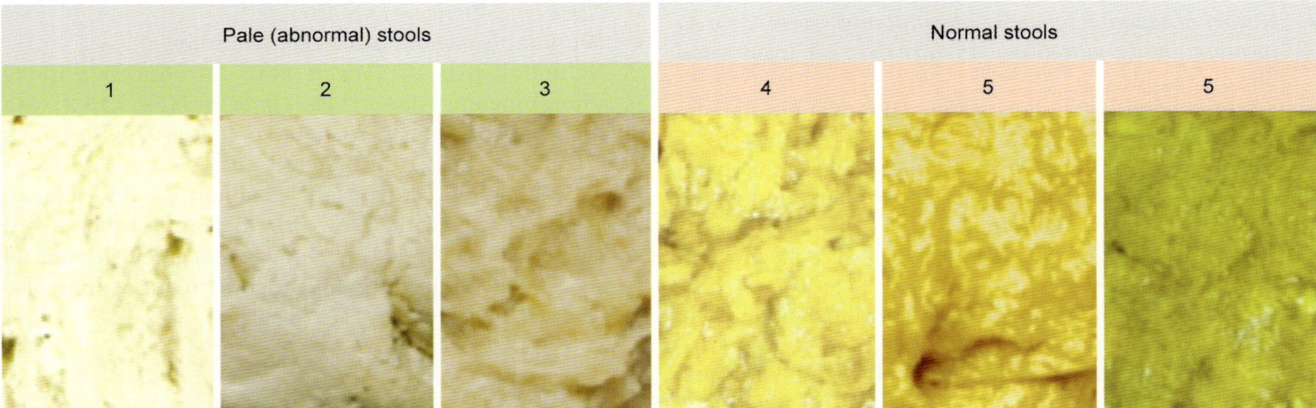

Fig. 9.15.2: Infant stool card.

- In medical cholestasis, the uptake is decreased, but the excretion into the gut is normal.
- In BA, the uptake is normal but excretion into gut is decreased, so that there is no radioactivity in the gut, even 24 hours later.
- The presence of radioactivity in the gut is a strong point against the diagnosis of BA.
- In the advanced stage of NH, the hepatocytes are so much damaged that they are not able to excrete the isotope and hence it may be mistaken for BA.

Magnetic Resonance Cholangiography

Nonvisualization of the common bile duct (CBD) and presence of small GB suggest BA.

Endoscopic Retrograde Cholangiopancreatography

Though useful, the need for high technical expertise and general anesthesia limits its usefulness.

Percutaneous Transhepatic Cholangiography

Here, dye is injected into the liver through a very thin Chiba needle and X-rays are taken. Visualization of a patent biliary tract with antegrade flow of the contrast medium into the duodenum excludes BA.

Near infrared reflectance spectroscopy of homogenized stool specimens for bilirubin and bile acids is both highly sensitive and specific for BA.

Liver Biopsy

If there is no excretion in the hepatobiliary scintigraphy scan, liver biopsy is the single most valuable test to distinguish BA from NH.

- The features of BA include:
  - Marked bile ductular proliferation and fibrosis
  - Minimal giant cell formation
  - Presence of bile lakes
- Features of NH include:
  - Very little bile ductular proliferation
  - Striking giant cell formation
  - Focal hepatocellular necrosis
- The characteristic findings of alpha-1 antitrypsin deficiency:
  - Diastase-resistant, periodic acid-Schiff (PAS) positive, magenta-colored, globular inclusions in the endoplasmic reticulum of periportal hepatocytes
- Intranuclear owl-eye bodies may be seen in CMV hepatitis
- *Electron microscopy of bile*: Coarse granular bile (Byler's bile) in PFIC-1.

MANAGEMENT OF NEONATAL CHOLESTASIS SYNDROME

Nutrition

Cholestasis leads to maldigestion and malabsorption of fat, and fat-soluble vitamins due to diminished bile acid secretion. This leads to steatorrhea that aggravates malnutrition. The other causes of malnutrition are anorexia, early satiety secondary to compression of abdominal viscera by the enlarged liver and spleen, and ascites, recurrent infections, etc.

- Breastfeeding should be encouraged.
- 200 cal/kg and 1–2 g/kg protein should be given.
- These children will be severely deficient in all fat-soluble vitamins, and also other nutrients, which should be supplemented.
- *Vitamin K*: 5 mg of vitamin K should be given daily for the first 3 days after diagnosis and then 5 mg weekly. Dose may be adjusted depending on prothrombin time done monthly.
- *Vitamin A*: Aquasol A 2,500–5,000 IU/day orally or 50,000 IU of vitamin A IM at the time of diagnosis and then 10,000 IU monthly till cholestasis resolves.
- *Vitamin D*: 30,000 IU of vitamin D2 IM at the time of diagnosis and then 10,000 IU monthly till cholestasis resolves or 3–5 µg/kg/day of 25-hydroxycholecalciferol orally
- *Vitamin E*: 50–400 IU/day or 25–50 IU/kg/day. Vitamin E absorption can be increased by binding tocopherol to polyethylene glycol succinate (TPEGS), as it can form micelles without the involvement of bile acids.
- *Water-soluble vitamins*: Excess doses of B complex vitamins should be given.
- *Minerals*:
  - *Oral elemental calcium*: 25–100 mg/kg/day
  - *Phosphorus:* 25–50 mg/kg/day
  - *Zinc*: 1 mg/kg/day
  - *Magnesium*: 1–2 mEq/kg/day
  - *Elemental iron*: 5–6 mg/kg/day.

Treatment of Pruritus

It is believed to be due to the deposition of bile acids in the skin or due to increased endogenous opioids like met-enkephalins synthesized in the gut. Some of the treatment options are:

- Cholestyramine
- Colestipol
- *Colesevelam hydrochloride*: This is a newer bile acid sequestrant. However, pediatric data are limited; adult dose is 625 mg once daily. It is a very potent

bile-acid-binding resin and may severely deplete the concentration of free luminal bile acids aggravating risk of fat-soluble vitamin deficiency.
- Phenobarbitone
- *Ursodeoxycholic acid*: Dose 15–30 mg/kg/day
- *Opioid antagonists*: IV naloxone or oral nalmefene
- Rifampicin
- Antihistamines
- Carbamazepine
- Plasmapheresis
- Ultraviolet B light
- External diversion of bile.

Immunization

In general, all routine vaccines including HB vaccine should be given to children with NCS. HA vaccine should be given to children of more than 1 year. Influenza, chickenpox and pneumococcal vaccines may be given in the absence of contraindications. Live vaccines are contraindicated in children who have undergone liver transplantation.

Antibiotic Policy

A combination of ampicillin and aminoglycosides like gentamicin or amikacin is the best, if septicemia is suspected. It is better to avoid ceftriaxone, as it tends to cause biliary sludge. Cefotaxime and ceftazidime are better choices.

Surgery

If Kasai portoenterostomy (KPE) is done before 2 months of age, 80% may improve. Results are very bad after 2 months **(Fig. 9.15.3)**. In the best of centers, the overall 5-year survival following Kasai ranges from 40% to 50%. Of these, 45% progress to cirrhosis and 55% have cholestasis on follow-up.

Recurrent cholangitis due to ascending bacterial colonization up the Roux limb toward the portal plate is a serious problem in infants with BA following Kasai operation. The common organisms responsible are *Klebsiella pneumoniae, Enterococcus, Escherichia coli*, and *Pseudomonas aeruginosa*. Some studies have shown that this may be prevented by prophylactic antimicrobials like neomycin or lactobacillus therapy.

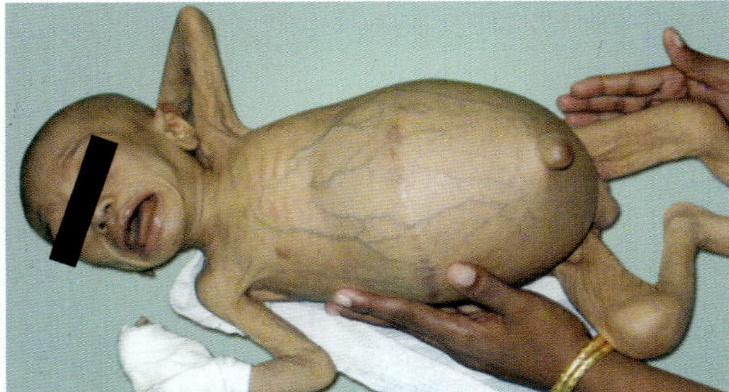

Fig. 9.15.3: Biliary atresia—failed Kasai portoenterostomy (KPE). Note severe PEM, ascites, umbilical hernia and dilated anterior abdominal wall veins.

Outcome of Kasai Portoenterostomy

- One-third of children who had undergone KPE at an appropriate age will not clear jaundice *(failed KPE)*
- One-third would clear jaundice but would develop jaundice in early childhood following disease progression/cholangitis requiring LT.
- The remaining one-third would clear jaundice and remain jaundice free until they enter adulthood *(Successful KPE)*

Successful Kasai Portoenterostomy

These children clear jaundice and pass cholic stools. Serum bilirubin levels should fall below 2 mg/dL within 3 months of KPE. However, it may not indicate a perfectly normal liver and safe transition to adulthood. Their transaminases continue to be high and they subsequently develop fibrosis, recurrent cholangitis, cirrhosis and its complications like gastrointestinal (GI) bleeding.

KEY MESSAGES

- In all neonates with conjugated jaundice, serious underlying liver disease should be ruled out.
- The key features of biliary atresia are persistent conjugated jaundice, pale stools and dark urine in an otherwise healthy term infant.
- Severe Rh/ABO incompatibility may lead to severe hemolysis and subsequently to inspissated bile syndrome, which mimics biliary atresia.
- Sick infants who require urgent treatment should be picked up at the earliest.
- Simple dietary measures like lactose elimination in galactosemia are rewarding.
- The immediate treatment of any child with cholestasis is vitamin K injection.
- The cholestatic syndromes with good prognosis are benign recurrent intrahepatic cholestasis (Summerskill syndrome) and Aagenaes syndrome
- Gold standard for confirming the diagnosis of BA is preoperative cholangiography.
- Association of NC and congenital heart disease—congenital rubella syndrome, Alagille syndrome, Smith-Lemli-Opitz syndrome.
- Kasai portoenterostomy for biliary atresia should be done before 2 months.
- The definitive treatment of biliary atresia is liver transplantation.

BIBLIOGRAPHY

1. Balistreri WF, Bezerra JA. Whatever happened to "Neonatal hepatitis?" Clin Liver Dis. 2006;10:27-54.
2. Poddar U, Thapa BR, Das A, et al. Neonatal cholestasis: differentiation of biliary atresia from neonatal hepatitis in a developing country. Acta Paediatr. 2009;98(8):1260-4
3. Ramachandran P, Safwan M, Reddy MS, et al. Recent trends in the diagnosis and management of biliary atresia in developing countries. Indian Pediatr. 2015;52(10):871-9.
4. Riyaz A. Cholestatic liver disorders. In: Riyaz A. Pediatric Gastroenterology and Hepatology. Hyderabad: Paras Publishers; 2019. pp. 390-427.
5. Shanmugam NP, Narasimhan G, Rajindrajith S. Living with biliary atresia: From Kasai portoenterostomy to liver transplantation Sri Lanka. J Child Health. 2016;45(2): 116-22.
6. Yachha SK. Indian Academy of Pediatrics. Pediatric Gastroenterology Subspecialty Chapter. Consensus report on neonatal cholestatic syndrome. Pediatric Gastroenterology Subspecialty Chapter of Indian Academy of Pediatrics. Indian Pediatr. 2000;37(8):845-51.
7. Zagory JA, Nguyen MV, Wang KS. Recent advances in the pathogenesis and management of biliary atresia. Curr Opin Pediatr. 2015;27(3):389-94.

9.16 Cholestatic Disorders in Older Children

B Bhaskar Raju

INTRODUCTION

Cholestasis is not a disease, rather, a symptom of many diseases due to a pathologic state of reduced bile formation or flow. The most common causes of chronic cholestatic liver disease in children are:

- Intrahepatic cholestasis, like neonatal hepatitis
- Inherited and genetic defects of bile formation and secretion like progressive familial intrahepatic cholestasis (PFIC)
- Extrahepatic biliary obstruction like biliary atresia, choledochal cyst.

They form the prime indications for liver transplantation also, in pediatrics.

DEFINITION

Cholestasis is defined as the failure of bile to reach duodenum due to pathology or block anywhere between the cytoplasm of the hepatocyte and ampulla of Vater. This may occur due to impairment in bile secretion or any condition where there is impediment to bile flow. Clinically, cholestasis is recognized by the presence of jaundice, high-colored urine, hypopigmented or frank acholic stools, with usually itching due to retention of pruritogenic substances that are normally excreted in bile. Cholestasis, however, is also defined pathologically and morphologically as the accumulation of bile and components of bile, in liver cells and biliary passages, along with generalized bile acid induced injury in a biopsy. At a biochemical level, cholestasis is defined as any condition in which substances normally excreted into bile are retained in blood. Elevated direct bilirubin is, hence, the usual marker for cholestasis, except in rare inherited syndromes of bilirubin transport defects, like Dubin Johnson and Rotor syndromes, where direct bilirubin may be elevated in blood but not, other components of bile.

EPIDEMIOLOGY

Biliary atresia, an important cause of neonatal cholestasis, occurs with estimated frequency of 1 in 8,000 to 15,000 live births. Exact prevalence of PFIC remains unknown, but the estimated incidence varies between 1/50,000 and 1/100,000 births. They exist worldwide with equal sex distribution. As per studies, PFIC represents 10–15% causes of cholestasis in children and 10–15% of liver transplantation indications in children. PFIC1 and PFIC2 represent two-thirds cases of PFIC, and PFIC3 one-third of cases. Choledochal cyst (CDC), the most common surgical cause of childhood cholestasis, has an incidence of one in 13,000 to 15,000 births. In Japan, however, it is much more common occurring 1 in 1,000

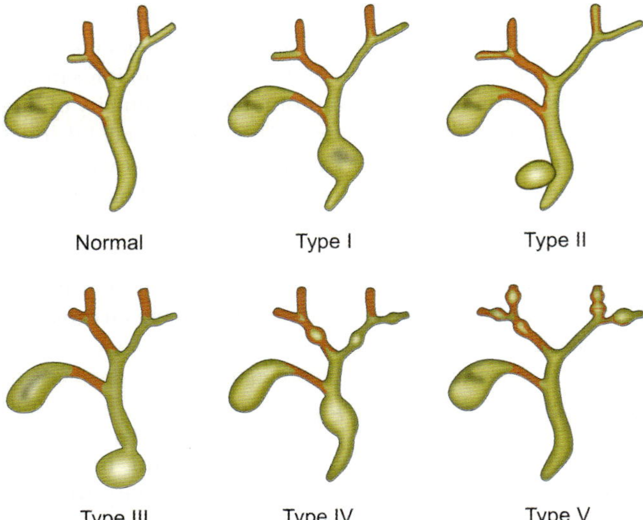

Fig. 9.16.1: Classification of choledochal cysts.
Courtesy: Dr Frank Gaillard, Royal Melbourne Hospital, Australia

Clinical Features

Clinical features vary according to age. When it is symptomatic in neonatal period (<5%), it presents like neonatal hepatitis/ biliary atresia. The classical clinical picture of jaundice with abdominal pain and lump at the right hypochondrium is seen, hardly in 15–20% of cases. Most, however, have at least two of the three above signs. Presentation can also be as pancreatitis, cholangitis, and perforation of bile duct and rarely as biliary cirrhosis with PHT.

Diagnosis

Ultrasonography is the most useful study to diagnose a CDC. The cystic dilatation can be easily visualized. Intrahepatic biliary radicular dilatation is however rare in CDC. Magnetic resonance cholangiopancreatography (MRCP) is currently the investigation of choice to study the extent of intra- and extrahepatic biliary involvement and in classification of the cyst.

Management

Surgical excision of the cyst with Roux-en-Y hepatico-jejunostomy gives excellent long-term results. Long-term follow-up is essential particularly after cysto-enterostomy as there is continued risk of recurrent cholangitis, lithiasis, pancreatitis and possible cholangiocarcinoma.

GALLSTONES AND CHOLEDOCHOLITHIASIS

Gallbladder (GB) calculi are relatively uncommon in children, but its incidence has dramatically increased following widespread use of USG, which picks up silent stones. Most gallstones picked up these days are in children where no pathology can be made out to explain the stones. The extensive use of ceftriaxone (which crystalizes in bile) in pediatric practice has contributed significantly to this increase incidence of GB stones in the absence of any GB pathology.

Cholelithiasis discovered in childhood needs evaluation for:

- Congenital malformation of bile ducts
- Hemolytic disease
- Lipid abnormalities
- Chronic liver disease

Other predisposing factors include obesity, trauma, intra-abdominal sepsis, and prolonged immobilization. Pigment stones are generally more common in children.

Most GB stones stay asymptomatic. Less than 5% are present with complications secondary to CBD or pancreatic ductal obstruction. Treatment would include long-term ursodeoxycholic acid (UDCA) for cholesterol stones, endotherapy for obstructing stones and elective cholecystectomy if stones persist into adolescence.

PORTAL BILIOPATHY

Portal biliopathy is a rare but serious complication of PHT of any cause, but commonly due to portal venous thrombosis, which results in development of varices around the gallbladder and CBD, where they cause pressure obstruction, strictures and rarely stones in CBD. Any icterus in extrahepatic portal venous obstruction (EHPVO) should raise suspicion of portal biliopathy, though it is very uncommon below 10 years of age.

Diagnosis is by biochemistry confirming cholestasis, and ultrasound. Ultrasonogram, especially color Doppler flow imaging, can visualize the varices around the GB and CBD well. Doubtful cases can be confirmed by MRCP.

Treatment would be endoscopic retrograde cholangiopancreatography (ERCP) with stent placement, balloon dilatation of strictures, stone removal, if present, and in intractable cases, decompression surgery for PHT and hepaticojejunostomy.

CLINICAL FEATURES OF CHOLESTASIS

Patients with cholestasis may present clinically in many different ways depending on the disease process.

- Prolonged neonatal jaundice
- Scleral icterus and high-colored urine
- *Pruritus*: Many conditions like Alagille have significant pruritus before icterus becomes obvious.
- Xanthomas and xanthalasmas
- Maldigestion, malabsorption, steatorrhea and failure to thrive due to low bile salt levels in intestinal lumen.
- Increase of copper in blood

Flowchart 9.16.1: Complications of cholestasis.

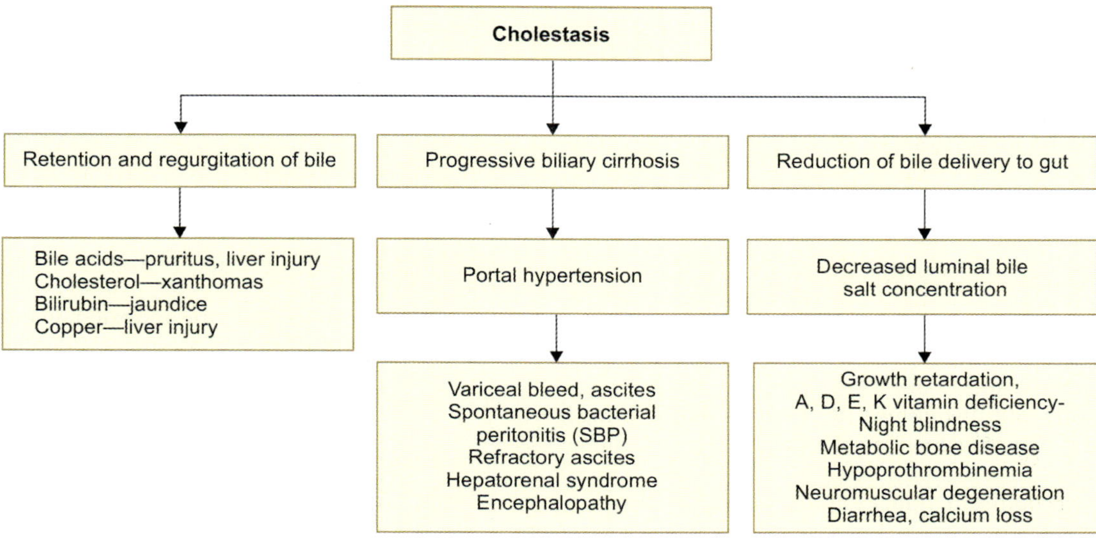

- In acute obstructive causes, the child can present with classic Charcot's triad of fever, severe abdominal pain and jaundice.
- Long-standing cholestasis results in chronic liver disease-biliary cirrhosis **(Flowchart 9.16.1)**.

DIAGNOSIS

Biochemical Investigations

- Increased serum direct bilirubin levels
- Increased total serum bile salt concentration
- Increased total serum cholesterol level (except PFIC 1 and 2)
- Increased AFP in PFIC3
- Increased serum lipoprotein-X, GGTP, serum alkaline phosphatase, 5′ nucleotidase. Patients with PFIC1 and PFIC2, however, have normal serum GGTP activity. GGTP is usually elevated in PFIC3.
- Increased fecal fat levels in virtually all cholestatic diseases.
- Screening for viral markers, especially hepatitis B, A and E, might be needed in short duration cholestasis.
- Rarely, one might have to consider mantoux, chest X-ray, HIV serology and investigations for other granulomatous conditions like sarcoidosis, granulomatous disease, etc.

Imaging

- Ultrasonography of liver and bile ducts is useful to detect causes of obstructive cholestasis like CDC, CBD stones, Caroli's disease and pancreatic causes of biliary obstruction.
- Associated renal anomalies might be picked up by USG, like polycystic kidneys (congenital hepatic fibrosis, Caroli's disease), single kidneys, and ureteric duplication (Alagille disease).
- Color flow and Doppler USG picks up varices around gall-bladder and CBD in portal biliopathy well.
- Abdominal CT, ERCP or MRCP scan, endo USG, if USG findings are equivocal.

Liver Biopsy

Histopathological evidence of cholestasis:

- Biliary duplication
- Bile within hepatocytes/canaliculi
- Cholate-induced hepatocellular injury
- Paucity of bile ducts in Alagille syndrome
- Relatively bland picture of cholestasis in PFIC1 compared to PFIC2 and -3
- Giant cell hepatitis.
- Peri-portal fibrosis and early cirrhotic changes.

MEDICAL CARE OF CHOLESTASIS

Treatment of cholestasis is disease specific but many do not respond well to therapy of any sort. In most, symptomatic treatment is all that medicine can offer, short of transplant.

Methods to Improve Bile Flow/Remove Toxic Bile Acids

- Ursodeoxycholic acid (20–30 mg/kg/day), to increase bile salt dependent bile formation and antagonize the effect of hydrophobic toxic bile acids in PFICs.

- Phenobarbitone (5 mg/kg/day) to improve bile salt independent bile flow.
- Biliary diversion, ileal diversion to remove toxic bile acids in PFIC.

Treatment of Pruritus

- Reduce the bile acid pool in the body by:
    - Decreasing ileal reabsorption of excreted bile acids using binding resins like cholestyramine 240 mg/kg/day or celestipol 500 mg/kg/day.
    - Increasing bile acid excretion using UDCA, phenobarbitone, and rifampicin (10 mg/kg/day).
- Reduce irritation of peripheral nerve endings by pruritogenic factors in bile using:
    - Sedative antihistamines (diphenhydramine 5 mg/kg/day, hydroxyzine 2 mg/kg/day) and short course steroids.
- Decrease propulsion of itch impulses through nerves to CNS using:
    - Opiate antagonists like naltrexone at a dose of 0.25–0.5 mg/kg.
    - Anti-serotonin drugs like ondansetron and its analogs.
    - Nonspecific neural transmission suppressants like carbamazepine.
- Central depressants like propofol given as slow subcutaneous infusions can be used in intractable pruritus. Plasmapheresis and biliary diversion are used as last resorts.
- Liver transplant is of course curative in pruritus.

Nutrition in Cholestasis

- Increased carbohydrate and protein intake.
- Replace fat with medium-chain triglycerides (MCT) oil or coconut oil with added essential fatty acid (EFA).
- Parenteral fat-soluble vitamin A, K, and D periodically or additional oral supplementation.
- Water soluble vitamin E orally (tocopherol polyethylene glycol succinate).
- Calcium 50–100 mg/kg/day, orally
- Phosphorus 25–50 mg/kg/day
- Iron 3–5 mg/kg/day
- Selenium 1–2 mg/kg/day
- Zinc 1 mg/kg/day, zinc sulfate, orally
- Water-soluble vitamins—two times recommended dietary allowance (RDA).

KEY MESSAGES

- Cholestasis is not uncommon problem in childhood.
- Common causes are: Choledochal cyst, children with neonatal hepatitis and post-Kasai biliary atresia, growing into childhood with the cholestasis.
- Alagille disease usually presents with pruritus and minimal jaundice and tends to have a chronic indolent course into adulthood.
- PFICs present like neonatal hepatitis, but are better picked up now with investigations. They respond better to choleretic therapy.
- Biliary blocks (stones, strictures and external compressions) are other rare causes of cholestasis in childhood.
- Diagnostic modalities have improved considerably last decade with USG, MRCP and biopsy clarify the cause of cholestasis very well.
- Treatment modalities have not kept pace with diagnostic facilities and many childhood medical causes of cholestasis are still not curable. Most require liver transplant.
- Advent of liver transplant has revolutionized the outlook for untreatable causes of cholestasis.

BIBLIOGRAPHY

1. Cies JJ, Giamalis JN. Treatment of cholestatic pruritus in children. Am J Health-Syst Pharm. 2007;64:1157-62.
2. Davit-Spraul A, Gonzales E, Baussan C, et al. Progressive familial intrahepatic cholestasis. Orphanet J Rare Dis. 2009;4:1.
3. Dhiman RK, Puri P, Chawla Y, et al. Biliary changes in extrahepatic portal venous obstruction: compression by collaterals or ischemic? Gastrointest Endosc. 1999;50:646-52.
4. Kamath BM, Loomes KM, Piccoli DA. Medical Management of Alagille Syndrome. J Pediatr Gastroenterol Nutr. 2010;50:580-6.
5. McEvoy CF, Suchy FJ. Biliary tract disease in children. Pediatr Clin North Am. 1996;43:75-98.
6. Sarin SK, Bhatia V, Makwane U. Portal biliopathy in extrahepatic portal vein obstruction. Indian J Gastroenterol. 1992;2:A82.
7. Tomer G, Shneider BL. Disorders of bile formation and biliary transport. Gastroenterol Clin North Am. 2003;32:839-55.
8. Mehl A, Bohorquez H, Serran MS, et al. Liver transplantation and management of progressive intrafamilial cholestasis in children. World J Transplant. 2016;6(2):278-90.
9. Srivatsava A. Progressive familial cholestasis. J Clin Exp Hepatol. 2014;4(1):25-36.
10. Khalaf R. Cholestasis beyond the neonatal and infancy periods. J Ped Gastroenterol Hepatol Nutr. 2016;19(1):1-11.

9.17 Fulminant Hepatic Failure

Rajiv Chandra Mathur

INTRODUCTION

Fulminant hepatic failure (FHF) is one of the important causes of death in hospitalized children in India. It presents acutely in previously healthy children and progresses rapidly, leading to multiorgan failure. Viral hepatitis A and E are the common causes of FHF in the developing world. Early recognition and timely intervention are needed to improve prognosis. Liver transplantation has improved survival in children.

DEFINITION

The Pediatric Acute Liver Failure Study Group proposed the following criteria:

- Hepatic coagulopathy not corrected by parenteral administration of vitamin K.
- No history of previous liver disease.
- Prothrombin time (PT) 15–19.9 seconds/international normalized ration (INR) 1.5–1.9 with encephalopathy; or PT ≥ 20 seconds/INR ≥ 2 without encephalopathy.

Hepatic encephalopathy is a state of disturbed neurological function associated with liver disease. Unlike in adults where encephalopathy is central it may be absent, late or unrecognized especially in neonates and infants.

Based on the time interval between the onset of jaundice and development of encephalopathy, International Association of Study of Liver proposed three subcategories of FHF.

- *Hyperacute liver failure*: Interval is less than 10 days. Risk of rapid development of coma is high but survival is better.
- *Acute liver failure*: Interval is between 10 days and 30 days. There is high risk of cerebral edema and it has a poor prognosis.
- *Subacute hepatic failure*: Interval is between 4 weeks and 24 weeks. There is least incidence of cerebral edema and prognosis is worst. Ascites is an important presentation.
- In certain conditions, there may be acute decompensation of the diseased liver. This is known as *acute-on-chronic liver failure;* e.g. acute decompensation with Wilson disease (WD), chronic autoimmune hepatitis and Budd-Chiari syndrome.

ETIOLOGY

Etiology varies with the age of presentation **(Table 9.17.1)**. The most common causes in neonates and infants are metabolic liver disease, septicemia, viral infections especially *Herpes simplex* 1 and 2, and neonatal hemochromatosis. In children older than 1-year, viral hepatitis (most common hepatitis A and E), drugs and systemic infections are the most common etiologies followed by unknown causes.

Table 9.17.1: Etiology of fulminant hepatic failure.

Neonates and infants	*Older children*

• Septicemia
• Inborn errors of metabolism
  – Tyrosinemia type 1
  – Galactosemia
  – Hemochromatosis
  – Hereditary fructose intolerance
• Mitochondrial disorders
• Severe birth asphyxia
• Perinatal herpes simplex infection
• Hemophagocytic lymphohistiocytosis
	• Viral hepatitis A, B, B + D, E
	• Other viral infections
	  – Parvovirus
	  – Adenovirus
	  – *Herpes simplex virus*
	  – Cytomegalovirus (CMV)
	  – Epstein–Barr virus (EBV)
	  – Dengue
	• Nonviral infections#
	• Hepatotoxic drugs*
	• Shock, ischemic hepatitis@
	• Hematological malignancies
	  – Hodgkin lymphoma
	  – Leukemic infiltrates
	• Autoimmune hepatitis type 2
	• Wilson disease
	• Inborn errors of metabolism
	• Industrial poisons

*Valproic acid, INH, paracetamol, halothane, phenytoin, ketoconazole, carbamazepine, cyclophosphamide, methotrexate, nonsteroidal anti-inflammatory drugs (NSAIDs), antiretroviral drugs, and herbal drugs.

@Budd–Chiari syndrome, portal vein thrombosis, and hepatic veno-occlusive disease.

#Leptospira, typhoid, and malaria.

PATHOPHYSIOLOGY

Fulminant hepatic failure is characterized by marked splanchnic and systemic arteriolar vasodilatation along with hyperdynamic circulation and low arteriovenous oxygen content difference. Tissue hypoxia develops despite adequate arterial oxygen and this contributes to the development of multiorgan failure and is a marker of poor prognosis.

- Microcirculatory plugging is caused by formation of microthrombias a consequence of activation and consumption of platelets along with the increased adhesion of leukocytes to the endothelial wall. Increased activity of cyclic guanosine monophosphate (cGMP) results in vasodilatation.

Table 9.17.2: Grades of hepatic encephalopathy in children.

Grades of encephalopathy	*Mental status*	*Behavior*	*Tone and reflexes*	*Pupils*
Grade I	Alert, oriented	Restless, irritable	Normal	Normal
Grade II	Lethargic confused, irritated, in attention to task, inconsolable crying	Combative, euphoric	Increased tone, brisk reflexes	Hyperactive
Grade III	Stupor, somnolence	Marked confusion	Decreased tone, hyperreflexia	Hippus
Grade IV	Unconscious			
Grade IVa IVb	Arousable with painful stimuli/not arousable Decerebration/decortication		Flaccid Absent reflexes	Dilated, sluggish

(*Source:* IAP Consensus Statement, 2013.)

- Encephalopathy results from the accumulation of nonmetabolized ammonia, mercaptans, fatty acids and gamma-aminobutyric acid (GABA). Production of false neurotransmitters is enhanced due to decreased aromatic and branched chain amino-acids in the blood. The cerebral metabolism is altered.
- Renal failure of various degrees occurs in FHF patients. Hypovolemia caused by vasodilatation, microcirculatory disturbances, and acute tubular necrosis are important contributing factors.
- Rapid deterioration in nutritional status with depletion of muscle and fat stores often occurs as a consequence of impaired gluconeogenesis and impaired glycogen storage. Hypoglycemia, hypophosphatemia and hypomagnesemia are common.
- Metabolic acidosis is relatively frequent due to tissue hypoxia, increased peripheral lactate production and renal failure.
- Reduced hepatic synthesis of clotting factors, increased consumption of clotting factors and platelets contribute to the coagulopathy associated with FHF.
- Children with FHF are susceptible to infections as a consequence of impaired neutrophil and Kupffer cell phagocytic function with reduced complement levels. Induced bacterial changes in the gut flora may also contribute to this. The common infections that occur are pneumonia, septicemia, urinary tract infections and spontaneous bacterial peritonitis (SBP).
- A vicious cycle of endotoxemia, circulatory collapse, tissue hypoxia, increased bacteria translocation, and leaky intestinal mucosa contribute to multiorgan failure.

CLINICAL MANIFESTATIONS

Fulminant hepatic failure affects previously healthy children with no recognized risk factors for liver disease. Children usually present with hepatitis and worsening of symptoms over a period of several days or weeks. Jaundice is the presenting symptom in most of the children and its day of onset should be noted. A prodrome of flu-like illness may precede jaundice. Fever, anorexia, vomiting, abdominal pain and fetor hepaticus are common. Altered consciousness and mental changes present later. Infants initially may present with poor feeding, irritability and disturbances in sleep rhythm. Hemorrhagic diathesis and ascites may develop later. A detailed history of mental changes, easy bruising, seizures, decreased urine output, contact with infections, injections, blood transfusion, drug intake, and family history of WD or autoimmune diseases should be elicited. For neonates and infants presenting with FHF an additional history of developmental delay, consanguinity, perinatal or antenatal infections and neonatal deaths should be sought.

Initial physical assessment should include growth, development and nutrition parameters, signs of chronic liver disease, liver and splenic span, ascites, signs of coagulopathy, urine output, and circulatory adequacy. Neurological assessment for grading of encephalopathy **(Table 9.17.2)** should be done several times a day.

Complications are often encountered in association with grade III and IV encephalopathy. They include cerebral edema, convulsions, hypoglycemia, hypophosphatemia, dyselectrolytemia, metabolic acidosis, hypotension, sepsis, gastrointestinal bleeding, coagulopathy, hepatorenal syndrome (HRS), and multiorgan failure.

INVESTIGATIONS

- Serum bilirubin, alanine aminotransferase (ALT), aspartate aminotransferase (AST), and PT should be performed to assess liver cell injury.
- PT $\geq$ 15 seconds and INR $\geq$ 1.5, which is not corrected by parenteral vitamin K in 6 hours along with the biochemical evidence of liver injury indicates liver failure.
- Laboratory monitoring should include complete blood counts with platelets (CBP), electrolytes, renal function tests, blood glucose, phosphorus, serum ammonia, lactate, arterial blood gases, coagulation profile, and blood culture for infection screening.
- Specific laboratory screening to identify the cause of FHF based on age of the child should be initiated simultaneously as early treatment results in better recovery.

- Serum copper, ceruloplasmin, viral serology, autoimmune markers, and metabolic screen should be performed as an initial etiology screen.

MANAGEMENT

Management in an intensive care is mandatory for all patients with more than grade I encephalopathy. Nursing in quiet environment is essential. Barrier nursing should be practiced. Specific therapies where treatable etiologies can be identified needs to be initiated early **(Table 9.17.3)**. Treatment is supportive but specific for multiorgan dysfunction **(Table 9.17.4)**.

Table 9.17.3: Specific therapy for treatable underlying disease causing fulminant hepatic failure (FHF).

Cause	*Treatment*
Acetaminophen poisoning	N-acetyl cysteine (NAC)
Acute hepatitis B	Lamivudine/Entecavir. Alpha-interferon-2 b
Autoimmune hepatitis	IV methylprednisolone
Herpes simplex virus	IV acyclovir
Neonatal hemochromatosis	Deferoxamine, selenium, NAC

Periodic monitoring of infants and children with FHF is essential for improving care and outcome. Vital signs and oxygen saturation should be continuously monitored. Neurological assessment and encephalopathy grading should be done every 12 hours. Blood sugar, electrolytes, PT, and blood gas analyses should be performed every 12 hours or more frequently if needed. Once a day, liver and renal function tests should be done till the child is stable. Calcium and phosphate should be monitored twice a week. Blood and urine cultures should be done for infection surveillance wherever warranted.

Orthotopic liver transplant using whole, split or auxiliary liver from either deceased donor or living related donors has greatly improved survival. It is indicated when there is acute deterioration in mental status, stage 3 or 4 encephalopathy, PT ≥ 100 sec/INR ≥ 4, serum bilirubin ≥ 17.6 mg/dL, worsening lactic acidosis, HRS or the disease is irreversible (Wilson disease with FHF).

Extracorporeal liver assist systems have been developed as abridge till the native liver regenerates or transplantation is possible. Molecular adsorbent recirculating system (MARS) involves usage of albumin-resin dialysate to remove protein bound and low molecular toxins.

Table 9.17.4: Supportive therapy in fulminant hepatic failure.

Goal	*Intervention*
Maintain hemodynamic stability and electrolyte balance	• Colloid, dopamine/dobutamine or epinephrine infusion • Avoid fluid overload • Calcium, phosphate, magnesium and potassium supplementation • Prevent hyponatremia
Prevention of stress ulcer	H2 blockers/Proton pump inhibitors
Sedation	Propofol
Optimize oxygen delivery	• Oxygen/ventilation for more than grade 2 encephalopathy • N-acetylcysteine and prostaglandin E1 infusions
Coagulopathy	• FFP in active hemorrhage, INR > 7. • *Recombinant factor VIIa, if unresponsive bleed*: 5–10 µg/kg • Packed-cell transfusion in hemodynamically destabilizing anemia • Platelet concentrates when platelet count becomes less than 20,000/µL or < 50,000 with bleed
Prevention and correction of hypoglycemia	• 10–20% dextrose 10–15 mg/kg/min
Prevention of hepatic encephalopathy (Decrease ammonia)	• Dietary protein restriction 0.5–1 g/kg/day • Lactulose 1 mg/kg/6 hourly till three loose motions per day in grade 1 encephalopathy (Avoid abdominal distention) • Rifaximin therapy for changing gut microbiota • Sodium benzoate 0.25 g/day • Ornithine phenylacetate as adjunctive therapy
Cerebral edema	• *Monitor ICP (subdural transducer or repetitive transcranial Doppler examination)*: Keep less than 20 mm Hg pressure • Quiet environment, 20–30° head elevation, pyrexia control, and sedation • 20% mannitol infusion • Elective ventilation • Induction of hypernatremia (145–150 mEq/L) by 3% NaCl • Fever management

Contd...

Contd...

Goal	Intervention
Subclinical or clinical seizures	• Phenytoin infusion, thiopental infusion
Diet	• Enteral nutrition/TPN • High calorie 150% of recommended allowance, 50% nonprotein calories • High-carbohydrate, protein restriction • Vegetable protein preferred
Prevention and treatment of infections	• Intravenous line care, infection surveillance • Prophylactic antibiotics (third generation cephalosporins, vancomycin/teicoplanin), anti-fungal agents (fluconazole) in Grade III and IV
Renal failure	• Maintain intravascular volume and pressure • Continuous peritoneal dialysis in established failure

(FFP: fresh frozen plasma; INR: international normalized ratio; ICP: intracranial pressure; TPN: total parenteral nutrition)

Newer modalities undergoing research are hepatocyte transplantation into portal vein and alginate encapsulated hepatocyte intraperitoneal transfusion.

PROGNOSIS

Prognosis depends upon the underlying cause. Various criteria have been established to prognosticate FHF. Some of the indicators for poor prognosis are INR more than 4, hypoglycemia, factor V concentration less than 25%, lactic acidosis, hyperphosphatemia, grade 4 encephalopathy, HRS, children less than 2 years of age and WD. Outcome varies with etiology. Prognosis is better with FHF due to hepatitis A and E, ischemic liver injury and paracetamol poisoning. The overall mortality exceeds 50%.

BIBLIOGRAPHY

1. Arya R, Gulati S, Deopujari S. Management of encephalopathy in children. Post Grad Med J. 2010;86(1011):34-41.
2. Bhatia V, Bavdekar A, Yachha SK. Pediatric Gastroenterology Chapter of Indian Academy of Pediatrics. Indian Academy of Pediatrics. Management of acute liver failure in infants and children: Consensus Statement of pediatric gastroenterology chapter, Indian academy of pediatrics. Indian Pediatr. 2013;50(5):477-82.
3. Bhatia V, Lodha R. Intensive care management of children with acute liver failure. Indian J Pediatr. 2010;77(11):1288-95.
4. Dhaliwal MS, Raghunathan V, Mohan N, et al. Acute Liver Failure in children–A Constant challenge for the treating intensivist. J Pediatr Crit Care. 2016;3(4):37-51.
5. EASL Clinical Practical guidelines on the management of acute (Fulminant) liver Failure. J Hepatology. 2017;66:1047-81.
6. Faraz W, Dar F, Bartlett A, et al. Auxiliary liver transplantation for acute liver failure in children. Ann Surg. 2010;251(2):351-6.
7. Kaur S, Kumar P, Kumar V, et al. Etiology and prognostic factors of acute liver failure in children. Indian J Pediatr. 2013;50(7):677-9.
8. Lufti R, Abulebda K, Nitu ME, et al. Intensive care management of pediatric liver failure. JPGN. 2017;64(5):660-70.
9. Shanmugam NP, Bansal S, Greenough A, et al. Neonatal liver failure: aetiologies and management—state of the art. Eur J Pediatr. 2011;170(5):573-81.
10. Squires RH, Dhawan A, Alonso E, et al. Intravenous N-acetylcysteine in pediatric patients with nonacetaminophen acute liver failure: a placebo-controlled clinical trial. Hepatology. 2013;57(4):1542-9.

9.18 Ascites

Balvir S Tomar

DEFINITION

The term "ascites" is derived from the Greek words "*askites*" and "*askhos*", which refer to a "bag", "bladder", "belly" or "sack". It describes pathologic fluid accumulation within the peritoneal cavity **(Fig. 9.18.1)**. Ascites can occur at any age, even in utero. In children it is usually the result of liver or renal disease. Detection and appropriate treatment of ascites is important to minimize morbidity from its complications.

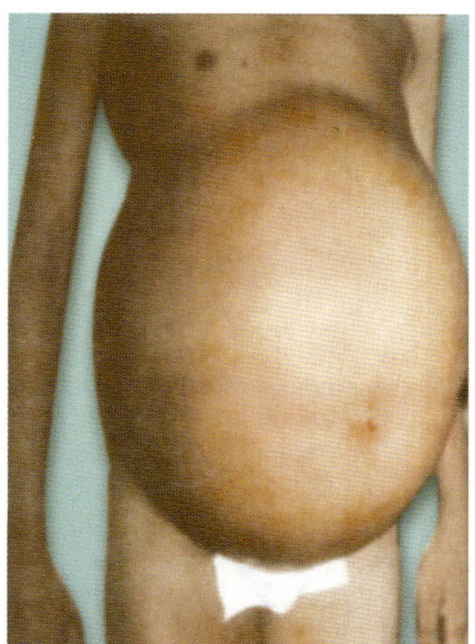

Fig. 9.18.1: Child with ascites.

BACKGROUND

The outer layer of peritoneum lines the abdominal wall and the inner layer covers the organs inside the abdominal cavity. The peritoneum produces a fluid that acts as a lubricant and allows the abdominal organs to glide smoothly over one another. Excess of this, fluid can build up between the two layers and results in ascites.

Ascites may be associated with portal hypertension. This means that there is an increased blood pressure in the veins draining the liver secondary to liver damage. The lymphatic system takes excess fluid and particles away from the liver. Ascites can thus be due to impaired drainage in the lymphatic system. Low levels of albumin and other proteins in the blood also contribute to ascites. The force that holds plasma water within the blood vessels is reduced. Plasma water is lost into the abdominal cavity. Albumin in the ascitic fluid pulls more fluid into this cavity.

Blood flow to the kidneys might be reduced leading to increased secretion of aldosterone resulting in retention of salt and water by the kidneys. Urinary output is decreased, and fluid is retained. In some cases, kidney disease contributes to impaired elimination of salt and water. Fluid may leak from capillaries, the pancreas, or the lymphatic system. Capillary fluid leakage may follow inflammation or infection.

PATHOPHYSIOLOGY

The accumulation of ascitic fluid represents a state of total body sodium and water excess; but the event that initiates the imbalance is unclear. Three theories of ascites formation have been proposed.

1. *Under-filling theory*: This suggests that the primary abnormality is inappropriate sequestration of fluid within the splanchnic vascular bed due to portal hypertension and the consequent decrease in effective circulating blood volume. This activates the plasma renin, aldosterone, and sympathetic nervous system, resulting in renal sodium and water retention.
2. *Overflow theory*: The primary abnormality is inappropriate renal retention of sodium and water in the absence of volume depletion. Thus, patients with cirrhosis have intravascular hypervolemia rather than hypovolemia.
3. *Peripheral arterial vasodilatation hypothesis*: This combines both the above theories. The portal hypertension leads to vasodilatation, which causes decreased effective arterial blood volume. As the disease progresses, neurohumoral excitation increases, more renal sodium is retained, and plasma volume expands. This leads to overflow of fluid into the peritoneal cavity. According to the vasodilatation theory, the under-filling theory is proposed to be operative early and the overflow theory is operative late in the natural history of cirrhosis **(Flowchart 9.18.1)**.

Although the sequence of events that occurs between the development of portal hypertension and the renal sodium retention is not entirely clear, portal hypertension apparently leads to an increase in nitric oxide levels. Nitric oxide mediates splanchnic and peripheral vasodilatation. Patients with ascites have greater hepatic artery nitric oxide synthase activity compared to patients without ascites.

Regardless of the initiating event, a number of factors contribute to the accumulation of fluid in the abdominal cavity. Elevated levels of epinephrine and norepinephrine are well-documented factors. Hypoalbuminemia and reduced plasma oncotic pressure favor the extravasation of fluid from the plasma to the peritoneal fluid and thus ascites is infrequent in patients with cirrhosis unless both portal hypertension and hypoalbuminemia are present. If the liver is damaged, it may produce less blood protein. This may upset the body's fluid balance, which causes fluid to build up in the body tissues, including the abdomen.

Cancer cells can block the lymphatic system. The lymphatic system is a network of fine channels, which runs throughout the body. One of its functions is to drain off excess fluid, which is eventually got rid of in the urine. If some of these channels are blocked, the system cannot drain efficiently and fluid can buildup. The pathophysiologic mechanism of ascites is shown in **Box 9.18.1 and Flowchart 9.18.2**.

ETIOLOGY

Fetal Ascites

Isolated ascites in the absence of hydrops fetalis is uncommon. Fetal ultrasound evaluation has become common even in a normal pregnancy; yet only a small number of isolated fetal ascites have been reported **(Box 9.18.2)**.

Cytomegalovirus (CMV) is the most common congenital infection of the fetus and can cause fetal ascites and liver

Flowchart 9.18.1: Pathophysiology of ascites.

'B' Increased water and sodium retention
Increased blood volume
'A' Increased sunusoidal pressure (Portal hypertension) and/or low oncotic pressure
Ascitic formation
Decreased effective blood volume
Increased renin-angiotensin-aldosterone and sympathetic nervous system activity
Increased splanchnic blood volume
Decreased peripheral vascular resistance
'C' Peripheral arterial vasodilatent

Box 9.18.1: Pathogenic mechanisms in ascites formation.

Increased hydrostatic pressure:
- Cirrhosis **(Flowchart 9.18.2)**
- Hepatic vein occlusion (Budd–Chiari syndrome)
- Inferior vena cava obstruction
- Constrictive pericarditis
- Congestive heart failure

Decreased colloid osmotic pressure:
- End-stage liver disease with poor protein synthesis
- Nephrotic syndrome with protein loss
- Malnutrition
- Protein-losing enteropathy

Increased permeability of peritoneal capillaries:
- Tuberculous peritonitis
- Bacterial peritonitis
- Malignant disease of the peritoneum

Leakage of fluid into the peritoneal cavity:
- Bile ascites
- Pancreatic ascites (secondary to a leaking pseudocyst)
- Chylous ascites
- Urine ascites

Miscellaneous causes:
- Myxedema
- Ovarian disease (Meigs syndrome)
- Chronic hemodialysis

Flowchart 9.18.2: Ascites formation in cirrhosis.

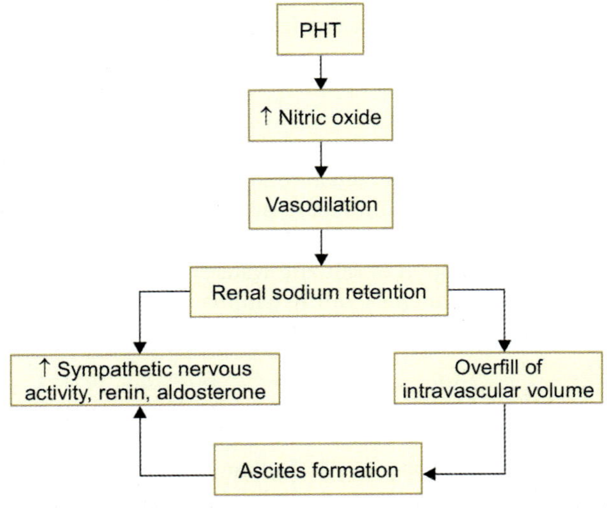

(PHT: portal hypertension)

disease. Ascites is typically detected at between 21 weeks and 30 weeks of gestation. The presence of ascites in utero does not necessarily indicate severe infection or a poor prognosis. Histologic examination of severely infected fetal liver shows

Box 9.18.2: Causes of fetal ascites.

Gastrointestinal disorders:
- Meconium peritonitis
- Intestinal malrotation
- Small intestinal or colonic atresia
- Intussusception
- Volvulus
- Cystic fibrosis
- Biliary atresia
- Portal venous malformations

Genitourinary disorders:
- Hydronephrosis
- Polycystic kidney
- Urinary obstruction
- Ovarian cyst

Cardiac disorders:
- Arrhythmia
- Heart failure

Metabolic diseases:
- Niemann-Pick type C
- Congenital disorders of glycosylation
- Lysosomal storage disease

Chylous ascites

Infections:
- Parvovirus
- Syphilis
- Cytomegalovirus
- Toxoplasmosis
- Acute maternal hepatitis

Hematologic disorders:
- Hemolytic anemia
- Neonatal hemochromatosis
- Homozygous alpha-thalassemia

Chromosomal abnormalities:
- Trisomy 13, 18 and 21
- Turner syndrome

Neoplasms

Miscellaneous:
- Maternal/fetal abuse
- Idiopathic

hepatocellular degeneration with extensive bridging fibrosis and intrahepatic calcifications.

Neonatal Ascites

The common causes of neonatal ascites are listed in **Box 9.18.3**. It may be iatrogenic as in extravasations of parenteral nutrition from femoral or umbilical venous catheters or perforation of the bladder or urachal remnant with extravasation of urine into the peritoneal cavity **(Fig. 9.18.2)**.

Ascites in Infants and Children

Cirrhosis from chronic liver disease is the most common hepatic cause of ascites in infants and children **(Box 9.18.4 and Fig. 9.18.3)**. Inflammatory conditions of the bowel that involve the serosal surface, such as eosinophilic enteropathy and Crohn's disease, may result in ascites. Vitamin A intoxication may also present with ascites, and measurement of retinol-binding protein is important in establishing the diagnosis.

Pancreatic ascites occurs is rare in children. One-third of cases occur in infants younger than 1 year old. Serum amylase and lipase levels may be normal and the diagnosis is often missed unless ascitic fluid is analyzed. Ascites appears to be an accurate independent predictor of severity of pancreatitis and pseudocyst formation.

Box 9.18.3: Causes of neonatal ascites.

1. Hepatobiliary disorders
- Cirrhosis
- Alpha-1 antitrypsin deficiency
- Congenital hepatic fibrosis
- Viral hepatitis
- Budd–Chiari syndrome
- Biliary atresia
- Bile duct perforation
- Portal venous malformation
- Ruptured mesenchymal hamartoma

2. Genitourinary disorders
- *Obstructive uropathy*:
  - Posterior urethral valves
  - Ureterocele
  - Lower ureteral stenosis
  - Ureteral atresia
  - Imperforate hymen
  - Bladder rupture
- Bladder injury from umbilical artery catheterization
- Nephrotic syndrome

3. Gastrointestinal disorders
- Intestinal malrotation
- Intestinal perforation
- Acute appendicitis
- Intestinal atresia
- Pancreatitis

4. Cardiac disorders
- Arrhythmia
- Heart failure

5. Hematologic disorders
- Neonatal hemochromatosis

6. Parenteral nutrition extravasation

7. Metabolic diseases
- Mucopolysaccharidosis VIII

8. Miscellaneous
- Cutis marmorata telangiectasia congenita
- Intravenous vitamin E
- *Pseudoascites*: Small bowel duplication
- Abdominal trauma
- Idiopathic

demonstrates deep acoustic enhancement. Free ascites does not displace organs but typically situates itself between them, contouring to organ margins and demonstrating acute angles at the point at which the fluid borders the organ.

The smallest amounts of fluid first tend to collect in the Morison pouch and around the liver as a sonolucent band. With massive ascites, the small bowel loops have a characteristic polycyclic, "lollipop", or arcuate appearance because they are arrayed on either side of the vertically floating mesentery.

Certain sonographic findings **(Tables 9.18.2 and 9.18.3)** suggest that the ascites may be infected, inflammatory, or malignant.

CT and MRI

Ascites is demonstrated well on computed tomography (CT) scan images. Small amounts of ascitic fluid localize in the right perihepatic space, the posterior subhepatic space (Morison pouch), and the Douglas pouch. A number of CT features suggest neoplasia. Hepatic, adrenal, splenic, or lymph node lesions associated with masses arising from the gut, ovary, or pancreas are suggestive of malignant ascites. Patients with malignant ascites tend to have proportional fluid collections in the greater and lesser sacs, whereas, in patients with benign ascites, the fluid is observed primarily in the greater sac and not in the lesser omental bursae.

Table 9.18.2: Ultrasonography findings in ascites.

Condition	*Findings*
Tuberculous	• Multiple septa, matting or clumping of bowel loops • Thickening of interfaces between fluid and adjacent structures
Blood	Coarse internal echoes
Chyle	Fine internal echoes
Malignant	Bowel loops do not float freely but may be tethered along the posterior abdominal wall plastered to the liver or other organs or surrounded by loculated fluid collection
Pseudomyxoma Peritonei	Multiple septa

Table 9.18.3: Minimum amount of fluid required.

Test	*Minimum fluid in mL*
Fluid thrill	1000–1500
Shifting dullness	500
Puddle sign	120
Ultrasound scan	100
Computed tomography scan	100
Diagnostic tap	10–20

Upper Gastrointestinal Endoscopy

This is done to confirm esophageal or fundal varices.

ASCITIC TAP (ABDOMINAL PARACENTESIS)

Abdominal paracentesis is the most rapid and perhaps the most cost-effective method of diagnosing the cause of ascites formation. Therapeutic paracentesis may be performed for refractory or tense ascites.

Position

- *For large volume ascites*: Supine position with head slightly elevated.
- *For low volume ascites*: Lateral decubitus position.
- *For small volume ascites:* Face down position or hand knee position **(Fig. 9.18.4)**.

Site

- *Midline site*: Below the umbilicus, this is avascular area.
- When midline site is inappropriate (e.g. presence of scar), a site two-finger breadth medial to the anterior superior iliac spine is chosen.
- *Ultrasonic guidance* is needed in specific indications.

Technique

Needle is inserted, using a Z tract to prevent leakage of fluid. This is achieved by retracting (with one glove hand) the skin approximately 2 cm caudal in relation to the deep abdominal wall and then slowly inserting the paracentesis needle. The skin is not released until the needle has penetrated the peritoneum or fluid flows. When the needle is finally removed at the end to procedure, the skin resumes its original position and seals the needle pathway **(Fig. 9.18.5)**.

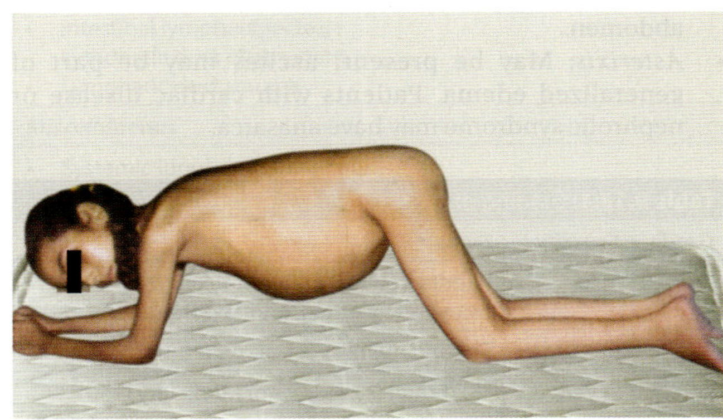

Fig. 9.18.4: Minimal ascites is tapped in knee chest position.

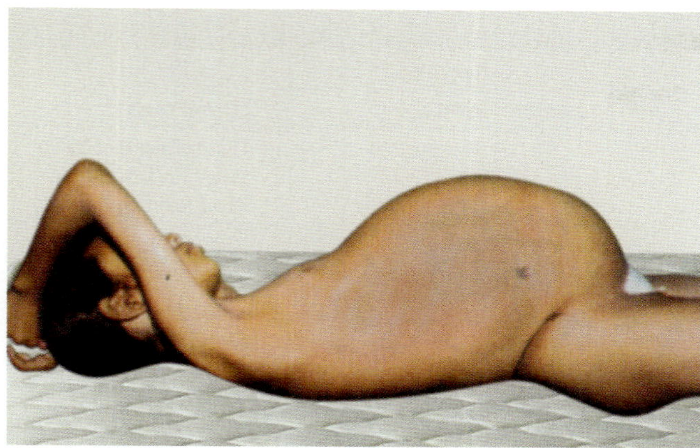

Fig. 9.18.5: Site of ascitic tap.

Gross Appearance

- Most ascitic fluids are *transparent and tinged yellow*. This may be attributed to either a traumatic tap or malignancy.
- *Bloody fluid* from a traumatic tap is heterogeneously bloody, and the fluid will clot. Nontraumatic bloody fluid is homogeneously red and does not clot because it has already clotted and lysed.
- *Purulent cloudy*: Neutrophil counts of more than 50,000 cells/mL have a purulent cloudy consistency and indicate infection. It may be *red* because of presence of red cells more than 10,000 cells/mm^3.
- *Milky* if it is lipid laden
- *Dark brown* in presence of bilirubin
- *Black or tea color* in pancreatic ascites.

Ascitic Fluid Analysis

- Cell count or cytology
- Gram stain and culture
- Acid-fast bacilli smear and culture
- Total protein (albumin or globulin ratio)
- Glucose
- Amylase
- Lactate dehydrogenase (LDH).

Ascitic Fluid Cell Count

- *White cell count*: Normal ascitic fluid contains less than 500 leukocytes/mL and less than 250 polymorphonuclear leukocytes (PMN)/mL. Any inflammatory condition can cause an elevated white blood cell count. White cell count when greater than 350/µL is suggestive of infection. A neutrophil count of more than 250/mL is highly suggestive of bacterial peritonitis. In tuberculous peritonitis and peritoneal carcinomatosis, a predominance of lymphocytes usually occurs. If most of the cells are polymorphonuclear, bacterial infection should be suspected. When mononuclear cells predominate, tuberculosis or fungal infection is likely to be present. This is the single most useful test. Only recent trauma gives false results. To correct this, one PMN is subtracted from absolute ascitic fluid PMN count for every 250 red blood cell (RBC). In old trauma, PMN would already have been lysed, so no correction is needed.
- *Red blood cell count*: When RBC count is greater than 50,000/µL; it denotes hemorrhagic ascites, which usually is due to malignancy, tuberculosis or trauma.

Cytopathology

Cytology smear results are reported to be 58% positive in peritoneal carcinomatosis. Sensitivity increased by centrifuging large volume, pH when less than 7 suggests bacterial infection.

Total Protein

In the past, ascitic fluid has been classified as an exudate if the protein level is greater than or equal to 2.5 g/dL. However, the accuracy is only approximately 56% for detecting exudative causes. The total protein level may provide additional clues when used with the serum-ascites albumin gradient (SAAG). An elevated SAAG and a high protein level are observed in most cases of ascites due to hepatic congestion. Those patients with malignant ascites have a low SAAG and a high protein level.

Gram Stain

It is only 10% sensitive for helping visualize bacteria in early-detected spontaneous bacterial peritonitis (SBP). Approximately, a bacteremia of about 10,000/mL are required for detection by Gram stain; the median concentration of bacteria in SBP is 1 organism/mL.

Microbiology/Culture

The common bacterial infections of ascitic fluid are monomicrobial with a very low bacterial concentration. The sensitivity with bedside inoculation of blood culture bottles with ascitic fluid results in 92% detection of bacterial growth in neutrocytic ascites.

Ascitic Fluid Biochemical Studies

- *Lactate dehydrogenase*: Estimation is often helpful in distinguishing SBP from gut perforation. LDH more than 225 mU/L, glucose less than 50 mg/dL, total protein more than 1 g/dL and multiple organisms on Gram stain suggest secondary bacterial peritonitis (ruptured viscus or loculated abscess).
- *Triglycerides*: A high level of triglycerides confirms chylous ascites.
- *Amylase*: In pancreatitis or gut perforation it is markedly elevated, usually greater than 2,000 IU.

Table 9.18.4: Characteristics of ascitic fluid in various disease states.

Condition	Gross appearance	Protein, g/dL	SAAG g/dL	Cell count		Other tests
				RBC >10,000/L	WBC/L	
Tuberculous peritonitis	Clear, turbid, hemorrhagic, or chylous	>2.5 (50%)	<1.1	7%	>1,000 (70%), Usually > 70% lymphocytes	Peritoneal biopsy stain and culture for acid fast bacilli
Neoplasm	Straw-colored, hemorrhagic, mucinous, chylous	>2.5 (75%)	<1.1	20%	>1,000 (50%); Variable cell types	Cytology, cell block Peritoneal biopsy
Cirrhosis	Chylous, straw-colored or bile-stained	<2.5 (95%)	>1.1	1%	<250 (90%); Predominantly mesothelial	Peritoneal biopsy stain and culture for acid fast bacilli
Nephrosis	Straw-colored or chylous	<2.5 (100%)	<1.1	Unusual	<250; Mesothelial mononuclear	If chylous, ether extraction Sudan staining
Congestive heart failure	Straw-colored	Variable	>1.1	10%	<1,000 (90%); Usually mesothelial mononuclear	
Pyogenic peritonitis	Turbid or purulent	If purulent >2.5	<1.1	Unusual	Predominantly polymorphonuclear leukocytes	Positive Gram stain culture
Pancreatic ascites (pancreatitis pseudocyst)	Turbid, hemorrhagic or chylous	Variable, often >2.5	<1.1	Variable, may be blood stained	Variable	Increased amylase in ascitic fluid and serum

(SAAG: serum-ascites albumin gradient; RBC: red blood cell; WBC: white blood cell)

- *Bilirubin*: An elevated bilirubin level suggests biliary or gut perforation.

Serum-ascites Albumin Gradient

The SAAG is the best single test for classifying ascites into portal hypertensive (SAAG > 1.1 g/dL) and nonportal hypertensive (SAAG < 1.1 g/dL) causes. It is calculated by subtracting the albumin concentration of the ascitic fluid from the albumin concentration of a serum specimen obtained on the same day.

Serum ascites albumin gradient (SAAG) = Serum albumin – Ascitic fluid albumin

It correlates directly with portal pressure. The accuracy of the SAAG results is approximately 97% in classifying ascites. High albumin gradient and low albumin gradient should replace the terms transudate and exudate, in the classification of ascites, as accuracy is not good in the latter. The test is accurate despite ascitic fluid infection, diuresis, therapeutic paracentesis, albumin infusion and etiology of liver disease **(Tables 9.18.4 and 9.18.5; Flowcharts 9.18.3 and 9.18.4)**.

Table 9.18.5: Interpretation of ascitic fluid protein and SAAG.

Condition	Differential diagnosis	Suggestive findings
Low SAAG, low protein	Nephrotic syndrome	High serum lipids Massive proteinuria
Low SAAG, high protein	Tuberculous (TB) ascites	Ascitic fluid lymphocytes increased High ADA
	Chylous ascites	High ascitic fluid TG
	Pancreatic ascites	High ascitic fluid amylase
	Peritoneal carcinomatosis	Malignant cells
High SAAG, low protein	Cirrhosis	Signs of CLD
High SAAG, high protein	Budd–Chiari syndrome Constrictive pericarditis	Veins in back JVP raised

(SAAG: serum-ascites albumin gradient)

Complications of Paracentesis

These include infection, electrolyte imbalances, bleeding and bowel perforation. Bowel perforation should be considered in any patient with recent paracentesis who develops a new onset of fever and/or abdominal pain. All patients with longstanding ascites are at risk of developing umbilical hernias. Large volume paracentesis often results in large intravascular fluid shifts. This can be avoided by administering albumin replacement, if more than 5 L is removed.

Contraindications of Paracentesis

- Disseminated intravascular coagulation
- Primary fibrinolysis

Flowchart 9.18.3: Types of ascites according to level of serum ascites albumin gradient (SAAG).

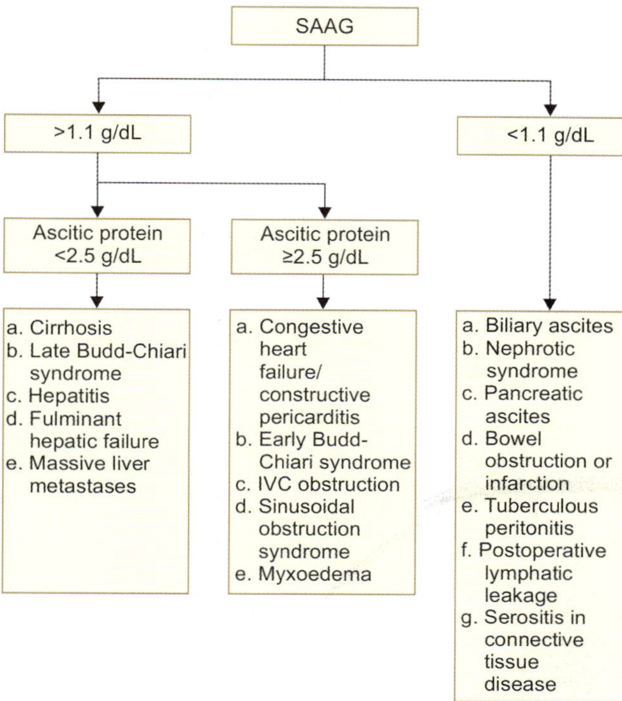

(IVC: inferior vena cava)

- Massive ileus with bowel distension
- Surgical scar at proposed site

Indications for Admitting Patients of Chronic Liver Disease with Ascites

- For investigating the cause of liver disease
- Child not responsive to appropriate OPD basis therapy
- For intensive education of the patient in preparing a diet limited to 88 mmol of sodium per day
- For careful monitoring of serum and urine electrolytes and serum concentration of urea nitrogen and creatinine
- Grade III ascites with respiratory difficulty or distress
- Ascites with suspected SBP
- If a child develops diuretic induced complications—electrolyte imbalances
  - *Hyponatremia*: Serum sodium less than 125 mEq/L
  - *Hypokalemia*: Serum potassium less than 3.0 mEq/L
  - *Hyperkalemia*: Serum potassium more than 6.0 mEq/L
- Hepatorenal syndrome (HRS)
  - Increase in baseline serum creatinine by more than 100% or an absolute value of 1.5 mg/dL (even if the patient is responding to diuretics)
  - Urinary Na+ less than 10 mEq/L
  - Creatinine clearance less than 0.75 mg/kg/min
- Hepatic encephalopathy
- Refractory ascites.

MANAGEMENT

Principles of Treatment

- Initial evaluation
- Diagnostic ascitic fluid tap
- Ascitic fluid analysis
- Identify and treat the underlying cause
- Treatment of diuretic-sensitive ascites
- Indications to stop diuretics
- Treatment of refractory ascites.

Nondrug Management

- *Bed rest*: Upright position increases renin-aldosterone activity and increased retention of sodium or water. Bed rest reduces this activity.
- *Medical care*: The goals of pharmacotherapy are to reduce morbidity and to prevent complications.
- *Diet*: Sodium restriction (20–30 mEq/d) and diuretic therapy constitute the standard medial management for ascites and are effective in approximately 95% of patients.
- *Fluid restriction*: It is the sodium restriction not the fluid restriction, which results in weight loss. Fluid restriction is only indicated when there is persistent hyponatremia and serum sodium less than 120 mEq/L (reduced renal free water clearance). Renal sodium retention is the phenomenon primarily responsible for fluid retention and ascites formation. It occurs months before impairment of renal free water clearance.

Measurements of 24 hours urinary sodium excretion (with measurement of creatinine to assess completeness of collection) are essential. A major goal of treatment is to increase urinary sodium excretion to more than 78 mmol/day **(Flowchart 9.18.5)**.

MEDICAL MANAGEMENT

Diuretics

Spironolactone

It is used for the management of edema resulting from excessive aldosterone excretion. It competes with aldosterone for receptor sites in distal renal tubules, increasing water excretion while retaining potassium and hydrogen ions. The peak effect of spironolactone is approximately 3 days.

- *Dose*: 2–3 mg/kg/day PO in divided doses q6–24h.
- *Contraindications*: Documented hypersensitivity, anuria, renal failure, and hyperkalemia.
- *Precautions*: Caution in renal and hepatic impairment; may cause gynecomastia and impotence in men.

Flowchart 9.18.4: Differential diagnosis of ascites (approach by abdominal paracentesis).

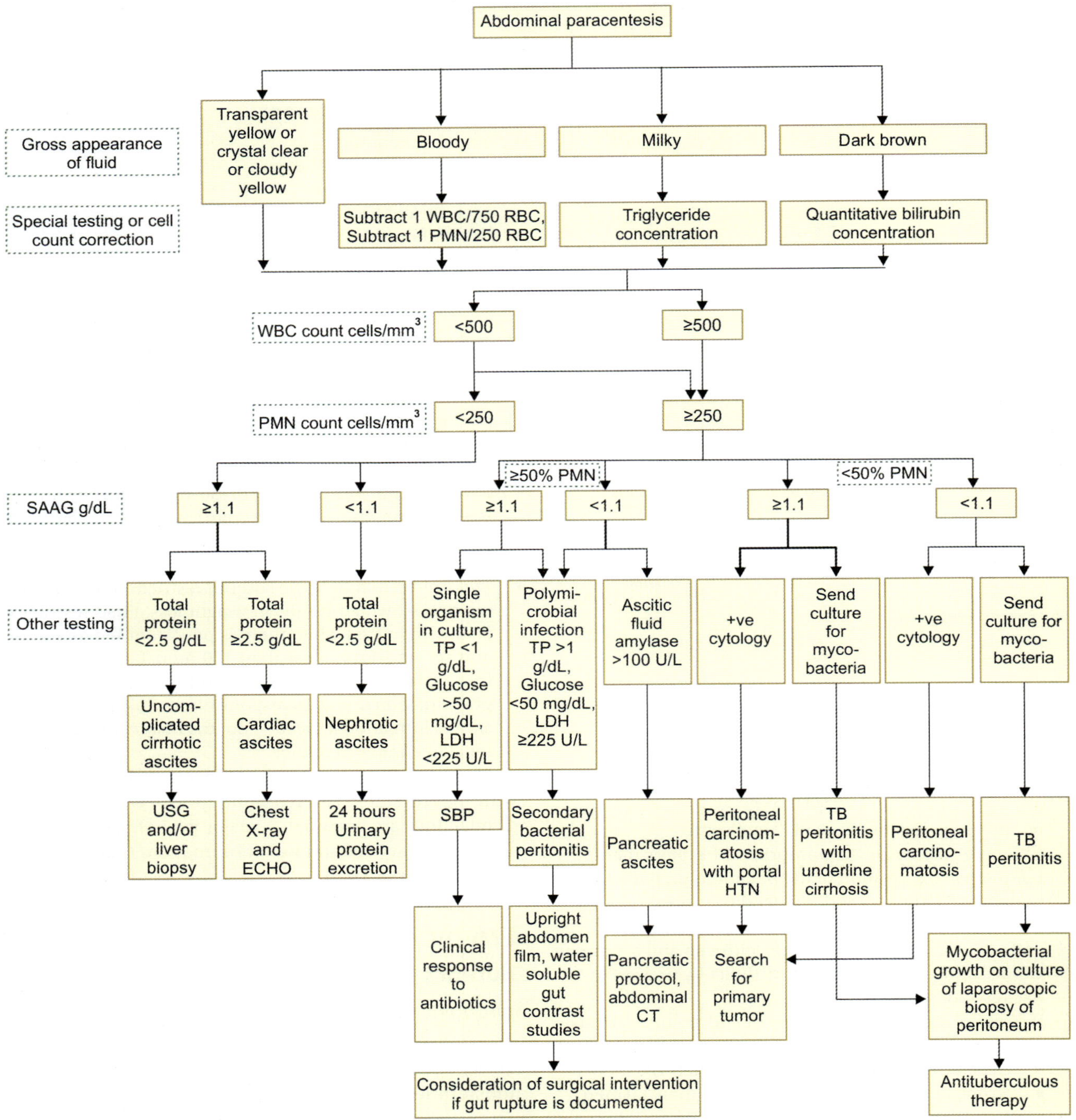

(SAAG: serum-ascites albumin gradient; RBC: red blood cell; WBC: white blood cell; PMN: polymorphonuclear leukocytes; TB: tuberculosis; ECHO: echocardiogram; SBP: spontaneous bacterial peritonitis; HTN: hypertension; UCG: ultrasonography; CT: computed tomography)

Flowchart 9.18.5: Approach to a patient with ascites.

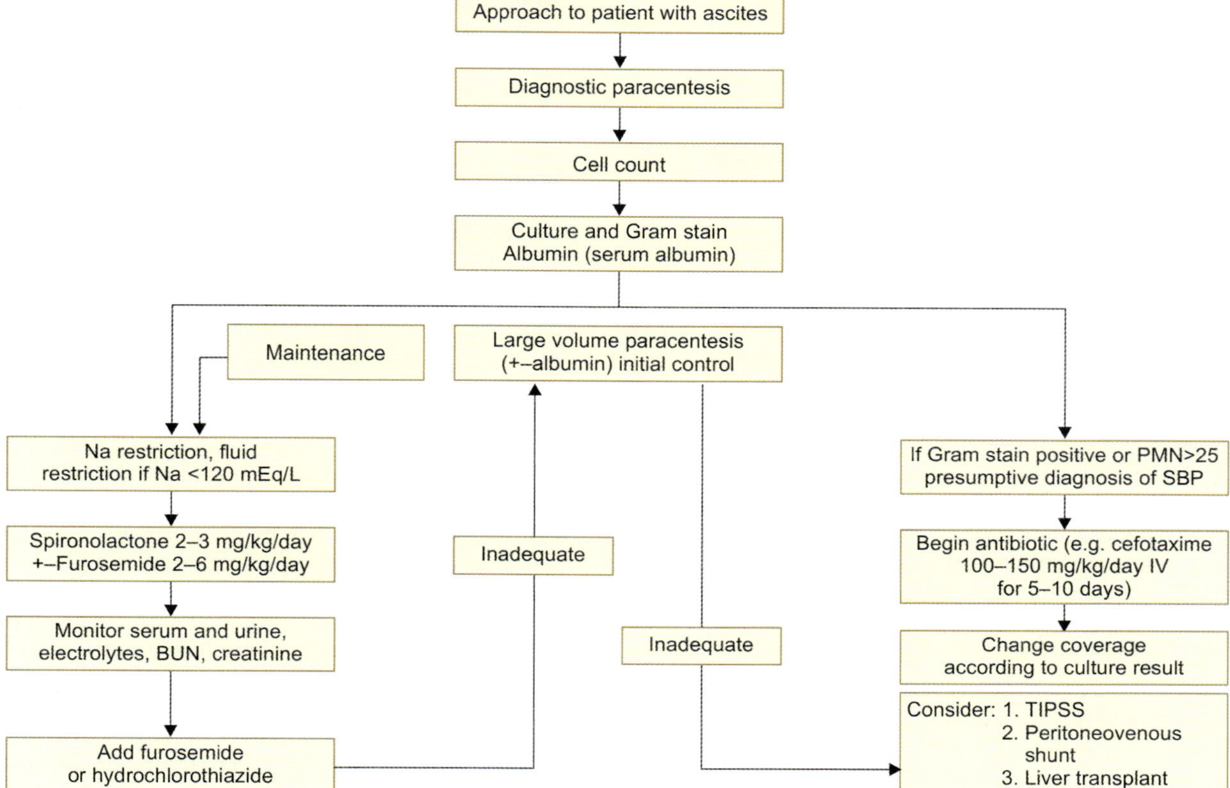

(PMN: polymorphonuclear leukocytes; SBP: spontaneous bacterial peritonitis)

Frusemide

- Increases excretion of water by interfering with chloride binding cotransporter system, which, in turn, inhibits sodium and chloride reabsorption in ascending loop of Henle and distal renal tubule. Dose must be individualized to patient.
- *Dose*: 1–2 mg/kg/dose PO; not to exceed 6 mg/kg/dose; do not administer more than q6h; 1 mg/kg IV/IM slowly under close supervision; not to exceed 6 mg/kg. When treating infants, titrate in increments of 1 mg/kg/dose until a satisfactory effect is achieved.
- *Contraindications*: Documented hypersensitivity; hepatic coma; anuria; state of severe electrolyte depletion.
- *Precautions*: Perform frequent serum electrolytes, carbon dioxide, glucose, creatinine, uric acid, calcium, and blood urea nitrogen (BUN) determinations during first few months of therapy and periodically thereafter.
- *Torasemide*: It is three times more potent and longer acting than furosemide.

Amiloride

- A pyrazine-carbonyl-guanidine unrelated chemically to other known antikaliuretic or diuretic agents. Potassium conserving (antikaliuretic) drug which, compared with thiazide diuretics, possesses weak natriuretic, diuretic, and antihypertensive activity.
- *Dose*: Not established fully in pediatric practice.
- *Contraindications:* Documented hypersensitivity; elevated serum potassium levels (>5.5 mEq/L); impaired renal function, acute or chronic renal insufficiency. Monitor electrolytes closely if evidence of renal functional impairment is present, BUN less than 30 mg/100 mL, or serum creatinine level more than 1.5 mg/100 mL.
- *Precautions*: Potassium retention accentuated in presence of renal impairment and may result in rapid development of hyperkalemia. Monitor serum potassium level. Mild hyperkalemia usually not associated with abnormal electrocardiogram (ECG) findings.

Metolazone

- Helps treat edema in congestive heart failure (CHF). Increases excretion of sodium, water, potassium, and hydrogen ions by inhibiting reabsorption of sodium in distal tubules. May be more effective in those with impaired renal function.
- *Dose*: 5–20 mg/dose PO q24h.

- *Contraindications*: Documented hypersensitivity; hepatic coma or anuria.
- *Precautions*: Caution in hepatic or renal disease, diabetes mellitus, gout, or lupus erythematosus.

Mannitol

- Inhibits tubular reabsorption of electrolytes by increasing osmotic pressure of glomerular filtrate. Increases urinary output.
- *Dose*: Mannitol (20%) 2 mL/kg every 6 hours for 2 days or 0.5–3.0 g/kg/dose 8 hourly.
- *Contraindications*: Documented hypersensitivity, anuria, severe pulmonary congestion, progressive renal damage, severe dehydration, active intracranial bleeding, and progressive heart failure.
- *Precautions*: Carefully evaluate cardiovascular status before rapid administration because a sudden increase in extracellular fluid may lead to fulminating CHF. Avoid pseudoagglutination. When blood is given simultaneously, add at least 20 mEq of sodium chloride to each liter of mannitol solution. Do not give electrolyte-free mannitol solutions with blood.

Which Diuretics in Pediatrics and when to Increase Dose?

Diuretics should be initiated in patients who do not respond to sodium restriction. A useful regimen is to start with spironolactone. The addition of loop diuretics may be necessary in some cases to increase the natriuretic effect. If no response occurs after 4–5 days, the dosage may be increased stepwise.

Duration of Diuretics Therapy

- *To treat*: Diuretic therapy is continued till ascites.
- *To prevent*: In certain conditions like cirrhosis effective doses of diuretics have to be continued for months to years, to prevent reaccumulation of fluid.

Indications to Stop Diuretics

- Encephalopathy
- Serum sodium less than 120 mmol/L despite fluid restriction
- Serum creatinine more than 2.0 mg/dL
- Clinically significant complications of diuretics
- Hyperkalemia and metabolic acidosis (spironolactone)
- Painful gynecomastia
- Muscle cramps.

Diuretic-resistant Ascites

For ascites resistant to medical therapy, treatment options include:

- Therapeutic paracentesis
- LeVeen or Denver (peritoneovenous) shunt
- Liver transplantation
- Extracorporeal ultrafiltration of ascitic fluid with reinfusion
- Transjugular intrahepatic portosystemic stent shunt.

Beta-blockers (Propranolol)

Lowers portal pressure and inhibits renin secretion or combination of these effects, results increased natriuresis.

Updated Guidelines for Management of Ascites

- Drugs that lower arterial pressure, including *angiotensin converting enzyme inhibitors, angiotensin-receptor blockers*, and even *beta-blockers,* should be avoided or, if used, should be accompanied by careful monitoring of blood pressure and renal function.
- *Vaptans,* which inhibit the action of vasopressin on its receptors, should be avoided in patients with cirrhosis.
- The use of *intravenous albumin infusion* after large-volume paracentesis has been controversial. Albumin infusion should be given at a rate of 6–8 g/L of fluid removed when more than 5 L of ascites is drained.
- *Terlipressin plus albumin* was shown to reduce mortality compared with albumin alone in patients with type 1 HRS. Until then, *octreotide plus midodrine* should be considered.
- The common use of quinolones to prevent SBP in high-risk patients with cirrhosis has led to an increase in multidrug-resistant organisms. To reduce the risk for resistance, prophylactic antibiotics should be used only when indicated and for a limited duration when possible. The spectrum should be narrowed once susceptibility results are available.

Drugs Contraindicated in Ascites

- *Nonsteroidal anti-inflammatory drugs* are contraindicated in patients with ascites because of risk of developing further sodium retention, hyponatremia, renal failure and diuretic resistance.
- Drugs that decrease arterial pressure or renal blood flow such as *angiotensin-converting enzyme (ACE) inhibitors, angiotensin II antagonist* or *alpha-1-adrenergic receptor blocker* are contraindicated because of increased risk of renal impairment.
- *Aminoglycosides* are associated with an increased risk of renal failure.

SURGICAL MANAGEMENT

Transjugular Intrahepatic Portosystemic Shunt

Transjugular intrahepatic portosystemic shunt (TIPSS) is a side-to-side portal-systemic shunt placed by an interventional radiologist **(Figs. 9.18.6 and 9.18.7)**. TIPSS is an

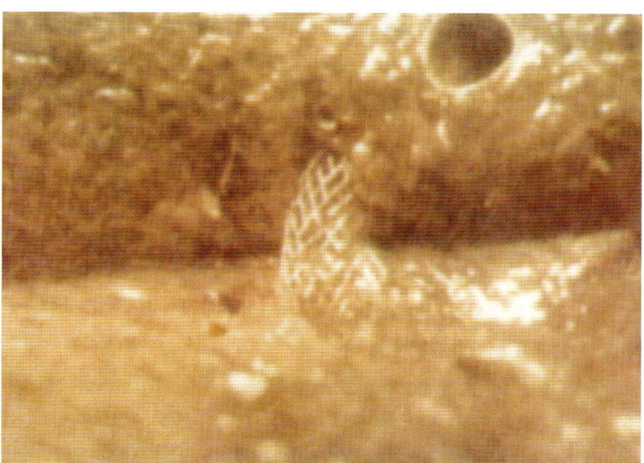

Fig. 9.18.6: Liver explain showing metal mesh of a transjugular intrahepatic portosystemic shunt (TIPSS).

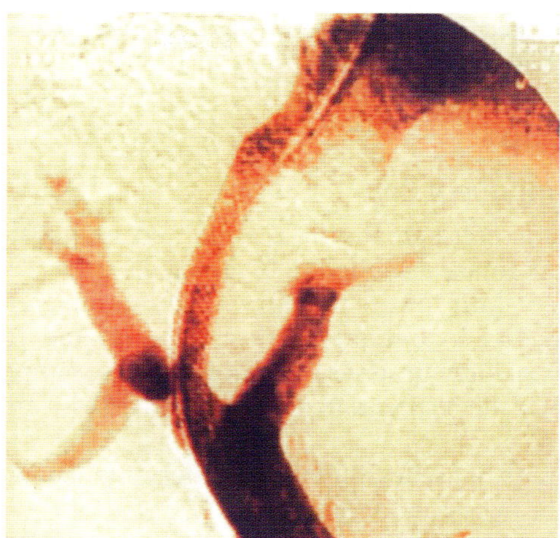

Fig. 9.18.7: Transjugular intrahepatic portosystemic shunt (TIPSS) from hepatic vein to portal vein.

efficacious treatment for patients with refractory ascites. Survival may be better than in patients treated with serial large volume paracentesis. TIPSS is associated with suppression of antinatriuretic systems, and an improvement in renal function and renal response to diuretics. Although the main indication for TIPSS remains variceal bleeding refractory to endoscopic therapy, the procedure reduces the activity of the renin-angiotensin-aldosterone system (RAAS) and increases natriuresis and glomerular filtration rate (GFR). Shunt dysfunction and development of encephalopathy remain the major concerns in this patient group.

Peritoneovenous Shunt

Peritoneovenous shunts [e.g. LeVeen **(Fig. 9.18.8)** or Denver] have been shown to have poor long-term patency. They are associated with excessive complications, including peritoneal fibrosis, and confer no survival advantage relative to standard therapy. It should be reserved for diuretic-resistant patients who are candidates for neither liver transplantation nor serial large-volume paracentesis (because of multiple surgical scars or distance from a physician able to perform paracentesis).

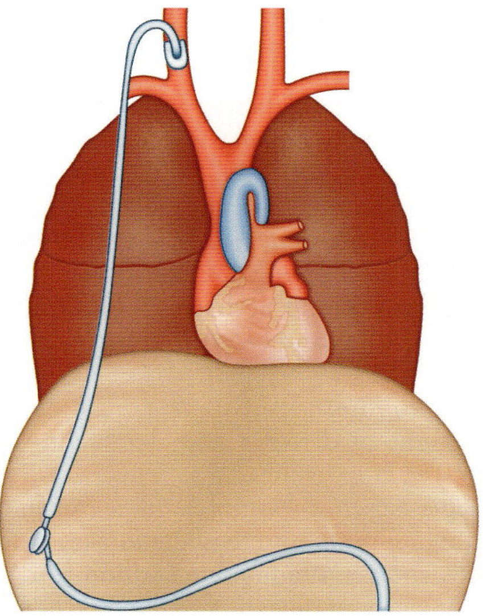

Fig. 9.18.8: Peritoneovenous (LeVeen) shunt.

Liver Transplantation

This is the ultimate treatment modality available for refractory ascites in end-stage liver disease. Replacement of cirrhotic liver corrects portal hypertension and its underlying mechanisms of ascites. Ideally transplantation should be done before HRS sets in. Scarcity of facility and exorbitant costs are currently the limiting factors in our country. The development of ascites refractory to standard medical therapy in a patient with cirrhosis is associated with an approximately 50% 6 months survival, and an approximately 25% 12 months survival.

Surgical Portosystemic Shunting

Portocaval shunt operation involves the anastomosis of the portal vein and the inferior vena cava, consequently reducing the portal pressure. The shunt also produces marked diuresis and natriuresis. However, despite reported efficacy, surgical portosystemic shunts are rarely used in the treatment of advanced cirrhotic ascites, because of the high incidence of postshunt encephalopathy. In addition, surgical shunts may cause technical difficulties during subsequent orthotopic liver transplantation.

Follow-up

Further Inpatient Care

- Patients can actually be maintained free of ascites if sodium intake is limited to 10 mmol/dL
- Twenty-four hours urinary sodium measurements are useful in patients with ascites related to portal hypertension to assess the degree of sodium avidity, monitor the response to diuretics, and assess compliance with diet
- For grade III ascites, therapeutic intermittent paracentesis may be necessary
- It is important to monitor body weight and the intake and output of fluids. Fluid restriction is necessary only if the serum sodium concentration drops below 120 mEq/L. It is also important to determine the sodium balance, which can be approximated by monitoring intake (diet, sodium containing medications and intravenous solutions) and urinary excretion because, a negative sodium balance is a predictor of weight loss.
- A reasonable goal for a patient without peripheral edema is a negative sodium balance with a weight loss of 0.5 kg/day.

Response to therapy is indicated by the following parameters:

- *Optimal decrease in body weight is 0.5–1% every 24 hours as compared to the previous day's weight.* Weight loss more than this would be harmful and indicates rapid shift of body fluids and calls for immediate reduction of diuretic dose.
- *Relief of abdominal distension* as evidenced by improvement of distress and decreasing abdominal girth.
- *Achieving a negative sodium balance* (when the patient is excreting more sodium than the intake) indicates good diuretic response. Inadequate sodium restriction is an important cause of diuretic resistant ascites and can be suspected if the patient does not lose weight and fluid despite an appropriate natriuresis.

Further Outpatient Care

- Daily weight recording.
- *The dose of diuretics* depends upon the degree of ascites and the severity of the liver disease. A usual regime is 2–3 mg/kg spironolactone (or 10–20 mg amiloride) daily with frusemide 2–6 mg/kg/day daily for the patient with more marked ascites initially, or with a poor response to spironolactone alone.
- *Serum electrolytes, creatinine, urea and LFTs* are monitored every 4 weeks for the stable outpatient. In a patient who has been treated initially as an inpatient, an earlier check at 1 week after discharge allows an adjustment to the management plan before electrolyte or clinical imbalance has occurred.
- As liver function improves and the edema and ascites resolve, it may be possible to stop the frusemide first and then the spironolactone.
- The *"no added salt"* (1–2 mEq/kg/day for infant and children, and 1–2 g/day adolescent) is maintained in the majority of patients.

COMPLICATIONS OF ASCITES

Umbilical Hernia

Some patients may develop or may show an increase in the size of already existent umbilical hernia. Most hernias recur after surgical repair unless the ascites is controlled.

Hydrothorax

Pleural effusion, particularly on the right side can develop in some patients with ascites. It occurs due to passage of fluid through small holes in the diaphragm. These effusions may be very large.

Spontaneous Bacterial Peritonitis

Spontaneous bacterial peritonitis is an infection of ascitic fluid in patients with cirrhosis and is defined by an ascitic PMN count of more than 250 cells/mm^3. SBP is thought to develop as a result of delayed intestinal transit and increased permeability of the intestinal wall. In this setting bacteria migrate from the intestinal lumen to the mesenteric lymph nodes, a process known as bacterial translocation.

Most patients present with fever, abdominal pain, chills, general malaise, loss of appetite, nausea or vomiting. A diagnostic paracentesis should be carried out in all patients with cirrhosis and ascites at hospital admission to rule out SBP. It should also be performed in patients with gastrointestinal bleeding, shock, fever, or other signs of systemic inflammation, gastrointestinal symptoms, as well as in patients with worsening liver and/or renal function, and hepatic encephalopathy.

Diagnosis

The diagnosis of SBP is based on neutrophil count in ascitic fluid of more than 250/mm^3 as determined by microscopy **(Table 9.18.6 and Flowchart 9.18.6)**. Ascitic fluid culture is frequently negative even if performed in blood culture bottles and is not necessary for the diagnosis of SBP, but it is important to guide antibiotic therapy. Blood cultures should be performed in all patients with suspected SBP before starting antibiotic treatment.

The most common isolated microorganisms are Gram-negative bacteria, most often *Escherichia coli* or *Klebsiella* species. Usually, only a single bacterial species is found. Recent studies suggest that diagnosis of SBP may be improved by using reagent strips. The principle of these strips is based on the detection of leukocyte esterase. The esterase in the fluid reacts with an ester on the test strip and in combination with a dye. It corresponds to the amount of leukocytes present. The main advantages of reagent strips are the fact that the results are immediately available and the costs are low.

Treatment

Antibiotic treatment should be started as soon as the diagnosis, based on the PMN count in ascites, is made. Empirical antibiotics should be started immediately following the diagnosis of SBP.

Table 9.18.6: Interpretation of ascitic fluid in spontaneous bacterial peritonitis (SBP).

Polymorphonuclear neutrophil count	***Ascitic culture***	***Interpretation***
>250 cells/mm^3	Positive	SBP
>250 cells/mm^3	Negative	False-negative culture
Normal	Positive	Contamination of culture/ early SBP*

*When polymorphonuclear neutrophil count is normal and ascitic culture is positive, it represents early SBP or transient bacterial ascites; a repeat paracentesis is helpful in interpreting results.

Since the most common causative organisms of SBP are Gram-negative aerobic bacteria, such as *E. coli*, the first line antibiotic treatment are third-generation cephalosporins. Alternative options include amoxicillin/clavulanic acid and quinolones such as ciprofloxacin or ofloxacin. However, the use of quinolones should not be considered in patients who are taking these drugs for prophylaxis against SBP, in areas where there is a high prevalence of quinolone-resistant bacteria or in nosocomial SBP.

SBP resolves with antibiotic therapy in approximately 90% of patients. Resolution of SBP should be proven by demonstrating a decrease of ascitic PMN count to less than 250/mm^3 and sterile cultures of ascitic fluid, if positive at diagnosis. A second paracentesis after 48 hours of start of treatment may help guide the effect of antibiotic therapy. Failure of antibiotic therapy should be suspected if there is worsening of clinical signs and symptoms and/or no marked reduction or increase in ascitic fluid PMN count compared to levels at diagnosis. Failure of antibiotic therapy is usually due to resistant bacteria or secondary bacterial peritonitis. Once secondary bacterial peritonitis has been excluded, antibiotics should be changed according to in vitro susceptibility of isolated organisms, or modified to alternative empiric broad-spectrum agents.

Hepatorenal syndrome occurs in approximately 30% of patients with SBP treated with antibiotics alone, and is associated with a poor survival. The administration of

Flowchart 9.18.6: Approach to the diagnosis and treatment of spontaneous bacterial peritonitis.

Diagnostic paracentesis
Ascitic fluid, cell count and differential
ascitic fluid bacterial culture

PMN ≥ 250 cells/mm^3

Signs and symptoms of infection

Culture positive?

Begin empiric antibiotic therapy for SBP

No antibiotics indicated

Bacterascites—repeat diagnostic paracentesis when culture growth is discovered

Presumptive SBP
Begin empiric antibiotic therapy (Cefotaxime 100–150 mg/kg/day) IV Albumin 1.5 g/kg on day 1 and 1 g/kg on day 3

Culture positive?

Confirmed SBP—Narrow antibiotic regimen based on susceptibility results to complete 5 days course

Complete 5 days antibiotic course

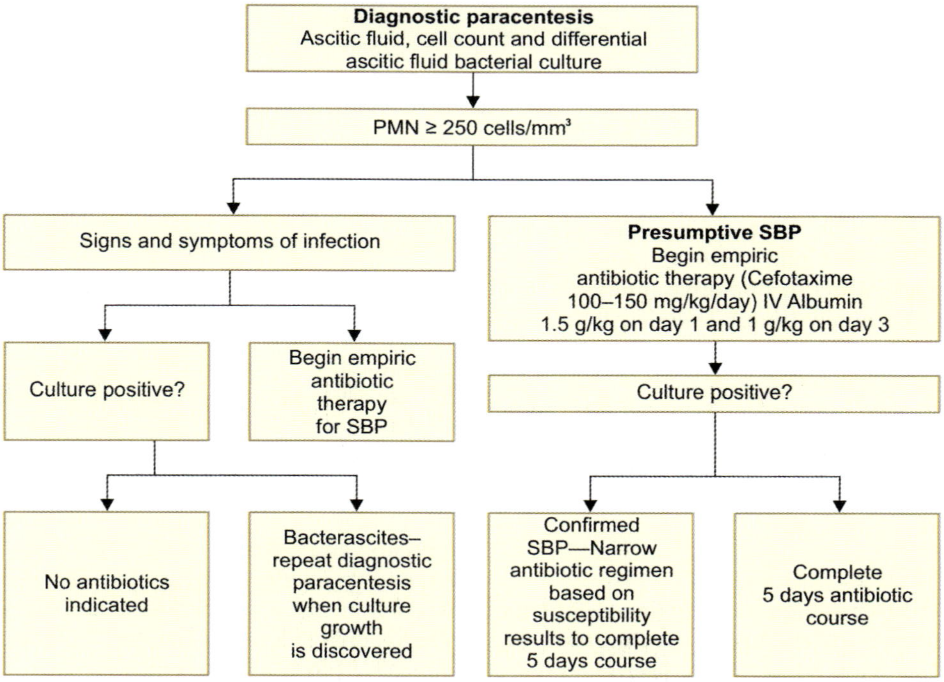

(SBP: spontaneous bacterial peritonitis; PMN: polymorphonuclear leukocytes)

albumin (1.5 g/kg at diagnosis and 1 g/kg on day 3) decreases the frequency of HRS and improves survival. It is unclear whether albumin is useful in the subgroup of patients with baseline serum bilirubin less than 68 μmol/L and creatinine less than 88 μmol/L. Until more information is available, we recommend that all patients who develop SBP should be treated with broad-spectrum antibiotics and intravenous albumin.

Follow-up Paracentesis

Necessary only if there are atypical features [symptoms, clinical setting, ascitic fluid analysis, organism(s), response to therapy] suggestive of secondary peritonitis.

Liver Transplantation

The prognosis in patients who develop SBP is so poor, that liver transplantation should be considered in all survivors of SBP.

Prevention

Cirrhotic patients, with low ascitic fluid total protein levels (<1 g/dL) or gastrointestinal hemorrhage or those who have recovered from an episode of SBP, are at high risk of developing SBP and are candidates for long-term prophylactic therapy with oral antibiotics. Oral antibiotic primary prophylaxis, with norfloxacin, ciprofloxacin or cotrimoxazole, appears to be effective in preventing an initial episode of SBP or a recurrence of SBP. The emergence of infections caused by bacteria resistant to specific antibiotics is a potential problem.

LOW ALBUMIN GRADIENT ASCITES

These patients usually do not have portal hypertension and do not respond to salt restriction and diuretics. Patients with "tuberculous peritonitis" are cured by antituberculous therapy. Pancreatic ascites may resolve spontaneously, require endoscopic stenting or operative intervention or need "somatostatin" therapy. Lymph leak usually resolves spontaneously or may require surgical intervention or peritoneovenous shunting: Chlamydial peritonitis requires tetracycline therapy. Nephrotic and lupus ascites may require steroids. Malignant ascites requires surgical debulking of malignancy and chemotherapy. Ascites may respond to aggressive dialysis.

Urinary Sodium

Twenty-four hours urinary sodium measurement is a helpful parameter. When patient has no urinary sodium excretion despite diuretics, recommend an alternative treatment of paracentesis.

REFRACTORY ASCITES

Definition

It is defined as ascites that cannot be mobilized or prevented from recurring by medical therapy. It is divided into diuretic resistant (ascites is not mobilized despite maximum diuretic dosage) and diuretic intractable ascites (development of diuretic induced complications that preclude use of an effective diuretic dosage). Dietary history, use of NSAID or angiotensin converting enzyme or angiotensin II receptor blockers and patient compliance with treatment regimen must be reviewed before confirming diagnosis.

Criteria

- Lack of response to maximal doses of diuretic for at least 1 week
- Diuretic-induced complications in absence of other precipitating factors
- Early recurrence of ascites within 4 weeks of fluid mobilization
- Persistent ascites despite sodium restriction
- Mean weight loss less than 0.8 kg over 4 days
- Urinary sodium excretion less than sodium intake.

Management

- *Serial large-volume paracentesis* (6–10 L) are safe and effective in controlling refractory ascites.
- Therapeutic paracentesis:
  - *The volume of fluid to be tapped*: Up to 100 mL/kg safely at any time
  - *How frequently one should tap?*: Large volume tap is indicated in one sitting then frequent taps.

Mechanism of Relief by Paracentesis

Taking out fluid from peritoneal cavity decreases systemic venous congestion, increases GFR and renal plasma flow, which helps in producing diuresis. Advanced cirrhosis is associated with a hyperdynamic circulation characterized by reduced systemic vascular resistance secondary to splanchnic vasodilatation, which leads to effective hypovolemia. Intense activation of the RAAS and the sympathetic nervous system, and nonosmotic release of vasopressin occur, with consequent renal hypoperfusion. This becomes more accentuated as patient's progress from decompensated cirrhosis to the HRS. In patients with no urinary sodium excretion and a dietary intake of 88 mmol sodium daily, the required frequency is about every two weeks. The frequency is influenced by the degree of compliance with the low sodium diet. The sodium content of ascitic fluid is about 130 mmol/L. Thus, a 6 L paracentesis removes 780 mmol sodium. Patients, who ingest 88 mmol sodium per day and excrete

10 mmol sodium in nonurinary losses and no sodium in the urine, retain 78 mmol sodium per day. Accordingly, a 6 L paracentesis removes the sodium retained over a period of 10 days, and a 10 L paracentesis removes the sodium retained over approximately 17 days.

Intravenous colloid replacement, e.g. albumin 6–8 g/L, is recommended immediately following a large-volume paracentesis (>5 L), to minimize intravascular hypovolemia, activation of vasoconstrictor and antinatriuretic systems, and impairment of renal function. Dextran 70 is less efficacious than albumin. If a paracentesis is less than 5 L, colloid replacement appears to be unnecessary.

Novel Treatments in Ascites

- *Atrial natriuretic peptide (ANP)*: It normally increases GFR and natriuresis. Patients with advanced cirrhosis and ascites have a reduced natriuretic response to ANP despite elevated levels. Exogenous ANP administration, together with the splanchnic vasoconstrictor terlipressin to counter the hypotensive effect of ANP, increases renal blood flow, GFR and natriuresis in patients with refractory ascites.
- *Other agents*: Although not tested specifically for refractory ascites, a number of agents have been tried in humans, which may increase diuresis in cirrhotic patients with ascites. These include the V2 receptor antagonist, OPC-3126, Niravoline, a k-opioid antagonist, and the adenosine-1-receptor antagonist FK352. Future studies using these novel agents may provide further information regarding their efficacy in refractory ascites.

CHYLOUS ASCITES

Chylous ascites is a turbid, milky or creamy peritoneal fluid due to the presence of thoracic or intestinal lymph having triglyceride (fat) concentration of more than 1,000 mg/dL. If patient has nothing by mouth, then milky color will fade and the fluid will look like transudate with predominance of lymphocytes (85%).

Causes

Congenital anomaly of lymphatics, lymphangiectasis, obstruction of duct within its abdominal portion from trauma, tumor, large lymph nodes, rupture of major lymphatic channel, tuberculosis, filariasis, nephrotic syndrome, cirrhosis, rheumatoid arthritis and other serositis.

The characteristic features of chylous ascites are listed in **Table 9.18.7**.

Table 9.18.7: Chylous ascites.

Color	*Milky and cloudy*
Triglyceride level	Above 200 mg/dL
Cell count	Above 500/mm^3 (lymphocytic predominance)
Total protein	Between 2.5 g/dL and 7.0 g/dL
SAAG	Below 1.1 g/dL
Cholesterol	Low (ascites/serum ratio <1)
Lactate dehydrogenase	Between 110 IU/L and 200 IU/L
Culture	Positive in selected cases of tuberculosis
Cytology	Positive in malignancy
Amylase	Elevated in cases of pancreatitis
Glucose	Below 100 mg/dL

PSEUDOCHYLOUS ASCITES

In chronic peritonitis/persistent ascites fluid have somewhat similar color, from the degeneration of inflammatory products (leukocytes/tumor cell), and may be confused with chylous fluid **(Table 9.18.8)**.

Table 9.18.8: Difference between true and pseudochylous fluid.

True chylous fluid	*Pseudochylous fluid*
Ether test—top thick layers becomes clear fluid	Turbidity is unchanged
Alkali test—no change in color	Becomes clear (dissolves cellular protein)
Fat globules stained by Sudan	Not stained

MANAGEMENT

- Dietary
- *Low fat diet*: Containing medium chain triglycerides, because these are absorbed directly into the portal circulation.
- High protein diet
- Parenteral nutrition supplementation.
- *Paracentesis*: Duration of treatment may require several months for effective medical management.
- *Surgical approach*: Abdominal exploration to detect the site of the leak.

PROGNOSIS

Prognosis depends on the underlying disorder, the degree of reversibility of a given disease process, and the response to treatment.

Patient Education

The most important aspect of patient education is determining when therapy is failing and recognizing the need to see a physician. Unfortunately, in most cases, liver failure has a dismal prognosis. All patients must be taught which complications are potentially fatal and the signs and symptoms that precede them. Abdominal distension and/or pain despite maximal diuretic therapy are common problems, and patients must realize the importance of seeing a physician immediately.

MONITORING OF THE PATIENT

The treatment of ascites depends on its cause. In the majority of patients, cirrhosis leading to portal hypertension is the major cause. A particular value of recognizing portal hypertension as a cause of ascites is that medical management using diuretics and salt restriction is often effective in portal hypertensive patients. Conversely, ascites due to peritoneal inflammation or malignancy alone does not respond to salt restriction and diuretics.

Monitoring during Diuretic Therapy

The main concern during diuretic therapy is whether there is too rapid fluid mobilization and diuretic induced complications. In OPD settings, the patient needs to be assessed after 1 week of starting therapy and thereafter every 2 weeks. At each visit compliance for low sodium diet, bed rest and diuretic doses should be ascertained. Examination for changes in weight, abdominal girth, and pedal edema, ascitic grading and subtle signs of spontaneous bacterial peritonitis should be done. Weight loss of more than 1% per day or 4–6% per week of the previous weight would indicate too rapid fluid mobilization and natriuresis. This cautions us to evaluate renal functions along with reduction in the dose of diuretics.

Evaluation of serum Na, K, blood urea and creatinine and LFTs would be useful in assessing diuretic response and its attendant complications. Serial measurement of fractional excretion of sodium is an objective measure of the effectiveness of the diuretic response. This requires simultaneous estimation of serum and spot urinary sodium and creatinine concentrations. At the earliest suspicion of spontaneous bacterial peritonitis, an ascitic tap should be performed and antibiotic therapy instituted. Admitted patients are usually those who have resistant ascites or have developed diuretic induced complications. Thus their monitoring is more intense and repeated every 48 hours.

SUMMARY

The circulatory disturbances seen in advanced cirrhosis lead to the development of ascites, which can become refractory to diet and medical therapy. These abnormalities may progress and cause a functional renal failure known as the HRS. Management of refractory ascites and HRS is a therapeutic challenge and if appropriate, liver transplantation remains the best treatment. New therapeutic options have recently appeared including the transjugular intrahepatic portosystemic shunt and selective splanchnic vasoconstrictor agents, which may improve renal function and act as a bridge to transplantation.

KEY MESSAGES

- Paracentesis is recommended in hospitalized patients with cirrhosis and ascites.
- Delayed paracentesis is associated with increased mortality in spontaneous bacterial peritonitis (SBP). Every hour delay in paracentesis is associated with 3 % increase in mortality.
- Early initiation of diuretic therapy lowers 90-day mortality. Pneumonia is associated with high mortality in those with new onset cirrhosis-related ascites.

BIBLIOGRAPHY

1. Achiron R, Gindes L, Kivilevitch Z, et al. Prenatal diagnosis of congenital agenesis of the fetal portal venous system. Ultrasound Obstet Gynecol. 2009;34(6):643-52.
2. Albornoz L, Motta A, Alvarez D, et al. Nitric oxide synthase activity in the splanchnic vasculature of patients with cirrhosis: relationship with hemodynamic disturbances. J Hepatol. 2001;35(4):452-6.
3. Arora NK, Mathur P, Ahuja A, et al. Acute liver failure. Indian J Pediatr. 2003;70(1):73-9.
4. Ben-Haroush A, Yogev Y, Levit O, et al. Isolated fetal ascites caused by Wolman disease. Ultrasound Obstet Gynecol. 2003;21(3):297-8.
5. Ginès P, Cárdenas A, Arroyo V, et al. Management of cirrhosis and ascites. N Engl J Med. 2004;350(16):1646-54.
6. Kim JJ, Tsukamoto MM, Mathur AK, et al. Delayed paracentesis is associated with increased in-hospital mortality in patients with spontaneous bacterial peritonitis. Am J Gastroenterol. 2014;109:1436-42.
7. Le S, Spelman T, Chong CP, el al. Could adherence to quality of care indicators for hospitalized patients with cirrhosis-related ascites improve clinical outcomes? Am J Gastroenterol. 2016;111:87-92.
8. Runyon BA. Practice Guidelines Committee, American Association for the Study of Liver Diseases (AASLD). Management of adult patients with ascites due to cirrhosis. Hepatology. 2004;39(3):841-56.
9. Suzumori N, Obayashi S, Hattori Y, et al. Prenatal diagnosis of persistent cloaca. Congenit Anom (Kyoto). 2009;49(3):116-7.
10. Wallerstedt S, Olsson R, Simrén M, et al. Abdominal tenderness in ascites patients indicates spontaneous bacterial peritonitis. Eur J Intern Med. 2007;18(1): 44-7.

9.19 Common Metabolic Liver Disorders

Ashish Bavdekar

INTRODUCTION

Liver plays a central role in innumerable metabolic processes in the body, and hence is affected primarily or secondarily in many inborn errors of metabolism; these are referred to as metabolic liver disorders (MLDs). MLDs now account for up to 40% of all chronic liver admissions to large medical centers in India. A strong index of suspicion is the key to make a definitive diagnosis. The most common MLDs seen in India are Wilson disease (WD), glycogen storage disease (GSD), and galactosemia. Not all of them have a specific therapy but in some like WD, GSD, galactosemia, etc. medical therapy or dietary manipulations, are important to sustain a normal life.

The possibility of a MLD should be considered, if any of the following are present:

- Family history of liver disease or consanguinity
- Unexplained hepatomegaly without jaundice
- Any unexplained chronic liver disease
- Associated rickets, failure to thrive and dysmorphism
- Associated renal, respiratory or neurological disease
- Recurrent episodes of liver disease
- Liver failure in early infancy, severe uncorrectable coagulopathy.

WILSON DISEASE

Wilson disease is an inborn error of metabolism characterized by toxic accumulation of copper in liver, brain, cornea and other tissues. It is an autosomal recessived is order and occurs worldwide with an estimated prevalence of 1 in 30–50,000. It is one of the leading causes of chronic liver disease in Indian children. The gene responsible has been identified as the *ATP7B* gene located on chromosome 13q.

Clinical Manifestations

The clinical manifestations are a result of the deposition of copper in various organs and the age of presentation can vary from 4 years to 60 years. The manifestations are more likely to be hepatic in early childhood and neurological in adolescents; however, other forms of presentation are also seen. The spectrum of hepatic manifestations includes all forms of chronic or acute liver disease. In Indian children, neurological manifestations can begin even in the first decade. They can be equally varied and include clumsiness, speech difficulties, scholastic deterioration, behavior problems, choreoathetoid, and dystonic movements. Other presentations are "osseomuscular" with bony deformities (knock knees) suggestive of resistant rickets. Hemolytic anemia can occur due to erythrocyte membrane injury from the free copper in the serum.

Diagnostic Challenges

No single test is diagnostic by itself, and a group of appropriate tests of copper metabolism need to be done in order to make the diagnosis.

- *Serum ceruloplasmin:* The level of ceruloplasmin in normal individuals is 20–40 mg/dL. Serum ceruloplasmin is reduced in most patients with WD. However, 5–40% of WD may have a normal ceruloplasmin.
- *Twenty-four*-hour *urine copper:* In symptomatic patients with WD, the 24-hour urinary copper excretion is more than 100 μg/day (normal < 40 μg/day). However, similar high values have also been documented in non-WD chronic hepatitis, Indian childhood cirrhosis, chronic cholestatic liver disease, acute liver failure of any etiology and copper contaminated urine samples.
- *Kayser-Fleischer (KF) ring:* It appears as a golden brown or greenish-yellow discoloration in the limbus of the cornea. As lit-lamp examination is necessary for detection. In India, KF ring is seen at an earlier age and also in a significant number of hepatic cases.
- *Hepaticcopper*: Normal values are less than 50 μg/g of dry weight of liver. It is the best predictive marker for WD and considered the gold standard, with values usually above 250 μg/g dry weight. Disorders like Indian childhood cirrhosis and chronic cholestatic disorders also give rise to high hepatic coppers but can be clinically differentiated from WD.
- *Genetic studies*: Direct genetic diagnosis is difficult because of the occurrence of more than 200 mutations, each of which is rare. The WD mutations in different regions of India suggest high genetic heterogeneity and the absence of a single or a limited number of common founder mutations.

Diagnostic Approach

In a eurological setting, diagnosis of WD is made by presence of KF ring with either a low ceruloplasmin or high urinary copper. In liver disease, WD is strongly suggested by any two of the following: Low ceruloplasmin, high urinary copper or presence of KF rings, and confirmed by a high hepatic copper.

Management

- *Diet*: It is advisable to avoid high copper-containing foods like organ meats (liver), chocolates, nuts, and dry fruits.
- *Drugs*: Continuous lifelong drug therapy is essential in the management of WD. Treatment comprises of an initial phase, where copper is reduced to subtoxic threshold. D-penicillamine (DP) or trientine with/without zinc is used as initial therapy, and a maintenance phase to maintain as lightly negative Cu balance so as to prevent copper accumulation and toxicity. DP, trientine or zinc has been traditionally used for this phase.
- *Liver transplant*: Liver transplant is the treatment of choice in children with acute liver failure or decompensated cirrhosis unresponsive to medical therapy. One-year survival ranges from 79% to 87%.

GLYCOGEN STORAGE DISEASES

Glycogen storage diseases are a heterogeneous group of entities classified on the basis of specific enzyme defects in various steps of glycogen synthesis or breakdown. Types I, III, IV, VI, and IX have liver involvement.

Glycogen Storage Disease Type I

Glucose-6-phosphatase deficiency is the most severe form of hepatic GSD and results in defective gluconeogenesis.

Patients present in infancy with doll-like facies, truncal obesity, massive hepatomegaly, nephromegaly, failure to thrive, hypoglycemia and lactic acidosis after short-fasting intervals. Serum triglycerides, cholesterol and uric acid are moderately elevated. The kidneys are enlarged on ultrasound due to increased glycogen content. Liver biopsy shows markedly increased fat and glycogen without fibrosis.

Glycogen Storage Disease Type III

Glycogen storage disease III is due to abnormal activity of debrancher enzyme—amylo-1-6 glucosidase. Type IIIa is associated with progressive cardiomyopathy while IIIb has mainly liver disease. In infancy, presentation is similar to GSD type I (GSDI), but milder with hepatomegaly and hypoglycemia. Gradually hepatomegaly decreases and fasting hypoglycemia improves. This is the most common GSD in India.

Glycogen Storage Disease Type IV

This rare disorder occurs due to a defecting lycogen-branching enzyme. Patients are normal at birth. Hepatomegaly and failure to thrive are seen in infancy. Cirrhosis and splenomegaly soon become manifest and death from liver cell failure usually occur before 3 years of age. Liver biopsy shows cirrhosis and abnormal glycogen, which is diastase resistant.

Glycogen Storage Disease Types VI and IX

These GSDs are due to defect in the hepatic phosphorylase system. The disorders are fairly benign and long-term outlook for growth and liver function are good.

Management of Glycogen Storage Disease

Treatment of GSDI is aimed at preventing hypoglycemia by frequent daytime feeding with slowly resorbed carbohydrates (starch, glucose polymers) and continuous nocturnal feeding. Liver transplant is the only available option for GSDIV but may not prevent progression of extrahepatic disease.

GALACTOSEMIA

It is an autosomal recessive disorder of galactose metabolism due to deficiency of enzymes galactokinase and galactose-1-phosphate uridyl-transferase (GALT) (which is the most common) or uridine diphosphate galactose-4-epimerase.

GALT deficiency should be suspected in any of the following presentations in neonatal period: Jaundice, hepatomegaly, hypoglycemia, cirrhosis, ascites, liver failure and coagulopathy, cataracts and *Escherichia coli* sepsis. If untreated, these children go on to develop liver failure or chronic liver disease.

The laboratory findings besides those of deranged liver function include elevated blood galactose and galactose-1-phosphate, hypoglycemia, hyperglycosuria, hyperchloremic metabolic acidosis, albuminuria and hyperaminoaciduria. Urine-reducing substances have been the traditional screening test, but there commended diagnostic method is red blood cell count gal-1-PUT, for which the Buetler screening test is widely used.

Elimination of dietary galactose is the only available treatment. Inneonates and small infants, the preparation used is lactose-free case in hydrolysates or soyabean milks. In older children, diets restricted to less than 125 mg galactose are advised.

KEY MESSAGES

- Metabolic liver diseases account for up to 40% of chronic liver diseases in Indian children.
- Presentation may be in early infancy or in childhood.
- Wilson disease, glycogen storaged is ease and galactosemia are the most common MLDs.
- Early diagnosis essential for appropriate treatment and favorable outcome.

BIBLIOGRAPHY

1. Bavdekar AR. Therapeutic and management challenges in Wilson's disease. J Gastroenterol Hepatol. 2004;19:S391-6.
2. Bavdekar AR, Tanner MS. Indian childhood cirrhosis and other metabolic liver diseases. In: Kumar D (Ed.). Genetic Disorders of the Indian subcontinent. Nederland, Dordrecht: Kluwer Academic Publishers; 2004. pp. 223-45.
3. Ghishan FK, Ballew MP. Inborn errors of carbohydrate metabolism. In: Suchy SJ, Sokol RJ, Balistreri WF (Eds). Liver Disease in Children, 2nd Edition. Philadelphia: Lippincott Williamsand Wilkins; 2001. pp. 565-72.
4. Gupta A, Chattopadhyay I, Dey S, et al. Molecular pathogenesis of Wilson disease among Indians: A perspective on mutation spectrum in ATP7B gene, prevalent defects, clinical heterogeneity and implication towards diagnosis. Cell Mol Neurobiol. 2007;27(8):1023-33.
5. Roberts EA, Schilsky ML. American Association for Study of Liver Diseases (AASLD). Diagnosis and treatment of Wilson's disease: Anupdate. Hepatology. 2008;47(6):2089-111.
6. Segal S. Komrower Lecture. Galactosemia today: The enigma and the challenge. J Inherit Metab Dis. 1998;21(5): 455-71.

9.20 Acute Pancreatitis

D Nirmala, Vandhanaa Natarajan

INTRODUCTION

Acute pancreatitis is a disorder of varied etiology with obscure pathogenesis presenting both as mild disease and multiorgan failure and is difficult to treat as there is no specific treatment and has an unpredictable outcome. It is relatively uncommon during childhood and there is a significant morbidity and mortality associated with it.

Acute pancreatitis is an acute inflammatory process of the pancreas resulting in edema, hemorrhagic or fatty necrosis of pancreatic acinar cells and peripancreatic tissues and even remote organ involvement, which are often reversible. Mild acute pancreatitis is the term reserved for pancreatitis with minimal or no organ dysfunction, whereas severe pancreatitis should be considered if there is evidence of life-threatening complications such as organ failure (shock, pulmonary insufficiency and renal failure) or local complications like necrosis, abscess or pseudocyst.

EPIDEMIOLOGY

The frequency and true incidence of pancreatitis in children are unknown due to limited case reporting and underdiagnosis, but recent studies have demonstrated that the incidence of acute pancreatitis has increased even in pediatrics. A review of pancreatitis in childhood over a 15 years period concluded that pancreatitis was not rare in childhood and had a significant overall mortality rate of 30% or greater as compared to 12% in adults. Pseudocysts complicate acute pancreatitis in approximately 10–23% of cases. The incidence of pancreatic pseudocysts is greater than 50% when associated with traumatic injury to the abdomen.

ETIOPATHOGENESIS

The causes of pancreatitis are as diverse or even more in children compared to adults as shown in the **Table 9.20.1**.

Drugs and blunt trauma were the leading causes for acute pancreatitis in children followed by gallstone disease, tuberculosis, mumps, viral hepatitis and hypertriglyceridemia, according to one Indian study and the cause was not known in 35% of cases according to this study.

Acute pancreatitis usually follows a complex cascade of events. The pancreas is protected from the harmful effects of its lytic enzymes by a series of highly compartmented systems. At each step of their formation and secretion the enzymes are totally sequestrated in a membrane-bound space.

The various potent inhibitors of proteolytic enzymes present in many body fluids, and tissues constitute a second line of protection, defending the organism against inappropriate activation of the digestive proenzymes of the pancreas. These inhibitors bind strongly to the proteases and render them inactive.

Till now, the exact mechanisms of the development of acute pancreatitis are a matter of debate. The most common and widely accepted theory is that pancreatitis develops because of an injury to the pancreatic acini or disruption of

Table 9.20.1: Etiology of acute pancreatitis.

Physical injury: • Abdominal trauma (blunt or penetrating) • Abdominal surgery • Endoscopic retrograde cholangiopancreatography • Posterior penetrating duodenal ulcer	*Metabolic disorders*: • Hyperlipidemia (primary type I and IV) • Diabetes mellitus • Hypercalcemia • Hyperparathyroidism • Uremia	*Pancreatic-flow obstruction disorders*: • Cystic fibrosis • Pancreas divisum • Pancreatic/ductal anomalies • Annular pancreas
Multisystem diseases: • Crohn's disease • Hemolytic uremic syndrome • Reye syndrome • Sepsis • Sarcoidosis • Shock (hypoperfusion)	*Toxins*: • Alcohol • Boric acid • Carbamate • Organophosphorus • Yellow scorpion sting *Nutritional problems*: • Hyperalimentation • Malnutrition • Rapid refeeding after starvation	*Biliary tract obstruction*: • Biliary tract anomalies • Choledochal cyst • Gallstones • Parasites (Ascaris) *Vasculitis*: • Henoch-Schönlein purpura • Kawasaki disease • Systemic lupus erythematosus
Drugs: • L-asparaginase • Azathioprine • Corticosteroids • Didanosine • Estrogens • Ethacrynic acid • Furosemide • Procainamide • Sulphasalazine • Sulphonamides • Tetracyclines • Thiazides • Valproate • Zalcitabine	*Infections*: • *Campylobacter* • *Cryptosporidium* • *Leptospira* • *Mycoplasma* • *Salmonella typhi* • *Toxoplasma* • Viruses such as mumps, coxsackie, cytomegalovirus, herpes simplex virus, hepatitis B and varicella-zoster virus	*Miscellaneous*: • Graft-versus-host disease • Hereditary • Idiopathic • Renal transplantation

the pancreatic duct, which permits the leakage of pancreatic enzymes (trypsin, chymotrypsin and elastase) into pancreatic tissue. The leaked enzymes become activated in the tissue, initiating autodigestion and acute pancreatitis. The activated proteases (trypsin and elastase) and lipase breakdown tissue and cell membranes, causing edema, vascular damage, hemorrhage, ischemia inflammation and necrosis with release of toxic factors in both pancreatic and peripancreatic tissues leading to systemic effects such as multiorgan failure. **Figure 9.20.1** illustrates the pathophysiology of acute pancreatitis.

CLINICAL FEATURES AND COMPLICATIONS

Abdominal pain with nausea and vomiting is the hallmark of pancreatitis in children as well as in adults. Abdominal pain is characteristically a sharp and steady epigastric pain of sudden onset, commonly aggravated by eating and improved by drawing the knees up to the chest. Radiation of pain to the back or pain in other sites of abdomen is rare in children unlike adults. The pain increases in intensity over 24–48 hours and the patient may require hospitalization. Infants and toddlers cannot verbalize abdominal pain, but vomiting, irritability and lethargy are common. In severe acute pancreatitis, children may initially present with shock, followed by symptoms of multiorgan failure, including dyspnea, oliguria, hemorrhage, and mental status changes.

On physical examination, the child usually appears anxious and uncomfortable, particularly with any movement. Tachycardia and fever are common; diffuse abdominal tenderness, more marked in the upper abdomen, and quiet bowel sounds are the rule. However, the diagnosis is not always obvious, and the symptoms can easily be attributed to other acute abdominal emergencies.

Other possible findings include signs of pancreatic ascites, an epigastric mass suggestive of phlegmon or a pseudocyst formation, and bluish flanks (Grey Turner's sign) or umbilicus (Cullen's sign), indicating hemorrhagic pancreatitis. Evidence of pleural effusion, more commonly on the left side or dyspnea in the presence of acute respiratory distress syndrome (ARDS) may be found on examination of the chest.

Severe acute pancreatitis is rare in children. In this life-threatening condition, the patient may be acutely ill with

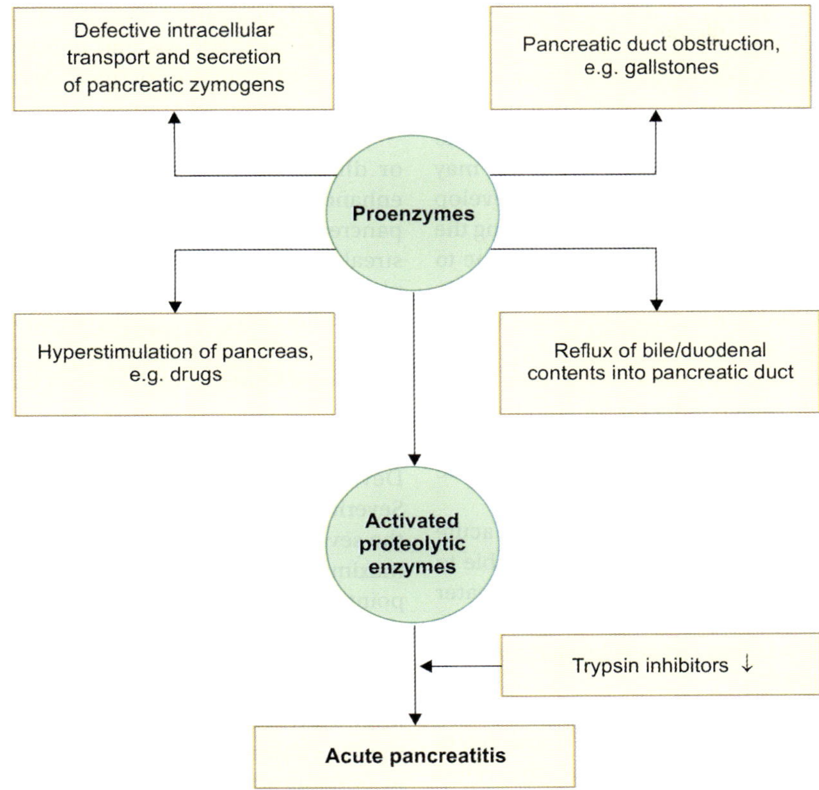

Fig. 9.20.1: Pathogenesis of acute pancreatitis.

severe abdominal pain and vomiting progressing to shock, high fever, jaundice, ascites and pleural effusion. The mortality is highly related to systemic inflammatory response syndrome with multiple organ dysfunctions like shock, renal failure, ARDS, disseminated intravascular coagulation (DIC) and systemic infection.

There are several scoring indices that have been used as predictors of survival. Two such scoring systems are the Ranson's criteria and Acute Physiology and Chronic Health Evaluation II (APACHE II) indices. Most but not all studies report that the APACHE score may be more accurate. These scoring systems are meant for adults and not well validated in children.

DeBanto Scoring

It is a prognostic scoring system to assess the severity of acute pancreatitis in children. The factors identified in this study were age less than 7 years, weight less than 23 kg, admission white blood cell (WBC) more than 18,500, an admission lactate dehydrogenase (LDH) more than 2,000, ionized calcium of less than 8.3 mg/dL at 48 hours, trough albumin less than 2.6 g/dL at 48 hours, 48 hours fluid sequestration more than 75 mL/kg/48 hours and a 48 hours rise in blood urea nitrogen (BUN) more than 5 mg/dL. When the cutoff for predicting a severe outcome was set at three or more the author's prediction rule was found to be more sensitive for predicting severe acute pancreatitis than Ranson scores (70% vs 30%).

COMPLICATIONS OF ACUTE PANCREATITIS

- *Local complications* include pancreatic pseudocyst, necrosis and phlegmon or abscess formation, splenic artery pseudoaneurysms, hemorrhage from erosions into splenic artery and vein, thrombosis of the splenic vein, superior mesenteric vein and portal veins (in descending order of frequency), duodenal obstruction, common bile duct obstruction and progression to chronic pancreatitis.
- *Systemic complications* include ARDS, DIC, hypocalcemia (from fat saponification), hyperglycemia, multiple organ dysfunction syndrome, and insulin-dependent diabetes mellitus (from pancreatic insulin-producing beta cell damage).

DIAGNOSIS

High index of suspicion with a history of abdominal (even if trivial) trauma, drugs or acute infections is stressed. Screening

prevent hypoxemia, ARDS, and cardiac complications like heart failure, myocardial infarction, cardiac arrhythmia, and shock.

Surgical Treatment

Surgical management of acute pancreatitis is rarely required. Surgical intervention is only needed if the symptoms are severe and prolonged or complicated by necrosis or abscess formation that requires debridement. Peritoneal lavage has been used in adults in an effort to reduce the incidence of secondary infection; however, its efficacy has not been confirmed through clinical trials in children. If underlying pancreatic obiliary disease is present, surgical intervention is required for cure. Surgery for pancreatic ductal disruption or compromise (i.e. acute traumatic pancreatitis with ductal injury) is indicated after medical failure.

Acute pancreatic pseudocysts, which are smaller than 5 cm in diameter, are managed with observation for 4–6 weeks. Most of them resolve spontaneously. Pancreatic pseudocysts larger than 5 cm in diameter may require surgical intervention.

Endoscopic sphincterotomy with stone extraction is the treatment of choice for pancreatitis secondary to obstruction of gallstone at the ampulla though it is found to be rare in children.

Cases of uncomplicated acute pancreatitis usually resolve within 2–4 days but severe acute pancreatitis may require parenteral nutrition for long. Diagnosis of the specific cause of pancreatitis is important to elucidate as there is a 9% recurrence rate, most of which are diagnosed with idiopathic recurrent pancreatitis or structural anomalies.

KEY MESSAGES

- Acute pancreatitis though rare in children, there is an increased incidence due to increased awareness among physicians.
- Causes are plenty but blunt trauma, systemic causes and drugs are common etiologies.
- Pathogenesis still remains obscure in spite of many theories.
- Diagnosis is possible in the presence of clinical suspicion with elevated amylase and lipase, which is then confirmed by imaging.
- Management is essentially medical consisting of supportive care and prevention of complications and surgery is rarely needed.
- Mild acute pancreatitis carries good prognosis though severe pancreatitis carries high mortality.

BIBLIOGRAPHY

1. Balthazar EJ. Acute pancreatitis: assessment of severity with clinical and CT evaluation. Radiology. 2002;223:603-13.
2. Coffey MJ, Nightingale S, Ooi CY. Serum lipase as an early predictor of severity in pediatric acute pancreatitis. J Pediatr Gastroenterol Nutr. 2013;56:602-8.
3. Das S, Arora NK, Gupta DK, et al. Pancreatic diseases in children in a North Indian referral hospital. Indian Pediatr. 2004;41:704-11.
4. DeBanto JR, Goday PS, Pedroso MR, et al. Acute pancreatitis in children. Am J Gastroenterol. 2002;97:1726-31.
5. Koizumi M, Takada T, Kawarada Y, et al. JPN Guidelines for the management of acute pancreatitis: Diagnostic criteria for acute pancreatitis. J Hepatobiliary Pancreat Surg. 2006;13:25-32.
6. Lautz TB, Chin AC, Radhakrishnan J. Acute pancreatitis in children: Spectrum of disease and predictors of severity. J Pediatr Surg. 2011;46:1144-49.
7. Manes G, Uomo I, Menchise A, et al. Timing of antibiotic prophylaxis in acute pancreatitis: A controlled randomized study with meropenem. Am J Gastroenterol. 2006;101:1348-53.
8. Peiró AM, Martínez J, Martínez E, et al. Efficacy and tolerance of metamizole versus morphine for acute pancreatitis pain. Pancreatology. 2008;8:25-9.

9.21 Chronic Pancreatitis

Seema Alam, Bikrant Bihari Lal, Prabir Maji

DEFINITION

Pediatric chronic pancreatitis (CP) has been defined as irreversible, structural changes in the pancreas such as diffuse or focal destruction, sclerosis, and pancreatic duct abnormalities/obstruction with:

- Some periods of consistent abdominal pain or lipase/amylase $\geq 3 \times$ ULN (upper limit of normal)
- Exocrine pancreatic insufficiency (EPI), and/or
- Endocrine pancreatic insufficiency.

Chronic pancreatitis is a progressive inflammatory disorder in which pancreatic secretory parenchyma is destroyed and replaced by fibrous tissue, eventually leading to malnutrition and diabetes. Earlier two forms were recognized—a large-duct calcifying type and a small-duct variant. Traditionally, CP has been classified as fundamentally different from acute pancreatitis—the latter is usually characterized by restoration of normal pancreatic histology after full clinical recovery. However, acute, recurrent, acute and CP are now regarded as a disease continuum and there is an overlap in causative factors, both genetic and environmental.

EPIDEMIOLOGY

As per the US national database, the incidence of CP has decreased over time in children (2.2/100,000 persons in 2007 to 1.9/100,000 persons in 2014). There is a linear increase in incidence with increasing age. The prevalence of pediatric CP (5.8/100,000 persons) was much less than in adults (91.9/100,000 persons). Although from the adult data it is apparent that the disease is uncommon in Europe, USA and Japan, the prevalence seems to be considerably high in south India (114–200 per 100,000) and most of these were chronic calcific pancreatitis (CCP). While Poddar et al. reported 156 cases of CP over a 12-year period among children from a north Indian center, Chowdhury et al. described 99 pediatric cases of CP over 5 years from a tertiary care center in south India.

ETIOPATHOGENESIS

It has been seen in experimental studies that an attack of pancreatitis begins as pancreastasis—prevention of apical exocytosis in the pancreatic acinar cell. The acinar cell quickly releases newly synthesized enzyme via the basolateral membrane into lymphatics, by way of the interstitium, and directly into the bloodstream. Some zymogen granules also release their stored enzyme basolaterally. These events result in inflammation. Reactive oxygen species (ROS) are the trigger of so-called pancreastasis and the potentiator of inflammation by activating signaling cascades that convert the damaged acinar cell into a factory for chemokines and cytokines. With time the secretory parenchyma is destroyed and replaced by fibrous tissue leading to malnutrition and diabetes. **Figure 9.21.1** depicts the natural history of CP and the interplay of the various etiological factors.

Unlike adults, most children have a single, self-limited episode of pancreatitis. It is clear that the etiologies of pancreatitis are quite varied in childhood. The most common causes of CP in children are genetic variations, obstruction, autoimmune, toxic, and metabolic diseases. Till a few years back, the etiology of CP used to remain elusive in majority of cases; however, with advent of next generation sequencing, as many as 60–82% of cases of CP have now been identified to harbor at least one disease associated mutation. **Table 9.21.1** lists the common etiologies/risk factors for development of pediatric CP from the largest series worldwide. Some children may have two or more risk factors at the same time. Most of our children with calcific pancreatitis had heterozygous mutation in *SPINK-1* gene. Nevertheless, *SPINK* mutation has been shown to predispose to pancreatic calculi formation.

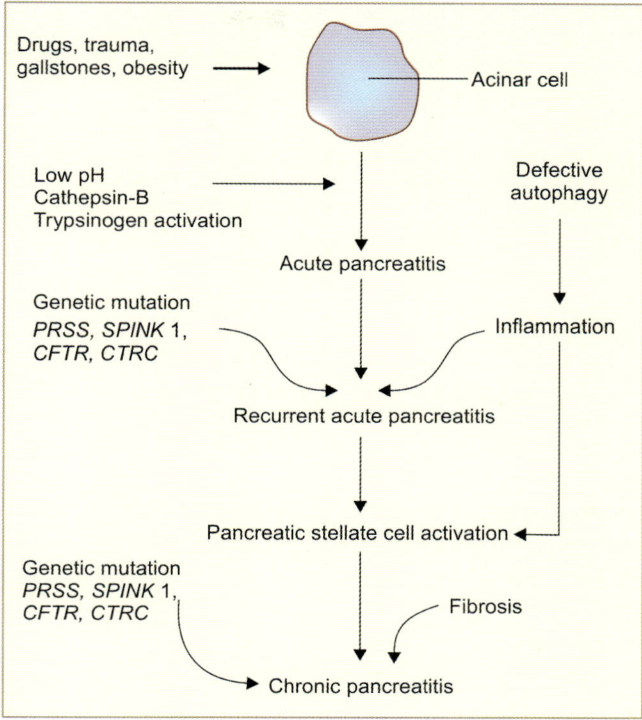

Fig. 9.21.1: Pathogenesis of chronic pancreatitis (CP). (PRSS: protease serine; SPINK1: serine protease inhibitor, Kazal type 1; CFTR: cystic fibrosis transmembrane conductance regulator gene; CTRC: chymotrypsin C)

Role of Genetics

A recent study analyzed 10 disease associated genes by next generation sequencing and found that 81.8% had at least 1 mutation and 19% had multiple disease causing mutations in cationic trypsinogen protease serine 1 (PRSS1), serine protease inhibitor, Kazal type 1 (SPINK1), cystic fibrosis transmembrane conductance regulator gene (CFTR), chymotrypsin C (CTRC), calcium-sensing receptor (CASR), cathepsin B (CTSB), and keratin 8 (KRT8). The INSPPIRE (International Study Group of Pediatric Pancreatitis: In Search for a Cure) data states that 75% of children with onset before 6 years of age had a genetic mutation in clinically relevant genes. It is important for practitioners to keep in mind that presence of genetic modifiers in isolation may not always be sufficient to cause disease. Isolated SPINK-1 mutations are frequent in general population (1–3%), hence, SPINK mutations should

Table 9.21.1: Common risk factors for chronic pancreatitis in children.

	ILBS, New Delhi, 2018	*INSPPIRE database 2016*	*CMC Vellore 2013*	*SGPGI Lucknow 2017*	*China, 2017*	*Poland, 2017*
Sample size (n)	59	146	99	156	55	276
Genetic PRSS1 SPINK1 CFTR CTRC CASR CTSB KRT8	22/53* (41.5%) 1 21 0	86/118* (73%) 24/104 (23%) 50/108 (46%) 25/99 (25%) 4/73 (5%)	NS	22/40* (55%) 0 19 4 0	45/55 (82%) 17 18 22 1 5 5 1	112 (40.6%) 34 66 20
Obstructive Pancreas divisum Gallstones Pancreatobiliary malunion	15 (25.4%) 9 3 3	47/144 (33%) 22/140 (16%) 6/139 (4%) 6/139 (4%)	8 (8.4%)	10(6.4%)	NS	74 (26.8%)
Autoimmune	1 (1.7%)	14/108 (13%)	NS	NS	NS	0
Toxic/Metabolic	4 (6.8%)	22/137 (16%)	NS	NS	NS	29 (10.5%)
Chronic calcific pancreatitis	11 (18.6%)	NS	68 (68.7%)	68(43.6%)	NS	NS
Posttraumatic	1 (1.7%)	NS	4 (4.0%)	3(1.9%)		0
Idiopathic	13 (22%)	14%	95 (95.9%)	134 (86%)	NS	107 (38.7%)

*Percentages denote the proportion of patients positive for particular risk factor among the patients tested.
(CASR: calcium-sensing receptor; CFTR: cystic fibrosis transmembrane conductance regulator; CTRC: chymotrypsin C; CTSB: cathepsin B; ILBS: Institute of Liver and Biliary Sciences; KRT8: Keratin 8; NS: not specified; PRSS1: cationic trypsinogen protease serine 1, SPINK1: serine protease inhibitor, Kazal type 1; INSPPIRE: International Study Group of Pediatric Pancreatitis: In Search for a Cure)

be considered significant if associated with other mutations, ductal obstruction or structural anomalies. Of the 21 patients with mutations in *SPINK1* gene at our center, 5 patients were homozygous and the rest were heterozygous for disease causing mutations. In a recent Indian study, 86% of cases of CP were initially labeled as idiopathic, but when evaluated by genetic analysis, 55% of them were found to be harboring disease associated mutations.

Structural Causes

It is controversial whether structural defects like pancreas divisum (PD) induce pancreatitis. Detection of PD was significantly higher in CP patients than for subjects in the community group (2.6%), but was not higher for acute pancreatitis (13%; $p = 0.357$). The mere presence of PD should not preclude genetic testing for other risk factors in children.

Tropical Calcific Pancreatitis

This is another entity, which is common in the second decade of life. Tropical calcific pancreatitis (TCP) is a juvenile form of chronic calcific, nonalcoholic pancreatitis, prevalent almost exclusively in the developing countries of the tropical world. Some of its distinctive features are younger onset, presence of large intraductal calculi, exocrine insufficiency, high prevalence of diabetes, accelerated course of the disease, and high susceptibility to pancreatic cancer.

Progression from Recurrent Acute Pancreatitis to Chronic Pancreatitis

Approximately, 40% children with recurrent acute pancreatitis (RAP) progress to CP at a median time of 25 months from first episode. Factors, which strongly predispose to progression, are idiopathic causes, presence of SPINK1 mutation and prolonged duration of illness.

CLINICAL FEATURES

Chronic pancreatitis can present with a combination of one or more of the following features:

- Recurrent or chronic abdominal pain
- Symptoms and signs of local complications of the disease (e.g. pseudocyst, obstruction of adjacent organs or vascular thrombosis)
- Symptoms suggestive of exocrine and/or endocrine dysfunction.

Pain is the most disabling feature of CP. In fact, Lord Moynihan described pancreatitis as a condition with illimitable agony. Pain of CP can be chronic or intermittent and at times child may be pain free but may present with other complications. The pain occurs in episodes that last about 1 week or may be constant. It starts in the epigastrium and moves through to the dorsal spine or localizes to the left hypochondrium, radiating to the left infrascapular region. The pain is sometimes associated with nausea and vomiting and can be partially eased by sitting up and leaning forward or by application of local heat or other counter irritants to the dorsal spine or epigastrium. The pain can be so severe that patient fears food and loses weight.

An epigastric swelling suggests a pseudocyst or an inflammatory mass. Multisystemic involvement is a feature of autoimmune pancreatitis. A family history of CP and presence of genetic mutations have been associated with early onset of disease.

In a series among Indian children, 9.1% of CP had diabetes mellitus. Of the 22 children tested for stool fat, 45.5% had steatorrhea. Chronic calcific pancreatitis was the most common presentation (69.7%) and was more commonly associated with diabetes mellitus and steatorrhea. Pseudocyst (17.1%) and ascites (9.1%) were the most common complications. Abdominal pain was reported by 77% within the past year. Children reporting constant pain were more likely to miss school, visit the emergency department, and experience hospitalizations compared with children with episodic pain.

Nutrition in Chronic Pancreatitis

As per INSPPIRE data, around one-third children with CP have EPI and a recent Polish study identified malnutrition in 25% children with CP. The pathogenesis of malnutrition in CP is multifactorial with key factors being EPI leading to maldigestion and malabsorption, increased resting energy expenditure (REE), dietary restrictions, surgical procedures, recurrent infections and impact of diabetes. Fat-soluble vitamin deficiencies are common, and their levels should be monitored at least annually and appropriate corrections should be given. Bone mineral density should be measured in children with malnutrition, hypovitaminosis D or history of fractures, especially in hip and vertebrae.

DIAGNOSTIC MODALITIES

Radioimaging

The typical morphological changes on imaging in CP include pancreatic calcification, duct dilatation, side duct ectasia and parenchymal atrophy.

Plain X-rays

An abdominal radiograph will show pancreatic calculi in at least 30% of patients overall and 90% patients with TCP.

Magnetic Resonance Cholangiopancreatography and Endoscopic Retrograde Cholangiopancreatography

Anomalies (congenital or acquired) in the PD system are best seen on magnetic resonance cholangiopancreatography (MRCP) and endoscopic retrograde cholangiopancreatography (ERCP); the former better at detecting small-duct disease than the latter. Both these modalities have technical issues in small children. In 143 children with CP, ERCP findings included a dilated and irregular main PD (64.3%), PD calculi (53%), dominant PD stricture (16%), PD leak (4.9%), pancreas divisum (24.5%) and common bile duct (CBD) stricture (2%). Secretin-stimulated MRI/MRCP is an upcoming imaging modality to evaluate pancreatic ductal abnormalities as well as exocrine pancreatic function. Endoscopic ultrasound is a good modality to pick up early changes of CP.

Multidetector CT

It can provide excellent images of the calcifications and pseudocyst **(Figs. 9.21.2A and B)** as well as main PD; but is not the ideal choice for side branches which are best seen on ERCP or secretin-enhanced MRCP which has a sensitivity of 73.3% in diagnosing PD.

Endoscopic Ultrasound

It identifies both parenchymal and ductal alterations but is observer dependent and could be difficult procedure for younger children. Endoscopic ultrasound (EUS) may detect very early changes of CP in children.

Major criteria for CP on EUS are:
- Hyperechoic foci with shadowing, main PD calculi, and
- Lobularity with honeycombing.

Minor criteria for CP are cysts, irregular and dilated ducts (3.5 mm), dilated side branches (1 mm), nonshadowing hyperechoic foci, and lobularity with noncontiguous lobules. Imaging demonstrates ductal abnormalities and pancreatic atrophy more commonly than calcifications in children with CP.

Genetic Studies

The clinician should keep a high index of suspicion for hereditary pancreatitis and its preferable to look for common disease causing genetic mutations (refer to etiopathogenesis).

Tests of Exocrine Pancreatic Function

Sudan Black Staining for Fat Globules in Stool

Microscopic demonstration of fecal increased amount of fat droplets in the fecal samples and their interpretation can be enhanced by Sudan Black staining (>2.5 droplets/high-power

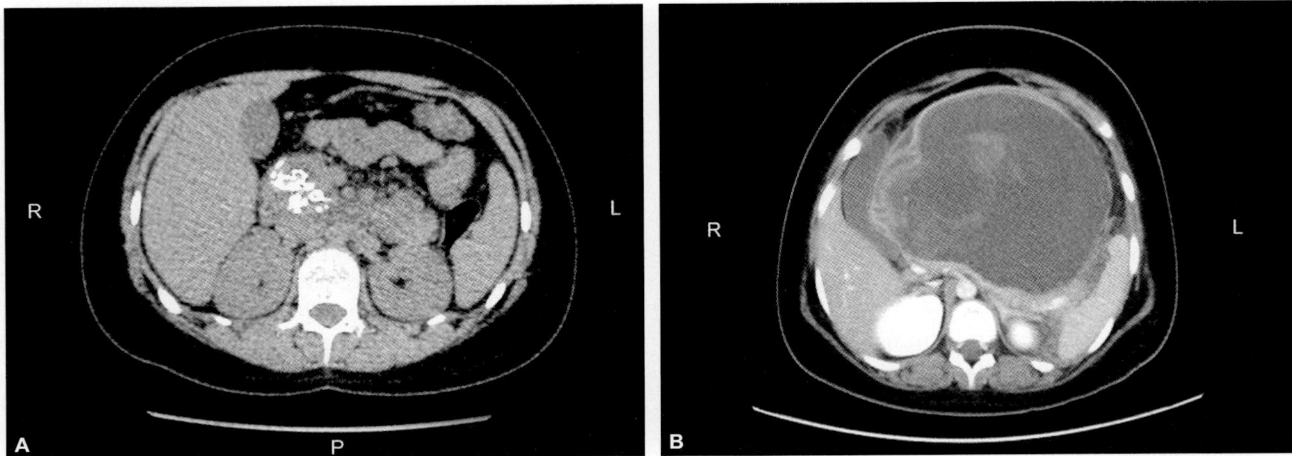

Figs. 9.21.2A and B: (A) Pancreatic calcifications in the head region of a 12-year-old boy with chronic pancreatitis (CP); (B) Pancreatic pseudocystin a 12-year-old girl with chronic pancreatitis (CP).

field). This is not specific for pancreatic insufficiency as high fat intake or malabsorption or even increased gut transit time may give positive results.

Fat Quantification in Stool

Fat quantification in stool by modified van de Kamer method of fat extraction is considered the gold standard for steatorrhea. Fecal fat measures the coefficient of fat absorption (CFA) using the formula:

CFA = Fat measured in stool (g) × 100 ÷ Fat intake (g)

In infants less than 6 months of age, reference values are more than 85%, and above that age, reference values are more than 93–95%. Diet for preceding 3 days should contain 100 g of fat per day for adolescents as well as adults and 2 g/kg in infants and younger children. The standardized stool collection time is 72 hours. If already on pancreatic enzyme replacement therapy (PERT), it should be withheld for 7 days before testing.

Fecal Elastase-1

The sensitivity of the fecal elastase-1 (FE-1) for proven cases of cystic fibrosis in children is between 86% and 100%. FE-1 as an indirect pancreatic function test offers following advantages:

- FE-1 is resistant to degradation by endoluminal bacteria and is biochemically stable over a wide range of pH and temperatures;
- FE-1 test uses monoclonal antibodies against human pancreatic elastase, which do not cross-react with elastase in pancreatic enzyme replacement therapy (PERT). Therefore, it is not necessary for patients to discontinue PERT when performing the FE-1 test.
- A spot sample is adequate.

The normal level is more than 200 mg/g of dry stool; less than 200 mg/g indicates EPI, and less than 100 mg/g correlates well with steatorrhea.

Fecal Chymotrypsin

Fecal chymotrypsin can be determined by a photometric assay, but it requires discontinuation of PERT. It can be used to assess compliance to PERT.

Steatocrit

The steatocrit is a ratio of stool fat to total stool from a spot sample. Half a gram of stool sample is collected, homogenized and centrifuged for 15 minutes. The height of the fat layer is measured in a column as a percentage of the height of the total solid layer. The advantage is that the method is simple, cheap and rapid.

^{13}C-mixed Triglyceride Breath Test

The most widely used test for EPI is the ^{13}C-mixed triglyceride breath test. The ^{13}C is a natural nonradioactive form of the carbon. The test measures ^{13}C-labeled CO_2, which is one of the breakdown products of digested triglycerides. Patient is given a combination of ^{13}C-labeled mixed triglycerides and butter on toast after an overnight fast. The ^{13}C is measured by mass spectrometry or near-infrared analysis. The amount of ^{13}C-labeled CO_2 is related to the activity of lipases present, and thus, the test indirectly measures pancreatic function.

Tests of Endocrine Pancreatic Function

These include glucose tolerance test and hemoglobin A1c (HbA1c).

Other Tests

Lipid profile and serum calcium for type-1 hyperlipidemia and hypercalcemia respectively should be looked for in patients with suspected CP.

An abnormal liver function profile suggests sclerosing cholangitis, gallstones or constriction of the intrapancreatic bile duct in autoimmune pancreatitis.

Tests for Possible Autoimmune Etiology

Autoimmune pancreatitis (AIP) is characterized by five cardinal features—lymphoplasmacytic inflammation, fibrosis and IgG4 immunostaining on histology; imaging findings (hypointense global or focal gland enlargement, MPD irregularity); positive serology; presence of other autoimmune diseases and prompt response to corticosteroids. The disease is usually seen in older children and presents with abdominal pain and/or obstructive jaundice. Elevated serum IgG4 levels are only seen in around 20% children. If autoimmune disease is suspected, serology may show raised (two times of the normal) concentrations of IgG4 (135 mg/dL), antilactoferrin, anticarbonic anhydrase, rheumatoid factor, and antinuclear antibody. Imaging tests show distinctive changes in autoimmune pancreatitis; although confirmatory diagnosis is through periampullary or pancreatic biopsy. An international consensus statement suggested two distinct variants:

1. *Type 1 AIP,* seen in approximately 85% of adult patients and characterized by elevated serum IgG4 concentrations and association with IgG4-related disease at extrapancreatic sites (e.g. sialadenitis and retroperitoneal fibrosis). Histologically, type 1 AIP shows massive infiltration by IgG4þ (IgG4-positive) plasma cells.
2. *Type 2 AIP,* in which the serological markers are usually absent with no systemic manifestations except for possible association with inflammatory bowel disease. It is characterized by neutrophilic infiltration with granulocytic epithelial lesions (GELs) and few, if any, IgG4þ plasma cells.

Predominant type of AIP in children appears to be type 2, given that more than a half of reported pediatric cases had GELs, whereas "definitive type 1 AIP" has never been described in children.

MANAGEMENT OF CHRONIC PANCREATITIS AND ASSOCIATED COMPLICATIONS

The goals of therapy for CP include providing adequate and sustained pain relief, preserve exocrine and endocrine functions, achieve normal growth and improve the quality of life. Multidisciplinary team consisting of pediatric gastroenterologist, endoscopist, intervention radiologist, surgeon, nutritionist and pain physicians are required to provide holistic treatment. **Flowchart 9.21.1** shows the widely accepted step-up approach in management of patients with CP. A step-up approach involves initial medical management followed by endotherapy in those refractory to medical therapy; and patients are offered surgery when endotherapy fails. Although, few studies are now favoring early surgery against endotherapy; and this is being further evaluated in the ESCAPE trial. The issues with step-up approach are:

- There is no clear-cut definition of treatment failure
- Medical management does not alter disease progression and may delay intervention
- Opioid scan leads to dependence, tolerance, hyperalgesia, and a negative impacton social functioning.

Despite these limitations, step-up approach remains the current preferred approach in most recommendations on management of CP, mostly because the approach is "least expensive, least invasive and more readily available" at all centers.

Alleviation of Pain

Modalities for pain relief are medical, endoscopic, interventional or surgical. Analgesics and pancreatic enzyme supplements are mainstay in relieving pain of pancreatitis.

Analgesics

Most CP patients need some form of analgesia in the form of nonopioid narcotics (acetaminophen or aspirin) but more often than not these agents fail. In the opioid group, agents with least potency should be used, e.g. propoxyphene, tramadol or meperidine. Tramadol is a dual action analgesic with μ-opioid and monoaminergic properties; higher doses produce analgesia similar to morphine. The dose is gradually increased to an acceptable pain level rather than complete pain relief.

Pancreatic Enzyme Replacement Therapy

The indication for pancreatic enzyme replacement therapy (PERT) in children with CP is presence of EPI, poor growth or chronic/recurrent abdominal pain. The basis for their use is ability to activate the feedback control to reduce pancreatic secretion. Randomized controlled trials (RCTs) in adults showed effectiveness in relieving pain with non-enteric-coated enzyme preparations, but no benefit with enteric-coated microsphere preparations. The basis for this difference is that feedback sensitive part of small bowel is the most proximal portion, and enteric-coated preparations may not release most of their proteases until they reach the more distal small bowel. As the nonenteric-coated preparations are destroyed by gastric acid, concomitant acid suppression with H2 receptor blockers (H2RA) (e.g. ranitidine 3–5 mg/kg/dose 2–3 times a day) or proton pump inhibitors (PPI,

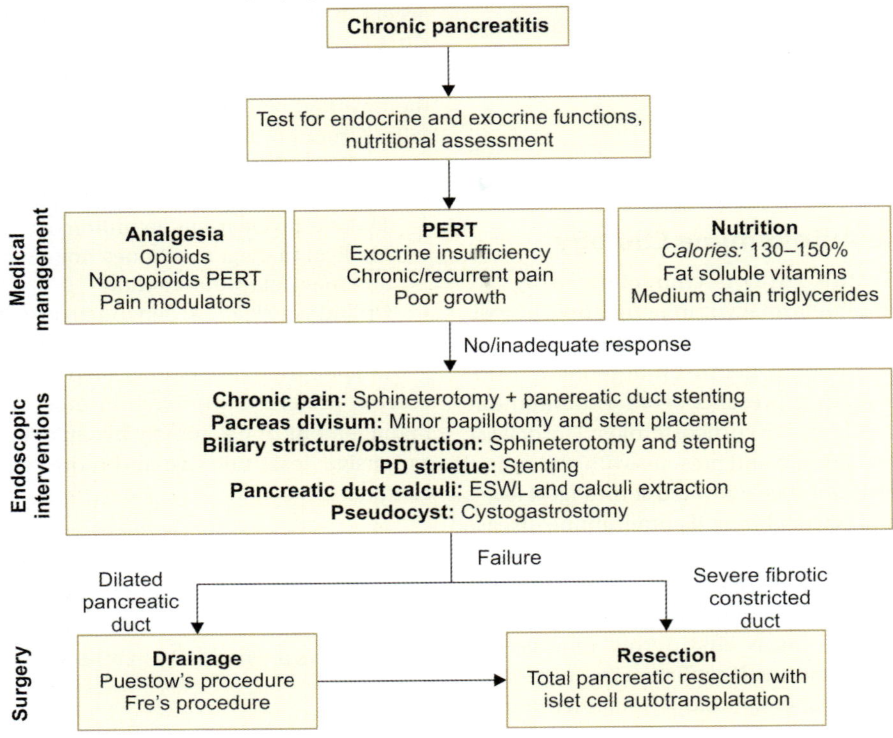

Flowchart 9.21.1: Step-up approach to management of pediatric chronic pancreatitis.

e.g. omeprazole 0.7–0.33 mg/kg/day in 1–2 divided doses) are recommended. Nonenteric-coated preparations are not available in India.

Pain relief is seen in around 56% of children with appropriate PERT. The dosing of PERT in children with CP is based on studies on cystic fibrosis. Children less than 4 years of age usually require 1,000 to 2,500 lipase units/kg/meal; and older children require 500–2,500 lipase units/kg/meal. Half the dose should be given with snacks. However, PERT is costly and as per a recent study, PERT contributed 54% of the annual INR 88,982 financial burden to an adult Indian patient.

Other medical therapies: These include antioxidants (selenium, β-carotene, vitamins C and E, and methionine) and octreotide. Octreotide acts by decreasing pancreatic secretion and reducing circulating cholecystokinin (CCK) levels. Steroids are indicated only in autoimmune pancreatitis in a dose of 30–40 mg/day (2 mg/kg/day) with gradual taper over 3 months period and a maintenance dose of 5–7.5 mg/day (0.1–0.2 mg/kg/day).

Endoscopic Therapy

The goal of ERCP is to improve pancreatic ductal drainage by relieving obstruction. Endotherapy is indicated in presence of ductal calculi, ductal obstruction, and presence of PD stricture or for pseudocyst. Endotherapy may include sphincterotomy, removal of calculi, stent insertion and stricture dilatation. ERCP and EUS have high technical success and low complications when performed in high volume pediatric centers. Usually a combination of modalities is needed in most of the patients. Patients with pancreas divisum presenting with CP and upstream ductal dilatation usually benefit from minor sphincter papillotomy and stent placement.

In a large study of 223 children undergoing endotherapy, there was significant decrease in the frequency of pancreatitis episodes (1.73 episodes/year to 0.23 episodes/year). Around 62% of patients undergoing endotherapy achieve resolution of pain. Therapeutic procedures included major (65%) and minor papilla sphincterotomy (22.3%), PD stenting (53.8%), and CBD stenting (2.2%). Extracorporeal shock wave lithotripsy (ESWL) is the procedure of choice for large pancreatic ductal calculi (≥5 mm) with complete clearance rates of 86% in a pediatric series.

Nerve Blocks and Neurolysis

These modalities are used in adults with intractable pain. Combination of glucocorticoids and bupivacaine is used for celiac plexus block, whereas absolute alcohol is used for neurolysis. The procedure can be done under CT or EUS guidance.

Surgery

Surgery is indicated only in children who have failed on medical and endoscopic therapy, especially if chronic pain persists and the child has narcotic or insulin dependence. The options for surgery include pancreatic drainage procedures, resection, or a combination of both. Two common surgical modalities in CP are Puestow's procedure and Frey's procedure. Puestow's surgery involves lateral pancreaticojejunostomy whereas Frey's procedure additionally involves removal of the diseased portions of the pancreatic head, better exposing the main pancreatic duct resulting in improved drainage. Appropriate and timely surgery has been shown to provide long-term relief in 50–80% of patients. While patients with dilated duct may benefit with drainage procedures, total pancreatectomy with islet cell autotransplant (TP-IAT) is indicated for those with severe fibrotic constricted ducts manifesting with intractable pain, opioid dependence and insulin dependence. While pancreatectomy removes the nidus of chronic pain, autologous islet transplantation aims to restore endocrine function. Review of current literature shows that TP-IAT provided sustained pain relief, insulin independence in 75% and improvement in quality of life in 90% of patients.

Nutritional Therapy

Nutrition management of CP has a threefold strategy involving:

- Supplementation using PERT
- Correction of nutrition deficiencies
- Maintenance of adequate dietary intake.

Patients with pancreatic exocrine insufficiency often have macronutrient and micronutrient deficiencies. A recent prospective study of 40 CP patients revealed that deficiency of vitamin K was more common, affecting 63% of the cohort, followed by vitamin D (53%), vitamin E (10%), and vitamin A (3%). Metabolic bone disease is a common consequence of malabsorption of calcium and vitamin D in CP.

Maintenance of Adequate Nutrition and Calorie Requirement

Patients with CP have higher resting energy expenditures (>30–50% of normal). The aim of nutrition management is to provide adequate nutrition, reduce maldigestion, and decrease malabsorption. Majority of patients can be treated adequately with a normal diet and PERT. A high-calorie diet is needed to match the increased resting energy expenditure.

- *Medium-chain triglycerides (MCTs):* They can be added to the diet in CP patients, because MCTs are absorbed through the mucosa of the jejunum and ileum without the need for lipase or bile salts, both of which are deficient in patients with CP. Sources of MCTs include coconut oil and palm kernel oil. MCTs can induce ketogenesis, hence should be taken with caution in diabetic patients.
- *Fiber:* Fiber in the diet can inhibit lipase activity; hence reduced fiber intake is recommended.
- *Frequency:* In patients who can tolerate an oral diet, the consumption of 6–8 small meals daily is recommended.
- *Exocrine pancreatic insufficiency:* If signs of exocrine insufficiency are present, 70–100 g of fat per day, 1–2 g/kg of protein, and PERT are recommended. After the onset of steatorrhea, medium chain triglycerides can be added to the diet. Most patients with CP can be managed by these dietary recommendations. Tube feeding is indicated in approximately 5% and parenteral nutrition in less than 1%.

Management of Pancreatic Exocrine Dysfunction

In malabsorption and steatorrhea with related nutritional deficits, PERT is advised with lipase (1,000–2,500 U/kg/meal; 30,000 U/meal for adults). Enteric coated preparations are preferred, along with H2RA or PPI and should be spread over each meal. Efficacy of treatment is assessed by change in stool consistency, loss of visible fat and improvement in weight. Fat soluble vitamins (A, D, E, and K) should be supplemented in a dose 2–3 times of recommended dietary allowance.

Management of Diabetes and its Complications

Diabetes in calcific pancreatitis usually develops before development of exocrine insufficiency and the severity is proportional to number and size of pancreatic calculi and calcifications. Management of diabetes is similar except that liberal caloric and protein intake is advised because of underlying malnutrition, and these patients are more prone to hypoglycemic episodes. Oral hypoglycemic agents may be used in the initial phase, but most patients ultimately require insulin. Microvascular complications of diabetes should be looked for in follow-up.

Management of Local Complications of Pancreatitis

Pancreatic Pseudocyst

Pseudocyst occurs in nearly 25% of cases of adults with CP, but the prevalence is not known in children. Complications include compression of surrounding viscera or vessels, infection, hemorrhage, pseudoaneurysm or pancreatic fistula formation with resultant pancreatic ascites and pleural effusion. Therapy is indicated for symptomatic, enlarging or complicated pseudocyst and includes CT-guided percutaneous or endoscopic drainage or surgery. Endoscopic drainage procedures may be done either through the papilla (transpapillary), or through the wall of stomach (cystogastrostomy) or small intestine (cystoduodenostomy or cystojejunostomy). Surgical drainage for cyst is usually combined with ductal drainage procedures.

Gastrointestinal Bleeding

Bleeding in the setting of CP may occur because of bleeding within pseudocyst, rupture of pseudoaneurysm, variceal bleed secondary to portal or splenic vein thrombosis or due to NSAID-related ulcer or gastric erosions. Bleeding within pseudocyst or rupture of pseudoaneurysm may be slow and intermittent or acute and massive, which may remain confined to peritoneal or retroperitoneal compartments or may manifest as hemosuccus pancreaticus (bleeding into PD presenting as pain, jaundice and melena). Therapeutic options are either embolization or surgery.

Other Complications

Rare complications like bile duct obstruction, duodenal obstruction or stenosis and pancreatic fistula may develop. Biliary obstruction is usually managed with endoscopic therapy and stent exchange. Surgery in the form of bypass is indicated for most of them as definite therapy. Pancreatic fistulas may be external or internal. External fistulas usually develop following surgery or percutaneous drainage and may take weeks to heal. Internal fistulas usually occur after rupture of pseudocyst and may track to peritoneal cavity (pancreatic ascites) or pleural space (pancreatic pleural effusion). Diagnosis is established through documentation of high amylase levels in respective fluids. Complete bowel rest, hyperalimentation and octreotide are indicated for management of both types of fistulas. Additionally, endoscopic stent placement across the site of ductal disruption effectively closes the fistula rapidly.

Other Measures

Healthy Lifestyles

Children should be educated to abstain from alcohol and smoking, as alcohol increases the pain and severity of CP and smoking doubles the risk of pancreatic malignancy in hereditary pancreatitis.

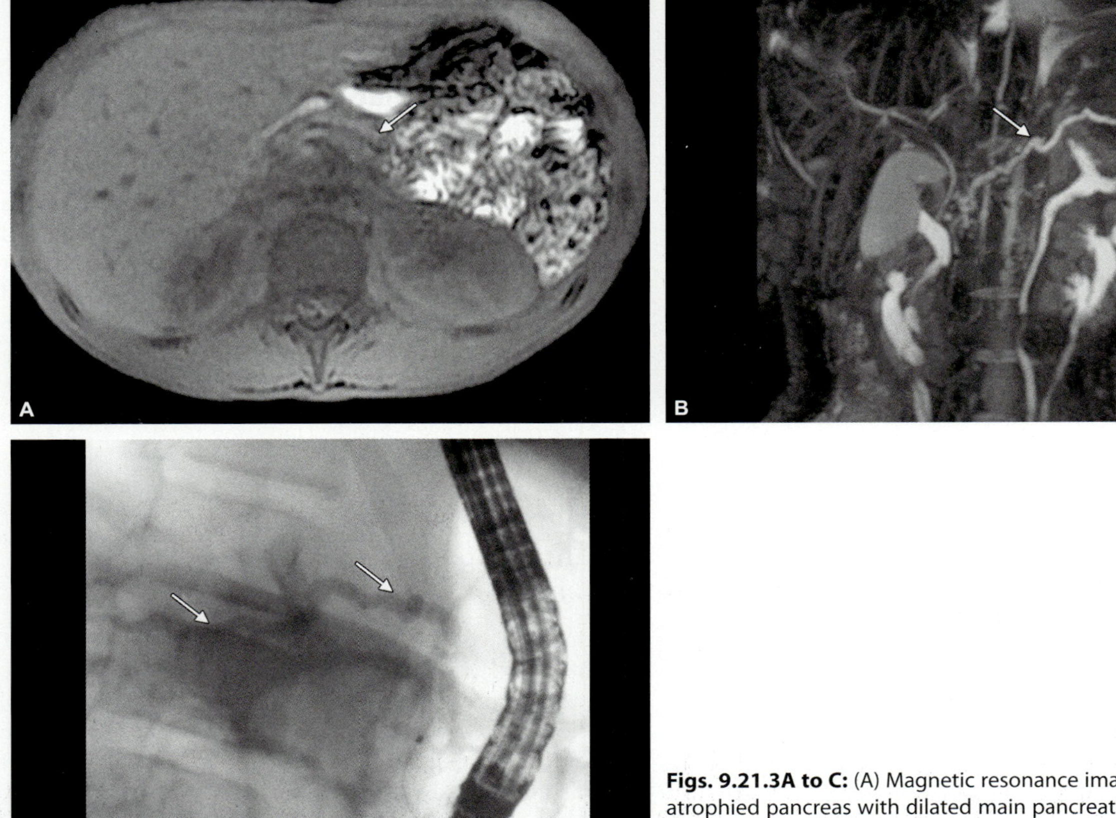

Figs. 9.21.3A to C: (A) Magnetic resonance imaging (MRI) showing atrophied pancreas with dilated main pancreatic duct (PD); (B) and (C) Magnetic resonance cholangiopancreatography (MRCP) and endoscopic retrograde cholangiopancreatography (ERCP) of the same patient showing a dilated main PD.

Screening for Malignancy

There is a 50- and 17-times increased risk of pancreatic cancer in hereditary and TCP respectively. Thus, children should be screened for malignancy in follow-up. The recommended age to start screening begins from 35 years of age or 10 years before onset of malignancy in cases with family history of pancreatic cancer. Diagnostic screening modality is either CT or EUS.

RECENT ADVANCES

- Genetic mutations are important to look for in idiopathic CP (for details see the etiopathogenesis).
- Newer radioimaging modalities [e.g. EUS, secretin-enhanced MRCP and multidetector computed tomography (MDCT)] would give better yield for diagnosis of CP and structural defects like PD.

CASE SCENARIO

A 14-year-old boy was referred with complaints of heaviness in abdomen after taking meals and weight loss of 20 kg in a year with normal stools. There was no history of trauma or jaundice. In a previous hospital admission 2 years back, his serum amylase (1,651 U/L) and serum lipase (1,726 U/L) were found to be raised. USG abdomen showed bulky pancreas with normal gallbladder. Multidetector CT abdomen revealed acute pancreatitis with bilateral pleural effusion with ascites with CT severity index 5. He was diagnosed as a case of mild acute pancreatitis and treated with antibiotics and intravenous fluids. Repeat USG showed reduction in size of pancreas with pleural effusion and ascites. He had two subsequent similar episodes.

On examination he was stable, but cachexic, with no icterus or pallor and a normal systemic examination. The serum amylase and lipase were normal; but the MRCP revealed atrophied pancreas with dilated main PD with no evidence of cholelithiasis or choledocholithiasis. ERCP done subsequently confirmed a dilated PD **(Figs. 9.21.3A to C)**. Serum calcium, lipid profile and glucose tolerance test were normal. The work-up for hereditary causes showed a normal sweat chloride level and SPINK 1 mutation was not found.

A diagnosis of idiopathic CP was made and he was managed with pancreatic enzyme replacement treatment. On follow-up he had gained weight with no further heaviness after meals.

KEY MESSAGES

- Chronic pancreatitis (CP) should be differential diagnosis of patients with recurrent/chronic abdominal pain of the upper abdomen especially where it is associated with weight loss.
- All these cases should undergo appropriate diagnosis and etiologic workup.
- All cases should be assessed for pancreatic exocrine and endocrine dysfunction.
- Nutrition and pancreatic enzyme replacement therapy are the backbone of the treatment.

BIBLIOGRAPHY

1. Abu-El-Haifa M, Cu A, Berlin SL, et al. Nutritional Considerations in Pediatric Pancreatitis: A Position Paper from the NASPHAN Pancreas Committee and ESPHAN Cystic Fibrosis/Pancreas Working Group. J Pediatr Gastroenterol Nutr. 2018;67(1):131-43.
2. Bellin MD, Forlenza GP, Majumder K, et al. Total Pancreatectomy With Islet Autotransplantation Resolves Pain in Young Children With Severe Chronic Pancreatitis. J Pediatr Gastroenterol Nutr. 2017;64(3):440-5.
3. Jawad ZAR, Kyriakides C, Pai M, et al. Surgery remains the best option for the management of pain in patients with chronic pancreatitis: A systematic review and meta-analysis. Asian J Surg. 2017;40(3):179-85.
4. Kumar S, Ooitz CY, Berlin S, et al. Risk Factors Associated With Pediatric Acute Recurrent and Chronic Pancreatitis: Lessons from INSPPIRE. JAMA Pediatr. 2016;170(6):562-9.
5. Lin TK, Abu-El-Haija M, Nathan JD, et al. Pancreas Divisum in Pediatric Acute Recurrent and Chronic Pancreatitis: Report From INSPPIRE. J Clin Gastroenterol. 2018.
6. Oracz G, Pertkiewicz J, Kierkus J, et al. Efficiency of pancreatic duct stenting therapy in children with chronic pancreatitis. Gastrointest Endosc. 2014;80(6):1022-9.
7. Poddar U, Yachha SK, Borkar V, et al. Clinical profile and treatment outcome of chronic pancreatitis in children: a long-term follow-up study of 156 cases. Scand J Gastroenterol. 2017;52(6-7):773-8.
8. Schwarzenberg SJ, Bellin M, Husain SZ, et al. Pediatric chronic pancreatitis is associated with genetic risk factors and substantial disease burden. J Pediatr. 2015;166(4):890-6.
9. Wejnarska K, Kolodziejczyk E, Wertheim-Tysarowska K, et al. The Etiology and Clinical Course of Chronic Pancreatitis in Children With Early Onset of the Disease. J Pediatr Gastroenterol Nutr. 2016;63(6):665-70.
10. Xiao Y, Yuan W, Yu B, et al. Targeted Gene Next-Generation Sequencing in Chinese Children with Chronic Pancreatitis and Acute Recurrent Pancreatitis. J Pediatr. 2017;191:158-63.e3.

9.22 Pediatric Liver Transplantation

Neelam Mohan

INTRODUCTION

Liver transplantation (LT) or hepatic transplantation is the replacement of a diseased liver with a healthy liver allograft. The most commonly used technique is orthotopic transplantation, in which the native liver is removed and the donor organ is placed in the same anatomic location as the original liver. The history of pediatric LT starts with the first human attempt at transplantation by Dr Thomas Starzl in 1963. Since then, new advances and techniques in both surgical and medical management have increased the incidence and improved the outcomes of LTs. While pediatric liver transplants account for small proportion of all LT, there exist sufficient differences between pediatric and adult patients seeking LT. These include but are not limited to distinct diseases, clinical susceptibilities, physiological responses, as well as neurocognitive and neurodevelopmental features. Children need specialized care from pediatric transplantation physicians and pediatric hepatologists who are well aware of the challenges of pediatric care.

INDICATIONS FOR LIVER TRANSPLANTATION IN CHILDREN

In general, LT is indicated when the risk of mortality from the native liver disease outweighs the overall risk of transplantation. The indications for LT in children have traditionally been an end-stage liver disease with a predicted life expectancy under 1 year, acute liver failure (ALF), nonresectable localized hepatic tumors and liver-based metabolic defects. With improved survival of these traditional indications, there had a surge of using LT for more nontraditional indications. These include growth failure, intractable pruritus or bone density loss from cholestatic disorders, intractable seizures from metabolic liver disease, and liver tumors in the absence of significant extrahepatic disease.

Broadly, the indications for LT can be divided into the following and the detailed causes are listed in **Box 9.22.1**.

- Cholestatic diseases
- Metabolic diseases
- Acute liver failure
- Malignancy
- Hepatitis: Infectious, autoimmune
- Other conditions.

Box 9.22.1: Indications for pediatric liver transplantation.

Cholestatic disease
- Biliary atresia
- Progressive familial intrahepatic cholestasis (Byler disease)
- Idiopathic neonatal hepatitis
- Alagille syndrome (bile duct paucity syndrome)
- Sclerosing cholangitis

Metabolic liver disease
- Wilson disease
- Tyrosinemia type I
- Glycogen storage disease types I, III and IV
- Crigler-Najjar syndrome type I
- Alpha1-antitrypsin deficiency
- Cystic fibrosis
- Urea cycle defects
- Primary hyperoxaluria
- Organic acidemia
- Familial hypercholesterolemia

Acute liver failure
- *Neonates*

Infectious: Herpes viruses, echovirus, adenovirus, hepatitis B virus (HBV)

Metabolic: Galactosemia, tyrosinemia, neonatal hemochromatosis, mitochondrial disease, fatty acid oxidation defects
- *Older children*

Infectious: Hepatitis A virus (HAV), HBV, herpes viruses, sepsis, other

Drugs: Acetaminophen, valproate, isoniazid, carbamazepine, halothane, propylthiouracil.

Toxins: Amanita phalloides, carbon tetrachloride, phosphorus.

Metabolic: Wilson's disease, hereditary fructose intolerance

Autoimmune: Types 1 and 2

Other cryptogenic

Hepatic tumors
- Nonresectable hepatoblastoma
- Nonresectable hepatocellular carcinoma
- Nonresectable large benign tumors (hemangioendothelioma)

Hepatitis
- Autoimmune hepatitis
- Chronic viral hepatitis (B and C)
- Cryptogenic cirrhosis
- Nonalcoholic steatohepatitis (NASH)

Others
- Budd–Chiari syndrome
- Polycystic liver disease
- Caroli's disease
- Traumatic/postsurgical biliary tract diseases
- Factor VII deficiency
- Primary immunodeficiency with cirrhosis (combined bone marrow and liver transplantation)

Cholestatic Liver Disease

Biliary atresia (BA) is the leading diagnosis of the pediatric transplant recipients across the globe. This disease is universally fatal if untreated. Diagnosis of BA and performance of a hepatoportoenterostomy within 6–10 weeks of age is optimal for transplant-free survival beyond early childhood. The majority of the patients following hepatoportoenterostomy fall into two groups: (1) those that develop end-stage liver disease or recurrent cholangitis over the course of the first 1–2 years of life, in literature only 16% of children with BA survive to 2 years with their native liver if the total serum bilirubin measured 3 months following hepatoportoenterostomy is over 6 mg/dL, compared to 84% for those with a total bilirubin less than 2 mg/dL and (2) those that have satisfactory biliary drainage but eventually develop cirrhosis and end-stage liver disease in late childhood or adolescence. Complications posthepatoportoenterostomy that require LT include failure of biliary drainage with progressive cholestasis, portal hypertension, refractory ascites or gastrointestinal bleeding, recurrent cholangitis or rarely hepatopulmonary syndrome.

Alagille syndrome is another cholestatic condition that may require LT due to end-stage liver disease and/or intractable pruritus. Progressive familial intrahepatic cholestasis (PFIC) is another inherited cholestatic disorder in which bile salt, phospholipid, or cholesterol transport genes are mutated such that protein function is either abnormal or absent. PFIC accounts for up to 15% of neonatal cholestatic disorders and is, therefore, one of the more common indications for pediatric LT, however, the outcomes in PFIC 1 patients have not been as favorable secondary to an aggravation of baseline high volume diarrhea, posttransplant steatosis, and eventual cirrhosis.

Metabolic Liver Disease

These disorders are typically a result of mutations that affect amino acid, metal, lipid metabolism or mitochondrial function. In general, LT in the setting of an inherited metabolic disorder is offered to those that can be cured or those patients whose medical management can be significantly facilitated with the transplant. In these patients, LT is not only lifesaving, it also accomplishes phenotypic and functional cure of the disease. Hepatic replacement to correct the metabolic defect should be considered before other organ systems are affected, or the consequences of the defect result in irreversible quality-of-life compromises or complications that would prove to be contraindications for transplantation. Thus, these patients should be referred to a transplant center early in course of their disease so that timely intervention can be done before the occurrence of irreversible damage. The indications of performing LT in inborn errors of metabolism have expanded from being life-saving to improving quality-of-life and avoiding long-term sequelae in other diseases.

Pediatric Acute Liver Failure

Pediatric acute liver failure (PALF) is defined as per PALF longitudinal research study criteria including:

1. Absence of a known, chronic liver disease
2. Liver-based coagulopathy that is not responsive to parenteral vitamin K
3. International normalized ratio (INR) between 1.5 and 1.9 with clinical evidence of encephalopathy or 2.0 and higher regardless of the presence of clinical encephalopathy.

It is a heterogeneous condition with many different etiologies and in this scenario, clinical deterioration sometimes makes the establishment of a primary diagnosis impossible before the need for urgent transplantation. The etiology of ALF varies depending on the age of the child, some of the etiologies have been attributed to viral hepatitis, drug toxicity like paracetamol overdose or toxin exposure, though a significant number is cryptogenic. Rarely mitochondrial disorder, fatty acid oxidation defects could be the underlying cause in young children and also neonatal hemochromatosis in newborns. Nevertheless, a significant proportion of children with ALF have spontaneous liver function recovery.

The decision to proceed with transplantation should be made at a point when there is no clinically significant evidence of liver regeneration or recovery of function. Selection of fulminant hepatic failure candidates for transplantation is difficult. The King's College Hospital criteria **(Box 9.22.2)** have been extensively used and are acknowledged to have a high degree of specificity but have been criticized for lack of sensitivity. More recent recommendation from the same group is to use an INR more than 4 or factor V concentration less than 25% as the best available criteria for listing for LT. Although these various criteria are helpful, careful observation for progression and clinical change is most rewarding and emergency referral to a transplant center is of paramount importance.

Box 9.22.2: The King's College criteria transplantation in pediatric acute liver failure.

(A) For acetaminophen poisoning:
- Arterial pH < 7.3
- Or the following three factors
  - Prothrombin time (PT) > 100 sec
  - Creatinine > 3.5 mg%
  - Grade III or IV encephalopathy

(B) For other causes:
- PT > 100 sec
- Or any three of the following
  - PT > 50 sec
  - Bilirubin > 17.5 mg%
  - Age < 10 years
  - Cryptogenic or drug induced
  - Jaundice for more than 7 days before onset of encephalopathy

Liver Tumors

Hepatoblastoma (HB) is the most common liver tumor in children and the incidence has been increasing over time. In patients with nonresectable and chemoresistant tumors, with no extra hepatic metastasis LT is a viable option. Patients with HB and pulmonary metastases can be considered for LT if, following chemotherapy, a chest computed tomography is clear of metastases or, if a tumor is identified, the pulmonary wedge resection reveal the margins are free of the tumor.

Others Conditions

Autoimmune hepatitis is a progressive inflammatory liver disorder characterized by increased aminotransferases, high serum levels of immunoglobulin G, and the presence of autoantibodies like antinuclear antibody, antismooth muscle antibody and antiliver-kidney microsomal antibody. LT is considered in patients with autoimmune hepatitis who present with ALF or those who develop complications of end-stage liver disease.

Budd-Chiari syndrome (BCS) is the result of hepatic venous outflow tract obstruction at any level from any mechanism exclusive of cardiac disease. Well-selected patients of BCS can benefit from LT with good long-term survival.

Inborn errors of metabolism can be divided into two types, those in which liver is the primary organ to be affected such as tyrosinemia, glycogen storage disease or Wilson disease and in those where the primary organ affected is not the liver but the enzyme defect is in liver, necessitating the need of LT, e.g. primary hyperoxaluria a rare autosomal recessive disorder of hepatic enzyme alanine-glyoxylate aminotransferase leading to excessive systemic oxalate, renal failure and ultimately death. These patients require both liver and kidney transplantation for correction of metabolic abnormality and oxalate excretion. In urea cycle defects and organic acidemias neurological involvement is seen but hepatic enzyme deficiency exists. The purpose of liver transplant in this group of diseases is to replace the missing hepatic enzyme to prevent or reverse extrahepatic disease. Other such conditions include Crigler-Najjar syndrome type 1, familial hypercholesterolemia and maple syrup urine disease.

In a large series of 200 pediatric LT reported by the author from India, the leading indications of LT were cholestatic liver disease (46%) followed by metabolic liver disease (33%) and ALF/acute on chronic liver failure (28.5%).

CONTRAINDICATIONS TO LIVER TRANSPLANTATION

Some absolute contraindications include mostly systemic disorders that cannot be cured or can be worsened by transplantation, such as ongoing infections, malignancies, severe metabolic disorders, or in advanced cardiopulmonary diseases such as seen in severe pulmonary disease or heart failure.

Box 9.22.3: Pretransplant assessment.

Nutritional status: Height, weight, triceps skinfold, midarm muscle area, midarm circumference
Identification of hepatic complications: Ascites, varices
Cardiac assessment: Electrocardiography, echocardiography, chest radiography, cardiac catheterization
Respiratory function: Oxygen saturation, ventilation-perfusion scan, lung function tests
Neurologic and developmental assessment: Electroencephalography, Bailey developmental scales, and Stanford–Binet intelligence scales
Renal function: Urea, creatinine, electrolytes, urinary protein-to-creatinine ratio, and chromium ethylene diaminetetraacetic acid (EDTA)
Serology: Cytomegalovirus; Epstein–Barr virus; varicella-zoster virus; herpes simplex virus; hepatitis A, B, and C; human immunodeficiency virus (HIV); measles
Hematology: Full blood count, platelets, and blood group
Radiology: Ultrasonography of liver and spleen for vascular anatomy, wrist radiography for bone age and rickets
Dental assessment

PRETRANSPLANT EVALUATION

The pretransplantation evaluation of the patient is particularly important and should include the following:

- Assessment of the severity of the liver disease and the possibility for medical management
- Assessment of the technical feasibility of the operation
- Consideration of any contraindications
- Psychological preparation of the family and child.

The assessment has been tabulated in **Box 9.22.3**.

PREPARATIONS FOR LIVER TRANSPLANTATION

Immunization

Most units consider live vaccines to be contraindicated after liver transplant because of the risk of dissemination, secondary to immunosuppression. It is therefore better to complete normal immunizations before transplant. Every effort should be made to immunize the patients as early as possible prior to transplant, using an accelerated schedule if needed. Ideally, transplant should not occur until at least 2–3 weeks following live vaccine administration.

Growth Monitoring

Growth failure is common in chronic liver disease. Children with a chronic liver disease are at risk for malnutrition, as they require 20–80% more calories than normal children to achieve adequate growth. It has been demonstrated with several studies that nutritional status at liver transplant is an important prognostic factor in survival. A high-calorie protein feed (150–200% of estimated average requirement) is required with high calorie supplements given orally or by nocturnal nasogastric enteral feeding or continuous enteral feeding. Special attention should be paid to fat-soluble vitamin deficiencies (A, D, E, and K) and should be supplemented accordingly. Even water-soluble vitamins need to be supplemented.

Management of Hepatic Complications

It is important to ensure that specific hepatic complications such as variceal bleeding, ascites, and spontaneous bacterial peritonitis are appropriately managed while the patient waits for transplant.

Psychological Preparation

Liver transplant is a major undertaking for the child and family; thus, psychological counseling, information giving and preparation of the child and family is an essential component of pretransplantation management.

LIVER TRANSPLANT SURGERY

The graft is either a cadaveric liver or a living related.

Cadaveric Liver Transplantation

Here, the liver of a brain-dead person is used for transplantation. Cadaveric transplants could be:

- *Whole graft:* The entire graft is transplanted in the recipient.
- *Reduced graft:* When only a part of the cadaveric liver (i.e. right/left/left lateral part) is used for the recipient **(Fig. 9.22.1)**.
- *Split graft:* The shortage of suitable organs for young children led to development of split livers. The liver of the cadaveric donor is divided and used for two patients usually the right lobe for adults and left lobe for children.

Living-related Liver Transplantation

This has been a further step to answer the shortage of organs for children. In living-related LT, a part of the liver from a living related donor is used in the child. This procedure is more popular in Eastern countries like Japan, Korea, and India where cadaveric LT has not been possible until recently. To carry out living related liver transplants, two-transplant surgeons' team is required as simultaneously surgery is being carried out on the donor and the recipient.

Mostly blood compatible transplants are done. However in living related liver transplant scenarios recently ABO incompatible transplants are also being done with preoperative use of plasmapheresis and modified immunosuppression.

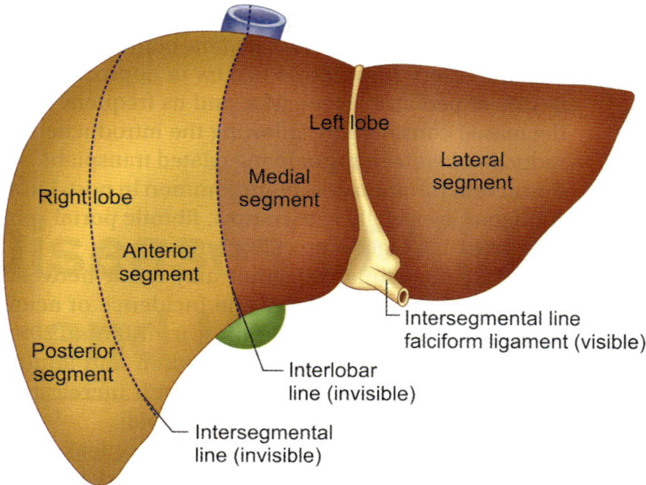

Fig. 9.22.1: Parts of liver

Auxiliary Liver Transplant

The term auxiliary liver transplant is referred when a part of the donor liver (usually segments 2 + 3) is implanted beside or in continuity with the native liver. The main purpose of this form of liver transplant is to ensure that the native liver is retained in the event of graft failure or for the future development of gene therapy. Auxiliary transplant is now accepted therapy for Crigler-Najjar syndrome type I and also for propionic acidemia and ornithine transcarbamylase deficiency while its role in the management of fulminant hepatic failure is more controversial.

Immunosuppression

Following liver transplant, the patient requires lifelong immunosuppression according to the present consensus. The most common immunosuppressive drugs used following LT are tacrolimus, mycophenolate mofetil, and steroids. Few centers use steroid-sparing induction regimen with basiliximab. Newer drugs like OKT3, sirolimus and everolimus are used in occasional patients.

POSTOPERATIVE COMPLICATIONS

Early Postoperative Complications

Primary graft non-function: Primary nonfunctioning of the transplanted liver occurs within 48 hours. The cause is unknown and may be related to cadaveric donor factor; this is not seen in living related transplant scenarios. The only appropriate management is retransplant.

Table 10.1.1: Tubular functions.

Sites	*Function*	
	Reabsorption	*Secretion*
Proximal tubule	Bicarbonate (80%) Calcium (70%) Phosphorus (80%) Magnesium (15%) Potassium (67%) Proteins as amino acids (100%) Sodium and chloride (67%) Urea (67%) Water (67%)	
Henle's loop • Thin descending limb • Thin ascending limb • Thick ascending limb	Water (15%) Sodium chloride (25%) Bicarbonate (10%) Calcium magnesium (60%) Potassium (20%) Ammonium (variable) Calcium (20%) Sodium chloride (25%)	Urea
Distal tubule	Bicarbonate (10%) Calcium (9%) Magnesium (5%) Phosphorus (10%) Sodium chloride (5%)	
Collecting duct	Bicarbonate (4%) Potassium (Nil) Sodium chloride (3%) Urea (variable) Water (variable)	Ammonium (variable) Bicarbonate in metabolic alkalosis Potassium (0–70%) Urea (variable)

Source: Koeppen BM, Stanton BA. Renal Physiology, 4th edition. Philadelphia: Mosby, Elsevier; 2007. pp. 19-30.

called "transporters". Active transporters include Na^+/K^+ ATPase, Ca^{2+} ATPase, H^+/K^+ ATPase and H^+ ATPase. The passive transporters are $Na^+/K^+/Cl^-$ and Na^+ glucose co-transporters and Ca^{2+}/Na^+ and H^+/Na^+ exchanger.

Almost all cells in the nephron have a single nonmotile primary cilium that protrudes into the tubular lumen. These cilia function as mechanosensors, sensing changes in flow rate of the tubule fluid, and chemosensors, sensing or responding to compounds in the surrounding fluids to initiate calcium-dependent signaling pathways including those that control nephron function, proliferation, differentiation and apoptosis.

Nephrons are classified by their location as superficial and juxtamedullary. The glomeruli of superficial nephrons are located in the outer cortex. These nephrons have short loops of Henle, and have efferent arterioles that branch into peritubular capillaries surrounding adjacent nephrons in addition to their own segments. This capillary network provides a pathway for the return of reabsorbed water and solutes to the circulatory system. The glomeruli of juxtamedullary nephron are located at the corticomedullary junction while their loops of Henle are long and extend deep into the medulla. Their efferent arterioles form a network of peritubular capillaries as well as several vascular loops called the vasa recta deep in the medulla. The long loops of Henle and their vasa recta help to concentrate the urine.

BIBLIOGRAPHY

1. Eaton DC, Pooler JP. Vander's Renal Physiology, 7th edition. New York: McGraw Hill; 2009.
2. Koepen BM, Stanton BA. Renal Physiology, 4th edition. Philadelphia: Mosby; 2009.

10.2 Diagnostic Evaluation of Kidney and Urinary Tract

RN Srivastava

INTRODUCTION

There are only a few specific manifestations of renal diseases in infants and children. Other clinical features are subtle or vague and may not lead to a suspicion of an underlying renal disorder. Kidney diseases should be considered in children with failure to thrive, unexplained fever, obscure anemia, rickets and dyselectrolytemia with acid-base abnormalities. A family history of renal disease should always be obtained. A meticulous urinalysis is the crucial diagnostic investigation and expert ultrasonography is required in most cases. Computed tomography (CT) and magnetic resonance imaging (MRI) and radionuclide studies must be used judiciously.

CLINICAL FEATURES

Common presenting features suggestive of an underlying renal disease include gross hematuria, edema, hypertension, dysuria, flank pain and decrease in urine output.

Hematuria

Urine color may vary from frank red to shades of brown, described as cola or tea colored. A small amount of blood (1 mL in 1 L of urine) is sufficient to change the urine color. Concentrated urine looks like mustard oil and is often mistakenly reported as hematuria. Myoglobinuria, porphyria or alkaptonuria may cause brown discoloration of urine, while administration of rifampicin and pyridium and ingestion of sugar beet or red dyes impart a reddish orange color. Hematuria should be confirmed by microscopy and differentiated from hemoglobinuria and methemoglobinuria. The Dipstick test identifies heme and thus is not specific for red blood cells (RBCs). Important causes of hematuria and steps of evaluation are listed in the chapter "Asymptomatic Hematuria".

Edema

Facial edema is an important feature of renal disease and is often ignored unless acute and associated with other abnormalities such as gross hematuria or oliguria. Nephrotic syndrome characteristically manifests with gradually increasing periorbital edema, which is often mistakenly attributed to an allergic or eye problem. In acute glomerulonephritis (GN), edema is turgid and persistent whereas in nephrotic syndrome, the swelling is soft and pits on pressure. Nephrotic syndrome is easily differentiated from other causes of edema such as severe malnutrition, congestive cardiac failure and cirrhosis of liver.

Oliguria

A decrease in urine volume denotes renal dysfunction. Oliguria is defined as a urine output less than 500 mL/day/1.73 m^2 or less than 0.5 mL/kg/hour (<1 mL/kg/hour in newborns). Anuria may result from severe dehydration and hypovolemia, complete obstruction of the urinary tract or profound renal parenchymal injury.

Polyuria

Urine volumes more than 4–6 mL/kg/hour reflect impaired urinary concentration. Polydipsia is often associated. Conditions causing excessive solute excretion (osmotic diuresis, e.g. diabetes mellitus) or reduced proximal tubular reabsorption (Fanconi syndrome and isolated hypercalciuria) lead to mild polyuria. Impaired distal concentration due to vasopressin deficiency (central diabetes insipidus) or lack of tubular response to vasopressin (nephrogenic diabetes insipidus) will lead to profound water losses. Distal tubular dysfunction may result from obstructive uropathy, chronic hypokalemia or interstitial nephritis. Polyuria and polydipsia are important features of nephronophthisis, a familial nephropathy that manifests during infancy.

Abdominal Pain

Flank pain is often present in acute pyelonephritis and nephrolithiasis. Young children may not be able to localize the pain. Ultrasonography is a useful tool for evaluation of the anatomy of kidneys and urinary tract.

Abnormalities of Micturition

Constant bedwetting, weak urinary stream, dribbling and crying during micturition are abnormal and require evaluation. Distal obstruction, most commonly from

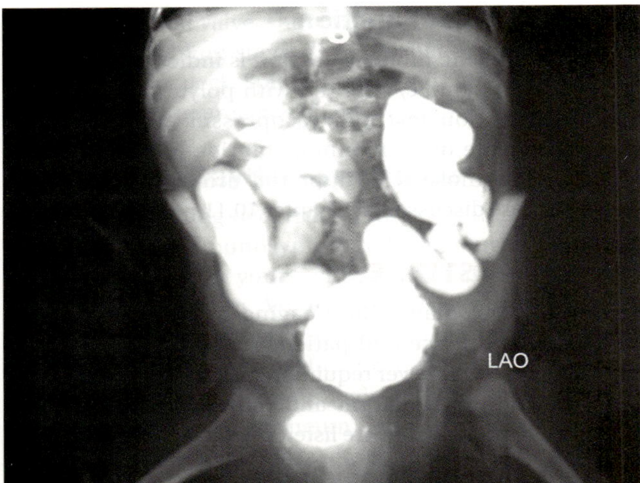

Fig. 10.2.1: Micturating cystourethrogram showing bilateral grade V vesicoureteric reflux in a 3-year-old boy with recurrent urinary tract infections. The urethra is not visualized.

(LAO: left anterior oblique view)

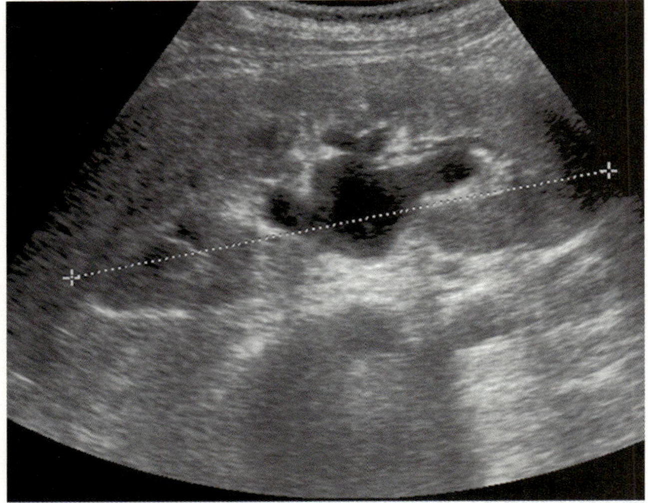

Fig. 10.2.2: Ultrasound study in a 6-year-old boy showing hydronephrosis; note enlarged kidney and dilated renal pelvis.

since it is painless, requires no sedation or radiocontrast administration, and can be repeated safely. Ultrasound is useful in guiding procedures such as renal biopsy or fine needle aspiration. The major limitation of ultrasonography is that it is operator dependent; interpretation in children requires considerable experience.

The renal cortical echotexture is compared with liver, spleen and renal medulla; nonspecific changes may occur with renal parenchymal disease. Measurement of renal size helps assess its growth. Doppler evaluation is useful for assessment of blood flow.

Antenatal Ultrasonography

Evaluation in antenatal period allows detection of common abnormalities such as unilateral or bilateral hydronephrosis and multicystic dysplastic kidney. Particular attention is directed toward the amount of amniotic fluid, anteroposterior diameter of renal pelvis and pelviectasis, renal echotexture, appearance of the ureters and urinary bladder. Distended bladder with bilateral hydronephrosis suggests distal obstruction as seen with posterior urethral valves, while unilateral hydronephrosis with normal ureters and bladder suggests pelviureteric junction obstruction.

Computerized Tomography

Noncontrast helical CT scanning is useful in identifying very small calculi, which might not be detected on ultrasonography. CT provides excellent anatomical details, which is especially useful in evaluating abdominal masses (e.g. tumor or abscess). The disadvantages include radiation exposure, the need for sedation and risks of contrast nephropathy.

Magnetic Resonance Imaging

Magnetic resonance imaging is used for the detection of spinal abnormalities such as tethered cord. MRI provides superior resolution and avoids radiation. Magnetic resonance urography is an alternative to IVP and provides clear information of renal function and excretion. However, the procedure requires sedation.

Radionuclide Imaging

Radionuclide methods are increasingly replacing conventional radiocontrast studies such as IVP and angiography, since they are noninvasive, highly sensitive and involve lower radiation exposures. They are used to assess differential renal function and renal perfusion, and to identify cortical scars, intrarenal masses and upper tract dilatation.

Renography

Renography or renal perfusion study monitors the arrival, uptake and elimination of a radiopharmaceutical by the kidney. Agents used include ^{99m}Tc-labeled diethylene triamine penta-acetic acid (DTPA), an agent excreted purely by glomerular filtration, and mercaptoacetylglycine (MAG-3) and LL-ethylene cysteine (LL-EC) dimer, excreted by glomerular filtration and tubular secretion.

Figures 10.2.3A and B show the three phases of a normal renogram. The peak of the curve depends on renal blood flow, renal function, tubular transit and excretion. Therefore, the peak is delayed in renal artery stenosis, renal parenchymal disease, oliguria and with obstruction. Dynamic scans are useful in identification of pelviureteric junction obstruction

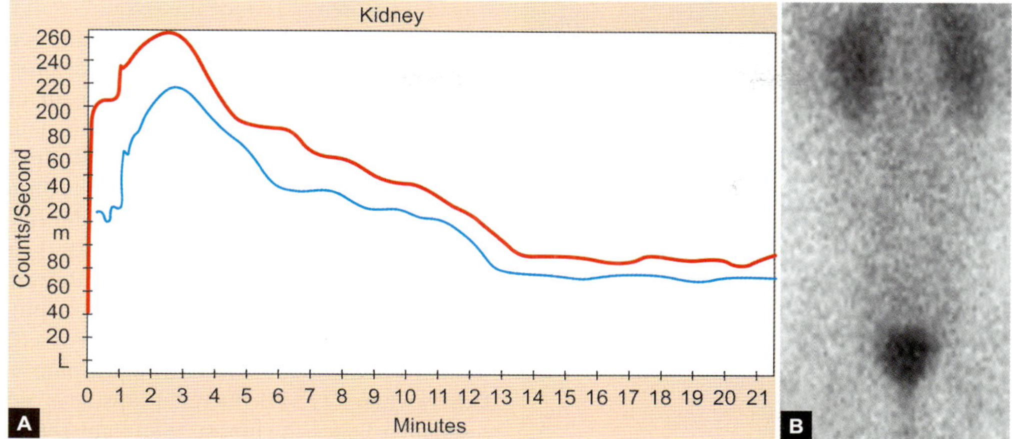

Figs. 10.2.3A and B: Diethylenetriamine penta-acetic acid renogram showing normal concentration and excretion of the radiolabeled agent through both kidneys. Note the three phases: (i) a rapid rise and fall due to first pass perfusion; (ii) slow rise to a peak due to arrival of the agent into the kidney and (iii) declining amplitude due to excretion. Delayed image shows clearing of the radionuclide from both kidneys and its presence in urinary bladder.

and renovascular stenosis, evaluation of differential and total renal function, assessment of allograft function and perfusion. A diuretic renogram helps differentiate obstructive dilatation of the upper urinary tract from nonobstructive hydronephrosis; in the latter, the radionuclide clears promptly following the injection of frusemide. Administration of captopril acutely reduces renal blood flow and GFR, thus accentuating the abnormalities, which facilitates the diagnosis of renal arterial stenosis.

Renal Static Imaging

Renal static imaging provides a two-dimensional depiction of the concentration and distribution of radionuclide. ^{99m}Tc labeled dimercaptosuccinic acid (DMSA) and glucoheptonate (GHA) provide excellent quality of images. ^{99m}Tc DTPA visualizes the pelvicalyceal collecting system and ureters well. Due to its concentration in the renal cortex and a slow rate of urinary excretion, DMSA is particularly useful for demonstration of renal scarring **(Fig. 10.2.4)**, identification of ectopic kidneys and in detecting damage from trauma. Imaging with GHA is useful when evaluating abnormalities in both the cortex and collecting system since it is filtered, partially reabsorbed and retained in proximal tubular cells.

Clearance Studies

Agents such as ^{51}Cr-ethylene-diamine-tetra-acetic acid (EDTA) and ^{99m}Tc DTPA are used for estimation of total and differential glomerular filtration. ^{131}I orthoiodohippurate helps determine effective renal plasma flow.

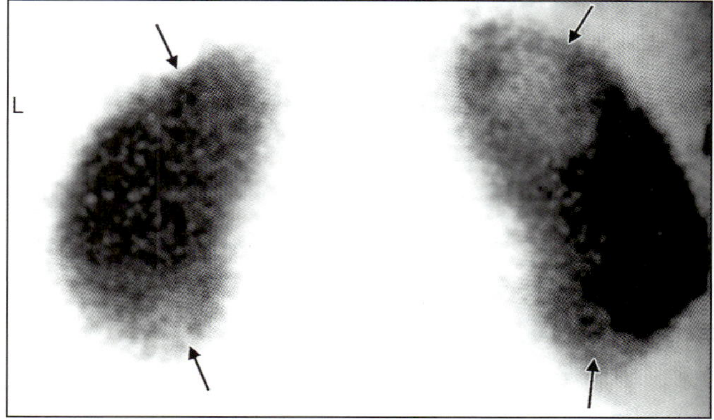

Fig. 10.2.4: Dimercaptosuccinic acid scan showing bilateral cortical scarring in a 7-year-old girl with recurrent urinary tract infections.

Direct Radionuclide Cystogram

Direct radionuclide cystography (DRNC) is a reliable and sensitive technique for the detection of VUR. It is performed by instilling radionuclide through a urethral catheter or by its injection into the bladder. Thereafter, rapid sequence images of the bladder are obtained while the patient voids. These provide a visual representation of the rate of bladder emptying, residual urine volume and evidence of reflux. Compared to MCU, the technique involves lower radiation exposure, making it suitable for repeated follow-up examinations.

RENAL BIOPSY

Evaluation of renal histology is an important tool for the diagnosis of various renal parenchymal diseases involving

Table 10.2.1: Indications for renal biopsy.
Common or usually indicated: • Steroid-resistant nephrotic syndrome • Acute renal failure of unknown cause • Rapidly progressive renal failure
Systemic disease (Henoch-Schönlein purpura, lupus, hemolytic uremic syndrome, immunoglobulin A nephropathy) • Inherited nephropathies, e.g. Alport syndrome • Renal allograft dysfunction • Detection of calcineurin toxicity
Less useful: • Chronic renal failure, to ascertain etiology • Non-nephrotic range proteinuria • Microscopic hematuria • Steroid-sensitive nephrotic syndrome

glomeruli or tubulointerstitium. Indications for kidney biopsy are listed under specific conditions in **Table 10.2.1**. A renal biopsy is not necessary in uncomplicated cases of poststreptococcal GN and corticosteroid-responsive nephrotic syndrome. The procedure should be performed early in case of rapidly progressive glomerulonephritis (RPGN), suspected SLE nephritis and renal vasculitis, where early institution of specific therapy may improve outcome.

The availability of disposable automatic devices (biopsy gun) and ultrasonographic guidance have improved the yield of the procedure, with relatively less risks. Prior to biopsy, a normal coagulation profile and normal blood pressure must be ensured to reduce the risk of bleeding. Patients with marked azotemia should be dialyzed and receive intranasal desmopressin 30–60 minutes prior to the procedure.

The procedure is performed on an empty stomach (4-hour fasting) under light sedation using intravenous midazolam with ketamine; atropine administration reduces the risk of secretions. The child lies in the prone position with a folded towel or bedsheet placed under his lower ribs and epigastrium to push the kidney posteriorly and stabilize its position. The biopsy site is the angle made by the lower edge of the 12th rib and the lateral border of sacrospinalis. The kidney is localized with a "probing" 23-gauge needle or visualized directly by ultrasound. The entry of the biopsy needle into the kidney when it pierces the renal capsule is indicated by slight resistance. Following biopsy, vital signs should be monitored closely for the next 6–8 hours. Complications include local pain, gross hematuria, perinephric hematoma, infection, and rarely, formation of traumatic arteriovenous fistula. Strenuous exercise should be avoided for a few days.

Renal histology is examined by light microscopy and immunofluorescence. Electron microscopic examination is useful for precise diagnosis of Alport syndrome, MPGN and thin glomerular basement membrane disease.

BIBLIOGRAPHY

1. Bagga A, Srivastava RN. Diagnostic evaluation. In: Srivastava RN, Bagga A (Eds). Pediatric Nephrology, 5th edition. New Delhi: Jaypee Brothers Medical Publishers (P) Ltd.; 2011. pp. 20-47.

10.3 Developmental Anomalies

Susan Uthup

INTRODUCTION

Congenital anomalies of the kidney and urinary tract (CAKUT) represent a broad range of disorders. Severe structural fetal anomalies occur in 1% of pregnancies and defects of renal development might account for 30% of chronic kidney failure in children. CAKUT is phenotypically variable and can affect the kidney(s) alone and/or the lower urinary tract. In young children, congenital anomalies are the leading cause of kidney failure and for kidney transplantation or dialysis. CAKUT can also lead to significant renal problems in adulthood including hypertension and/or proteinuria. Congenital renal anomalies can be sporadic or familial, syndromic or nonsyndromic. Anomalies of other organ systems may occur in association with renal anomalies. Clues suggesting renal anomalies are given in **Table 10.3.1**.

The development of kidneys begins at the 5th week of gestation from the intermediate mesoderm, which differentiates into pronephros, mesonephros and metanephros. Pronephros and mesonephros degenerate. The definitive fetal kidneys develop from the metanephros. The ureteric bud, originating from the mesonephric (Wolffian) duct, penetrates the metanephric blastema and induces its differentiation into renal parenchyma. In the absence of ureteric bud, metanephric kidneys will not form. The kidneys

Table 10.3.1: Clues suggesting renal anomalies.

- Oligohydramnios
- Fetal compression syndrome (Potter sequence: Flat facies, low set malformed ears, pulmonary hypoplasia, limb anomalies)
- Chromosomal disorders: Trisomy 13; trisomy 18; Turner syndrome
- Tuberous sclerosis
- Prune Belly syndrome (absent abdominal muscles, cryptorchidism)
- Meningomyelocele
- Anorectal malformations
- Aniridia (Wilms' tumor)
- Family history of renal disease (Alport syndrome, polycystic kidney disease)

ascend from sacral to lumbar region, and nephrogenesis is complete by 36 weeks of gestation. Embryologically, the ureter begins development as a solid cord. As the collecting system lengthens and canalizes, anomalies can lead to transient or permanent, partial or complete obstruction to urine flow. This obstructive process, if significant and persistent, results in varying degrees of cystic dysplasia and renal dysfunction. The fetal kidneys start producing urine by the 9th week of gestation and contribute to the amniotic fluid. An adequate amniotic fluid volume is essential for normal lung development. Patients with oligohydramnios show pulmonary hypoplasia, deformities of the skeleton and soft tissues.

Developmental anomalies of kidneys include malformation of the renal parenchyma, abnormalities of migration or in the development of collecting system. Derangements in cellular, molecular and morphogenic mechanisms that direct normal renal system development are the major causes of CAKUT.

RENAL AGENESIS

Renal agenesis is the complete absence of identifiable renal tissue due to failure of development of ureteric bud or metanephros. It may be unilateral or bilateral. Renal agenesis occurs in 1 in 500–1,000 births. Typically, the ureter and ipsilateral trigone of urinary bladder are absent. In unilateral renal agenesis, the contralateral normal kidney hypertrophies. Bilateral renal agenesis, with an incidence of 1 in 3,000 births, is incompatible with life. It is associated with pulmonary hypoplasia and facial appearance characterized by wide set eyes, squashed flattened nose, receding chin, large low set ears, small mandible and deficiency of cartilage. The absent renal echoes and urinary bladder can be detected at 12 weeks of gestation on ultrasound. Death occurs in the perinatal period due to respiratory insufficiency.

RENAL HYPOPLASIA

The hypoplastic kidney is small but the shape and structure are normal. The functioning renal parenchyma is reduced as there is reduction in the number of nephrons. Hypoplastic kidney may be unilateral or bilateral. Bilateral renal hypoplasia is an important cause of kidney failure in the first decade of life.

RENAL DYSPLASIA

There is abnormal differentiation of renal parenchyma with development of cysts, undifferentiated mesenchymal tissue, cartilage, primitive glomeruli and primitive tubules. Dysplasia may be unilateral or bilateral and may be associated with other developmental abnormalities of the urinary tract. Intrauterine obstruction of the urinary tract may cause severe bilateral renal dysplasia. Severe bilateral dysplasia presents as Potter sequence and is incompatible with life.

CYSTIC LESIONS

Multicystic Dysplastic Kidney

This is the most common renal cystic disease. The kidney is enlarged and presents as an abdominal mass in neonates. There is severe cystic renal dysplasia with no functioning renal tissue. The cysts are randomly arranged. Multicystic dysplastic kidneys may be associated with developmental abnormalities of the urinary tract. Surgical removal is seldom necessary as the dysplastic kidney usually involutes.

Polycystic Kidney Disease

Inherited polycystic kidney disease is an important cause of end-stage renal disease. Two distinct patterns of inheritance have been described, autosomal dominant and recessive, each with different characteristics.

Autosomal Dominant Polycystic Kidney Disease

Autosomal dominant polycystic kidney disease (ADPKD) is one of the most common inherited human disorders and the most frequent genetic cause of renal failure in adults. It often presents in adults but can occasionally be detected in children. Chief manifestations include palpable kidneys, hematuria, hypertension, urinary tract infections and renal stones. The genetic loci are on chromosomes 16 and 4. The kidneys are enlarged with multiple cysts. Hepatic cysts, cysts in pancreas, spleen and cerebral aneurysms may also occur. End-stage kidney disease occurs in the 5th or 6th decade. Screening ultrasound examination of parents and siblings should be done.

Autosomal Recessive Polycystic Kidney Disease

Autosomal recessive polycystic kidney disease, linked to chromosome 6, has a more severe clinical course than ADPKD. It may present as Potter sequence with pulmonary hypoplasia, chronic kidney disease during childhood or with liver disease in older survivors. The kidneys are enlarged with multiple cysts. The reniform shape is maintained.

ABNORMALITIES IN POSITION

Renal Ectopia, Malrotation

During development, kidneys ascend and rotate so that renal pelvis faces medially. Renal ectopia occurs in 1 in 800 births. Pelviureteric junction obstruction and vesicoureteral reflux may occur in kidneys that fail to ascend.

Horseshoe Kidney

In horseshoe kidneys, the lower poles of kidneys commonly fuse in the midline. This anomaly occurs in 1 in 400 births. One-third of patients with Turner syndrome have horse-shoe kidneys. Reflux, obstruction, infection and stone formation are common; there is increased risk of Wilm's tumor. Skeletal, cardiovascular, neural tube defects and anorectal malformations are associated.

Crossed Fused Ectopia

During the ascent, one kidney may cross the midline and fuse with the other. Patients with this condition often show anomalies of the collecting system, including reflux and obstruction.

ANTENATAL HYDRONEPHROSIS

Antenatal ultrasonography can detect anomalies of kidneys as early as 16 weeks of gestation. Hydronephrosis is the most common renal anomaly detected on ultrasound in 3–5% pregnancies. The dilatation may involve the calyces (caliectasis) or pelvis (pelviectasis) or both. Antenatally detected hydronephrosis may be the result of obstruction or nonobstructive causes **(Table 10.3.2)**. Obstructive lesions, particularly bilateral lesions are harmful to the developing kidneys.

The anteroposterior diameter of the fetal renal pelvis more than 4 mm below 20 weeks, and more than 7 mm above 20 weeks of gestation, is considered significant. In most cases (60%), antenatal hydronephrosis is physiological and resolves by the first year of life.

Table 10.3.2: Causes of antenatal hydronephrosis.

- Physiological
- Obstructive lesions
- Pelviureteric junction obstruction
- Posterior urethral valve
- *Vesicoureteric reflux*:
  - Primary
  - Secondary to duplex collecting system, ectopic ureter and prunebelly syndrome
- Nonobstructive nonrefluxing ureters
- Primary megaureter

Amniotic fluid volume is the chief determinant of fetal survival in these babies, oligohydramnios being associated with pulmonary hypoplasia. Oligohydramnios beyond the second trimester indicates urinary obstruction or renal failure in the fetus. The presence of bilateral upper tract dilatation and persistently distended bladder suggest the possibility of posterior urethral valves. Oligohydramnios and brightly echogenic kidneys if detected on ultrasound prior to 24 weeks of gestation predicts fetal end-stage renal disease syndrome and poor postnatal survival. In such cases, termination of pregnancy may be contemplated. Careful postnatal follow-up is needed in all children with CAKUT.

BIBLIOGRAPHY

1. Elder JE. Congenital anomalies and dysgenesis of kidneys. In: Nelson Textbook of Pediatrics, 18th edition. Saunders; 2007. pp. 2221-3.
2. Goodyer P. Renal dysplasia/hypoplasia. In: Avner E, Harmon W, Niaudet P (Eds). Pediatric Nephrology, 5th edition. Philadelphia: Lippincott Williams and Wilkins; 2004. pp. 83-92.
3. Nammalwar BR, Vijayakumar M. Genetic and developmental renal disease. In: Principles and Practice of Pediatric Nephrology. New Delhi: Jaypee Brothers Medical Publishers (P) Ltd.; 2004. pp. 424-34.
4. Pohl M, Bhatnagar V, Mendoza SA, et al. Toward an etiological classification of developmental disorders of the kidney and upper urinary tract: Perspectives in Basic Science. Kidney Int. 2002;61:10-9.
5. Song R1, Yosypiv IV. Genetics of congenital anomalies of the kidney and urinary tract. Pediatr Nephrol. 2011;26(3):353-64.
6. Toka HR, Toka O, Hariri A, et al. Congenital anomalies of kidneys and urinary tract. Semin Nephrol. 2010;30(4):374-86.

10.4 Glomerulonephritis

Kamran Afzal

INTRODUCTION

Glomerulonephritis (GN) refers to disorders in which an immunologic insult triggers inflammation and proliferation of glomerular tissue with damage to the glomerular basement membrane (GBM), mesangium, or capillary endothelium. GN may be primary (confined to the kidney) or secondary (part of a systemic disorder). Depending on duration of disease onset and the rate of progression, GN could be acute, rapidly progressive or chronic.

ACUTE GLOMERULONEPHRITIS

Acute GN, or the acute nephritic syndrome, is defined as sudden onset of hematuria and proteinuria, accompanied by hypertension, edema and impaired renal function.

Postinfectious GN is the most common cause, and nearly 80% cases are poststreptococcal glomerulonephritis (PSGN) **(Table 10.4.1)**. Immunoglobulin A (IgA) nephropathy is the most common primary GN worldwide; the disease is frequent in Japan and Korea.

Table 10.4.1: Etiology of acute glomerulonephritis.

Postinfectious:
- *Bacteria*: Streptococci (group A, beta-hemolytic), staphylococci, pneumococci, meningococci, *Treponema pallidum, Salmonella typhi, Leptospira*
- *Viruses*: Hepatitis B and C, cytomegalovirus, parvovirus, Ebstein-Barr virus, coxsackie virus, echovirus, varicella, rubella, rickettsiae and mumps
- *Parasites*: *Plasmodium malariae, P. falciparum, Toxoplasma filariasis, Schistosoma mansoni*
- *Others*: Infection of shunts and prosthesis, infective endocarditis

Noninfectious:
- *Primary renal diseases*
  - IgA nephropathy
  - Membranoproliferative glomerulonephritis
  - Mesangial proliferative glomerulonephritis
  - Hereditary nephropathy
- *Systemic diseases:*
  - *Vasculitis*: Henoch-Schönlein purpura, microscopic polyangiitis, Wegener's granulomatosis
  - *Collagen vascular disorder*: Systemic lupus erythematosus

Pathogenesis

Most cases of GN are due to an immunologic response to a variety of etiologic agents. PSGN is associated with throat or skin infection with nephritogenic strains of group A streptococci. Their nephritogenicity is related to the M-protein serotype: Types 2, 49, 56 and 60 are associated with pyoderma and PSGN, while 1, 4, 12 and 25 are associated with throat infection and PSGN. The process of renal injury begins with deposition of immune complexes formed either in the circulation or *in situ* by binding of antibodies to antigens trapped in the glomerulus or native glomerular components. The immune complexes and streptococcal antigens activate the complement pathways with recruitment of leukocytes and macrophages, and release of growth factors and cytokines that together initiate and propagate glomerular inflammation and injury. The early phase of PSGN is associated with C3 nephritic factor activation of alternate pathway and depletion of plasma C3.

Pathology

Light microscopy shows diffuse proliferative and exudative changes with polymorphonuclear infiltrate and variable mesangial matrix expansion. There is endothelial and mesangial cell proliferation, resulting in obliteration of glomerular tuft. Severe injury results in proliferation of parietal and visceral epithelial cells resulting in crescents.

Immunofluorescence reveals irregular IgG and C3 deposits along the capillary wall in early stages (starry sky appearance) and the mesangium later. Garland pattern of confluent deposits along capillaries correlates with heavy proteinuria.

Clinical Features

Poststreptococcal glomerulonephritis affects children in the age group of 5–12 years (rare below 2 years), with male preponderance. Asymptomatic disease is 4–5 times more common among sporadic PSGN, although less frequently during epidemics. Subclinical cases have microscopic hematuria, and low complement with or without hypertension. Symptomatic cases have an abrupt onset with hematuria, proteinuria and variable edema and hypertension. History of streptococcal infection may precede clinical disease onset by 1–2 weeks for throat infections and 3–4 weeks for skin infections. Anuria is rare, though transient oliguria may be noted.

The occurrence of similar symptoms within 3–4 days of a respiratory or gastrointestinal infection suggests IgA nephropathy or Alport syndrome. The presence of rash, arthralgia, abdominal pain and hemoptysis suggests diagnoses other than postinfectious GN **(Table 10.4.2)**. Family history of renal disease suggests hereditary nephropathies such as Alport syndrome or thin basement membrane disease. Systemic features are seen with systemic vasculitis and systemic lupus erythematosus.

Complications

An occasional patient may present with nephrotic range proteinuria or hypertensive emergency. The latter is characterized by stage 2 hypertension, with clinical evidence of heart failure, pulmonary edema or encephalopathy. Rarely, there is progressive worsening of renal functions with hypertension and oligoanuria.

Diagnosis

Dilutional anemia (normocytic, normochromic) correlates with expansion of the extracellular fluid. The presence of thrombocytopenia requires investigations for lupus or hemolytic uremic syndrome (HUS). On urinalysis, gross hematuria is present; dysmorphic red cells, and red cell and hyaline casts may be seen. While proteinuria is often mild, occasionally nephrotic range proteinuria may be observed. The finding of neutrophils on microscopy does not suggest a urinary tract infection.

Although most patients have mild-to-modest elevations in the serum concentrations of creatinine and urea, the spectrum could range from severe azotemia to even normal levels at presentation. Hyperkalemia, metabolic acidosis and hyponatremia are only present in patients with significant renal function impairment.

Antistreptolysin O titers are elevated in up to 80% of cases suggesting preceding streptococcal infection, although antibiotic treatment may attenuate this response. Total hemolytic complement and some components are low during acute PSGN suggesting activation of the alternative pathway of the complement system. The concentration of C3 has been found to be low in more than 90% patients and normalizes by 6–8 weeks. The level of C3 does not have any prognostic significance, but persistent hypocomplementemia suggests an alternative diagnosis such as lupus, membranoproliferative glomerulonephritis (MPGN) or postinfectious GN, bacterial endocarditis, visceral abscess and shunt nephritis.

Kidney biopsy is not needed to confirm the diagnosis of PSGN. It is indicated in those with heavy proteinuria, suspected crescentic GN or significant deviation from the natural course of the disease **(Table 10.4.3)**.

Table 10.4.2: Clues to underlying etiology of glomerulonephritis.

Clinical presentation	***Investigations***	***Diagnosis***
Preceding sore throat/skin infection, abscess, endocarditis, infected shunt, prosthetic valves, indwelling catheters	Hematuria; high blood creatinine; low serum C3, C4; ASO, anti-DNase B, antihyaluronidase	Postinfectious GN
Purpura, joint pain, abdominal pain, nausea, vomiting	*Skin biopsy*: Leukocytoclastic vasculitis, IgA and C3 deposits *Renal biopsy*: Proliferative GN; mesangial IgA deposits	Henoch-Schönlein purpura
Recurrent hematuria, proteinuria, following respiratory tract infection	Mesangial IgA deposits	IgA nephropathy
Hematuria following respiratory infections; sensorineural deafness; lenticonus, retinopathy; family history	*Electron microscopy*: Irregular thickening, splitting and lamination of glomerular basement membrane	Alport syndrome
Arthralgia, malar rash, nephritis	Positive ANA, dsDNA; low C3	SLE
Sinusitis, pulmonary infiltrates and nephritis	Positive for c-ANCA *Biopsy*: Pauci-immune necrotizing GN	Wegener's granulomatosis
Nephritis, fever, weight loss; rash, arthralgia, pulmonary hemorrhage	Positive for p-ANCA *Biopsy*: Pauci-immune necrotizing GN	Microscopic polyangiitis
Hemoptysis; pulmonary hemorrhage	Anti-GBM antibody in serum, biopsy	Goodpasture syndrome

(ANA: antinuclear antibody; ANCA: antineutrophil cytoplasmic antibody; ASO: antistreptolysin O; dsDNA: double-stranded DNA; GN: glomerulonephritis; SLE: systemic lupus erythematosus)

Table 10.4.3: Indications for renal biopsy in acute glomerulonephritis.

During early phase of disease:
- Latent period between streptococcal infection and acute glomerulonephritis of less than 1 week; no serologic evidence of streptococcal infection; normal serum complement C3
- Extrarenal manifestations of systemic disease: Rash, joint pain, fever, hepatosplenomegaly, lymphadenopathy, hemoptysis
- Anuria and/or rapidly deteriorating renal function

During recovery phase:
- Persistent hypertension or nephrotic range proteinuria beyond 2 weeks
- No improvement or continued decrease in the glomerular filtration rate beyond 2 weeks
- Persistent hypocomplementemia beyond 12 weeks
- Persistent gross hematuria more than 1-month, microscopic hematuria more than 18 months

Treatment

Therapy is essentially symptomatic with mild cases of PSGN, requiring home-based treatment. Hospital admission is required for those with oligoanuria, moderate-to-severe edema or hypertension and impaired renal functions. Penicillin for 7 days may be used in those with residual pharyngitis or pyoderma, prevents spread of streptococci to others but does not alter disease course in the index case. Those with oliguria or anuria require strict control of fluid intake to insensible water losses along with replacement of urine output. Prudent use of diuretics (furosemide 1–3 mg/kg) helps to manage fluid overload and circulatory congestion. Salt and fluid intake should be limited in those with significant hypertension, edema or renal failure. Dialysis is required in patients with refractory or worsening acute renal failure. Mild hypertension is treated with oral diuretics, β-adrenergic blockers or angiotensin-converting enzyme inhibitors. Severe hypertension requires oral/IV furosemide and oral or sublingual nifedipine. For those presenting with hypertensive emergencies, IV short-acting antihypertensive (sodium nitroprusside, labetalol or nicardipine) are used for controlled reduction in blood pressure.

Specific therapy is not available for most other causes except infections. Those with heavy proteinuria or rapidly progressive glomerulonephritis (RPGN) require prompt therapy (see below). Patients with IgA nephropathy and microscopic or recurrent gross hematuria but subnephrotic range proteinuria (<1 g/1.73 m^2) do not require specific treatment.

Course

Attempts to identify the etiology of postinfectious GN are prudent. Although the course and prognosis for PSGN is well-known and almost always favorable, this is not always so with nonstreptococcal forms of the condition. Edema usually resolves in 5–10 days, and the blood pressure returns to normal after 2–3 weeks, though persistence of elevated blood pressure for up to 6 weeks is compatible with complete resolution. Urinary abnormalities resolve at various times after onset: gross hematuria and proteinuria resolve early but microscopic hematuria could continue for 6–12 months. C3 concentration returns to normal in more than 95% patients by 8–10 weeks. Clinical manifestations of the disease rarely recur, and second episodes of PSGN are rare.

RAPIDLY PROGRESSIVE (CRESCENTIC) GLOMERULONEPHRITIS

Acute GN can rarely show RPGN characterized by hematuria, edema, hypertension, oligoanuria and azotemia. Extensive crescents on renal biopsy are the histological hallmark. Crescents are two or more layers of segmental to circumferential proliferation of parietal or visceral epithelial cells that completely or partially obliterate the Bowman's space. Crescentic GN is labeled when 50% or more glomeruli have crescents. Crescents can evolve rapidly from cellular to fibrocellular and fibrous especially in the event of delayed treatment.

Crescentic GN is rare in children. Its causes are categorized based on findings on renal immunofluorescence: Immune, pauci-immune and anti-GBM disease, reflecting different mechanisms of glomerular injury **(Table 10.4.4)**. Immune complex GN is common in children.

Clinical Features

There is variable degree of gross hematuria, hypertension, oligoanuria and edema. Systemic complaints (cough, sinusitis, vasculitic rash, arthritis and neurological manifestations) are more common with pauci-immune disease. Hemoptysis and pulmonary hemorrhage are seen in anti-GBM disease, but may occur in lupus, Henoch-Schönlein purpura (HSP), Wegener's granulomatosis or any GN with pulmonary edema.

Diagnosis

Investigations include blood counts, urinalysis (hematuria, proteinuria and red cell casts), and blood levels of urea, creatinine and C3 (low in PSGN, lupus and MPGN). Serology includes antistreptolysin-O in preceding streptococcal infection; and antinuclear and anti-dsDNA autoantibodies in lupus. Antinuclear cytoplasmic antibodies (ANCA) with specificity for proteinase-3 produce cytoplasmic staining on immunofluorescence (cANCA), e.g. Wegener's granulomatosis. Myeloperoxidase specific ANCA produces perinuclear staining on immunofluorescence (pANCA) in

Table 10.5.1: 2012 Revised International Chapel Hill Consensus Conference Nomenclature of Vasculitides.

Vessel size	***Disease***
Large (LVV)	• Takayasu arteritis (TAK) • Giant cell arteritis (GCA)
Medium (MVV)	• Polyarteritis nodosa (PAN) • Kawasaki disease (KD)
Small (SVV)	Antineutrophil cytoplasmic antibody (ANCA)-associated vasculitis (AAV) • Microscopic polyangiitis (MPA) • Granulomatosis with polyangiitis (Wegener granulomatosis) (GPA) • Eosinophilic granulomatosis with polyangiitis (Churg-Strauss) (EGPA) *Immune complex SVV* • Antiglomerular basement membrane (anti-GBM) disease • Cryoglobulinemic vasculitis (CV) • IgA vasculitis (Henoch-Schönlein) (IgAV) • Hypocomplementemic urticarial vasculitis (HUV) (anti-C1q vasculitis)
Variable vessel vasculitis (VVV)	• Behçet disease (BD) • Cogan syndrome (CS)
Single-organ vasculitis (SOV)	• Cutaneous leukocytoclastic angiitis • Cutaneous arteritis • Primary central nervous system vasculitis • Isolated aortitis • Others
Vasculitis associated with systemic disease	• Lupus vasculitis • Rheumatoid vasculitis • Sarcoid vasculitis • Others
Vasculitis associated with probable etiology	• Hepatitis C virus-associated cryoglobulinemic vasculitis • Hepatitis B virus-associated vasculitis • Syphilis-associated aortitis • Drug-associated immune complex vasculitis • Drug-associated ANCA-associated vasculitis • Cancer-associated vasculitis • Others

Table 10.5.2: Selected definitions for common vasculitides in children (as adopted by the 2012 International Chapel Hill Consensus Conference).

Disease	***Criteria***
Takayasu arteritis (TK)	Arteritis, often granulomatous, predominantly affecting the aorta and/or its major branches. Onset usually in patients younger than 50 years.
Kawasaki disease (KD)	Arteritis associated with the mucocutaneous lymph node syndrome and predominantly affecting medium and small arteries. Coronary arteries are often involved. Aorta and large arteries may be involved. Usually, occurs in infants and young children.
Polyarteritis nodosa (PAN)	Necrotizing arteritis of medium or small arteries without glomerulonephritis or vasculitis in arterioles, capillaries, or venules, and not associated with antineutrophil cytoplasmic antibodies (ANCAs).
IgA vasculitis (Henoch-Schönlein purpura) (IgAV)	Vasculitis, with IgA-dominant immune deposits, affecting small vessels (predominantly capillaries, venules, or arterioles). Often involves skin and gastrointestinal tract, and frequently causes arthritis. Glomerulonephritis indistinguishable from IgA nephropathy may occur.
ANCA-associated vasculitis (AAV)	Necrotizing vasculitis, with few or no immune deposits, predominantly affecting small vessels (i.e. capillaries, venules, arterioles, and small arteries), associated with myeloperoxidase (MPO) ANCA or proteinase 3 (PR3) ANCA. Not all patients have ANCA.
Microscopic polyangiitis (MPA)	Necrotizing vasculitis, with few or no immune deposits, predominantly affecting small vessels (i.e. capillaries, venules, or arterioles). Necrotizing arteritis involving small and medium arteries may be present. Necrotizing glomerulonephritis is very common. Pulmonary capillaritis often occurs. Granulomatous inflammation is absent.
Granulomatosis with polyangiitis (Wegener, GPA)	Necrotizing granulomatous inflammation usually involving the upper and lower respiratory tract, and necrotizing vasculitis affecting predominantly small-to-medium vessels (e.g. capillaries, venules, arterioles, arteries and veins). Necrotizing glomerulonephritis is common.

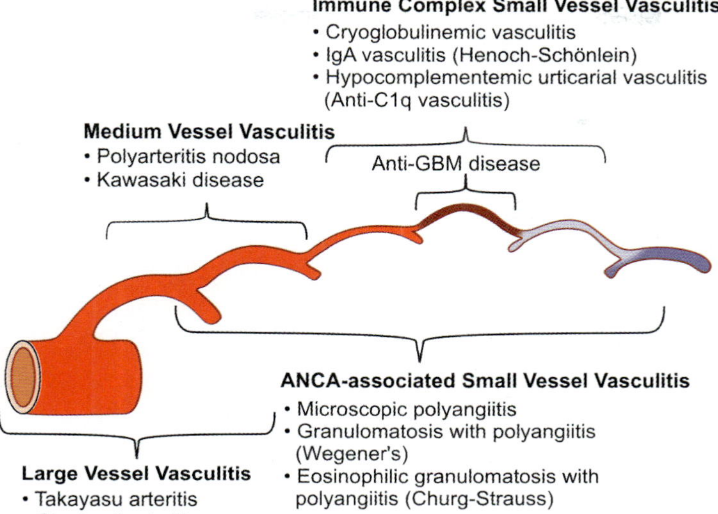

Fig. 10.5.1: The nomenclature of vasculitides by vessel size.

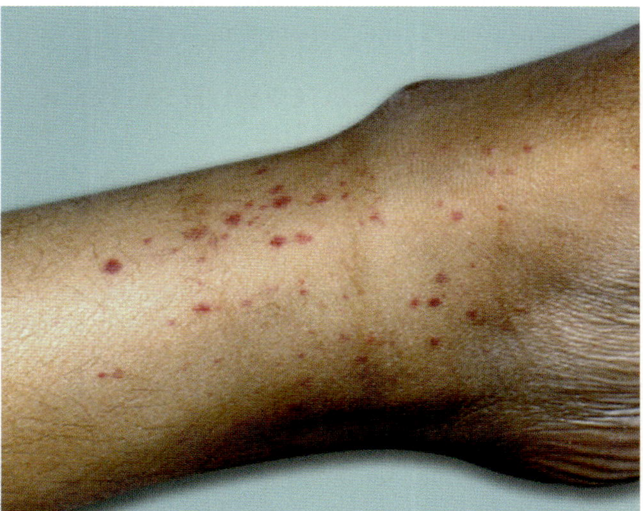

Fig. 10.5.2: Henoch-Schönlein purpura.

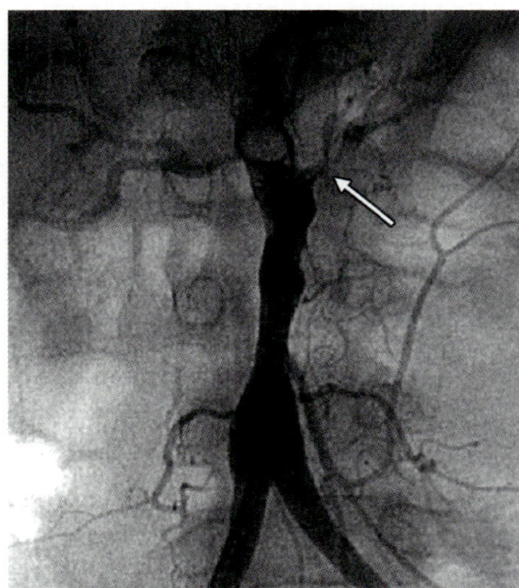

Fig. 10.5.3: Takayasu arteritis with left renal artery stenosis.

Urinalysis might show active sediment with hematuria, proteinuria, and casts. Urea and creatinine may be raised. ANA, anti-dsDNA and ANCA serology, and complement levels are useful in ascertaining the diagnosis. In ANCA-associated vasculitis, renal biopsy shows pauci-immune crescentic GN **(Fig. 10.5.5)**.

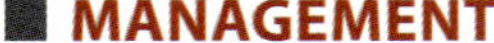

MANAGEMENT

Supportive management with antipyretics, antibiotics, and antihypertensive agents are used as required. Renal failure is managed with salt, potassium and fluid restriction and dialysis when indicated. Management of extrarenal symptoms is done simultaneously. The specific management of the renal disease in the majority of these conditions (PAN, Takayasu disease, SLE and ANCA-related vasculitis) involves therapy with steroids and other immunosuppressive agents with regular monitoring to keep disease activity (clinical and serological) under control and for adverse effects of therapy. Renal revascularization procedures (stenting, grafting or autotransplantation) may be required in patients developing arterial stenosis or dilatation.

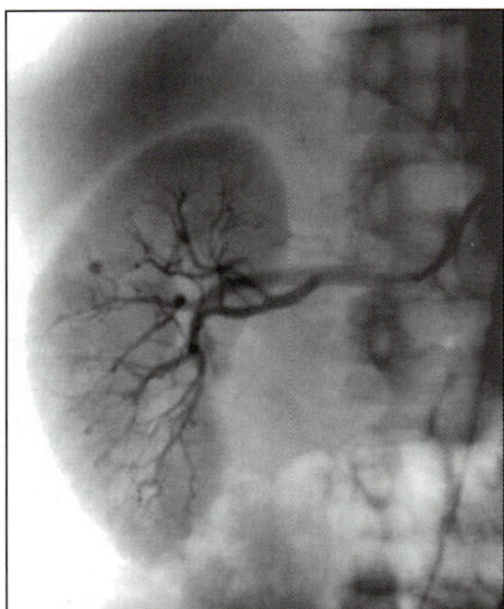

Fig. 10.5.4: Renal aneurysms in polyarteritis nodosa.

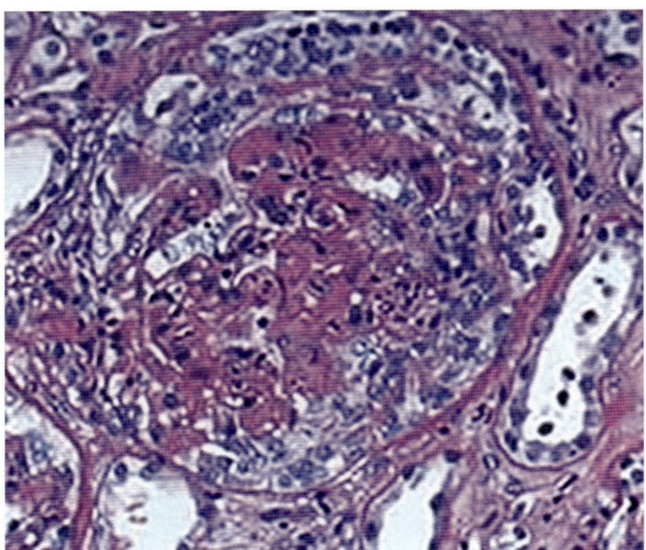

Fig. 10.5.5: Crescentic glomerulonephritis.

IGA VASCULITIS/HENOCH-SCHÖNLEIN PURPURA NEPHRITIS

Henoch-Schönlein pupura (HSP) is the most common childhood vasculitis. Renal involvement is reported to occur in 30–50% patients with risk of progression to ESRD in 1–3%. Renal manifestations in the majority, occur within 4–6 weeks after onset of rash but may occur up to six months. Occasional late progression up to 2 years after onset has been documented in patients who have initially improved, making long-term follow-up essential.

The chief renal finding is microscopic hematuria or minor proteinuria, which are generally self-limiting. The presence of renal insufficiency, hypertension or significant proteinuria indicates a poorer prognosis with increased likelihood of persistence and progression. Renal biopsy findings are classified according to International Study for Kidney Diseases in Children (ISKDC) criteria and vary from mesangial and/or endocapillary proliferation to severe involvement with crescentic GN. Predominant IgA mesangial deposits on immunofluorescence, indistinguishable from IgA nephropathy, are characteristic.

A short course of corticosteroids is recommended in patients with severe abdominal symptoms. The presence of microscopic hematuria alone does not warrant specific treatment. Prophylactic therapy with corticosteroids does not reduce the risk of HSP nephritis but may improve outcome in established cases. Patients with severe HSP nephritis, particularly RPGN, are treated with combinations of oral or IV corticosteroids, immunosuppressive agents (azathioprine, cyclophosphamide, mycophenolate mofetil), antiplatelet and anticoagulant agents, IVIG and plasma exchange. HSP nephritis may recur after renal transplant.

NEPHRITIS ASSOCIATED WITH SYSTEMIC LUPUS ERYTHEMATOSUS

Systemic lupus erythematosus is a multisystem disease with renal involvement occurring in 50–75% children, the majority within the first two years of presentation. Lupus nephritis is characterized by variable grades of hematuria, proteinuria, hypertension and renal functional impairment. Renal tubular dysfunction occurs rarely. The Systemic Lupus International Collaborating Clinics (SLICC) 2012 Criteria for renal involvement in SLE are, the equivalent of 24-hour urine protein more than 500 mg, or RBC casts.

Multiple ANA are found in SLE, of which anti-dsDNA is the most specific. Activation of the classical pathway of complement results in low levels of C3 and C4 and the deposition of C3, C4 and C1q in renal tissue.

A renal biopsy is indicated in all patients with renal involvement, as there might be unsatisfactory correlation of clinical findings, serology, and pathology. The deposition of IgG, IgA and IgM immune-complexes, C3, C4 and C1q indicates a full house on immunofluorescence, characteristic of SLE nephritis. Histological grading influences management and prognosis **(Box 10.5.1)**. Class IV or diffuse proliferative GN is most common and may have a rapidly progressive course with devastating consequences if untreated.

Class I–II lupus nephritis is treated with corticosteroids, with management aimed more at extrarenal disease. Patients with class IV nephritis with high activity indices

Box 10.5.1: Histopathological grading of systemic lupus erythematosus nephritis.

- *Class I*: Minimal changes on light microscopy
- *Class II*: Mesangial proliferative glomerulonephritis
- *Class III*: Focal proliferative glomerulonephritis (<50% glomeruli involved)
- *Class IV*: Diffuse proliferative glomerulonephritis with or without crescents (>50% glomeruli involved)
- *Class V*: Membranous changes
- *Class VI*: Sclerosed lesions

Subclassifications:
- Segmental (<50% glomerular tuft involved) versus global (≥50% glomerular tuft involved) glomerular lesions
- Chronic disease (fibrosis/sclerosis) versus active disease (thickened capillary walls creating the wire-loop lesion, necrosis, and cellular crescent formation)

are treated aggressively with combinations of high dose steroids and cytotoxic agents. Commonly used protocols include induction agents such as high dose IV or oral corticosteroids, cyclophosphamide and mycophenolate mofetil (MMF). Maintenance therapy with azathioprine or MMF may be effective and associated with fewer side effects. Hydroxychloroquine should be administered in all patients. Treatment options in patients with refractory illness include plasmapheresis, IV immunoglobulin and rituximab. Other biological agents are also under trial in severe disease.

ANCA-ASSOCIATED NEPHRITIS

The common ANCA-associated renal diseases are GPA (formerly known as Wegener granulomatosis) and microscopic polyangiitis (MPA), while Churg-Strauss syndrome is rare in children. The former are severe diseases that have a fulminant course with high-risk of ESRD and mortality. Renal disease presents with a nephritic-nephrotic syndrome, acute renal failure and rapidly progressive glomerulonephritis.

Circulating antineutrophil cytoplasmic antibodies have a role in pathogenesis and correlate with disease activity. Immunofluorescence detects protoplasmic ANCA (p-ANCA or perinuclear pattern of staining) or cytoplasmic ANCA (c-ANCA with diffusely granular, cytoplasmic staining). ELISA may show antimyeloperoxidase (anti-MPO) specificity or antiprotease 3 (anti-PR3) specificity.

Renal histopathology reveals a necrotizing, pauci-immune glomerulonephritis with crescents. Aggressive immunosuppression is required, the most common agents used are steroids and cyclophosphamide. Methotrexate, MMF, azathioprine have been used as maintenance therapies. Plasmapheresis, IVIG, rituximab and other biological compounds are used in severe and resistant cases.

BIBLIOGRAPHY

1. Batu ED, Ozen S. Vasculitis: do we know more to classify better? Pediatr Nephrol. 2015;30(9):1425-32.
2. Bertsias GK, Tektonidou M, Amoura Z, et al. EULAR/ERA-EDTA recommendations for the management of adult and pediatric lupus nephritis. Ann Rheum Dis. 2012;71(11):1771-82.
3. Brogan P, Eleftheriou D, Dillon M. Small vessel vasculitis. Pediatr Nephrol. 2010;25:1025-35.
4. Dillon MJ, Eleftheriou D, Brogan PA. Medium-size-vessel vasculitis. Pediatr Nephrol. 2010;25:1641-52.
5. Gulati A, Bagga A. Large vessel vasculitis. Pediatr Nephrol. 2010;25:1037-48.
6. Jennette JC, Falk RJ, Bacon PA, et al. 2012 revised International Chapel Hill Consensus Conference Nomenclature of Vasculitides. Arthritis Rheum. 2013;65(1):1-11.
7. Jennette JC, Nachman PH. ANCA glomerulonephritis and vasculitis. Clin J Am Soc Nephrol. 2017;12(10):1680-91.
8. Kawasaki Y, Ono A, Ohara S, et al. Henoch-Schönlein purpura nephritis in childhood: pathogenesis, prognostic factors and treatment. Fukushima J Med Sci. 2013;59(1):15-26.
9. Pohl M. Henoch-Schönlein purpura nephritis. Pediatr Nephrol. 2015;30(2):245-52.
10. Sinha R, Raut S. Pediatric lupus nephritis: Management update. World J Nephrol. 2014;3(2):16-23.

10.6 Acute Kidney Injury

Sumantra Kumar Raut, Arvind Bagga

INTRODUCTION

Acute renal failure (ARF) or acute kidney injury (AKI) is present when there is a rapid decline in kidney function. The Kidney Disease: Improving Global Outcome (KDIGO) Consensus Conference in 2012 defined AKI as an absolute increase in serum creatinine of either more than or equal to 0.3 mg/dL, a percentage increase in serum creatinine of more than or equal to 50% over 7 days or less, and/or reduction in urine output to less than 0.5 mL/kg/h for more than 6 hours. The inclusion

Table 10.6.1: Staging of acute kidney injury.*

Stage	Serum creatinine criteria	Urine output criteria
1	Increase in serum creatinine by ≥ 0.3 mg/dL from baseline within 48 hours or to 150–200% (1.5 to 2-fold) of baseline within 7 days	Less than 0.5 mL/kg/h for 6–12 hours
2	Increase in serum creatinine to more than 200–300% (>2 to 3-fold) from baseline	Less than 0.5 mL/kg/hour for > 12 hours
3	Increase in serum creatinine to > 300% (>3-fold) of baseline or increase in serum creatinine, by ≥4** mg/dL from baseline, with acute increase of ≥ 0.5 mg/dL. ≤ or initiation of renal replacement therapy, or decrease in estimated glomerular filtration rate to <35 mL/min/1.73 m^2	Less than 0.3 mL/kg/hour for 24 hours, or anuria for 12 hours

*Only one criterion (creatinine or urine output) is required for staging
**2.5 mg/dL in case of neonates

of a percentage change in creatinine accommodates variations in creatinine related to age, gender and body mass index (BMI) and reduces the need for a baseline level of serum creatinine. If the diagnosis of AKI is based on the urine output criterion alone, urinary tract obstruction and other reversible causes of oliguria (dehydration, diuretic use), should be excluded. Patients meeting the definition of AKI can be staged from stage 1 to stage 3 based on KDIGO criteria **(Table 10.6.1)**.

ETIOLOGY

Acute kidney injury occurs in a variety of settings with clinical features ranging from mild elevation in serum creatinine to anuric renal failure. The etiology of AKI is conventionally classified as prerenal, intrinsic renal or postrenal **(Table 10.6.2)**. The index most useful in helping differentiate prerenal from renal azotemia is the fractional excretion of sodium. Patients with prerenal illness show a low fractional excretion of sodium (<1%); higher values are seen with acute tubular necrosis (ATN). The chief causes of AKI include ATN secondary to hypovolemia, sepsis and nephrotoxic agents, acute glomerulonephritis (GN) and hemolytic uremic syndrome (HUS). Recent multicenter reports indicate that AKI, chiefly ATN, is quite common in sick hospitalized children and is associated with risk factors such as sepsis, hypotension, ventilation and surgery; AKI was observed in 26% of critically ill children ("AWARE" study), 30% of sick neonates ("AWAKEN" study), and in 30–65% patients following cardiac surgery for congenital heart disease.

Table 10.6.2: Important causes of acute kidney injury.

Prerenal failure
- Hypovolemia (dehydration, blood loss, diabetic ketoacidosis, nasogastric drainage, burns)
- Third space losses (septicemia, nephrotic syndrome)
- Congestive heart failure
- Hepatorenal syndrome
- Perinatal asphyxia
- *Drugs*: ACE inhibitors, diuretics, NSAIDs, calcineurin inhibitors

Intrinsic renal failure
- *Acute tubular necrosis*
  - Prolonged prerenal insult (see above)
  - *Medications:* Aminoglycosides, radiocontrast agents, cisplatin, amphotericin B, drugs causing prerenal insult
  - Disseminated intravascular coagulation
  - *Exogenous toxins:* Diethylene glycol, methanol, heavy metals
  - Intravascular hemolysis, hemoglobinuria, tumor lysis syndrome
  - *Infections:* Malaria, leptospirosis, dengue hemorrhagic fever; pyelonephritis
- *Rapidly progressive glomerulonephritis*
  - *Immune complex*: Postinfectious glomerulonephritis; IgA nephropathy; membranoproliferative glomerulonephritis; lupus nephritis, Henoch-Schönlein purpura
  - *ANCA-associated vasculitides*: Microscopic polyangiitis
  - Antiglomerular basement membrane nephritis
- Hemolytic uremic syndrome (infection associated, secondary and atypical forms); thrombotic thrombocytopenic purpura
- *Vascular causes*
  - Renal artery stenosis
  - Renal artery or vein thrombosis
- *Interstitial nephritis*: Drug-induced, idiopathic

Postrenal failure
- Posterior urethral valves, urethral stricture
- Bilateral pelviureteric junction obstruction
- Ureteral obstruction (stenosis, stone, ureterocele)
- Neurogenic bladder

(ACE: angiotensin-converting enzyme; ANCA: antineutrophilic cytoplasmic antibodies; NSAIDs: nonsteroidal anti-inflammatory drugs)

Perinatal asphyxia and respiratory distress syndrome are leading causes of AKI in neonates. In developing countries, AKI is chiefly community acquired and usually secondary to a single cause like acute gastroenteritis or infections such as malaria.

EVALUATION

A careful history provides clues to the underlying cause. A history of diarrhea, vomiting, fluid or blood loss should be sought and an assessment of fluid intake in the previous 24 hours be made. Important investigations in patients with AKI include:

- Complete blood counts, urea, creatinine, sodium, potassium, calcium, phosphate, pH, bicarbonate.

- Urinalysis (for red cells, casts, proteinuria); culture (if febrile); sodium, osmolality, fractional excretion of sodium.
- *Chest X-ray*: For fluid overload, cardiomegaly.
- *Abdominal ultrasonography*: To identify urinary tract dilatation or obstruction.
- *Complement (C3)*: Suspected atypical HUS or rapidly progressive GN.
- Peripheral smear examination, platelet and reticulocyte count, lactate dehydrogenase levels: Suspected HUS.
- Stool culture (suspected typical or shiga toxin-associated HUS).
- Blood antistreptolysin O (ASO), antinuclear antibody (ANA), antineutrophil cytoplasmic antibody (ANCA): Suspected acute or rapidly progressive GN.
- Ultrasonography (for kidney size and structure).
- *Doppler ultrasound*: Suspected arterial or venous thrombosis.
- Screening for malaria, leptospirosis or dengue, if suspected.

A kidney biopsy is not required in most patients with AKI. Indications for kidney biopsy are: rapidly progressive or non-resolving GN; AKI associated with systemic lupus erythematosus or Henoch-Schönlein purpura; suspected interstitial nephritis; or if the underlying cause of AKI is not apparent on clinical features and investigations.

Various biomarkers that have been tested for role in the early detection or timely prediction of AKI but are yet to show clinical utility in pediatric patients, include: insulin-like growth factor binding protein 7 (IGFBP-7), tissue inhibitor of metalloproteinase-2 (TIMP-2), neutrophil gelatinase-associated lipocalin (NGAL), kidney injury molecule-1 (KIM-1), interleukin-18 (IL-18) and liver-type fatty acid-binding protein (L-FABP).

MANAGEMENT

Specific management of the underlying disorder is possible in some cases (**Table 10.6.3**). Fluid resuscitation in patients with septic shock or dehydration improves renal perfusion and improves urine output. Patients with urinary tract obstruction need catheterization. It is important to manage life-threatening complications including hyperkalemia, pulmonary edema, hypertensive emergencies, and severe acidosis **(Table 10.6.4)**.

Hyperkalemia is a serious emergency. Urgent treatment is instituted depending on blood potassium levels and electrocardiography (ECG) changes. Concomitant metabolic acidosis should be corrected. While sodium bicarbonate, glucose, insulin, and salbutamol reduce the extracellular concentration of potassium by moving the ion into the cells, calcium infusion decreases membrane irritability without altering serum potassium levels. The action of Kayexalate (sodium polystyrene sulfonate) or calcium resonium, which exchanges potassium for sodium or calcium ions, is slow and not useful in emergencies. Peritoneal or hemodialysis is the most effective method to remove excess potassium from the body.

Hypertension is commonly observed in cases of GN and HUS. The symptoms of hypertensive encephalopathy are related to rapidity of rise rather than absolute value of the blood pressure. These include headache, blurring of vision, convulsions, papilledema, cranial nerve palsies, vomiting, and altered sensorium. Blood pressure should be reduced slowly and carefully with sodium nitroprusside or labetalol infusion. In asymptomatic hypertension, oral nifedipine, amlodipine, prazosin and labetalol may be used.

Hyponatremia (sodium < 130 mEq/L) is usually the result of excessive fluid administration rather than salt loss. Patients with blood sodium concentration more than 125 mEq/L are rarely symptomatic. Hyponatremia is best managed by fluid restriction; patients with resistant hyponatremia can be satisfactorily managed by dialysis. Treatment with hypertonic saline (3%) is reserved for those with symptomatic hyponatremia (encephalopathy, lethargy and seizures), but should be used cautiously because of potential complications of fluid overload, hypertension, and intraventricular hemorrhage.

Table 10.6.3: Management of conditions causing acute kidney injury (AKI).

Prerenal AKI	Administer fluids and/or vasopressors to correct dehydration and maintain blood pressure; avoid NSAIDs, ACE inhibitors and radiocontrast agents
Acute tubular necrosis	Supportive care; treat infections or underlying cause (e.g. circulatory failure)
Glomerulonephritis	Supportive care; plasma exchange; immunosuppression
Hemolytic uremic syndrome	Supportive care; plasma exchanges/infusions or eculizumab for atypical forms
Vasculitis	Immunosuppression (IV methylprednisolone, cyclophosphamide)
Interstitial nephritis	Discontinue offending drug; consider oral corticosteroids
Renal artery or vein occlusion	Anticoagulation; thrombolysis or surgery
Urinary tract obstruction	Bladder catheter; nephrostomy; surgical treatment

(ACE: angiotensin-converting enzyme; IV: intravenous; NSAIDs: nonsteroidal anti-inflammatory drugs)

Table 10.6.4: Management of complications.

Complication	*Treatment*
Fluid overload	*Fluid restriction*: Insensible losses (400 mL/m^2/day, as 5% dextrose) plus urine output and other losses (as N/5 saline); consider dialysis
Pulmonary edema	Oxygen; fluid restriction; furosemide 2–4 mg/kg IV; monitor CVP; consider dialysis
Hypertension	*Symptomatic*: Sodium nitroprusside 0.5–8 µg/kg/min or labetalol 0.25–3 mg/kg/hour as infusion; furosemide 1–4 mg/kg IV, if fluid overload; nifedipine 0.3–0.5 mg/kg oral/sublingual; reduce blood pressure by 25% of the desired reduction during first 8 hours and the remainder over the next 12–24 hours *Asymptomatic*: Amlodipine, prazosin, labetalol, clonidine
Metabolic acidosis	Sodium bicarbonate (IV or oral) if bicarbonate levels < 18 mEq/L; monitor for hypernatremia, hypocalcemia and fluid overload; consider dialysis
Hyperkalemia	Calcium gluconate (10%) 0.5–1 mL/kg over 5–10 minutes IV Salbutamol 5–10 mg nebulized over 10 minutes Sodium bicarbonate (7.5%) 1–2 mL/kg over 5–15 minutes Dextrose (10%) 0.5–1 g/kg and insulin 0.1–0.2 U/kg Calcium or sodium resonium (Kayexalate) 1 g/kg orally or rectally every 4–6 hours
Hyponatremia	Fluid restriction; if sensorial alteration or seizures, give 3% saline 6–12 mL/kg over 30–90 minutes
Severe anemia	Packed red cells 3–5 mL/kg; monitor for hypertension, hyperkalemia and fluid overload; consider exchange transfusion
High phosphate	Reduce dietary phosphate; consider phosphate binders (calcium carbonate; aluminum hydroxide)

(CVP: central venous pressure; IV: intravenous)

FLUID AND NUTRITION

Fluid and electrolyte intake in a patient with AKI should be regulated based on a clinical examination of extracellular fluid volume status, urine output, and daily weights. The daily fluid requirement amounts to insensible water losses (300–400 mL/m^2), urinary output, and extrarenal fluid losses. Insensible fluid losses are replaced with 5-10% dextrose or glucose solution. Urine output should be measured without resorting to catheterization. Urinary losses and those from extrarenal sources should have their composition analyzed and replaced accordingly. It is preferable to administer the required amounts of fluid by mouth, whenever feasible. If there is persistent vomiting, intravenous route may be necessary. Potassium-containing fluids should not be given to patients with oliguria.

Ongoing treatment is guided by intake output analysis, daily weight, physical examination, and serum sodium. If fluid in an appropriate volume and composition has been given, the patient should lose 0.5–1% of his weight every day. This weight loss is the result of caloric deprivation and not inadequate fluid therapy. Serum sodium concentrations should be maintained within the normal range. A rapid weight loss and increasing level of serum sodium suggest inadequate free water replacement. On the other hand, an absence of weight loss and hyponatremia indicate excessive free water replacement.

The types of fluids used are mostly crystalloids, e.g. saline or Ringer's lactate. There is no conclusive evidence that crystalloids are better or worse than colloids in resuscitating patients with sepsis.

Adequate nutritional support is preferred with maximization of caloric intake. A diet containing 1.2–2 g/kg of protein in infants and 0.8–1.2 g/kg in older children, and 60–80 Cal/kg should be given. Once dialysis is initiated, dietary protein, fluid, and electrolyte intake should be increased.

DIURETICS AND DRUGS

Diuretics may be useful in instances where high urine flow is required to prevent intratubular precipitation as with intravascular hemolysis, hyperuricemia, and myoglobinuria.

Drugs that increase severity of renal damage, delay recovery of function or reduce perfusion, e.g. aminoglycosides, radiocontrast media, nonsteroidal anti-inflammatory drugs (NSAIDs), amphotericin B, angiotensin-converting enzyme (ACE) inhibitors and indomethacin, should be avoided. Standard charts are used for modifying the dose and dosing interval of antibiotics, depending on the severity of renal injury.

There is no beneficial effect of dopamine infusion on the outcome of AKI. Its routine use for prevention or treatment of ATN is therefore not recommended. The role of other medications, including fenoldopam, atrial natriuretic peptide, calcium-channel blockers (CCBs) and other medications is investigational.

RENAL REPLACEMENT THERAPY

Indications for initiating renal replacement therapy (RRT) include severe or persistent hyperkalemia (>7 mEq/L), fluid overload (pulmonary edema, severe hypertension), uremic encephalopathy, severe metabolic acidosis (TCO_2 < 10–12 mEq/L), severe (<120 mEq/L or symptomatic hyponatremia, or severe hypernatremia).

The initial RRT of choice in sick and unstable patients is often intermittent peritoneal dialysis (PD) as it is technically less challenging, is readily performed in all settings and requires limited expertise. It is easy to initiate in children of all ages including neonates. Peritoneal access can be obtained using a stiff catheter and trocar. While PD can be effectively performed with these catheters, these should be removed after 48–72 hours beyond which the risk of infection is very high. If the duration of AKI is prolonged, chronic PD may be performed, either manually (continuous ambulatory PD) or with the use of an automated device (continuous cycling PD).

Hemodialysis is more efficient for correction of fluid and electrolyte abnormalities. However, it is expensive to institute, requires expertise and skilled nursing and is not available at most centers in our country. It is not suited for patients with hemodynamic instability, bleeding tendency and in very young children where vascular access might be difficult. Continuous renal replacement therapy (CRRT) is useful when RRT is necessary in sick and unstable patients. Special equipment and trained staff are necessary to provide CCRT in children. Hemodialysis is less expensive than CRRT and should be the first RRT of choice in centers where it is available.

HEMOLYTIC UREMIC SYNDROME

Hemolytic uremic syndrome characterized by microangiopathic hemolytic anemia, thrombocytopenia, and renal impairment is one of the most common causes of AKI in children. The diarrhea-associated (classic) HUS occurs in childhood, usually caused by shiga toxin (verotoxin) producing bacteria (*Escherichia coli* 0157:H7, *Shigella dysenteriae*) and is associated with a satisfactory prognosis. More than 90% children recover normal renal function with supportive therapy. Atypical (nondiarrheal) HUS is a heterogeneous disorder with less favorable outcome. This condition is distinguished from classic HUS by absence of diarrheal prodrome, a chronic and relapsing course, high mortality and risk of end-stage renal disease (ESRD). Certain conditions (e.g. malignancy, systemic lupus erythematosus, hematopoietic stem cell transplantation) and drugs (e.g. cyclosporine, tacrolimus, ticlopidine) are also known to be associated with HUS, termed secondary HUS.

The diagnosis of HUS is made in presence of azotemia, thrombocytopenia (<100,000/mm^3) and hemolysis, occurring with or without history of preceding diarrhea or dysentery. The underlying histological lesion is a thrombotic microangiopathy (TMA) involving capillaries and small arterioles in the kidney. While histological changes are most marked in the kidneys, evidence of TMA might be present in the brain, heart, lungs, gastrointestinal tract, and pancreas.

Activation of the alternative complement pathway is important in an important proportion of cases. Defects in the genes for multiple components have been identified. These include loss of function mutations in complement factor H (*CFH*), membrane cofactor protein (*MCP*, CD46), complement factor I (*CFI*), factor H-related proteins 1-5 (*CFHR1-5*) and thrombomodulin, and gain of function mutations in *factor B* and *C3*. About 10–15% cases have been associated with autoantibodies against factor H (anti-CFH antibodies), particularly in the background of mutations in CFHR1/3 genes. Deficiencies of metalloproteinase with thrombospondin motifs 13 (ADAMTS13) and defective cobalamin metabolism are also rarely pathogenic.

Enterohemorrhagic *E. coli* (EHEC) or *S. dysenteriae* is the likely cause of HUS in patients older than 6 months with history of diarrhea or bloody diarrhea in the preceding 2 weeks. Serum levels of complement factors C3 and C4 should be estimated. A low level of C3 in a patient with normal C4 indicates selective activation of the alternative pathway. Where possible, blood samples are taken for estimation of FH, FI, complement factor B (FB), CD46 and anti-FH antibodies, before instituting plasmapheresis or infusing blood products.

Therapy for HUS includes the management of AKI. Specific management includes treatment of hematological complications, avoiding antidiarrheal drugs and monitoring for extrarenal involvement. Transfusion of packed red blood cells (RBC) is needed in patients with severe anemia (hemoglobin < 6 g/dL). Careful monitoring of blood pressure, urine output, and respiratory rate is necessary. Platelet transfusions are limited to children with active bleeding since they might contribute to microthrombi formation and promote tissue ischemia.

While recent evidence-based guidelines on therapy for atypical HUS recommend the use of eculizumab, a monoclonal antibody against C5 that prevents terminal complement cascade formation, the drug is expensive and not yet marketed in India. In absence of complement blockade, therapeutic plasma exchanges form the standard of care. Where this is not feasible, infusion of fresh-frozen plasma may be considered. Patients with anti-FH autoantibodies additionally benefit from administration of immunosuppressive medications.

BIBLIOGRAPHY

1. Bagga A, Bakkaloglu A, Devarajan P, et al. Improving outcomes from acute kidney injury: report of an initiative. Pediatr Nephrol. 2007;22(10):1655-8.
2. Noris M, Remuzzi G. Atypical hemolytic uremic syndrome. N Engl J Med. 2009;361(17):1676-87.
3. Ricci Z, Cruz D, Ronco C. The RIFLE criteria and mortality in acute kidney injury: a systematic review. Kidney Int. 2008;73(5):538-46.
4. Mehta R, Bagga A, Patibandla R, et al. Detection and management of AKI in the developing world: the 18th Acute Disease Quality Initiative (ADQI) International Consensus Conference. Kidney Int Rep. 2017;2(4):515-8.
5. Mian AN, Askenazi DJ, Mhanna MJ. Therapeutic options for neonatal acute kidney injury (AKI). Curr Treat Options Pediatr. 2016;2(2):69-81.
6. Blanco FC, Ortega G, Qureshi FG. Renal replacement therapy in children. Semin Pediatr Surg. 2015;24(1):25-31.
7. Honore PM, Jacobs R, Hendrickx I, et al. Prevention and treatment of sepsis-induced acute kidney injury: an update. Ann Intensive Care. 2015;5(1):51.
8. Ciccia E, Devarajan P. Pediatric acute kidney injury: prevalence, impact and management challenges. Int J Nephrol Renovasc Dis. 2017;10:77-84.
9. Fakhouri F, Zuber J, Fremeaux Bacchi V, Loirat C. Hemolytic uremic syndrome. Lancet. 2017;390(10095):681-96.

10.7 Nephrotic Syndrome

Arvind Bagga, Aditi Sharma

INTRODUCTION

Nephrotic syndrome is characterized by heavy proteinuria (more than 40 mg/m^2 per hour), hypoalbuminemia (albumin < 2.5 g/dL), hyperlipidemia (cholesterol > 200 mg/dL) and edema. It is a rare disease, with incidence of 1–6 per 100,000 children, varying by ethnicity and region. The large majority is primary (idiopathic); a secondary cause [amyloidosis, lupus, Henoch-Schönlein purpura (HSP)] is rare.

The therapy and outcome of nephrotic syndrome is determined by corticosteroid responsiveness and frequency of relapses. Most (>80%) children with idiopathic nephrotic syndrome show remission following therapy with oral corticosteroids (steroid-sensitive disease). The prognosis in these cases is favorable, contrasted to patients who do not respond (steroid resistance). The disease course in patients with steroid sensitive nephrotic syndrome is variable. While a few children have no relapses (20%) or 1–2 relapses a year (20–25%), about 40–50% patients show frequent relapses. A small proportion shows resistance after initial steroid responsiveness (late steroid resistance). **Table 10.7.1** lists definitions that clarify the course of nephrotic syndrome.

Table 10.7.1: Important definitions.

- *Remission*: Urine albumin nil or trace (or proteinuria < 4 mg/m^2/hour or spot protein: creatinine ratio < 0.2 mg/mg) for three consecutive early morning specimens and no edema.
- *Relapse*: Urine albumin 3+ or 4+ by dipstick (or proteinuria > 40 mg/m^2/hour or spot protein: creatine ratio > 2 mg/mg) for three consecutive early morning specimens, having been in remission previously.
- *Frequent relapses*: Two or more relapses within 6 months of discontinuing initial treatment or four or more relapses in any 12 months.
- *Steroid dependence*: Two consecutive relapses when on prednisolone on alternate days or within 14 days of its discontinuation.
- *Steroid resistance*: Absence of remission despite therapy with daily prednisolone at a dose of 2 mg/kg or 60 mg/m^2 for ≥ 4 weeks, in absence of significant infection.

CLINICAL PRESENTATION AND EVALUATION AT ONSET

Patients typically present between 2 years and 5 years of age, with progressive edema, initially periorbital and noticed in the morning. There may be an antecedent infection. Urine appears frothy or foamy; output may be reduced. Abdominal pain is usually attributed to mesenteric ischemia but may be secondary to bacterial peritonitis. Evaluation of a patient with suspected nephrotic syndrome includes history and physical examination, with attention to etiology, prior therapies, edema, blood pressure, anthropometry, and evidence of infections. Heavy (nephrotic range) proteinuria is presence of 3–4 + (300–1,000 mg/dL) urine protein by dipstick on early morning urine for three consecutive days, a spot urine

Table 10.7.2: Investigations at the first episode of nephrotic syndrome.

Essential
- Urinalysis: Proteinuria, red cells, casts
- Blood levels of urea, creatinine, albumin, cholesterol
- Complete blood counts
- Tuberculin test

If required
- C3 and antistreptolysin O (gross or persistent microscopic hematuria)
- Chest X-ray (positive tuberculin test; history of contact with tuberculosis)
- Hepatitis B surface antigen (if recent jaundice, raised levels of transaminases)
- Antinuclear antibodies (if features of systemic lupus erythematosus)
- Urine culture (if clinical features of urinary tract infection)

protein/creatinine ratio more than 2 mg/mg, or protein excretion more than 40 mg/m^2 per hour on a timed sample. A precise quantitative assessment of proteinuria is not necessary. Relevant investigations are listed in **Table 10.7.2**.

Indications for Biopsy

Most children with nephrotic syndrome do not require a biopsy during the disease course. A biopsy is indicated at the onset of nephrotic syndrome, if a cause other than minimal change nephrotic syndrome is likely:

- Age at onset less than 1 year or more than 16 years
- Gross or persistent microscopic hematuria, or low C3
- Renal failure, not attributed to hypovolemia
- Suspected secondary cause, and
- Sustained hypertension.

A biopsy is considered later in steroid resistance and prior to proposed use of calcineurin inhibitors.

MANAGEMENT OF THE INITIAL EPISODE

The adequacy of treatment of the initial episode, in terms of dose and duration of corticosteroids, is an important determinant of long-term course.

Agents

Prednisolone and prednisone are of proven benefit in patients with nephrotic syndrome. Other agents such as deflazacort, methylprednisolone, dexamethasone or triamcinolone should not be used. Prednisolone is given after meals to reduce gastrointestinal (GI) side effects; administration of antacids is usually not required.

Dose and Duration

Prednisolone is given at a dose of 2 mg/kg or 60 mg/m^2 daily (maximum 60 mg) in single or divided doses for 6 weeks, followed by 1.5 mg/kg or 40 mg/m^2 (maximum 40 mg) as a single morning dose on alternate days for the next 6 weeks. Therapy with corticosteroids is then stopped.

Evidence from controlled studies suggests that adequate initial steroid therapy (for 8–12 weeks or longer) is associated with reduced risk for relapses than shorter regimens. Recent studies indicate that further prolongation of initial therapy is not useful in ameliorating disease course; they also carry risk of steroid adverse effects. Based on available evidence and opinion from prospective studies, initial therapy with oral steroids is recommended for 12 weeks. Failure to achieve remission of proteinuria despite treatment with prednisolone in adequate doses for 4–8 weeks is labeled as steroid resistant nephrotic syndrome (SRNS).

THERAPY FOR RELAPSE

Relapses are often triggered by minor infections. Symptomatic therapy of infectious illness often results in remission of 1+/2+ proteinuria. However, persistence of 3+/4+ proteinuria with infections denotes a disease relapse that requires therapy. Prednisolone is given at a dose of 2 mg/kg/day until urine protein is trace or nil for three consecutive days (remission), and subsequently as a single morning dose of 1.5 mg/kg on alternate days for 4 weeks. Treatment for a relapse thus usually lasts for 5–6 weeks. Shorter regimens for treatment of relapses are being examined in controlled studies. The subsequent management of a patient with steroid sensitive nephrotic syndrome depends on the course of the illness.

Infrequent Relapses

Patients suffering from three or fewer relapses a year should receive treatment for each disease relapse as described earlier, i.e. prednisolone at 2 mg/kg/day (single or divided doses) until remission, followed by the same agent given in a single morning dose of 1.5 mg/kg on alternate days for 4 weeks. Therapy is then discontinued.

Frequent Relapses and Steroid Dependence

These patients require prolonged treatment to maintain disease remission. The strategies are summarized here. Patients are initially managed with low-dose prednisolone on alternate days; therapy with steroid-sparing agents is initiated when low-dose alternative-day steroid therapy fails or when severe adverse effects of steroids develop.

Long-term, Alternate Day Steroids

Following treatment of a relapse, prednisolone is tapered to a dose of 0.5–0.7 mg/kg on alternate days, which is given for 9–18 months. Relapses are often triggered by upper respiratory tract or other minor infections. Recent studies suggest that the risk of relapses is reduced, if prednisolone is administered daily for 5–7 days at the onset of infection in patients receiving corticosteroids on alternate days.

Steroid-sparing Agents

Alternative agents are recommended, if:

- Prednisolone threshold more than 0.5–0.7 mg/kg on alternate days; and
- Features of corticosteroid toxicity (growth failure, hypertension and cataract) appear.

The agents used are listed here:

Levamisole

- *Dose and duration*: 2–2.5 mg/kg on alternate days for 12–24 months.
- *Adverse effects*: Flu-like symptoms, neutropenia, hepatotoxicity, convulsions, skin rash.
- *Monitoring*: Total and differential leukocyte count, every 3–4 months.
- *Concomitant steroid therapy*: The dose of prednisolone is tapered to 0.25–0.5 mg/kg on alternate days and may be discontinued.

Cyclophosphamide

- *Dose and duration*: 2–2.5 mg/kg/day for 8–12 weeks (cumulative dose should not exceed 168 mg/kg; repeat courses are avoided).
- *Adverse effects*: Leukopenia, alopecia, vomiting, hemorrhagic cystitis, gonadal toxicity, malignancies.
- *Monitoring*:
  - Leukocyte counts are monitored every 2 weeks; cyclophosphamide is stopped, if the total leukocyte count is less than 4,000/mm^3; and
  - Fluid intake should be increased; patients are encouraged to void frequently.

Concomitant steroid therapy: Cyclophosphamide has a potent steroid-sparing potential, allowing discontinuation of steroids. The dose of prednisolone is maintained at 1 mg/kg during cyclophosphamide therapy; subsequently prednisolone is tapered and discontinued over 2–3 months.

Mycophenolate mofetil

- *Dose and duration*: 600–1,000 mg/m^2/day or 20–30 mg/kg/day for 12–36 months.
- *Adverse effects*: Uncommon; GI discomfort, diarrhea, leukopenia.
- *Monitoring*
  - Leukocyte counts are monitored every 1–2 months; treatment is withheld if count falls below 4,000/ mm^3; and
  - Side-effects mimic infectious gastroenteritis.

Concomitant steroid therapy: The agent has moderate steroid-sparing potential; prednisolone is tapered and discontinued over 3–6 months.

Calcineurin inhibitors [cyclosporine (CsA), tacrolimus]

These agents are indicated in patients with steroid dependence that fails to benefit with levamisole, cyclophosphamide and/or mycophenolate mofetil (MMF).

- *Dose and duration*: CsA 4–5 mg/kg/day; tacrolimus 0.1–0.2 mg/kg/day for 12–24 months.
- *Adverse effects*: Nephrotoxicity; hirsutism, gum hyperplasia; hypertension; hypercholesterolemia; hyperglycemia; headache and seizures; diarrhea.
- *Monitoring*: Monitor
  - Renal function every 3 months; and
  - Trough levels (CsA 80–120 ng/mL; tacrolimus 3–7 ng/mL), particularly if response is unsatisfactory, noncompliance is suspected and if nephrotoxicity; lipid profile and blood sugar
  - Repeat biopsy after 2–3 years of therapy, particularly, if further therapy is planned.

Relapses during therapy are treated with daily steroids, followed by tapering doses of prednisolone on alternate days. The occurrence of frequent relapses despite use of alternative agent is an indication for use of another agent.

Rituximab

Rituximab, a monoclonal antibody that depletes B cells, is shown to have considerable steroid-sparing efficacy that is comparable to calcineurin inhibitors. This biological agent is administered intravenously at 375 mg/m^2 in 2–3 doses one week apart, targeting CD19 depletion. The drug is effective in most patients with steroid-dependent nephrotic syndrome, allowing corticosteroid withdrawal and sustained remission for 9–24 months. Adverse effects are limited to mild infusion reactions (e.g. chills, rigors, rash) that are minimized by appropriate premedication, but severe complications such as acute lung injury and anaphylaxis are reported.

Flowchart 10.7.1 summarizes the protocol for management of patients with frequent relapses and steroid dependence.

STEROID-RESISTANT NEPHROTIC SYNDROME

Initial resistance is defined by the lack of remission at the first episode of nephrotic syndrome, and late resistance is considered in patients who are steroid sensitive initially but show steroid resistance during a subsequent relapse.

All children with steroid resistance (initial or late) should undergo renal biopsy before instituting specific treatment. Histology shows minimal change disease (MCD) and focal segmental glomerulosclerosis (FSGS) in 30–40% patients each, and mesangioproliferative glomerulonephritis (MesPGN) in a small group. Patients with MCD show a satisfactory response to therapy; FSGS with chronic

Flowchart 10.7.1: Management of in steroid-sensitive nephrotic syndrome.

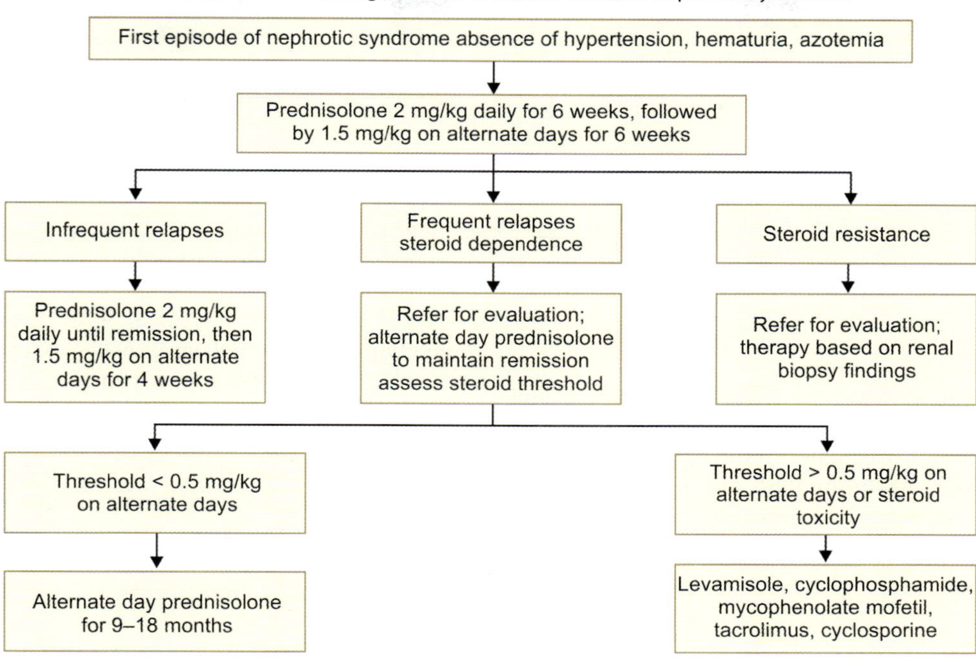

tubulointerstitial changes is associated with less satisfactory outcomes on the long-term.

Genetic Studies

About one-third patients with initial steroid resistance might show mutations in genes encoding podocyte proteins. While defects in over 75 genes are recognized, genes-encoding podocin (*NPHS2*), nephrin (*NPHS1*) and Wilms' tumor *(WT1)* are most commonly implicated. Such illness is unresponsive to immunosuppressive medications, progresses rapidly to end-stage renal disease (ESRD), and unlike nongenetic FSGS (which recurs after transplantation in 80%), does not recur. Where facilities exist, mutational analysis should be offered to patients with:

- Congenital nephrotic syndrome
- Family history of SRNS
- Sporadic initial resistance that does not respond to therapy with cyclophosphamide or calcineurin inhibitors
- Girls with steroid resistant FSGS (may have Frasier syndrome with *WT1* mutations).

Management

Patients with idiopathic SRNS secondary to MCD, FSGS or MesPGN are treated similarly. The chief factor predicting outcome is the response of proteinuria to therapy rather than the renal histology.

The aim of therapy in patients is to induce and maintain remission of proteinuria, while avoiding medication adverse effects. Most regimens use a combination of an immunosuppressive agent with prednisolone and enalapril **(Table 10.7.3)**. Significantly higher rates of remission are seen with calcineurin inhibitors as compared to other agents.

Calcineurin Inhibitors

Treatment with CsA or tacrolimus results in complete or partial remission of SRNS in almost 70–75% children. Adverse effects require close monitoring **(Table 10.7.3)**.

Cyclophosphamide

Oral cyclophosphamide has limited efficacy in inducing remission. Intravenous (IV) cyclophosphamide has modest success, when given monthly for six doses with tapering doses of prednisolone, inducing remission in 30–40%.

Pulse Corticosteroids with Cyclophosphamide

Pulses of IV methylprednisolone or dexamethasone were previously used in combination with oral cyclophosphamide with some efficacy. The risk of steroid toxicity is high, and patients show systemic infections, hypertension, and electrolyte abnormalities. Most expert guidelines do not recommend following this therapy.

Table 10.7.3: Agents used in the management of steroid resistant nephrotic syndrome.

Agent	*Dose*	*Duration*	*Efficacy*	*Adverse effects*
Cyclosporine (CsA)	4–5 mg/kg/day	12–36 months	60–70%	Acute and chronic nephrotoxicity; hirsutism and gum hyperplasia (CsA > Tac); hypertension; hypercholesterolemia (CsA > Tac); hyperglycemia (Tac); elevated transaminases; neurotoxicity (headache, seizures; Tac > CsA)
Tacrolimus (Tac)	0.1–0.2 mg/kg/day		70–75%	
Intravenous cyclophosphamide	500–750 mg/m^2	6 pulses	30–40%	Leukopenia; alopecia; nausea and vomiting; gonadal toxicity; hemorrhagic cystitis

Other Options

Therapies with limited efficacy in patients with SRNs include rituximab, combination of CsA and MMF, abatacept (CTLA-4 agonist), anti-tumor necrosis factor-alpha antibodies, adrenocorticotropic hormone, and plasmapheresis. Very recently, low-density lipoprotein apheresis using Liposorber has been successfully used patients with refractory FSGS.

Prednisolone

Prednisolone is a component of all regimens used in therapy of SRNS. The agent is given on alternate days at 1 mg/kg/day for 2–3 months, following which the dose is tapered.

Angiotensin-converting Enzyme Inhibitors, Angiotensin Receptor Blockers

Therapy with angiotensin-converting enzyme inhibitors (ACEIs, enalapril 0.3–0.6 mg/kg/day; ramipril 6 mg/m^2 q24h) is associated with decrease in proteinuria and control of hypertension. Adverse effects include dry cough, hyperkalemia and decline in renal function. Angiotensin receptor blockers (losartan, valsartan) may be used in case of persistent dry cough or as add-on for better antiproteinuric effect.

Monitoring

Patients are monitored for proteinuria (dipstick, spot samples), blood levels of creatinine and albumin, and edema every 2–3 months. While the aim of treatment is complete remission, the occurrence of partial remission is satisfactory. Most patients who respond to treatment do so within 6 months. Therapy is considered not effective and discontinued, if nephrotic range proteinuria persists beyond 6 months. Patients that fail therapy with one regimen may show response to different agents.

Monitoring for drug levels is recommended when using CsA or tacrolimus, because variable bioavailability might result in either subtherapeutic or toxic levels. Trough level (sample drawn 15–30 minutes prior to due dose) is estimated 2 weeks after introduction of therapy or suspecting toxicity or poor compliance. Trough levels of 80–120 ng/mL for CsA and 4–7 ng/mL for tacrolimus are acceptable.

Examination of renal histology may be useful in patients with persistent decline in renal function (creatinine > 50% above baseline) despite reduced dose or discontinued treatment. Since prolonged therapy might show histological nephrotoxicity, in presence of normal levels of creatinine, biopsy is advised in patients receiving therapy with CsA or tacrolimus for longer than 3 years.

CONGENITAL NEPHROTIC SYNDROME

Congenital nephrotic syndrome is defined as the presence of nephrotic syndrome within the first 3 months of life. This condition has diverse etiologies. While inherited defects in genes encoding key podocyte proteins underlie almost 80% cases, rare causes include intrauterine infections and maternal drugs. Genomic sequencing of *NPHS1* enables diagnosis of the Finnish nephrotic syndrome. Mutations in other genes (*NPHS2, WT1, PLCE* and *LAMB2*) might be important in other cases. A correct diagnosis is important for prognosis, therapy, and genetic counseling. Immunosuppression has no role in managing infants with congenital nephrotic syndrome. ACEIs (enalapril 0.2–0.5 mg/kg/day) are effective in reducing proteinuria. Supportive care includes adequate nutrition, supplementation of vitamin D, thyroxine and multivitamins, judicious use of diuretics, and regular administration of IV albumin. Progression of ESRD is usual during the first decade of life and parents should be counseled about the imminent need for renal replacement therapy.

SUPPORTIVE CARE AND MANAGEMENT OF COMPLICATIONS

Edema

Daily administration of corticosteroids results in diuresis within 2–4 days. Therapy for edema is therefore not required in most patients with steroid sensitive nephrotic syndrome. Patients with significant edema require treatment with diuretics. Anasarca results in discomfort and an increased risk of infections and should be avoided.

Short-term therapy with furosemide (1–3 mg/kg/day, in 1–2 doses) is effective; therapy beyond 3–4 days is rarely necessary. Edema that does not respond to maximal doses of furosemide requires coadministration of a thiazide. If furosemide is used for prolonged duration or at high doses, therapy with spironolactone (2–4 mg/kg/day) prevents the occurrence of hypokalemia. Patients with refractory edema are hospitalized and given IV furosemide either as bolus injections (1–3 mg/kg/dose, infused over 15–20 minutes) or as infusion (0.1–1 mg/kg/hour), under close monitoring.

Infusions of albumin (20% albumin, 0.5–1 g/kg over 2–4 hours), with IV furosemide, administered at the end of the infusion, are useful in patients with evidence of hypovolemia (see below) or severe hypoalbuminemia (albumin < 1.5 g/dL). The effect is transient and repeat administration of albumin is often required. Albumin infusions should be given carefully in patients with respiratory distress, hypertension, and impaired kidney function.

Hypovolemia

Hypovolemia may occur during a disease relapse or following administration of diuretics, particularly in children with poor oral intake, diarrhea, and vomiting. Patients complain of abdominal pain, lethargy, dizziness, and leg cramps. Signs include the presence of tachycardia, hypotension, delayed capillary refill, low volume pulses, and cold peripheries. An elevated ratio of blood urea to creatinine, rising hematocrit and urine sodium less than 20 mEq/L suggest the presence of hypovolemia. Patients require admission and rapid infusion of normal saline (10–20 mL/kg) over 20–30 minutes. Patients who do not respond to two saline boluses should receive infusion of 5% albumin (10–15 mL/kg) or 20% albumin (0.5–1 g/kg).

Infections

Table 10.7.4 provides a summary of management of common bacterial infections in patients with nephrotic syndrome. During serious infections, steroids should be administered daily at stress doses **(see Table 10.7.4)**.

Varicella may be life-threatening illness in immunocompromised patients. All patients should receive oral acyclovir (80 mg/kg/day in four doses) for 7 days; severe illness requires admission and administration of IV acyclovir. Administration of varicella zoster immunoglobulin (in a single dose within 96 hours of exposure), or IV immunoglobulin (400 mg/kg, single dose) might prevent or lessen the severity of the disease in susceptible individuals exposed to varicella.

Children with nephrotic syndrome and positive tuberculin test in absence of evidence of tuberculosis should receive prophylaxis with isoniazid for 6 months.

Thrombosis

Children with nephrotic syndrome are predisposed to venous thrombosis during relapses, due to loss of antithrombin III, low-intravascular volume, immobilization, indwelling vascular catheters, and puncture of deep vessels. Cerebral venous sinus thrombosis is the most common site; children usually present with headache, interfering with daily activities and/or sleep, during the first episode of untreated relapse. The use of diuretics in a child with intravascular volume depletion due to low intake and/or diarrhea or vomiting predisposes to thrombosis. Diagnosis requires confirmation with magnetic resonance imaging (MRI) with venography. Therapy is with low molecular weight heparin initially, followed by oral warfarin. Patients with persistently low serum albumin levels (e.g. congenital nephrotic syndrome, patients refractory to calcineurin inhibitors) may benefit from prolonged therapy with aspiring/or oral anticoagulants.

Hyperlipidemia

Patients with steroid resistance may show persistent dyslipidemia due to abnormalities in lipid metabolism, leading to hypercholesterolemia, hypertriglyceridemia, and various lipoprotein abnormalities. Treatment is usually with

Table 10.7.4: Management of systemic bacterial infections in nephrotic syndrome.

Infection	*Drug (dose)*	*Duration*
Peritonitis	Intravenous (IV) cefotaxime (100–150 mg/kg/day) or IV ceftriaxone (75–100 mg/kg/day)	7–10 days
Cellulitis	IV cloxacillin (100–200 mg/kg/day) + IV ceftriaxone (50–100 mg/kg/day) *or* IV co amoxiclav (100 mg/kg/day) amoxicillin) Shift to oral cloxacillin (100 mg/kg/day) or coamoxiclav (30–40 mg/kg/day) once erythema and induration resolve	10 days
Pneumonia	Coamoxiclav (30–40 mg/kg/day) or cephadroxil (30 mg/kg/day)	7–10 days
	Atypical, nonsevere: Azithromycin (10 mg/kg/day), if atypical pathogens likely	3–5 days
	Severe: IV cefotaxime (100–150 mg/kg/day) or ceftriaxone (75–100 mg/kg/day)	7–10 days
	Severe infection with S aureus: Teicoplanin (10 mg/kg/day) or vancomycin (40–60 mg/kg/day) with or without amikacin (15 mg/kg/day)	10–14 days

atorvastatin (10–20 mg/day) with monitoring of liver function and creatinine kinase.

Vaccination

Live vaccines (oral polio, varicella) are deferred until the child is off immunosuppressive medications for at least 4 weeks. Two doses of the varicella vaccine are given 4 weeks apart, while the child is in remission and off immunosuppressive medications. Injectable polio vaccine should be administered to children with nephrotic syndrome and their siblings.

The administration of pneumococcal vaccine is desirable. Children below 2 years of age should receive the pneumococcal conjugate vaccine. Above 2 years of age, one dose of the conjugate vaccine is given, followed 2 months later by the polysaccharide vaccine (PPV23). Children who continue to have relapses of nephrotic syndrome may receive one repeat dose of PPV23, 5 years after the primary vaccination. Patients on prolonged immunosuppression should receive the killed influenza vaccine annually.

Nutrition

During remission, children should eat a balanced and nutritious diet. Salt restriction is advised in patients with anasarca; undue restrictions that make food unpalatable are not required. Patients with persistent or recurrent proteinuria should increase their daily intake of proteins to 2–2.5 g/kg. Those receiving prolonged (>3 months) steroid therapy should receive supplements of calcium carbonate (250–500 mg) and vitamin D (125–250 IU).

Stress Doses of Steroids

Patients who have received steroids at high doses for more than 2 weeks in the past year are at risk of suppression of the hypothalamic-pituitary-adrenal axis. These children require steroid supplements during surgery, anesthesia or serious infections, which are given as parenteral hydrocortisone (2–4 mg/kg/day) followed by oral prednisolone (0.3–0.6 mg/kg/day). The medications are given for the duration of stress and tapered rapidly.

Parent Education and Counseling

The parents are explained the natural history of the disease, and the likely adverse effects of repeated courses of high-dose corticosteroids and other medications. The patient should return for follow-up at 2 and 4 weeks of therapy of the initial episode, and during disease relapses. The need to examine urine protein at home (by either dipstick or boiling method) is emphasized. Parents should maintain a diary, recording urine protein excretion, intake of medications, and intercurrent illnesses. The record provides useful assessment of patient's disease status and course, including steroid threshold for relapses.

BIBLIOGRAPHY

1. Bagga A, et al. Indian Pediatric Nephrology Group, Indian Academy of Pediatrics, Management of steroid sensitive nephrotic syndrome: revised guidelines. Indian Pediatr. 2008;45(3):203-14.
2. Bagga A, Mantan M. Nephrotic syndrome in children. Indian J Med Res. 2005;122(1):13-28.
3. Gulati A, Bagga A, et al. Indian Society of Pediatric Nephrology. Management of steroid resistant nephrotic syndrome. Indian Pediatr. 2009;46(1):35-47.
4. Hodson EM, Hahn D, Craig JC. Corticosteroids for the initial episode of steroid-sensitive nephrotic syndrome. Pediatr Nephrol. 2015;30(7):1043-6.
5. Hodson EM, Wong SC, Willis NS, et al. Interventions for idiopathic steroid-resistant nephrotic syndrome in children. Cochrane Database Syst Rev. 2016;10:CD003594.
6. Lombel R, Gipson DG, Hodson EM. Treatment of steroid-sensitive nephrotic syndrome: New Guidelines from KDIGO. Pediatr Nephrol. 2013;28(3):415-26.
7. Noone DG, Iijima K, Parekh R. Idiopathic nephrotic syndrome in children. Lancet. 2018;392(10141):61-74.
8. Pravitsitthikul N, Willis NS, Hodson EM, et al. Noncorticosteroid treatment for nephrotic syndrome in children. Cochrane Database Syst Rev. 2013;(10):CD002290.
9. Tullas K, Webb H, Begga A. Steroid-resistant nephrotic syndrome. Lancet Child Adolsc Hlth. 2018; 2(12):880-90.

10.8 Urinary Tract Infection, Vesicoureteric Reflux, and Reflux Nephropathy

Aditi Sinha

URINARY TRACT INFECTIONS

Urinary tract infections (UTIs) are among the most common infections of childhood. About 2–8% of children develop UTI by the age of 14 years; the risk being approximately 1–3% in boys and 3–10% in girls. During infancy, the male to female ratio is 3–5:1. However, beyond 1–2 years, there is a female preponderance with male to female ratio of 1:10. The diagnosis of UTI is often missed in infants and young children since symptoms are nonspecific. Prompt identification and adequate management are mandatory to prevent renal cortical scarring, which can lead to progressive parenchymal damage and hypertension. Young age, delayed or inadequate antibacterial therapy, recurrent infections, voiding dysfunction and associated high grades of vesicoureteric reflux (VUR) are risk factors for renal scarring in young children.

Clinical Features

Newborns with UTI present with septicemia, jaundice, vomiting, and shock. In infancy, symptoms are nonspecific, such as unexplained fever, diarrhea, vomiting, and failure to thrive. UTIs are an important cause of fever without focus in children below 2 years of age. Older children have dysuria, increased frequency, and suprapubic pain. Fever, flank pain, and toxic appearance suggest renal parenchymal involvement (complicated UTI). Any febrile UTI in a young child should be considered as pyelonephritis.

Examination should include evaluation for features suggesting underlying structural abnormalities, such as distended bladder, palpable enlarged kidney(s), tight phimosis in a boy, vulval synechiae in a girl, palpable fecal lump(s) in the abdomen, patulous anus, neurological deficit in lower limbs, urinary incontinence, and evidence of previous surgery of the urinary tract, anorectal malformation or meningomyelocele.

Etiology and Pathogenesis

Urinary tract infections are usually caused by ascending infection from the urethra to the bladder and/or kidneys. Infections spread by the hematogenous route are common in newborns. The most common cause of UTI in children is *Escherichia coli* (60–80%). Other organisms, such as *Proteus, Klebsiella, Staphylococcus saprophyticus, Streptococcus faecalis, Enterococcus* and *Enterobacter*, are chiefly isolated in immunocompromised children, nosocomial setting or following prolonged urinary catheterization. Preterm infants, immunocompromised children and those receiving prolonged antibiotics are at risk of *Candida* UTI.

Diagnosis

Urinary tract infection is suggested by the presence of leukocytes at more than 5 white blood cells (WBCs) per high power field (HPF) in centrifuged urine (spun at 2,000 rpm for 10 minutes), and bacteria on microscopic examination of a carefully collected fresh sample of urine. Presence of bacteriuria on noncentrifuged urine indicates more than 10^4 bacteria/mL. Presence of white cell casts is highly suggestive of UTI. Enhanced urinalysis includes evaluation of noncentrifuged urine for leukocyturia (>10 WBC/mm^3 in Neubauer counting chamber) along with Gram staining (any bacteria per 10 oil immersion fields).

The nitrite test, based on the bacterial enzyme nitrate reductase that converts urinary nitrate to nitrite, is 98% specific for UT, it may be falsely negative in children with urinary frequency resulting in insufficient time for incubation of bacteria in urine, or during infection with bacteria lacking nitrate reductase, e.g. *Streptococcus*. Staining for the neutrophil enzyme leukocyte esterase detects leukocyturia; however, white cells may be excreted in urine in diverse conditions such as interstitial nephritis and glomerulonephritis. The combination of these two rapid tests has high sensitivity and specificity in making a diagnosis of UTI, particularly when combined to positive enhanced urinalysis.

The gold standard for diagnosis of UTI is urine culture. The threshold bacterial colony count for making a diagnosis of UTI depends on the method of collection of urine. UTI is diagnosed in presence of a colony count of more than 10^5 colony-forming units (CFUs)/mL when urine is collected by a standard midstream clean catch specimen. On samples collected by urethral catheterization, a colony count of more than 5×10^4 CFU/mL indicates UTI. A lower colony count usually indicates urinary contamination unless the child has received antimicrobial therapy. If urine sample is obtained by suprapubic aspiration (e.g. infants), any number of pathogens can indicate UTI. Urine culture is not recommended on samples collected from the urinary bag.

Other investigations at evaluation of UTI should include complete blood counts, blood urea, serum creatinine, and electrolytes. Leukocytosis and raised C-reactive protein and procalcitonin are nonspecific findings that do not confirm the diagnosis of UTI.

Definitions

The diagnosis of UTI requires demonstration of significant bacteriuria on urine culture in the presence of symptoms. Important definitions are listed here:

- *Significant bacteriuria*: Count of more than 10^5 CFU/mL of a single bacterial species in a midstream clean catch sample of urine.
- *Asymptomatic bacteriuria*: Significant bacteriuria without symptoms of UTI.
- *Recurrent UTI*: Occurrence of two or more episodes of UTI.
- *Complicated UTI*: Fever more than 39°C, systemic toxicity, persistent vomiting, dehydration, renal angle tenderness or raised serum creatinine.
- *Simple UTI*: Dysuria, frequency or urgency with or without fever, and none of the symptoms of complicated UTI.

The term complicated UTI implies upper tract infection or acute pyelonephritis, while dysuria and frequency indicate lower tract involvement (cystitis, urethritis).

Management

Prompt treatment is needed to reduce the morbidity of infection and minimize renal damage and subsequent complications. Hospital admission is required in young infants (<3 months), patients with systemic toxicity (complicated UTI), dehydration or inability to retain orally, and if noncompliance is likely. Useful empirical parenteral antibiotics, used as monotherapy, include ceftriaxone, cefotaxime, amikacin, gentamicin, and coamoxiclav. Treatment is modified later according to antimicrobial sensitivity. After 48–72 hours of parenteral therapy, once the patient improves, therapy is switched over to oral medications. Useful choices include cefixime, coamoxiclav, ciprofloxacin, ofloxacin, and cephalexin. Patients older than 3 months with simple UTI are treated with oral antibiotics from diagnosis. With adequate therapy, fever resolves and symptoms reduce by 48–72 hours. Failure to respond to therapy may be due to resistant pathogens, complicating factors or noncompliance, and requires evaluation. The optimal duration of therapy is not established; no difference in efficacy is demonstrated when given for 7, 10 or 14 days. Therapy is administered for 7–10 days in simple UTI and for 10–14 days in complicated UTI; therapy for even 3–5 days may suffice in lower tract infections.

Supportive therapy includes maintenance of adequate hydration and control of fever. Parenteral fluids are indicated in febrile children within adequate oral intake or dehydration. A repeat urine culture is not necessary, unless there is persistence of fever and toxicity despite 72 hours of adequate antibiotic therapy.

Chemoprophylaxis

Following treatment of UTI, prophylactic antibiotic therapy is initiated in children below 1 year of age, until appropriate imaging of the urinary tract is completed. Drugs used include cotrimoxazole (1–2 mg/kg/day), cephalexin (10 mg/kg/day), cephadroxil (5 mg/kg/day) or nitrofurantoin (1–2 mg/kg/day), administered in a single dose at bedtime. The chief intent is to keep urine sterile, particularly in patients with VUR. Chemoprophylaxis is administered for 12–48 months, depending upon associated anomalies and UTI recurrence.

Imaging Studies

The aim of imaging following the diagnosis of UTI is to identify urinary tract abnormalities that predispose to UTI and to detect renal scarring **(Flowchart 10.8.1)**. All children presenting for the first time with UTI should undergo an ultrasonography, which may demonstrate renal anomalies, dilated or irregular pelvicalyceal system and severe parenchymal scarring. However, an ultrasound is insensitive to detecting mild hydronephrosis or ureteric dilatation associated with VUR, acute pyelonephritis, and mild renal scarring.

Demonstration of reduced cortical uptake during ^{99}Tc-dimercaptosuccinic acid (DMSA) scan during the acute phase of UTI is sensitive and specific in detecting

Flowchart 10.8.1: Evaluation following the first febrile urinary tract infection.

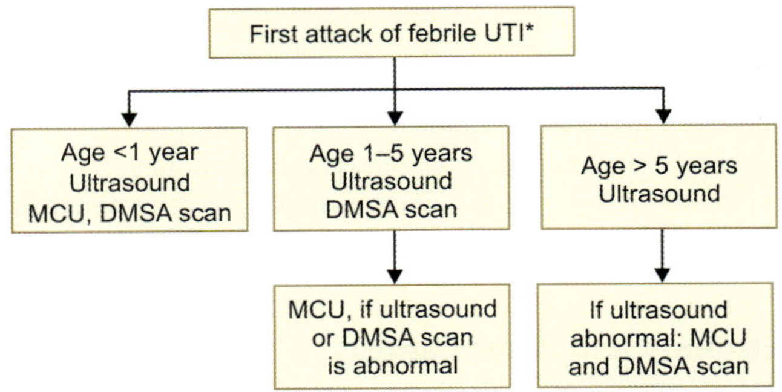

*All children with recurrent UTI need detailed evaluation with ultrasonography, DMSA scan, and MCU.
(DMSA: dimercaptosuccinic acid; MCU: micturating cystourethrogram; UTI: urinary tract infection)

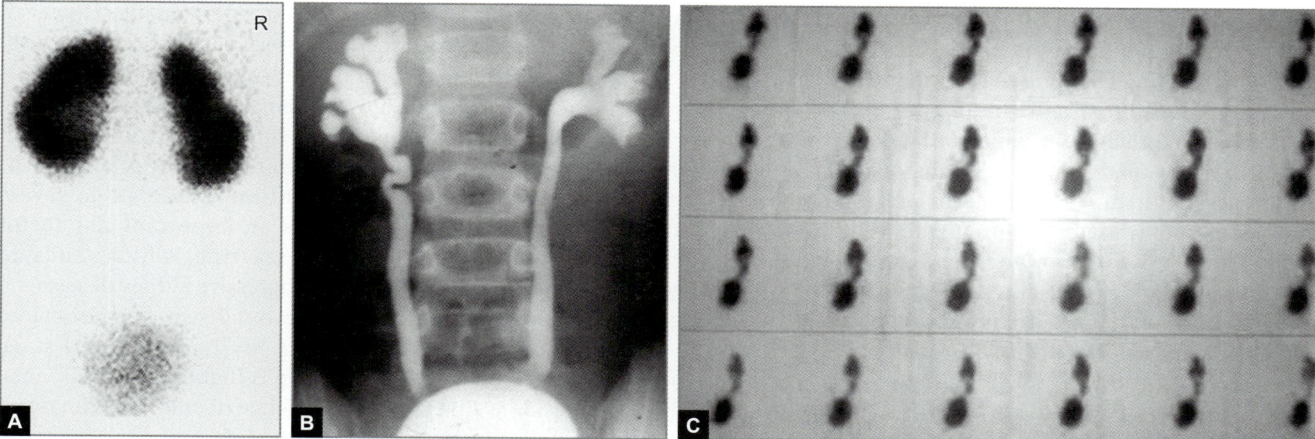

Figs. 10.8.1A to C: Imaging studies in an 18-month-old girl with recurrent urinary tract infections since 6 months of age. (A) Dimercapto-succinic acid shows multiple scars and loss of volume in the right kidney while the left kidney is normal; (B) Micturating cystourethrography showed bilateral grade V vesicoureteric reflux; the ureters appear dilated and tortuous while the calyces show cupping; and (C) Direct radio-nuclide cystourethrography (DRCG) at 4 years of age shows persistence of severe reflux on the right side.

pyelonephritis. More often, DMSA is used at 2–4 months of follow-up to identify cortical scars **(Fig. 10.8.1A)**. An abnormal DMSA suggests underlying significant VUR.

Cystourethrography is an invasive procedure that requires catheterization, risking UTI, and exposes the child to radiation. Micturating cystourethrography (MCU) involves filling the bladder up with radiocontrast, followed by capturing of images during voiding. MCU is the gold standard for diagnosing and staging VUR **(Figs. 10.8.1B and 10.8.2)**. The anatomy of bladder and urethra are defined well during an MCU, helping detect bladder abnormalities due to lower tract dysfunction caused by neurogenic bladder or obstruction by posterior urethral valves. Both MCU and ultrasound allow the assessment of residual urine. An MCU should be performed only after adequate control of infection.

As compared to MCU, direct radionuclide cystourethrography (DRCG) is more sensitive at detecting VUR at a lower radiation exposure. It is a useful alternative to MCU for repeat evaluations for persistence of VUR during follow-up **(Fig. 10.8.1C)**. It is not recommended for initial screening as it does not detail the anatomy of bladder and urethra.

The approach to radiological evaluation following the first episode of UTI is based on the balance between risks with investigations and benefits of improving outcome by detecting abnormalities such as significant VUR **(Flowchart 10.8.1)**. The likelihood of underlying significant abnormalities as well as the opportunity for improving outcomes through early detection is highest for UTI presenting in infancy. Hence, the Indian Society of Pediatric Nephrology recommends that infants presenting with the first episode of UTI should undergo an ultrasound, DMSA scan, and MCU. Children between 1 year and 5 years should undergo ultrasonography and DMSA scan following the first episode of UTI, and an MCU if ultrasound or DMSA scan is abnormal. Children above 5 years of age with the first attack should be evaluated with an ultrasound alone; MCU and DMSA are needed if the ultrasound is abnormal. All children with recurrent UTI need detailed evaluation with ultrasonography, DMSA scan, and MCU.

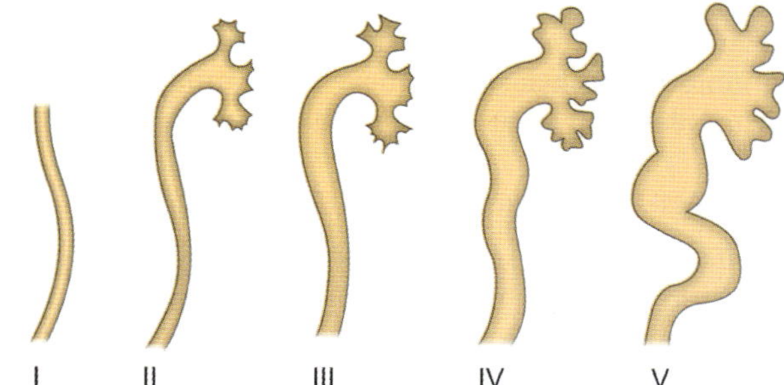

Fig. 10.8.2: Graphic representation of the grading of vesicoureteric reflux on micturating cystourethrogram.

RECURRENT UTI AND VOIDING DYSFUNCTION

About 30–50% children with UTI show recurrence of symptoms, usually within 3 months of the first UTI, and usually with the same pathogen as previously. Any child with recurrent UTI should undergo thorough clinical examination and review of imaging studies to evaluate for risk factors such as VUR, obstruction of the urinary system, neurogenic bladder, constipation, and bowel bladder dysfunction (voiding dysfunction).

Features that suggest bowel bladder dysfunction include constipation, impacted stools, and maneuvers to postpone voiding (holding maneuvers, e.g. Vincent curtsy, squatting) and infrequent voiding (<4 times a day). Other abnormalities include straining or poor urinary stream, and thickened bladder wall (>2 mm), significant post void residue (>20 mL) and spinning top configuration of bladder on ultrasound or MCU. Children with VUR, bowel bladder dysfunction, obstruction, and neurogenic bladder require multidisciplinary approach to their management, involving consultations with both urology and nephrology, retraining of toilet habits and therapy of constipation.

There is limited benefit from long-term daily administration of a low dose of antibiotic to prevent UTI. However, while awaiting clear demonstration of benefit or harm, antibiotic prophylaxis is administered in patients with (i) VUR; and (ii) recurrent febrile UTI, even if VUR or other significant predisposing factors have been excluded. The drugs most commonly used include nitrofurantoin and cotrimoxazole, given at bedtime daily; cephalexin is preferred in young infants (<6 months old) and in those with deficiency of glucose 6-phosphate dehydrogenase. Patients on antibiotic prophylaxis may have breakthrough UTI due to noncompliance or development of bacterial resistance.

ASYMPTOMATIC BACTERIURIA

Screening of normal school children may reveal significant bacteriuria in 0.05% boys and 1% girls. In most cases, the organism is *E. coli* of low virulence that colonizes the lower tract. Treating such colonization may lead to symptomatic infections with more virulent organisms. Hence, asymptomatic bacteriuria does not merit any treatment, even in the presence of VUR.

VESICOURETERIC REFLUX AND REFLUX NEPHROPATHY

Vesicoureteric reflux implies passage of urine into the ureter during micturition. Normally, the long submucosal and intravesical segment of the ureter at the ureterovesical junction closes when the bladder contracts, effectively preventing VUR. Incompetence of ureterovesical junction due to shortening and lack of obliquity of the submucosal and intravesical segments results in VUR. Primary VUR is an isolated defect that has a genetic basis and may occur in siblings. VUR may be secondary to bladder outflow obstruction (e.g. posterior urethral valves), neurogenic bladder or a functional voiding disorder.

During micturition, VUR allows the rise in intravesical pressure to be transmitted to the ureter and renal pelvis, which enables urine to enter papillary collecting ducts and renal tubules (intrarenal reflux). Thus, pathogenic organisms present in the bladder can reach the renal parenchyma and initiate inflammation and subsequent scarring. However, renal damage may occur even in sterile urine, possibly due to the transmitted pressure or by immunological mechanisms.

One-third of children with febrile UTI have underlying VUR. VUR is present in 30–50% of children with recurrent febrile UTI and renal cortical scarring. Low grades (I-III) of VUR are likely to resolve over time. Moderate-to-severe VUR, particularly if bilateral, is an important risk factor for pyelonephritis and renal scarring, which leads to hypertension, proteinuria and progressive kidney disease.

Reflux nephropathy refers to renal scarring associated with primary VUR. It accounts for 7–17% of end-stage renal disease. The risk of scarring is highest among infants. Intrauterine VUR, even in the absence of infection, can result in renal dysplasia or hypoplasia. Most patients with renal dysplasia have severe VUR and no documented UTI.

Clinical Features

Children with VUR may present with recurrent febrile UTI with or without structural anomalies of the urinary tract. VUR may be detected following evaluation of antenatally detected hydronephrosis or during screening of offsprings or siblings of patients with VUR (see below). Patients with reflux nephropathy may present with chronic acidosis, hypertension, and renal failure.

A high proportion of patients with VUR have bladder bowel dysfunction. Symptoms to be enquired include urgency, holding maneuvers, nocturnal and diurnal incontinence, frequency and constipation. Spinal dysraphism should be ruled out as a cause of secondary VUR.

Diagnosis

The severity of VUR is graded from I to V based on the appearance of the urinary tract on contrast MCU, using the International Study Classification **(Fig. 10.8.2)**. Mild-to-moderate VUR (grades I-III) is characterized by reflux in to nondilated or dilated ureter and upper collecting system. In severe VUR (grades IV–V), there is reflux in to grossly dilated and distorted ureter(s), pelvis, and calyces.

While DRCG is more sensitive and specific for the detection of VUR than MCU, it cannot delineate anatomic abnormalities, and the grading is not reliable. Hence, the use of DRCG is limited to follow-up studies **(Figs. 10.8.1A to C)**.

The DMSA scan is a sensitive technique to detect renal scarring in reflux nephropathy. Patients with imaging evidence of scars on the background of VUR require evaluation for evidence of hypertension or proteinuria.

Management of Vesicoureteric Reflux

Children with VUR and otherwise normal urinary tract are treated with long-term prophylaxis with nitrofurantoin, cotrimoxazole, cephalexin or cefadroxil while awaiting spontaneous resolution of VUR. Infants with VUR grades I and II receive antibiotic prophylaxis up to 1 year of age and continue to be followed up till 5–7-years of age. Children with grades III-V VUR should receive antibiotic prophylaxis up to 5 years of age. Beyond 5 years, prophylaxis is continued, if there is bowel bladder dysfunction. In all categories, antibiotic prophylaxis is restarted if breakthrough febrile UTI is noted. Training the child for double or triple voiding reduces the residual urine and is beneficial. Urine microscopy and culture are performed, whenever UTI is suspected.

Surgery for reflux is indicated in patients with:

- Recurrent breakthrough febrile UTIs while on prophylaxis;
- Nonresolution of grades III-V VUR by 5 years of age;
- Vesicoureteric reflux grades III-V associated with bilateral renal scarring beyond 2 years of age; and
- By parental choice (remote residence, anxiety).

There are two surgical options for correction of VUR. Subureteric injection of dextranomer/hyaluronic acid polymer (Deflux) is a day care technique, which is 70% effective in eliminating VUR in patients with grade III or IV VUR. A daycare minimal access extravesical ureteric reimplantation technique is also suitable for grades III or IV VUR. The cost of the implant and risk of failure, particularly in inexperienced hands or with bladder bowel dysfunction, limit its utility. The most effective method of reflux elimination is open surgical ureteric reimplantation.

Voiding dysfunction is an important reason for recurrences of UTI, particularly in children with VUR. Failure to manage this entity is a common cause of failure of antibiotic prophylaxis and/or surgery. Treating constipation and voiding dysfunction is an important component of the management of VUR in children.

Patients with renal scarring should be monitored for hypertension, proteinuria, and for physical growth. Investigations during follow-up include serum creatinine and electrolytes, urinalysis and ultrasound for renal growth. Radionuclide cystography can be repeated every 1–2 years to assess for resolution of VUR, especially in patients with VUR grades III-V. DMSA scan may be done to understand the prognosis. Most cases of grades I-III VUR resolve; higher grades of reflux may disappear in a small percentage of patients.

Screening of Siblings and Offspring

Vesicoureteric reflux is inherited in an autosomal dominant manner with incomplete penetrance. About 25% of siblings and 25–50% of offsprings of patients may have reflux. Majority of inherited VUR is low grade and not associated with UTI. Ultrasonography is the modality of choice to screen these individuals. Further imaging is required, if ultrasonography is abnormal or on occurrence of febrile UTI.

Long-term Follow-up

Children with renal scars (reflux nephropathy) are counseled regarding the need for early diagnosis and therapy of UTI, and regular follow-up. Physical growth and blood pressure should be monitored every 6–12 months through adolescence. Investigations include urinalysis for proteinuria and estimation of serum creatinine. Yearly ultrasound examinations are done to monitor renal growth. Patients with proteinuria and hypertension benefit from treatment with angiotensin-converting enzyme inhibitors (ACEIs) and angiotensin II receptor blockers.

BIBLIOGRAPHY

1. Balighian E, Burke M. Urinary tract infections in children. Pediatr Rev. 2018;39:3-12.
2. Garcia-Roig ML, Kirsch AJ. Urinary tract infection in the setting of vesicoureteral reflux. F1000Res. 2016:30:5.
3. Korbel L, Howell M, Spencer JD. The clinical diagnosis and management of urinary tract infections in children and adolescents. Paediatr Int Child Health. 2017;37:273-9.
4. Okarska-Napierała M, Wasilewska A, Kuchar E. Urinary tract infection in children: diagnosis, treatment, imaging: comparison of current guidelines. J Pediatr Urol. 2017;13:567-73.
5. Traisman ES. Clinical management of urinary tract infections. Pediatr Ann. 2016;45:e108-11.
6. Vijayakumar M, Kanitkar M, et al. Indian Society of Pediatric Nephrology, Revised statement on management of urinary tract infections. Indian Pediatr. 2011;48:709-17.
7. Yeung CK, Chowdhary SK, Sreedhar B. Minimally invasive management for vesicoureteral reflux in infants and young children. Clin Perinatol. 2017;44:835-49.

10.9 Disorders of Micturition and Obstructive Uropathy

Madhuri Kanitkar

INTRODUCTION

The continuous process of urine formation ends in an intermittent act of micturition due to the storage capacity of the urinary bladder. The bladder can empty to completion at an appropriate time and place, once control is achieved by 5 years of age. An aberration of this function results in a wet child, or a child who cannot void to completion. The disorders are classified as *primary functional voiding disorders,* which occur in the presence of an intact neuronal pathway and no congenital or anatomical abnormality of the urinary tract; or may be *secondary* to a neurological or structural anomaly.

Disorders of micturition are associated with recurrent urinary tract infections (UTIs) and vesicoureteric reflux (VUR). High bladder pressures combined with poor emptying result in stasis and infection, and back-pressure changes affect the pelvicalyceal system and the kidneys, which is an important cause for chronic kidney disease (CKD) in children.

NOMENCLATURE

The urinary bladder functions as a compliant compartment with adequate capacity and a competent sphincter. This process is controlled by the somatic and autonomic nervous system and the brain. The nomenclature for symptoms has been recently standardized **(Table 10.9.1)**. While continuous incontinence is almost always due to an underlying anatomical or neurological anomaly, intermittent incontinence is mostly functional.

The common embryological origin of the bladder and rectum (from the cloaca) results in functional disorders that affect both organs, termed bowel bladder dysfunction (BBD). Functional voiding disorders may be either overactive bladder when it is a filling phase disorder or dysfunctional voiding when it is an evacuation phase disorder due to bladder sphincter dyssynergia. A long-standing dyssynergic bladder may result in an overstretched low-pressure underactive

Table 10.9.1: Classification of disorders of micturition.

Term	***Definition***
Incontinence	Uncontrollable leakage of urine
Continuous	Constant leakage of urine usually due to anatomical/neurological causes
Intermittent	Urine leak in discrete amounts: daytime (functional voiding disorder); night-time (enuresis)
Storage symptoms	
Frequency	Increased if more than 8 times/day; decreased if less than 3 times/day
Urgency	Sudden and unexpected experience of immediate need to void
Nocturia	Child wakes up at night to void
Voiding symptoms	
Hesitancy	Difficult initiation of voiding or child waits a considerable period before voiding starts
Weak stream	Passage of urine with a weak force, relevant from infancy
Straining	Child applies abdominal pressure to initiate and maintain voiding
Intermittency	Micturition in several discrete spurts
Holding maneuvers	Strategies used to postpone voiding or suppress urgency such as standing on tiptoe, forcefully crossing the legs or squatting with the heel pressed into the perineum
Voiding postponement	Daytime incontinence with habitual postponement of micturition
Vaginal reflux	Toilet trained prepubertal girls who experience incontinence in moderate amounts, consistently occurring within 10 minutes after normal voiding

bladder leading to overflow incontinence. Severe bladder sphincter dyssynergia is noted in the Hinman syndrome where the urinary bladder is trabeculated, develops high pressure with bilateral VUR akin to neurogenic bladder without any obvious structural abnormality. Constipation is a major aggravating factor for bladder dysfunction.

Enuresis

More than 85% children have complete bladder control by 5 years of age. A child having bedwetting at least twice a month after the 5th year has enuresis and warrants attention. It is termed *primary* when the child has never been dry and *secondary* when bedwetting starts after a minimum period of 6 months of dryness at night. It is termed *monosymptomatic* if it is not accompanied by any lower urinary tract symptoms. This should be differentiated from voiding disorders when enuresis is accompanied with daytime urge symptoms.

Some of the factors responsible for enuresis are maturational delay, deep sleep and a loss of circadian rhythm of the antidiuretic hormone (ADH) secretion. A child may have nocturnal polyuria, with nocturnal urine output more than 130% of expected bladder capacity for age, resulting in enuresis. A genetic basis is well-known. Less than 5% children with primary monosymptomatic enuresis have an organic basis and most require no evaluation other than a urinalysis. History and clinical examination exclude an anatomical or neurological cause for incontinence. A voiding diary helps rule out voiding dysfunction, since the history of daytime symptoms may not be forthcoming.

TREATMENT

Timely treatment of nocturnal enuresis prevents psychological distress. Dry bed training includes emptying the bladder before retiring to bed, encouraging bedtime resolution and keeping a chart of wet and dry nights. The child should be rewarded for active cooperation in the therapy and not just for dry nights. Behavioral changes significantly improve the outcome and advice is given to drink more water during the daytime, avoid extra fluids after dinner, prevent constipation and increase physical activity. The child is encouraged for timely voiding. Studies have shown that neither bladder holding nor stretching exercises are efficacious.

The alarm device is used to elicit a conditioned response of awakening to the sensation of a full bladder. Several medications are used for treatment of nocturnal enuresis **(Table 10.9.2)**. Therapy once initiated is continued for 2 weeks before assessing efficacy and adjusting the dose. Once the child is dry the dose is maintained for 3–6 months and then weaned over 3–4 weeks. Anticholinergic drugs are useful in children who manifest urge symptoms. Desmopressin [1-deamino-8-D-arginine vasopressin (DDAVP)] is used in

Table 10.9.2: Medications used for enuresis.

Drug	*Dose*	*Side effects*	*Age for use*
DDAVP nasal spray	10–40 µg/day	Nasal stuffiness, hyponatremia, seizures	Any if supervised
DDAVP tablets	0.2–0.6 mg/day	Headache, epistaxis, nausea	Any
DDAVP lyophilisate	60–240 µg/day		
Oxybutynin	5–20 mg/day	Dryness of mouth, flushing, palpitations blurring of vision	Any
Tolterodine	2 mg at bedtime	Like oxybutynin but milder	>5 years
Imipramine	0.9–1.5 mg/kg/day	Anxiety, personality change palpitations	>7 years

(DDAVP: 1-deamino-8-D-arginine vasopressin)

patients showing high nocturnal urine production. The spray should be administered under the supervision to prevent accidental or intentional overdose.

Water restriction is recommended when using DDAVP to prevent hyponatremia. The oral tablet and the lyophilisate preparation now available in India have been found to be more effective with better compliance. Tricyclic antidepressants may be used if other therapeutic options have failed; however they are best avoided in young children.

The use of alarm is preferred in patients who do not respond to dry bed training and behavioral modifications. If the child is unresponsive to the alarm, DDAVP may be used as an adjunct. The latter is used initially if short-term benefits are necessary.

FUNCTIONAL VOIDING DISORDERS

A functional voiding disorder presents with daytime wetting or recurrent UTI. Children with enuresis refractive to therapy or a persistent VUR may also have voiding dysfunction.

A wet child requires systematic evaluation in a stepwise manner **(Flowchart 10.9.1)**. Clinical examination should include the lower back to look for clues suggesting spinal and sacral anomalies and the abdomen for palpable bladder and kidneys. The lower limbs are assessed for tone, power and sensations, and the perineum for ectopic ureters or epispadias.

A voiding diary is requested to include a frequency volume charting of urine output and oral fluid intake for 2–3 days with record of accidents/wetting. The voided volume of urine

Flowchart 10.9.1: A stepwise systemic evaluation of a wet child.

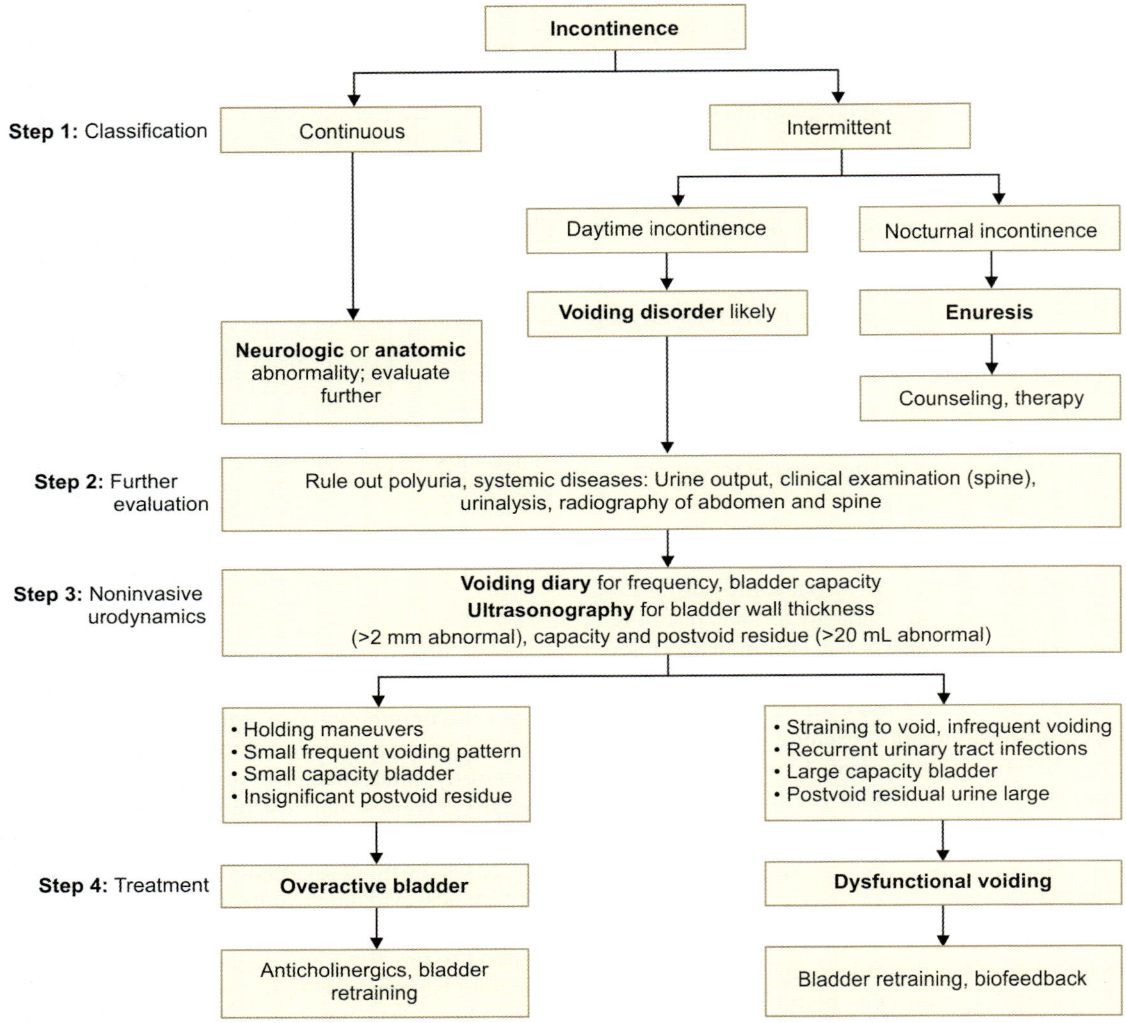

Incontinence

Step 1: Classification

- Continuous → **Neurologic** or **anatomic** abnormality; evaluate further
- Intermittent
  - Daytime incontinence → **Voiding disorder** likely
  - Nocturnal incontinence → **Enuresis** → Counseling, therapy

Step 2: Further evaluation

Rule out polyuria, systemic diseases: Urine output, clinical examination (spine), urinalysis, radiography of abdomen and spine

Step 3: Noninvasive urodynamics

Voiding diary for frequency, bladder capacity
Ultrasonography for bladder wall thickness (>2 mm abnormal), capacity and postvoid residue (>20 mL abnormal)

- • Holding maneuvers
  • Small frequent voiding pattern
  • Small capacity bladder
  • Insignificant postvoid residue
- • Straining to void, infrequent voiding
  • Recurrent urinary tract infections
  • Large capacity bladder
  • Postvoid residual urine large

Step 4: Treatment

- **Overactive bladder** → Anticholinergics, bladder retraining
- **Dysfunctional voiding** → Bladder retraining, biofeedback

each time is then compared to the expected capacity of the bladder. Ultrasonography of the abdomen is done to examine for dilatation of the upper tract, bladder wall thickness and the presence of postvoid residual urine. A magnetic resonance imaging (MRI) scan of the spine helps to detect an occult problem of the spinal cord, which might result in a neurogenic bladder. A micturating cystourethrogram (MCU) helps to determine the presence of and severity of VUR and delineates the posterior urethra if the patient has recurrent UTI. Urodynamic study may be required in some cases, especially those with daytime symptoms, holding maneuvers and abnormal voiding pattern with postvoiding residue. Uroflow study combined with electromyography (EMG) for pelvic floor muscles is less invasive and can delineate most children requiring further evaluation.

Treatment of UTI and (re) institution of structured voiding patterns with appropriate hydration, hygiene and timed voiding is important. Constipation should be corrected. In patients with overactive bladder, an anticholinergic medication (e.g. oxybutynin) is effective. Biofeedback therapy and computer games help in training children to develop relaxed voiding. In children with dysfunctional voiding with large postvoid residues, clean intermittent catheterization is advised.

OBSTRUCTIVE UROPATHY

This term is used to refer to a group of disorders characterized by either prevesical or bladder outlet obstruction (anatomical or functional) resulting in pelvicalyceal dilatation, increased

Table 10.9.3: Etiology and diagnosis of obstructive uropathy.

Bladder outlet obstruction	***Suspect***	***Diagnosis***
Posterior urethral valves	Antenatal hydronephrosis, weak stream, dribbling, recurrent urinary tract infections (UTI), palpable kidneys, urinary bladder, postvoid residue	Micturating cystourethrogram (MCU), cystoscopy
Urethral strictures/atresia	Straining, weak stream, history of urethral manipulations and/or trauma	Cystoscopy, MCU
Urogenital sinus anomalies, bladder agenesis, anorectal malformations	Continuous incontinence, abnormal external genitalia, recurrent UTI	MCU, cystoscopy, magnetic resonance urography
Neurogenic bladder	Sacral dimple, tuft of hair or pad of fat, meningomyelocele, neurological deficits, incontinence, weak urinary stream	Magnetic resonance imaging (MRI) spine, MCU, urodynamic studies
Prune belly syndrome	Poorly developed abdominal muscles	MCU
Supravesical obstruction	***Suspect***	***Diagnosis***
Pelviureteric junction obstruction, vesicoureteric junction obstruction	Antenatal hydronephrosis, recurrent UTI, abdominal mass	DTPA scintigraphy, intravenous pyelography (IVP)
Recurrent ureteric calculi	Ureteric colic, hematuria, recurrent UTI	DTPA scintigraphy, IVP, high resolution CT

(CT: computed tomography; DTPA: diethylenetriaminepentacetate)

back-pressure and renal damage. Stasis due to postvoid residual urine results in recurrent UTI leading to progressive increased renal damage. The long-term outcome depends on timing and severity of the obstruction and its relief. Common causes for obstructive uropathy are enumerated in **Table 10.9.3**.

The aim of treatment is preservation of renal function and prevention of UTI. Long-term follow-up is necessary and should comprise annual ultrasound, physical examination for growth, controlling blood pressure, urinalysis for proteinuria and estimation of blood creatinine.

BIBLIOGRAPHY

1. Kanitkar M. Disorders of micturition. In: Srivastava RN, Bagga A (Eds). Pediatric Nephrology, 5th edition. New Delhi: Jaypee Brothers Medical Publishers (P) Ltd.; 2011. pp. 464-90.
2. Kanitkar M, Ramamurthy HR. Bed wetting—silent suffering: an approach to enuresis and voiding disorders in children. Indian J Pediatr. 2013;80(9):750-3.
3. Nevéus T, von Gontard A, Hoebeke P, et al. The standardization of terminology of lower urinary tract function in children and adolescents: report from the standardization committee of the International Children's Continence Society. J Urol. 2006;176(1):314-24.
4. Nunes VD, O'Flynn N, Evans J, et al. Management of bedwetting in children and young people: summary of NICE guidance. BMJ. 2010;341:c5399.
5. Ramamurthy HR, Kanitkar M. Noninvasive urodynamic assessment in children—are they reliable? Indian J Pediatr. 2010;77(12):1400-4.
6. VandeWalle J, Rittig S, Bauer S, et al. Practical consensus guidelines for the management of enuresis. Eur J Pediatr. 2012;171(6):971-83.

10.10 Chronic Kidney Disease and Renal Replacement Therapies

Saumil Gaur, Kishore Phadke

CHRONIC KIDNEY DISEASE

Introduction

Chronic kidney disease (CKD) is an abnormality of kidney function or structure as determined by laboratory tests, urinalysis or imaging tests, with or without reduced glomerular filtration rate (GFR) less than 60 mL/min/1.73 m^2, which has been present for at least 3 months. It is usually of gradual onset; irreversible and has a progressive course irrespective of etiology. CKD results in significant societal burden due

Table 10.10.1: Stages of chronic kidney disease [National Kidney Foundation: Kidney Disease Outcome Quality Initiative (NKF-KDOQI)].

Stage	*Description*	*GFR (mL/min/1.73 m²)*
1	Kidney damage with normal or increased GFR	≥90
2	Kidney damage with mild decrease in GFR	60–89
3	Moderate decrease in GFR	30–59
4	Severe decrease in GFR	15–29
5	Kidney failure, end-stage renal disease	<15 (or dialysis)

(GFR: glomerular filtration rate)

Box 10.10.1: Features suggesting chronic kidney disease.

- Failure to thrive, not explained by malnutrition
- Unexplained anemia
- Bony deformities
- Unexplained polyuria
- Recurrent urinary tract infections
- Positive family history of renal disease
- Exposure to nephrotoxic drugs
- Systemic disease with known renal involvement
- Hypertension
- Persistent proteinuria, abnormal urinalysis
- Abnormal renal imaging

to its complications, disability, and economic implications. Early recognition and appropriate management of CKD can reduce its morbidity and retard the rate of progression.

The staging of CKD as proposed by National Kidney Foundation-Kidney Disease Outcome Quality Initiative (NKF-KDOQI) is useful to standardize definitions **(Table 10.10.1)** based on GFR. GFR is estimated by the modified Schwartz formula:

$$[k \times \text{height (cm)}/\text{creatinine (mg/dL)}]$$

Where, k is a constant (0.413 for all children from 1 year to 18 years irrespective of age and sex).

Patients with stage 5 CKD may have life-threatening biochemical abnormalities requiring renal replacement therapies (RRT), such as dialysis or transplantation for survival.

Etiology and Prevalence

The incidence and prevalence is underdiagnosed owing to lack to regional registries. Data from North America and European registries suggest the incidence to be 11–12 per million age-related population (PMARP) and prevalence of 50–60 pmarp for CKD stages 3–5. The causes of CKD in children are quite different in children compared to adults, whereas in adult's diabetes mellitus and hypertension are the leading causes, in children congenital causes are in forefront. Congenital malformations of the kidneys (e.g. hypoplastic or dysplastic kidneys, obstructive uropathy and posterior urethral valves) or genetic disorders (e.g. hyperoxaluria, polycystic kidney disease, congenital nephrotic syndrome and Wilms' tumor) are causes of CKD in young children. Glomerular diseases [nephrotic syndrome with focal segmental glomerulosclerosis (FSGS), hemolytic uremic syndrome (HUS), chronic glomerulonephritis, and Alport disease] or tubulointerstitial diseases (e.g. tubulointerstitial nephritis, cystinosis, nephronophthisis, and nephrotoxic drugs) predominate in older children.

Clinical Features

Chronic kidney disease may be asymptomatic especially in the early stages. The manifestations may be subtle, posing challenges in recognition **(Box 10.10.1)**.

Evaluation

Urine Tests

Urine analysis helps in establishing the glomerular or tubular nature of the primary disease, which leads to CKD. The degree of proteinuria and hematuria increases as CKD progresses. Urinary specific gravity is usually fixed at value of 1.010 due to loss of concentrating capacity of renal tubules in CKD known as isosthenuria.

Blood Tests

Blood urea and creatinine are commonly used to screen and monitor CKD. As function deteriorates, blood levels of these markers rise. Disproportionately high blood urea levels are seen during dehydration, high protein intake or hypercatabolic states (high fever, gastrointestinal bleed, steroid therapy, and sepsis). Serum calcium, phosphate, alkaline phosphatase and parathyroid hormone (PTH) levels assess the mineral bone disease (MBD). Serum electrolytes and bicarbonate levels are useful to assess electrolyte and acid-base disturbances. Serum cystatin C levels can be used instead of serum creatinine as these are independent of muscle mass. They are currently used only in research settings. GFR is estimated with help of serum creatinine, using the modified Schwartz formula. Radiolabeled iothalamate, diethylenetriamine penta-acetate (DTPA) or ethylene diaminetetra-acetic acid (EDTA) are exogenous biomarkers that may be used to estimate GFR.

Imaging Studies

Renal ultrasound is a noninvasive technique that provides useful information about the size, shape, echotexture, presence of cysts, evidence of obstruction, and renal stones. Renal scans are used to diagnose specific conditions, e.g. renal scars and differential renal functions.

Renal Biopsy

A percutaneous renal biopsy may be indicated in early course of CKD. In advanced stages of CKD, renal histopathology is not useful in determining the etiology as findings of glomerulosclerosis, tubular atrophy and interstitial fibrosis are nonspecific and fail to highlight the primary disease.

Management

The aims of conservative management are:

- Correct reversible component of renal dysfunction
- Slow the rate of progression of renal disease
- Treat metabolic derangements
- Optimize growth and development
- Prepare for treatment of end-stage renal disease (ESRD), plan RRT.

The clinical action pyramid for various stages of CKD is summarized in **Figure 10.10.1**.

Dietary Management

The diet aims at controlling hypertension, edema and electrolyte disturbances, and retarding progression of renal failure while promoting growth and development. The diet should provide recommended dietary allowances (for age and height) of calories and high biological value proteins. Restriction of sodium and fluid is necessary in oliguric or anuric renal failure. Children with polyuric renal failure often require sodium and water supplementation. Potassium restriction is required for children with CKD stage 5 to prevent hyperkalemia.

Anemia

The anemia of CKD is normocytic and normochromic. Causative factors include reduced erythropoietin synthesis, iron and folate deficiencies, occult blood losses, bone marrow suppression, decreased lifespan of red cells and secondary hyperparathyroidism. Anemia results in fatigue, anorexia, exercise intolerance, and poor cognitive performance and is an important cardiovascular risk factor. Oral iron is poorly absorbed in CKD. As GFR declines, parenteral iron may be needed to maintain the transferrin saturation index above 30%. The hemoglobin target should be selected in the range of 11–12 g/dL. The initial dose of recombinant human erythropoietin is 50–150 IU/kg/dose thrice a week given subcutaneously. The dose is titrated to obtain the desired response, while maintaining adequate iron stores. Darbepoetin-alpha has a longer half-life, allowing administration once in 1–2 weeks. Blood transfusions are avoided for fear of exposure to infectious agents and to avoid sensitization, increasing the risk of rejection following transplantation.

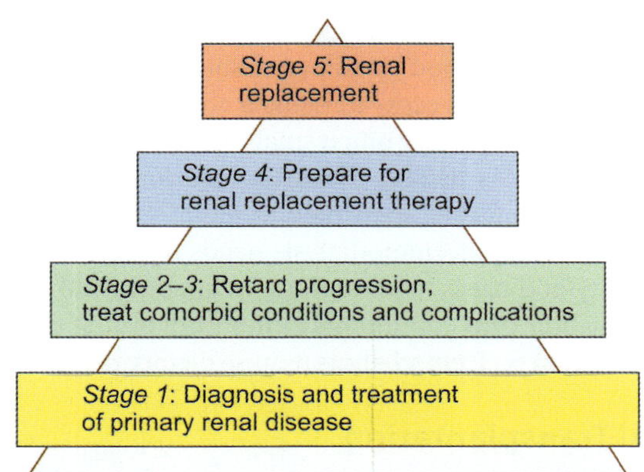

Fig. 10.10.1: Clinical action pyramid for chronic kidney disease.

Chronic Kidney Disease-Mineral Bone Disease

Causes of CKD-MBD include phosphate retention, hypocalcemia, hyperparathyroidism, impaired renal calcitriol synthesis, and aluminum toxicity. Controlling serum phosphorus requires dietary intervention and use of phosphate binders, which may be either calcium-containing (carbonate or acetate) or calcium free (sevelamer and lanthanum carbonate). Aluminum-based phosphate binders are avoided for fear of its toxicity. The product of calcium and phosphorus should not exceed 65 in older children and 55 in children less than 12 years. Calcium supplements and vitamin D and its analogs such as calcitriol or paricalcitol are used to suppress PTH. Calcimimetic agents (cinacalcet) act on calcium-sensing receptors and reduce levels of PTH. They are generally not used in routine practice.

Growth Failure

Factors contributing to growth failure include inadequate nutrition, secondary hyperparathyroidism, anemia, metabolic acidosis, salt depletion (in polyuric states) and abnormalities of the growth hormone-insulin like growth factor (GH-IGF) axis. Short stature is therefore managed by nutritional rehabilitation and correction of acidosis, anemia, and bone disease. If growth retardation persists, these children are offered human recombinant GH; its cost is a limiting factor for routine use.

Cardiovascular Disease

Cardiovascular disease is the leading cause of death in CKD with 1,000 times more risk than age matched non-CKD population. Cardiovascular disease (CVD) anomalies begin early in CKD and remain progressive with stage progression due to endothelial dysfunction of medium and large sized vessels. Dyslipidemia, atherosclerosis, hypertension, and abnormal glucose intolerance are traditional risk factors, which combine along with CKD-related risk factors such as hyperparathyroidism, abnormal calcium or phosphorus metabolism and left ventricular hypertrophy to increase morbidity. Regular monitoring and rectification of above risk factors can significantly reduce morbidity and improve the outcome in pre- and post-transplant periods of CKD.

Other Issues

Control of hypertension helps to slow down the progression of renal disease. Angiotensin-converting enzyme (ACE) inhibitors and receptor blockers have the advantage of reducing intraglomerular hypertension; renal functions, and potassium levels need to be monitored. Other drugs that may be used for control of hypertension include calcium-channel blockers, beta-adrenergic or alpha-blockers, and clonidine.

Metabolic acidosis should be corrected to maintain bicarbonate levels at around 20 mEq/L. Patients with CKD should receive complete vaccinations to prevent infection associated morbidity. Drugs should be used with appropriate dosage modification and nephrotoxic agents should be avoided.

The management of a child with CKD requires a team approach. It is helpful to have a medical social worker involved in the care of the child and the family. The social worker will address issues such as compliance, adherence to treatment, regular follow-up visits, financial issues, preparing the child and the family for the future and discussing options for RRT. The child should be encouraged to participate in age appropriate activities and attend regular school.

Slowing Down the Progression

The modifiable factors for retarding progression of CKD include hyperfiltration, proteinuria, hypertension, hyperparathyroidism, dyslipidemia, and nephrotoxic drugs. Every effort should be made to control these modifiable factors. Lowering blood pressures to target systolic and diastolic blood pressures below 90th percentile is important. ACE inhibitors and angiotensin receptor blockers (ARBs) have renoprotective effects by reducing proteinuria, lowering intraglomerular pressure and by their antifibrotic effects.

RENAL REPLACEMENT THERAPIES

End-stage renal disease is the term used when the child in stage five CKD needs RRTs for survival. It generally corresponds to the level of GFR less than 10–15 mL/min/1.73 m^2. RRTs aim at removal of endogenous metabolites in absence of normal functioning kidneys and maintain a near normal metabolic hemostasis. Renal transplantation is the preferred modality of RRT in children. Dialysis treatment should be used as a bridge toward transplantation; awaiting transplantation, or if transplantation cannot be performed.

Dialysis Treatment

Dialysis should be initiated when the GFR is below 10 mL/min/1.73 m^2 or when symptoms of uremia appear. Two types of dialysis are available: peritoneal dialysis (PD) and hemodialysis (HD).

Peritoneal Dialysis

Peritoneal dialysis is the preferred modality of dialysis in young children. The peritoneum functions as a semipermeable membrane across which exchange of solutes and fluids occurs across the osmotic gradient. The dialysate fluid is filled in the peritoneal compartment and allowed to dwell for few hours. During this period, gradual exchange of solutes occurs according to the concentration gradient. Hence, the serum levels of urea, creatinine, and potassium fall. This is a continuous form of RRT where the exchange occurs for almost 16–18 hours a day in contrast to intermittent HD, which is usually 4 hours per session 3 times a week. The development of automated PD using a cycler has made home dialysis possible. The main complication of PD is peritonitis. The child and the parents are trained to perform the exchanges and child can take part in his daily activities of school and home. The diet for a child on PD is much more liberal than on HD.

Hemodialysis

Hemodialysis is performed in a dialysis center. It is usually of 4 hours duration and 3 times a week; hence also referred to as "intermittent HD". It is conducted using a HD machine at a dialysis center in a hospital. The blood is run through extra-corporeal circuit from a central vein or arteriovenous (AV) fistula to a dialyzer filter (artificial kidney). In the dialyzer filter, the blood flows in opposite direction to the flow of dialysate fluid (exchange fluid). Due to this counter-current flow, rapid exchange of the metabolites occurs in a short duration of time with attainment of good clearance of solutes such as urea and creatinine. Vascular access remains a challenge in small children, as blood vessels are much smaller in size. The HD double lumen catheter is usually placed in internal jugular veins. AV fistula or grafts are attempted in older children weighing more than 15–20 kg. Hemodialysis needs technical expertise, availability of dialysis machines, dialyzers (artificial kidneys), heparinization, and continuous monitoring during the procedure. Children on Hemodialysis require dietary restrictions.

Renal Transplantation

Every child who has CKD stage 5 or ESRD should be offered renal transplantation as the preferred modality of treatment.

An adult kidney can be successfully transplanted into a child who is more than 10 kg. The choice of a kidney donor is either "living related" from a close blood relative (usually parent or grandparent < 65 years of age) who is medically fit or a deceased brain-dead donor. The Indian Government has passed a Transplantation of Human Organ Act in 1994, defining brain death, paving the way for deceased donor organ transplantation. The recipient needs life-long immunosuppressive medications to prevent rejection of the allograft. Complications after transplantation include acute tubular necrosis, rejection of graft, infections, vascular thrombosis, and recurrence of original disease, hypertension, drug toxicities, and malignancy. The results of pediatric transplantation in experienced centers are excellent with 1 year and 5 years graft survival of more than 90% and 70% respectively. Excellent rehabilitation is expected in children with functioning grafts. The living-related kidney donors are expected to lead a normal life. Renal transplantation provides children with ESRD a good quality of prolonged life.

BIBLIOGRAPHY

1. KDOQI Work Group. KDOQI Clinical Practice Guideline for Nutrition in Children with CKD: 2008 update. Am J Kidney Dis. 2009;53(3 Suppl 2):S11-104.
2. KDOQI, National Kidney Foundation. III. Clinical practice recommendations for anemia in chronic kidney disease in children. Am J Kidney Dis. 2006;47(5 Suppl 3):S86-108.
3. Klaus G, Watson A, Edefonti A. Prevention and treatment of renal osteodystrophy in children on chronic renal failure: European guidelines. Pediatr Nephrol. 2006;21(2):151-9.
4. Phadke KD, Goodyer P, Iyengar AA. Renal transplantation. In: Phadke KD, Goodyer P, Bitzan M (Eds). Manual of Pediatric Nephrology. Berlin, Heidelberg: Springer-Verlag; 2014. pp. 429-44.
5. Sinha A. Chronic kidney disease. In: Srivastava RN, Bagga A (Eds). Pediatric Nephrology, 5th edition. New Delhi: Jaypee Brothers Medical Publishers (P) Ltd.; 2011. pp. 360-85.

10.11 Renal Tubular Diseases

Aditi Sinha

INTRODUCTION

In comparison to glomerular diseases, tubular disorders are less common. A high index of suspicion and correct diagnosis allow specific management in many patients. Tubulopathies should be suspected in children presenting with symptoms listed in **Box 10.11.1**. The diagnosis of a primary tubular disorder implies that there is no significant impairment of glomerular function or tubulointerstitial inflammation. The disorder may be congenital or acquired and involve a single tubular function (renal glucosuria, nephrogenic diabetes insipidus) or multiple functions (Fanconi syndrome). Most disorders can be diagnosed following careful interpretation of specific urine and plasma biochemical tests.

Box 10.11.1: Presenting features of tubular disorders.

- Growth retardation, failure to thrive
- Delayed gross motor milestones
- Polyuria, excessive thirst
- Recurrent episodes of dehydration, vomiting, fever
- Rickets, bone pains
- Episodic weakness
- Constipation
- Craving for salt and savory foods

RENAL TUBULAR ACIDOSIS

Renal tubular acidosis (RTA) include conditions characterized by a defect of renal acidification resulting in impaired capacity for net acid excretion and hyperchloremic metabolic acidosis, in the presence of normal glomerular function. Transport defects are usually secondary to reduced proximal tubular reabsorption of bicarbonate (HCO_3^-)[3], as in proximal RTA, or the distal secretion of protons (hydrogen ion, H^+), as in distal RTA. A third variety called type IV RTA is distinguished by the presence of hyperkalemia. These conditions may be primary, with or without known genetic defects, or secondary to other causes **(Table 10.11.1)**.

Pathophysiology

The excretion of acid and the reabsorption of filtered bicarbonate are mediated by tubular secretion of hydrogen ions (H^+). In the proximal tubule, filtered HCO_3^- is reabsorbed through carbonic anhydrase in the tubular brush border. The primary defect in proximal (type II) RTA is reduced renal threshold for HCO_3^- reabsorption leading to bicarbonaturia.

Table 10.11.1: Inherited and acquired forms of renal tubular acidosis (RTA).

Type of RTA	*Inherited*	*Acquired*
Type 1 (distal) RTA	Autosomal dominant Autosomal recessive With or without hemolytic anemia or hearing loss	Systemic lupus erythematosus, Sjögren syndrome Obstructive uropathy, reflux nephropathy Sickle cell anemia Amphotericin B toxicity
Type 2 (proximal) RTA: isolated Multiple tubular dysfunction (Fanconi syndrome)	Autosomal dominant Autosomal recessive (with ocular abnormalities: band keratopathy, cataracts or glaucoma; defective dental enamel; intellectual impairment; basal ganglia calcification) Autosomal dominant, autosomal recessive X-linked (Dent's disease) *Syndromic*: Cystinosis; galactosemia; tyrosinemia; Wilson disease; hereditary fructose intolerance; Lowe syndrome; glycogen storage disease type I; mitochondrial disorders*	Carbonic anhydrase inhibitors (acetazolamide) Vitamin D dependent rickets Primary hyperparathyroidism Acute tubulointerstitial nephritis with uveitis *Drugs*: Ifosfamide, cisplatin, aminoglycosides *Toxins*: Lead, cadmium, mercury, toluene
Type 3 (combined)	Autosomal recessive (with osteopetrosis; blindness, deafness)	
Type 4 (hyperkalemic)	Pseudohypoaldosteronism types 1 and 2 Congenital adrenal hyperplasia	*Aldosterone deficiency without renal disease* (Addison disease; adrenal tuberculosis; necrosis) *Chronic renal insufficiency* (obstructive uropathy, interstitial nephritis) *Aldosterone resistance* (amiloride, spironolactone)

*Syndromic forms of Fanconi show autosomal recessive inheritance, except Lowe syndrome which has X-linked recessive inheritance

Fanconi syndrome refers to a generalized proximal tubular dysfunction characterized by tubular proteinuria, aminoaciduria and variable bicarbonaturia, phosphaturia, and glucosuria.

In the distal tubule, secreted H^+ ions combine with sodium hydrogen phosphate (Na_2HPO_4) and ammonia to form NaH_2PO_4 and NH_4^+, measured as titratable acidity and urinary ammonium ion, respectively. Additional factors that influence H^+ secretion and HCO_3^- reabsorption include extracellular fluid volume, potassium balance and plasma aldosterone. Distal RTA is characterized by decreased distal tubular secretion of H^+ ions, leading to low rates of excretion of ammonium (NH_4^+) ions and titratable acidity. Hypokalemic distal (classic or type 1) RTA occurs due to a secretory (rate) defect, with decreased secretion of H^+ due to impaired function of anion channel [H^+ adenosine triphosphatase (ATPase), H^+/K^+ ATPase or Cl^-/HCO_3^- exchanger], or a gradient (permeability) defect, where an increased backleak of normally secreted protons dissipates the pH gradient. In both forms, the urine pH cannot reach maximal acidity (i.e. remains > 5.5) despite acidemia. Hypokalemia is attributed to increased urinary losses of K^+, partially secondary to hyperaldosteronism in response to volume contraction and urinary losses of Na^+.

Distal RTA with hyperkalemia may result from a voltage defect (hyperkalemic distal RTA), secondary to insufficient negative intraluminal potential in the cortical collecting duct, or a rate defect, due to aldosterone deficiency or resistance (type 4 RTA). Other than normokalemia or hyperkalemia, the findings in hyperkalemic distal RTA resemble classic distal RTA. Aldosterone resistance or deficiency decreases distal reabsorption of Na^+, which lowers the transtubular potential gradient for H^+ secretion. In addition, lack of aldosterone action decreases urinary excretion of K^+. Hyperkalemia in turn reduces ammoniagenesis. In type 4 RTA, maximally acidic urine (<5.5) can be formed, indicating intact ability to establish a maximal H^+ gradient.

Clinical Features

Features that suggest RTA are listed in **Box 10.11.1**. Children with proximal RTA present with failure to thrive, irritability, anorexia, listlessness, and uncommonly, with symptoms of hypokalemia (weakness, paralysis). Patients with Fanconi syndrome may have features of the underlying disorder **(Table 10.11.1)**, as in patients with cystinosis (presentation in infancy, photophobia, hepatosplenomegaly, blond hair) or Lowe syndrome (presentation in infancy with severe rickets, cataract, buphthalmos, hypotonia and developmental delay).

Features in distal RTA include impaired growth, polyuria, nephrocalcinosis **(Fig. 10.11.1)** or nephrolithiasis, symptoms of hypokalemia and/or hearing loss. Children with type 4 RTA have milder acidosis without nephrocalcinosis, urolithiasis or bone lesions. Underlying tubulointerstitial disease may be evident. The autosomal recessive form of pseudohypoaldosteronism (PHA) type 1 is an important differential diagnosis in infants presenting with salt loss, hypotension, hyperkalemia, and metabolic acidosis. The autosomal dominant form of PHA type 1 involves only the kidney and is less severe than the recessive form, which is systemic, affecting sweat and salivary glands and colon.

Evaluation

Metabolic acidosis may result from either increased endogenous acid synthesis (e.g. ketoacidosis, lactic acidosis) or enhanced bicarbonate losses (diarrhea, intestinal tube drainage or fistula, ureterosigmoidostomy, cholestyramine).

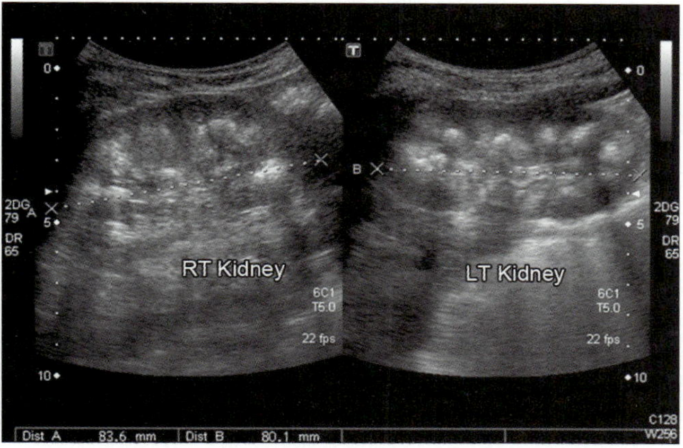

Fig. 10.11.1: Nephrocalcinosis in a 6-year-old girl with distal renal tubular acidosis, presenting with polyuria and failure to thrive.

Since all types of RTA are associated with hyperchloremic metabolic acidosis, the initial step is the determination of the plasma anion gap, which is normal (8–12 mEq/L) in all types of RTA. **Table 10.11.2** lists important steps of evaluation.

Elevated excretion of urinary NH_4^+ in patients with metabolic acidosis suggests extrarenal HCO_3^- losses (diarrhea), while low excretion points to RTA. Since the difference between urinary unmeasured anions (sulfates, phosphates, organic anions) and cations (calcium, magnesium) is relatively constant (at ~80 mEq/L), the measurement of important ions as urine anion gap (UAG; urine net charge) effectively estimates NH_4^+ excretion.

Loading with sodium bicarbonate, performed orally (2–4 mEq/kg/day for 3 days) or intravenously (0.5 mEq/mL at 3 mL/min) to achieve urine pH more than 7.5 and normal serum HCO_3^- (>22 mEq/L), allows simultaneous measurement of fractional excretion of bicarbonate and urine to blood CO_2 gradient, reflecting proximal bicarbonate handling and distal tubular acidification, respectively.

Table 10.11.3 summarizes the differences among various types of RTA. Additional tests are required depending on the type suspected. In patients with proximal RTA, other proximal functions are evaluated, including for aminoaciduria, glucosuria, low molecular weight proteinuria, and calculation of fractional excretion of phosphate ($FEPO_4$) and tubular maximum for phosphate. Patients are screened for cystinosis, Lowe syndrome, galactosemia and Wilson disease. Evaluation in patients with distal RTA includes ultrasonography (nephrocalcinosis, renal calculi) and measurement of urinary calcium and citrate excretion. All

Table 10.11.2: Evaluation in patients with suspected renal tubular acidosis (RTA).

Step	*Test*	*Comment*
1	Plasma anion gap	Calculated as $[Na^+ - (Cl^- + HCO_3^-)]$ Normal (8–12 mEq/L) in RTA and diarrhea Elevated in patients with ketoacidosis, lactic acidosis, inborn errors of metabolism, poisoning or uremia
2	Urine anion gap (UAG) or urine net charge	UAG = Urinary $Na^+ + K^+ - Cl^-$ Urinary NH_4^+ = 80 – UAG Is positive in normal conditions; during systemic acidosis, negative UAG suggests extrarenal (diarrheal) HCO_3^- losses and positive UAG reflects impaired urinary acidification (RTA)
3	Urine pH	Is measured on fresh voided specimen with pH meter, not dipstick Estimates < 1% of urinary proton excretion During systemic acidosis, pH > 5.5 suggests distal RTA; value < 5.5 suggests extrarenal cause or RTA type 2 or 4
4	Fractional excretion of bicarbonate ($FEHCO_3$)	$FEHCO_3\ (\%) = \frac{\text{Urine bicarbonate} \times \text{Plasma creatinine}}{\text{Plasma bicarbonate} \times \text{Urine creatinine}} \times 100$ After bicarbonate loading, value is >15% in proximal RTA; <5% in normal persons and distal RTA
5	Urine to blood pCO_2 gradient (U-B CO_2)	Urine pCO_2 sensitively reflects distal H^+ secretion, rising to >70 mm Hg during alkalosis U-B CO_2 = Urine pCO_2 – blood pCO_2 After bicarbonate loading, value <10 mm Hg suggest classic distal RTA; value is >20 mm Hg in normal individuals; patients with permeability and voltage defects; types 2 and 4 RTA

(U-B pCO_2: urine to blood pCO_2 gradient)

patients should undergo hearing evaluation; older children are evaluated for secondary (e.g. autoimmune) causes.

Workup in patients with type 4 RTA should include renal function tests and ultrasonography to identify structural or parenchymal disease. Measurements of plasma renin activity and aldosterone levels are required. Transtubular potassium gradient is a useful test in diagnosing type 4 RTA. When coupled to a mineralocorticoid challenge, this test allows distinction between aldosterone deficiency and resistance.

Treatment

Management of RTA involves correction of acidosis through administration of alkali supplements (Uriliser, Polycitra, Shohl solution) and provision of adequate nutrition, fluids and deficient electrolytes. Patients with distal RTA require 2–3 mEq/kg/day of alkali. Urinary potassium losses decrease with correction of acidosis, but some patients require prolonged potassium supplementation. Similarly, rickets improves with management of acidosis. Urinary calcium excretion should be monitored; patients with persistent hypercalciuria require thiazides.

The requirement of alkali supplements is higher (5–20 mEq/kg/day) in patients with proximal RTA. This is given as a combination of sodium and potassium citrate, with restriction of dietary sodium. Administration of hydrochlorothiazide causes contraction of extracellular fluid volume and increased proximal HCO_3^- reabsorption. Supplements of phosphate (neutral phosphate, Joulie solution) are necessary in Fanconi syndrome. Small doses of vitamin D may enable healing of rickets. Specific treatment may be useful, such as therapy with cysteamine in patients with cystinosis, penicillamine in Wilson disease, nitisinone in tyrosinemia, and dietary interventions (galactosemia, hereditary fructose intolerance, and tyrosinemia).

Table 10.11.3: Investigations to differentiate types of renal tubular acidosis.

Investigation	*Proximal RTA*	*Distal RTA*		*Type 4 RTA*
		Classic	*Hyperkalemic*	
Plasma K^+	Normal/low	Normal/low	High	High
Urine pH	<5.5	>5.5	>5.5	<5.5
Urine anion gap	Positive	Positive	Positive	Positive
Urine NH_4^+	Low	Low	Low	Low
Fractional HCO_3^- Excretion	>10–15%	<5%	<5%	>5–10%
U-B pCO_2 mm Hg	>20	<20	</>20	>20
Urine calcium	Normal	High	High	Normal/low
Other tubular defects	Often present	Absent	Absent	Absent
Nephrocalcinosis	Absent	Present	Present	Absent
Bone disease	Common	Often present	Uncommon	Absent

(RTA: renal tubular acidosis; U-B pCO_2: urine to blood pCO_2 gradient)

TUBULOPATHIES WITH URINARY CHLORIDE WASTING

Bartter and Gitelman syndromes are caused by defects in ion transporters resulting in increased urinary losses of chloride, accompanied by potassium and sodium wasting.

Bartter Syndrome

Patients present with failure to thrive, polyuria, polydipsia and recurrent episodes of dehydration. The neonatal form is particularly severe with maternal polyhydramnios, polyuria, dehydration, hypercalciuria, and nephrocalcinosis. Hypokalemia is marked with hypochloremic metabolic alkalosis and increased levels of plasma renin and aldosterone.

Bartter syndrome is differentiated from other conditions with persistent hypokalemic metabolic alkalosis by the presence of normal blood pressure, and high urinary excretion of chloride and calcium. Further characterization of the molecular defect is based on genetic testing. Differences in presentation may help characterize the defect **(Table 10.11.4)**.

Management of Bartter syndrome includes fluid replacement and supplementation of potassium chloride (1–3 mEq/kg/day). Administration of indomethacin (2–3 mg/kg/day) or ibuprofen (30 mg/kg/day) decreases elevated prostaglandins and ameliorates polyuria. Potassium-sparing diuretics and angiotensin-converting enzyme (ACE) inhibitors may aid potassium retention.

Table 10.11.4: Tubular diseases presenting with hyperchloremic metabolic alkalosis with hypokalemia and normal or low blood pressure.

Disorder	*Presentation*
Antenatal Bartter syndrome (aBS): Types 1, 2 and 4	Polyhydramnios, prematurity *Neonatal*: Failure to thrive, nephrocalcinosis Sensorineural deafness in type 4 Bartter syndrome
Classic Bartter syndrome (cBS; type 3)	Growth retardation, hypercalciuria, no nephrocalcinosis, normal serum magnesium
Type 5 Bartter syndrome	As classic; hypomagnesemia; hypocalcemia
Gitelman syndrome	Episodic muscle weakness; mild polyuria; hypocalciuria, hypomagnesemia, chondrocalcinosis

Inherited in autosomal recessive manner, except type 5 Bartter syndrome that is autosomal dominant

Gitelman Syndrome

Patients with Gitelman syndrome have abnormalities similar to Bartter syndrome, including hypokalemia, metabolic alkalosis, and hypomagnesemia. However, symptoms, including polyuria and growth retardation, are milder and appear in older children. Episodes of weakness, vomiting, abdominal pain, and tetany may occur. The underlying mechanism is a defect in the thiazidesensitive, sodium chloride cotransporter in the distal tubule. Urinary calcium excretion is low but magnesium wasting is prominent. Treatment is with supplementation of potassium and magnesium (as oral magnesium oxide, chloride, gluconate, oxide or hydroxide).

POLYURIA

Polyuria is defined as urine output exceeding 6 mL/kg/h or 2 L/m^2 in children. Polyuria may accompany structural renal disorders including juvenile nephronophthisis, renal dysplasia (reflux nephropathy, obstructive uropathy) and chronic tubulointerstitial nephritis, or solute losses (RTA, Bartter-like syndromes and diabetes mellitus).

Nephrogenic diabetes insipidus is a rare condition characterized by tubular unresponsiveness to the antidiuretic hormone (ADH, vasopressin). Most cases are inherited in an X-linked recessive pattern with mutations in the gene for the arginine vasopressin V2 receptor (AVPR2); 10% cases are inherited autosomally through mutations in the aquaporin 2 gene. Infants present with irritability, failure to thrive, recurrent episodes of dehydration and intermittent fever. Nephrogenic diabetes insipidus may be acquired, as with obstructive uropathy, analgesic nephropathy, sickle cell disease, chronic pyelonephritis, hypercalcemia, hypokalemia, sarcoidosis and with use of lithium and tetracyclines.

Diagnosis of diabetes insipidus requires confirmation of polyuria and exclusion of differential diagnoses. Useful investigations include measurement of urine osmolality, electrolytes, sugar and ketones; blood electrolytes, pH, bicarbonate, sugar, calcium and creatinine, and renal ultrasonography. Upon water deprivation, diabetes insipidus is suggested by plasma sodium of more than 145 mEq/L, plasma osmolality more than 295 mEq/kg and urine osmolality less than 300 mEq/kg. A rise in urine osmolality to more than 150% of baseline following administration of desmopressin (DDAVP) suggests complete central diabetes insipidus, while no change (<110% of baseline) suggests complete nephrogenic diabetes insipidus.

Patients with diabetes insipidus require adequate intake of water. Restriction of dietary sodium to 1 mEq/kg/ day and administration of hydrochlorothiazide (2–4 mg/kg/day), with or without amiloride (0.3 mg/kg/day) help reduce polyuria in patients with nephrogenic diabetes insipidus. Indomethacin (2 mg/kg/day) is also useful.

REFRACTORY RICKETS

Rickets results from a lack of adequate mineralization of growing bones. The diagnosis is based on clinical findings, radiological features **(Fig. 10.11.2)** and blood biochemistry. The term refractory rickets is used for patients who fail to show radiological healing and normalization of biochemical abnormalities despite therapy with two large doses of vitamin D; alternatively, it is diagnosed in presence of rickets despite normal serum 25-hydroxy vitamin D levels. The causes of refractory rickets are grouped into two categories according to the underlying defect, abnormal vitamin D metabolism or impaired renal tubular phosphate handling **(Box 10.11.2)**. The former is characterized by low serum levels of calcium and phosphate, aminoaciduria and high parathyroid hormone (PTH). The latter shows hypophosphatemia with normal serum calcium and PTH. Rickets in distal RTA is attributed to impaired renal hydroxylation of calcidiol and a negative calcium balance secondary to persistent metabolic acidosis. Presentation varies by cause and severity. Patients

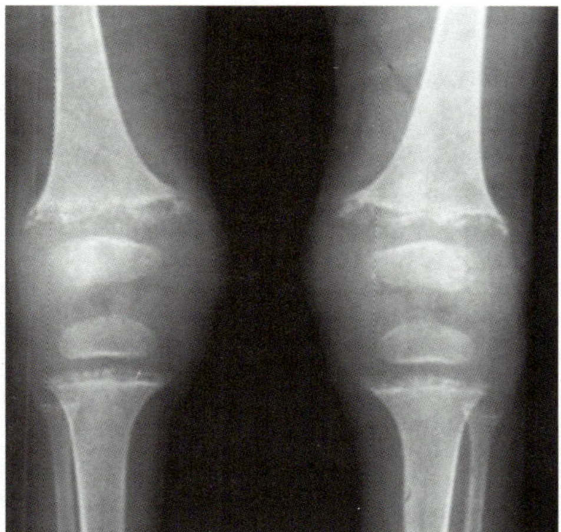

Fig. 10.11.2: Radiograph of both knees in a 4-year-old boy showing widening, flaring and irregularity of the metaphyseal ends of long bones. Serum 25-hydroxyvitamin D levels were above normal limits due to past treatment and a diagnosis of refractory rickets was made.

Box 10.11.2: Causes of refractory rickets.

Calcipenic rickets
- Vitamin D dependent rickets, types 1 and 2

Hypophosphatemic rickets
- X-linked familial
- Autosomal dominant
- Autosomal recessive
- Hypophosphatemic rickets with hypercalciuria
- Dent's disease
- Fanconi syndrome

Distal renal tubular acidosis

Chronic kidney disease mineral bone disease

Flowchart 10.11.1: Evaluation in patients with refractory rickets.

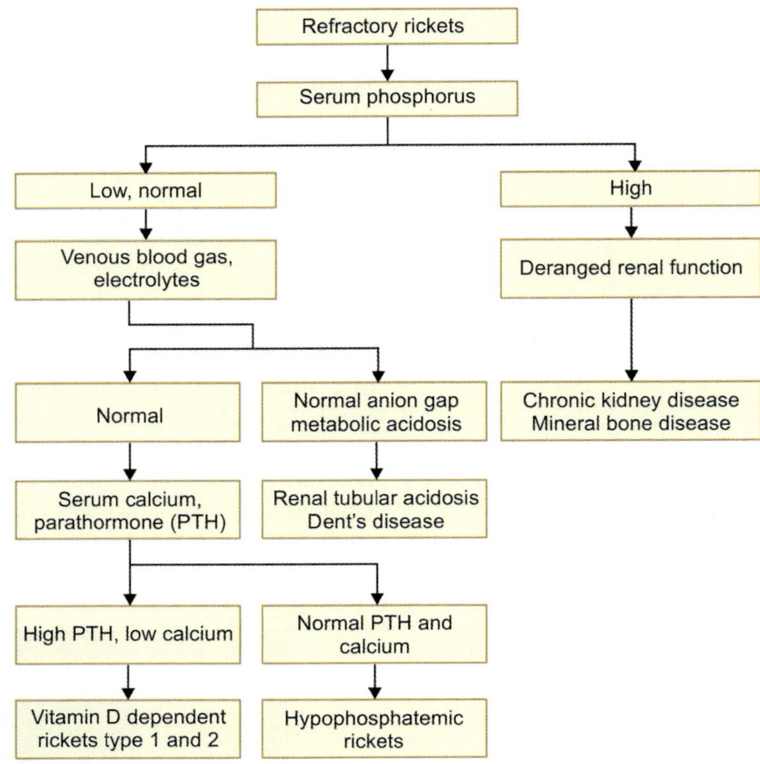

with vitamin D dependent rickets (VDDR) have onset in infancy with tetany, seizures, delayed dentition and hypocalcemia. Patients with VDDR type 1 show enamel hypoplasia; those with VDDR type 2 may have alopecia and ectodermal defects (oligodontia, epidermal cysts). Presentation of hypophosphatemic rickets includes short stature, lower limb deformities, and dental abnormalities (pulp deformities, abscess). Patients with hypercalciuric variant of hypophosphatemic rickets, distal RTA or Dent's disease may show nephrocalcinosis or nephrolithiasis. Presentation of RTA and Fanconi has been discussed.

Evaluation should include estimation of blood levels of calcium, phosphorous, alkaline phosphatase, creatinine, pH, electrolytes, bicarbonate, 25-hydroxyvitamin D and PTH; urinalysis; estimation of timed excretion of calcium, phosphate, protein and creatinine; and ultrasonography of kidneys. **Flowchart 10.11.1** provides an approach to diagnosis.

The therapy of rickets is tailored to the underlying cause. Patients with VDDR type1 are treated with calcidiol or calcitriol (1–2 µg daily) and supplements of calcium and phosphate. Requirement of calcitriol is higher (0.05–0.2 µg/kg/day) in patients with VDDR type 2. These patients may benefit from administration of high-dose calcium infusions.

The rickets in RTA responds satisfactorily to correction of acidosis; patients with proximal RTA additionally require supplements of oral phosphate with or without vitamin D. Management of hypophosphatemic rickets involves supplementation of phosphate (30–50 mg/kg/day) as neutral phosphate or acid phosphate (Joulie solution).

Patients with X-linked hypophosphatemic rickets also require small doses of calcitriol (25–50 ng/kg/day; 0.25–0.5 µg daily). Management of mineral bone disease associated with chronic kidney disease relies on control of hyperphosphatemia (dietary restriction, use of oral phosphate binders) and therapy with active vitamin D analogs.

BIBLIOGRAPHY

1. Bagga A, Bajpai A, Menon S. Approach to renal tubular disorders. Indian J Pediatr. 2005;72:771-6.
2. Bagga A, Sinha A. Evaluation of renal tubular acidosis. Indian J Pediatr. 2007;74:679-86.
3. Berend K. Review of the diagnostic evaluation of normal anion gap metabolic acidosis. Kidney Dis (Basel). 2017;3:149-59.

4. Goldsweig BK, Carpenter TO. Hypophosphatemic rickets: lessons from disrupted FGF23 control of phosphorus homeostasis. Curr Osteoporos Rep. 2015;13:88-97.
5. Lowenstein J, Grantham JJ. The rebirth of interest in renal tubular function. Am J Physiol Renal Physiol. 2016;310: F1351-5.
6. Santos F, Ordóñez FA, Claramunt-Taberner D, et al. Clinical and laboratory approaches in the diagnosis of renal tubular acidosis. Pediatr Nephrol. 2015;30:2099-107.
7. Tasic V, Gucev Z. Nephrolithiasis and nephrocalcinosis in children: metabolic and genetic factors. Pediatr Endocrinol Rev. 2015;13:468-76.

10.12 Asymptomatic Hematuria

Indira Agarwal

INTRODUCTION

Microscopic hematuria is often detected on routine urinalysis. Gross hematuria though uncommon, may be more serious, as it often originates from glomeruli or the urinary tract and needs immediate attention. The persistent finding of five or more red cells per high power field (HPF) on a centrifuged urine specimen performed over 2–3 weeks warrants evaluation.

Dipsticks have a sensitivity of 100% and specificity of 99% in detecting 1–5 red blood cells (RBCs)/HPF but need confirmation by microscopy of the centrifuged specimen. Presence of dysmorphic RBC and granular casts with proteinuria more than 2+ suggests a glomerular cause. A positive dipstick reaction in the absence of RBC and RBC casts in the urine suggests hemoglobinuria or myoglobinuria. This can be differentiated from hematuria by centrifugation where a clear pink supernatant with minimal or no deposits suggests hemoglobinuria while cloudy red or dark brown supernatant suggests hematuria. Phase-contrast microscopy helps to determine the site of origin of the bleeding.

EPIDEMIOLOGY

The prevalence of gross hematuria is 0.1% with more than half being due to identifiable causes. Asymptomatic microscopic hematuria is ten-fold as prevalent as gross hematuria; most often it is transient and on repeated evaluation the prevalence decreases to less than 0.5%.

The first step is to identify the site of bleeding: glomerular or nonglomerular. If bleeding occurs in the upper tract the color of the urine is "cola-colored" or "tea-colored" and shows dysmorphic RBC (>30% by phase contrast microscopy). Urine from the lower tract is bright red, has clots and eumorphic RBC. Beets, dyes, medications (phenazopyridine), uric acid and porphyrins can color urine red or pink.

Causes of glomerular hematuria include postinfectious glomerulonephritis (GN), immunoglobulin (IgA) nephropathy, systemic lupus, Henoch-Schönlein purpura (HSP), hemolytic uremic syndrome (HUS), membranoproliferative glomerulonephritis (MPGN), infections (malaria, leptospirosis, and endocarditis), benign familial hematuria, and Alport syndrome. Nonglomerular causes include nephrolithiasis, hypercalciuria, viral hemorrhagic cystitis, urinary tract infection (UTI), and vascular abnormalities.

CLINICAL FEATURES

A history of facial puffiness, oliguria, hypertension, and impaired renal function suggests a glomerular disease. IgA nephropathy can mimic postinfectious GN but can be differentiated by symptoms being "synpharyngitic", normal C3 and recurrent episodes with normal urine in between.

Presence of fever, rash, joint pains with or without abdominal pain suggests an underlying systemic disorder. Patients with collagen vascular disorders may occasionally present with rapidly progressive glomerulonephritis (RPGN) and require urgent intervention **(Flowcharts 10.12.1 and 10.12.2)**.

In the absence of systemic signs and symptoms, conditions such as benign familial hematuria or Alport syndrome should be considered. Urinalysis of family members, and eye (anterior lenticonus) and hearing assessments (high-tone hearing deafness) are advised. Hematological conditions such as sickle cell disease and trait, coagulopathies, and thrombocytopenia may occasionally present with hematuria.

Loin pain hematuria syndrome (LPHS) presents with recurrent episodes of loin pain (unilateral, bilateral) and hematuria (microscopic, gross) where investigations do not reveal any abnormality. Nutcracker syndrome due to entrapment of left renal vein between aorta and superior

Flowchart 10.12.1: Gross hematuria.

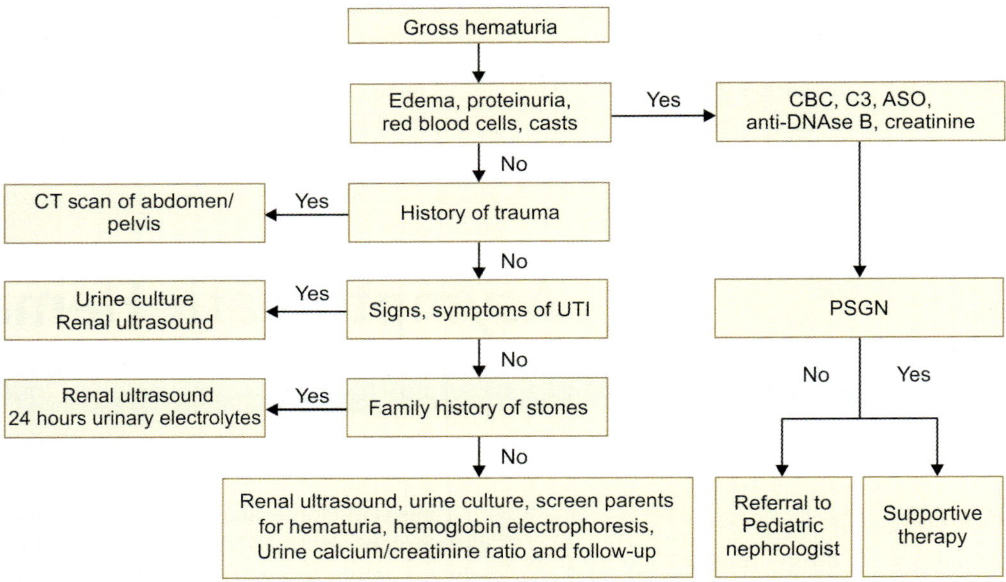

(ASO: antistreptolysin O; CBC: complete blood count; CT: computed tomography; PSGN: poststreptococcal glomerulonephritis; UTI: urinary tract infections)
Source: Evaluation of hematuria. In: Kaplan BS, Kevin EC (Eds). Pediatric Nephrology and Urology: The Requisites in Pediatrics. Philadelphia: Elsevier Mosby; 2005. pp. 95-102.

Flowchart 10.12.2: Microscopic hematuria.

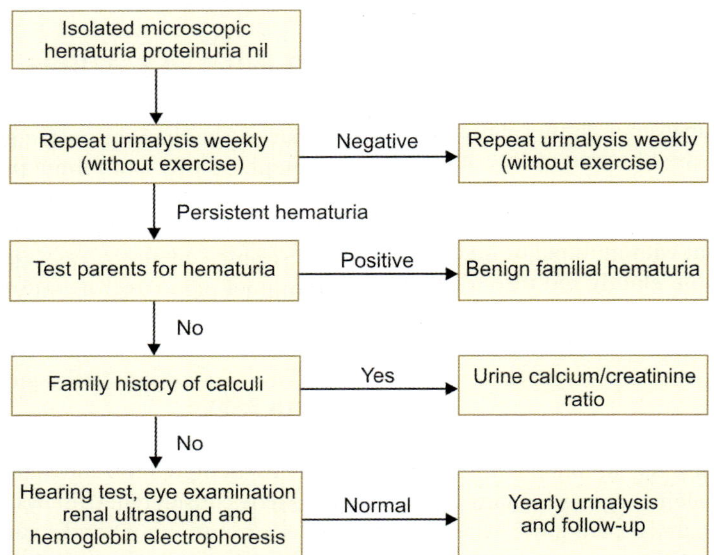

Source: Evaluation of hematuria. In: Kaplan BS, Kevin EC (Eds). Pediatric Nephrology and Urology: The Requisites in Pediatrics. Philadelphia: Elsevier Mosby; 2005. pp. 95-102.

mesenteric artery presents similarly. Patients with hematuria due to a disorder in the lower tract have symptoms of dysuria, burning, frequency or hesitancy. Terminal hematuria suggests cystitis, while at initiation suggests urethritis. UTI present with fever; adenovirus infection may result in hemorrhagic cystitis. Children with nephrolithiasis present with renal colic, gross or asymptomatic microhematuria while those with hypercalciuria have hematuria without evident calculi.

Interstitial nephritis may present with malaise, fatigue, and variable volumes of urine output.

INVESTIGATIONS

Urinalysis and complete blood count (CBC) is the first step in evaluation, followed by electrolytes, creatinine, complement levels (C3, C4) and antistreptolysin O (ASO). Low C3 and evidence of streptococcal infection confirms the diagnosis of poststreptococcal GN. C3 levels are low in lupus nephritis, MPGN, and cryoglobulinemia. If there is no evidence of streptococcal infection, other infections or alternative glomerular disease needs to be considered. If hematuria is persistent and accompanied by heavy proteinuria and reduced renal function, renal biopsy with electron microscopy differentiates glomerular disease from an inherited nephropathy.

Minor trauma can precipitate hematuria in children with renal cysts and hydronephrosis. Arteriovenous malformations and hemangiomas, which cause episodic gross hematuria, may be difficult to diagnose even by cystoscopy or angiography.

Eumorphic RBC suggests nonglomerular hematuria. If white cells are present, a clean-catch urine culture is indicated. If genitourinary tuberculosis is suspected, then urine is cultured for acid-fast bacilli. Urine calcium/creatinine ratio is estimated for hypercalciuria. If calculi are not visualized by ultrasound abdomen, a spiral computed tomography (CT) scan should be done. Stone analysis is useful but a metabolic workup is necessary to determine the underlying cause.

Cystoscopic evaluation rarely reveals a cause for hematuria but should be considered, if bladder pathology is suspected and is best done when there is active bleeding. In young girls with recurrent gross hematuria, child abuse or insertion of vaginal foreign body should not be forgotten. Genital examination should be carefully done in these situations.

BIBLIOGRAPHY

1. Diven SC, Travis LB, A practical primary care approach to hematuria in children. Pediatr Nephrol. 2000;14(1):65-72.
2. Meyers KE. Evaluation of hematuria in children. Urol Clin North Am. 2004;31(3):559-73.
3. Moore GP, Robinson M. Do urine dipsticks reliably predict microhematuria? The bloody truth! Ann Emerg Med. 1988;17(3):257-60.
4. Phadke KD, Vijayakumar M, Sharma J, et al. Consensus statement on evaluation of hematuria. Indian Pediatr. 2006;43(11):965-73.

10.13 Nephrolithiasis

Uma Ali

INTRODUCTION

Stones in the kidneys and urinary tract are not uncommon in childhood. Children are at a high risk for recurrent stone formation and an underlying metabolic disorder may be found in 50–75% cases. A family history of renal stones is present in approximately 40% patients.

ETIOLOGY

Nephrolithiasis may result from varied causes, including inherited metabolic defects, infections, structural urological abnormalities, and drugs **(Table 10.13.1)**.

PATHOGENESIS

Crystals may form due to supersaturation of urine with solutes due to their excessive excretion (calcium oxalate, sodium urate or cystine), a decrease in urinary volume (poor water intake; excessive intestinal or renal losses) or a decrease in the urinary inhibitors of crystallization (citrate, magnesium or pyrophosphate). Damage to the uroepithelial lining with formation of calcium phosphate plaques leading to crystal adherence and growth is another mechanism of stone formation. Irrespective of the etiology, high protein or salt intakes increase the risk of nephrolithiasis.

Table 10.13.1: Causes of nephrolithiasis.

Etiology	*Cause*
Metabolic	
Hypercalciuria	*With hypercalcemia*: Vitamin D overdose; hyperparathyroidism *With normal serum calcium*: Idiopathic; distal renal tubular acidosis; Dent's disease; familial hypophosphatemia with hypercalciuria
Hyperoxaluria	Primary hyperoxaluria types 1 and 2; increased intestinal absorption
Hyperuricosuria	Lesch-Nyhan syndrome; glycogen storage disease type 1
Others	Cystinuria; xanthinuria
Struvite	Urinary tract infections, usually in the presence of a structural abnormality (pelviureteric obstruction, vesicoureteric reflux, neurogenic bladder, bladder exstrophy)
Drugs	Indinavir, ceftriaxone

CLINICAL FEATURES

Nephrolithiasis is often silent and detected incidentally during imaging for unrelated symptoms. Presentations include gross hematuria and complications such as urinary tract infection (UTI) or obstruction. Pain is a feature of ureteric calculi; it may radiate from loin to groin, or mimic appendicitis or diverticulitis. Bladder stones present with dysuria, urgency, incontinence, interrupted stream, strangury and, rarely, acute retention of urine.

INVESTIGATIONS

Investigations for nephrolithiasis include: (a) imaging studies; (b) urinalysis and culture; (c) urine and serum biochemistry; and (d) stone composition.

Imaging Studies

The aim of imaging is to confirm the presence, size and location of the stone, and to identify underlying urological abnormalities or associated obstruction.

Ultrasonography

Ultrasonography is the modality of choice since it is safe, easily available, and lacks radiation exposure. It is also useful for the evaluation of renal anatomy and for obstruction, and a convenient method for follow-up monitoring. Ultrasound has a sensitivity of 96% and specificity of almost 100% for stones above 5 mm; however, the sensitivity and specificity are lower for ureteric stones.

Radiography of the Kidney Ureter Bladder

Radiography of kidney ureter bladder (KUB) is a poor modality for detecting stones with a sensitivity of 77% and specificity of 87%. Its chief role is in differentiating radiolucent from radiopaque stones, which may suggest stone composition; while calcium oxalate and phosphate stones are radiopaque, uric acid and drug stones are radiolucent.

Intravenous Urography

Intravenous urography formerly considered the gold standard for the diagnosis of nephrolithiasis has high specificity (92–100%) but low sensitivity (as low as 51% in some studies). Its utility is restricted to defining anatomical abnormalities preoperatively, if required.

Noncontrast Computed Tomography

Noncontrast computed tomography (NCCT) is the current gold standard for the diagnosis of nephrolithiasis since its sensitivity and specificity are close to 100%. Uric acid and xanthine stones that are radiolucent on KUB can be diagnosed on NCCT. Chief limitations include cost and radiation. While anatomic delineation is excellent, radiation dose is very high with an enhanced CT. The risk from radiation is reduced by using low doses of contrast. Anatomical and functional delineation is limited in absence of contrast.

Magnetic Resonance Urography

Magnetic resonance urography cannot identify calculi but can provide good anatomical delineation without radiation exposure. Its use is limited by cost and availability.

Caution should be exercised in minimizing radiation exposure during repeated imaging done for monitoring for recurrence of nephrolithiasis.

Urinalysis and Culture

Routine urinalysis may show hematuria, pyuria or crystals. Pyuria or fever suggests UTI but requires confirmation by culture. While crystals of calcium oxalate, calcium phosphate or uric acid are often present in urine of normal individuals, the finding of crystals such as hexagonal cystine crystals or drug crystals may provide clues to etiology.

Urine and Serum Biochemistry

Biochemical investigations are required to evaluate renal function and to identify underlying metabolic abnormalities with an excess of solutes [e.g. hypercalcemia, hyperuricosemia, renal tubular acidosis (RTA)] or decrease in inhibitors of crystallization (e.g. hypocitraturia). Blood investigations include urea, creatinine, calcium, phosphorous, alkaline phosphatase, uric acid, magnesium, venous blood pH, bicarbonate, and electrolytes. Timed (12 or 24 hours) urine collection is required to estimate the excretion of calcium, oxalate, uric acid, cysteine, and citrate. In younger children in whom timed collections are difficult, spot samples of urine solute/creatinine can be used (**Table 10.13.2**).

Stone Analysis

Stones excreted in the urine or removed surgically should be analyzed using X-ray diffraction or near infrared spectroscopy. Analysis is useful in the identification of rare stones such as cystine, uric acid, and drug-induced stones and has implications for management.

TREATMENT

Medical Management

Acute Management

Children presenting with renal colic are managed with antiemetics, nonsteroidal anti-inflammatory drugs, and in severe pain, opioids. Forced intravenous hydration may facilitate nonsurgical expulsion of stone in distal ureteric stones less than 4 mm in size. The efficacy of alpha-blockers and calcium-channel blockers (CCBs), used in adults to facilitate stone expulsion, has not been established in children.

Long-term Management

Pharmacological and nonpharmacological measures are used to prevent recurrence of stones and prevent renal damage. General measures include increasing fluid intake and dietary modifications. Increasing urine volume reduces supersaturation of crystals, while urine output of over 1 mL/kg/h prevents formation of calcium crystals; larger outputs are required for insoluble substances such as cystine and xanthine.

Patients with hypercalciuria should take calcium within the accepted recommended daily allowance; medications containing calcium are avoided. Restricting the intake of animal proteins and salt reduces the rate of calcium excretion as natural sources of citrate, fruits, and vegetables are beneficial. Patients with hyperoxaluria should restrict the intake of foods rich in oxalate, such as chocolates, tea, coffee, green leafy vegetable, and nuts.

Pharmacological measures are targeted to the underlying cause. The solubility of the incriminated solute may be modified by altering the urine pH, e.g. alkalinization enhances the solubility of uric acid and cystine. Increasing urinary citrate may enhance the solubility of calcium. Drugs may decrease production of solutes, e.g. allopurinol for uric acid stones (**Table 10.13.3**).

Table 10.13.2: Normal values of solutes in 24 hours urine.

Chemical	*Value*
Calcium	<4 mg/kg
Oxalate	<40 mg/1.73 m^2; <2 mg/kg
Uric acid	<800 mg/1.73 m^2; <35 mg/kg
Cystine	<60 mg/1.73 m^2
Xanthine	30–90 μg
Citrate	>180 mg/g creatinine

Surgical Management

Stone removal may be indicated as an emergency due to acute obstruction or performed electively. The choice of modality for stone removal depends on the size, number and location of stone and the presence of obstructive uropathy or underlying urological abnormalities.

Extracorporeal Shock Wave Lithotripsy

Extracorporeal shock wave lithotripsy focuses shock wave energy at the calculus. It is the preferred treatment in children with calculi below 20 mm in size. Success rates are lower with hard cystine stones and stones in the lower calyx.

Ureterorenoscopy

Ureterorenoscopy is ideally suited for calculi in the mid and distal ureter. With the availability of smaller scopes, it is now feasible in children.

Table 10.13.3: Medications used in the treatment of nephrolithiasis.

Medication	*Dose*	*Indication*
Allopurinol	10 mg/kg/day in 2–3 divided doses	Hyperuricosuria
Captopril	0.5–2 mg/kg dose 2–4 times a day	Cystinuria
Hydrochlorothiazide	1–2 mg/kg/day in 1–2 divided doses	Hypercalciuria
Potassium citrate	0.5–2 mEq/kg/day in 3 doses	Hypercalciuria, hyperuricosuria
Pyridoxine	3–5 mg/kg/day in one daily dose	Primary hyperoxaluria
D-Penicillamine	30 mg/kg/day divided in 4 doses	Cystinuria

Percutaneous Nephrolithotomy

Percutaneous nephrolithotomy (PCNL) is a more invasive procedure and is reserved for children with larger and more complex calculi. Stones above 1.5 cm or lower pole stones above 1 cm benefit with PCNL. The calyx is punctured under ultrasonic guidance and the instrument inserted under fluoroscopic guidance to fragment and remove the stones.

Surgical Approaches

Including laparoscopic or open surgery are required in more than 5% cases, chiefly for large stones, multiple stones and those associated with structural abnormalities.

BIBLIOGRAPHY

1. Alon US. Medical treatment of pediatric urolithiasis. Pediatr Nephrol. 2009;24(11):2129-35.
2. Gurgoze MK, Sari MY. Results of medical treatment and metabolic risk factors in children with urolithiasis. Pediatr Nephrol. 2011;26:933-7.
3. Straub M, Gschwend J, Zorn C. Pediatric urolithiasis: the current surgical management. Pediatr Nephrol. 2010;25(7): 1239-44.
4. Turk C, Knoll T, Petrik A, et al. EAU Clinical Guidelines—Guidelines on Urolithiasis. Arnhem, The Netherlands: European Association of Urology; 2011.

10.14 Hypertension

Jitendra Meena, Pankaj Hari

INTRODUCTION

The prevalence of hypertension has increased in children. Approximately 3–4% children and adolescents have hypertension while elevated blood pressure present in 10%. Essential hypertension is less common in younger children but it is being increasingly recognized in adolescent. Children with persistent severe hypertension are at increased risk of adverse outcomes, such as hypertensive encephalopathy, retinopathy, congestive heart failure, and renal failure.

DEFINITIONS AND STAGING OF HYPERTENSION

New normative reference data for blood pressure is provided, in recent clinical practice guidelines (CPGs) for screening and management of high blood pressure in children and adolescents by American Academy of Pediatrics (AAP). These new tables have been developed, from previous normative data of fourth report, after excluding data of overweight and obese children, as adiposity is strongly associated with higher blood pressure. New tables provide blood pressure values, based on gender, age and height percentiles, at 50th 90th, 95th and 95th+12 mm Hg, and should be used to define and stage the high blood pressure **(Table 10.14.1)**. Based on new normative blood pressure data, **Figures 10.14.1 and 10.14.2** provide charts for screening and staging of hypertension in boys and girls respectively. **Table 10.14.2** provides screening blood pressure cutoffs for identification of the children who require further evaluation and it is based on 90th centile blood pressure for age and gender at 5th centile of the stature.

Table 10.14.1: Definition and staging of hypertension in children.

Elevated blood pressure	≥90th percentile to < 95th percentile or 120/80 mm Hg to < 95th percentile (whichever is lower)*
Hypertension	SBP or DBP ≥ 95th percentile or > 130/80 mm Hg*
Stage 1 hypertension	SBP or DBP between ≥ 95th percentile to <95th percentile +12 mm Hg, or 130/80 to 139/89 mm Hg (whichever is lower)*
Stage 2 hypertension	SBP or DBP ≥ 95th percentile +12 mm Hg, or ≥ 140/90 mm Hg (whichever is lower)*

(DBP: diastolic blood pressure; SBP: systolic blood pressure)
*For adolescent aged ≥ 13 years.
Source: Adapted from 2017 clinical practice guideline by American Academy of Pediatrics

- White coat hypertension refers to high office blood pressure in a child who has normal blood pressures in familiar setting.
- Masked hypertension refers to situations where office blood pressures are normal but the child is actually hypertensive.

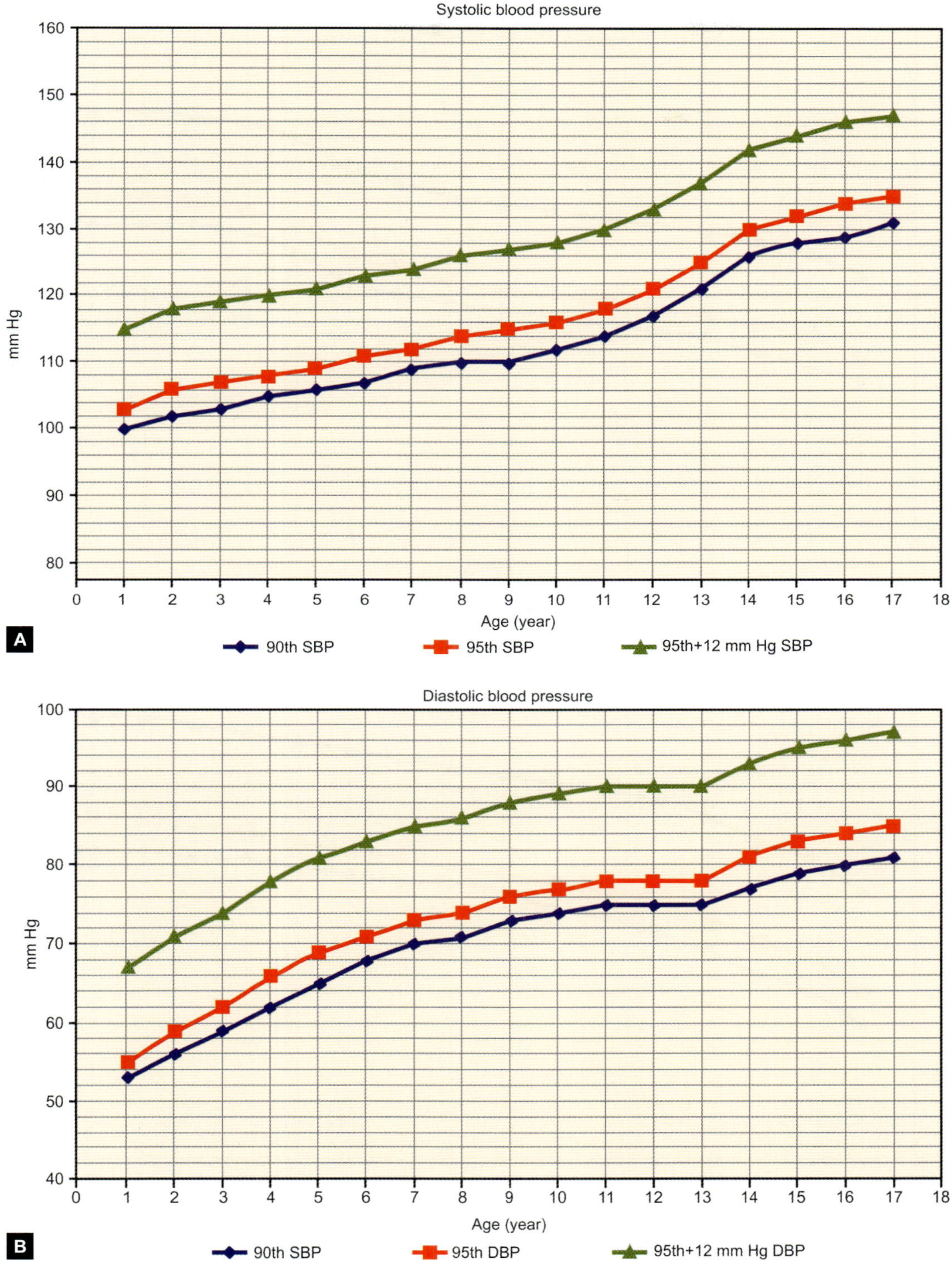

Figs 10.14.1A and B: Blood pressure levels for boys at 50th percentile for height. Chart depicting 90th (closed diamonds), 95th (open squares) and 95th +12 mm Hg (closed triangles) percentile values for (A) systolic and (B) diastolic blood pressures, representing cut-off values for the diagnosis of elevated blood pressure, stage 1 and stage 2 hypertension respectively in boys (based on AAP clinical practice guideline for screening and management of high blood pressure in children and adolescents 2017).

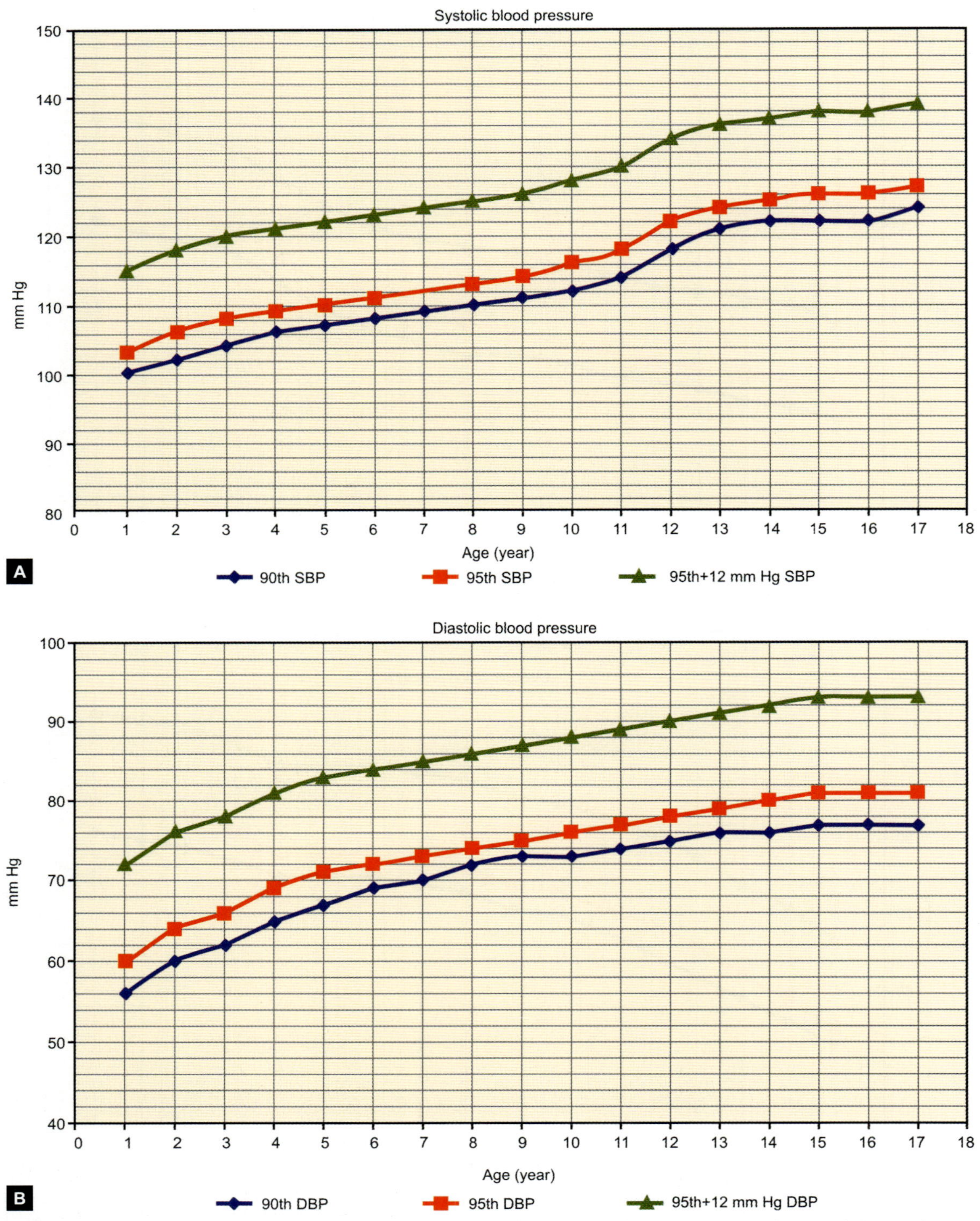

Figs. 10.14.2A and B: Blood pressure levels for girls at 50th percentile for height. Chart depicting 90th (closed diamonds), 95th (open squares) and 95th +12 mm Hg (closed triangles) percentile values for (A) systolic and (B) diastolic blood pressures, representing cut-off values for the diagnosis of elevated blood pressure, stage 1 and stage 2 hypertension respectively in girls (based on AAP clinical practice guideline for screening and management of high blood pressure in children and adolescents 2017).

Table 10.14.2: Screening blood pressure for children.

Age (year)		1	2	3	4	5	6	7	8	9	10	11	12	≥13
Girls	SBP (mm Hg)	98	101	102	103	104	105	106	107	108	109	111	114	120
	DBP (mm Hg)	54	58	60	62	64	67	68	69	71	72	74	75	80
Boys	SBP (mm Hg)	98	100	101	102	103	105	106	107	107	108	110	113	120
	DBP (mm Hg)	52	55	58	60	63	66	68	69	70	72	74	75	80

(DBP: diastolic blood pressure; SBP: systolic blood pressure)

Table 10.14.3: Blood pressure monitoring techniques.

Technique	***Advantages***	***Drawbacks***
Auscultatory (mercury sphygmomanometer)	• Most evidence based • Noninvasive • Quick to perform • Easily available	• White coat effect • Observer bias • Terminal digit preference • *Safety hazard*: Mercury spill
Aneroid manometer	• Easily portable • Mercury free	Needs frequent calibration
Oscillometric devices	• Easy to use • Useful in infants, where auscultation is difficult • No observer bias	• Limited reference data • Values of diastolic pressure derived from mean pressure; may be inaccurate • Requires repeated validation • Cost and availability
Ambulatory blood pressure monitoring (ABPM)	For white coat, masked hypertension, data on diurnal variability	• Considerable cost • Needs patient cooperation and training

DIAGNOSIS OF HYPERTENSION

To diagnose hypertension blood pressure either systolic or diastolic more than the 95th percentile should be documented on at least three separate occasions, unless patient is symptomatic. Blood pressure should be measured, annually in all children and adolescents more than or equal to 3 years of age and at every healthcare visit in all children, if they have specific conditions associated with increase risk of hypertension. These conditions include prematurity, obesity, renal disease, heart disease, diabetes, systemic illnesses associated with hypertension (neurofibromatosis, tuberous sclerosis, sickle cell disease), history of solid organ transplant, and taking drugs that are known to raise blood pressure.

MEASUREMENT OF BLOOD PRESSURE

Table 10.14.3 shows a comparison of various techniques for measurement of blood pressure. Blood pressure measurement by auscultation should be the preferred method for confirmation of abnormal blood pressure as normative data is based on auscultated measurements. Blood pressure measurement in children should be performed after adequate rest of 3–5 minutes while sitting in an upright position with the back supported, feet uncrossed on the floor and the cubital fossa at the level of the heart. The right arm is preferred to avoid falsely low readings in patients with coarctation of the aorta and for consistency.

At least three measurements are taken on a visit, for confirming reproducibility of the result and for decreasing the effect of white coat hypertension. An appropriate cuff size with an inflatable bladder width that is at least 40% of the arm circumference, and bladder length sufficient to cover 80–100% of the arm circumference should be used.

Ambulatory blood pressure monitoring (ABPM) refers to the continuous recordings of blood pressure over 24-hour; it is believed to reflect true blood pressures accurately, is more reproducible and correlates with target organ damage. Data are assessed in terms of mean blood pressure load (percentage of readings above the ambulatory 95th percentile) and nocturnal dipping (percent day-night difference). ABPM is indicated for diagnosis of masked hypertension, white coat hypertension, and nocturnal hypertension and to assess the effectiveness of antihypertensive therapy for control of hypertension.

ETIOLOGY

Sustained hypertension in children is often secondary to an underlying etiology **(Box 10.14.1)**; in approximately 90% of patients secondary hypertension is due to renal

Box 10.14.1: Causes of hypertension.

Transient hypertension

- Acute renal failure; acute glomerulonephritis
- Increased intracranial pressure
- Acute intermittent porphyria
- Guillain–Barré syndrome
- Hyperthyroidism

Persistent hypertension

Renal parenchymal disease:
- Glomerulonephritis
- Hemolytic uremic syndrome
- Reflux nephropathy; obstructive uropathy
- Polycystic kidney disease, renal dysplasia
- Post-kidney transplantation

Renovascular:
- Renal vein thrombosis
- Renal artery stenosis
- Fibromuscular dysplasia
- Takayasu arteritis
- Tumors compressing on renal vessels
- Syndromes (William, Turner, neurofibromatosis type 1)

Cardiovascular:
Coarctation of aorta

Primary (essential) hypertension:
- Isolated
- With metabolic syndrome

Endocrine:
- Cushing syndrome
- Congenital adrenal hyperplasia
- Primary hyperaldosteronism
- Hyperthyroidism, hypothyroidism
- Liddle syndrome
- Syndrome of apparent mineralocorticoid excess
- Glucocorticoid remediable aldosteronism

Tumors
Renal:
- Wilms' tumor
- Reninoma
- Hemangiopericytoma
- Hamartoma

Extrarenal:
- Pheochromocytoma
- Neuroblastoma
- Paraganglioma

Medications/Iatrogenic:
- Corticosteroids
- Substance abuse
- Nasal decongestants (phenylephrine, pseudoephedrine, oxymetazoline)
- Nonsteroidal anti-inflammatory drugs
- *Others*: Erythropoietin, calcineurin inhibitors, theophylline, caffeine, antidepressants

parenchymal or renovascular abnormalities. In recent years, essential hypertension has become an important health concern. Patients with essential hypertension are usually postpubertal and overweight and typically show stage 1 hypertension.

CLINICAL FEATURES

Patients with elevated blood pressure and stage 1 hypertension are usually asymptomatic. Symptoms are more common in patients with secondary hypertension. Symptoms such as headache, dizziness, vomiting, irritability, epistaxis, flush, visual disturbances, and vertigo usually occur with significant elevation of blood pressure.

Hypertensive crisis: Some patients with stage 2 hypertension may present with hypertensive crises, which are classified as emergencies or urgencies. Hypertensive emergencies are associated with acute target organ damage such as encephalopathy, intracranial hemorrhage, acute left ventricular failure with pulmonary edema, dissecting aortic aneurysm, papilledema, and acute renal failure (ARF). Hypertensive urgency is severe hypertension without end organ damage. The occurrence of these complications is related to the rate of rise and duration of hypertension, rather than absolute blood pressure values.

Complications of sustained hypertension include hypertensive retinopathy, albuminuria, left ventricular hypertrophy, diastolic dysfunction and premature atherosclerosis as evidenced by increased carotid intima media thickness.

EVALUATION

Careful history and physical examination may provide important clues to the underlying etiology **(Table 10.14.4)**. Family history is taken for hypertension, diabetes, dyslipidemia, obesity, premature cardiovascular or cerebrovascular disease and renal disorders. Assessment of body mass index and measurement of blood pressure in all four limbs are necessary.

INVESTIGATIONS

Since the majority of patients with hypertension have underlying renal or renovascular etiology, screening tests (urinalysis, blood urea and creatinine, electrolytes, lipid profile and renal ultrasound) are designed to evaluate for these conditions **(Box 10.14.1)**. Patients with hypertension should also be screened for target organ damage. Based on clinical features and initial evaluation, a cause for hypertension is suggested in most instances. Confirmation of the diagnosis of underlying etiology requires specific investigations tailored to specific needs **(Tables 10.14.4 and 10.14.5)**. However recent AAP guideline recommends that children more than 6 years of age, who are obese or overweight and if they have family history of hypertension, do not require comprehensive investigation in the absence of physical finding suggestive of a cause for secondary hypertension.

MANAGEMENT

Management of high blood pressure should begin with therapeutic lifestyle modification, especially in children who have modifiable risk factors. The indications for pharmacological therapy are listed in **Box 10.14.2**.

Table 10.14.4: Clinical features and investigations for secondary hypertension.

Condition	*Clinical features*	*Investigations*
Glomerulonephritis	Facial puffiness, edema, hematuria and oligoanuria	Urinalysis, 24-hour urine protein, C3, antinuclear antibody, antineutrophil cytoplasmic antibody, renal biopsy
Reflux nephropathy	Dysuria, frequency, history of urinary tract infections	Renal ultrasound, micturating cystourethrography, renal scintigraphy
Renovascular disease	Asymmetric pulses, abdominal/neck bruit, weak femoral artery pulses	Doppler ultrasound, captopril renography, computed tomography (CT), magnetic resonance imaging angiography or digital subtraction angiography (DSA)
Coarctation of aorta	Weak femoral artery pulses	Echocardiography, DSA
Metabolic syndrome	Adolescent age, obesity	Blood sugars, HbA1c, lipid profile, aspartate transaminase and alanine transaminase
Endocrine	Muscle weakness, cramps, episodic fever, flushing, tachycardia, polyuria, polydipsia, failure to thrive, ambiguous genitalia	Plasma renin, aldosterone, plasma and urinary cortisol, plasma and urine metanephrines, metaiodobenzyl guanidine (MIBG) scan, CT/MRI scan

Table 10.14.5: Diagnostic workup.

Evaluation for etiology	*Screen for target organ damage*
Hemogram	Retina fundus examination
Blood urea, creatinine, electrolytes	Urinalysis, urine spot protein to creatinine ratio
Lipid profile, uric acid, HbA1c (if patient is obese)	Chest X-ray
Urinalysis, culture 24-hour protein	Electrocardiogram (ECG)
Renal ultrasonography and Doppler	Echocardiography

Target Blood Pressure

American Academy of Pediatrics (2017) CPGs recommend lowering systolic and diastolic blood pressure to below 90th percentile in all children and less than 130/80 mm Hg in adolescent more than 13 years old. However guidelines recommend that in hypertensive children with chronic kidney disease target blood pressure should be less than 50th percentile of mean 24-hour ambulatory blood pressure to reduce the rate of decline in kidney function.

Elevated Blood Pressure

These patients are managed by lifestyle modifications (see later) and reevaluated 3–6 months later. Medications are not required unless the patient has comorbid conditions.

Essential Hypertension

Patients with essential hypertension are initially managed with lifestyle modifications, and pharmacological therapy is initiated later. Thiazide diuretics and beta-blockers, especially in combination, should be avoided due to their significant diabetogenic potential. Therapy may be initiated with a calcium-channel blockers (CCB) or angiotensin-converting enzyme inhibitor (ACEI). Screening for dyslipidemia, fatty liver and impaired glucose tolerance should be done.

Box 10.14.2: Indications for drug therapy.
• Stage 2 hypertension without modifiable risk factors
• Symptomatic hypertension
• Secondary hypertension
• Hypertension in patient with diabetes and chronic kidney disease
• Persistent hypertension despite nonpharmacological measures
• Hypertension with additional risk factors (i.e. obesity, hyperlipidemia)

Secondary Hypertension

Patients with sustained secondary hypertension require therapy with antihypertensive agents. The treatment plan should incorporate nonpharmacological measures in all patients.

Nonpharmacological Therapy

Major lifestyle modification recommended for management of hypertension is weight reduction, improving physical activity, stress reduction and dietary approach to stop hypertension (DASH). Weight reduction in overweight and obese patient with hypertension results in significant reduction in blood pressure as well as also reduces other cardiovascular risk factors, i.e. hyperlipidemia and insulin resistance. Recent CPGs recommend 30–60 minutes per session of moderate-to-vigorous aerobic physical activity 3–5 days per week with limitation of sedentary activity to 2 hours per day. Children with hypertension may benefit from DASH, which includes increasing the intake of fresh fruit, fiber, low fat dairy product and whole grains with reduction in sugar and salt consumption.

Pharmacological Therapy

Study of antihypertensive drugs regarding safety and their impact on cardiovascular outcomes is limited in children. Pharmacological therapy should be initiated with single medication at low end of dosing range while continuing lifestyle modification. Dosing recommendations are shown in **Table 10.14.6.** Drugs with a longer duration of action are preferred for better compliance. When required, dose should be increased every 2–4 weeks until blood pressure is controlled or adverse effects occur. Patient should have a

Table 10.14.6: Commonly used drugs for treatment of hypertension in children.

Agents	*Dose*	*Side effects/Comments*
Angiotensin-converting enzyme inhibitors (ACEIs)		
• Captopril	0.05–6 mg/kg/day	• Use cautiously if glomerular filtration rate (GFR) < 30 mL/min/1.73 m^2
• Enalapril	0.08–0.6 mg/kg/day	• Avoid in renal artery stenosis
• Lisinopril	0.06–0.6 mg/kg/day	• Use smaller doses in neonates
• Ramipril	1.6–6 mg/m^2	• Monitor serum potassium, creatinine, contraindicated in pregnancy
Angiotensin receptor blockers (ARBs)		Similar to ACEI; cough, angioedema not seen
• Losartan	0.75–1.4 mg/kg/day	
• Olmesartan	10–40 mg/day	
• Valsartan	1.3–2.7 mg/kg/day	
• Candesartan	0.02–0.4 mg/kg/day	

Contd...

Contd...

Agents	***Dose***	***Side effects/Comments***
Calcium-channel blockers • Amlodipine • Nifedipine • Isradipine	0.05–0.6 mg/kg/day 0.25–3 mg/kg/day 0.15–0.6 mg/kg/day	• Headache, flushing, tachycardia, edema, dizziness • May increase proteinuria
Beta-blockers • Atenolol • Labetalol • Metoprolol	0.5–2.0 mg/kg/day 1–40 mg/kg/day 1–6 mg/kg/day	• Avoid in asthma, heart failure • Reduce dose of atenolol in renal dysfunction
Central alpha-agonist Clonidine	5–25 μg/kg/day	Rebound hypertension when withdrawn
Peripheral alpha-antagonists Prazosin	0.05–0.5 mg/kg/day	Syncope
Diuretics • Hydrochlorothiazide • Furosemide • Amiloride • Spironolactone	1–2 mg/kg/day 0.5–6 mg/kg/day 0.4–0.6 mg/kg/day 1–3 mg/kg/day	*Thiazide*: Hyperuricemia, hyperlipidemia, hyperglycemia, hypokalemia, ineffective at GFR < 30 mL/min/1.73 m^2 *Loop diuretics*: Alkalosis, hypokalemia *Potassium-sparing diuretics*: Hyperkalemia especially with ACEI, ARB
Vasodilators • Hydralazine • Minoxidil	1–8 mg/kg/day 0.1–1.0 mg/kg/day	• Headache, palpitation • Hypertrichosis, fluid retention, pericardial effusion

clinic visit every 4–6 weeks until blood pressure is normalized. A second medication with a complementary mechanism of action should be added if blood pressure control is still not achieved and dose increased to maximum, if necessary. If blood pressure not controlled, a third antihypertensive drug of a different class may be added. Therapy in children is often started with a CCB or ACEI. The choice of initial medication often depends on the cause of hypertension and associated comorbidities and complications. In hypertensive children with chronic kidney disease, proteinuria and diabetes ACEI are the preferred drugs unless there is an absolute contraindication.

Follow-up and Monitoring

After initiation of drug therapy, follow-up visits should be frequent (every 4–6 weeks) until blood pressure is controlled. Once blood pressure is controlled patient can be followed up once in every 3–4 months. At every follow-up visit adherence to medication, home blood pressure monitoring and assessment for side effects should be done. ABPM can be used to assess the control of blood pressure especially in a patient with chronic kidney disease and/or target end organ damage. After successful blood pressure control, "step down" of therapy may be attempted. Monitoring for target organ damage should be done at regular intervals.

MANAGEMENT OF HYPERTENSIVE CRISES

Hypertensive emergency requires immediate reduction in blood pressure in order to prevent or limit target organ damage. These patients require constant monitoring and supportive care, necessitating hospitalization. A hypertensive emergency is treated with a potent intravenous antihypertensive titrated to produce a controlled reduction in blood pressure, with the ultimate aim of reducing the blood pressure up to ~95th percentile. Up to 25% of the planned reduction should be done over the first 8 hours of presentation and then remainder reduction gradually over next 12–24 hours. Overly rapid reduction of blood pressure may compromise blood flow to important organs causing ischemic damage, especially since autoregulation may be impaired or altered. Therapy with oral antihypertensive drugs should be commenced as soon as patient can take orally, in order to permit withdrawal of intravenous therapy. The drug therapy of hypertensive emergency is summarized in **Table 10.14.7**. Intravenous nitroprusside and labetalol are the preferred antihypertensive drugs for management of the hypertensive emergency. Alternatively intravenous nicardipine or esmolol may be used. Hypertensive urgency can be treated with oral medications over 24–48 hours.

Table 10.14.7: Commonly used drugs for hypertensive emergency.

Drug	*Onset*	*Route*	*Dose*	*Side effects*
Labetalol	5–10 min	Intravenous (IV) infusion	0.25–3 mg/kg/hour	• Orthostatic hypotension, bradycardia, pallor, abdominal pain, diarrhea • Asthma and overt heart failure are relative contraindication
		IV bolus	0.2–1 mg/kg/dose q 5–10 min (maximum 40 mg)	
Sodium nitroprusside	30 sec	IV infusion	0.5–10 µg/kg/min (in 5% dextrose)	Nausea, vomiting, headache, tachycardia, cyanide toxicity (dizziness, confusion, seizures, jaw stiffness and lactic acidosis)
Nicardipine	1–10 min	IV infusion	0.5–4 µg/kg/min (maximum 5 mg/hour)	Flushing, reflex tachycardia, phlebitis, edema, headache, nausea, vomiting
		IV bolus	30 µg/kg (max 2 mg/dose) q 15 min	
Esmolol	60 sec	IV infusion	Loading with 100–500 µg/kg over 1–2 min; then maintain at 25–100 µg/kg/min	Bradycardia, orthostatic hypotension, pallor
Hydralazine		IV bolus or intramuscular Oral	0.1–0.2 mg/kg/dose, maximum 0.4 mg/kg Bolus dose every 4 hour 0.25 mg/kg/dose every 6–8 hour	Tachycardia
Sodium nitroglycerin	2–5 min	IV infusion	1–3 µg/kg/min	Methemoglobinemia, headache, tachycardia
Nifedipine	10–30 min	Oral	0.2–0.5 mg/kg (maximum 10 mg) q 4–6 hour	Excessive hypotension, peripheral edema
Minoxidil		Oral	0.1–0.2 mg/kg/dose up to 10 mg per dose; every 8–12 h	

BIBLIOGRAPHY

1. Bagga A, Jain R, Vijayakumar M, et al. Evaluation and management of hypertension. Indian Pediatr. 2007;44(2):103-2.
2. Constantine E, Linakis J. The assessment and management of hypertensive emergencies and urgencies in children. Pediatr Emerg Care. 2005;21(6):391-6.
3. Falkner B. Changes in the 2017 pediatric hypertension clinical guidelines. Am J Hypertens. 2017;31(1):18-20.
4. Flynn JT, Daniels SR, Hayman LL, et al. Update: Ambulatory blood pressure monitoring in children and adolescents: a scientific statement from the American Heart Association. Hypertension. 2014;63(5):1116-35.
5. Flynn JT, Kaelber DC, Baker-Smith CM, et al. Subcommittee on screening and management of high blood pressure in children. Clinical practice guideline for screening and management of high blood pressure in children and adolescents. Pediatrics. 2017;140(3):e20171904.
6. Whelton PK, Carey RM, Aronow WS, et al. Guideline for the prevention, detection, evaluation, and management of high blood pressure in adults: Executive Summary: A report of the American College of Cardiology/American Heart Association Task Force on Clinical Practice Guidelines. Hypertension. 2018;71(6):1269-324.

Section 11

Diseases of Blood

11.1 An Approach to Anemia in the Newborn

Ved Prakash Choudhry

INTRODUCTION

Anemia is a unique problem in neonates. Development of anemia within 7 days of life is termed as "early onset anemia", while anemia occurring after 7 days is called "late onset anemia". The causes of anemia in these two groups are quite different and so is the treatment.

Etiology

The three major causes of anemia are:
1. Blood loss
2. Hemolysis
3. Reduced red cell production.

Blood loss leading to anemia may occur prenatally, during delivery or over the first 7 days **(Box 11.1.1)**.

FETOMATERNAL TRANSFUSION

Fetomaternal transfusion occurs in nearly 50% of pregnancies, and in most cases, it is minimal without any consequences. But in conditions like abruptio placentae and manual extraction of placenta, there is significant fetomaternal transfusion.

CLINICAL PRESENTATION

It depends upon the amount of hemorrhage and rapidity of bleed. In acute hemorrhage, the neonate is pale and sluggish, develops gasping respiration and signs of circulatory shock **(Fig. 11.1.1)**. Clinical presentation of acute and chronic blood loss along with treatment are given in **Table 11.1.1**.

Box 11.1.1: Hemorrhage in newborn (blood loss).

- Obstetric causes
  - Cesarean section
  - Placenta previa, abruptio placentae, and rupture of umbilical cord
  - Intrauterine manipulation or placenta removal
- Fetomaternal transfusion
- Amniocentesis in the third trimester
- External cephalic version
- *Fetofetal transfusion*: Transfusion from one twin to other
- Spontaneous hemorrhage
- *Internal hemorrhage*: Intracranial or retroperitoneal, rupture of organs
- *Iatrogenic*: Multiple sampling

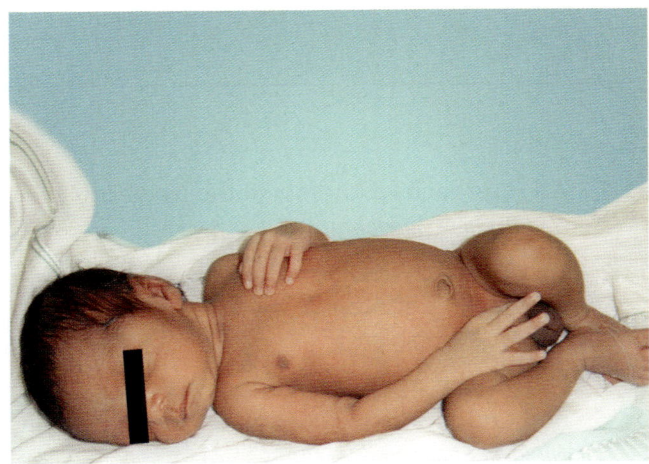

Fig. 11.1.1: Anemia in newborn.
Courtesy: Dr MR Lokeshwar, Mumbai, Maharashtra and Dr Ved Prakash Choudhry, New Delhi, India.

Table 11.1.1: Acute and chronic blood loss in neonates.

Clinical features	*Acute blood loss*	*Chronic blood loss*
Physical signs	• Pallor • Shallow rapid and irregular breathing • Tachycardia • No organomegaly	• Significant pallor • Hepatomegaly • Signs of congestive failure depending upon the Hb level
Venous pressure	Low	Normal or elevated
Hemoglobin level	Normal initially and decreases within 24 hours	Low at birth
Red cell morphology	Normocytic, normochromic	Microcytic, hypochromic
Coomb's test	Negative	Negative
Fetal cells in maternal blood	Present	Significantly present
Treatment	Pack cell transfusion	Pack cell transfusion, if anemia is severe
Iron therapy	Later	Immediate

(Hb: hemoglobin)

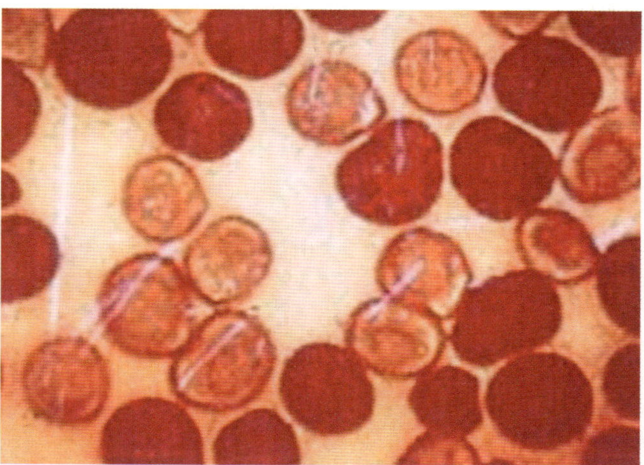

Fig. 11.1.2: A fetomaternal transfusion: Kleihauer-Betke test on mother's blood.

The Kleihauer–Betke test is a blood test used to measure the amount of fetal hemoglobin (Hb) transferred from a fetus to a mother's bloodstream **(Fig. 11.1.2)**. Even though, it is usually done as a positive screening test on all Rhesus (Rh)-negative mothers of Rh-positive infants, it is indicated in all the cases of maternal trauma.

FETOFETAL TRANSFUSION

It occurs in monozygotic twins with monochorial placenta. Nearly 20% of these transfusions are associated with twin-to-twin transfusion. Donor neonate has anemia, while recipient twin is polycythemic. Clinical presentation depends upon the volume of blood transfusion and whether the process has been acute or chronic. The anemic twin may develop pallor and congestive heart failure. Plethoric twin may develop hyperviscosity, hyperbilirubinemia, or disseminated intravascular coagulopathy.

INTERNAL HEMORRHAGE

Neonates may develop anemia within 24 hours of birth in the absence of jaundice, often secondary to internal hemorrhage. These forms of bleed occur in difficult deliveries following vacuum or forceps extraction. These deliveries are associated with subdural and subarachnoid hemorrhage or cephalhematoma. Breech deliveries are associated with internal hemorrhage of kidneys, spleen, liver, or other organs. Bleeding is severe in the presence of vitamin K deficiency.

Subarachnoid or intraventricular bleeding has been observed in half of babies with birth weight below 1,500 g. Many neonates are asymptomatic. These babies may be lethargic and have poor sucking, sluggish neonatal reflexes, and pallor, and/or breathing problems. Bleeding can be confirmed by computed tomography of head.

IATROGENIC HEMORRHAGE

A major cause of anemia in critically ill neonates in intensive care unit (ICU) is secondary to frequent blood sampling, especially in very low birth weight (LBW) babies (<1,500 g). About 1 mL of blood represents 1% of total blood volume in these neonates. Approaches used to reduce the amount of blood drawn in ICU include the following:

- Use of micromethods
- Use of close method to allow return of initial sample drawn
- To draw the minimum blood required for tests
- Special culture media requiring minimal blood
- Use of transcutaneous monitoring techniques (analysis of blood gases, electrolytes, etc.).

HEMOLYTIC ANEMIA IN NEWBORN

Normal red cell survival in term neonate is 60–80 days, while it is 20–30 days in preterm neonate born between 30 weeks and 32 weeks. Most neonates with hemolytic anemia develop jaundice as liver is unable to conjugate and excrete the bilirubin. Symptoms depend upon the level of Hb as described earlier. High reticulocyte counts are seen in the absence of hemorrhage. The common causes of hemolytic states in newborn are given in **Box 11.1.2 and Figures 11.1.3A and B**.

Hemolytic Disease of the Newborn

Among the various causes of hemolytic anemia, immune-mediated disorders are most common, such as Rh and ABO incompatibility. Most infants have hyperbilirubinemia, which usually does not exceed 12 mg/dL.

Rhesus hemolytic disease is due to Rh incompatibility between mother and neonate. Its prevalence in Indian neonates is about 5%. It occurs as fetal red cells from Rh-positive neonate cross into maternal circulation in an Rh-negative mother. She produces antibody response to fetal red cells (Rh-positive), and these antibodies cross the

Box 11.1.2: Causes of neonatal hemolytic states.

- Drug induced
- *Red cell enzyme deficiencies*: Glucose-6-phosphate dehydrogenase deficiency, pyruvate kinase deficiency
- *Disorders of red cell membrane*: Hereditary spherocytosis, hereditary elliptocytosis, hereditary stomatocytosis
- *Hemoglobinopathies*: α-thalassemia, β-thalassemia, and sickle cell anemia
- *Infection or septicemia*: Gram-positive and Gram-negative, intrauterine infections (TORCH), malaria **(Figs. 11.1.3A and B)**
- Disseminated intravascular coagulopathy
- Galactosemia

(TORCH: toxoplasmosis, rubella, cytomegalovirus, herpes simplex, and HIV)

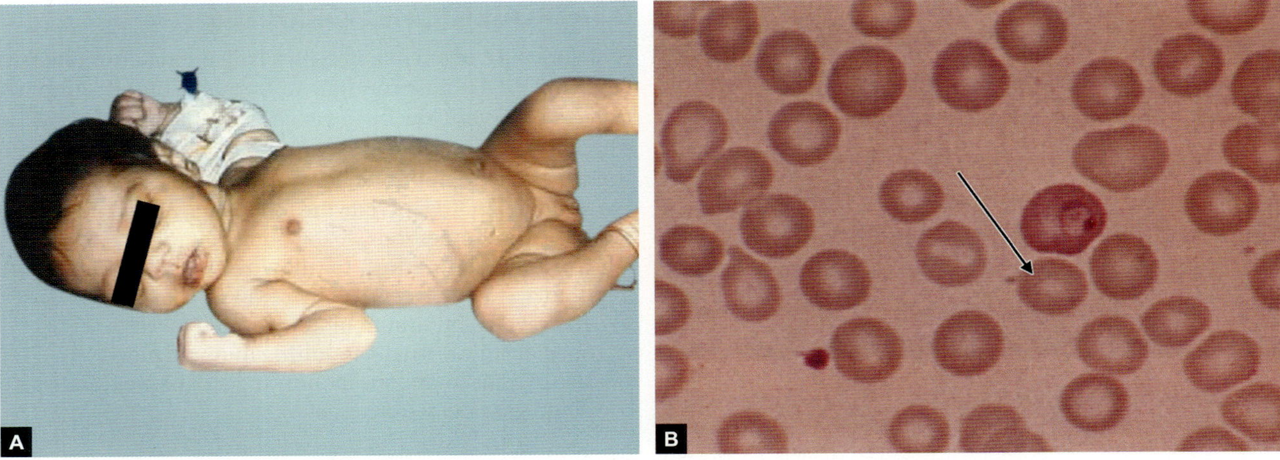

Figs. 11.1.3A and B: (A) Anemia in a neonate following malarial infection due to *Plasmodium vivax* and (B) the peripheral smear shows the malarial parasite.
Courtesy: Dr MR Lokeshwar, Mumbai, Maharashtra and Dr Ved Prakash Choudhry, New Delhi, India.

placenta resulting in fetal red cell hemolysis. The neonate develops jaundice, high reticulocyte count, and positive direct Coomb's test.

ABO hemolytic disease in India is common but the disease is generally milder. The mother has usually O blood group, while fetus has A or B blood group. Hemolysis is more severe in OA incompatibility than OB incompatibility. Fetomaternal incompatibility has been observed in nearly 25% of pregnancies. However, significant hemolysis occurs only in 10% of such cases.

The diagnosis can be suspected by high serum bilirubin levels in cord blood and confirmed by the presence of maternal immunoglobulin G anti-A or anti-B antibodies, antibody-dependent cell-mediated cytotoxicity along with high retic count, the presence of spherocytes on peripheral blood smear, and increased fragility of red cells. Direct Coomb's test is generally negative or only weekly positive.

LATE ONSET OF ANEMIA

Anemia developing after 7 days of life is termed late onset anemia. The causes of anemia during this period include:

- Physiological anemia of prematurity
- Reduced red cell production
- Hemolytic anemia
- Mild form of Rh isoimmune hemolytic anemia and ABO incompatibility. [These may manifest before 7 days, while other causes of hemolytic anemia **(Box 11.1.2)** often present after 7 days].

Septicemia causes anemia by two mechanisms, viz.

1. Hemolysis
2. Inhibiting erythropoietic activity.

Repeated blood sampling during neonatal period is also a major cause of late onset of anemia.

HEMOGLOBINOPATHIES IN NEWBORN PERIOD

Among various hemoglobinopathies, alpha and gamma chain defects are more frequent in neonatal period than β chain defects. Alpha chain disorders are common as it is a part of all Hbs at birth. These disorders are detected on routine neonatal screening. In newborns, hemolytic disease occurs with homozygous α-thalassemia. It occurs with defect in two genes or more. Mean corpuscular volume (MCV) is generally low along with the presence of the hemoglobin H (HbH) disease. It presents as late onset of anemia.

Hemoglobin H disease is more severe and is a result of inheritance of three gene deletions. Neonates with HbH disease have high levels of Hb Barts with anemia and jaundice. Hydrops fetalis is a result of four-gene deletion and results in death of the affected fetus or soon after birth. Peripheral blood shows marked hypochromia, poikilocytosis, and target cells. A negative Coomb's test and the presence of intracellular crystals of the Hb Barts with supravital staining confirm the diagnosis. Anemia in this condition is of early onset.

The β-chain mutations often do not present in newborn period.

Sickle cell hemoglobinopathies may present in neonatal period. In homozygous form, sickle cell concentration at birth is around 20%. These neonates may present with fever, jaundice, pallor, and respiratory distress. Hyperbilirubinemia is more common among neonates with sickle cell anemia. Sickle cell disease can be diagnosed by Hb electrophoresis.

RED CELL ENZYME DEFICIENCY

Glucose-6-phosphate Dehydrogenase Deficiency

Deficiency of glucose-6-phosphate dehydrogenase (G6PD) in red cells is common among Asians and accounts for 5–20% in different ethnic groups. This deficiency is inherited as X-linked recessive state. Hemolysis often occurs following exposure to drugs or infections. Neonate may receive the offending drug transplacentally or through breast milk. In addition to hemolysis, there is reduced glucuronidation of bilirubin in the presence of G6PD deficiency in hepatocytes.

Methemoglobin reduction is a simple screening test. However, G6PD levels can be measured. During acute episodes, the test is negative (normal activity) as G6PD-deficient cells have been hemolyzed. Anemia with high reticulocyte count along with jaundice may occur during neonatal period. Usually, its course is mild but may be severe enough to require exchange transfusion.

Pyruvate kinase deficiency is uncommon but its clinical course is mild.

DISORDERS OF RED CELL MEMBRANE

Hereditary spherocytosis is the most common form but usually it presents in later life. It presents with pallor, high reticulocyte count, and high bilirubin levels along with mild splenomegaly. Peripheral smear shows spherocytosis. Another cause of spherocytosis and splenomegaly is ABO incompatibility in the newborn.

REDUCED RED CELL PRODUCTION

Several conditions, such as pure red cell aplasia, Diamond-Blackfan syndrome, and Pearson syndrome, are uncommon disorders characterized by reduced erythropoiesis but with normal white cells and platelets. Low birth weight is observed in 10% of these cases:

- Babies with Diamond-Blackfan syndrome have microcephaly, cleft palate, and anomalies of eye, web neck, and thumb. It has autosomal recessive inheritance pattern. Neonates are likely to respond to steroids if diagnosed early.
- The Pearson syndrome is characterized by the presence of vacuoles in bone marrow precursor cells along with sideroblastic anemia and exocrine pancreatic dysfunction.
- Impaired red cell production has also been observed in intrauterine infections with rubella, cytomegalovirus, adenovirus, and human parvovirus.
- Congenital leukemia and Down syndrome have been associated with impaired erythropoiesis and are uncommon causes of late onset of anemia in the neonate.

PHYSIOLOGICAL ANEMIA OF PREMATURITY

Hemoglobin level in term infants decreases over the first few weeks of life. Premature neonates have greater fall in Hb resulting in "physiological anemia of prematurity". The Hb levels may decrease to 8 g/dL at 4–8 weeks of life in premature neonates with birth weight of less than 1,500 g. The decrease in Hb is primarily due to decrease in red cell mass rather than Hb dilutional effect. Other factors which contribute to the development of anemia include:

- Reduced red cell survival
- Reduced hematopoietic activity as evident by decrease in reticulocyte count
- The premature neonates are able to make physiological adjustments to such a low Hb levels by:
  - Increasing the cardiac output
  - Improving oxygen unloading capacity; and
  - Redistribution of blood flow
- Increased oxygen extraction by increase in 2,3-diphosphoglycerate levels of red cells
- Gradual rightward shift in the oxyhemoglobin dissociation curve by decrease in fetal Hb levels.

DIAGNOSTIC APPROACH TO ANEMIA IN NEWBORN

The causes of anemia in the neonate are variable with different pathogenesis:

- A detailed history of antenatal events, including the presence of anemia along with the treatment received by the mother is essential.
- Detailed family history of hemoglobinopathies is helpful.
- Physical examination particularly the presence of congenital anomalies and hepatosplenomegaly, stigmata of intrauterine infections, birth weight and development of jaundice, etc. are helpful for correct diagnosis.
- Initial laboratory studies should include complete blood counts along with red cell indices (MCV and mean corpuscular Hb), reticulocyte count, examination of peripheral blood smear, and Coomb's test (direct and indirect).
- A simple algorithm based on reticulocyte count and red cell indices is given in **Flowchart 11.1.1**.
- Subsequently specific tests can be undertaken for the confirmation of diagnosis.
- Correct diagnosis and prompt appropriate treatment plays a major role for survival.

RECENT ADVANCES

Autologous Transfusion

It has been observed that cord blood contains 75–125 mL of blood at birth (one-third of fetal blood). Autologous

Flowchart 11.1.1: Diagnostic approach to neonatal anemia.

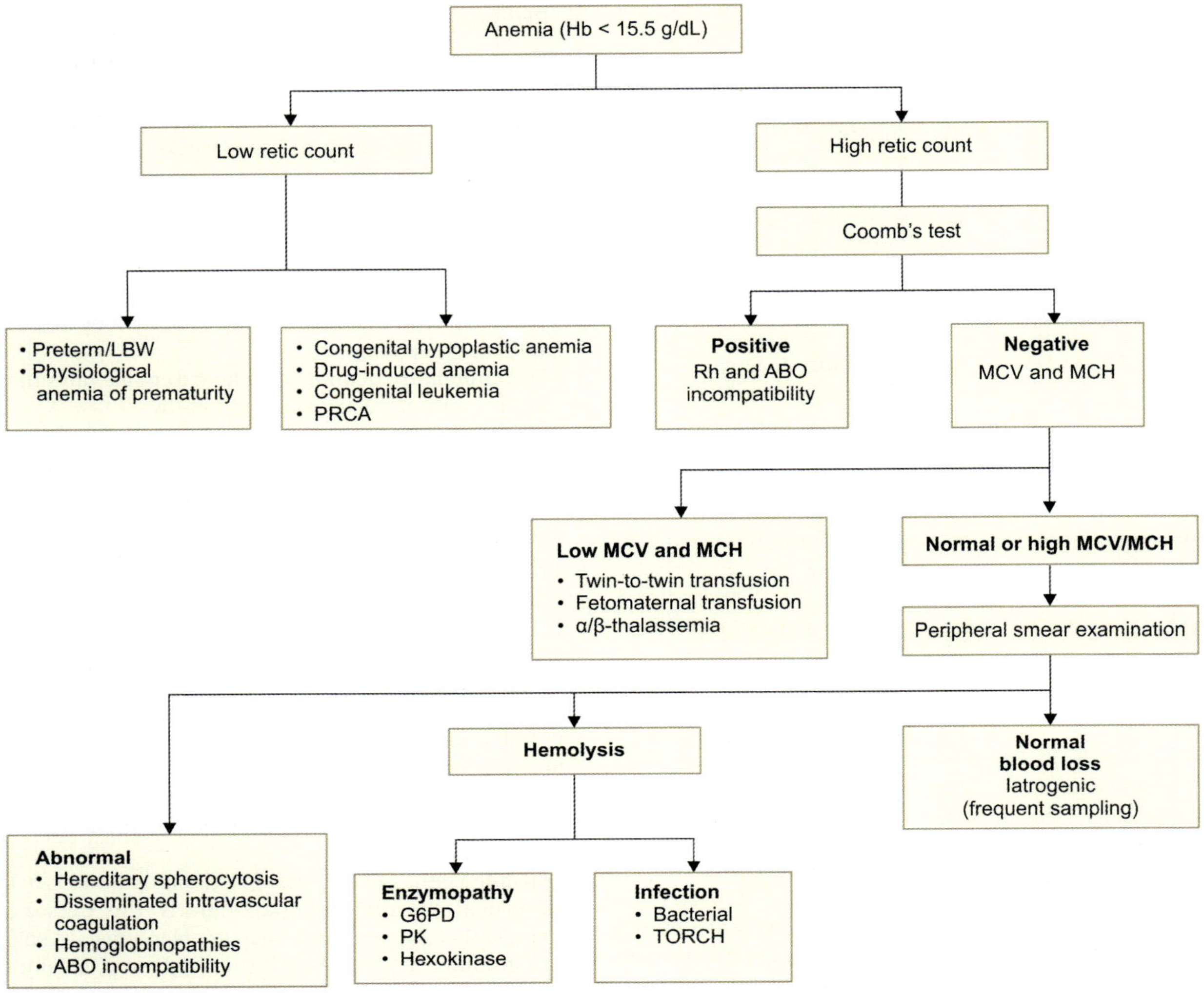

- Anemia (Hb < 15.5 g/dL)
  - Low retic count
    - • Preterm/LBW • Physiological anemia of prematurity
    - • Congenital hypoplastic anemia • Drug-induced anemia • Congenital leukemia • PRCA
  - High retic count
    - Coomb's test
      - **Positive** Rh and ABO incompatibility
      - **Negative** MCV and MCH
        - **Low MCV and MCH** • Twin-to-twin transfusion • Fetomaternal transfusion • α/β-thalassemia
        - **Normal or high MCV/MCH**
          - Peripheral smear examination
            - **Abnormal** • Hereditary spherocytosis • Disseminated intravascular coagulation • Hemoglobinopathies • ABO incompatibility
            - **Hemolysis**
              - **Enzymopathy** • G6PD • PK • Hexokinase
              - **Infection** • Bacterial • TORCH
            - **Normal blood loss** Iatrogenic (frequent sampling)

(G6PD: glucose 6-phosphatase dehydrogenase; LBW: low birth weight; MCH: mean corpuscular hemoglobin; MCV: mean corpuscular volume; PK: pyruvate kinase; PRCA: pure red cell aplasia; TORCH: toxoplasmosis, rubella, cytomegalovirus, herpes simplex, and HIV)

transfusions are safe, provided red cells are collected aseptically and stored properly in the blood bank. Autologous transfusions are useful in premature babies requiring neonatal intensive care facilities, iatrogenic anemia, and septicemia.

Delayed Clamping of Cord

Several studies have shown that neonates with delayed cord clamping tend to have high Hb levels than those in whom clamping was not delayed. Reduced blood volume is associated with increased mortality among premature infants who develop respiratory distress syndrome. Similarly, it has been observed that delayed cord clamping in premature infants is associated with reduced blood transfusion requirements and better survival.

Recombinant Erythropoietin and Anemia of Prematurity

Several studies have clearly shown that the use of erythropoietin in anemia of prematurity reduces the need of red cell transfusions in the premature or neonates with birth weight of 1,000 g at birth. However, in our country, the use of erythropoietin may not be cost effective. However, neonates receiving blood transfusions are at higher risk of developing transfusion-transmitted infections.

KEY MESSAGES

- Anemia in the neonatal period is quite common, especially in premature, LBW babies, and sick neonates requiring intensive care.
- Anemia in neonatal period is associated with high morbidity and mortality.
- Causes of neonatal anemia are variable. Detailed history of prenatal events, history of maternal diseases and drug intake is essential along with complete clinical evaluation of the newborn.
- Use of reticulocyte count, red cell indices, and peripheral smear examination along with Coomb's test is useful for an approach to neonatal anemia.
- Prompt treatment of underlying cause of anemia plays a major role for better survival.

BIBLIOGRAPHY

1. Luban NL. Management of anemia in the newborn. Early Hum Dev. 2008;84(8):493-8.
2. Nathan DG, Oski SH. Anemia in the newborn. In: Nathan DG, Orkin SH (Eds). Nathan and Oski's Hematology of Infancy and Childhood, 5th edition. Philadelphia, PA: WB Saunders; 1997. pp. 34-52.
3. Singh M. Anemia. In: Singh M (Ed). Care of the Newborn, 7th edition. New Delhi: Sagar Publications; 2010. pp. 362-5.

11.2 An Approach to Diagnosis of Anemia in Children

Ved Prakash Choudhry

INTRODUCTION

A person is considered anemic when the amount of hemoglobin (Hb), the oxygen-carrying pigment of the red blood cells (RBCs), is reduced from the normal value for that age and gender. Anemia is characterized by abnormally low levels of healthy RBCs, reduced Hb, or red cell blood volume (hematocrit). The reduction of any or all the three blood parameters affects the oxygen-carrying capability of blood adversely. **Table 11.2.1** provides the mean Hb concentration levels along with 2 standard deviations below the mean for normal population for gender and age, defined as normal blood levels by the "World Health Organization (WHO)," the United Nations Children's Fund, and the United Nations University.

The levels of Hb below which child is considered to have anemia as per the WHO criteria are given in **Table 11.2.2**.

EPIDEMIOLOGY

Anemia is widely prevalent and is a major cause of morbidity. Globally, anemia affects 1.62 billion people which correspond to 24.8% of the population. The highest prevalence is seen in preschool-age children (47.4%), and the lowest prevalence is seen in men (12.7%). Various surveys, including the "National Family Health Survey" have revealed that anemia is highest in children below 6–35 months of age. The data given in **Table 11.2.3** indicates that the prevalence of anemia in India has

Table 11.2.1: Normal hemoglobin, hematocrit, or packed cell volume at different ages.

	Hb (g/dL)		*PCV (%)*		*RCC (10^{12}/L)*	
Age	*Mean*	*±2 SD*	*Mean*	*±2 SD*	*Mean*	*±2 SD*
Birth (cord blood)	16.5	13.5	51	42	4.7	3.9
1–3 days	18.5	14.5	56	45	5.3	4.0
7 days	17.5	13.5	54	42	5.1	3.9
14 days	16.5	12.5	51	39	4.9	3.6
1 month	14.0	10.0	43	31	4.2	3.0
2 months	11.5	9.0	35	28	3.8	2.7
6 months	11.5	9.5	35	29	3.8	3.1
1 year	12.0	10.5	36	33	4.5	3.7
2–6 years	12.5	11.5	37	34	4.6	3.9
6–12 years	13.5	11.5	40	35	4.6	4.0
12–18 years:						
Girls	14.0	12.0	41	36	4.6	4.1
Boys	14.5	13.0	43	37	4.9	4.5

(Hb: hemoglobin; PCV: packed cell volume; RCC: red cell count; SD: standard deviation)

Table 11.2.2: World Health Organization criteria for hemoglobin below which person is anemic.

Age/gender groups	***Hb (g/dL)***
Children 6 months to 5 years	<11
Children 6–14 years	<12
Adult males	<13
Females (nonpregnant)	<12
Females (pregnant)	<11

(Hb: hemoglobin)

Table 11.2.3: Prevalence of anemia in different groups as per surveys in India.

Group	***Reference***	***Prevalence (%)***
Early childhood	NFHS II, 1998–99	74
Preschool children (6–35 months)	NFHS III, 2006–7	79
Adolescent girls	Seshadri, 1999, Rural Gujarat	62
	Seshadri, 1999, Urban affluent	22
	ICMR, 2001, Rural India	90

(ICMR: Indian Council of Medical Research; NFHS: National Family Health Survey)

increased over the last decade. It is more common in rural areas as compared to urban population.

ETIOLOGY

The etiology of anemia is variable. It may occur because of:

- Decreased erythropoiesis either due to the deficiency of nutrition or the defect in erythropoiesis
- Increased blood loss
- Diminished red cell survival as result of immune disorders and chronic infections.

The etiology of anemia is given in **Table 11.2.4**.

CLASSIFICATION

It is preferable to classify anemia based on the pathophysiologic effects for its better understanding **(Table 11.2.5)**. The classification based on red cell morphology (red cell size and Hb content) is useful in determining the etiology and is helpful in investigating the cause of anemia with minimal investigations **(Flowcharts 11.2.1 to 11.2.4)**.

CLINICAL FEATURES

Presence of anemia is associated with significant morbidity and mortality. The symptoms depend on the severity of

Table 11.2.4: Etiology of anemia.

1.	Inadequate dietary intake of iron and other nutrients (vitamin B_{12} and folic acid)
2.	*Inadequate supply of iron at birth:* Prenatal or maternal nutrition deficiency, prematurity, low birth weight, or multiple births and prenatal blood loss
3.	*Inadequate absorption of iron:* Gluten-induced enteropathy, atrophic gastritis, and postgastrectomy, presence of phytates and calcium in the diet, and presence of recurrent or chronic diarrhea
4.	Excessive physiological demands of iron associated with rapid growth periods—Prematurity, preschool period, and adolescence
5.	Hemolytic anemias: a. *Extracorpuscular*: Autoimmune hemolytic anemia, microangiopathic hemolytic anemia, toxic effects due to infection, due to splenomegaly, paroxysmal nocturnal hemoglobinuria, hematopoietic disorders (e.g. leukemia, aplastic anemia, myelodysplastic anemia), blood loss (acute or chronic), chronic illnesses, such as juvenile rheumatoid arthritis, renal disease, heart diseases, poisoning (lead, arsenic, and other heavy metals.) b. *Intracorpuscular:* Red cell membrane disorders (hereditary spherocytosis, hereditary elliptocytosis, hereditary stomatocytosis), red cell enzyme deficiencies (G6PD deficiency, PK deficiency), thalassemia, and hemoglobinopathies
6.	Hematopoietic disorders (leukemia, aplastic anemia, and myelodysplastic anemia)
7.	Blood loss (acute or chronic), secondary to parasitic infections such as hookworm, giardiasis, gastritis, peptic ulcer, polyps, etc.
8.	Chronic illnesses like juvenile rheumatoid arthritis, renal disease, heart diseases, etc.
9.	*Poisoning:* Lead, arsenic, and other heavy metals

(G6PD: glucose-6-phosphate dehydrogenase; PK: pyruvate kinase)

Table 11.2.5: Pathophysiologic classification of anemia.

Anemia due to increase blood loss	• Acute posthemorrhagic anemia • Chronic blood loss due to some chronic disease, e.g. hookworm infestation, ulcerative colitis, polyps, etc.
Anemia due to impaired red cell production	• *Deficient heme synthesis:* Iron-deficiency anemia • Vitamin B_{12} or folic acid deficiency (megaloblastic anemia) • *Deficient globin synthesis:* Thalassemia • Aplastic anemia (acquired or hereditary) • Pure red cell aplasia • Anemia of chronic disorders (chronic renal failure, cardiac disorders)
Anemia due to increased red cell destruction (hemolytic anemia)	• Sickle cell anemia, thalassemia, hemoglobinopathies • Autoimmune hemolytic anemia • Hereditary spherocytosis • Paroxysmal nocturnal hemoglobinuria

Flowchart 11.2.1: Clinical approach to a child with anemia.

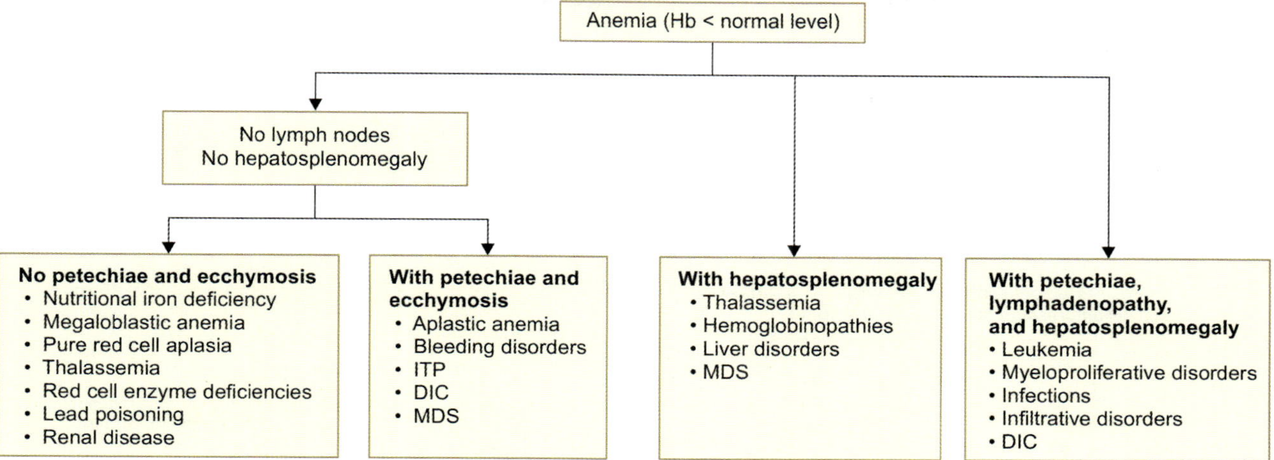

(DIC: disseminated intravascular coagulopathy; Hb: hemoglobin; ITP: immune thrombocytopenic purpura; MDS: myelodysplastic syndrome)

anemia and whether it develops over a short or long period of time. Children may remain asymptomatic for long duration if the onset of anemia is insidious. When the onset of anemia is acute, children develop significant pallor, exertional dyspnea, and restlessness. Severe anemia also leads to cardiac enlargement, flow murmurs, and even chronic heart failure.

The tongue papillae are atrophied. The structural changes in the intestine may result in malabsorption and even protein enteropathy. Nails may become brittle and flat with longitudinal ridges (koilonychia). The work capacity or the activity of the child gets impaired. Persistence of anemia leads to neurophysiological and developmental deficits. Children may have reduced motor development, muscle power, and coordination with behavioral effects. The intelligence quotient of children may be reduced by 5–7 points.

Persistence of anemia has adverse impact on the bactericidal activity of neutrophils and impairs cell immunity leading to recurrent infections. In addition, children may develop lymph node enlargement, petechiae, ecchymosis, or bleeding symptoms. Presence of liver and spleen enlargement should be observed during the examination of child.

Clinical Approach to Anemia

The causes of anemia are variable; hence, family history of anemia, jaundice, race, and area of origin should be recorded. Detailed clinical history should be taken, including dietary habits and chronic diarrhea. Evaluation of growth retardation and organomegaly is of utmost importance. A simple algorithm for clinical diagnosis is given in **Flowchart 11.2.1**.

Laboratory Approach to Anemia

The objectives of laboratory tests are to determine the type, severity, and the etiology of anemia. The severity of anemia is determined by the Hb level. The examination of peripheral blood film identifies the morphological type of anemia. Based on the red cell morphology and red cell indices, such as mean corpuscular volume (MCV), the anemia has been classified as microcytic hypochromic, macrocytic and normocytic normochromic. Simple algorithms toward the diagnosis of various etiological conditions are given in **Flowcharts 11.2.2 to 11.2.4**.

Reticulocyte count indicates the erythropoietic activity and serves as a useful indicator for diagnosis. Recently red cell distribution width (RDW) is provided by most cell counters. RDW along with MCV helps in differentiating various etiological conditions **(Table 11.2.6)**.

Detailed peripheral smear examination is of utmost importance. This not only helps in the classification of anemia but the presence of red cell abnormalities gives clue to the underlying diagnosis.

- Presence of spherocytes in high number (15–20/100 RBC) is suggestive of hereditary spherocytosis or immune hemolytic anemia, while the presence of a few spherocytes is suggestive of other states **(Table 11.2.7)**.
- Presence of schistocytes suggests life-threatening conditions, such as disseminated intravascular coagulopathy or hemolytic uremic syndrome.
- Presence of basophilic stippling is suggestive of various types of hemolytic anemia, lead or arsenic poisoning, and sideroblastic anemia **(Table 11.2.7)**.

Based on the peripheral blood examination, one may proceed to undertake specific tests to confirm the etiology of the disease process.

Detailed history, clinical examination, and complete blood counts along with a peripheral blood examination and various algorithms aid in reaching a diagnosis. These children may be subjected to few additional tests for the confirmation of etiology of anemia **(Table 11.2.8)**.

Flowchart 11.2.2: Algorithm for microcytic and hypochromic picture on peripheral blood.

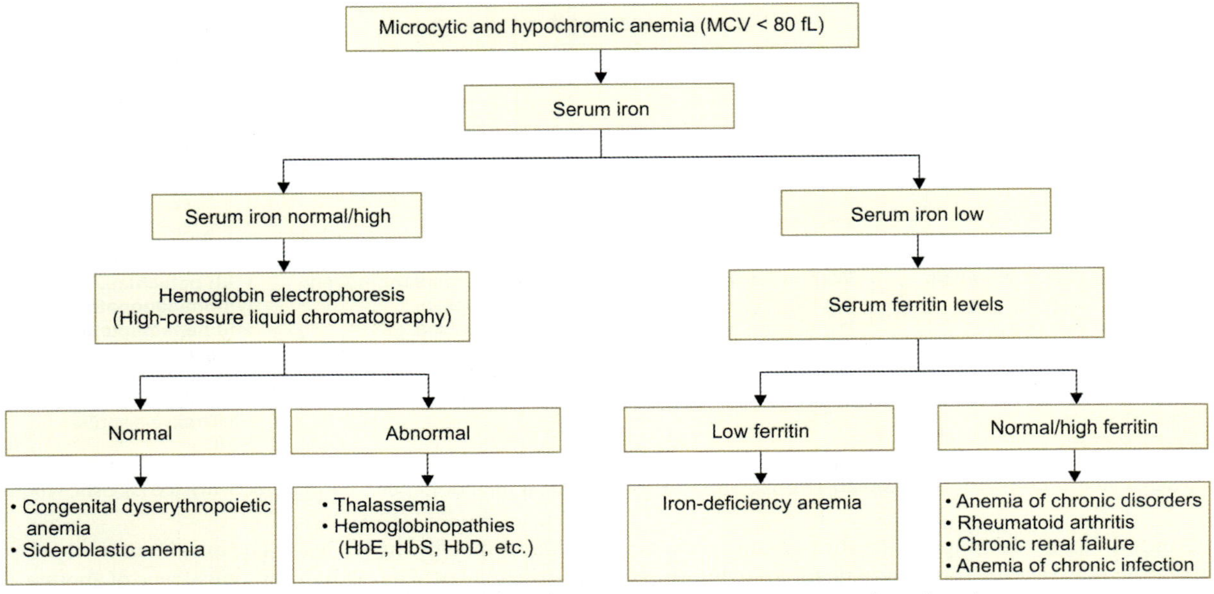

(HbE: hemoglobin E; HbS: hepatitis B surface; MCV: mean corpuscular volume)

Flowchart 11.2.3: Algorithm for macrocytic picture on peripheral blood.

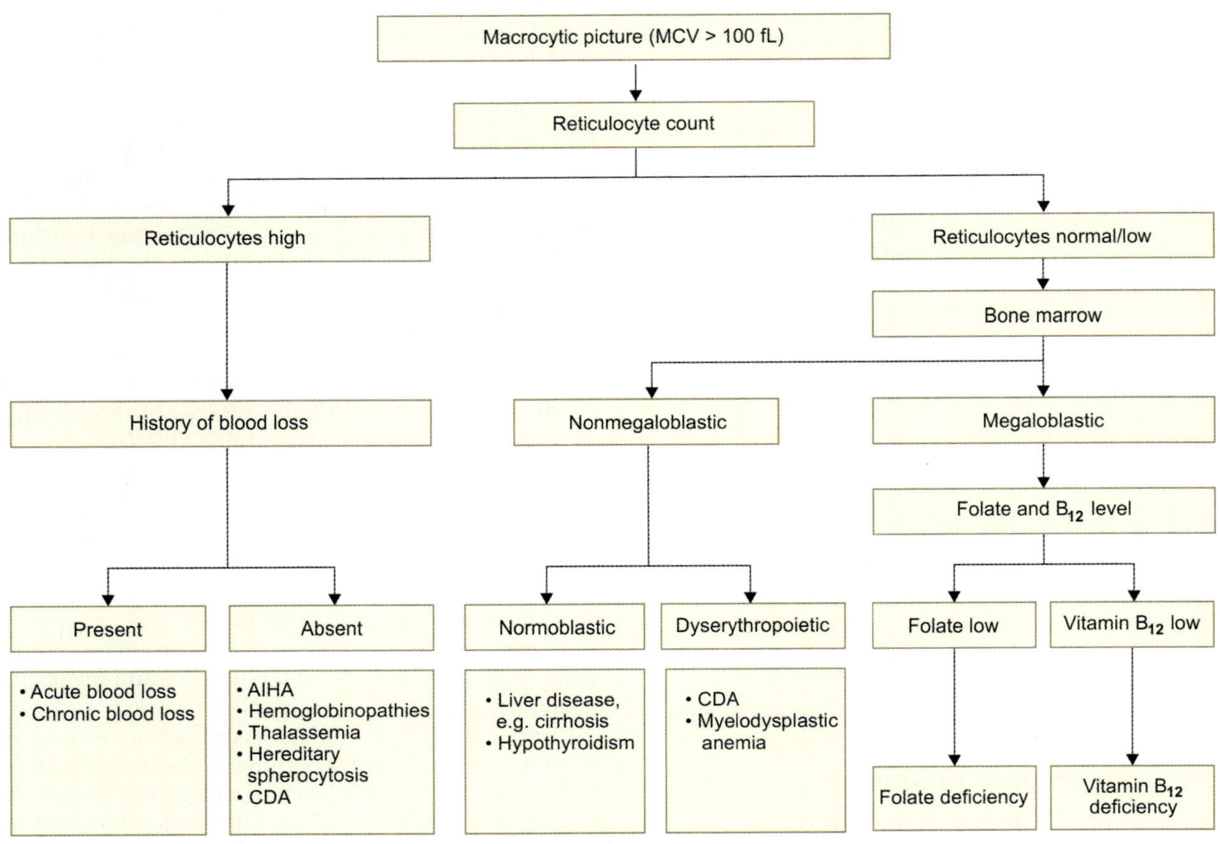

(AIHA: autoimmune hemolytic anemia; CDA: congenital dyserythropoietic anemia)

Flowchart 11.2.4: Algorithm for normocytic and normochromic picture on peripheral blood.

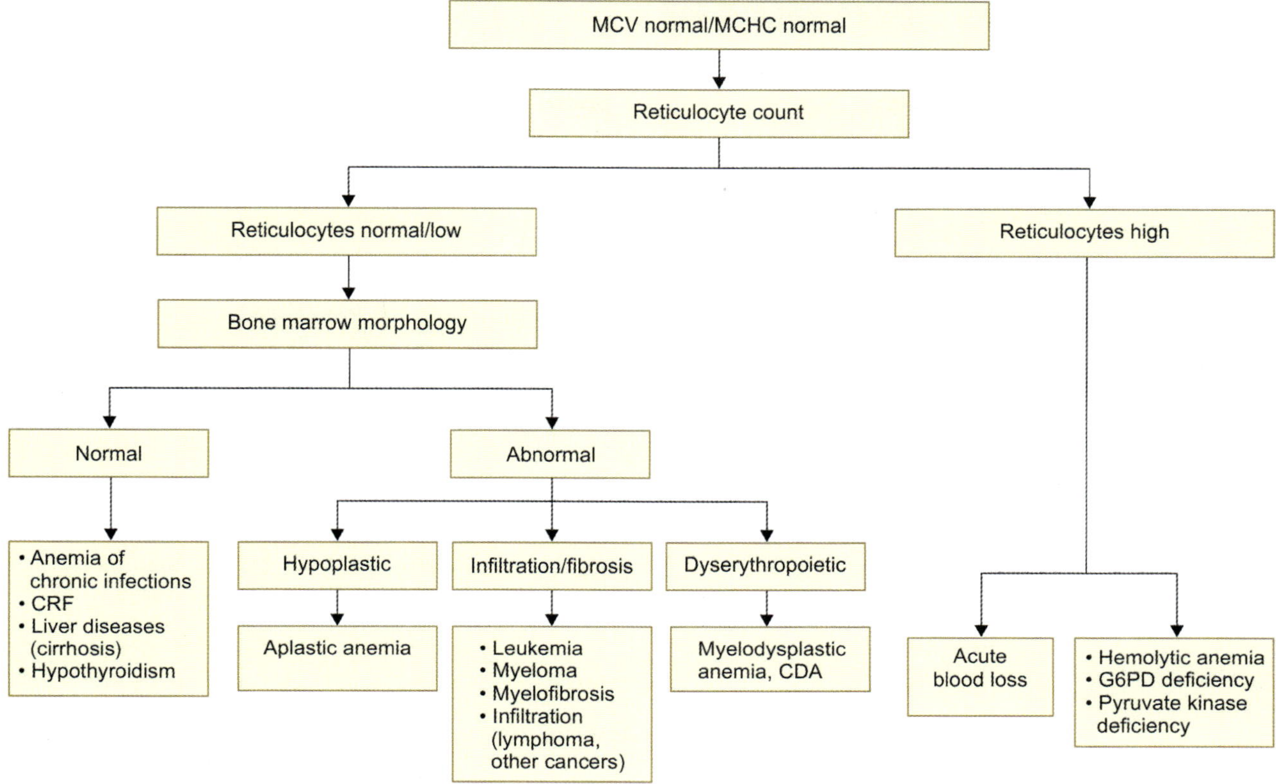

(CDA: congenital dyserythropoietic anemia; CRF: chronic renal failure; G6PD: glucose-6-phosphate dehydrogenase; MCHC: mean corpuscular hemoglobin concentration)

Table 11.2.6: Diagnosis of anemia on mean corpuscular volume and red cell distribution width.

RDW	*Low MCV*	*Normal MCV*	*High MCV*
RDW < 15	• Thalassemia trait • Heterozygous HbE, HbC, etc. • ACD	• ACD • Heterozygous HbE, HbS, HbC, etc. • Hereditary spherocytosis • Acute hemorrhage	• Aplastic anemia • MDS • Myeloma • Liver disease • Hyperthyroidism
RDW > 15	• Iron-deficiency anemia • Thalassemia intermedia • Sideroblastic anemia • ACD • RBC fragmentation	• Early nutritional deficiency • Myelodysplasia • Myelophthisic anemia • Sickle cell disease	• B_{12} deficiency • Folate deficiency • AIHA • *Drugs:* Hydroxyurea

(ACD: anemia of chronic disease; AIHA: autoimmune hemolytic anemia; MCV: mean corpuscular volume; MDS: myelodysplastic syndromes; RBC: red blood cell; RDW: red cell distribution width)

RECENT ADVANCES

Role of Hepcidin in Iron Metabolism

Several studies have demonstrated that hepcidin controls the release of iron from variety of cells, such as macrophages, hepatocytes, and enterocytes into plasma. However, the recycling of iron from RBC lysis and release of iron from tissue iron stores are carried by the interaction of hepcidin with ferroportin which is a cellular iron exporter in vertebrates. It has been shown that the release of ferroportin is primarily expressed by enterocytes and macrophages, which is also controlled by hepcidin.

Iron homeostasis in the body is controlled by very complex mechanism, and the main components include:

- Erythropoietic activity
- Hypoxia
- Iron stores
- Inflammation.

Table 11.2.7: Abnormal cells on peripheral smear and underlying disorders.

Characteristics	*Underlying disorders*
Spherocytes	• Hereditary spherocytosis • Autoimmune hemolytic anemia • Hemolytic transfusion reactions • Severe burns • Hypersplenism • *Clostridium welchii* septicemia
Target cells	• Hemoglobinopathies S, C, D, and E • Thalassemia • Postsplenectomy
Elliptocytes	• Hereditary elliptocytosis • Thalassemias • Myelofibrosis • Myelophthisic anemia
Schistocytes and fragmental red cells	• Disseminated intravascular coagulopathy • Hemolytic uremic syndrome • Prosthetic heart valve • Malignant hypertension
Basophilic stippling	• Thalassemia • Poisoning (arsenic or lead) • Sideroblastic anemia • Unstable hemoglobins • Hemolytic anemias

All these components act through common pathways of hepcidin. Enhanced erythropoiesis and the presence of tissue hypoxia decrease the hepcidin production by the liver, resulting in enhanced iron absorption. In contrast, increased iron stores and the presence of infection reduce the hepcidin production by the liver, which causes internalization and degradation of ferroportin by the target cells, leading to decrease or total inhibition of iron absorption by the enterocytes and release of iron by the macrophages and other cells. Thus hepcidin primarily controls the iron absorption.

Infections and Anemia

Children, particularly infants, living in the developing countries are highly vulnerable to infectious diseases. Iron deficiency is associated with the impairment of innate (natural) immunity and cell-mediated immunity, thereby contributing to increased risk of infections. The iron acquisition by the microbes and their virulence is determined by various host and microbial mechanisms which are given here:

- Reduced neutrophil function with decreased enzymatic activity
- Impaired natural killer cell activity and impaired bactericidal activity
- Depression of T-lymphocyte numbers/defective T-lymphocyte response, impaired interleukin-2 production
- Reduced production of macrophage migration inhibition factor
- Impaired delayed cutaneous hypersensitivity tuberculin reactivity.

Table 11.2.8: Diagnostic tests to confirm the etiology of anemia.

Bone marrow aspiration	Type of erythropoiesis (normocytic or megaloblastic), leukemia, hemolytic anemia, etc. and marrow iron stores
Bone biopsy	Aplastic anemia, infiltrative disorders (lymphoma or secondaries), myelofibrosis
Iron-deficiency anemia	• Serum iron, total iron-binding capacity • Percent saturation transferrin • Serum ferritin • Serum transferrin receptor assays • Red cell protoporphyrin levels
Megaloblastic anemia	• Serum folate levels • Serum vitamin B_{12} levels • Schilling test of vitamin B_{12} absorption
Pernicious anemia	• Estimation of intrinsic factor in gastric juice • Intrinsic factor antibodies levels • Parietal cell antibodies • Plasma (or serum) vitamin B_{12}-binding capacity
Hemolytic anemia	• Estimation of serum haptoglobin levels • Demonstration of hemosiderin in urine • Serum bilirubin, total and indirect, serum urobilinogen • Serum lactic dehydrogenase levels
Hereditary hemolytic anemia	• Detection of enzyme deficiency, such as G6PD assay, pyruvate kinase assay • Glutathione stability test for G6PD-deficient patients • Coomb's test (direct and indirect) • Hemoglobin electrophoresis (high-pressure liquid chromatography) • Hemoglobin fetal and hemoglobin A2 estimation
Acquired hemolytic anemia	• Warm and cold autoantibodies detection • Detection of incomplete antibodies by the Coomb's test • Ham test for paroxysmal nocturnal hemoglobinuria • Flow cytometry evaluation of G-PI-linked proteins on neutrophils • CD-55 and CD-59 markers

(CD: clusters of differentiation; G6PD: glucose 6-phosphate dehydrogenase; G-PI: glycophosphatidylinositol)

Developmental and Neurophysiological Deficits in Iron Deficiency

Recently iron deficiency has been shown to have effect on brain metabolism, neurotransmitter function, and myelination. These changes lead to neurophysiological and developmental deficits in infants and children, which may have adverse effect even during adulthood. Motor development and coordination are reduced. In addition, there is impaired language development, scholastic achievement, psychological and behavioral effects, such as insecurity, fatigue, poor attention, etc. These children have decreased physical activity. Changes in brain iron content caused by early iron deficiency are not reversible on iron therapy in animals in spite of correction of anemia and other tissue iron deficits. These observations provide explanation why some effects of iron deficiency are irreversible even after complete correction of iron deficiency. Thus the timing of iron deficiency during infancy and its severity have critical impact even in adult life.

KEY MESSAGES

- Anemia is widely prevalent in the world. It is more common in the developing countries.
- Children and women are worst affected.
- Iron-deficiency anemia (IDA) is the most common cause of anemia.
- Persistence of severe IDA has adverse effects in adult life.
- Detailed history, examination, and use of simple tests are essential for early diagnosis.
- Simple algorithms are helpful for early diagnosis of anemia.

BIBLIOGRAPHY

1. Choudhry VP. Hematological disorders. In: Ghai OP, Gupta P, Paul VK (Eds). Essential Pediatrics, 6th edition. New Delhi: CBS Publishers and Distributors; 2004. pp. 298-307.
2. Choudhry VP. Hepcidin and its role in iron metabolism. Indian J Pediatr. 2010;77(7):787-8.
3. Kumar V, Choudhry VP. Iron deficiency and infection. Indian J Pediatr. 2010;77(7):789-93.
4. Madan N, Rusia U, Sikka M, et al. Developmental and neurophysiologic deficits in iron deficiency in children. Indian J Pediatr. 2011;78(1):58-64.
5. NFHS-3. National Family Health Survey-3 (2005-2006). Status of Children in India. Mumbai: Institute for Population Sciences (IIPS) and Macro International; 2007.
6. Oski FA, Brugnara C, Nathan DG. A diagnostic approach to the anemic patient. In: Nathan DG, Orkin SH (Eds). Hematology of Infancy and Childhood, 5th edition. Philadelphia, PA: WB Saunders; 1997. pp. 375-84.
7. World Health Organization. Nutritional anemia: report of WHO scientific group. WHO technical report series no. 405. Geneva: WHO; 1968.
8. Yadav S, Chandra J. Iron deficiency: beyond anemia. Indian J Pediatr. 2011;78(1):65-72.

11.3 Nutritional Anemias in Infancy and Childhood

Niranjan Shendurnikar

INTRODUCTION

Nutritional anemias are conditions in which hemoglobin (Hb) concentration of a given individual is below the normal level for the age, due to the deficiency of one or more nutrients needed for hematopoiesis, and the Hb can be increased by the supplementation of the deficient nutrient(s).

World Health Organization (WHO) criteria for the diagnosis of anemia are Hb levels less than 11 g/dL in children between 6 months and 6 years and below 12 g/dL in children between 6 years and 14 years. The main nutrients are iron, folate, vitamin B_{12}, proteins, and vitamin E.

IRON-DEFICIENCY ANEMIA

Iron-deficiency anemia (IDA) is currently the most widespread micronutrient deficiency and affects nearly 1.5 billion people globally. Presently, available data have shown that about one-third of world population suffers from IDA of which 90% lives in the third-world countries. Infants, preschool children, adolescents, and women of child-bearing age are at the greatest risk of developing iron deficiency and its resultant anemia. Around 74% of children between the ages of 6 months and 35 months are anemic.

The WHO estimates that roughly 50% of anemia prevalence can be attributed to iron deficiency. The Third

National Family Health Survey (NFHS-3) in 2005–2006 found that the prevalence of anemia among under-five children approaches 70%. The high prevalence of IDA is accounted for by the combination of limited iron stores at birth, timing of umbilical cord clamping at birth, delayed introduction of complementary foods, and the frequency of infections. If not corrected, it leads to increasing severity of anemia, reduced work capacity, increased susceptibility to infections, and greater risk of death associated with pregnancy and child birth.

Iron Requirements during Childhood

Understanding the requirements, intake and bioavailability of iron is essential to explain the vulnerability of some individuals to develop IDA. The iron released from senescent red cells during the first 8–12 weeks of life (a period of quiescent erythropoiesis) is stored in the body and helps to maintain erythropoiesis up to 4–6 months in a normal term baby and up to 2 months in a low-birth-weight baby.

- Normal infants have about 75 mg of iron per kg body weight, two-thirds of which is present in red blood cells (RBCs).
- Infants and young children should continue to absorb 0.8–1.0 mg of iron daily to reach the adult level of stores of 4–5 g.
- The majority of body iron is in the form of Hb with about 10% in iron-containing proteins in nonheme tissues (myoglobin and cytochromes).
- Further 10–15% is stored intracellularly as ferritin or its degradation product, hemosiderin.
- Iron requirements are highest in infancy during the period of rapid growth, and these are also increased during adolescence, menstruation, pregnancy, and lactation.

Normal body loss of iron is about 20 μg/kg/day, but this may increase manifold during the episodes of diarrhea, dysentery, and parasitic infestations. Factors, such as preferential delivery of iron to fetus during the third trimester, delayed cord clamping, and exclusive breastfeeding in the first 6 months of life, protect infants from becoming iron deficient. Malnutrition, chronic infections, and worm infestations also contribute to a high prevalence of anemia.

ETIOLOGY

The causes of IDA are listed in **Box 11.3.1**.

Box 11.3.1: Causes of iron deficiency.

Decreased iron stores:
- Preterm
- Small-for-date babies
- Twins

Decreased intake/assimilation:
- Delayed introduction of complementary feeds
- Malnutrition/iron-poor diet/malabsorption syndromes
- Chronic infection/chronic diarrhea
- Gastrointestinal surgery

Increased losses:
- GI bleeding
- Malaria
- Hookworm infestation
- Peptic ulcer
- Diverticulitis
- Bleeding diathesis
- Fetomaternal hemorrhage
- Repeated venous sampling

Increased demands:
- Prematurity
- LBW babies
- Recovering from PEM
- Adolescents

(GI: gastrointestinal; LBW: low birth weight; PEM: protein-energy malnutrition)

Source of Iron

The dietary iron comes from two sources: heme and nonheme iron. The major source of iron is in the diet and is found in variable degrees in the foods of plant origin. Heme iron is present in meat, fish, and poultry but the intake of these products is generally low. Heme iron is better absorbed than nonheme iron and is not influenced by dietary factors. Breast milk in spite of low levels of iron (0.5 mg/L) has a better absorption and bioavailability as compared to cow's milk. Good sources of iron in the diet include pulses, dals, green leafy vegetables, bajra, dates, nuts, jaggery, meat, and fish. The administration of 50 mg of vitamin C daily increases iron absorption by twofold.

CLINICAL MANIFESTATIONS

Iron deficiency is a systemic disorder involving multiple systems rather than being an isolated hematological condition associated with anemia. The peak incidence of iron deficiency in children occurs between 6 months and 3 years, followed by adolescents 11–17 years. Children between 6 months and 24 months are a particularly high-risk group for the development of iron deficiency due to the low content of bioavailable iron in the weaning foods in the developing countries.

The appearance of symptoms depends upon the rate of fall of Hb and hemostatic adjustment of various organs systems. As the fall of Hb is often gradual, the onset of symptoms is insidious. Given the gradual development of IDA, pediatric patients rarely exhibit significant physiological consequences of decompensation.

Initial manifestations include irritability, anorexia, and pallor. Later hyperdynamic circulation leads to palpitation, the shortness of breath, easy fatigability, reduced exercise

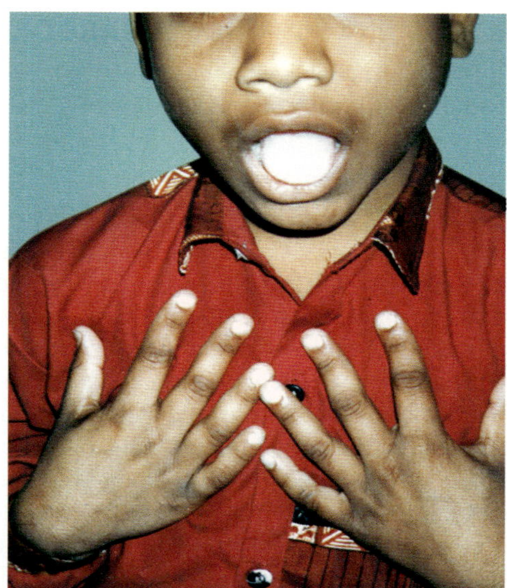

Fig. 11.3.1: Pallor in iron-deficiency anemia.
Courtesy: Dr MR Lokeshwar, Mumbai, Maharashtra, India.

tolerance, and heart failure. Gradual onset of pallor may escape notice even when the Hb falls to 4 g/dL. Platonychia, koilonychias, glossitis, stomatitis, and angular cheilitis may be observed, especially with long-standing anemia **(Fig. 11.3.1)**. Pica is a well-documented feature of anemia in children and manifested as craving for inedible things, such as dirt, clay (geophagia), ice (pagophagia), laundry starch (amylophagia), salt, cardboard. Pica is seen in almost 70–80% of patients and is usually cured by prompt iron therapy.

Growth retardation and altered host immune responses are other associated features of IDA in children. Blue sclera is also occasionally observed in iron deficiency in children and adolescents.

Iron-deficiency anemia is associated with impaired performance on a range of mental and physical functions, including physical coordination and capacity, mental development, cognitive abilities, social and emotional development. Iron deficiency leads to impaired growth, compromises cognitive development, and contributes to shortened attention span and scholastic failure **(Box 11.3.2)**.

Other health consequences include reduced immunity, increased morbidity, and increased susceptibility to heavy metal (including lead) poisoning. These changes may be related to functional changes in iron-containing enzymes at cellular level. Iron-deficiency anemia at the time of crucial brain growth and development may produce permanent and irreversible abnormalities in these functions.

The triad of dysphagia due to esophageal webs, koilonychia, and splenomegaly with IDA is known as Plummer-Vinson or Paterson-Kelly syndrome and is not common in children. Mild hepatosplenomegaly is also not uncommon in IDA.

Box 11.3.2: Nonhematologic features of iron deficiency in children.

- Koilonychia, glossitis, esophageal web
- Pica
- Reduced work capacity
- Reduced exercise performance
- Decrease attention span/cognition

Box 11.3.3: Summary of laboratory tests in iron-deficiency anemia.

- Depletion of stainable iron from BM
- Reduction of serum ferritin levels (<15 ng/mL)
- Increased RDW (>14.5%)
- Low serum iron (<75 mg/dL)
- Increased TIBC (>470 μg/dL)
- Low transferrin saturation (<12% and 14% for infants and children)
- Increased red cell protoporphyrin concentration

(BM: bone marrow; RDW: red cell distribution width; TIBC: total iron-binding capacity)

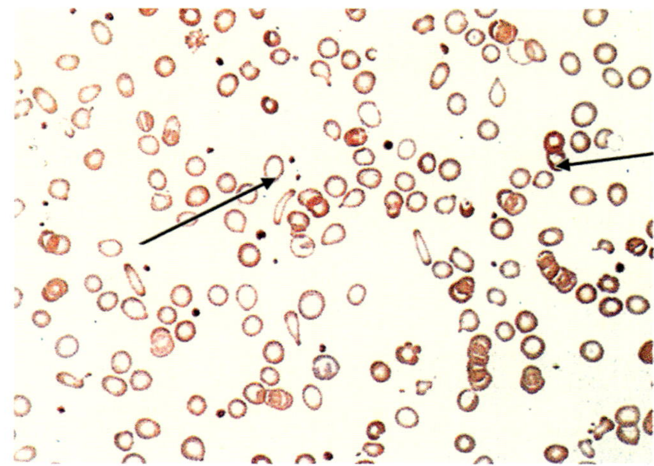

Fig. 11.3.2: Hypochromia and microcytosis in iron-deficiency anemia.

Laboratory Tests in Iron Deficiency

Iron-deficiency anemia develops sequentially from the depletion of iron stores, iron-deficient erythropoiesis to IDA **(Box 11.3.3)**. Laboratory tests in IDA are required to diagnose IDA and to establish its cause.

- Hemoglobin, RBC count, and hematocrit are decreased in IDA along with low mean corpuscular volume (MCV), mean corpuscular Hb (MCH), and MCH concentration.
- Blood smear shows hypochromia, microcytosis, poikilocytosis, and target cells **(Fig. 11.3.2)**.
- Reticulocyte count is usually normal unless the child has an acute or recent blood loss or has received hematinics. However, in mild iron deficiency, RBC morphology and indices are not altered.

- Low serum iron, increased total iron-binding capacity (>470 µg/dL), and low transferrin saturation.
- Serum ferritin levels may be normal, if there is an associated illness as ferritin is an acute phase reactant.
- A low MCV with an elevated red cell distribution width (RDW) is strongly suggestive of IDA. Red cell distribution width is highly sensitive (>90%) but low in specificity (50–70%) in detecting IDA.
- Soluble transferrin receptor measures the severity of IDA, and values more than 9 mg/L are considered abnormal.
- Depletion of stainable iron from bone marrow (BM) (routinely BM examination not required).

Diagnosis

An algorithm for the diagnosis of microcytic hypochromic anemia in a child is shown in **Flowchart 11.3.1**. Differential diagnosis of microcytic hypochromic anemia includes the following:

- Iron-deficiency anemia
- Anemia of chronic infection
- Thalassemias
- Lead poisoning
- Sideroblastic anemia.

Flowchart 11.3.1: An algorithm for child with microcytic hypochromic anemia.

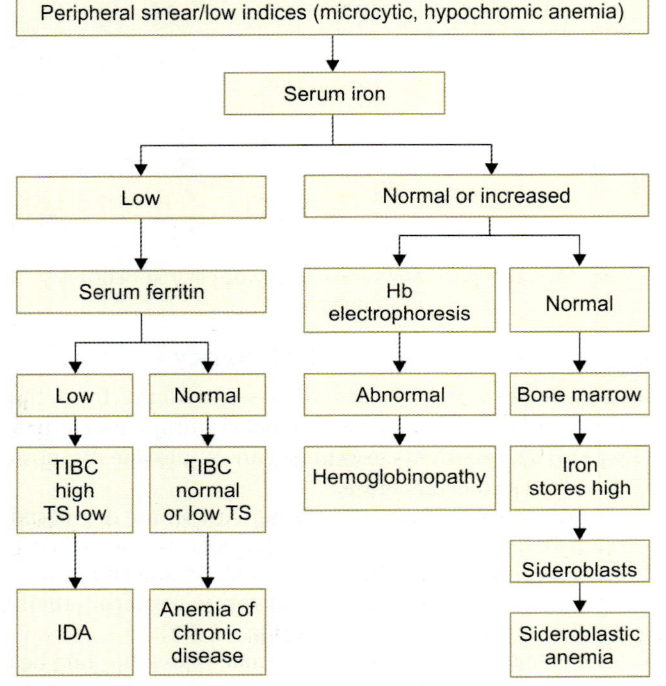

MANAGEMENT

The basic principle of management of IDA is the correction of anemia and the eradication of underlying cause.

Oral Iron Therapy

It is an effective, safe, and economical mode for the treatment of IDA. Bivalent iron salts, such as ferrous sulfate, fumarate, gluconate, succinate, and lactate, are preferred over ferric preparations as these are 4–10 times better absorbed than ferric compounds. The bioavailability of iron from ferric salts is 3–4 times less than that of ferrous sulfate. Ferrous sulfate (20% elemental iron) is commonly used for tablet preparations. Iron salts of carbonate, citrate, choline citrate, and pyrophosphates are not efficiently absorbed. Hb-containing preparations do not offer additional advantage over simple ferrous salts.

Many new iron preparations are now available that are not affected by the dietary factors and have less gastrointestinal side effects. These are iron polymaltose complex, iron amino acid chelates, and carbonyl iron. Newer iron preparations, such as ferrous ascorbate and ferrous bisglycinate, have a high bioavailability and are less affected by the dietary factors and have fewer gastrointestinal side effects.

The recommended dosage of elemental iron is 3 mg/kg/day as higher doses are unnecessary. Higher doses may increase side effects and reduce patient compliance. Single daily doses are as effective, but 2–3 divided doses are better tolerated by children.

It is recommended that 20 mg of elemental iron along with 100 µg of folic acid be used for prophylaxis in children between 6 months and 36 months in National Nutritional Anemia Control Program.

Adolescents require 60 mg of elemental iron per day in the case of mild anemia and 120 mg/day (60 × 2) for moderate and severe anemia.

Iron therapy needs to be continued for 3 months after the blood values have returned to normal to replenish the iron stores. Suboptimal response to iron therapy may be due to poor compliance, inadequate dosage, associated infections, occult blood loss, or other causes of microcytic hypochromic anemia. Knowing the elemental iron content of the preparation is very important to ensure the adequate intake of therapeutic dose of iron and get an optimal response.

The assessment of response to treatment is made by reticulocyte count which rises in 2–4 days of therapy **(Table 11.3.1)**. Approximately 2 months are required to achieve a normal Hb level.

Once-weekly or twice-weekly therapies are also effective as human intestine has mucosal turnover between 5 days and 6 days, and greater iron absorption may be achieved

Table 11.3.1: Response to iron therapy in iron-deficiency anemia.	
12–24 hours	Replacement of iron enzymes, subjective improvement, decreased irritability, increased appetite
36–48 hours	Initial bone marrow response, erythroid hyperplasia
48–72 hours	Reticulocytosis, peaking at 5–7 days
1–3 months	Repletion of stores

by iron administration to new gut cells. Twice-weekly dose is considered cost effective with a need of lesser number of doses, with fewer side effects and better compliance. Twice-weekly iron-folic acid (IFA) supplementation is found to be comparable to daily IFA.

Parenteral Iron Therapy

Indications

- Intolerance to oral iron
- Persistent noncompliance
- Gastrointestinal bleed aggravated by oral iron therapy.

There are four commercially available intravenous (IV) iron preparations:

1. Iron dextran
2. Iron sucrose
3. Iron ferric gluconate
4. Ferric carboxymaltose injection.

Iron dextran is a complex of ferric hydrochloride and high molecular weight dextran. This needs to be given by IV route either by infusion or bolus (single total) dose. The dosage is calculated as:

$$\text{Iron (mg)} = \text{Weight in kg} \times \text{Hb deficit (g/dL)} \times 4$$

Life-threatening anaphylactic reactions may occur; and hence, parenteral iron should be given in hospital setting only. Other side effects may include fever, abdominal cramps, pain, skin rash, arthralgia, and serum sickness like illness. The use of iron dextran has been decreased because of the risk of anaphylaxis.

Ferric carboxymaltose injection has a better safety and tolerability profile than existing products and has little toxicity. High doses can be administered with good local tolerance.

Table 11.3.1 shows the response to iron therapy in IDA with iron therapy.

Blood transfusion may be needed in most severe cases of IDA when the Hb level is below 3–4 g/dL or when superimposed infection may interfere with optimal therapeutic response. Packed red cells may be slowly given, preferably 2–3 mL/kg at one time.

Prevention of Iron Deficiency

Appropriate nutritional strategies are important factors in the prevention of IDA. These include:

- Protection and promotion of breastfeeding with timely introduction of complementary feeding at 6 months.
- Low-birth-weight infants need iron supplementation from the age of 2 months.
- Dietary modification and consumption of habitual foods increases consumption by 5–30%.
- Processes, such as germination (sprouting of green grams) and intake of green leafy vegetables, are also helpful in prevention of IDA.
- Periodic deworming should be considered in endemic areas.
- Administration of one pediatric (small) tablet containing 20 mg of iron and 100 µg of folic acid daily for 100 days every year has been recommended by National Nutritional Anemia Control Program.
- Food and salt fortification would be the most effective strategy to control IDA. Salt fortification gives an iron content of 1 mg/g of salt in preparation. Common salt fortified with iron orthophosphate and sodium hydrogen sulfate with ascorbic acid has been found stable and effective in field trials in India.
- Microencapsulated iron sprinkles are a novel approach, and this can be sprinkled on any complementary food at the table and does not change the color or the taste of the food.
- Various contact points, such as measles (9 months) and diphtheria-tetanus-pertussis booster (16–18 months) in Integrated Child Development Services scheme, should be utilized for the distribution of iron.

NUTRITIONAL MEGALOBLASTIC ANEMIAS

Megaloblastic anemia is caused by the deficiency of either folate or vitamin B_{12}, or both. The recommended dietary allowance for vitamin B_{12} is 0.3–0.5 and 1–1.5 µg/day for infants and children, respectively. These deficiencies are due to:

- *Decreased intake*: Vitamin B_{12} deficiency is observed with strict vegetarian diets, malnutrition, and in breastfed infants of mothers with low serum B_{12} levels. Folate content of goat's milk is extremely low, and cooking of vegetables for long time in boiling water also reduces the folate content of the item.
- *Impaired absorption*: Failure to secrete intrinsic factor, intestinal diseases, such as celiac disease, or surgical resection leads to vitamin B_{12} deficiency.
- *Defective utilization*: Drugs, such as phenytoin and pyrimethamine, interfere with folic acid metabolism.
- *Increased demands*: Preterm babies, infants recovering from protein-energy malnutrition and chronic hemolytic anemia have an increased demand for vitamin B_{12} and folic acid.

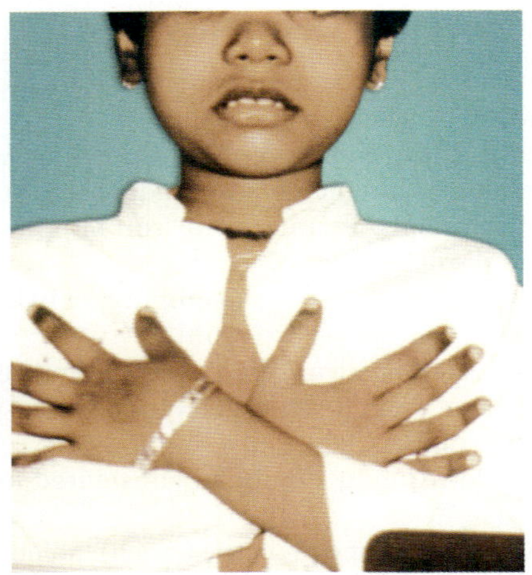

Fig. 11.3.3: Hyperpigmentation of dorsum of hands and knuckles.

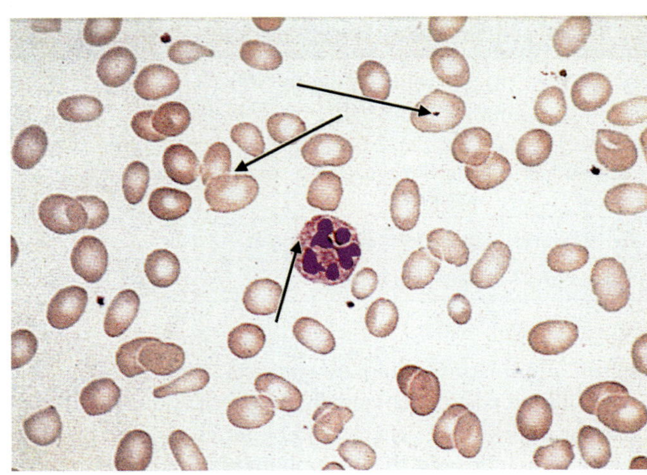

Fig. 11.3.4: Peripheral smear showing macroovalocytes and hypersegmented neutrophils.

CLINICAL FEATURES

These children appear sicker than the degree of anemia warrants. Anorexia, mental apathy, and fatigability are early symptoms, while glossitis and diarrhea can also occur. Hyperpigmentation of dorsum of hands and knuckles are important findings **(Fig. 11.3.3)**. Tremors, failure to thrive, and developmental regression are also observed. Vitamin B_{12} deficiency causes neurological manifestations, such as degeneration of peripheral nerves, selected columns in spinal cord, and defective cerebral function. Folate deficiency does not cause neuropathy.

LABORATORY DIAGNOSIS

Peripheral blood smear is one of the best indicators of megaloblastic anemia with the presence of macroovalocytes, hypersegmented neutrophils (3% with more than five lobes), and a raised MCV **(Fig. 11.3.4)**. There may be evidence of leukopenia and thrombocytopenia in severely deficient cases. Macrocytosis precedes anemia, and the MCV may be in the range of 110–130 fL. However, it may be masked by the presence of IDA. Red blood cells folate level and low B_{12} levels more accurately reflect the folate and vitamin B_{12} balance, respectively.

MANAGEMENT

Treatment of folate deficiency needs 100–200 µg of folate daily; however, it is given in a daily dose of 1–5 mg for 14–21 days for therapeutic response and then needs to be continued for 1–2 months for the replenishment of the body stores.

Different vitamin B_{12} replacement regimens are used to treat vitamin B_{12} deficiency in infants and children with B_{12} deficiency. About 500–1,000 µg of vitamin B_{12} is given intramuscularly on alternate days for a period of 2–3 weeks.

This should be followed by 100–250 µg/dose once every month given intramuscularly as a maintenance therapy to prevent recurrence. Vitamin B_{12} given orally is not universally effective due to poor patient compliance and an erratic absorption.

Treatment with folate alone can produce hematologic response in vitamin B_{12} deficiency but does not correct neurological impairment caused by B_{12} deficiency.

Anemia unresponsive to folate or B_{12} may be caused by certain rare metabolic diseases (homocystinuria) or antimetabolic drugs.

KEY MESSAGES

- Iron-deficiency anemia is the most prevalent micronutrient deficiency and affects nearly 70% of under-five children as per NFHS-3 survey.
- Iron requirements are highest in infancy during the period of rapid growth, and these are also increased during adolescence, menstruation, pregnancy, and lactation.
- Iron-deficiency anemia is a systemic disorder affecting multiple systems rather than being only a hematological condition.
- A low MCV with an elevated RDW is strongly suggestive of IDA.
- Oral iron therapy is an effective, safe, and economical mode for the treatment of IDA. Ferrous salts are most commonly used preparations for IDA.
- Newer iron compounds, such as iron polymaltose complex and amino acid chelates, have an improved tolerance and are not affected by dietary factors.

- Protection and promotion of breastfeeding with timely introduction of complementary feeding at 6 months forms an important strategy in the prevention of IDA.
- The megaloblastic anemia should always be treated with adequate doses of both folate and vitamin B_{12}.

BIBLIOGRAPHY

1. Awasthi S, Verma T, Vir S. Effectiveness of biweekly versus daily iron folic acid administration on anemia status in preschool children. J Trop Pediatr. 2005;51(2):67-71.
2. Choudhury P. Iron deficiency anemia. In: Lokeshwar MR, Shah N, Agarwal B, Sachdeva A (Eds). IAP speciality series on pediatric hematology and oncology. Mumbai: Indian Academy of Pediatrics; 2006. pp. 28-35.
3. Davis I. Iron deficiency anemia. In: Zaoutis LB, Chiang VW (Eds). Comprehensive pediatric hospital medicine. Philadelphia, PA: Mosby, Elsevier; 2007. pp. 723-4.
4. Desai M. The big fight: conventional versus new oral preparations vs. parenteral iron therapy. Blood. 2010;116:4754-61.
5. Nagpal J, Choudhury P. Iron formulations in pediatric practice. Indian Pediatr. 2004;41(8):807-15.
6. Naithani R, Saxena R. Hematinics in children. Indian J Pract Pediatr. 2008;10:96-105.
7. National Rural Health Mission. (2013). Guidelines for the control of iron deficiency anemia. National iron + initiative. Adolescent Division, Ministry of Health and Family Welfare, Govt. of India. [online] Available from: http:www.unicef.org/india/10 [Accessed October, 2018].
8. Sen A, Kanani SJ. Impact of iron-folic acid supplementation on cognitive abilities of school girls in Vadodara. Indian Pediatr 2009;46(2):137-43.
9. WHO/UNICEF/UNU. (2001). Iron deficiency anemia: assessment, prevention and control. Geneva: WHO (WHO/NHD/01.3). [online] Available from: http:www.who.int/nut/documents/ida_assessment_prevention_control.pdf [Accessed November, 2018].

11.4 Bone Marrow Failure Syndrome

Nitin Shah

INTRODUCTION

Aplastic anemia (AA) is an uncommon but potentially serious hematological disorder caused due to pancytopenia with a hypocellular bone marrow (BM) without infiltration or fibrosis with annual incidence of about 2–6/million population. It affects all the age-groups, and a small peak occurs at the age of 5–6 years due to inherited causes of AA. It results in decreased production of one or more hematopoietic lineages—mature red cells, granulocytes, and platelets leading to pancytopenia, i.e. AA or mono- or bicytopenia (e.g. agranulocytosis, red cell aplasia)—and is characterized by hypocellular (or fatty) marrow.

Aplastic anemia is defined as the presence of any two peripheral blood criteria [absolute neutrophil count (ANC) less than 1,500/mm^3, platelet count less than 40,000/mm^3, and reticulocyte count less than 40,000/mm^3] in the presence of BM hypocellularity on BM biopsy. Severe AA is characterized by the presence of any two of the peripheral blood criteria (ANC < 500/mm^3, platelet count < 20,000/mm^3, corrected reticulocyte count <1%) along with the presence of either of the marrow criteria—severe hypocellularity (<25%), moderate cellularity with less than 30% of hematopoietic cells. All nonsevere AA cases are defined as moderate AA. If left untreated, 80–90% of patients with severe AA will die within a year.

ETIOLOGY

Aplastic anemia is classified as acquired or inherited. Inherited cases may or may not be present at birth (congenital). The etiological classification of AA is shown in **Table 11.4.1**. There is also a genetic predisposition for the development of marrow aplasia seen in patients with human leukocyte antigens (HLA) class II antigens DR2 and DPW3 **(Table 11.4.1)**.

ACQUIRED APLASTIC ANEMIA

Pathophysiology

Seed Theory

Hematopoietic stem cell has tremendous proliferative capacity and has potential, not only to differentiate into various cell lineages, but also has property of self-renewal.

Table 11.4.1: Etiology of aplastic anemia.
A. Acquired
a. Idiopathic b. Secondary 1. Drugs: Sulfa, anticancer drugs, antiepileptic agents, chloramphenicol, gold, carbamazepine, indomethacin, phenylbutazone 2. Chemicals: Benzene, sniffing glue, insecticides, dyes 3. Radiation 4. Viruses: Hepatitis, Epstein-Barr virus, parvovirus 5. Pregnancy 6. PNH 7. Miscellaneous: Hypogammaglobulinemia, thymoma, eosinophilic fasciitis, preleukemic syndromes
B. Inherited
1. Fanconi anemia 2. Dyskeratosis congenita 3. Reticular dysgenesis 4. Shwachman syndrome 5. Diamond–Blackfan syndrome
C. Miscellaneous
1. Familial aplastic anemia 2. Monosomy 7 3. Down syndrome 4. Amegakaryocytic thrombocytopenia

(PNH: paroxysmal nocturnal hemoglobinuria)

It has been observed that primitive progenitor cell number is significantly reduced in all patients with severe AA. Seed theory contemplates that AA is caused due to the lack of pluripotent stem cells/progenitor cells or a qualitative defect of common stem cell population.

Soil Therapy

Survival and proliferation of hematopoietic cells are dependent on stroma cells. Lack of surrounding microenvironment or stromal support (a soil or microenvironment deficiency) leads to AA. Success of BM transplant favors seed theory, whereas success of immunotherapy proves that in some patients it is the soil which is at fault. Probably there are different mechanisms of damage in different patients.

Clinical Presentation

Symptoms and signs depend on cell line involved. The onset is usually insidious.

- Thrombocytopenia will lead to bleeding manifestations, such as skin bleeds, mucosal bleeds, gastrointestinal (GI) tract bleeding, hematuria, menorrhagia, and rarely intracranial hemorrhage **(Figs. 11.4.1A and B)**.
- Neutropenia will lead to infection and fever with or without localization of infection.
- Anemia appears last and if severe will lead to fatigue, breathlessness, puffiness, edema of feet, and congestive cardiac failure. One should look for evidence of etiological factors, such as hepatitis, past history of drugs use **(Fig. 11.4.2)**.
- Presence of hepatomegaly, splenomegaly, lymphadenopathy, bone pains, etc. usually rules out AA and suggests more sinister disease, such as leukemia.

The differential diagnosis of pancytopenia is shown in **Box 11.4.1**.

Diagnosis

Diagnosis of AA is one of exclusions, and proper examination of BM is essential.

Peripheral Blood

- Anemia with normal red cell distribution width, normocytic normochromic red blood cells (RBCs), occasional macrocytosis with low-corrected reticulocyte count.
- Leukopenia with decreased ANC.
- *Thrombocytopenia*: Decreased platelet count with normal mean platelet volume.
- *Stress erythropoiesis*: Raised fetal hemoglobin (HbF) and I antigen in some patients.
- Coagulation parameters are generally normal.
- Pancytopenia without blasts in the blood is most likely due to marrow aplasia, but diagnosis requires aspirate and trephine biopsy of BM.
- Iron study may show iron overload.

The first sign of recovery after successful therapy is a rise in reticulocyte count, followed by increase in hemoglobin (Hb) levels, then neutrophils, while platelets slowest to recover if at all.

Bone Marrow and Trephine Biopsy

It is mandatory to do BM trephine biopsy as well as an aspiration to diagnose AA. It will show hypocellular marrow with empty spicules, increased fats spaces, hypoplasia may be patchy, especially early in the disease. Marrow consists of little more than fat, stromal cells, lymphocytes, and plasma cells; mast cells may be prominent. Because of diminution in the erythron, storage iron and sideroblasts may be increased; ring sideroblasts are not seen, except in rare specific syndromes **(Fig. 11.4.1B)**.

- *Stress cytogenetics*: It should always be done to rule out Fanconi anemia (FA) which will show increased spontaneous and clastogen-induced chromosomal breaks.
- *Others*: This includes tests to find out etiological factors, such as LFT.

Treatment

Curative Therapy

Curative therapy for AA involves the use of stem cell transplant (SCT), immunomodulating therapy, and rarely other modalities of treatment.

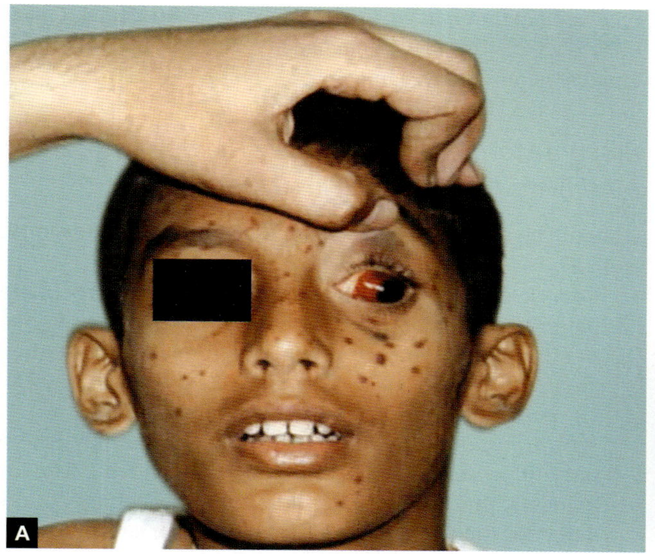

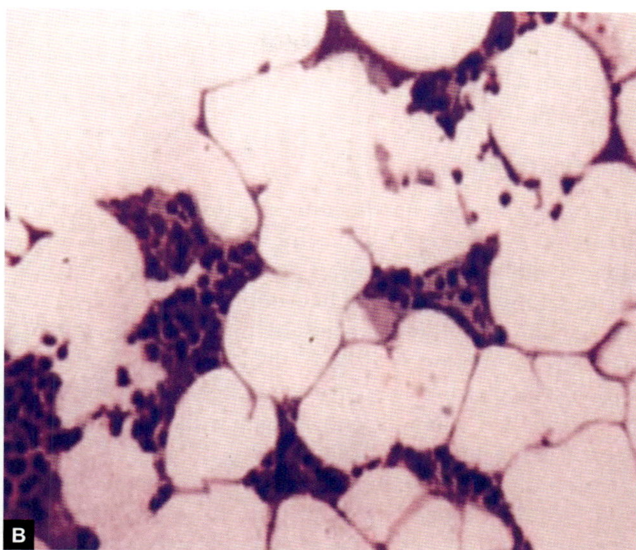

Figs. 11.4.1A and B: Trephine biopsy in aplastic anemia.
Courtesy: Dr MR Lokeshwar and Dr Nitin Shah.

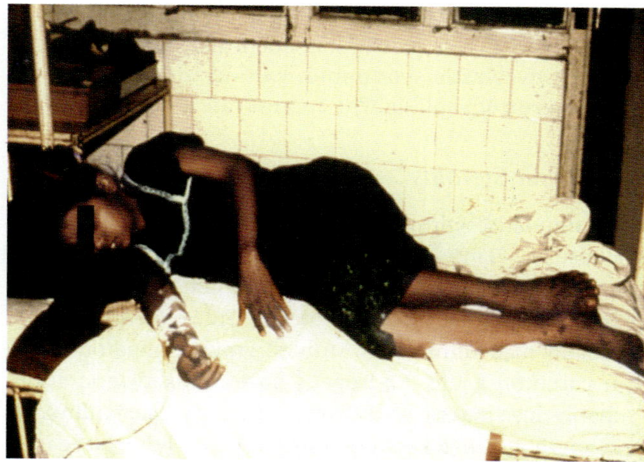

Fig. 11.4.2: Aplastic anemia. Sick-looking child, anemia, ecchymosis, petechiae, purpura, bleeding tendency, no hepatosplenomegaly, or bony tenderness.
Courtesy: Dr MR Lokeshwar and Dr Nitin Shah.

Supportive Therapy

Supportive care provides the backbone of any therapy. It includes the use of appropriate antimicrobial therapy and occasional use of colony-stimulating factors for the control of infections, use of blood components to tackle anemia and thrombocytopenia, and management of iron overload.

- *Anemia*: Leukodepleted packed cell transfusion should be given to maintain Hb above 7–8 g% avoiding the use of relative donor for the fear of HLA sensitization and graft-versus-host disease (GVHD). Iron chelation is started when serum ferritin level is more than 500–1,000 ng/mL.

Box 11.4.1: Differential diagnosis of pancytopenia in children.

- *Artifact*: Clot in sample
- *Genuine*: Central (bone marrow involved)
- *Replacement*: As in leukemia, and other malignancies
- *Infections*: Kala-azar, severe malaria
- Myelosclerosis, osteopetrosis, myelofibrosis, HLH, severe megaloblastic anemia
- *Peripheral*: Sequestration, hypersplenism (portal hypertension)
- *Destruction of mature elements*: Infection (most commonly viral), immune (SLE), complement mediated (paroxysmal nocturnal hemoglobinuria, PNH)
- *Mechanism obscure*: Organic acidemias

(HLH: hemophagocytic lymphohistiocytosis; PNH: paroxysmal nocturnal hemoglobinuria; SLE: systemic lupus erythematosus)

- *Bleeding*: Platelet transfusion is given when the patient has acute mucosal bleeds or severe internal bleeding. Isolated skin bleeds do not merit use of platelets, howsoever, grotesque and frequent they may be.

Prophylactic platelets may be used when the platelet count falls below less than 5,000/mm^3. However, misuse of platelets for minor or skin bleeds may lead to refractoriness. General measures, such as local pressure, use of epsilon-aminocaproic acid or tranexamic acid, dental care, avoiding use of nonsteroidal anti-inflammatory drugs, also help prevent bleeding.

Infections

Standard protocols of febrile neutropenia should be followed in patients with AA who develop fever.

One can use 5–10 days of granulocyte-colony-stimulating factor (G-CSF) in 5 µg/kg/day subcutaneous to tide over crisis in a sick severely neutropenic child with fever.

Asepsis precautions, such as sterile diet, chlorhexidine mouthwashes, betadine bath, clean drinking water, and hand sanitization, go a long way in preventing infections in neutropenic patients.

Stem Cell Transplant

Stem cell transplant has become treatment of choice for patients with severe AA who are young and have HLA-matched sibling donor. However, problem of SCT include nonavailability of HLA-matched donor with small family size, nonaffordability of procedure, higher complications, especially in greater than 40-year-old patients and poor response in previously heavily transfused patients and high mortality in patients who are sick with uncontrollable infection at the time of transplant.

Cure rates in young patients with HLA-matched donor are over 80%. Complications of procedure include acute and chronic GVHD, interstitial pneumonia, other infections, veno-occlusive disease.

Other long-term problems secondary to SCT are those due to chemotherapy and radiation. These include poor pulmonary function, endocrine dysfunction, including infertility, cognitive disorders, leukoencephalopathy, and occurrence of second malignancy.

Immunomodulatory Therapy

It involves use of drugs, such as cyclosporine A (CsA), antithymocyte globulin, antilymphocyte globulin, and steroids used in combination. One can use these agents alone if the patient cannot afford all the drugs; however, the response is not as well as when used in combination.

Antithymocyte Globulin/Antilymphocyte Globulin

They are used in doses of 10–40 mg/kg/day given for 5–10 days (follow the manufacturer's recommendations). Antithymocyte globulin/antilymphocyte globulin can lead to anaphylaxis but fortunately it is rare. One should run the infusion slowly initially to look for hypersensitivity. Premedication with antihistamines will help reduce other minor sensitivity reactions, such as fever, chills, and urticaria. Serum sickness after about 10 days of therapy is also common. 1 mg/kg of prednisolone is started on day 5 till 15 days and tapered over the next 7 days to counter these side effects.

Cyclosporin A

It is usually started on day 21 after steroids are stopped to avoid overlapping toxicities, such as hypertension. It is used in the doses of 5–10 mg/kg/day to keep a trough level of 100–150 ng/mL and continued for up to 6 months. Nephrotoxicity can be dose limiting. All patients on CsA must receive *Pneumocystis carinii* prophylaxis. Side effects, such as electrolyte disturbance, renal toxicity, liver toxicity, hirsutism, gingival hypertrophy, can occur.

Response to Immunosuppressive Therapy (Antithymocyte Globulin Plus Cyclosporine A)

It should be assessed after 3–4 months of treatment. Response is divided as follows:

- *Complete response*: Defined as response to therapy where patient is free from transfusion support, Hb is maintained at normal level for age and gender, ANC is maintained greater than 1.5×10^9/L, and platelets greater than 150×10^9/L on repeated counts 4 weeks apart.
- *Partial response*: Defined as response to therapy where patient is transfusion independent for RBC and/or platelets but does not have complete recovery of counts and does not anymore meet the criteria for severe AA.
- *No response*: Patient continues to fulfill criteria for severe AA. Overall long-term survival after immunomodulatory therapy is comparable to SCT in Western world for moderate AA. However, late clonal hematological diseases, such as paroxysmal nocturnal hemoglobinuria, myelodysplastic syndromes, can occur after apparent recovery from aplasia. The success rate is 60–70%.

Androgenic Steroids

They stimulate erythropoiesis. Nandrolone enanthate is used in a dose of 2–5 mg/kg/day as injectable form once in 10 days and continued till response is evident. Some response is seen in 20–30% of patients of moderate AA. Side effects are many, especially masculinization, stunted growth, hepatotoxicity, liver carcinoma, etc. Androgens have a mixed reputation. Probably dose makes the difference. One can use nandrolone decanoate at 5 mg/kg/week intramuscularly for at least 3 months. The advantage of this preparation is freedom from hepatotoxicity.

Corticosteroids

Steroids stimulate erythropoiesis. It also stabilizes capillary membrane and decrease bleeding. They are useful to counteract side effects of androgenic steroids on growing epiphysis and the serum sickness of immunotherapy.

Oral prednisolone is used in the dose of 0.5–1 mg/kg/day and tapered to a minimum effective dose.

Pulsed intravenous methylprednisolone in doses of 30 mg/kg has been used by some with limited success.

Side effects include hypertension, fluid electrolyte imbalance, infections, suppression of neuroendocrine axis, psychosis, avascular necrosis of femur, etc.

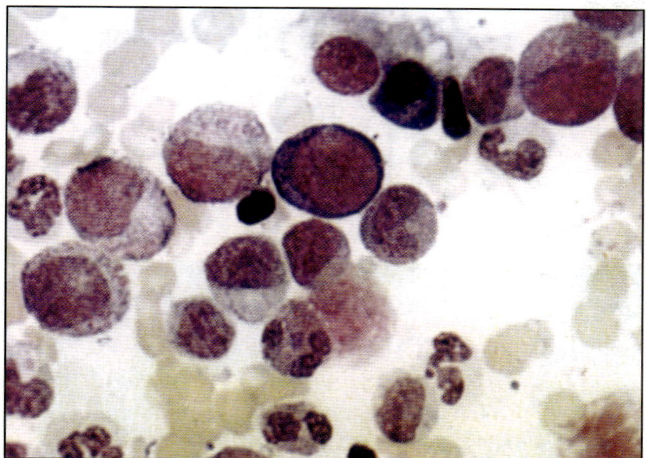

Fig. 11.4.6: Diamond–Blackfan syndrome cellular marrow with profound erythroid hypoplasia.
Courtesy: Dr MR Lokeshwar and Dr Nitin Shah.

profound erythroid hypoplasia with markedly increased M:E ratio. HbF is elevated in most cases as also I antigen on the red cell surface. Mainstay of treatment is transfusion therapy and corticosteroid.

Hemosiderosis is unavoidable complication and may also eventually lead to portal hypertension and hypersplenism; and hence, chelation therapy and splenectomy may be required. Dose of steroid is 1–2 mg/kg of Prednisolone for 4–6 weeks, and if unsuccessful, then may be discontinued. Steroid therapy may have to be maintained to the minimal required dose for years. Successful SCT have been reported in patients' refractory to above therapy and having HLA identical sibling. Intravenous gammaglobulin has been found to be useful. In most of the patients, carefully adjusted steroid therapy has been found successful.

BIBLIOGRAPHY

1. Bhatnagar SK, Chandra J, Narayan S, et al. Pancytopenia in children: etiological profile. J Trop Pediatr. 2005;51(4):236-9.
2. Chandra J, Naithani R, Ravi R, et al. Antithymocyte globulin plus cyclosporin in children less than 12 years with acquired aplastic anemia. Br J Haematol. 2006;133 (Suppl 1):118.
3. Davies JK, Guinan EC. An update on the management of severe aplastic anaemia in children. Br J Haematol. 2007;136(4):549-64.
4. Frickhofen N, Heimpel H, Kaltwasser JP, et al. Antithymocyte globulin with or without cyclosporin A: 11-year follow-up of a randomized trial comparing treatments of aplastic anemia. Blood. 2003;101(4):1236-42.
5. George B, Mathews V, Viswabandya A, et al. Fludarabine and cyclophosphamide based reduced intensity conditioning (RIC) regimens reduce rejection and improve outcome in Indian patients undergoing allogeneic stem cell transplantation for severe aplastic anemia. Bone Marrow Transplant. 2007; 40(1):13-8.
6. Kutler DI, Singh B, Satagopan J, et al. A 20-year perspective on the International Fanconi Anemia Registry (IFAR). Blood. 2003;101(4):1249-56.
7. Marsh JC, Ball SE, Darbyshire P, et al. Guidelines for the diagnosis and management of acquired aplastic anaemia. Br J Haematol. 2003;123(5):782-801.
8. Marwaha RK, Bansal D, Trehan A, et al. Androgens in childhood acquired aplastic anemia in Chandigarh, India. Trop Doct. 2004;34(3):149-52.
9. Young NS, Calado RT, Scheinberg P. Current concepts in the pathophysiology and treatment of aplastic anemia. Blood. 2006;108(8):2509-19.

11.5 Thalassemia Syndromes

MR Lokeshwar

INTRODUCTION

Thalassemia was first clinically described nearly a century ago, and the treatment of this genetic disease has greatly advanced during this period. During the nine decades following the first clinical description of thalassemia, there have been revolutionary changes in the field of science and medicine, which have impacted on the understanding and treatment of the thalassemia.

HISTORICAL REVIEW

The disease was first described by Thomas B Cooley **(Fig. 11.5.1)** and Pearl Lee in 1925 and hence was known as "Cooley's anemia." Whipple and Bradford first used the term "Thalassemia" in 1932, *thalassa* in Greek meaning *sea* and *-emia*, meaning anemia around the sea. It was also known as "Mediterranean anemia" as it was initially described around Mediterranean countries. However, it was soon realized that

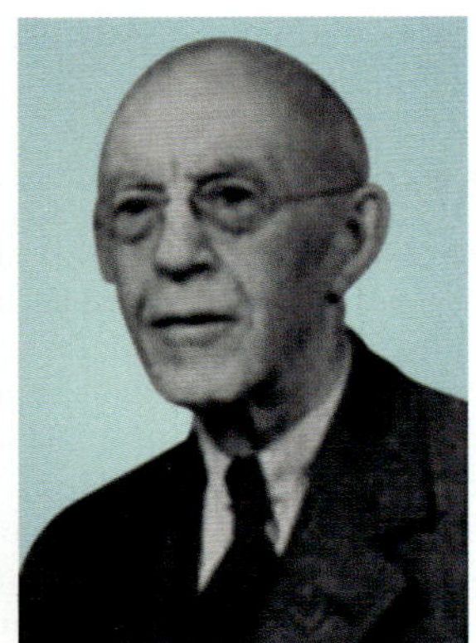

Fig. 11.5.1: Thomas B Cooley.

it also occurs not only around Mediterranean regions but also in Southeast Asia, Indian subcontinent, and Middle East. The first case of Thalassemia was reported from India by Dr M Mukherjee from Campbell Medical School Calcutta in 1938. Dr PK Sukumaran from Mumbai did pioneering works in the field of diagnosis of thalassemia syndromes in India.

CLASSIFICATION

The hemoglobin (Hb) consists of two pairs of amino acid chains: A pair of (1) α-chain and (2) non-α-chains. Adult Hb (HbA) consists of pair of α-chains and a pair of β-chains (α_2 β_2). Fetal Hb (HbF) is constituted by a pair of α-chains and a pair of ϒ chains (α_2 ϒ2). HbA_2 is constituted by pair of α-chains and a pair of δ chains (α_2 δ_2) **(Table 11.5.1)**. Deficiency or abnormalities in any of the Hb chains leads to thalassemia syndromes or hemoglobinopathies.

Thalassemia is caused by a defect/reduction in Hb chain synthesis due to various mutations of genes which code for the globin chain.

It is characterized by decreased synthesis of one of the polypeptide chains α or non-α, which form Hb molecule. α-globin chains are represented by four genes, while β-globin is encoded by two genes.

The α-gene is present on chromosome 16, and β-gene is represented on chromosome 11. Both are inherited in an autosomal recessive manner.

Table 11.5.1: Classification based on the chain affected.

• α-thalassemia—α-chain is affected	• β-thalassemia—β-chain is affected
• β^0-thalassemia—β-chain is absent	• β^+-thalassemia—β-chain is partially present
• Double heterozygous states	• Sickle thalassemia, HbE thalassemia, HbD thalassemia, etc.

(HbD: hemoglobin D; HbE: hemoglobin E)

Thalassemia is classified depending on the deficiency of type of globin chain of Hb.

In α-thalassemia, α-chain synthesis is affected. They are classified into four different categories depending upon the number of genes affected **(Table 11.5.2)**.

Alpha-globin chains are represented by four genes, while β-globin is encoded by two genes. Both are inherited in an autosomal recessive manner.

In β-thalassemia, β-chain is involved. If β-chain is absent, it is termed β^0-thalassemia, if partially produced, then β^+-thalassemia **(Table 11.5.3)**.

INHERITANCE

Thalassemia is inherited as an autosomal recessive disease. There is 25% chance that children born in each pregnancy will develop thalassemia major (TM). However, it is not unusual to see consecutive children being born with TM, emphasizing 25% chance in each pregnancy **(Figs. 11.5.2A to C)**.

Thalassemia minor (trait or carrier) is due to single gene mutation (heterozygous), and in homozygous state, both genes are mutated, which may be *thalassemia intermedia* or *TM*. β-thalassemia is also classified as transfusion dependent (TM) and transfusion independent (thalassemia intermedia) **(Figs. 11.5.3A to C)**.

More than 200–250 mutations have been described in patients with β-thalassemia. The common mutations responsible for more than 90% of thalassemia mutations in our country include 619-bp deletion, IVS 1-5 (G-C), IVS1-1 (G-T), FS8/9 (+G), and FS 41/42 (–CTTT).

Rarer mutations have been described and include codon 4/5 and 6 (ACT CCT GAG-ACA TCTTAG), codon 47/48

Table 11.5.2: Classification of α-thalassemia syndromes.

Syndrome	*Clinical features*	*Hemoglobin pattern*	*α-globin genes affected*
Silent carrier	No anemia, normal red cells	1–2% Hb Bart's (γ^4) at birth	1
α-thalassemia trait	Mild anemia, hypochromic microcytic red cells	5–10% Hb Bart's (γ^4) at birth	2
HbH disease	Moderate anemia, hypochromic, microcytic, red cells	5–30% HbH (β^4) At birth	3
Hydrops fetalis	Death in utero caused by severe anemia	Mainly Hb Bart's, small amounts of HbH	4

(Hb: hemoglobin; HbH: hemoglobin H)

Table 11.5.3: Classification of β-thalassemia syndromes.

Syndrome	*Clinical features*	*Hemoglobin pattern*	*β-globin genes affected*
Silent carrier	Asymptomatic No anemia	Normal, diagnosed by chain synthesis or identification of mutation	Heterozygous state
Thalassemia trait	Mild anemia, hypochromic microcytic red cells	Elevated HbA_2 > 3.4%	Heterozygous state
Thalassemia intermedia	Moderate, not dependent on blood transfusion for their survival May require transfusion occasionally	HbF and/or HbA_2 elevated	Homozygous/Double heterozygous state
Thalassemia major	Dependent on regular blood transfusion for survival	HbF markedly elevated	Homozygous state

(HbA_2: hemoglobin A_2; HbF: fetal hemoglobin)

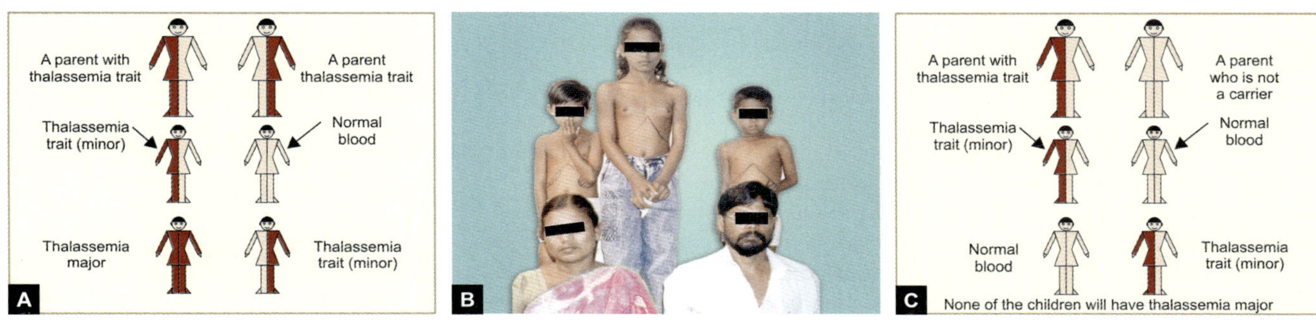

Figs. 11.5.2A to C: Inheritance of thalassemia major: 25% inheritance means 25% in each pregnancy. All the above three children are thalassemia major.
Courtesy: MR Lokeshwar, Anupam Sachdeva, and Mamta Manglani.

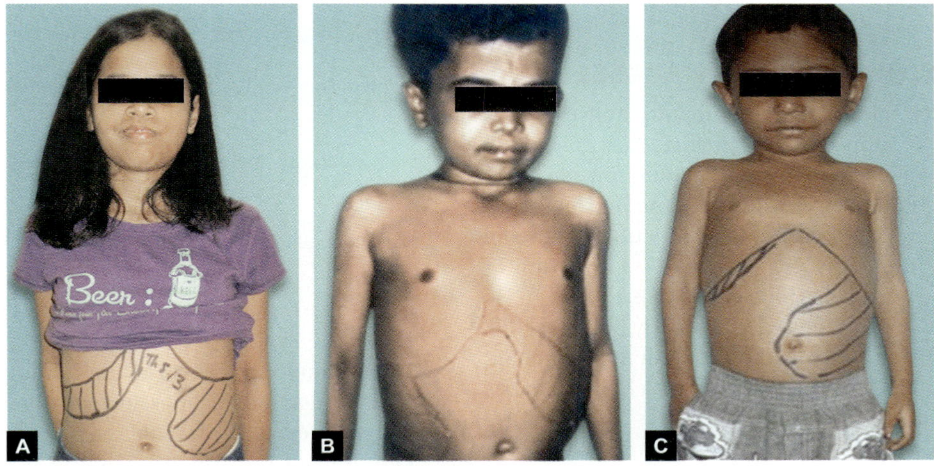

Figs. 11.5.3A to C: (A and B) Anemia and hepatosplenomegaly in thalassemia intermedia and (C) child with thalassemia major.
Courtesy: Dr MR Lokeshwar and Dr Mamta Manglani.

(+ATCT), codon 55 (+A), IVS2-837 (T to G), codon 88 (+T), codon 5 (–CT), IVS1-110 (G-A), and codon 15 (TGG-TAG).

Thalassemia Incidence: World Scenario

Thalassemia belt stretches across African continent, Mediterranean regions, Middle East, Indian subcontinent, Southeast Asia, Southern China, and Melanesia. The prevalence of thalassemia and falciparum malaria was similar, suggesting that nature developed genetic mutation to overcome mortality and morbidity of malaria. However, population migration has not restricted the gene frequency to above tropical areas and hence seen all over the world **(Figs. 11.5.4A and B)**.

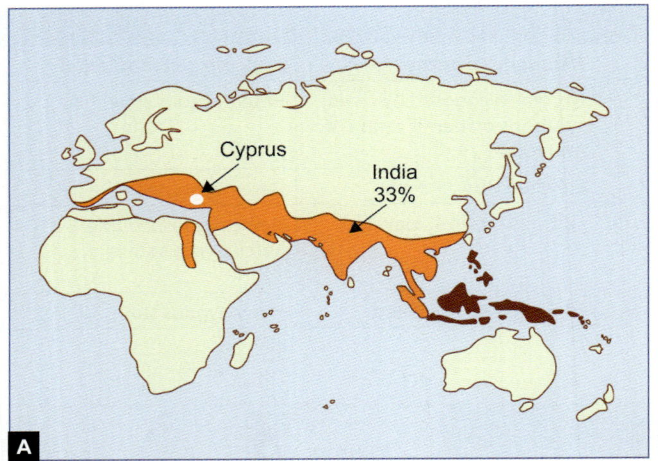

A higher frequency is noted in certain communities in India:

- Sindhis, Punjabis from North
- Migrants from Pakistan to north India such as Khatris and Khukrejas
- Bhanushalis, Lohanas, Kutchis, Baniyas from Gujarat
- Neo-Buddhists, Mahars, Chamars, Buddhists, Kolis, Agris, Kunbis from Maharashtra
- Reddys, Gowdas, Lingayats, Kurgs from Andhra Pradesh and Karnataka
- Goud Saraswats from Goa

B

Figs. 11.5.4A and B: (A) Thalassemia incidence: world scenario thalassemia belt; (B) Frequency in certain communities in India.

All over the world, there are more than 250 million (1.5% of world population) carriers of β-thalassemia gene, and in Southeast Asia, there are 40 million carriers of this gene. In India, prevalence of the β-gene (trait) varies from 1% to 17%. Thalassemia incidence varies in various communities, religions, and ethnic groups in India. All over the world around 100,000 children are born each year with severe homozygous state of these diseases. With the birth rate of 22.8 per 1,000 in India, it is estimated that there are about 9,000–10,000 cases being added every year, and there are around 65,000–67,000 β-thalassemia patients in our country at given time.

PATHOPHYSIOLOGY OF β-THALASSEMIA

Excess α-chains that have no complementary non-α-chains with which to pair form insoluble inclusions that precipitate on red cell membrane and damage it leading to premature destruction of red blood cells (RBCs) in bone marrow (BM) and peripheral circulation, particularly reticuloendothelial system of spleen (ineffective erythropoiesis) resulting in persistent progressive anemia **(Flowchart 11.5.1)**.

Due to reduced production of HbA in early postnatal life, the normal switch mechanism leading to reduction in γ-chain synthesis does not occur. In β-thalassemia, γ-chain synthesis persists after fetal life.

Extramedullary erythropoiesis results in expansion of BM spaces producing characteristic hemolytic facies—frontal, parietal, and occipital bossing; malar prominence and malocclusion of teeth—along with distortion and osteoporosis of ribs and vertebrae, pathological fracture of long bones; splenomegaly with its complications hypersplenism, hepatomegaly, gallstones, and chronic leg ulcers.

Flowchart 11.5.1: Pathophysiology of β-thalassemia.

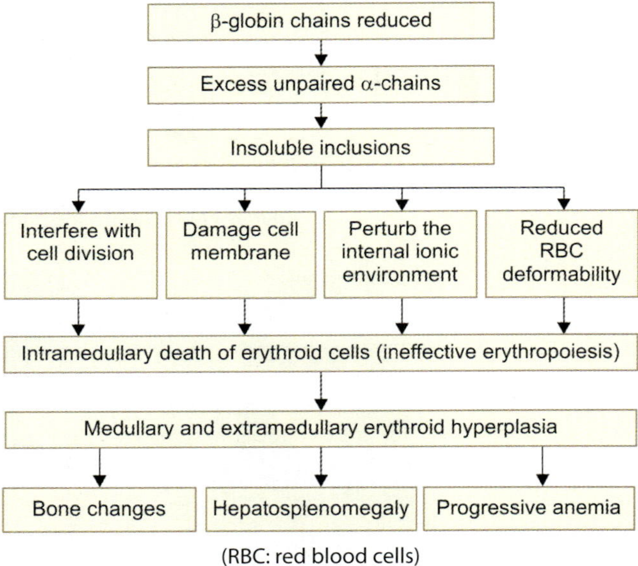

(RBC: red blood cells)

CLINICAL MANIFESTATIONS

Severe β-thalassemia usually manifests in the first year of life (6–18 months) when the HbF declines normally. In India, many children born with TM die undiagnosed, due to the lack of investigation facilities and treatment. The spectrum of clinical manifestation of β-thalassemia varies widely.

One end of the spectrum is the serious homozygous form (TM) that presents in early infancy (6–18 months) with gradually increasing pallor, poor feeding, failure to thrive, irritability, fatigability, intercurrent infections, and develops hepatosplenomegaly. Affected children grow well for initial few months (2–4 months) after birth. No anemia is observed during newborn period. If undiagnosed and untreated, more than 90% do not survive beyond 3–4 years of age without transfusion. Untreated or irregularly treated children develop significant hemolytic facies, including frontoparietal bossing with a hot cross bun appearance of the skull (caput

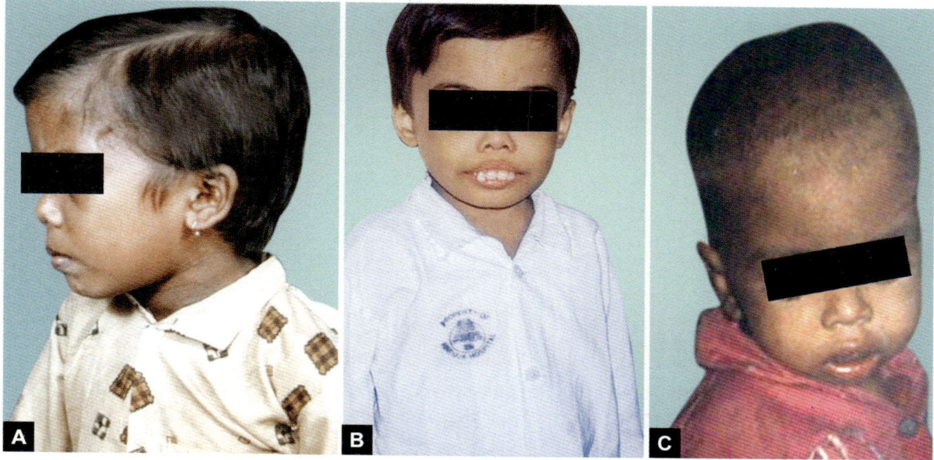

Figs. 11.5.5A to C: Characteristic features of thalassemia major: (A) Occipital bossing; (B) Malar prominence and malocclusion of teeth, and (C) Caput quadratum.
Courtesy: Dr MR Lokeshwar and Dr Mamta Manglani.

quadratum), depressed bridge of nose, malar prominence, and malocclusion of teeth with protrusion of maxillary teeth **(Figs. 11.5.5A to C)**.

Siderosis iron overload follows in various endocrine glands—pituitary, thyroid, and parathyroid glands—as well as pancreas and heart. As a result, the child develops various secondary endocrine problems **(Fig. 11.5.6)** (growth retardation, delayed or absent puberty), diabetes mellitus, and cardiac complications (congestive failure, intractable arrhythmias). In older children, liver and spleen may be enlarged due to extramedullary erythropoiesis and hemosiderosis and may develop hypersplenism. Unless supported by regular transfusion, severe and progressive anemia and retardation of growth and development are the rule. The other end of the spectrum is the heterozygous form thalassemia minor where children can lead relatively normal life except for mild persistent anemia not responding to hematinic and have normal life span. They can pass on their genes to their siblings. Occasionally, some of them may not even have elevated HbA_2 and are termed as silent gene carriers.

In between these two extremes, there are forms with varying degree of clinical manifestations of anemia, hepatosplenomegaly, and bone changes. They also maintain their life fairly comfortably and are not dependent on blood transfusions for their survival and are called thalassemia intermedia and are homozygous.

DIAGNOSIS

For detection of hemoglobinopathies, it is advisable to correlate clinical profile and ethnicity of the individuals, with the blood count and blood film evaluation and do further investigations to confirm the diagnosis.

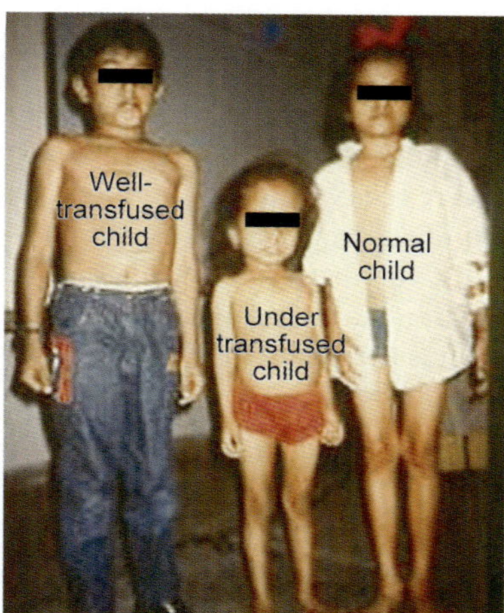

Fig. 11.5.6: Growth retardation in thalassemia children.

Complete Blood Count

This includes red cell indices, peripheral blood film (PBF) examination, and reticulocyte count. Complete blood count and PBF examination is sufficient to postulate the diagnosis of thalassemia.

Peripheral blood film examination is diagnostic and has a characteristic bizarre picture with microcytic, hypochromic red cells with striking number of normoblasts. In addition, there may be target cells, macrocytosis, poikilocytosis, polychromasia, moderate basophilic stippling, Cabot rings, and fragmented erythrocytes.

Reticulocyte count ranges from 2% to 4%. It is characteristically low (often less than 1%) in TM due to severe significant ineffective erythropoiesis in the BM, whereas in thalassemia intermedia, it may be elevated to 3–6% due to less

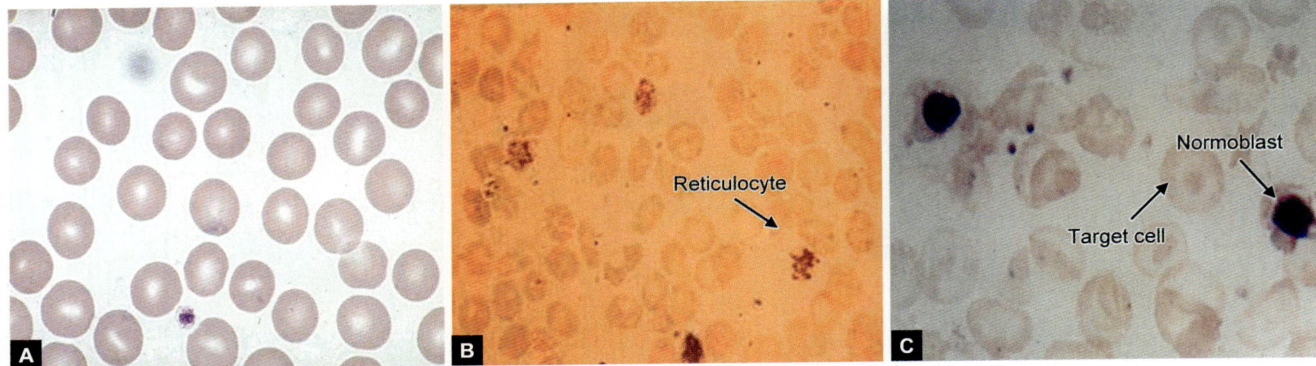

Figs. 11.5.7A to C: (A) Normal smear; (B) Reticulocyte count; and (C) Bizarre picture with microcytic, hypochromic red cells with smear showing target cell and normoblast.

severe ineffective erythropoiesis. Normoblasts are increased on peripheral smear **(Figs. 11.5.7A to C)**.

Mean corpuscular volume is reduced in both iron-deficiency anemia (IDA) as well as thalassemia minor.

Red blood cell count: In thalassemia minor, high red cell count relative to Hb concentration and hematocrit is seen. In IDA, there is marked fall in RBC count, MCV, and mean cell Hb.

Red cell distribution width (RDW): RDW is the coefficient of the variation of red cell volume distribution. It is the objective documentation of subjective anisocytosis. It is significantly high suggesting a very high degree of anisocytosis. RDW is normal in thalassemia trait as well as in anemia of chronic infection, while it is increased in IDA. Normal range of RDW is 11.5–14.5%.

Naked Eye Single Tube Red Cell Osmotic Fragility Test

The test has a high sensitivity of 95%, but its poor precision, intertechnician variability, and low specificity have precluded it from becoming a practical procedure **(Figs. 11.5.8)**. It is a reasonable specific test for the detection of β-thalassemia trait. This test is economical, as the cost of performing a single test is less than a rupee, quick, easy to perform, and does not require any sophisticated equipment. The solution once prepared has got a long shelf life. A high negative predictive value can reasonably rule out β-thalassemia trait cases. So, it should be adopted as a screening test for β-thalassemia trait, as it is not practical or feasible to employ HbA_2 in every case of anemia in childhood.

Tests for Iron Status

- *Serum iron and transferrin saturation:* Decreased in IDA; increased/normal in thalassemia depending upon iron overload
- *Serum total iron-binding capacity:* Increased in IDA and normal in thalassemia and anemia of chronic infection

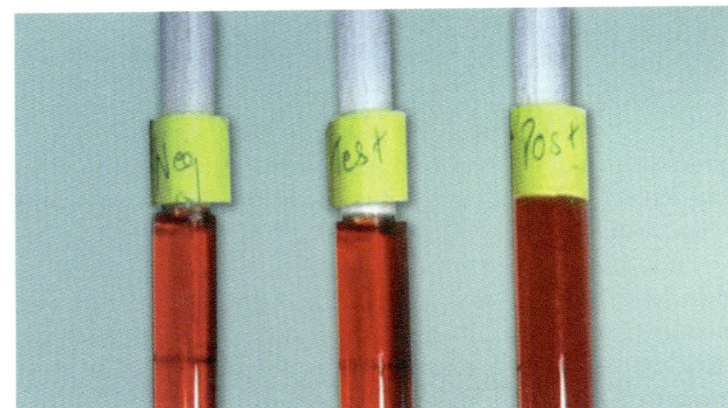

Figs. 11.5.8: Naked eye single tube red cell osmotic fragility test.

- *Serum ferritin:* Decreased in IDA, whereas increased in thalassemia, and is proportionate to iron overload and increased in infection
- *Osmotic fragility:* Reduced.

Other Methods of Iron Estimation

Liver iron concentration (keep level below 7 mg/g of liver, levels above 15 mg/g is associated with cardiac problems), *superconductive quantum interference device (SQUID)*, *biomagnetic liver spectrometry*, magnetic resonance imaging (MRI), and urine iron content.

Bone marrow examination: This is not required for diagnosis. It shows normoblastic erythroid hyperplasia, and iron staining of BM shows increased store of iron in the form of hemosiderin in thalassemia.

Measurement of Hemoglobin A2

Cellulose acetate electrophoresis: Quantitation of HbA_2 is the gold standard for the diagnosis of thalassemia trait and confirmatory investigation for the diagnosis of thalassemia syndrome. Hemoglobin electrophoresis in nontransfused patients with TM shows HbF 20–100% and 2–7% of HbA_2, and HbA 0–80% depending upon the genotype. Thalassemia minor is characterized by elevated HbA_2 more than 3.4% **(Figs. 11.5.9A and B)**.

Other methods: Isoelectric focusing, microcolumn chromatography, automated high-performance liquid chromatography (HPLC), and Biorad variant machine **(Figs. 11.5.10A and B)**.

Radiological Changes

These changes can be observed on X-rays of skull as "hair-on-end" appearance and osteopenia and osteoporosis of the long bones **(Figs. 11.5.11A to D)**.

MANAGEMENT OF THALASSEMIA MAJOR

Principles of Therapy

Management of TM should be preferably done at a comprehensive thalassemia care center with outdoor transfusion facilities. A team approach includes pediatric hematologist, pediatrician, blood transfusion specialist, endocrinologist, psychologist, and social worker.

Management of TM should include

- Correction of anemia—packed red cell transfusions
- Management of complications of blood transfusions
- Management of transfusion-transmitted diseases—hepatitis B, hepatitis C, human immunodeficiency virus (HIV), malaria, cytomegalovirus (CMV), and *Yersinia*
- Removal of excess iron—chelation therapy
- Management of endocrine and cardiac complications
- Curative treatment—BM transplant (BMT)/stem cell transplant;
- Hypersplenism—role of splenectomy
- Management of other complications—gallstones/anemia/hypoxia/leg ulcers
- Pharmacological methods to increase γ-chain synthesis
- Future treatment—Gene replacement therapy, intrauterine BMT

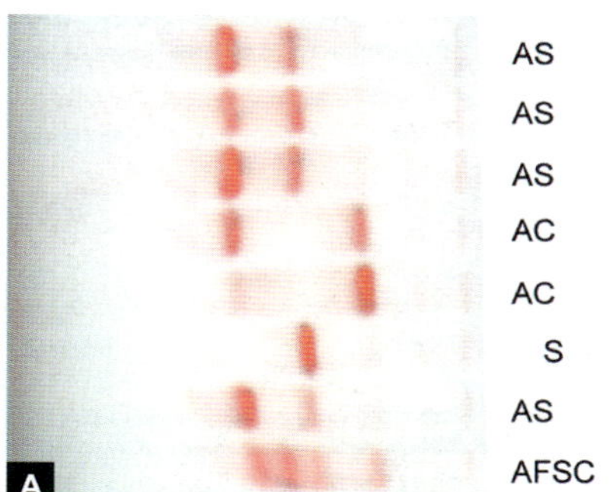

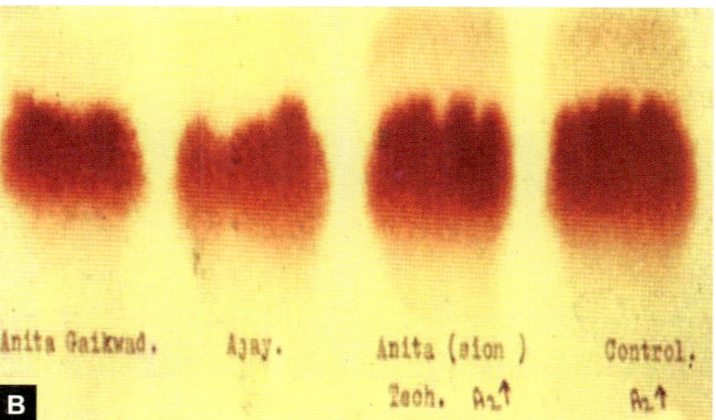

Figs. 11.5.9A and B: Elevated HbA2: (A) cellulose acetate electrophoresis and (B) paper electrophoresis. (HbA2: hemoglobin A2)
Courtesy: Dr MR Lokeshwar and Dr Ajit C Gorakshakar.

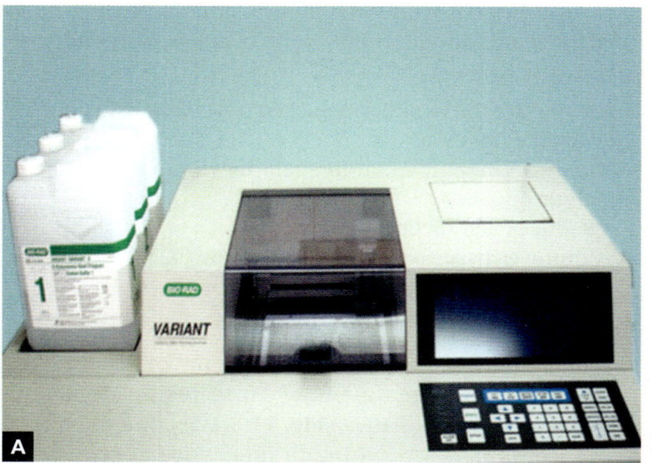

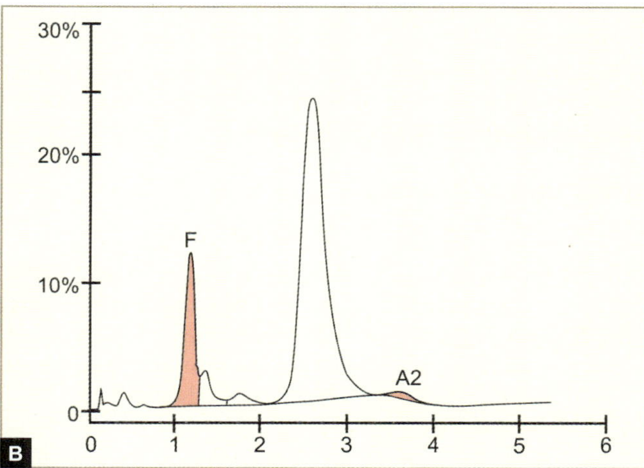

Figs. 11.5.10A and B: Automated high-performance liquid chromatography (HPLC) and Bio-rad variant machine.

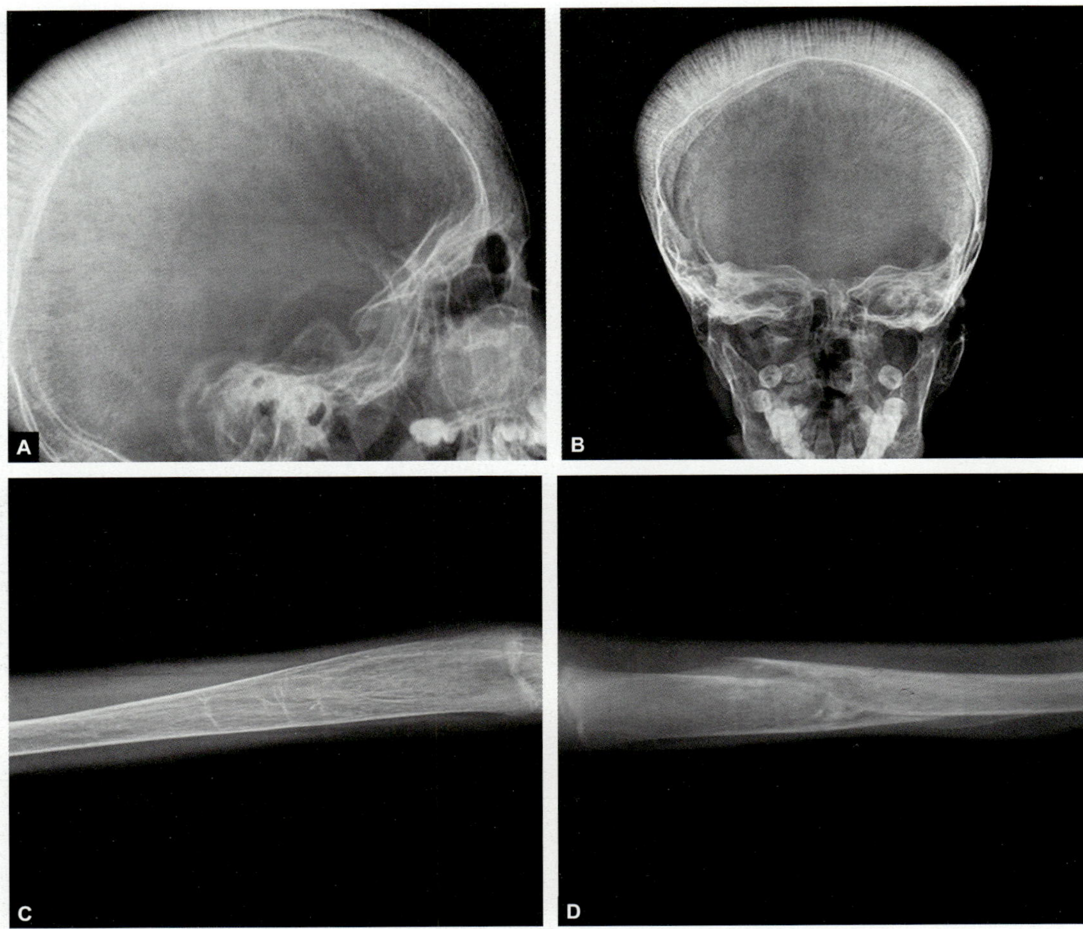

Figs. 11.5.11A to D: (A and B) Thalassemia major: Skull X-ray showing "hair-on-end" appearance; (C and D) Osteopenia and osteoporosis of the long bone.
Courtesy: Dr MR Lokeshwar and Dr Mamta Manglani.

- Newer chelating agents
- Prevention of disease by antenatal diagnosis and genetic counseling

It is not only necessary to suspect thalassemia and confirm the diagnosis but also important to anticipate complications due to iron overload/blood transfusion.

Correction of Anemia

Transfusion Therapy in Thalassemia

Transfusion-dependent β-thalassemia is managed with regular leukocyte depleted, packed red cell transfusions preferably with a complete red cell genotype match (at least for C, c, D, E, e, and Kell) or at least after Coomb's crossmatching.

Packed Red Cell Transfusions

Packed red cell transfusion remains the cornerstone of therapy in TM. The decision to initiate lifelong regular transfusion in patients with β-thalassemia should be based on the molecular defect, severity of symptoms, clinical criteria, such as failure of growth and development, bone changes, and endocrine glands involvement.

Following are the benefits of packed red cell transfusion:
- Obviates anemia
- Reduces hepatosplenomegaly by reducing ineffective erythropoiesis
- Reduces hemolytic facies
- Improves tissue oxygenation and growth.

Types of Transfusion

Palliative transfusion: Aimed at maintaining the Hb at 8.5 g/dL.

Conventional treatment of "transfusion-dependent β-thalassemia" is palliative **(Fig. 11.5.12A)** and often leads to noncompliance, resulting in ineffective control of the manifestations and complications.

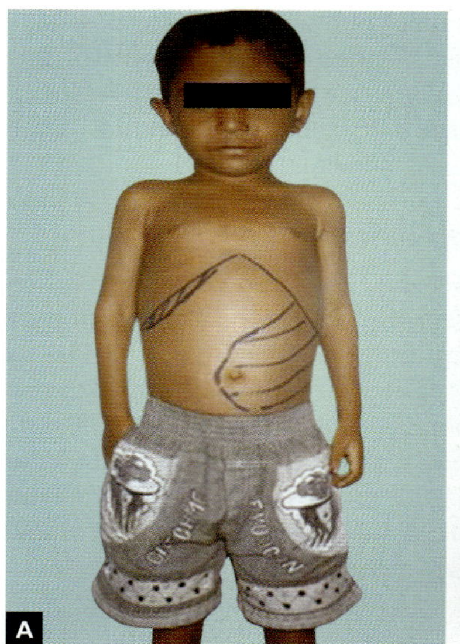
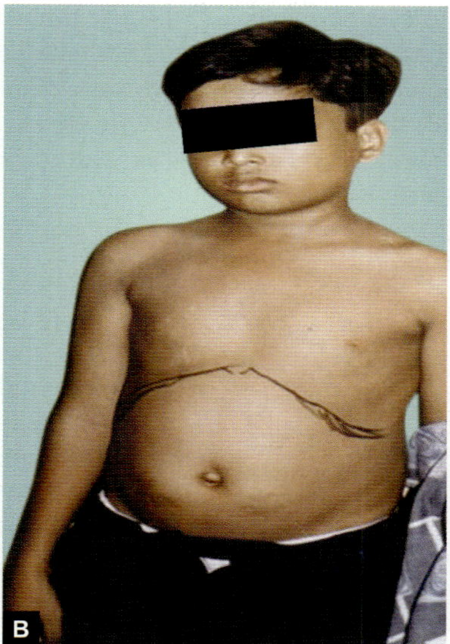
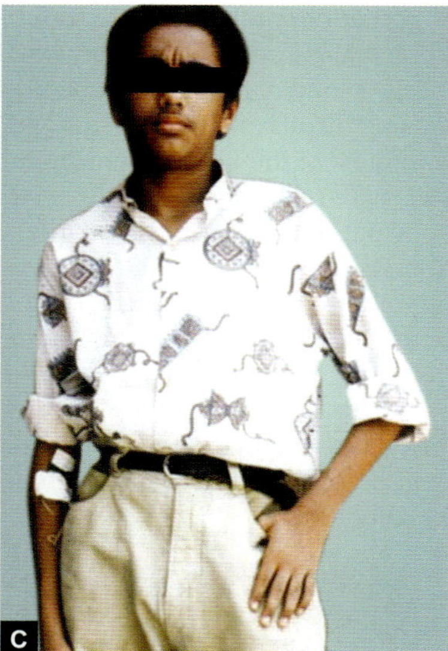

Figs .11.5.12A to C: (A) Palliative transfusion; (B) Moderate transfusion; and (C) Hypertransfusion.

This leads to improved survival, but the chronic illness, bone disease, and cardiomyopathy persist.

It causes significant psychological trauma to the patients as well as the family, leading to a poor quality of life. Hence, there is a need to have alternative and/or improved treatment for β-TM and transfusion-dependent thalassemia. It is also expensive, causing a huge burden to the individual family as well as the nation.

Moderate transfusion or normotransfusion ***(Fig. 11.5.12B)****:* In Europe, a newer regimen has been recommended by the Thalassemia International Federation.

In this regimen, pretransfusion Hb is maintained between 9 g/dL and 10.5 g/dL. It promotes normal growth and development, prevents the onset of severe hepatosplenomegaly and hemolytic facies, lowers the absorption of gastrointestinal (GI) iron, and reduces the anemia/cardiomyopathy changes **(Fig. 11.5.11)**.

Hypertransfusion: Maintaining the pretransfusion Hb above a minimum of 10 g/dL and posttransfusion Hb above 12 g/dL. Hypertransfusion **(Fig. 11.5.12C)** seems to be a promising treatment that should be recommended as first-line approach and promotes normal growth and development.

Supertransfusion: Maintain pretransfusion Hb of above 12 g/dL.

However, this is not significantly superior to hypertransfusion and given up.

Initiation of Transfusion Therapy

The diagnosis of thalassemia intermedia can be ascertained by observing the rate of fall of Hb without transfusions. If the Hb drops to below 7 g/dL without transfusion, in the absence of any concurrent illness, it is imperative to put the child on a regular transfusion program. It is important to know the complete genotype of the red cells to prevent red cell alloimmunization. The alternative to this is Coomb's crossmatch for each transfusion to prevent alloimmunization. The most ideal way to transfuse thalassemia is by using group and type-specific packed red cells that are compatible by direct antiglobulin test.

Leukodepletion Filters at Bedside

The prestorage leukodepleted packed red cell is the ideal method of leukodepletion **(Fig. 11.5.13)**. This helps to almost

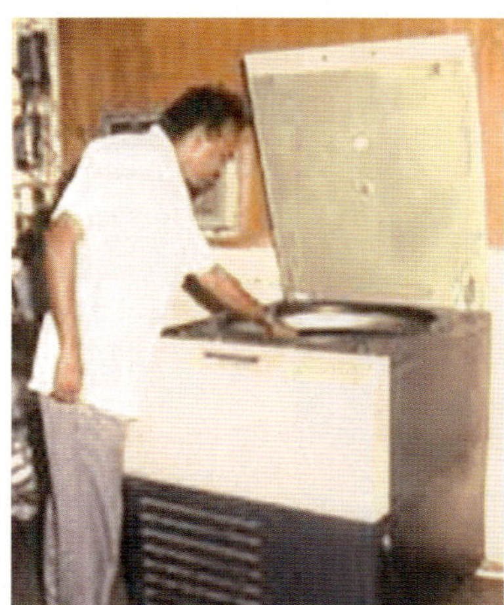

Fig. 11.5.13: Cold centrifuge.

eliminate the nonhemolytic febrile transfusion reactions as it would prevent the cytokine release, which happens during storage of the blood, which cannot be prevented in bedside filtration using disposable filters. However, this facility is not available in most of the blood banks in our country and cost of the filter (600–1,000/disposable filter) is not affordable for most of our patients alternatively triple saline-washed red cells and bedside filtration **(Fig. 11.5.14)** using disposable filters and frozen cells may be used.

The red cells should be fresh, not more than 4–5 days old.

Nucleic acid amplification testing-tested packed red cells are now common in the developed world and is rare in the majority of the centers in India; it further shortens the window period of various transfusion-transmitted infections and makes blood safer.

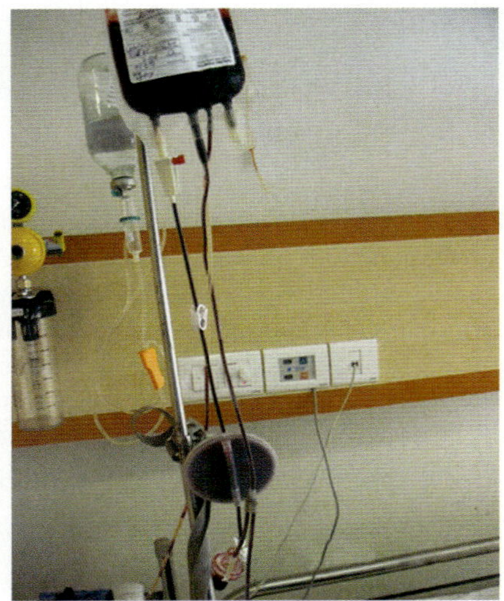

Fig. 11.5.14: Leukodepletion filters.

Those thalassemic children anticipating possibility of BM transplantation transfusing irradiated units help in prevention of posttransplant graft-versus-host disease (GVHD).

With the shortage of availability of blood, "artificial red cell substitutes" is the hope for future.

Amount and Rate of Transfusions

Approximately 180 mL/kg of red cells are required to be transfused per year in nonsplenectomized, nonsensitized patients to maintain the Hb above 10 g/dL, whereas splenectomized patients require 133 mL/kg/year. Even without hypersplenism, the requirement is 30% higher in nonsplenectomized patients. Red cells should be transfused at the rate of 3–4 mL/kg/h, every 2–4 weeks to maintain the Hb above 10 g/dL. Patients with cardiac decompensation should be given red cells at the rate of not more than 1–2 mL/kg/h.

In the daycare outdoor transfusion center, the following steps are followed:

- Transfusions are given on an OPD basis and hence no hospitalization is required.
- Children are more comfortable with the familiar staff members.
- There is less school absenteeism, and parents lose fewer workdays.

When the patient is hospitalized and transfused in the ward of the hospital, the average expenditure is much more as compared to when treated on an outdoor basis **(Figs. 11.5.15A and B)**.

- There is threat of contacting infections from other patients in the wards.
- Parents and children are happy to be with other children and parents who share the same feelings.

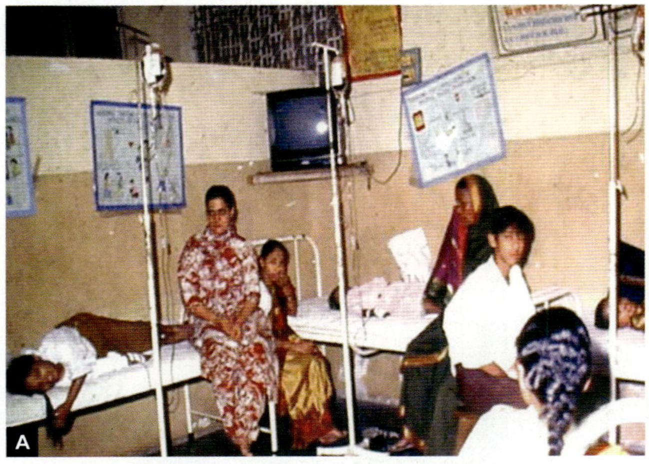

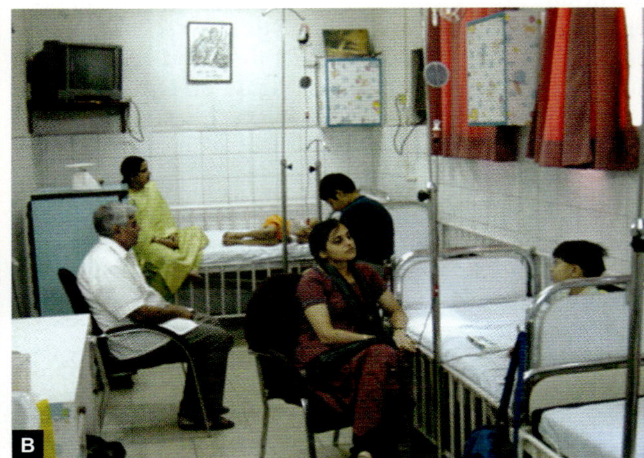

Figs. 11.5.15A and B: Daycare outdoor transfusion center.
Courtesy: Dr MR Lokeshwar, Dr Mamta Manglani, and Dr Anupam Sachdeva.

Transfusion-related Complications

- Transfusion-transmitted infections
- Iron overload and other complications.

Iron Overload and Chelation Therapy

Iron overload is due to:

- Treatment with multiple transfusions—a bottle of blood transfusion given adds 200–250 mg of iron to the body store
- Ineffective erythropoiesis leading to excessive dietary absorption of iron from gut
- Lack of physiologic excretory mechanisms for the removal of excess iron from the body
- Iron overload leads to the damage of various organs:
  - *Liver damage* starting at 2 years; fibrosis of liver at 10 years and earlier, if hepatitis B and C infection are present
  - *Cardiac damage* at about 10 years age and overt failure at about 15 years
  - *Delayed pubertal development* due to iron deposition in pituitary
  - *Diabetes mellitus*
  - *Damage to thyroid and parathyroid glands.*

Chelation Therapy

Most of the complications of β-thalassemia are attributable to iron overload. Excess iron is toxic to the heart, liver, and various endocrine glands. In β-thalassemia, 70% of deaths are due to cardiac complications. Growth failure is seen in 30% of patients in the western world and nearly all patients in our country and is due to various factors including endocrine dysfunction.

The goal is to reduce the iron store and maintain at low ferritin level to below 1,000–2,000 ng/mL and hepatic iron concentration below 268 mmol/g of dry weight of liver.

The optimal time to start chelation therapy is:

- Serum ferritin level 2,000 ng/mL or above
- After receiving more than 15–20 transfusions
- Hepatic iron concentration greater than 3.2 mg/g dry weight.

Though several hundred compounds have been developed and tried, desferrioxamine (DFO) is the gold-standard therapy. It is the most effective and safe iron chelator.

Desferrioxamine

This was introduced in the early 1960s, but its impact on the survival curves in thalassemic patients was recognized 15–20 years later.

This is a hexadentate chelator. About 1 g will bind 93 mg of iron. It cannot easily mobilize iron from intracellular compartment due to its high molecular weight. Other disadvantages include the following:

- Desferrioxamine cannot be given orally.
- Given for severe iron load and cardiac involvement, DFO slowly binds iron to form ferrioxamine.
- Desferrioxamine does not bind with iron from transferrin.
- It has a short half-life of 5–10 minutes.
- For routine use, DFO has to be given as a continuous subcutaneous infusion with the help of a Desferal pump in a dose of 20–40 mg/kg/day (not to exceed more than 100 mg/kg) over 8–10 hours for 5–6 nights a week **(Figs. 11.5.16A and B)**.
- Giving DFO only during transfusion is not recommended, and it should never be added directly to the blood unit.
- Vitamin C helps convert Fe^{3+} to Fe^{2+} which is chelatable and thus increases the iron excretion. It is recommended in a dose not more than 2–3 mg/kg/day; 50 mg for children less than 10 years and 100 mg greater than 10 years. Dose should not increase greater than 200 mg.

Toxicity of Desferrioxamine

Desferrioxamine has minimal side effects. When given parenterally, there may be liberation of histamine leading

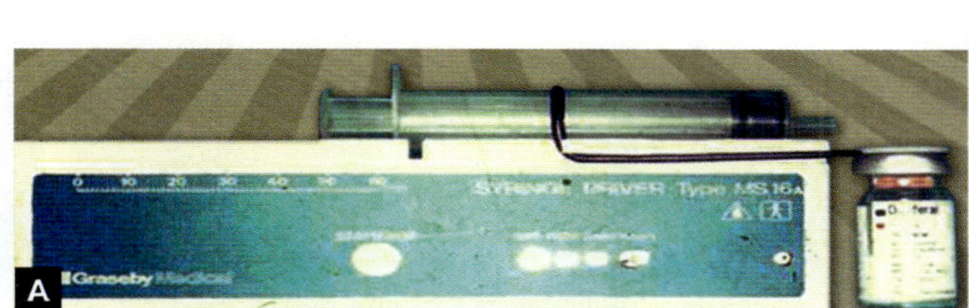

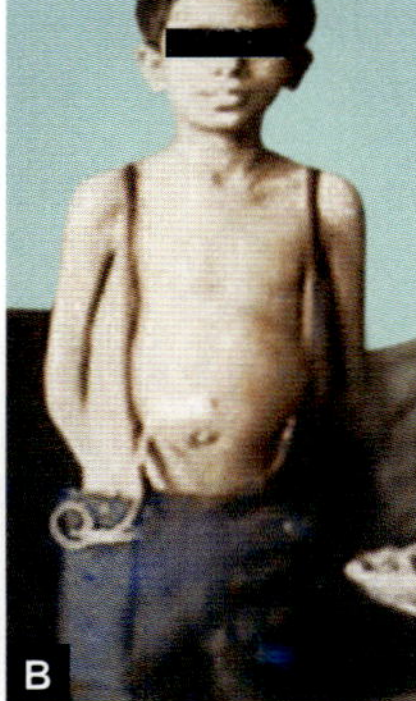

Figs. 11.5.16A and B: Continuous subcutaneous infusion with the help of a Desferal pump.

to bradycardia, hypo/hypertension, rigors, rash, headache, photophobia, feeling cold and hot, etc.

Local reactions: Local pain, redness, indurations, erythema may appear at the site of injection, and hence, it is important to rotate the site of injection.

- *Visual abnormalities:* Decreased acuity of vision, peripheral field vision defects, defective dark adaptation, and cataracts
- *Hearing:* High frequency sensory-neural hearing loss
- *Growth retardation and slowed growth:* Delayed linear growth may be seen in children less than 3 years of age treated with DFO and may be accompanied by mild skeletal abnormalities, such as short trunk, sternal protrusion, and genu valgum
- *Caution:* As the auditory and visual toxicity is reversible, regular slit-lamp eye examination **(Fig. 11.5.17)** and audiometric evaluation (brain-evoked response audiometry) are recommended annually.

Continuous Intravenous Infusion

Intravenous Desferal can be given particularly in those with very high iron overload through port-a-cath (central line). However, it is not easy to maintain the central catheter, and infections are common.

Continuous intravenous infusion significantly enhances iron excretion, presumably due to exchange between DFO and tissue iron pools.

- *Indications:* Children with very high levels of ferritin, cardiac complications, during pregnancy, prior to BM transplant (BMT) and persistent local reaction at injection site.
- *Dose:* For intravenous DFO is 50–100 mg/kg body weight. Given for severe iron load with cardiac involvement and for IV therapy.

Oral Chelating Agents

Though DFO is a gold standard in the management of iron overload in TM, it has not become popular, particularly in the developing countries. The high cost of DFO and the need for continuous subcutaneous injection over 6–8 h resulted in poor compliance, particularly in the adolescent group which has prompted the need for simpler oral chelators.

Deferiprone (Kelfer): Deferiprone (L1) **(Fig. 11.5.18)** or 1,2-dimethyl-3-hydroxypyridin-4-one. Kelfer is a water-soluble, bidentate molecule. It mobilizes iron from transferrin, ferritin, and hemosiderin. Results show that it is 70–100% as effective as DFO, is less expensive, and is given orally. The recommended dose of deferiprone is 75 mg/kg to 100 mg/kg body weight/day in 2–3 divided doses.

Deferiprone/L1 has a better protective effect on myocardial tissue as shown in various studies. It also chelates zinc in addition to iron.

Toxicity: No evidence of ear or eye toxicity. Kidney and liver parameters do not show any alteration. Few children develop GI symptoms, such as nausea, vomiting, pain in abdomen, and diarrhea. Around 20–30% children had arthropathy, which is reversible after reducing the dose or on stopping deferiprone. Antinuclear antibody, double-stranded deoxyribonucleic acid (DNA), antihistone antibodies may be positive in few cases. Absolute neutropenia and thrombocytopenia also have been reported in occasional cases.

Caution: Physical examination, particularly of the joints and complete blood count including platelet count, must be done regularly.

Deferasirox (ICL670, Exjade): Deferasirox (ICL670) (4-[3,5-bis(2-hydroxyphenyl)-1,2,4-triazol-1-yl] benzoic acid) (Asunra, Desirox, Exjade Defrijet, Desifer) is a new class

Fig. 11.5.17: Slit-lamp eye examination.

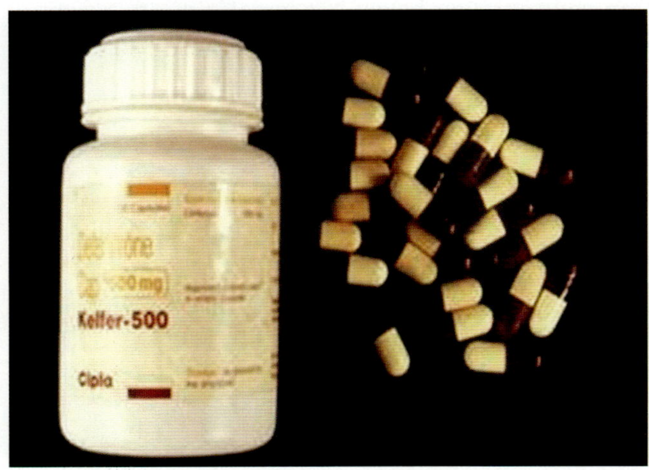

Fig. 11.5.18: Deferiprone (Kelfer).

of tridentate chelators with a high specificity for iron. It is an orally active chelating agent developed for the treatment of chronic iron overload. It is twice as effective as subcutaneous DFO. It mobilizes iron from both the hepatocellular and reticuloendothelial source. It prevents myocardial cell iron uptake and removes iron directly from myocardial cells. In liver, it removes iron from the intracellular labile iron pool and from the surface of reticuloendothelial cells at the location where iron is handed over to transferrin.

- *Metabolism:* The plasma half-life (11–19 hours) supports the once-daily oral dosing regimen. Excretion is mainly via feces and is dose dependent.
- *Dose and administration:* It is available as dispersible tablets containing 125 mg, 250 mg, and 500 mg. Dose is 20–30 mg/kg. It is to be taken on empty stomach at least 30 minutes before food, preferably at the same time each day. The tablets are to be dispersed in water, orange juice, or apple juice prior to administration.
- *Side effects:* It is neither mutagenic (teratogenic), nor carcinogenic. Side effects include skin rashes and pigmentation, GI disturbances (abdominal pain, diarrhea, nausea, vomiting, and constipation), hearing loss, nephropathy, and transient asymptomatic increase of liver enzymes.

Combination Therapy

The shuttle hypothesis: Combination of chelators has shown considerable success. Combination therapy has been tried to bring down the cost, improve the compliance, increase the efficacy of the chelation therapy, and to reduce the side effects. Combination of deferasirox and DFO has additive and synergistic effect. Deferasirox acts as intracellular chelator, and DFO acts as powerful extracellular chelator. A bidentate (L1) or (Kelfer) a tridentate ligand with access to a variety of tissues acts as a "shuttle" to mobilize the iron from tissue compartments to the bloodstream, where most exchanges with a larger hexadentate (DFO) "sink." The sink binds this iron irreversibly, promoting its excretion. Combination therapy is more effective with hydroxybenzyl-ethylenediamine-diacetic acid (HBED), and L1; ICL670A [*Deferasirox (ICL670, Exjade)*] and DFO also have been successfully tried. *Oral deferiprone 75 mg/kg/day for 5 days during weekdays, and DFO 40–50 mg/kg/day subcutaneously on weekends (2 days) is a good acceptable regimen.*

Similarly, several studies have proven the superiority of the efficacy of deferiprone and deferasirox in combination over the drugs given singly.

Pharmacologic Manipulation of Fetal Hemoglobin

Three classes of HbF-inducing agents have introduced several drugs which modulate the levels of HbF and have been successfully tried in thalassemia syndromes. They are *hypomethylating* agents, such as (HU) hydroxyurea, decitabine, and 5-azacytidine; *histone deacetylase inhibitors* (such as sodium phenylbutyrate and isobutyrate); and finally *recombinant erythropoietin***.**

Hydroxyurea has been found to be useful particularly in thalassemia intermedia, double heterozygotes and sickle cell disease (dose 10–20 mg/kg/day).

All these agents have shown promising results in sickle cell disease and non-transfusion-dependent thalassemia, but to a lesser extent in TM or transfusion-dependent thalassemia. HU is the Food and Drug Administration-approved drug recommended for use in thalassemia and sickle cell disease as an HbF-elevating drug.

Drugs Under Trial (Newer Iron Chelators)

Various other drugs under trial include desferrithiocin (DFT), HBED, NaHBED, pyridoxal isonicotinoyl hydrazone (PIH), etc.

Desferrithiocin caused kidney damage in rats on prolonged oral DFT. The damage was believed to be due to toxic effects of the Fe^{3+} complex, ferrithiocin. One of its analogs, 4-OH-desaza-desmethyl-DFT, appears to be less toxic iron chelator in animal studies.

GT56-252: It is a novel orally available iron chelator derived from DFT that forms a 2:1 complex with Fe^{3+}.

SSP-004184: *SSP-004184*, previously termed FBS0701, is a DFT derivative, a tridentate chelator. It is currently in phase 2/3 trials in several centers. It was found to be safe at four escalating doses and may be recommended as once-daily dose.

Deferitrin is a tridentate chelator being developed. However, the drug was stalled when the animal models developed severe nephrotoxicity. Its newer derivatives are currently being developed.

Pyridoxal isonicotinoyl hydrazone is an effective iron chelator. It is a tridentate chelator with a selectivity for iron comparable to that of DFO. Various PIH analogs have been synthesized, and some of them, such as pyridoxal-benzoyl hydrazones, were much more effective than PIH. The latter studies have shown that the orally administered analogs are about two to six times more effective than intraperitoneally administered DFO in mobilizing liver iron in rats.

40SD02 (CHF1540): 40SD02 is a new entity synthesized by chemically attaching DFO to a modified starch polymer. Single doses of up to 600 mg/kg of the compound were safe and well tolerated and stimulated a clinically significant amount of iron excretion. It is high molecular weight chelator and has prolonged half-life.

Folic acid: Folic acid (1 mg/day) should be given to nontransfused or low-transfused patients because they have increased folate consumption and may develop folic acid deficiency.

Amlodipine: In TM patients with cardiac siderosis, amlodipine combined with chelation therapy reduced cardiac iron more effectively than chelation therapy alone; oral dose-amlodipine 5 mg/day.

Monitoring Iron Overload

Serum Ferritin

Maintain values of *less than 2,000 ng/mL*. However, serum level of ferritin can be affected by various factors, such as inflammation, infection, ascorbate status, and hepatitis.

Liver iron concentration of less than 7 mg/g dry weight of liver is associated with reduced cardiac or liver complications.

Magnetic resonance imaging (MRI) and SQUID can also measure liver iron concentration noninvasively. But these technologies are less widely available.

MANAGEMENT OF COMPLICATIONS

Hypersplenism

Hypersplenism may occur due to inadequate transfusions, alloimmunization, and rarely autoimmune hemolysis complicating TM and chronic liver disease.

Splenectomy (Fig. 11.5.19)

Splenectomy should be considered when:

- Annual blood requirement exceeds 1.5 times the basal requirement for a patient maintaining pretransfusion Hb about 10 g/dL (transfusion requirement increases to more than 200–220 mL/kg/year of packed red cells)
- Massive spleen enlargement posing a risk of splenic rupture or when splenic enlargement is associated with the left upper quadrant pain
- Presence of leukopenia or thrombocytopenia
- Splenectomy should be deferred till the patient is 5 years of age as there is a risk of overwhelming sepsis below this age.

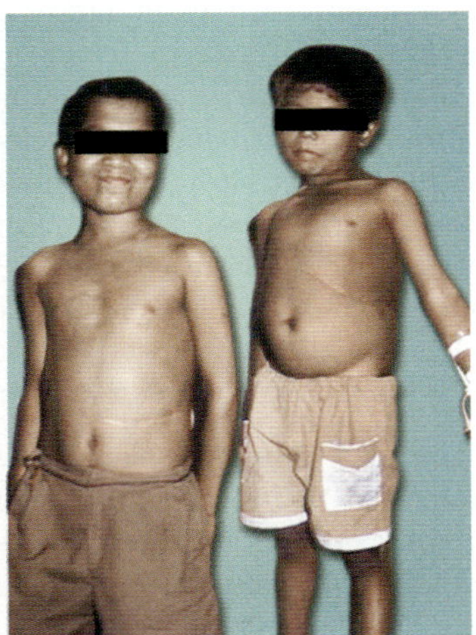

Fig. 11.5.19: Splenectomy.

Prophylaxis: All patients undergoing splenectomy should receive immunization to protect against capsulated organisms. These include pneumococcal, *Haemophilus influenzae* type B, meningococcal vaccines, *Salmonella typhi*, which should be given at least 4 weeks before surgery. Lifelong postsplenectomy penicillin prophylaxis *125 mg twice a day for children up to 2 years and 250 mg twice a day for children 2 years and above is recommended.* Chemoprophylaxis is recommended for at least 2 years, while some advocate this for whole life. In the presence of early signs of infection, treatment should be started immediately with broad spectrum antibiotics without waiting for the result of laboratory tests. Postsplenectomy, there may be transient or persistent thrombocytosis. Aspirin 50–100 mg/day is recommended for patients whose platelet count exceeds 800,000/mm^3.

Cardiac Complications

Cardiovascular disease resulting from iron accumulation is still a major cause of death in patients with TM. Iron overload causes deposition of iron in the ventricular walls, mainly in the left, relatively sparing the atria and the conduction system. Cardiac failure and ventricular arrhythmias are the main cause of death in patients with TM. Other cardiac complications include decrease in left ventricular ejection fraction, overt cardiomyopathy, left atrial dilatation, and aortic root dilatation. Early detection of cardiac involvement is done by the evaluation of ferritin level regularly along with cardiac function tests, such as electrocardiography, two-dimensional echocardiogram, stress test, and Holter monitoring. T2 cardiac MRI is the method of accessing accurately the severity of cardiac iron overloading.

Deferiprone/L1 has better protective effect on myocardial tissue. Continuous subcutaneous/intravenous high-dose DFO can reverse the ventricular dysfunction and can improve progressive heart failure and complicate arrhythmias.

Oral dose—amlodipine 5 mg/day. Amlodipine treatment did not cause any serious adverse events. In TM patients with cardiac siderosis, amlodipine combined with chelation therapy reduced cardiac iron more effectively than chelation therapy alone.

Thalidomide

Thalidomide is a synthetic glutamic acid derivative; however, due to severe teratogenic effects observed in pregnant women administered thalidomide, it was completely withdrawn. However, it was reintroduced for its antiangiogenic properties and is now used in various inflammatory disorders and in malignancies, such as multiple myeloma.

Thalidomide has not yet undergone adequate trials for its routine use in thalassemia syndromes.

It has significant adverse events including serious life-threatening ones. Thrombosis has already been reported recently even with a single course of thalidomide in a patient of TM.

There have only been anecdotal reports of its use in those patients, in whom transfusions were near impossible due to alloimmunization, and other immunomodulators failed to improve the situation. Even in such patients, it is mandatory to explain to the patients and their families the need for use of a nonapproved drug with its inherent life-threatening adverse effects. Only if they then consent, should it be used.

Transfusion-transmitted Infections

The common transfusion-transmitted infections seen in these multiply transfused thalassemic children include the following:

- Hepatitis B and C
- Human immunodeficiency virus
- *Yersinia* spp.
- Malaria
- Cytomegalovirus

Hepatitis B

Hepatitis B has been reported in 5–30.6% among multiply transfused individuals in various studies.

- Stringent screening of donors and testing of all blood bags for HIV, hepatitis B virus surface antigen (HBsAg), and anti-hepatitis C virus (HCV) has reduced the rate of these transfusion-transmitted infections.
- In addition, it has been possible to effectively control hepatitis B through transfusions by vaccinating with hepatitis B vaccine, all children at diagnosis, *with double dose, intense regimen (0 month, 1 month, 2 months, and 12 months).*
- Boosters may be given at 5-year intervals.

Hepatitis C

The prevalence of hepatitis C is quite high and has been reported in 11–69% of transfused thalassemic (before it was mandatory to screen all blood bags for HCV antibodies).

The treatment of these patients is difficult, as it is highly expensive. Interferons and Ribavirin are the commonly used therapies. Pegylated interferons are obtained by conjugating Intron A with polyethylene glycol. This prolongs the activity of interferon allowing weekly dosing instead of the conventional thrice-weekly dosing.

Human Immunodeficiency Virus

The occurrence of transfusion-transmitted HIV has ranged from 0% to 70%. Children with transfusion-transmitted HIV progress to AIDS over a period of 5–10 years unlike perinatally infected children, who progress quite rapidly. They can be managed with antiretroviral therapy, as per the national guidelines for children and adults.

Other infections commonly seen in these children include malaria and CMV infections. CMV infection can be prevented by reducing the leukocyte content of packed red cells, either by prestorage filtration or using bedside leukocyte filters. Moreover, use of red cells from CMV-negative donors and frozen red cells are other alternatives in the developed world.

Malaria

Malaria must be treated as and when it occurs, as despite screening blood bags for malaria, it would not be possible to identify all donors harboring the parasite due to a low-sensitivity and interobserver variability of peripheral blood smear evaluation.

Yersinia Infection

Yersinia enterocolitica is known to occur in iron overloaded and deferoxamine-treated patients. If a patient on deferoxamine comes with the symptoms of abdominal pain, diarrhea, and vomiting, deferoxamine should be stopped immediately, appropriate stool culture or blood serology undertaken and treatment with cotrimoxazole or aminoglycoside is given.

Endocrine Evaluation

Growth and Development

The commonly affected endocrine glands include pituitary, pancreas, thyroid, parathyroid glands and gonads. Clinically, they may remain latent. Hence, investigations should be done in all thalassemic children from time to time to detect these disorders and treat them appropriately.

- Short stature is commonly noted at 10–11 years of age.
- Diabetes may be seen as early as 5 years of age and particularly seen in adolescent children.
- Dysfunction of thyroid and parathyroid glands may be subclinical initially.
- Glucose tolerance test and thyroid functions, particularly T4 and thyroid-stimulating hormone, should be done.
- Serum calcium, phosphorus, and alkaline phosphatase should be done frequently, if possible every year, beginning at the age of 5 years.
- Height, weight, growth velocity, cardiac work-up, endocrine study, and bone studies evaluation are required from 10 years of age onward. This helps in early detection and better management.

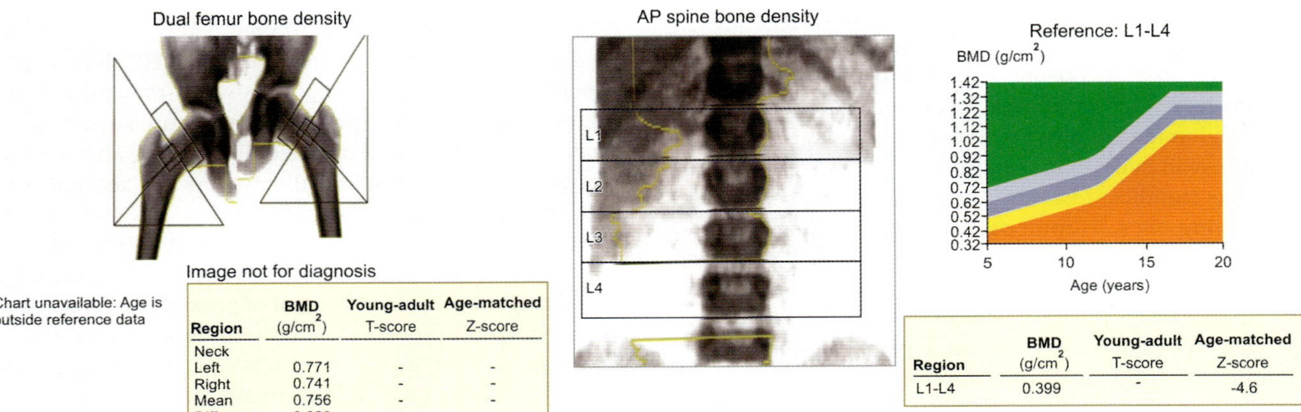

Region	BMD (g/cm^2)	Young-adult T-score	Age-matched Z-score
Neck			
Left	0.771	-	-
Right	0.741	-	-
Mean	0.756	-	-
Diffrence	0.029	-	-

Region	BMD (g/cm^2)	Young-adult T-score	Age-matched Z-score
L1-L4	0.399	-	-4.6

Fig. 11.5.20: Dual-energy X-ray absorptiometry (DEXA).

Hepatic Dysfunction

Liver dysfunction is secondary to plasma-borne infections and iron overload. It is thus necessary to do the liver function tests and hepatitis markers, particularly HBsAg and HCV antibodies every 6 months.

Osteopenia and Osteoporosis

Osteopenia and osteoporosis are major causes of morbidity in aging thalassemic population more in women. Osteoporosis as defined by WHO is a "progressive systemic skeletal disease characterized by low bone mass and micro architectural deterioration of bone tissue, with consequent increase in bone fragility and susceptibility to fracture". This can be diagnosed by *dual-energy X-ray absorptiometry* **(Fig. 11.5.20)** scan for bone density and biochemical studies of serum calcium, inorganic phosphate, alkaline phosphatase, urinary calcium/creatinine ratio (>0.2), and urinary phosphorus/creatinine ratio (>0.6).

Treatment of Osteopenia and Osteoporosis

- Hormone replacement therapy for endocrinal abnormalities
- Calcitonin inhibitor of osteoclasts
- Hydroxyurea
- Bisphosphonates
- Moderate- and high-impact activities—walking, ballet dancing, aerobics jogging, etc.
- Diet, rich in calcium and vitamin D.

Leg Ulcers

Leg ulcers ***(Fig. 11.5.21)****:* Ulceration around the ankles is commonly seen in thalassemia intermedia, thalassemia minor, and inadequately transfused TM. This occurs due to venous stasis, vaso-occlusion, anemia, and local trauma.

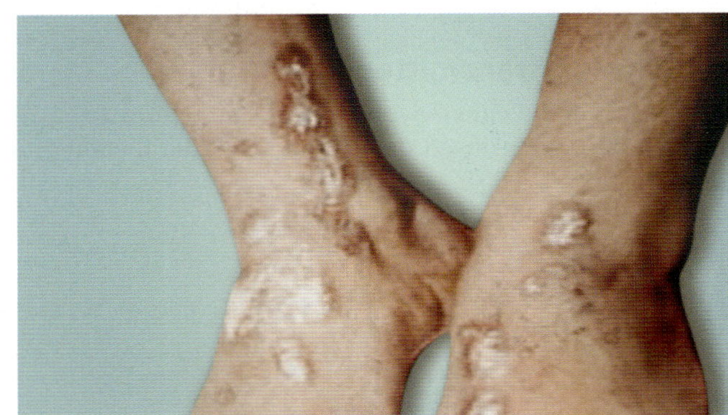

Fig. 11.5.21: Chronic leg ulcers.

Treatment includes bed rest, increased transfusions, wound care, and the use of local tissue factors. Local irrigation of the wound with granulocyte-colony stimulating factor—one vial diluted in normal saline has been found beneficial.

Gallstones

Gallstones are more commonly seen in children receiving irregular treatment as well as in thalassemia minor. In asymptomatic cases, no active treatment is required. However, they may be removed along with splenectomy (if splenectomy is indicated).

CURATIVE TREATMENT

Stem Cell Transplantation (Fig. 11.5.22)

This is only the curative therapy available today for TM. BM transplantation is effective and offers the potential permanent cure if a human leukocyte antigen-matched sibling donor is available when compared with the long-term ideal treatment. The sources for stem cells include BM, cord blood, peripheral

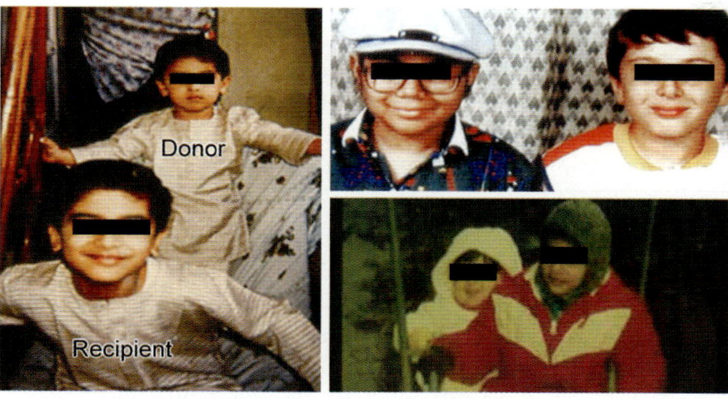

Fig. 11.5.22: Stem cell transplantation.

blood, and fetal liver. Though expensive, it is cost effective as compared to yearly cost of regular packed red cell transfusions, chelation therapy, and treatment of complications. Multiple pricks, blood transfusion hospitalization, can be averted.

The outcome of this procedure depends upon the three factors:

1. Hepatomegaly—more than 2 cm
2. Hepatic fibrosis
3. Irregular chelation.

According to these factors, patients are classified into three classes which are as follows:

1. *Class I:* None of the above factors
2. *Class II:* One or two factors
3. *Class III:* All the above.

For those with none of these factors (Class I), the success rate is about 93%, with one or two factors (Class II), it is 85% and with all three factors (Class III), it drops to a very low figure of 60 %. Umbilical cord stem cells have good results in most centers. Lower GVHD and longer engraftment have been reported. However, some have found higher early morbidity.

Bone Marrow Transplantation In Utero

Research is underway on BM transplantation (BMT) in utero, at 14 weeks of gestation. Since the immune system is not developed at that time, there would be no rejection, and mother's purified stem cells could be used, although the risk of GVHD would have to be looked into **(Fig. 11.5.23)**.

FUTURE PERSPECTIVES

Gene Therapy

Gene therapy is an exciting prospect for thalassemic children. Aim of therapy is the addition of a normal copy of the human β-gene along with key regulatory sequences into lentivirus vectors, a group of retroviruses. These are still experimental and hopefully will become available in near future. But this approach has been impeded by a difficulty of attaining high-titer vectors. Recent advances in vector construction have circumvented some of the problems limiting gene transfer efficiency and regulation of transgene expression. However, it will be some time before clinical application of this therapy becomes a reality.

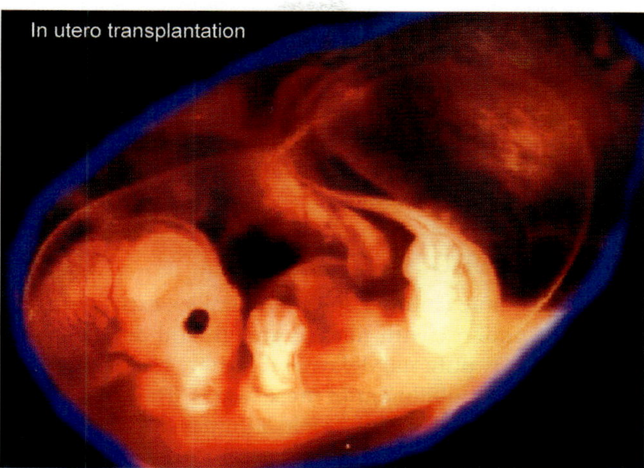

Fig. 11.5.23: Bone marrow transplantation *in utero*.

PREVENTION OF THALASSEMIA

The birth of a thalassemic child thus places considerable strain not only on affected child and family but also on society at large. Therefore, there is an emphasis for shift from treatment to prevention of birth of such children in future. Not even 5–10% of thalassemic children born in India receive optimal treatment. Cost of treatment of a 4-year-old thalassemic child is around 100,000 annually. BM transplantation as a curative treatment is out of reach for the majority of children, which costs around 10–20 lakhs.

Carrier Screening

The various strategies for career screening include the following:

- Population education
- Mass screening—screening of target population of high-risk communities
- Genetic counseling of "minor" couples and of those who test positive for thalassemia minor
- Genetic counseling
- Prenatal diagnosis of thalassemia
- Methods used for screening include measurement of RBC indices, naked eye single tube red cell osmotic fragility test, HPLC analysis of Hb, and genetic counseling.

Prenatal Diagnosis of Thalassemia

The incidence of misdiagnosis in prenatal testing is less than 1%. The reasons for failure include technical failure to amplify target DNA fragment, doubtful paternity, maternal contamination of samples, and sample exchange.

Both preimplantation diagnosis and preconception diagnosis are available especially for couples who do not wish to undergo medical termination of pregnancy. However, the procedures are technically demanding, difficult to organize, and involve enormous cost.

FUTURE PROSPECTS

Most thalassemic children and their families expect to reach the age of puberty, with normal growth and development. Growth failure, pubertal delay, and fertility represent major obstacles to the fulfillment of these hopes. They also expect same attainment as those of their healthy peers—in education, employment, and a well-adjusted social and sexual life.

Until the last few decades, thalassemia was regarded as uniformly fatal disease, and death was expected during the second decade of life before adulthood. However, progress in the understanding and management of the disease has brought brighter prospects of survival extending into the third and fourth decades of life, provided, they receive the latest treatment with good compliance. This has opened a new chapter in the management of thalassemia beyond blood transfusion and chelation therapy. The advent of advanced technology, with better management modalities and facilities, have metamorphosed TM from a fatal to a preventable, manageable as well as a curable disease.

BIBLIOGRAPHY

1. Agarwal MB. ICL 670: a new oral chelator: a major breakthrough in treatment of thalassemia. Indian J Hematol Blood Transfusion. 2003;31:26-8.
2. Anderson LJ, Wonke B, Prescott E, et al. Comparison of effects of oral deferiprone and subcutaneous desferrioxamine on myocardial iron concentrations and ventricular function in beta-thalassemia. Lancet. 2002;360(9332):516-20.
3. Colah RB, Mohanty D. Beta-thalassemia: expression, molecular mechanisms and mutations in Indians. Indian J Pediatr. 1998;65(6):815-23.
4. Giardina PJ, Grady RW. Chelation therapy in β-thalassemia: an optimistic update. Semin Hematol. 2001;38(4):360-6.
5. Lokeshwar MR, Shah N, Kanika S, et al. IAP Textbook of Pediatrics, 3rd edition. New Delhi: Jaypee Brothers Medical Publishers (P) Ltd.; 2006. pp. 622-30.
6. Manglani M, Lokeshwar MR, Vani VG, et al. 'T': an effective screening test for β-thalassemia trait. Indian Pediatr. 1997;34(8):703-8.
7. Orkin SH, Nathan DG. Thalassemia. In: Nathan DG, Orkin SH, Ginsburg D, Look AT (Eds). Nathan and Oski's Hematology of Infancy and Childhood, 6th edition. Philadelphia, PA: WB Saunders Co; 2003. pp. 842-919.
8. Vaz FE, Thakur CB, Banerjee MK, et al. Distribution of beta-thalassemia mutations in the Indian population referred to a diagnostic center. Hemoglobin. 2000;24(3):181-94.
9. Weatherall DJ, Clegg JB. The Thalassemia Syndromes, 4th edition. Oxford: Blackwell Scientific Publications; 2001.

11.6 Sickle Cell Disease

Vibhawari S Dani

INTRODUCTION

Sickle cell disease (SCD) is a term used for a group of genetic disorders characterized by production of hemoglobin S (HbS). Sickle cell hemoglobinopathy occurs due to mutation of β-globin gene situated on the short arm of chromosome 11, where thymine replaces adenine in the deoxyribonucleic acid (DNA) encoding the β-globin gene. This leads to an amino acid change in β-chain of hemoglobin (Hb) molecule, from glutamic acid to valine at the sixth position. The result is a profound change in the molecular stability and solubility of HbS. Minor variations in noncoding nucleotide sequences of gene are also seen.

These polymorphic variations are called haplotypes, responsible for variability in presentation of SCD in the different parts of the world. Four such haplotypes have been found. Arab-Indian haplotype is found in eastern Saudi Arabia and Indian subcontinent. The Benin and Bantu haplotypes are prevalent in Africa, Mediterranean countries, North and South America. Senegal haplotype is prevalent in Africa. **Figure 11.6.1** shows the prevalence of sickle cell gene as reported from India.

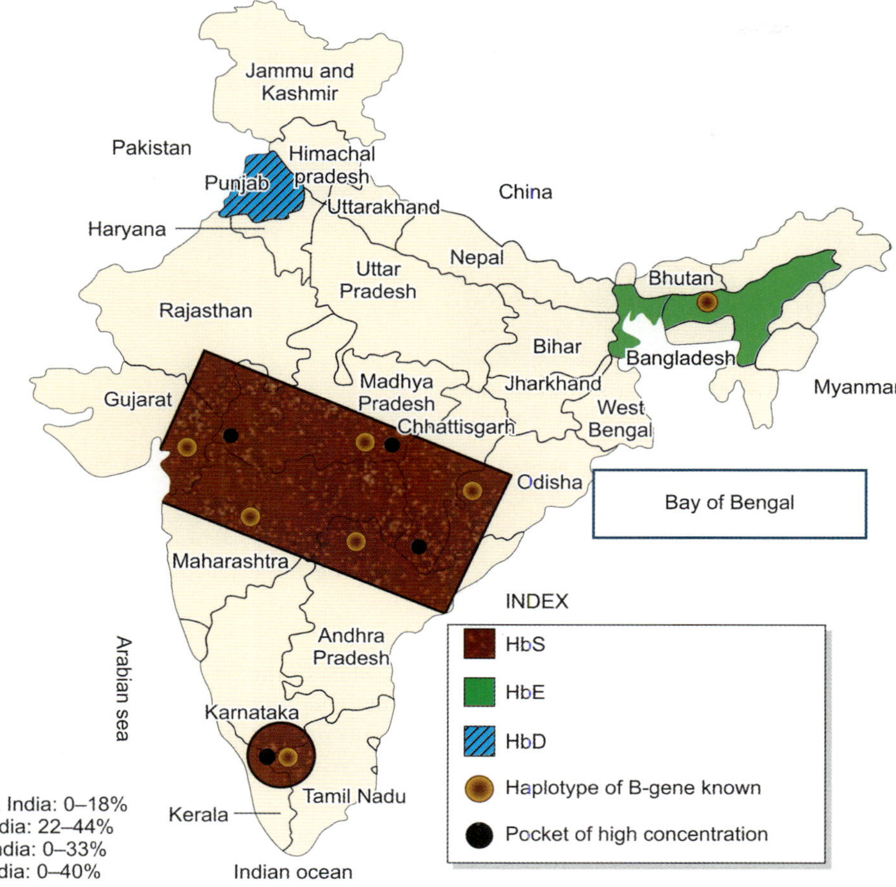

Fig. 11.6.1: Prevalence of sickle cell gene in India.
Source: Reproduced with permission from Gupta P, Menon PSN, Ramji S, Lodha R (Eds). PG Textbook of Pediatrics. New Delhi: Jaypee Brothers Medical Publishers (P) Ltd.; 2015.

SICKLE CELL GENOTYPES

Sickle cell disease includes several distinct genotypes:

- Homozygous SCD (SS)—α2β2val 6 α2β2val 6.
- Sickle cell anemia, heterozygous form (AS)—α2β2val 6 α2β2Glu 6. This is a benign condition. Red cells survival is not decreased, and there is no anemia.
- Sickle β-thalassemia (SB0)—Clinical severity depends on the output of thalassemia β-gene.

Less commonly seen forms are as follows:

- SD Punjab disease—α2β2val 6 α2β2Glu 121. It has a severe clinical presentation.
- SO Arab disease—α2β2val 6 α2β2lys 121. It has a severe clinical presentation.
- SC disease—α2β2val 6 α2β2lys 6. It has milder clinical presentation than SCD.
- *Sickle alpha-thalassemia*: Primary effect of alpha-thalassemia is to reduce the cellular content of HbS. There is microcytosis. Reduction in mean cell Hb concentration prolongs the time required for HbS polymerization. The red cells are less rigid. Life expectancy is increased in association of alpha-thalassemia with SCD. However, there is no protection from stroke, and increased incidence of avascular necrosis of femur is observed.

Hemoglobin F

Hemoglobin F (HbF) level in SCD may vary from 0.5% to 30%. HbF reduces polymerization of HbS molecule, thereby reducing severity of clinical picture. HbF is heterogeneously distributed in red blood cells. Number of red cells with HbF and amount of HbF in red cells also varies in individuals. This results in variable preferential survival of F cells over non-F cells.

Pathophysiology

- The "sol" (soluble) form of Hb changes to "gel" form, when HbS is deoxygenated. In gel form the Hb crystallizes to

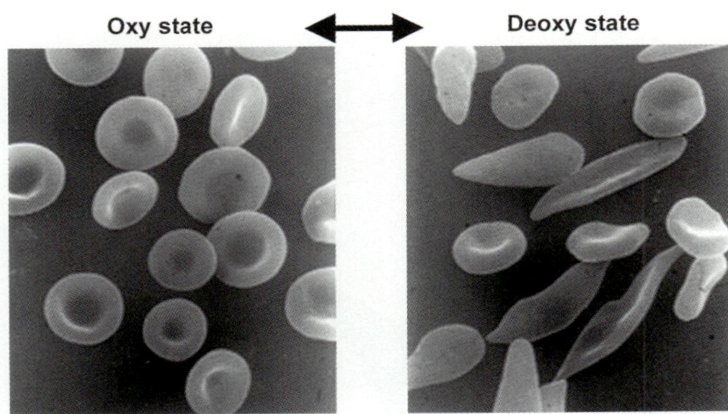

Fig. 11.6.2: Deoxygenation of "SS" erythrocytes lead to intracellular hemoglobin polymerization, loss of deformability, and changes in cell morphology.
Source: Reproduced with permission from Gupta P, Menon PSN, Ramji S, Lodha R (Eds). PG Textbook of Pediatrics. New Delhi: Jaypee Brothers Medical Publishers (P) Ltd.; 2015.

small, rigid, and boat-shaped objects known as "tactoids." These spectrin-Hb complexes polymerize forming insoluble structure, deforming the red blood cells to sickle shape. The red cell membrane becomes more fragile **(Fig. 11.6.2)**.

- The polymerization is facilitated by increased concentration of HbS, acidic pH, low oxygen saturation, stasis of blood flow, and decreased levels of HbF.
- Autooxidation of HbS generates free radicals (e.g. superoxide and peroxide) and hydroxyl radicals leading to the damage of red cell membrane.
- Upon reoxygenation the sickle cell initially resumes normal configuration, but with repeated cycles of sickling and unsickling, fixation of membrane occurs in sickle configuration, leading to irreversible sickle cell formation, and hemolysis. This hemolysis is responsible for anemia.
- In SCD the red cells have increased adherence to endothelium. CD44 and integrin present on red cell membrane adhere to endothelial protein, "vascular cell adhesion molecule-1" and "integrin." Leukocytes adhere to "intercellular adhesion molecule-1" and "E-selectin," present on endothelium. This infiltration causes narrowing of vessels.
- Platelets aggregate over the adherent red cells and damaged endothelium, causing the blockage of microvasculature and ischemia of the tissue.
- During vaso-occlusive crisis, there is activation of coagulation and fibrinolytic system.
- Nitric oxide levels are depleted in SCD leading to vasoconstriction.

CLINICAL FEATURES

Clinical manifestations of SCD are extremely varied. Some patients are entirely asymptomatic and stable, whereas others are constantly troubled by painful episodes.

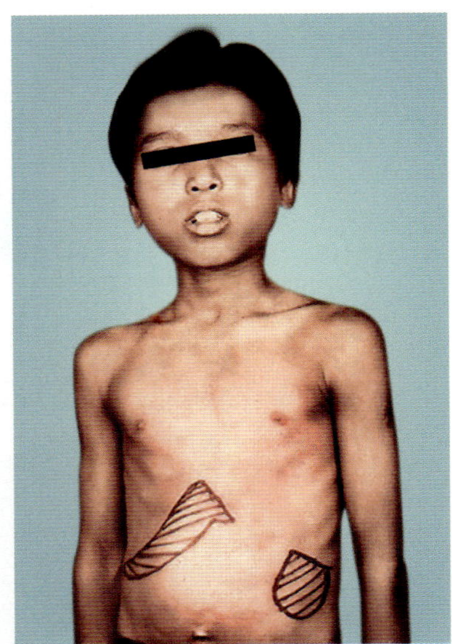

Fig. 11.6.3: Splenohepatomegaly in homozygous SS disease in a 12-year-old child.

Most of the patients fall in two extreme categories and experience intermittent clinical crisis. Splenohepatomegaly is usually present. In Indian children, persistent splenomegaly, till 12 years of age, is frequently seen **(Fig. 11.6.3)**.

Vaso-occlusive Crisis

Hand-foot Syndrome

- This occurs due to obstruction to microvascular circulation. Obstruction of capillaries of bone marrow causes ischemic necrosis and death of bone marrow and initiates inflammatory response and increasing intramedullary pressure.
- Clinically, there is swelling over the affected bones with severe pain and tenderness.
- In younger children, this process is most marked in small bones of hands and feet, causing "hand-foot syndrome" or dactylitis **(Fig. 11.6.4)**. Hand-foot syndrome disappears coincidently with physiological regression of active bone marrow from the small bones of hands and feet in children above 5 years. The pain distribution reflects the articular areas of long bones.

Avascular Necrosis

- Avascular necrosis of bone occurs secondary to vaso-occlusion of nutrient artery.
- Femoral head, humerus, and the upper third of tibia can be affected, but weight-bearing makes femoral head necrosis more likely resulting in severe disability **(Figs. 11.6.5A and B)**.

Painful Abdominal Crisis

Painful abdominal crisis occurs due to localized areas of bowel dysfunction caused by vaso-occlusion. There is severe abdominal pain and signs of peritoneal irritation. Persistence of bowel sound differentiates it from acute abdomen requiring surgical exploration. It usually resolves in 3–5 days. The management consists of bowel rest and maintenance of hydration by intravenous fluids.

Acute Chest Syndrome

It occurs due to vaso-occlusion of pulmonary vessels leading to infarction and pulmonary sequestration. Superadded infection complicates the issue. It is an important cause of mortality and morbidity in children under 3 years of age.

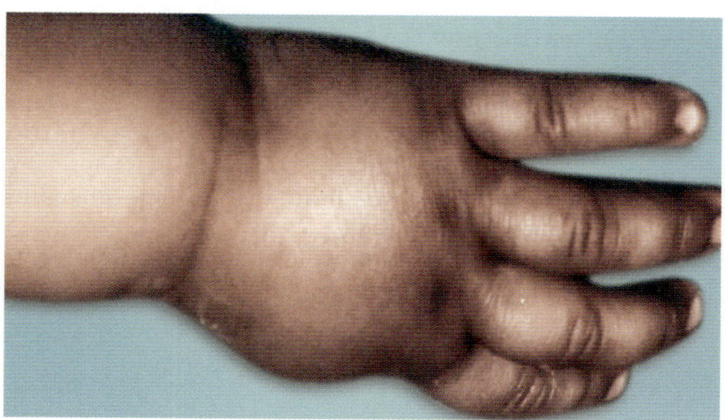

Fig. 11.6.4: Dactylitis of hand-foot syndrome.

Stroke

Stroke occurs in 6–17% patients in Benin and Bantu haplotypes. In our series, we have found it to be 2.5%. This could be due to high levels of fetal Hb in our Arab-Asian haplotype. Common age-group for stroke is 3–10 years. Around 70–90% of patients experience repeated episodes of stroke within 36 months unless they are on transfusion regimen maintaining HbS level below 30%.

Priapism

Priapism is persistent painful penile erection **(Fig. 11.6.6)**. Recurrent acute episodic attacks last from few minutes to several hours. It usually subsides spontaneously. Impotence may be a sequel. Blood transfusion is indicated if pain and engorgement persist for 24–48 hours.

Sequestration Crisis

The event is characterized by sudden trapping of large amount of blood in spleen or less commonly in liver. These patients present with profound anemia and shock. Enormously enlarged spleen fills the abdomen. Dramatic regression of splenomegaly and increase in Hb level occur with prompt correction of hypovolemia and blood transfusion.

Splenic dysfunction occurs due to obstruction of sinusoidal blood flow, causing diversion of blood through intrasplenic shunts, bypassing phagocytic reticuloendothelial element of the spleen. Children with palpable spleen at 6 months of age are at high risk of pneumococcal septicemia.

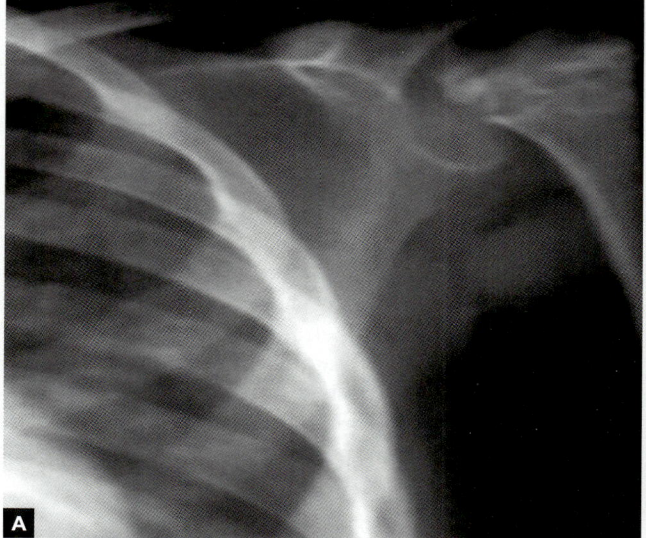

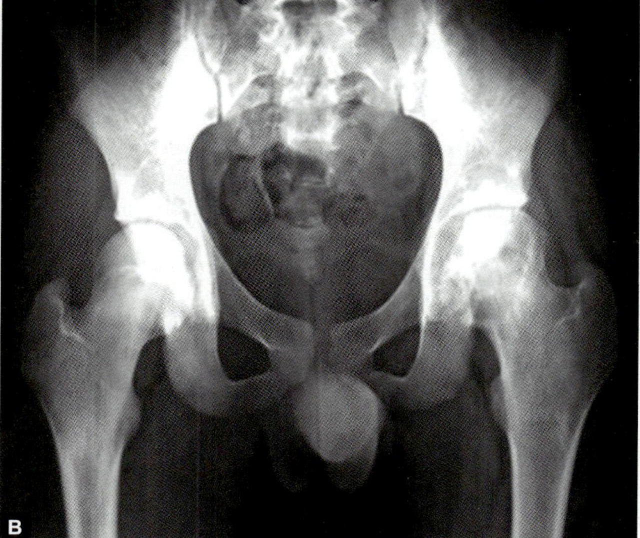

Figs. 11.6.5A and B: (A) Avascular necrosis of humerus; and (B) Avascular necrosis of head of femur.
Source: (B) Reproduced with permission from Gupta P, Menon PSN, Ramji S, Lodha R (Eds). PG Textbook of Pediatrics. New Delhi: Jaypee Brothers Medical Publishers (P) Ltd.; 2015.

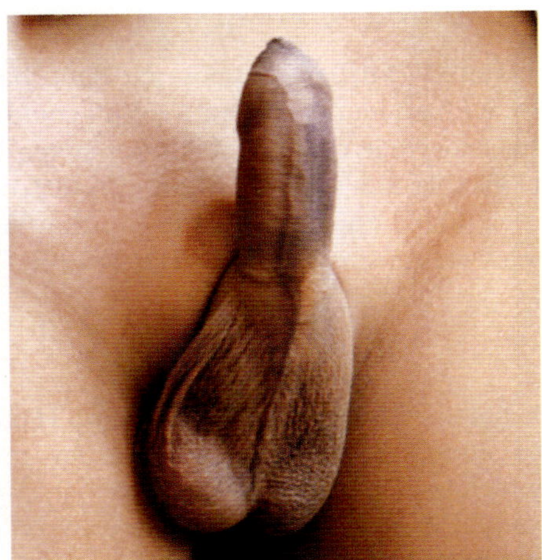

Fig. 11.6.6: Priapism.
Courtesy: MR Lokeshwar.

Aplastic Crisis

The causative organism is parvovirus B19, leading to the destruction of erythroid precursors in bone marrow. The child presents with acute anemia, without reticulocytosis. The condition is always self-limiting with the duration of 7–10 days. Blood transfusions during this period prevent mortality.

Megaloblastic Crisis

It occurs due to sudden arrest of erythropoiesis due to folate depletion. Chronic erythroid hyperplasia drains the folate reserve, and folate deficiency occurs. The Hb level can drop to 2–3 g/dL. Treatment is by oral folate supplementation.

Infections

The patients of SCD are more prone to infections. *Streptococcus pneumoniae* and *Haemophilius influenza B* are common causes of respiratory infections. Salmonella osteomyelitis may occur. Parvovirus B_{19} causes red cells aplasia and reticulocytopenia leading to aplastic crisis.

Chronic Organ Damage

Cardiovascular system: Chronic anemia and compensatory increase in cardiac output may occur. Pulmonary hypertension is the most severe cardiovascular complication.

Renal system: Sickle cell nephropathy includes papillary necrosis, nephrotic syndrome, renal infarction, hyposthenuria, and renal medullary carcinoma. The presentation could be hematuria (microscopic or gross), proteinuria, and renal insufficiency.

Hepatobiliary system: Cholelithiasis and hepatic infarction may occur. Only symptomatic gallstones should be subjected to surgery.

Eyes: Proliferative and nonproliferative retinopathy can lead to vitreous hemorrhage and retinal detachment.

Growth: Somatic and sexual growth is delayed in SCD. Age of menarche is delayed by 2.5 years. Zinc deficiency has been suggested as a cause for poor growth. It has been observed that zinc supplementation augments sexual growth but does not affect somatic growth.

Enuresis: It is common in SCD. It is probably secondary to hyposthenuria, associated with small bladder capacity up to 8–10 years of age. Eventually, it always resolves.

DIAGNOSIS AND SCREENING

- Community screening for SCD can be done by sodium metabisulfite slide test and solubility test. These are screening tests and cannot differentiate between sickle cell trait and disease. These tests should not to be used in the first year of life as high level of HbF is present.
- The diagnosis can be confirmed by Hb electrophoresis, isoelectric focusing, high-performance liquid chromatography, and globin DNA analysis. Diagnostic test for SCD should not be done within 3 months after receiving blood transfusion.
- Diagnosis of a neonatal screening of high-risk population should be done for SCD. Prenatal diagnosis can be done at 8–10 weeks of gestation, with chorionic villus biopsy, or amniocentesis.

MANAGEMENT

Treatment of Painful Crisis

- For mild pain—codeine, aspirin, ibuprofen, acetaminophen, and naproxen can be used.
- For severe pain—meperidine, ketorolac, tolmetin, and oxycodone may be useful.
- Vasodilators, such as pentoxifylline, nifedipine, and buflomedil, increase microvascular circulation.
- Blood transfusion leads to increase in oxygen saturation, thereby reversing sickling process and relieving obstruction to microvascular bed.
  - *Indications*: Sequestration crisis, aplastic crisis, stroke, and hypoxia with acute chest syndrome.
  - A standard simple transfusion is necessary in sequestration crisis and aplastic crisis, while in all other situation, exchange transfusion is preferable.

Chronic transfusion program is used in children with recurrent stroke, to reduce number of HbS-containing cells.

Management of Infections

All newborns with SCD should be given oral penicillin 125 mg, twice a day, up to the age of 3 years, followed by oral penicillin 250 mg, twice a day, up to the age of 5 years.

Episode of fever in SCD should be evaluated for bacterial infections and treated promptly. Third-generation cephalosporins may be given.

Hydroxyurea

It leads to increase in HbF. It also decreases hemolysis by improving hydration of red cells, hampering sickling mechanism, which ameliorates the severity of SCD.

Indications

- Child more than 5 years of age having more than three painful episodes in a year
- Single episode of acute chest syndrome
- Stroke
- Avascular necrosis of bone

Dose

Starting dose is 15–20 mg/kg with an incremental dose every 8 weeks of 2.5–5 mg/kg if no toxicity occurs, up to a maximum of 35 mg/kg. Strict monitoring for hematological toxicity by complete blood counts, reticulocyte count should be done in every 2 weeks. In Indian setup, it is found that fixed low dose of 10–15 mg/kg, without escalating, is as effective as the recommended schedule.

Zinc

Supplementation of 10–15 mg of elemental zinc seems to be beneficial. It prolongs red cell life span. Zinc has membrane-modifying effect, thus it reduces irreversibly sickled cells. It decreases the adherence of red cells to endothelium, thereby reducing vascular obstruction. Zinc also causes maturation of gonads and may be of help in delayed sexual growth.

Bone Marrow Transplant

Autologous bone marrow transplant has been found successful in very severe SCD. It needs expertise and is very expensive.

PREVENTION

- Exposure to hypoxia, dehydration, extreme cold, extreme heat, change in altitude, and infections are precipitating factors for crisis. They should be avoided.
- Dehydration and loss of electrolytes may lead to red cell dehydration precipitating sickling process. Fluid requirement is usually increased by 50% of the usual requirement.
- Parent's education for recognizing specific complication at the earliest should be done.
- *Immunization*: Pneumococcal vaccine at the age of 6 weeks, 10 weeks, and 14 weeks; booster at 18 months. Influenzae (*Haemophilus influenzae* type b) vaccine at 6 weeks, 10weeks, and 14 weeks; booster at 18 months. Hepatitis B vaccine at birth, 6 weeks, 6 months, and booster every 5 years.
- Hemoglobin levels should be maintained at 10–12 g/dL.
- Folate supplementation should be given, as there is rapid turnover of bone marrow.
- Behavior change communication for genetic counseling of high-risk communities should be done to avoid marriages between homozygous or heterozygous persons, to reduce prevalence.

RECENT ADVANCES

- Drugs, such as 5-azacytidine, hydroxyurea, and sodium butyrate, lead to increase in HbF, which ameliorate the severity of SCD.
- Benzyl esters increase the solubility of Hb and prevent polymer formation. These drugs are still under experimental trial.
- *Gene therapy*: It is still in experimental stage. Random insertion of normal β-gene, or correction of the defective gene by genetic engineering in hematopoietic cell, is still on horizon.

PRACTICE POINTS/TIPS

- Once diagnosed, a child should be under regular follow-up.
- Maintain Hb level above 10 g/dL.
- In our country's hot climate, child should be given plenty fluids to avoid dehydration.
- Splenectomy may be considered in the case of repeated attacks of sequestration crisis.

KEY MESSAGES

- In Indian patients, spleen remains enlarged in pediatric age-group.
- Quality of life can be much better if Hb level is maintained above 10 g/dL.

BIBLIOGRAPHY

1. Atweh GF, Sutton M, Nassif I, et al. Sustained induction of fetal hemoglobin by pulse butyrate therapy in sickle cell disease. Blood. 1999;93(6):1790-7.
2. Brawley OW, Cornelius LJ, Edwards LR, et al. National Institutes of Health Consensus Development Conference statement: hydroxyurea treatment for sickle cell disease. Ann Intern Med. 2008;148(12):932-8.
3. Italia K, Jain D, Gattani S, et al. Hydroxyurea in sickle cell disease—a study of clinicopharmacological efficacy in the Indian haplotype. Blood Cells Mol Dis. 2009;42(1):25-31.
4. Mashon RS, Dash PM, Khalkho J, et al. Higher fetal hemoglobin concentration in patients with sickle cell disease in eastern India reduces frequency of painful crisis. Eur J Haematol. 2009;83(4):383-4.
5. Saunthararajah Y, Vichinsky EP, Embury SH. Sickle cell disease. Clinical features and management. In: Hoffman R, Benz EJ, Shattil SS (Eds). Hematology: Basic Principles and Practice, 5th edition. Philadelphia, PA: Churchill Livingston; 2008. Chapter 43.

11.7 Red Cell Membrane Disorders

Rashmi Dalvi

INTRODUCTION

The erythrocyte membrane structure comprises an outer lipid bilayer of phospholipids and glycolipids, with integral proteins which penetrate or span this bilayer. These include glycoproteins and glycophorins for MNS blood group and others interacting with the inner cytoskeleton. Important among these are the band three proteins, which are vital for anion transport in cellular respiration and contain ABO blood group antigens on their outer surface. Inner to the lipid bilayer is a separate network of proteins forming a membrane cytoskeleton, viz. spectrin, ankyrin, actin, protein 4.1, protein 4.2, actin, and many others. A normal intact membrane structure is critical to red cell deformability, stability, and membrane permeability. A hereditary or acquired defect in any of these structural components destabilizes the cytoskeleton, alters red cell morphology, and shortens the red cell lifespan resulting in variable degrees of anemia.

HEREDITARY SPHEROCYTOSIS

This is the most common of red cell membranopathies, characterized by the following:

- Hemolysis, intermittent jaundice, splenomegaly with the spherocytes in the peripheral smear being its morphologic hallmark.
- It is inherited as an autosomal dominant trait in most patients, although de novo sporadic mutations are also seen and rarely may be recessively inherited.
- Hereditary spherocytosis (HS) results from a deficiency or defect in spectrin or its anchoring proteins, ankyrin, band 3 protein, or protein 4.2. Molecular defects causing these deficiencies are now known **(Fig. 11.7.1)**.
- However, most mutations though common within a family almost always vary between families.
- Deficient cytoskeleton results in the loss of membrane lipids and converts red cells into rigid, osmotically fragile spherocytes which get sequestered in the spleen. In the process, they undergo various metabolic changes, nutrient loss and lose other membrane components. These deformed red blood cells (RBCs) are susceptible to destruction by splenic macrophages.

CLINICAL FEATURES

There is marked heterogeneity of clinical presentation from the asymptomatic to a transfusion-dependent hemolytic anemia:

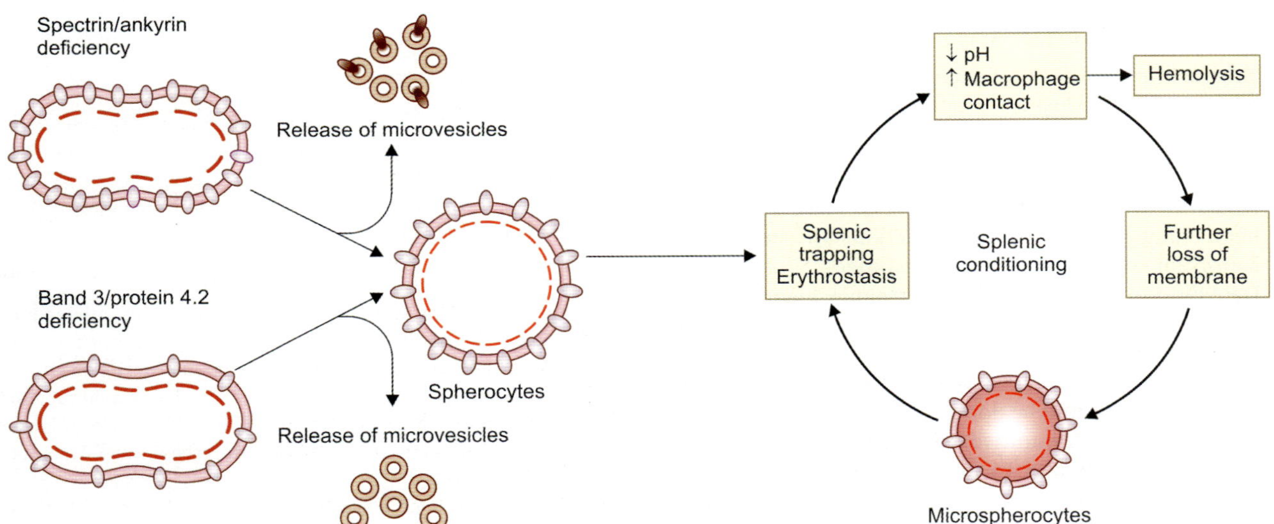

Fig. 11.7.1: Molecular defects and pathogenesis in hereditary spherocytosis.

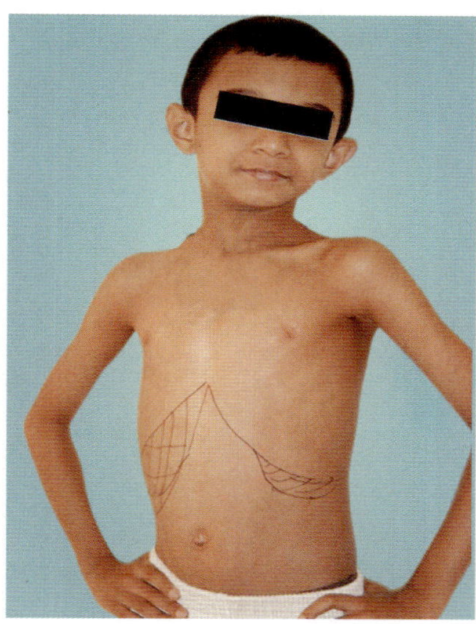

Fig. 11.7.2: Anemia with hepatosplenomegaly, jaundice (indirect type), and hereditary spherocytosis.

- Most patients present during infancy or childhood with anemia, although presentation in the fourth or fifth decade is also known.
- Typically, there is a history of mild jaundice, mild or absent anemia, or intermittent anemia and jaundice.
- However, mild-to-moderate splenomegaly is always present **(Fig. 11.7.2)**.
- More severe forms may present in the newborn period with anemia and severe hyperbilirubinemia necessitating exchange transfusion.
- As in other hemolytic anemias, they are prone to aplastic crisis following parvovirus infection, or megaloblastic crisis due to folate deficiency.
- Some patients may develop or rarely even present with symptomatic gallstones.
- Rarely leg ulcers and growth retardation can also complicate the course.

LABORATORY FEATURES

- The hemoglobin (Hb) is usually mildly decreased or normal, with normal mean corpuscular volume (MCV) and typically high mean corpuscular Hb (MCH) content.
- Most patients however exhibit marked reticulocytosis indicating compensatory erythroid hyperplasia.
- Red cell morphology is distinctive with 15–20% being hyperchromatic spherocytes lacking central pallor **(Fig. 11.7.3)**. There is variable polychromatophilia and even spherocytosis in peripheral smear. Poikilocytosis in severe HS is due to combined spectrin-ankyrin deficiency or in recessive variants.

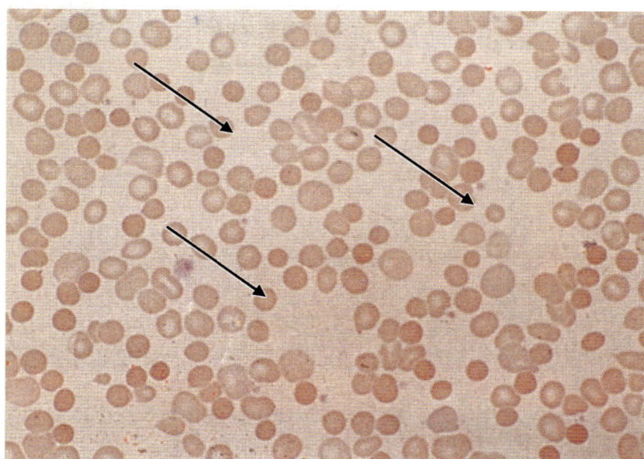

Fig. 11.7.3: Peripheral smear showing microspherocytes.

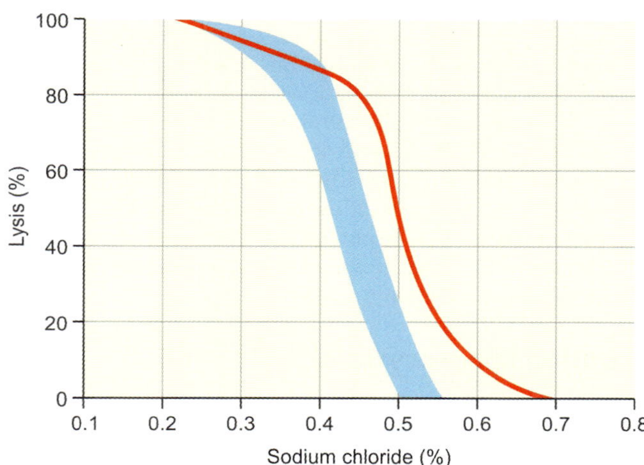

Fig. 11.7.4: Osmotic fragility curve.

The most common diagnostic screening test used is osmotic fragility test. Red cells in HS show increased osmotic fragility when incubated with hypotonic NaCl solutions in vitro, yielding a diagnostic osmotic fragility curve **(Fig. 11.7.4)**.

- In most cases, a definitive diagnosis of HS can be made based on family history, red cell indices and morphology, and a positive screening test.
- However, quantitation of membrane proteins, especially spectrin content, is possible by flow cytometric or gel electrophoretic analysis, and characterization of molecular lesions is done in the research setting.
- Patients can be classified into clinical severity phenotypes based on Hb, reticulocyte count, serum bilirubin, and spectrin content **(Box 11.7.1)**.

Box 11.7.1: Differential diagnosis of spherocytes.

Spherocytes are also seen in other states, such as:
- ABO incompatibility
- Immune-mediated hemolytic anemia
- Burns
- *Clostridium perfringens* sepsis

Clinically HS should be differentiated from other inherited disorders presenting with episodic anemia, jaundice, and splenomegaly, such as other red cell membranopathies, enzymopathies, unstable Hb, and autoimmune hemolytic anemia.

MANAGEMENT

Basic supportive care is advised to all patients in the form of:
- Lifelong folate supplementation.
- Prevention of iron deficiency.
- Prompt treatment of infections.
- Blood transfusion may be required on a regular basis in severe phenotypes, in individuals in a steady state during the episodes of acute hemolysis, or during aplastic crisis.
- Regular follow-up is recommended to monitor growth, spleen size, Hb trend, and occurrence of gallstones.
- Splenectomy prolongs RBC survival to almost 80% of normal and prevents other complications, however, is recommended only in clinically severe phenotype.
- Because of the higher risk of postsplenectomy sepsis, it should be postponed to at least 5 years of age.

Acquired Spherocytosis

Certain acquired conditions may also cause reduction in membrane surface area with resultant spherocyte formation, such as
- Immune adherence and thermal injury
- Mechanical injury (microangiopathic anemia)
- Clostridial sepsis
- Certain snake, bee, and spider venoms

HEREDITARY ELLIPTOCYTOSIS SYNDROMES

- Hereditary elliptocytosis (HE) designates a group of inherited disorders that have in common the presence of elliptical RBCs.
- Characterized by defects in spectrin binding with other membrane proteins.
- In most patients, it is inherited as an autosomal dominant trait with a striking molecular heterogeneity, having a variable clinical spectrum ranging from the asymptomatic trait to a life-threatening hemolysis.

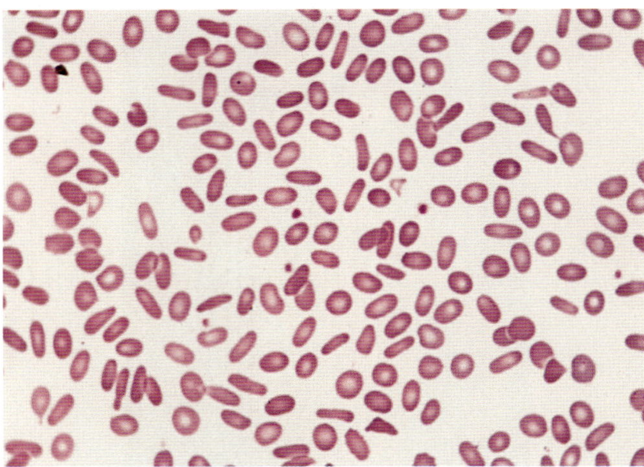

Fig. 11.7.5: Ovalocytes in peripheral smear.

- Members of the same family may exhibit different clinical courses, and an individual's frequency and severity may change with time.
- Although mutations of alpha-spectrin are responsible for most cases of dominantly inherited common HE, it is also seen due to deficiencies in protein 4.1 or glycophorin C or with defects in band 3 protein/beta-spectrin impairing ankyrin binding.
- These defects in the cytoskeleton make the red cells less tolerant to shear stress during circulation. Red blood cell precursors here are round initially but become more elliptical as they age.
- In children and adults, common HE is usually asymptomatic often discovered accidentally on a peripheral smear showing 15–20% elliptocytes.
- Others many have a mild hemolytic anemia and splenomegaly, sometimes with gallstones.
- Common HE is asymptomatic in the neonatal period with elliptocytes appearing only by 4–6 months of age.

HEREDITARY PYROPOIKILOCYTOSIS

Hereditary pyropoikilocytosis (HPP) is a recessively inherited form of hemolytic anemia biochemically related to common HE, having a severe clinical phenotype. They typically present in the newborn period with severe anemia and neonatal jaundice, with red cell fragmentation, poikilocytosis, elliptocytosis, and microspherocytosis.

South East Asian ovalocytosis is another variant of HE seen in malaria-endemic regions of South East Asia and is characterized by red cells with a broad oval shape and the presence of stomatocytes. It is clinically a benign disorder **(Fig. 11.7.5)**.

Laboratory Diagnosis

Hemoglobin may be normal or decreased, and the reticulocyte count will reflect the severity of hemolysis. Other evidence of hemolysis may be present, such as reduced serum haptoglobin, elevated serum lactate dehydrogenase, serum bilirubin, and urinary urobilinogen levels.

Osmotic fragility testing is not required although it is increased in severe HE/HPP. Red cells in HPP also show increased thermal instability as red cells undergo lysis at lower temperatures.

Management

- Treatment is rarely indicated for mild HE or its variants.
- Daily folate supplementation is recommended in patients with significant hemolysis.
- Acute hemolysis during viral infections or other febrile illnesses may need attention.
- Vigilance for gallstones is required.
- Splenectomy may be indicated in severe HE/HPP wherein it results in increase in Hb, decrease in reticulocyte counts, and improved symptoms.

RED CELL PERMEABILITY DISORDERS

Hereditary Stomatocytosis

It is a rare heterogeneous group of autosomal dominant hemolytic anemia characterized by marked increase in RBC membrane permeability to sodium and an increase in red cell water content.

This results in cup-shaped red cells that have a mouth, such as slit in place of the normal central pallor on stained blood films.

Most patients have a very mild hemolytic anemia and jaundice with variable reticulocyte increase, high MCV, 10–50% red cells as stomatocytes, and an increased osmotic fragility.

Splenectomy is contraindicated as these stomatocytic red cells are abnormally adherent, thereby increasing the risk of thrombosis in conjunction with postsplenectomy thrombocytosis.

Hereditary Xerocytosis

It is a rare autosomal dominantly inherited hemolytic anemia characterized by increased red cell permeability to potassium ions and thereby leakage of potassium and water out of the cell. This results in cellular dehydration and is also known as dehydrated stomatocytosis. Laboratory features are characterized by elevated MCH content and mildly elevated MCV.

DISORDERS OF RED CELL MEMBRANE LIPID BILAYER

Red blood cell membrane lipid disorders are characterized by the presence of acanthocytes, echinocytes, and target cells.

Acanthocytic Disorders

Acquired acanthocytes are seen in hypothyroidism, anorexia nervosa, postsplenectomy, severe hepatocellular disease, vitamin E deficiency (especially in neonates/ preterms), and inherited neurological disorders, such as abetalipoproteinemia and McLeod syndrome.

Echinocytes are seen in hemolytic anemia associated with hypophosphatemia, pyruvate kinase deficiency, uremia, and long-distance runners.

Target cells are formed due to increased ratio of cell surface compared to volume and are seen in thalassemia, HbC disease, familial lecithin-cholesterol acyltransferase deficiency, and obstructive liver disease.

BIBLIOGRAPHY

1. Abdullah F, Zhang Y, Camp M, et al. Splenectomy in hereditary spherocytosis: review of 1,657 patients and application of the pediatric quality indicators. Pediatr Blood Cancer. 2009;52(7):834-7.
2. Golan DE. Hemolytic anemias: red cell membrane and metabolic disorders. In: Goldman L, Ausiello D (Eds). Cecil Medicine, 23rd edition. Philadelphia, PA: Saunders Elsevier; 2007.
3. Hassoun H, Palek J. Hereditary spherocytosis: a review of the clinical and molecular aspects of the disease. Blood Rev. 1996;10(3):129-47.
4. Maciag M, Płochocka D, Adamowicz-Salach A, et al. Novel beta-spectrin mutations in hereditary spherocytosis associated with decreased levels of mRNA. Br J Haematol. 2009;146(3):326-32.
5. Perrotta S, Della Ragione F, Rossi F, et al. A truncated beta-chain responsible for dominant hereditary spherocytosis. Haematologica. 2009;94(12):1753-7.
6. Perrotta S, Gallagher PG, Mohandas N. Hereditary spherocytosis. Lancet. 2008;372(9647):1411-26.

11.8 Red Cell Enzymopathies

Jagdish Chandra

INTRODUCTION

Defects in various enzymes associated with the red blood cell (RBC) glycolytic pathway, hexose monophosphate shunt, or pentose phosphate pathway (PPP), leading to the development of hemolytic anemias of varying severity, are defined as red cell enzymopathies or erythroid enzymopathies (EEPs). These anemias are mostly congenital nonspherocytic hemolytic anemias. The enzymopathies are linked to the prevention of oxidative damage or the generation of energy in the RBCs.

INHERITANCE

Glucose-6-phosphate dehydrogenase (G6PD) deficiency and phosphoglycerate kinase deficiency is chromosome X-linked recessive, and the other EEPs are usually inherited in an autosomal recessive manner.

PENTOSE PHOSPHATE PATHWAY (HEXOSE MONOPHOSPHATE SHUNT)

Glucose-6-phosphate dehydrogenase is the first enzyme involved in the PPP and controls the flux through this pathway. **Figure 11.8.1** depicts the PPP, and **Figure 11.8.2** shows the glutathione cycle and synthetic pathways along with the various enzymes involved in different reactions.

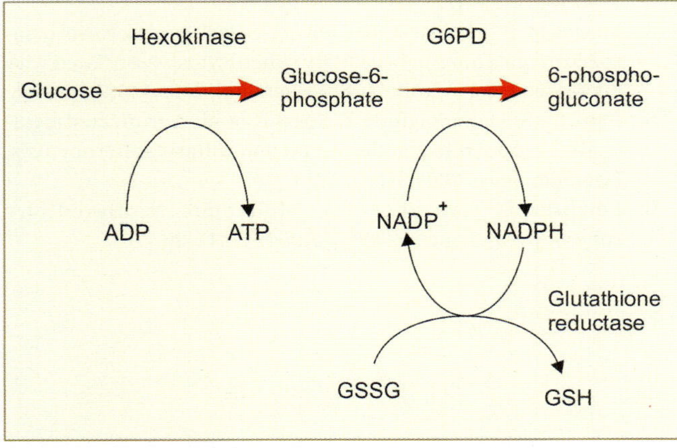

Fig. 11.8.1: Pentose phosphate pathway.

GLUCOSE-6-PHOSPHATE DEHYDROGENASE DEFICIENCY

Glucose-6-phosphate dehydrogenase deficiency is the most common genetically determined enzymopathy in the world, with approximately 440 million people being affected. At least 127 enzyme variants and numerous other polymorphisms that do not affect enzyme activity have been described. The gene for G6PD is located on the X-chromosome at Xq28 and comprises 13 exons and 12 introns. It helps in the conversion of glucose-6-phosphate to 6-phosphogluconate through the reduction of nicotinamide adenine dinucleotide phosphate ($NADP^+$) to nicotinamide adenine dinucleotide phosphate-oxidase (NADPH).

The 6-phosphogluconate is also a substrate for the glycolytic pathway. Under normal conditions, only 10% glucose is metabolized by the PPP, and its activity is governed by the availability of nicotinamide adenine dinucleotide (NAD^+) and its feedback inhibition by adenosine triphosphate (ATP).

Nicotinamide adenine dinucleotide phosphate availability is dependent on the activity of the glutathione pathway, which is linked to the PPP through the enzyme glutathione reductase. The availability of $NADP^+$ is the major rate-limiting step for PPP. Nicotinamide adenine dinucleotide phosphate-oxidase is required to keep glutathione in reduced form, which prevents red cells from oxidative damage. The clinical consequences of G6PD deficiency are virtually limited to the RBCs, with occasional malfunction of the leukocytes, in some variants, as RBCs cannot generate NADPH in any other way. Majority of the mutations affect the stability of the transcribed enzyme so that the activity declines rapidly in the mature enucleate RBCs.

Being an X-linked disorder, males are commonly affected, and females are heterozygous carriers **(Fig. 11.8.2)**. These heterozygous females are often susceptible to oxidative stress because of the effects of X-inactivation and marked lyonization in leaving a significant population of deficient red cells.

Epidemiology

Glucose-6-phosphate dehydrogenase deficiency is widely disseminated throughout Africa, the Mediterranean basin,

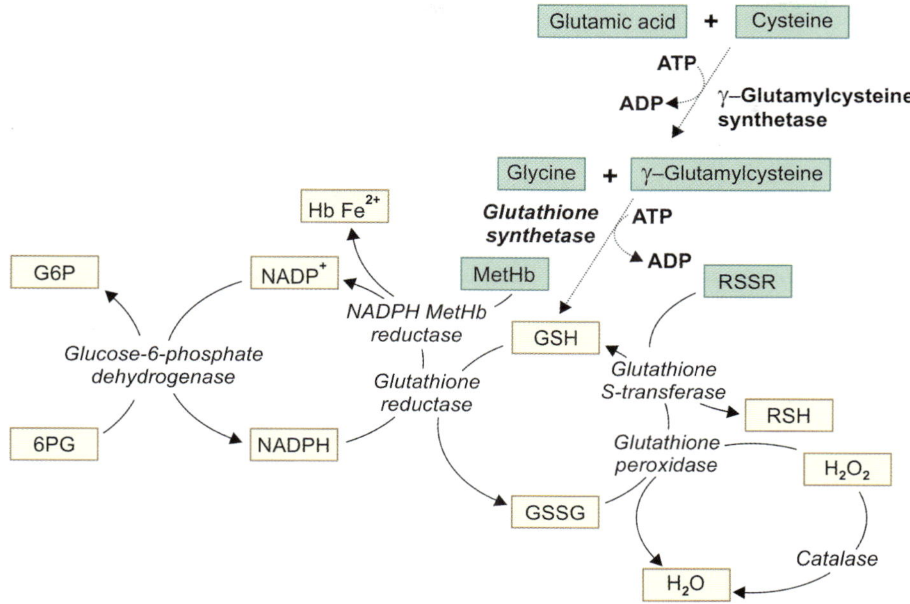

Fig. 11.8.2: The glutathione cycle and synthetic pathways.

the Middle East, South East Asia, and among the indigenous populations of the Indian subcontinent. In South East Asia the prevalence varies widely in different ethnic groups—10–20% in certain Cambodian groups to 1–3% in Vietnamese population groups. Glucose-6-phosphate dehydrogenase deficiency was reported about 40 years ago from India, and varying prevalence rates of 0–27% have been reported from diverse ethnic, caste, linguistic, and tribal groups. The most common variants are:

- Mediterranean variant among the caste groups
- Odisha variant among the Indian tribal
- Kerala-Kalyan is the third most common variant seen in India.

A higher incidence of G6PD deficiency has been observed in north and west India (15% in Parsees to 27% in Angami Nagas), as compared to the south (1–2%), except in the tribal belt of Tamil Nadu and Andhra Pradesh (5–13%).

Glucose-6-phosphate Dehydrogenase and Malaria

It has been hypothesized that the distribution of G6PD deficiency equates with areas where *Plasmodium falciparum* malaria is common, and this is thought to be the evolutionary drive that produced such widespread polymorphisms. It has subsequently been confirmed that G6PD deficiency does indeed protect against lethal falciparum malaria, particularly in childhood. This hypothesis has been called G6PD/malaria or "malaria hypothesis." Malarial parasite grows less well in red cells deficient in G6PD. Decreased parasitemia has been documented in these individuals in various studies.

Variants of Glucose-6-phosphate Dehydrogenase

Based upon biochemical and other characterization, 442 different variants of G6PD have been identified. Of them, 299 have been characterized with the methods recommended by World Health Organization (WHO). About 100 biochemical variants are thought to be polymorphic in human populations. A total of 13 biochemically characterized variants have been reported from India. These variants are grouped to five classes by WHO scientific working group depending upon the residual enzymatic activity and clinical presentation, as given in **Table 11.8.1**.

- *Polymorphic variants*: These variants have achieved a high frequency in some populations and represent

Table 11.8.1: Variants of glucose-6-phosphate dehydrogenase seen in India.

Class	*Enzyme activity*		*Clinical presentation*
I	Severe deficiency	(<20%)	Congenital nonspherocytic hemolytic anemia, acute exacerbations
II	Severe deficiency	(<10%)	Favism, AIVHA (drug-induced), neonatal jaundice
III	Moderate-to-mild deficiency	(10–60%)	AIVHA (drug-induced) neonatal jaundice
IV	Mild or none	(60–100%)	None
V	Increased activity	(>2 Xn)	None

(AIVHA: avian influenza virus hemagglutinin)

balanced polymorphisms, e.g. G6PD Mediterranean, G6PD African, and oriental variants.

- *Sporadic variants*: These are characterized by chronic nonspherocytic hemolytic anemia (CNSHA) and get exacerbated by oxidant stress. These are not limited to a particular population alone. A total of 13 such variants have been reported from the Indian subcontinent, though all of these have not been characterized at the molecular level.
- *Glucose-6-phosphate dehydrogenase mutations in India*: Mutations in the Indian subcontinent in the G6PD are seen in exon 6 and 7, which is near G6PD-binding site.

Glucose-6-phosphate dehydrogenase Mediterranean (563 C-T) is the most common polymorphism in India, and it is a severely deficient variant associated with drug-induced hemolytic anemia, favism, and neonatal jaundice (NNJ); G6PD Kerala-Kalyan (949 G-A) and G6PD Odisha (131 C-G) are the other common variants in India. Glucose-6-phosphate dehydrogenase Chatham (1003 G-A) with undetectable enzyme activity and G6PD Insuli (989 G-A) with normal enzyme activity are very rare in Indian population.

CLINICAL PRESENTATION

There are four main syndromes associated with G6PD deficiency. In G6PD-deficient individuals, hemolysis is aggravated by exposure to oxidative stress through infection or ingestion of oxidative foods or drugs.

The four syndromes are:

1. Neonatal jaundice
2. Favism
3. Chronic nonspherocytic hemolytic anemia
4. Drug-induced hemolytic anemia.

The NNJ syndrome has been described in class I, II, and III variants; favism in mainly, although not exclusively, class II; CNSHA in class I; and the drug-induced hemolysis in mainly class III.

Neonatal Jaundice and Glucose-6-phosphate Dehydrogenase Deficiency in Infancy

Neonatal jaundice is a severe manifestation of G6PD deficiency, and resultant kernicterus is the main cause of morbidity and mortality. Most common variants have been associated with NNJ, including the A- and Mediterranean variants. The jaundice probably starts in utero in the perinatal period, but the clinical problem becomes apparent only about the second day or third day after birth. Between 10% and 50% of the deficient infants are affected. Phototherapy or exchange transfusion (ET) may be required to prevent neurological sequelae. Anemia is usually absent, and it is thought that this is a manifestation of liver enzyme deficiency, along with the physiological underdevelopment of neonatal liver function or the coinheritance of uridine diphosphate glucuronyl transferase 1 deficiency of Gilbert's syndrome though the Gilbert association has not been consistently observed to increase the severity. Acute hemolytic crises may occur in G6PD-deficient infants, usually through exposure to oxidative stress, including nitrites or nitrates in water or the ingestion of fava beans by the mother, which may result in severe intrauterine hemolysis and hydrops fetalis. In some cases, idiopathic severe and sometimes fatal hemolysis has been reported. In an Indian series, in 12 out of 100 neonates with jaundice, G6PD deficiency was the cause, of them 10 being G6PD Mediterranean type.

Acute Intravascular Hemolysis

Glucose-6-phosphate dehydrogenase was first described during investigation for "primaquine sensitivity." Since then many drugs have been incriminated to result in intravascular hemolysis in individuals with G6PD deficiency. Children with certain variants of G6PD deficiency are clinically in a steady state till they develop anemia of sudden onset under the effect of some oxidative stress. Within 24–48 hours of exposure to such stress, the child suddenly becomes pale and has cola-colored or dark colored urine. Depending upon the severity of hemolysis and the resultant anemia, the child may present with incipient or frank congestive cardiac failure. Depending upon the degree of extravascular hemolysis, splenic enlargement may be noticed. Hemolysis occurs after the exposure to stressor but does not continue with continued exposure. This is thought to be because of older RBCs being damaged first as they have most severe deficiency of enzyme. Once the population of deficient RBC is hemolyzed, the juvenile RBC and reticulocytes withstand the stress as they have typically higher levels of enzyme activity. Hemoglobinemia and hemoglobinuria may result in azotemia and/or acute renal failure.

Laboratory findings during intravascular hemolysis include moderate-to-severe anemia which is usually normocytic-normochromic. Red blood cell morphology shows anisocytosis due to increased number of juvenile red cells and contracted cells. Poikilocytosis with the presence of "bite cells" may be seen. Intense reticulocytosis is present. Plasma hemoglobin (Hb) level is increased and so is unconjugated bilirubin level. Haptoglobin and other Hb-binding proteins are decreased.

Box 11.8.1 lists the drugs that need to be avoided in G6PD-deficient individuals and the risk of hemolysis associated with these drugs. In an Indian series, bacterial sepsis, malaria, and hepatitis were identifiable triggers other than drugs. Alpha hydroxy acids following ingestion of soft drink containing ascorbate have also been reported from India.

Box 11.8.1: Drugs to be avoided in patients with glucose-6-phosphate dehydrogenase deficiency.

- Acetanilide
- Acetylphenylhydrazine (2-phenyl-acetohydrazide)
- Aldesulfone sodium (sulfoxone)
- Aminophenazone (aminopyrine)
- Antazoline (antistine)
- Arsine
- Ascorbic acid
- Beta-naphthol (2-naphthol)
- Chloramphenicol
- Chloroquine
- Ciprofloxacin
- Colchicine
- Dapsone (diaminodiphenyl sulfone)
- Dimercaprol
- Diphenhydramine
- Dopamine (L-dopa)
- Doxorubicin
- Furazolidone
- Glibenclamide
- Glucosulfone sodium
- Isobutyl nitrite
- Isoniazid
- Menadiol sodium sulfate
- Menadione (menaphtone)
- Menadione sodium bisulfite (vitamin K_3 sodium bisulfite)
- Mepacrine (quinacrine)
- Mesalazine 5-aminosalicylic acid (paraminosalicylic acid)
- Methylthioninium chloride (methylene blue)
- Nalidixic acid
- Naphthalene, pure (naphthalene)
- Niridazole
- Nitrofural (nitrofurazone)
- Nitrofurantoin
- Norfloxacin
- *O*-acetylsalicylic acid (acetylsalicylic acid)
- Oxidase, urate (urate oxidase)
- Phenazopyridine
- Phenylbutazone
- Phenytoin
- Pamaquine
- *Para*-aminobenzoic acid (4-aminobenzoic acid)
- Paracetamol (acetaminophen)
- Pentaquine
- Phenacetin (acetophenetidin)
- Phenylhydrazine
- Phytomenadione (vitamin K_1)
- Primaquine
- Probenecid
- Procainamide
- Proguanil (chlorguanidine)
- Pyrimethamine
- Quinidine
- Quinine
- Stibophen
- Streptomycin
- Sulfacetamide
- Sulfacytine
- Sulfadiazine

Contd...

Contd...

- Sulfadimidine
- Sulfafurazole (sulfafurazole, sulfisoxazole)
- Sulfaguanidine
- Sulfamerazine
- Sulfamethoxazole
- Sulfamethoxypyridazine
- Sulfanilamide (sulfanilamide)
- Sulfapyridine
- Sulfasalazine
- Salazosulfapyridine (salazopyrin)
- Thiazosulfone (thiazolesulfone)
- Tiaprofenic acid
- Tolonium chloride, tolonium chloride (toluidine blue)
- Trihexyphenidyl (benzhexol)
- Trimethoprim
- Trinitrotoluene (2,4,6-trinitrotoluene)
- Tripelennamine

Favism

Favism is the term given to the G6PD syndrome when acute intravascular hemolysis may be precipitated by exposure to the broad bean *Vicia faba*. Pallor, jaundice, and hemoglobinuria are the clinical hallmarks. Fresh, dried, or frozen beans or even exposure to pollen may precipitate the crisis. The offending agent is divicine, or its aglycone isouramil, which can produce free oxygen radicals on autoxidation. The extent of hemolysis is related to the extent of exposure. In children, acute hemolysis, sometimes life-threatening, is common, but renal failure is uncommon although there may be systemic symptoms of fever and loin pain.

Renal failure occurs more often in adults, possibly because of comorbidity. Favism is usual in class II variants, e.g. Mediterranean and Canton, but may occur in others, including the African A-variant. Some other chemicals and compounds, such as topical henna, and some of the pulses used to make up local sweetmeats can also precipitate hemolysis. Patients with favism are G6PD deficient, but not all G6PD-deficient patients develop favism when they ingest fava beans.

Chronic Nonspherocytic Hemolytic Anemia

Chronic anemia with normal/near normal red cell morphology is the most severe form of G6PD deficiency and is usually seen in infancy or childhood. Chronic nonspherocytic hemolytic anemia develops in a minority of cases with G6PD deficiency (class I variants). Most of the mutations causing CNSHA are seen on exon 10 and affects the formation of dimers and tetramers. Clinical presentation is variable. Chronic nonspherocytic hemolytic anemia affects only male patients, and these patients usually have history of NNJ necessitating therapeutic intervention. The patient presents later with anemia and jaundice. Splenomegaly is variable. Anemia is normocytic, normochromic, and slight macrocytosis may be observed due to reticulocytosis. Unconjugated hyperbilirubinemia, increased levels of lactate dehydrogenase, and decreased levels of haptoglobin are present. Hemolysis is usually extravascular, although additional oxidant stress may precipitate intravascular hemolysis. Continuous hemolysis in these patients results from red cell membrane damage due to oxidation of sulfhydryl group of Hb resulting in its precipitation.

Association with other Hemolytic States

In the cases with sickle cell disease, the presence of G6PD deficiency has been found to be an independent risk factor for abnormally high cerebral velocities as assessed by transcranial Doppler assessment. In another study, association of G6PD deficiency did not influence the severity and frequency of painful crisis, anemic episodes, or infections in patients with sickle cell disease.

Laboratory Diagnosis

The acute intravascular hemolysis raises the suspicion of G6PD deficiency. The peripheral blood smear shows red cells with contracted Hb in "ghost" membrane. Hemoglobinuria may be gross, producing almost black urine without red cells in the centrifuge deposit. Several screening tests have been devised to identify G6PD deficiency in RBCs. The most widely used tests are the brilliant Cresyl blue decolorization test, the methemoglobin reduction test, and an ultraviolet spot test. These are good qualitative tests that can differentiate between the deficient and nondeficient cases but do not provide quantitative data. If a screening test indicates deficiency or is doubtful, the ideal follow-up test for definitive diagnosis is quantification of G6PD activity by spectrophotometric assay. The quantification is essential in the case of hemolytic attack, wherein the oldest red cells (with the least G6PD activity) are destroyed selectively, and the surviving red cells have a relatively higher (but still deficient) G6PD activity. This increases further as the reticulocyte response evolves. During this time, a screening test might yield a false-normal result and, rarely, even a quantitative test might do so. In such cases, it is best to repeat the test a couple of weeks later. The oldest remaining cells can be isolated by differential centrifugation, and they can be shown to have a low G6PD activity.

Quantitative estimation is also important for the diagnosis of heterozygous females; the probability of clinically significant hemolysis in a heterozygote roughly correlates with the proportion of G6PD-deficient red cells in her blood. Thus the demonstration of a normal level of G6PD activity in a heterozygote makes it unlikely that the affected individual will be at risk of G6PD-related hemolysis. In regions where G6PD has a high prevalence and the main variants are known, DNA analysis is the most effective way of identifying heterozygotes.

Enzyme-linked immunosorbent assay-based methods have been developed for field use. A recent study reported a good sensitivity and specificity of this test and recommended for use in resource-limited settings. Another test for field studies is NADPH fluorescence test on paper (NFP test). This test was compared with polymerase chain reaction (PCR)-based G6PD genotyping also using blood samples on filter papers. There was good agreement between the NFP test results and the PCR findings. The estimate of the sensitivity of the NFP test was 98.2% (95.8–99.6%), and the specificity was 97.1% (94.2–99.2%).

Preventive and Therapeutic Strategies

Preventing the development of hemolysis is of key importance in managing patients with G6PD deficiency, along with appropriate treatment of acute and chronic anemia and NNJ. World Health Organization recommends screening all newborns for G6PD deficiency population groups with prevalence rates of 3–5% or more in males. Identifying the affected newborns early makes it easier to take due precautions for preventing the development of NNJ. Avoidance of the known oxidative stresses and drugs in G6PD-deficient individuals can help prevent the development of hemolytic anemia.

Management of NNJ should be as per the standard protocols, including phototherapy and ET. Phototherapy in these neonates may be started at a lower level than otherwise recommended.

A novel approach is the use of heme-oxygenase inhibitor—Tin-mesoporphyrin—which reduces bilirubin production and has shown promising results in preventing the development of significant hyperbilirubinemia in G6PD-deficient neonates. Treatment of acute episode of intravascular hemolysis includes transfusion support to correct anemia and supportive care. Adequate fluid therapy during hemolytic episodes is crucial for prevention and treatment of acute renal failure.

Patients with CNSHA require meticulous monitoring. In most cases, occasional exacerbation may require blood transfusion. During steady state, administration of folic acid is recommended to meet the increased demands due to increased red cell turnover. Occasional patient may need to be started on chronic transfusion therapy. Splenectomy may be required due to large size, development of hypersplenism, or to decrease the transfusion requirement.

OTHER ENZYMOPATHIES OF THE GLUTATHIONE PATHWAY

- *Gamma-glutamyl cysteine synthetase deficiency*: It is the rate-limiting enzyme in glutathione biosynthesis. Patients may present with CNSHA, oxidative hemolytic anemia, basophilic stippling, and spinocerebellar degeneration in adulthood. The genetic locus is identified on chromosome 6p12.

- *Glutathione peroxidase deficiency*: This enzyme is responsible for the elimination of hydrogen peroxide from the erythrocytes, and its production depends on adequate selenium supply. Moderate deficiency may result in nonspherocytic hemolytic anemia in infants or self-limited NNJ, and Heinz bodies. Oxidizing drugs need to be avoided. The genetic locus is localized to chromosome 3p21.3.
- *Glutathione synthetase deficiency*: Mutations in the glutathione synthetase gene lead to low levels of this enzyme in the RBCs, leading to 5-oxoprolinemia and oxoprolinuria. The classical triad of presentation is hemolysis, metabolic acidosis, and mental deterioration. The affected gene is located at chromosome 20q11. Treatment is to supplement vitamin C, vitamin E, bicarbonate, and avoidance of oxidative drugs.
- *Glutathione reductase deficiency*: This enzyme is responsible for the reduction of oxidized glutathione in the presence of flavin adenine dinucleotide, and its deficiency leads to increased susceptibility to drug-induced hemolysis and favism. Its activity increases with dietary riboflavin supplementation in a few patients. In patients with a 2,246 base pair gene deletion in the glutathione reductase gene, riboflavin supplementation does not lead to its increased activity.
- *Enzymopathies of the glycolytic pathway*: Pyruvate kinase (PK) deficiency is the well-recognized enzymopathy of glycolytic pathway, and along with G6PD deficiency **(Fig. 11.8.3)**. It is the most common cause of CNSHA. In contrast to G6PD deficiency, patients with deficiency of enzymes of glycolytic pathway usually have CNSHA with the onset in neonatal period. Drug-induced hemolytic anemia is not a common problem in these patients. **Table 11.8.2** lists the important features of important enzymopathies of the glycolytic pathway.

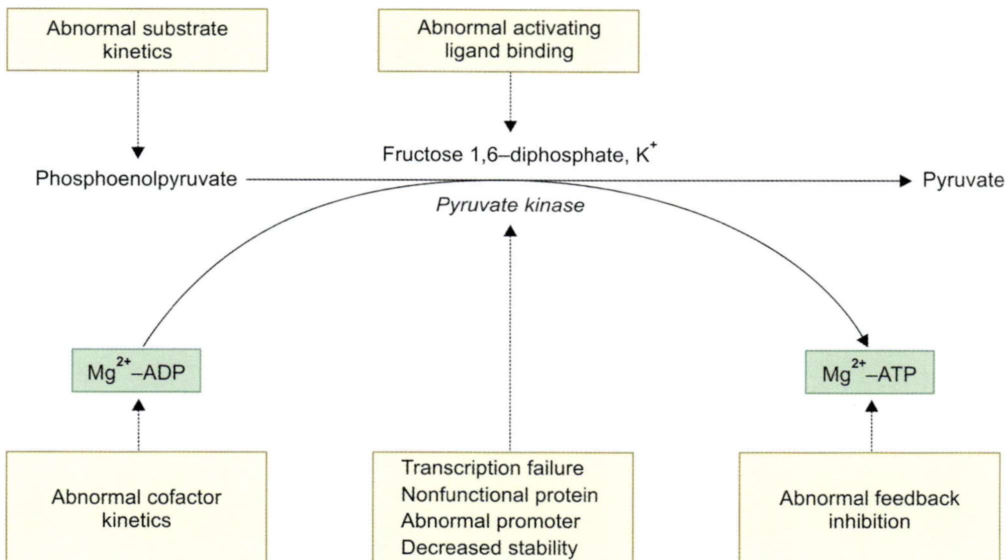

Fig. 11.8.3: The reactions of pyruvate kinase and the sites affected by various mutations in pyruvate kinase deficiency.

Table 11.8.2: Enzymopathies of the glycolytic pathway.

S. no.	*Enzyme*	*Genetics (chromosome/ inheritance)*	*Clinical features*	*Other systems affected*	*Hematological/ other laboratory findings*	*Treatment*	*Comments*
1.	Hexokinase	10q11.2/AR	• NNJ • Anemia • Splenomegaly • CNSHA • Gallstones, • Hyperhemolytic episodes • High O_2 affinity	None directly	Red cell morphology unremarkable	• Packed RBC transfusions • Folic acid • Splenectomy	• Very rare • Occasional AD

Contd...

Contd...

S. no.	Enzyme	Genetics (chromosome/ inheritance)	Clinical features	Other systems affected	Hematological/ other laboratory findings	Treatment	Comments
2.	Glucose phosphate isomerase	19 cen-q12/AR	• NNJ • Hydrops • CNSHA • Hyperhemolytic episodes	None directly	Erythrocytosis very high Reticulocyte count High MCV	• Packed RBC transfusions • Folic acid • Splenectomy	Most common after PK deficiency
3.	Phosphofructokinase	1(M) and 21(L)/ complex	• Erythrocytosis (Type VII glycogen storage disease) • Mild hemolytic anemia	Dominant myopathy	No lactate production in "ischemic arm test" Muscle biopsy	Unsatisfactory	Tarui's disease, subunit genes
4.	ALDOA	16q22–q24/AR	Severe CNSHA	Myopathy, dysmorphism, mental retardation	Normal red cell morphology	Undefined	Very few cases
5.	TPI	12p13/AR	• Moderate-to-severe CNSHA • Neonatal anemia	Neuromuscular, cardiac	Very high reticulocyte count	• Transfusions, folic acid • Splenectomy	Sudden death
6.	Glyceraldehyde-3-phosphate dehydrogenase	12p13/AD	None/associated with other defects, such as hereditary spherocytosis	None	Nonspecific	Nonspecific	Gene syntenic with TPI, membrane protein band 6
7.	Phosphoglycerate kinase	Xq13/X-linked	CNSHA NNJ	CNS, myopathy, rhabdomyolysis	Reticulocytosis	Splenectomy	Rare, variable systems involved
8.	2,3-DPG mutase	7q23-q34/AR	• Polycythemia • Neonatal onset of progressive anemia described with 50% activity	None	Erythrocytosis	Phlebotomy for symptomatic polycythemia	Very rare
9.	Enolase		• Shortened red cell survival not necessary • Nitrofurantoin-induced hemolysis	None	Spherocytosis	Undefined	
10.	Pyruvate kinase	1q21-q22 (PKLR)/AR rarely AD	See text				Most common CNSHA
11.	Lactate dehydrogenase		Decreased levels not associated with anemia				

(AD: autosomal dominant; ALDOA: fructose diphosphate aldolase; AR: autosomal recessive; CNS: central nervous system; CNSHA: chronic nonspherocytic hemolytic anemia; DPG: diphosphoglycerate; MCV: mean corpuscular volume; NNJ: neonatal jaundice; PK: pyruvate kinase; PKLR: pyruvate kinase, liver, and RBC; RBC: red blood cell; TPI: triose phosphate isomerase)

PYRUVATE KINASE DEFICIENCY

Pyruvate kinase enzyme catalyzes the final step of the glycolytic pathway, leading to overall net gain of ATP from this pathway. This enzyme is a tetramer with four tissue specific subunits: R (RBC), L (liver), M1-muscle, and M2 for platelets and leukocytes. Genetic control is separate for R-L subunit and M1-M2 subunits. Deficient PK activity leads to the accumulation of substrates upstream, including

2,3-diphosphoglycerate, which shifts the oxygen dissociation curve to the right, indicating low oxygen affinity. Pyruvate kinase activity decreases during RBC aging, as the enzyme is gradually denatured, and after the activity falls below a critical level, glycolytic failure and ATP depletion result. Over 150 genetic mutations are associated with PK deficiency. Most patients are compound heterozygotes for the two most common mutant forms of the enzyme. This deficiency is common in people of northern European lineage. Prevalence of PK deficiency has varied from 0.14% to 6%. Pyruvate kinase deficiency provides some protection against malaria. Figure 11.8.3 depicts the biochemical role of PK.

Clinical Features

Chronic nonspherocytic hemolytic anemia with extravascular hemolysis is the hallmark of clinical presentation in PK deficiency. Around one-third of patients present with jaundice in the newborn period, and one-third of these cases are severe enough to warrant packed RBC transfusions and/or ET.

Severe anemia and hydrops are the usual cause of death during this period. Milder variants usually present in late childhood with nonsevere anemia, unconjugated hyperbilirubinemia and splenomegaly, which may be massive at times. Chronic leg ulcers are a complication in some individuals. Aplastic crisis due to parvovirus infection can occur. Gallstones are increasingly seen after the first decade. The prognosis is confounded by the lack of good correlation between PK activity level and the severity of clinical hemolysis.

Laboratory Features

Red cell morphology is normocytic-normochromic. Active regeneration of RBCs leading to macrocytosis and acanthocytosis may be observed. Reticulocyte count is increased but not proportionate to the extent of hemolysis, due to selective sequestration of young RBCs and reticulocytes in the spleen. A paradoxical rise in reticulocytes after splenectomy therefore is commonly seen. Hepatic PK deficiency leads to elevated liver enzymes. Iron overload disproportionate to transfusions is sometimes observed and has been explained based on associated hemochromatosis mutations.

Treatment

Treatment of PK deficiency includes transfusion support, folate supplementation, splenectomy, and cholecystectomy for gallstones. The use of salicylates may lead to hyperhemolytic crisis in patients with PK deficiency. The role of splenectomy as a therapeutic measure is not well established, and variable response rates are reported.

ENZYMOPATHIES OF THE NUCLEOTIDE METABOLISM

Pyrimidine 5′ Nucleotidase (Uridine 5′ Monophosphate Hydrolase) Deficiency

It is probably the third most common EEP, probably equal to glucose phosphate isomerase deficiency. Pyrimidine 5′ nucleotidase deficiency is inherited in an autosomal recessive manner, and the gene is located on chromosome 7p15–14. The accumulation of pyrimidine nucleotides in high concentration leads to marked basophilic stippling in the RBCs. Diagnosis is confirmed by a decrease in the nucleotide OD260:OD280 ratio and decreased enzymatic activity. Patients present with hemolysis of varying severity and its sequelae. Splenectomy is usually of little value, though some cases have reported benefit.

Adenosine Deaminase Excess

Adenosine deaminase (ADA) is a purine catabolic enzyme that leads to the conversion of adenosine to inosine. Its deficiency leads to severe combined immunodeficiency, while its excess due to increased amplification of the ADA, messenger ribonucleic acid, produces hemolytic anemia.

OTHER ENZYMOPATHIES ASSOCIATED WITH HEMOLYSIS

Heme-oxygenase-1 Deficiency

Heme-oxygenase-1 converts heme to bilirubin and is protective against oxidative stresses. Clinical presentation is in early childhood with hemolytic anemia, abnormal coagulation/fibrinolytic system, asplenia, and marked growth retardation. It can present as intravascular hemolysis with RBC fragmentation in the absence of hyperbilirubinemia and decreased haptoglobin.

Lecithin Cholesterol Acyltransferase Deficiency

This enzyme is involved in lipoprotein metabolism, and its deficiency leads to erythroid membrane defects due to excess of unesterified cholesterol. These patients may have renal disease with proteinuria and corneal opacifications, and the lipid profile shows decreased high-density lipoprotein levels.

Clinical Approach

The diagnosis of enzymopathy should be suspected in all cases with chronic hemolysis and unexplained unconjugated hyperbilirubinemia, particularly if red cell morphology is unremarkable. Intense reticulocytosis supports the diagnosis of various enzymopathies. In the cases presenting with acute intravascular hemolysis, history of exposure to trigger drugs helps in the diagnosis. Family history of jaundice, anemia, splenectomy, and cholelithiasis may also point toward such a disease. In the absence of such history, the diagnosis may be difficult. The diagnosis can be confirmed by appropriate enzyme assays or by the demonstration of, accumulation of proximal or depletion of distal intermediary compounds of the glycolytic pathway. The diagnostic tests need to be made available more widely, and a high index of suspicion is needed to suspect these conditions.

BIBLIOGRAPHY

1. Bernaudin F, Verlhac F, Chevret S, et al. G6PD deficiency, absence of alpha thalassemia and hemolytic rate at baseline are significant independent risk factors for abnormally high cerebral velocities in patients with sickle cell anemia. Blood. 2008;112;4314-7.
2. Frank JE. Diagnosis and management of G6PD deficiency. Am Fam Physician. 2005;72(7):1277-82.
3. Ip S, Chung M, Kulig J, et al. An evidence-based review of important issues concerning neonatal hyperbilirubinemia. Pediatrics. 2004;114(1):e130-53.
4. Memon MJ, Gahine R, Hussain N, et al. Influence of glucose-6-phosphate-dehydroginase (G-6-PD) deficiency upon clinic-haematological and biochemical expression of patients with sickle cell disease. Int J Adv Med. 2017;4:573-80.
5. Mohanty D, Mukherjee MB, Colah RB. Glucose-6-phosphate dehydrogenase deficiency in India. Indian J Pediatr. 2004;71(6):525-9.
6. Mohanty D, Sukumar S, Mukherjee MB, et al. G6PD deficiency and malaria in India. Am J Hematol. 2003;72(2): 150-1.
7. National Institute of Diabetes and Digestive and Kidney Diseases. Hembase. (2014). [online] Available from: http://www.niddk.nih.gov/research-funding/at-niddk/labs-branches/MMB/Hembase/Pages/about.aspx. [Accessed October, 2018].
8. Steiner LA, Gallagher PG. Erythrocyte disorders in perinatal period. Semin Perinatol. 2007;31(4):254-61.
9. Sukumar S, Mukherjee MB, Colah RB, et al. Molecular basis of G6PD deficiency in India. Blood Cells Mols Dis. 2004;33(2):141-5.
10. Zanella A, Fermo E, Bianchi P, et al. Red cell pyruvate kinase deficiency: molecular and clinical aspects. Br J Haematol. 2005;130(1):11-25.

11.9 Autoimmune Hemolytic Anemia

Bharat Agarwal

INTRODUCTION

In children, hemolytic anemia is usually caused by intrinsic red cell defect leading to hemolysis and anemia as seen typically in membranopathy or red cell enzymopathy, and most of these are inherited in nature. At times hemolytic anemia can result due to factors extrinsic to red cell and most of these causes are acquired in nature. Autoimmune hemolytic anemia (AIHA) is one such cause resulting from interaction of red cell with the immune system. It is characterized by shortened red cell life, hemolysis, and anemia. It is caused by autoantibody to red cell antigens.

Keen clinical observation led to the concept of AIHA as a disease different from the congenital causes, such as hereditary spherocytosis (HS). Invention of Coomb's reagent and testing led to detection of the "incomplete" autoantibodies seen in AIHA.

The detection of complement components on red cell membrane in AIHA further expanded the understanding of the pathophysiology. Improved understanding of the spleen and its functions help understand the mechanism of red cell clearance in AIHA. Focus for current research, as in any autoimmune disorder, is on the role of T-cell and B-cell in AIHA, reasons of failure of self-tolerance and uncontrolled production of autoantibodies, and possible therapeutic options based on molecular pathophysiology.

CLASSIFICATION

Autoimmune hemolytic anemia can be classified in various ways depending on the type of autoantibody, site of hemolysis, or the precipitating illness.

However, the most practical classification of AIHA is whether it is primary or secondary as shown in **Box 11.9.1**.

Primary Autoimmune Hemolytic Anemia

Primary AIHA is not uncommon in children and is next to immune thrombocytopenic purpura in its occurrence as immune hematological disorder.

Box 11.9.1: Classification of autoimmune hemolytic anemia.

Primary autoimmune hemolytic anemia
- Warm-reactive antibody (mainly IgG)
- Cold agglutinin disease (mainly IgM and complements)
- Paroxysmal cold hemoglobinuria (mainly IgG and complements)

Secondary AIHA
- Underlying autoimmune disorders, e.g. systemic lupus erythematosus, Evan's syndrome
- Drug induced, e.g. penicillin
- Immunodeficiency, e.g. HIV, primary immunodeficiency
- Specific infections, e.g. mycoplasma infection
- Malignancies, e.g. lymphomas, leukemia

(AIHA: autoimmune hemolytic anemia; HIV: human immunodeficiency virus; IgG: immunoglobulin G; IgM: immunoglobulin M)

- Primary AIHA occurs without any baseline immune disorder or obvious precipitating factors, though many of the primary AIHA cases occur following nonspecific viral infections, and cold agglutinin disease in children usually follows specifically mycoplasma infection.
- In west, it is more common than hypoplastic anemia, but in our country, hypoplastic anemia is more common due to rampant misuse of drugs and highly prevalent viral infections.

Secondary Autoimmune Hemolytic Anemia

- Secondary AIHA occurs as a part of some systemic illness or wider baseline immune disease.
- It occurs more common in adolescents and young adults and is more common in females, as are other immune disorders.
- Cold agglutinin disease has abrupt onset of symptoms, short history, need aggressive short-term treatment, and ultimately recover.

Paroxysmal cold hemoglobinuria (PCH) is caused by autoantibody of immunoglobulin G (IgG) class that binds red cell antigen at below 37°C, efficiently fixes complements, and leads to intravascular hemolysis.

CLINICAL FORMS OF AUTOIMMUNE HEMOLYTIC ANEMIA

Warm-reactive Autoantibody

- Caused by autoantibody of IgG class that binds the red cell antigens at 37°C, sometimes fixes complements, and leads to extravascular hemolysis.
- Autoantibody IgG molecule binds firmly to red cell antigens which may or may not fix complements. The reticuloepithelial (RE) system recognizes the fragment crystallizable (Fc) segment of the bound IgG through its interaction with the Fc receptor present on the surface of the RE cells. The sensitized red cell if engulfed completely is removed from circulation leading to extravascular hemolysis. However, if only a part of the red cell membrane is bitten off, it will form a spherocyte which will return to circulation.
- Warm-reactive IgG antibody-sensitized red cells are preferentially removed in spleen. If IgG antibody also fixes and activated complements, it will be recognized by the macrophages with receptor to C3b, mainly in the liver.

Cold Reactive Autoimmune Hemolytic Anemia

- Caused by autoantibody of IgM class that binds red cell antigen at below 37°C efficiently fixes complements and leads to intravascular hemolysis and rarely IgG (in PCH).
- It reacts with the red cell antigen at 40°C and fixes complements; however, at body temperature, the antibody dissociates, and there is hardly any antibody attached to red cells. However, the complement activation continues. If the complement activation is complete, the red cell will lyse and lead to intravascular hemolysis. If the complement activation stops at C3b, it will be recognized by the receptor to C3b present on the surface of the macrophages of the RE system, preferentially in liver.
- Often have chronic illness with intermittent relapses and remissions, need long-term therapy, and develop treatment-associated complications. However, overall mortality in children with AIHA is usually less than 10%. Children between 2 years and 12 years seem to have best prognosis.

Paroxysmal cold hemoglobinuria caused by autoantibody of IgG class that binds red cell antigen at below 37°C efficiently fixes complements and leads to intravascular hemolysis.

CLINICAL EVALUATION

- Patients with AIHA usually have typical history and physical findings. The patient will present with anemia, acholuric jaundice, and organomegaly. There may be the presence of fever in some patients.
- History suggestive of nonspecific viral infection in recent past. Being an acquired disorder, the family history is usually not contributory.
- Anemia will present with fatigue, lassitude, and giddiness.
- Acholuric jaundice due to indirect hyperbilirubinemia following hemolysis (icterus in eyes without dark urine). The presence of dark urine is usually due to intravascular hemolysis [cola-colored urine with the presence of hemoglobin (Hb) without the presence of red cells on urinalysis].
- Organomegaly in the form of enlarged liver and spleen, which occur due to hyperplasia of RE system, the site of extravascular hemolysis. Marked hepatosplenomegaly should arouse suspicion of some other disease like leukemia. Always look for secondary cause, such as systemic lupus erythematosus (SLE), malignancy, human

immunodeficiency virus (HIV), recent ingestion of certain drugs.

LABORATORY WORKUP

Investigations are targeted to look for
- Presence of hemolysis
- Presence of autoantibody
- Presence of secondary cause, if any.

Complete Blood Count

- *Hemoglobin* may fall as low as 3–5 g/dL without many symptoms or cardiac failure as there is adequate cardiovascular compensation.
- *White blood cell (WBC) count and platelet count* should be normal as low platelet count may suggest microangiopathic anemia, and the presence of low WBC counts and platelet counts will suggest other cause like aplastic anemia; though in rare cases of Evan's syndrome, the platelet count as well as Hb may be low due to autoimmune pancytopenia.
- *The red cell indices*: The red cell indices, such as mean corpuscular volume and mean corpuscular Hb concentration (MCHC), will be normal as the large reticulocytes are balanced by the presence of microspherocytes; however, the red cell distribution width will be high due to the presence of marked anisocytosis. High MCHC should arouse suspicion of HS.
- *Reticulocyte count*:
  - Reticulocyte count will be high indicating the presence of hemolysis with normal marrow response. It will be seen as polychromasia on peripheral smear (PS) stained with Wright's stain. Very high reticulocyte count with the presence of nucleated red cells on smear may suggest more severe disease with propensity to chronicity.
  - Reticulocyte count may be low due to autoantibody also affecting the red cell precursors in bone marrow (BM) or due to associated parvovirus B19 infection.

Peripheral Smear

Peripheral smear will show the presence of macrocytosis, polychromasia, anisocytosis, nucleated red cells, and microspherocytes. In extreme cases, there may be the presence of autoagglutination. Features of microangiopathy, such as schistocytes and helmet cells, will be absent differentiating it from other causes of hemolytic anemia (microangiopathic hemolytic anemia). The presence of significant target cells would suggest hemoglobinopathy.

Others

- There will be other markers of hemolysis, such as high *serum lactate dehydrogenase* (LDH) levels and increased *serum bilirubin* with high indirect component.
- *Intravascular hemolysis* will lead to hemoglobinuria with the presence of Hb in urine without red cells, hemoglobinemia, low hemalbumin and low hemopexin levels, and in long run hemosiderinuria.
- Bone marrow is not indicated in the clinical setup of suspected hemolytic anemia. However, if BM study is done, it will show erythroid hyperplasia.
- *Presence of autoantibody*: The direct evidence of AIHA is to detect the presence of autoantibody and/or complement component C3 on red cell. This is done by direct antiglobulin test (DAT) also known as Coombs' test **(Fig. 11.9.1)**.
- While IgM antibody-coating red cell membrane can be detected by saline agglutination tests, IgG antibody is an incomplete antibody not detectable easily. In DAT, polyspecific sera containing antihuman IgG and anticomplement rabbit globulin are added. This helps "bridge" the autoantibodies present on the red cell and leads to agglutination. Once DAT is positive, one can characterize the presence of autoantibody or complement C3, or both by using monospecific test. This will also help characterize cold agglutinin disease where the IgM may no more be attached to red cell at 37°C or the presence of Donath-Landsteiner antibody.
- Direct antiglobulin test is usually reported on a scale of 1–4 depending on the strength of reaction. One can estimate titers of the autoantibody involved. Direct antiglobulin test may be false negative, if the steps of the tests are not followed properly.
- In 10% of patients of AIHA, DAT may be truly negative either due to scanty number of autoantibodies or due to the presence of IgA antibody.
- Direct antiglobulin test may also be false positive in some otherwise normal patients who never progress to develop AIHA. It can also be positive following recent blood transfusion. However, in both these cases, it is weakly positive.

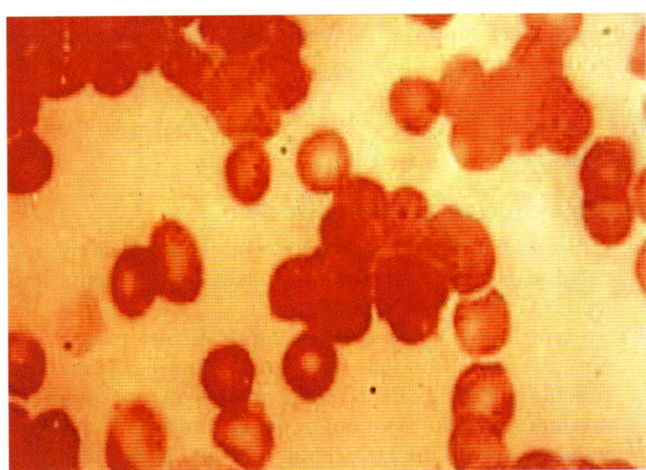

Fig. 11.9.1: Positive direct antiglobulin test.

DIFFERENTIAL DIAGNOSIS

- The presence of anemia, acholuric jaundice, splenohepatomegaly, reticulocytosis, PS showing changes of hemolysis with positive DAT clinches the diagnosis of AIHA.
- *Hereditary spherocytosis*: The presence of microspherocytes may lead to confusion with HS. Clinical settings are totally different in these conditions. Microspherocytes are not the prominent feature in AIHA, and DAT is negative in HS. In addition, MCHC will be high in HS. Microspherocytes may also be seen in other conditions.
- Microangiopathy may be confused with AIHA; however, platelets will be low and DAT negative in microangiopathic hemolytic anemia.
- Secondary cause of AIHA should be looked for, such as SLE, malignancies, immunodeficiency syndromes, especially HIV, and incriminating drugs. Autoimmune hemolytic anemia with low reticulocyte count should be investigated for parvovirus B19 infection.

PATHOPHYSIOLOGY

Both primary and secondary AIHA are caused by the presence of autoantibodies that bind the red cell antigens. This leads to intravascular hemolysis (as in cold agglutinin disease or PCH) or extravascular clearance of the sensitized red cells in spleen or liver (as in warm-reactive antibody). Hence, it is important to understand the role of the autoantibody and the RE system in AIHA.

- *Autoantibody*: It is important to understand the characteristics of the autoantibody, including its isotype, thermal range, capacity to fix complements, binding affinity, and antigenic specificity.
- *Antibody isotype*: In most cases of AIHA, the antibody is of IgG class. Most of the IgG autoantibodies are warm reactive, though some may be cold reactive as seen in PCH or rarely cold agglutinin disease. In others the autoantibody is of IgM type as seen classically in cold agglutinin diseases following mycoplasma infections seen in children. Rarely the autoantibody is of IgA class, which is not detectable by standard DAT. The essential characteristics of these different autoantibody isotypes seen in the three clinical forms of primary AIHA are shown in **Table 11.9.1**.

In 70% of the cases with IgG autoantibody, IgG1 is the only subtype, in 20%, it is IgG1 plus some other subtype. In rest, subtypes other than IgG1 are involved. IgG1 and IgG2 are better capable to bind complement than IgG3 or IgG4.

Thermal Amplitude

Warm-reactive IgG autoantibody has thermal reactivity at 37°C, which means that it shows activity at body temperature.

Table 11.9.1: Essential characteristics of different autoantibody isotypes seen in autoimmune hemolytic anemia.

Characteristic	*Warm reactive*	*PCH*	*Cold agglutinin*
Isotype	IgG	IgG	IgM
Temperature	37°C	4°C	4°C
Complement fixation	Variable	Yes	Yes
Antigen specificity	Rh	P	I/i
Site of destruction of RBC	Extravascular	Intravascular	Intravascular/ liver
DAT			
At 37°C	IgG ± C3	C3	C3
At 4°C	No need	IgG ± C3	C3
Titers of antibody	Low	Moderate	High
Treatment	Steroids/ intravenous immunoglobulin splenectomy	Avoid cold Steroids	Avoid cold
Plasmapheresis outcome	Chronic	Short term	Short term

(DAT: direct antiglobulin test; IgG: immunoglobulin G; IgM: immunoglobulin M; PCH: paroxysmal cold hemoglobinuria; RBC: red blood cell; Rh: Riemann hypothesis)

Cold reactive IgG autoantibodies of PCH show thermal reactivity at 4°C. They bind the red cell antigen at 4°C and bind complements. At body temperature the IgG antibody dissociates and cannot be detected by DAT at 37°C, but the complement cascade gets amplified leading to hemolysis. Hence this antibody is demonstrated by a special biphasic test. IgM autoantibody seen in cold agglutinin disease has thermal activity below 37°C and is best at 4°C. The clinical disease also depends on the antigenic specificity and the complement-binding capacity.

Complement-binding capacity, red cell antigen specificity, and antibody-binding affinity: Bound immunoglobulin binds complement C1q via its Fc portion. This leads to further cascade effect up to the formation of C3b. At this juncture, either the red cell is cleared by the RE system that recognizes the C3b via specific surface receptor leading to extravascular hemolysis, or the complement cascade activation continues till the red cell is destroyed leading to intravascular hemolysis. As IgG autoantibody has specificity to Rhesus (Rh) system which has sparse distribution on red cell surface, and as two molecules of IgG antibodies are needed nearby to bind C1q, the complement capacity binding of IgG autoantibody is inefficient leading to extravascular hemolysis, whereas IgM autoantibody being a pentamer binds complement efficiently leading to intravascular hemolysis. IgM antibody has antigen specificity against I/i antigen. Similarly, as the cold reactive IgG autoantibody has specificity against P antigen, which is densely present on the red cell membrane, it binds the complements efficiently leading to intravascular hemolysis. IgG antibody binds the red cell antigen with high affinity as compared to IgM antibody.

MANAGEMENT

General Management

- Patients with mild disease who are otherwise comfortable are better observed alone without much therapy.
- Most patients are usually very sick looking in the first few days. They may go into severe intravascular hemolysis with renal involvement.
- It is important to maintain good urine output.
- As there is rapid turnover of red cells, folic acid should be replaced in therapeutic doses.
- Packed red blood cell (PRBC) transfusion:
  - Packed red blood cells can be lifesaving in patients with severe AIHA and should never be withheld with fear of hemolytic reactions.
- Hemoglobin levels should be maintained at 6–8 g/dL. If the Hb is allowed to drop lower than that, it can lead to cardiovascular decompensation.

Two problems may occur with transfusion in patients with AIHA:

1. There is usually a problem with cross-matching the unit.
2. There are chances of hemolysis following transfusion.

As most of the warm-reactive antibodies are against Rh system, they are pan reactive and will react with all the units of PRBC. One can use the pack that is found to be "least incompatible" on cross-matching and start the transfusion at very slow rate initially to see for hemolytic reaction.

Always watch for hemolysis, which will be evident with fever, restlessness, loin pain, hemoglobinuria (dark urine), and check for hemoglobinemia in plasma and hemoglobinuria in urine tests.

Steroids

Corticosteroids are the first line and the mainstay in the definitive therapy of AIHA. It is indicated for moderate-to-severe disease. They are effective in 80% of warm-reactive antibodies and occasionally even in cold agglutinin disease. For initial few days, one can use intravenous (IV) methylprednisolone in the dose of 1–2 mg/kg 6–8 hourly. Once the patient is stable, one can switch over to high-dose oral prednisolone in the dose of 2 mg/kg/day for 2–4 weeks, followed by gradual tapering over 3 months based on the symptoms, Hb levels, evidence of hemolysis, serum LDH levels, reticulocyte count, and DAT grade.

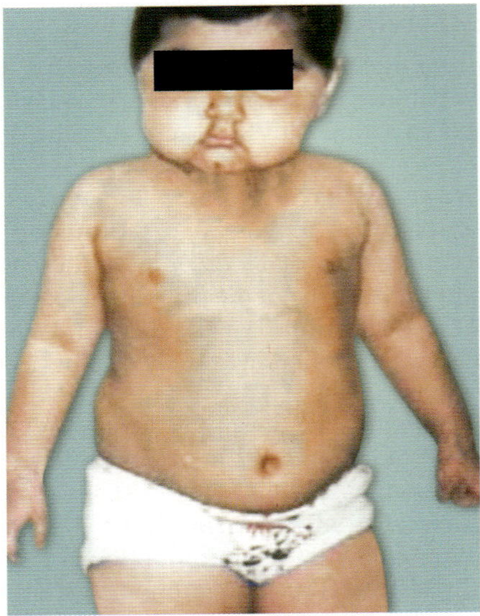

Fig. 11.9.2: Autoimmune hemolytic anemia on steroid therapy.
Courtesy: Dr MR Lokeshwar and Dr Bharat Agarwal, Mumbai, Maharashtra, India.

While tapering, one may switch over to daily or alternate single dose of steroids. Steroids work by blocking the Fc receptor as well as suppressing the antibody production. Hence the effect is usually seen in few days of therapy. One should regularly monitor with blood pressure, blood sugar, and weight recordings for common side effects **(Fig. 11.9.2)**.

Intravenous Immunoglobulin

Intravenous immunoglobulin (IVIg) in high doses of 2–5 g/kg has only limited response and is exorbitantly expensive and has potential side effects. It has shown benefit only in 30–50% of AIHA treated with IVIg. It is not the standard of care as the first-line therapy in AIHA.

- *Exchange transfusion*: Exchange transfusion is beneficial as it removes the antibody, complements, and the sensitized red cells. However, it is labor intensive and hazardous.
- *Plasma exchange*: Plasma exchange is found to be very successful in IgM antibody-induced AIHA. IgM being a large molecule stays in the circulation and does not leak into the tissues. As IgM does not bind to red cells at body temperature, it is likely to be free in plasma available for exchange, especially in warm atmosphere.

Splenectomy

Warm-reactive AIHA is likely to be chronic despite steroids and IVIg use. Many such patients who are perpetually sick and need repeated admissions and packed red cell transfusions with its own therapy-related complications, and splenectomy is the ultimate therapy of choice and works better in patients with IgG-induced AIHA than IgM-induced AIHA. Nearly

60% respond very well, and another 20% have satisfactory response. All the precautions, such as immunization against capsulated organisms before splenectomy and penicillin prophylaxis for life after splenectomy, must be followed. Splenectomy is avoided as far as possible till the age of 5 years.

Other Modalities Tried

- High-dose dexamethasone.
- Cytotoxic drugs, such as vincristine, cyclophosphamide, and azathioprine.
- Immunomodulators, such as danazol, cyclosporine.
- Rituximab, the monoclonal anti-CD20 antibody, has been used as off label in many autoimmune disorders, including AIHA with anecdotal reports of success. There is limited experience to use these drugs in children with AIHA. They also have limited success and are toxic in children.

SECONDARY AUTOIMMUNE HEMOLYTIC ANEMIA

Autoimmune hemolytic anemia can occur as a part of underlying autoimmune disease or because of a specific precipitating cause, which must be looked for in every case. Secondary AIHA can occur in patients with underlying autoimmune disease, such as SLE, scleroderma, Sjögren syndrome, dermatomyositis. It can occur as a part of autoimmune cytopenias—Evan's syndrome where one sees antibody to platelets and at times to neutrophils. Evan's syndrome is potentially severe and fatal and hence needs aggressive management.

It can also occur in malignancies, such as acute leukemia and lymphoma. The main problem in such patients is of course the malignancy and not AIHA. It is also seen in patients with immunodeficiency including HIV because of immune dysregulation.

Cold agglutinin disease in children usually follows mycoplasma infection. Bacterial sepsis can lead to exposure of the cryptic T antigen and immune hemolysis. Drugs, such as penicillin including cephalosporins, can induce AIHA.

Secondary AIHA needs twofold therapy, treatment of AIHA and treatment of the baseline disease. Attention should be paid to remove the offending drugs. Steroids are equally useful in secondary AIHA as in primary AIHA and can be used without fear even in the cases of immunodeficiency.

BIBLIOGRAPHY

1. Collins PW, Newland AC. Treatment modalities of autoimmune blood disorders. Semin Hematol. 1992;29(1):64-74.
2. Engelfriet CP, Overbeeke MAM, von dem Borne AE. Autoimmune hemolytic anemia. Semin Hematol. 1992;29(1): 3-12.
3. Heidemann SM, Sarnaik SA, Sarnaik AP. Exchange transfusion for severe autoimmune hemolytic anemia. Am J Pediatr Hematol Oncol. 1987;9(4):302-4.
4. Hilgartner MW, Bussel J. Use of intravenous gamma globulin for the treatment of autoimmune neutropenia of childhood and autoimmune hemolytic anemia. Am J Med. 1987;83(4A):25-9.
5. Kowal-Vern A, Jacobson P, Okuno T, et al. Negative direct antiglobulin test in autoimmune hemolytic anemia. Am J Pediatr Hematol Oncol. 1986;8(4):349-51.
6. Salama A, Berghofer H, Mueller-Eckhardt C. Red blood cell transfusion in warm-type autoimmune haemolytic anaemia. Lancet. 1992;340(8834-8835):1515-7.
7. Salama A, Mueller-Eckhardt C. Autoimmune haemolytic anemia in childhood associated with non-compliment binding IgM autoantibodies. Br J Haematol. 1987;65(1):67-71.
8. Ware RE. Autoimmune hemolytic anemia. In: Nathan DG, Ginsburg D, Orkin SH, Look AT (Eds). Hematology of infancy and childhood. Philadelphia, PA: Saunders; 2003. pp. 521-59.

11.10 Coagulation Disorders and Hemophilia

Sunil Gomber

INTRODUCTION

Coagulation disorders are disruptions in the body's ability to control blood clotting, an essential function of the body designed to prevent blood loss. Coagulation disorders are usually discovered when an injury or surgery initiates bleeding, and bleeding does not stop spontaneously.

Coagulation is a complex process (called coagulation cascade) that involves 12 coagulation factors found in blood plasma and several other blood components. A deficiency

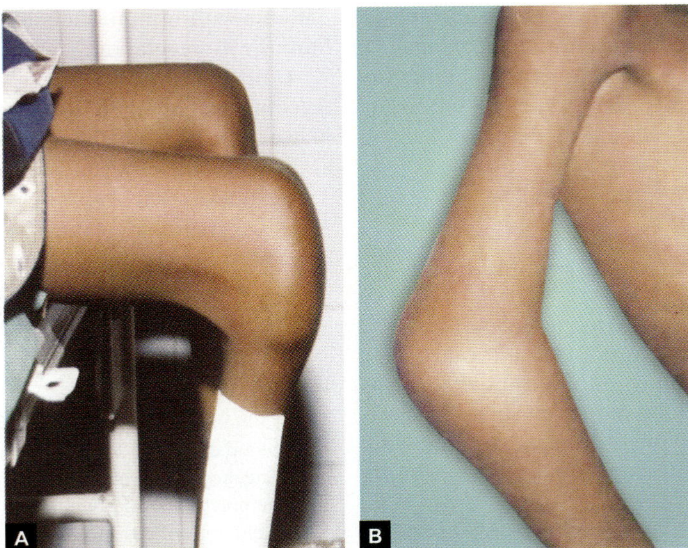

Figs. 11.10.1A and B: Coagulation disorders.
Courtesy: Dr MR Lokeshwar, Mumbai, Maharashtra and Dr Sunil Gomber, New Delhi, India.

in clotting factors or a disorder that affects one of the many steps in the entire process can disrupt clotting and severely complicate blood loss from injury, surgery, or spontaneously **(Figs. 11.10.1A and B)**.

DIAGNOSTIC APPROACH IN BLEEDING DISORDER CHILD

History

Clinical evaluation of bleeding patients begins with a careful history, considering the child's age, gender, clinical presentation, past history, and family history while a bleeding history is being elicited; attention should be directed to the type of bleeding present as given in **Table 11.10.1**.

Age and Gender of the Patient

Inherited bleeding disorders should be strongly considered when the onset of bleeding manifestations occurs in infancy or early childhood and is associated with a positive family history. However, a negative family history does not exclude an inherited coagulation disorder, as up to the one-third of the patients with hemophilia have a negative family history.

Laboratory Testing

The usual initial screening tests in a bleeding child include quantitation of platelets, examination of peripheral blood smear, and coagulation tests. Routine test of blood coagulation, such as prothrombin time (PT), activated partial thromboplastin time (aPTT), and thrombin time (TT), are frequently ordered to assess clotting function in patients.

Table 11.10.1: Clinical presentation past history and family history of bleeding patients.

Clinical finding	*Coagulation disorders*	*Purpuric disorders (disorder of platelets and blood vessels)*
Skin petechiae	Not usually seen	Characteristic
Ecchymosis	Common large one or more	*Characteristic*: Small or many scattered
Soft-tissue hematoma	Characteristic	Rare
Joint hemorrhages	Characteristic: Hallmark of disease	Not usually seen
Delayed bleeding	Common	Rare
Bleeding from superficial skin abrasion	Uncommon	Common and persistent
Family history of bleeding	Common	Rare

- *Prothrombin time*: This is used to assess the extrinsic pathology of clotting, which consists of tissue factor and factor VII and coagulation factors in the common pathway (factors II, V, X, and fibrinogen).
- *Activated partial thromboplastin time*: This is used to assess the integrity of the intrinsic coagulation pathway (prekallikrein; high-molecular-weight kininogen; and factors XII, XI, IX, and VIII) and final common pathway.
- *Thrombin time*: The TT measures the final step of the clotting pathway, the conversion of fibrinogen to fibrin.

Box 11.10.1: Interpretation of mixing studies

NS—corrected	NS—not corrected	NS—not corrected
Ads—not corrected	Ads—corrected	Ads—not corrected
↓	↓	↓
Diagnosis Factor IX deficiency	*Diagnosis:* Factor VIII deficiency von Willebrand disease (↑ BT)	*Diagnosis:* Factor XI or XII deficiency
	Factor assay	Factor assay

(NS: normal serum; Ads: aluminum hydroxide adsorbed plasma; BT: bleeding time).

- *Reptilase time*: Reptilase, a thrombin-like enzyme obtained from snake venom, differs from thrombin by generating fibrinopeptide A but not fibrinopeptide B from fibrinogen and by resisting inhibitor by heparin via antithrombin III.
- *Mixing studies*: After an abnormality in a clotting test (PT or aPTT) has been detected, it is important to distinguish between a clotting factor deficiency and an inhibitor against clotting factors. This is accomplished by performing a mixing study, in which the patient's plasma is mixed in a 1:1 ratio with normal serum (NS) or aluminum hydroxide adsorbed plasma (Ads), and the abnormal tests are repeated. Normal serum contains factors IX, X, XI, and XII, and Ads contains factors V, VIII, XI, and XII. Mixing studies (with prolonged aPTT) are interpreted as given in **Box 11.10.1**.

Diagnostic Test

- *Fibrin* D-dimer: Plasmin cleaves fibrin at multiple sites and releases fibrin degradation products (FDPs). One of the major FDPs is D-dimer. An elevated plasma concentration of D-dimer indicates recent or ongoing intravascular blood coagulation.
- *Clot solubility in urea*: Fibrin is cross-linked through the action of factor XIII, making the final fibrin clot insoluble in 5-M urea. The ability of urea to solubilize the mature clot reflects a deficiency of factor XIII.

HEMOPHILIA A AND HEMOPHILIA B

Hemophilia A [factor VIII (FVIII) deficiency] and hemophilia B [factor IX (FIX) deficiency] are the most common and serious congenital coagulation factor deficiencies. The clinical findings in hemophilia A and hemophilia B are virtually identical. Hemophilia A is more common than hemophilia B.

Diagnosis of Hemophilia

Hemophilia should be suspected in patients presenting with a history of:

- Easy bruising in early childhood
- Spontaneous bleeding (particularly into joints and soft tissue)

Table 11.10.2: Severity of bleeding in relation to clotting factor level.

Severity	*Clotting factor level (% activity)*	*Bleeding episodes*
Mild	5–40	Severe bleeding with major trauma or surgery
Moderate	1–5	Occasional spontaneous bleeding, severe bleeding with trauma and surgery
Severe	<1	Spontaneous bleeding predominantly in joints and muscles

Table 11.10.3: Severity and site of bleeding.

Severity	*Site of bleeding*
Serious	• Joint • CNS • Muscle/soft tissue • Mouth/gum/nose • Hematuria
Life-threatening	• GIT • Neck/throat

(CNS: central nervous system; GIT: gastrointestinal tract)

- Excessive bleeding, following trauma or surgery.

The severity of bleeding manifestation in hemophilia is generally corrected with the clotting factor level as shown in **Table 11.10.2**.

The bleeding manifestations in hemophilia can be graded as serious or life threatening depending on the site of bleeding **(Table 11.10.3)**.

The incidence of different sites of bleeding is as follows:

- *Hemarthrosis*: 70–80%
- *Muscle/soft tissue*: 10–20%
- *Other major bleed*: 5–10%
- *Central nervous system bleed*: Less than 5%.

Chronic complications of hemophilia include the following:

- Musculoskeletal complications
- Chronic hemophilic arthropathy
- Chronic synovitis
- Deforming arthropathy
- Contractures
- Pseudotumor formation (soft tissue or bone)
- Fracture
- Inhibitors against FVIII or FIX
- Transfusion-related infections.

Management of Hemophilia

Principles of Care

Prevention of bleeding should be the goal:

- Acute bleeds should be treated early (within 2 hours if possible).

Table 11.10.4: Treatment of some common types of hemorrhage in patients with hemophilia.

Type of hemorrhage	*Hemophilia A*	*Hemophilia B*
Hemarthrosis	FVIII concentrate 40 IU/kg on day 1 Followed by 20 IU/kg on day 2, day 3, day 5 until joint functions are normal or back to baseline	FIX concentrate 60–80 IU/kg on day 1 Followed by 40 IU/kg on day 2, day 4
Muscle or subcutaneous hematoma	FVIII concentrate 20 IU/kg; may need every other day treatment until hematoma resolves	FIX concentrate 40 IU/kg; may need treatment every 2–3 days until hematoma resolves
Mouth and tooth extraction	FVIII concentrate 20 IU/kg Antifibrinolytic therapy	FIX concentrate 40 IU/kg Antifibrinolytic therapy
Iliopsoas hemorrhage	FVIII concentrate 50 IU/kg Followed by 25 IU/kg every 12 hours until asymptomatic Followed by 20 IU/kg every other day for a total of 10–14 days	FIX concentrate 120 IU/kg Followed by 50–60 IU/kg every 12–24 hours until asymptomatic Followed by 40–50 IU/kg every other day for a total of 10–14 days

- Home therapy should be used to manage only uncomplicated, mild, or moderate bleeding episodes.
- All severe bleeds should be managed in the hospital settings.
- Patients should avoid trauma by adjusting their lifestyle.
- Intramuscular injection and arterial puncture must be avoided.
- Regular exercise should be encouraged to promote strong muscle.

Management of Bleeding

When mild-to-moderate bleeding occurs, levels of FVIII or FIX must be raised to hemostatic levels in the 35–50% range. For life-threatening or major hemorrhages the dose should aim to achieve levels of 100% activity. Calculation of the dose of FVIII and FIX is as follows:

- Dose of FVIII (IU) = % desired (rise in FVIII) × body weight × 0.5
- Dose of FIX (IU) = % desired (rise in FIX) × body weight × 1.0

Treatment of some common types of hemorrhage in patients with hemophilia has been listed in **Table 11.10.4**.

Desmopressin

It is a synthetic analog of antidiuretic hormone. It boosts the plasma levels of FVIII after administration and is useful in the treatment of mild hemophilia. This is not effective in the treatment of moderate or severe hemophilia A and hemophilia B.

Adjunctive Management

- Rest, ice, compression, and elevation are important adjunctives in the management of bleeding in muscle or joints in addition to increasing factor level with clotting factor concentrate or desmopressin in mild hemophilia A.
- Antifibrinolytic drugs (e.g. tranexamic acid, epsilon-aminocaproic acid) for 5–10 days are effective as adjunctive treatment for mucosal bleeds and are used to decrease the use of coagulation products in dental extractors.

Prophylaxis

Prophylaxis is the administration of clotting factors at regular intervals to prevent bleeding and must be the goal of all hemophilic care programs until a cure is available.

- *Primary prophylaxis*: Usually such programs are initiated with the first joint hemorrhage. Such programs, although expensive, are highly effective in preventing or greatly limiting the degree of joint pathology. Treatment is usually provided every 2–3 days to maintain a measurable plasma level of clotting factor (1–2%) when assayed just before the next infusion. At present, the most commonly suggested protocol for prophylaxis is the infusion of 25–40 IU/kg of clotting factor concentrate three times a week and twice a week for those with hemophilia A and hemophilia B, respectively.
- *Second prophylaxis*: In patients with repeated bleeding, particularly, into specific joints (target joints), short-term secondary prophylaxis for 4–8 weeks can be used to interrupt the bleeding cycle. This may be combined with intensive physiotherapy or synoviorthesis.

Comprehensive Care

Today, patients with hemophilia are best managed through comprehensive hemophilia care centers. Such centers are dedicated to patients and family education as well as to the prevention and/or treatment of the complications of hemophilia, including chronic joint disease and inhibitor development as well as infection, such as hepatitis C and human immunodeficiency virus. Such centers involve a team of physicians, nurse, orthopedists, physical therapists, and psychosocial workers, among others.

11.11 Platelet and Vascular Disorders

Sunil Gomber

INTRODUCTION

Platelets play a pivotal role in vascular hemostasis. They are present in blood in a concentration of 150–400 × 10^9/L. Any derangement in platelet number or function leads to the loss of vascular hemostasis.

PHYSIOLOGY OF HEMOSTASIS

Platelet plug formation occurs after a sequence of events starting from vascular wall injury, resulting in exposure to collagen and endothelial protein. Initial platelet adhesion is mediated via von Willebrand factor and collagen binding to platelet glycoproteins, Gp1b/9 and Gp2b/3a, fibrinogen, and calcium. Platelet adhesion results in intracellular signaling, and platelet activation brings about degranulation, activation of Gp2b/3a complex, exposure of anionic phospholipids, and generation of procoagulant microvesicles. The release of various granules and proteins leads to collagen binding to glycoprotein Gp6, resulting in cellular activation and firm adhesion. This leads to further platelet aggregation. Exposure of anionic phospholipids results in thrombin generation and fibrin production, leading to hemostatic plug stabilization. The actin-myosin complexes within the platelet shorten leading to clot retraction. Thromboxane A2 (TXA2) generation induces further platelet aggregation, blood vessel contraction, and vasoconstriction.

DISORDERS OF PLATELETS AND BLOOD VESSELS

Disorders of vascular hemostasis can be broadly classified as:

- *Primary*: Qualitative/quantitative defect in platelet number and function and vascular disorders.
- *Secondary*: Clotting factor defect.

Primary defects predominantly present with superficial bleeding, whereas secondary defects often lead to deep visceral bleeding.

Primary platelet disorders may be due to quantitative or qualitative defects. Quantitative platelet disorders are divided into neonatal or postneonatal depending on the time of onset.

NEONATAL THROMBOCYTOPENIA

As discussed before, there are many causes of neonatal thrombocytopenia, but the most common cause of significance includes alloimmune and autoimmune platelet disorders. The common causes are listed in **Table 11.11.1**. There are many causes of neonatal thrombocytopenia, but the most common cause of significance includes alloimmune and autoimmune platelet disorders.

Neonatal Alloimmune Thrombocytopenia

- Most common cause of severe thrombocytopenia.
- Occurs in 10–20% babies with neonatal thrombocytopenia.
- Commonest antigen responsible: Human platelet antigen 1-a [platelet antigen (PLA)-1].
- The severity of disease increases with subsequent pregnancies.
- *Pathogenesis*: Maternal sensitization to the paternally derived antigens expressed on fetal platelets, occurs during early gestation—production of immunoglobulin G antibodies—crosses placenta, and attaches to fetal platelets leading to platelet destruction.
- Any systemic disease in baby and mother should be ruled out.
- Typically, healthy infants present with petechiae, purpura, ecchymosis, and bleeding; 10–15% may present with intracranial bleed.
- About 90% have a platelet count less than 50 × 10^9/L.

Table 11.11.1: Neonatal quantitative platelet disorders.

Immune disorder	*Autoimmune/alloimmune*
Prenatal	• Preeclampsia/eclampsia • Abruptio placentae • Dead twin fetus • Congenital infections
Natal	• Breech delivery
Postnatal	• Infections • Respiratory distress syndrome • Hypoxia • Indwelling catheters
Drugs	• Prolonged antibiotics • Thiazides in mother
Bone marrow disorders	• Fanconi syndrome • Osteopetrosis • Congenital leukemia
Inborn error of metabolism	• Isovaleric acidemia • Propionic acidemia
Isolated megakaryocytic hypoplasia	

- Mainstay of treatment includes PLA-negative platelet transfusion, intravenous (IV) immunoglobulin (IVIg), and steroids. Recovery of platelet count occurs in 2–3 weeks.

Neonatal Autoimmune Thrombocytopenia

- Passive transfer of antibodies from the mother to baby.
- Noted in maternal conditions, including systemic lupus erythematosus, hypothyroidism, lymphoproliferative states, and idiopathic thrombocytopenic purpura (ITP).

Table 11.11.2: Neonatal autoimmune thrombocytopenia.

Increased platelet destruction	*Decreased platelet production*	*Platelet pooling*
Idiopathic (immune)	*Drugs*: Chlorothiazide, tolbutamide	Hypersplenism
Infections	Megaloblastic anemia	Hypothermia
Drug induced	Inborn errors of metabolism	
Autoimmune	Aplastic anemia: Idiopathic/acquired	
HUS TTP	Marrow infiltration	
DIC	*Infections:* Rubella	
Hemophagocytic syndrome	Constitutional	
Kasabach–Merritt syndrome		
Lymphoreticular malignancy		

(DIC: disseminated intravascular coagulation; HUS: hemolytic uremic syndrome; TTP: thrombotic thrombocytopenic purpura)

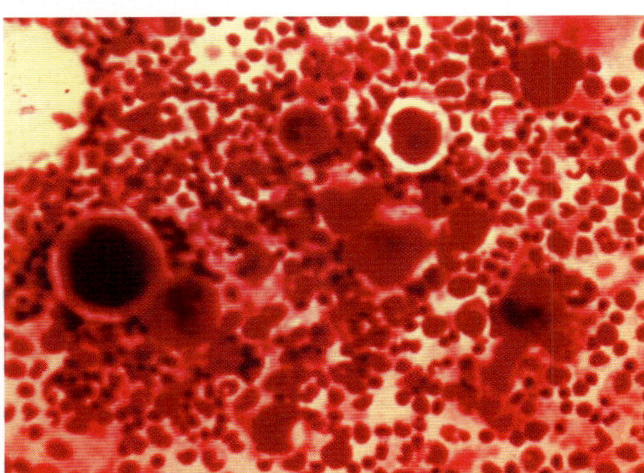

Fig. 11.11.1: Bone marrow examination in immune-mediated thrombocytopenia.
Courtesy: Dr MR Lokeshwar and Dr Sunil Gomber.

- Autoimmune thrombocytopenia is less severe than alloimmune thrombocytopenia.
- Gestational thrombocytopenia does not lead to neonatal thrombocytopenia.
- Antibody formed against an antigen presents on maternal platelet as well as fetal platelet.
- Commonest antigens: Gp2b/3a, Gp1b/9.
- Mainstay of treatment includes platelet transfusion, IVIg, and steroids.
- Recovery occurs in nearly 3 weeks **(Table 11.11.2)**.

IDIOPATHIC THROMBOCYTOPENIC PURPURA

Idiopathic thrombocytopenic purpura is the most common cause of thrombocytopenia in healthy children **(Figs. 11.11.1 to 11.11.3)**.

- Peak age of occurrence: Between 2 years and 5 years
- *Mechanisms*: Antibody-mediated destruction directed against Gp2b/3a, Gp1b/9, and Gp1a/2a; impaired megakaryopoiesis mediated by immune cell-derived cytokines; and antibody and cellular cytotoxicity.

Clinical Presentation

- It commonly presents 1–3 weeks after a viral infection; implicated virus: human immunodeficiency virus, rubella, hepatitis C, cytomegalovirus, chickenpox, and following administration of live viral vaccines.
- Predominant clinical manifestations are petechiae, purpura, and ecchymosis. Idiopathic thrombocytopenic purpura may present with bleeding. Intracerebral hemorrhage is noted in 0.2–0.8%.

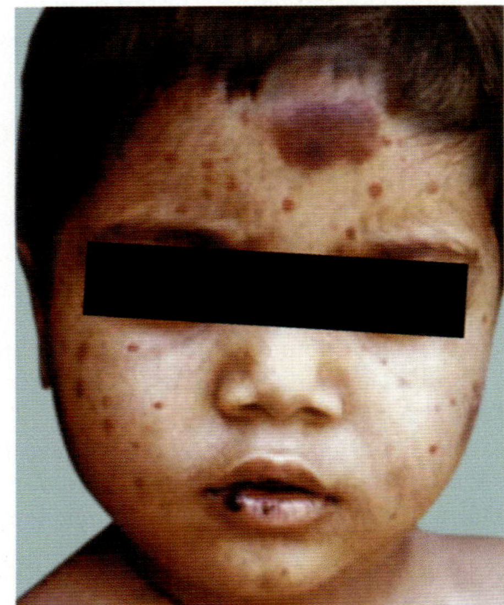

Fig. 11.11.2: Idiopathic thrombocytopenic purpura.
Courtesy: Dr MR Lokeshwar and Dr Sunil Gomber.

- Atypical presentation includes isolated thrombocytopenia, with normal counts in otherwise healthy child without any hepatosplenomegaly, lymphadenopathy, and bony tenderness, following a viral infection 1–3 weeks earlier.

Investigations

Complete blood count should be done in all cases. Bone marrow (BM) examination shows normal or increased megakaryocytes with normal or erythroid and myeloid maturation. In a typical case, BM examination is unnecessary.

Indications for Bone Marrow Examination

- Presentation suggestive of leukemia/aplastic anemia
- Sick child
- Persistent thrombocytopenia beyond 6 months
- Presence of generalized lymphadenopathy or bony tenderness

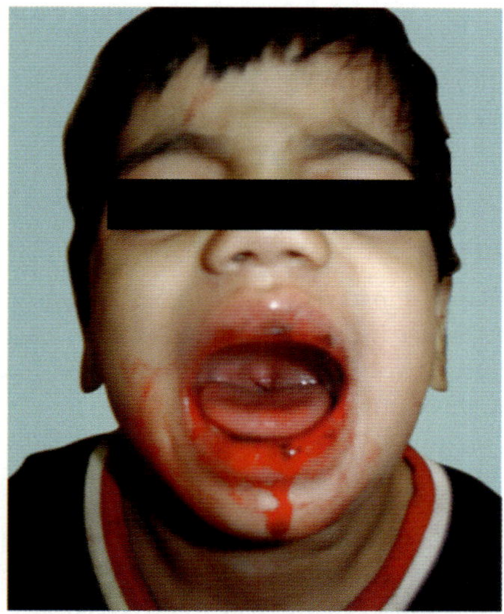

Fig. 11.11.3: Glanzmann's thrombasthenia.
Courtesy: Dr MR Lokeshwar and Dr Sunil Gomber.

Table 11.11.3: Other modalities of treatment.	
Nonsteroidal immunosuppressive therapy (vincristine, cyclosporine, rituximab)	Some benefit in chronic immune-mediated thrombocytopenia
Plasmapheresis	Some benefit as emergency measure
Splenectomy	Acute immune-mediated thrombocytopenia with uncontrolled bleed Chronic immune-mediated thrombocytopenia persisting at least 12–24 months

- Anemia disproportionate to the severity of bleeding
- Presence of weight loss
- Before starting corticosteroids.

Management

The majority (80%) of the children with ITP remit within 6 months. Hence, only reassurance is necessary in most cases. However, danger signs should be explained to the child and family members if platelet count is greater than 20,000/mm^3 with no bleeding.

Platelet transfusion should be given if count is less than 10,000/mm^3 irrespective of whether bleeding is present or not. The Working Party of British Committee for Standards in Hematology recommends the following:

- Treat mild cases with supportive advice and a 24-hour contact program.
- Intervention reserved only for children with organ or life-threatening bleeding irrespective of the platelet count.
- Any serious bleed should be managed with platelet support.

Drugs

Prednisolone (oral): 4 mg/kg/day for 4 days, followed by 2 mg/kg/day for 10 days, followed by tapering over the next 10 days. In a randomized controlled study, group receiving oral prednisolone (60 mg/m^2/day for 21 days) had a significantly faster platelet rise than the group receiving a placebo. Around 90% of the children achieved a platelet count of 30 × 10^9/L within the first 10 days.

Methylprednisolone (IV): 30 mg/kg/day for 3–5 days. It seems wise to use high-dose corticosteroids regimens for as short a time as necessary to achieve a meaningful end point.

Intravenous immunoglobulin: 1 g/kg for 2 days. High-dose IVIg blocks the fragment crystallizable receptors on macrophages in the reticuloendothelial system, especially spleen, causing

Table 11.11.4: Qualitative platelet disorders.	
Adhesion defects	Bernard–Soulier syndrome von Willebrand disease
Primary aggregation defects	Glanzmann's thrombasthenia Congenital afibrinogenemia
Platelet secretion disorders	Storage pool diseases Hermansky–Pudlak Chediak–Higashi Gray platelet syndrome
Arachidonic acid pathway defects	Cyclooxygenase deficiency Thromboxane synthetase deficiency
Others	Platelet factor 3 deficiency Idiopathic afibrinogenemia

dramatic increase in platelets. The randomized controlled trial by Blanchette et al. showed IVIg equivalent to oral steroids in the early rise of platelet count to greater than 20 × 10^9/L and superior to oral steroids in the rise of platelet count to greater than 50 × 10^9/L.

Anti-D globulins (IV rhesus immune globulin): A single dose of 75 µg/kg of anti-D globulin can be recommended as standard dosing for treatment of children with acute ITP, who are rhesus (D) positive. Beneficial effect is due to the competitive inhibition of reticuloendothelial function by preferential sequestration of immunoglobulin-coated autologous red blood cells. In a randomized clinical trial in 101 children by Tarantino et al., IV anti-D 75 µg/kg was found to be superior to IV anti-D 50 µg/kg but was equivalent to IVIg given in a dose of 0.8 g/kg with respect to platelet count greater than 20 × 10^9/L at 24 hours after therapy.

Table 11.11.3 lists other modalities of treatment which are less commonly used.

QUALITATIVE PLATELET DISORDERS

Qualitative platelet defects are not common and are enlisted in **Table 11.11.4**.

11.12 Evaluation of a Child with Thrombosis

Tulika Seth

INTRODUCTION

Thrombosis can cause significant morbidity and mortality in newborns and children. Excessive coagulation or abnormal hemostasis leading to the formation of a thrombus can potentially obstruct blood flow. Thrombosis may be venous or arterial. This is a relatively uncommon emergency in pediatrics. However, it is important to ensure early diagnosis and a proper management to reduce permanent sequelae.

EPIDEMIOLOGY

- Critically ill children may develop thrombosis due to inflammation, infection, disseminated intravascular coagulation (DIC), and impaired liver function and from central venous or arterial catheters.
- Sick newborns are at higher risk as children till 6 months of age have lower levels of the vitamin K-dependent coagulation factors II, IX, and X, compared to adults.
- Thrombin inhibitors, such as antithrombin and heparin cofactor II, and proteins C and S are low at birth. Protein S levels reach adult levels by 1 year of age, but protein C levels remain low throughout childhood.
- Plasminogen levels are low in newborns and infants.
- Thrombin generation is decreased (due to low prothrombin levels) and delayed in newborns compared with adults.
- The incidence of thrombosis peaks in infants younger than 1 year and again during adolescence.

ETIOPATHOGENESIS

The process of hemostasis is divided into a *cellular* and *fluid* phase. The former involves platelets and the vascular wall, while the latter involves plasma proteins. The *fluid phase* is divided into three processes:

1. The multiple-step zymogen pathway that leads to thrombin generation
2. Thrombin-induced formation of fibrin clot
3. Complex fibrinolytic mechanisms which limit clot propagation.

Current evidence suggests that there is an overlap between the previously described intrinsic and extrinsic pathways and an important interaction between cells directly involved in hemostasis [i.e. tissue factor (TF)-bearing cells and platelets] and the coagulation factors. Tissue factor-VIIa complex activates factors in both extrinsic and intrinsic systems. The cell-based model of coagulation identifies the membranes of TF-bearing cells and platelets as the site of activation of specific coagulation factors. It has three phases:

1. Initiation
2. Amplification
3. Thrombin production and action.

The *initiation* occurs after a vascular injury, with the binding of cells that bear tissue, which activate factor VII. This produces a small amount of thrombin, which activates platelets and cofactors in the *amplification* phase. The prothrombinase complex (factor Xa + cofactors bound to activated platelets) is responsible for the burst of *thrombin production*, which leads to the third phase of *clot formation*.

The coagulation cascade is triggered after injury to a blood vessel allowing exposure to TF-bearing cells. The factor Xa and activated factor V (Va) as a cofactor propagate coagulation by converting prothrombin (factor II) to thrombin (factor IIa). Factor Xa is central to the amplification of this process. This process may be set off by inherited prothrombotic factors **(Box 11.12.1)** but are more commonly due to inflammation, vasculitis, infection, malignancy, etc.

Box 11.12.1: Risk factors for thrombosis in children.

- *Time-limited risk factors:*
  - Indwelling catheters
  - Infections
  - Surgery
  - Disseminated intravascular coagulation
  - Postinfectious transient antiphospholipid antibodies
  - Surgically correctable congenital heart disease (risk decreases once corrected)
    - Ongoing risk factors
    - Inherited thrombophilias
  - Factor V Leiden
  - Deficient antithrombin, protein C, protein S
  - Elevated homocysteine level
  - Elevations in lipoprotein (a)
  - Other less common genetic disorders of coagulation regulation or fibrinolysis
- *Acquired thrombophilias and prothrombotic states:*
  - Primary antiphospholipid antibody
  - Acquired decrease in coagulation regulatory proteins (nephrotic syndrome, protein-losing enteropathy)
  - Indwelling catheters
  - Leukemia, solid tumors, and chemotherapy (e.g. L-asparaginase)
  - Inflammatory diseases (e.g. Systemic lupus erythematosus, inflammatory bowel disease)
  - Prosthetic cardiac valves
  - Sickle cell anemia
  - Thalassemia intermedia
  - Diabetes mellitus

CLINICAL FEATURES

- Symptoms of thrombosis vary with the site and type—whether venous or arterial **(Figs. 11.12.1A and B)**.
- In deep vein thrombosis (DVT), there may be pain and swelling of the limb. Pulmonary embolism (PE) may present with anxiety, breathlessness, pleuritic chest pain, fever, and cough; and a high index of suspicion is required to identify this early.
- Symptoms of central nervous system (CNS) thrombosis include vomiting, lethargy, seizures, or weakness in an extremity.
- Stroke may occur in utero, in newborns may present with seizures and lethargy. In older children the presentation is with headaches and acute onset of weakness in an extremity/hemiplegia, with a preceding episode of infection, dehydration, or trauma.
- Patients with renal vein thrombosis may present with flank pain and hematuria.
- Signs, such as limb edema, erythema, and tenderness on dorsiflexion of the foot (positive Homan's sign), are present in DVT but are difficult to elicit in young children.
- Thrombosis of the inferior vena cava (IVC) and/or renal vein can cause flank tenderness.
- Signs of PE are nonspecific and include diaphoresis, tachycardia, and tachypnea.

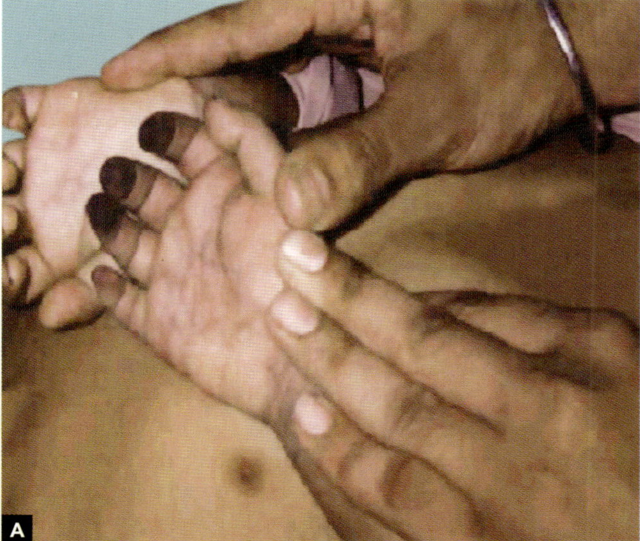

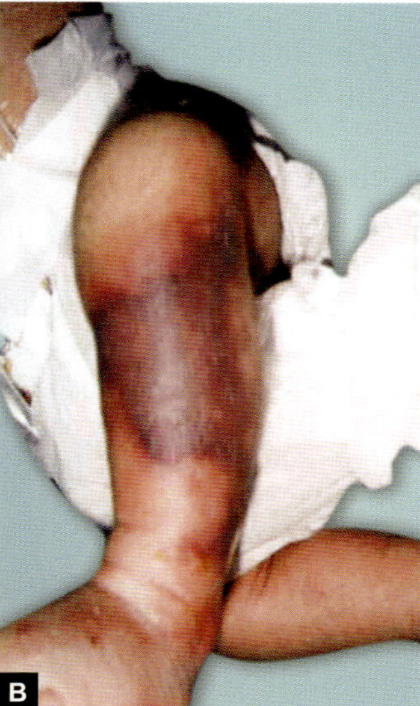

Figs. 11.12.1A and B: Children with thrombosis. (A) Gangrene following microvascular thrombosis; (B) Purpura fulminans.
Courtesy: Dr MR Lokeshwar, Mumbai, Maharashtra and Dr A Sachdeva, New Delhi, India.

- Signs of arterial thrombosis include diminished or absent peripheral pulses and a coolness of extremity skin, with ischemic changes if not diagnosed early.

Some important sites and their clinical features and risk factors are described below.

Cerebral Sinovenous Thrombosis

The cerebral sinovenous system comprises superficial cortical veins, superior sagittal sinus, lateral sinuses and deep, straight sinus, vein of Galen, internal cerebral and jugular veins. The important risk factors for thrombosis are infection and trauma of the head and neck. Other factors include perinatal complications in newborn infants (e.g. hypoxia and placental abruption), bacterial sepsis, connective tissue disorders, hematologic disorders (e.g. sickle cell disease, leukemia, pediatric myelodysplasia, and paroxysmal nocturnal hemoglobinuria), solid tumors, cardiac disease, indwelling vascular catheter, prothrombotic states (antiphospholipid antibodies or lupus anticoagulant; factor V Leiden or prothrombin G20210A; acquired deficiency of protein S, protein C, or antithrombin III), procoagulant drugs (e.g. L-asparaginase). A small percentage of patients (2%) will not have any identifiable risk factor.

Renal Vein Thrombosis

Neonates may develop thrombosis of a renal vein. Risk factors are polycythemia, dehydration, gestational diabetes (as it is associated with polycythemia and respiratory distress), asphyxia, sepsis, and hypercoagulable states (protein C deficiency, antithrombin III deficiency). The newborn presents with flank mass, hematuria, hypertension, thrombocytopenia, and oliguria. Diagnosis requires a high clinical suspicion with appropriate diagnostic tests, e.g. ultrasonography. The infant should be evaluated for a hypercoagulable state if no other causative factor is identified.

Protein C Deficiency

This usually presents in early infancy or childhood. There may be a history of consanguinity in the family. The parents are heterozygous for the protein C defect. A marked deficiency of protein C (<1% of normal) is usually associated with a homozygous or double heterozygous deficiency. Recurrent episodes of purpura fulminans and/or DVT will occur unless anticoagulation therapy is given. It may be difficult to differentiate this from DIC in a newborn.

Activated Protein C Resistance Ratio

Activated protein C (APC) normally has an anticoagulant effect. Some patients with recurrent venous thrombosis do not show the expected anticoagulant effect when APC is added to clotting tests, and these persons are termed "resistant" to the anticoagulant effect of APC. This is usually due to an autosomal dominant inherited mutation in factor V (factor V Leiden), which resists proteolysis by APC when activated to factor Va.

Antiphospholipid Syndrome

Antiphospholipid syndrome (APS) is a disorder that manifests clinically as recurrent venous or arterial thrombosis and/or fetal loss. If either lupus anticoagulants or increased anticardiolipin antibodies levels are present, APS should be suspected. The diagnosis should not be made on a single abnormal test. It is important to demonstrate that the antibody is persistent in a patient with appropriate clinical findings, with at least two positive values at least 6 weeks apart.

The diagnosis of the APS (according to the Sydney criteria or Sapporo classification) requires at least one of the clinical criteria and one of the four laboratory criteria listed below.

Clinical Criteria

- One or more vascular thrombosis in any artery, vein, or small vessel in the absence of vasculitis
- Three or more unexplained consecutive abortions before the 10th week of gestation with normal maternal and paternal cytogenetics and normal maternal anatomy
- One or more unexplained fetal death after the 10th week of gestation with normal fetal morphology
- One or more premature birth before the 34th week of gestation because of eclampsia or severe preeclampsia
- One or more premature birth before the 34th week of gestation with placental insufficiency.

Laboratory Criteria

- Lupus anticoagulant on two or more occasions 12 or more weeks apart
- Immunoglobulin G (IgG) and/or IgM anticardiolipin antibody at moderate-to-high titers (>40 G phospholipids or M phospholipids units) on two or more occasions 12 or more weeks apart
- Immunoglobulin G and/or IgM anti-beta-2-glycoprotein antibody on two or more occasions 12 or more weeks apart
- Mixed (more than one of the above).

Portal Vein Thrombosis

In children, portal vein thrombosis is rare, it may occur if certain risk factors are present. These may involve the liver, the portal vein, or the intra-abdominal structures drained by the portal vein. Known risk factors are intra-abdominal infection or inflammation; decreased blood flow due to cirrhosis with portal hypertension or fibrosis; mass lesion interfering with blood flow including congenital anomalies; hypercoagulable states—protein S or protein C deficiency, antithrombin III deficiency, or factor V Leiden; vascular injury from blunt abdominal trauma, catheterization, infusion of drugs or hyperosmolar glucose into the umbilical vein and exchange transfusion via umbilical vein.

MODALITIES OF DIAGNOSIS

- If venous thrombosis is present, look for fever, recent surgery, trauma, central venous catheter use, nephrotic syndrome, varicella, and other infections.
- Elicit a history of any previous thrombosis. Obtain a thorough family history to suggest inherited thrombophilia states **(Box 11.12.2)**.
- Inquire for a history or symptoms suggestive of congenital heart disease and/or recent cardiac catheterization, which are the most common causes of arterial thrombosis in children.

Laboratory Studies

- Many clotting factors are consumed in the clot formation, and some tests are hindered by the concomitant use of heparin or warfarin, and the reported low protein C and protein S level may be the result of the existing thrombosis. Hence, tests need to take account of the current status and type of antithrombotic medications being given.
- The child should be evaluated to rule out DIC, complete blood counts with peripheral blood smear, prothrombin time (PT), activated partial thromboplastin time (aPTT), and fibrinogen level **(Box 11.12.2 and Fig. 11.12.2)**.

Box 11.12.2: Initial workup for thrombosis to evaluate for hypercoagulable state.

- Complete hemogram (Hb/TLC/platelet count, DLC, peripheral blood film)
- PT/aPTT
- Radiology as indicated by symptoms
- Activated protein C resistance and/or factor V Leiden mutation
- Antithrombin
- Lupus anticoagulant (which may be screened by using the dilute Russell viper venom test)
- Anticardiolipin antibodies
- Ipoprotein (a) level
- Plasma homocysteine values
- Prothrombin gene *20210A* mutation (infrequent in India)
- Protein C (usually decreased in acute thrombosis)
- Free and total protein S (usually decreased in acute thrombosis)
- Warfarin therapy affects protein C, protein S, and antithrombin assay
- Heparin therapy (both unfractionated and low molecular weight) affects antithrombin, protein C, protein S, and APC resistance assays
- Neither drug affects the results of anticardiolipin antibodies, factor V Leiden, the prothrombin mutation, lipoprotein (a) nor homocysteine levels

(APC: activated protein C; aPTT: activated partial prothrombin time; DLC: differential leukocyte count; Hb; hemoglobin; PT: prothrombin time; TLC: total leukocyte count)

Imaging Studies

Imaging studies are difficult as the child requires sedation, and the small size of blood vessels makes the imaging even more complex.

- *Color Doppler imaging* is performed in vessels with thrombosis. The Doppler signals are absent, and the lumen cannot be compressed with direct pressure in a thrombosed vessel. However, this may not be sufficiently sensitive to detect thrombosis in certain vessels, such as subclavian veins, superior vena cava, or brachiocephalic veins.
- *Echocardiography* is of great utility in detecting vena caval and proximal subclavian vein thrombosis.
- *Central nervous system imaging*: A contrast-enhanced head computed tomography (CT) is useful for detecting venous sinus thrombosis. However, both magnetic resonance imaging (MRI) and magnetic resonance angiography are better at detecting early arterial ischemic strokes and suspected CNS thrombosis.
- *Chest radiography* can show the classic findings of PE, including small pleural effusions with a wedge-shaped pleural-based opacity of pulmonary infarction, but frequently the X-ray of chest may be normal.
- *Pulmonary imaging*: Multirow detector CT pulmonary angiography and pulmonary CT angiography studies are successful in visualizing arteries to the level of segmental pulmonary arteries, but the evaluation of subsegmental pulmonary arteries is limited to 80% visualization.
- *Ventilation-perfusion (V/Q) scanning* is the procedure of choice in children with suspected PE. As an alternative, if D-dimer levels are elevated and if the V/Q scan indicates intermediate probability, spiral CT may be useful.

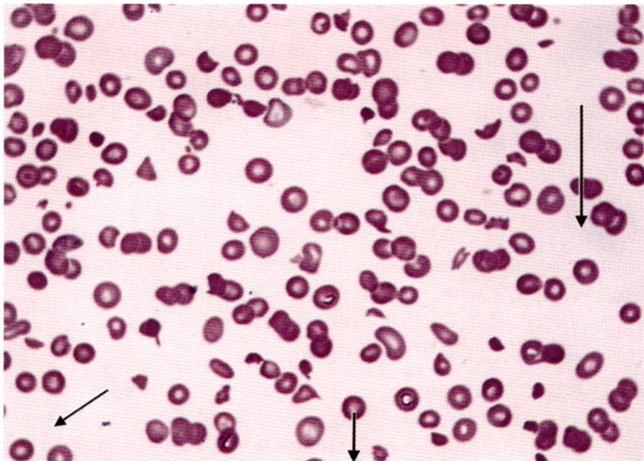

Fig. 11.12.2: Picture of DIC. This picture shows decreased platelets, spherocytes, and fragmented red cells.
(DIC: disseminated intravascular coagulation)

Table 11.12.1: Dosage for antithrombotic therapy in children.

Age	Dose	Monitoring
Oral warfarin		
Age	***Dose***	***Monitoring***
Infants younger than a year Older children	Up to 0.5 mg/kg/day 0.1–0.15 mg/kg/day	The *INR* is first measured after 3–5 days of therapy Warfarin should be overlapped with heparin. Heparin should not be discontinued until the INR is in therapeutic range for two consecutive readings INR between 2 and 3 is therapeutic range
LMWH (enoxaparin) q12h subcutaneous route		
Age	***Dose***	***Monitoring (necessary in neonates and to be avoided if renal dysfunction)***
Newborns less than 1-month-old Infants between 1 month and 1 year of age Children 1–5 years of age Children 6–18 years of age	1.625 mg/kg 1.5 mg/kg 1.375 mg/kg 1.25 mg/kg	Antifactor Xa activity 0.5–1.0 U/mL
UFH by continuous intravenously *(Loading dose, U/kg initial maintenance dose)* (Used less due to risk of heparin-induced thrombocytopenia and safety and experience with LMWH)		
Age	***Loading (maintenance dose)***	***Monitoring***
Neonates 28–37 weeks of gestation Infants at least 37 weeks of gestation Infants and children older than 1 month	50 U/kg (15 U/kg/h) 100 U/kg (28 U/kg/h) 75 U/kg (20 U/kg/h)	Baseline aPTT is prolonged in neonates and infants, may be difficult to monitor Therapeutic range aPTT is 2× of normal

(aPTT: activated partial thromboplastin time; INR: international normalized ratio; LMWH: low-molecular-weight heparin; UFH: unfractionated heparin)

MANAGEMENT

Once a diagnosis of thrombosis is made, the child needs urgent management to prevent mortality and late sequelae. If sick, stabilization is required, and if respiratory distress or neurological problems exist, management in an intensive care unit is required. Screening tests for hypercoagulable state should be sent prior to initiating anticoagulation therapy if possible. Initial therapy requires heparin [unfractionated heparin (UFH) or low-molecular-weight heparin (LMWH)], followed by oral warfarin therapy **(Table 11.12.1)**.

Close monitoring is required to prevent overdosage and the risk of bleeding. Underdosing will hamper resolution of the thrombus; most early recurrent thrombosis is due to inadequate therapy. The decision for long-term thrombosis depends on the risk of recurrence; this can be assessed by testing for thrombophilia status after 3 months of event and after stopping anticoagulants. The *international normalized ratio (INR)*, which is the ratio of PT of patient to standard, is the most useful test for monitoring oral anticoagulation. The INR therapeutic range is 2–3. Because the effects of LMWH on thrombin are minimal, the aPTT prolongation by LMWH is also correspondingly small. Hence, aPTT can be used for the monitoring of UFH only, and for LMWHs, the antifactor Xa assay may be needed in the presence of renal compromise or extreme obesity, and in newborns.

Box 11.12.3: Contraindications to antithrombotic treatment in infants and children.

For unfractionated heparin:
- Known allergy to heparin
- History of heparin-induced thrombocytopenia

For low-molecular-weight heparin:
- Known allergy to low-molecular-weight preparation
- History of heparin-induced thrombocytopenia
- Plan to perform an invasive procedure within 24 hours
- Thrombolysis by interventional radiology
- Limitations due to small size of involved vessels
- Known allergy
- Systemic tissue plasminogen activator
- Active bleeding
- Central nervous system ischemia/hemorrhage/surgery (includes birth asphyxia) in last 7–10 days
- Seizures within the last 48 hours
- Had an invasive procedure within the last 3 days

History of heparin-induced thrombocytopenia:
- Argatroban (not available in India) or Fondaparinux may be used—this product available in India

Newer guidelines recommend UFH also be monitored by anti-Xa activity; however, this is available in only few hospitals in India. Thrombolytic agents can be administered systemically or locally. The most relevant monitoring during thrombolytic therapy is clot lysis as determined by objective imaging. Clots should be imaged prior to and at the end of thrombolytic therapy.

Some children may need special care in the selection of anticoagulant medication or may need alternative therapy due to contraindications to anticoagulation; these children may benefit from the placement of a temporary IVC filter **(Box 11.12.3)**. Any IVC filter should be removed as soon as possible, as prolonged placement may make removable impossible and require lifelong anticoagulation due to the IVC filter.

Antithrombin activity is necessary to mediate the anticoagulant effect of heparin. This is decreased physiologically in well-term infants, more so in sick preterm infants, and low in children with extensive thromboses, nephrotic syndrome, or on L-asparaginase chemotherapy. A baseline aPTT within the normal range for age can be used to monitor UFH with a target aiming for a prolongation to 2–3 times the baseline value. If LMWH used in newborns, it is essential to monitor with the specific assays, else best to use UFH in these cases.

COMPLICATIONS

The sequelae can be devastating and permanent; they will depend on the site, extent, and duration of thrombosis.

- In utero, CNS thrombosis or placental thrombosis may lead to severe, irreversible neurologic damage.
- Superior sagittal vein thrombosis, if managed early, may have only slight residual weakness which may resolve.
- Arterial thrombosis may lead to vascular compromise and even loss of limb.
- Postphlebitic syndrome is characterized by persistent swelling, skin discoloration, and pain. It is very common if delayed treatment of DVT and is difficult to treat. This may cause significant stress and impairment in the quality of life.

PROGNOSIS

Predictors of a poor outcome in a child with thrombosis can be evaluated by factor VIII and D-dimer levels. The factors found to correlate with a poor thrombotic outcome are:

- The presence of residual thrombosis at 3 months or 6 months after onset
- Recurrent thromboembolism within 2 years in a previously unaffected venous system
- Development of postthrombotic syndrome.

Children with elevated factor VIII and/or D-dimer at presentation with thrombosis or persisting after 3–6 months after standard duration of anticoagulant therapy need close follow-up and longer therapy.

Recent Advances

- Factor Xa activates clotting over a wider concentration range than thrombin. New *direct factor Xa inhibitors or direct acting oral anticoagulants* (DOAC) possess many properties of an ideal anticoagulant, including oral administration, rapid onset of action, and predictable pharmacokinetics and pharmacodynamics, with reduced need for monitoring. These include rivaroxaban, apixaban, and edoxaban. Rivaroxaban, apixaban, etc. have been approved in Europe for the management and prevention of venous thromboembolism in adult patients.
- Parenteral direct *thrombin inhibitors* are currently available for clinical use—lepirudin, bivalirudin, dabigatran, and argatroban. However, even though they have been available for some time, pediatric use is limited due to safety issues and lack of approval for children. Bleeding episodes can be as severe as with other agents and are difficult to control; Dabigatran has a specific antidote—idarucizumab (a monoclonal antibody); others will need prothrombin complexes to control bleeding.
- Thrombin has a central role in the coagulation cascade. Produced in small amounts in the initiation phase and large amounts in the propagation phase, thrombin is essential for the amplification of coagulation and fibrin formation. Parenteral direct *thrombin inhibitors* currently available are argatroban or fondaparinux and can be used for anticoagulation in patients with heparin-induced thrombocytopenia.
- However, DOACs/novel oral anticoagulants are still not routinely used in children; they are not well studied in children with cancer. Risk of bleeding is present, and they are difficult to reverse; this makes these agents less useful for sick children.
- An anticoagulant protein isolated from mosquito saliva inhibits thrombosis by blocking platelet adhesion. *Anopheline antiplatelet protein* interferes with the link between collagen and the platelet glycoprotein VI receptor.
- Adenosine diphosphate (ADP) is the ligand for both P2Y1 and P2Y12 receptors. Stimulation of P2Y1 receptors initiates platelet activation and aggregation. Activation of P2Y12 amplifies the process. *The P2Y12 receptor* is the target for the thienopyridines group of drugs—clopidogrel and ticlopidine. Prasugrel, a new thienopyridine, binds P2Y12 more avidly than clopidogrel.
- A different approach to platelet inhibition involves the hydrolysis of ADP into inactive adenosine monophosphate, thereby removing this potent stimulant from the platelet's microenvironment. Cluster of differentiation (CD) 39, found on epithelial surfaces, has a hydrolytic function that confers both anti-inflammatory and anti-thrombotic properties. Recombinant human CD39 has been shown to inhibit platelet aggregation in vivo.

CASE SCENARIO

A 15-month-old boy presented with lethargy and seizures after 3–4 days low-grade fever, vomiting, and diarrhea. Initial examination showed responsiveness only to painful stimuli, extensor posturing, and hyperreflexia of the lower extremities (left greater than right) with bilateral clonus. Hemoglobin was 12.9 g/dL, total leukocytes count 5,000/mm^3, and platelet count was 325,000/L. Cerebrospinal fluid showed normal white and red cell counts and glucose and a protein level of 262 g/dL. An MRI showed thrombosis of the straight sinus and internal cerebral veins, hemorrhage in the posterior limb of the left internal capsule. The patient was started on continuous UFH infusion. Increased intracranial pressure was treated with dexamethasone and mannitol.

A partial workup for hypercoagulable disease was performed. Factor V Leiden, anticardiolipin antibodies, beta-2 glycoprotein, and serum homocysteine were within normal limits. The patient was discharged on warfarin, with regular monitoring of INR from the outpatient department. On follow-up, after 6 months of oral anticoagulation, his complete thrombophilia workup was performed. Protein C, protein S, and antithrombin were found to be normal. Repeat MRI showed resolution, and anticoagulation was stopped. On follow-up at 4 years of age, the child had a normal neurologic examination, except for a slight terminal tremor in the right upper extremities.

PRACTICE GUIDELINES

- Early initiation of treatment is required for good outcome.
- Standard dosing and monitoring is essential.
- Lifelong anticoagulation is not needed in all children.
- Consultation with a hematologist for severe thrombosis and to get the appropriate thrombophilia tests performed, as this may be a life-threatening condition.
- The baseline aPTT is prolonged in neonates and infants.
- Unfractionated heparin does not result in a linear prolongation of the aPTT, and regular monitoring is essential.

PRACTICE POINTS/TIPS

- Inadequate dosing results in recurrent thrombosis and frequent boluses may put the child at risk for hemorrhage.
- Unfractionated heparin and LMWH have similar results; the clinical scenario will dictate which will be used.
- The need for monitoring depends on the underlying disease and risk for bleeding in the individual case.
- Due to fear of bleeding complications associated with anticoagulants, clinicians are reluctant to treat neonates and children with thrombosis aggressively, despite a high prevalence of short- and long-term sequelae in this age-group.

KEY MESSAGES

- Thrombosis needs treatment.
- Investigate to find the underlying cause.
- Treat other comorbid factors.
- Initial thrombophilia workup prior to anticoagulation (if possible).
- Repeat thrombophilia workup after 3–6 months.

BIBLIOGRAPHY

1. Ghosh K, Ghosh K. Advances in haematological pharmacotherapy in 21st century. Indian J Hematol Blood Transfus. 2010;26(2):30-40.
2. Goldenberg NA, Knapp-Clevenger R, Manco-Johnson MJ, et al. Elevated plasma factor VIII and D-dimer levels as predictors of poor outcome of thrombosis in children. N Engl J Med. 2004;351(11):1081-8.
3. Hoffman M, Monroe DM. Coagulation 2006: a modern view of hemostasis. Hematol Oncol Clin North Am. 2007;21(1):1-11.
4. Kearon C, Akl EA, Ornelas J, et al. Antithrombotic therapy for VTE disease: CHEST guideline and expert panel report. Chest. 2016;149(2):315-52.
5. Manco-Johnson MJ. How I treat venous thrombosis in children. Blood. 2006;107(1):21-9.
6. Miyakis S, Lockshin MD, Atsumi T, et al. International consensus statement on an update of the classification criteria for definite antiphospholipid syndrome (APS). J Thromb Haemost. 2006;4(6):295-306.
7. Sharma SK, Kumar S, Seth T, et al. Eosinophilia: rare cause of arterial thrombosis and cardioembolic stroke in childhood. World J Cardiol. 2012;4(4):128-9.
8. Seth T. Thrombosis in neonates and children. East J Med. 2009;14:36-45.
9. Tormene D, Gavasso S, Rossetto V, et al. Thrombosis and thrombophilia in children: a systematic review. Semin Thromb Hemost. 2006;32(7):724-8.

11.13 Disseminated Intravascular Coagulation

Anupam Sachdeva

INTRODUCTION

Disseminated intravascular coagulation (DIC) is a syndrome characterized by massive activation of coagulation that occurs inside the blood vessels, leading to widespread deposition of fibrin in the small vessels, thus compromising blood supply to major organ systems. At the same time the ongoing coagulation consumes platelets and coagulation factors, leading to severe bleeding. Disseminated intravascular coagulation is never a disease per se; it is always secondary to an underlying disorder that causes activation of coagulation in vivo.

ETIOLOGY

- Disseminated intravascular coagulation is seen in 0.4–1% of hospitalized children. In children, 95% of the cases are due to underlying infections.
- Disseminated intravascular coagulation is a clinical diagnosis, based on deranged laboratory values in a patient with an underlying disease that is known to be associated with DIC. It is usually a rare complication of many of the diseases listed in **Table 11.13.1**.

PATHOGENESIS

Initiating Disseminated Intravascular Coagulation

The various stimuli that initiate DIC act on the normal processes that activate coagulation, viz. platelet adhesion and aggregation, and activation of coagulation process either by contact factor activation (intrinsic pathway) or tissue factor (TF) activation (extrinsic pathway). However, unlike in normal coagulation, these activating stimuli drive the coagulation process unchecked, thus preventing the normal compensatory processes. As a result, thrombin gets generated persistently, and fibrin strands are generated in the small blood vessels. Fibrinolytic pathways also get activated, thus leading to the formation of fibrin degradation products (FDPs), which per se impair the hemostatic function. Bleeding occurs because of the consumption of coagulation factors and platelets, whereas microvascular occlusion due to fibrin generation leads to organ dysfunction. This process perpetuates as a vicious cycle, and ultimately the interplay between various compensatory mechanisms (e.g. fibrin generation versus fibrinolysis, coagulation factor consumption versus repletion) dictates the clinical manifestation and course of the disease.

What Initiates Disseminated Intravascular Coagulation?

- In Gram-negative infections, endothelial injury occurs due to circulating endotoxins, resulting in collagen exposure, activation of platelets, and activation of TF. Any factor that increases the propagation of sepsis (e.g. immunosuppression) can foster DIC. There is no difference in the incidence of DIC in patients with Gram-negative or Gram-positive sepsis.
- In diseases, such as cancers, tissue injury, etc., there is the release of procoagulant tissue extracts into the circulation which then results in TF activation and generation of thrombin.
- Promyelocytes in acute promyelocytic leukemia (APML) express annexin II that results in increased plasmin production and increased fibrinolytic activity. Leukemic blasts also release TF-containing vesicles into the circulation.
- In obstetric complications, such as placental abruption, release of decidual fragments results in a similar process.
- In giant hemangiomas as in Kasabach-Merritt syndrome, there are large gaps in the endothelium that expose the subendothelial collagen which initiates the coagulation process.
- Disseminated intravascular coagulation is commonly observed with venomous snakebites worldwide. Hematological toxicity is observed commonly in viper envenomation. These venoms contain proteinases that activate the coagulation process; phospholipases that cause hemolysis of red cells and polypeptides that disrupt the endothelial lining. These result in the consumption of coagulation factors, fibrinolysis, and DIC.
- Further for the activation of coagulation is the release of cytokines, such as endotoxins, interleukin (IL)-1, IL-6, IL-8, platelet-activating factor, and tumor necrosis factor.

Table 11.13.1: Conditions associated with disseminated intravascular coagulation.

Infections: • Bacterial sepsis (gram-negative organisms, e.g. meningococcemia) • Viruses (HIV, CMV, varicella, herpes, rubella, acute hepatitis, Reye syndrome) • Fungal (histoplasma, aspergillosis) • Protozoal (malaria, kala-azar) • Rickettsial	*Tissue injury/organ failure:* • Polytrauma, massive head injury, and crush injury • Hypoxia/hypoperfusion and shock • Cardiac arrest • Hypothermia • Heat stroke • Extensive surgical intervention • Fat embolism • Extracorporeal circulation • Severe pancreatitis • Liver cell failure
Immunological conditions: • SLE • Autoimmune hemolytic anemia • Crohn's disease/ulcerative colitis • Transfusion reactions (ABO incompatibility) • *Transplant rejections*: Graft-versus-host disease	*Vascular abnormalities:* • Kasabach-Merritt syndrome • Large vascular aneurysms • Coarctation of aorta • Large prosthetic arterial grafts
Cancer: • Acute promyelocytic leukemia • Acute monoblastic leukemia • Lymphoproliferative disorders • Hemophagocytic lymphohistiocytosis • Solid tumors (neuroblastoma)	*Gastrointestinal disorders:* • Fulminant hepatitis • Severe inflammatory bowel disease
Neonatal conditions: • Maternal toxemia • Maternal infections • Dead twin • Abruptio placentae • Amniotic fluid embolism • Necrotizing enterocolitis • Perinatal hypoxia • Congenital infections • Respiratory distress syndrome • Erythroblastosis fetalis	
Thrombotic disorders: • Homozygous protein C deficiency • Antithrombin III deficiency • Heparin-induced thrombosis	*Miscellaneous:* • Snakebites • Insect bites • Recreational drugs • *Poisoning*: Acute iron toxicity • Massive transfusions • Infusion of activated prothrombin complex concentrates

(CMV: cytomegalovirus; HIV: human immunodeficiency virus; SLE: systemic lupus erythematosus)

Propagation of Disseminated Intravascular Coagulation

Once initiated, there is accelerated turnover of platelets and coagulation factors. Natural anticoagulants, such as antithrombin and protein C, are also diminished in DIC. Impaired protein C pathway contributes to the procoagulant manifestation seen in this disease. The end result of coagulation pathway activation is the formation of strands of fibrin in the small blood vessels. Circulating red blood cells (RBCs) get injured while passing through microvasculature with intravascular fibrin strands, thus forming schistocytes. Fibrin deposition on endothelial surfaces activates the process of fibrinolysis thus resulting in the formation of FDPs **(Flowchart 11.13.1)**.

Chronic Disseminated Intravascular Coagulation

Otherwise known as compensated DIC, it occurs when the trigger is either a weak stimulus or is intermittent. Chronic DIC has been observed in giant hemangiomas, various vasculitis, aneurysms, and some forms of cancers. In such conditions the destruction and coagulation of clotting factors are balanced.

Flowchart 11.13.1: Pathophysiology clinical features in disseminated intravascular coagulation.

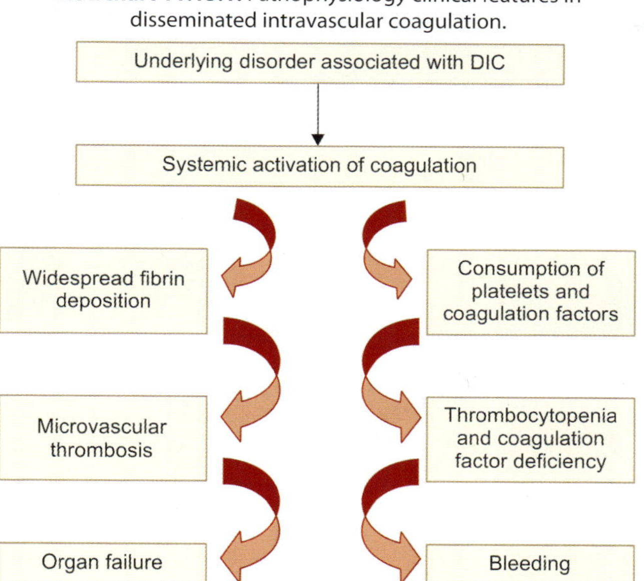

(DIC: Disseminated intravascular coagulation)

CLINICAL FEATURES

Bleeding

Typically seen in acute DIC, it is often abrupt, massive, and occurring from multiple sites. Bleeding, occurring from intravascular access sites, venipuncture sites, surgical wounds, is the early indications of DIC. Mucocutaneous bleeding in the form of petechiae, purpura, gum bleeding, and epistaxis may be noticed. Bleeding may also be noticed from tracheal tubes while suctioning. In advanced disease, gastrointestinal (GI) bleeding, hematuria leading to hemodynamic compromise, and intracranial bleeding leading to increased intracranial pressure; herniation of brain leading to respiratory compromise have been observed. Bleeding is often severe enough to lead to hypovolemia and hypoperfusion **(Figs. 11.13.1A and B)**.

Thrombosis

Generalized microvascular thrombosis leads to the development of purpura fulminans, peripheral acrocyanosis, and gangrenous changes in digits, genitalia, nose, and ears **(Figs. 11.13.1C and D)**. Sharply demarcated ecchymoses areas can occur due to thrombotic occlusion of dermal vessels. In advanced disease, microvascular occlusion leads to multiorgan failure **(Table 11.13.2)**.

In a recent study of the profile of DIC in over 5,000 hospitalized children, it was observed in 1.12% of the patients. The underlying etiology was infection in over 95% and major trauma in around 5% of the patients. Bleeding and thrombosis were observed in 48% and 4.8%, respectively. Multiorgan dysfunction was observed in 85% of these patients with DIC.

INVESTIGATIONS

There is no single laboratory test that can either confirm or rule out the diagnosis of DIC. Hence, it is of utmost importance to consider both the clinical background and the various laboratory variables while coming to a decision. Laboratory investigations are aimed at

- Identifying the underlying etiology.
- Demonstrating the evidence of consumption coagulopathy and increased activation of fibrinolytic cascade.
- Disseminated intravascular coagulation is a dynamic process. Laboratory values change rapidly; and hence, frequent monitoring is necessary to guide therapeutic decisions. The International Society for Thrombosis and Hemostasis Scientific Standardization, Subcommittee on DIC, proposed a scoring system based on four laboratory values: (1) prothrombin time (PT); (2) platelet count; (3) fibrin-related markers; and (4) fibrinogen level.

Complete blood Count

- *Thrombocytopenia* suggests thrombin-induced platelet aggregation leading to consumption of platelets. Platelets counts are usually in the range of 50,000–100,000/μL. Platelet count of less than 50,000/μL is noticed in around 50% of the cases. A single normal platelet count does not rule out DIC. A persistent downward trend in platelet count is a sensitive indicator of DIC.
- *Peripheral smear* shows fragmented RBCs or schistocytes. The percentage of schistocytes, however, does not correlate to clinical severity. Schistocytes are neither sensitive nor specific for the diagnosis of DIC. It may be seen in other cases of microangiopathy, such as thrombotic thrombocytopenic purpura (TTP).
- *Prothrombin time, activated partial thromboplastin time (aPTT), and thrombin time (TT)* are prolonged in around 50% of the cases of DIC due to the consumption of coagulation proteins. The other factors that lead to similar prolongation are liver disease, vitamin K deficiency, and massive bleeding per se. In some cases, PT and aPTT may be shortened or be normal, due to the presence of circulating activated coagulation factors, such as thrombin. Hence, normal PT and aPTT do not rule out DIC. Thrombin time is prolonged in greater than 50% of the cases due to low serum fibrinogen and high levels of circulating FDPs. Thrombin time per se again does not have a role in the diagnosis of DIC, but is helpful along with reptilase test to rule out heparin contamination.

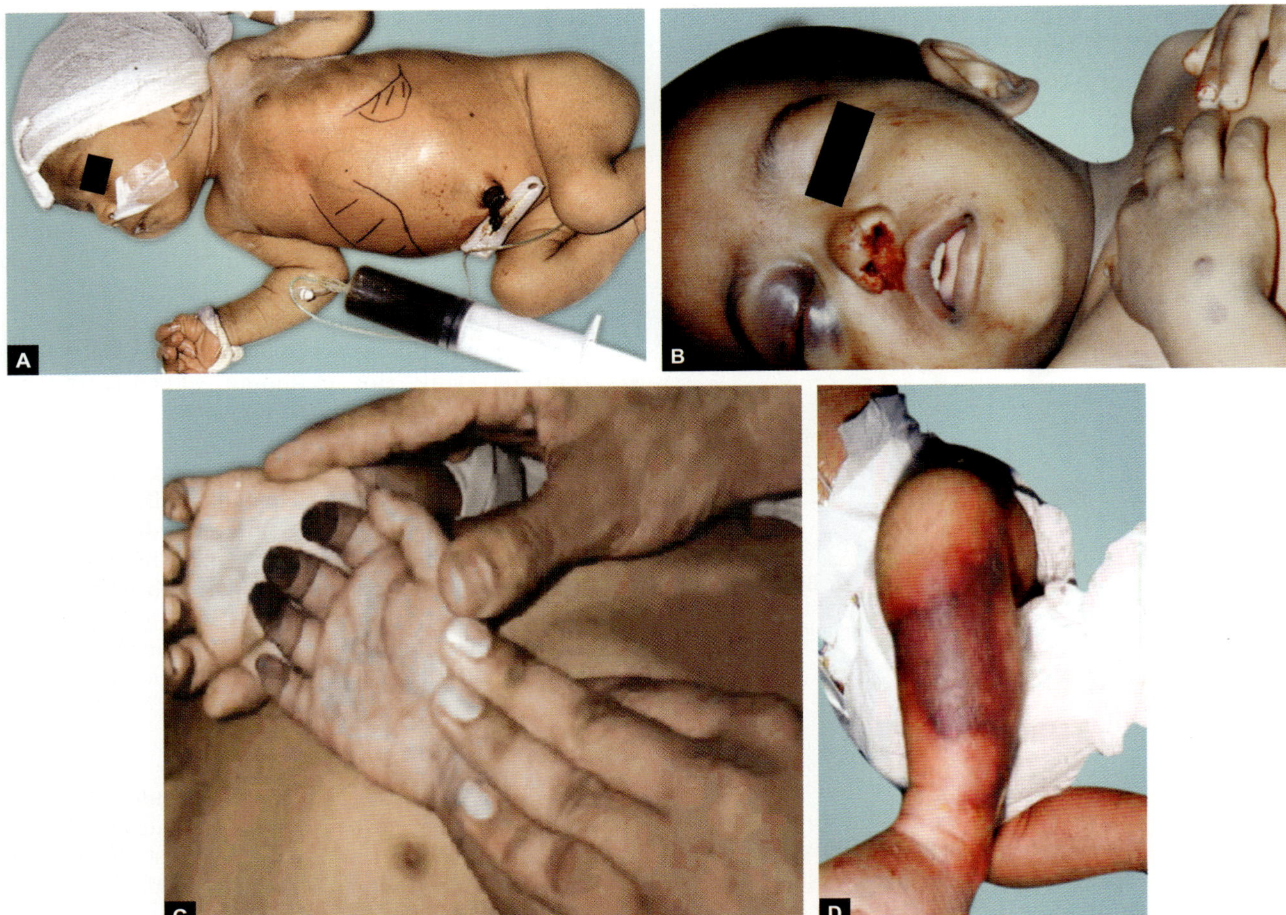

Figs. 11.13.1A to D: Clinical features of disseminated intravascular coagulation. (A) Disseminated intravascular coagulation in a newborn with hematuria; (B) Disseminated intravascular coagulation in a child; (C) Gangrene following microvascular thrombosis; and (D) Purpura fulminans.
Courtesy: MR Lokeshwar and Anupam Sachdeva.

- *Fibrin degradation products/D-dimer*: Fibrinolytic activity, measured as FDPs, is increased in DIC. D-Dimer assay, which measures cross-linked FDPs, is a sensitive test for the detection of DIC. Semiquantitative assays are used now. However, increased D-dimer levels are not specific for DIC and may be observed in trauma, recent surgery, and in venous thromboembolism (VTE). Hence, elevated levels should always be interpreted in the light of the clinical scenario and associated changes in platelet count and coagulation profile. Moreover, D-dimer helps in differentiating DIC from liver disease which is also associated with low platelet counts and altered coagulation profile, but is associated with normal D-dimer levels.
- *Serum fibrinogen*: Although being used as a marker for evidence of DIC, the levels of serum fibrinogen remain normal for a long period of time, as it is an acute phase reactant. Inflammatory conditions lead to the elevation of serum fibrinogen. Hence, a drop in fibrinogen to normal values in DIC may be interpreted as normal, unless monitored serially.

Table 11.13.2: Clinical manifestations.

Hemorrhagic	Skin and mucous membrane bleeding, hemorrhage from surgical incisions, drains, intravascular catheters, and venipuncture sites
Thrombotic	Peripheral acrocyanosis, purpura fulminans, gangrenous changes in digits, nose, and genitalia
Multiorgan dysfunction in disseminated intravascular coagulation	Deranged hepatic, renal, and cardiac function; jaundice; arrhythmias; oliguria; respiratory distress; gastrointestinal ulcerations; adrenal insufficiency; and CNS abnormalities

(CNS: Central nervous system)

Table 11.13.3: Scoring system for disseminated intravascular coagulation.
Risk assessment: Does the patients have an underlying disorder known to be associated with overt DIC? • *If yes*: Proceed • *If no*: Do not use this algorithm
Scoring system
1. *Platelet count*: – 100 × 10^9/L = 0 – <100 × 10^9/L = 1 – <50 × 10^9/L = 2
2. *Elevated fibrin marker (D-dimer, fibrin degradation products)*: – No increase = 0 – Moderate increase = 2 – Strong increase = 3
3. Prolonged PT – <3 seconds = 0 – 3 seconds but <6 seconds = 1 – >6 seconds = 2
4. Fibrinogen level – 1 g/L = 0 – <1 g/L = 1
Cumulative score
• *5*: Compatible with overt DIC. Advised to repeat score daily • *<5*: Suggestive for nonovert DIC. Advised to repeat every 1–2 days

(DIC: disseminated intravascular coagulation; PT: prothrombin time)

- *Other investigations*: Thrombin–antithrombin complexes and plasmin–antiplasmin complexes are often elevated in sepsis-associated DIC. Abnormal light transmission of aPTT is a recent investigation that has been shown to be a simple and rapid indicator of DIC.

Scoring System for Diagnosis of Disseminated Intravascular Coagulation

The International Society for Thrombosis and Hemostasis Scientific Standardization, Subcommittee on DIC has proposed a scoring system for the diagnosis and monitoring of DIC in 2001 **(Table 11.13.3)**.

A five-step diagnostic algorithm has been proposed that utilizes common investigations available in most hospitals. It is found to be useful in both acute and chronic DIC. The clinical setting for DIC is a must to use this algorithm. Score of greater than or equal to 5 has 91% sensitivity and 97% specificity for the diagnosis of DIC. For each point increase in DIC score, the odds ratio for mortality increases by 1.29.

DIFFERENTIAL DIAGNOSIS

- *Thrombotic thrombocytopenic purpura*: Patients present with thrombocytopenia, microangiopathic hemolysis, and multiorgan dysfunction. Differentiating features are the rarity of petechiae, purpura, and normal coagulation functions (PT, aPTT, TT, and FDP) in TTP.
- *Fulminant hepatic failure*: Decreased synthesis of coagulation factors along with thrombocytopenia due to portal hypertension with hypersplenism leads to laboratory values that suggest DIC. Moreover, FDP may be elevated due to reduced clearance in liver disease. However, the generalized bleeding tendency is less in liver disease compared to DIC. Bleeding is often due to varices, gastritis, or GI ulcers.

MANAGEMENT

The most important aspect of managing a patient with DIC is to identify the underlying disorder and control it. In few situations, resolution of the underlying condition leads to complete resolution of DIC by itself. Usually, supportive measures are required to control DIC until the underlying condition is resolved.

Treatment of Underlying Disorder

Although the replacement of coagulation factors and platelets helps in controlling DIC, identification and treatment of the underlying trigger for DIC is of utmost importance. In few situations, treatment of the underlying disorder itself will help reverse DIC.

Replacement Therapy

Rational therapy in patients who are bleeding or are at risk of bleeding is to attempt restoring the consumed platelets and coagulation factors.

- This is ensured by platelet transfusions and restoring coagulation factor by transfusing fresh frozen plasma (FFP), cryoprecipitate, and fibrinogen. Fears in the past of "feeding the fire" and worsening thrombosis by transfusing platelets and coagulation factors in patients with active DIC is no longer considered true.
- The decision for transfusion should be always based on the clinical condition and should not be based on the laboratory values alone.
- *Platelet transfusion*: A threshold of less than 50 × 10^9/L is used for platelet transfusion in patients with bleeding. In nonbleeding patients, a lower cutoff of 10–20 × 10^9/L may be used. However, in patients at high risk of bleeding, it is prudent to use a higher cutoff.
- *Plasma transfusion*: FFP may be administered at a dose of 15 mL/kg.
- The main aim of replacement therapy should be to replenish the fibrinogen. This can be achieved by administering cryoprecipitate (1 U = 250 mg fibrinogen), FFP, or purified fibrinogen concentrates when available.
- There are few case reports of the successful use of recombinant factor VIIa in the management of life-threatening hemorrhage in DIC.

- Therapy should never be instituted based on laboratory results alone and should always be guided by the clinical indications. So also, response should be monitored by both improvements in the clinical condition as well as normalization of laboratory variables.

ANTICOAGULATION

Anticoagulation with heparin is a rational approach to inhibit the activation of intravascular coagulation in DIC. Treatment with heparin should be considered in the cases where the thrombotic manifestations predominate, such as venous or arterial thromboembolism, peripheral ischemia, purpura fulminans, etc. It is beneficial in chronic DIC.

- In patients at high risk for bleeding, unfractionated heparin is preferred due to its short half-life and rapid reversibility. Small doses of 10 µg/kg/h may be used without targeting aPTT prolongation. It would be difficult to monitor heparin anyway due to the underlying coagulopathy.
- Again, anticoagulants are indicated for the prophylaxis of VTE in patients with DIC who are not bleeding.
- Use of heparin has been established in the cases of chronic DIC where recurrent thrombosis ensues.
- Anticoagulant factor concentrates, such as antithrombin concentrates and activated protein C concentrates, have been evaluated in DIC. There are no randomized trials to prove the efficacy of antithrombin supplementation. Activated protein C concentrates have been found to be beneficial in patients with DIC due to sepsis. However, there is a high risk of major bleeding, including intracranial hemorrhage.

ANTIFIBRINOLYTIC AGENTS

Antifibrinolytic agents that are used commonly in other bleeding diathesis, such as tranexamic acid, have limited benefit in patients with bleeding. As formation of fibrin predominates in the pathogenesis of consumptive coagulopathy, the use of fibrinolysis inhibitors has been debated. In some conditions, where there is a component of hypofibrinolysis (as in APML) to the DIC, it may be used. However, recent studies have failed to show any benefit in APML-associated DIC. Moreover, severe thrombosis may be observed when tranexamic acid is used along with differentiating agents, such as all transretinoic acid used in APML.

CONCLUSION

Disseminated intravascular coagulation results from continuous activation of hemostasis leading to pathological circulation of thrombin and fibrin. Clinical manifestations of DIC include bleeding or thrombosis, or both. Successful therapy of DIC hinges on identifying the triggering factor and switching off the activation of coagulation pathways. Valuable time should not be wasted trying to correct the abnormal laboratory values without attempting to correct the underlying disorder.

BIBLIOGRAPHY

1. Franchini M, Lippi G, Manzato F. Recent acquisitions in the pathophysiology, diagnosis and treatment of disseminated intravascular coagulation. Thromb J. 2006;4:4.
2. Labelle CA, Kitchens CS. Disseminated intravascular coagulation: treat the cause, not the lab values. Cleve Clin J Med. 2005;72(5):377-8.
3. Levi M, Opal SM. Coagulation abnormalities in critically ill patients. Crit Care. 2006;10(4):222.
4. Levi M, Toh CH, Thachil J, et al. Guidelines for the diagnosis and management of disseminated intravascular coagulation. British Committee for Standards in Haematology. Br J Haematol. 2009;145(1):24-33.
5. Oren H, Cingöz I, Duman M, et al. Disseminated intravascular coagulation in pediatric patients: clinical and laboratory features and prognostic factors influencing the survival. Pediatr Hematol Oncol. 2005;22(8):679-88.
6. Rodgers GM. Acquired coagulation disorders. In: Pine JW (Ed). Wintrobe's clinical hematology, 12th edition. Philadelphia, PA: Lippincott Williams and Wilkins; 2008. pp. 1425.

11.14 Transfusion Medicine and Component Therapy

Deepak Bansal, Rekha Hans

INTRODUCTION

Blood is categorized as a drug as per "Drugs and Cosmetic Act 1940," Government of India and rules therein, because of its use in treating diseases. The demand for this life-sustaining drug invariably exceeds the amount collected. Despite this, one third of the country's annual collection is wasted as single unit whole blood transfusions **(Table 11.14.1)**. Advances in transfusion therapy have improved blood preservation techniques and enabled separation of whole blood into its components. Component therapy has enabled the optimal use of every donation as specific components can be transfused selectively to different patients, depending on the actual need of an individual patient.

BLOOD COMPONENTS AND SEPARATION TECHNIQUES

Whole blood is made up of cellular elements [red blood cells (RBCs), leukocytes, and platelets] and plasma. Whole blood can be separated into its components depending on their specific gravity, by centrifugation techniques, as illustrated in **Flowchart 11.14.1**.

Apheresis is a specialized procedure, wherein, whole blood is removed from the donor and is then separated into its components by centrifugation in a cell separator **(Fig. 11.14.1)**. The desired components (e.g. platelets) are collected, and the remainder returned to the donor. The procedure allows selective collection of platelets or granulocytes in sufficient amounts from a single matched, ABO-compatible donor. Volume, storage temperature, and shelf life of different blood components are tabulated in **Table 11.14.2**.

Table 11.14.1: Blood component use in various countries.

Country	*% Used as whole blood*	*% Used as components*
India	31	69
South Korea	1	99
Sri Lanka	5	95
Nepal	30	70
Thailand	20	80

Whole Blood

There are very few indications for the use of whole blood. The major indication would be in some cases of cardiac surgery or

Flowchart 11.14.1: Separation of components from blood.

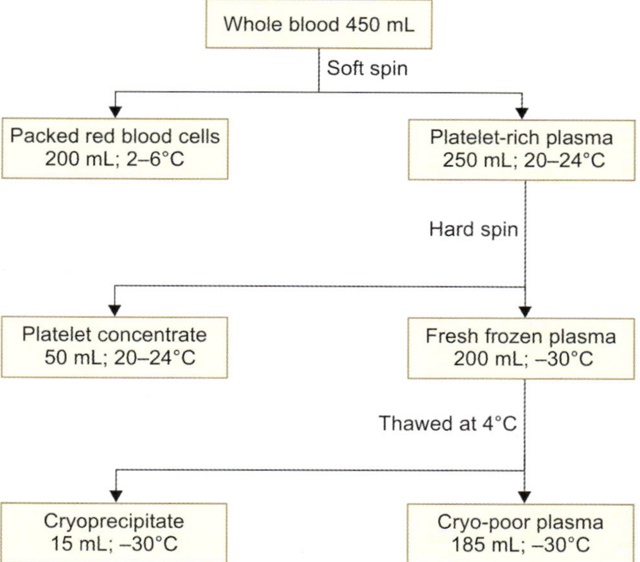

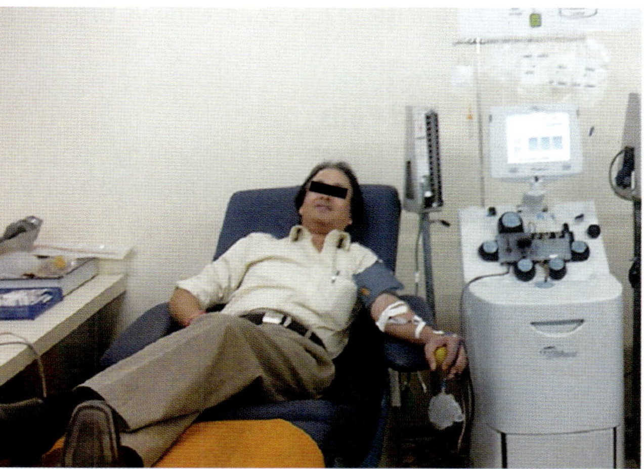

Fig. 11.14.1: Cell separator for the collection of specific components from whole blood or for plasmapheresis.

Table 11.14.2: Volume, storage temperature, and shelf life of blood and components.

	Volume (mL)	***Storage temperature (°C)***	***Shelf life***
Whole blood	400–500	2–6	35 days
Packed RBC (CPDA-1)	200–300		
Packed RBC–SAGM (nutrient solution)	250–350	2–6	42 days
Platelet concentrates	50–90	20–24	5 days
Fresh frozen plasma	150–220	<–30	1 year
Cryoprecipitate	15–20	<–30	1 year

(CPDA: citrate phosphate dextrose adenine; RBC: red blood cell; SAGM: saline, adenine, glucose, mannitol)

massive hemorrhage as in trauma. It may be the only choice for life-threatening hemorrhage when RBC component therapy is not available. For exchange transfusions in neonates, whole blood or reconstituted whole blood may be used.

Fresh Whole Blood

It is a myth that whole blood collected within 24 hours is the best. It is often requisitioned in bleeding disorders in the erroneous belief that it provides platelets and clotting factors. Almost 90% of platelets and 40% of activity of factor VIII are lost within 24 hours of storage at 4°C. In addition, time is required for mandatory screening for infections. This age old practice, therefore, has no role in modern times. Specific blood component therapy should be requested depending on the etiology of bleeding. For neonatal exchange transfusion, blood up to 7-10 days old is good enough to prevent hyperkalemia.

Packed Red Blood Cells

The usual dose for packed RBCs (PRBCs) is 10–15 mL/kg but varies greatly on the clinical indication **(Boxes 11.14.1 and 11.14.2)**.

- In severe [hemoglobin (Hb) <5 g/dL] chronic anemia, child should receive 2–3 aliquots of 3–5 mL/kg over 2–3 hours, separated by a few hours.
- A partial exchange transfusion may be considered in those presenting with overt features of congestive heart failure. This corrects the anemia rapidly and isovolumetrically.

Each unit of transfused PRBC is expected to increase the Hb level by 1 g/dL and hematocrit level by 3% in a 70-kg adult. In a pediatric patient, a dose of 10–15 mL/kg will increase the Hb by about 2–3 g/dL or hematocrit by 6–9%.

Box 11.14.1: Indications for packed red blood cells transfusion for neonates.

- *PCV < 36% and requiring:*
  - >35% supplemental oxygen
  - Mean airway pressure ≥ 6–8 cm H_2O by CPAP/IMV
- *PCV < 31% and:*
  - Requiring <35% supplemental oxygen or MAP < 6 cm H_2O by CPAP/IMV
  - >9 episodes of apnea and bradycardia in 12 hours or 2 episodes in 24 hours, requiring bag and mask ventilation while on methylxanthine
- *PCV < 40%* and
  - HR > 180 per minute or RR > 80 per minute, persisting for > 24 hours
  - Weight gain <10 g/day for 4 days, while on 120 kcal/kg/day
  - Undergoing surgery
- *PCV < 21%* and
  - Asymptomatic with reticulocytes < 2%
- Hypovolemic shock associated with acute blood loss

(CPAP: continuous positive airway pressure; HR: heart rate; IMV: intermittent mandatory ventilation; MAP: mean airway pressure; PCV: packed cell volume; RR: respiratory rate)

Box 11.14.2: Indications for PRBC transfusion for children more than or equal to 4 months of age.

- In deficiency anemia, with features of overt CHF. Often children with iron deficiency anemia are treated with oral iron alone, even with Hb < 5 g/dL
- *Thalassemia major*: Attempt should be made to maintain a pretransfusion Hb > 9–10 g/dL
- *Aplastic anemia*: Children often do well with Hb > 6 g/dL. Leukocyte filters (Fig. 11.14.2) should be utilized to prevent alloimmunization and graft rejection, if a BMT is planned
- *Malignancies*: Hb < 8 g/dL. Factors influencing decision include the intensity of chemotherapy and timing (counts expected to rise or fall)
- *Significant preoperative anemia*: Individual approach is necessary; most children who do not have cardiorespiratory disease do not require Hb > 8 g/dL
- Postoperative Hb < 8 g/dL with symptoms/signs of anemia. Most children can quickly restore Hb with oral iron. There should be a compelling reason to administer a postoperative red cell transfusion
- *Pediatric ICU*: Restrictive strategy is gaining favor in the PICU. It has been demonstrated that in stable, critically ill children, an Hb of 7 is as good as 9.5 g/dL (children with severe hypoxia, hemodynamic instability, and cyanotic heart disease were excluded in the study). Blood is immunosuppressive. Cytokines released following the transfusion may contribute to enhanced inflammatory response and increased morbidity

(BMT: bone marrow transplant; CHF: congestive heart failure; Hb: hemoglobin; ICU: intensive care unit; PICU: pediatric intensive care unit; PRBC: packed red blood cell)

Caution: PRBC transfusion should be started within 30 minutes of removal of unit from refrigerator, and transfusion should be complete within 4 hours of commencement.

Washed Red Blood Cells

Patients who have severe allergic reactions to RBC transfusion may benefit from washed RBCs, as washing removes plasma, the cause of allergy. Washed RBCs should be used within 6–24 hours.

Platelet Transfusion and Plateletpheresis

The process of obtaining platelet-rich plasma and platelet concentrate is outlined in **Flowchart 11.14.1**.

Platelets derived from whole blood are known as random donor platelets (RDPs). Random donor platelets must contain at least 5.5×10^{10} platelets. The alternative approach involves the collection of single-donor platelets by apheresis using a cell separator **(Fig. 11.14.1)**. A single unit obtained from apheresis has 3×10^{11} platelets which equals to 5–6 RDPs. The yield is higher with single-donor platelets; in addition, the donor exposure is reduced. Platelets are stored at 20–24°C, under constant agitation for 5 days. Beyond this duration, the risk of bacterial contamination increases excessively. The dose of RDP is 1 U/10 kg of body weight or 5–10 mL/kg for newborns. Indications include disseminated intravascular coagulation (DIC) with bleed (50×10^9/L), major surgery (50–100 × 10^9/L), leukemia, aplastic anemia (10×10^9/L; each unit may have own policy; lower threshold if concomitant fever or sepsis), and platelet function defects with severe bleeding. Indications in neonates are listed in **Box 11.14.3**.

Fresh Frozen Plasma

Indications

- Coagulopathy with bleeding (e.g. hemorrhagic disease of newborn, liver disease)
- Hemophilia A/B (if factors unavailable or cannot be afforded)
- Deficiency of antithrombin III, protein C/S
- Warfarin overdose
- Factor XI deficiency
- Vitamin K deficiency
- Massive transfusion
- Replacement fluid for plasma exchange in the cases of thrombotic thrombocytopenic purpura and hemolytic uremic syndrome.

The use of fresh frozen plasma (FFP) is not justified for hypovolemia (use crystalloids), prolonged international normalized ratio in the absence of bleeding, and for hypoalbuminemia (use albumin). The dose is 10–20 mL/kg for infants/children and 5–10 mL/kg for newborns. Fresh frozen plasma must normally be ABO compatible to avoid risk of hemolysis in the recipient and should be transfused within 6 hours of thawing.

Box 11.14.3: Indications of platelet transfusion in neonates.

- *<50 × 10^9/L:*
  - Preterm infant (<33 weeks): First week of life
  - Clinically unstable term infants: First week of life
  - Invasive procedure (e.g. ventricular tap)
  - Preterm neonate
    - To be started on ibuprofen or indomethacin
    - Recent onset grade 3 or 4 IVH
- *<20 × 10^9/L:*
  - Stable infants beyond the first week of life without active bleeding

(IVH: intraventricular hemorrhage)

Box 11.14.4: When to ask for irradiated blood products?

- Donations from relatives (directed donation)
- Intrauterine transfusion
- *Exchange transfusion:*
  - If there is previous intrauterine transfusion
  - Related donor
  - *Routine cases*: Only if it does not unduly delay the procedure
- *Immunocompromised patients*: SCID, BMT, Hodgkin disease
- Granulocyte transfusion

(BMT: bone marrow transplant; SCID: severe combined immunodeficiency)

Cryoprecipitate

The contents include fibrinogen, von Willebrand factor, factors VIII and XIII. The corresponding indications are fibrinogen less than 1.0 g/L (e.g. DIC with bleeding), hemophilia A (*Note*: It does not contain factor IX and, thus, not indicated in hemophilia B), von Willebrand disease, and factor XIII deficiency. The average dose is 1 U for 5–10 kg body weight.

Cryoprecipitate can be transfused across ABO barrier (as it contains scant amount of RBCs) and should be transfused immediately after thawing.

Irradiated Blood Products

Under normal circumstances, T-lymphocytes in donor blood are destroyed by the recipient. They can survive and proliferate if they are not recognized as foreign (e.g. related donor) or if recipient is immunocompromised. The proliferating T-cells cause graft-versus-host disease (GVHD). It is a rare, however, a frequently fatal complication that occurs 3–30 days following blood transfusion. As there is no effective treatment, aim is to recognize high-risk patients and to administer blood products with T-cells that have been rendered ineffective **(Boxes 11.14.4 and 11.14.5)**. This is done by exposing blood bag to ionizing radiation. Facilities for irradiating blood are gradually increasing at centers in India.

Box 11.14.5: Conditions where irradiated blood is not required.

- Newborns for top up transfusion
- HIV, AIDS
- Solid organ transplant
- Autoimmune diseases

(AIDS: acquired immune deficiency syndrome; HIV: human immunodeficiency virus)

Leukoreduction

It refers to the removal of white cells from a blood product. Deleterious effects caused by leukocytes include:

- Febrile nonhemolytic reactions
- Human leukocyte antigen (HLA) alloimmunization
- Platelet refractoriness
- Transmission of cytomegalovirus (CMV), Epstein-Barr virus, human immunodeficiency virus (HIV), human T-cell lymphotropic virus (HTLV)
- Possibly organ dysfunction and increased mortality.

A unit of whole blood contains approximately 2×10^9 leukocytes. These can be removed soon after collecting blood (prestorage), or at the bedside. Prestorage leukoreduction is superior, as inflammatory cytokine accumulation following release from white blood cells (WBCs) during storage is avoided. It is likely that leukoreduction (residual leukocytes less than 5×10^6) will prevent GVHD, but is not certain. In Indian circumstances, bedside leukocyte filters **(Fig. 11.14.2)** should be considered for patients receiving multiple transfusions, e.g. thalassemia major.

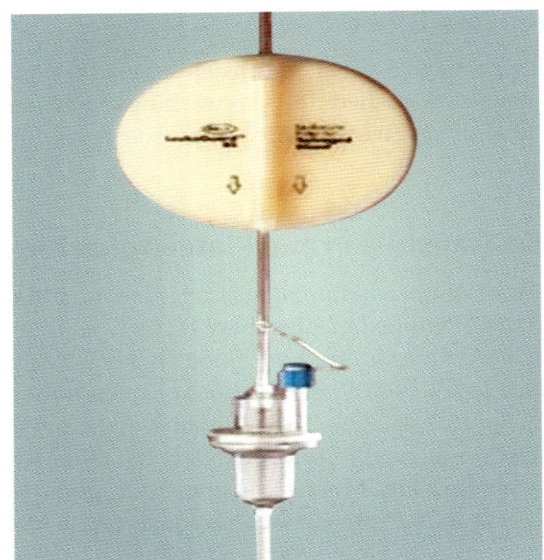

Fig. 11.14.2: A bedside leukocyte filter.

Autologous Blood

It is the collection and reinfusion of the patient's own blood. It is possible for some children who have to undergo elective surgery for which transfusion is anticipated. Advantage is reduction in the risk of transfusion-transmitted viral diseases. Blood, proportionate to the size of the child, is collected 4–5 weeks prior to surgery. The Hb should be >11 g/dL before the collection of blood. Oral iron is supplemented. All risks are not avoided: the stored unit could still be contaminated with bacteria or a wrong unit could be inadvertently transfused.

Hazards of Blood Transfusion

Adverse reactions to blood transfusion can be subdivided according to whether they are immediate or delayed and whether they are immunologically mediated **(Table 11.14.3)**. Acute hemolytic reaction is the dreaded complication of blood transfusion, one of the common causes being clerical errors of mislabeling or misidentification, resulting in the infusion of a wrong patient's blood. Signs and symptoms include fever, chills, back/chest pain, flushing, nausea, and hemoglobinuria. These can progress to shock with acute renal failure. Management is outlined in **Box 11.14.6**. Two

Table 11.14.3: Adverse effects of transfusion.

Adverse effect	***Usual cause***
Immunological	
Hemolysis	Red cell incompatibility
Anaphylaxis	Antibody to IgA in donor plasma
Febrile, nonhemolytic	Antibody to donor leukocyte antigen
Urticaria	Antibody to donor plasma proteins
Transfusion-related acute lung injury	Donor antibody to leukocyte of patient
Graft-versus-host disease	Functional lymphocytes in blood
Nonimmunological	
Transfusion-associated circulatory overload	Volume overload
Fever with shock	Bacterial contamination
Hypothermia	Rapid infusion of cold blood
Air embolus	Air infusion in line
Hyperkalemia	Rapid infusion of multiple units of stored blood
Hypocalcemia	Massive transfusion of citrated blood
Disease transmission	HIV, hepatitis B and C, CMV, malaria, syphilis
Iron overload	Multiple transfusions in chronically anemic patients without blood loss

(CMV: cytomegalovirus; HIV: human immunodeficiency virus; IgA: immunoglobulin A)

Box 11.14.6: Management of acute hemolytic transfusion reaction.

- Discontinue blood transfusion, however, maintain IV access
- Alert blood bank and send back unit of blood along with BT set
- Draw clotted and anticoagulated blood specimens from a vein other than the one being used for transfusion. Send anticoagulated sample to blood bank with compatibility form, mentioning details of transfusion reaction. Request the following tests: DCT, plasma Hb, blood counts, urea, creatinine, and bilirubin
- Collect urine sample for urinary Hb
- Investigate for DIC; blood culture if fever is a prominent feature
- Monitor urine output
- *Treatment is largely supportive*: Infusion of normal saline to maintain adequate urine output, furosemide to enhance renal cortical perfusion. Dialysis may be required if acute tubular necrosis develops

(BT: blood transfusion; DCT: direct Coombs' test; DIC: disseminated intravascular coagulation; Hb: hemoglobin; IV: intravenous)

common, but less known adverse effects are detailed here. All the transfusion reactions should be recorded and reported to the blood transfusion services.

Bacterial Contamination of Blood Products

This is a relatively common, however a poorly recognized complication. The source of contamination could be the donor (skin commensals or unrecognized bacteremia), environment, or improper handling of product. Clinical profile often resembles an acute hemolytic reaction. Platelets are most commonly implicated as they are stored at room temperature. Broad-spectrum antibiotics should be initiated at the earliest suspicion.

Transfusion-related Acute Lung Injury

It is currently the most common cause of transfusion-related death reported in western literature. The incidence is 1:1200 to 1:190000 plasma-containing transfusions (RBCs, platelets, or FFP) and typically occurs during or within 6 hours of completion of a transfusion. It is characterized by acute onset hypoxemia in the absence of circulatory overload. Chest X-ray shows bilateral lung infiltration. It usually resolves in 24–72 hours. Management is supportive. Mechanical ventilation may be required. There is no role of steroids or diuretics. Mortality is 5–10%. Antibodies (HLA or WBC) from donor are implicated in causing pulmonary capillary leak. Prevention is by deferral of donors who are commonly multiparous females.

CASE SCENARIOS AND FREQUENTLY ASKED QUESTIONS

Q.1. 1.5 kg preterm neonate; 5 days old; Hb: 9 g/dL; on ventilator, has to be given packed red cells: 25 mL. What should be done with the remaining bag?

Ans. The best option is to request the blood bank to issue blood in a pediatric bag. One red cell unit can be divided into several pediatric bags to be used for a single neonate/infant, over an extended period of time **(Figs. 11.14.3A and B)**. It reduces donor exposure and prevents wastage. Remaining unit should never to be stored in a refrigerator **(Fig. 11.14.4)**.

Q.2. I requested blood for an anticipated use; however, the unit was not administered. Can the blood be returned to the blood bank?

Ans. Every blood bank should have a policy for unused products. Ideal policy is that the blood components that have

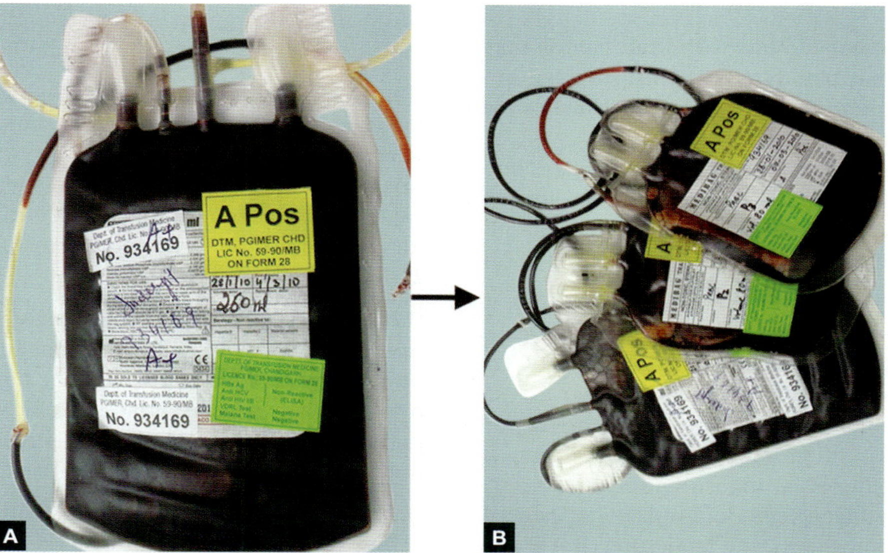

Figs. 11.14.3A and B: The use of blood can be optimized in neonates and infants by the use of pediatric bags.

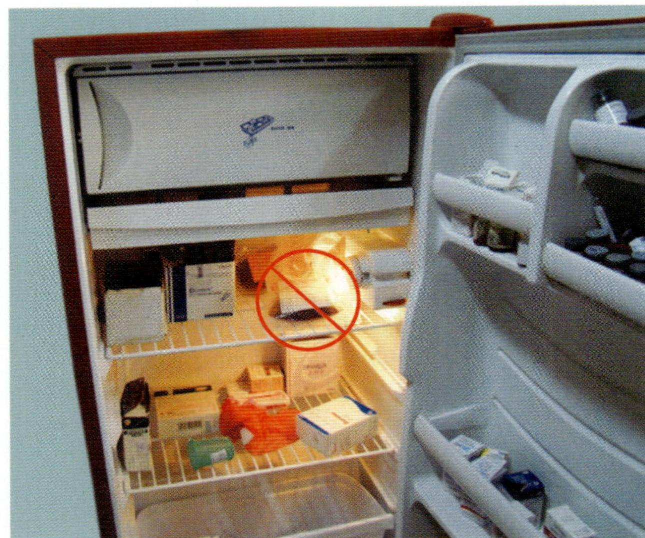

Fig. 11.14.4: Blood is never to be stored in the fridge.

been outside of a temperature-controlled environment for greater than 30 minutes must be discarded.

Q.3. Red cell transfusion is on flow for a child. He develops fever of 39°C after 30 minutes. What should be done?
Ans. The algorithm is illustrated in **Flowchart 11.14.2**.

Q.4. How late can one wait to start a blood transfusion after obtaining the bag from the blood bank?
Ans. If transfusion is not initiated within 30 minutes of removal from blood bank or an approved temperature-controlled blood product refrigerator, the unit should be returned immediately to prevent wastage.

Q.5. There is an 11-year-old boy with thalassemia major. He receives 3–4 weekly blood transfusions. Hb is 8 g/dL on a visit for transfusion to the hospital. How slowly should one transfuse a unit of packed red cells?
Ans. It is appropriate to transfuse over a period of 2–3 hours. No diuretic is required, unless the Hb has been low for a prolonged duration. No transfusion should take greater than 4 hours, because of the risk of bacterial proliferation at room temperature.

Q.6. Platelets were transfused to a patient; however, the posttransfusion count did not increase significantly. What are the common causes and remedial measures?
Ans. Sepsis, fever, idiopathic thrombocytopenic purpura (ITP), DIC, splenomegaly, amphotericin, and alloimmunization. Remedial measures include ordering ABO-compatible product, single-donor platelets, increasing the number of units transfused, and requesting HLA or cross-matched platelets.

Flowchart 11.14.2: Algorithm for management of fever while a blood transfusion is running.

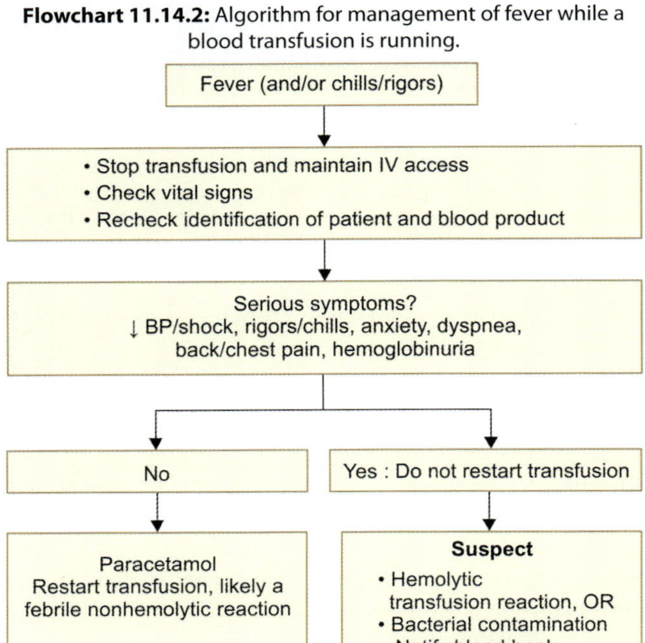

Q.7. I ordered platelets at 9 PM but subsequently decided to transfuse them the next morning. In which compartment of the fridge should I store them until the next day?
Ans. Platelets are stored under continuous agitation to prevent clumping, at 20–24°C (room temperature). Do not store in refrigerator.

Q.8. A child has A+ blood group. Can he be transfused B+ platelets?
Ans. Same blood group is preferred. Alternate group can be transfused, if the plasma volume is limited.

Q.9. B+ platelets are transfused to a B– patient inadvertently. The patient is asymptomatic. Does anything need to be done?
Ans. Rhesus (Rh) immunoglobulin should be administered, especially to females of childbearing age to prevent Rh-alloimmunization from the transfused red cells **(Table 11.14.4)**.

Q.10. How should fresh frozen plasma (FFP) be thawed?
Ans. Ideally by a plasma thawer (nonaqueous) as it may not be available in the majority of units; the bag may be thawed by placing over a clean surface. If using water, ensure that the ports are above the water level. Blankets, body surface (e.g. arm pits), or heaters should not be used.

Q.11. I diagnosed a 7-month infant with thalassemia major. Is there anything that should be requested from the blood bank prior to the first transfusion?

Table 11.14.4: Requirement of ABO and Rh compatibility for transfusing blood components.

	ABO compatibility	*Rh compatibility*
Red cells	Must	Must
Platelets	Preferred	Preferred
Plasma	Must	No
Cryoprecipitate	Preferred, but not required	

(Rh: Rhesus)

Ans. Extended red cell phenotyping (Rh, K, Kidd, and Duffy) should ideally be performed. Attempt should be made to match minor blood group antigens in patients who receive multiple transfusions.

Q.12. A child develops urticarial lesions while blood is running. Should I hold or discontinue the transfusion?
Ans. The algorithm is illustrated in **Flowchart 11.14.3**.

Q.13. A child with thalassemia major has frequent "reactions" to blood. What can be done?
Ans. Prophylactic antihistaminic and paracetamol can be given. Leukocyte filter should be used, if affordable. Request blood matched for C, E, and Kell antigens. Washed red cells may be required (saline washing removes plasma proteins).

Q.14. A child needs blood transfusion. Father is an engineer. Fearing risk of transmission of human immunodeficiency virus (HIV), the concerned father offers to donate blood for his baby. Should such a directed donation be encouraged?
Ans. No, there is a risk of transfusion-associated GVHD from products obtained from close relatives. Such transfusions, if given, must be irradiated.

Q.15. What are the tests mandatory for infection screening of blood in India?
Ans. HIV 1 and 2, hepatitis B and C, syphilis, and malaria.

Q.16. What are the additional tests performed in the developed world?
Ans. Nucleic acid testing for HIV and hepatitis C virus, HTLV, CMV, West Nile virus, etc.

Q.17. A child develops dyspnea during transfusion. What are the possible causes?
Ans. Transfusion-related acute lung injury, circulatory overload, and anaphylaxis.

Q.18. A 3-year-old child is diagnosed with idiopathic thrombocytopenic purpura (ITP). He has widespread skin bleeds and epistaxis. Platelet count is 2×10^9/L. Decision is taken to administer anti-D. Should platelets be transfused?
Ans. No, it is a common error to transfuse platelets for ITP. Transfused platelets are rapidly destroyed due to circulating antibodies. Platelet transfusion is rarely indicated for life-threatening situations (e.g. intracranial bleed) along with steroids/intravenous immune globulin.

Flowchart 11.14.3: Algorithm for management of allergic reactions while blood is being transfused.

Allergic reactions: Urticaria, facial edema

- Stop transfusion and maintain IV access
- Check vital signs
- Recheck identification of patient and blood product

Serious symptoms?
↓ BP/shock, dyspnea, tachycardia, wheezing, chest pain, widespread rash > 2/3 body

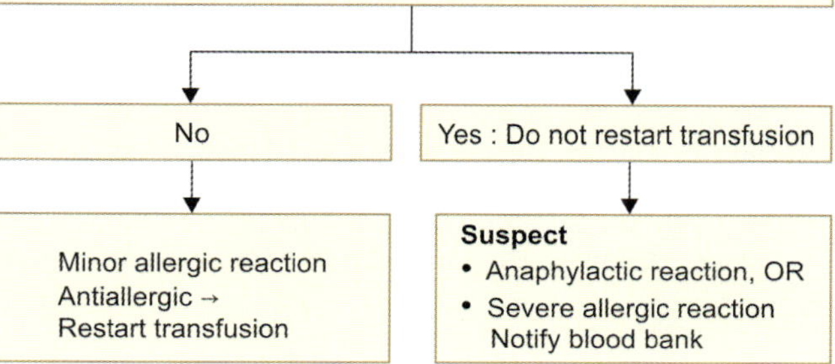

Q.19. What are the prerequisites for a plateletpheresis procedure? How long does it take?
Ans. Request patient's attendants to arrange 2–3 donors (excluding first-degree relatives) of the same blood group as that of the patient. Counsel the attendants for the cost of the disposable kit for the procedure (₹ ~8,000 in a government hospital). The donors are asked to contact blood bank along with a requisition for plateletpheresis. The procedure takes ~2–3 hours.

Q.20. How can I improve transfusion practice in my unit?
Ans. Cordial and regular communication with the blood bank personnel is the key. Avoid blame game. Accept limitations and frame guidelines after mutual discussion.

Q.21. Why it is necessary to report adverse transfusion reactions to blood banks?
Ans. Under "Hemovigilance program of India," blood banks need to report data regarding adverse transfusion reactions to a central reporting authority.

Q.22. I need to transfuse a patient. What are the prerequisite documentations needed?
Ans. Document the indication(s) and type of blood component(s) to be transfused in the patient's file. Prior to sending the blood requisition to the blood bank, obtain a written consent from the patient or the guardian (in the case of a minor) after explaining the indication and the associated risks.

SUMMARY

Blood and blood products should be transfused only when there are clear and specific therapeutic indications. The risk of transfusion reactions and transfusion-related infections deserve careful consideration. Specific blood component therapy suited to the requirements of an individual patient must be recommended, whenever possible.

BIBLIOGRAPHY

1. Bansal D, Totadri S. Common hematological disorders in children. Indian J Pediatr. 2014;81(1):42-50.
2. Carless PA, Henry DA, Carson JL, et al. Transfusion thresholds and other strategies for guiding allogeneic red blood cell transfusion. Cochrane Database Syst Rev. 2010;(10):CD002042.
3. Funk MK, Grossman BJ, Westhoff CM (Eds). Technical Manual, 18th edition. Bethesda MD. AABB Press; 2014.
4. Gupta A, Bansal D, Dass R, et al. Transfusion associated graft versus host disease. Indian Pediatr. 2004;41(12):1260-4.
5. Jain A, Kaur R. Hemovigilance and blood safety. Asian J Transfus Sci. 2012;6:137-8.
6. Kennedy MS. Transfusion therapy. In: Harmening DM (Ed). Modern Blood Banking and Transfusion Practices, 6th edition. New Delhi: Jaypee Brothers Medical Publishers (P) Ltd.; 2013. pp. 352-66.
7. Lacroix J, Hébert PC, Hutchison JS, et al. Transfusion strategies for patients in pediatric intensive care units. N Engl J Med. 2007;356:1609-19.
8. Marwaha N. Whole blood and component use in resource poor settings. Biologicals. 2010;38(1):68-71.
9. National AIDS Control Organisation, Ministry of Health and Family Welfare, Government of India. Annual report 2016–2017. [online]. Available from http://naco.gov.in/NACO/Quick_Links/Publication/Annual_Report/NACO_Annual_Report/Annual_Report_NACO_2016-17_English/ [Accessed October, 2018].
10. Sloan SR, Friedman DF, Kao G, et al. Transfusion medicine. In: Orkin SH, Nathan DG, Ginsburg D, et al. (Eds). Nathan and Oski's Hematology of Infancy and Childhood, 7th edition. Philadelphia, PA: Saunders Elsevier; 2009. pp. 1623-62.
11. Treleaven J, Gennery A, Marsh J, et al. Guidelines on the use of irradiated blood components prepared by the British Committee for Standards in Haematology Blood Transfusion Task Force. Br J Haematol. 2011;152(1):35-51.

Section 12

Pediatric Malignancies

12.1 Malignancies in Children: An Introduction

Purna A Kurkure

The recent understanding and advances in the total management of pediatric cancers form one of the most exciting chapters in the entire field of oncology. With increasing control of infectious diseases, eradication of malnutrition, and the rapid strides of the pediatric surgeons in correcting benign surgical problems, more children are now living to be diagnosed with cancer.

In the United States of America, cancer is second to accidents as a cause of mortality in children beyond first year of life. There is a paucity of accurate statistics in our country. Children constitute approximately one-third of India's population, which is more than 1.2 billion. Annual incidence rates of cancer are about 75 and 80 per 100 men and women respectively or around 8,00,000 new cancers per year. Approximately, 5% of these are in pediatric age group as estimated by population-based cancer registries. Thus, approximately 40,000 new pediatric cancers are estimated to be diagnosed annually. Leukemias and lymphomas comprise nearly half of the pediatric cancers followed by tumors of the central nervous system (CNS), sympathetic nervous system, soft tissues, kidney, bone, eye, liver, and germ cells. "Child is not a miniature adult." The types of childhood cancers and response to therapy totally differ from those in adults.

The hallmark of success in pediatric oncology is the multidisciplinary approach executed through carefully orchestrated multimodality team comprising a pediatric oncologist, a pediatric surgeon/pediatric oncosurgeon, a radiation oncologist, various diagnostic specialists (pathologist, hematopathologist, molecular pathologist, and radiologist), and supportive care services (registered dietician, physical therapist, occupational therapist, and psychologist). Burchenal succinctly characterized the basic tenet of multidisciplinary approach by stating "the pride of discipline must be put aside." All the experts should work together, keeping well-being of the child as the focus.

First chance is the best chance and giving optimum treatment at the outset is the most important factor in deciding the outcome. Any advances in health care are only as valuable as its availability and accessibility to those who need it. It has been well-documented that organized and coordinated treatment programs carried out by experienced pediatric oncologists in well-staffed and well-equipped pediatric cancer units are the most effective. But, the community pediatrician's role is crucial for a prompt diagnosis, early referral, and to ensure efficient follow-up.

The National Training Project in Practical Pediatric Oncology (NTPPPO) has been initiated under the auspices of Pediatric Hematology Oncology (PHO) chapter of Indian Academy of Pediatrics (IAP) in collaboration with the International Society of Pediatric Oncology (SIOP) since 1998 with the aim to train, educate, and encourage pediatricians to participate in shared care of childhood cancer patients.

Advances in the treatment of childhood cancers have dramatically increased survival rates to more than 70% in the developed countries. It has been estimated that by the year 2020, approximately 1 in 750 young adults in the society will be a survivor of childhood cancer in the United States of America. In India, children treated at comprehensive pediatric cancer units also stand equal chance of being survivors. Childhood cancer survivors are unique and precious. Their contributions to the future are priceless. For each child who survives cancer, on average, 71 years of life will be saved.

Although this constitutes a remarkable medical achievement, the late morbidity in this growing survivor population has become an area of concern. The need to predict the future impact of current therapeutic strategies is a major challenge for the pediatric oncologist. A balance of reassurance to the survivor and vigilance in monitoring for late relapse, second malignancies, and other sequel is required. Recent concept of a truly "cured child" in pediatric oncology envisages not only a biological cure of the disease but also a child on par with peers in growth and development physically and in achievements and aspirations, both mentally and emotionally.

12.2 Leukemia

Anupama S Borker, Pooja Balasubramanian

INTRODUCTION

Leukemias are malignant neoplasms arising from the uncontrolled proliferation and loss of differentiation of hematopoietic stem cells. Depending on the lineage of the progenitor stem cell involved, they are classified as lymphoid or myeloid. Depending on the natural history of the leukemia, they are classified as acute or chronic.

Acute leukemias account for about 40% of childhood cancers. Acute lymphoblastic leukemia (ALL) comprises about 70–80% and acute myeloid leukemia (AML) comprises about 10–15% of childhood leukemias. The remaining subset consists of the uncommon childhood leukemias, viz. chronic myeloid leukemia and juvenile myelomonocytic leukemia.

ETIOPATHOGENESIS

The exact etiology of acute leukemia is unknown. Several genetic conditions are known to predispose to leukemia. These include Down syndrome (Trisomy 21), Fanconi syndrome, Bloom syndrome, Shwachman syndrome, Klinefelter syndrome, Turner syndrome (45, XO), neurofibromatosis, ataxia telangiectasia, severe combined immunodeficiency, and Li-Fraumeni syndrome (p53 deletion). Exposure to ionizing radiation, benzene, and certain drugs such as alkylating agents, nitrosourea, and epipodophyllotoxins have been clearly associated with the development of leukemia. Certain environmental factors, viral infections, and immunodeficiency disorders may also predispose to leukemia.

Leukemia arises following certain carcinogenic stimuli that lead to the malignant transformation of hematopoietic cells rendering them capable of unregulated proliferation (self-renewal) coupled with loss of differentiation and loss of apoptosis (programmed cell death). The uncontrolled proliferation of these malignant cells leads to the expansion of marrow cavity with resultant suppression of normal cell lines.

CLASSIFICATION OF LEUKEMIA

Acute leukemias in children are classified according to their lineage as ALL and acute myeloblastic leukemia. The further subclassification of ALL and AML keeps evolving as does our understanding of the characteristics of leukemia cells at the cytogenetic and molecular level. Beginning from the morphologic classification as L1, L2, and L3, authors now classify ALL on the basis of the surface markers as those derived from "B" or "T" cell precursors **(Table 12.2.1)**.

Cytogenetic analysis further characterizes leukemia on the basis of chromosomal aberrations that are known to influence outcomes **(Table 12.2.2)**. Similarly, the morphologic classification of AML has given way to the World Health Organization (WHO) classification based on morphology, cytogenetic features, etiology, and preceding myelodysplasia **(Table 12.2.3)**.

CLINICAL FEATURES

The common age group for acute leukemia is 2–5 years, and males are often slightly more affected than females. Fever is the most common presenting feature of acute leukemia. The other features usually reflect the suppression of one or more hematopoietic cell lines. Anemia may present with progressive pallor, weakness, fatigue, lethargy, refusal to feed, or shortness of breath. Thrombocytopenia leading to petechiae, ecchymosis, or gum bleeds is common. Neutropenia with resultant infections may present with fever, pneumonia, otitis, skin, soft tissue, and perianal infections. Mucositis with oral ulcers and thrush is a common finding in neutropenic patients. Hepatosplenomegaly and lymphadenopathy, secondary to leukemic infiltration,

Table 12.2.1: Classification of acute lymphoblastic leukemia.

ALL subtype	Surface markers	Significance
Pre-B-cell	$CD10^+$, $CD19^+$, $CD20^+$, $CD21^+$, HLA DR+	The most common subtype with good prognosis
B-cell	$CD19^+$, $CD20^+$, $CD21^+$, sIg^+	Burkitt leukemia (L3), good prognosis with short duration intensive chemotherapy
T-cell	$CD3^+$, $CD5^+$, $CD7^+$	Common in older boys, associated with high WBC counts, mediastinal mass, and CNS involvement

(ALL: acute lymphoblastic leukemia; CD: cluster of differentiation; HLA: human leukocyte antigen; WBC: white blood cell; CNS: central nervous system)

Table 12.2.2: Common chromosomal abnormalities in acute lymphoblastic leukemia.

Chromosomal abnormality	*Fusion protein*	*Clinical significance*
t(9;22)	BCR/ABL	Considered very high risk. Therapy with imatinib along with chemotherapy has improved survival
t(4;11)	MLL	Common in infantile leukemia, associated with high tumor burden, intrinsically drug resistant. Connotes poor prognosis
t(1;19)	PBX1/E2A	Associated with higher rates of CNS relapse
t(12;21)	TEL/AML-1	Good prognosis, needs minimal therapy
t(8;14)	MYC/IgL	Burkitt leukemia, needs short duration intensive chemotherapy

(BCR: B-cell receptor; MLL: mixed lineage leukemia; PBX1: pre-B-cell leukemia transcription factor 1; AML-1: acute myeloid leukemia-1; IgL: immunoglobulin L; CNS: central nervous system)

are common. The lymphadenopathy can be generalized and sometimes massive. Mediastinal lymphadenopathy mostly occurs in T-cell ALL. The resultant obstruction of the superior vena cava and the airway can present as medical emergencies. Children and adolescents with the superior vena cava syndrome present with edema and suffusion of the face and upper extremities, headache, and dilated neck veins. The superior mediastinal syndrome resulting from compression of the trachea leads to cough, breathlessness, and air hunger; and if untreated may progress to hypoxia with cyanosis, altered sensorium, and seizures.

Children with large tumor burden may sometimes develop spontaneous tumor lysis syndrome leading to acute renal failure, secondary to uric acid nephropathy.

Less common presenting features include bone and joint pains with tenderness, and rash or eruption, which may be due to cutaneous involvement. About 5–10% patients have central nervous system (CNS) involvement at diagnosis, and may present with cranial nerve palsies or seizures. Signs of raised intracranial pressure such as headache and papilledema may be present. Painless testicular enlargement suggestive of testicular involvement is extremely rare at diagnosis.

Gum hypertrophy is rather a common presentation of AML, especially M4 subtype. Extramedullary myeloid cell tumors or chloromas can occur at a variety of locations and may sometimes precede the development of marrow involvement in AML. Disseminated intravascular coagulation is more common in AML especially in M3 subtype or acute promyelocytic leukemia (APML).

Table 12.2.3: Classification of acute myeloid leukemia.

French–American–British (FAB) Classification	
M0	Minimal differentiation
M1	Myeloblastic leukemia without maturation
M2	Myeloblastic leukemia with maturation
M3	Promyelocytic leukemia
M4	Myelomonocytic leukemia
M5	Monocytic leukemia
M6	Erythroleukemia
M7	Megakaryocytic leukemia
World Health Organization Classification	
Acute myeloid leukemia with recurrent chromosomal translocations: • Acute myeloid leukemia with t(8;21) (q22;q22) AML-1/CBF-α/ETO • *Acute promyelocytic leukemia*: Acute myeloid leukemia with t(15;17) (q22;q12) and variants PML/RAR-α • Acute myeloid leukemia with abnormal bone marrow eosinophils and inv (16)(p13;q22) and t(16;16)(p13;q22) CBF-β/MYH-1 • Acute myeloid leukemia with 11q23 MLL abnormalities	
Acute myeloid leukemia with multilineage dysplasia: • With prior MDS • Without prior MDS	
Acute myeloid leukemia with myelodysplastic syndrome, therapy related: • Alkylating agent related • Epipodophyllotoxin related • Other types	
Acute myeloid leukemia, otherwise categorized: • Acute myeloid leukemia minimally differentiated • Acute myeloid leukemia without maturation • Acute myeloid leukemia with maturation • Acute myelomonocytic leukemia • Acute monocytic leukemia • Acute erythroid leukemia • Acute megakaryocytic leukemia • Acute basophilic leukemia • Acute panmyelosis with myelofibrosis	

(AML-1: acute myeloid leukemia-1; CBF-α: core-binding factor-alpha; PML: promyelocytic leukemia; RAR-α: retinoic acid receptor-alpha; CBF-β: core-binding factor-beta; MLL: mixed lineage leukemia; MDS: myelodysplastic syndrome)

DIFFERENTIAL DIAGNOSIS

The differential diagnosis of ALL is several benign and malignant conditions. Viral infection-induced cytopenias are the most common conditions, which mimic leukemia. Infectious mononucleosis, cytomegalovirus infection, and a host of other viral infections may present with fever and lymphadenopathy along with anemia, thrombocytopenia, and/or neutropenia with atypical lymphocytosis. Immune thrombocytopenia presents with sudden onset of thrombocytopenia with petechiae, purpura, and ecchymosis, in an otherwise healthy child. The presence of atypical features such as fever, lymphadenopathy, or anemia may warrant a bone marrow examination to rule out leukemia. Drug-induced cytopenias can be suspected by a detailed history and withdrawal of the offending drug usually leads to the recovery of concerned cell lines. Bone marrow failure syndromes, myelodysplastic syndromes, and hypoplastic/aplastic anemia usually have a longstanding history and need a bone marrow biopsy for confirmation. Some collagen vascular disorders such as rheumatoid arthritis and systemic lupus erythematosus can present with symptoms of leukemia. Langerhans cell histiocytosis with or without marrow involvement is another common differential.

Malignant conditions that mimic acute leukemia include metastases from solid tumors such as neuroblastoma and rhabdomyosarcoma and marrow involvement in non-Hodgkin lymphoma (NHL).

LABORATORY FEATURES AND DIAGNOSIS

The complete blood count may reveal anemia and/or thrombocytopenia. The white cell count may be increased or decreased; in either case, it is characterized by neutropenia. Hyperleukocytosis [white blood cell (WBC) count greater than 100,000/mm^3] is seen more commonly in ALL than AML. The peripheral blood smear may or may not reveal blasts. Often, they may be reported as atypical lymphocytes or immature cells. Coagulopathy may be present with elevated prothrombin time (PT), partial thromboplastin time (PTT), and fibrinogen degradation products.

The diagnosis of leukemia is established by a bone marrow aspiration. The presence of 25% blasts confirms the diagnosis of ALL (20% in case of AML). In case of dry tap, a bone marrow biopsy may be rarely needed.

In patients with high WBC, there may be elevation of uric acid and lactate dehydrogenase (LDH). Tumor lysis syndrome is characterized by elevated potassium, phosphorus, uric acid, and depressed calcium. In severe cases, renal function may be compromised with elevation of blood urea nitrogen and creatinine. Elevated transaminases and hyperbilirubinemia may, occasionally, be present in cases of extensive liver involvement.

Chest X-ray may reveal a mediastinal mass, more often, in T-cell ALL. Hepatosplenomegaly and, occasionally, nephromegaly may be documented by a sonography.

Box 12.2.1 shows the investigations needed at the diagnosis of acute leukemia.

Box 12.2.1: Investigations recommended for the diagnosis of acute leukemia.

- Complete blood counts with peripheral smear
- *Bone marrow aspiration*: Morphology, immunophenotyping, cytogenetic analysis, FISH or PCR for specific translocations
- Bone marrow biopsy, if dry tap
- *Cerebrospinal fluid examination*: To look for the presence of blasts
- *Serum electrolytes*: Serum sodium, potassium, chloride, calcium, phosphorus, magnesium
- Renal function tests
- Liver function tests
- Serum lactate dehydrogenase
- Serum uric acid
- *Coagulation profile*: Prothrombin time, activated partial thromboplastin time, fibrinogen, D-dimer
- Serology for HIV, HBsAg, anti-HBsAb, anti-HCV
- Blood grouping
- Quantitative serum immunoglobulin
- Chest X-ray
- Ultrasound of abdomen

(FISH: fluorescence *in situ* hybridization; PCR: polymerase chain reaction; HIV: human immunodeficiency virus; HBsAg: hepatitis B surface antigen; HBsAb: hepatitis B surface antibody; HCV: hepatitis C virus)

MANAGEMENT

The treatment of acute leukemia involves specific antileukemic therapy and supportive care. Specific antileukemic therapy depends on the subtype of the leukemia. At diagnosis, the leukemic tumor burden approximates to 10^{12} cells. Chemotherapy given in phases reduces the leukemia cells exponentially with each cycle.

Acute Lymphoblastic Leukemia

In ALL, antileukemic therapy is given in phases with specific aims.

- *Induction chemotherapy* refers to the first 4–6 weeks of chemotherapy designed to induce a clinical and morphological remission in the marrow. It typically uses 3–4 drugs including a steroid (prednisone or dexamethasone), vincristine, and daunorubicin or L-asparaginase along with weekly doses of intrathecal methotrexate. About 90–95% patients achieve a remission at the end of induction chemotherapy.
- *Consolidation chemotherapy* has 16–20 weeks of intensive chemotherapy administered to further decrease the leukemic cell burden in the body. It uses combinations of drugs including cyclophosphamide, cytosine arabinoside, methotrexate, vincristine, and daunorubicin.
- *Central nervous system-directed therapy* is aimed at eliminating the leukemic cells from within the CNS, which are usually shielded by the blood-brain barrier. The components of CNS-directed therapy include cranial

irradiation, intrathecal chemotherapy, and high-dose systemic chemotherapy. Although an effective means of CNS therapy, cranial irradiation is associated with serious long-term toxicity including neurocognitive dysfunction and secondary malignancies. Newer protocols have documented equivalent results with prolonged intrathecal chemotherapy and high-dose systemic chemotherapy thus eliminating the use of radiotherapy (RT).

- *Maintenance chemotherapy* is low-dose oral chemotherapy administered for 24–30 months after completion of intensive chemotherapy, and is necessary to clear the marrow of residual leukemic cells. Methotrexate and 6-mercaptopurine are used for the maintenance therapy.

Acute Myeloid Leukemia

In acute myeloid leukema (AML), induction chemotherapy uses 2–3 drugs: daunorubicin, cytosine arabinoside with or without etoposide. The remission rate is approximately 70% and then followed by 2–4 cycles of consolidation chemotherapy usually with cytosine arabinoside. Intrathecal chemotherapy with methotrexate or cytosine arabinoside is used for CNS therapy. There is no established role of the maintenance chemotherapy in AML.

Acute Lymphoblastic Leukemia with t(9;22)

Acute lymphoblastic leukemia with t(9;22), also known as Philadelphia chromosome positive ALL, was conventionally considered very high risk in ALL due to its chemoresistant nature, and needed bone marrow transplantation (BMT) for cure. Since the advent of the targeted drug, imatinib, its prognosis has vastly improved. Imatinib is a tyrosine kinase inhibitor (TKI) that binds the adenosine triphosphate (ATP)-binding site of the tyrosine kinase molecule and disrupts its downstream enzymatic activity, thereby inhibiting cell division. Given in combination with chemotherapy, imatinib induces lasting remissions in patients.

Acute Promyelocytic Leukemia

Acute promyelocytic leukemia is a type of AML with a distinct cytogenetic abnormality t(15;17) with the promyelocytic leukemia (PML)/retinoic acid receptor-alpha (RAR-α) fusion. It is characterized by the proliferation of promyelocytes rich in granules that result in disseminated intravascular coagulation. Treatment with all-trans-retinoic acid (ATRA) results in the differentiation of promyelocytes into mature neutrophils leading to the resolution of coagulopathy and to remission.

Minimal Residual Disease

Minimal residual disease (MRD) is the presence of residual leukemic cells below the threshold that can be detected by light microscopy. These low levels of leukemic blasts can be detected by immunophenotyping using flow cytometry technique or by reverse transcription polymerase chain reaction (RT-PCR). The presence of positive MRD at the end of induction calls for augmentation of therapy to get rid of these persistent leukemic cells. The cut-off level to define MRD positivity is 0.01% in ALL and 0.1% in AML. Risk stratification of the patients on the basis of MRD status is now considered a standard of care in treatment of ALL.

Hematopoietic Stem Cell Transplantation

Most children with leukemia can be cured with chemotherapy. The indications for hematopoietic stem cell transplantation in childhood leukemia are as follows:

1. *Very high risk ALL*: Those with poor cytogenetic features or those who fail induction therapy
2. Early relapse of ALL
3. Late relapse of ALL who fail to respond to chemotherapy
4. Second or subsequent relapses of ALL
5. Acute myeloid leukemia with poor cytogenetic features or failure of induction therapy.

An HLA-matched sibling is the best possible donor for an allogeneic transplant. In the absence of a matched sibling donor, matched unrelated donor from donor registries can be used. Haploidentical bone marrow transplant using either of the parents is now being practiced in many centers abroad and also in India. The success rate of BMT for relapsed leukemia is about 50%.

Recent Advances

Targeted Therapy

- Cytotoxic chemotherapy kills rapidly dividing cancer cells by various mechanisms. Targeted therapy recognizes and attacks certain targets on the surface of tumor cells such as certain receptors or chromosomal alterations. As a result the action is very specific and it spares normal cells.
- The use of TKI imatinib which targets the BCR/ABL1 gene rearrangement in the Philadelphia chromosome in patients with chronic myeloid leukemia revolutionized the treatment of this disease and set the stage for the discovery of hundreds of such new drugs.
- Imatinib has been used successfully along with chemotherapy in the treatment of Ph+ ALL.
- The development of second-generation TKIs (dasatinib and nilotinib) have helped to overcome imatinib resistance.
- Other new agents with potential role in ALL therapy include FLT3 (FMS-like tyrosine kinase receptor 3) inhibitors, farnesyltransferase inhibitors, proteasome inhibitors, demethylating agents (decitabine), and histone deacetylase inhibitors (vorinostat). Rituximab (anti-CD20), inotuzumab (anti-CD22), epratuzumab

(anti-CD22), and gemtuzumab (anti-CD33) have been incorporated in trials.

Immunotherapy

Our body's immune surveillance mechanism is responsible for suppressing thousands of potentially carcinogenic events every day. Since cancer is caused by the failure of the immune surveillance to thwart these events, immunotherapy aims to activate the immune system and eliminate the cancer cells from the body.

In chimeric antigen receptor (CAR) T-cell technology, patients T-cells are collected and modified in vitro to modify its antigen receptor in such a way that when reintroduced in the patient's body, it recognizes the leukemic cells and mounts an immune reaction to eliminate them.

This has been tried most successfully in B-cell ALL by targeting surface antigen CD19. Blinatumomab, a bispecific anti-CD19/CD3 chimeric antibody (BiTE) helps to bring malignant cell and T-cell in close proximity resulting in cell lysis. It has shown encouraging results in relapsed/refractory disease and those with persistent MRD.

SUPPORTIVE CARE

Supportive care involves the management of emergencies that the patient may present with at diagnosis and the management of complications during therapy.

Emergencies at diagnosis include obstructive conditions such as the superior vena cava syndrome and the superior mediastinal syndrome, metabolic conditions such as tumor lysis syndrome and hematological conditions such as severe anemia and bleeding.

Children with superior vena cava and superior mediastinal syndrome need prompt care in the intensive care unit (ICU) with close monitoring. Patients should be kept in the propped-up position to prevent the mediastinal mass from further compressing the airway and the great vessels. If patient has high WBC with circulating blasts, definitive diagnosis can be established by morphology and immunophenotyping of the peripheral blood, thereby obviating the need for a marrow examination. If there is an associated pleural effusion, thoracocentesis can be diagnostic as well as therapeutic as flow cytometry of pleural fluid can clinch the diagnosis. If bone marrow study is mandatory, it should be performed with the patient in the propped-up position without sedation or general anesthesia to prevent hypoxia, as these patients are difficult candidates for endotracheal intubation. Intravenous (IV) hydration should be started using a leg vein to avoid aggravating the congestive symptoms in the upper body. Once a diagnostic specimen has been obtained, the patient can be started on steroids, which give rapid relief by shrinking the mass.

Patients with hyperleukocytosis (WBC count > 100,000/mm^3) may present with symptoms of thrombosis or with tumor lysis syndrome with hyperkalemia, hyperuricemia, hyperphosphatemia, and hypocalcemia. If untreated, this condition can rapidly progress to azotemia and acute renal shutdown. Tumor lysis syndrome occurs usually within 7 days of starting cytotoxic therapy but can occur due to spontaneous cell lysis even before starting the treatment. Patients with hyperleukocytosis need rigorous monitoring with electrocardiogram (ECG) and electrolytes to prevent complications such as arrhythmias and acute renal failure. IV hydration with twice maintenance potassium-free fluids is recommended. The urine pH should be maintained between 7 and 8 to prevent precipitation of uric acid and phosphate crystals. Allopurinol, a xanthine oxidase inhibitor, helps to prevent the formation of uric acid. Rasburicase, a urate oxidase helps in degrading uric acid converting it into the water-soluble allantoin, which is easily excreted by the kidneys.

Supportive care during therapy includes blood component therapy and aggressive management of infectious complications. Packed red blood cell (RBC) transfusions are indicated to maintain hemoglobin over 8 g/dL in healthy children and over 10 g/dL in patients with fever and infection. Platelet transfusions are indicated, if platelet count is less than 10,000/mm^3 or in the case of overt bleeding, especially in patients with fever and infection. Every episode of febrile neutropenia should be treated aggressively with broad-spectrum antibiotics after drawing blood cultures. All patients should receive prophylaxis for *Pneumocystis carinii* pneumonia with cotrimoxazole and for oral candidiasis with clotrimazole lozenges. Maintenance of oral and perianal hygiene reduces the risk of infections to a significant extent. The use of hematopoietic growth factors [granulocyte colony-stimulating factor (GCSF) and granulocyte-macrophage colony-stimulating factor (GM-CSF)] reduces the period of neutropenia, but they are expensive and do not improve the overall outcome of the patients.

In ALL, BMT is indicated for very high-risk patients, those who fail induction therapy, and those who have early relapse while still on therapy. In AML, BMT is indicated for patients with unfavorable cytogenetic features and those who relapse.

PROGNOSIS AND OUTCOME

Acute lymphoblastic leukemia is a heterogeneous disease and treatment outcomes depend on several factors. These factors are divided as those pertaining to the patient such as age, sex, ethnicity, and underlying immunodeficiency; those pertaining to the disease such as presenting WBC and tumor burden, CNS involvement, lineage, subtype, chromosomal abnormality, and ploidy; and those pertaining to therapy such as chemotherapy regimens and their intensity.

The early response to treatment as judged by the clearance of blasts from the peripheral blood by day 7 of therapy and

Table 12.2.4: Risk stratification of acute lymphoblastic leukemia.

Risk stratification	Features
Low risk	Age 1–9 years, WBC count < 50,000/mm^3, Pre-B ALL, trisomy 4 and 10, hyperdiploidy, t(12;21)
Standard risk	Age 1–9 years, WBC count < 50,000/mm^3, Pre-B ALL, normal cytogenetics
High risk	Age < 1 year and > 9 years, WBC count
	> 50,000/mm^3, T-cell ALL, CNS involvement, hypodiploidy, positive MRD after induction
Very high risk	t(9;22), t(4;11), induction failure

(WBC: white blood cell; ALL: acute lymphoblastic leukemia; CNS: central nervous system)

from the marrow by day 14 of therapy was considered one of the best predictors of outcomes. The presence of MRD at the end of induction is now considered the best predictor of outcome. Risk stratification based on the above features helps to tailor therapy to ensure the best results with the least toxicity. **Table 12.2.4** shows risk stratification of ALL.

Presently, the cure rates in ALL in developed countries are as high as 79–86% using intensive protocols. Few studies published from tertiary institutes in India have reported cure rates of 40–60%. Cure rates for AML are about 60–80% in developed countries and around 30–40% in developing countries.

PRACTICE GUIDELINES

- Always establish a complete and accurate diagnosis before committing a patient to therapy.
- Treat the patient according to published protocols without undue deviations to ensure the best outcomes.
- Promptly initiate broad-spectrum antibiotics during febrile neutropenia treating it as a medical emergency.
- Lifelong follow-up of leukemia survivors is important to monitor for late effects and secondary malignancies.

KEY MESSAGES

- The incidence of leukemia is high enough for all pediatricians to maintain a high index of suspicion in children with unusual symptoms.
- Refer a suspected case of leukemia early to a tertiary center, as early diagnosis can make a significant difference in the outcome of this curable disease.
- Be wary of administering steroids to a patient suspected of having leukemia. It can precipitate tumor lysis syndrome, and sometimes, mask the diagnosis.
- If a patient is severely anemic, packed RBC transfusion can be given before transfer to a tertiary center as it can be lifesaving.

BIBLIOGRAPHY

1. Bajel A, George B, Mathews V, et al. Treatment of children with acute lymphoblastic leukemia in India using a BFM protocol. Pediatr Blood Cancer. 2008;51(5):621-5.
2. Campana D. Role of minimal residual disease monitoring in adult and pediatric acute lymphoblastic leukemia. Hematol Oncol Clin North Am. 2009;23:1083-98.
3. Hunger SP, Raetz EA, Loh ML, et al. Improving outcomes for high risk ALL: translating new discoveries into clinical care. Pediatr Blood Cancer. 2011;56(6):984-93.
4. Kulkarni KP, Marwaha RK, Trehan A, et al. Survival outcome in childhood ALL: experience from a tertiary care center in North India. Pediatr Blood Cancer. 2009;53(2):168-73.
5. Magrath I, Shanta V, Advani S, et al. Treatment of acute lymphoblastic leukemia in countries with limited resources; lessons from use of a single protocol in India over a twenty year period [corrected]. Eur J Cancer. 2005;41(11):1570-83.
6. Margolin JF. Molecular diagnosis and risk adjusted therapy in pediatric hematologic malignancies: a primer for pediatricians. Eur J Pediatr. 2011;170(4):419-25.
7. Pui CH, Carroll WL, Meshinchi S, et al. Biology, risk stratification, and therapy of pediatric acute leukemias: an update. J Clin Oncol. 2011;29(5):551-65.
8. Schultz KR, Prestidge T, Camitta B. Philadelphia chromosome positive acute lymphoblastic leukemia in children: new and emerging treatment options. Expert Rev Hematol. 2010;3(6): 731-42.
9. Shi H, Sun M, Liu L, Wang Z. Chimeric antigen receptor for adoptive immunotherapy of cancer: latest research and future prospects. Mol Cancer. 2014;13:219.
10. Urayama KY, Ma X, Selvin S, et al. Early life exposure to infections and risk of childhood acute lymphoblastic leukemia. Int J Cancer. 2011;128(7): 1632-43.

12.3 Lymphoma

Brijesh Arora

INTRODUCTION

Lymphomas are the third most common group of cancers in children and adolescents after leukemias and brain tumors, accounting for 10–15% of newly diagnosed cancers in this age group. They are neoplasms of lymphocytes or their precursors, which arise as a consequence of genetic aberrations that influence their proliferation, differentiation, and ability to undergo apoptosis (or programmed cell death). They usually present with distinct clinical syndromes reflecting the histological subtype. About 60% of all childhood lymphomas have been classified as NHLs representing 3% of all childhood malignancies for children younger than 5 years and 8–9% in children and adolescents between 5 years and 19 years of age. Hodgkin lymphoma comprises 6% of childhood cancers. Both of these major lymphoma subtypes have distinct origins, clinical presentations, biology, treatment approaches, and outcome **(Table 12.3.1)**, and hence, they are discussed separately in the following sections.

HODGKIN DISEASE

Hodgkin disease (HD) occurs in 5–7 per 100,000 population. The incidence is highest in late childhood and early adulthood (15–35 years). It is very uncommon under 5 years of age and almost never seen under 2 years of age. In Asian population, HD is common even at younger ages. The sex ratio varies from male preponderance of 10:1 under the age of 7 years falling to 1:1 after the age of 12 years.

Table 12.3.1: Comparative clinical features of Hodgkin and non-Hodgkin lymphoma.

Clinical feature	*Hodgkin disease*	*Non-Hodgkin lymphoma*
Nodal spread	Continuous	Discontinuous
Localized	Yes	Rare
Extranodal disease	Rare	Common
CNS disease	Rare	Common
Bone marrow	Rare	Common
Constitutional or class B symptoms	Common	Uncommon
Abdominal disease	Uncommon	Common
Subtype-based therapy	Not important	Crucial
Cure rates	85–95%	70–80%

(CNS: central nervous system)

ETIOLOGY

Variation in the incidence of HD in different ethnic groups and association with human leukocyte antigens (HLA) suggest that inherited susceptibility plays an important role in the pathogenesis. Environmental factors such as Epstein–Barr virus (EBV) infection, familial clustering of cases, and higher incidence in twins may be some of the other contributing factors.

PATHOBIOLOGY

All cases of Hodgkin lymphoma arise from germinal center B-cells that cannot synthesize immunoglobulin and are characterized by a variable number of characteristic multinucleated giant cells [Reed–Sternberg (R–S) cells] or large mononuclear cell variants [lymphocytic and histiocytic (L and H) cells] in an inflammatory background of small lymphocytes, histiocytes, neutrophils, eosinophils, plasma cells, and fibroblasts in different proportions depending on the histologic subtype **(Table 12.3.2)**. It has been conclusively shown that R–S cells and/or L and H cells represent a clonal population. Also, EBV genetic material can be detected in R–S cells from some patients with Hodgkin lymphoma. Hodgkin lymphoma can be divided into two broad pathologic classes:

1. Nodular lymphocyte-predominant Hodgkin lymphoma and
2. Classical Hodgkin lymphoma

Nodular Lymphocyte-Predominant Hodgkin Lymphoma

This pathologic class of Hodgkin lymphoma is characterized by large cells with multilobed nuclei, referred to as popcorn cells. Nodular lymphocyte-predominant Hodgkin lymphoma (NLPHL) is most common in males younger than 10 years of age. Patients with NLPHL generally present with localized, non-bulky disease usually in the mediastinum. Almost all patients are asymptomatic.

Table 12.3.2: Histopathologic classification of classical Hodgkin disease.

REAL subgroups	*Distinctive features*	*Relative frequency (%)*
Lymphocyte-rich (LR)	Benign appearing lymphocytes with or without histiocytes. Few R–S cells. No fibrosis	10–15
Nodular sclerosis (NS)	Thickened capsule with proliferation of orderly collagenous bands that divide lymphoid tissue in nodules: lacunar variant of R–S cells	20–50
Mixed cellularity* (MC)	5–15 R–S cells/high power field. Fine fibrosis in interstitium. Focal necrosis may be present	20–40
Lymphocyte depletion (LD)	• Abnormal cells with relative paucity of lymphocytes • Fibrosis and necrosis common but diffuse	5–16

(REAL: Revised European–American lymphoma; R–S cells: Reed–Sternberg cells)
*Most common in developing countries and in children

Classical Hodgkin Lymphoma

The hallmark of classical Hodgkin lymphoma is the R–S cell that is often characterized by a bilobed nucleus, with two large nucleoli, giving an owl's eye appearance to the cells. The classical subtypes are defined according to the number of R–S cells, characteristics of the inflammatory milieu, and the presence or absence of fibrosis. A striking characteristic is the rarity (about 1%) of the malignant R–S cells in specimens and the abundant reactive cellular infiltrate. The histologic features and clinical symptoms of Hodgkin lymphoma have been attributed to the numerous cytokines secreted by the R–S cells, which include interleukin-1, interleukin-6, and tumor necrosis factor. Classical HD is divided into four subtypes as detailed in the **Table 12.3.2**.

STAGING

Current Hodgkin lymphoma staging is based on Cotswold's modification of Ann Arbor staging proposed in 1998, which is detailed in **Table 12.3.3**.

Table 12.3.3: Modified Ann Arbor classification of Hodgkin disease.

Stage	*Description*
I	Involvement of single lymph node region (I) or of a single extralymphatic organ or site (IE) by direct extension
II	Involvement of two or more lymph node regions on the same side of diaphragm or localized involvement of an extralymphatic organ or site and of one or more lymph node regions on the same side of the diaphragm (IIE)
III_1	• Involvement of lymph node regions on both sides of the diaphragm • Abdominal disease is limited to the upper abdomen (i.e. spleen, splenic hilar nodes, celiac nodes, porta hepatitis nodes)
III_2	• Involvement of lymph node regions on both sides of the diaphragm • Abdominal disease includes para-aortic, mesenteric, and iliac involvement with or without disease in the upper abdomen
IV	Disseminated involvement of one or more extralymphatic organs or tissues with or without associated lymph node disease
A	No symptoms
B	Fever, night sweats, or weight loss of more than 10% of body weight in the previous 6 months
X	Bulky disease (>10 cm in maximum dimension; >1/3rd of the internal transverse diameter of the thorax at the level T5/T6)
E	Limited involvement of a single extranodal site
CS	*Clinical stage*: When based solely on physical examination and imaging technique
PS	*Pathologic stage*: When based on biopsies

CLINICAL PRESENTATION

Hodgkin disease has an insidious onset. The most frequent presentation in up to 80% of patients is painless cervical or supraclavicular lymphadenopathy, of which 60% have asymptomatic involvement of the mediastinum. Enlarged nodes are generally firm and have a rubbery texture. Constitutional or class "B" symptoms such as fever, night sweats, and weight loss are more common with advanced disease (stage I—5%, stage IV—81%) and are associated with a poorer outcome. Approximately 20% of patients have bulky adenopathy (maximum mediastinal diameter greater than one-third of the chest diameter and/or a node or nodal aggregate larger than 10 cm). About 15–20% of patients have noncontiguous extranodal involvement (stage IV) of lung, liver, bones, and bone marrow. A reduced cell-mediated immunity results in an increased susceptibility to infections.

EVALUATION OF A PATIENT

- History and physical examination
- Complete blood count
- Liver and renal function tests, serum lactate dehydrogenase (LDH), and serum albumin
- Lymph node biopsy
- *Bone marrow aspiration and biopsy*: This is done in patients with advanced disease (stage III/IV), B-symptoms, and bony involvement or abnormal counts.
- *Radiological studies*: Chest X-ray; computed tomography (CT) scan of neck, chest, abdomen, and pelvis; imaging of other sites as and when indicated.
- *Positron-emission tomography scan of the whole body*: Positron-emission tomography (PET) scanning may identify more sites of initial disease than conventional imaging and is more accurate in detecting viable Hodgkin lymphoma in post-therapy residual masses. Rapid early response documented by significant reduction in disease volume and PET negativity at an early stage (after one or two cycles of chemotherapy) is associated with a favorable outcome. PET scanning should be performed at baseline and a minimum of 3 weeks postchemotherapy completion and 8–12 weeks postradiation.

PROGNOSTIC FACTORS

Several factors influence the success and choice of therapy. Pretreatment factors associated with an adverse outcome include advanced stage of disease, presence of symptoms, bulky disease, extranodal extension, male sex, and elevated erythrocyte sedimentation rate. These factors are interrelated in the sense that disease stage, bulk, and biologic aggressiveness are frequently co-dependent. There is some controversy as to whether histology is an important prognostic factor. The rapidity of response to initial cycles of chemotherapy based on PET is also prognostically important and is being used to determine subsequent therapy in current trials.

MANAGEMENT

Treatment of HD in pediatric population is different in certain respects from adults. Devising the ideal therapeutic approach for children with HD is complicated by their increased risk for late adverse effects. In particular, radiation therapy can cause profound musculoskeletal growth retardation and increase the risk for cardiovascular disease and secondary solid malignancies in children. Further complicating the treatment of children are gender-specific differences in chemotherapy-induced gonadal injury. The desire to cure young children with minimal side effects has stimulated attempts to reduce the intensity of chemotherapy (particularly alkylating agents) and radiation dose or volume. In general, the use of combined chemotherapy with radiation broadens the spectrum of potential toxicities, while reducing the severity of individual drug- or radiation-related toxicities. Current approaches use chemotherapy alone with or without low-dose (15–25 Gy) involved-field radiation therapy (LD-IFRT). The volume of radiation and the intensity/duration of chemotherapy are determined by risk grouping based on prognostic factors at presentation, including presence of constitutional symptoms, disease stage, and bulk. The current therapeutic strategy and outcome for children with HD is outlined in **Table 12.3.4**.

Table 12.3.4: Treatment modalities and results in Hodgkin disease.

Risk group	*Treatment modality*	*Overall survival (%)*
Low risk (stage I, IIA, no bulk, no B-symptoms)	VAMP/ABVE/ABVD 2–4 cycles + low-dose (15–25 Gy) IFRT	96–98
High risk (IIB, III, IV, bulky disease)	COPP-ABV/ABVE-PC/ ABVD/ BEACOPP 6 cycles + LD (15–25 Gy) IFRT	85–90

(ABV: adriamycin, bleomycin, and vincristine; ABVD: adriamycin, bleomycin, vincristine, and dacarbazine; ABVE: adriamycin, bleomycin, vincristine, and VP16; BEACOPP: bleomycin, VP16, adriamycin, cyclophosphamide, oncovin (vincristine), prednisone, and procarbazine; COPP: cyclophosphamide, oncovin (vincristine), procarbazine, and prednisone; IFRT: involved field radiotherapy; VAMP: vincristine, adriamycin, methotrexate, and prednisone)

Principles of Chemotherapy

All children generally receive combination chemotherapy as the initial treatment. While regimens containing alkylating agents are associated with an increased risk for infertility and therapy-related leukemia; in nonalkylator-containing regimens, doxorubicin (DOX) is associated with cardiac damage and bleomycin can produce pulmonary fibrosis. Common regimens currently utilized for the treatment include nonalkylator-containing regimens such as adriamycin DOX, bleomycin, vinblastine, and dacarbazine (ABVD) or hybrid regimens with lower total cumulative doses of alkylators, DOX, and bleomycin such as cyclophosphamide, oncovin [vincristine (VCR)], procarbazine, and prednisone (COPP) or adriamycin, bleomycin, and vinblastine (ABV); adriamycin, bleomycin, VCR, and etoposide (VP16; ABVE); bleomycin, VP16, adriamycin, cyclophosphamide, oncovin (VCR), prednisone, and procarbazine (BEACOPP); and VCR, adriamycin, methotrexate, and prednisone (VAMP).

Principles of Radiotherapy

Most newly diagnosed children are treated with risk-adapted chemotherapy alone or in combination with LD-IFRT. Low-dose involved-field radiation therapy involves the use of meticulous and judiciously designed fields to achieve local control of disease and to minimize damage to normal tissue. The low-dose radiation therapy (LDRT) treatment volume includes the initially involved lymph node region(s). In general, doses of 15–25 Gy are used, with modifications based on patient's age, the presence of bulk or residual (postchemotherapy) disease, and normal tissue concerns. Transposition of ovaries to midline and midline pelvic block to protect ovarian function and testicular shield or sperm banking in male children is routinely considered.

Nodular Lymphocyte-Predominant Hodgkin Lymphoma

Children with nodular lymphocyte-predominant Hodgkin lymphoma (NLPHL) have a favorable outcome, particularly when the disease is in early stage. Thus, treatment for NLPHL focuses on reducing initial therapy to reduce long-term treatment-related morbidity and mortality. Although, current standard therapy for children with NLPHL is chemotherapy plus LD-IFRT; patients have also been successfully treated with either chemotherapy alone or complete resection of isolated nodal disease. Anti-CD20 monoclonal antibody, rituximab is increasingly being used as a single agent or in combination with chemotherapy in relapsed NLPHL and is being evaluated as a frontline therapy in clinical trials.

LATE EFFECTS

Survivors of Hodgkin lymphoma are at risk for numerous late complications of treatment. Alkylating agents and VP16 have been associated with acute myelocytic leukemia (AML) and myelodysplastic syndromes. Doxorubicin can lead to cardiomyopathy and bleomycin can cause pulmonary fibrosis. Steroid use can produce avascular necrosis. Radiation therapy can lead to thyroid dysfunction, increased risk for myocardial atherosclerotic heart disease, and is associated with solid tumor development in radiation fields. All these potential complications mandate a close long-term follow-up after completion of therapy.

CONCLUSION

Hodgkin disease is one of the most curable cancers in children. Current use of appropriate staging techniques and risk-adapted treatment, protocols have resulted in an excellent overall survival. The formidable challenge is to maintain high cures and ameliorate treatment sequelae.

KEY MESSAGES

- Hodgkin lymphoma comprises 6% of childhood cancers and 40% of all childhood lymphomas.
- It is of two distinct pathologic subtypes: nodular lymphocyte-dependent and classical Hodgkin lymphoma with presence of hallmark malignant R–S cells.
- It usually presents with painless cervical lymphadenopathy with contiguous spread and B-symptoms in advanced stages.
- It is diagnosed on lymph node biopsy and staged based on modified Ann Arbor staging system.
- Risk-stratified treatment based on the use of multiagent chemotherapy with LD-IFRT achieves cure in 80–90% children.
- The current focus is on maintaining high cure rates with minimal chemoradiotherapy and minimization of long-term late effects.

BIBLIOGRAPHY

1. Hudson M, Constine LS. Hodgkin's disease. In: Halperin EC, Constine LS, Tarbell NJ (Eds). Pediatric Radiation Oncology, 4th edition. Philadelphia, PA: Lippincott Williams and Wilkins; 2004. pp. 223-60.
2. Hudson MM, Donaldson SS. Hodgkin's disease. In: Pizzo PA, Poplack DG (Eds). Principles and Practice of Pediatric Oncology, 5th edition. Philadelphia, PA: Lippincott Williams and Wilkins; 2006. p. 695.
3. Re D, Thomas RK, Behringer K, et al. From Hodgkin disease to Hodgkin lymphoma: biologic insights and therapeutic potential. Blood. 2005;105(12):4553-60.
4. Schwartz CL. The management of Hodgkin disease in the young child. Curr Opin Pediatr. 2003;15(1):10-6.
5. Thomson AB, Wallace WH. Treatment of paediatric Hodgkin's disease: a balance of risks. Eur J Cancer. 2002;38(4):468-77.

NON-HODGKIN LYMPHOMA

Non-Hodgkin lymphoma (NHL) is neoplasm of a wide range of cell types that comprise the immune system. It is generalized disease from the outset and has patterns of spread that mimic the migration patterns of their normal cellular counterparts. It accounts for approximately 7% of cancers in children less than 20 years of age. Approximately 2,500 cases of childhood NHL are estimated to occur annually in India. It occurs most commonly in the second decade of life, and occurs less frequently in children younger than 3 years of age. Immunodeficiency, both congenital (e.g. Ataxia-telangiectasia, Wiskott-Aldrich syndrome) and acquired [human immunodeficiency virus (HIV) infection or post-transplant], increases the risk of NHL. Indeed, NHL is the most frequent malignancy in children with acquired immunodeficiency syndrome (AIDS). With current treatments, about 80% of children and adolescents with NHL will survive at least 5 years.

CLASSIFICATION AND CLINICAL PRESENTATION

In children, NHL is distinct from the more common forms of lymphoma observed in adults. While lymphomas in adults are more commonly low- or intermediate-grade, are dominantly

Table 12.3.5: Major histopathological categories of pediatric NHL as per World Health Organization classification.

NHL type	*Immunophenotype*	*Clinical presentation*	*Chromosome translocation*
Burkitt and Burkitt-like lymphomas	Mature B-cell (CD10, CD19, CD20) and kappa and lambda light chains	Intra-abdominal (sporadic), head and neck (non-jaw, sporadic), jaw (endemic)	t(8;14)(q24;q32), t(2;8)(p11;q24), t(8;22)(q24;q11)
Diffuse large B-cell lymphoma	Mature B-cell (CD19, CD20, CD22, CD38, and CD79a)	Nodal, abdomen, bone, primary CNS, mediastinal	No consistent cytogenetic abnormality identified
Lymphoblastic lymphoma (precursor T-cell or precursor B-cell)	Pre-T-cell	Mediastinal, bone marrow	t(1;14)(p34;q11), t(11;14) (p13;q11)
	Pre-B-cell	Skin, bone	
Anaplastic large cell lymphoma (systemic)	CD30, Alk, EMA$^+$	Lymph node, skin, bones, visceral, soft tissues	t(2;5)(p23;q35)
	T-cell or null-cell		

(CD: cluster of differentiation; CNS: central nervous system; NHL: non-Hodgkin lymphoma)

nodal, have variable growth fraction and poor long-term outcome; almost all NHL that occurs in children is high-grade, extranodal, has higher growth fraction, and good outcome.

Non-Hodgkin lymphoma of childhood currently falls into three therapeutically relevant categories **(Table 12.3.5)**:

1. B-cell NHL [Burkitt lymphoma/leukemia (BLL) and diffuse large B-cell lymphoma (DLBL)]
2. Lymphoblastic lymphoma (LL) primarily precursor T-cell lymphoma, and less frequently, precursor B-cell lymphoma
3. Anaplastic large cell lymphoma (ALCL; T-cell or null-cell lymphomas)

Each type of childhood NHL is associated with distinctive clinical presentation, immunophenotype, and molecular biological characteristics. Distribution of NHL subtypes among children and adolescents in India differs from the rest of the world, namely a higher prevalence of DLBL and LL and a lower frequency of BLL.

CLINICAL FEATURES

Burkitt Lymphoma

Burkitt lymphoma accounts for about 50% of childhood NHL and exhibits consistent, aggressive clinical behavior. The malignant cells show a mature B-cell phenotype, and tumor has "starry sky" appearance. Burkitt lymphoma expresses a characteristic chromosomal translocation, usually t(8;14) and more rarely t(8;22) or t(2;8). Each of these translocations juxtaposes the *c-myc* gene to immunoglobulin locus regulatory elements, resulting in the inappropriate expression of *c-myc*, the gene involved in cellular proliferation. The two most common primary sites of disease are: (1) abdomen and (2) head-neck region. In India, these patients usually present with abdominal pain, vomiting, abdominal distension, palpable mass, intussusception, ascites, obstructive jaundice, or hepatosplenomegaly (sporadic presentation). Endemic Burkitt lymphoma is common in Africa, presents as jaw mass in majority of cases and is usually associated with EBV infection. Other sites of involvement include testes, bone, peripheral lymph nodes, skin, bone marrow, and central nervous system (CNS).

Diffuse Large B-Cell Lymphoma

Diffuse large B-cell lymphoma (DLBCL) is a mature B-cell neoplasm that represents 10–20% of pediatric NHL. Diffuse large B-cell lymphoma occurs more frequently during the second decade of life than during the first. Pediatric DLBCL may present clinically similar to Burkitt, though it is more often localized and less often involves the bone marrow or CNS. Outcomes for children with DLBCL are more favorable than those observed in adults, with overall 5-years event-free survival (EFS) rates of approximately 90% at 5 years. About 20% of pediatric DLBCL present as primary mediastinal disease [primary mediastinal B-cell lymphoma (PMBCL)]. This presentation is more common in older children and adolescents, and is associated with an inferior outcome compared with other pediatric DLBCL.

Lymphoblastic Lymphoma

Lymphoblastic lymphoma (LL) makes up approximately 20% of childhood NHL. More than 75% of LLs have a T-cell immunophenotype and the remainder has a precursor B-cell phenotype.

Nearly 75% of patients with LL present with anterior mediastinal mass, and symptoms of dyspnea, wheezing, stridor, dysphagia, or swelling of the head and neck suggestive of superior vena cava syndrome (SVCS). Pleural effusions may be present and the involvement of lymph nodes, usually above the diaphragm, may be a prominent feature.

There may also be involvement of bone, skin, bone marrow, CNS, abdominal organs (but rarely bowel), and occasionally, other sites such as lymphoid tissue of Waldeyer's ring and testes. Patients with more than 25% marrow blasts are considered to have leukemia, and those with fewer than 25% marrow blasts are considered to have lymphoma.

Anaplastic Large Cell Lymphoma

Anaplastic large cell lymphoma accounts for approximately 10% of childhood NHL. While the predominant immunophenotype of ALCL is mature T-cell; null-cell disease [i.e. no T-cell, B-cell, or natural killer (NK)-cell surface antigen expression] does occur. More than 90% of ALCL cases have the translocation t(2;5)(p23;q35) leading to the expression of the fusion protein nucleophosmin (NPM)/anaplastic lymphoma kinase (ALK). Clinically, ALCL has a broad range of presentations, including involvement of lymph nodes and a variety of extranodal sites, particularly skin, bone, gastrointestinal tract, lung, pleura, and muscle. Involvement of the CNS and bone marrow is uncommon. Anaplastic large cell lymphoma is often associated with systemic symptoms (e.g. fever, weight loss) and a prolonged waxing and waning course, making diagnosis difficult and often delayed.

EVALUATION OF CHILDREN WITH NON-HODGKIN LYMPHOMA

Pediatric NHL is a high-grade and a very rapidly growing tumor; hence, rapid diagnosis is imperative to prevent complications. **Box 12.3.1** lists the diagnostic tests required in the evaluation of NHL. Determination of the histologic subtype and immunophenotype on lymph node/tissue guides therapy. Patients with large mediastinal masses and SVCS are at risk of cardiac or respiratory arrest during general anesthesia or heavy sedation. Due to these risks, the least invasive available procedure to establish the diagnosis of lymphoma such as bone marrow examination, thoracocentesis, a lymph node biopsy under local anesthesia, or a CT-guided core needle biopsy should be contemplated.

STAGING, PROGNOSTICATION, AND RISK STRATIFICATION

The modified Ann Arbor staging classification does not adequately reflect prognosis in childhood NHL. The most widely used staging scheme for childhood NHL is that of the St Jude Children's Research Hospital (Murphy's staging), which is outlined in **Table 12.3.6**. In general, treatment for childhood NHL depends on localized versus disseminated disease. Localized disease is usually defined as stage I or II disease, while stage III or IV disease is generally considered disseminated. Currently, B-cell non-Hodgkin lymphoma (B-NHL) is risk stratified further for treatment planning, which incorporates stage, LDH, extent of surgical resection, and extent of bone marrow or CNS involvement. Similarly, ALCL is classified further based on visceral, skin, and mediastinal involvement **(Table 12.3.7)**.

Box 12.3.1: Evaluation of patient with non-Hodgkin lymphoma.

- History and physical examination
- Complete blood count with peripheral smear for blasts
- *Biochemistry*: Blood urea, uric acid, creatinine, liver function tests, serum electrolytes, serum lactate dehydrogenase, calcium, and phosphorus.
- *Imaging*: X-rays, ultrasound, CT scan or MRI of primary site and for staging, PET scan (optional)
- Adequate surgical biopsy for immunophenotyping, cytogenetics/molecular studies
- Bone marrow aspiration and biopsy
- CSF for cytology

(CSF: cerebrospinal fluid; CT: computed tomography; MRI: magnetic resonance imaging; PET: positron-emission tomography)

MANAGEMENT

Childhood NHL is an extremely chemosensitive disease. Surgery plays a very limited role, mainly for arriving at a diagnosis or for emergency management of obstruction or perforation. Radiation of primary sites is used very rarely in emergency situations. Hence, multiagent chemotherapy directed to the histologic subtype and stage of the disease remains the cornerstone of therapy.

Emergency Management

Pediatric NHL has very high growth fraction and short doubling time, sometimes as short as 24 hours seen with Burkitt lymphoma. Life-threatening complications may develop as a result of physical compression of tumor masses on vital structures or because of high cell turnover in a large tumor with resultant biochemical disturbances. The following complications can occur and which must be anticipated early and addressed immediately:

Table 12.3.6: St Jude's staging system for childhood non-Hodgkin lymphoma.

Stage	*Definition*
I	• Single tumor (extranodal) • Single anatomic area (nodal) excluding mediastinum or abdomen
II	• Single tumor (extranodal) with regional node involvement • Primary gastrointestinal tumor with or without involvement of mesenteric node or • *On same side of diaphragm*: – Two or more nodal areas – Two single extranodal tumors with or without regional node involvement
III	• All primary intrathoracic tumors • All extensive primary intra-abdominal disease • Two or more nodal or extranodal areas on both sides of diaphragm
IV	• Any of the above with CNS or bone marrow involvement

(CNS: central nervous system)

Table 12.3.7: Pediatric non-Hodgkin lymphoma (NHL): new risk grouping.

Protocol	*Group*	*Definition*	*5-year EFS*
B-NHL (FAB)	A B C	Completely resected stage I and abdominal stage II Unresected stage I, nonabdominal stage II All stages III and IV B-ALL < 70%, Blast CNS –ve B-ALL > 70%, Blast CNS +ve	98% 92% 84%
B-NHL (German group)	R1 R2 R3 R4	Stage I/II initial complete resection Stage I/II unresected, stage III with LDH < 500 U/L Stage III with LDH > 500–999 U/L, BM +ve and LDH < 1000 U/L LDH > 1000 U/L and/or CNS +ve	94% 94% 85% 81%
ALCL	• Low risk • Standard risk • High risk	Stage I completely excised No skin, mediastinal, liver, spleen, lung involvement Biopsy-proven skin, mediastinal, liver, spleen, lung involvement	90% 90% 60%

(ALCL: anaplastic large cell lymphoma B-ALL: B-cell acute lymphoblastic leukemia; B-NHL: B-cell non-Hodgkin lymphoma; CNS: central nervous system; EFS: event-free survival; FAB: French-American-British; LDH: lactate dehydrogenase)

- Superior vena cava obstruction and esophageal compression from mediastinal masses seen with LL
- Tumor lysis syndrome due to metabolic disturbances seen with LL and BLL
- Airway obstruction from pharyngeal or intrathoracic masses
- Respiratory or cardiac compromise from massive serous effusions related to involvement of pleura/peritoneum or pericardium
- Paraplegia from epidural tumor or raised intracranial pressure and neurological deficits from intracranial lymphoma/CNS involvement
- Obstructive jaundice and pancreatitis from compression of bile/pancreatic ducts
- Gastrointestinal bleeding, obstruction of bowel, and rarely perforation from intestinal involvement

In patients with SVCS at risk of cardiac or respiratory arrest, least invasive available procedure to establish the diagnosis of lymphoma should be used and the treatment started immediately in intensive care unit (ICU) as discussed earlier. Tumor lysis syndrome results from the rapid breakdown of malignant cells resulting in a number of metabolic abnormalities, most notably hyperuricemia, hyperkalemia, and hyperphosphatemia. Hyperhydration and allopurinol or rasburicase (urate oxidase) are essential components of the therapy.

Definitive Therapy of Pediatric Non-Hodgkin Lymphoma

Localized (low-risk) NHL in children: Stage I and II patients with grossly resected (>90%) disease regardless of histology have low-risk disease and an excellent prognosis, with 90% or better disease-free survival (DFS). For localized B-NHL (Burkitt or DLBL), use of short, intensive, pulsed chemotherapy for 2–3 months with aggressive CNS-directed chemotherapy without cranial radiation is standard. Common drugs used are dexamethasone, cyclophosphamide, methotrexate, cytarabine, prednisolone, and intrathecal (IT) methotrexate, ifosfamide (IFOS), VP16, and DOX. For localized LL (grossly resected, i.e. more than 90% stage I/II disease), a leukemia-like approach with induction, consolidation, CNS-directed therapy, and maintenance for a total of 18–24 months leads to more than 90% DFS. For localized ALCL, pulsed chemotherapy similar to B-NHL therapy is preferred.

Disseminated Childhood B-cell Non-Hodgkin Lymphoma

Patients with disseminated B-lineage NHL (Burkitt or DLBCL) have an 80–90% long-term survival through the use of short, intensive, pulsed chemotherapy using above-mentioned drugs for 5–6 months with aggressive CNS-directed IT chemotherapy without cranial radiation. The use of high-dose methotrexate (>5 g/m^2), cytarabine, and VP16 have appeared to be helpful in addition to the drugs mentioned above. Patients with Burkitt leukemia should be treated with protocols designed for Burkitt lymphoma. Multiagent chemotherapy protocols associated with excellent outcome include continuous Children's Hospital of Philadelphia (CHOP)/Childhood Obesity Prevention Mission Project (COMP) (American protocol), French-American-British lymphoma malignancy B (FAB-LMB-96) protocol, Berlin-Frankfurt-Munster (BFM) protocols (German multicentric protocol), and MCP-842 (Indian protocol). Rituximab is a mouse/human chimeric monoclonal antibody targeting the CD-20 antigen and is routinely used against DLBCL in adults. In children, rituximab in combination with the intensive chemotherapy regimen is being evaluated.

Disseminated Childhood Lymphoblastic Lymphoma

Patients with disseminated LL have long-term survival rates higher than 80%. As opposed to other pediatric NHL, LL responds much better to ALL-like therapy with induction, consolidation, CNS-directed therapy (IT drugs), reinduction, and maintenance for a total of 2 years than with shorter, intensive, pulsed chemotherapy regimens used for B-NHL. Common drugs used are prednisone, dexamethasone, vincristine (VCR), daunorubicin, DOX, L-asparaginase, cyclophosphamide, cytarabine, methotrexate, 6-mercaptopurine, and 6-thioguanine. Cranial radiation is currently used only for patients with CNS disease at diagnosis. Commonly used protocols include BFM (German multicentric protocol) and LSA2L2 (American protocol).

Disseminated Childhood Anaplastic Large Cell Lymphoma

Children and adolescents with disseminated ALCL have a DFS of approximately 60–75%. Both short pulse-intensive as well as LL-like strategies are effective for the treatment of disseminated ALCL. However, B-NHL-like short pulse-intensive regimens incorporating vinblastine is being preferentially used.

Role of Hematopoietic Stem Cell Transplantation

Hematopoietic stem cell transplantation (HSCT) is currently considered for children with recurrent or refractory NHL. Among relapsed patients with B-NHL and LL, despite current salvage chemotherapy and autologous HSCT, only about 10–30% patients survive long term. However, in ALCL, with salvage chemotherapy and/or autologous or allogenic HSCT, more than half of children become long-term survivors.

CONCLUSION

Non-Hodgkin lymphoma presents with distinct clinical syndromes reflecting the histological subtype. The prognosis for childhood NHL has improved significantly over the past two decades. The management includes supportive care to prevent tumor lysis syndrome, anticipation and management of oncologic emergencies, and multiagent chemotherapy. Intensive combination chemotherapy regimens with optimal supportive care have been shown to be feasible and curative for most children with NHL. The current focus is now on risk-stratified therapy to reduce chemotherapy and associated complications for low-risk disease and intensifying treatment for high-risk NHL for optimum long-term survival. Management of relapses continues to be a challenge and warrants high-dose chemotherapy with stem cell rescue in selected cases.

KEY MESSAGES

- Non-Hodgkin lymphoma is the third most common cancer in children.
- Childhood NHL is high-grade and aggressive requiring rapid confirmation of diagnosis, staging, and prompt initiation of therapy.
- Prevention and appropriate management of oncologic emergencies is a must.
- Multiagent combination chemotherapy direct to histologic subtype is the mainstay of treatment and has improved the cure rate of childhood NHL to more than 75%.
- Children with LL are treated with protocols designed for ALL, which provide EFS rates up to 80%.
- Children with B-NHL are treated with a strategy of short, rapidly repeated, pulse-intense regimens, which leads to EFS rates of up to 90%.
- In patients with ALCL, comparable results are achieved with either strategy. Although, ALCL has the highest relapse rate but many relapses can be salvaged with vinblastine-based regimens with or without HSCT.

BIBLIOGRAPHY

1. Gore L, Trippett TM. Emerging nontransplant-based strategies in treating pediatric non-Hodgkin's lymphoma. Curr Hematol Malig Rep. 2010;5(4):177-84.
2. Gross TG, Termuhlen AM. Pediatric non-Hodgkin's lymphoma. Curr Oncol Rep. 2007;9(6):459-65.
3. Magrath IT. Malignant non-Hodgkin's lymphomas in children. In: Pizzo PA, Poplack DG (Eds). Principles and Practice of Pediatric Oncology, 4th edition. Philadelphia, PA: Lippincott Williams and Wilkins; 2002. pp. 661-705.
4. Pinkerton R. Continuing challenges in childhood non-Hodgkin's lymphoma. Br J Haematol. 2005;130(4):480-8.
5. Shukla NN, Trippett TM. Non-Hodgkin's lymphoma in children and adolescents. Curr Oncol Rep. 2006; 8(5):387-94.

12.4 Wilms Tumor

Purna A Kurkure

INTRODUCTION

Wilms tumor (WT) is the most common renal tumor encountered in childhood. It develops as a result of abnormalities in the development of metanephric blastema. It is the paradigm for multidisciplinary treatment of pediatric malignant solid tumors. Large randomized controlled trials by various collaborative groups, including the National Wilms Tumor Study Group (NWTSG), Societe Internationale D'oncologie Pediatrique or International Society of Pediatric Oncology (SIOP), and the United Kingdom Children's Cancer Study Group (UKCCSG), have facilitated WT treatment to be customized to minimize morbidity for low-risk disease and to maximize the prognosis for high-stage, high-risk patients. Consequently, the outcome for patients with WT has improved remarkably in the past few decades.

EPIDEMIOLOGY

The median age at presentation is 4 years for unilateral tumors and 2.5 years for bilateral tumors. About 1.5% cases of WT are familial. It constitutes 6% of all childhood cancers.

Wilms tumor has been reported to be associated with various anomalies. Genitourinary anomalies are the most common and account for incidence of 4–8%. These include fused kidney, renal dysplasia, cryptorchidism, hypospadias, duplication of the collecting system, and WT, aniridia, genitourinary abnormalities, and mental retardation (WAGR) syndrome. Wilms tumor is also featured in many disorders of overgrowth including Beckwith-Wiedemann syndrome (BWS), Perlman syndrome, and isolated hemihypertrophy. Although most patients with WT are karyotypically normal, genomic studies have led to the localization and subsequent cloning of *WT* genes in two regions: (1) 11p13 and (2) 11p15. The former is *WT1* gene and is associated with WAGR syndrome and the latter is *WT2* gene, which is associated with BWS.

PATHOLOGY

The classic triphasic WT [favorable histology (FH)] is made up of varying proportions of three cell types:

1. Blastemal
2. Stromal
3. Epithelial

Unfavorable histology (UH) is characterized by qualitative variation from the classical type. Presence of focal or diffuse anaplasia, clear cell sarcoma, and rhabdoid tumor (RT) is considered to be unfavorable histologic features.

Most WTs are unicentric, 11% are multicentric but unilateral, and 7% are bilateral.

The SIOP trials recognized three prognostic groups of renal tumors of childhood:

- Low-risk tumors
- Intermediate-risk tumors
- High-risk tumors **(Table 12.4.1)**

Table 12.4.1: International Society of Pediatric Oncology working risk stratification of renal tumors of childhood (2001).

Pretreated cases	***Primary nephrectomy cases***
Low-risk tumors	*Low-risk tumors*
• Mesoblastic nephroma • Cystic partially differentiated nephroblastoma • Completely necrotic nephroblastoma	• Mesoblastic nephroma • Cystic partially differentiated nephroblastoma
Intermediate-risk tumors	*Intermediate-risk tumors*
• Nephroblastoma—epithelial type • Nephroblastoma—stromal type • Nephroblastoma—mixed type • Nephroblastoma—regressive type • Nephroblastoma—focal anaplasia	• Nonanaplastic nephroblastoma and its variants • Nephroblastoma—focal anaplasia
High-risk tumors	*High-risk tumors*
• Nephroblastoma—blastemal type • Nephroblastoma—diffuse anaplasia • Clear cell sarcoma of the kidney • Rhabdoid tumor of the kidney	• Nephroblastoma—diffuse anaplasia • CCSK • RT of the kidney

(RT: rhabdoid tumor; CCSK: clear cell sarcoma of the kidney)

Table 12.4.2: Investigations to be done in Wilms tumor.

Investigation	*Purpose*
Abdominal ultrasonogram	• Organ of origin • Identify contralateral kidney • Presence/absence of tumor thrombus in IVC (may need Doppler ultrasonogram)
CT scan (with contrast)	• Further evaluation of extent of tumor • Extension into adjoining structures such as liver, spleen, and colon • Visualization and function of contralateral kidney
Chest X-ray/CT scan (with contrast)	Pulmonary metastasis
Bone scan and skeletal survey	Bone metastasis in clear cell sarcoma of kidney (CCSK)
Brain imaging (MRI/CT scan)	Intracranial metastasis in rhabdoid tumor (RT) and CCSK
Retroperitoneal image-guided fine-needle core biopsy of renal mass	Cytological confirmation of diagnosis and risk stratification (presence of anaplasia) prior to prenephrectomy chemotherapy

(CT: computed tomography; MRI: magnetic resonance imaging; IVC: inferior vena cava; USG: ultrasonography)

CLINICAL FEATURES

- Asymptomatic flank mass
- Pain in abdomen
- Others—hematuria and hypertension

INVESTIGATIONS

These are listed in **Table 12.4.2**.

STAGING

Table 12.4.3 provides the staging system of the National Wilms Tumor Study Group (upfront surgery) and **Table 12.4.4** provides the staging system of the SIOP (upfront chemotherapy).

Table 12.4.3: Staging system of the National Wilms Tumor Study Group (upfront surgery).

Stage I	*Tumor limited to the kidney and completely excised:* • The tumor was not ruptured before or during removal • The vessels of the renal sinus are not involved beyond 2 mm • There is no residual tumor apparent beyond the margins of excision
Stage II	*Tumor extends beyond the kidney but is completely excised:* • No residual tumor is apparent at or beyond the margins of excision • Tumor thrombus in vessels outside the kidney is Stage II, if the thrombus is removed en bloc with the tumor *Although tumor biopsy or local spillages confined to the flank were considered stage II by NWTSG in the past, such events will be considered Stage III in upcoming COG studies.*
Stage III	*Residual tumor confined to the abdomen:* • Lymph nodes in the renal hilum, the periaortic chains or beyond are found to contain tumor • Diffuse peritoneal contamination by the tumor • Implants are found on the peritoneal surfaces • Tumor extends beyond the surgical margins either microscopically or grossly • Tumor is not completely resected because of local infiltration into vital structures
Stage IV	Presence of hematogenous metastases or metastases to distant lymph nodes
Stage V	Bilateral renal involvement at the time of initial diagnosis

(COG: Children's Oncology Group; NWTSG: National Wilms Tumor Study Group)

MANAGEMENT

Overall management plan has been represented in **Flowcharts 12.4.1 and 12.4.2**.

Surgery

The timing of surgery with regards to preoperative therapy has varied between the European and the North American groups. Nevertheless, surgical resection is an important constituent in the multimodal management of WT. Debates about the exploration of contralateral kidney at surgery exist but evidence now suggests that it can be omitted. Data from NWTS 4 study showed that omission of routine exploration does not affect the outcome or management of newly diagnosed WT, if adequate preoperative computed tomography (CT) or magnetic resonance imaging (MRI) is obtained.

A transperitoneal approach is preferred to provide adequate exposure for complete staging, which includes inspection for local tumor extension, hilar and regional lymph nodes, liver metastases, and peritoneal seedings. Prevention of tumor spillage should be of prime concern as this has a bearing in upstaging the tumor; hence, gentle handling and careful removal is mandatory. The inferior vena cava (IVC) and the renal vein should be palpated for the presence of tumor thrombus, which if present should be removed en bloc with the kidney.

Generally, WT does not infiltrate the adjoining structures; hence, a radical en bloc resection is rarely needed. However, a wedge resection, if performed safely, may help in downstaging the tumor to stage II. As regards to lymph node dissection,

Table 12.4.4: Staging System of International Society of Pediatric Oncology (upfront chemotherapy).

Stage I	Tumor is limited to kidney or surrounded with fibrous pseudocapsule if outside of the normal contours of the kidney, the renal capsule or pseudocapsule may be infiltrated with the tumor, but it does not reach the outer surface, and is completely resected (resection margins "clear"): • The tumor may be protruding into the pelvic system and "dipping" into the ureter (but it is not infiltrating their walls) • The vessels of the renal sinus are not involved. • Intrarenal vessel involvement may be present. Fine-needle core biopsy does not upstage the tumor. The presence of necrotic tumor or chemotherapy-induced changes in the renal/sinus fat and/or outside of the kidney should not be regarded as reason for upstaging a tumor
Stage II	Tumor extends beyond the kidney but is completely excised or penetrates through the renal capsule and/or fibrous pseudocapsule into perirenal fat but is completely resected (resection margins "clear"): • The tumor infiltrates the renal sinus and/or invades blood and lymphatic vessels outside the renal parenchyma but is completely resected. • The tumor infiltrates adjacent organs or vena cava but is completely resected.
Stage III	• Incomplete excision of the tumor, which extends beyond resection margins (gross or microscopical tumor remains postoperatively) • Any abdominal lymph nodes are involved • Tumor rupture before or intraoperatively (irrespective of other criteria for staging) • The tumor has penetrated through the peritoneal surface • Tumor implants are found on the peritoneal surface • The tumor thrombi present at resection margins of vessels or ureter, transected or removed piecemeal by surgeon • The tumor has been surgically biopsied (wedge biopsy) prior to preoperative chemotherapy or surgery *The presence of necrotic tumor or chemotherapy-induced changes in a lymph node or at the resection margins should be regarded as Stage III*
Stage IV	Hematogenous metastases (lung, liver, bone, brain, etc.) or lymph node metastases outside the abdomen–pelvic region
Stage V	Bilateral renal tumors at diagnosis Each side should be substaged according to the above criteria

(FNAC: fine-needle aspiration cytology)

Flowchart 12.4.1: National Wilms Tumor Study Group (NWTS) management plan.

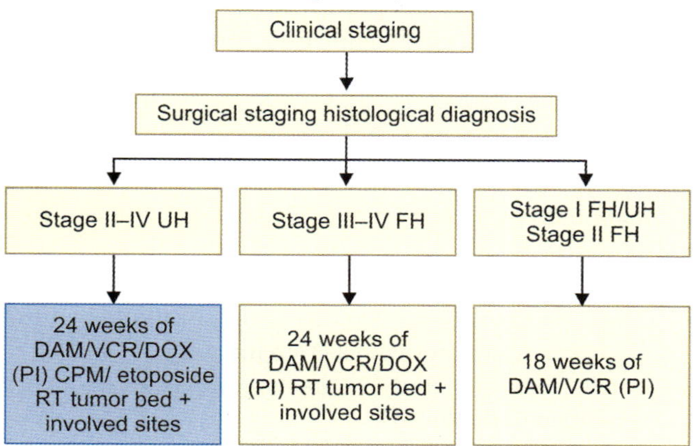

(CPM: cyclophosphamide; DAM: dactinomycin; DOX: doxorubicin; FH: favorable histology; PI: pulse intensive; RT: radiotherapy; UH: unfavorable histology; VCR: vincristine)

Flowchart 12.4.2: International Society of Pediatric Oncology (SIOP) management plan.

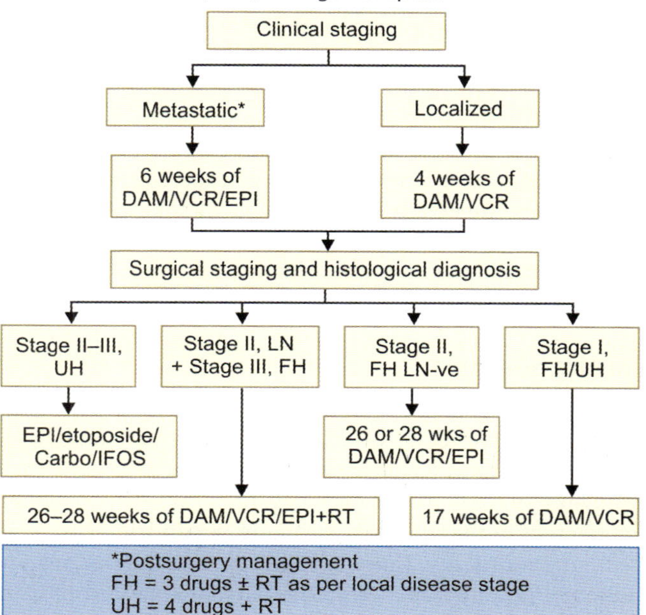

(Carbo: carboplatin; CPM: cyclophosphamide; DAM: dactinomycin; DOX: doxorubicin; EPI: epirubicin; IFOS: ifosfamide; RT: radiotherapy; SIOP: International Society of Pediatric Oncology; VCR: vincristine)

sampling of suspicious lymph node is recommended instead of a formal lymph node dissection.

Partial nephrectomy in the routine management of WT has not gained popularity. The reasons being most WT are large or centrally located, making only less than 5%

eligible for partial nephrectomy at presentation and even after preoperative chemotherapy only about 10% would be feasible for a nephron-sparing surgery. These surgeries carry a risk of leaving behind nephrogenic rest in addition to other procedure-related complications. Hence, partial nephrectomy is recommended for patients with synchronous or metachronous bilateral tumors, tumors in solitary kidneys, renal insufficiency of any etiology, and children with risk of multiple neoplasm's such as in BWS.

Chemotherapy

The current first-line drugs for WT are vincristine (VCR), dactinomycin (DAM), and doxorubicin (DOX). The second-line drugs for high-risk, relapse disease are ifosfamide (IFOS), etoposide, carboplatin (Carbo), and cyclophosphamide (CPM). Large cooperative groups have different chronology for deliverance of chemotherapy, drug combination, and duration, which have been refined over successive trials to optimize survival rates while minimizing acute and long-term toxicities. Despite these differences, the survival results among all the groups are similar. The SIOP and UKCCSG groups have favored the use of preoperative chemotherapy in an attempt to downstage the tumor, whereas the NWTSG advocates upfront nephrectomy without preoperative therapy in order to precisely identify the tumor stage.

Absolute Indications for Prenephrectomy Chemotherapy

- Large tumor, technically, is difficult to deliver at surgery
- Presence of major tumor thrombus in the IVC
- Bilateral WT
- Wilms tumor in a solitary kidney or horse-shoe kidney

Bilateral tumors and tumors considered inoperable at first should receive 4–6 weeks of chemotherapy followed by second-look surgery. In case of bilateral tumors, effort should be made to preserve as much of each kidney as possible. In such cases, chemotherapy may have to be given for a longer period to enable partial nephrectomy to be done.

Radiotherapy

As a result of the NWTSG and SIOP studies, the role of surgery has been customized though not eliminated. Radiation was an important treatment modality in preoperative and adjuvant settings in the earlier studies. With subsequent refinement in therapy with an aim in maximizing cure and reducing morbidity, there are now precise indications for adjuvant radiotherapy (RT). The current standard of care includes flank/abdominal irradiation (10.8 Gy in six fractions) for stage III FH tumors and stage II–III diffuse anaplastic WT.

Table 12.4.5: National Wilms Tumor Study V treatment results (favorable histology).

Stage	*4 years EFS (%)*	*4 years OS (%)*
I	92.4	98.3
II	81.4	97.6
III	88.7	94.8
IV	74.6	86.3

(EFS: event-free survival; OS: overall survival)

Table 12.4.6: National Wilms Tumor Study V treatment results (unfavorable histology).

Stage	*4 years EFS (%)*	*4 years OS (%)*
I	69.5	82.6
II	82.6	81.2
III	64.7	66.7
IV	33.3	33.3

(EFS: event-free survival; OS: overall survival)

The role of lung irradiation in metastatic disease is unresolved with difference among the groups. The NWTSG continues to administer whole lung irradiation (12 Gy in eight fractions) in patients with pulmonary metastases, while the SIOP group advocates omission of RT for patients whose lung metastases disappear completely after 6 weeks of prenephrectomy chemotherapy with VCR, DAM, and DOX. The role of pulmonary irradiation in children with pulmonary metastases visible on CT but not chest radiograph is further mystified.

Principles of Radiation Therapy

- Radiotherapy should be planned starting within 10 days of surgery.
- No change of RT dose for FH and UH.
- *Target volume:* Volume should encompass tumor bed and site of excised kidney with 2–3 cm margin.
- Entire vertebral body to be encompassed to avoid disproportionate growth.

The results of FH WT and UH WT are given in **Tables 12.4.5 and 12.4.6**, respectively.

CONCLUSION

Since WT is one of the most curable malignancies of childhood, special emphasis needs to be laid on the need for surveillance for late effects of therapy in terms of cardiotoxicity, musculoskeletal development, fertility, and second malignant neoplasm.

KEY MESSAGES

- The survival of patients with WT has dramatically improved from 30% several decades ago to almost 90%.
- A long-standing difference of opinion about the timing of nephrectomy in management of children with unilateral WT remains unresolved.
- Upfront versus delayed nephrectomy results in similar tumor control rates but a different overall burden of treatment.
- The improved survival has brought into focus important late sequelae of treatment; therefore, the emphasis is now shifting from successful treatment to reducing the burden of treatment.

BIBLIOGRAPHY

1. Dome JS, Cotton CA, Perlman EJ, et al. Treatment of anaplastic histology Wilms tumor: results from the Fifth National Wilms Tumor Study. J Clin Oncol. 2006;24(15):2352-8.
2. Graf N, van Tinteren H, Bergeron C, et al. Characteristics and outcome of stage II and III non-anaplastic Wilms tumour treated according to the SIOP trial and study 930-1. Eur J Cancer. 2012;48(17):3240-8.
3. Pritchard-Jones K, Moroz V, Vujanic G, et al. Treatment and outcome of Wilms tumour patients: an analysis of all cases registered in the UKW3 trial. Ann Oncol. 2012;23(9):2457-63.
4. Tongaonkar HB, Qureshi SS, Kurkure PA, et al. Wilms tumor: an update. Indian J Urol. 2007;23(4):458-66.

12.5 Neuroblastoma

ATK Rau

INTRODUCTION

Neuroblastomas are malignant embryonal tumors of precursor cells of the sympathetic ganglia and adrenal medulla. These are essentially tumors of infancy, which if detected at this age itself is associated with excellent prognosis. However, these tumors are also seen in later childhood when, due to various reasons, not the least being due to different tumor biology, the outcome is poor.

EPIDEMIOLOGY

Neuroblastomas constitute 8% of all neoplasia in childhood and are the most frequent solid malignant tumors in infancy. The mean age at diagnosis in various studies has been estimated to be between 2 years and 3 years, while the cumulative age distribution has been noted as follows:

- Less than 1 year—35%
- Less than 2 years—50%
- Less than 4 years—75%
- Less than 10 years—90%

The tumor occurs with equal incidence in girls and boys and is rarely observed in adolescents and adults.

ETIOPATHOGENESIS

The etiology of the tumor is as yet unknown. However, there are reports of a 40 times higher than expected incidence of neuroblastic precursor cells in the autopsies of infants less than 3 months of age who have died of other causes, implying that though the presence of neuroblastic cells is common in the first few months of life, all of them do not become malignant. Other reports have suggested an association between alcohol and drugs in pregnancy, parental occupation, and viral infections. Familial occurrence, association with other diseases such as neurofibromatosis and Hirschsprung disease, and features such as heterochromia iridis have been reported.

MOLECULAR CHARACTERISTICS

MYCN oncogene amplification, expression of neurotropic receptors, the deoxyribonucleic acid (DNA) index, and chromosomal abnormalities are commonly observed and help in prognostication. MYCN gene amplification, seen usually in older children, suggests a uniformly poor survival rate, while hyperdiploidy, common in infants, indicates excellent survival (95%). Increased expression of tyrosine kinase (TRK) 1, a neurotropic receptor, indicates increased susceptibility to chemotherapy and better chances of survival.

CLINICAL FEATURES

Sites

The tumor can occur in any area where sympathetic tissue exists. However, some sites are more often involved than others which in order of frequency are as given as follows:

- Abdomen—65% (adrenal medulla—46%, rest—19%)
- Posterior mediastinum—25%
- Pelvis—4%
- Head and neck—3%
- Others—3%

Symptomatology

It can be broadly classified under four categories:

1. *Those due to tumor*: Pallor, lassitude, weight loss, fever, abdominal pain, irritability, and bone pains.
2. *Those due to increased catecholamine secretion*: Paroxysmal attacks of sweating, pallor, flushing, headache, palpitations, and hypertension.
3. *Paraneoplastic features*, which may manifest as the opsoclonus-myoclonus syndrome or the vasoactive intestinal peptide (VIP) syndrome associated with diarrhea and hypokalemia or persistent anemia and thrombocytopenia due to bone marrow infiltration.
4. *Localized symptoms*, pertaining to various organ systems are as follows:
   - *Eyes:*
     - Periorbital edema and ecchymoses **(Fig. 12.5.1)**—the so-called "raccoon eyes."
     - Proptosis, exophthalmos, strabismus.
     - Retinal hemorrhage, optic atrophy.
   - *Neck:*
     - Cervical lymphadenopathy.
     - Horner syndrome.
     - Supraclavicular mass.
   - *Chest, mediastinum, and vertebra:*
     - Superior mediastinal syndrome (SMS) and superior vena cava syndrome (SVCS).
     - Infiltration into the intervertebral spaces—the "dumb-bell" tumor.
     - *Nerve compression*: Gait disturbances, paresthesia, and bowel and bladder dysfunction.
   - *Abdomen:*
     - Abdominal mass, usually detected by an enthusiastic clinician during routine immunization. Frequently crossing the midline, this characteristic differentiates it from a WT, which is also a tumor seen predominantly in this age group.
     - Hepatomegaly—the "pepper liver."
   - *Skin:*
     - Subcutaneous nodules, which rapidly change color from an initial blue to bright red color as it becomes more vascular. These nodules are seen mainly in neonates and younger infants with disseminated neuroblastoma.
   - *Bone and bone marrow:*
     - Lytic lesions on X-ray of skull and long bones.
     - Marrow infiltration occurs in about 50% of patients and may be the only organ involved other than the primary tumor, which is then designated as stage IV-S.

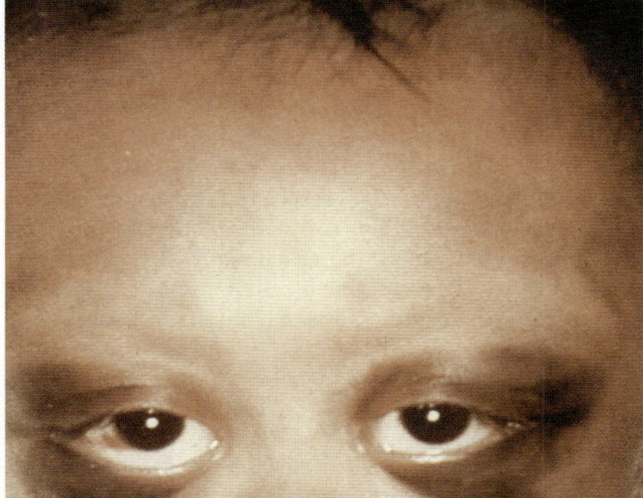

Fig. 12.5.1: The typical "raccoon eyes" of neuroblastoma.

Metastatic Spread

The tumor spreads through the lymphatics and blood. Metastasis at diagnosis is present in 40–50% of children below 1 year of age and in 70% of older children. Sites of metastasis include the bone, bone marrow, liver, skin, brain, spinal cord, and lungs.

PATHOLOGICAL FEATURES

Gross

These tumors are pale gray and soft with varying amounts of necrosis and calcification within. Most are noted to be highly adherent to the underlying structures.

Microscopy

One of the so called "round blue cell tumor," these tumors vary widely ranging from the undifferentiated neuroblastoma to the moderately differentiated ganglioneuroblastoma to the well-differentiated ganglioneuroma. The characteristic histopathological feature is the pseudorosette also called the "Homer-Wright" pseudorosettes as seen in **Figure 12.5.2**. However, in many instances, it becomes very difficult to distinguish the tumor from other members of the round blue cell tumor family and requires immunohisto-chemistry (IHC) to confirm the diagnosis. **Table 12.5.1** denotes the various differential diagnoses and their characteristic reactions to IHC.

EVALUATION

Laboratory tests for diagnosis include elevated levels of vanillyl-mandelic acid (VMA), homovanillic acid (HVA), and 3-methoxy-4-hydroxyphenylglycol (MHPG) seen in over 90%

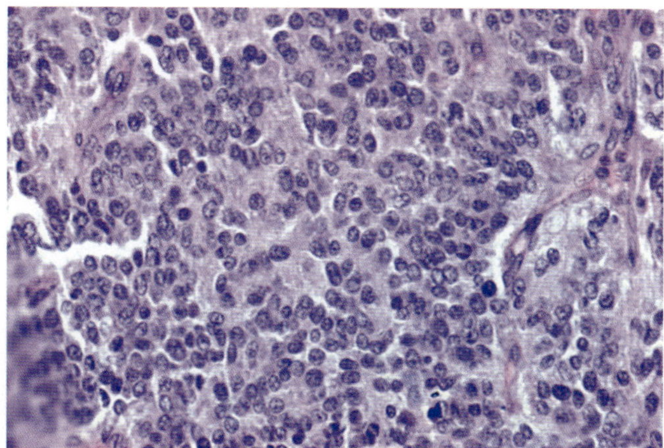

Fig. 12.5.2: Typical morphology of neuroblastoma showing the Homer-Wright pseudorosettes.

Table 12.5.1: Immunohistochemistry in pediatric "round blue cell" tumors.

Tumor	*IHC markers*
Neuroblastoma	Neuron-specific enolase, chromogranin, synaptophysin, TRK A, ganglioside GD2
Rhabdomyosarcoma	Myogenin, desmin, muscle-specific actin, dystrophin, vimentin, MyoD1
Ewing sarcoma/primitive neuroectodermal tumors (PNET)	CD99, β_2-microglobulin, synaptophysin, vimentin
Synovial sarcoma	Epithelial membrane antigen (EMA), cytokeratin, Bcl-2, TLE 1
Desmoplastic small round cell tumors	Desmin, cytokeratin, WT-1, EMA, CD57
Lymphoma	CD34, CD45, CD3, CD5, CD7, CD19, CD20, Sig, HLA-DR
Wilms tumor	WT-1, EMA, cytokeratin

(CD 99: cluster of differentiation; IHC: immunohistochemistry; MyoD1: myogenic differentiation 1; TLE 1: transducin-like enhancer of split 1; TRK A: tyrosine kinase A)

of patients. These tests are also useful as follow-up tumor markers. The bone marrow biopsy analysis confirms primary or metastatic involvement and is essential for staging the disease.

Imaging

- *Conventional radiography* often reveals mediastinal widening or calcification in an abdominal tumor **(Fig. 12.5.3)**. A complete body bone scan is useful in detecting bone metastasis and is necessary for staging.
- *Ultrasound scan, computed tomography (CT;* ***Fig. 12.5.4****) and magnetic resonance imaging (MRI)* all help to delineate the primary tumor and detect metastasis.

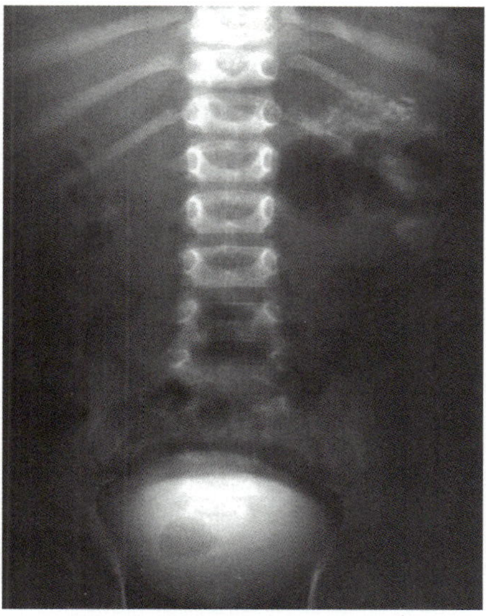

Fig. 12.5.3: Typical plain X-ray abdomen showing left-sided paraspinal calcification.

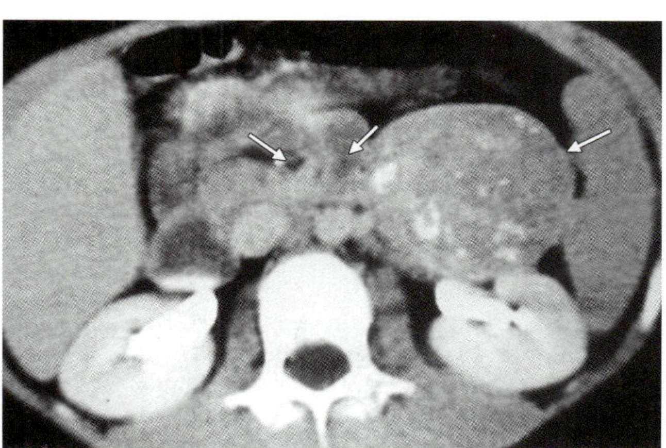

Fig. 12.5.4: Computed tomography film of a left-sided abdominal mass with calcification—typical of neuroblastoma.

- The *methylisobenzoyl guanidinium (MIBG) scintigraphy scan* ***(Fig. 12.5.5)*** is a radiolabeled, specific, and very sensitive method for evaluation and follow-up of primary and metastatic disease. Recent reports also suggest its very useful therapeutic role in the treatment of advanced and relapsed disease.
- *Myelography* is very important in the evaluation of primary or metastatic spinal disease and if performed early can diagnose the exact location and site of lesions causing impending motor weakness of the limbs. However, safer modes of investigations (e.g. MRI) are preferred.

DIFFERENTIAL DIAGNOSIS

All malignant tumors with the characteristic "round blue cell" morphology have to be differentiated from neuroblastoma

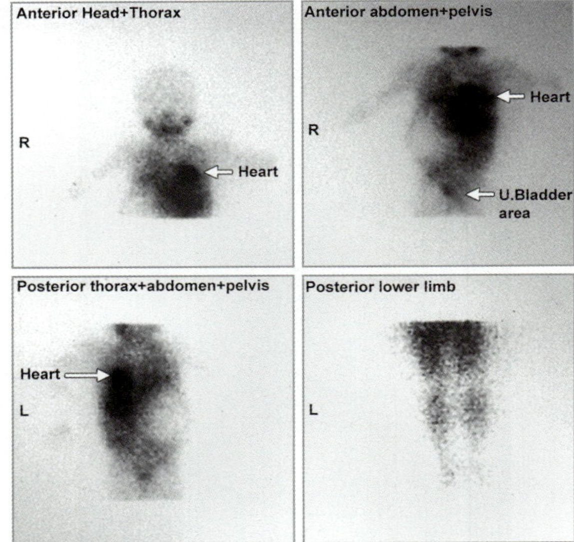

Fig. 12.5.5: Methylisobenzoyl guanidinium (MIBG) scan of an infant with neuroblastoma showing increased uptake by the tumor tissue.

and these include lymphoma, primitive neuroectodermal tumors (PNET), undifferentiated rhabdomyosarcoma (RMS), Ewing sarcomas and retinoblastomas, and Wilms tumor in older children. Nonmalignant differentials include osteomyelitis, rheumatoid arthritis, cerebellar ataxia, and other causes of pyrexia of unknown origin.

STAGING

Accurate staging is one of the keys to tailoring therapy in these children. Faulty understaging results in inadequate therapy and subsequent relapse while faulty upstaging results in unacceptable toxicity of therapy. The International Neuroblastoma Staging System (INSS) is presently used **(Table 12.5.2)** in all tertiary centers around the world in those cases where surgery is performed upfront and histopathology details are available. This system of staging is accurate and useful for prognosis.

In those children in whom surgery is not feasible at the beginning of therapy, the older but simpler Evan's clinical staging [Children's Cancer Study Group (CCSG)] system **(Table 12.5.3)** is used to stage the disease and start therapy accordingly.

Table 12.5.2: International Neuroblastoma Staging System.

Stage	*Description*
I	Localized tumor with complete gross excision, with or without microscopic residual disease with ipsilateral representative lymph nodes (IRLs) negative for tumor microscopically (nodes attached to the tumor itself may be positive)
IIA	Localized tumor with incomplete gross excision; IRL negative microscopically
IIB	Localized tumor with or without complete gross excision. Ipsilateral representative lymph nodes are positive for tumor. Representative contralateral nodes are negative for disease
III	Unresectable unilateral tumor infiltrating across the midline with or without regional lymph node involvement; or localized unilateral tumor with contralateral node involved or midline tumor with bilateral extension or lymph node involvement
IV	Primary tumor with distant metastasis to bone, bone marrow, liver, skin, or other organs (except stage IV-S disease as given below)
IV-S	Localized primary tumor (stage I, IIA, or IIB) with dissemination to bone marrow, liver, or skin (restricted to infants < 1 year of age)

Table 12.5.3: Evan's Clinical Staging System.

Stage	*Description*
I	Tumor limited to organ or structure of origin
II	Tumor with regional spread not crossing the midline
III	Tumor crossing the midline; bilateral nodes involved
IV	Distant metastasis
IV-S	Localized primary tumor with disseminated disease to liver; skin, and/or bone marrow (in infants < 1 year of age)

RISK STRATIFICATION AND THERAPY

Neuroblastomas are classified as low-risk, intermediate-risk, and high-risk, based on 13 prognostic factors including age, stage, histology, MYCN status, DNA ploidy, and others.

Low risk: Surgery alone is the treatment of choice in a majority of patients in this group but in some symptomatic patients 6–12 weeks of chemotherapy with cyclophosphamide (CTx), doxorubicin (DOX), etoposide (VP16), and carboplatin (carbo) may be added. These include cases with spinal cord compression, respiratory distress due to hepatic infiltration and infants with large stage IV-S disease. Selected cases of low-risk neuroblastomas (small tumors incidentally detected in neonates and infants with low VMA and HVA levels and without spinal cord or great vessel involvement) may safely be observed without either obtaining a definitive histological diagnosis or subjecting the child to surgery thus, avoiding potential complications of therapy.

Intermediate risk: Patients with intermediate risk are treated with surgery and 12–24 weeks of chemotherapy using the same drugs as in low-risk cases.

High risk: High-risk patients are aggressively treated with a combination of high-dose chemotherapy with cisplatin (Cis), ifosphamide (IFOS), VP16, DOX, and CTx. After preliminary

Table 12.5.4: Risk stratification.

Risk	*Stage*	*Age (months)*	*MYCN*	*Therapy*	*Survival*
Low	I IIA/IIB IV-S	Any Any <1 year	Non-amp Non-amp Non-amp	Surgery Surgery + LDCT Observation/CT or RT	>90% >80%
Intermediate	III IV IV-S	<18 months Any Any	Non-amp Non-amp Non-amp	CT (CTx + Cis + VP16 + DOX) RT to tumor bed, if residual disease + /second look surgery	>75%
High	II/III/IV/IV-S	>12 months	Amp	Multiagent CT + Autologous SCT + maintenance Cis RA	50%

(Cis: cisplatin; Cis RA: 13-*cis*-retinoic acid; CT: chemotherapy; CTx: cyclophosphamide; DOX: doxorubicin; LDCT: low-dose chemotherapy; RT: radiotherapy; SCT: stem cell transplant; VP16: etoposide)

chemotherapy (neoadjuvant chemotherapy), "second look" surgery is performed after which consolidation with near myeloablative chemotherapy is instituted. Radiation, with or after chemotherapy, is offered in some cases. Maintenance chemotherapy thereafter with 13-*cis*-retinoic acid (*cis*-RA) improves chances of survival in these children. **Table 12.5.4** delineates risk stratification and therapy recommended for each category.

Relapse: Newer drugs such as topotecan, paclitaxel, irinotecan, and MIBG have been used with varying success in relapsed cases.

Newer Therapies

Monoclonal antibodies, *cis*-retinoic acid, and its newer synthetic analogs as well as MIBG are all promising in a therapeutic role. These are at present undergoing trials and are awaiting approval before being introduced to newer protocols. Autologous stem cell transplants (SCTs) with high-dose MIBG administration are promising (40% increase in survival) in the management of high-risk/relapsed disease.

PROGNOSIS

- *Low risk*: 90% long-term event-free survival (EFS).
- *Intermediate and high risk*: 60–70% respond to initial therapy with partial or complete remission but a large number relapse with conventional chemotherapy. However, if consolidation includes very high-dose chemotherapy with autologous stem cell rescue, the chances of survival in this group are about 50–60%.

KEY MESSAGES

- Neuroblastomas are primitive blastemal tumors that are usually seen in infants and young children.
- Infants and young children with the disease have excellent prognosis while older children do not do as well despite adequate therapy.
- Recent advances in the therapy promise a great deal in the treatment of advanced and relapsed neuroblastomas, especially in older children.
- Early diagnosis and adequate therapy are still the cornerstones to successful outcome.

BIBLIOGRAPHY

1. Arceci RJ. Proceedings of the 42nd Congress of the SIOP, Boston. J Pediatr Blood Cancer. 2010;55:55-9.
2. Brodeur GM, Hogarty MD, Mosse YP, et al. Neuroblastoma. In: Pizzo PA, Poplack DG (Eds). Principles and Practice of Pediatrics Oncology, 6th edition. Philadelphia PA: Lippincott Williams and Wilkins; 2011. pp. 886-922.
3. Coppes MJ, Fry TJ, Mackall CL. Hematopoietic stem cell transplantation. Pediatr Clin North Am. 2010;57(1):1-352.

12.6 Retinoblastoma

Amita Trehan, Richa Jain

INTRODUCTION

Retinoblastoma (RB) is the most common primary intraocular malignancy of childhood affecting around 8,000 children annually and accounting for 1% of tumors in infancy. When the disease is diagnosed in its early intraocular stages, as is usual in developed countries, the probability of disease-free survival is around 90%. In developing countries, the diagnosis of RB is frequently made at later stages of the disease when extraocular dissemination has occurred resulting in poor survival rates, estimated to be 60% and 30% in low-middle and low-income countries, respectively.

EPIDEMIOLOGY

The incidence of sporadic RB is 1 in 15,000–20,000 live births, with no gender or racial predilection. It typically presents in the first 2–3 years of life, the median age being 12 months in heritable cases and around 24 months in sporadic cases. Presentation after 6 years of age is rare.

GENETICS AND INHERITANCE PATTERN

The tumor arises from primitive cells of the developing retina with the loss of function of the RB tumor suppressor gene (*RB1*), which is located within the q14 band of chromosome 13 (Ch13q14). There are two copies (alleles) of the *RB* gene in every cell in the body. At least one functioning allele is required to prevent the development of RB in a retinal cell. Loss of both the alleles results in RB tumors. Identification of the genetic mutation is important to enable screening of family members for the mutation. In addition to *RB* gene mutation, p53 pathway is also affected in approximately 66% patients.

Retinoblastoma may be inherited or occur sporadically and may occur unilaterally or bilaterally. Approximately 60% cases are nonhereditary and unilateral; 15% are hereditary and unilateral; and 25% are hereditary and bilateral. The inheritance is autosomal dominant with incomplete penetrance and is identified by the presence of a germline mutation of the *RB1* gene. The significance of germline mutations lies in the possibility of transmission to the next generation, and the need for genetic testing of the affected family members. Over 90% of children carrying the *RB* gene defect will develop RB. Inherited form of RB is seen at a younger age and these children are also at the risk of developing new tumors over time.

Mutation analysis in the index case can be performed in the blood or the tumor tissue; it should ideally be done in all patients of RB regardless of the pattern of presentation. This is essential for genetic counseling and testing in future pregnancies. Patients who have germline *RB* gene mutation are at a later risk of sarcomas including osteosarcoma, soft tissue sarcomas, melanoma, and other malignancies. This may be further potentiated by the use of radiotherapy (RT). Patients with nonheritable RB, on the other hand, do not have an increased risk of secondary malignancies.

ANATOMY

The tumor arises from the retina and grows toward the vitreous. This is known as endophytic growth, and is associated with vitreous seeding. Occasionally there is growth in the subretinal space, and this is called exophytic growth. Progression of the tumor results in the involvement of ocular coats and optic nerve, which may subsequently lead to scleral, orbital, and central nervous system (CNS) involvement. It progresses through the choroid and can invade the bloodstream with resultant distant metastasis.

CLINICAL FEATURES

The most frequent presenting symptoms are leukocoria, a white reflex in the pupil followed by squint, noted by family members or the child's pediatrician. Other clinical features include redness and pain, secondary to tumor deposits and increased intraocular pressure. Bilateral cases often present with poor vision, and nystagmus or searching eye movements as a result of tumor involving the central part of the retina (macula) in both the eyes. Massive proptosis or a fungating mass with lymphadenopathy is frequently seen at presentation in developing countries (including India) because of late presentation **(Fig. 12.6.1)**. Metastases occur by spreading of the tumor along the optic nerve to involve the CNS, or through the choroid resulting in hematogenous spread to bones, bone marrow, lungs, and liver. Rarely trilateral RB (with the involvement of pineal gland) or quadrilateral RB (pineal and suprasellar region involvement) may occur; they are associated with a dismal prognosis.

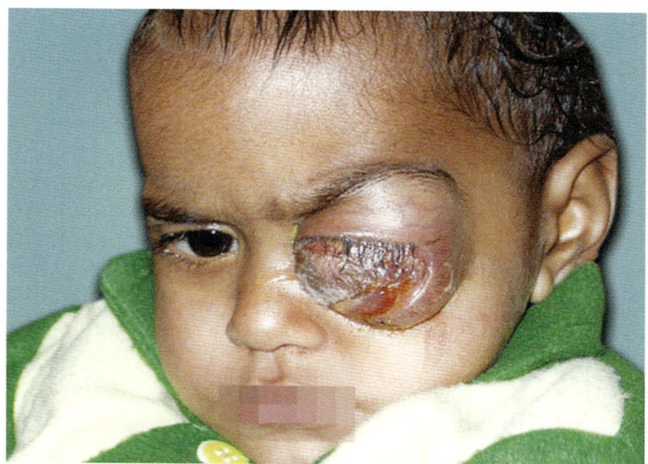

Fig. 12.6.1: Large mass is the presenting feature in developing countries.

Categorization

Retinoblastoma is categorized as intraocular or extraocular:

- *Intraocular:* Localized to the eye and may be confined to the retina. It may involve the choroid, ciliary body, anterior chamber, and optic nerve head. However, there should not be any evidence of disease at the optic nerve resection margin, or beyond the sclera.
- *Extraocular:* Tumor has extended beyond the eye. It may be localized to the tissues around the eye (orbital RB); it may have spread to the CNS or may have spread systemically (metastatic RB).

DIFFERENTIAL DIAGNOSIS

The important differential diagnosis includes:

- Coats' disease
- Persistent fetal vasculature
- Toxocariasis
- Cellulitis
- Metastasis
- Cataract
- Coloboma
- Retinopathy of prematurity
- Retinal detachment.

INVESTIGATIONS

The diagnosis is essentially clinical, with the support from imaging. Intraocular RB typically does not require tissue diagnosis.

- *Indirect ophthalmoscopy:* This is generally performed under anesthesia. This includes assessment of intraocular pressure. A manual examination is aided by real-time retinal imaging systems such as retcam, which can provide digital recording.
- *B-scan ultrasonography:* This confirms the presence of masses in the posterior segment of the eye. Calcification is characteristic of this tumor.
- *Computed tomography (CT)/magnetic resonance imaging (MRI) scan:* Imaging is done for visualization of the globe, orbit, CNS, and the pineal region (to look for pinealoblastoma, trilateral RB). MRI is preferred, as there is limited radiation exposure and improved visualization of the periorbital structures and orbital portion of the optic nerve.
- *CSF examination for malignant cytology:* This is indicated in microscopic or overt extraocular disease or presence of optic nerve thickening on neuroimaging. It is not required in intraocular RB.
- *Bone marrow:* This is performed in patients with extraocular disease (stage II and above) and/or those with altered complete blood counts (CBC). Typically, a bilateral trephine along with bone marrow aspirate is done.
- *Abdominal ultrasound*: This is performed when there is suspicion of metastasis to liver.
- *Biopsy or fine-needle aspiration cytology (FNAC):* This is a contraindication; occasionally FNAC or vitreous tap may be performed when there is doubt in the primary diagnosis.

STAGING

There are separate staging systems for intraocular RB and extraocular RB. The current staging system for intraocular RB is known as the International Classification of Intraocular Retinoblastoma **(Table 12.6.1)**. It is based on the extent of tumor seeding in the vitreous and subretinal space, and helps in predicting success of therapy. The prior Reese-Ellsworth classification has fallen in disuse. Another staging system exists for patients undergoing enucleation. This system is known as the International Retinoblastoma Staging System (IRSS); it also helps in defining and prognosticating extraocular RB **(Table 12.6.2)**.

Table 12.6.1: International Classification of Intraocular Retinoblastoma.

Group A	No tumor greater than 3 mm in dimension; away from fovea and optic nerve
Group B	Any eye not in Group A with no vitreous seeding, subretinal fluid is less than 5 mm from the base of the tumor
Group C	Tumors with focal fine vitreous seeding or subretinal fluid (less than one quadrant)
Group D	Massive or diffuse vitreous seeding, extensive subretinal masses
Group E	Unsalvageable eyes; neovascular glaucoma, tumor touching the lens, anterior segment tumor, phthisis, diffuse-infiltrating retinoblastoma

Table 12.6.2: Staging: International Retinoblastoma Staging System (IRSS).

Stage 0	Patients treated conservatively
Stage I	Eye enucleated, completely resected histologically
Stage II	Eye enucleated, microscopic residual tumor
Stage III	• Regional extension • Overt orbital disease • Preauricular or cervical node extension
Stage IV	*Metastatic disease:* *Stage IVa:* Central nervous system extension (with or without any other site of regional or metastatic disease) • Prechiasmatic lesion • Central nervous system mass • Leptomeningeal and cerebrospinal fluid (CSF) disease *Stage IVb:* Hematogenous metastasis [without central nervous system involvement] • Single lesion • Multiple lesions

TREATMENT

The therapy aims at:
1. Eradication of disease
2. Preservation of vision.

Limited stage intraocular disease may be treatable only by focal therapy (detailed below). In case of advanced stage (Group D or E) intraocular disease, enucleation may be required. Alternative therapies include combination of chemotherapy and focal therapies, intra-arterial chemotherapy, and newer modalities in a bid to preserve the eye.

Treatment of extraocular RB, which has locoregional extension, includes initial neoadjuvant chemotherapy followed by enucleation, further chemotherapy, and RT. Metastatic disease has poor outcome, and patients with CNS metastasis fare the worst, with dismal survival despite multimodality therapy and autologous stem cell transplantation.

Types of Focal Therapy

- *Photocoagulation* is the primary treatment in smaller tumors. It may also be used after chemoreduction. The argon laser is used for photocoagulation. Laser treatment is not effective for vitreous seeds.
- *Cryotherapy:* A special probe is applied through the sclera to produce temperatures as low as –60°C to –80°C resulting in cryonecrosis of the tumors. This is suitable for tumors smaller than 4 disc diameters close to the retina.
- *Thermotherapy:* Diode laser is used for thermotherapy, at temperatures just below the photocoagulation range.

Intra-arterial Chemotherapy

Intra-arterial chemotherapy is a modality used for advanced stage intraocular disease. This involves direct delivery of chemotherapy into the eye via cannulation of the ophthalmic artery. Typically one to six courses of such therapy may be required. Melphalan is the most commonly used chemotherapeutic agent. Intra-arterial chemotherapy helps in preserving the eye, though vision may not always be salvaged. Other agents, such as topotecan and carboplatin, are also being tested and administered as single agents or in combination. This has shown high success in intraocular unilateral tumors.

Chemotherapy

The main role of chemotherapy is in the treatment of extraocular disease; it is also used for intraocular advanced stage disease. It helps to shrink the tumors to a size where local treatment can be effective. The most commonly used drugs include carboplatin, etoposide, vincristine, anthracyclines, and cyclophosphamide. In intraocular disease only high-risk cases are candidates for chemotherapy. High risk includes presence of anterior chamber involvement with or without buphthalmos, choroidal involvement, postlaminar optic nerve or scleral involvement. Extraocular disease including metastatic RB is treated with a multimodality approach consisting of combination chemotherapy, delayed surgery, and adjuvant high-dose chemotherapy with/without a hematopoietic stem cell transplant.

Surgery

Enucleation is the common surgical modality. It is the treatment of choice for advanced uniocular disease with no hope for vision or the worse eye of bilateral cases. The eye is removed with a long segment of optic nerve. Chemotherapy may be required in cases with high-risk features. Orbital exenteration is almost never used in the current scenario.

Radiotherapy

Retinoblastoma is a radiosensitive tumor. In combination with chemotherapy, radiation is used for the treatment of extraocular disease. This is in the form of external beam RT. Brachytherapy can be used to treat small intraocular tumors, which have not responded well to chemotherapy or other forms of focal therapy. Proton beam therapy, though not available widely, has a role in the treatment of bilateral disease, as there is less chance of secondary malignant neoplasm.

Newer Modalities

1. *Subtenon (subconjunctival) chemotherapy:* Periocular injections of carboplatin/other agents to increase levels of

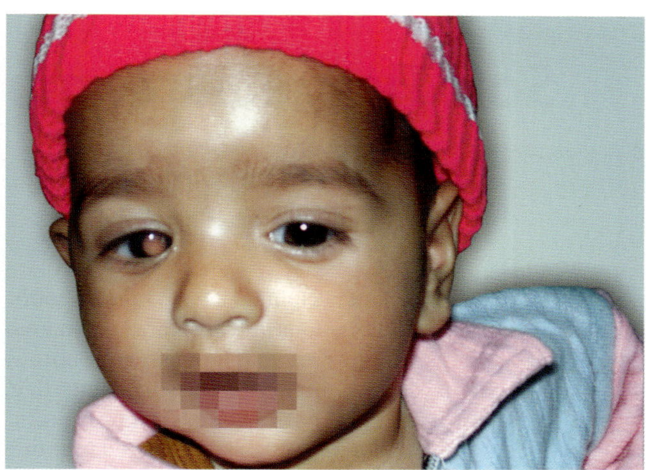

Fig. 12.6.2: White eye reflex along with squint in a case of intraocular retinoblastoma.

the drug and enhance efficacy, particularly in high-tumor burden.

2. *Intravitreal chemotherapy:* Direct injection of drugs into the vitreous cavity has been attempted. Pilot studies suggest that direct intravitreal injection of melphalan may be effective in controlling active vitreous seeds.
3. *Gene therapy:* "Suicide gene therapy" has been tried in early clinical trials in children with advanced intraocular disease **(Fig. 12.6.2)**.

OUTCOME

While outcome of intraocular and nonmetastatic RB ranges from 40% to 80%; presence of metastatic disease is associated with exceedingly poor prognosis. These patients have outcomes in the range of 10–15% despite intensive multimodality therapy. The important problems associated with RB in the developing countries are advanced stage of presentation, poor socioeconomic status of majority of patients and most importantly, treatment abandonment due to fear of enucleation. Early detection of RB, and emphasis on regular screening the other eye of the patient as well as siblings of patients with RB are modalities, which would help improve outcomes.

KEY MESSAGES

- Retinoblastoma has a good prognosis when the tumor is intraocular at diagnosis.
- Advanced stage of presentation is frequent in developing countries.
- Essentially, it is a clinical diagnosis; biopsy or FNAC are contraindicated.
- Small intraocular tumors may be cured by focal therapy.
- Chemotherapy helps shrink tumors.
- Almost 40% tumors are inherited.

BIBLIOGRAPHY

1. Chantada GL, Dunkel IJ, Abrams DH. Management of high-risk retinoblastoma. Expert Rev Ophthalmol. 2012;7:61-72.
2. Chevz-Barrios P, Gimbos DS. Clinical features, diagnosis, pathology. In: Rodriguez-Galindo C, Wilson MW (Eds). Retinoblastoma, 1st edition. New York: Springer; 2010. pp. 25-40.
3. Hurwitz R, Shields CL, Shields JA. Retinoblastoma. In: Pizzo PA, Poplock DG (Eds). Principles and Practice of Pediatric Oncology, 6th edition. Philadelphia: Lippincott Williams and Wilkins; 2011. pp. 809-37.
4. Parulekar MV. Retinoblastoma—current treatment and future direction. Early Hum Dev. 2010;86(10):619-25.
5. Rodriguez-Galindo C. Chemotherapy in the treatment of retinoblastoma. In: Rodriguez-Galindo C, Wilson MW (Eds). Retinoblastoma, 1st edition. New York: Springer; 2010. pp. 67-90.
6. Rodriguez-Galindo C, Orbach DB, VanderVeen D. Retinoblastoma. Pediatr Clin North Am. 2015;62:201-23.
7. Shields CL, Bianciotto CG, Jabbour P, et al. Intra-arterial chemotherapy for retinoblastoma report No. 1, control of retinal tumors, subretinal seeds, and vitreous seeds. Arch Ophthalmol. 2011;129(11):1399-406.
8. Wilson MW. Treatment of intraocular retinoblastoma. In: Rodriguez-Galindo C, Wilson MW (Eds). Retinoblastoma, 1st edition. New York: Springer; 2010. pp. 91-101.

12.7 Soft Tissue Sarcoma

Gauri Kapoor

INTRODUCTION

Pediatric soft tissue sarcomas (STS) are a group of malignant tumors that originate from primitive mesenchymal tissues and account for 7% of all childhood tumors. Rhabdomyosarcomas (RMS) are the most common of these and constitute about half of all cases of STS in children. The remaining nonrhabdomyosarcomatous soft tissue sarcomas (NRSTS) account for approximately 3% of all childhood tumors. The latter constitute a heterogeneous group of tumors and are rare in children. They include fibrosarcoma, neurofibrosarcoma, leiomyosarcoma, liposarcoma, synovial sarcoma, hemangiopericytoma, alveolar soft part sarcoma, and malignant fibrous histiocytoma, of which the synovial sarcomas, fibrosarcomas, and malignant peripheral nerve sheath tumors predominate in pediatric patients.

EPIDEMIOLOGY

- About 3% of all childhood cancers are RMS.
- About 350 new cases of RMS occur each year in the United States of America. The number of new cases has not changed much over the past few decades.
- Most RMS cases are diagnosed in children and teenagers. About 6 out of 10 of these tumors are diagnosed in children under the age of 10 years.
- These tumors are usually embryonal RMS and occur in the head and neck area or in the genital and urinary tracts.
- Adolescents and adults are more likely than younger children to have alveolar RMS, found more often in the arms, legs, or trunk.
- This disease is slightly more common in boys than in girls.
- There is no particular geographic location or ethnic group that has an unusually high rate of RMS.

ETIOPATHOGENESIS

No known environmental factors are known to cause RMS in children. Some genetic and environmental factors have been associated with the development of NRSTS: Li-Fraumeni syndrome and neurofibromatosis type 1 (NF1). Members of the Li-Fraumeni families have an increased risk of developing soft tissue tumors, bone sarcomas, breast cancers, brain tumors, and acute leukemias and have heritable mutations in the p53 tumor suppressor gene. Approximately 4% of patients with NF1 develop malignant peripheral nerve sheath tumors. Patients with familial adenomatous polyposis are at increased risk for developing desmoid tumors. The malignant fibrous histiocytoma can develop within a previously irradiated site; others (e.g. leiomyosarcoma) have been linked to Epstein-Barr virus (EBV) infection in patients with acquired immune deficiency syndrome (AIDS).

CLINICAL FEATURES

The most common sign of childhood STS is a painless lump or swelling, which may occur anywhere in the body. There may be no other symptoms at first; however, as the sarcoma grows, it may manifest with pressure symptoms on adjacent organs, nerves, muscles, or blood vessels, leading to pain or weakness, etc. Systemic symptoms (e.g. fever, weight loss, and night sweats) are rare. Hypoglycemia and hypophosphatemic rickets have been reported in cases of hemangiopericytoma, whereas hyperglycemia has been noted in patients with fibrosarcoma of the lung.

- *Rhabdomyosarcomas* may originate in different sites of the body depending upon the age of the child. Most head and neck tumors occur in children under the age of 8 years, while those of the extremity are most commonly found in adolescents. Less common primary sites for this cancer are the genitourinary tract, including the bladder and prostate in the male and the vagina in the female.
- The *NRSTS* arise most commonly in the trunk and extremities. These neoplasms can present initially as an asymptomatic solid mass, or they may be symptomatic because of local invasion of adjacent anatomical structures. Synovial sarcomas, the most common NRSTS, reported in children, most commonly occur in the lower extremity followed by upper extremity, trunk, abdomen, and head and neck. Approximately 30% of patients with synovial sarcoma are younger than 20 years. The most common site of metastasis is the lung.

DIAGNOSIS

The first step is to establish a confirmed histological diagnosis. Often an imaging, a computed tomography (CT) scan or magnetic resonance image (MRI), of the tumor is done followed by fine-needle aspiration cytology (FNAC) prior to planning a biopsy. These results determine type of biopsy—Tru-cut needle biopsy, incisional biopsy, or excisional biopsy. RMS is a malignant round cell tumor, and can appear very similar to other childhood cancers at the microscopic level, and immunohistochemistry (IHC) and molecular genetic tests may be required to establish a firm diagnosis. Hence, obtaining adequate tissue for histology and IHC is very important.

Biopsy

Technique of biopsy is critically important in the diagnosis and management of STS. Tissue may be obtained by core-needle biopsy, incisional biopsy, or excisional biopsy. Adequate material is essential for routine histopathological studies as well as panel of immunohistochemical markers and molecular characterization of the tumor particularly in the case of NRSTS. It is recommended that planning of biopsy be done by the surgeon who will perform the definitive resection as poorly planned biopsies may affect the performance of the primary resection.

STAGING

Once histological diagnosis is confirmed, further tests are done to determine the stage of the disease. Clinical staging has an important role in predicting the clinical outcome and determining the most effective therapy for pediatric STS. In RMS, bone marrow aspiration and biopsy, CT chest, and bone scan are done to look for metastatic disease at these sites while for NRSTS, only CT chest is usually required. Whole body positron-emission tomography (PET) scan may also be done as a single imaging to look for metastatic disease. The staging systems used are the intergroup RMS study Intergroup Rhabdomyosarcoma Study Group (IRSG), tumor, node, metastases (TNM) for RMS, and the Children's Oncology Group (COG) staging system for children with NRSTS **(Tables 12.7.1 to 12.7.3)**.

PROGNOSIS

The treatment outcome for pediatric RMS depends on anatomic site, patient age, stage, and histology, on the basis of which they are risk stratified. The various unfavorable prognostic factors include older age, metastatic disease, large tumor, alveolar histology, and primary tumor in trunk or pelvis. Low-risk, intermediate-risk, and high-risk patients have a 3-year failure-free survival rate of 88%, 55–75%, and less than 30%, respectively **(Table 12.7.4)**.

MANAGEMENT

The treatment for childhood STS requires a multidisciplinary oncology team comprising pediatric oncologists, surgeons, and radiotherapists.

Rhabdomyosarcoma

Chemotherapy

Rhabdomyosarcoma is a chemosensitive disease, and micrometastatic disease is believed to be present from its onset. Hence, all children with RMS receive chemotherapy, which forms the backbone of treatment, and the dose and duration depend on various risk factors. The most effective drugs include cyclophosphamide, vincristine, dactinomycin, doxorubicin, ifosphamide, and etoposide. The total duration of treatment ranges from 6 months to 12 months.

Surgery

All children diagnosed with RMS also require surgery, either to remove all or part of the primary tumor or to perform an

Table 12.7.1: Classification of soft tissue sarcomas (STS) according to histological type with corresponding chromosomal aberration.

Group	*Histological type*	*Chromosomal aberration*
Rhabdomyosarcomas (RMS)	• Pleomorphic RMS	
	• Embryonal RMS	LOH of 11q15
	• Alveolar RMS	t(2;13)(q35;q14), t(1;13)(p36;q14)
Nonrhabdomyosarcomas soft tissue sarcomas (NRSTS)	• Fibrosarcoma	
	• Neurofibrosarcoma	Deletion 17q11.2
	• Infantile fibrosarcoma	t(12;15)(p13;q25)
	• Malignant fibrous histiocytoma	(qp+, ring chromosome)
	• Dermatofibrosarcoma protuberans	t(17;22)(q22;q13)
	• Kaposi sarcoma	
	• Hemangioendothelioma	t(12;14)
	• Leiomyosarcoma	
	• Liposarcoma	t(x;18)(p11.2;q11.2)
	• Angiosarcoma	t(x;17)(p11.2;q25)
	• Synovial sarcoma	
	• Alveolar soft part sarcoma	
	• Epithelioid sarcoma	

Table 12.7.2: Children's oncology group-soft tissue sarcomas (COG-STS) pretreatment staging system for rhabdomyosarcoma (RMS).

Stage	*Sites of primary tumor*	*T stage*	*Tumor size*	*Regional lymph nodes*	*Distant metastasis*
I	Favorable sites Orbit Head and neck Genitourinary	T1 or T2 T1 or T2 T1 or T2 T1 or T2	Any size	N0 or N1 or NX	M0
II	Unfavorable sites Bladder/prostate Extremity Cranial Parameningeal	T1 or T2 T1 or T2 T1 or T2 T1 or T2 T1 or T2	*a*, ≤5 cm	N0 or NX	M0
III	Other Unfavorable sites Bladder/prostate Extremity Cranial Parameningeal	T1 or T2 T1 or T2 T1 or T2 T1 or T2 T1 or T2	*a*, ≤5 cm *b*, >5 cm	N1 N0 or N1 or NX	M0
IV	Other Any site All	T1 or T2 T1 or T2	Any size	N0 or N1 or NX	M1

(M0: absence of metastatic spread; M1: presence of metastatic spread beyond the primary site; N0: absence of nodal spread; N1: presence of nodal spread beyond the primary site; NX: unknown N status)

Table 12.7.3: Children's oncology group-soft tissue sarcomas (COG-STS) surgicopathologic group system for rhabdomyosarcoma (RMS).

Group	*Definition*
I (Approximately 13% of all patients are in this group)	A localized tumor that is completely removed with pathologically clear margins and no regional lymph node involvement
II (Approximately 20% of all patients are in this group)	A localized tumor that is grossly removed with: a. Microscopic disease at the margin b. Involve, grossly removed regional lymph nodes - Both (a) and (b)
III (Approximately 48% of all patients are in this group)	A localized tumor with gross residual disease after incomplete removal or biopsy only
IV (Approximately 18% of all patients are in this group)	Distant metastases are present at diagnosis

incisional/needle biopsy to reach a definitive diagnosis. Only about 10% of newly diagnosed children have tumors that can be completely removed. Every attempt should be made to resect the primary tumor with negative margins before or after chemotherapy (second-look surgery) and while causing minimum cosmetic and functional impairment.

Table 12.7.4: Children's oncology group-soft tissue sarcomas (COG-STS) rhabdomyosarcoma risk group classification.

Risk group prognosis (event-free survival)	*Histology*	*Stage*	*Group*
Low-risk Excellent (70–≥85%)	Embryonal	1	I, II, III
	Embryonal	2, 3	I, II
Intermediate-risk Good (50–70%)	Embryonal	2, 3	III
	Alveolar	1, 2, 3	I, II, III
High-risk Poor (≤30%)	Embryonal or alveolar	4	IV

Radiotherapy

Radiotherapy is an important local control measure for all children with RMS except those with completely resected Stage I and II disease. Total radiation dose ranges from 4,000 cGy to 5,500 cGy over a period of 4–6 weeks. It is usually planned approximately 9 weeks after chemotherapy has begun and earlier for those with parameningeal disease. With the use of both surgery and radiation therapy, local control of the primary tumor can be achieved in more than 80% of patients.

Outcome

With appropriate treatment, the 5-year survival of low-, intermediate-, and high-risk RMS is 90%, 70%, and 30%, respectively.

Nonrhabdomyosarcomatous Soft Tissue Sarcomas

Surgery

For NRSTS, surgery is the cornerstone of the treatment. Ideally, an attempt is made to completely remove the mass with wide margins (portions of the surrounding tissue) to ensure that no microscopic disease remains. The most important prognostic factor is the ability to completely remove the primary tumor.

Radiation Therapy

Radiation therapy is indicated for patients with inadequate surgical margins and for larger, high-grade tumors. This is particularly important in high-grade tumors with tumor margins less than 1 cm. Brachytherapy and intraoperative radiation may be applicable in select situations.

Chemotherapy

Chemotherapy is sometimes used to shrink large tumors to make them operable. The two most active agents are ifosphamide and Adriamycin. The role of adjuvant (postoperative) chemotherapy remains controversial for NRSTS.

Targeted Therapy

The role of antiangiogenesis agents and mTOR inhibitors has been explored in adults but not in children.

Outcome

Long-term survival is dependent on the presence of metastatic disease and completeness of the surgical excision.

LATE EFFECTS

Improved outcomes with multimodality therapy in children with STS have caused increasing concern about the potential long-term side effects of therapy, especially when considering the expected longer life-span of children. Late effects including consequences on growth and development, cardiac function, second malignancy, etc. all need to be considered when planning the treatment.

KEY MESSAGES

- Soft-tissue sarcomas comprise the fifth most common type of childhood solid tumor, of which RMS is the most common.
- It can arise at any site and in any tissue in the body except bone, hence may present as a mass or lump.
- Confirmation of histology and staging work-up are essential prior to starting the therapy.
- The treatment for childhood STS is a coordinated multidisciplinary team effort comprising pediatric oncologists, surgeons, and radiotherapists.
- Chemotherapy is an essential component of therapy for RMS along with surgery and/or RT for local control. Survival depends on the risk group.
- For NRSTS, surgery is the mainstay of treatment with or without RT.

BIBLIOGRAPHY

1. American Cancer Society. (2018). Rhabdomyosarcoma. [online]. Available from *www.cancer.org/Cancer/Rhabdomyosarcoma/DetailedGuide/rhabdomyosarcoma-key-statistics* [Accessed October, 2018].
2. National Cancer Institute. Childhood rhabdomyosarcoma treatment (PDQ®). [online]. Available from www.cancer.gov/cancertopics/pdq/treatment/childRMS/HealthProfessional [Accessed October, 2018].
3. National Cancer Institute. Soft tissue sarcoma. [online]. Available from www.cancer.gov/cancertopics/types/soft-tissue-sarcoma [Accessed October, 2018].
4. Okcu MF, Pappo AS, Hicks J, et al. The nonrhabdomyosarcoma soft tissue sarcoma. In: Pizzo PA, Poplack DG (Eds). Principles and Practice of Pediatric Oncology, 6th edition. Philadelphia, PA: Lippincott Williams and Wilkins; 2011. pp. 953-86.
5. Wexler LH, Meyer WH, Helman LJ. Rhabdomyosarcoma. In: Pizzo PA, Poplack DG (Eds). Principles and Practice of Pediatric Oncology, 6th edition. Philadelphia, PA: Lippincott Williams and Wilkins; 2011. pp. 923-53.

12.8 Pediatric Bone Marrow Transplantation

Satya Prakash Yadav

INTRODUCTION

Hematopoietic stem cell transplant (HSCT), a term that covers bone marrow transplant (BMT), peripheral blood stem cell transplant (PBSCT), and cord blood transplant (CBT), is a well-recognized therapy for diverse malignancies, both blood cancers and some solid tumors, in addition to selected nonmalignant diseases.

HISTORY

In 1956, George Mathe treated four physicists exposed to high-dose radiation, following an accident at nuclear plant at Vinca (then Yugoslavia), with intravenous (IV) infusions of allogeneic bone marrow cells harvested from family donors. In 1977, Donnall (Don) Thomas and his colleagues reported the results of human leukocyte antigen (HLA)—identical sibling transplants in 100 patients with "end-stage" leukemia. Thomas was awarded the Nobel Prize in Medicine in 1990 for his substantial contributions to this research. The past two decades have seen a rapid development in HSCT, as the procedure has become safer and more widely used.

TYPES OF HEMATOPOIETIC STEM CELL TRANSPLANT

An allogeneic stem cell transplant (SCT) is a transplant between two individuals—a donor and a recipient. When individuals are identical twins, the transplant is known as syngeneic; when the donor and recipient are not related, the transplant is known as matched unrelated donor (MUD); and when the donor and the recipient are HLA-matched siblings, then it is called matched sibling donor (MSD). An autologous SCT is a transplant by which patient's own stem cells are harvested (collected), stored, and later returned intravenously.

Role of Human Leukocyte Antigen Typing

The molecules encoded by Class I and II major histocompatibility complex are called HLA, and these constitute a major component of the immunological barriers. The currently known Class I genes are *HLA-A*, *HLA-B*, and *HLA-C*, and are found on virtually all nucleated cells and they are for recognition of self. Class II genes are expressed only on lymphocytes and a few other cells and the most important genes are *HLA-DR*, *HLA-DQ*, and *HLA-DP*; these are necessary for cross-talk between immunological cells and self-antigens.

Selection of the Donor

The best donors are HLA-identical sibling donors because they are not only phenotypically matched for HLA antigens, but also have genotypic identity. The chances of finding an MSD are about 30%. Most current studies suggest that a "perfect" donor is one who is fully molecularly matched for HLA-A, B, C, DRB1, and DRQB1. Such a donor is referred to as 10/10 match. In general, mismatches of two or more HLA subtypes are associated with a considerably poorer outcome. Matched unrelated donor SCT is offered to those who do not have an MSD available. National marrow donor program has a facility for searching a worldwide donor register consisting of over 13 million HLA-typed volunteers. This pool is currently able to provide suitable donors for about 80% of recipients for a Caucasian; the corresponding figures for patients from ethnic minorities drop below 30%. When an MUD is not available, other sources such as unrelated cord blood (CB) units from many public cord banks worldwide are used.

INDICATIONS FOR BONE MARROW TRANSPLANTATION

Indications for allogeneic HSCT are given in **Box 12.8.1**. Indications for autologous HSCT are described in **Box 12.8.2**.

SOURCES OF HEMATOPOIETIC STEM CELLS

Bone Marrow

From the earliest efforts to offer HSCT to humans until about 1993, all donations were collected from the bone marrow. Bone marrow is harvested from the patient (for autologous SCT) or the donor (for allogeneic SCT) under general anesthesia by aspiration from the pelvic bones (iliac crests) **(Fig. 12.8.1)**.

Box 12.8.1: Indications for allogeneic hematopoietic stem cell transplantation for pediatric diseases.

- Acute lymphoblastic leukemia (ALL) in CR1 for patients with very high-risk ALL (prednisone poor response on day 7 with T-immunophenotype or total leukocyte count more than 100,000/µL; t(9;22); not in remission at the end of induction phase) and CR2 or later complete remission
- Acute myeloid leukemia in CR1 except those with presence of t(15;17), t(8;21), and inv16 or those who are relapsed cases
- Chronic myeloid leukemia
- Myelodysplastic syndromes
- Relapsed or refractory Hodgkin and non-Hodgkin lymphoma
- Severe acquired aplastic anemia
- Inherited bone marrow failure syndromes (Fanconi anemia, dyskeratosis congenita, Diamond-Blackfan anemia)
- Hemoglobinopathies (thalassemia major, sickle-cell disease)
- Congenital immunodeficiency syndromes (severe combined immunodeficiency, Wiskott-Aldrich syndrome, hyperimmunoglobulin M (HIgM) syndrome, leukocyte adhesion defects, Chédiak-Higashi syndrome, Kostmann syndrome, chronic granulomatous disease, and other neutrophil defects)
- X-linked lymphoproliferative disorder (Duncan syndrome)
- Familial hemophagocytic lymphohistiocytosis
- Infantile malignant osteopetrosis
- Selected types of mucopolysaccharidosis (Hurler) or other liposomal/peroxisomal disorders (X-linked adrenoleukodystrophy)
- Selected severe variants of platelet function disorders (Bernard-Soulier syndrome and Glanzmann's thrombasthenia)

(CR: complete remission)

Box 12.8.2: Indications for autologous hematopoietic stem cell transplantation for pediatric diseases.

- Acute myeloid leukemia in CR1 or CR2
- Acute lymphoblastic leukemia after an isolated extramedullary relapse
- Relapsed Hodgkin or non-Hodgkin lymphoma
- High-risk, relapsed, or resistant brain tumors
- High-risk neuroblastoma
- Relapsed/refractory rhabdomyosarcoma
- Relapsed/refractory Ewing sarcoma
- Life-threatening autoimmune diseases resistant to conventional treatments (systemic lupus erythematosus, juvenile rheumatoid arthritis)

(CR: complete remission)

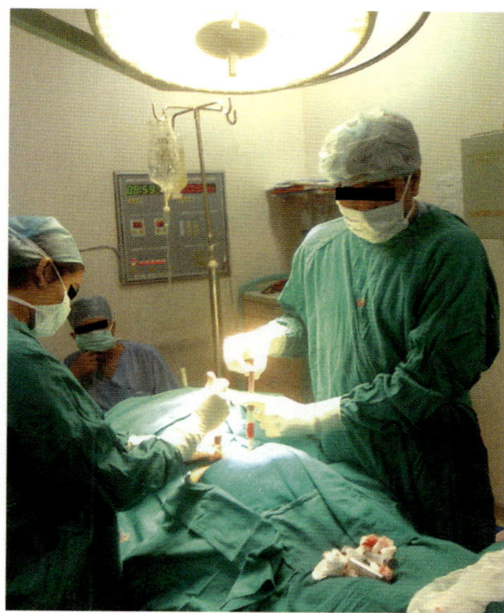

Fig. 12.8.1: Bone marrow harvest from bilateral iliac crests from a donor under general anesthesia.

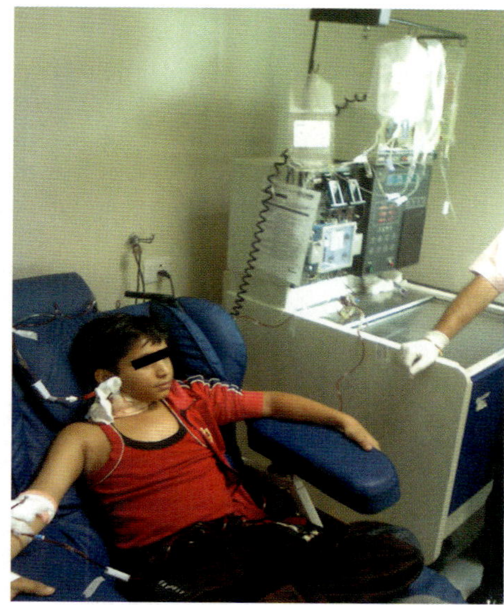

Fig. 12.8.2: Peripheral blood stem cell harvest by leukapheresis.

Peripheral Blood Stem Cells

Since 1993, transplanters have been increasingly using peripheral blood for harvesting stem cells. Hematopoietic stem cell (HSC) may be mobilized from the peripheral blood following administration of granulocyte colony-stimulating factor (G-CSF) and harvested using cell separators **(Fig. 12.8.2)**.

Cord Blood Stem Cells

The use of umbilical cord blood (UCB)-derived HSC **(Fig. 12.8.3)** has been pioneered by Eliane Gluckman in Paris, since 1989. The major drawback has been the low stem cell dose leading to delayed engraftment. The major advantages are the abundant supply of CB units with no risk to mother or infant and immaturity of immune cells reduces the risk of

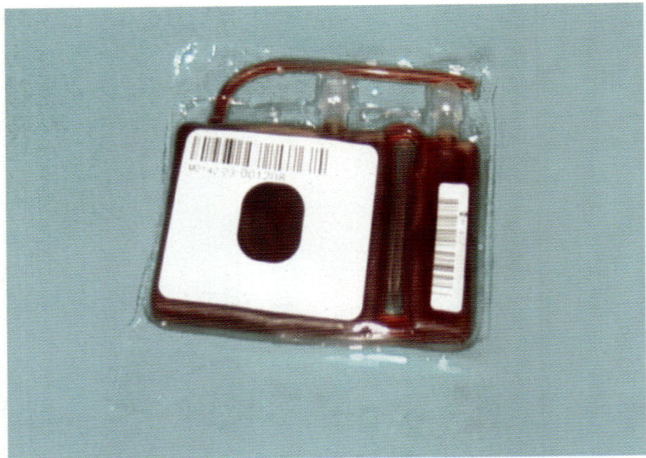

Fig. 12.8.3: Umbilical cord blood unit after thawing.

HLA mismatch (even 4/6 and 5/6 matches are acceptable) and subsequent graft-versus-host disease (GVHD) incidence is low.

CONDITIONING

Most conditioning treatment regimens comprise chemotherapy, immunotherapy, and sometimes radiotherapy. The principal function of this treatment is to kill all cancer cells that might still be present at the time of SCT, to reduce disease to a minimal level and make "space" in the bone marrow "niches" for the donor stem cells, and to suppress the host immune system so that the donor cells (graft) are unlikely to be rejected.

MANAGEMENT OF PATIENTS UNDERGOING STEM CELL TRANSPLANT

Conditioning is administered over a period of 7–10 days. On day 0, stem cells are infused to the recipient from the donor. A rising neutrophil count followed by rising platelet count over the next 15–45 days is the evidence of engraftment. Donor engraftment can be confirmed by polymerase chain reaction (PCR)-based chimerism studies, fluorescence *in situ* hybridization (FISH) for XX/XY in sex mismatch SCT or change of blood group of recipient to donor group in ABO mismatched SCT. The patient is transferred out of the BMT unit when his neutrophil count is over 500/mm^3 and discharged when there are no IV medications to be administered. Following HSCT for a patient who has no GVHD, cyclosporine is given as prophylaxis at full doses for 6 months after which it is tapered and stopped 1 year post-transplant.

Table 12.8.1: Glucksberg's criteria for staging and grading of acute graft-versus-host disease.

Organ	*Stage*	*Extent of organ involvement*
Skin	1 2 3 4	<25% 25–50% Generalized erythema Desquamation, bullous
Liver bilirubin	1 2 3 4	2–3 mg/dL 3.1–6 mg/dL 6.1–15 mg/dL >15 mg/dL
Gastrointestinal	1 2 3 4	10–15 mL stool/kg/day 16–20 mL stool/kg/day 21–25 mL stool/kg/day >25 mL stool/kg/day; severe pain with or without ileus
Overall clinical grade	***Organ system***	***Clinical stage***
I (mild)	Skin Liver Gastrointestinal	1–2 0 0
II (moderate)	Skin Liver Gastrointestinal	1–3 1 1
III (severe)	Skin Liver Gastrointestinal	2–3 2–3 2–3
IV (life-threatening)*	Skin Liver Gastrointestinal	2–4 2–4 2–4

*With severe constitutional symptoms.

COMPLICATIONS

Graft-versus-host disease, infection, and interstitial pneumonia are the major complications of HSCT.

Graft-versus-Host Disease

This is one of the most devastating complications of HSCT and is termed as acute **(Table 12.8.1)**, if it occurs in the first 100 days following transplantation and chronic **(Box 12.8.3)**, if it continues or develops after this period.

Other Short-term and Long-term Complications

Short-term and long-term complications of HSCT are described in detail in **Box 12.8.4**.

Box 12.8.3: Staging of chronic graft-versus-host disease.

Limited chronic GVHD

- Localized skin involvement
- Hepatic dysfunction secondary to chronic GVHD

Extensive chronic GVHD

- Generalized skin involvement or
- Localized skin involvement or hepatic dysfunction (or both) as a result of chronic GHVD plus
  - Liver histology showing chronic aggressive hepatitis, bridging necrosis, cirrhosis, or
  - *Eye involvement:* Schirmer's test (<5 mm wetting), or
  - Involvement of minor salivary glands or oral mucosa demonstrated by buccal biopsy, or
  - Involvement of any other target organ

(GHVD: graft-versus-host disease)

Box 12.8.4: Short-term and long-term complications of hematopoietic stem cell transplant.

Short-term

- Graft rejection
- Infection
- Bleeding
- Acute graft-versus-host disease
- Veno-occlusive disease of the liver
- Idiopathic pneumonitis
- Side effects of radiation therapy, chemotherapy, and immunosuppressive therapy (e.g. pancytopenia, mucositis)

Long-term

- Late graft failure
- Chronic graft-versus-host disease and its sequelae (e.g. bronchiolitis obliterans)
- Pulmonary disorders
- Infection
- Altered intellectual and growth development in children
- *Endocrine dysfunction:*
  - Hypothyroidism
  - Growth retardation
  - Pubertal delay, gonadal failure
  - Sexual dysfunction
- Complications secondary to radiation therapy (e.g. cataracts, radiation nephritis)
- Complications secondary to immunosuppressive therapy (e.g. aseptic necrosis of bone)
- Dental problems
- Psychosocial problems
- Increased risk for second malignancies

HEMATOPOIETIC STEM CELL TRANSPLANT IN INDIA

In September 2005, data from six transplant centers in India were collected and a total of 1,540 transplants have been performed in a country of over 1 billion population.

At the center in Vellore, Tamil Nadu, a total of 626 transplants have been performed in 595 patients. At Sir Ganga Ram Hospital, New Delhi from January 2006 to August 2009, authors have performed 39 transplants (16 allogeneic and 23 autologous) in 34 patients.

RECENT ADVANCES

There are key developments happening in the field of haploidentical SCT, natural killer cell immunotherapy, infusing T-regulatory cells to control GVHD, and gene therapy for severe combined immunodeficiency and thalassemia, etc.

BIBLIOGRAPHY

1. Chandy M. Stem cell transplantation in India. Bone Marrow Transplant. 2008;42(Suppl 1):S81-4.
2. Haining WN, Duncan C, Lehmann LE. Principles of bone marrow and stem cell transplantation. In: Orkin SH, Nathan DF, Ginsburg D, Look AT, Fisher DE, Lux SE (Eds). Nathan and Oski's Hematology of Infancy and Childhood, 7th edition. Philadelphia: Saunders. 2009. pp. 397-452.
3. Yadav SP, Kalra M, Sachdeva A, et al. The experience of hematopoietic stem cell transplantation from an emerging center in North India. Blood. 2009;114:4317.

12.9 Late Effects of Treatments in Survivors of Childhood Cancers

Purna A Kurkure

INTRODUCTION

Improvements in cancer therapy with multimodality approach have dramatically increased the survival rates in childhood cancers in the developed countries. The number of subjects that have successfully completed the treatment for cancer diagnosis during childhood and are entering adulthood is increasing over time. It has been estimated that 0.1% of individuals 20 years of age are survivors of childhood cancer. Although this constitutes a remarkable medical achievement, the late morbidity in this growing survivor population has become the area of current concern. Curing more children and, even more importantly, without recurrence, has become the goal to be achieved. The concept of a truly "cured child" in pediatric oncology envisages not only eradication of the cancer but a surviving child at par with peers in growth and development, physically, mentally, and emotionally.

SURVIVORS, LONG-TERM EFFECTS AND LATE EFFECTS

It is often difficult for the cancer patients and his or her family to make the transition from active patient to survivorship, the fear of relapse being always intense despite counseling. While some risk of relapse is always present, it is safe to say that for most childhood cancers "cure" means disease-free survival of 2 years from cessation of therapy or 5 years after the diagnosis. A review of 5-year survivors of childhood cancers revealed that 92% of patients who were relapse-free at 5 years were alive at 15 years after diagnosis. Any side effect that does not resolve after completion of treatment is a "long-term effect of therapy." "Late effects" refer specifically to those unrecognized toxicities that are absent or subclinical at the end of therapy but manifest later with the unmasking of unseen injury because of multiple factors such as developmental processes, failure of compensatory mechanisms with time, organ senescence, etc.

CURRENT KNOWLEDGE OF LATE EFFECTS

The problems seen in the survivors fall into two broad categories: medical and psychosocial. Medical problems can be assessed by the interplay of type of primary cancer and specific therapy (radiotherapy, chemotherapy, surgery) on one hand and vulnerable organ system on the other hand. Almost all organ systems are vulnerable. Organs which are most commonly or most seriously affected include: musculoskeletal, cardiopulmonary, central nervous system (CNS), renal/genitourinary system, endocrine system, GI system, and immune system **(Table 12.9.1)**. Another major concern is the risk of developing second malignant neoplasm (SMN). It has been estimated that 3–12% of children treated for cancer will develop SMN within 20 years from diagnosis. Psychosocial problems are more diverse and include issues of mental illness (depression, anxiety disorder), school performance, vocational training, employment opportunities, marriage, reproduction, and intrafamily interaction.

SURVEILLANCE OF LATE EFFECTS

There is no disagreement that childhood cancer survivor should have a long-term follow-up. As these late effects can have delayed onset and/or can be potentially progressive in nature of some of the medical/psychosocial problems such evaluation needs to be continued for long-term and should be based on the risk for late effects development. Continued surveillance of childhood cancer survivors is a good medicine. It is important for the pediatrician and family practitioner to know what are the most common sequelae and when a thorough investigative work-up is warranted. The frequency of clinical and laboratory evaluation are individualized according to problems anticipated by the oncologist based on the therapeutic and disease history.

Routine Evaluation

Routine evaluation of the survivors includes the following:

Clinical Evaluation

- Measurement of height, weight, and maintaining growth charts
- Assessment of pubertal development
- Monitoring for relapse/second malignancy
- Assessment of neuropsychological, social status, and rehabilitation needs.

Table 12.9.1: Summary of the commonly encountered late effects.

Organ system	***Late effect of chemotherapy***	***Late effect of radiotherapy***
Bone and soft tissues	Avascular necrosis (steroids)	Short stature, limb length discrepancy, scoliosis, osteonecrosis, soft tissue atrophy, second cancers
Cardiovascular	Cardiomyopathy (anthracyclines, high-dose cyclophosphamide)	Pericardial effusion, pericarditis, early onset coronary artery, and peripheral vascular disease
Pulmonary	Pulmonary fibrosis (bleomycin), interstitial pneumonitis (methotrexate)	Pulmonary fibrosis, decreased lung volumes
CNS	Neuropsychiatric manifestations, hemiplegia, seizures (methotrexate), peripheral neuropathy (vincristine, cisplatin), hearing loss (cisplatin)	Neuropsychologic deficits, structural changes (atrophy, ventricular enlargement, calcifications)
Renal, Genitourinary	Renal dysfunction (cisplatin, methotrexate, ifosphamide), hemorrhagic cystitis, bladder fibrosis (cyclophosphamide)	Hypertension, reduced creatinine clearance, bladder fibrosis
Endocrine	Metabolic syndrome (steroids), Drug-induced diabetes (steroids, L-asparginase)	Hypothyroidism, thyroid nodule, thyroid cancer, growth hormone deficiency, pituitary failure, abnormal pubertal development
Gonadal	*Male:* Sterility, *Female:* premature ovarian failure (alkylating agents)	*Male:* Sterility, Leydig cell dysfunction *Female:* Premature ovarian failure, early menopause, infertility due to decrease in egg count
Ophthalmologic	Cataracts (steroids)	Cataracts, retinopathy, keratoconjunctivitis

(CNS: central nervous system)

Investigations

- Investigations for confirmation of disease-free status to designate survivor status
- Screening for transfusion transmitted diseases, viz. hepatitis B virus (HBV), hepatitis C virus (HCV), and human immunodeficiency virus (HIV)
- Baseline complete blood count
- Baseline biochemical profile
- X-ray chest
- Late-effect screening based on previous therapeutic exposure and organs/organ systems at risk of developing these late effects

Screening tests as depicted in **Table 12.9.2** may help to detect subclinical late effects that could become clinically relevant in the future. A balance of reassurance to the survivor and his/her family and vigilance in monitoring recurrence such as SMN and late relapse are of utmost importance.

AFTER COMPLETION OF TREATMENT

Drawing inspiration from the model of care established at St Jude Children Research Hospital (SJCRH), USA, a follow-up clinic for long-term survivors of childhood cancer was initiated at Tata Memorial Hospital (TMH) in February, 1991. This clinic was appropriately named *After Completion of Treatment (ACT)* clinic to emphasize that ACTs are needed beyond therapy treatment to achieve "cure" in its full dimensions. The aim of this clinic is to monitor growth, development, sexual maturation, and late effects of therapy and to apply corrective measures whenever feasible. Other objective is to rehabilitate survivors for useful, productive adult life, and collect data for future protocol modifications so as to obviate/minimize late effects. A team approach is adapted with pediatric oncologist, clinical psychologist, and medical social worker as a core group interacting with array of specialists from medical and rehabilitation field to deal with issues effectively. From February 1991 to February 2015, 1,750 survivors (off therapy and disease-free for >2 years) have been enrolled in ACT clinic. These survivors are followed up regularly in a systematic manner.

The training and resources for survivorship care are lacking. No national or state-level policy addresses ongoing medical care, employment, or health insurance barriers for survivors of childhood cancer. Several initiatives aim to improve this scenario: Indian Cancer Society's Project PICASSO (Partnership in Cancer Survivorship Optimization) promotes and facilitates hospital-based ACT clinics at high-volume centers. *Ugam,* an advocacy and support group for survivors of childhood cancers created under the umbrella of the Indian Cancer Society, currently engages and works with Mumbai-based survivors for their rehabilitation and advocacy; and the Indian Pediatric Oncology Group and Pediatric Hematology Oncology Group of Indian Academy of Pediatrics has formed a late-effects study group to promote survivorship research.

Table 12.9.2: Organ/organ system-specific late-effects screening.

Organ/organ system at risk	*Screening tests*	*Previous therapeutic exposure*
Musculoskeletal	Physical examination annually to include height, weight, and growth velocity X-ray as and when needed (p.r.n.)	Local radiotherapy (RT) + Surgery
Cardiac	2 D-echo baseline for all; at 1 year, then q 2–5 yearly (p.r.n.)	Anthracyclines + Cardiotoxic chemotherapy ± Mediastinal RT
Pulmonary	PFT baseline, then q 3–5 years (p.r.n.)	Bleomycin ± Mediastinal RT
CNS	• Neurocognitive testing at baseline, then q 3–5 years (p.r.n.) • MRI brain (p.r.n.)	Cranial RT
Neuroendocrine	• Growth curve q 1 year, bone age (age 9) Free T3,T4, and TSH at baseline q 2–5 year (p.r.n.) • LH, FSH, testosterone/estradiol, prolactin (baseline; p.r.n.) • GH stimulation test, morning cortisol (p.r.n.)	Hypothalamic-pituitary RT RT to thyroid (neck, craniospinal)
Renal	• Creatinine clearance baseline and q 3–5 years (p.r.n.) • Urea, creatinine, serum electrolytes, Ca^{2+}, $MgPO_4$ 1–2 years, Urinalysis 1–2 years	Cisplatin, carboplatin, ifosfamide RT
Ovary	Menstrual history annually, LH, FSH, estradiol baseline, AMH (age >12) and (p.r.n.)	Alkylating agents, RT
Testes	• LH, FSH, testosterone baseline (age >12) and (p.r.n.) • Sperm analysis (p.r.n.)	Alkylating agents, RT
Breast	• Breast examination • Mammography beginning age 25–30 years	Mediastinal RT

(CNS: central nervous system; PFT: pulmonary function tests; FSH: follicle-stimulating hormone; LH: luteinizing hormone; AMH: anti-Müllerian hormone; p.r.n.: "when necessary" (from the Latin "prorenata," for an occasion that has arisen, as circumstances require, as needed)

CONCLUSION

Pediatric oncologists, in developing countries, are currently preoccupied with refining delivery of care to attain survival rates, which are comparable to the developed countries. However, they have an obligation to remember the lessons learned from the developed countries and actively build long-term follow-up and survivorship programs as an integral part of pediatric oncology initiative.

Cancer survivors will be increasing in number as the time passes. In spite of their overall wellness, they are at risk of complications and need close supervision. It will be the responsibility of health professionals, both at primary care and tertiary level, to assess and care for these long-term issues and aid these survivors in realizing their optimum potential.

BIBLIOGRAPHY

1. DeSantis CE, Lin CC, Mariotto AB, et al. Cancer treatment and survivorship statistics, 2014. CA Cancer J Clin. 2014;64:252-71.
2. Kurkure PA, Achrekar S, Uparkar U, et al. Surviving childhood cancer: what next? Issues under consideration at the After Completion of Therapy (ACT) clinic in India. Med Pediatr Oncol. 2003;41(6):588-9.
3. Kurkure PA, Achrekar S, Dalvi N, et al. Childhood cancer survivor; living beyond cure. Indian J Pediatr. 2003;70(10):825-8.
4. Li FP, Myers MH, Heise HW, et al. The course of five-year survivors of cancer in childhood. J Pediatr. 1978;93(2):185-87.
5. Maeda M. Late effects of childhood cancer: life-threatening issues. J Nippon Med Sch. 2008;75(6):320-4.
6. Meadows AT, Krejmas NL, Belasco JB. The medical cost of cure: sequelae in survivors of childhood cancer. In: Van Eys J, Sullivan MP (Eds). Status of the curability of childhood cancers. New York: Raven Press; 1980. pp. 263-76.
7. Neglia JP, Friedman DL, Yasui Y, et al. Second malignant neoplasms in five-year survivors of childhood cancer: childhood cancer survivor study. J Natl Cancer Inst. 2001;93(8):618-29.
8. Oeffinger KC, Hudson MM. Long-term complications following childhood and adolescent cancer: foundations for providing risk-based health care for survivors. CA Cancer J Clin. 2004;54(4):208-36.
9. Tonorezos ES, Barnea D, Cohn RJ, et al. Models of care for survivors of childhood cancer from across the globe: advancing survivorship care in the next decade. J Clin Oncol. 2018;36(21):2223-30.
10. Ward E, DeSantis C, Robbins A, et al. Childhood and adolescent cancer statistics, 2014. CA Cancer J Clin. 2014;64:83-103.

Section 13

Endocrinology

13.1 Disorders of Growth

PSN Menon

SHORT STATURE

Introduction

A child is diagnosed to have short stature when his or her height is below the 3rd percentile or below 2 SD (standard deviation) of the mean height for that age and gender. Even when the current height measurements are within normal ranges, the child should be regarded as short, if the height velocity is less than the 25th percentile for age and gender over 6–12 months of observation or the child is very short for midparental or target height. Children with a very slow growth trajectory crossing two lower major percentile lines between the age of 2 years and puberty also need to be evaluated even if the current height is in the normal range. Assessment of stature should take into account the previous records of stature, stage of pubertal development, height of parents, and the ethnic background of the population.

Rationale of Clinical Evaluation

Measurement of Growth

Supine length is measured by an infantometer in infants and children less than 2 years and standing height by a stadiometer in older children. The techniques for measuring height are detailed in Chapters 3.1 and 3.2. Measurements of weight, body mass index, waist circumference, waist/hip ratio, midarm circumference, skinfold thickness, and head circumference are often helpful in diagnosis.

The height and weight can be expressed as SD scores (SDS or *Z* score). *Z* score is calculated using the formula: (The child's height minus mean height for age) divided by 1 SD of height for that age.

Height Velocity

Estimation of height velocity is essential for optimal decision-making. On an average, most infants measure 50 cm in length at birth, and gain approximately 25 cm in the first year of life, 12.5 cm in the second year, 6–7 cm each in the third and fourth years, and subsequently, 5 cm every year until pubertal growth spurt. The peak height velocity during adolescence is about 9–11 cm/year for boys and about 7–9 cm/year for girls. Retardation of height is significant if height velocity is low or decreasing. On the other hand, if the child has a normal height velocity and is growing along his/her percentiles, the parents can be reassured. Height velocity can also be expressed in *Z* scores.

Growth Charts

The growth pattern of child should be recorded both numerically as well as graphically using appropriate growth charts (refer to Chapters 3.3 and 3.4 for details). In addition to the normal growth charts for age and gender, there are disease-specific growth charts for some selected diseases such as Turner syndrome, Noonan syndrome, Down syndrome, Prader-Willi syndrome, and achondroplasia.

Predicting Adult Height

A crude way to assess the genetic potential is to plot the height of the parents on the adult equivalent (e.g. at 18–20 years) on a standard growth chart. The target height or midparental height is calculated by the formula—for boys: average of father's height and mother's height plus 6.5 cm; for girls: average of mother's and father's height minus 6.5 cm. The range is ±10.5 cm in boys and ±8 cm in girls. Midparental height should be plotted on the adult equivalent on the growth chart. It provides the target height for the child and the percentile he/she is likely to follow **(Fig. 13.1.1)**.

Body Proportions

The body proportions employed in clinical decision-making are upper segment:lower segment ratio (US:LS ratio) and arm-span-to-height ratio. They vary with age. The US:LS ratio is approximately 1.7 at birth, 1.3 at 3 years, 1.1 by 6 years, and 1 by 10 years. Arm span is less than length at birth by 2.5 cm and equals height at about 11 years, and, thereafter it is greater than height. An abnormal US:LS ratio or arm-span-to-height ratio indicates disproportionate short stature. Children with achondroplasia have a normal-sized trunk with short limbs, while spondyloepiphyseal dysplasia gives rise to short trunk and normal limbs.

Pubertal Assessment

Pubertal assessment has an important role in the diagnosis and prognosis of short stature. Onset of puberty is associated with the height spurt seen during adolescence. Delayed or

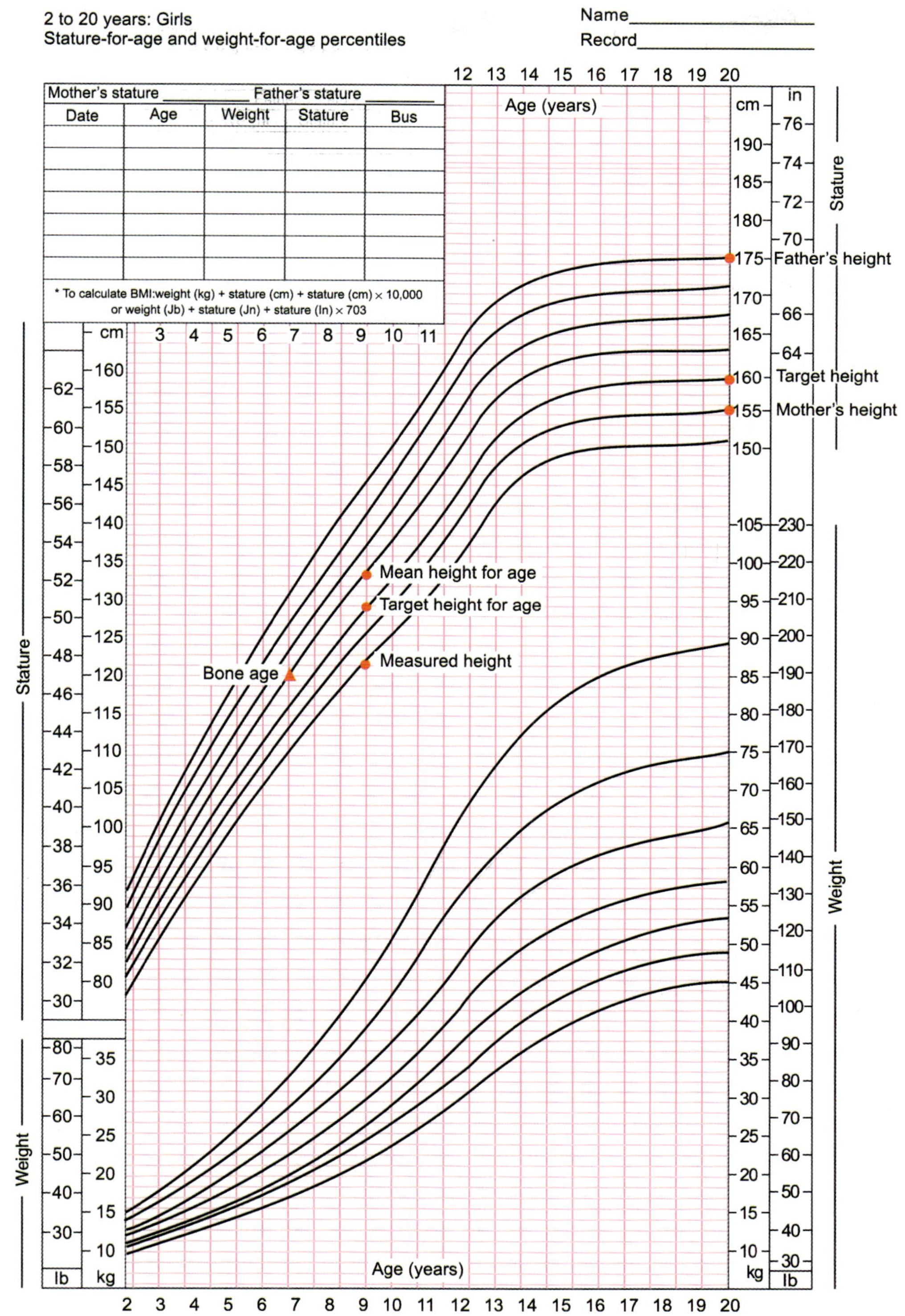

Fig. 13.1.1: Growth chart showing how to record a child's height. The actual height of a 9-year-old girl is recorded as 120 cm as "measured height". The father's height, mother's height, and the target or midparental height are recorded at 20 years on the growth chart. She is expected to follow the 25th percentile according to the target height but is short for her target height for age. The mean height for the age is recorded at the 50th percentile. Bone age, recorded, as a triangle, is further behind her chronological age, but equal to her "height age", the point where the actual height crosses the 50th percentile.

precocious puberty thus has an important role in stature (*see* Chapter 13.4). The stage of puberty is assessed by the Tanner's method of sexual maturity rating detailed in Chapter 3.5. Testicular volume is measured by an orchidometer.

Bone Age Assessment

An essential investigative tool for evaluating short stature is bone age assessment. This is conventionally done from X-rays of wrist and elbow. The bone age is computed from the appearance of epiphyseal centers and fusion of epiphysis with metaphysis using Greulich-Pyle or Osman-Ratib atlas. Tanner-Whitehouse method (TW2 or TW3) scores the maturity of each epiphysis, and the bone age is derived from a total score. Alternately, it may be computed by online apps such as Bone Xpert. A child with delayed bone age has a better prognosis for future height gain than those with appropriate or advanced bone age. Children with familial genetic short stature (FGSS) have bone age appropriate for chronological age, whereas those with constitutional delay in growth and puberty (CDGP) or an endocrine disorder such as growth hormone (GH) deficiency (GHD) or hypothyroidism have delayed bone age. Adult height can be predicted by computing chronological age and bone age using the Bayley-Pinneau charts.

Etiology of Short Stature

Short stature may be due to a variety of disorders **(Table 13.1.1)**. Common endocrine causes include hypothyroidism, hypopituitarism, diabetes mellitus, Cushing syndrome, pseudohypoparathyroidism, and hypogonadism. A significant number of children who turn up for evaluation of short stature have no pathological abnormality and have a physiological cause for their short stature.

Table 13.1.1: Differential diagnosis of short stature.

A. Normal variants
• Familial genetic short stature (FGSS) • Constitutional delay in growth and puberty (CDGP)
B. Disproportionate short stature
• *Skeletal dysplasia*: Achondroplasia, hypochondroplasia, spondyloepiphyseal dysplasia • *Rickets*: Nutritional, metabolic • Congenital hypothyroidism (missed at birth or infancy) • Mucopolysaccharidosis type 4 (morquio)
C. Proportionate short stature of prenatal onset
• *Intrauterine growth restriction:* – *Placental insufficiency disorders*: Maternal toxemia, diabetes mellitus – *Intrauterine infections*: TORCH complex – *Teratogens*: Alcohol, nicotine, drugs • *Dysmorphic syndromes*: Russell-Silver syndrome (RSS), Seckel syndrome, 3-M syndrome • *Chromosomal anomalies*: Down syndrome, Turner syndrome, Noonan syndrome, Prader-Willi syndrome, DiGeorge syndrome, Aarskog syndrome
D. Proportionate short stature of postnatal onset
• *Nutritional disorders*: Malnutrition, nutritional anemia • *Chronic infections*: Tuberculosis, chronic malaria, giardiasis, persistent worm infestations, HIV infection • *Gastrointestinal disorders*: Celiac disease, chronic diarrhea, malabsorption syndromes, chronic liver disease, inflammatory bowel disease • *Hematological disorders*: Hemolytic anemia • *Renal disorders*: Chronic renal failure, tubular disorders • *Cardiac disorders*: Congenital cyanotic heart disease, chronic congestive cardiac failure • *Pulmonary disorders*: Cystic fibrosis, chronic asthma • *Endocrine disorders*: Hypothyroidism, growth hormone deficiency and insensitivity, Cushing syndrome, hypogonadism, pseudohypoparathyroidism, diabetes mellitus • Psychosocial short stature

(HIV: human immunodeficiency virus)

Clinical and Laboratory Evaluation

An algorithmic approach to diagnosis of short stature is given in **Flowchart 13.1.1**.

Clinical History

The time of onset of short stature has great relevance in the differential diagnosis. Thus history of antenatal care and birth of the child (including maternal illness during pregnancy, birth weight, length, gestational age, and signs of congenital anomalies), development, puberty, psychosocial behavior, and nutrition are important. Details of consanguinity, family history of short stature, and pubertal development are indispensable.

- Short stature with normal height velocity with the growth trajectory parallel to 3rd percentile and positive family history suggest FGSS.
- Children with CDGP have growth failure noted from the age of 2–3 years with delayed onset of puberty, family history of short stature, and/or delayed puberty in parents or siblings.
- When the growth failure is noted postnatally, environmental causes such as malnutrition, chronic infections, and emotional disturbances in the family should be probed.
- Social history is important to detect psychosocial short stature.
- Malnutrition starting from early life causes weight loss and stunting often accompanied by cognitive and behavioral deficits. Role of nutrients including vitamins and minerals such as iron, calcium, and zinc in growth and development are detailed in Section 4.
- All systems including endocrine, renal, and gastrointestinal should be reviewed carefully to identify a cause for

Flowchart 13.1.1: An algorithmic approach to diagnosis of short stature.

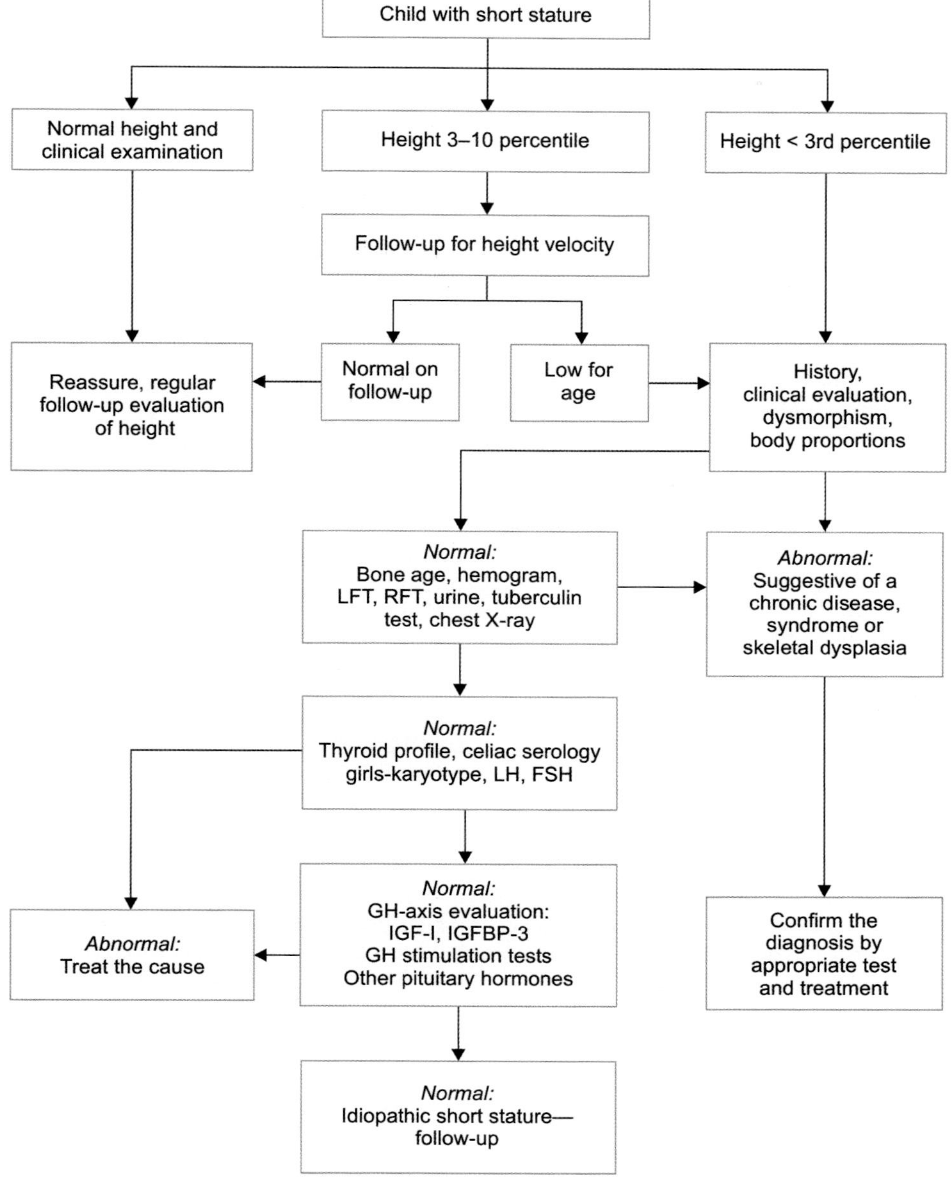

(FSH: follicle-stimulating hormone; GH: growth hormone; IGF-I: insulin-like growth factor-I; IGFBP-3: insulin-like growth factor-binding protein-3; LFT: liver function tests; LH: luteinizing hormone; RFT: renal function tests)

deceleration of growth even in the absence of any specific history.

- Short stature is common in chronic nutritional and hemolytic anemia. Look for history of multiple blood transfusions and presence of hemolytic facies.
- Short stature is also seen in survivors of childhood malignancies. Signs of pituitary insufficiency, delayed puberty, obesity with abnormal body proportions are common following cranial and/or spine radiation for childhood malignancies.

Physical Examination

The presence of characteristic physical signs of an endocrine/systemic disorder or dysmorphic syndrome greatly facilitates the diagnostic workup. Children with endocrine disorders generally have a weight percentile better than that of height, whereas those with systemic disorders usually lose weight first and are thin by the time they are short. Disproportions of body are seen in skeletal dysplasia, rickets, hypothyroidism, and some dysmorphic syndromes. Pallor and signs of vitamin deficiencies are frequent in many nutritional disorders, malabsorption, chronic anemia, hypothyroidism, and renal failure. It is also important to evaluate the genitalia and grade the pubertal development.

- Constitutional delay in growth and puberty is defined as a delay of growth and puberty in an otherwise healthy child, usually an adolescent, with a standing height below the expected for chronological age, but not for his/her bone age. It tends to affect boys more often than girls. It is a diagnosis of exclusion. The final adult height is within the normal range. These children are short from 23 years of age. Growth is below but parallel to the 3rd percentile initially with further deviation as the adolescent height spurt is delayed. Bone age is delayed. There is a familial tendency for short stature and delayed catch-up. The spine length may be relatively short compared to limb length.
- Children with FGSS are short with a height appropriate for the parent's height with normal height velocity. The growth curve is below but parallel to the 3rd percentile. Body proportions are normal and pubertal development is appropriate for age. Bone age is appropriate for his/her age. Again this is a diagnosis of exclusion.
- Children with congenital GHD are short and have a cherubic appearance, doll-like face, and micropenis. Presence of midline anomalies, such as cleft lip, cleft palate or single central incisor tooth and crowding of midfacial structures, and abdominal adiposity, suggests the possibility of hypopituitarism. Visual field defects, optic atrophy, optic nerve hypoplasia, and papilledema are often associated with septo-optic dysplasia and tumors of the pituitary-hypothalamic region (Chapter 13.2).
- Children with GH insensitivity have almost all the features of GHD with more pronounced short stature and features of GHD.
- Acquired hypothyroidism often manifests as short stature. Coarse facies, myxedema, dry rough skin, macroglossia, lethargy, bradycardia, constipation, cold intolerance, and developmental delay with delayed relaxation of deep tendon reflexes characterize hypothyroidism (Chapter 13.5).
- Growth retardation may sometimes be the only presenting feature of Cushing syndrome in childhood. Cushing disease is characterized by central obesity, striae, hypertension, and proximal muscle weakness.
- Pseudohypoparathyroidism manifests with short stature, round facies, central obesity, short fourth metacarpals and mental subnormality, hypocalcemic tetany or seizures, cataract, and calcification in the basal ganglia.
- Celiac disease may often present with short stature without any other evidence of malabsorption or jejunal pathology.
- Turner syndrome may present in girls as isolated short stature. It is characterized by the presence of short webbed neck, shield chest, widely placed nipples, lymphedema with characteristic cardiac, renal, and skeletal defects.
- Down syndrome, a common cause of mental retardation, has short stature with characteristic facies with mongoloid slant of eyes.
- Russell-Silver syndrome (RSS) is characterized by intrauterine growth restriction (IUGR), small triangular facies, hemihypertrophy, clinodactyly, occasionally a large penis and precocious puberty, and sometimes GHD.

Investigations

If the clinical workup suggests a cause for short stature, the appropriate confirmatory test should be performed. Many a time children with short stature present with no other abnormality on history and examination. Thus in all cases of significant short stature with a low growth velocity and/or delayed bone age, it is advisable to perform a battery of screening investigations to diagnose some of the important causes **(Box 13.1.1)**.

Box 13.1.1: Laboratory evaluation for short stature.

- *Radiology*: X-ray for bone age; for deformities, sella, X-ray chest if tuberculosis or cardiorespiratory disease is suspected
- *Hematological tests*: Hemoglobin, hematocrit, red cell indices, total and differential leukocyte counts, peripheral blood cell morphology, ESR
- *Urinalysis*: pH, specific gravity, osmolality, microscopy, protein, glucose estimations
- *Stool examination*: Microscopy for parasitic infections, fat globules for malabsorption, glucose, or reducing substances
- *Blood chemistry*: Fasting blood sugar, renal function (urea, creatinine, sodium, potassium, chloride), bone profile (calcium, phosphorus, alkaline phosphatase), liver function (total protein, albumin, and transaminases), iron profile, venous CO_2
- *Special tests*: Tuberculosis (tuberculin, chest X-ray, microbiology screen), hypothyroidism (thyroid hormones T4 and TSH), celiac disease (IgA, antiendomysial and tissue transglutaminase antibodies and jejunal biopsy), malabsorption (bone profile, vitamin D, appropriate biopsy), Turner syndrome (FSH and karyotype), RTA (arterial blood gases, studies of calcium axis, and appropriate X-rays), skeletal dysplasia (skeletal survey and genetic testing)
- *Tests for hypothalamic-pituitary axis*: IGF-I, IGFBP-3, and dynamic GH testing, X-ray skull for sellar abnormalities, and suprasellar calcification, CT/MRI brain, tests for other pituitary hormones

(CT: computed tomography; ESR: erythrocyte sedimentation rate; FSH: follicle-stimulating hormone; GH: growth hormone; IgA: immunoglobulin A; IGFBP-3: insulin-like growth factor-binding protein 3; IGF-I: insulin-like growth factor-I; MRI: magnetic resonance imaging; RTA: renal tubular acidosis; TSH: thyroid-stimulating hormone)

Estimation of bone age is the first vital step in the diagnosis of short stature. Most children with CDGP, nutritional disorders, chronic diseases have mild delay, whereas endocrinopathies such as GHD and hypothyroidism have significantly delayed bone age. Cushing syndrome and precocious puberty cause an advancement of bone age. Metacarpal shortening may be present in Turner syndrome and pseudohypoparathyroidism. Madelung deformity (dorsal and radial bowing of the radius) may be present in some cases of short stature associated with homeobox gene (*SHOX*) mutations and Turner syndrome.

- If the screening tests are normal, tests to exclude relatively silent causes of short stature should be performed. These include tests to exclude hypothyroidism, GHD, renal tubular acidosis (RTA), Turner syndrome, and celiac disease.
- Celiac disease and RTA are two commonly missed causes of short stature on routine diagnostic evaluation. RTA is associated with polyuria, failure to thrive, and bony deformities.
- It is a policy in some pediatric endocrine centers to do thyroid function in all children and chromosome studies (for Turner syndrome) in all girls referred for short stature. Elevated gonadotropins, especially follicle-stimulating hormone, point toward the diagnosis of Turner syndrome.
- Those with disproportionate short stature require skeletal survey, and evaluation for hypothyroidism and RTA. Low bicarbonate levels suggest RTA.
- Measurement of insulin-like growth factor-I (IGF-I) is useful when the cause of short stature is uncertain. In some centers, IGF-binding protein-3 (IGFBP-3) is also estimated as a screening tool. Low levels (below 2 SD of the mean) of IGF-I and IGFBP-3 suggest the probability of GHD.
- Measurement of GH in a random blood sample is not a reliable test for GHD, as GH levels are usually low during day and spontaneous peaks are brief and unpredictable. The most practical method is a dynamic GH stimulation test using insulin, clonidine, or other agents. A GH level less than 10 ng/mL following stimulation indicates impaired pituitary secretion. The cutoff levels for diagnosis differ from center to center. Details of GHD and insufficiency are given in Chapter 13.2.
- Other investigations for hypopituitarism include thyroid functions, basal gonadotropins (especially in older children), prolactin, and morning cortisol along with pituitary magnetic resonance imaging.
- Specialized genetic testing should be considered if a genetic cause is suspected.

Management

After the initial visit, the family should be counseled regarding the importance of a balanced diet with adequate calories and proteins including macro- and micronutrients, coupled with regular physical exercises. Supplemental hematinics and vitamins are prescribed if indicated. Height and weight should be recorded and height gain assessed every 2–3 months. Counseling of the child and the family is essential in conditions such as FGSS, CDGP, skeletal dysplasia, and IUGR. The importance of regular follow-up and monitoring of therapy should be stressed. The child should receive all immunizations as recommended.

Treatment of short stature essentially depends on the cause. He/she should receive the optimal treatment for an underlying systemic disorder. There is no specific treatment for FGSS and most cases of IUGR. Constitutional delay in growth and puberty can cause enormous anxiety, and peer-group pressure may lead to psychological distress. In such a situation, induction of puberty should be considered as a treatment option. They may benefit from a short course of low-dose testosterone (50 mg testosterone intramuscularly every 3–4 weeks) for boys or estrogen (2.5 µg of ethinyl estradiol daily) for girls given for 3–6 months followed by reevaluation. This will trigger the secondary sexual characteristics and the pubertal growth spurt.

Hypothyroidism should be managed with replacement by levothyroxine. Low-dose estrogens are useful in girls with Turner syndrome and delayed puberty. Anabolic steroids (oxandrolone) have been tried with some success in Turner syndrome and a few children with CDGP. They act by increasing GH secretion. A low-dose daily regimen will induce growth spurt, which continues even after the steroids are stopped.

Specific therapy for chronic systemic disorders, e.g. RTA and celiac disease, is associated with good catch-up growth. For most skeletal dysplasias, there is no medical treatment, even though GH has been shown to benefit some selected groups. Limb lengthening surgery is an option for some skeletal dysplasias.

Growth hormone is indicated in children with GHD. The recombinant GH is given in a dose of 0.25–0.3 mg/kg/week (1 mg = 3 IU) given daily subcutaneously, preferably at night, till adult height is reached. There are very few side effects reported in children, who have received GH for GHD. Contrary to earlier suggestions, there is no report of increased susceptibility to tumors or leukemia in treated children. Children gain on an average 10–12 cm in the first year of therapy and 6–8 cm/year thereafter every year. However, the high cost of therapy has limited its use in the subcontinent. Addition of gonadotropin-releasing hormone agonist analogs to delay puberty during GH therapy is recommended in some centers.

Growth hormone has been used to increase height in a number of other disorders with limited success. These include Turner syndrome, SHOX haploinsufficiency, end-stage chronic renal failure, and a group of children with small for gestational age with poor catch-up growth. It is also used in children with Prader-Willi syndrome and RSS. It has been shown to be effective in some groups of children with CDGP and idiopathic short stature. The dose of GH used is higher than that used in GHD.

In Turner syndrome, a combination of GH with low-dose estrogen and/or oxandrolone has been shown to produce excellent height gain. The chances for development of side effects are higher in these children. Hence, regular monitoring of therapy with recording of height is essential to obtain good results. Recently, aromatase inhibitors such as anastrozole and letrozole have been tried with some success in adolescent boys with short stature. These aromatase inhibitors delay the tempo of bone age acceleration by estrogen blockade.

Primary IGF-I deficiency is the only indication for recombinant IGF-I treatment.

TALL STATURE

Introduction

Children who have a height above 99.6th percentile or > 2 SD above the population mean for age and gender using country-specific growth references and/or above their parental target height percentile are considered to be exceptionally tall for the reference population. Compared to short stature, referrals for tall stature are uncommon.

Etiology and Clinical Features

A list of common causes for tall stature is given in **Box 13.1.2**.

- Some children have constitutional tall stature with tall parents. Tall stature is usually evident early in childhood. They have a high growth velocity and often a slightly advanced bone age. If the tall stature is a matter of psychological concern, sex steroids appropriate for the gender may be given at the onset of puberty to achieve early epiphyseal fusion.
- Many children with exogenous obesity appear tall, but the adult height is normal.
- Children with precocious puberty appear to be taller than peers due to the growth enhancing action of gonadal steroids. However, early epiphyseal fusion makes them short as adults, unless treated early.
- Hyperthyroidism is associated with tall stature, neurobehavioral changes, and rarely eye signs. *See* Chapter 13.5 for details.
- Gigantism is due to excessive production of GH by an acidophil adenoma of the pituitary gland or a hypothalamic tumor. It is characterized by tall stature with prognathism, increased soft tissue of hands and feet, broad root of nose, profuse sweating, hypertension, and glucose intolerance. The diagnosis is confirmed by detection of raised IGF-I levels and lack of suppression of GH (levels < 1 ng/mL) following administration of oral glucose, 1.75 g/kg. Treatment is done by transsphenoidal pituitary surgery. Recurrence can be managed by octreotide, a somatostatin analog.
- Sotos syndrome (cerebral gigantism) is characterized by increased birth weight and length, macrocephaly and dolichocephaly, hypertelorism, and mental retardation. It is caused by the mutations in *NSD1* gene.
- Marfan syndrome is characterized by tall stature, arachnodactyly (long thin fingers) and long thin limbs with an abnormally long LS, resulting in arm span more than height. In addition, there may be hypotonia, hyperextensible joints, scoliosis, flexion contractures, dislocation of the lens, and cardiac anomalies. It is caused by mutations in the fibrillin gene *FBN1*.
- Homocystinuria is an inborn error of metabolism of the amino acid methionine caused by the deficiency of cystathionine β-synthase and characterized by developmental delay, ectopia lentis, skeletal abnormalities, and clinical features of Marfan syndrome.
- Beckwith-Wiedemann syndrome is an overgrowth syndrome characterized by macrosomia, macroglossia, visceromegaly, renal abnormalities, and embryonal tumors. Adults with this syndrome are not unusually tall.
- Klinefelter syndrome is associated with tall stature, abnormally long legs, gynecomastia, mental retardation, and behavioral abnormalities with a karyotype of 47,XXY. Other sex chromosome variants associated with tall stature include 47,XYY, 47,XXX, 48,XXXY, and 48,XXYY.
- Fragile X-syndrome has characteristic physical features such as long and narrow face, large ears, prominent jaw, hyperflexible fingers, enlarged testicles along with delayed development and mild-to-moderate intellectual disability, and hyperactive behavior. It is due to mutations in the *FMR1* gene.

Box 13.1.2: Etiology of tall stature in children.

- Constitutional tall stature
- Exogenous obesity
- Precocious puberty (at initial manifestation)
- Hyperthyroidism
- Growth hormone excess—Gigantism
- *Adrenal:* Adrenal tumor, congenital adrenal hyperplasia (at initial presentation)
- *Overgrowth syndromes:* Sotos syndrome, Weaver syndrome, Beckwith-Wiedemann syndrome
- *Genetic syndromes with tall stature:* Marfan syndrome, multiple endocrine neoplasia 2B
- *Metabolic:* Homocystinuria
- *Sex chromosome abnormalities:* Klinefelter syndrome, Fragile X-syndrome

Management

The management of constitutional tall stature includes reassurance to alleviate anxiety. Medical intervention is usually not necessary. Exogenous sex steroids are used to induce puberty to reduce final height if the predicted adult height is more than 2.5 SD.

BIBLIOGRAPHY

1. Allen DB. Growth hormone therapy for short stature: is the benefit worth the burden? Pediatrics. 2006;118(1):343-8.
2. Badada SK, Bhansali A, Ravikumar P, et al. Changing scenario in aetiological profile of short stature in India—growing importance of celiac disease: a study from tertiary care centre. Indian J Pediatr. 2011;78:41-4.
3. Cook DM, Rose SR. A review of guidelines for use of growth hormone in pediatric and transition patients. Pituitary. 2012;15:301-10.
4. Desai MP, Menon PSN, Bhatia V. Pediatric Endocrine Disorders, 3rd edition. Hyderabad: Universities Press; 2014. pp. 47-119.
5. Drop SL, Greggio N, Cappa M, et al. Current concepts in tall stature and overgrowth syndromes. J Pediatr Endocrinol Metab. 2001;14(Suppl 2):975-84.
6. Farber RS, Kerrigan JR. The multiple indications for growth hormone treatment of pediatric patients. Pediatr Ann. 2006;35(12):926-32.
7. Menon PSN. Use of growth hormone (GH) in non-GH deficient short stature. Indian J Pediatr. 2008;75(Suppl):S14-9.
8. Ranke MB, Lindberg A, Chatelain P, et al. Prediction of long-term response to recombinant human growth hormone in Turner syndrome: development and validation of mathematical models. KIGS International Board. Kabi International Growth Study. J Clin Endocrinol Metab. 2000;85(11):4212-8.
9. Rogol AD, Hayden GF. Etiologies and early diagnosis of short stature and growth failure in children and adolescents. J Pediatr. 2014;164(5 Suppl):S1-14
10. Rosenthal S, Cohen P, Clayton P, et al. Treatment perspectives in idiopathic short stature with a focus on IGF-I deficiency. Pediatr Endocrinol Rev. 2007;4(Suppl 2):252-71.

13.2 Disorders of Pituitary

PSN Menon

INTRODUCTION

The anterior pituitary develops from the Rathke's pouch and the posterior pituitary from the infundibulum, which is a downgrowth from the floor of the diencephalon. The principal hormones produced by the anterior pituitary are:

- Thyroid-stimulating hormone (TSH)
- Adrenocorticotropic hormone (ACTH)
- Follicle-stimulating hormone (FSH)
- Luteinizing hormone (LH)
- Growth hormone (GH)
- Prolactin (PRL).

These hormones act on target glands and a variety of tissues in the body. The hypothalamus produces a number of hormones, which regulate pituitary hormone secretion. These include:

- *Growth hormone-releasing hormone (GHRH)* regulates GH release.
- *Gonadotropin-releasing hormone (GnRH)* regulates LH and FSH release.
- *Thyrotropin-releasing hormone* regulates TSH and PRL release.
- *Corticotropin-releasing hormone* regulates ACTH release.
- *Somatostatin or GH release inhibiting hormone* which inhibits GH release.
- *Prolactin-inhibiting factor* inhibits release of PRL, TSH, and GH.
- *Ghrelin* regulates GH release.
- *Arginine vasopressin (AVP)* has a role in ACTH release in addition to water homeostasis.

PHYSIOLOGY

Growth hormone has specific growth-promoting actions on protein synthesis, skeletal growth, and intermediary metabolism. A number of regulatory proteins or transcription factors are important for the development and function of the pituitary. They act at different stages of pituitary development and trigger the expression of specific genes involved in hormone release and action. These transcription factors include *HESX1, POU1F1 (PIT-1), PROP-1, LHX3, LHX4, GLI2,* and *SOX3*.

The GH-binding proteins (GHBP) act as a reservoir for circulating GH. Their levels reflect the GH receptor concentration, with the GHBP constituting the extracellular domain of the GH receptor. A single molecule of GH released from circulation binds to two GH receptors to form a dimer complex. The actions of GH are mediated through synthesis of insulin-like growth factor-I (IGF-I). Insulin-like growth factor-I in turn circulates bound to binding proteins called

IGF-binding proteins (IGFBP); the major one being IGFBP-3. The GH-IGF axis plays a key role in regulating growth, and the growth-promoting effects of IGF-I can be both GH-dependent and GH-independent.

GROWTH HORMONE DEFICIENCY

Growth hormone deficiency (GHD) is characterized by short stature. The growth impairment starts within a few months after birth, but a clinical diagnosis is usually not obvious till the child is about 1 year or 2 years old.

Etiology

The spectrum of GHD varies from complete to milder grades of insufficiency. Incidence varies from 1 in 4,000–10,000 worldwide. The common causes of GHD are given in **Box 13.2.1**. The most common form however is idiopathic.

Clinical Features

The height is usually less than the 3rd percentile for the age, and the height gain is often as low as 1 cm/year. These children have normal body proportions and are somewhat overweight for their height with increased subcutaneous fat, truncal obesity, and normal body proportions. Bone age is delayed to a variable extent. The height age is less than the bone age, and both are less than chronological age.

The typical child with GHD is very short and plump with immature facies and prominent forehead **(Fig. 13.2.1)**. They look much younger than their actual age. Some of the features of congenital hypopituitarism include midline facial abnormalities, such as cleft palate and lip, single central upper incisor tooth, and prominent philtrum. The eyes appear very prominent with a depressed nasal bridge with a saddle-shaped nose. In addition, there may be underdeveloped mandible and chin, crowding of teeth, nystagmus with impaired vision, and a high-pitched voice. The hands and feet are small with slowly growing nails and hair. The skin is thin, with a tendency for premature wrinkling.

Most children with GHD have normal length at birth. Only 2–5% of children with GHD have suggestive clinical signs in early infancy and present by the age of 2 years. Thus, regular height monitoring may help in early detection. Hypoglycemia and prolonged jaundice in neonatal period are early pointers to the diagnosis of GHD. Neonatal hypoglycemia and convulsions are often associated with ACTH deficiency. Hypogonadism may be evident in boys as small-sized genitalia **(Fig. 13.2.2)**. Pubertal growth spurt is less than normal. Mental development and intelligence are normal.

Box 13.2.1: Causes of growth hormone deficiency.

- *Congenital:* Developmental defects of the hypothalamus and/or pituitary:
  - Anencephaly, holoprosencephaly
  - Septooptic dysplasia (de Morsier's syndrome), Hall-Pallister syndrome
  - *Midline brain and facial abnormalities:* Single central incisor tooth, cleft lip/palate
  - *Associated with abnormal pituitary morphology on MRI:* Aplasia or hypoplasia of anterior pituitary, thin or absent pituitary stalk, interruption or hypoplasia of stalk, ectopic posterior pituitary, empty sella syndrome
- Defects in genes necessary for pituitary development and function:
  - *Isolated GHD:* Autosomal recessive, autosomal dominant, X-linked (mutations of *GH-1*, *GHRHR*, *SOX3*, *HESX1*)
  - *Combined pituitary hormone deficiencies:* Autosomal recessive [mutations of *PIT-1* (*POUF1*), *PROP 1*, *LHX3*, *LHX4*, *HESX1*]; autosomal dominant [mutations of *PIT-1* (*POUF1*), *PROP 1*]; and X-linked, Rieger's syndrome
- *Acquired:*
  - *Tumors within the hypothalamic-pituitary axis:* Craniopharyngioma, germinoma, teratoma
  - *Cranial irradiation:* Leukemia, medulloblastoma, astrocytoma/glioma, ependymoma, rhabdomyosarcoma
  - *Trauma to the hypothalamic-pituitary region:* Perinatal (breech, forceps) or postnatal
  - *Infiltration:* Langerhans cell histiocytosis, hemochromatosis, thalassemia major
  - *Central nervous system infections:* Tuberculosis, meningitis

(GHD: growth hormone deficiency; MRI: magnetic resonance imaging)

Diagnosis

Children with a height below the 3rd percentile and height gain less than 4 cm/year over a period of observation for at least 6 months, with a bone age below the chronologic age, need evaluation for GHD. The diagnosis of GHD depends on demonstration of absent or low levels of GH in response to stimulation. Since GH levels fluctuate during day and night

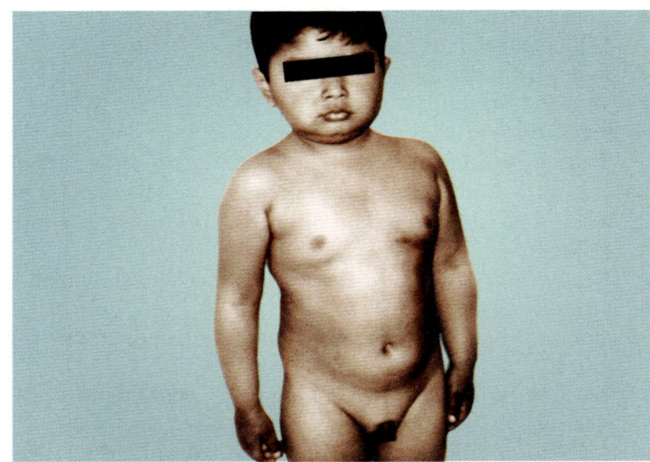

Fig. 13.2.1: A 9-year-old boy with growth hormone deficiency. Note immature facies, hypoplastic scrotum, and micropenis.

because of its pulsatile nature, random or fasting blood GH level measurements are not helpful in diagnosis.

Pharmacological stimuli are preferred to physiological stimuli. Tests that are based on the physiological stimuli include physical exercise and deep sleep **(Table 13.2.1)**. They are not preferred in clinical settings.

- Standard provocation tests use insulin, clonidine, arginine, L-3,4-dihydroxyphenylalanine, glucagon, or GHRH. Of these, insulin (0.05–0.1 IU/kg IV) and clonidine (0.15 mg/m^2 orally) are the most preferred stimuli.
- Blood samples are collected before and at 15–30 minutes intervals for 2 hours. Diagnosis of GHD is suspected when the peak GH level is less than 10 ng/mL following stimulation. The cutoff varies from center to center.
- The tests are not foolproof, and there is often an overlap between normal short children and children with GHD. Hence, two standard provocative tests are usually suggested before recommending GH therapy.
- Insulin administration carries the risk of hypoglycemia and seizures. Hence, in infancy, glucagon test is preferred.
- Priming with sex steroids is required in short children with delayed puberty and a bone age of 10 years or more (*Boys:* Depo-testosterone 100 mg intramuscular 3–5 days before the test; *Girls:* Premarin 5 mg orally the night before and morning of the test). Euthyroid state is essential before GH testing.
- The spontaneous secretion of GH can be evaluated by measuring GH levels every 15–20 minutes during a 12- or 24-hour period. However, this is not practiced in India.
- Insulin-like growth factor-I and IGFBP-3 are increasingly used for initial screening in the diagnosis of GHD. There are technical limitations to IGF-I assays. Their levels vary with age, nutritional status, and certain disease states. Insulin-like growth factor-I is low in infancy and less dependable in young children (<5 years of age), and there may be an overlap with GHD. It is not dependable in GHD associated with brain tumors and/or cranial irradiation. IGFBP-3, not IGF-I, is helpful for diagnosis during infancy and can be used in suspected neonatal GHD. The IGFBP-3 assay is technically simple, and plasma concentrations vary much less with age and nutritional status. It is a good predictor of GHD in a child with short stature.
- Growth hormone deficiency may be associated with deficiencies of other anterior pituitary hormones. Hence, a complete evaluation of anterior pituitary function is undertaken in each patient with GHD.
- Computed tomography (CT) or magnetic resonance imaging (MRI) of brain is useful in the evaluation of GHD to rule out organic causes and study pituitary morphology—ectopic posterior pituitary, anterior pituitary hypoplasia, interruption or absence of pituitary stalk, midline anomalies, and tumors. Approximately 15% of children with GHD have an abnormality of pituitary on imaging.
- Molecular genetic testing provides an additional useful diagnostic tool. Inherited forms of genetic abnormality may be the probable underlying cause of GHD in 10–15% of all patients.
- Increased serum concentrations of GH, both basal and stimulated, together with low IGF-I and low IGFBP-3 levels, suggest GH insensitivity. Estimation of GHBP is helpful in the diagnosis of GH insensitivity.

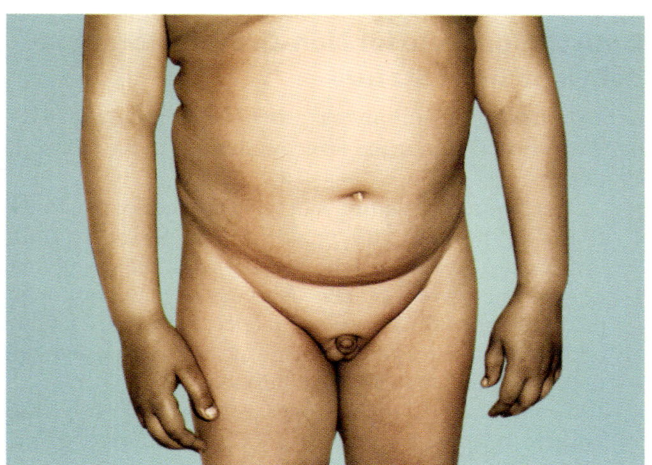

Fig. 13.2.2: A 10-year-old boy with growth hormone deficiency—please note micropenis and hypoplastic scrotum.

Table 13.2.1: Commonly employed growth hormone stimulation tests.

Test	*Dose*	*Blood collection timings (minutes)*	*Side effects*
Insulin	0.1 U/kg IV	0, 15, 30, 45, 60, 75, 90, 120	Hypoglycemia
Clonidine	0.15 mg/m^2 PO	0, 30, 60, 90	Hypotension
L-DOPA	<10 kg: 125 mg; 10–35 kg: 250 mg PO	0, 30, 60, 90	Headache, nausea
Glucagon	20 µg/kg IV	0, 30, 60, 90, 120, 150, 180	Nausea
GHRH	1 µg/kg IV	0, 15, 30, 45, 60, 90, 120	Flushing
Arginine	0.5 g/kg IV	0, 15, 30, 45, 60	Hypotension

(GHRH: growth hormone-releasing hormone; IV: intravenous; PO: per os)

Treatment

It is important to observe the child with regular growth records for 6 months to 1 year. A child who gains more than 4 cm/year is unlikely to have hypopituitarism. If GH levels are low, the child may be given recombinant GH in a dose of 0.25–0.5 mg/kg/week or 0.7–1 mg/m^2/day (1 mg = 3 IU) subcutaneously, till adequate growth is achieved. Dosage is titrated with the growth rate, pubertal stage, bone age, and serum IGF-I levels. Long-acting GH preparations are under trials now.

Growth hormone therapy in children with GHD induces rapid catch-up growth during the first 2–3 years of treatment, increasing the height gain two- to fourfold above the pretreatment rate. The child on an average gains a height of 10–14 cm in the first year of therapy and 6–8 cm/year thereafter every year for 2–3 years. In subsequent years, the height gain typically declines and follows normal patterns of growth. Younger children and those receiving a higher dose show a better response than older children with conventional dose.

Growth hormone is administered daily by subcutaneous injection in the evening (six times a week was recommended earlier), varying the site of injection. Pen devices and prefilled syringes are available, which simplify daily administration. Many centers start GH therapy at half the normal replacement dose and increase the dose during the first month to avoid the possible adverse effects of fluid retention. In addition to growth, serum IGF-I levels also help as a guide during GH dose titration. If IGF-I levels are low, assessment of injection technique and compliance might be necessary before dose adjustment. If IGF-I levels are above the normal range and height gain is adequate, a reduction in dose should be considered.

The cessation of GH therapy at the end of linear growth is guided by the following criteria:

- Height gain decreasing to 1 cm/year
- Attainment of an acceptable height close to target height
- Bone age is over 16 years in boys and 14 years in girls.

After final height has been achieved, GH therapy should be discontinued and GH status reassessed to identify those with persistent severe GHD (peak GH < 5 ng/mL). Discontinuation of GH therapy is recommended for a period of 1–3 months or longer before retesting.

Growth hormone therapy is relatively safe. Contrary to earlier suggestions, there is no report of increased susceptibility to tumors or leukemia in treated children. Salt and water retention occurs within the first few months of initiation. Treatment with GH increases the risk for prepubertal gynecomastia, slipped capital femoral epiphysis, pseudotumor cerebri, and worsening of scoliosis. Impaired glucose tolerance may develop in a few; hence, blood glucose and glycated hemoglobin estimations are recommended periodically.

There is also need for regular monitoring of thyroid function during therapy with GH, as some patients develop reversible hypothyroidism. Poor growth in a child with GHD on treatment with GH should prompt evaluation of thyroid hormone status. Pituitary- thyroid axis should be checked annually. The dose required to maintain euthyroid status is lower than in children with primary hypothyroidism. Hypothyroidism due to associated TSH deficiency is treated with replacement by sodium levothyroxine in a dose of 10 μg/kg along with regular thyroid hormone monitoring. Supplementation of other pituitary/hypothalamic hormones along with GH depending upon concomitant pituitary deficiencies is important. ACTH deficiency is managed by hydrocortisone replacement with doses usually not exceeding 10 mg/m^2/24 hours. Excessive doses of glucocorticoids given for ACTH deficiency can decrease the effectiveness of GH. Sex steroid replacement should be started at the normal age around 11–12 years in girls and 12–13 years in boys. Concurrent treatment with GH and a GnRH analog (leuprolide) or aromatase inhibitor (anastrozole or letrozole) is recommended in peripubertal children presuming that interruption of puberty will delay epiphyseal fusion allowing prolonged growth to give a better final height.

Growth Hormone for Non-Growth Hormone-deficient Short Stature

Growth hormone enhances growth of many non-GH-deficient short children and is recommended in the following situations:

- *Turner syndrome:* A number of early studies demonstrated that GH therapy with or without anabolic steroids accelerated growth velocity and led to an improved final height. The current practice is to use GH approximately 0.35 mg/kg/week. In clinical practice, it may be useful to add oxandrolone as a synergistic agent if response to GH becomes attenuated in late childhood.
- *Chronic renal insufficiency prior to undergoing renal transplantation:* Food and Drug Administration, United States have approved GH (0.3 mg/kg/week) in children with chronic renal insufficiency with poor height gain over 6 months, prior to undergoing renal transplantation.
- *Small for gestational age:* Small-for-gestational age children aged 4 years or older with failure to catch up, height below 2.5 standard deviation (SD), and height SD scores (SDS) more than 1 SD below midparental height SDS are eligible for GH treatment in United States since 2001 and in Europe since 2003. The recommended dose is 0.23–0.35 mg/kg/week.
- *Prader-Willi syndrome:* The indications for GH therapy in Prader-Willi syndrome are for the improvement of both growth and body composition. The recommended dose is 0.16–0.25 mg/kg/week.

- *Idiopathic short stature:* Idiopathic short stature (ISS) is a heterogeneous group of disorders with two common features: (1) short stature (height less than 2 SD or below the 3rd percentile for age and gender) and (2) normal GH response to stimulation tests. The tempo of growth may be slow or normal. It is a diagnosis of exclusion. Long-term GH therapy (0.25–0.37 mg/kg/week) can lead to increased adult height in children with ISS, but the degree and predictability of height gain are uncertain.

Insulin-like Growth Factor-I Deficiency and Growth Hormone Insensitivity

Insulin-like growth factor-I deficiency can result from genetic or nongenetic defects and has been found to be an important underlying cause of short stature in children. Laron and colleagues reported one of the first examples of insensitivity to GH in 1966 in three Israeli Jewish siblings presenting with hypoglycemia, and a clinical phenotype of GHD, but with marked elevation of immunoreactive serum GH. Similar cases have been reported from India. This is a hereditary disorder with primary resistance to actions of GH due to a molecular defect in the GH receptor.

The primary genetic form of GH intensity (GHI) is associated with abnormalities of the GH receptor, required to mediate actions of GH. It may also follow post-GH receptor defects or molecular defects in IGF-I. Children with primary GH insensitivity have the classic clinical phenotype of severe isolated GHD in its most severe form. The craniofacial features may be more prominent with characteristic midfacial hypoplasia, depressed nasal bridge, and protruding forehead. Height age is more severely retarded in relation to bone age.

Basal serum GH concentration may be normal or elevated, with excessive GH response to provocative stimuli. Typically these children have low levels of IGF-I, IGFBP-3, and very low or absent GHBP. Administration of GH does not bring about a rise in IGF-I levels, which forms the basis of the IGF-I generation test. The final diagnosis of GHI is based on the demonstration of the specific molecular defect in GH receptor gene, in the presence of clinical phenotype and laboratory criteria.

Initial results of treatment with recombinant IGF-I appear to be promising, but there are a number of limitations.

ACROMEGALY AND GIGANTISM

Excess secretion of GH in children, usually due to a pituitary adenoma, results in somatic overgrowth or gigantism. When hypersecretion of the hormone occurs after the fusion of skeletal epiphyses, it causes acromegaly, which is seen in adults.

Clinical Features

There is rapid linear growth, and the child is taller than his/her peers. Peripheral parts of the body, hands, feet, nose, and mandible appear disproportionately large. The head circumference is increased. Facial features are characteristic with coarse with prominent jaw, broad nose, enlarged tongue, and bushy eyebrows. Skin and subcutaneous tissue are thick with dorsal kyphosis. Muscle weakness, bony and cartilaginous overgrowth, cardiomyopathies, and pigmentation of skin may be present. Diffuse or nodular goiter or hyperthyroidism may be present. Involvement of other endocrine organs may lead to hypogonadism, hypocortisolism, or diabetes mellitus. Headaches, visual field defects including bitemporal hemianopia, papilledema followed by optic atrophy, and external ophthalmoplegia are common. Behavioral problems may be present. GH-secreting adenoma may occur in association with McCune-Albright syndrome or multiple endocrine neoplasia type 1.

Diagnosis

The diagnosis is based on clinical examination, periodic growth assessment, and investigations. Enlarged sella turcica with erosion of margins is seen on X-ray. Tufting of phalanges and increased heel-pad thickness may be present. Skeletal maturation is normal. CT or MRI scan of brain should be done to determine the extent of the tumor. The diagnosis is confirmed by the detection of raised IGF-I levels and lack of suppression of GH (levels <1 ng/mL) following administration of oral glucose, 1.75 g/kg. Secretion of ACTH, TSH, LH, and FSH may be impaired.

Treatment

Treatment of adenoma includes surgery, irradiation, and medical therapy. The pituitary microadenoma is resected by transsphenoidal route, if there is evidence for raised intracranial tension. Larger tumors can be removed by transcranial route. Conventional or high-voltage radiotherapy may halt the progress of the disease but may not cause clinical improvement. Pituitary radiation can also be carried out by implanting radioactive isotopes. A long-acting somatostatin analog, octreotide has been found to be better than bromocriptine in suppressing the levels of GH, IGF-I, and IGFBP-3 and reducing the size of tumor mass.

DIABETES INSIPIDUS

Diabetes insipidus (DI) results from the lack of antidiuretic hormone, also known as AVP. Arginine vasopressin is secreted from the supraoptic and paraventricular nuclei of the hypothalamus. It is transported through axons to posterior pituitary where it is stored until release. It acts on receptors (V_1 and V_2), especially in the collecting ducts of kidney. Binding of AVP to the V_2 receptor leads to a cascade of actions through the G-protein-adenylyl cyclase system and release of a second messenger known as aquaporin 2, which allows transport of water. AVP release is primarily controlled by alterations in plasma osmolality.

Etiology

The deficiency may be partial, complete, or transient.

- Central DI results from various abnormalities of AVP synthesis and/or action due to lesions of neurohypophysis, such as suprasellar tumors (craniopharyngioma, optic glioma), histiocytosis, reticuloendotheliosis, encephalitis, tuberculosis, granulomas, and trauma. DI can occur in the newborn following asphyxia, intracranial bleeding, and meningitis. DI with diabetes mellitus, optic atrophy, and deafness is known as Wolfram or DI, diabetes mellitus, optic atrophy, and deafness syndrome.
- Nephrogenic DI is due to the inability of the kidney tubules to respond to AVP—failure to increase renal water reabsorption in the presence of adequate AVP. It is often due to abnormalities in kidney function and structure affecting collecting duct or mutations that affect the V_2 receptors.
- There is a psychogenic form of polydipsia with associated polyuria due to compulsive water drinking.

In central and nephrogenic DI, diffusion of water from the distal tubules and collecting ducts is reduced due to lack of AVP. Since sodium and water transport from the loop of Henle and distal tubule remains unchanged, urine becomes hypotonic and cannot be concentrated beyond 150 mOsm/kg.

Clinical Features

These children are thirsty and pass large quantities of urine and often report with nocturnal enuresis. The symptoms are often not recognized by the parents. Infants with DI thus may present with intermittent high fever, irritability, weight loss, poor feeding, dehydration, and collapse. Abnormal behavior and hyperactivity are common. In children, who have acquired bladder control, enuresis may be the first symptom. Signs and symptoms of causative lesions may be present and include growth retardation, cachexia, obesity, sleep disturbances, precocious puberty, visual disturbances, and emotional disorders.

Diagnosis

Polyuria and polydipsia should be confirmed by 24-hour intake and output records. Urinary specific gravity varies from 1.001 to 1.005 and osmolality 50–200 mOsm/kg. Serum osmolality may vary depending on the degree of dehydration. Other renal function studies are normal. Often DI is suspected in the presence of life-threatening hypernatremia. Serum AVP levels are helpful in establishing the diagnosis with the child in a hyperosmolar state with voiding hypoosmotic urine.

Often the distinction between central and nephrogenic DI requires a water deprivation test or desmopressin (DDAVP) test. During water deprivation test for a minimum of 3–6 hours, children with central and nephrogenic DI fail to concentrate urine and plasma more than 300 mOsm/kg, whereas there is urinary concentration in children with compulsory water drinking. The interpretation of water deprivation test is given in **Box 13.2.2**. If there is concentration of urine following DDAVP administration, the cause is primary AVP deficiency. Failure to concentrate urine and absence of response to DDAVP indicate nephrogenic DI.

Radiologic studies including MRI may reveal evidence for intracranial tumor, such as calcification, enlargement of sella, erosion of clinoid process, and increased width of suture lines or evidence of reticuloendotheliosis, such as rarefaction. MRI of brain also can demonstrate the absence of the bright hyperintense spot in hypothalamic-pituitary lesions.

Treatment

Central DI can be treated by administration of DDAVP, an analog of AVP given as a nasal spray, nasal solution, or oral or sublingual tablets. The usual dose is 5–10 µg daily either as a single dose or divided into two doses. Children under 2 years require lesser doses (0.15–0.50 µg/kg). Oral administration of chlorpropamide 20 mg/kg/24 hours in two divided doses may reduce polyuria and polydipsia in partial deficiency. Hydrochlorothiazide and indomethacin may offer some relief in nephrogenic DI.

Box 13.2.2: Interpretation of water deprivation test.

- *Initial evaluation*:
  - Serum sodium
  - Plasma osmolality
  - Urine osmolality
  - Weight (calculate 5% weight)
- Test not required if urine osmolality greater than 750 mOsm/kg or plasma osmolality greater than 300 mOsm/kg
- *Monitoring*:
  - Urine osmolality and plasma osmolality hourly
  - Urine output and weight hourly
  - Look for features of dehydration
- *Termination of test*:
  - Weight loss greater than 5%
  - Urine osmolality greater than 750 mOsm/kg
  - Plasma osmolality greater than 300 mOsm/kg
- *Vasopressin response test*:
  - Aqueous vasopressin (0.1–0.5 U/kg, IM)
  - DDAVP (1–2 mg subcutaneously)
  - Avoid intranasal DDAVP
- *Classification:* Increase in urine osmolality:
  - *Less than 50% of baseline:* Nephrogenic DI
  - *Greater than 50% of baseline:* Central DI

Note: Conversion of urine osmolality to urine specific gravity: 300 mOsm/kg greater than or equal to 1.005; 750 mOsm/kg greater than or equal to 1.010.

(DAVP: desmopressin; DI: diabetes insipidus; IM: intramuscular)

BIBLIOGRAPHY

1. Bajpai A, Kabra M, Gupta AK, et al. Growth pattern and skeletal maturation following growth hormone therapy in growth hormone deficiency: factors influencing outcome. Indian Pediatr. 2006;43(7):593-9.
2. Bajpai A, Menon PS. Insulin like growth factors axis and growth disorders. Indian J Pediatr. 2006;73(1):67-71.
3. Carr M, Gill D. Polyuria, polydipsia, polypopsia: "Mummy I want a drink". Arch Dis Child Educ Pract Ed. 2007;92(5):139-43.
4. Dabrowski E, Kadakia R, Zimmerman D. Diabetes insipidus in infants and children. Best Pract Res Clin Endocrinol Metab. 2016;30(2):317-28.
5. Desai MP, Menon PSN, Bhatia V (Eds). Pediatric endocrine disorders, 3rd edition. Hyderabad: Universities Press; 2014. pp. 81-119.
6. Growth Hormone Research Society. Consensus guidelines for the diagnosis and treatment of growth hormone (GH) deficiency in childhood and adolescence: summary statement of the GH Research Society. GH Research Society. J Clin Endocrinol Metab. 2000;85(11):3990-3.
7. Rivkees SA, Dunbar N, Wilson TA. The management of central diabetes insipidus in infancy: desmopressin, low renal solute load formula, thiazide diuretics. J Pediatr Endocrinol Metab. 2007;20(4):459-69.
8. Rosenfeld RG. Molecular mechanisms of IGF-I deficiency. Horm Res. 2006;65(Suppl 1):15-20.
9. Rosenthal S, Cohen P, Clayton P, et al. Treatment perspectives in idiopathic short stature with a focus on IGF-I deficiency. Pediatr Endocrinol Rev. 2007;4(Suppl 2):252-71.
10. Saenger PH, Mejia-Corletto J. Long acting growth hormone: an update. Endocr Dev. 2016;30:79-97.

13.3 Obesity

Anju Virmani

INTRODUCTION

The problem of obesity is increasing among children and adolescents across the world, from 5% in the 1970s to over 15% now. World Health Organization (WHO) estimated that in 2013, the number of overweight children under the age of 5, globally, was over 42 million, of which 31 million were from the developing countries. Similarly, in urban and semiurban India, prevalence is rising rapidly, with 5–15% urban Indian adolescents overweight or obese. Increasingly, low socioeconomic status (SES) is correlated with obesity, due to several factors, such as high intake of energy-dense foods (which are often cheaper); reduced physical activity for lack of safety, time, or other factors; higher screen time; and lesser access to quality medical care and awareness campaigns. Low SES populations, especially in the developing countries, are even worse equipped to handle this epidemic. On the other hand, since 2008, prevalence appears to be plateauing in the United States, France, Switzerland, Australia, and the other developed countries, perhaps due to aggressive preventive measures. This gives hope that the problem can be controlled if tackled at several levels: societal, environmental, and individual.

Obesity is now recognized as not just cosmetic but a disease which causes impaired mobility and interference with daily living activities, serious morbidity **(Box 13.3.1)**, and even mortality. Almost 50% obese children become obese adolescents, and almost 80% of them become obese adults. With onset in childhood, and thus longer duration, the health burden of obesity and its consequences will rise in the coming decades. This in turn would have severe economic consequences for individuals as well as societies.

Much of the morbidity is related to visceral rather than peripheral fat and can be reversed with weight loss. However, established obesity is very frustrating to manage, as sustained weight loss is difficult to achieve, and lost weight returns rapidly. It is critical that the entire family be involved in the weight loss process; if family members are unwilling to change their habits, the child alone should not be forced to make drastic changes. The goal of management is not attainment of ideal body weight, which may be near impossible, but achieving and maintaining steady weight loss to the extent possible. Even 5% weight loss results in a significant improvement in the metabolic parameters. Because loss is difficult, prevention is crucial. Pediatricians

Box 13.3.1: Comorbidities of obesity.

- *Type 2 diabetes mellitus (T2DM):* With hyperinsulinemia and insulin resistance, presentation may range from asymptomatic and picked up on screening to frank diabetic ketoacidosis
- *Hypertension:* Rises from about 4–6% in under 5 years to 15% in adolescents
- *Dyslipidemia:* Generally, low high density lipoproteins (HDL), raised low density lipoproteins (LDL) and triglycerides—in up to 20% obese adolescents
- *Polycystic ovarian syndrome:* With hyperandrogenemia and hyperinsulinism
- *Abnormal puberty:* Early puberty and short final height in some girls
- *Renal dysfunction:* Higher rate of glomerulosclerosis; proteinuria and focal segmental glomerulosclerosis; and end-stage renal disease
- *Hepatic dysfunction:* Higher rate of raised transaminases, fatty liver on ultrasound, nonalcoholic fatty liver disease, gallstones, and even progression to cirrhosis
- *Sleep apnea:* Rate much higher; apnea in turn can worsen hypertension, behavior and school performance
- *Mechanical problems:* Slipped capital femoral epiphysis, genu valgum, tibia vara, Legg-Calvé-Perthes disease, low back pain, scoliosis, and osteoarthritis
- Vitamin D deficiency
- *Psychological problems and eating disorders:* Feelings of inadequacy and being different; being stereotyped as greedy, clumsy, lazy, stupid, or worthless
- *Skin:* Acanthosis nigricans, skin tags, intertriginous infections
- *Miscellaneous:* Hyperuricemia, increased risk of malignancies

must be vigilant in preventing obesity, while trying to reduce the health impact in those already obese.

DEFINITIONS

The definitions given by WHO and International Obesity Task Force using body mass index [BMI = (weight in kg)/(height in m^2)] are most commonly used to quantify obesity. In adults, obesity is defined as BMI greater than 25 kg/m^2, morbid obesity as BMI greater than 40, and super obesity as BMI greater than 60. South Asians tend to be "fat-thin" (i.e. having more body fat for the same BMI and more adverse body fat patterning, including abdominal adiposity), so their recommended cutoff is 23 kg/m^2.

In children, normal BMI changes with age, so the BMI for age should be looked at, using the Center for Disease Control charts which provide percentiles or by calculating the *z*-score for BMI, using the standard norms given on the WHO website. The child is "overweight" if the BMI is 85–95 percentiles for age and gender, and "obese" if BMI is greater than 95 percentile. Weight for height can be calculated ("overweight": up to 120% of ideal, "obese": > 120%) and is often used for children under 5 years, but it can also be useful in older children to help the family understand the severity of the problem. Body mass index or weight-for-height norms may sometimes be misleading, e.g. in muscular persons or those with early or delayed puberty. However, they are relatively robust and widely used.

Other parameters are waist circumference, measured at the level of the iliac crest, and waist-hip ratio, interpreted according to age, gender, and ethnicity. They have the additional benefit of emphasizing abdominal obesity, which is better correlated with insulin resistance (IR) and cardiovascular (CV) risk.

PATHOGENESIS

The basic reason for obesity and the consequent metabolic diseases is a disordered energy balance, i.e. energy (food) intake chronically exceeds energy expenditure. The excess weight is stored in adipose tissue, which is not just a passive storage depot but an active endocrine organ. Several hormones (e.g. insulin and leptin) and nutrients (glucose and fatty acids) link the brain and gastrointestinal tract with the adipose tissue, influencing appetite, energy expenditure, and growth. A number of orexicants (including ghrelin, cholecystokinin, cortisol, agouti-related protein, neuropeptide Y, gamma-aminobutyric acid, melanin-concentrating hormone, and endocannabinoids) and anorexiants [leptin, α-melanocyte stimulating hormone, proopiomelanocortin (POMC), insulin, serotonin, dopamine, and glucagon-like peptide 1 (GLP-1) and glucose-dependent insulinotropic peptide] are involved in the complex processes of energy intake and expenditure and maintenance of body weight. Many of them act via the melanocortin-4 receptor (MC4R) in the arcuate nucleus of the hypothalamus. Loss-of-function mutations of MC4R cause severe obesity by disrupting hypothalamic appetite control centers, and promoting binge eating. Leptin, produced by adipose tissue, suppresses food intake and increases energy expenditure, but early hopes of therapeutic possibilities were belied as obese individuals are relatively leptin resistant. Other compounds are being explored for possible therapeutic use.

Adipose tissue also metabolizes sex steroids (e.g. converts androstenedione to testosterone and estrone to estradiol), which in turn may play a role in fat distribution. Adolescence is a particularly difficult period characterized by IR (and also more defiant and risk-taking behavior, more body image and self-esteem issues). Increased fat deposits are seen in hypogonadal states, such as Turner and Klinefelter syndromes. Adipose tissue also secretes inflammatory cytokines (e.g. tumor necrosis factor-α, interleukin-6, plasma activator inhibitor type 1, adiponectin, and visfatin), linking central or visceral obesity with CV disease.

In addition to these well-described processes, the recent recognition of the roles played by different adipocytes is opening fresh areas for therapeutic intervention in obesity, diabetes, and other metabolic diseases. Brown adipose tissue

(BAT) possesses uncoupling protein-1 and has long been known, especially in newborns, to transform chemical energy into heat (nonshivering thermogenesis). BAT can generate 300 times more heat than any other tissue, using lipids and glucose as fuel, and it has been shown in experimental models to modulate obesity and diabetes. Positron emission tomography scans have shown that small but significant amounts of classical BAT continue to exist in adults; methods which augment it would reduce weight and hyperglycemia. In addition, newly recognized beige (or brite: brown in white) fat cells (seen in white fat depots under certain conditions) can increase whole-body energy expenditure and are perhaps easier to get activated. Several centers are trying to explore how to induce formation of these beige adipose cells, thus increasing whole-body metabolic rates and protecting against obesity and diabetes.

ETIOLOGY

Obesity is caused by an imbalance of energy intake and output; exact mechanisms are becoming better understood. With greater industrialization, the environment is becoming more obesogenic, whether at the level of the individual (e.g. differences in food choices, levels of physical activity, attitudes to food, activity, body image, etc.) or of the environment (town planning and building architecture, e.g. availability of safe areas to play, side roads so that walking and cycling are possible, etc.). The total calorie intake is increasing, in addition to the wrong kind of calories being consumed. Use of processed foods is increasing; most packaged foods have low fiber, high simple carbohydrate (fructose, sucrose, and refined cereals), high fat (often *trans*-fat), and low micronutrient content. Food labels are often inadequate, deliberately difficult to read, or even misleading. Awareness levels of good nutrition are low, drowned out by aggressive advertising and attempts to target taste at the cost of nutrition. Consistently strong correlations are seen specifically with the consumption of sweetened beverages and with television (TV) viewing (reduces activity, increases calorie intake, pushes wrong messages about food, and encourages intake of junk foods). Increased screen time is correlated with decreased physical fitness, increased CV risk, decreased self-esteem, and lower school performance.

Genetic influences also exist, as shown by studies on adopted children and twins. In general, obesity runs in families, as they share both genes and environment; parental obesity is a strong risk factor. Eighty percent of children of both obese parents and 40% of one obese parent are overweight. Maternal weight, weight gain during the prenatal period, and diabetes are important predictors. Low birth weight (LBW) with subsequent obesity confers high risk for hyperinsulinemia and CV disease. The "developmental origins of adult disease" concept links periconceptual, fetal, and early infant phases of life and explains the higher risk of obesity and metabolic consequences in adulthood. Keeping these factors in mind, health personnel must start delivering appropriate messages early, e.g. encouraging preconception normalization of weight, warning obese parents to increase activity and reduce calorie intake themselves and aim for normal weight rather than chubby children, discouraging force feeding especially of LBW babies, educating parents about healthy diets and need for activity on an ongoing basis. Pathologic causes account for less than 1% of all cases **(Table 13.3.1)**. Corticosteroid or other drug therapy is most common. Endocrine causes are almost universally associated with decreased height velocity. In Cushing syndrome, obesity distribution is truncal, but in infants, distribution can be generalized **(Fig. 13.3.1)**. Several single-gene mutations can result in variable degrees of obesity syndromes, such as Prader-Willi, Laurence-Moon-Biedl, pseudohypoparathyroidism type 1A, Alstrom, Carpenter, Cohen, and POMC deficiency.

Table 13.3.1: Laboratory evaluation for short stature.

Endocrine: • Hypothyroidism • Growth hormone deficiency • Cushing syndrome
Hypothalamic: • Laurence-Moon-Biedl syndrome • Prader-Willi syndrome • Craniopharyngioma
Drugs: • Corticosteroids • Sodium valproate
Miscellaneous: • Achondroplasia • Muscular dystrophy • Severe mental retardation

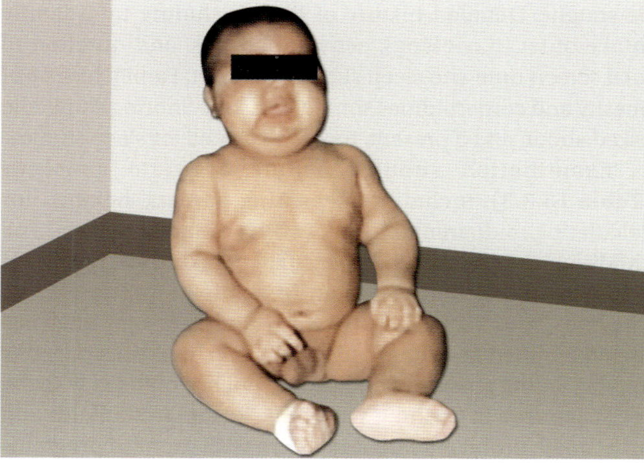

Fig. 13.3.1: An infant with Cushing syndrome: please note that unlike children, in infants, the obesity may be generalized.

Table 13.3.2: History.

Early influences: • Maternal diabetes, parental obesity; family history of obesity, diabetes, hypertension, dyslipidemia, heart disease • Weight gain during pregnancy • Birth weight, growth measurement • Duration of breastfeeding • Early obesity rebound
Diseases: • Central nervous system disease • Drug intake • Polyuria, nocturia, polyphagia • Menstrual history, acne, hirsutism
Environment: • Details of activity patterns • Availability of safe play areas • Duration of TV viewing • Diet details, including total fat intake • Attitudes toward food • Mental development and school performance • Past attempts at dieting (child or parents)

In craniopharyngioma, obesity is multifactorial and tends to worsen after surgery.

Clinical Evaluation

The most important clinical feature, which distinguishes pathological from exogenous obesity, is height. Children with exogenous obesity are taller than expected for age and family; those with pathology are shorter than expected (unless they also have precocious puberty or virilization). Detailed history is necessary **(Table 13.3.2)**.

Parents and/or the child may be concerned about appearance, easy fatigability, darkening of skin (acanthosis), or small penile size. Gestational history (e.g. diabetes, obesity, and hypertension during pregnancy) and birth weight should be sought. Detailed history of diet (including total family intake of fat in cooking), activity patterns, and duration of total screen time and sleep should be taken. Family history of obesity and comorbidities should be taken. Snoring should be asked about, and if present, indicates a need for sleep studies.

Examination should include accurate auxology **(Table 13.3.3)**, including measuring parents' heights [for calculating midparental height (MPH) or target height]. The child's height age should be calculated, taking age and MPH into account. Acanthosis seen in skinfolds [neck, axillae, knuckles, and groin **(Fig. 13.3.2)**] and skin tags suggests hyperinsulinemia. With rapid weight gain, pinkish striae may appear, fading gradually, and should not be confused with the red striae seen in Cushing syndrome. Rashes in skinfolds and orthopedic problems might interfere with exercise programs unless treated.

Careful genital examination is needed, including stretched penile length (SPL) in boys, since the penis is usually buried in abdominal fat. The small looking penis may be misinterpreted by parents concerned about small genitalia and even doctors as "hypogonadism". True micropenis (SPL <2 SD for age) may be seen in growth hormone deficiency (GHD) and some syndromes. Adolescent boys may also be brought to medical attention for large breasts, which could be due to gynecomastia, lipomastia, or both. The child's behavior should be assessed, as those who are embarrassed, withdrawn, or depressed are less likely to exercise and may be more prone to binge eating.

Table 13.3.3: Examination.

Auxology: • Height, weight, BP • Waist circumference, waist-hip ratio (WHR) • Pattern of fat distribution • Parents' height, weight
General physical: • *Skin*: Striae, acanthosis, acne, hirsutism, rashes in skin folds • Dysmorphism, features of any syndromes • Features of endocrine disease (Cushing, hypothyroidism)
Systemic: • Pubertal staging, including stretched penile length (SPL) in boys • Fundus examination • Orthopedic problems • Self-esteem, behavior • Mental development and school performance

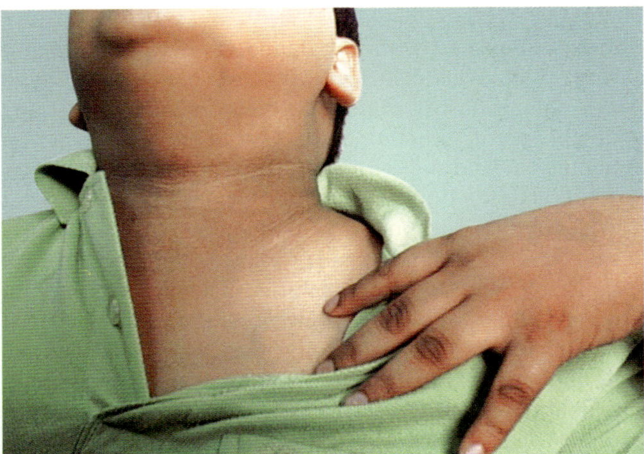

Fig. 13.3.2: Acanthosis nigricans seen as dark velvety area at the folds of the neck and knuckles in an obese boy.

LABORATORY EVALUATION

Investigations are guided by the clinical presentation. The tall child, with normal growth velocity, normal blood pressure (BP) or mild hypertension, no clinical evidence of dysmorphism or pathology, somewhat advanced bone age (usually close to height age), is likely to have exogenous obesity. The Endocrine

Society's guidelines recommend against routine testing for endocrinopathies in such children. Blood glucose (fasting and 2 hours after oral glucose load of 1.75 g/kg, up to a maximum of 75 g), lipids, transaminases, thyroid-stimulating hormone (TSH), and insulin should be tested; and fatty liver looked for with ultrasound. Fasting insulin greater than 20 IU/mL denotes hyperinsulinemia (normal < 15 IU/mL). Homeostasis model assessment (HOMA)-estimated IR (HOMA-IR) index can be calculated as a marker of IR (IR, significant > 4.39). [HOMA-IR = (fasting insulin in μU/mL × fasting glucose in mmol/L)/22.5]. Glycosylated hemoglobin for diagnosis of diabetes poses several difficulties, especially in children, and if tested, should be interpreted with caution. Further workup is hardly ever required.

If tested in exogenous obesity, mildly raised TSH [TSH < 10 μU/mL with normal thyroxine (T4) is not an indication for T4 replacement] and cortisol (easily suppressible with overnight dexamethasone) may be seen; urinary free cortisol is normal. Similarly, growth hormone (GH) may be low in stimulation tests, but insulin-like growth factor (IGF)-1 and IGF-binding protein-3 are normal. Changes of polycystic ovary syndrome (PCOS) may be seen in the adolescent girl [raised testosterone and/or dehydroepiandrosterone sulfate, altered luteinizing hormone (LH)/follicle-stimulating hormone (FSH) ratio, polycystic changes in the ovaries]. Other findings include proteinuria, fatty liver, raised serum T3, decreased sex hormone-binding globulin, and pubertal levels of FSH in 7–9-year-old girls (with no increase in LH). In adults, serum parathyroid hormone may be raised and is an independent predictor of obesity. Sleep studies, if the child has marked snoring, may reveal sleep apnea (obstructive, central, or combined).

The short or slowly growing child (bone age retarded) needs serum T4, TSH, 8 AM cortisol, and other tests as guided by the clinical examination. If features of any genetic syndrome are present, evaluation by a geneticist and appropriate tests are needed. Children with steady weight gain from early infancy may have MC4R mutations, but the test is positive in less than 5% obese children and does not change the management.

PREVENTION

Prevention of obesity and metabolic problems before and during pregnancy and promoting breastfeeding are safe ways to reduce pediatric obesity. All children should have weights and heights measured and plotted on a growth chart annually till growth is complete. Those showing rapid weight gain (crossing percentile lines), especially in high-risk groups (LBW, one or both obese parents, obese sibling/s, maternal age greater than 35 years at birth, single child, single parent, precious child, taking certain medications), need early family attention. The three windows of opportunities for obesity prevention are—the first year of life, the period of adiposity rebound (age 3–7 years), and puberty, especially menarche. Diet control by the entire family (discussed in greater detail in management), not "dieting," along with regular physical activity, is needed on a sustained basis **(Table 13.3.4)**. Diet changes alone, or exercise alone, will not prevent or manage obesity. Consistency is critical.

Table 13.3.4: Prevention of obesity.
Family: • Adequate breastfeeding, no force feeding • Ensure low-fat milk and products; keep cooking fat low • Avoid junk food, sweetened drinks and fried foods • Encourage fruits, salads, whole dals, and grilled/steamed animal products • Encourage water as drink • No missed meals • Look for calorie and carbohydrate content of packaged foods • Encourage physical activity • *Controlled screen time*: TV, computers, video games • Avoid tuitions, academic overcompetitiveness • Express affection or approval in nonfood ways • Avoid shaming behavior
Schools: • No sugary or sports drinks, juices, fried snacks available in or near school • No high-calorie foods or snacks in school meals • Offer fruits, low-fat dairy drinks • Make exercise mandatory, ensure all children participate • Identify, counsel those at risk • Specific counseling for those already obese • Avoid shaming behavior • Early referral if there is rapid weight gain
Community: • Provide adequate, safe spaces for play • Ensure cycle tracks on roads

Recent unhealthy trends in urban areas include leaving few open places for play, forbidding games in even the few which exist, and discouraging walking and cycling (crowded roads without cycle tracks). Parents and schools encourage sedentary lifestyles (pressure on academics, after school tuitions) and expose early to screens, often using phones, TV, and iPads as babysitter substitutes; children are attracted to mobile phones and games. Pediatricians must lobby actively against such trends with schools and society in general, to ensure children are given enough space and time to play outdoors, and reduce exposure to unhealthy foods and eating patterns.

MANAGEMENT

Management of pathological obesity depends on the underlying cause, e.g. replacement of T4 in hypothyroidism, GH in GHD, or gonadal replacement in hypogonadism, treatment of Cushing syndrome, etc.

In exogenous obesity, not only weight loss but also maintenance of loss is critical. Efforts to motivate the entire family to make long-term diet and activity changes are needed. Small, permanent changes are more useful than drastic, short-lived changes. Very-low-calorie diets should be planned only in lifesaving situations, i.e. extreme obesity, severe sleep apnea, or cardiopulmonary manifestations (Pickwickian syndrome) under careful supervision. Dietary measures and increased activity, supported by behavioral modification techniques, should be advised. Considerable psychological support for the child and family may be needed; e-health methods often work with adolescents for awareness, motivation, recording, goal setting, and other behavior changes. Drug therapy and bariatric surgery are less frequently advised in childhood and adolescence. Comorbidities should be adequately managed.

Diet Therapy

Standard diet therapy restricts calories, while maintaining a normal balanced pattern—fat intake less than 25% of total calories, protein 15–20%, rest 55% as complex carbohydrates, with adequate fiber, micronutrients, and plenty of liquids. Even with severe obesity, calorie restriction should be moderate, aiming for weight loss of 0.5 kg/week, while ensuring adequate protein (0.8–1 g/kg/day). Nutritional deficiencies (iron, calcium, vitamin D, etc.) should be corrected and ongoing minimal supplementation given as required. Cooking and food purchase patterns should be discussed in detail and restriction on processed foods and excess cooking fat advised. Principles of prevention **(Table 13.3.4)** should be strongly advocated, including encouraging intake of foods with low glycemic index (GI)—whole fruits (avoid peeling), salads, brown rice, whole wheat products, other coarse grains (e.g. millets), whole legumes, low-fat milk and dairy products (unsweetened), nuts in small quantities; drinking plenty of water; and discouraging undesirable and "diet foods" or "health foods". Sweetened drinks including diet drinks, juices, sugar-free desserts, chocolates, baked chips, etc. often have very high-calorie content and should be discouraged. Large meals with long gaps, and missed meals, should also be avoided—"grazing" is better than "gorging". Children should be involved in cooking and food choices, and family meal times (without TV) should be encouraged. Care must be taken to make small changes initially, and not to overrestrict fat intake. Foods low in fat, high in carbs, have high GI (e.g. polished rice, potatoes, packaged cereals, bread and other maida products, zero-fat milk) and cause sharp insulin spikes, which actually promote weight gain. At no time should diet restrictions be viewed as punishments.

Very-low-calorie diets (400–800 cal/day) for 2–6 weeks result in rapid weight loss and marked improvement in BP and levels of blood glucose, insulin, leptin, and lipids. However, they are dangerous unless closely monitored and adequately supplemented with minerals and vitamins. Long-term results are poor, with weight gain returning within 1–5 years. Stringent dieting can cause poor height gain, slowed pubertal development, osteopenia, irritability, behavioral problems, and a weight loss plateau because of a slower metabolic rate.

Exercise

All physical activity (purposeful exercise or nonexercise activity thermogenesis) increases energy expenditure and is essential for good health and healthy weight loss. Other benefits include psychological well-being, lesser irritability, better academic performance, lesser acne and hirsutism, more regular menses, better lipid profiles/BP/insulin levels, reduced appetite, and increased metabolic rate (while calorie restriction alone causes decreased metabolic rate).

For compliance, ensure activity is incorporated into daily life (e.g. walking to school, classes on different floors), and active games are viewed as fun (walking with friends, swimming, dancing, and sports). Initially low impact, moderate-intensity exercise (30 min × 5 days/week) should be advised; later, the time and intensity of exercise should be increased to an hour or more daily.

Screen time of less than 2 hours/day has been recommended.

Adequate sleep is essential, as inadequate (or excessive) sleep has been shown to result in weight gain. Parents, teachers, and the child must understand that play and adequate sleep are not time wasted; instead they are crucial for physical, mental, and academic well-being.

Behavior Modification and Social Support

These are absolutely critical, especially maintaining diaries of food intake, activity and screen time, motivational techniques and group activities. Children respond well to small, zero calorie awards (hug, stationery or sports item, star on a chart); adolescents may be more enthusiastic about e-techniques, such as mobile apps for diet or exercise monitoring, motivational messaging, and so on. Such devices can also be used for tracking behaviors and providing personalized feedback. Several techniques (**Box 13.3.2**) may be used in various combinations. Reasonable, clear goals must be set by the family and health personnel working together.

Occasional treats should be given so that frustration and dysfunctional behavior do not occur. Unhealthy family habits and disparagement of the child should be strongly discouraged. Initially monthly reviews with reinforcement may be necessary. Yo-yo weight patterns are undesirable because each weight loss or gain cycle causes metabolic and psychological changes which make subsequent weight loss more difficult.

Treatment of Comorbidities

Associated problems—hypertension, type 2 diabetes mellitus (T2DM), dyslipidemia, PCOS, psychological, orthopedic and

Box 13.3.2: Behavior modification techniques.

- Monitoring
- Goal setting
- Contracting
- Stimulus control
- Social reinforcement
- Reward and punishment
- Aversion therapy
- Managing high-risk situations
- Relapse prevention

skin problems, sleep apnea—are often paid inadequate attention by health personnel (***See* Box 13.3.1**). This not only impacts general health but also interferes with weight loss. Comorbidities should be actively looked for, and adequately treated.

MEDICATIONS

Several anorexic agents (amphetamines, nonamphetamine appetite suppressants) and antidepressants have come into the market, become popular, and then been banned because of adverse effects. Medication options are limited and should be considered only after significant efforts at diet, exercise, and behavior control have failed, only as an add-on to these efforts. Orlistat, approved by the Food and Drug Administration for use in children over 12 years of age, is a potent reversible inhibitor of gastrointestinal lipases. It must be given at mealtimes; the adult dose is 120 mg thrice daily. It decreases fat absorption by 30%, causing weight loss, and improving lipid and glycemic profiles, but the benefit is not marked in severe obesity, and side effects include oil spotting, flatulence, frequent stools, and deficiency of fat-soluble vitamins, such as vitamins A and D.

In PCOS and T2DM, metformin, an insulin sensitizer, has been shown to safely achieve modest weight loss, decrease body fat, and decrease plasma leptin/insulin/lipids, but it is not approved for use in obesity. Other drugs such as thiazolidinones, sibutramine, lorcaserin, topiramate, GLP-1 analogs, and octreotide have lesser safety profiles/lesser efficacy/little pediatric data and are not approved.

Surgery

Surgical treatment, only considered for morbid obesity after intensive lifestyle modification and medication have failed, is relatively contraindicated in patients less than 18 years old. Body mass index greater than 50 kg/m^2, or severe complications, such as sleep apnea with BMI greater than 40 kg/m^2, not responding to nonsurgical treatment, may call for bariatric surgery, after suitable psychological preparation. An experienced surgeon should be available, and the child and family should be willing to continue following a healthy diet and exercise pattern. It should not be offered if there is an uncontrolled psychiatric illness, unresolved eating disorder, or Prader-Willi syndrome. Side effects can be significant—pulmonary embolism, wound infection, micro- and macronutrient malabsorption, diarrhea, anemia, cholecystitis, and dumping syndrome. Some patients may regain lost weight within 1–5 years.

SUMMARY

Pediatric and adolescent obesity is increasing worldwide, due to lifestyle alterations, and has major health and economic implications. Efforts at prevention at all levels are crucial. Health-care givers should push for societal changes at the community level, while actively educating all parents about healthy lifestyles, focusing especially on high-risk groups (LBW babies, obese parents, single parent, only or precious child, chronic illnesses, and drug intake, etc.). Weight loss may be difficult to achieve and sustain, but a loss of even 5–10% results in substantial metabolic improvement, so high relapse rates should not discourage as intensive attempts at weight loss as possible to every family. Comorbidities should be actively treated.

BIBLIOGRAPHY

1. August GP, Caprio S, Fennoy I, et al. Prevention and treatment of pediatric obesity: an Endocrine Society Clinical Practice Guideline based on expert opinion. J Clin Endocrinol Metab. 2008;93(12):4576-99.
2. Bhargava SK, Sachdev HS, Fall CH, et al. Relation of serial changes in childhood body-mass index to impaired glucose tolerance in young adulthood. N Engl J Med. 2004;350(9):865-75.
3. Bhatia V. IAP National Task Force for Childhood Prevention of Adult Diseases: insulin resistance and Type 2 diabetes mellitus in childhood. Indian Pediatr. 2004;41(5):443-57.
4. Dennison BA, Erb TA, Jenkins PL. Television viewing and television in bedroom associated with overweight risk among low-income preschool children. Pediatrics. 2002;109(6):1028-35.
5. Dubey S, Kabra M, Bajpai A, et al. Serum leptin levels in obese Indian children relation to clinical and biochemical parameters. Indian Pediatr. 2007;44(4):257-62.
6. Keiss W, Wabitsch M, Maffeis C, et al. Metabolic syndrome and obesity in childhood and adolescence. Pediatr Adolesc Med. 2015;19:166-70.
7. Laxmaiah A, Nagalla B, Vijayaraghavan K, et al. Factors affecting prevalence of overweight among 12- to 17-year-old urban adolescents in Hyderabad, India. Obesity (Silver Spring). 2007;15(6):1384-90.
8. Marwaha RK, Tandon N, Singh Y, et al. A study of growth parameters and prevalence of overweight and obesity in school children from Delhi. Indian Pediatr. 2006;43(11):943-52.
9. Reinehr T, Hinney A, de Sousa G, et al. Definable somatic disorders in overweight children and adolescents. J Pediatr. 2007;150(6):618-22.
10. Singh R, Bhansali A, Sialy R, et al. Prevalence of metabolic syndrome in adolescents from a north Indian population. Diabet Med. 2007;24(2):195-9.

13.4 Disorders of Puberty

Prisca Colaco

INTRODUCTION

The term "puberty" is derived from the Latin word "puberatum" which means age at maturity or adulthood. What triggers the onset of puberty is still hypothetical. The onset of puberty is associated with an increase in the frequency and amplitude of gonadotropin-releasing hormone (GnRH) pulses, which precedes the rise in luteinizing hormone (LH) and follicle-stimulating hormone (FSH).

There is a wide range of normal age at which puberty usually begins. The age at onset is controlled by both genetic and extrinsic factors and therefore may occur earlier or later than normal. The 4–5 years of physiological variation in age at onset of puberty that is observed among normal individuals involves genetic factors, ethnicity, and environmental factors such as nutrition, light, stressors, and endocrine disruptors.

ASSESSMENT OF PUBERTY

Pubertal development is usually assessed by Tanner stages also known as sexual maturity rating. Tanner stage 1 is prepubertal, whereas Tanner stage 5 is adult maturity (*see* Chapter 3.3 for details). In boys, penis and testis development, as well as pubic hair growth are assessed. In girls, breast development and pubic hair growth are assessed. In girls, puberty usually begins with breast development (thelarche), but occasionally with the appearance of pubic hair (pubarche). Menarche usually occurs about 2 years after breast development begins. In boys, testicular enlargement (>3 mL) marks the onset of puberty and is followed by the appearance of pubic hair and development of the external genitalia. The pubertal growth spurt is an early event in girls usually at Tanner stage B2, while in boys, the growth spurt occurs late, usually at the time when a testicular volume of 10 mL is achieved.

PRECOCIOUS PUBERTY

Definition

The age threshold for the definition of precocious puberty is controversial. Puberty is considered precocious if its onset is before the lower limits of normal (the age at which 95% of children achieve Tanner stage 2 or 2 standard deviation below the mean age of pubertal onset in normal children). This was considered to be 8 years in girls and 9 years in boys. Based on the findings of a large study in the United States, it was recommended that puberty be considered precocious if the onset is before the age of 7 years in white girls and 6 years in black girls. However, as a significant incidence of underlying pathology was found in girls in the 6–8-year-age group, many still use the traditional threshold of 8 years to define precocious pubertal development in girls. For boys, the onset of puberty before the age of 9 years is considered precocious.

Classification

Box 13.4.1 depicts the classification and causes of precocious puberty.

Box 13.4.1: Causes of precocious puberty.

A. *Central or gonadotropin-dependent precocious puberty (due to the premature activation of the HPG axis and therefore isosexual)*
- Idiopathic
- *Neurogenic:*
  - *Tumors*: Hypothalamic hamartoma, glioma, astrocytoma, ependymoma, germ-cell tumor, pinealoma
  - Infections
  - Cerebral malformations
  - Perinatal insults, trauma
  - Cranial irradiation

B. *Peripheral or gonadotropin-independent precocious puberty (results from the production of sex steroids independent of the HPG axis. May be isosexual or heterosexual)*
- *Autonomous gonadal activation*:
  - Ovarian cysts
  - McCune-Albright syndrome
  - Familial male limited precocious puberty (testotoxicosis)
- *Tumors of the ovary or testis*:
  - Granulosa cell tumor, androgen-producing ovarian tumor, testicular Leydig cell tumors, hCG-producing tumors
- *Adrenal disorders*:
  - Congenital adrenal hyperplasia, adrenal tumor
- Exposure to exogenous sex steroids
- Severe, untreated primary hypothyroidism

C. *Pubertal variants:*
- Premature thelarche
- Premature pubarche
- Premature menarche.

(hCG: human chorionic gonadotropin; HPG: hypothalamic pituitary gonadal)

Central Precocious Puberty

Central precocious puberty (CPP) is the most common form of precocious puberty and is about five times more common in girls than in boys **(Fig. 13.4.1)**.

- Central precocious puberty in girls is most often idiopathic (about 75%). In contrast to girls, in about two-thirds of boys, CPP is secondary to central nervous system (CNS) pathology.
- The younger the child, the greater is the likelihood of underlying pathology.
- In idiopathic CPP, the appearance of sexual characteristics is merely a normal event occurring early and puberty progresses normally.
- Hypothalamic hamartomas are the most common tumors causing precocious puberty.
- In India, CNS infections, particularly tuberculous meningitis, are important causes of neurogenic CPP.

Peripheral Precocious Puberty

Peripheral precocious puberty (PPP) is only about one fifth as common as CPP. While CPP is always isosexual, PPP may be iso- or heterosexual and may be due to adrenal or gonadal causes. Adrenal disorders, most commonly congenital adrenal hyperplasia (CAH), are the most common causes of PPP in boys **(Fig. 13.4.2)**. PPP is therefore much more common in boys as compared to girls. The prepubertal size of the testes suggests the diagnosis.

- Some forms of PPP predominate in boys, such as chorionic gonadotropin-secreting tumors and familial gonadotropin-independent precocious puberty or testotoxicosis, which is caused by activating mutations of the LH receptor.
- Ovarian, rather than adrenal, disorders are much more likely in girls with isosexual PPP.
- McCune-Albright syndrome (MAS) consists of fibrous bony dysplasia, skin pigmentation, and precocious puberty, and predominantly affects girls.
- Autonomous secreting follicular cysts of the ovary without any evidence of MAS may also result in sexual precocity. These cysts are often more than 2 cm in diameter in contrast to the smaller cysts, which may be normally present in the prepubertal ovary or in CPP. Pubertal signs often develop rapidly. Subsequent atresia of the cysts results in withdrawal bleeding.
- Adrenal disorders, CAH, and tumors result in heterosexual puberty in girls.
- Hypothyroidism, untreated or inadequately treated, is sometimes associated with precocious puberty. The cause is not clear, but it is thought to be due to the effect of markedly elevated thyroid-stimulating hormone (TSH) levels on the FSH receptor.

Pubertal Variants

The incomplete forms of sexual precocity can be differentiated from precocious puberty by the absence of other signs of puberty and a normal growth rate.

Premature thelarche: Breast development persists beyond 6 months of age or occurs anew. It usually occurs before 3 years of age and rarely after 4 years. There is no other evidence of estrogen effects such as increase in uterine size,

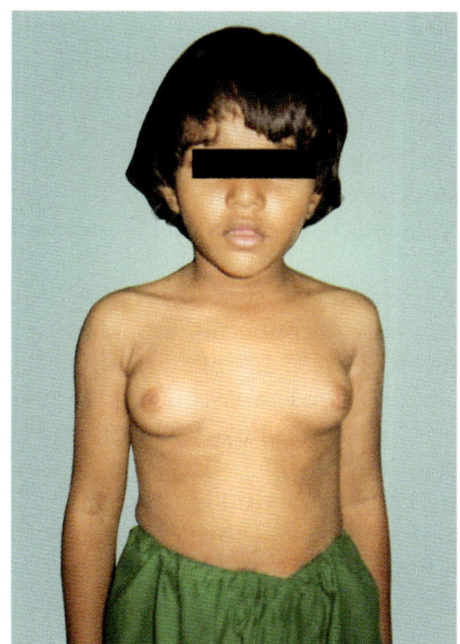

Fig. 13.4.1: A 4-year-old girl with idiopathic central precocious puberty.

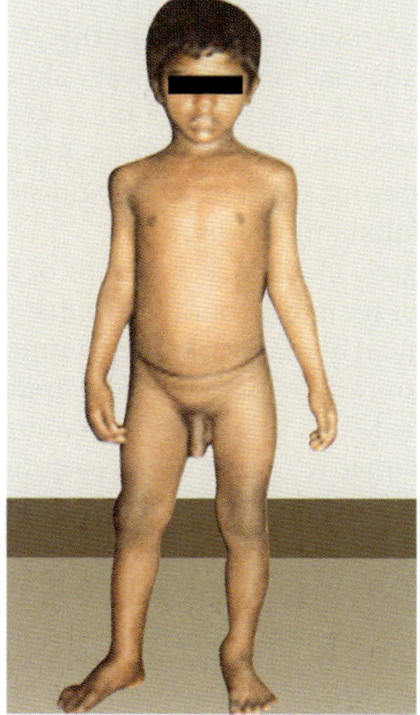

Fig. 13.4.2: A 3-year-old boy with peripheral precocious puberty due to congenital adrenal hyperplasia. Sexual maturity rating stage 4. Testicular volume 2 mL. Note the generalized hyperpigmentation.

changes in external genitalia, growth acceleration, or bone age advancement. The cause is unknown. It could be caused by transient estrogen secretion by follicular cysts of the ovary. Exogenous estrogens in food or environmental exposure could also lead to breast development.

Premature pubarche: This is due to increased adrenal dehydroepiandrosterone sulfate (DHEAS) secretion (adrenarche), which results in the appearance of pubic hair. It is more commonly seen in girls in the 3–8-year-age group. Pubarche is not progressive. Occasionally these children may develop slight acne, axillary hair, and adult-type body odor but no other secondary sexual characteristics. Skeletal maturation and linear growth are at upper normal limits. Signs of severe androgen excess should prompt a search for a virilizing condition such as an adrenal tumor or CAH.

Premature menarche: This is a rare condition and local lesions must be ruled out. It is due to transient ovarian activity resulting in an isolated follicular cyst. It may occasionally be the first sign of puberty.

EVALUATION

A detailed history and clinical evaluation are helpful in arriving at a diagnosis and directing investigations.

History

- *Age at onset:* Idiopathic CPP usually presents between 6 years and 7 years of age. The earlier the onset, the greater is the likelihood of an underlying organic cause. Hypothalamic hamartoma and familial testotoxicosis present very early in the first 3–4 years of life.
- *Pubertal progression*: In idiopathic CPP, the rate of progression may sometimes be very slow with menarche occurring up to 5 years after breast development. Very rapid progression of puberty is seen in androgen-producing tumors, ovarian cysts, and some CNS tumors such as hypothalamic hamartoma.
- *Accelerated growth:* This is a feature of both central and PPP but is not seen in pubertal variants.
- Irregular vaginal bleeding is more common in functioning ovarian tumors and hypothalamic hamartoma.
- History of past CNS infection, headaches, visual disturbances, personality changes, developmental delay, and seizures would suggest a neurologic disorder.
- Drug exposure should be enquired into.
- Symptoms suggestive of hypothyroidism should be looked for.
- A family history of precocious puberty would suggest constitutional precocious puberty or familial testotoxicosis. A history of precocious puberty in boys and genital ambiguity in girls of the same family would suggest CAH.

Clinical Examination

Evaluate

- *Androgen effects:* Acne, hirsutism, increased muscle mass, and clitoromegaly.
- *Estrogen effects:* Breast development and changes in vaginal mucosa.
- *Pubertal staging:* According to Tanner.
- *Abdominal and rectal examination:* For uterine size, ovarian masses, and adrenal tumors.
- *Testicular palpation:* A testicular volume greater than 3 mL indicates the onset of CPP. Scrotal masses suggest testicular tumors or adrenal rests.
- *Inspection of the skin:* Is helpful in MAS, neurofibromatosis, and tuberous sclerosis.
- *Neurologic examination:* Should include fundus examination and perimetry.
- Examination for signs of *hypothyroidism*.

Investigations

It is recommended that all boys with precocious pubertal development and all girls with the following features should be evaluated for the mechanism and potential for progression of puberty:

- Precocious puberty stage 3 or higher
- Stage 2 with additional criteria such as increased growth velocity
- Evidence of CNS dysfunction or PPP.

Hormonal Evaluation

- *Sex steroids:*
  - In girls, serum estradiol levels are not very helpful in determining the stage of puberty. Levels overlap between normal prepuberty, early puberty, precocious puberty, and premature thelarche. Levels greater than 20 pg/mL suggest that puberty has started. Markedly elevated levels (>100 pg/mL) are seen in estrogen secreting ovarian tumors and sometimes in follicular cysts.
  - In boys, serum testosterone levels less than 30 ng/mL are generally prepubertal, though in some laboratories, levels of 10–30 ng/mL may indicate early puberty. Testosterone levels may be very high related to the stage of puberty in boys with primary gonadotropin excess.
- *Serum gonadotropins*: Gonadotropin levels are elevated in CPP and suppressed in PPP. Basal serum FSH and LH are of limited value in early puberty. But random LH estimated by sensitive third-generation assays is a good screening test for CPP. A level of less than 0.1 IU/L is prepubertal and 0.3 IU/L or more is pubertal. Random FSH levels are not helpful in discriminating between prepubertal and pubertal children.

- *Gonadotropin-releasing hormone stimulation test* is more helpful in distinguishing CPP from PPP. In CPP, an LH predominant response is seen. An increase in FSH levels much more than LH indicates that the child is prepubertal. In PPP, gonadotropin levels do not rise in response to GnRH stimulation.
- *Serum DHEAS levels* are elevated in premature adrenarche and can be very high in virilizing adrenal problems.
- *Serum 17-hydroxyprogesterone* and the response to adrenocorticotropic hormone or serum 11-deoxycortisol may be required to rule out CAH.
- *Serum human chorionic gonadotropin (hCG) levels,* if a hCG-secreting tumor is suspected in boys.
- Thyroid hormone studies in suspected hypothyroidism.

Radiology

- *Bone age:* Skeletal maturation is advanced in all cases of precocious puberty, except if associated with hypothyroidism, but remains normal in the incomplete forms. It is also helpful in predicting adult height.
- *Computed tomography or magnetic resonance imaging of brain:* To determine the etiology of CPP.
- *Pelvic and abdominal sonography:* To evaluate the size and morphology of the uterus, ovaries, and adrenals. This is essential in PPP to find the cause. In CPP, the size of the uterus is increased (>2 mL in volume or >3.4 cm in length) and an endometrial shadow is seen. The ovaries will also be enlarged bilaterally and may show multiple small follicular cysts.
- *Testicular sonography:* If a tumor is suspected.
- *Skeletal survey:* In suspected cases of MAS.

Management

Surgery

- Any underlying cause should be identified and treated, e.g. intracranial, gonadal, and adrenal tumors.
- Surgery of hypothalamic hamartoma is hazardous and not recommended, because they do not grow or become malignant.
- Ovarian cysts greater than 3 cm in size should be explored surgically. Smaller cysts require repeated evaluation.

Medical Treatment

Not all children with precocious puberty need to be treated. The only long-term complication of CPP is compromised adult height, which may improve with treatment. Treatment of progressive CPP is indicated if:

- There is evidence that adult height may be significantly compromised.
- Menarche occurs before 6 years of age.
- Pubertal development is psychologically distressing to the child.
- Pubertal development progresses rapidly over an observation period of about 6 months.

Gonadotropin-releasing Hormone Analog Therapy

Therapy aims at reversing the development of sexual characteristics and decreasing the acceleration of growth and bone age by using GnRH analog (GnRHa) therapy. A suppressed LH response to GnRH or GnRHa indicates that the therapy is having the desired effect. Mean gains over predicted height in several studies ranged from 3 cm to 10 cm. Factors which affect height gain include baseline bone age and duration of treatment. Discontinuation of therapy at 11 years is associated with optimum height outcomes. Pubertal manifestations reappear within months of stopping treatment with a mean time to menarche of 16 months.

Antigonadotropic and antiandrogen drugs, such as medroxyprogesterone and cyproterone acetate cause regression of pubertal signs but have no effect on growth acceleration and bone age progression.

Treatment of PPP includes treatment of the cause as in hypothyroidism or CAH. Drugs used in gonadotropin-independent precocious puberty include androgen and estrogen receptor blockers, and aromatase inhibitors.

Psychological Support

Psychological support for the child and parents is an essential part of the general management scheme. The child's psychological development corresponds with the chronologic age. No major psychopathology is associated with precocious puberty. Future fertility is maintained.

DELAYED PUBERTY

Definition

Puberty is considered to be delayed if sexual maturation is not apparent by 14 years of age in boys or 13 years in girls. The absence of menarche by age 16 years or within 5 years of pubertal onset is also included in the diagnosis.

Classification

Delayed puberty results from inadequate gonadal steroid secretion caused by hypothalamic, pituitary, and gonadal disorders, and is classified according to the circulating levels of the gonadotropins, FSH, and LH as shown in **Table 13.4.1**.

Evaluation

- *History:* We should focus on a review of symptoms, which may indicate a chronic systemic disease, prolonged drug therapy, poor nutrition, head trauma, and anosmia. Family history of delayed puberty or hypogonadism and

Table 13.4.1: Causes of delayed puberty.

Hypergonadotropic (primary gonadal failure)
A. *Congenital*: • Sex chromosome anomalies, e.g. Turner, XO/XY, Klinefelter syndromes • Anomalies of testosterone synthesis or action • Pure gonadal dysgenesis • Associated with other syndromes, e.g. Noonan's, Alstrom, Smith-Lemli-Opitz syndromes
B. *Acquired*: • Surgical or traumatic castration • Orchitis/oophoritis • Chemotherapy, radiotherapy • Idiopathic
Hypogonadotropic (secondary hypogonadism)
C. *Temporary causes (functional):* • *CDGP*: Sporadic or familial • Nutritional disorders • Chronic systemic disease • Hormonal disturbances, e.g. hypothyroidism, isolated GHD, excess glucocorticoids
D. *Permanent causes*: • *Congenital:* – Isolated gonadotropin deficiency – LH deficiency – Associated with syndromes, e.g. Kallmann, Prader-Willi syndromes – Panhypopituitarism • *Acquired:* – Tumors, surgery – Irradiation – Trauma – Hyperprolactinemia

(CDGP: constitutional delay in growth and puberty; GHD: growth hormone deficiency; LH: luteinizing hormone)

a history of parental consanguinity should be enquired into. In constitutional delay in growth and puberty (CDGP), a history of delayed puberty is often obtained in either a parent or sibling.

- *Growth assessment:* It often helps in distinguishing the causes of delayed puberty and is an important part of the evaluation. The height of those with primary gonadal failure is usually normal unless associated with specific syndromes **(Fig. 13.4.3)**. Children with temporary delay are commonly short. In CDGP, the growth velocity is appropriate for bone age while in growth hormone (GH) deficiency (GHD), it is subnormal. In isolated gonadotropin deficiency, childhood growth is normal, but the pubertal growth spurt does not occur. Growth is subnormal if there is associated GHD or secondary hypothyroidism.
- *Body proportions:* Children with isolated gonadotropin deficiency and Klinefelter syndrome have eunuchoid proportions due to delayed epiphyseal closure because of subnormal conversion of serum testosterone to estradiol.

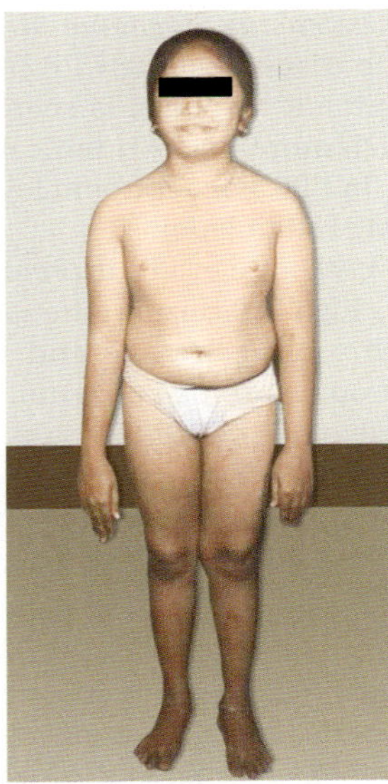

Fig. 13.4.3: A 14-year-old girl with hypergonadotrophic hypogonadism—Turner's syndrome.

- *Weight related to height:* It is decreased in malnutrition and chronic disease and increased in most hormonal disorders. Obesity is a feature of many syndromes associated with hypogonadism.
- *Pubertal assessment:* Signs of puberty should be staged according to Tanner staging. In gonadotropin deficiency, pubertal development is absent or incomplete. Slow progression suggests a partial gonadotropin deficiency. In CDGP, the rate of pubertal progression is normal.
- Search for the presence of chronic disease, malnutrition, anosmia, midline defects, endocrine disorders, and dysmorphic syndromes.
- *Neurological assessment:* It includes fundus examination and evaluation of visual fields.
- Male babies born with congenital gonadotropin deficiency have normal sexual differentiation but micropenis.

Investigations

Hormonal Evaluation

- *Serum gonadotropin levels:* FSH and LH distinguish between hypogonadotropic and hypergonadotropic hypogonadism.
- *Serum gonadotropin response to GnRH stimulation:* It may show a pubertal response in CDGP but is not usually helpful in distinguishing it from isolated gonadotropin deficiency.
- *Serum testosterone/estradiol.*
- *Serum DHEAS levels:* They are usually normal for chronologic age in hypogonadotropic hypogonadism but are low

for age and correspond with the bone age in CDGP, where the tempo of maturation is delayed.

- Serum thyroxine, TSH, prolactin, insulin-like growth factor-1 (IGF-1), and GH stimulation tests if indicated.

Radiographic Investigations

- *Bone age evaluation:* To distinguish CDGP from gonadotropin deficiency. In CDGP, the bone age corresponds with the height, age, and stage of puberty and evidence of sexual maturation should be evident by a bone age of 13 years. In isolated gonadotropin deficiency, bone age is usually slightly delayed. But with multiple pituitary hormone deficiency, the bone age is markedly delayed.
- *Pelvic ultrasonography:* It provides information about the development of the uterus and ovaries.
- *Computed tomography/magnetic resonance imaging:* If indicated.

Management

Treatment of the cause whenever possible will result in subsequent pubertal development. Patients with CDGP require reassurance that there is nothing wrong and that puberty though delayed will progress normally. In few cases of profound delay, short-term low-dose hormonal treatment with testosterone or estrogens for 3–6 months may occasionally be required if the patient is psychologically stressed. Permanent hypogonadism (primary or secondary) requires long-term replacement therapy with gradually increasing doses of sex steroids over 2–3 years.

BIBLIOGRAPHY

1. Carel JC, Eugster EA, Rogol A, et al. Consensus statement on the use of gonadotropin-releasing hormone analogs in children. Pediatrics. 2009;123(4):e752-62.
2. Carel JC, Leger J. Clinical practice: precocious puberty. N Engl J Med. 2008;358(22):2366-77.
3. De Luca F, Argente J, Cavallo L, et al. Management of puberty in constitutional delay of growth and puberty. J Pediatr Endocrinol Metab. 2001;14(Suppl 2):953-7.
4. Kaplowitz PB, Oberfield SE. Reexamination of the age limit for defining when puberty is precocious in girls in the United States: implications for evaluation and treatment. Drug and Therapeutics and Executive Committees of the Lawson Wilkins Pediatric Endocrine Society. Pediatrics. 1999;104(4 pt 1): 936-41.
5. Klein KO. Precocious puberty: who was it? Who should be treated? J Clin Endocrinol Metab. 1999;84(2):411-4.
6. Rosen DS, Foster C. Delayed puberty. Pediatr Rev. 2001;22(9): 309-15.

13.5 Disorders of Thyroid Gland

Meena P Desai, Ruchi Parikh

INTRODUCTION

The actions of thyroid hormones to a large extent are age and target tissue dependent, and their effects on growth, development, maturation, and brain functions are unique to pediatric age-group. Thyroid hormones influence physical growth and maturation, play a crucial role in fetal and early postnatal brain development, and govern various biologic and metabolic functions of the body. They increase oxygen consumption; stimulate protein synthesis; affect carbohydrate, lipid, and vitamin metabolism; influence enzyme systems; affect growth factors; and promote growth and cell differentiation.

Congenital and acquired disorders of thyroid gland predominate among children and adolescents, constituting nearly 25–30% of all endocrinopathies in this age-group. The three major clinical forms of thyroid disorders are primary *hypothyroidism* (75%) with insufficient secretion of thyroid hormones, *goiters* (thyromegaly), of which nearly 20% have no associated alterations in thyroid function, and *hyperthyroidism or thyrotoxicosis* in 5% with excessive thyroid hormone secretion. Thyroid neoplasia is uncommon. Endemic cretinism or hypothyroidism is more common in certain endemic regions of iodine deficiency.

Undiagnosed or suboptimally treated congenital hypothyroidism (CH) in early infancy can lead to irreversible impairment in neurocognitive function emphasizing the role of thyroid hormones in brain development in fetal and early postnatal life. Frequently, CH may be associated with mortality due to cardiac failure in fetuses and in neonates.

THYROID DEVELOPMENT, PHYSIOLOGY, ACTIONS, AND REGULATORY CONTROL

The human thyroid originates embryologically from an invagination of the pharyngeal epithelium with cellular contributions from the lateral pharyngeal pouches around 4 weeks, followed by its descent to the neck between 5 to 7 weeks and 7 weeks of embryonic life, with occasional persistence of the remnants along the tract as "lingual thyroid", ectopic thyroid, thyroglossal cyst, or nodule. Thyroid embryogenesis is completed by 10–12 weeks, and thyroglobulin (Tg) can be detected in thyroid follicles by 12 weeks. There is progressive increase in Tg and thyroxine (T4) production throughout gestation but fetal and neonatal triiodothyronine (T3) tend to be low as placental type 3 deiodinase activity which converts the prohormone T4 to T3, and inactive reverse T3 (rT3) and diiodothyronine, is low. This is a protective mechanism controlling in utero thermogenesis. Thyroid-specific transcription factors, thyroid transcription factor (TTF)-1, TTF-2, and paired box gene 8, are important for thyroid gland morphogenesis and differentiation. PIT-1 and PROP-1 are important for growth and differentiation of pituitary thyrotropes secreting thyroid-stimulating hormone (TSH).

The thyroid gland concentrates iodine from blood and synthesizes and secretes T4 along with smaller amount of 3,3′,5-T3. The capacity to concentrate iodine appears by about 12 weeks, followed by synthesis and secretion of thyroid hormones through a series of enzyme-dependent steps. The Tg so formed is stored in colloid thus permitting storage of thyroid hormones and iodine. Thyroid hormones are released in circulation as and when required.

Thyroxine and T3 are bound to transport proteins—the T4-binding globulin, T4-binding prealbumin and albumin. Seventy-five percent of circulating T3 in blood is derived by monodeiodination of T4 in liver, kidney, and other peripheral tissues with the simultaneous formation of rT3, which is metabolically inactive. There is a certain amount of tissue autonomy in the production of T3 from T4. The concentrations of free T4 (FT4) and free T3 (FT3), active at the cellular level approximate 0.03% and 0.30%, respectively, of the total hormone concentration. T3 is almost four times more potent than T4, and 85% of the bioactivity of T4 is attributed to T3. Approximately 100 µg of T4 is secreted by the thyroid gland daily, and about 90 µg of iodide (15 µg/kg) is the recommended daily dose during infancy with higher requirements in preterm.

Thyroid gland is under the regulatory control of the pituitary thyrotropin or TSH, which in turn is regulated by the hypothalamic, thyrotropin-releasing hormone (TRH) which can be recognized in the fetus at around 18 weeks. The fetal thyroid gland and the hypothalamic-pituitary-thyroid axis function largely independent of the mother. Maternal TRH can cross the placenta but not TSH. Placenta is less pervious to the passage of maternal thyroid hormones normally, but presence of T4 in cord blood of athyreotic fetus suggests passage of maternal T4 in third trimester which is an important source of neuroprotective factor, T3 for fetal brain. During first half of pregnancy, maternal euthyroid status and optimal levels of maternal thyroid hormones seem to be neuroprotective for the fetus. Simultaneous presence of maternal and fetal hypothyroidism is detrimental to neurocognitive outcome as in endemic iodine deficiency or in presence of other abnormalities of thyroid function. This justifies biochemical screening of women with a personal or family history of thyroid disease prior to contemplating pregnancy.

After birth, there is an acute surge in TSH level within 30 minutes in response to relative hypothermia, followed by rise in serum T3 and T4 levels by 24 hours, with a gradual decline by the end of the first week. If TSH is the primary neonatal screening procedure, sample collection should be done from cord blood, or after 72 hours of birth to prevent problems in interpretation. Thyroid-stimulating hormone and/or T4 screening is often undertaken between 3 days and 5 days of birth. Thyroid-stimulating hormone surge in the premature infant is of a lesser magnitude with a greater decline in T4 concentration in the following 2 weeks. Hence, appropriate interpretation of TSH, T3, and T4 values obtained in neonatal period is important for correct diagnosis and management. T3 and T4 levels are higher in the pediatric age-group as compared to adults with TSH levels up to 10 µU/mL considered normal in early infancy, provided serum T4 is in upper normal range. The usual mean T4 level in infancy is 10.5 µg/dL, with mean T3 of 1.68 ng/mL and TSH of 2.1 µU/mL. Thereafter, there is not much variation till adulthood.

HYPOTHYROIDISM

Etiology and Epidemiology

Hypothyroidism in infancy can be congenital or acquired, permanent or transient, and secondary or tertiary **(Box 13.5.1)**.

Congenital form of primary hypothyroidism due to thyroid dysgenesis is most common. About 80–90% of cases with permanent primary CH have thyroid dysgenesis. It denotes developmental abnormalities of the thyroid gland ranging from agenesis, hypoplasia to ectopia. Recent studies indicate the role of genetic factors in some cases. Occasionally, lingual or sublingual thyroid or thyroglossal cyst may be the only source of thyroid hormone production.

Hypothyroidism acquired later in childhood or adolescence is usually due to autoimmune thyroid disease (AITD) or less frequently due to other causes listed in **Box 13.5.1**. A variety of inherited biosynthetic defects causing

Box 13.5.1: Causes of hypothyroidism in childhood and adolescence.

A. *Primary hypothyroidism*
- *Thyroid dysgenesis*:
  - Aplasia, hypoplasia
  - Ectopic or lingual thyroid gland
- Inborn errors of thyroid hormone synthesis, secretion, or utilization
- Endemic iodine deficiency
- Autoimmune thyroiditis
- *Iatrogenic*:
  - Antithyroid drugs and goitrogens
  - Irradiation
  - Post-thyroidectomy

B. *Secondary/tertiary hypothyroidism (pituitary/hypothalamic)*
- *Congenital*:
  - Isolated or panhypopituitarism
- *Acquired*:
  - Trauma
  - Infection
  - Neoplastic/postsurgical
  - Irradiation

C. *Transient congenital hypothyroidism*
- *In utero exposure to goitrogens*:
  - Iodides
  - Antithyroid drugs
  - Maternal antibody induced
  - Idiopathic

Box 13.5.2: The American Academy of Pediatrics Guidelines and Recommendations for neonatal screening.

- *Initial workup*:
  - Detailed history and physical examination
  - Referral to pediatric endocrinologist
  - Recheck serum TSH and FT4
  - Thyroid ultrasonography and/or thyroid scan
- *Medications*:
  - *Levothyroxine*: 10–15 µg/kg by mouth once daily in infancy
- *Monitoring (Recheck T4, TSH)*:
  - Around 2–4 weeks after initial treatment is begun
  - Every 1–2 months in the first 6 months
  - Every 3–4 months between 6 months and 3 years of age
  - Every 6–12 months from 3 years of age to end of growth
- *Goal of therapy*:
  - Normalize TSH and maintain T4 and FT4 in upper half of reference range
- *Assess permanence of CH*:
  - If initial thyroid scan shows ectopic/absent gland, CH is permanent
  - If initial TSH is less than 50 µU/mL, and there is no increase in TSH after newborn period, then trial off therapy at 3 years of age
  - If TSH increases off therapy, consider permanent CH

(CH: congenital hypothyroidism; FT4: free T4; T4: thyroxine; TSH: thyroid-stimulating hormone)

dyshormonogenesis leading to hypothyroidism with varying degrees of goitrous enlargement of thyroid gland have been identified. AITD is a common cause of hypothyroidism beyond mid-childhood and in adolescents. Endemic iodine deficiency remains an important cause of endemic cretinism and hypothyroidism in some parts of the world as in Europe and in north and northeastern regions of India. Pituitary or hypothalamic disease can cause secondary or tertiary forms of hypothyroidism, respectively, which may be congenital or acquired. It is less common and is usually associated with deficiency of other pituitary hormones.

Neonatal Screening for Congenital Hypothyroidism

Among all neonatal screening programs, screening for CH is the most cost-effective. Clinical recognition of CH in the newborn and during early infancy may be difficult. Less than 5–10% of newborns detected on screening can be diagnosed clinically. As classical symptoms and signs evolve gradually, a high index of clinical suspicion is important in early life in the absence of routine neonatal screening. In the neonatal period, serum T4 less than 6.5 µg/dL and TSH greater than 10 µU/mL (new generation assay) may be suggestive of CH. Large majority of newborns with primary CH have TSH values between 30 µU/mL and 50 µU/mL.

Serum Tg and imaging studies, such as ultrasonography and technetium-99m, scan delineating thyroid gland help in confirming the diagnosis and prognosticate the outcome.

The worldwide incidence of CH on neonatal screening is about 1:3,500 to 4,000 with racial and ethnic differences. Studies from the United Kingdom indicate higher prevalence in Asians. Studies from India have reported higher prevalence of 1:2,600 in 1994 and recently 1 in 1,172 amongst 100,000 newborns in Indian Council of Medical Research sponsored multicenter study in 2013. Recent higher incidence is ascribed to many factors including improved testing strategies and higher number of preterm births. Now almost all neonatal screening programs are based on obtaining filter paper (FP) TSH, T4, or T4/TSH concentrations. Threshold value for TSH differs but usually less than 10 µU/mL is considered normal. Confirmation with venous serum samples is essential when FP values are abnormal. Management strategies are also described in **Box 13.5.2**. Thyroid imaging may be undertaken, if feasible.

Clinical Manifestations

Symptoms and signs of CH in neonatal period and early infancy are vague, nonspecific, with difficulties in clinical diagnosis. In early infancy, symptoms often predominate over signs. Growth retardation so characteristic of CH in postnatal life is not seen at birth, some of them being large and postmature. Prolonged physiological jaundice, constipation, feeding difficulties, inactivity, macroglossia, constipation, wide fontanelles, dry and mottled skin, hypothermia, and hoarse cry should arouse suspicion. Over the following weeks, coarse hypothyroid facies, puffiness of eyes, protruding tongue, pallor, lethargy, fullness in supraclavicular regions, altered skin and hair texture, hypotonia, distended abdomen with umbilical hernia, and low-pitched irritable prolonged cry are features, which combine to give a characteristic appearance **(Fig. 13.5.1)**. Bradycardia, muffled heart sounds, delayed relaxation while eliciting deep tendon reflexes are the helpful signs. Growth failure and delayed milestones become increasingly obvious. Children with dyshormonogenesis may present with goiter at birth, or later. Careful thyroid palpation should be routinely done. The incidence of other associated congenital abnormalities with CH is around 8%.

Hypothyroidism in older children is usually caused by AITD but occasionally children with hypoplastic or ectopic thyroid gland or dyshormonogenesis may present late. Symptoms and signs may be subtle. Lassitude, growth failure/short stature, excess weight gain, scholastic problems, delayed sexual maturation or uncommonly sexual precocity, muscular hypertrophy, and goiter with insidious onset may be noted. Small goiter which is firm in consistency with a pebbly surface favors the possibility of thyroiditis as opposed to dyshormonogenesis where the goiter may be small or large, with soft to firm consistency and occasional presence of a bruit **(Fig. 13.5.2)**. Dyshormonogenesis with autosomal recessive transmission can be familial with sibling involvement; familial occurrence with AITD in parents and other family members is also well known. Hence, family history is important in both these conditions.

Diagnosis

The diagnosis of primary hypothyroidism is confirmed by the presence of low serum T4 and elevated serum TSH values. Estimation of FT4 and FT3 is also available. Thyroid-stimulating hormone is an extremely sensitive index of primary hypothyroidism. Presence of Tg in the serum is also indicative of functioning thyroid tissue. Significant delay in skeletal maturation and epiphyseal dysgenesis on X-rays are very helpful. The skeletal age can indicate the approximate age of the onset of hypothyroidism. Imaging studies, such as ultrasonography and radioisotope scans, help in delineating the anatomical and functional status of the gland but are not mandatory. Thyroid antibody studies—anti-Tg (ATG) and antimitochondrial (AMA) or antiperoxidase (APO) antibodies in particular—help in identifying autoimmune basis of the disease.

In secondary and tertiary forms of disease, which may be congenital or acquired **(*see* Box 13.5.1)**, the TSH concentration may be low or undetectable with subnormal levels of T3/FT3 and T4/FT4. It is usually associated with deficiency of other pituitary hormones.

Treatment

Once the diagnosis is established, the need for lifelong therapy in CH should be adequately stressed. The goal of therapy

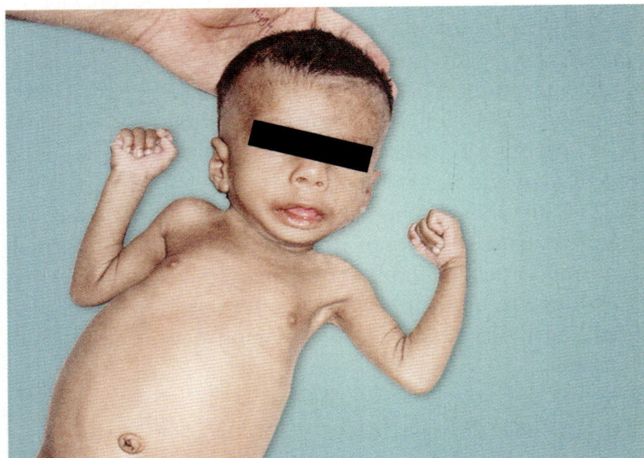

Fig. 13.5.1: A 5-month-old male child with congenital hypothyroidism presented for constipation, feeding difficulty, and failure to grow. Note the protruding tongue, distended abdomen, and small umbilical hernia (with permission of parents).

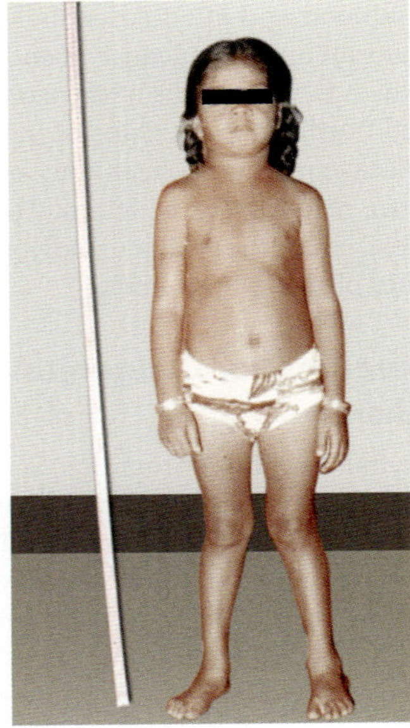

Fig. 13.5.2: An 8-year-old girl with goitrous hypothyroidism due to dyshormonogenesis. Note hypothyroid facies, puffiness of eyes, and goiter. She had two more siblings with similar clinical picture (with kind permission of parents).

is to maintain the circulating serum T4 level in the upper normal range and normalize the elevated TSH. The preferred preparation is sodium-levothyroxine because of its uniform potency, reliable absorption, and good bioavailability. In newborns detected on screening and in early infancy, 10 µg/kg/day has been recommended. Full replacement therapy can be initiated promptly. In long-standing thyroid deprivation where the diagnosis is delayed for months or occasionally for years, one fourth of the daily dose can be administered initially and stepped up gradually to full replacement dose, in 3–6 weeks. The daily requirement is about 100 µg/m^2, with the required dose administered as one single dose, preferably at a convenient fixed time daily on empty stomach to maximize absorption. Regular therapy is extremely important. Therapeutic monitoring is recommended with blood samples obtained at periodic intervals for TSH, T3, and T4 estimations in all children permitting individualization of treatment. Clinical evaluation and growth monitoring during therapy are important.

Prognosis

The outcome in CH is closely related to the nature and severity of the underlying thyroid abnormality, the age at diagnosis and onset of treatment, adequacy and regularity of therapy with the required degree of clinical and laboratory follow-up. Worldwide neonatal screening programs for CH have had a significant impact on reducing intellectual deficits in hypothyroid infants diagnosed and treated early.

HYPERTHYROIDISM

Hyperthyroidism (thyrotoxicosis) is an uncommon disorder of childhood and adolescence. The most common cause in children is autoimmune Graves' disease (GD). Genetic studies indicate involvement of genes controlling immune regulation. It results from excessive secretion of thyroid hormones. Occasionally, chronic lymphocytic thyroiditis (CLT) leads to transient hyperthyroid state before hypothyroidism supervenes. Other uncommon causes are thyrotoxicosis factitia (ingestion of thyroid hormones), iodine-induced hyperthyroid state, McCune-Albright syndrome, toxic adenoma, and multinodular goiter or very rarely TSH-producing pituitary tumors. In infants born of mothers with GD, hyperthyroidism may occur as a transitory phenomenon during neonatal period due to transplacental passage of thyroid-stimulating immunoglobulin. Very rarely germline mutations of the TSH receptor due to gain of function mutation can cause familial or sporadic hyperthyroidism and can manifest very early in life.

Clinical Manifestations

About 5–10% of all patients with hyperthyroidism are under 15 years of age with peak incidence in adolescence. The incidence is almost five times higher in girls. Family history of thyroid disease is often present in nearly 50–60% of these children. The clinical course is variable but less severe than in adults. The onset of symptoms is often insidious with the interval between the onset of the disorder and diagnosis ranging between 3 months and 12 months.

Emotional disturbances and behavioral changes characterized by excitability, irritability, and tendency to emotional outbursts may herald the onset of the disease. Motor hyperactivity and restlessness may be misdiagnosed as chorea. Increased appetite with no increase in weight or actual loss of weight, diarrhea, heat intolerance, excessive sweating, and mild fever are some of the other findings. Tremors of the hands become evident with further progression. Exophthalmos may be present but not severe. Lid lag on looking downward, impairment of convergence, and retraction of upper eyelids with infrequent blinking may be noticeable. Accelerated linear growth and advanced skeletal maturation may be noted. Craniosynostosis may occur in infants. The degree of thyroid enlargement is variable but never marked with presence of soft goiter in almost 90%. It may escape detection. Bruit may be heard. Palms may be warm and moist. Muscular weakness is uncommon. Patient may complain of feeling of weakness, tiredness, and palpitations. Tachycardia is appreciable, and a wide pulse pressure is often noted. Dyspnea, cardiac decompensation, and rarely atrial fibrillation may occur. Thyroid "crisis" or "storm" and the apathetic, cachectic type of hyperthyroidism are uncommon in childhood.

Neonatal thyrotoxicosis involves 2–3% of infants born to mothers with active or history of GD, due to transplacental passage of thyroid receptor antibodies (TRAb). It tends to be transient but can be severe in some babies. Persistent fetal tachycardia may be indicative and can be controlled by treating mothers with antithyroid drugs.

Laboratory Data

Serum levels of T4, T3, FT4, and FT3 are elevated. In some patients, T3 may be higher with T4 levels in the upper normal range or minimally elevated (T3 toxicosis). Thyroid-stimulating hormone is suppressed much below normal and thyroid antibodies APO/AMA or ATG are present. TRAb are positive in more than 90% of these children. Radioiodine uptake and assay for TRAb may not be easily available and are not essential for diagnosis but helpful. Radioisotope (iodine-131) uptake is not essential but helps to rule out subacute thyroiditis which is uncommon in children and usually transient not requiring antithyroid medication.

Treatment

The therapy is directed toward reducing the production of thyroid hormones and blunting their effects. Medical therapy is the preferred modality of treatment in children rather than subtotal thyroidectomy or radioiodine therapy. The thionamide drugs in use are propylthiouracil (PTU), methimazole, and carbimazole. Use of PTU is not recommended in children because of danger of acute liver failure. Methimazole is administered in a dose of 0.5–1 mg/kg in children. Therapy should be continued for 1–2 years or longer to prevent relapses. Periodic therapeutic monitoring is essential. Toxic reactions such as agranulocytosis, hepatic dysfunction, and lupus-like syndrome do occur. Transient urticarial rashes are most common. Beta blocker such as propranolol (0.5–2 mg/kg/day in 8 hourly doses for 4–6 weeks) helps in controlling symptoms due to hyperactivity of the sympathetic nervous system, such as palpitation and tremors. Other modalities of therapy, such as radioiodine thyroid ablation or subtotal surgical excision, are indicated if medical therapy fails after adequate trial.

GOITER

Presence of goiter may be the initial complaint for which children and adolescents may seek medical attention. In these patients, underlying cause of the thyromegaly needs to be determined; and the functional status of the thyroid gland whether euthyroid, hypothyroid, or hyperthyroid needs to be ascertained.

Common causes which lead to goitrous enlargement in this age-group are simple goiter or physiological enlargement, CLT, dyshormonogenesis, iodine deficiency, thyroid hormone resistance, or rarely malignancy. Raised serum TSH with high T3 and T4, and presence of goiter are suggestive of thyroid hormone resistance syndrome. Occasionally, it also involves other family members. It may be asymptomatic or cause mild hypothyroidism. World Health Organization has defined goiter as a thyroid gland where the size of the lateral lobes exceeds the size of the terminal phalanx of the thumb of the subject examined. Prevalence of small asymptomatic goiters in school children to the extent of 6% have been noted though the incidence is higher in regions of endemic iodine deficiency.

Strategies for management are based on the functional status of the thyroid gland and the underlying cause of goiter. Nodular goiter or single nodules need careful evaluation for the presence of thyroid malignancy. In addition to the laboratory investigations, imaging studies and fine needle aspiration cytology may be undertaken to rule out possibility of papillary or follicular carcinoma which are uncommon in childhood. Surgical intervention and/or radioiodine ablation are needed.

KEY MESSAGES

- In neonates and infants, high index of suspicion is required in the absence of neonatal screening.
- Confirmation of diagnosis is needed in neonates detected on screening by laboratory evaluation and imaging, if feasible. If diagnosis seems doubtful then therapy should be initiated and can be withdrawn by 3 years of age. Hormonal profile can be reassessed after 6 weeks; if TSH is high and T4/FT4 is low then lifelong therapy is advisable.
- Prompt optimal therapy is to be initiated with levothyroxine 10 μg/kg in newborns and infants. Per kg dose reduces to 8–6 μg/kg in early childhood, 6–5 μg/kg or 4 μg/kg in later childhood; 3–2 μg/kg during adolescence (100 $\mu g/m^2$ applicable at all ages).
- In CH, emphasize the need for lifelong, regular treatment. Also explain consequences of lack of compliance.
- Periodic clinical and laboratory monitoring is essential.
- Beyond early childhood, gradual stepping up of levothyroxine dose over 3–6 weeks is advisable.
- In AITD with mild hypothyroidism, therapy can be withdrawn after 3 years of age for a period of 6 weeks to ascertain the need for continuation.
- In hyperthyroidism, therapy may be needed for 2–3 years based on severity. Periodic monitoring and adjustment of dose are necessary. Monitoring complete blood counts and liver function tests is essential.
- Simple goiters with no thyroid dysfunction need observation and follow-up. Repeat laboratory evaluation, if necessary. Therapy will depend on underlying cause.

BIBLIOGRAPHY

1. Brown RS. The thyroid. In: Brook CGD, Clayton PE, Brown RS (Eds). Brook's Clinical Pediatric Endocrinology, 6th edition. New Jersey, United States: Wiley-Blackwell; 2009. pp. 250-82.
2. Delange F. Iodine deficiency as a cause of brain damage. Postgrad Med J. 2001;77(906):217-20.
3. Desai MP. Disorders of the thyroid gland. In: Desai MP, Menon PSN, Bhatia V, (Eds). Pediatric Endocrine Disorders, 3rd edition. Hyderabad: Universities Press; 2014. pp. 187-220.
4. Fisher DA. Disorders of the thyroid in the new born and infants. In: Sperling MA (Ed). Pediatric Endocrinology. Philadelphia, PA: WB Saunders; 2002. pp. 161-86.
5. Halac I, Zimmerman D. Thyroid nodules and cancers in children. Endocrinol Metab Clin North Am. 2005;34(3):725-44.
6. ICMR. (2013). ICMR releases results of study on congenital hypothyroidism;March15, 2013. Chennaionline News. Mht. [online]. Available from <http://www.news.chennaionline.com/chennai/ICMR> [Accessed October, 2018].
7. Koch CA, Sarlis NJ. The spectrum of thyroid diseases in childhood and its evolution during transition to adulthood: natural history, diagnosis, differential diagnosis and management. J Endocrinol Invest. 2001;24(9):659-75.
8. Kraiem Z, Newfield RS. Graves' disease in childhood. J Pediatr Endocrinol Metab. 2001;14(3):229-43.
9. Luton D, LeGac I, Vuillard E, et al. Management of Graves' disease during pregnancy: the key role of fetal thyroid gland monitoring. J Clin Endocrinol Metab. 2005;90(11):6093-8.
10. Rose SR, Brown RS, Foley T, et al. Update of newborn screening and therapy for congenital hypothyroidism. Pediatrics. 2006;117:2290-303.

13.6 Mineral Metabolism and Disorders of Parathyroid Glands

Anju Seth

INTRODUCTION

Calcium (Ca) is not only a major component of bone where 99% of body Ca is stored; it also has a critical role in many biological processes. The bone thus acts as a reservoir for homeostasis of Ca and inorganic phosphorus (P). Physiology of Ca and other minerals involved in its metabolism is closely related to bone physiology and disorders pertaining to both are also interrelated.

Serum Ca exists in equilibrium with Ca present in extracellular and intracellular spaces and in the recently accumulated surface bone. Though accounting for only 1% of total body Ca, these Ca pools are responsible for modulating vital body functions including neural transmission, blood clotting, intracellular signal transduction, maintenance of cardiac rhythm, muscle contractility, etc. Thus serum level of Ca, especially that of its metabolically active ionized form, is tightly regulated. The chief mechanisms involved in regulation of serum Ca levels involve Ca-sensing receptor (CaSR) located on the chief cells of parathyroid gland (PTG) and renal tubules, parathyroid hormone (PTH) and its receptor, and vitamin D hormone system.

REGULATION OF CALCIUM AND PHOSPHORUS HOMEOSTASIS

Parathyroid Glands and Hormone

The four PTGs produce PTH, the main hormone responsible for regulating serum ionized Ca (iCa) level. The stimulus for PTH production is a fall in serum iCa level, its most important function being to maintain serum iCa level within a narrow physiological range. Low serum iCa level inhibits the CaSR, leading to increase in PTH release, which in turn increases serum Ca level. Conversely, high iCa level stimulates CaSR, inhibiting PTH production. Both activating and inactivating mutations of CaSR are known to occur, which can lead to pathological hypo- and hypercalcemia, respectively.

Parathyroid hormone acts on its target tissues—bone and kidney. In the physiological state, it stimulates osteoblasts to promote bone mineralization. During hypocalcemia, elevated PTH levels induce bone mineral release, thereby increasing circulating Ca and P. In the kidney, PTH increases tubular Ca reabsorption and P excretion. The net effect of actions of PTH on bone and kidney is to increase plasma Ca and decrease plasma P. PTH also stimulates conversion of 25-hydroxyvitamin D [25(OH)D] to its active form, 1,25-hydroxyvitamin D [1,25$(OH)_2$D] (calcitriol), which increases intestinal Ca and P absorption. A fall in iCa concentration also directly enhances renal Ca reabsorption by inhibition of CaSR located in renal tubules **(Flowchart 13.6.1)**.

Vitamin D Hormone System

Vitamin D plays a crucial role in Ca and bone metabolism. The dietary sources of this vitamin are few and an individual obtains most of his/her vitamin D by dermal synthesis of cholecalciferol by action of ultraviolet rays on 7-dehydrocholesterol present within the dermal cells. This undergoes hydroxylation in the liver under influence of the enzyme vitamin D 25-hydroxylase. The resultant compound 25(OH)D gets stored in fat and muscle and circulates in the plasma with a half-life of 2–3 weeks. Serum levels of this compound are indicative of vitamin D status of an individual. The 25(OH)D undergoes another hydroxylation in the kidney to form 1,25$(OH)_2$D. The activity of the enzyme catalyzing this conversion is stimulated by PTH and low serum P. The synthesis of this active form of vitamin D is tightly controlled by plasma iCa levels through PTH. The 1,25$(OH)_2$D induces absorption of Ca and P from intestine. It also influences growth plate mineralization and exerts a negative influence on PTH secretion.

Calcitonin

Calcitonin is a polypeptide secreted by the C cells of the thyroid. It is secreted in response to hypercalcemia and its main role is to lower plasma Ca level. It may have some role in promoting fetal skeletal mineralization, but has unclear physiological role in postnatal life.

Fibroblast Growth Factor-23

Fibroblast growth factor-23 (FGF-23) is a hormone secreted by osteocytes, in response to rising serum P. Its synthesis is also influenced by several factors including phosphate-regulating

Flowchart 13.6.1: Normal calcium homeostasis.

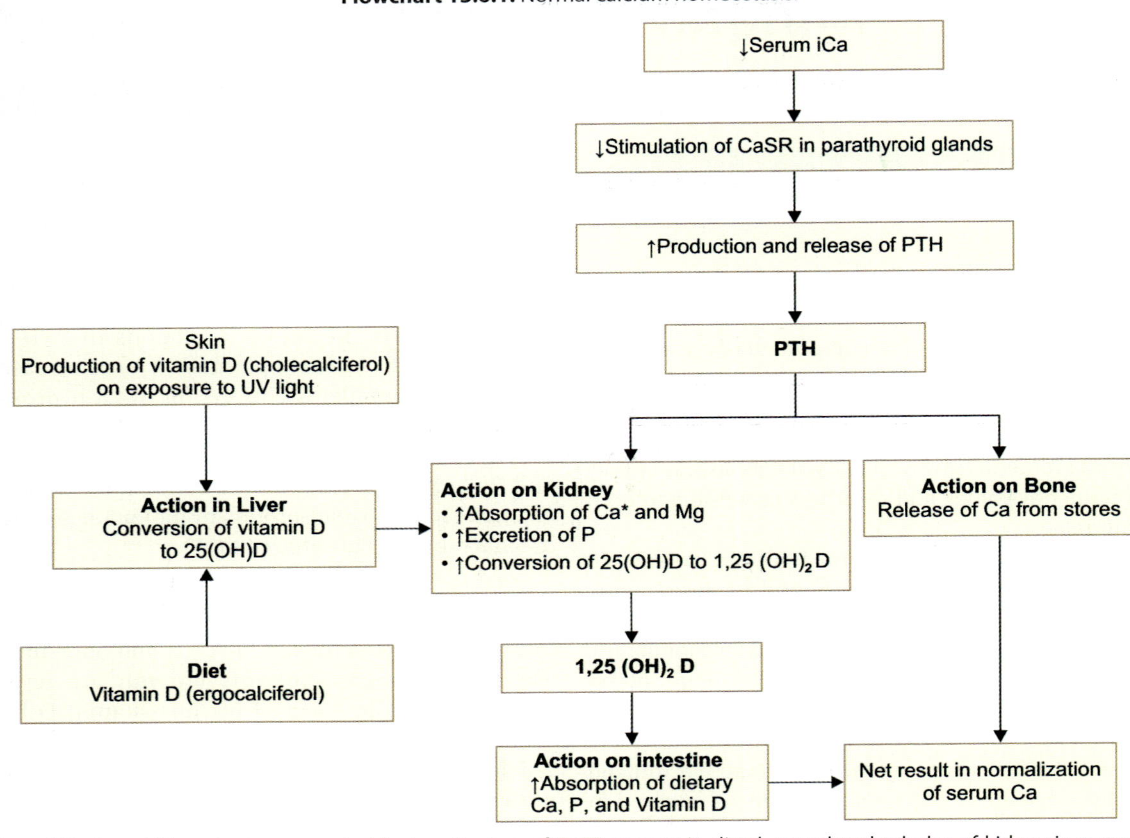

*Absorption of Ca from kidney is also promoted by inactivation of CaSR present in distal convulated tubules of kidney in response to low serum iCa.

(PTH: parathyroid hormone; Ca: calcium; iCa: ionized calcium; Mg: magnesium; UV: ultraviolet; 25(OH)D: 25-hydroxyvitamin D; 1,25(OH)$_2$D: 1,25-dihydroxyvitamin D)

gene with homologies to endopeptidases on the X chromosome (PHEX), dentine matrix protein-1 (DMP1), and bone morphogenic protein-1. The actions of FGF23 include renal P excretion coupled with sodium absorption, and impaired 1-hydroxylation of 25(OH)D. The resultant lower levels of 1,25(OH)$_2$D lead to decreased absorption of P from intestine.

Parathyroid Hormone-related Peptide

Parathyroid hormone-related peptide (PTHrP) is a polypeptide with PTH-like biologic activity. It is considered to have some role in promoting positive Ca gradient across placenta in the fetus. In postnatal life, its principal importance is as a cause of malignancy-related hypercalcemia.

Serum Calcium

Intestinal absorption of dietary Ca is stimulated by 1,25(OH)$_2$D. About half of plasma Ca exists in metabolically active ionized form (iCa), while the remaining is bound to albumin (40%) or other molecules. Total serum Ca (tCa) level is age-dependent. Normal tCa for 1–5 years is 9.4–10.8 mg/dL, 6–12 years is 9.4–10.2 mg/dL, and more than 20 years is 8.8–10.2 mg/dL. Ca binding to albumin is affected by many factors, such as alkalosis, increase in free fatty acids in serum, lipid infusion, etc. Therefore it is desirable to measure iCa while diagnosing hypocalcemia in a setting of acute illness or hypoalbuminemia. Normal serum iCa level ranges between 4.4 mg/dL and 5.2 mg/dL (1.1–1.3 nmol/L).

Serum Inorganic Phosphorus

Phosphorus is abundantly available in foods and is readily absorbed through small intestine. About 85% of body P is present in the bone, and the remainder is in the extracellular and intracellular compartments. In serum and extracellular fluid (ECF), P exists almost entirely in ionized form as PO_4. The regulation of serum P occurs primarily through kidney. Usually, about 85–95% of the filtered P load is reabsorbed in the proximal tubule. The most important factor affecting proximal renal tubular reabsorption of P is *FGF23*. Mutations in *PHEX*, *DMP1*, and *FGF23* genes, which lead to unregulated increase in FGF23 levels cause hypophosphatemic rickets. Along with FGF23, the renal reabsorption is affected by the glomerular filtration rate (GFR), plasma P level, and PTH, which has a phosphaturic effect. In addition to homeostatic mechanisms influencing long-term changes, short-term changes in serum P can occur due to redistribution between ECF and bone/cells. Thus cell lysis or acidosis causes release of P into plasma, while insulin, respiratory alkalosis, and rapid bone mineralization decrease serum P.

Assessment of renal excretion of phosphate is an important tool for evaluation of P wasting states. It is done by measuring simultaneously plasma and urinary phosphate and creatinine (Cr) levels in a timed collection and calculating fractional excretion of phosphate as follows:

$$FePO_4 = \frac{U_{PO4}/P_{PO4}}{U_{Cr}/P_{Cr}}$$

Tubular reabsorption of P is derived as $(1 - FePO_4) \times 100\%$.

The renal tubular threshold for P expressed, as tubular maximum reabsorption of phosphate (TMP)/GFR, is a more sensitive measure of phosphaturia relative to serum P. This can be calculated using serum P and tubular reabsorption of phosphate levels using the nomogram of Bijvoet and Walton.

Serum Alkaline Phosphatase

Circulating alkaline phosphatase (ALP) is largely derived from liver and bone. Serum ALP levels are a measure of osteoblastic activity and bone turnover and are physiologically elevated during periods of rapid growth, infancy, and adolescence. They are also raised in rickets.

Serum Magnesium

Magnesium (Mg) is intimately involved in Ca metabolism. Its clinical relevance lies in the fact that adequate Mg level is needed for PTH secretion as well as action.

HYPOCALCEMIA IN NEONATAL PERIOD

CALCIUM HOMEOSTASIS IN THE NEWBORN

There is a physiological dip in serum Ca levels soon after birth in neonates due to sudden interruption of supply from the placenta. Plasma tCa and iCa concentrations fall rapidly in first 6–12 hours to reach a nadir from 12 mg/dL at delivery to 9 mg/dL by 24–72 hours of age. Immaturity of the PTGs, poor establishment of feeding in the first few days of life, and certain perinatal conditions compound this physiological dip and may lead to hypocalcemia in vulnerable newborns.

Hypocalcemia is defined as serum tCa < 7 mg/dL in a preterm newborn, < 8 mg/dL in a full-term newborn, and < 8.8 mg/dL in postneonatal age group. For iCa, the corresponding figures are < 4.4 mg/dL for newborns and < 4.7 mg/dL for children beyond neonatal age group.

CAUSES OF HYPOCALCEMIA

Hypocalcemia is commonly observed in the neonatal period. Depending upon the time of occurrence, neonatal hypocalcemia is classified as early (occurring within 72 hours of birth) or late (occurring > 72 hours of birth).

Early neonatal hypocalcemia (ENH) is usually secondary to maternal illness or certain perinatal conditions, which exaggerate the physiological dip in serum Ca level that occurs soon after birth, resulting in transient hypocalcemia. A combination of factors including blunting of physiological postnatal rise in PTH level, relative resistance of renal tubules to PTH-mediated P excretion, increased P load due to cellular injury, decreased Ca intake, and hypercalcitoninemia contribute to this dip.

Causes of late neonatal hypocalcemia (LNH) include vitamin D deficiency, high-dietary phosphate load as might occur in infants on cow milk, and hypoparathyroidism (**Box 13.6.1**).

CLINICAL MANIFESTATIONS

Early neonatal hypocalcemia is often asymptomatic. When present, the symptoms are neither specific for hypocalcemia, nor related to its severity. These include jitteriness, irritability, tremulousness of limbs, and focal or generalized seizures. On the other hand, LNH is often symptomatic and presents in full term, usually healthy newborns toward the end of first week of life or beyond, with convulsions. Other uncommon features include stridor due to laryngospasm, apnea and cyanosis, and disturbances of cardiac rhythm.

Box 13.6.1: Causes of hypocalcemia in newborns.

I. *Causes of hypocalcemia in infants <72 hours:*
   1. *Neonatal illness:*
      - Prematurity
      - Birth asphyxia
      - Intrauterine growth retardation
      - Sepsis
      - Respiratory distress
      - Citrated blood/alkali
      - Phototherapy
   2. *Maternal illness:*
      - Diabetes mellitus
      - Toxemia of pregnancy
      - Hyperparathyroidism

II. *Causes of hypocalcemia in infants >72 hours:*
   - High dietary phosphate load
   - Maternal vitamin D deficiency
   - *Hypomagnesemia:* Transient/metabolic disorder
   - *Hypoparathyroidism:* Transient/permanent
   - Chronic renal insufficiency
   - Pseudohypoparathyroidism

DIAGNOSTIC APPROACH

Important issues in history: Age at onset of symptoms (early/late hypocalcemia), gestational age (prematurity), perinatal events (birth asphyxia, jaundice, and respiratory distress), type of feeding (high phosphate load), maternal illness (diabetes, hypoparathyroidism, and toxemia) and drug intake, and family history of hypocalcemic seizures (hypoparathyroidism).

Examination: Gestation, systemic sickness, facial dysmorphism, other malformations especially cardiac (DiGeorge syndrome).

Investigations

- *All cases*:
  - Serum tCa, iCa, Mg, P, ALP, total protein, and albumin
  - Venous blood gas analysis, kidney function test, X-ray chest (thymic shadow, cardiac disease)
- Second-line investigations (required in almost all cases of LNH and some of ENH depending upon initial evaluation):
  - Serum PTH, 25(OH)D, 1,25$(OH)_2$D
  - Maternal Ca, P, PTH, 25(OH)D
  - Urinary Ca/Cr ratio, P, creatinine

Key biochemical findings in important causes of hypocalcemia are presented in **Box 13.6.2**.

TREATMENT

Asymptomatic hypocalcemia in the newborn should be treated at tCa level < 6 mg/dL in preterm and < 7 mg/dL in full-term infant with oral Ca supplements 75 mg/kg/day given 6 hourly for 3–4 weeks. Patients with hypocalcemic seizures require therapy with 1–2 mL/kg of intravenous (IV) 10% Ca gluconate given slowly under cardiac monitoring over a period of 10–20 minutes. This is followed by infusion of Ca gluconate at a rate of 50 mg/kg/day titrated to achieve eucalcemia. Once eucalcemia is achieved, the infusion is tapered over a period of 48 hours with simultaneous introduction of oral Ca 50–75 mg/kg/day. Serum Ca levels should be monitored 12 hourly during Ca infusion and its tapering.

Box 13.6.2: Characteristic biochemical features of important disorders leading to hypocalcemia.

↓Ca, ↓P, ↑PTH, ↑ALP, ↓25(OH)D	Vitamin D deficiency
↓Ca, ↑P, ↑creatinine, ↑PTH	Renal failure
↓Ca, ↑P, →creatinine, ↓PTH	Hypoparathyroidism
↓Ca, ↑P, ↓ PTH, ↓Mg	Hypomagnesemia
↓Ca, ↑P, →creatinine, ↑PTH:	High dietary P load/PHP

(ALP: alkaline phosphatase; Ca: calcium; 25(OH)D: 25-hydroxyvitamin D; Mg: magnesium; P: phosphorus; PHP: pseudohypoparathyroidism; PTH: parathyroid hormone)

A secure IV line is mandatory while administering intravenous Ca to avoid subcutaneous necrosis from extravasation. Ca infusions should not be mixed with solutions containing phosphates and bicarbonates to avoid precipitation.

Further treatment depends upon underlying etiology. Newborns with ENH usually require no further therapy. Most patients with hypomagnesemia, apart from those rare subjects with Mg-wasting states, respond well to two doses of 50% magnesium sulfate 0.2 mL/kg given 12–24 hours apart. Patients with hypoparathyroidism require 20–60 ng/kg/day of calcitriol with oral Ca supplements 30–75 mg/kg/day. These patients require careful, ongoing monitoring of therapy to prevent hypercalcemia and hypercalciuria. Neonatal hypoparathyroidism is often transient in which case treatment can be stopped after 6 weeks and PTH levels assessed to ascertain the same.

Neonates with vitamin D deficiency require to be given 2,000 IU vitamin D/day for 90 days with oral Ca supplements for 2–4 months. A preventive dose of 400 IU should be given subsequently to prevent recurrence of deficiency and building up of body stores. Daily vitamin D rather than a single mega dose should be given to newborns and infants, since there is insufficient evidence of safety of large doses of vitamin D in this age group.

HYPOCALCEMIA BEYOND NEONATAL PERIOD

CAUSES

Beyond neonatal period, chronic hypocalcemia is most often due to deficiency of PTH or 1,25$(OH)_2$D or to resistance to their biological effects (**Box 13.6.3**).

Transient hypocalcemia may often be observed during acute and critical illness, such as sepsis, acute pancreatitis, and toxic shock.

CLINICAL FEATURES

Most children with mild or long-standing hypocalcemia are asymptomatic. Abrupt decreases in serum iCa, on the other hand, predispose children to more severe symptoms, mostly neurological in nature, including muscle spasms and anticonvulsant-resistant seizures. Older children with hypocalcemia may have numbness, tingling in circumoral region, fingers or toes, or frank tetany. Chronic hypocalcemia may lead to dental hypoplasia, basal ganglia calcification, and cataract, if associated with hyperphosphatemia (as in hypoparathyroidism or PTH resistance), and skeletal changes of rickets if associated with hypophosphatemia (as in vitamin D deficiency). Clinical examination may reveal twitching of ipsilateral angle of mouth on gently tapping the facial nerve

Box 13.6.3: Causes of hypocalcemia in older children and adolescents.

1. *Parathyroid-related:*
   - *Congenital hypoparathyroidism:*
     - Congenital agenesis/hypoplasia of PTGs
     - *Defect in PTH production and processing:* DiGeorge and other syndromes, CaSR gene mutation
   - *Acquired hypoparathyroidism:*
     - Autoimmune polyglandular syndrome, infiltrative diseases such as thalassemia major and Wilson disease, neck irradiation
   - *Target organ resistance*: Hypomagnesemia or pseudohypoparathyroidism
2. *Vitamin D-related:*
   - Deficiency of vitamin D
   - Malabsorption states
   - *Increased losses:* Anti-epileptics
   - *Metabolic defects in vitamin D action:* VDDR type I
   - *End organ resistance:* VDDR type II
3. *Calcium deficiency:*
   - Nutritional deprivation
4. *Hypomagnesemia:*
   - Malabsorption states
   - Bartter syndrome
   - Renal tubular acidosis
   - Diuretics
5. *Hyperphosphatemia:*
   - Renal failure
   - Tumor lysis
   - Phosphate administration

*Other contributing factors in renal failure include inadequate PHT response and low $1,25(OH)_2D$.

($1,25(OH)_2D$: 1,25-hydroxyvitamin D; PTG: parathyroid glands; PTH: parathyroid hormone; VDDR: vitamin D-dependent rickets)

just below the maxilla (Chvostek sign). Carpopedal spasm may be elicited by inflating a blood pressure cuff around an arm and maintaining pressure at 10 mm Hg above systolic for 3 minutes (Trousseau sign, **Fig. 13.6.1**).

EVALUATION

Transient hypocalcemia is seen during acute sickness, which is obvious on clinical examination. **Table 13.6.1** gives the pointers on clinical evaluation of a child with documented hypocalcemia. Important biochemical parameters to be measured include serum iCa, P, ALP, PTH, Mg, and creatinine. Further evaluation depends upon the results obtained on these tests **(Box 13.6.2)**. Hypomagnesemia is an infrequent but important cause of hypocalcemia. It leads to both impaired PTH release and a resistance to PTH action. It is therefore routinely assessed in evaluation of a child with hypocalcemia. ALP is a sensitive marker of bone turnover, being increased in disorders related to vitamin D and within normal range when hypocalcemia is secondary to hypoparathyroidism. Among the second-level tests, estimation of serum 25(OH)D is important since disorders of

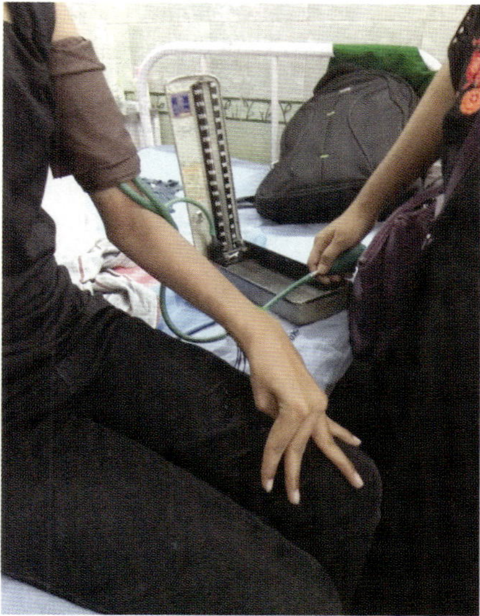

Fig. 13.6.1: Demonstration of Trousseau sign in hypocalcemia.

Table 13.6.1: Clinical pointers to etiology of hypocalcemia.

Clinical evaluation	***Possible etiology***
Bony deformities	Rickets
Alopecia, epidermal cysts along with bony deformities of rickets	VDDR II
Recurrent infections, typical facies (mandibular hypoplasia, hypertelorism, short philtrum, low set ears), heart murmur	DiGeorge syndrome
History of neck surgery/ irradiation, cataract, deafness	Hypoparathyroidism, PHP
Mucocutaneous candidiasis, alopecia, vitiligo	APS-I
Family history, short stature, brachydactyly, round facies, obesity	Albrights hereditary osteodystrophy

(APS: autoimmune polyendocrine syndrome; PHP: pseudohypoparathyroidism; VDDR: vitamin D-dependent rickets)

vitamin D and its metabolism frequently cause hypocalcemia. Serum PTH is the most critical investigation in determining etiology of hypocalcemia; a high PTH in the setting of hypocalcemia usually indicates a compensatory response. A low PTH on the other hand indicates hypoparathyroidism or hypomagnesemia. A normal PTH in presence of hypocalcemia is likely in activating mutation involving CaSR wherein PTH secretion gets inhibited at a relatively lower level of serum Ca.

MANAGEMENT

The primary goal in treatment of hypocalcemia is to increase serum Ca to a level that renders patient asymptomatic and as close to lower range of normal as possible. Specific management in accordance with the underlying cause is then instituted. Asymptomatic hypocalcemia (tCa > 7.5 mg/dL) does not require immediate intervention. Lower levels or symptomatic hypocalcemia would require intravenous administration of 0.2–0.5 mL/kg (maximum 10 mL) of 10% Ca gluconate given slowly under cardiac monitoring over a period of 10–20 minutes. This is followed by infusion of Ca gluconate at a rate of 20 mg/kg/day titrated to achieve eucalcemia monitored 12 hourly. Once eucalcemia is achieved, the infusion is tapered over a period of 48 hours with simultaneous introduction of oral Ca 50–75 mg/kg/day.

Further treatment depends upon underlying etiology. Treatment of hypomagnesemia and hypoparathyroidism has been described earlier in the section on neonatal hypocalcemia. Infants with vitamin D deficiency will require 2,000 IU/day of vitamin D for 3 months while older children and adolescents require 3,000–6,000 IU/day for 3 months along with Ca supplements of 500 mg daily. A single dose of 150,000 IU for children 1–12 years and 300,000 IU for older children can be given as an alternative to daily therapy. In all cases, response to therapy should be reassessed at 3 months and further treatment given as required. Once normal serum 25(OH)D levels are achieved, a preventive dose of 400 IU/day for infants and 600 IU for older children should be given subsequently to prevent recurrence of deficiency.

Box 13.6.4: Causes of hypercalcemia in children.

Neonates and Infants
- *Neonates:* Maternal vitamin D excess, maternal hypoparathyroidism
- Hypervitaminosis D
- *Dietary:* High-calcium load, low-phosphate diet (breast milk/standard formula in preterm babies, total parenteral nutrition)
- Subcutaneous fat necrosis (birth trauma, birth asphyxia)
- Neonatal severe hyperparathyroidism (homozygous inactivating CaSR mutation)
- Williams syndrome
- Jansen metaphyseal dysplasia
- Bartter syndrome

Older children
- Hypervitaminosis D
- Hyperparathyroidism
  a. Familial hypocalciuric hypercalcemia (heterozygous inactivating CaSR mutation)
  b. Parathyroid adenoma (sporadic)
  c. Multiple endocrine neoplasia type I, II
  d. McCune-Albright syndrome
- Malignancy (ectopic production of PTHrP)
- *Others:*
  a. Immobilization
  b. Williams syndrome
  c. Hypophosphatasia
  d. Jansen metaphyseal dysplasia (activating PTH receptor mutation)
  e. *Drugs*: Thiazides, vitamin A

(CaSR: calcium-sensing receptor; PTH: parathyroid hormone; PTHrP: parathyroid hormone-related peptide)

HYPERCALCEMIA

Serum Ca levels are higher in children compared to adults, and age-appropriate cutoffs should be considered to diagnose hypercalcemia. In neonates and infants, serum Ca > 10.8–11.3 mg/dL and in older children and adolescents, values > 10.3 mg/dL are considered as hypercalcemia.

DIFFERENTIAL DIAGNOSIS

Hypercalcemia is much less encountered than hypocalcemia in children. The causes vary by age (**Box 13.6.4**).

- *Iatrogenic*: Most common cause in pediatric practice is hypervitaminosis D [serum 25(OH)D level > 100 ng/mL], due to administration of excessive vitamin D, usually to a child with nonnutritional or misdiagnosed rickets.
- *Low dietary phosphate intake*, such as associated with exclusive breast milk in preterm babies or total parenteral nutrition, stimulates 1α-hydroxylase activity in the kidney and can result in hypercalcemia.
- *Calcium-sensing receptor loss-of-function mutation*: Heterozygous mutation causes familial hypocalciuric hypercalcemia (FHH), an autosomal-dominant disorder. This inactivation of CaSR results in continued PTH secretion even in the face of high serum Ca. The hypercalcemia in FHH is generally mild and asymptomatic. A homozygous loss-of-function mutation of CaSR results in life-threatening hypercalcemia in the newborn called neonatal severe hyperparathyroidism (NSHPT).
- *Primary hyperparathyroidism (PHPT)* is mostly sporadic in children and results from a parathyroid adenoma. Inherited autosomal-dominant genetic syndromes, such as multiple endocrine neoplasia (MEN), can also lead to PHPT.
- *Secondary hyperparathyroidism* can be present in patients with chronic renal failure.
- *Malignancy*: Patients with malignancy (leukemia, lymphoma, and neuroblastoma) can rarely have hypercalcemia because of production of humoral factors such as PTHrP.
- *Williams syndrome* is a rare genetic disease characterized by growth retardation, facial dysmorphism, cardiac defect, developmental delay, and hypercalcemia.
- *Jansen metaphyseal dysplasia*, a rare skeletal disorder consisting of disproportionate short stature and bony deformities, can manifest with hypercalcemia.
- *Prolonged immobilization* results in disuse atrophy and decreased bone deposition with increased resorption, resulting in hypercalcemia.

MANIFESTATIONS OF HYPERCALCEMIA

Symptoms are generally seen when serum Ca exceeds 12 mg/dL and consist of vomiting, irritability, hypotonia, constipation, polyuria, and dehydration. Patients with chronic hypercalcemia have failure to thrive, abdominal pain, bone pains, and nephrocalcinosis. A serum Ca and P product exceeding 56 can cause soft tissue and vascular calcification (manifesting with hypertension). Serum tCa > 14 mg/dL can lead to cardiac arrest.

DIAGNOSTIC APPROACH

The *history* includes review of symptoms of hypercalcemia, intake of vitamin D and Ca, symptoms of malignancy, family history of renal stones, MEN, and parathyroid surgery.

Examine for bony deformities (Jansen metaphyseal dysplasia and rickets in hypophosphatasia), dysmorphism (Williams syndrome), and features of other endocrinopathies (adrenal insufficiency and pheochromocytoma). Radiography of limbs can help diagnose metaphyseal dysplasia.

Laboratory tests indicated include evaluation of Ca, P, 25(OH) D, $1,25(OH)_2D$, PTH, and urinary Ca level **(Table 13.6.2)**. High PTH levels are suggestive of PTH-dependent causes, such as hyperparathyroidism or CaSR inactivating mutation. Low PTH on the other hand suggests vitamin D or Ca excess and malignancy. Family members should be screened for hypercalcemia and hypocalciuria. Radionuclide Sestamibi technetium-99m scan is a useful imaging modality to localize parathyroid adenomas preoperatively.

TREATMENT

Mild asymptomatic hypercalcemia as in benign FHH requires no treatment. Urgent treatment is required when symptoms occur with serum Ca > 12 mg/dL and all patients with levels > 14 mg/dL. All vitamin D supplements and Ca should be discontinued and a diet with low Ca and P content given.

Serum Ca can be lowered by parenteral rehydration with normal saline and loop diuretics. For severe hypercalcemia, bisphosphonates and calcitonin can be used. Calcitonin inhibits Ca resorption from bone, while bisphosphonates are extremely helpful in controlling hypercalcemia due to increased osteoclastic activity (PHPT, malignancy, and immobilization). Surgical removal is indicated in parathyroid adenoma. Parathyroidectomy may be required in cases with hyperparathyroidism or NSHPT.

HYPOPHOSPHATEMIA

Transient hypophosphatemia is common in children with severe malnutrition and those critically ill. This is due to a combination of factors that lead to shift of P from extracellular to intracellular space. These include glucose infusion, insulin infusion, refeeding syndrome, mechanical ventilation or

Table 13.6.2: Differential diagnosis of hypercalcemia.

Disorder	*Serum calcium*	*Serum phosphate*	*Serum PTH*	*Serum 25(OH)D*	*Serum $1,25(OH)_2D$*	*Urinary calcium*
Low phosphate diet	↑	↓	↓	N	↑	↑
Hypervitaminosis D	↑	↑	↓	↑↑	N	↑
Granulomatous disease/ subcutaneous fat necrosis	↑	↑	↓	N	↑↑	↑
Immobilization	↑	↑	↓	N	↓	↑
FHH*	↑	N-↓	N-↑	N	↑	↓
NSHPT†	↑↑↑	↓	↑↑	N-↓	↑	↓
William syndrome	↑		↓		N-↑	↑
Jansen metaphyseal dysplasia	↑	↓	↓	N	↑	↑
Primary hyperparathyroidism	↑	↓	↑	N	↑	↑
Malignancy	↑↑	↓/↑‡	↓	N	↑/↓‡	↑

*FHH—Familial hypocalciuric hypercalcemia due to calcium-sensing receptor (CaSR) loss-of-function mutation.
†NSHPT—Neonatal severe hyperparathyroidism.
‡Depending upon production of PTHrP or osteolytic bone invasion.
[25(OH)D: 25-hydroxyvitamin D; $1,25(OH)_2D$: 1,25-hydroxyvitamin D; PTH: parathyroid hormone]

not been given to supplementation of all minerals), as dietary sources of phosphorus are common. In India, vitamin D deficiency is particularly encountered in the neonate or infant, due to poor maternal stores. Thereafter, it is prominent during adolescence, especially in girls, who cannot take advantage of the sunshine due to modest clothing and poor outdoor activity. In toddlers and mid-childhood (and also in older age groups), dietary calcium deficiency plays a predominant role. Nutritional rickets is discussed in detail in Chapter 4.6 on fat soluble vitamins.

Nonnutritional Rickets

When vitamin D and calcium supplementation have been given in adequate doses for at least 2 months without onset of radiological healing or improvement in serum alkaline phosphatase, nonnutritional or resistant rickets should be suspected. Alternatively, in the presence of clues to a nonnutritional cause, rickets may be investigated for without waiting. Such clues include alopecia, features of malabsorption, hypokalemia, nephrocalcinosis, polyuria, or dense bones, among others **(Fig. 13.7.1)**. Resistant rickets may be categorized into calcium deficiency or phosphorus deficiency rickets for ease of differential diagnosis and investigative pathway **(Table 13.7.1)**.

Etiology and Presentation

Children with renal tubular acidosis (RTA) may present with polyuria, failure to thrive, hypokalemia, and in the case of distal RTA, with dental enamel hypoplasia, nephrocalcinosis, or nephrolithiasis. In proximal RTA, additional features include glycosuria, proteinuria, and sometimes phosphaturia leading to hypophosphatemic rickets. Anemia, abdominal pain, diarrhea, Bitot's spots, night blindness, or hypoalbuminemia may alert the pediatrician to the presence of malabsorption. Hypophosphatemic rickets typically presents at the end of the first year of life. Rachitic features predominantly affect the skull and lower limbs, with relative sparing of upper limbs and chest.

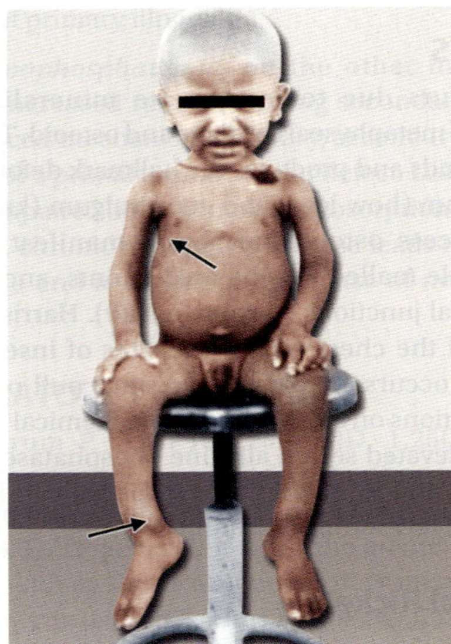

Fig. 13.7.1: Clinical photograph of a child with calcitriol receptor abnormality (vitamin D-resistant rickets type 2), showing alopecia, rachitic rosary, and widened malleoli at the ankles (highlighted by arrows).

Diagnosis

Typical clinical differentiating features of calcium versus phosphorus deficiency rickets are highlighted in **Table 13.7.2**. If a good clinical examination does not provide a clue to etiology, then PTH should guide further workup. Primary and secondary hyperparathyroidism result in increased phosphorus leak from the proximal tubule. Thus, a child with any cause of calcipenic rickets, such as malabsorption or distal RTA, due to concomitant secondary hyperparathyroidism, may appear to have hypophosphatemic rickets or proximal RTA. Serum PTH is a useful investigation at this juncture, being only marginally elevated in hypophosphatemic rickets and significantly raised in calcipenic rickets.

Cases with high PTH should be investigated for distal RTA by serum potassium, blood and urine pH, ammonium chloride loading test if necessary, and ultrasound of kidneys for nephrocalcinosis.

Malabsorption tests include erythrocyte sedimentation rate, antiendomysial or tissue transglutaminase antibodies, D-xylose test, and endoscopic duodenal biopsy. If these are negative, serum 25(OH)D (25-hydroxycholecalciferol) and

Table 13.7.1: Causes of rickets.

Calcipenic rickets	*Phosphopenic rickets*
Vitamin D/calcium deficiency	Prematurity (calcium plus phosphorus deficiency)
Anticonvulsant induced	Fanconi syndrome (proximal renal tubular acidosis)
Malabsorption	Congenital hypophosphatemic rickets—X-linked/autosomal dominant/autosomal recessive (mutations in *PHEX, FGF 23, DMP1*, or *ENPP1* genes)
Distal renal tubular acidosis	Hypophosphatemic rickets with hypercalciuria (*SLC34A3* gene mutation)
Chronic renal failure	Tumor-induced (mesenchymal tumor, epidermal nevus)
1α-hydroxylase defect	McCune-Albright-syndrome-associated rickets
Calcitriol receptor defect	–

adrenal hyperplasia. CD due to ectopic ACTH production is extremely rare in children.

Autonomous secretion of cortisol from adrenal glands accounts for nearly 15% cases of CS. Adrenocortical carcinoma (ACC) has bimodal distribution with peak incidence at 3 years of age and the other peak in the fourth to fifth decade. In children, ACC may be associated with Li-Fraumeni or Beckwith Weidman syndrome. Primary pigmented nodular adrenal hyperplasia is due to usually mutations in the *PRKR1A* gene, regulatory alpha subunit of protein kinase A. It is associated with Carneys complex, multiple endocrine neoplasia, myxomas, and lentigenes. McCune-Albright syndrome due to a somatic mutation of G protein alpha subunit may present with ACTH-independent CS due to constitutional activation of ACTH receptor. It is associated with fibrous dysplasia, *café-au-lait* spots, and other endocrinopathies, including precocious puberty and hyperthyroidism.

Clinical Features

The classical features, such as central obesity, striae, moon facies, and buffalo hump, are uncommon in children. Growth failure coupled with weight gain is the most common feature. However, it is an extremely rare cause of childhood obesity. The fat distribution is often centripetal with accumulation on the face, neck, and abdomen. The extremities appear wasted with muscle weakness **(Figs. 13.8.1 and 13.8.2)**.

Other clinical features include hypertension, delayed puberty, lethargy, bone pain, and obsessive-compulsive behavioral disorders. There may be thinning of skin with violaceous striae (frequently seen on the abdomen, buttocks, thighs, and axillae) and easy bruising. ACTH-dependent CS is characterized by hyperpigmentation. Androgen excess leads to hirsutism, acne, deepening of voice, and rarely clitoral hypertrophy.

Children with ectopic ACTH production usually present with hypertension and hypokalemic alkalosis.

Diagnosis

The evaluation of children with CS after exclusion of an adrenal tumor is more complex because most of the diagnostic tests are based on studies in adults, and then extrapolated for children. An algorithmic approach to diagnosis of CS is given in **Flowchart 13.8.1**.

Step 1: The first step in the evaluation of a child suspected to have CS is to exclude exogenous CS, by detail history and estimation of 8.00-am basal serum cortisol. If serum cortisol is undetectable, ACTH stimulation test is required to document suppression of HPA axis.

Step 2: Second step is to document autonomous cortisol production. Two out of the following screening tests, namely 24-hours urinary free cortisol (UFC), late-night salivary cortisol, 1-mg overnight dexamethasone suppression test, or low-dose longer dexamethasone suppression test, should be abnormal for a diagnosis of CS.

- Loss of diurnal rhythm is the earliest biochemical marker of hypercortisolism. Usually cortisol is highest at 9 am and lowest at midnight. The normal plasma cortisol levels range between 5 µg/dL and 25 µg/dL (140–690 nmol/L) in the early morning, which is reduced to less than half by 11 pm. Morning cortisol levels are not elevated in many patients with CS, whereas late-night cortisol is usually increased.

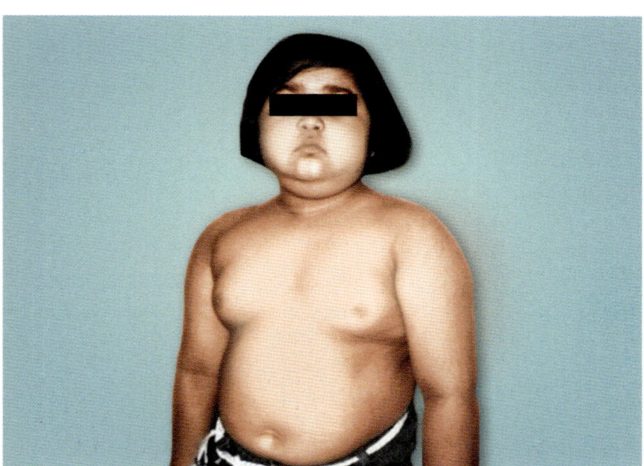

Fig. 13.8.1: An 8-year-old girl with Cushing syndrome (CS) due to pituitary microadenoma. Note central obesity and moon facies.

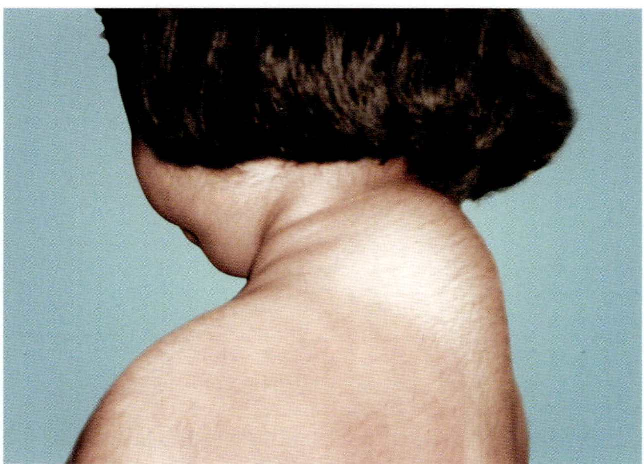

Fig. 13.8.2: An 8-year-old girl with Cushing syndrome (CS). Note buffalo hump and hypertrichosis.

Flowchart 13.8.1: Approach to a child with Cushing syndrome.

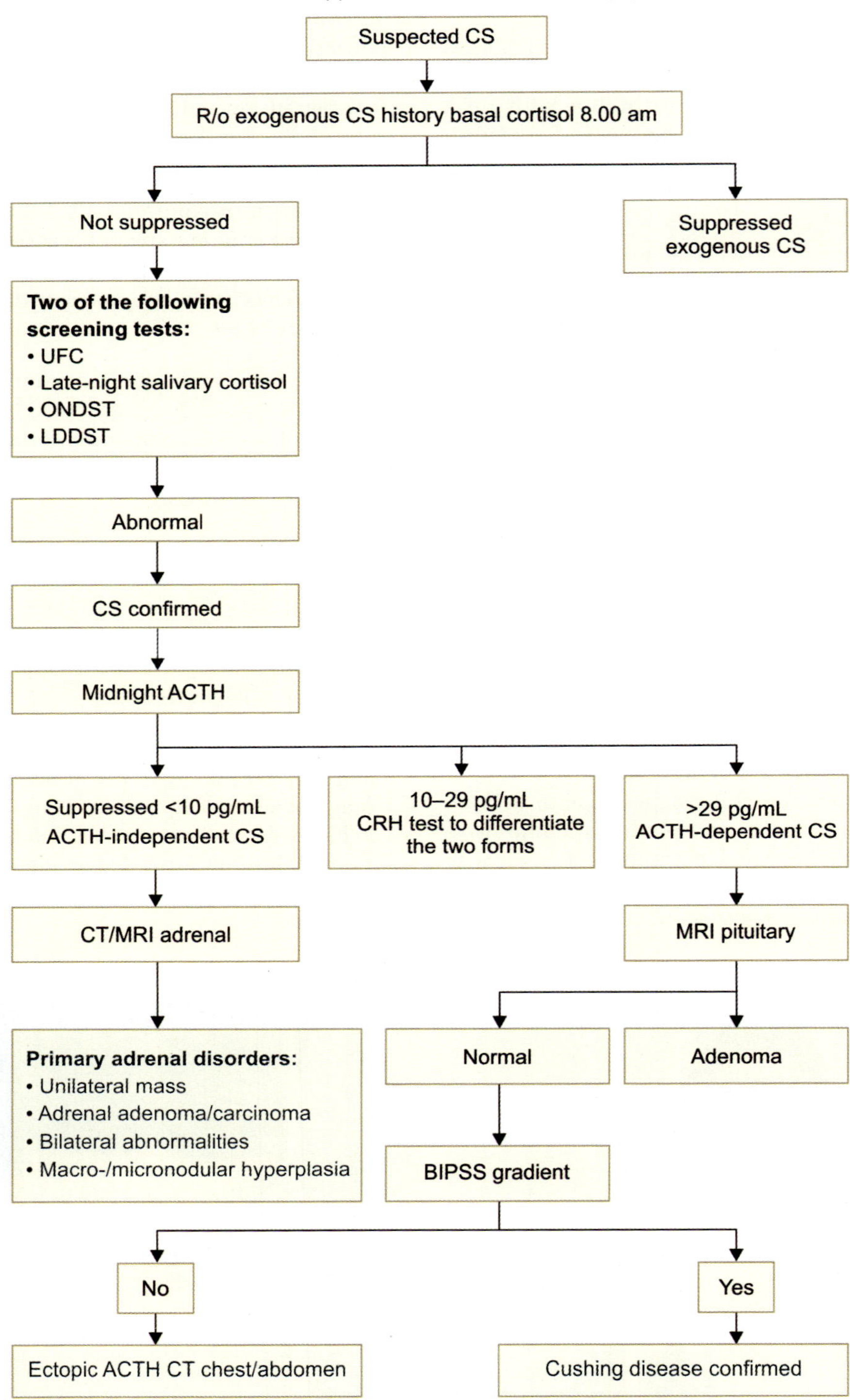

(ACTH: adrenocorticotropic hormone; BIPSS: bilateral inferior petrosal sinus sampling; CRH: corticotropin-releasing hormone; CS: Cushing syndrome; CT: computed tomography; LDDST: low-dose dexamethasone suppression test; MRI: magnetic resonance imaging; ONDST: overnight dexamethasone suppression test; UFC: urinary free cortisol)

- Estimation of excretion of UFC is a good screening test for CS. Normal levels vary between 25 μg/m^2/day and 75 μg/m^2/day, and UFC levels greater than 75 μg/m^2/day are suggestive of CS.
- Salivary cortisol is a better alternative and cortisol level greater than 8.6 nmol/L is suggestive of CS.
- *Overnight dexamethasone suppression:* Following administration of 1 mg of dexamethasone at 11 pm to 12 midnight, plasma cortisol is estimated in the morning sample. Cortisol levels above 1.8 μg/dL are suggestive of CS.
- Low-dose dexamethasone suppression test is based on the principle that dexamethasone will suppress ACTH, and hence cortisol release in normal subjects, whereas patients with autonomous cortisol production will not suppress below a specified cut-off. This test involves the measurement of serum cortisol or UFC before and after oral dexamethasone (5 μg/kg/dose, every 6 hours for 2 days or 1.25 mg/m^2/day divided into four doses given over 2 days). Serum cortisol levels greater than 1.8 μg/dL is diagnostic of CS.

Step 3: Third step is to decide whether CS is ACTH-dependent or independent by the estimation of plasma ACTH.

- If circulating ACTH is suppressed to less than 10 pg/mL, it suggests ACTH-independent CS, most likely due to adrenal cause.
- Plasma ACTH value greater than 10 pg/mL suggests ACTH-dependent CS due to pituitary lesion or ectopic production of ACTH. There is a wide overlap in ACTH values in pituitary and ectopic ACTH production. A morning ACTH value of more than 29 pg/mL in the case of confirmed CS has a sensitivity of 70% of identifying children with a corticotrophin-dependent etiology of CS.
- Children with ACTH levels between 10 pg/mL and 29 pg/mL are best evaluated by the CRH stimulation test. Mean increase in cortisol level of 20% from baseline, 30 minutes to 45 minutes and ACTH level of at least 35%, 15 minutes to 30 minutes after IV CRH (1 μg/kg, maximum 100 μg, sampling basal and after 30 minutes and 60 minutes) is suggestive of pituitary ACTH-dependent etiology while no increase is seen in children with adrenal pathology or ectopic ACTH production.

Step 4: Fourth step is to determine the anatomical site of lesion by radiological investigations.

- Once ACTH-independent CS is confirmed, adrenal CT or MRI should be performed to detect the type of adrenal lesion: unilateral or bilateral, or benign adenoma or carcinoma.
- Pituitary MRI is recommended for ACTH-dependent CS. The use of dynamic MRI (with IV gadolinium) with spoiled gradient sequences may increase the sensitivity.
- Inferior petrosal sinus sampling is the test available for identifying the source of ACTH production and is performed in children with ACTH-dependent CS with normal neuroimaging. The experience with children is limited.
- Computed tomography or MRI of chest abdomen or rarely neck is required to determine the source of ectopic ACTH production.
- Labeled octreotide scanning or Gallium-68 labeled positron emission tomography CT imaging is useful in localizing ectopic ACTH source.

Radiological evaluation usually shows retarded bone age but may be advanced in children with virilization. Osteoporosis and pathological fractures may be present.

Management

Resection of adrenal lesion—unilateral adrenalectomy for adenoma or carcinoma and bilateral adrenalectomy for bilateral lesion is recommended. Prolonged cortisol excess causes suppression of the normal contralateral adrenal. This mandates close monitoring for adrenal insufficiency in the perioperative period. Recovery of HPA axis may be delayed up to 6 months after surgery. Transsphenoidal resection of pituitary adenoma is recommended for children with CD. The success rate varies from 66% to 80%. Pituitary irradiation or bilateral adrenalectomy is recommended in children with failed pituitary surgery or recurrent disease.

Nelson syndrome characterized by the enlargement of sella and hyperpigmentation is a dreaded complication after bilateral adrenalectomy in these patients. Lifelong follow-up is required after pituitary surgery.

Adrenal carcinoma is highly malignant and has a high rate of recurrence. Combination of cisplatin, etoposide, and doxorubicin with surgery has shown good results in stage III ACC, in a recent trial by Children's Oncology Group. Chemotherapy with mitotane is ineffective in children with recurrence of the disease.

Medical management of childhood CS with inhibitors of steroidogenesis (ketoconazole, cyproheptadine, and mitotane) has been tried but is largely disappointing.

HYPERALDOSTERONISM

Primary hyperaldosteronism due to increased adrenal aldosterone production is extremely rare in children. These include aldosterone-producing adrenal adenoma, familial primary hyperaldosteronism, and much rarely adrenal carcinoma. Secondary hyperaldosteronism results from factors that activate renin–angiotensin system. The most common clinical features of primary hyperaldosteronism are due to hypertension and hypokalemic alkalosis manifesting as fatigue, muscle cramps and weakness, polyuria, nocturia, and poor growth. This condition needs to be differentiated from Bartter syndrome, in which PRA is elevated with normal blood pressure.

Hyperaldosteronism should be managed with salt restriction and antialdosterone agent, spironolactone. Surgery is indicated only if an aldosterone-producing adenoma has been conclusively proven.

PHEOCHROMOCYTOMA

Pheochromocytoma is a catecholamine-secreting tumor, which arises from the chromaffin cells of adrenal medulla. It can also arise from abdominal sympathetic chain, periadrenal area, urinary bladder, thoracic cavity, or cervical region. It is rare in children and accounts for only 2% of cases of secondary hypertension. It usually coexists with other familial syndromes or tumors, such as neurofibromatosis (von Recklinghausen disease and von Hippel-Lindau disease) and multiple endocrine neoplasia type II. Mutations in the rearranged during transfection proto-oncogene and succinate dehydrogenase enzyme gene have been reported in these patients. Genetic screening for mutation detection in the genes associated with these familial syndromes is recommended in childhood pheochromocytoma.

Clinical Features

Clinical features are due to hypersecretion of catecholamines. These include hypertension, sustained more often than paroxysmal. There may be associated headache, palpitation, pallor, sweating, nausea, vomiting, visual disturbances, polyuria, and polydipsia. Convulsions due to hypertensive encephalopathy may occur. Unexplained fever and weight loss due to hypercatabolism are seen more commonly in children than adults.

Diagnosis

Demonstration of increased plasma catecholamine levels or urinary excretion of catecholamines and their derivatives confirms the diagnosis. Abdominal imaging with ultrasound, CT scan, or MRI is done to localize the lesion. Radionuclide imaging with iodine 123-metaiodobenzylguanidine is also used for localization of the tumor. Often the tumors are multiple.

Family screening is required, if stigmata of syndromes are present.

Management

Surgical removal of the tumor is the choice of treatment after adequate alpha-blockade with phenoxybenzamine or prazosin. Recently calcium-channel blocking agent, nifedipine, has been tried with some success.

BIBLIOGRAPHY

1. Bista B, Beck N. Cushing syndrome. Indian J Pediatr. 2014;81(2):158-64.
2. Bornstein SR, Allolio B, Arlt W, et al. Diagnosis and treatment of primary adrenal insufficiency: an endocrine society clinical practice guideline. J Clin Endocrinol Metab. 2016;101(2):364-89.
3. Desai MP, Menon PSN, Bhatia V. Pediatric endocrine disorders, 3rd edition. Hyderabad: Universities Press; 2014. p. 221-67.
4. Lenders JW, Duh QY, Eisenhofer G, et al. Pheochromocytoma and paraganglioma: an endocrine society clinical practice guideline. Endocr Soc J Clin Endocrinol Metab. 2014;99(6):1915-42.
5. Lodish MB, Keil MF, Stratakis CA. Cushing's syndrome in pediatrics: an update. Endocrinol Metab Clin North Am. 2018;47(2):451-62.
6. Nieman LK, Biller BM, Findling JW, et al. The diagnosis of Cushing's syndrome: an Endocrine Society Clinical Practice Guideline. J Clin Endocrinol Metab. 2008;93(5):1526-40.
7. Nieman LK, Biller BM, Findling JW, et al. Treatment of Cushing's syndrome: an endocrine society clinical practice guideline. J Clin Endocrinol Metab. 2015;100(8):2807-31.
8. Pivonello R, De Martino MC, De Leo M, et al. Cushing's syndrome. Endocrinol Metab Clin North Am. 2008;37(1):135-49.
9. Raff H. Cushing syndrome: update on testing. Endocrinol Metab Clin North Am. 2015;44(1):43-50.
10. Storr HL, Chan LF, Grossman AB, et al. Paediatric Cushing's syndrome: epidemiology, investigation and therapeutic advances. Trends Endocrinol Metab. 2007;18(4):167-74.

13.9 Disorders of Adrenocortical Biosynthesis

P Raghupathy

INTRODUCTION

The adrenal cortex produces several steroid hormones, such as cortisol, aldosterone, and androgens. The ability to convert cholesterol into steroidal hormones (steroid biosynthesis) is present only in the adrenal cortex, gonads of both genders, and the placenta. An enzymatic defect of steroidogenesis may not affect the adrenal cortex and gonads equally. Hence, disorders of sex development may result from the biosynthetic pathway defects in the adrenal cortex or the gonads, or both.

STEROIDOGENESIS

The adrenal cortex functions as two separate units because of the enzymatic differences between the zona glomerulosa and the inner two zones—zona fasciculata and zona reticularis. The zona glomerulosa lacks 17α-hydroxylase activity and, therefore, cannot synthesize 17α-hydroxypregnenolone and 17α-hydroxyprogesterone (17-OHP), the precursors of cortisol and androgens. The synthesis of aldosterone by this zone is totally regulated by the renin-angiotensin system and by potassium.

The two inner zones produce cortisol, androgens, and small quantities of estrogens. These two zones are directly controlled by adrenocorticotropic hormone (ACTH). They lack 18-dehydrogenase and so cannot synthesize aldosterone.

The various enzymes involved in the biosynthetic pathway of cortisol are given in **Flowchart 13.9.1**. Corticotropin-releasing factor produced by the hypothalamus regulates ACTH. ACTH in turn induces synthesis and secretion of steroids within minutes. The conversion of cholesterol to pregnenolone is the major site of ACTH action on the adrenal cortex and is the rate-limiting step.

CONGENITAL ADRENAL HYPERPLASIA

In congenital adrenal hyperplasia (CAH), cortisol synthesis from cholesterol is affected due to deficiency of one of the several enzymes in the adrenal cortex **(Flowchart 13.9.1)**. ACTH elevation is secondary to plasma cortisol deficiency via the negative feedback mechanism. Overproduction of the hormonal precursors proximal to the block and deficiency of the hormones distal to the blocked enzymatic step are responsible for the clinical features encountered. The enzymatic defects are inherited by an autosomal recessive mode and produce characteristic clinical and biochemical pictures. The genes and enzymes involved in adrenal steroidogenesis are listed in **Table 13.9.1**.

21-HYDROXYLASE DEFICIENCY

The 21-hydroxylase deficiency (21-OHD) is the most common enzyme deficiency seen in more than 90% of individuals with CAH. The exact incidence of 21-OHD in India is unknown. In the West, the incidence is reported to be 1 in 10,000 to 1 in 20,000. The absence of 21-hydroxylase causes decreased synthesis of glucocorticoid and mineralocorticoid with elevated precursors. The 17-OHP accumulates in serum because it is not converted to 11-deoxycortisol. Similarly, progesterone accumulates following lack of conversion to 11-deoxycorticosterone (DOC) **(Flowchart 13.9.1)**. The ultimate effects are: (1) cortisol deficiency and ACTH elevation giving rise to adrenocortical hyperplasia, and (2) mineralocorticoid deficiency causing salt loss, dehydration, and shock. As the formation of mineralocorticoids and glucocorticoids from cholesterol is blocked, the conversion of cholesterol flows largely into the androgen pathway without hindrance because adrenal androgen synthesis is not blocked. The classic clinical varieties of this deficiency are as follows:

- *Salt-wasting type* in nearly 75% of 21-OHD. This is the classic disorder presents usually between 1 week and 1 month of age occurring with cortisol deficiency along with salt wasting and hypovolemia arising from aldosterone deficiency and the natriuretic effect of accumulated precursors, such as 17-OHP. The effects of this enzyme deficiency begin in the intrauterine period. Hence, the accumulation of excessive adrenal androgens causes virilization of the external genitalia of a female infant seen at birth, in both the salt-wasting and simple virilizing types.
- *Simple virilizing type* without salt loss. Nonsalt losers with virilization account for nearly 25% of cases. The absence of salt loss can be explained by a partial defect in 21-OHD, since only a minimal 21-hydroxylase activity is needed for mineralocorticoid production. Virilization is seen at birth in girls.
- *Non-classic (late onset) type,* wherein 50% of enzyme activity is retained. The presentation may also be varied,

Flowchart 13.9.1: Scheme of adrenal steroidogenesis. Chemical names of enzymes are shown next to the arrows; enclosed numbers indicate traditional names of the enzymes: (1) 20,22-desmolase; (2) 3β-hydroxy steroid dehydrogenase/isomerase; (3) 17α-hydroxylase; (4) 17,20-lyase; (5) 21-hydroxylase; (6) 11β-hydroxylase; (7) 18-hydroxylase; (8) 18-oxidase; (9) 17β-hydroxysteroid dehydrogenase; (10) aromatase.

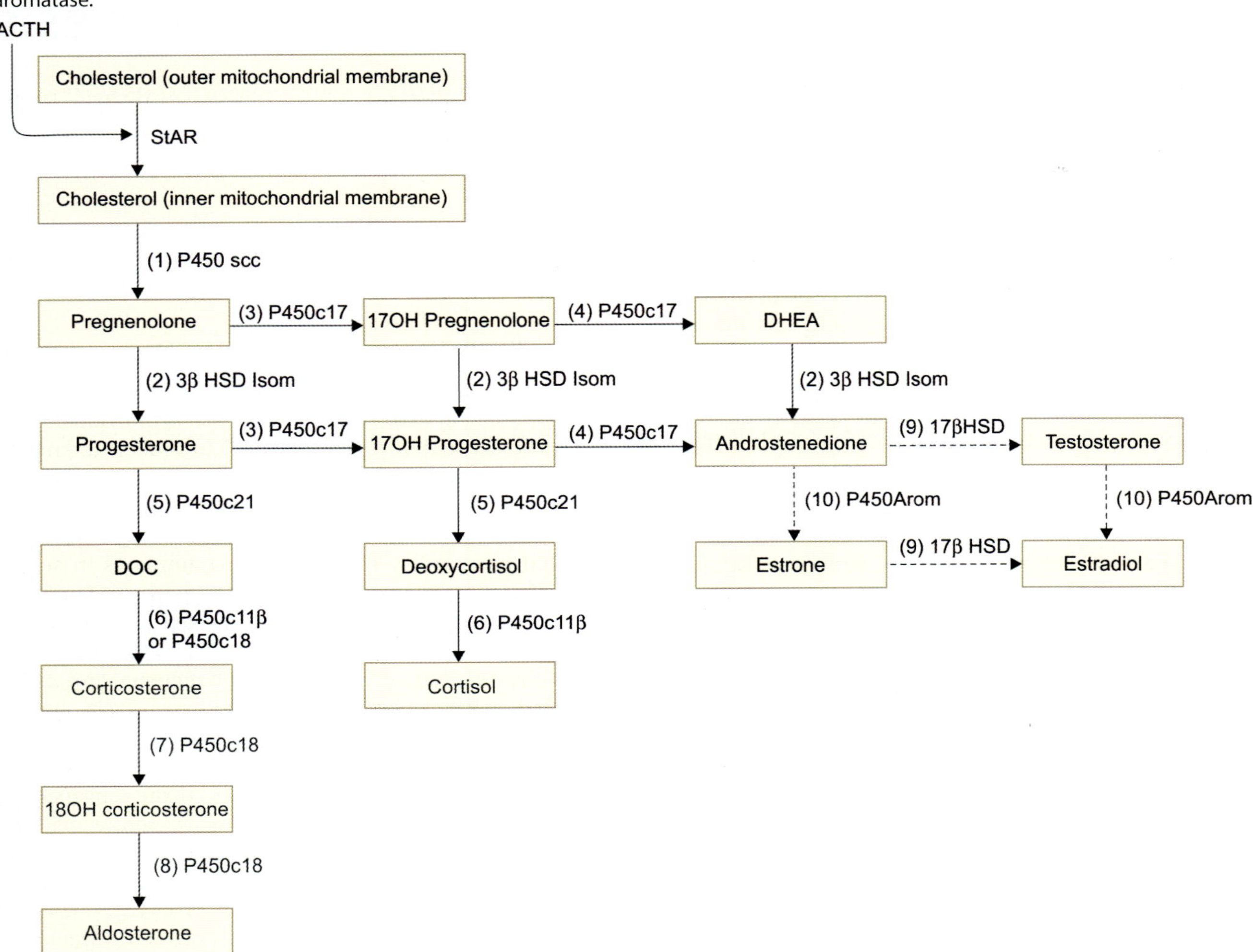

(ACTH: adrenocorticotropic hormone; DHEA: dehydroepiandrosterone; DOC: 11-deoxycorticosterone; StAR: steroidogenic acute regulatory protein)

Table 13.9.1: Genes and enzymes involved in adrenal steroidogenesis.

Gene	*Chromosomal location*	*Enzyme*	*Enzymatic activity*	*Cellular location*
CYP11A1	15q23–q24	P450scc (*CYP11A1*)	Cholesterol desmolase (side chain cleavage)	Mitochondrion
HSD3B2	1p13.1	3βHSD (*3βHSDII*)	3β-hydroxysteroid dehydrogenase	Endoplasmic reticulum
CYP17	10q24.3	P450c17 (*CYP17*)	17α-hydroxylase/17,20-lyase	Endoplasmic reticulum
CYP21A2	6p21.3	P450c21 (*CYP21A2*)	21-Hydroxylase	Endoplasmic reticulum
CYP11B1	8q21-22	P450c11 (*CYP11B1*)	11β-Hydroxylase	Mitochondrion
CYP11B2	8q21-22	P450c18 (*CYP11B2*)	Aldosterone synthase (corticosterone 18-methylcorticosterone oxidase/lyase)	Mitochondrion

such as adrenarche, early growth spurt, or accelerated skeletal maturation. The manifestations can also occur for the first time during adulthood as hirsutism in women or reduced fertility in both sexes.

There is no hypertension. Use of appropriate sized cuffs for measurement of blood pressure is essential. If siblings are affected, then they tend to have the same clinical type.

- *Salt loss:* It may present as hypovolemic shock, especially as unexplained dehydration, and may also occur beyond neonatal period in cases infection induced stress situations.
- *Virilization:* The diagnosis of 21-OHD is easily identified in girls because of genital ambiguity. In boys with simple virilizing form, however, the condition can go unnoticed when androgen excess causes increased height velocity, increase in the size of the external genitalia, appearance of pubic hair, and other signs of male secondary sexual characteristics are observed. Hyperpigmentation involving external genitalia, nipples, and umbilicus with a "tanned appearance" of skin may be a very important clue for early diagnosis in these children.

The degree of genital ambiguity does not correlate with the form of 21-OHD. Virilization in the female may present as mild clitoral hypertrophy, varying degrees of ambiguity, or complete masculinization with normal-looking male genitalia but with an empty scrotum. Thus, the absence of testes would be helpful in diagnosis.

Apart from the external virilizing and biochemical features, there are no abnormalities in genetic sex, gonadal differentiation, or development of the internal genitalia. The female infant will have normal ovaries, fallopian tubes, uterus, and proximal vagina. Postnatally, in untreated cases, there will be continued virilization effects with clitoromegaly or penile enlargement, accelerated growth, advanced skeletal maturation far in excess of the height age, and premature appearance of secondary sexual characteristics. Untreated males will have advancing penile enlargement with disproportionately small testes. Untreated females have clitoromegaly, hirsutism, male-type baldness, menstrual irregularities, and impaired fertility. Short adult height resulting from premature epiphyseal fusion is a regular feature in all untreated cases. Even with regular therapy and good control, predicted adult height is not always achieved in CAH, and bone age may be advanced.

Laboratory Features

Hyponatremia, hyperkalemia, increased urinary sodium losses due to renal salt wasting, high plasma renin activity (PRA), accompanied by low serum and urinary aldosterone levels, acidosis, and uremia are the biochemical features in salt-wasting type. Hypoglycemia may also be present. Elevated serum 17-OHP, markedly lowered serum cortisol, elevated levels of serum dehydroepiandrosterone sulfate (DHEAS), and testosterone are diagnostic. On short Synacthen (also ACTH) stimulation test, serum 17-OHP and DHEAS rise more than two to threefold but there is no significant elevation of serum cortisol. Urinary estimation of steroid metabolites is not preferred nowadays. The difficulty experienced in the 24-hour urine collection from an infant with ambiguous genitalia is considerable. The results are quite often difficult to interpret.

Nonclassic 21-OHD (also known as cryptic CAH) may be totally asymptomatic and presents only with hormonal abnormalities as in the classic cases and may be picked up only during family studies. Prenatal virilization is absent, and postnatal virilization is variable. Nonclassic cases may have only milder elevation of 17-OHP, especially when performed in the afternoon or late forenoon. Hence, it is preferable to get the hormonal profile always in the mornings. Salt wasting is absent and cortisol deficiency is rare.

Treatment

The essential principles of treatment are to replace the deficient hormones and to suppress the overproduction of precursor hormones. Hydrocortisone is required in the dose of 8–15 mg/m^2/day in two or three divided doses. Constant monitoring is required to arrive at the right dose to facilitate normal growth and also the lowest possible dose in order to prevent central obesity, growth retardation, and decreased bone mineral density. Salt wasters require, in addition, 9a-fluorohydrocortisone 0.1–0.3 mg (50–200 µg) per day and need to be monitored for hypertension, edema, and suppressed PRA. Sodium chloride supplementation up to 1–2 g daily may be needed along with feeds in the infants and young children. This is generally not required beyond infancy but may be encouraged in hot weather conditions and in situations with excessive sweating.

In the newborn period at presentation, a large dose of hydrocortisone and fluorohydrocortisone may be required. Dosages are modified by monitoring serum sodium and potassium daily and ideally, by frequent serum 17-OHP and PRA estimations. Dose of hydrocortisone is gradually reduced and changed over to 5 mg twice a day orally.

The hormonal profile reverts to the normal range with appropriate treatment, which is monitored 3–6 monthly by estimating 17-OHP and PRA values and when appropriate dosage adjustment is affected. The daily dose of hydrocortisone may be doubled or tripled during acute stress periods, such as fever, gastrointestinal illness, surgery, or trauma.

In the newborn period at presentation, a large dose of hydrocortisone and fluorohydrocortisone may be required. Dosages are modified by monitoring serum sodium and potassium daily and ideally, by frequent serum 17-OHP and PRA estimations. Dose of hydrocortisone is gradually reduced and changed over to 5 mg twice a day orally. In older children, when higher dosage is given, a few endocrinologists advise a larger dose at night, e.g. if the child needs 12.5 mg of hydrocortisone per day, 5 mg is given in the morning, and 7.5 mg in the evening. This is done with a view to suppress ACTH pulses during the night, although insufficient data exist to recommend this as a routine.

In stress situations, e.g. febrile infections, major trauma, surgery, or shock, large amounts of glucocorticoids are required to combat the stress. The daily dose of hydrocortisone is doubled or tripled and given orally or intramuscularly, if oral administration is not tolerated. Fludrocortisone dose remains unchanged.

Nonclassic CAH does not always require treatment but when treatment is required at puberty or later, lower glucocorticoid doses are used.

Appropriate Sex Assignment

Assigning the appropriate sex is of paramount importance. The affected female with CAH has the potential for a normal fertile female role. Surgical correction of the genital abnormality (feminizing genitoplasty) is carried out in girls at around 1 year of age by doing reduction clitoroplasty. Definitive vaginoplasty with routine dilatation will also be required in late adolescence.

It is very important that the parents understand the nature of the disease, chronicity of the treatment required lifelong, the complication arising from poor compliance, and how steroids play an essential role in stress situations, such as surgery, infection, or shock, which can be life threatening, if inappropriately managed. Early epiphyseal fusion in both sexes will eventually cause short stature, if treatment is irregular and incomplete with the disease being poorly controlled. The parents are given adequate health education regarding this condition. They are advised that daily dose of hydrocortisone must be doubled or tripled for a few days during stress situations. If oral doses are not tolerated, intramuscular injections are given.

Prenatal Treatment

In families with an affected infant, prenatal treatment of the mother has been tried in subsequent pregnancies for nearly three decades. The aim of prenatal treatment is to prevent external genital deformity in the female fetus due to virilization. This mode of treatment is best considered experimental at present, as long-term effects of prenatal dexamethasone are unknown and several fetal effects have been described.

Neonatal Screening

Screening of all newborns with filter paper 17-OHP is carried out in many developed nations. It is not yet determined whether this is mandatory. This newborn screening is helpful:

- To identify infants with the classic form 21-OHD who carry the risk of developing life-threatening salt-wasting crisis
- To make a rapid diagnosis in cases of female infants with ambiguous genitalia.

11β-HYDROXYLASE DEFICIENCY

In this disorder, which accounts for nearly 5% of cases of CAH, cortisol and corticosterone are deficient with low aldosterone and overproduction of 11-deoxycortisol and 11-deoxycorticosterone. The precursor hormones are shunted into the androgen pathway causing prenatal and postnatal virilization. The accumulation of DOC results in sodium and water retention, increased plasma volume, and hence causes hypertension. Serum level of 11-deoxycortisol elevation is diagnostic. PRA is suppressed, serum aldosterone is lowered, and hypokalemia may be present. Glucocorticoid therapy is effective in reversing all the abnormalities causing remission.

17-HYDROXYLASE/17,20-LYASE DEFICIENCY

This is a rare disorder occurring with cortisol deficiency, ACTH excess, overproduction of DOC causing hypertension and hypokalemia. Affected males are incompletely virilized (undervirilized male) owing to diminished androgen production and may be phenotypically female or ambiguous. In addition, ACTH excess driven by cortisol deficiency causes mineralocorticoid excess with sodium retention, hypokalemia, and hypertension. Both sexes present with female external genitalia at birth and usually manifest at puberty with absence of secondary sexual characteristics. PRA and aldosterone are low. Glucocorticoid therapy suppresses overproduction of the hormones.

3β-HYDROXYSTEROID DEHYDROGENASE/4,5 ISOMERASE DEFICIENCY

Classic and nonclassic forms are seen in this disorder. Salt wasting, deficiency of cortisol, and aldosterone are the usual manifestations of this condition. In the nonclassic form, there is no aldosterone deficiency. Males with this condition may show undervirilization with ambiguity of external genitalia owing to underproduction of testosterone in utero. Pseudovaginal hypospadias may be present in the males due to absence of potent androgens. But the excessive collection of the weak androgen, DHEAS, may cause clitoral enlargement in the female. Most of them have aldosterone deficiency with elevation of PRA. Hyperpigmentation is seen, and serum ACTH level is high. Treatment is with glucocorticoids.

P450 OXIDOREDUCTASE DEFICIENCY

Several enzymes including 17OH, 21OH, and aromatase depend on P450 oxidoreductase (POR) for their catalytic activity. The action of POR at multiple sites of steroidogenesis **(Flowchart 13.9.1)** explains multiple hormonal deficiencies. The action of POR at nonadrenal sites further explains the occurrence of skeletal dysplasia, which is seen as an associated finding in some patients. 17-Hydroxylase deficiency may cause hypertension.

LIPOID ADRENAL HYPERPLASIA

In this rare steroidogenic acute regulatory protein deficiency disorder which affects adrenal cortex and gonads, there is a global deficiency of all adrenal hormones, glucocorticoids, mineralocorticoids, and sex hormones, which affects adrenal cortex and gonads. Gonadal steroids are also absent. Clinical presentation is very early in life with salt-wasting crisis. Females have no abnormality of internal or external genitalia. Males are phenotypically female but may have inguinal gonads. Sex-hormone replacement will be necessary in those with undervirilization or in those with delayed puberty with the objective of achieving normal pubertal development, normal sexual function, and fertility. Later presentation up to 1 year of age has also been described.

CONCLUSION

Knowledge regarding CAH is widening constantly. The chromosomal locations and nature of the genes encoding the various enzymes needed for adrenocortical biosynthesis, the cellular locations, functions and abnormalities of these enzymes, the pathophysiology of adrenocortical disorders, the clinical features, and laboratory parameters have been documented further. Prenatal diagnosis and treatment as well as newborn screening are practiced widely. However, the ideal way of keeping the disease under good control in an effort to mimic normal physiology has always been difficult and requires enormous effort.

BIBLIOGRAPHY

1. Ahmed SF, Rodie M. Investigation and initial management of ambiguous genitalia. Best Pract Res Clin Endocrinol Metab. 2010;24(2):197-218.
2. El-Maouche D, Arlt W, Merke DP. Congenital adrenal hyperplasia. Lancet. 2017;390(10108):2194-210.
3. Nimkarn S, Lin-Su K, New MI. Steroid 21 hydroxylase deficiency congenital adrenal hyperplasia. Endocrinol Metab Clin North Am. 2009;38(4):699-718.
4. Speiser PW, Azziz R, Baskin LS, et al. Congenital adrenal hyperplasia due to steroid 21-hydroxylase deficiency: an endocrine society clinical practice guideline. J Clin Endocrinol Metab. 2010;95(9): 4133-60.
5. White PC. Update on diagnosis and management of congenital adrenal hyperplasia due to 21-hydroxylase deficiency. Curr Opin Endocrinol Diabetes Obes. 2018;25(3):178-84.

13.10 Disorders of Sex Development

P Raghupathy

NORMAL SEX DETERMINATION AND DIFFERENTIATION

The undifferentiated human embryos of the two genders differ only by their karyotypes. The gender of the individual is normally determined by factors that direct the gonads as early as the third gestational week in the male to differentiate along male line, and the process is continued in turn, by gonadal hormones which determine the development of the phenotypic sex. The *SRY* (sex-determining region on the Y-chromosome) gene residing in the Y-chromosome has now been documented as the mammalian sex-determining gene, which actively induces the formation of the testis and the male phenotype during embryonic life. The gonads, internal genitalia (genital ducts), and the external genitalia, which are all bipotential, are influenced by several genes and other factors necessary for sex differentiation.

Gonads

The gonads in the embryo remain undifferentiated until the 6th week of gestation. Subsequent development into either a testis or ovary is directed by the genetic sex (XY or XX). The testis develops more rapidly than the ovary. Fetal testicular differentiation begins in the 7th week of gestation, whereas ovarian development begins not earlier than the 16 weeks of gestation. Female sex differentiation is not dependent on ovarian hormones, but there is evidence that *Wnt* signaling molecules play a role in Müllerian duct development and suppression of Leydig cell differentiation in ovary.

Testicular Differentiation

The *SRY* gene (with 204 amino acids) located on the short arm of Y-chromosome (Yp11.3) is the trigger for testicular differentiation, by inducing the development of Sertoli cells, and subsequently, seminiferous tubules and Leydig cell formation in that order. *SRY* activates *SOX9* (SRY-homeobOX-like gene), an autosomal gene (chromosome 17q24), and *SF1* (steroidogenic factor 1) to induce differentiation of the bipotential gonad into a testis. *SRY* suppresses dosage-sensitive sex reversal, adrenal hypoplasia critical region, on chromosome X, gene 1(*DAX1*), which normally inhibits *SOX9*. The testis induces male sex differentiation including testicular descent through a hormone-mediated process.

Ovarian Differentiation

DAX1, *SOX3*, and *Wnt4* are the three candidate genes currently known to suppress testicular differentiation. *DAX1* and *SOX3* inhibit *SF1* and *SOX9*, preventing Sertoli cell differentiation, favoring granulosa cell development. *Wnt4* arrests the Leydig cell precursors and induces development of Müllerian ducts into fallopian tubes, uterus, cervix, and upper third of vagina. Though the effects of these genes have been considered to result in ovarian differentiation, it should be remembered that active testicular differentiation occurs much earlier when compared to the ovarian.

Internal Genitalia

Testosterone initially under the control of human chorionic gonadotropin (hCG) is produced locally (paracrine) by Leydig cells of the fetal testis on either side. It helps in ipsilateral differentiation of the Wolffian ducts into epididymis, vas deferens, seminal vesicles, and ejaculatory ducts. Anti-Müllerian hormone (AMH), secreted by the Sertoli cells, causes ipsilateral involution of the Müllerian structures.

In female fetuses, Wolffian structures regress in the absence of testosterone, and Müllerian ducts persist in the absence of AMH. However, *Wnt4* gene appears to play an important role in Müllerian duct differentiation and fetal ovarian function.

External Genitalia

From the initial undifferentiated stage of the external genitalia, masculinizing features develop in the male under the influence of dihydrotestosterone formed peripherally from testosterone by the action of 5α-reductase. This process is dependent on an adequate number of functioning androgen receptors in the pubic skin. Formation of the female external genitalia does not require any active process and will persist with normal ovaries, in androgen insensitivity or even in the absence of gonads, sex chromosome abnormalities, streak gonads, or nonfunctioning testes.

ABNORMALITIES OF SEX DEVELOPMENT

Terms, such as intersex, hermaphroditism, pseudohermaphroditism, sex reversal and gender-based diagnostic conditions, are currently recommended to be avoided. These terms may be deemed derogatory and confusing to parents and practitioners as well. Hence, changes in terminology have been proposed **(Table 13.10.1)**.

It is advisable to use terminology that are precise, descriptive, clear in expressing the genetic, etiologic or diagnostic condition, and at the same time, sensitive to the concerns of parents. The revised classification of disorders of sex development (DSD) is presented in **Table 13.10.2**.

When *SRY* gene undergoes mutation in its high-mobility group box protein, testicular failure or genital ambiguity will result. *SOX9* mutation in 46,XY males leads to a female phenotype and streak ovarian-like gonads. Chromosomal abnormalities may lead to disorders of male gonadal differentiation or give rise to ovotesticular differentiation.

Wolffian development and Müllerian regression on each side are dependent on the ipsilateral production or testosterone and AMH, respectively. Hence, abnormalities of the internal genitalia will be encountered, based on the presence of gonadal elements on that side. A streak gonad,

Table 13.10.1: Revised nomenclature.

Previous	***Revised***
Intersex	Disorders of sex development (DSD)
Male pseudohermaphrodite: Undervirilization of an XY male Undermasculinization of an XY male	46,XY DSD
Female pseudohermaphrodite: Virilization of an XX female Masculinization of an XX female	46,XX DSD
True hermaphrodite	Ovotesticular DSD
XX male or XX sex reversal	46,XX testicular DSD
XY sex reversal	46,XY complete gonadal dysgenesis

Table 13.10.2: Revised classification of disorders of sex development.

Sex chromosome DSD	*XY DSD*	*XX DSD*
45,X (Turner syndrome and variants) 47,XXY (Klinefelter syndrome and variants) 45,X/46,XY (Mixed gonadal dysgenesis, ovotesticular dysgenesis) 46,XX/46,XY (Chimeric, ovotesticular dysgenesis)	*Disorders of gonadal (testicular) development*: • Complete gonadal dysgenesis • Partial gonadal dysgenesis • Gonadal regression • Ovotesticular DSD *Disorders in androgen synthesis or action:* • Androgen biosynthesis defect (e.g. 17β-hydroxysteroid dehydrogenase deficiency, 5α-reductase deficiency, *StAR* mutations) • Defects of androgen action (e.g. CAIS, PAIS) • LH receptor defects (e.g. Leydig cell hypoplasia, aplasia) • Disorders of AMH and AMH receptor (persistent Müllerian duct syndrome) • Others (e.g. Severe hypospadias, cloacal exstrophy)	*Disorders of gonadal (ovarian): Development*: • Ovotesticular DSD • Testicular DSD (e.g. SRY, dup SOX9) • Gonadal dysgenesis *Androgen excess:* • Fetal (e.g. 21-hydroxylase deficiency, 11β-hydroxylase deficiency) • Fetoplacental (aromatase deficiency, POR) • Maternal (luteoma, exogenous, etc.) *Others* (e.g. cloacal exstrophy, vaginal atresia, MURCS, other syndromes)

(AMH: anti-Müllerian hormone; CAIS: complete androgen insensitivity syndrome; DSD: disorders of sex development; LH: luteinizing hormone; MURCS: Müllerian, renal, cervicothoracic somite dysplasia; PAIS: partial androgen insensitivity syndrome; POR: P450 oxidoreductase; SOX: SRY-homeobOX-like gene: SRY: sex-determining region on the Y-chromosome; StAR: steroidogenic acute regulatory protein)

which produces neither testosterone nor AMH, will give rise to poorly formed Müllerian structures, such as a hypoplastic or hemiuterus on the side of the defective gonad.

Variable degrees of virilization of the female external genitalia leading to gender ambiguity will result when exposed to androgens, either from the mother (intake or excessive production of androgens in her body) or from the fetus [congenital adrenal hyperplasia (CAH), aromatase deficiency, ovotesticular DSD, or mixed gonadal dysgenesis]. Partial virilization producing ambiguity of the external genitalia or complete virilization with normal-looking male external genitalia (penis and a fully formed but empty scrotum) may occur in a genetic female with CAH due to 21-hydroxylase deficiency. A normal-looking female external genitalia (with testes in the labioscrotal folds) may be a case of complete androgen insensitivity syndrome. A genetic male may have undervirilization and present with underdeveloped and ambiguous genitalia as in 17α-hydroxylase deficiency or 3β-hydroxysteroid dehydrogenase deficiency. The appearance of the external genitalia does not always give any diagnostic clinical clues, e.g. an infant with ovotesticular DSD and a virilized female with genital ambiguity may look similar.

Ambiguous Genitalia

Ambiguous genitalia may be defined as discordance between the external genitalia and the gonads. If the genotype is XX, and the impalpable gonads are ovaries, but the external genitalia are virilized partially or fully, this is likely to be due to the exposure of a female fetus to excessive androgens during the period of sex differentiation in early gestation, e.g. CAH due to 21-hydroxylase deficiency, 11β-hydroxylase deficiency, 3β-hydroxysteroid dehydrogenase deficiency or maternal androgen excess due to a tumor or therapy **(Figs. 13.10.1 and 13.10.2)**. If the genotype is XY, the gonads which are palpable are testes, and the external genitalia is incompletely virilized or ambiguous; this may be due to a testosterone biosynthetic defect, or if the external genitalia is completely female, this may be a case of complete androgen insensitivity syndrome. If both ovarian and testicular tissues are present either in the same gonad (ovotestis) or opposite gonads—one gonad may be palpable or both gonads impalpable—this may be a case of ovotesticular DSD.

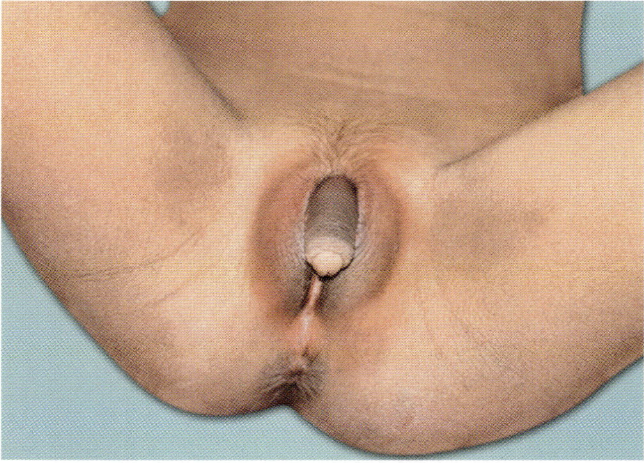

Fig. 13.10.1: A 3-year-old girl with marked clitoromegaly due to untreated congenital adrenal hyperplasia—21-hydroxylase deficiency (nonsalt-loser).

CLINICAL APPROACH TO AN INFANT WITH A DISORDER OF SEX DEVELOPMENT

Clinical evaluation of the infant with a suspected DSD should be done to decide assignment of sex and to plan the long-term management of the infant's condition. However, it is highly essential to rule out associated life-threatening metabolic conditions, such as adrenal insufficiency.

History taking should include details regarding parental consanguinity, maternal drug intake, history of previous sibling deaths due to salt loss in the neonatal period, affected siblings or family members with DSD, history of low birth weight or intrauterine growth retardation, and X-linked mode of inheritance (in the cases of androgen insensitivity).

Physical assessment should include examination for dysmorphic features, midline defects in the cases of microphallus due to pituitary defects **(Figs. 13.10.3 and 13.10.4)**; hypo- or hypertension, dehydration, virilization in the case of girls; undervirilization in the case of boys; presence or absence of gonads, hyperpigmentation of the skin, etc.

Severe hyponatremia, hyperkalemia, dehydration, hypotension, and shock usually in the second week after birth, with increased pigmentation of the skin in a virilized female infant or an infant with normal male genitalia strongly suggests the possibility of CAH due to salt-losing 21-hydroxylase deficiency **(Fig. 13.10.1)**. Non-salt-losers with this condition will present with the combination of increased pigmentation and virilization but without the dramatic signs of salt loss.

Female infants presenting with increased pigmentation, hypokalemia, hypertension, and virilization are most likely to have 11β-hydroxylase deficiency **(Fig. 13.10.2)**. These signs may not be present universally, especially during infancy. Boys with this condition will exhibit subtle changes in the external genitalia. Low cortisol and rennin values are encountered.

If physical examination reveals the presence of a gonad, it is most often a testis, and the infant is a case of 46,XY DSD. If there is no gonad palpable, the genetic sex cannot be identified clinically, and further workup is essential.

The phallus is measured for its length and width of erectile tissue and examined for chordee. Presence of separate openings of vagina and urethra should be looked for as also pigmentation and rugosity of labioscrotal folds.

It is often the responsibility of the pediatric endocrinologist or primary-care physician to inform the parents of an infant born with uncertain gender and to discuss with them in detail about the nature of the defect observed, the need for the investigations to establish the diagnosis, the gender of

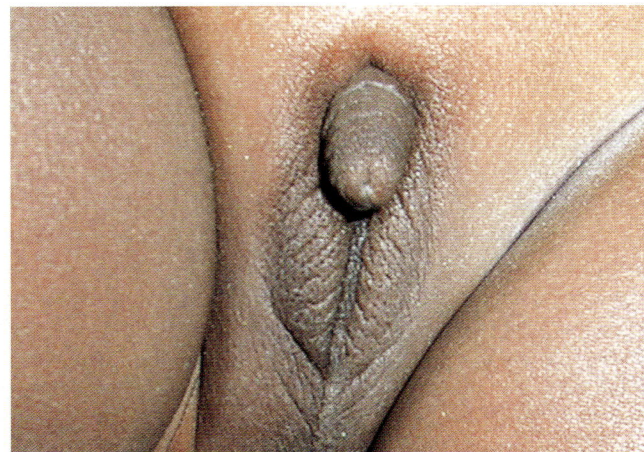

Fig. 13.10.3: Hypogonadism with microphallus in a 2-year-old boy with panhypopituitarism.

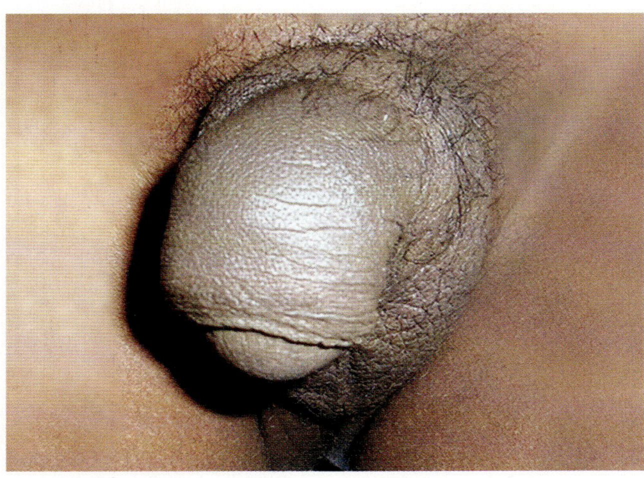

Fig. 13.10.2: Marked virilization external genitalia in a 4-year-old girl with 11β-hydroxylase deficiency.

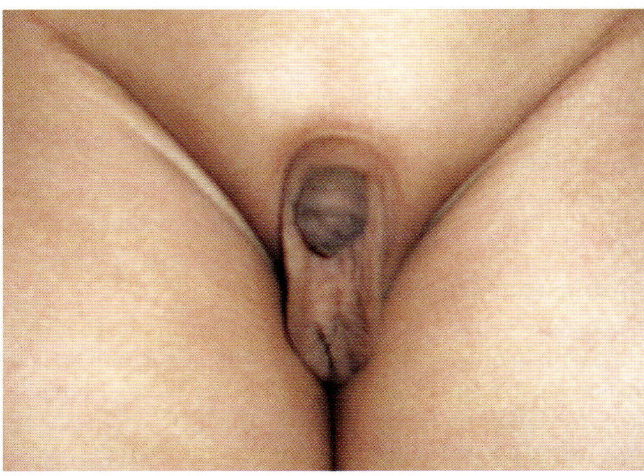

Fig. 13.10.4: A 1-year-old boy with severe hypogonadism due to panhypopituitarism.

rearing best suited for the infant. It is important to allay the anxiety and guilt of the parents and other family members in repeated sessions and to explain the available modalities and plan of treatment. To deal with the DSD optimally, a full team is ideal, viz. pediatric endocrinologists, neonatologists, family pediatricians, pediatric surgeons or urologists, gynecologists, radiologists, ultrasonologists, biochemists, cytogeneticists, pediatric psychologist/psychiatrists as well as nursing colleagues, and social workers. Support group of parents with similarly affected children will also be helpful. Most importantly, the parents should be included in all discussions concerning the evaluation and management of the infant with a DSD. It is always important to collect together all possible evidence for arriving at a diagnosis and then have discussions with the parents. Although urgency is still necessary, most parents will be willing to wait for a few days longer before making their decision about their child's future. Until the decision is made, it is better to refer to the infant as "baby," and not as "he" or "she."

INVESTIGATIONS

- Serum sodium, potassium
- Blood glucose
- Arterial blood gases
- Serum 17-hydroxyprogesterone
- Plasma renin activity (PRA)
- Serum cortisol
- Serum dehydroepiandrosterone sulfate
- Serum testosterone
- Ultrasound pelvis and abdomen
- Retrograde genitogram
- Karyotype
- Laparoscopy
- Urine analysis for albumin.

MANAGEMENT

The most common cause of ambiguous genitalia is 21-hydroxylase deficiency in genetic females. Nearly 75% present with salt loss typically during the second week of life. Hyperpigmentation of the skin, especially the nipples, umbilicus, and external genitalia should alert one to the diagnosis even before salt-losing manifestations appear. This clinical sign is particularly useful in males with CAH as they do not present with any abnormality of the external genitalia but have a high risk of shock due to salt loss. In the presence of the history of a previous sibling or family member involved, biochemical investigations may be performed earlier to hasten the diagnosis.

Virilized females with CAH having a uterus and ovaries are assigned the female gender. Clitoral reduction and genitoplasty are usually undertaken around 1 year of age, and care is taken to preserve the glans and the neurovascular bundle. Recommendations for assignment of gender in an individual with fully virilized male external genitalia and presence of female internal sex structures are still controversial. Reconstructive surgery for hypospadias is needed in those with 5α-reductase deficiency at the time of puberty. Assignment of a female gender to an individual with microphallus and fused scrotum is being reconsidered and not always accepted today by many. Testosterone therapy is recommended for microphallus and fused scrotum. In summary, there are no easy answers always for the assignment of gender in DSD.

BIBLIOGRAPHY

1. Brown J, Warne G. Practical management of the intersex infant. J Paediatr Endocrinol Metab. 2005;18(1):3-23.
2. Dreger AD, Chase C, Sousa A, et al. Changing the nomenclature/taxonomy for intersex: a scientific and clinical rationale. J Pediatr Endocrinol Metab. 2005;18(8):729-33.
3. Hughes IA, Houk C, Ahmed SF, et al. LWPES Consensus Group; ESPE Consensus Group. Consensus statement on management of intersex disorders. Arch Dis Child. 2006;91(7):554-63.
4. Lee PA, Nordenstrom A, Houk CP, et al. Global disorders of sex development update since 2006: perceptions, approach and care. Horm Res Paediatr. 2016;85:158-80.

13.11 Diabetes Mellitus

Vijayalakshmi Bhatia

INTRODUCTION

Diabetes mellitus is a common disorder of fuel metabolism. In children, it is most frequently due to an absolute deficiency of insulin secretion, due to destruction of the beta cells of the pancreatic islets. The disease is associated with many short- and long-term complications, many of which are linked with the degree of blood glucose (BG) control. In addition, diabetes in childhood and adolescence affects growth and puberty, and often psychological well-being. Diabetes is best managed by a team of personnel including a diabetes nurse/educator, dietician, and psychologist in addition to the physician.

CLASSIFICATION AND DIAGNOSTIC CRITERIA

Diabetes mellitus is not a single entity. It is a group of disorders of varying etiologies and pathogenesis, resulting in the same metabolic syndrome. The World Health Organization (WHO) in 1997 published a classification of diabetes based on etiology (**Box 13.11.1**). The typical insulin-dependent, ketosis-prone patient is classified as having type 1 diabetes. The non-insulin-requiring, non-ketosis-prone, usually, obese patient seen during adolescence is classified as type 2 diabetes. Pediatricians in India may occasionally encounter an additional type of diabetes that is due to a calcific chronic pancreatitis, which may clinically be insulin dependent or noninsulin dependent, which is classified under "diseases of the pancreas." Another type of diabetes presentation seen in the developing countries is that of a nonobese patient requiring insulin for glucose control but not exhibiting ketosis when off insulin. This was earlier termed "protein-deficient pancreatic diabetes" by the WHO. This terminology has largely been discarded now, as no direct role of protein deficiency in the etiology of permanent diabetes has been found. This entity has not found a place in the current classification because its etiology is not clear.

The cut-off limits for the diagnosis of diabetes mellitus have also been lowered in the last decade (**Box 13.11.2**). Most children with diabetes present with classical symptoms, and hence need only two random BG values to confirm the diagnosis.

Only type 1 diabetes will be further discussed.

Box 13.11.1: Etiological classification of diabetes mellitus.

- *Type 1 diabetes*:
  - Immune mediated
  - Idiopathic
- Type 2 diabetes
- *Other specific types*:
  - *Genetic defects of beta-cell function*:
    - HNF-1 alpha, 4 alpha, and 1 beta; glucokinase; IPF-1; and NeuroD1 (formerly MODY3, 1, 5, 2, 4, and 6)
    - Mitochondrial DNA, KCNJ11 (Kir 6.2)
  - *Genetic defects in insulin action*:
    - Type-A insulin resistance, leprechaunism, Rabson-Mendenhall syndrome, lipoatrophic diabetes
  - *Diseases of exocrine pancreas*:
    - Fibrocalcific pancreatopathy, cystic fibrosis, hemochromatosis, pancreatitis
  - *Endocrinopathies*:
    - Cushing syndrome, pheochromocytoma, hyperthyroidism, gigantism/acromegaly
  - *Drug or chemical induced*:
    - Pentamidine, glucocorticoids, phenytoin, thiazides, diazoxide, interferon-alpha, nicotinic acid, thyroid hormone, beta-adrenergic agonist, l-asparaginase
  - *Infections*
    - Congenital rubella, cytomegalovirus, enterovirus
  - *Uncommon forms of immune-mediated diabetes*:
    - IPEX and APECED syndromes, Stiffman syndrome, anti-insulin receptor antibodies
  - *Other genetic syndromes associated with diabetes*:
  - Down, Klinefelter, Turner, Wolfram, Friedreich ataxia, Laurence-Moon-Biedl, Prader-Willi, myotonic dystrophy
- Gestational diabetes mellitus

(HNF: hepatocyte nuclear factor; IPF: insulin promoter factor; MODY: maturity onset diabetes of young; KCNJ: potassium voltage-gated channel subfamily member 11; Kir: potassium inward rectifier; IPEX: immune dysregulation, polyendocrinopathy, enteropathy, X-linked syndrome; APECED: autoimmune polyendocrinopathy candidiasis ectodermal dysplasia)

TYPE 1 DIABETES MELLITUS

Epidemiology

The prevalence of diabetes among school children (up to 18 years of age) in the USA is approximately 1 in 500. Reliable prevalence and incidence data from India are not available. The incidence of new cases varies with geographical location, being highest in Finland and Sweden (40 per 100,000 children per year) and lowest in Japan (less than 1 per 100,000 children

Box 13.11.2: Diagnostic criteria for diabetes mellitus.

- Symptoms of diabetes plus random plasma glucose ≥ 200 mg/dL (on two separate occasions, if symptoms not typical or hyperglycemia not unequivocal) or
- Fasting plasma glucose ≥ 126 mg/dL on two occasions or
- Two-hour plasma glucose ≥ 200 mg/dL during oral glucose tolerance test on two occasions (glucose load 1.75 g/kg) or
- HbA_{1c} > 6.5% (taking care the laboratory reporting the HbA_{1c} uses an NGSP-certified technique standardized to the DCCT) (since HbA_{1c} alone as a criterion is not yet well documented in children, this may be considered along with one of the above criteria)

(DCCT: Diabetes Control and Complications Trial; HbA_{1c}: glycosylated hemoglobin; NGSP: National Glycohemoglobin Standardization Program)

per year). Boys and girls are equally at risk. The incidence in the European countries is increasing at the rate of 3% per year.

Etiology and Pathogenesis

Type 1 diabetes is a chronic autoimmune disease involving only the beta cells, with gradual loss of insulin secretion. Patients have a genetic predisposition to the disease, though only a few subjects so predisposed develop the disease. It is thought that an environmental factor is necessary to trigger the onset of autoimmunity. Autoimmune destruction is a slow process, and the decline in insulin production occurs over a period of months to years, overt diabetes becoming manifest when beta-cell reserve is below 20% of normal.

Genetics of Type 1 Diabetes

The inheritance of diabetes is polygenic. In comparison to a 0.6% lifetime risk (for a white Caucasian) to develop diabetes, a sibling of a proband may be said to have a 3–6% risk of developing diabetes, and an offspring a 2–6% risk (with a diabetic father conferring greater risk than a diabetic mother). The major susceptibility loci are the human leukocyte antigen (HLA) class II genes, and the insulin gene. Other important loci are the cytotoxic T-lymphocyte antigen 4 (CTLA4), protein tyrosine phosphatase *N22 (PTPN22)*, and the interleukin 2 receptor alpha *(IL2RA* or *CD25)* genes. Genome-wide association studies have shown that greater than 14 loci contribute to the risk of type 1 diabetes. In almost all races, HLA-DR3-DQ2 and DR4-DQ8 antigens are associated with increased risk of type 1 diabetes, whereas HLA-DR15/DQ6 confers protection.

Environmental Factors

Viruses, especially coxsackie and other enteroviruses, are the most commonly implicated environmental factor. Evidences include seasonal differences in the incidence of diabetes and episodes of viral infection frequently preceding the onset of diabetes. However, the only viral infection directly predisposing to diabetes is congenital rubella infection, in which 20% of affected children develop diabetes. Other proposed environmental agents include the role of early weaning to cow's milk (through albumin/casein), toxins (e.g. nitrosamines), and stress. Environmental factors may induce autoimmunity by molecular mimicry or by directly stimulating cytokine production.

Pathogenesis of Autoimmune Destruction

Numerous evidences exist for an autoimmune etiology of type 1 diabetes. Diabetes is frequently associated with conditions of known autoimmune etiology, such as Hashimoto thyroiditis, pernicious anemia, and Addison disease. It is also associated with the presence of many autoantibodies. About 80–90% of newly diagnosed type 1 diabetes patients (30–40% in India) have islet cell antibodies. A similar number is also positive for antibodies against glutamic acid decarboxylase, an enzyme present in the islet and other neuroendocrine tissue. Anti-insulin autoantibodies are present in 30–40% of newly diagnosed patients. Other important islet antibodies include islet antigen 2 (against tyrosine phosphatase) and zinc transporter 8 (against a zinc transporter). Studies in siblings of type 1 diabetes probands have shown that 60–80% of first-degree relatives positive for more than two autoantibodies go on to develop diabetes within 5 years. Lastly, abnormalities in "T" lymphocyte function exist in type 1 diabetes patients and animal models. With these evidences, a clearer picture of the pathogenesis is emerging. Some crucial antigen(s) of the beta cell, presented by the antigen presenting cells of the immune system, are presented to specific "T" lymphocytes in conjunction with specific HLA-D locus molecules. The activation of "T" lymphocytes sets off a series of responses including cytokine production, which amplify the immune response, ultimately resulting in beta-cell destruction.

The evidence of the autoimmune nature of type 1 diabetes, together with the possibility, albeit imperfect, of predicting which siblings of a proband will go on to develop diabetes, have led to the commencement of many trials (using insulin, nicotinamide, etc.) for the prevention of type 1 diabetes. A discussion of these is beyond the scope of this book. It may be said that all trials for the prevention of type 1 diabetes are at best experimental at present.

Pathophysiology

Insulin acts mainly on three tissues: liver, muscle, and adipose tissue. It induces glucose uptake, glycogen synthesis, and lipogenesis in the liver and stops gluconeogenesis. In muscle, insulin brings about glucose uptake and oxidation, and glycogen synthesis. In adipose tissue, glucose uptake and lipid synthesis occur. Thus in diabetes mellitus, hyperglycemia results due to glycogenolysis, gluconeogenesis, lipolysis, and absence of glucose uptake. Concomitant rise in the counterregulatory hormones (glucagon, epinephrine, cortisol, and growth hormone) aggravates hyperglycemia and ketogenesis. While lipolysis is caused by insulin deficiency, enhanced oxidation of the fatty acids so produced is induced by glucagon. Glucagon induces the carnitine palmitoyl transferase system of enzymes, which translocates fatty acids into mitochondria for beta oxidation, and thus causes ketogenesis.

When BG exceeds the renal threshold of 180 mg/dL, glycosuria, diuresis, electrolyte loss, dehydration, and hyperosmolality result. Untreated, dehydration and acidosis cause cerebral obtundation as well as circulatory failure.

Clinical Features

Diabetes in childhood typically presents with polyuria, polydipsia, polyphagia, weight loss, and weakness. Ketoacidosis is heralded by vomiting, dehydration, abdominal pain, deep and rapid (Kussmaul) respiration, and the fruity odor of acetone in the breath. Ketoacidosis may mimic an abdominal surgical emergency. Severe acidosis is accompanied by decreasing consciousness and hypotension. The presence of fever is an important clue to infection.

Laboratory findings include glycosuria, hyperglycemia, ketonemia, and ketonuria. Leukocytosis may be present without infection. Hypertriglyceridemia is typical. Diabetic ketoacidosis (DKA) is usually characterized by normal serum sodium, normal, low or initially raised serum potassium, significant ketonemia (blood ketone >0.6 mmol/L), blood pH < 7.3, and bicarbonate < 15 mEq/L. The metabolic acidosis of DKA exhibits an increased anion gap (>10 mmol), due to unmeasurable anions of ketoacids.

Diagnosis

In a patient who presents with the classical symptoms of polyuria, thirst, and weight loss, the diagnosis of diabetes is straightforward and requires only the demonstration of hyperglycemia. In a child with an accidental finding of glycosuria, one must differentiate diabetes mellitus from renal glycosuria or Fanconi syndrome. In a sick child with a severe systemic illness, such as sepsis, stress-induced (temporary) hyperglycemia may be encountered. Ketonuria can occur in starvation and, in adolescents, after an alcohol binge on an empty stomach. Both these conditions will not be accompanied by hyperglycemia, and ketonemia will be mild.

The child presenting with acidosis must be differentiated from other causes of metabolic acidosis with increased anion gap, such as uremia, lactic acidosis, and salicylate poisoning. Every child presenting in a coma must have a BG and urine ketone test to detect DKA.

MANAGEMENT

Management of diabetes mellitus includes treatment of DKA, postacidosis therapy in hospital, and management of diabetes at home.

Treatment of Ketoacidosis

Initial laboratory evaluation should include BG, blood and/or urine ketone, serum sodium, potassium, chloride, bicarbonate, calcium, phosphorus, arterial blood gas analysis, electrocardiogram, and blood culture and urine microscopic examination. The bladder should be catheterized in comatose patients.

In mild DKA (with BG 200–250 mg/dL, mild dehydration, pH 7.2–7.3, and bicarbonate 10–15 mmol/L), the child can be given oral rehydration with appropriate (sugar-free) fluid and subcutaneous insulin therapy started as below (see postacidosis insulin therapy).

Treatment of Severe Diabetic Ketoacidosis

Fluid and Electrolytes

The child in DKA is usually moderately to severely dehydrated. Therefore the quantity of deficit fluid to be replaced is 75–85 mL/kg of current weight. Of this, 10 mL/kg is given over the first hour if the child is hypotensive, and a higher rate of 20 mL/kg within the first hour is given to establish circulatory stability. The remainder of the deficit fluid is given evenly over the next 48 hours, along with the maintenance for the period.

Sudden introduction of hypoosmolal fluids has been implicated in the etiology of cerebral edema, a dreaded complication of DKA. The most commonly used approach in children is to start therapy with normal saline, but to switch to half normal saline (N/2) after the first 6 hours or so. Potassium (40 mEq/L) should be added to the infusion as soon as urine formation is ascertained, after the first hour of fluids, as body potassium is severely depleted in DKA. It may be temporarily delayed, if there is evidence of hyperkalemia on the electrocardiogram.

Though total body phosphorus is also depleted in DKA, and acute severe hypophosphatemia can have serious consequences, administration of phosphorus has not been shown to alter the course of the patient, on critical evaluation of available studies. Recent recommendations advise phosphorus administration in the form of potassium phosphate for half the potassium replenishment, taking care to monitor serum calcium frequently.

Alkali Therapy

Unnecessary alkali therapy in DKA is dangerous. It can precipitate cerebral edema by increasing central nervous system acidosis, precipitating hypokalemia, shifting the oxygen dissociation curve to the left, and causing alkalosis. Treatment of shock and adequate fluid therapy will automatically take care of acidosis. Sodium bicarbonate may be indicated for symptomatic hyperkalemia or if the blood pH persists at less than 6.9 after the first hour of rehydration, with cardiovascular instability. The dose to be infused is calculated by the formula: (mL of sodium bicarbonate = 0.15 × base deficit × kg-body weight). The amount (usually 40 mL) is never given as a bolus, but added to an N/2 infusion over 2 hours. Alkali therapy should be stopped when pH is greater than 7.0.

Insulin Therapy

The continuous low-dose insulin infusion is the method of choice for treating children with DKA. Regular insulin, 0.1 U/kg, is given as a continuous normal saline infusion at the rate of 0.1 U/kg/h (recent recommendations do not advise an insulin bolus for children). The goal is to slowly decrease the BG by 50–100 mg/dL every hour. The infusion of insulin is stopped only when acidosis has normalized, not just after normalization of hyperglycemia. Therefore when BG decreases to 200–250 mg/dL, 5% dextrose is added to the intravenous fluid infusion.

After correction of acidosis (which may take 24 hours or longer in severe DKA), the child is ready to be started on subcutaneous insulin therapy. An initial dose (0.2–0.4 U/kg) of regular insulin is given, half an hour after which the insulin infusion is stopped and the child allowed eating. Such a regimen of insulin plus meal is carried out every 6–8 hours until the child can be reliably predicted to eat, after which twice daily doses of regular plus intermediate-acting [neutral protamine Hagedorn (NPH)] insulin before breakfast and dinner are started, with a lunchtime dose of regular insulin and a small dose at evening snack time, if needed.

Monitoring during Diabetic Ketoacidosis

Clinical parameters such as vital signs, hydration, sensorium, pupils, urine output, fluid infused, insulin infusion rate, etc., must be monitored every hour, and a flow sheet should be carefully maintained. Capillary BG by finger prick should be done at the bedside every hour initially and later every 2 hours. Serum sodium, potassium, and bicarbonate should be measured every 4 hours initially and later 6 hourly. Urine ketones, serum phosphorus, and calcium may be done every 8–12 hours. Urine ketones may seem to worsen or persist for long, despite clinical improvement. This is because with insulin therapy, β-hydroxybutyrate, an unmeasured ketone present in larger quantities in DKA, is converted to acetone and acetoacetate, the measured ketones. This should not be interpreted as indicative of worsening.

Complications of Diabetic Ketoacidosis

Cerebral edema: Clinically symptomatic cerebral edema occurs in 1–2% of children with DKA and has a high mortality of 50%. It usually occurs during insulin therapy, when the child appears to be responding to treatment. The etiology is not clear but has been linked to too rapid correction of hyperosmolality, excessive use of alkali, high initial blood urea and greater hypocapnia, and lack of rise of serum sodium during treatment. Early signs include change in sensorium (drowsiness or agitation), headache, vomiting, comparative decrease in heart rate, or increase in blood pressure. Pupillary changes, papilledema, and upgoing plantar reflex are late signs. Prompt therapy with mannitol (without necessarily waiting for a confirmatory computed tomography scan) is indicated at the earliest suspicion.

Others: These include acute gastric dilatation or erosive gastritis, cerebral venous thrombosis, and respiratory distress syndrome.

POSTACIDOSIS THERAPY

After stabilization of the acidotic state, the following issues must be addressed:

- Management of precipitating factor for DKA, such as infection or emotional stress
- Subcutaneous insulin therapy
- Nutrition
- Education of the family for home management of diabetes
- Psychological and social support for the patient and the family.

Subcutaneous Insulin Therapy

Subcutaneous insulin therapy should be started when acidosis subsides. A mixture of regular and intermediate-acting (NPH) insulin can be given twice a day, half an hour before breakfast and dinner, with additional regular insulin doses at lunchtime and evening snack. Premixed insulin (e.g. 30/70 or 50/50) is not suitable for use in type 1 diabetes. This least expensive schedule may be modified if the (costlier) insulin analogs are used. The total daily dose (0.5–1.0 U/kg) is roughly divided into half to be given as NPH insulin, and half as regular insulin. These are just initial guidelines. From the next day, doses should be titrated according to BG responses, obtained the previous day. In most instances, for the first 1–2 months, much higher doses of insulin (1.5–2 U/kg) are needed, which automatically comes down to about 0.5–1 U/kg, subsequently.

Insulins available in India contain 40 U/mL or 100 U/mL. Care must be taken to administer U40 insulin only with a U40 syringe, and likewise, U100 insulin must be matched with a U100 syringe. The two insulins (regular and NPH) can be drawn into the same syringe, first regular, followed by NPH, to be given as a single subcutaneous injection. Disposable insulin syringes have clearer markings and less dead space than glass syringes. Suitable sites for insulin injection are the back of upper arm, front of thigh, abdomen, and buttocks. The injection site must be different each time, to avoid lipodystrophy. Insulin is ideally stored in a refrigerator (never frozen). Families who do not have the facility can store it in a damp cloth in the coolest portion of the house, or in a clay pot with water.

In addition to insulin, analogs of insulin are now available, which have unique features providing greater flexibility and lower chances of hypoglycemia. Insulin lispro, aspart, and glulisine, which have minor amino acid differences from insulin, have a quicker onset and shorter duration of action than regular insulin. This makes them suitable for use in toddlers, who cannot be depended upon to eat at a particular time, as the injection can be given after the child has actually started eating. The analogs glargine and detemir are poorly soluble at the pH of subcutaneous tissue and hence are peakless. They provide basal 24-hour blood levels, without the extent of hypoglycemia found with NPH. Unfortunately, these analogs are costlier than regular and NPH insulins at the time of writing.

Nutrition

The ideal diet for a child with diabetes is nothing but a healthy meal plan for any member of the family, with the additional requirement of avoidance of simple sugars. The total daily calories should be calculated from age, weight, pubertal status, and recommended dietary allowance calculations, tempered with the knowledge of the child's dietary pattern before the illness. A rough guideline is 1,000 cal at 1-year age, and additional 100 cal/year of age after that, up to puberty. Approximately, 55–65% of calories should derive from carbohydrates, 15% from protein, and 20–30% from fat. Foods rich in fiber (whole pulses, whole grain cereal, vegetable, and fruit) should be encouraged as they have a low glycemic index. Foods rich in fat, especially saturated fat, are to be limited and trans fats to be avoided. The day's meal plan should be divided into three meals (breakfast, lunch, and dinner) and 2–3 snacks (midmorning, evening, and bedtime). However, these schedules can be tailored according to the individual needs of the child and family, with insulin doses adjusted accordingly. It must be borne in mind that the patient is a child, for whose emotional well-being, we must accept some flexibility in the *do's and don'ts* of dietary management. Hence, items with simple sugar or excess fat must be allowed on special occasions such as birthdays or festivals.

Monitoring

The importance of excellent BG control in minimizing, preventing, or delaying long-term complications of diabetes is now well established. To this end, it is essential for BG to be monitored frequently so as to take steps to prevent or treat high BG levels.

Home Monitoring

With the advent of glucose oxidase strips, BG can be measured at home using strips with a reflectance meter. Urine glucose (positive only when BG rises above 180–200 mg/dL) is less informative than BG testing. Unfortunately, BG testing is expensive, and for some families, it may be necessary to accept a profile of 3–4 days' BG values once or twice a month.

Ideally, capillary BG should be tested daily fasting, premeals and 2-hour postmeals, and midnight on many nights. Where cost of strips and compliance are major issues, postmeal BG may be tested on 1 day or 2 days a week. BG should also be tested to confirm symptoms of hypoglycemia, whenever possible. A high BG before a meal may be dealt with by taking a small additional dose of regular insulin. When BG is persistently high (>300 mg/dL) and on days of fever/other sickness, serum or urine must be tested for ketones. This rigorous schedule of testing requires a motivated patient and supportive family interested in excellent BG control. The pediatrician must be careful to individualize these instructions. **Box 13.11.3** describes the BG goals for intensive therapy as well as less intensive therapy.

Laboratory Monitoring

Home glucose monitoring does not give an integrated picture of BG control over the long term. This deficiency is made up by performing glycosylated hemoglobin measurement once in 3 months. It represents the fraction of hemoglobin to which glucose has got attached, over the lifespan of a red blood cell. The normal value in people without diabetes is 4–6%. A value of up to 7% in a patient indicates excellent BG control, particularly if it can be achieved without excessive swings of BG from high to low. A value between 7% and 8% is regarded as good, and greater than 8% indicates scope for much improvement.

Education of the Patient and Family

Blood glucose patterns in diabetes are not necessarily stable from day to day. Variations are brought about by changes in exercise and meal pattern, emotional status, etc. Thus successful therapy of diabetes is not possible without the patient and/or family assuming responsibility for day-to-day care. This requires that the family be educated in diabetes management techniques. Diabetes management, as well as teaching, is best carried by a team consisting of the doctor, diabetes nurse/educator, dietician, psychologist, and social worker. In addition to insulin therapy, nutrition, monitoring, and hypoglycemia, patients must be taught the importance of exercise as well as management during days of unrelated sickness. Perhaps the

Box 13.11.3: Goals of intensive therapy.

- HbA1c 6.0–7.5% (or even < 6% if using insulin pumps and continuous glucose-monitoring sensors)
- Premeal blood glucose and midnight 70–145 mg/dL
- Postmeal (2 hours) blood glucose 90–180 mg/dL
- Bedtime 120–180 mg/dL
- Nocturnal 80–160 mg/dL

(HbA1c: glycosylated hemoglobin)

single most important message for patients, in relation to sick days, is that insulin must not be stopped. On the other hand, insulin requirement may actually rise during illness.

COMPLICATIONS OF DIABETES

Hypoglycemic Reaction

Mismatch between insulin dose on the one hand, and meal and exercise on the other, results in hypoglycemia quite frequently in the life of a child with diabetes. Defined as a BG of less than 70 mg/dL, it is heralded by adrenergic symptoms, such as sweating, pallor, trembling, and tachycardia. Patients are taught to recognize these symptoms and institute treatment. If unrecognized, BG levels may drop further, leading to neuroglycopenic symptoms, such as drowsiness, confusion, coma, or seizures. Most often, though, the release of counter-regulatory hormones at a level of 55–60 mg/dL leads not only to the warning (adrenergic) signs but also to a rebound rise in BG.

Treatment of Hypoglycemia

It is always advisable to first confirm the symptoms of hypoglycemia with a BG test. For immediate rise in BG, simple sugar (5–10 g) in the form of sugar, glucose, fruit juice, or a carbonated drink must be taken. In addition, a small snack of protein plus carbohydrate must be eaten. The unconscious child with hypoglycemia can be treated at home with 0.5 mg (1.0 mg in the adolescent) of glucagon given subcutaneously. If glucagon is not available, the child should receive intravenous glucose in the nearest emergency center.

After an episode of severe hypoglycemia is treated, the family must assess the reasons for its happening. Preventable factors such as missed meals or exercise uncompensated with food, must be recognized. Necessary reductions in insulin dosage must be instituted, if hypoglycemia shows a recurring pattern.

Long-term Complications

Microvascular (affecting the eye, kidneys, and nerves) and macrovascular (causing cerebrovascular and coronary heart disease) complications are responsible for long-term morbidity and mortality in diabetes mellitus. Growth retardation and pubertal delay are additional issues in childhood and adolescent diabetes. Pathogenetic mechanisms implicated include glycosylation of proteins, abnormalities in the polyol pathway, growth factors, platelet function defects, hyperinsulinemia, and free radical-induced damage. While the pathogenesis of each is not yet perfectly clear, large follow-up studies such as the Diabetes Control and Complications Trial, have clearly established a strong correlation between poor BG control and frequency of complications. Thus the onus is on all those who care for children with diabetes, to encourage the best possible metabolic control. Intensive insulin therapy aimed at maintaining near normal BGs is, however, associated with three times greater risk of severe hypoglycemia (coma/convulsions) than conventional insulin therapy. Therefore it may not be advisable in young children in those families where frequent BG testing is not possible, for those with hypoglycemia unawareness, or for those who do not have constant access to emergency care.

Complications of diabetes usually do not set in before duration of diabetes of at least 3–5 years. Background retinopathy occurs in almost 90% after 15 year's duration, but vision-threatening (proliferative) retinopathy occurs in only 25% patients after 25 years. Similarly, end-stage renal disease occurs in 15–20% of patients after a similar duration. These figures have almost halved in the last three decades, the fall in complication rate being attributable to improved BG control due to availability of home BG testing strips. It has been hitherto believed that complications do not occur in the prepubertal diabetic child, irrespective of duration of diabetes. However, recent prospective studies indicate that this may not be entirely true, and that prepubertal children must be screened for complications after duration of diabetes of 3–5 years.

BIBLIOGRAPHY

1. American Diabetes Association (2018). Clinical practice recommendations. [online]. Available from www.diabetes.org. [Accessed October, 2018].
2. Atkinson MA, Bluestone JA, Eisenbarth GS, et al. How does type 1 diabetes develop?: the notion of homicide or β-cell suicide revisited. Diabetes. 2011;60(5):1370-9.
3. Daneman D. Type 1 diabetes. Lancet. 2006;367(9513):847-58.
4. Dunger DB, Sperling MA, Acerini CL, et al. ESPE/LWPES consensus statement on diabetic ketoacidosis in children and adolescents. Arch Dis Child. 2004;89(2):188-94.
5. Glaser N. Treatment of diabetic ketoacidosis: new perspectives on intravenous fluid protocols and risk of cerebral injury. Pediatr Diabetes. 2017;18(Suppl. S25):4.
6. Indian Society for Pediatric and Adolescent Endocrinology Type 1 diabetes mellitus in children and adolescents in India: clinical practice guidelines 2011. [online]. Available from http://www.ispae.org.in/download_docs/Diabetes_guideline_for_Web.pdf [Accessed October, 2018].
7. ISPAD. (2018). ISPAD clinical practice consensus guidelines 2018 compendium. [online]. Available from www.ispad.org. [Accessed October, 2018].
8. Rachmeil M, Perlman K, Daneman D. Insulin analogues in children and teens with type 1 diabetes: advantages and caveats. Pediatr Clin North Am. 2005;52(6):1651-75.
9. Reichard P, Nilsson BY, Rosenqvist U. The effect of long-term intensified insulin treatment on the development of microvascular complications of diabetes mellitus. N Engl J Med. 1993;329(5):304-9.

Section 14

Genetics

14.1 Basic Genetics

VH Sankar

INTRODUCTION

Genetics is the science of human biologic variation. Medical genetics is the application of this knowledge for understanding health and disease, while clinical genetics is the application for diagnosis, prevention and management of patients with genetic disorders.

Deoxyribonucleic acid (DNA) is the hereditary material, which is present in the nucleus of the cell. The DNA is packaged into 23 pairs of chromosomes in each cell. Nucleic acid is composed of a long polymer of individual molecules called nucleotides. Each nucleotide is composed of a nitrogenous base, a sugar molecule and, a phosphate molecule. The nitrogenous base falls into two types:

1. Purines (adenine and guanine) and
2. Pyrimidines (cytosine, thymine and uracil).

Gene, which is the fundamental unit of heredity, is a segment of DNA molecule, which codes for a polypeptide. Each human is estimated to have approximately 24,000 genes. Alterations in these genes alone or in combinations of them can produce genetic disorders. These disorders are classified into the following major groups:

- *Chromosomal disorders:* Entire chromosome or segments of them are missing, duplicated or altered. Examples: Down syndrome (DS), Turner syndrome.
- *Single gene disorders (also known as monogenic disorders):* Disorders in which single genes are altered—often called "Mendelian" conditions since they follow Mendelian mode of inheritance. Examples: thalassemia, spinal muscular atrophy, hemophilia.
- *Mitochondrial disorders:* A relatively small number of diseases are caused by alterations in the small cytoplasmic mitochondrial DNA and are inherited in a non-Mendelian fashion.
- *Multifactorial disorders:* Results from a combination of multiple genetic and environmental causes. Examples: Birth defects like cleft palate/cleft lip, neural tube defect, and common diseases like diabetes, psychiatric illnesses and hypertension.
- *Somatic cell genetic disorders:* Cancers are caused by additive effects of mutations in several genes in a somatic cell. Other disorders included in this group are autoimmune disorders and aging process.

IMPACT OF GENETIC DISEASES

The incidence of genetic disorders and their impact on health can be gauged from the following observations:

- A chromosomal abnormality is present in 40–50% of all recognized first trimester pregnancy losses
- In neonates, 2–3% have at least one major congenital malformation
- The incidence of chromosomal abnormalities and single gene disorders in neonates are approximately 0.5% and 1% respectively
- As per the neonatal perinatal database of the National Neonatology Forum (NNF), congenital malformations were the second most common cause (9.9%) of stillbirths and the fourth most common cause (9.6%) of neonatal mortality.
- Genetic disorders account for 50% of all cases of mental retardation and 50% cases of childhood deafness
- Approximately 5–10% of common cancers such as breast, colon and ovary have a strong genetic component
- All common disorders like hypertension, psychiatric illnesses, diabetes and coronary artery disease have a strong genetic susceptibility factor.

CHROMOSOMES AND CELL DIVISION

At conception, human cell zygote consists of a single cell. This undergoes rapid division leading ultimately to the mature human adult, consisting of approximately one hundred trillion (10^{14}) cells. This process of cell division is called mitosis. During mitosis, each chromosome divides into two daughter chromosomes and one will segregate to each cell. Mitosis is a continuous process lasting for 1–2 hours. However, for convenience of description, it is divided into five distinct stages:

1. Prophase,
2. Prometaphase,
3. Metaphase,
4. Anaphase, and
5. Telophase **(Fig. 14.1.1)**.

Meiosis is a specialized cell division process in which a diploid cell gives rise to haploid gametes. This occurs only in the final division of gametogenesis. In contrast to mitosis, meiosis occurs as two rounds of cell division (meiosis I and meiosis II) **(Fig. 14.1.2)**.

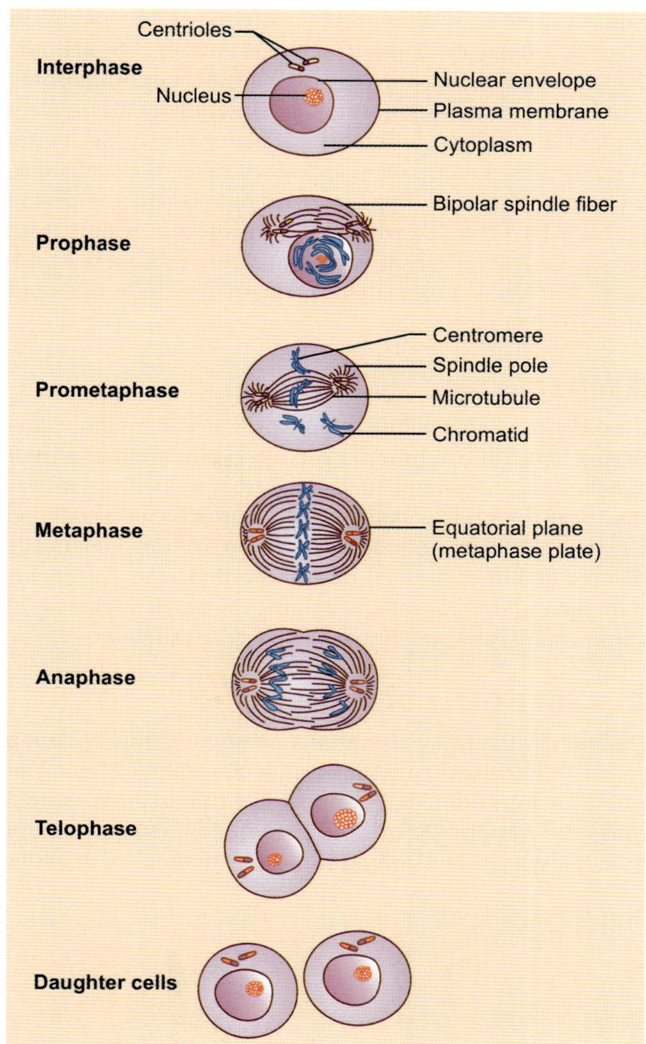

Fig. 14.1.1: The stages of mitosis resulting in two identical diploid cells formed from one original diploid cell.

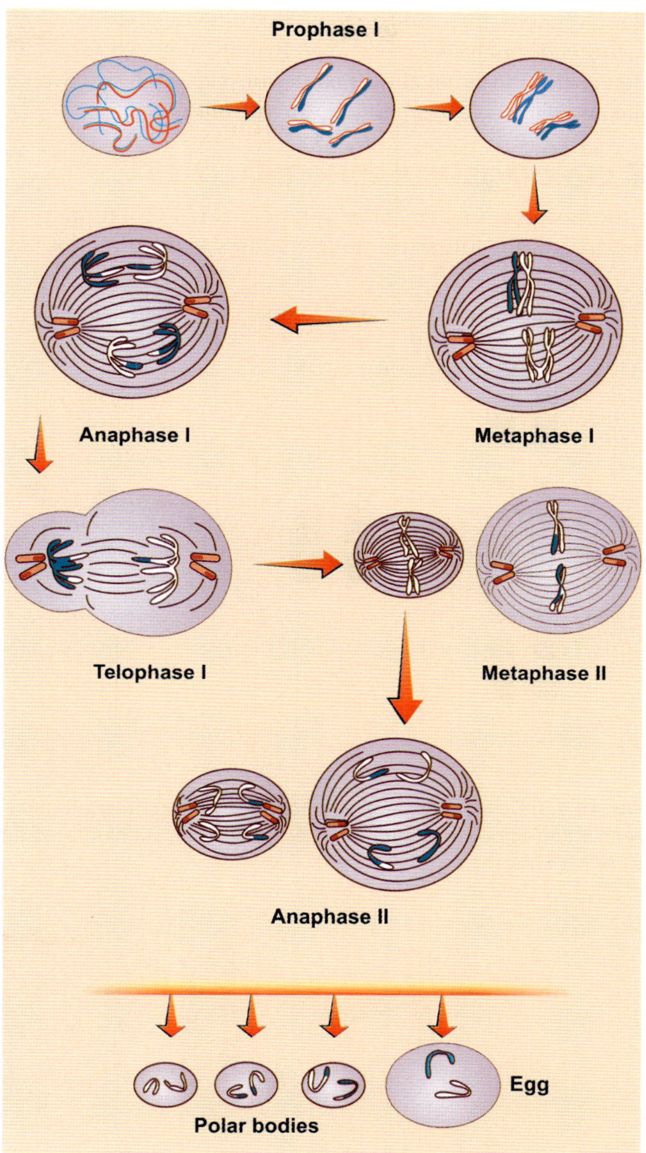

Fig. 14.1.2: The stages of meiosis during which haploid gametes are formed from a diploid cell.

The word "chromosome" is derived from the Greek words for "colored body". Human cells contain 46 chromosomes comprising 22 pairs of autosomes numbered from 1 to 22 and a pair of sex chromosomes (two X chromosomes in females and one X and one Y in males). The numbers are assigned in descending order of lengths of chromosomes and are classified into groups depending on the sizes of chromosomes and position of centromere in each chromosome. Each chromosome is made up of a short "p" arm and the longer "q" arm joined at the centromere. Various types of chromosomes are shown in **Figure 14.1.3**. The study of chromosomes is referred to as *cytogenetics.*

Karyotype refers to the orderly arrangement of chromosomes of one cell starting from the largest chromosome 1 to chromosome 22 followed by sex chromosomes. Chromosomes can be analyzed from any actively dividing cells. **Figure 14.1.4** shows a G-banded normal *karyotype*. The word "*karyotype*" is also used to describe the chromosome complement of an individual. For example, 46 XY means the individual has normal 46 chromosomes with one X and one Y chromosome. Newly developed molecular cytogenetic techniques such as fluorescent *in situ* hybridization (FISH) and microarray-based *cytogenetic* analysis do not need live dividing cells and can detect chromosomal abnormalities of very small size, which are not detectable by traditional *karyotyping*.

CHROMOSOME ABNORMALITIES

Chromosome abnormalities can be divided into numerical or structural. Numerical abnormalities involve the loss or gain of one or more chromosome, referred as aneuploidy. In trisomy, a single extra chromosome is present (DS—trisomy 21) whereas in monosomy, there is a loss of one chromosome (Turner syndrome—monosomy X). The addition of complete haploid set of chromosomes is called polyploidy. Structural chromosomal abnormalities include translocation, deletions, inversions, insertions, ring chromosome and isochromosome **(Table 14.1.1)**. A Robertsonian translocation results from breakage of two acrocentric chromosomes (numbers 13, 14, 15, 21 and 22) at or close to the centromere, with subsequent fusion of their long arms.

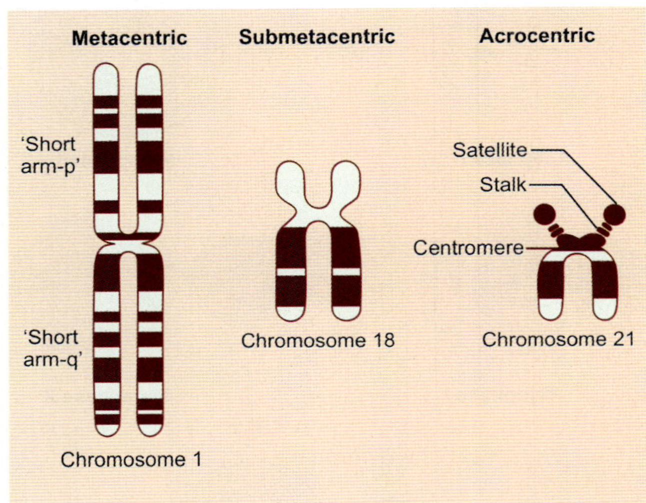

Fig. 14.1.3: *Different types of chromosomes:* Metacentric, submetacentric and acrocentric chromosomes. The classification is based on the location of the centromere.

MOSAICISM

Mosaicism is being defined as the presence in an individual or in a tissue of two or more cell lines, which differ in their genetic constitution but are derived from a single zygote, i.e. they have the same genetic origin. Chimeras can be defined as the presence in an individual of two or more genetically distinct cell lines derived from more than one zygote, i.e. they have different genetic origins. Mosaicism can be of chromosomal abnormality or a single gene mutation.

SINGLE GENE DISORDERS

Disorders caused by alterations in single genes are often called "Mendelian" conditions since they follow Mendelian mode of inheritance. Examples are thalassemia, spinal muscular atrophy (SMA) and hemophilia. Gregor Johann Mendel, who is considered to be the "father" of genetics

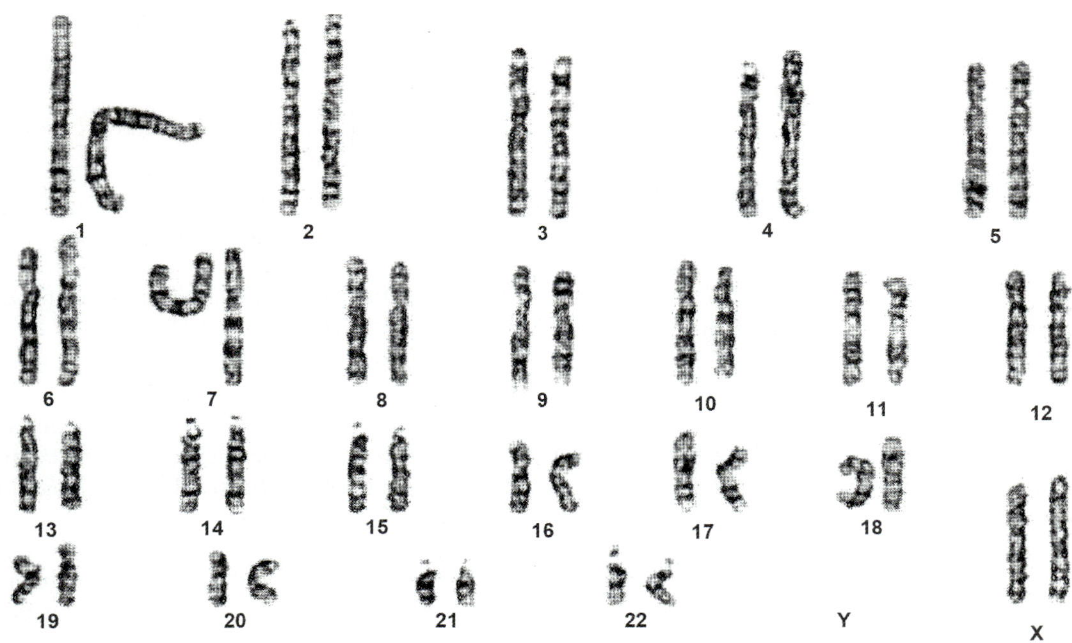

Fig. 14.1.4: G-banded karyotype of a normal female.

Table 14.1.1: Structural chromosomal abnormalities.

Type	*Description*	*Examples*
Deletions	A deletion involves loss of part of a chromosome results in monosomy for that segment of the chromosome	• Wolf-Hirschhorn syndrome (partial monosomy involving short arm of chromosome 4) • Cri du chat syndrome (partial monosomy involving short arm of chromosome 5)
Robertsonian translocation	This results from breakage of two acrocentric chromosomes (13, 14, 15, 21 and 22) at or close to the centromere with subsequent fusion of their long arms	Down syndrome due to translocation between chromosomes 14 and 21
Reciprocal translocation	This involves breakage of at least two chromosomes with exchange of the fragments	Ph chromosome: Involving chromosomes 9 and 22
Insertion	An insertion occurs when segment of one chromosome becomes inserted into another chromosome	
Inversion	An inversion is a two-break rearrangement involving a single chromosome in which a segment is reversed in position, i.e. inverted	Inversion can be *pericentric inversion* (involving centromere) or *paracentric inversion* (only one arm of the chromosome)

designed experiment on garden peas and formulated a series of fundamental principles of heredity. Two important principles include:

1. Principle of segregation, which states that sexually reproducing organisms possess genes that occur in pairs and that only one member of this pair is transmitted to the offspring (i.e. alleles on homologous chromosomes segregate).
2. Principle of independent assortment states that genes at different loci are transmitted independently.

BASIC CONCEPTS

Pedigree

Diagrammatic representation of family history is known as a pedigree. The symbols are used to depict males, females, their relationships and disease status **(Fig. 14.1.5)**. The affected individual who brings the family to notice is called as "proband" and the one who comes for genetic counseling is the "consultand".

Genotype and Phenotype

The term "genotype" has been defined as an individual's genetic constitution at a locus. The "phenotype", which is physically observable, results from interaction of genotype and environment.

Locus and Allele

The site of a gene on a chromosome is locus and allele is the alternative form of a gene found at the same locus on homologous chromosomes.

Dominance and Recessive

Dominance is not a property intrinsic to a particular allele but describes the relationship between it and the corresponding allele on the homologous chromosomes.

Heterozygote and Homozygote

An individual who possesses two different alleles (different versions of a gene) at one particular locus on a pair of homologous chromosomes is called *heterozygote*, whereas an individual who possesses two identical alleles at a particular locus on a pair of homologous chromosomes is called *homozygote*.

MENDELIAN INHERITANCE

A trait or disorder which is determined by a gene on an autosome is said to be followed an autosomal inheritance, whereas a trait or disorder determined by a gene on one of the sex chromosomes is said to be sex-linked disorder. Autosomal dominant (AD) disorders are those in which both heterozygous and homozygous individuals show the abnormal phenotype, and the disease is transmitted from one generation to the other **(Fig. 14.1.6)**. One copy of the mutant gene is sufficient for expression of the abnormal phenotype. An autosomal recessive disorder manifests only when both the copies of a gene are mutated in an individual and manifestations are seen in both male and female progeny of unaffected individuals. The autosomal recessive disorders usually manifest in the siblings and there is no clinically affected individual in generations above and below **(Fig. 14.1.7)**. Though, clinically normal both the parents of an individual with an autosomal recessive disorder are always

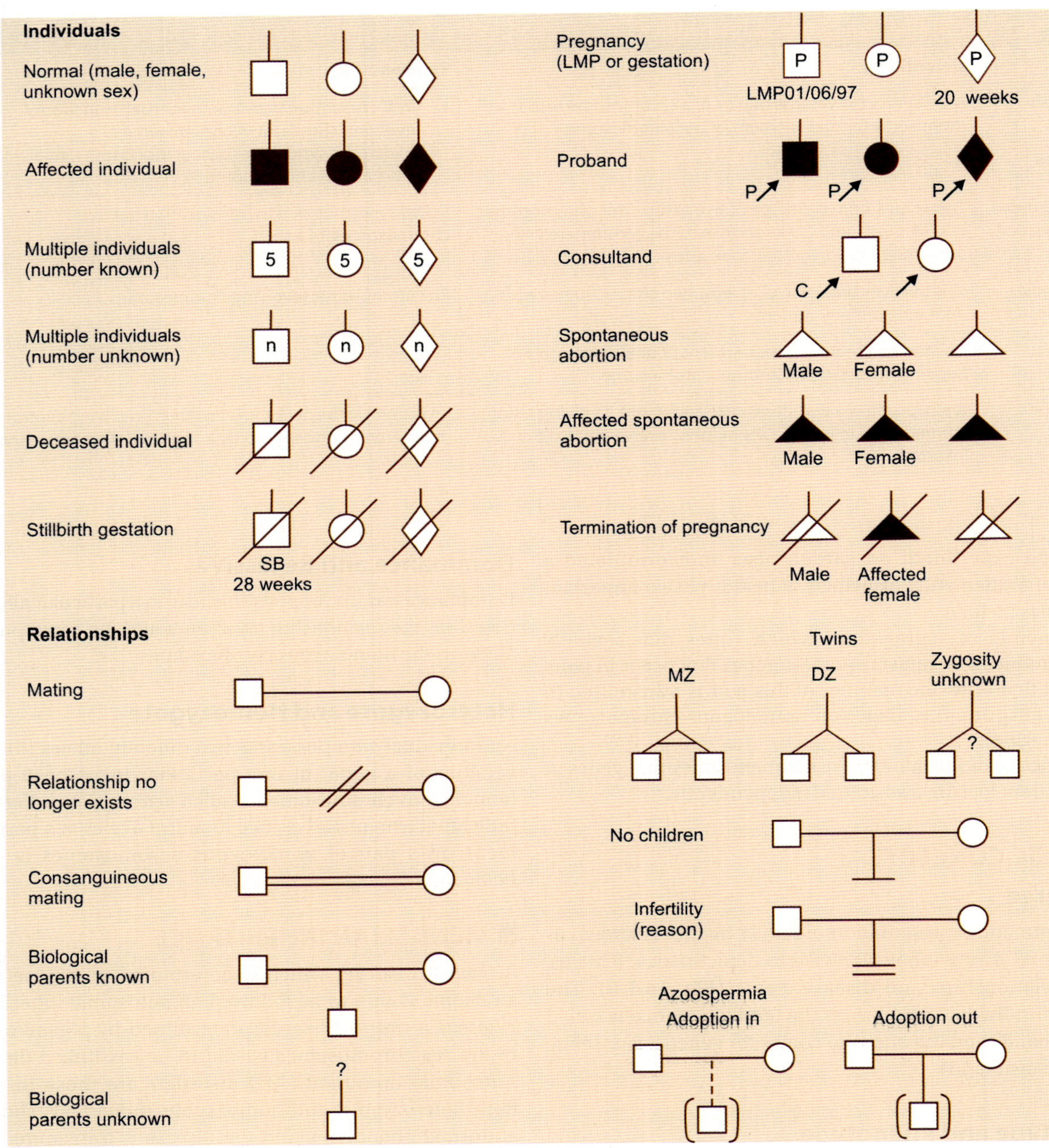

Fig. 14.1.5: Symbols for pedigree drawing.

heterozygous carriers. X-linked recessive inheritance is due to a gene present on the X chromosome, and manifest only in males **(Fig. 14.1.8)**. Affected males are related through carrier females. The X-linked disorders which manifest in heterozygous males and females are called X-linked dominant disorders **(Fig. 14.1.9)**. In this mode of inheritance, males and females are both affected, but the severity of disorder is usually less in females than males. The number of affected females is more than that of affected males. The Y-linked (holandric inheritance) implies that only males are affected (e.g. hairy ears). The characteristic pattern of each mode of inheritance is explained in the **Tables 14.1.2 and 14.1.3**.

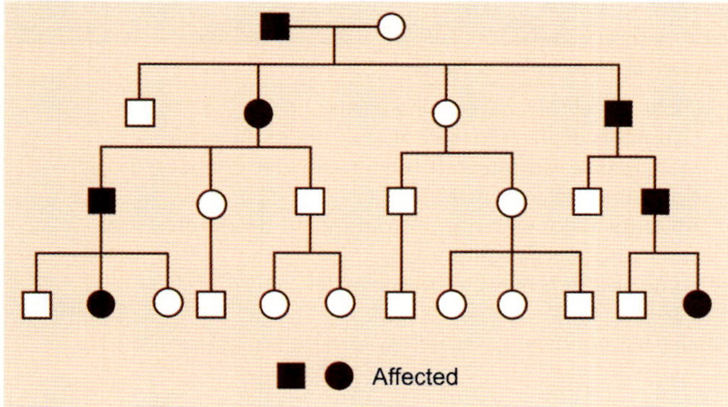

Fig. 14.1.6: A pedigree showing the inheritance of an AD inheritance. Solid symbols represent affected individuals.

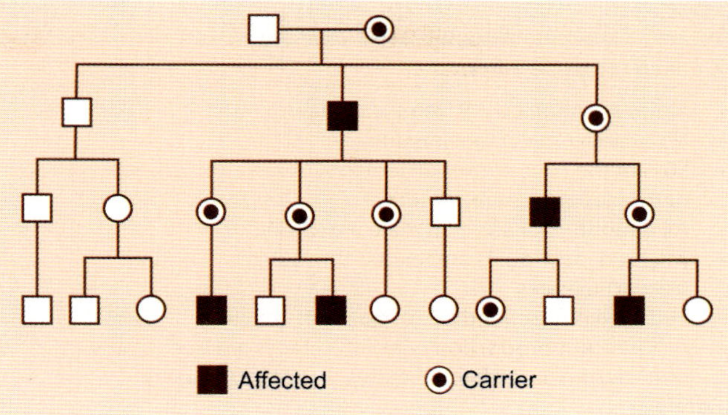

Fig. 14.1.8: A pedigree showing the inheritance of an X-linked recessive inheritance. Solid symbols represent affected individuals and dotted symbol represent heterozygous carriers. Note the oblique transmission.

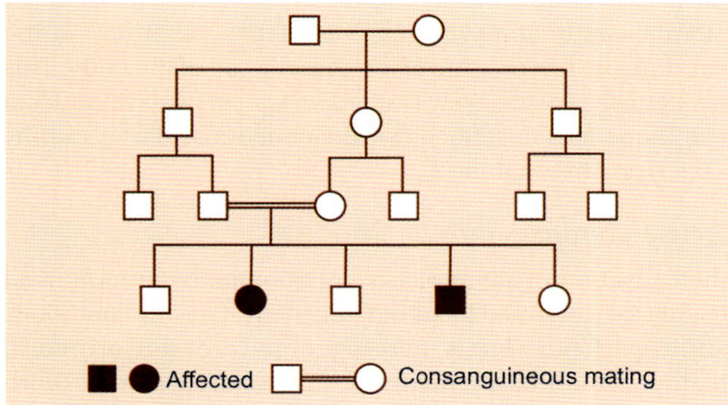

Fig. 14.1.7: A pedigree showing the inheritance of an autosomal recessive inheritance. Solid symbols represent affected individuals, double line indicates consanguinity. Note the horizontal transmission.

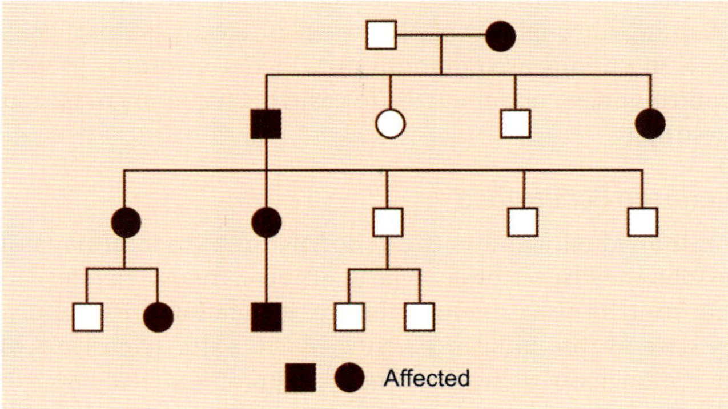

Fig. 14.1.9: A pedigree showing the inheritance of an X-linked dominant inheritance. Solid symbols represent affected individuals. Almost similar to AD but no male to male transmission.

Table 14.1.2: Characteristics of autosomal dominant inheritance and autosomal recessive inheritance.

Autosomal dominant inheritance	***Autosomal recessive inheritance***
• Successive or multiple generations in a family are affected • Males and females are both affected in approximately equal proportions • Males and females can both be responsible for transmission • There is at least one instance of male-to-male transmission *Examples:* • Neurofibromatosis (NF) • Tuberous sclerosis (TS) • Marfan syndrome • Familial hypercholesterolemia	• The disorder normally occurs in only one generation, usually within a single sibship • Both males and females are affected • The parents may be consanguineous *Examples:* • Thalassemia • Spinal muscular atrophy • Mucopolysaccharidosis

Mendelian Inheritance Pattern: Some Issues

New Mutation

A child may be born with an AD disorder without any similar diseases in parents or other family members (a sporadic case). This is usually due to new mutation in the affected child. A large proportion of observed AD disorders are due to new mutation. For example, it is estimated that 7 out of 8 cases of achondroplasia are caused by a new mutation. The recurrence risk for the individual's sibling is very low if the parents are

Table 14.1.3: Characteristics of X-linked recessive and X-linked dominant inheritance.

X-linked recessive inheritance	*X-linked dominant inheritance*
• Males are affected and females are carriers • No male-to-male transmission • 50% of the sons of the carrier females are affected; 50% of the daughters are carriers • All daughters of affected male are carriers • Affected individuals are related through transmitting (carrier) females • Pedigree is described as oblique transmission • A significant proportion of isolated cases are due to new mutations (some affected males do not reproduce) *Examples:* Hemophilia, Duchenne muscular dystrophy (DMD), Hunter syndrome	• Looks like autosomal dominant (AD) • Daughters of affected male always inherit the disorder • More females are affected, but have milder phenotype • No male-to-male transmission • Affected males with normal mates have no affected sons • and no normal daughters • Some disorders may be lethal in males *Examples:* Familial hypophosphatasia, Rett syndrome, Aicardi syndrome

normal, but it will be substantially high for the individual's offspring (50% in case of AD disorders like achondroplasia). New mutations are common in X-linked disorders as well contributing to about one-third cases of Duchenne muscular dystrophy.

Reduced Penetrance

An individual who has the genotype for a disease may not exhibit the disease phenotype at all, even though he/she can transmit the disease gene to the next generation. For example, in case of retinoblastoma, 10% of the obligate carriers of mutation in the retinoblastoma susceptibility gene do not get the disease and penetrance of the gene is then said to be 90%. Some genetic conditions like Huntington chorea, a delay in the age of onset of the disease may occur which is described as age-dependent penetrance.

Variable Expression

Here, penetrance may be complete, but the severity of the disease among affected family members may vary. The classical example is of tuberous sclerosis where a parent with milder manifestations like adenoma sebaceum may not be aware of the disease till his or her offspring develops seizures or *rhabdomyosarcoma*, which are severe manifestations of the same disease. The cause of variable expression may be environmental effects, or modifier gene (interaction of other genes).

Germline Mosaicism

Mosaicism describes presence of more than one genetically distinct cell lines in the body. When two or more offspring presented with an AD or an X-linked disease in family with no history of similar genetic disorder or carrier parent, the mechanism most likely to be responsible is germline mosaicism. During the embryonic development of one of the parents, a mutation occurred that affected all or part of the germline but few or none of the somatic cell of the body. This mechanism is extensively studied in osteogenesis imperfecta type II and also described in Duchenne muscular dystrophy (DMD) and hemophilia A.

Locus Heterogeneity

The causation of same disease phenotype by mutations at distinct loci is termed locus heterogeneity. Genetic conditions with significant locus heterogeneity are sensorineural deafness, retinitis pigmentosa, and Charcot-Marie-Tooth disease.

Pleiotropy

Genes that have more than one discernible effect on the body are said to be pleiotropic. A classic example of pleiotropic effects is Marfan syndrome: gene mutation affects eye, skeletal system and cardiovascular system.

Consanguinity

Because relatives share disease causing genes inherited from common ancestor, consanguinity is likely to be more frequent among the parents of an individual with an autosomal recessive disorder; especially so if the disorder in concern is rare. For genetic counseling, it is considered that prevalence of genetic diseases is roughly one to two times in the offspring of first-cousin marriages as compared to nonconsanguineous population. Quantification of sharing of genes between two relatives can be done by estimating the coefficient of relationship. This shows that sibling share ½ of their genes (first-degree relatives), uncle/aunt share ¼ of their gene (second-degree relatives) and first cousins share ⅛ of their genes (third-degree relatives), and so on.

Manifesting Female Carriers of X-linked Recessive Disorders

Although, female carriers of X-linked recessive disorders are usually asymptomatic, they can manifest the disease in following situations:

- *Homozygous for X-linked recessive disorders:* Female offspring of an affected father and a carrier mother.
- *Numerical X chromosome abnormalities:* Female carrier with only one X chromosome (Turner syndrome).
- *Female carrier with nonrandom or skewed X-inactivation:* In this situation, there is a departure from the normal random process of X-inactivation, with a greater proportion of normal X chromosome getting inactivated than the other one with a mutation of an X-linked disease.
- X-autosome translocation when the breakpoint of the translocation disrupts a gene on the X chromosome.

X-Inactivation (Lyon Hypothesis)

This states that one X chromosome in each cell is randomly inactivated early in the embryonic development of females. This would result in dosage compensation, an equalization of X-linked gene products in males and females.

Non-Mendelian Inheritance

Genomic Imprinting

One of the Mendel's law states that the phenotype is the same whether a given allele is inherited from father or the mother. Now, it has been recognized that different clinical features can result depending on whether the gene is inherited from the father or the mother. This "parent of origin" effect is referred to as genomic imprinting. Evidence of genomic imprinting has been classically observed in two dysmorphic syndromes associated with learning difficulties known as the Prader-Willi syndrome and Angelman syndrome. Prader-Willi syndrome is caused by absence of a small part of chromosome 15 of paternal origin, whereas the deletion of the same region on chromosome 15 from maternal origin gives rise to Angelman syndrome.

Uniparental Disomy

An individual normally inherits one of the pair of homologous chromosomes from each parent. On the contrary, if an individual inherits two copies of the same homologue from one parent, through an error in meiosis, this is called uniparental disomy (UPD). This mechanism has been identified as molecular pathology from a situation where a child with cystic fibrosis had only one parent who was carrier of cystic fibrosis mutation and the other parent was not carrier of cystic fibrosis. This mechanism is a cause in disorders of growth disturbances like Beckwith-Wiedemann syndrome (UPD of chromosome 11) and Silver-Russell syndrome (UPD chromosome 7).

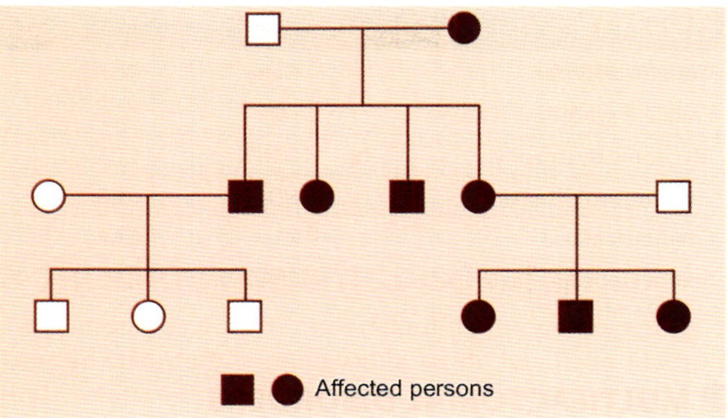

Fig. 14.1.10: A pedigree showing the inheritance of a disease caused by mitochondrial DNA mutation.

Mitochondrial Inheritance

Each human cell contains several hundreds of mitochondria in the cytoplasm. Mitochondria produce adenosine triphosphate (ATP), the energy source essential for cellular metabolism. They are having their own DNA molecule (mtDNA). Some important principles in mitochondrial inheritance are as follows:

- Since mtDNA is present in the cytoplasm, it is exclusively derived from the maternal side. The pattern of inheritance shown in the pedigree **(Fig. 14.1.10)** suggests that only females can transmit the disease to their offspring.
- The mutation rate in mitochondrial DNA is 10 times higher than that of nuclear DNA. The reason for this is high replication rate, lack of DNA repair and damage by oxygen-free radicals in mtDNA.
- Heteroplasmy indicates a cell with heterogeneous population of mitochondria with or without mutations. It often results in incomplete penetrance of mitochondrial inheritance.
- At the cellular level, the proportion of mutated mtDNA (mutation load) determines phenotypic expression called threshold of expression. Central nervous system (CNS) and heart need high energy are commonly involved in mitochondrial disorders.

Triplet Repeat Disorders

One assumption of Mendelian genetics is that mutant allele which is transmitted from parent to offspring unchanged. Recently, increasing number of disorders were identified in which the underlying mutation is an expansion of a triplet nucleotide repeat sequence that is unstable and can change in size on transmission from parent to offspring. The disorders with triplet repeat disorder are summarized in **Table 14.1.4**.

BIBLIOGRAPHY

1. Gardner RJM, Amor DJ. Chromosome Abnormalities and Genetic Counseling, 5th edition. Oxford: Oxford University Press; 2018.
2. Jorde LB, Carey JC, Bamshad MJ. Medical Genetics, 5th edition. Missouri: Mosby; 2015.
3. Keagle MB, Gersen SL. Principles of Clinical Cytogenetics, 2nd edition. New Jersey: Humana Press; 2005.
4. Koene S, Smeitink J. Mitochondrial medicine. J Inherit Metab Dis. 2011;34(2):247-8.
5. Phadke SR. Genetics for Clinicians, 1st edition. Bangalore: Prism Books; 2007.
6. Strachan T, Read AP. Human Molecular Genetics, 4th edition. Oxford: Garland Publishing; 2010.
7. Turnpenny PD, Ellard S. Emery's Elements of Medical Genetics, 15th edition. London: Churchill Livingstone; 2017.
8. Nussbuam RL, McInnes RR, Willard HF. Thompson & Thompson Genetics in Medicine, 7th edition. Philadelphia: Saunders Elsevier; 2007.

14.2 Clinical Dysmorphology

ML Kulkarni

INTRODUCTION

Dysmorphology is a word coined by Dr David W Smith in 1966 and is derived from the Greek words *"dys"* (disordered, abnormal) and *"morph"* (shape, form). Simply, it is the study of human congenital defects—abnormalities of body structure that originate before birth.

Individual birth defects are rare, but together they account for a large proportion of childhood mortality and morbidity. More than 4,000 dysmorphic; multiple congenital anomalies and mental retardation syndromes have been reported with more being added with time. About 1–3% of children are born with multiple or serious congenital defects. Knowledge and expertise are needed not only for identification of these serious defects but also other minor anomalies, which may give clues to a more serious underlying pathology. Prompt recognition of the condition helps in prognostications, investigations, treatment and also helps the family by way of genetic counseling about recurrence risk and prevention.

CLASSIFICATION OF DYSMORPHIC DEFECTS

It is probably impossible to know all the congenital defects and the associated conditions by heart; hence it is necessary to categorize them into manageable subdivisions. A *dysmorphic feature or anomaly* is an abnormality of shape, size or structure. These features are traditionally classified as *major* or *minor* anomalies. A *major anomaly* is one that has severe medical or cosmetic consequences if untreated, such as a congenital heart defect or a cleft lip. A *minor anomaly* represents a medically insignificant departure from normal development, such as wide-set eyes or a single palmar crease. Three or more minor malformations are associated with multiple major anomalies in 90% of the patients and hence warrant a thorough evaluation. Before ascribing an anomaly to be significant an astute clinician should first take into consideration the ethnical background and the familial occurrence.

Based on the pathogenesis birth defects can be classified as following:

- *Malformation:* Early embryological developmental error (e.g. Cleft palate)
- *Deformation:* Internal or external mechanical forces alters normally forming structure (e.g. Club foot)
- *Disruption:* Breakdown of a previously normal tissue (e.g. Amniotic band sequence) **(Fig. 14.2.1)**
- *Dysplasia:* Abnormal cellular organization within a tissue resulting in structural changes of organs containing the tissue involved (e.g. Achondroplasia).

When multiple birth defects are encountered, it is useful to classify them first in order to arrive at an appropriate diagnosis. The most commonly used system for classification is as follows:

- *Syndrome ("running together" in Greek):* A pattern of features, often with a unifying underlying cause that arise from several different errors in morphogenesis (e.g. Down syndrome). Most dysmorphic syndromes are a constellation of major and minor anomalies. The presence of only one feature is never diagnostic, but the unique combination gives the diagnosis of a syndrome.

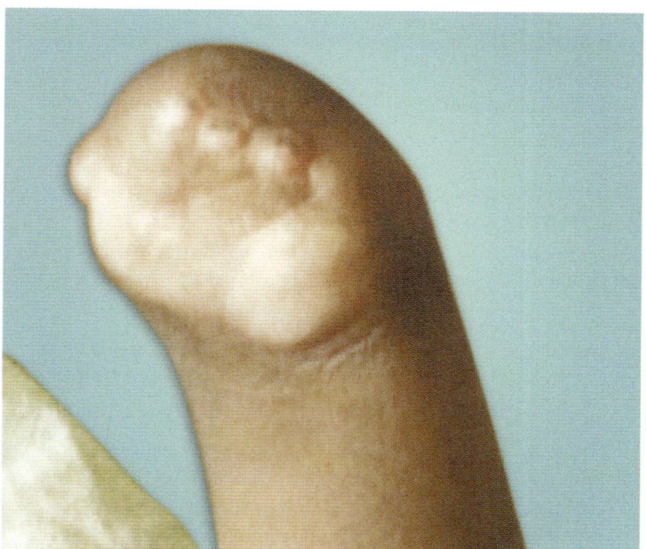

Fig. 14.2.1: Amnion rupture sequence; note the amputation and disruption of the finger morphogenesis.

- *Sequence:* A pattern of multiple anomalies derived from a single prior anomaly or mechanical factor
  - *Example:* In case of the Pierre-Robin sequence (micrognathia, glossoptosis and U-shaped cleft palate); the primary anomaly is the early mandibular hypoplasia, which results in a posteriorly located tongue (secondary anomaly) thereby impairing the closure of palatal shelves resulting in a cleft palate (tertiary anomaly) **(Figs. 14.2.2A and B)**. Roughly 17% of Pierre-Robin sequence cases are isolated and nonsyndromic; in remaining cases, it is a part of syndromes such as Stickler syndrome, velocardiofacial syndrome and Beckwith-Wiedemann syndrome.
- *Association:* Non-random tendency of some malformations to occur together more commonly than would be expected by chance, without being part of a syndrome.
  - *Examples:* VATERR association (Vertebral defects, anal atresia, cardiovascular anomalies, tracheoesophageal fistula, esophageal atresia, radial dysplasia, renal dysplasia) and MURCS association (Müllerian duct aplasia, renal aplasia, cervicothoracic Somite dysplasia)
  - Many cases of CHARGE association (coloboma of the eye, heart defects, atresia of the nasal choanae, retardation of growth and/or development, genitourinary abnormalities, and ear abnormalities and deafness) have recently found to be caused by *CHD7 gene* and hence, CHARGE is now grouped as a syndrome and not an association.

APPROACH TO A CHILD WITH MULTIPLE ANOMALIES

Suspicion

The first step in evaluation of dysmorphic child is "suspicion of genetic etiology", which should be suspected in any child who presents with:

- *Congenital anomalies*: Major anomaly or more than two minor anomalies
- *Growth deficit:* Short stature or failure to thrive
- Developmental delay, mental subnormality or developmental regression
- Failure to develop secondary sexual characteristics

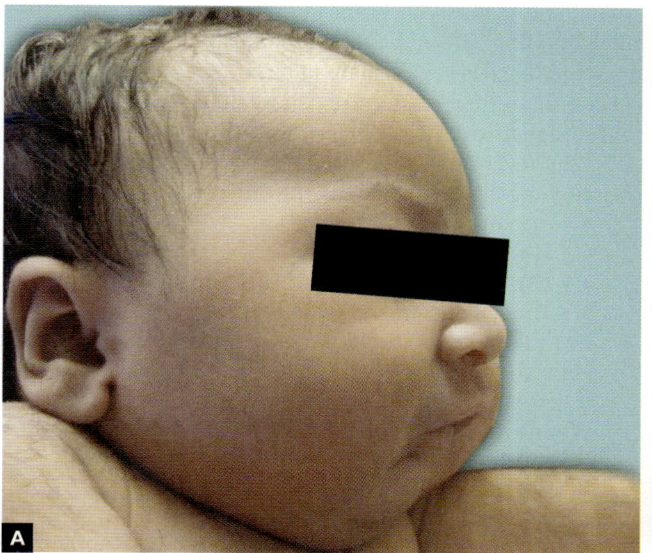

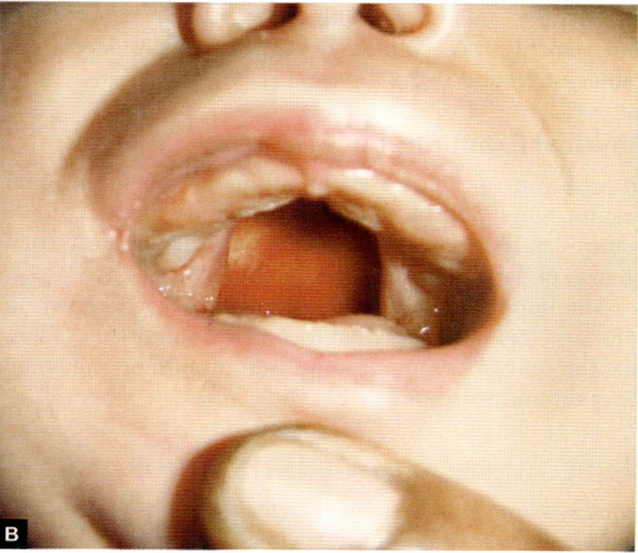

Figs. 14.2.2A and B: Pierre-Robin sequence. Note the micrognathia and unusual round-shaped palatal cleft unique to this sequence.

Table 14.2.1: Personal/family history.

History	*Significance*
Three generation pedigree chart using standard symbols	Indicates pattern of inheritance
Elderly mother (> 35 years)	Chromosomal aneuploidy *Example*: Down syndrome
Elderly father (> 45 years)	New AD mutation *Examples*: Achondroplasia and Marfan syndrome
Maternal disease *Example*: Diabetes mellitus	Known associated fetal abnormalities Diabetic embryopathy (Caudal regression, congenital heart defects, ear anomalies)
Poor social history	Possible alcohol/drug ingestion
Racial origin of parents	Known genes of high frequency in certain racial groups *Example*: Ellis-van Creveld syndrome in the Amish population
Parental consanguinity	Autosomal recessive disorders
Possible maternal uterine abnormalities	Deformations
Other affected family members or multiple single gene or chromosomal disorder	For diagnostic purpose and to know the pattern of inheritance

Table 14.2.2: Pregnancy history.

History	*Significance*
Antenatal ultrasound	Aids prenatal diagnosis, holds clues to the diagnosis and to assess fetal growth
Maternal drug or alcohol ingestion *Examples*: Warfarin, anticonvulsants, cocaine	Teratogenic effects *Examples*: Warfarin—hypoplasia of nasal cartilage, CNS abnormality Valproate—Spina bifida, craniofacial dysmorphism Cocaine—vascular disruptions
Exposure to radiation (especially therapeutic)	Possible mutagenic or teratogenic effects
Early rupture of membranes	Possible fetal compression leading to deformation
Oligohydramnios	Renal agenesis or outflow obstruction with Potter sequence
Polyhydramnios	Esophageal atresia, neuromuscular disorders
Poor fetal movements	Fetal compression, neuromuscular disorders
Breech presentation	Neuromuscular disorders

- Ambiguous genitalia
- Or simply does not look right.

History

Any mystery can be solved with a proper history. Some of the important historical points to be elicited are mentioned in the **Tables 14.2.1** and **14.2.2**.

Physical Examination

In addition to routine examination certain additional examination should be performed in a child with dysmorphic features. **Table 14.2.3** lists some of the salient features that point to underlying dysmorphic syndrome.

The importance of major anomalies is well known in syndrome delineation. When it comes to minor anomalies, presence of two or more features warrant further evaluation for syndrome association.

RECOGNITION OF GENETIC SYNDROMES

Some syndromes are so striking to the eye of the pediatrician that a diagnosis is made instantaneously based on the general gist of the patient. This termed as "gestalt diagnosis" is exemplified in the diagnosis of a patient with Rubinstein-Taybi syndrome **(Figs. 14.2.3A to E)**, wherein multiple minor anomalies make a combination so unique that a diagnosis is rarely missed. In order to have expertise in this mode of "gestalt diagnosis" one has to have a vast experience in seeing similar patients previously in order to create a mental snapshot of the condition. Given the rarity of individual syndromes, such an experience is seldom gained but by a few, hence repeated visual scanning of pictures of various syndromes from authoritative resources will have to suffice.

- Whenever an anomaly is noted, it should be described keeping in mind the following directives:
  - Appropriate terminology
  - Minor or major anomaly
  - *Etiology*: Malformation/disruption/deformation
  - Time of onset.
- Examination should not be restricted to the patient but should be extended to include all the available family members.
- Whenever feasible objective criteria should be used in diagnosing anomalies. The reader can refer to various Indian and foreign data useful in anthropometry.
- Cross-consultation should be taken from specialists of other fields in medicine when dealing with a child with multiple anomalies (e.g. ophthalmology consults in Reiger syndrome).

Table 14.2.3: Findings that suggest underlying genetic etiology.

General	• Short stature or tall stature • Failure to thrive or obesity • *Unusual head circumference*: Microcephaly or macrocephaly • *Unusual head shape*: Brachycephaly, scaphocephaly, trigonocephaly • *Altered body proportion*: Short spine, short limbs, long limbs
Facial features	• Synophrys (fused eyebrows) • Hypotelorism or hypertelorism* • Palpebral fissures that are up-slanting or down-slanting* • Short palpebral fissures (normally the length of palpebral fissure is equal to the distance between two eyes) • Short or long nose (the nose is usually 2/3 to 3/4 the length of the distance between the nasal bridge and the upper lip) • Ears that are low set or posteriorly rotated* • Ears that are simple or abnormally shaped • Lips that are thin/full, tented, down turned or cleft • Philtrum that is long or smooth • Palate that is high arched or cleft • Uvula that is bifid or absent • Prognathia or micrognathia*
Hands and feet	• Brachydactyly (short fingers) • Arachnodactyly (long fingers) • Clinodactyly (incurved fingers, usually the fifth)* • Syndactyly (fusion of digits) • Polydactyly (extra digits) • Dysplastic nails • Abnormal creases*
Skin and hair	• Abnormal skin pigmentation, e.g. hemangioma, cafe-au-lait • Spots, streaks or whorls • Abnormal amounts of hair, e.g. alopecia, hirsutism or hypertrichosis • Abnormal hair line, e.g. low hairline (posteriorly or anteriorly) or receding hairline • Altered hair color, e.g. white forelock
Musculoskeletal	• Short neck • Abnormal chest shape or size, e.g. pectus carinatum, pectus excavatum, short sternum • Abnormalities of nipples, e.g. widely spaced, supernumerary* • Inverted nipples • Abnormalities of the spine, e.g. anencephaly, encephalocele • Myelomeningocele or stigmata of spina bifida occulta (hair, lipoma, deep dimple*) • Unusual joint shape, e.g. flaring • Abnormal joint mobility, e.g. hypermobility or reduced range of motion
Abdomen	• Abdominal wall defects, e.g. omphalocele, gastroschisis • Hepatosplenomegaly • Nephromegaly • Ambiguous genitalia

**Indicate minor anomalies.*

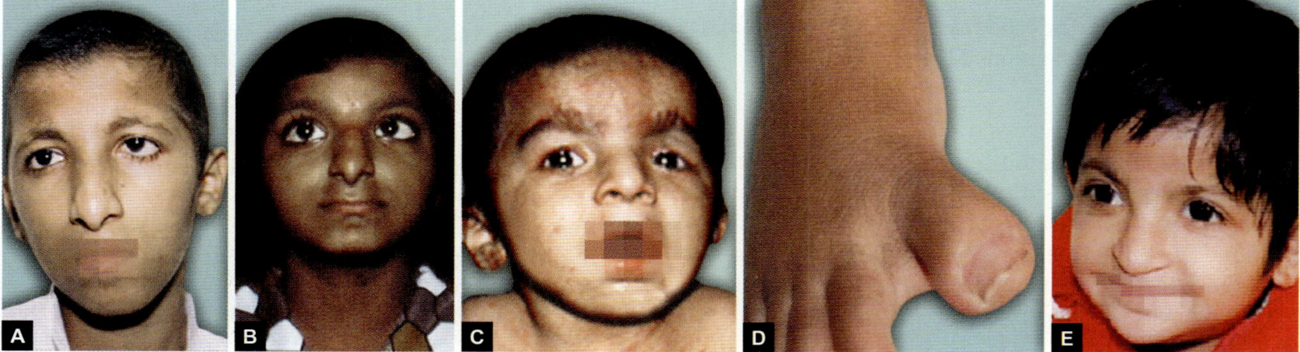

Figs. 14.2.3A to E: Unrelated children with Rubinstein-Taybi syndrome. Note the facial characteristics—down-slanting palpebral fissures, overhanging columella of nose. Great toe is broad and medially rotated.

Table 14.2.4: Some clinical features which suggest specific diagnosis.

Clinical sign	*Specific diagnosis*
Pursed lips	Whistling face syndrome
Broad thumbs and great toes	Rubinstein-Taybi syndrome
Absent clavicle	Cleidocranial dysostosis
Heterochromia iridis	Waardenburg syndrome
Mitten hands	Apert syndrome
Inverted nipples	Congenital disorder of glycosylation
Webbing of neck	Turner and Noonan syndromes
Eversion of the lateral third of lower eyelid	Kabuki make-up syndrome

- Consultation with a specialist in the field of dysmorphology is of utmost importance in the field of dysmorphology for the prompt diagnosis and for further evaluation.
- The camera plays the role of a stethoscope in the field of dysmorphology. Pictures are not only useful for record purposes and second opinions, but also help in the appraisal of the morphological evolution of a syndrome.
- Radiography goes hand in hand with physical examination when it comes to anomalies, since they are diagnostic in several conditions such as the group of skeletal dysplasia.

When immediate recognition is not possible, it is necessary to identify one or more features (handles), which might lead to syndrome diagnosis. The best handle or anomaly to be taken to consideration is one, which is least likely to be a normal variant. Features such as mental retardation, microcephaly, simian crease, clinodactyly are nonspecific and act as poor handles for syndrome delineation. The anomalies, which are less common but more specific are more useful for the search of diagnosis. Examples are microphthalmia, preaxial polydactyly, midline cleft lip, etc. Once a suitable handle is identified, reference should be made to standard monograph on syndromology or computer databases.

Sometimes some clinical features suggest specific diagnosis, which could be called as "Pearls of dysmorphology" and few examples are mentioned here **(Table 14.2.4)**.

Databases

Databases have become an integral aspect of practice in clinical genetics and dysmorphology. Some of the important textbooks and online catalogues of genetic syndromes are mentioned in **Table 14.2.5**. When using these databases one should keep in mind, that they are systems for experts and not expert systems.

"The Smith's approach" to a child with multiple malformations is a way of classifying syndromes based on the combination of major handles. The author considers this particular approach to be extremely effective and time tested. The following is the major list of classification that is used in "the Smith's approach".

- Very small and proportionate stature, not skeletal dysplasia (e.g. Seckel syndrome) **(Fig. 14.2.4)**
- Moderate short stature, facial ± genital (e.g. Aarskog syndrome, Williams syndrome) **(Figs. 14.2.5 and 14.2.6)**
- Senile-like appearance (e.g. Cockayne syndrome, Werner syndrome) **(Figs. 14.2.7A and B)**

Table 14.2.5: Important textbooks and online databases of genetic syndromes.

*Reference texts**	*Online and computerized databases*
Smith's recognizable pattern of human malformations (*Editor: Jones KL*)	Online Mendelian inheritance in man (*www.ncbi.nlm.nih. gov/omim*)
Atlas of skeletal dysplasias (*Editors: Wynne-Davies, Hall and Apley*)	GeneClinics and GeneTests (*www.geneclinics.com*)
Syndromes of the head and neck (*Editors: Gorlin, Cohen and Hennekam*)	London dysmorphology database (*www.lmdatabases.com*)
Management of genetic syndromes (Authors: Cassidy and Allanson)	POSSUM (Pictures of Standard Syndromes and Undiagnosed Malformations) (*www.possum.net*)
	TERIS (The teratogen information system) (*depts.washington.edu/terisweb/teris*)

*See Bibliography for details.

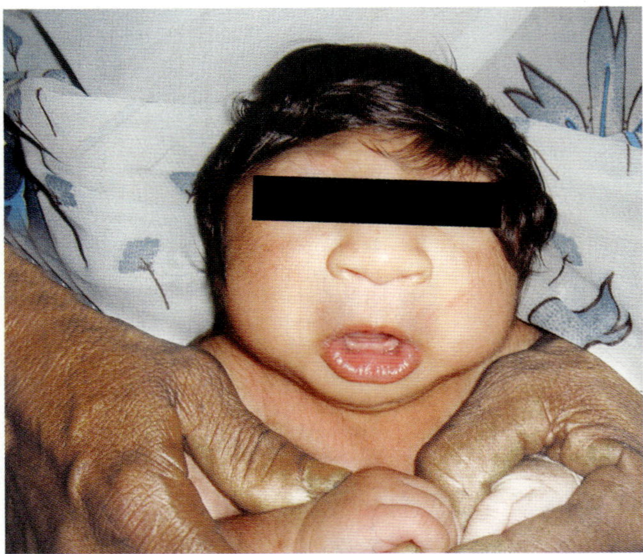

Fig. 14.2.4: Seckel syndrome, note the sever microcephaly with prominent nose.

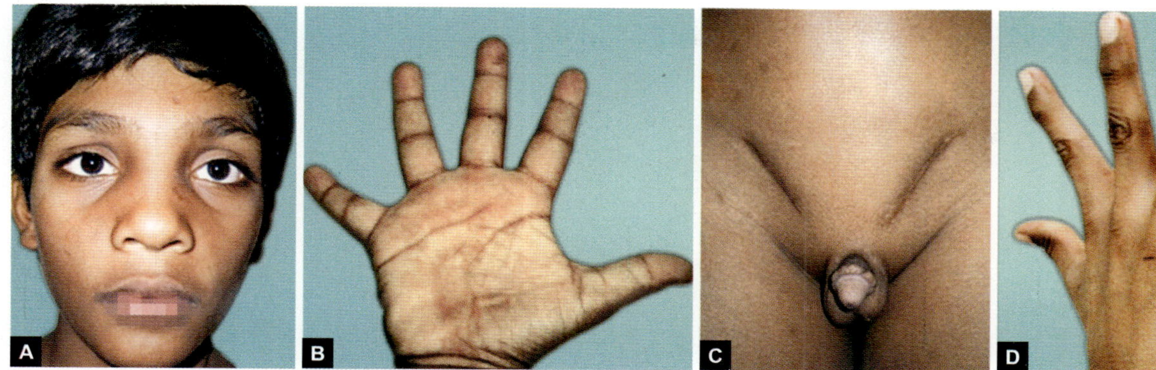

Figs. 14.2.5A to D: Aarskog syndrome. Note the hypertelorism and broad philtrum, hand showing brachydactyly with mild interdigital webbing (arrow), swan neck deformities of fingers and characteristic shawl scrotum. Scars due to operation for bilateral inguinal hernia are also seen. Patient was of moderate short stature.

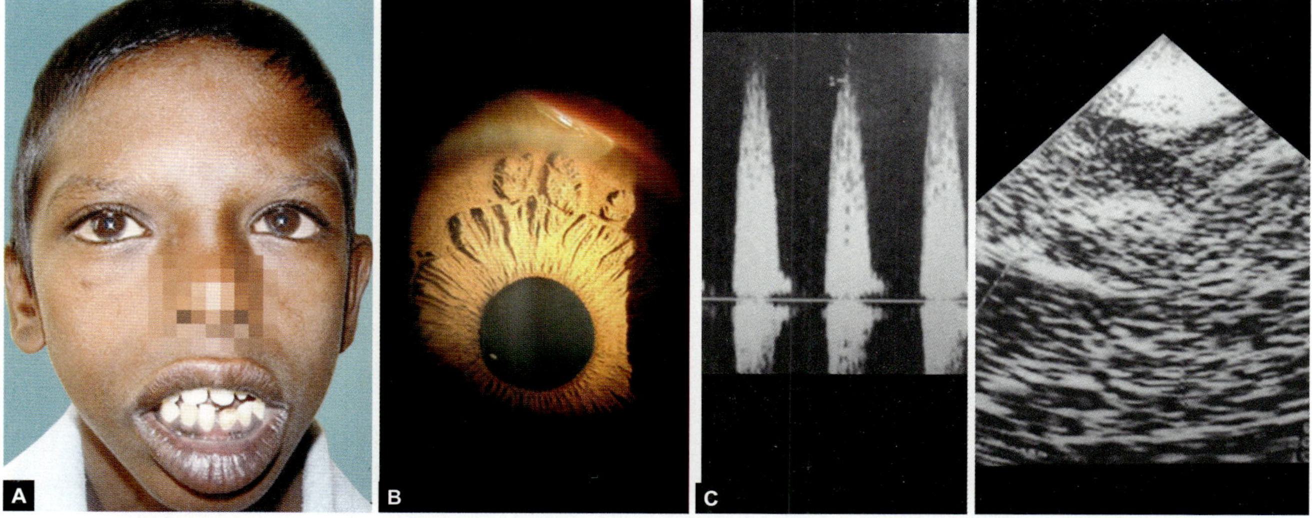

Figs. 14.2.6A to C: Williams syndrome. Note the periorbital fullness with medial eyebrow flare, prominent lips with an open mouth. Slit-lamp examination revealed characteristic stellate iris pattern. Echocardiogram confirmed the diagnosis of supravalvular aortic stenosis.

- Unusual brain and/or neuromuscular findings, with associated defects (e.g. Acrocallosal syndrome) **(Figs. 14.2.8A and B)**
- Early overgrowth with associated defects (e.g. Sotos syndrome) **(Fig. 14.2.9)**
- Facial defects as major feature (e.g. Frontonasal dysplasia syndrome) **(Fig. 14.2.10)**
- Facial-Limb defects as major feature (e.g. Hay-Wells syndrome of ectodermal dysplasia) **(Fig. 14.2.11)**
- Limb defects as major feature (e.g. Femoral hypoplasia) **(Fig. 14.2.12)**
- Craniosynostosis syndromes (e.g. Apert syndrome) **(Figs. 14.2.13A and B)**.

A special mention is warranted in the case of skeletal dysplasia, since the huge list and the varied presentations of this group of enigmatic condition is a challenge even to the astute clinician. The following approach based on that suggested by Bryan D Hall is considered to be extremely effective in reaching a diagnosis:

- Diagnosing short stature
- Diagnosing disproportionate short stature
- Diagnosing what causes this disproportion, is it short trunk (e.g. Spondyloepiphyseal dysplasias) or short limbs (e.g. Achondroplasia)
- If short-limbed, which part of the limbs are affected:
  - *Rhizomelia:* Proximal shortening, i.e. humerus and femur (e.g. Chondrodysplasia punctata)
  - *Mesomelia:* Shortening of the middle segment, i.e. radius, ulna, tibia and fibula (e.g. Mesomelic dysplasia)

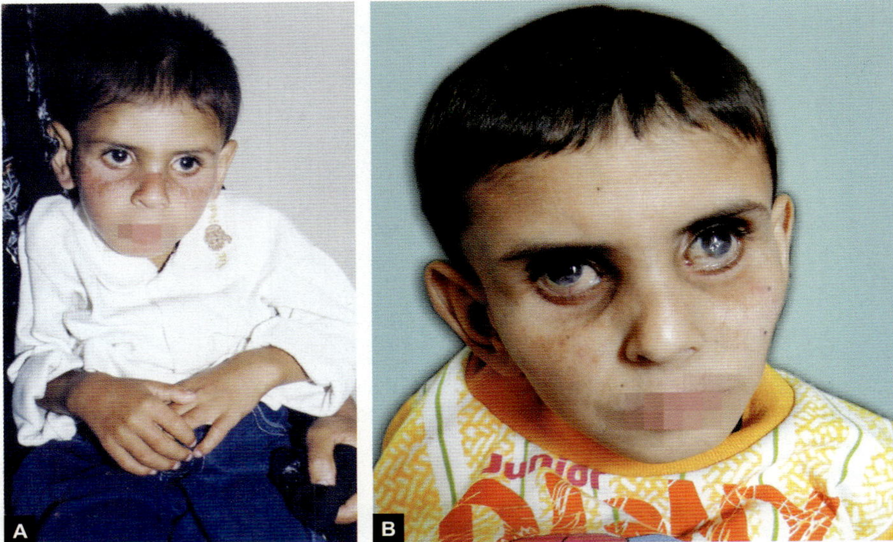

Figs. 14.2.7A and B: Cockayne syndrome: Deep set eyes, rash on cheeks and changes of premature aging. The same child at (A) 5 years and (B) 12 years of age.

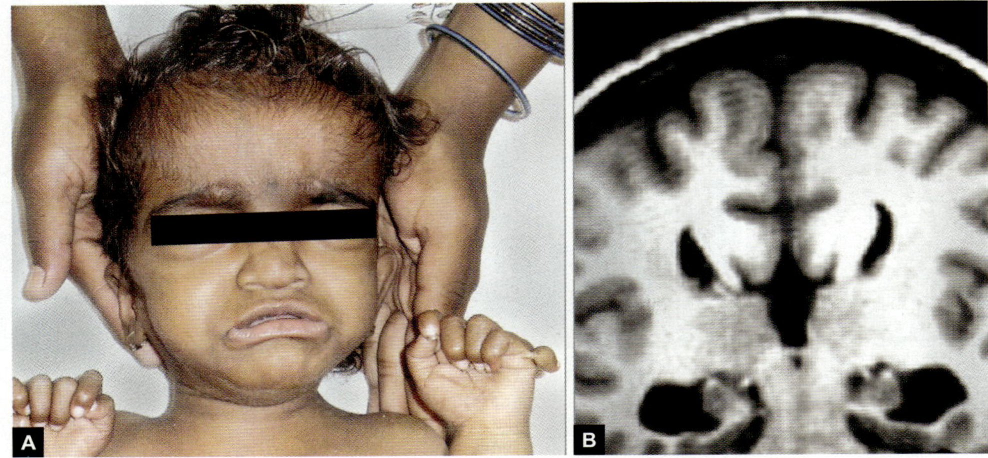

Figs. 14.2.8A and B: Acrocallosal syndrome: The hypertelorism, downslanting palpebral fissures, broad nasal bridge and short philtrum. (A) Postaxial polydactyly is seen in both the upper limbs. (B) Magnetic resonance imaging revealed absent corpus callosum.

    - *Acromelia:* Distal shortening, i.e. hand and foot (e.g. Acromesomelic dysplasia)
    - Combination: Ellis-van Creveld syndrome, Achondroplasia
- Diagnosing deformations caused by the osseous abnormalities (e.g. Craniosynostosis in thanatophoric dysplasia)
- Diagnosing associated malformations, which herald a clue to the actual condition (e.g. Heart defects in Ellis-van Creveld syndrome)
- *Categorizing based on the areas involved radiologically*: Epiphyseal dysplasias, diaphyseal dysplasias, metaphyseal dysplasias, spine involvement, cranial involvement, hand involvement
- *Categorizing based on clinical and radiological grounds*: Pure skeletal dysplasia (e.g. Achondroplasia):
    - Malformations associated (e.g. Stickler syndrome)
    - Malformation/Mental retardation associated (e.g. Campomelic dysplasia).

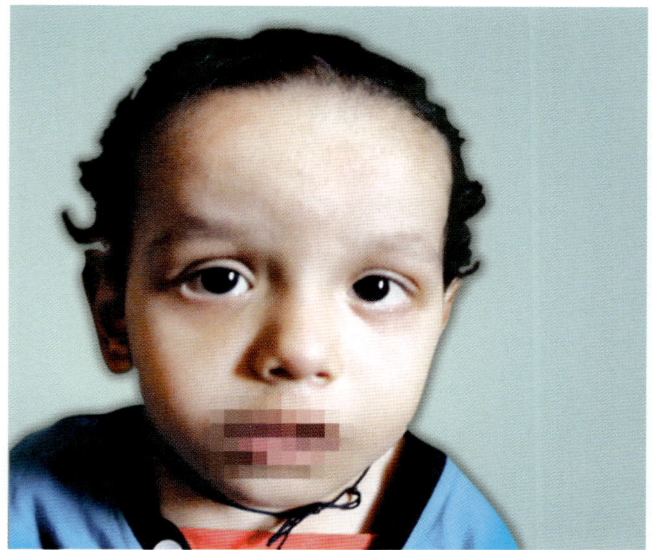

Fig. 14.2.9: Sotos syndrome: Macrocephaly, mild hypertelorism, prominent forehead and chin.

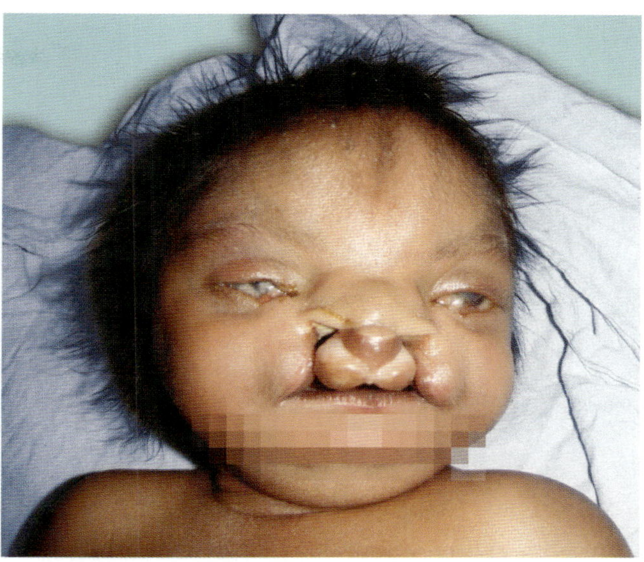

Fig. 14.2.11: Hay-Wells syndrome of ectodermal dysplasia: The obvious ankyloblepharon, broad nasal bridge with bilateral cleft lip and palate. Child had associate dystrophic nails and supernumerary nipples.

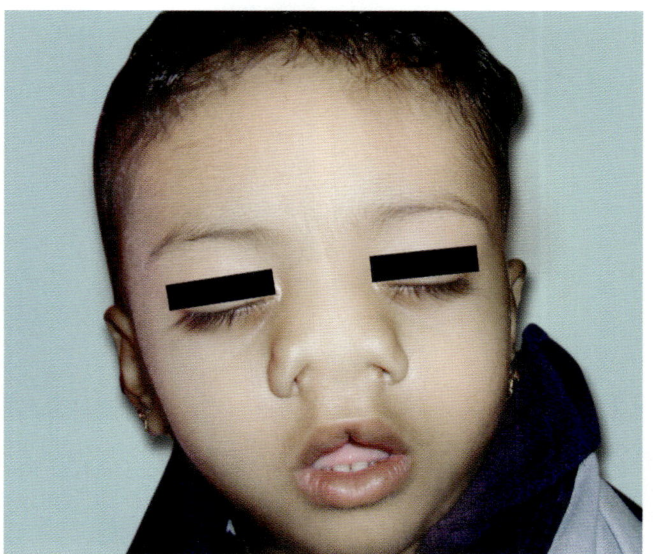

Fig. 14.2.10: Frontonasal dysplasia sequence: The completely divided nostrils with hypoplasia of the prolabium with a median cleft lip.

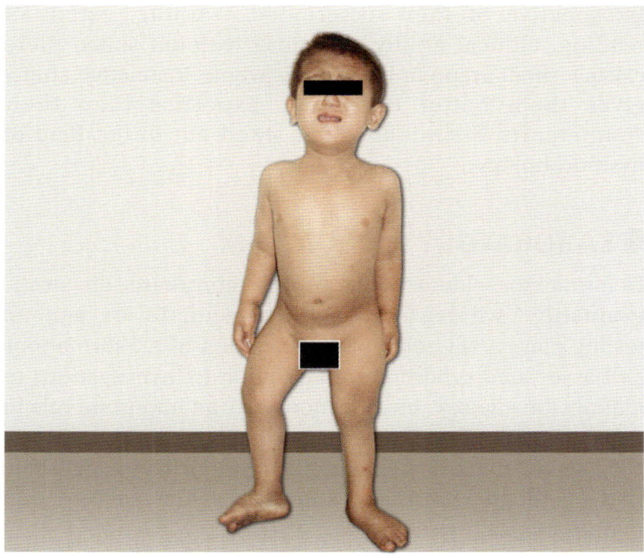

Fig. 14.2.12: Femoral hypoplasia—unusual facies syndrome: The short lower limbs; up-slanting palpebral fissures with a short nose, hypoplastic alae nasae, set ears.

Attributes of a Dysmorphologist

- He/she should be a meticulous and keen observer and must record any deviation from the norms
- He/she must see a number of cases and if not possible, must visually scan photographs and pictures
- Always use objective criteria and appropriate terminology
- As in any field a person interested in dysmorphology should be a learner forever
- One has to be honest in his/her approach, hungry for knowledge and humble in acquiring it.

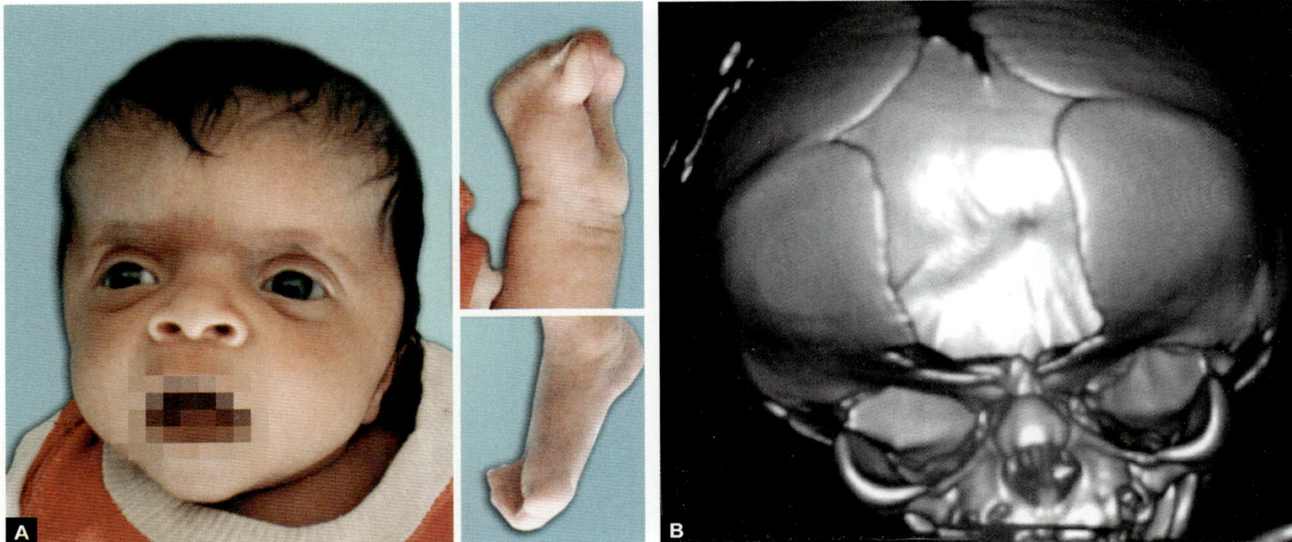

Figs. 14.2.13A and B: Apert syndrome: (A) High full forehead, hypertelorism and down-slanting palpebral fissures. Limbs show varying degree of syndactyly (Mitten hand); (B) Computed tomography (CT) head reconstruction shows bilateral coronal suture synostosis.

Intusion (the Unteachable and the Undefinable)

Irrespective of their experience, training, extent of reading, clinical ability and observational skills, there exists a small group of individuals whose instinctive ability gives them better diagnostic expertise than their counterparts. Such individuals stand out in the field of dysmorphology.

LABORATORY EVALUATION

Deformations seldom require any laboratory based diagnostic evaluation, whereas in this post-genomic era genetic testing plays a key role in the evaluation of malformations and associated syndromes. In addition to investigations to identify the etiology, investigations play an important role in detecting internal malformations of heart, brain, kidneys, etc. Diagnosis of malformation is not only useful in providing clue to the etiology but it is also important as the malformation may be surgically treatable.

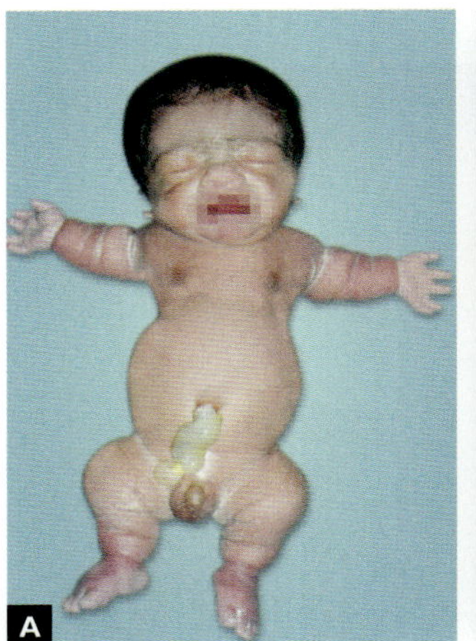

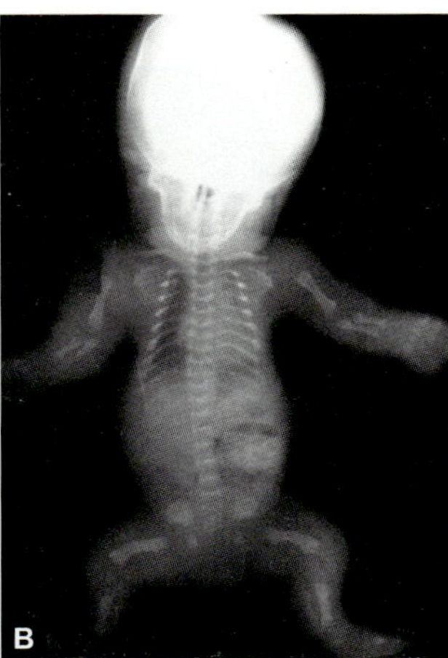

Figs. 14.2.14A and B: (A) Thanatophoric dysplasia, severe shortening of the limbs, i.e. acromesorhizomelic, loose folds of skin, macrocephaly with low nasal bridge, narrow thorax. (B) Curved femora and flat vertebrae are seen in the radiograph.

Karyotyping

Unless a non-chromosomal etiology is apparent in a child with multiple malformations, it is a useful diagnostic approach to start with a karyotype (chromosome analysis). It is the definitive diagnostic test for aneuploidy syndromes such as Down syndrome, Turner syndrome and other structural abnormalities of chromosomes.

Fluorescent *in Situ* Hybridization

The fluorescent *in situ* hybridization (FISH) technique has revolutionized the field of cytogenetics having tremendous implications in the diagnosis of malformation syndromes. FISH probes by their ability to attach to specific locus on a chromosome bring to light microdeletions that are not visible in the standard karyotype **(Figs. 14.2.14A and B)**. **Table 14.2.6**

Table 14.2.6: Microdeletion syndromes commonly diagnosed using the FISH technique.

Syndrome	*Chromosomal region*	*Clinical features*
Angelman syndrome	15q11–q13	Magnetic resonance (MR), spastic gait, happy temperament
Prader-Willi syndrome	15q11–q13	MR, hypotonia, hypogonadism, obesity, almond shaped eyes
Williams syndrome	7q11.2	Aortic stenosis, facial dysmorphism, friendly behavior
Cri-Du-Chat syndrome	5p15.2	MR, cat-like cry in infancy, microcephaly
Miller-Dieker syndrome	17p13.3	MR, microcephaly, lissencephaly, furrowing of forehead while crying
Rubenstein-Taybi syndrome	16p13.3	MR, beaked nose, broad thumbs and toes
Velocardiofacial syndrome	22q11.2	Conotruncal heart defects, cleft palate, prominent nose

(FISH: fluorescent in situ hybridization)

lists the more commonly used and available FISH probes for syndrome delineation. As FISH can look at only a specific area of a chromosome, it is important to clinically suspect the condition before ordering the FISH test.

New Genetic Tests

Comparative Genomic Hybridization

Comparative genomic hybridization combined with microarray technique is a newer addition to the armamentarium of the dysmorphologists. It can detect very small deletions/duplications anywhere in the genome in one test. The microarray based cytogenetic analysis has been advocated as a first-line of test for cases with mental retardation/malformation without obvious cause and the diagnostic yield of the test is 7–10%.

Biochemical Testing

Many biochemical genetic defects are associated with dysmorphic features such as mucopolysaccharidosis, Zellweger syndrome and Smith-Lemli-Opitz syndrome. Testing for specific enzyme defect may be diagnostic in these conditions and can be supplemented by finding the underlying genetic defect.

Mutation Detection

Genes for many malformation syndromes such as Cornelia de Lange syndrome, Apert syndrome, Treacher-Collins syndrome, etc. are known and many others are getting identified. However, due to large size of genes and large number of mutations observed in each syndrome use of mutation detection by DNA based techniques in clinical practice is not easy. For some disorders such as Apert syndrome, achondroplasia only one common mutation is identified in most of the cases. That is why mutation detection for such disorders is easy and available in India.

Now the sequencing of whole genome has become possible and if there are 2–3 patients of a disorder in a family, the causative gene can be identified using DNA samples of such a few cases.

Table 14.2.7 provides a summary of the approach to diagnosis and management of common genetic disorders in children.

PRENATAL DIAGNOSIS

In essence, it is determination of the status (genetic or otherwise) of the fetus by a variety of techniques [ultrasonography (USG), chromosomal, biochemical, DNA, etc.], using a variety of procedures. These include chorionic villus sampling (CVS) (8–11 weeks), amniocentesis (11–16 weeks) and blood analysis by cordocentesis. Radiological investigations such as antenatal ultrasound, fetal magnetic resonance imaging (MRI) and fetal echocardiogram (ECHO) play an important role in prenatal diagnosis of malformations.

GENETIC COUNSELING

Genetic counseling is the process of helping people understand and adapt to the medical, psychological and familial implications of genetic contributions to the disease. The counselor offers investigations, options and support whereas the "consultand" (the person who seeks the advice) makes his/her own decision, which is known as non-directive counseling. The essential steps include accurate diagnosis of the affected member in the family, risk assessment, proper communication, discussion of options and long-term contact and support. Assistance in enrolment of the patient in support groups may be paramount in this era of global communication.

DIFFICULTIES IN DYSMORPHOLOGY

Neonatal Period

It is a common occurrence in India, to be faced with a neonate with no antenatal ultrasound presenting with gross dysmorphic

Table 14.2.7: Summary of approach to dysmorphic child.

Suspicion	***Analysis***	***Previous laboratory and X-ray studies***	***Physical examination***
Congenital abnormalities Growth problems Mental deficit	• History • Pedigree • Family • Pregnancy and birth • Health • Growth and development		• Anatomic regions • Organ systems • Measurements • Photographs
Other	***Synthesis***	***Confirmation***	***Intervention***
Family investigation Watchful waiting	• "Pivotal" findings • Pattern recognition • Comparison with known cases: – Personal experience – Literature	• Laboratory • Clinical course • Birth of affected relatives	• Treatment • Counseling
Follow-up	• Lack of diagnosis • Counseling other family members • New diagnostic technique • Natural history		

features. This is exemplified in cases such as thanatophoric dysplasia **(Fig. 14.2.15)**, where early neonatal death is the rule. The attending pediatrician should be able to quickly assess such condition so as to stop futile resuscitation measures. Neonatal presentation of certain conditions such as Pierre-Robin sequence may be with feeding difficulties or failure to thrive with metabolic encephalopathy in cases such as Smith-Lemli-Opitz syndrome or Zellweger syndrome. Adequate expertise is needed for anticipation of difficulties in these conditions.

Evolution of Morphology

Some phenotypes evolve with time, such as *Proteus* syndrome; and it is the rule in many of the metabolic conditions such as the group of mucopolysaccharidosis and hence a diagnosis is rarely made in the neonatal period, whereas in certain conditions such as the Beckwith-Wiedemann syndrome the phenotype tends to dissolve as the age progress. These caveats reinforce the need for proper documentation and photography to study the evolving nature of the condition.

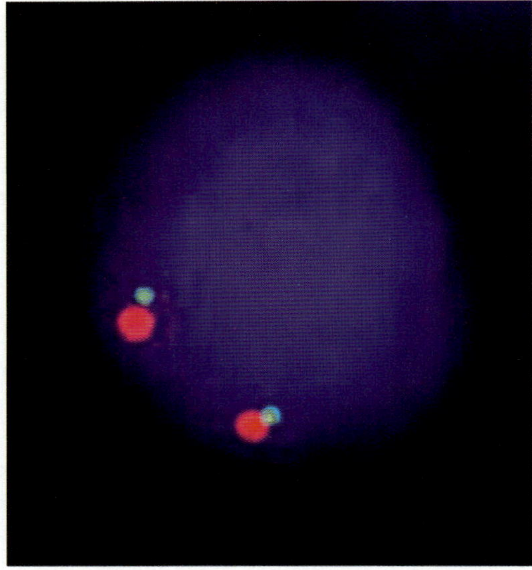

Fig. 14.2.15: Normal result of FISH technique. Two red (target region) and green (control probe) signals indicate the presence of two copies of a particular region of interest in the interphase nucleus and absence of microdeletion.

RECENT ADVANCES

Three-dimensional Face Shape Modeling

Human tendency to give objective criteria for subjective intuition has not overlooked the field of dysmorphology. A new modality of three-dimensional (3D) models of facial morphology is showing potential in objective syndrome delineation and discrimination.

Behavioral Phenotypes

A well-known phenomenon is the unique behavior associated with specific syndrome. This is exemplified in the friendly social nature of patients with Williams syndrome, tendency to overeat in case of Prader-Willi syndrome, self-mutilating and destructive behavior of Lesch-Nyhan syndrome, autistic behavior in Fragile-X syndrome and Rett syndrome, happy nature of Angelman syndrome and the lovable, friendly and music loving nature of Down syndrome. This old phenomenon termed as the "behavioral phenotype" is gaining more interest, not only as an aid to diagnosis but also in the comprehensive treatment of the patient.

BIBLIOGRAPHY

1. Allanson JE, Biesecker LG, Carey JC, Hennekam RC. Elements of morphology: introduction. Am J Med Genet A. 2009;149A(1):2-5.
2. Cassidy SB, Allanson JE. Management of Genetic Syndromes, 3rd edition. New York: Willey Blackwell; 2010.
3. Falk MJ, Robin NH. The primary care physician's approach to congenital anomalies. Prim Care. 2004;31(3):605-19.
4. Gorlin RJ, Cohen MM, Hennekam RCM. Syndromes of the Head and Neck, 4th edition. New York: Oxford University Press; 2001.
5. Hall J, Allanson J, Gripp K, Slavotinek A. Handbook of Physical Measurements, 2nd edition. New York: Oxford University Press; 2006.
6. Jones KL. Smith's Recognizable Pattern of Human Malformation, 6th edition. Philadelphia: Elsevier Saunders; 2006.
7. Kulkarni ML. An Atlas of Neonatology. New Delhi: Jaypee Brothers Medical Publishers (P) Ltd; 2005.
8. Kulkarni ML. Clinical Methods in Paediatrics. New Delhi: Jaypee Brothers Medical Publishers (P) Ltd; 2005.
9. Peter Hammond. The use of 3D face shape modelling in dysmorphology. Arch Dis Child. 2007;92(12):1120-6.
10. Toriello HV. Role of the dysmorphic evaluation in the child with developmental delay. Pediatr Clin North Am. 2008;55(5):1085-98.

14.3 Common Genetic Disorders

Madhulika Kabra

INTRODUCTION

With the increasing recognition that almost all disorders have a probable genetic basis; no clinician can escape learning about diagnosis and management of common genetic disorders. The fact that some of these disorders are now amenable to therapy and most of the severe/lethal disorders can be prevented; it is all the more important that the pediatricians, who are usually the first contact expand their knowledge and interest in this field.

Genetic disorders can be classified as follows:

- Chromosomal disorders.
- Single-gene disorders.
- Polygenic or multifactorial disorders.
- Mitochondrial disorders.
- Somatic cell (genetic) disorders (resulting in cancer).

In this chapter, we have discussed the clinical features, diagnosis, management and counseling issues of common genetic disorders encountered in clinical practice.

CHROMOSOMAL DISORDERS

These accounts for approximately 6% of all recognized congenital abnormalities and can be divided into numerical and structural, with a third category consisting of different chromosome constitutions in two or more cell lines, i.e. mosaicism. The presence of an extra chromosome is referred to as *trisomy*. Common trisomies seen in live-born infants include trisomy 21 (Down syndrome), trisomy 18 (Edward syndrome) and trisomy 13 (Patau syndrome). They differ in phenotype and course of disease. Other trisomies are not observed in live-born infants because they are lethal in early embryonic life and are not compatible with life at birth. The presence of an additional sex chromosome (X or Y) has only mild phenotypic effects.

The presence of only 1 chromosome of the pair is referred to as *monosomy*. Monosomy for an autosome is almost always incompatible with survival to term. Monosomy X (karyotype 45, X or Turner syndrome) is a frequent chromosomal aberration diagnosed in postnatal period. Structural chromosome rearrangements result from chromosome breakage with subsequent reunion in a different configuration. These can be balanced or unbalanced.

Down Syndrome

Down syndrome (DS) is the most common chromosomal anomaly present at birth. The incidence varies from 1 per 800–1,200 live births. Down syndrome is also known as trisomy 21 since chromosome 21 is present in triplicate. There is a strong association between the incidence of DS and advancing maternal age and studies have shown that this arises most commonly as a result of nondisjunction in maternal meiosis I.

Clinical Features

Clinical phenotype is easily identifiable clinically though diagnosis may be difficult in a neonate, especially a preterm one. **Table 14.3.1** provides a short checklist of clinical features. **Figures 14.3.1A to C** show a child with DS with characteristic facies.

Table 14.3.1: Checklist for clinical diagnosis of Down syndrome.

System/organ affected	*Abnormality detected*
Head	Brachycephaly with flat occiput, wide open fontanel
Face	Flat facial profile,* flat nasal bridge
Mouth	Habitually open furrowed/protruding tongue
Ears	Dysplastic,* small, low set
Eyes	Upward slant of palpebral fissures,* epicanthic folds, squint, speckled iris
Neck	Short and broad, abundant neck skin*
Hands	Short and broad, small fingers especially 5th finger, hypoplastic middle phalanx of 5th finger*(clinodactyly), Simian crease*
Feet	Increased space between 1 and 2 toes*, furrow on the sole extending from space between 1 and 2 toes
Joints	Hypotonia*
Muscles	Hyper-extensibility/hyper-flexibility*
Heart	Murmur, cyanotic or acyanotic defect
Reflexes	Lack of Moro reflex*

*Useful for making a diagnosis in the newborn.

Associated Problems

- *Congenital heart disease:*
  - About 40% of children with DS have congenital heart disease (CHD). Endocardial cushion defects account for about 40–60%. Presence of CHD is the most significant factor in determining survival.
  - All children with DS should have a cardiac evaluation during neonatal period or as early as possible and it should ideally include an ECHO.
- *Gastrointestinal malformations:*
  - Look for atresia (present in around 12% of cases), especially duodenal and Hirschsprung disease.
  - Manage accordingly.
- *Eye problems:*
  - Increased risk of cataract, nystagmus and squint, abnormalities of visual acuity
  - Routine evaluation in first year (or earlier if indicated) and then every year.
- *Hearing defect:*
  - About 40–60% of patients have conductive hearing loss and are also prone to serous otitis media (50–70% during first year).
  - Routine evaluation in first year and then every year.
  - Examine for otitis media at each visit.
  - Audiologic evaluation at least once between 5 years and 13 years and then every year is recommended.
- *Thyroid dysfunction:*
  - About 15–30% of children with DS have hypothyroidism
  - Thyroid function tests [T4 and thyroid-stimulating hormone (TSH)] are recommended once in the neonatal period/at first contact, twice a year in the first year and then once every year.
- *Atlanto-occipital subluxation:*
  - Variable incidence—reported in 10–30%.
  - Evaluation by CT scan is recommended before surgery, for participation in special games or if signs and symptoms suggest cord compression.
- *Physical growth:*
  - Regular follow-up for height and weight.
  - Linear growth is retarded as compared to normal children and these children tend to become obese with age.
  - Special growth charts for DS children should ideally be used.
  - Special growth charts for Indian children with DS are not available; charts published in western literature may be used.
- *Malignancy:*
  - Hematological malignancies are more common in DS than in general population.
  - In newborns and infants transient myeloproliferative disorder can be seen.
  - Increased incidence of acute leukemia during the first decade of life is reported.
- *Immunity and infections:*
  - Pneumonia and other infections are more common in DS.
  - Respiratory tract infections are more frequent due to associated CHD and hypotonia.
  - Defects in immunological system, both in B-cells and T-cells function contribute to infections.
- *Sexual development:*
  - Both males and females with DS display fairly normal sexual development.
  - The girls attain menarche and can be fertile but males are always infertile.

Laboratory Diagnosis

Diagnosis is confirmed by karyotype testing, i.e. chromosomal analysis. In about 94% of cases, the cause of Down syndrome is trisomy 21 **(Fig. 14.3.1D)**, about 1% of cases are mosaics and the rest 4% are due to translocations, most commonly involving chromosomes 21 and 14. Karyotyping of the parents is only required if baby has DS due to translocation.

Management

Apart from the investigations and monitoring as described above early stimulation and counseling are important components of management.

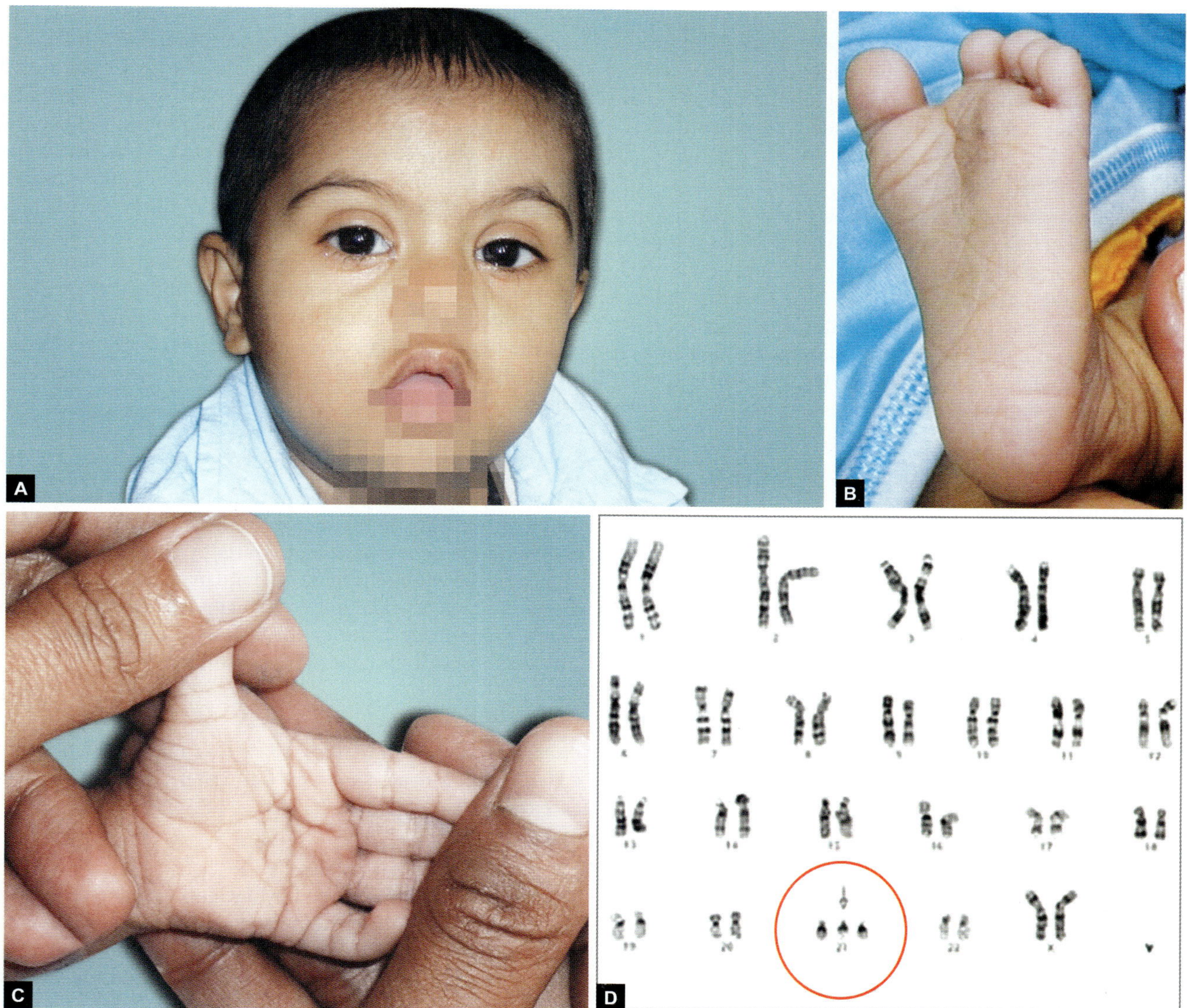

Figs. 14.3.1A to D: (A) Facial phenotype of Down syndrome (DS); (B) Increased gap in between first and second toes; (C) Single palmar crease; (D) Karyotype of DS.

Early stimulation: Early stimulation is recommended for all children with DS and should be started as soon as possible. Ideally should be done by a child psychologist but any pediatrician can guide the parents for the same. There has to be active involvement of the parents. The basic objectives of early stimulation are as follows:

- To involve parents for effectively teaching the relevant skills in different areas of development.
- To individualize the training program.
- To impart basic knowledge and change unfavorable altitudes of parents toward children with Down syndrome.

Counseling

Counseling of parents having a child with Down syndrome varies with the age at presentation for consultation and preparedness of the parents. The counselor has to be passionate and truthful. It is also important to discuss the attributes of patients, not only the problems. Diagnosis should be disclosed as early as one is sure, preferably after karyotyping particularly in a neonate. It is important to discuss with both parents together using simple language and giving sufficient time. It is usually not necessary to discuss about rare complications such as malignancies. One should give hope and emphasize need for early stimulation and its benefits. Counseling regarding risk of recurrence is important but may be postponed for a future date if the baby is very young. Parents should be encouraged to join a local parent group if existing. A regular follow-up needs to be ensured.

Risk of Recurrence

Women 35 years of age or less who have a child with trisomy have a 1% risk of having another, which is significantly greater than the general population. The risk is little increased, if any, over the usual maternal age-dependent frequency if the mother at risk is 35 years or older. For translocations inherited from the mother, the risk is about 10%, whereas it is about 4–5% when father is the carrier. The risk is 100% if either of the parents is a carrier of translocation between two chromosomes 21.

Prenatal Diagnosis

Mothers having a child with DS and those conceiving after the age of 35 years can opt for definite prenatal diagnosis by invasive techniques. Chorionic villus sampling is done at 10–12 weeks of gestation or amniocentesis around 16–18 weeks of pregnancy can be offered to determine the chromosomal status of the fetus. In other women with less risk, or who do not wish to go for invasive testing, biochemical screening for chromosomal abnormality can be carried out. Second trimester maternal serum screening includes alpha-fetoprotein (MSAFP), human chorionic gonadotropin (hCG) and estriol assays. In DS pregnancies AFP and estriol are low whereas hCG is high. Second trimester screen (16–20 weeks of gestation) gives a detection rate of about 70%. Quadruple screen, which includes Inhibin A increases detection rates further. First trimester screening by β-hCG and pregnancy associated plasma protein A (PAPP-A) are very promising with higher detection rates. Another screening modality for DS is fetal ultrasonography (USG). Important markers in first trimester are increased nuchal translucency and absent nasal bone. Second trimester stigmata include nuchal fold thickness, short femur, duodenal atresia, renal pyelectasis, etc. Software is used to calculate the risk of DS and the couple is offered prenatal diagnosis if the risk cut-off is high.

A recent noninvasive test referred to as noninvasive prenatal testing (NIPT) is presently being used extensively in high-risk cases with a very high negative predictive value (close to 98%). This technique utilizes next generation sequencing technologies on fetal DNA isolated from maternal blood for detecting common aneuploidies involving chromosomes 21, 18, 13, and sex chromosomes. Presently, the cost is prohibitive for the test to be used as a screening test universally.

Prenatal karyotyping can be done by various invasive procedures. Chorionic villus sampling can be carried out between 10 weeks and 12 weeks of pregnancy (transcervical or transabdominal). This allows diagnosis in the first trimester. The options for the couples coming late or opt for the initial screening with serum markers and USG are karyotyping by amniocentesis (16–18 weeks) or transabdominal placental biopsy, or cordocentesis (after 18 weeks). The karyotype results are available within a week with cord blood samples and direct CVS preparations. Amniotic fluid cultures take about 2–3 weeks for the results. The risk of fetal loss after CVS is about 1% and with cordocentesis it is about 3%. Amniocentesis poses the lowest risk of about 0.5% or less. Rapid prenatal diagnosis of trisomy 21 can be done by FISH or quantitative fluorescent polymerase chain reaction (QF-PCR) on amniotic fluid sample, as these test results are available in 2 days.

Edward Syndrome or Trisomy 18

Edward syndrome is the second most common autosomal trisomy, with an incidence of about 1 in 3,000 newborn babies. These babies have high mortality early in life. Half of them may die within the first week and many of the remaining die in the next 1 year. Only 5–10% survives the first year as severely mentally handicapped individuals. Most of the surviving individuals have partial trisomies.

Cytogenetics

Most cases have full trisomy 18, higher maternal age being a risk factor. Mosaicism or partial trisomy or translocation cases are rare.

Clinical Features

This disorder is characterized by developmental retardation, hypertonia, occipital prominence, low set and malformed ears, micrognathia, shield-shaped chest and short sternum, joint abnormalities including flexion deformity of fingers, limited hip abduction and short dorsiflexed hallux. Congenital heart disease is also common mostly ventricular septal defect and patent ductus arteriosus.

Recurrence Risk

The recurrence risk is lower than the 1% unless one of the parents is a carrier of balanced chromosomal rearrangement involving chromosome 18 and most trisomy 18 fetuses are spontaneously aborted.

Prenatal Diagnosis

Biochemical screening in first and second trimester is useful for detecting mothers having high risk for trisomy 18. Classically, all three markers are low in the maternal blood. Definitive prenatal diagnosis can be offered using same (including NIPT) modalities as for Down syndrome.

Patau Syndrome or Trisomy 13

The incidence is about 1 in 5,000 births. Most babies would die in first few days of life. Only 5% survive the first 6 months and have severe mental defects, often have seizures and fail to thrive.

Cytogenetics

Most cases have full trisomy 13; mosaicism or partial trisomy or translocation cases are rare.

Clinical Features

It is characterized by severe developmental and physical retardation, microcephaly with sloping forehead and holoprosencephaly type of defect with varying degrees of incomplete development of forebrain, olfactory and optic nerves. There may be microphthalmia, coloboma of iris, retinal dysplasia and hypertonia. Malformations of ears and cleft lip with or without cleft palate are common and many children are deaf. Capillary hemangiomas are characteristic. There are frequent abnormalities of fingers and toes such as polydactyly, flexion deformities and long and hyperconvex nails. Congenital heart defects are present in almost 80% of cases and the common defects are ventricular septal defect, patent ductus arteriosus, and atrial septal defect.

Recurrence Risk

Risk of recurrence in subsequent pregnancies is less than 1%.

Prenatal Diagnosis

Prenatal screening by biochemical screening and NIPT and confirmatory is possible by doing karyotype on CVS or amniotic fluid sample.

Turner Syndrome

Turner syndrome has an incidence of about 1 in 5,000 live births but is much more common at conception and in spontaneous abortions.

Clinical Features

Clinical picture is highly variable; at birth, these girls may be totally normal or may show nonpitting edema of hands and feet, neck webbing, deep-set nails, etc. **Box 14.3.1** gives list of suggestive clinical features. Common features include short stature, gonadal dysgenesis, low posterior hairline, webbing of neck, shield chest, cubitus valgus, behavioral problems, etc. All short prepubertal girls and girls with primary amenorrhea should be investigated for Turner syndrome.

A girl with Turner syndrome with a characteristic phenotype is shown in **Figures 14.3.2A to C**.

Box 14.3.1: Clinical features of Turner syndrome.

- Retarded growth and reduced final height
- *Gonadal dysgenesis*:
  - No pubertal development
  - Infertility
- *Endocrine disturbances:*
  - Glucose intolerance (adults)
  - Noninsulin-dependent diabetes mellitus
  - Insulin-dependent diabetes mellitus
  - Autoimmune hypothyroidism (adults)
  - Thyroid autoantibodies
- *Physical abnormalities:*
  - *Mouth:*
    - Triangular facies
    - Micrognathia (small mandibular bone)
    - High-arched palate
    - Abnormal dental development
  - *Eyes:*
    - Epicanthic folds
    - Near sightedness
    - Strabismus
    - Ptosis
  - *Ears:*
    - Prominent anomalous ears
    - Hearing impairment
    - Infection of middle ear
  - *Neck:*
    - Low posterior hair line
    - Short broad appearing neck
    - Pterygium colli (webbed neck)
    - Excess loose skin in the back of the newborn
  - *Thorax:*
    - Broad chest (shield chest) with widely spaced nipples
    - Inverted nipples
  - *Skin, nail and hair:*
    - Lymphedema of hands and feet at birth or later
    - Multiple pigmented nevi
    - Nail hypoplasia, deep set nails
    - Vitiligo
    - Alopecia
  - *Skeleton:*
    - Bone age retardation
    - Decreased bone mineral content
    - Cubitus valgus
    - Short IV metacarpal
    - Genu valgum
    - Congenital hip subluxation
    - Scoliosis
    - Madelung deformity
  - *Heart:*
    - Bicuspid aortic valve
    - Coarctation aorta
  - *Kidneys:*
    - Horseshoe kidney
    - Abnormal positioning or duplication of renal pelvis, ureter or vessels
    - Renal aplasia or hypoplasia
- Psychological problems
- *Others:*
  - Failure to thrive during first year of life

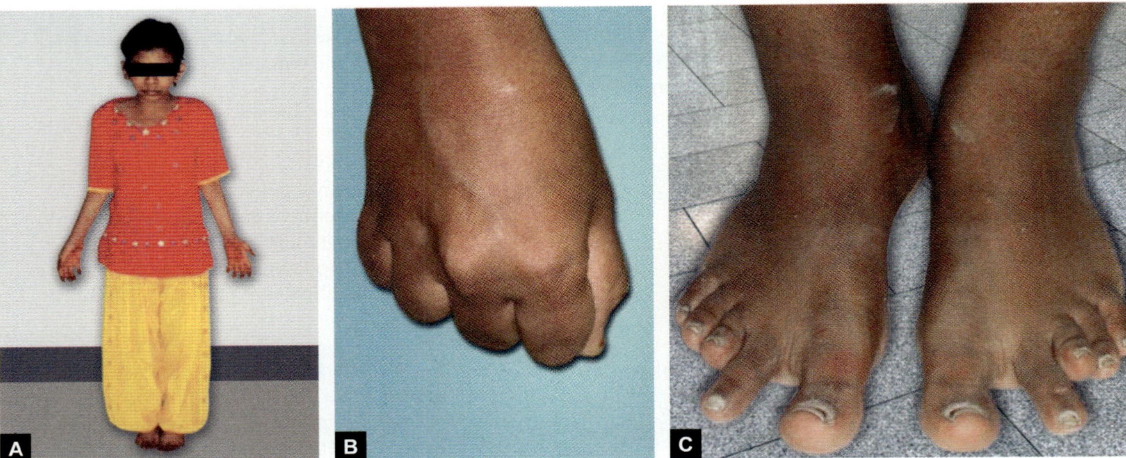

Figs. 14.3.2A to C: Girl with Turner syndrome: (A) Short stature, neck webbing and increased carrying angle; (B) Short 4th and 5th metacarpals; (C) Short 4th and 5th metatarsals.

Diagnosis

Investigations include hormonal profile, which shows a high follicle-stimulating hormone (FSH) and luteinizing hormone (LH) that suggest hypergonadotropic hypogonadism. Ultrasonography of pelvis commonly shows hypoplastic uterus and ovaries. Renal abnormalities may also be identified. Karyotype from peripheral blood is diagnostic which commonly shows 45,X. Other karyotype abnormalities could be 46,X,i(Xq); 45,X/46,XX; 45,X/46XY; 45,X/46,X,i(Xq). Search for Y cell line is warranted, especially if masculinization is present or mosaicism, unidentified marker or ring chromosome X is found in karyotype. Routine scoring of 20 metaphases is recommended but if karyotype is normal and there is high index of suspicion score 100 metaphases.

Management

- *Height monitoring* to check height velocity.
- Cardiac evaluation baseline and every year. Measurement of blood pressure, echocardiography—baseline and every year.
- Growth hormone therapy has been found to be beneficial and has been recommended by food and drug administration (FDA). Decision to treat should be left to the parents as the cost of treatment is high and height gain may be up to 10 cm.
- Counsel regarding *behavioral problems* due to short stature, amenorrhea and sterility (usually).
- *Evaluation for thyroid dysfunction:* Infancy and early childhood especially after 10 years of age. Hypothyroidism is often autoimmune. Replacement therapy should be given accordingly.
- *Ovarian hormone replacement:*
  - Start at 14 years [12 years, if patient has received and completed growth hormone (GH) therapy].
  - Start with conjugated estrogen at 0.3 mg/day or ethinyl estradiol 5–10 μg/day for 36 months; then increase to 0.625 mg or 1.25 mg (conjugated estrogen) or 20–50 μg/day (ethinyl estradiol)
  - *After 6 months to 1 year*: Cyclical therapy with adding progesterone.
- Regular audiometry in adults or earlier, if indicated.
- Evaluation for renal malformation by USG, and if abnormal manage accordingly.
- Prophylactic gonadectomy in Turner syndrome patients with Y chromosome.

Prenatal Diagnosis

Risk of recurrence in subsequent pregnancy is low (< 1%). Diagnosis of Turner syndrome can be suspected prenatally on first trimester USG scan with increased nuchal translucency or in second trimester showing cystic hygroma, generalized hydrops, or swelling localized to the neck (increased nuchal pad). Confirmation can be done by karyotype of fetal sample collected by CVS, amniocentesis or cordocentesis (blood from umbilical cord).

Klinefelter Syndrome

It is one of the most common causes of hypogonadism and infertility, affecting about 1.32 per 1,000 among newborns. There is failure of development of secondary sex characters and increased gonadotropin levels. The testis and penis are smaller in size for the age and they tend to have tall and slim stature with low upper and lower segment ratio. Pubertal development is delayed. The growth of pubic and facial hair is often late, while the pubic hair is generally feminine in distribution. Infertility is present, with hyalinization and fibrosis of seminiferous tubules. Virilization is partial and inadequate, with gynecomastia occurring in one-third of adolescents.

Chromosomal Analysis

Chromosomal analysis reveals 47,XXY karyotype. Errors in paternal meiosis I account for about one-half of 47,XXY males while the remainders are due to maternal meiosis II errors, and in a very small number of cases to a postzygotic mitotic error. Individuals with XXY/XY mosaicism have a better potential prognosis.

Structural Abnormalities

There can be partial deletion or duplications involving any part of any chromosome. These patients usually present with multiple major or minor malformations and developmental delay or mental retardation. Hence, karyotype of all children presenting with mental retardation with or without malformations is indicated especially if no other cause is detected.

SINGLE GENE DISORDERS

To date over 5,000 single gene traits and disorders have been identified. Each of these single gene disorders often called Mendelian traits or diseases, is relatively uncommon. Most Mendelian diseases are rare, affecting about 1/10,000 to 1/100,000 live births as an order of magnitude estimate. In total, they will add to the 1% of live births. Since only a single gene is involved in each case, these diseases generally have simple inheritance patterns in family pedigrees. This means they can be traced through families and their occurrence in later generations can be predicted. The defective version of the gene responsible for the disease is known as a mutant allele or a disease allele. The mode of inheritance is recognized by the pedigree chart. Details of Mendelian inheritance are discussed elsewhere. At minimum, a pedigree includes first-degree relatives (parents and siblings), second-degree relatives (aunts and uncles) and third-degree relatives (cousins and grandparents).

- Autosomal dominant trait is one, which manifests in the heterozygous state, i.e. in a person possessing both an abnormal or mutant allele and the normal allele. Examples are NF, achondroplasia, Marfan syndrome, etc.
- Autosomal recessive disorders only manifest when the mutant allele is present in a double dose, i.e. homozygosity. Examples of autosomal recessive disorders are: thalassemia, SMA, sickle cell anemia and almost all IEM.
- Sex-linked inheritance refers to the pattern of inheritance shown by genes, which are located on either of the sex chromosomes. X-linked dominant inheritance although is uncommon; there are disorders which manifest in the heterozygous female as well as in the male who has the mutant allele on his single X chromosome. Examples include hypophosphatemic type of vitamin D-resistant rickets, orofaciodigital syndrome, etc.
- X-linked recessive diseases usually manifest only in males. A male with a mutant allele on his single X chromosome is said to be hemizygous for that allele. Examples include: hemophilia A and B, Duchenne muscular dystrophy, etc.
- Mitochondrial inheritance is due to mutation in a mitochondrial gene; it is passed from a mother to all her children; sons will not pass it on, but daughters will pass it on to all of their children and so on. Examples include mitochondrial encephalopathy, lactic acidosis and stroke like syndrome (MELAS), Leber hereditary optic neuropathy (LHON).

In this chapter, we will discuss clinical features and management of some of the commoner single gene disorders.

AUTOSOMAL DOMINANT DISORDERS

Achondroplasia

Achondroplasia is an autosomal dominant (AD) disorder. More than half of the cases are due to *de novo* mutations. This disorder is caused by a common point mutation in Fibroblast Growth Factor Receptor 3 *(FGFR3)* gene. The mutations in the same gene also cause a lethal dysplasia called thanatophoric dysplasia and a relatively mild dysplasia known as hypochondroplasia.

Clinical Manifestations

The clinical manifestations include short stature with predominant short limbs. There is rhizomelic shortening, large head, frontal bossing, depressed nasal bridge, short and broad trident shaped hands, lumbar lordosis and hypotonia, and delayed motor development. Cognitive development is usually normal.

Complications include hydrocephalus, otitis media and hearing loss in adulthood, lumbar cord and nerve root compression syndromes. **Figures 14.3.3A to C** show typical phenotype of achondroplasia.

Characteristic radiological findings are small cuboid-shaped vertebral bodies with short pedicles and progressive narrowing of lumbar interpedicular distance (normally there is caudal widening), rectangular iliac wings, narrow greater sciatic notches, horizontal acetabular roofs, anterior breaking of lower thoracic or upper lumbar vertebrae, small foramen magnum, metaphysical flare, short and wide tubular bones of the hands and feet. **Figures 14.3.4A to D** show characteristic radiological findings of achondroplasia. Although, the diagnosis is essentially clinical-radiological, molecular testing is easily available and is confirmatory.

Risk of Recurrence

Risk of recurrence is 50% if either of the parents is affected but is very low if the disorder is caused by a de novo mutation.

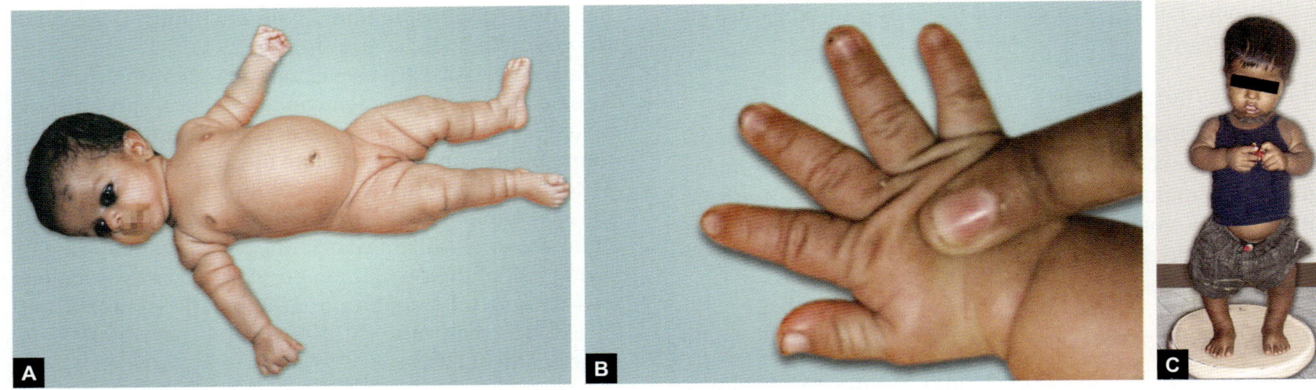

Figs. 14.3.3A to C: Achondroplasia: Short limbed short stature large head with frontal bossing, depressed nasal bridge and trident hand. (A) Folds on thighs and arms; (B) Trident hand; (C) Genu varus.

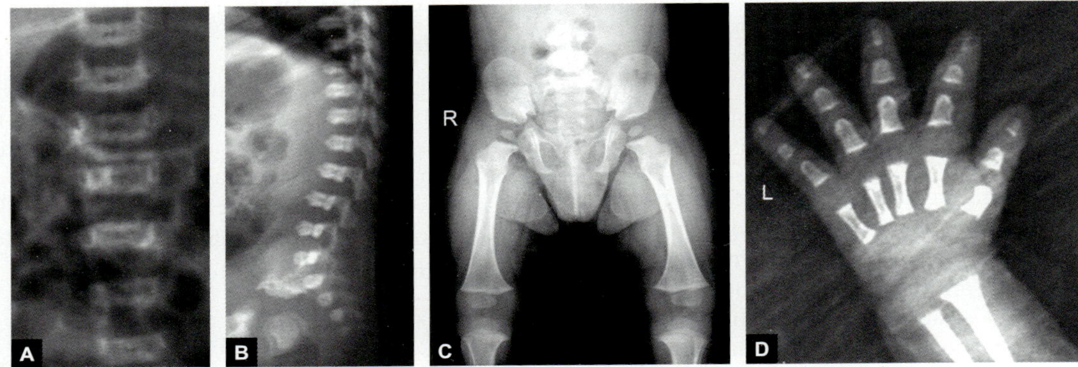

Figs. 14.3.4A to D: Radiological features of achondroplasia: (A) Small cuboid-shaped vertebral bodies with short pedicles and progressive narrowing of lumbar interpedicular distance (normally there is caudal widening); (B) Scalloping of posterior borders of vertebrae and anterior breaking of lower thoracic or upper lumbar vertebrae; (C) Rectangular iliac wings, narrow greater sciatic notches, horizontal acetabular roofs, metaphysical flare; (D) Short and wide tubular bones of the hands with trident appearance.

Management

There is no specific treatment. Prompt recognition and appropriate treatment of complications, management of psychological problems due to unusual appearance and prevention of obesity is important. Growth hormone therapy though may add a few inches to the final height but is not routinely recommended. Limb lengthening though very cumbersome has been tried to improve height.

Marfan Syndrome

Marfan syndrome is an AD disorder caused by mutations in the fibrillin gene located on chromosome 15q21.1. It has a high penetrance but expression may be variable.

Clinical Manifestations

The diagnosis of Marfan syndrome is suspected on clinical evaluation. Some scoring criteria, e.g. Ghent's criteria have also been proposed. The disorder primarily includes skeletal system, eyes and cardiovascular system. Common skeletal manifestations include tall stature, long limbs with increased arm span, arachnodactyly, joint laxity, scoliosis, kyphosis, decreased subcutaneous fat, pectus deformities (excavatum/carinatum), flat feet, etc. Characteristic eye abnormality is lens subluxation. Myopia, increased axial length of the globe and retinal detachment may be present. Cardiovascular defects include dilatation and aneurysm of aorta (commonly ascending), aortic and mitral regurgitation, mitral valve prolapse, etc. **Figures 14.3.5A to C** show a patient with Marfan syndrome.

Diagnosis

Molecular studies are not routinely done for diagnostic purposes as the gene is very big.

Management

Patients with Marfan syndrome need regular follow up for early detection and prevention of complications,

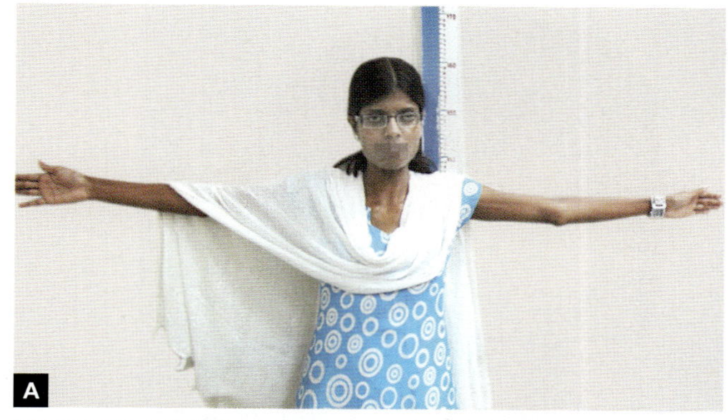

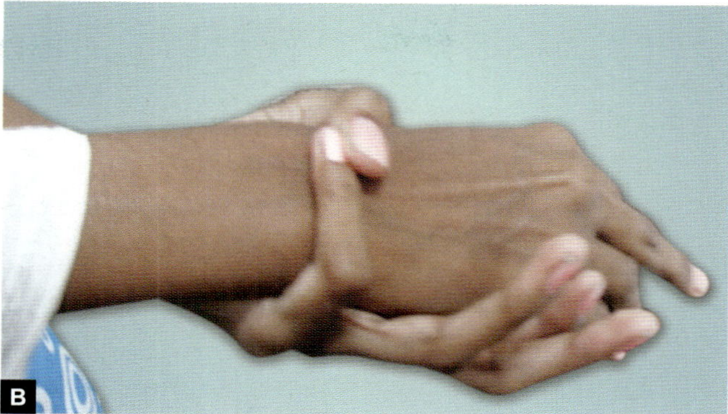

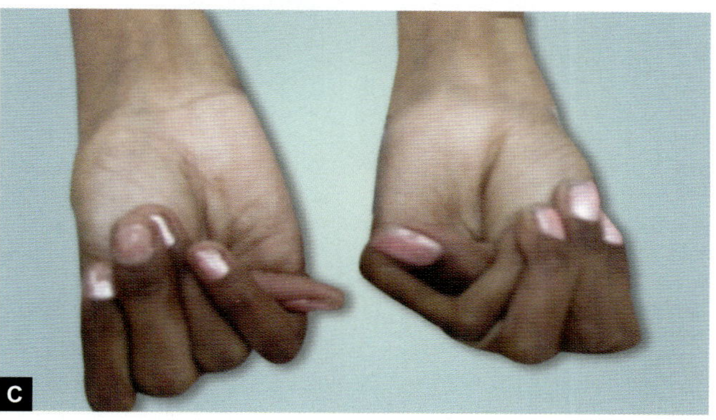

Figs. 14.3.5A to C: Marfan syndrome: (A) Increased arm span; (B) Wrist sign; (C) Thumb sign.

primarily cardiac. Beta-blockers are used to reduce cardiac complications. Recently, antagonist of the angiotensin II type 1 receptor-losartan has been found useful to prevent cardiac complications of Marfan syndrome.

Risk of Recurrence

Risk of recurrence in subsequent pregnancies is 50% if either of the parents is affected.

Tuberous Sclerosis

Tuberous sclerosis is an AD neurocutaneous syndrome with multisystem involvement. The disorder can include brain, skin, kidney, eyes and cardiovascular system. Tuberous sclerosis type 1 *(TSC1)* and tuberous sclerosis type 2 *(TSC2)* are the genes for TS.

Clinical Features

Major criteria include facial angiofibromas, subungal fibromas, hypomelanotic macules typically described as "ash leaf", Shagreen patch (flesh-colored elevated orange peel-like lesions), retinal hamartomas, cortical tubers (on neuroimaging), subependymal nodules, astrocytomas, cardiac rhabdomyoma, renal angiomyolipoma and pulmonary lymphangiomyomatosis. Half of the patients have developmental delay. Seizures are difficult to control, behavioral problems and autistic features are common. **Figures 14.3.6A and B** show skin manifestations in a patient with TS.

The unique skin lesions and neuroimaging findings are most helpful for confirming diagnosis. Confirmation of diagnosis can be made by mutation testing for the two genes: (1) *TSC1* and (2) *TSC2,* but it is very expensive. For detailed discussion, please refer to **Chapter 6.4.**

Management

Treatment of TS is largely symptomatic. Seizures may be refractory to treat. Some patients show a good response to vigabatrin therapy. Surgical interventions may be required for some patients.

Risk of Recurrence

Risk of recurrence is 50% if one of the parents is affected. Parents should be examined carefully and investigated for stigmata of TS as some of them may have very few features.

Neurofibromatosis

Neurofibromatosis is a common AD neurocutaneous syndrome with variable expression. It is classified in two types: (1) NF1 and (2) NF2.

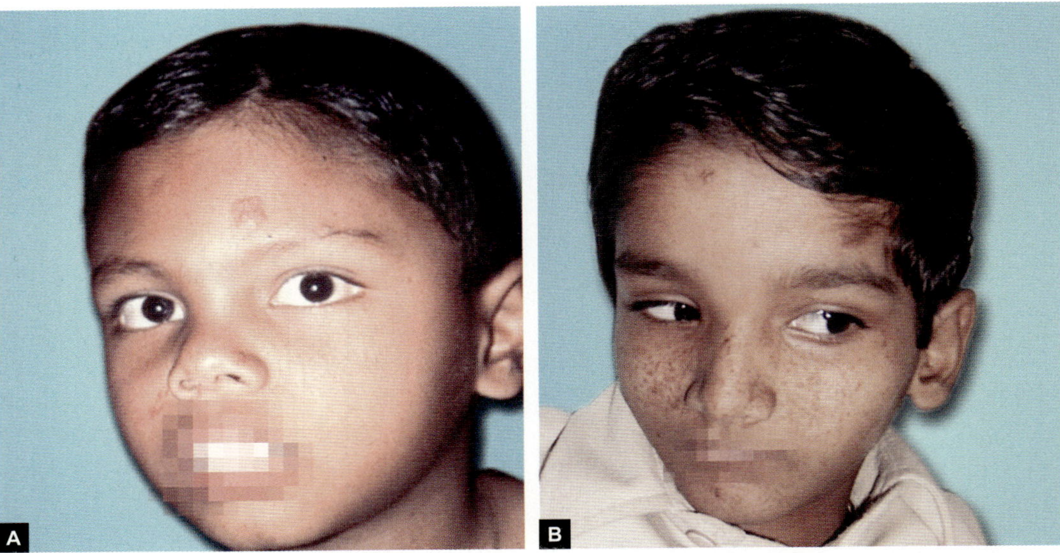

Figs. 14.3.6A and B: Skin lesions in a patient with TS: (A) Hyperpigmented thickened (Shagreen) patch on forehead; (B) Adenoma sebaceum on cheeks in butterfly distribution.

Clinical Features

Clinical features of NF1 include Café-au-lait spots (six or more, 1.5 cm or larger in postpubertal patients, 0.5 cm or larger in prepubertal patients), two or more neurofibromas, freckling of axillary or inguinal regions, optic pathway tumors, iris hamartomas (Lisch nodules), pseudoarthrosis of tibia and family history of affected first degree relative. For labeling as NF two or more of these features should be present. **Figure 14.3.7** shows a patient with NF1.

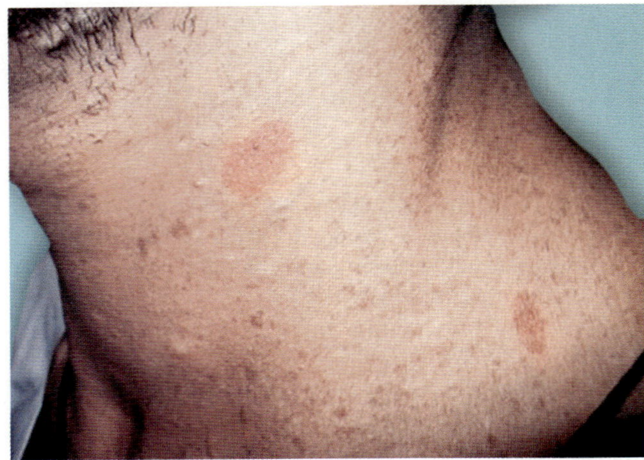

Fig. 14.3.7: Skin lesions in NF1 (Café-au-lait spots).

Diagnosis

Diagnosis is invariably clinical but can be confirmed by molecular studies.

Management

There is no specific treatment for NF1 and management consists of regular follow-up and evaluation for complications such as focal neurological dysfunction, optic gliomas, skeletal abnormalities, cognitive/learning problems, hypertension, etc. and provision of symptomatic therapy.

In NF2, skin manifestations may be there are less common. The most characteristic feature of NF2 is the development in early adult life of tumors involving 8th cranial nerves commonly called acoustic neuromas, which may require surgical intervention.

For detailed discussion, please refer to **Chapter 6.4.**

Autosomal Recessive Disorders

β-Thalassemia

β-thalassemia is an inherited autosomal recessive blood disorder. It is probably the most common autosomal recessive disorder in North India, the carrier frequency (about 3%) is approximately comparable to cystic fibrosis in Caucasians. In thalassemia, the genetic defect results in reduced rate of synthesis of one of the globin chains that make up hemoglobin. Reduced synthesis of one of the globin chains can cause the formation of abnormal hemoglobin molecules, and this in turn causes the anemia, which is the characteristic presenting symptom. These children usually become symptomatic in first year of life and present with severe anemia and splenomegaly. Repeated blood transfusions are required for survival. Details are discussed in **Chapter 11.5**.

β-thalassemia is due to mutations in the hemoglobin beta *(HBB)* gene on chromosome 11 (also inherited in an autosomal-recessive fashion). The severity of the disease depends on the nature of the mutation. If only *one* β-globin allele bears a mutation, the individual is clinically asymptomatic and is called β-*thalassemia minor* (or sometimes called β-*thalassemia carrier*). If both alleles have thalassemia mutations, the disease is β-*thalassemia major* or *intermedia* depending on the severity of anemia.

Risk of Recurrence and Prenatal Testing

Risk of recurrence in the siblings of a patient with thalassemia major is 25%. Prenatal diagnosis is possible as early as 10–11 weeks by molecular studies on chorionic villus tissue. Before doing prenatal diagnosis, the mutations in the family need to be identified by testing the affected child or both the parents who are obligate carriers. In view of high frequency, carrier screening should be recommended to all either early in pregnancy or preferably before planning pregnancy.

Spinal Muscular Atrophy

Spinal muscular atrophy is an autosomal recessive disorder and is a term applied to a number of different disorders, all having in common a genetic cause and the manifestation of weakness due to loss of the motor neurons of the spinal cord and brainstem. Infantile SMA (type 1) is the most severe form. These babies present in first few weeks/months of life with motor delay and floppiness. Characteristic tongue fasciculation's are seen in most cases. Patients with type I SMA die in early infancy. Spinal muscular atrophy types II and III are milder forms.

Diagnosis and Management

Electromyography (EMG) shows neurogenic pattern, and muscle biopsy shows group atrophy. In most cases (> 95%) diagnosis can be made by the survival motor neuron (SMN) gene test, which shows homozygous deletion of exon 7 of *SMN1* gene. Recently, a drug spinraza (nusinersen), which contains an antisense oligonucleotide, and selectively binds and targets RNA and regulates gene expression has been approved by the FDA. It has the potential to enhance the amount of functional SMN protein in infants and children with SMA and has shown promising results in recent trials. The cost is prohibitive. Risk of recurrence is 25% in subsequent pregnancies and prenatal diagnosis is possible using chorionic villus tissue. Details of SMA are discussed in **Chapter 6.15.**

X-LINKED DISORDERS

Duchenne/Becker Muscular Dystrophy

Muscular dystrophies form a group of genetically determined progressive disorder primarily involving the muscles. The various forms of muscular dystrophies are distinguished by a combination of clinical, pathological features and genetic investigations. The common muscular dystrophies following X-linked pattern of inheritance are Duchenne muscular dystrophy (DMD) and Becker muscular dystrophy (BMD).

Duchenne muscular dystrophy is a severe muscle wasting disorder, and BMD is a milder form of the disease with later onset and slow progression. In DMD, children usually present around 3–4 years of age with calf hypertrophy and proximal muscle weakness. Gower's sign is characteristically seen. Duchenne muscular dystrophy is also discussed in **Chapter 6.15.**

Dystrophin gene responsible for DMD/BMD maps to the short arm of the X chromosome at band Xp21. DMD being a severe form, there is little or no functional dystrophin protein. In BMD, a milder form, dystrophin may be reduced in amount or altered in size. Approximately 60% of the affected males have a deletion of one or more exons while the remaining patients have duplications and point mutations.

Recently therapy using Exon skipping technique for Exon 51 has been approved by FDA and long-term outcomes are being studied. Other kinds of therapies acting on stop-codon mutations are being explored.

Risk of Recurrence

Risk of recurrence in subsequent pregnancies is 50% for male offspring, if mother is a carrier. There are 50% chances of the daughters being carriers. Prenatal diagnosis is possible on chorionic villus tissue using molecular techniques.

Fragile X Syndrome

Fragile X syndrome (FXS) is an X-linked semi-dominantly inherited disorder with reduced penetrance and does not follow a classical Mendelian pattern of inheritance. Initially it was thought to be a chromosomal disorder because of presence of a fragile site at Xq27.3. Fragile X syndrome is the most common heritable form of moderate mental retardation and is second only to DS among all causes of moderate mental retardation in males. It is due to a mutation in a gene on X chromosome leading to expansion of a trinucleotide repeat sequence.

This disorder is caused by the expansion of the (CGGn) repeat in the 5′ untranslated region of the first exon of a gene called fragile X mental retardation 1 *(FMR1)*. Inheritance of this X-linked disorder is unusual, where it is passed on by an unaffected transmitting male but only can be expressed after being passed through a female. The normal repeat size is less than 50. In permutation carriers of FXS, the number of repeated CGG sequences is greater than 50 but less than 200. In full mutation, the number of repeats is more than 200. In general, the expression of phenotypic manifestation is less severe in females, as seen in X-linked dominant inheritance.

Clinical Features

Clinical features are nonspecific and include overgrowth, large dolichocephalic head, large ears, joint hyperextensibility,

14.4 Genetic Metabolic Disorders

Shubha Phadke

INTRODUCTION

The body of a living organism is a biochemical factory with complex metabolic pathways working simultaneously and maintaining life processes in an efficient manner. The metabolism proceeds in steps—each step being governed by an enzyme. Usually there is one gene for one enzyme. If a gene gets mutated, the enzyme will not be synthesized or will lose its function and the disease will manifest. These diseases are collectively known as "inborn errors of metabolism (IEM)". The enzymes are required in a very small quantity and hence most of the genetic metabolic disorders manifest only when both copies of a gene for an enzyme are mutated or abnormal. Thus, most genetic metabolic disorders are inherited in autosomal recessive mode indicating that both the parents of an affected individual are clinically normal but carry one mutated copy of the gene in concern, i.e. they are carriers of the disease. Some types of porphyria due to abnormalities in heme metabolism are inherited in an autosomal dominant fashion.

Genes for few enzymes are located on X chromosome. Examples of IEMs transmitted in X-linked manner include mucopolysaccharidosis type II (Hunter syndrome), Fabry disease, ornithine transcarbamylase deficiency, and Lesch-Nyhan syndrome. The X-linked IEMs usually manifest only in males, and females usually are asymptomatic carriers who can transmit the disorder to the sons. The rare cases of manifesting females are due to unusual situations such as a girl with Turner syndrome (having only one X chromosome) or nonrandom lyonization leading to preferential inactivation of X chromosome with a normal copy of gene in disproportionately more cells of the body.

The first IEM was described by Sir Archibald Garrod in 1902. The disorder was alkaptonuria, in which nappies of children suffering from the disease turned black on exposure to air. This was due to excretion of homogentisic acid in urine due to a block in the metabolism of tyrosine **(Flowchart 14.4.1)**. Later inborn errors of various pathways involving metabolism of amino acids, carbohydrates, fatty acids, lipids, trace minerals and various complex molecules such as lipoproteins, mucopolysaccharides and oligosaccharides were identified. The clinical manifestations are either due to accumulation of metabolic products of the substrate (as in phenylketonuria) or deficiency of the downstream product of the enzymatic reaction (as in albinism or hemophilia). In lysosomal storage disorders the intracellular accumulation of complex molecules due to lack of their degradation leads to signs and symptoms of the disease.

Flowchart 14.4.1: Metabolism of phenylalanine and tyrosine. On the left is an enzyme catalyzing the step and on the right is the disease *(Italics)* caused by deficiency of the enzyme.

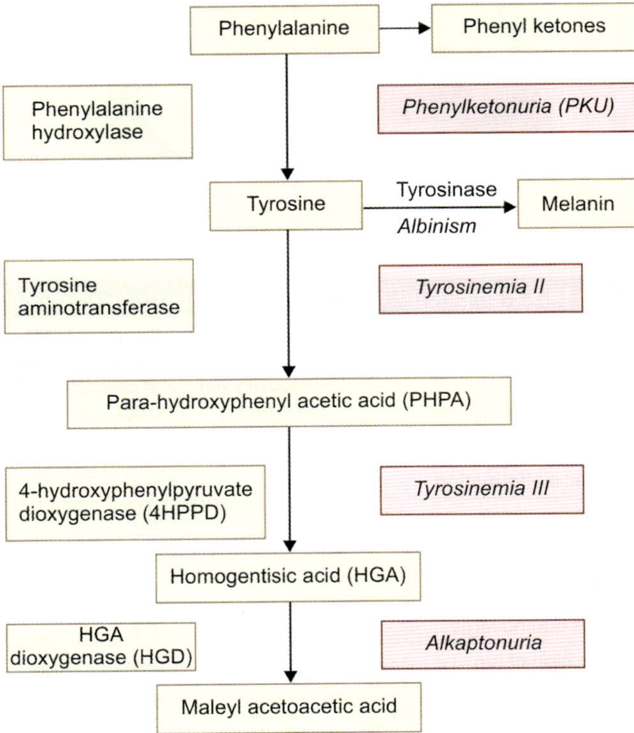

CLASSIFICATION

In addition to enzyme deficiencies, biochemical abnormalities of various proteins such as transport proteins, hormones, immunoglobulins, coagulation factors also give rise to diseases. The metabolic disorders are classified into the following categories **(Table 14.4.1)**:

CLINICAL FEATURES

The clinical features of category I group of genetic metabolic disorders depend on the function of the organ or system

Table 14.4.1: Classification of genetic metabolic disorders.

Category	*Group*	*Clinical manifestations*	*Examples*
I. Disorders that involve only one functional system or one organ		Symptoms characteristic for the system/organ involved	Immunodeficiency disorder, hemophilia, renal tubular acidosis
II. Diseases due to defects in the basic metabolic pathway common to a large number of cells or organs, or the pathway is restricted to one organ but has systemic effects	1. Defects affecting the synthesis or catabolism of complex molecules; defects of intracellular trafficking and processing	Progressive manifestations not affected by diet, or environmental factors	Lysosomal storage disorders such as Gaucher disease, Hunter syndrome, peroxisomal disorders, alpha I antitrypsin deficiency
	2. Defects of intermediary metabolism that leads to acute or progressive intoxication due to accumulation of toxic compounds proximal to the block	Acute or intermittent manifestations. Onset may be late. Central nervous system involvement is frequent	Amino acidurias, urea cycle defects
	3. Disorder due to deficiency in energy production or utilization	Hypoglycemia, lactic acidosis, involvement of heart muscles, brain, liver and multiple organs	Mitochondrial disorders, disorders associated with lactic acidosis, defects of neoglucogenesis

Source: Saudubray JM, Charpentier C. Clinical phenotype diagnosis/Algorithms. In: Scriver CR, Beaudet AL, Sly WS (Eds). The Metabolic and Molecular Bases of Inherited Disorders, 8th edition. New York: McGraw-Hill Medical; 2001. pp. 1329-30.

Table 14.4.2: Diagnostic approach to an acute sick neonate or child.

Acidosis	*Ketosis*	*Lactic acidosis*	*Hypoglycemia*	*Hyperammonemia*	*IEM*
–	+++	–	–	+/–	Maple syrup urine disease
+++	++	+++	+/–	+/–	Organic acidemia
++	–	+	++	+	Fatty acid oxidation defect
+	+	+++	+/–	–	Lactic acidosis
–	–	–	–	+++	Urea cycle defects

involved. The category II disorders are traditionally described as IEM and this chapter discusses this group of disorders. The clinical features of IEMs are varied and usually involve many systems. Involvement of nervous system is common. Many of these disorders manifest in neonatal period, infancy or early childhood. However, many disorders, e.g. hyperlipidemias, Fabry disease and some mitochondrial disorders may present at a later part of life. Adult onset variants of diseases clinically manifesting during infancy such as Tay-Sachs disease and metachromatic leukodystrophy (MLD) are known. Manifestations can be intermittent as well dependent on exposure to offending agent as in porphyria and some cases of urea cycle disorders. Acute illness with neurological deterioration in a neonate or an infant is a presentation of many IEMs such as aminoacidopathies, organic acidemias, galactosemia, disorders with lactic acidosis, glycogen storage disorders, and fatty acid oxidation defects. As neonates have limited manifestations and respond to any type of insult in the same way, the clinical picture of IEM, septicemia, birth asphyxia, and intracranial hemorrhage may superficially look similar. It is important to consider IEM in any acutely sick infant or neonate; especially if septicemia screen is negative, the delivery was uneventful, and manifestations start 2–3 days after a normal course in a neonate. Other indicators to point towards IEM are presence of consanguinity in parents and history of neonatal death(s) in previous siblings. The basic investigations of an acutely sick child or a neonate can give clue to the type of IEM **(Table 14.4.2)**.

In addition to acute presentation, some of the clinical manifestations suggestive of IEM are given in **Table 14.4.3**. Some disorders have intermittent acute presentation due to exposure to precipitating causes such as high protein diet or fasting. Many storage disorders have a chronic progressive course.

DIAGNOSIS

Inborn errors of metabolism are many, rare and the manifestations are overlapping. These make diagnosis difficult. Clinical diagnosis is not possible and diagnostic tests

Table 14.4.3: Common clinical presentations of IEMs.

Presentations	***Diseases***
Development delay, seizures, regression of milestones, tone abnormalities	• Biotinidase deficiency • Tay-Sachs disease • Metachromatic leukodystrophy • Krabbe disease • Neuronal ceroid lipofuscinosis • Canavan disease • Peroxisomal disorders
Coarse facies, hepatosplenomegaly, joint contractures, corneal clouding	• Mucopolysaccharidosis • Mucolipidosis • Oligosaccharidosis
Hepatosplenomegaly, neonatal cholestasis	• Alpha I antitrypsin deficiency • Galactosemia • Tyrosinemia • Niemann-Pick disease • Peroxisomal disorder • Cystic fibrosis • Hemochromatosis • Defects of bile acid synthesis
Hepatosplenomegaly	• Glycogen storage disease • Gaucher disease • Niemann-Pick disease
Cardiomyopathy	• Pompe disease • Mitochondrial diseases
Extrapyramidal manifestation and neuroregression	• Wilson disease
Hepatic failure	• Fatty acid oxidation defects • Mitochondrial disorder
Vomiting, diarrhea, failure to thrive	• Lysinuric protein intolerance • Wolman disease • Abetalipoproteinemia • Lactase deficiency • Acrodermatitis enteropathica

Table 14.4.4: Characteristic manifestations of some IEMs.

Manifestations	***Disorder***
Cherry red spot in fundus of eye	• Tay-Sachs disease • Niemann-Pick disease • Generalized gangliosidosis
Cataract	• Galactosemia • Lowe syndrome • Zellweger syndrome
Inverted nipple, abnormal fat distribution on buttocks	• Congenital defects of glycosylation
Corneal opacities	• Tyrosinemia type II • Cystinosis • Fabry disease • Mucopolysaccharidosis
Alopecia, skin rash	• Biotinidase deficiency
Pale, brittle, steely hair	• Menkes kinky hair disease
Macrocephaly (large head)	• Tay-Sachs disease • Canavan disease • van der Knapp disease • Glutaric aciduria type I • Alexander disease
KF ring in cornea	• Wilson disease
Retinitis pigmentosa	• Mitochondrial disease • Refsum disease • Neuronal ceroid lipofuscinosis
Muscle pain and myoglobinuria	• Glycogen storage disease V • Fatty acid oxidation defect
Rickets	• Tyrosinemia type I • Renal tubular acidosis
Macrocytic anemia	• Abnormalities of folate and cobalamin metabolism

are often not easily available. History and clinical examination are hence extremely important to search for diagnostic clues **(Fig. 14.4.1)**. **Table 14.4.4** lists some characteristic features of common IEMs.

Routine investigations can also help to reach diagnosis. For example, in a hypotonic infant with enlarged liver, presence of cataract, punctate ossifications of epiphyses in radiographs lead to the diagnosis of Zellweger syndrome. MRI brain is useful especially if white matter disease of brain is suspected **(Figs. 14.4.2A and B)**. Bone marrow examination may help in diagnosis of Gaucher and Niemann-Pick diseases. However, confirmation of diagnosis is needed using specialized tests like enzyme assays, metabolite profile of plasma and urine using tandem mass spectrometry (TMS) and gas chromatography mass spectrometry (GCMS). Quantification of very long chain fatty acids and plasmalogen is necessary for diagnosis

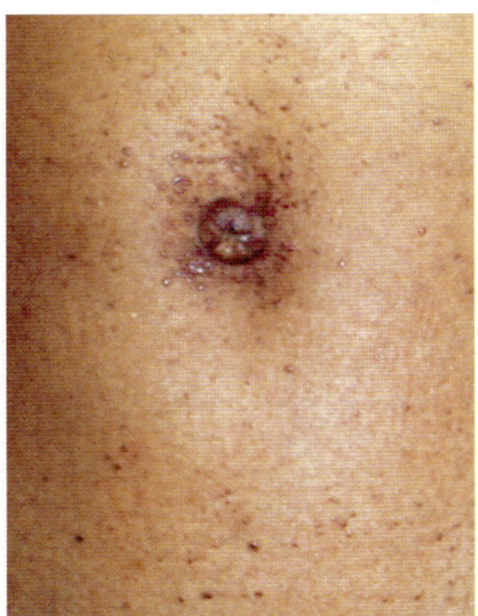

Fig. 14.4.1: Angiokeratomas characteristic of Fabry disease (also seen in fucosidosis).

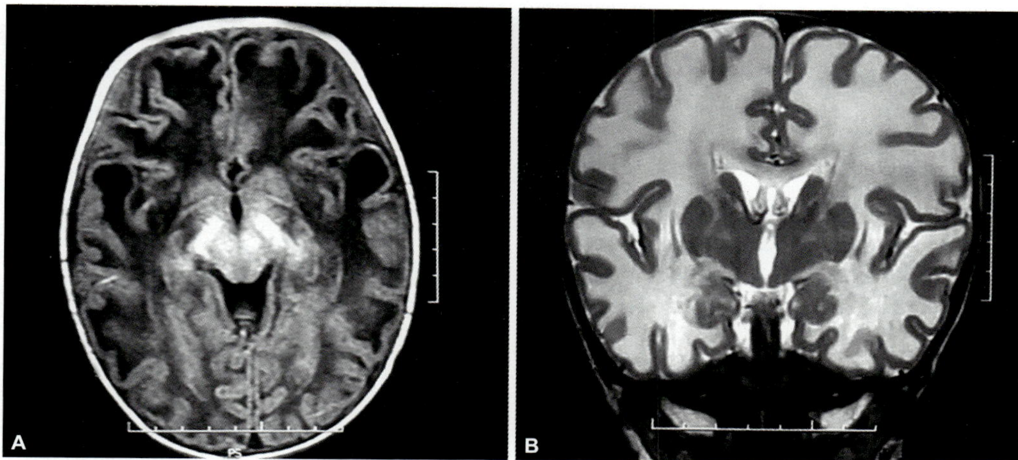

Figs. 14.4.2A and B: MRI brain showing cystic changes and leukodystrophy characteristic of van der Knapp disease. (A) Axial T1 Flair image showing cystic changes in both temporal regions; (B) Coronal T2 images shows extensive involvement and hyperintensity of central and peripheral white matter.

of peroxisomal disorders. Specific enzyme assays on white blood cells or cultured fibroblasts are necessary for confirmation of diagnosis of lysosomal storage disorders. Causative genes are known for most the IEMs and mutation detection helps in confirmation of diagnosis. It also helps in providing prenatal diagnosis. Genetic test for identification of disease causing mutation was previously done only after clinical and biochemical testing provided a diagnosis or a possible diagnosis. Now the situation has changed and genetic testing can be used as a first tier testing to provide rapid diagnosis and can help in the management of babies in the neonatal care unit. Deoxyribonucleic acid (DNA) based testing is done by a next generation sequencing (NGS) based testing which can sequence all genes or the whole genome in one go. This also can provide diagnosis when biochemical profile is not characteristic due to sample collection at inappropriate time or the secondary metabolic changes complicating the scenario. NGS is a powerful technology but the results should be carefully evaluated and correlated with clinical and biochemical phenotype.

Table 14.4.5: Treatment of inborn errors of metabolism.

Disorder	*Treatment*
Phenylketonuria	Phenylalanine restricted diet, tetrahydrobiopterin
Galactosemia	Lactose free diet
Biotinidase deficiency	Biotin
Tyrosinemia I	NTBC
Mucopolysaccharidosis	BMT, ERT
Wilson disease	Penicillamine, zinc
Pompe disease	ERT
Gaucher disease	BMT, ERT
Fatty acid oxidation defects	Prevent fasting, carnitine
Cobalamin metabolism disorder	Vitamin B_{12}
Homocystinuria	Pyridoxine
Porphyria	Load of glucose and acid hematin
Glycogen storage disorder type I	Corn starch

[BMT: bone marrow transplantation; ERT: enzyme replacement therapy; NTBC: 2-(2-nitro-4-trifluoromethyl benzoyl)-1,3-cyclohexanedione]

MANAGEMENT

Successful treatments with various strategies have been available for some disorders for decades **(Table 14.4.5)**. Over last few decades the number of disorders for which partial improvement is possible is increasing. However, there is no curative treatment for many IEMs. Successful enzyme replacement therapy (ERT) as in Gaucher disease **(Figs. 14.4.3A to D)**, mucopolysaccharidosis I SH, mucopolysaccharidosis II, glycogen storage disease type II (Pompe disease) and Fabry disease has brought hope that similar success stories may be repeated for other 40 lysosomal storage disorders. ERT cannot prevent neurological involvement yet as the modified enzymes cannot cross the blood brain barrier. Bone marrow transplantation (BMT) is successful in preventing central nervous system involvement if done in early stages. Similarly, liver transplantation to replace the damaged liver or as a source of enzyme, is successful in some disorders. Long-term success of gene therapy in more than 20 children with immunodeficiency disorders and recent success reported in gene therapy for beta thalassemia has shown the hope that the gene therapy may be an option for many disorders soon.

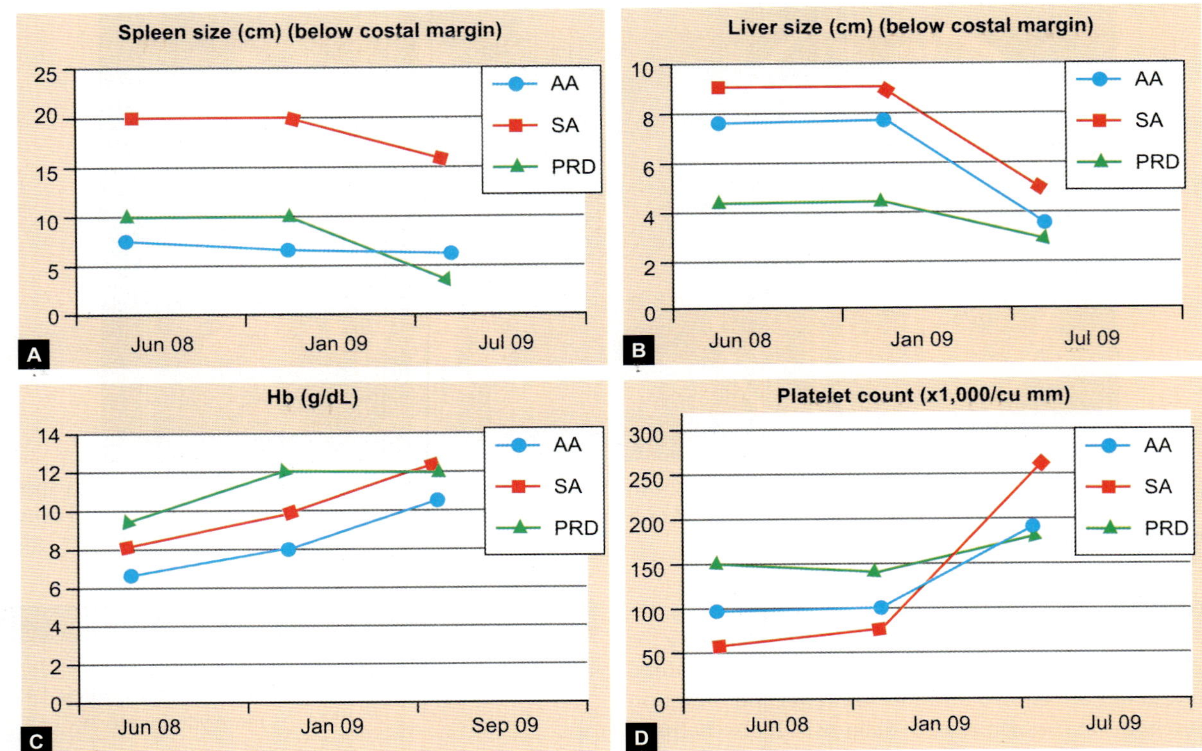

Figs. 14.4.3A to D: Response to enzyme replacement therapy (ERT) in three patients with Gaucher disease type I (different colors are used for different patients).

Lack of curative treatment, difficult, lifelong, costly treatment, and poor outcomes in many IEMs make genetic counseling and prenatal diagnosis important components of management. Accurate diagnosis of the affected patient in the family is the prerequisite for prenatal diagnosis. Hence, even if the child appears to be too serious to survive; all attempts should be made to confirm the diagnosis. Urine, plasma and blood for DNA should be stored for future analysis even if the affected child dies before diagnosis.

Deoxyribonucleic acid test for mutation in the chorionic villi is the best option for prenatal diagnosis. But for lack of mutation detection, metabolite estimation in amniotic fluid or enzyme assay on chorionic villi can be used for prenatal diagnosis. DNA-based mutation analysis has very minimal error rate as compared to prenatal diagnosis using biochemical tests.

SOME REPRESENTATIVE INBORN ERRORS OF METABOLISM

Phenylketonuria

Phenylketonuria (PKU) is one of the best studied IEMs. Still there is limited understanding of pathology about how phenylalanine metabolites lead to neurological abnormalities. The history of PKU starting from diagnosis, diet therapy, newborn screening, and fetal effects of maternal PKU reflects the developments in IEM. The recent treatment with biopterin as a molecule which modulates folding of protein molecule and improves function of mutated protein, opens up similar options for many other genetic disorders caused by mutations leading to abnormal folding, and hence decreased function of the protein.

Phenylketonuria is an autosomal recessive disorder caused by deficiency of phenylalanine hydroxylase (PAH); an enzyme, which converts phenylalanine to tyrosine **(Flowchart 14.4.2)**. The enzyme is coded by PAH gene which expresses in hepatic cells.

Tetrahydrobiopterin (BH4) is a cofactor for PAH gene which expresses in hepatic cells. In the absence of PAH, the phenylalanine accumulates in body and some of it gets metabolized by alternate pathways to produce increased amount of phenylpyruvic acid (a keto acid) which gets excreted in urine. That is why the name "phenylketonuria". The disease was described by Folling in 1934. In 1950, Horst Bickel performed successful intervention with dietary phenylalanine restriction in a patient with PKU. The phenylalanine levels in blood reduced and there was clinical improvement. However soon it became obvious that the treatment unless started

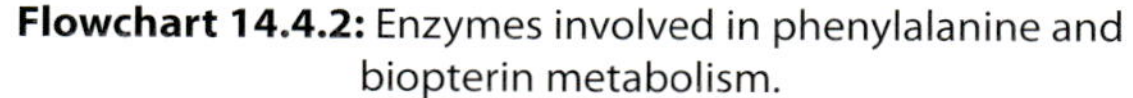

Flowchart 14.4.2: Enzymes involved in phenylalanine and biopterin metabolism.

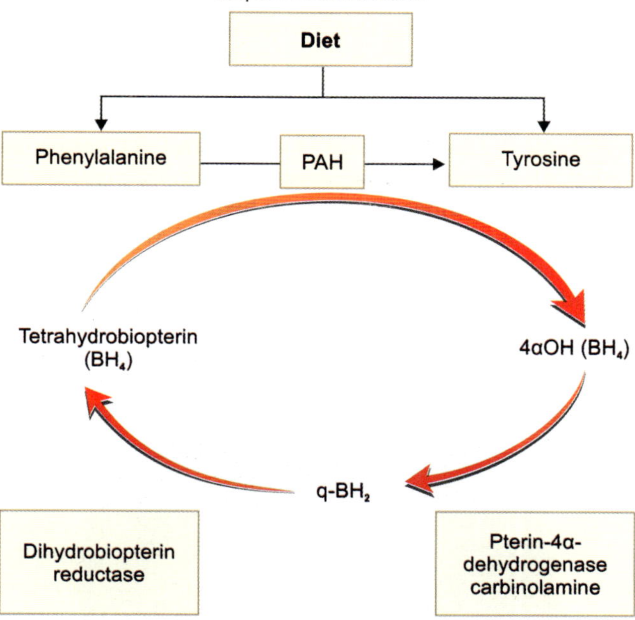

(PAH: phenylalanine hydroxylase)

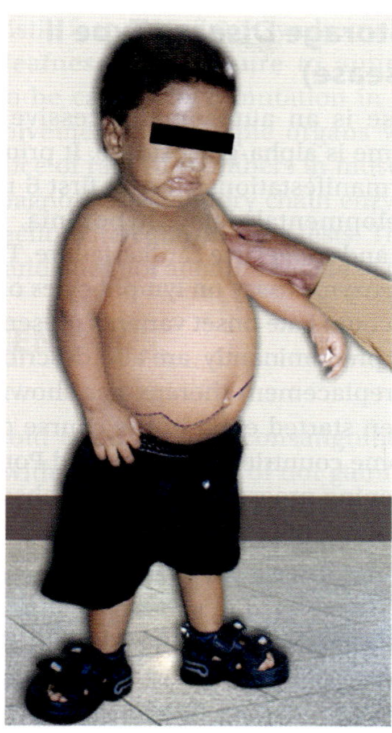

Fig. 14.4.4: An 18-month-old child with glycogen storage disease I (GSD I). A doll-like faces is characteristic feature.

during neonatal period could not prevent mental retardation. This led to the beginning of newborn screening in early 1960s. The prevalence of PKU varies from 1 in 10,000–100,000. Identification of PKU neonates through newborn screening and institution of diet therapy successfully prevented mental retardation. However if diet therapy is relaxed after childhood hyperphenylalaninemia leads to dysfunction of adult brain and lifelong continued control of phenylalanine levels in blood is necessary. Strict diet control is also necessary during pregnancy as hyperphenylalaninemia invariably leads to microcephaly, mental retardation, and cardiac malformation in the baby. One to two percent cases of hyperphenylalaninemia are due to abnormalities of BH4 synthesis or recycling. They do not respond to phenylalanine restricted diet.

The success of restriction of substrate in diet was completely or partially repeated in many other IEMs such as galactosemia, urea cycle disorders, maple syrup urine disease, etc. The special diets are costly and to maintain compliance is difficult. It was found that 10–20% of cases of PKU respond partially or completely to BH4 treatment. The response to biopterin was correlated with type of mutation in PAH gene. The BH4 treatment is effective in patients with mutations which lead to misfolding of protein and hence, loss of functional activity. Biopterin available as sapropterin for patient therapy acts as chaperone and stabilizes tertrameric form of mutated PAH in some cases and eliminates or reduces the need of phenylalanine restricted diet. Neonates diagnosed to have PKU need to be tested for biopterin response and it is indicated in biopterin responsive case. Long-term effects of biopterin use are yet to be evaluated. The other new option of treatment of PKU is phenylalanine ammonia lyase (PAL). PAL metabolizes phenylalanine in the gut to harmless cinnamic acid and insignificant amount of ammonia. This has shown great promise to avoid the need of special PKU diets. Clinical trials of pegylated molecule of PAL (PEG-PAL) have shown its efficacy in reduction of phenylalanine levels.

Glycogen Storage Disease IA (von Gierke Disease)

Glycogen storage disease IA (GSD-IA) is an autosomal recessive disorder caused by deficiency of glucose-6-phosphatase. Affected children present with hepatomegaly and episodes of seizures, sweating, and tachycardia due to hypoglycemia **(Fig. 14.4.4)**.

The patient may have severe lactic acidosis during an episode of minor infection. Liver biopsy shows storage of glycogen. Enzyme assay can be done on liver biopsy sample. In appropriate clinical setting enzyme assay and mutation detection is not necessary for starting treatment. Treatment is simple with frequent day time feeds and a diet rich in uncooked corn starch (to release glucose slowly) at night to prevent hypoglycemia. Associated hyperuricemia and hyperlipidemia may also need treatment. GSD-IB has similar presentation and may have associated neutropenia. It is caused by mutation in glucose-6-phosphate transporter gene, which is an important component of glucose-6-phosphate activity.

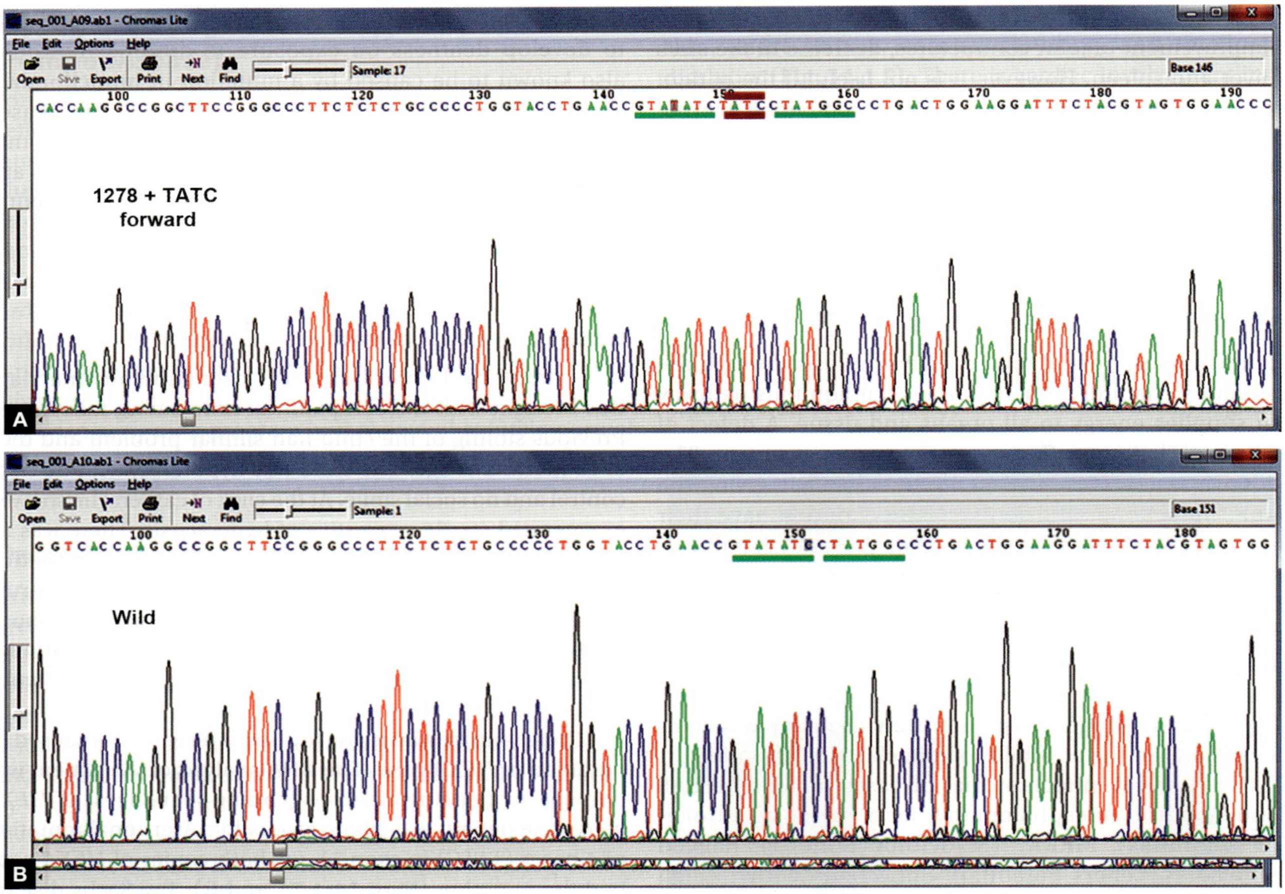

Figs. 14.4.7A and B: Sequencing results of part of exon 11 HEXA gene [Patient (A) and normal individual (B)]: The green line shows normal sequences flanking the region of mutation. Red line shows the extra 4 nucleotides inserted in the patient.
Source: Dr Parag Tamhankar.

pregnant. They had a 17-month-old daughter with spasticity and scissoring of both lower limbs **(Fig. 14.4.8)**. The child was normal till one year of age and had started standing and walking with support. She stopped that and the tone increased in lower limbs. The MRI brain showed demyelination of white matter consistent with leukodystrophy. The child was being followed up by a neurologist as a case of metachromic leukodystrophy (MLD). The clinical features, history of regression of milestones after normal development up to 1 year and MRI picture were consistent with MLD.

Metachromatic leukodystrophy is a progressive disease with no curative treatment. The risk of recurrence in sibs of affected child is 1 in 4 or 25%. For counseling and prenatal diagnosis, confirmation of the diagnosis by assay of arylsulphatase A enzyme on the white blood cells of the proband (affected child in the family) is necessary. The enzyme assay was done, which was very low confirming the diagnosis of MLD. As mutation detection would have taken long time, prenatal diagnosis in the current pregnancy was attempted by estimation of enzyme in the CVS. The enzyme

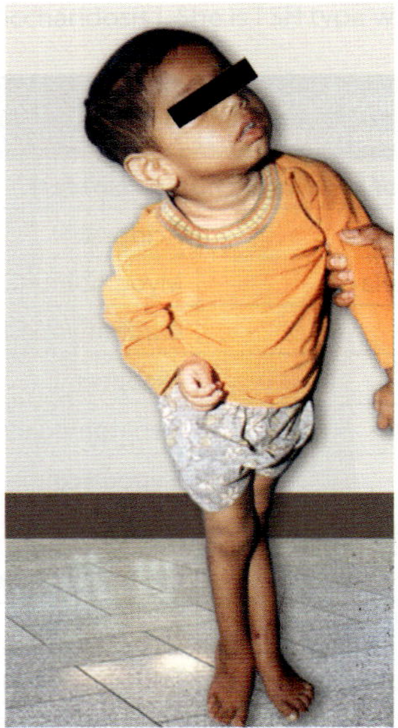

Fig. 14.4.8: A child with metachromatic leukodystrophy, superficially looking like cerebral palsy.

level in CVS was normal and the family continued the pregnancy. It was informed to the family that there is a small error rate of prenatal diagnosis test. It is more for the test based on enzyme assay than the DNA-based testing.

Case III

An 18-year-old medical student was admitted in intensive care unit with coma and acute renal failure. She was alright a week ago and then developed diarrhea and was given intravenous fluids. During childhood she was frequently hospitalized with documented attacks of hypoglycemia. Her brother also had attacks of hypoglycemia and died at 3 years of age. After early childhood, she stopped getting hypoglycemia. After 24 hours of IV fluids, she was discharged and then was readmitted in serious condition.

With this past history and family history the most likely diagnosis is a fatty acid oxidation defect. There are many types of fatty acid oxidation defects and the treatment is to prevent fasting and give carnitine supplementation during attacks. She recovered with supportive treatment and was advised tandem mass spectrometry of plasma to study acylcarnitine profile. Later the enzyme assays may be needed to confirm the type of fatty acid oxidation defect. These groups of disorders are included in newborn screening programs of developed countries.

Case IV

A 12-year-old boy was referred to the Department of Clinical Immunology with 6–7 years history of fever off and on and limb pains. He used to get fever almost every evening and had severe pain in limbs. The symptoms were so incapacitating that he had stopped going to school and was going from doctor to doctor in search of cure. There was no positive family history; there were no signs and symptoms of infection, or an autoimmune disorder. Erythrocyte sedimentation rate was normal. He was about to get the label of neurosis before the referral to Department of Medical Genetics. The only positive finding was documented fever of 100°F (37.78°C) in evening and agony on his face. The diagnosis of Fabry disease was suspected. Slit-lamp examination of his eyes showed corneal deposits. Enzyme assay for alpha-galactosidase A showed low levels and confirmed the diagnosis of Fabry disease. He was put on agalsidase beta (enzyme replacement therapy) which reduced his pain, requirement of carbamazepine regularly; and quality of life improved greatly.

Fabry disease is an X-linked disease and difficult to diagnose because of vague complaints and lack of signs. Average duration between onset of symptoms and diagnosis is 10–20 years. This patient did not have characteristic angiokeratomas. In addition to neuropathic pain, there is increased risk of early stroke, cardiomyopathy and development of chronic renal failure. There is no involvement of central nervous system except secondary to stroke. Enzyme replacement therapy (ERT) with recombinant enzyme has become available since 2003. It not only improves quality of life by reducing pain but is also supposed to decrease risk of involvement of heart, brain and kidneys. ERT increases excretion of ceramide deposited in blood vessels and various organs, thus it prevents organ damage.

Follow-up

His brother was brought with complaints of short stature and chronic diarrhea; the symptoms could be due to Fabry disease. On investigation his alpha-galactosidase was low. This means that the mother of these two boys is an obligate carrier. Her serum creatinine was normal but urine analysis showed protein in traces. Her corneas also showed some opacity. Though Fabry disease is an X-linked recessive disease, many of the carrier females show manifestation of varying severity. The mother and the brother need follow-up and are likely candidates for ERT. They have a clinically normal sister who can be tested for carrier status by DNA analysis and offered genetic counseling.

Case V

A 3-months-old child was admitted with uncontrolled seizures. He had development delay, alopecia and erythematous rash on face. His blood sample was collected for biotinidase assay and he was started on tablet biotin 10 mg per day. The convulsion stopped on second day. The biotinidase deficiency was confirmed by enzyme assay. This is an easily treatable disorder with oral biotin administration. If treated from neonatal period, the outcome for neurological function is very good. Hence, the disorder is included in the newborn screening program of many countries. This child showed dramatic improvement and was developing normally.

It is important to be aware of rare genetic disorders so that these disorders can be suspected in appropriate situations. Presence of alopecia and seizures suggested the diagnosis of biotinidase deficiency. Even if the disorder is treatable for successful long-term treatment, patient education and compliance are important. Communication with local primary care physician and his/her support can play an important role in such situations. Biotinidase deficiency is also an autosomal recessive disorder; and the family can be offered prenatal diagnosis or newborn screening and treatment of an affected child.

Case VI

A couple came with the history that their two sons died of septicemia during first month of life. The mothers of the husband and wife were sisters. There were no investigation reports of the babies. No blood or any other sample of the babies were available. Presence of consanguinity and recurrence in two children suggested the possibility of autosomal recessive inborn error of metabolism in the children and septicemia as the sole cause may be less likely. Hence the option of sequencing all coding regions of known disease-related genes (Clinical Exome Sequencing) by NGS was discussed with the family. This also covers the genes for immunodeficiency disorders and many other disorders presenting during neonatal period. The wife's 2 mL blood sample was sent for testing. Testing both was also an option but the test being costly only wife was tested as the possibility of X-linked genes as a cause of IEM cannot be denied. She was detected to harbor a known disease causing mutation (pathogenic sequence variation) in *BCKDHB* gene known to cause maple syrup urine disease, type Ib. The same mutation was tested in the husband and he was also found to be a carrier (heterozygote) for the same mutation. They were informed that the possibility that the next baby is not affected with the same disease is 75% and the possibility that the baby will have the same disease will be 25%. The family decided that during the next pregnancy they will get prenatal testing done and if the baby is found to be affected (homozygous for the same mutation); they will avoid the birth of the child by opting termination of the pregnancy. As the disease causing mutations in the carrier parents has been identified; definite prenatal diagnosis can be done by chorionic villus sampling.

It should be noted that for sick babies, a small amount of blood sample in EDTA tube should be stored and it may turn out to be very useful later for reaching correct etiological diagnosis even after the demise of the child.

KEY MESSAGES

- Though individually rare, IEMs contribute significantly to childhood mortality and morbidity.
- High level of suspicion of inborn errors of metabolism is necessary especially in acutely sick neonates and children.
- As new therapies have become available for IEMs, timely diagnosis is important.
- In addition to biochemical techniques such as GCMS, MSMS, enzyme assays and NGS-based testing should be used as a complementary and adjunct technique.
- NGS-based techniques have an advantage of looking at all genes in one go and stability of sample.
- NGS-based testing can also be done on obligate carrier parents, even if the affected child is not alive.
- Newborn screening for treatable disorders should be incorporated in care of children as prevention is better than cure.
- Sequencing of whole genome of all neonates is technically possible and is being done in research mode to evaluate the efficacy and many other ethical issues involved.
- Genetic counseling should be a part of management of any child with IEM.

BIBLIOGRAPHY

1. Anderson KE, Bloomer JR, Bonkovsky HL, et al. Recommendations for the diagnosis and treatment of the acute porphyrias. Ann Intern Med. 2005;142(6):439-50.
2. Borghesi A, Mencarelli MA, Memo L, et al. Intersociety policy statement on the use of whole-exome sequencing in the critically ill newborn infant. Ital J Pediatr. 2017;43(1):100.
3. Burton BK. Urea cycle disorders. Clin Liver Dis. 2000;4(4): 815-30.
4. Das AM, Steuerwald U, Illsinger S. Inborn Errors of Energy Metabolism Associated with Myopathies. J Biomed Biotechnol. 2010;2010:340849.
5. Ferreira CR, Gahl WA. Lysosomal storage diseases. Transl Sci Rare Dis. 2017;2(1-2):1-71.
6. Nakamura K, Hattori K, Endo F. Newborn screening for lysosomal storage disorders. Am J Med Genet C Semin Med Genet. 2011;157C(1):63-71.
7. Puri RD, Kapoor S, Kishnani PS, et al. Diagnosis and Management of Gaucher Disease in India—Consensus Guidelines of the Gaucher Disease Task Force of the Society for Indian Academy of Medical Genetics and the Indian Academy of Pediatrics. Indian Pediatr. 2018;55(2):143-53.
8. Staretz-Chacham O, Lang TC, LaMarca ME, et al. Lysosomal storage disorders in the newborn. Pediatrics. 2009;123(4):1191-207.
9. Tarailo-Graovac M, Wasserman WW, Van Karnebeek CD. Impact of next-generation sequencing on diagnosis and management of neurometabolic disorders: current advances and future perspectives. Expert Rev Mol Diagn. 2017;17(4):307-9.
10. Wang RY, Bodamer OA, Watson MS, et al. Lysosomal storage diseases: diagnostic confirmation and management of presymptomatic individuals. Genet Med. 2011;13(5):457-84.

Section 15

Adolescent Health

15.1 Why Adolescent Care Counseling?

MKC Nair

Adolescence is that period in our life where nothing seems to go smoothly and yet our best memories are about those wonderful days. The present-day adolescent is considered to be more knowledgeable about world affairs, thanks to the onslaught of the media. On the other hand, some feel disillusioned about the way things are going, and hence, point out the futility of any intervention program at this level.

Adolescence is also that period in our lives where contradictions are the rule and not the exception. A period when they demand independence, yet are mostly dependent; a period when maximum hostility is shown to the parents, but they want to be loved and cared for; a period with maximum rebellion shown, yet want to be the pet baby of their mothers; a period when they reject advice outright, yet love to be guided through difficulties. Surely any conventional approach is likely to fail with this group. Then, what do we do? Special problems of vulnerable and marginalized groups and problems of adolescent boys have to be addressed separately. Apart from these, we need to have a strategy for adolescents as a group in India, which should focus on:

- Malnutrition, anemia, iodine deficiency, etc.
- Obesity, diabetes, hypertension, all foundation for future heart problems
- Adolescent reproductive sexual health service delivery
- Scholastic backwardness issues and improving study habits
- Adolescent counseling services in the community **(Fig. 15.1.1)**
- Life skill and career guidance (employability training)
- National capacity building for delivery of services.

Child, adolescent, and youth mental health is probably a continuum from a child development perspective—normal and abnormal, evolution of problems, causative and risk factors, and ultimately the outcome. It is said that many of the

Name: ________ **Age (completed years):** ________ **Sex:** 1. Male 2. Female
Place/area: ________ **Phone no:** ________

Mental health section

1. Have you ever felt?
0. No 1. Anxious 2. Sad 3. Angry/irritable 4. Stressed/tension

2. Do you feel your symptoms are out of proportion to the cause?
0. No 1. Yes 2. Not applicable

3. Do you frequently have any of the following symptoms in the recent past?
0. None 1. Palpitations 2. Excessive sweating 3. Appetite significantly less/more
4. Sleep significantly less/more 5. Sexual interest significantly less?

4. Do the above symptoms disturb or affect daily activities?
0. No 1. Studies 2. Job 3. Other

5. Have you lost interest in things that you always enjoyed?
0. Never 1. Sometimes 2. Often

6. Have you often felt that?

(a) You are good for nothing (worthlessness)	0. Never	1. Sometimes	2. Often
(b) There is no future for you (hopelessness)	0. Never	1. Sometimes	2. Often
(c) You can do nothing in life (helplessness)	0. Never	1. Sometimes	2. Often
(d) Life is not worth living	0. Never	1. Sometimes	2. Often
(e) Want to harm yourself	0. Never	1. Sometimes	2. Often

7. Any other:--------

8. Clinical impression:
1. Anxiety 2. Depression 3. Suicidal tendency 4. Others (specify)

Fig. 15.1.1: CDC screening for adolescents' problems teen screen questionnaire-mental health (abridged). (CDC: Child Development Center, Kerala)

adult psychiatric disorders have their onset in adolescence. Mental health issues of adolescents have to be addressed in the primary-care setup itself, because there are far too many adolescents with behavioral and emotional problems in the community and with only a limited number of psychiatrists, clinical psychologists, and trained counselors being available. An adolescent pediatrician can screen the adolescents for mental health problems using teen screen questionnaire for mental health (TSQ-M), a simple screening tool and making both parents and adolescents comfortable in a non-stigmatizing way. TSQ-M short has an overall diagnostic accuracy better than the original TSQ-M. Although the original version includes symptoms for more mental health disorders, providing a wider screen, the short version would prove useful in big community studies.

All of us have fond memories of our adolescence. Traditionally, the societal norms were such that we mostly tried to limit our activities within the acceptable norms of the society. Our parents and teachers tried to instill in us the correct moral values as it was thought appropriate for the day. Time has changed. Very little societal control is perceived now, and whatever is still left is not appreciated. Present-day parents themselves often feel inadequate to cope with the fast-changing norms of society, and hence, they are not sure about how to guide the youngster. Teachers, our traditional source of wisdom, are often confused about their role in society at least vis-à-vis the problems of adolescence. Yet, they have the best opportunity to guide the destiny of millions of youngsters, only if we could empower them their legitimate role in the society.

BIBLIOGRAPHY

1. Nair MKC, Rajaraman V, Chacko D, et al. Comparison of the diagnostic accuracy and validity of a short version of teen screen questionnaire-mental health (TSQ-M-Short) for use in community. Indian J Psychol Med. 2015;37(2):201-4.
2. Nair MKC, George B, Indira MS, et al. Adolescent counseling. New Delhi: Jaypee Brothers Medical Publishers (P) Ltd; 2016.

15.2 Family Life Education

Manorama Verma, Jugesh Chhatwal

INTRODUCTION

In the vast population of India, nearly one fifth is comprised of adolescents (10–19 years old). Adolescents stand at the threshold of adulthood with all its attendant responsibilities and rights. The young adults, coming out of the teenage period, are eager to go out in the world and "live life." Very often, the urges and feelings of living life influence the adolescents in their teenage years, pushing them to experiment and take risks with their lives. As they evolve from teenagers to youth, the usual sources of information and guidance are peers and media, and rarely parents or teachers or doctors. In India, the social backgrounds are diverse. On one hand are the urban, well-educated parents usually working and on the other hand either illiterate or uneducated, conservative background parents. In either scenario, the parents are either not available or capable or comfortable talking to their children on various aspects of family life and sexual development. As a result, the adolescent is sandwiched between traditional parental controls and increasingly promiscuous media giving easily available unregulated information. The formal education provides little or no information or guidance on issues concerning family life. With this background, the adolescents experiment, make mistakes, and learn their societal lessons or enter adulthood ill-equipped to deal with many social issues.

WHAT IS FAMILY LIFE EDUCATION?

Family life education is a comprehensive program to educate the growing children, especially the adolescent age-group regarding various aspects of living in a society and interacting with other individuals at different levels and in different ways along with imparting age appropriate knowledge of biological and sexual development. It can help in providing accurate and sufficient information for the youth to be able to make sensible choices and become responsible adults and citizens. It should not be considered a mere euphemism for sex education. Family life education for adolescents addresses the two important kinds of needs: (1) their current normative needs associated with changing physical, sexual, cognitive, social, and emotional development and (2) their anticipatory or future family-related needs to help prepare them for adult roles and responsibilities in marriage and parenting.

CURRENT SCENARIO

The third National Family Health Survey (NFHS-3) conducted in 2005–2006 looked at adolescent sexual health and risk-taking behavior, and also, at family life education for the first time. This survey reported that among girls aged 15–19 years, 27.8% have had their first sexual encounter and in 8% earlier than 15 years of age. Most of these are within the marital context as the median age for marriage for girls is 17.2 years. Early marriage leads to early childbirth as well and this is evident from the fact that 53% of women had their first childbirth by 20 years of age. Among boys aged 15–19 years, 14.8% had two or more sexual partners in the preceding 12 months, 63% indulged in high-risk behavior, and only 31.3% used condoms. About 10% of both girls and boys reported symptoms suggestive of sexually transmitted infections. Although awareness about human immunodeficiency virus (HIV) or acquired immunodeficiency syndrome (AIDS) was present in nearly two thirds of the girls and 86.4% of boys, comprehensive knowledge regarding HIV even among those with 12 years of education was seen to be about 55% for girls and 62% for boys. Awareness regarding condoms use was still lacking in 10–20% men and women even with 12 years of education. It is apparent that the adolescent sexual activity whether within the framework of marriage or otherwise is a reality. With the above facts and the social scenario, there is a definite need to address the issues of lack of awareness, ignorance, or inappropriate knowledge among the youth so as to promote healthy behaviors and practices.

GOALS OF FAMILY LIFE EDUCATION

Family life education can help in:

- Providing knowledge, skills, and attitudes to the adolescents for healthy family life
- Equipping the adolescents with the ability to make responsible decisions about social and sexual behavior
- Increasing their awareness about their own health and personal development
- Enhancing their life skills.

Curriculum Guidelines

The curriculum for family life education should be appropriate for the targeted age-group. An advisory board should be formed at the school level to formulate the guidelines, decide on the content and implementation. Such a board should include the school principal, teachers, school management board members, parent representatives, medical professionals, and some other members like religious leaders, etc. The educators should have received training to conduct such sessions. An interactive approach and small group sessions are better for engaging the students. It has been shown that role play exercises also enhance the learning experience. Gender separation may be required for some sessions.

Given here are some of the topics, which can be included for adolescents' family life education program:

- *Adolescent development:* Physiological changes including growth and sexual development, emotional changes and responses, positive health practices.
- *Human relationships:* Appropriate friendship or group activities, assertiveness, recognizing danger signs in interpersonal interactions, future family roles.
- *Values, morals, ethics:* Honesty, trust, self-control, and discipline.
- *Family as a basic unit of society:* Family interactions, personality development within the family, preparing for adulthood, and family support.
- *Decision-making and problem-solving:* In the context of personal or social or peer pressure and messages from other sources like media, etc.
- *Career goals and planning:* Career choices, requirements, procedures.
- *Sexual activity:* Problems of premarital or nonmarital sex, consequences of unplanned pregnancy, viz. effects on educational goals, reputation, mental health, financial problems, sexually transmitted diseases, abstinence as a 100% effective method for preventing pregnancy.
- *Contraception:* Emergency contraceptives, temporary methods, permanent methods.
- *Pregnancy and childbirth:* Normal changes, care during pregnancy, dangers of teenage pregnancy, delivery, postnatal care, care of the newborn, breastfeeding.
- *Parenting skills:* Age-group, infant feeding, child development.
- *Preventing and coping with violence:* Misuse or possession of firearm and other weapons, dealing with violence or assault, child abuse, sexual assault and abuse, family violence, electronic media threats.
- *Stress management:* Coping with stress, e.g. examination stress, family-related problems, peer pressure, body image issues.
- *Substance abuse:* Smoking and tobacco use, alcohol, drugs, etc.
- *Sexually transmitted diseases:* Infections, HIV/AIDS—prevention, early signs, and management.
- *Diet and fitness:* Obesity, undernutrition, eating disorders.

IMPACT AND CHALLENGES

Family life education or sex education is an important factor in the context of first sex, and later sexual health and programs should continue to equip young as they make immediate sexual behavior decisions and further sexual health-related decisions throughout their lifespan. The protective effect of middle school comprehensive sex education program with family involvement was noted by Grossman et al., especially for boys. Many of the myths and fears associated with this education have been shown to be unfounded but challenges still exist. The parental and social acceptability is a major issue. In a nationwide survey, NFHS-3 assessed the acceptability of providing information in schools regarding moral values, body changes in boys and girls, sexual behavior, contraception, and HIV/AIDS. Majority of the men and women approved of teaching these topics, especially moral values and HIV/AIDS, and then in decreasing percentages for sexual behavior, body changes, and contraception. The preferred age at which most of these topics should be taught was about 15–16 years as per the opinion of the respondents. It is apparent that the social acceptability has increased, and with additional efforts, this education can be included in the curriculum for teenagers.

CONCLUSION

Adolescents by nature experiment, make mistakes, and learn their societal lessons. Otherwise they enter adulthood ill-equipped to deal with many social issues. Family life education is a means by which adolescents learn to cope with situations. It provides knowledge, skills, and attitudes for healthy family life; make them equipped with the ability to make responsible decisions about social and sexual behavior, increase their awareness about their own health and personal development. It also enhances their life skills.

BIBLIOGRAPHY

1. Boduszek D, Kelleher C, Mcbride O, et al. Sex education, sex and sexual health outcomes in adulthood: findings from a nationally representative health survey. Sex Educ Sex Soc Learn. 2014;14:299-309.
2. Brindis CD. A public health success: understanding policy changes related to teen sexual activity and pregnancy. Annu Rev Public Health. 2006;27:277-95.
3. Grossman JM, Tray AJ, Chormaraman L, et al. Protective effects of middle school comprehensive sex education with family involvement. J Sch Health. 2014;84:739-47.
4. International Institute for Population Sciences (IIPS), Macro International. National Family Health Survey (NFHS-3), 2005-06, India: key findings. Mumbai: International Institute for Population Sciences; 2007.
5. Nair MKC. Adolescence and Family Life Education. Bengaluru, Karnataka, India: Prism Books Private Limited; 2002.
6. USAID, Family Health International, Interagency Youth Working Group. Family Life Education: a Handbook for Adults Working with Youth. USA: Family Health International; 2008.

15.3 Adolescent Nutrition

Jugesh Chhatwal

INTRODUCTION

The hallmark of adolescent period is growth. It is apparent that for adequate and appropriate growth, nutrition is the most important factor. The major growth tasks that are to be completed during adolescence are as follows:

- *Increase in height:* Nearly one-fifth (20%) of the adult height is gained during adolescence.
- *Weight gain:* About 25–50% of the final adult, ideal weight is gained during adolescence.
- *Muscles mass:* A little less than half (45%) of skeletal muscle mass is added.
- *Bone mass:* Almost 50% of bone mass is accumulated and by the end of the second decade of life, 90% of total bone mass is gained.

In addition to the growth tasks, the adolescent nutrition is of significant importance as it has implications for future adult eating patterns. Moreover, in children entering the adolescent phase with a growth deficit secondary to childhood malnutrition, this period of growth provides another opportunity to catch up and improve their growth. The impact of inadequate or inappropriate dietary intake, at this phase of life, is also visible later in adult life. In addition to retarded physical growth, there can be delayed sexual maturation and effect on intellectual functioning. Associated micronutrient deficiencies can cause anemia, stunting, and poor bone health. These eventually affect the outcome as an adult and lead to diminished work capacity, skills, and cognitive functioning. In addition, in females, there is an increased obstetrical risk with poor pregnancy outcome and increased maternal morbidity and mortality.

ADOLESCENT NUTRITION: CURRENT STATUS

Various surveys have shown that the dietary intakes of Indian adolescents are significantly inadequate. The National Nutrition Monitoring Bureau Survey (2002) had shown that 30–40% of girls and 33–66% of boys consume less than 70% of the recommended daily allowance (RDA) for calories. Protein intake is also significantly less in more than half of the adolescent girls and boys. The intake of micronutrients is much more seriously reduced with the majority taking less than 50% of RDA for iron and more than 80% taking grossly inadequate amounts of vitamin A. A study on the beneficiaries of the adolescent girl scheme in six rural blocks found that the intake for milk or milk products, pulses, vegetables, and fruits was grossly inadequate, while it was better for cereals, oils or fats, and sugar. The National Family Health Survey (2015–2016) has revealed that among the adolescent girls aged 15–19 years, 53.8% have a normal body mass index (BMI) and the mean BMI is 19.4 kg/m^2. Among boys, 50.4% have normal BMI and mean BMI is 19.3 kg/m^2. The prevalence of any anemia in this age-group is reported to be 54% among girls and 29.1% among boys. In a study in Uttar Pradesh, the mean height and BMI of 11–18 years olds of both sexes were found to be significantly lower than the World Health Organization reference standards (2013).

Parallel to the problems of inadequate food intake is the situation of excessive consumption causing the obesity and overweight in significant proportion of the population, especially among urban youth. Prevalence of these disorders has been reported to range from 5% to 14% in the different parts of the country.

ADOLESCENT NUTRITIONAL NEEDS

Early adolescence is marked by rapid growth phase and pubertal changes during which time the nutrient requirement is different as compared to late adolescence when growth has stabilized and the micronutrients have an important role. The current weight, gender, growth phase, and the level of physical activity have a significant bearing on energy needs of the teenager. Daily requirements for adolescent age-group as per the revised Indian Council of Medical Research Guidelines (2010) are given in **Table 15.3.1**.

Micronutrient Requirements

The most important micronutrients during adolescent period are iron, calcium, and zinc. At the onset of puberty, the preadolescent child may already have a preexisting iron deficiency, and most Indian diets, even if adequate otherwise, are not a good source of iron. Iron is essential for both girls and boys. Girls with menarche will have additional requirements. Boys require iron as they are adding muscle bulk (myoglobin) and also increase in red cell mass increases the demand for iron (hemoglobin). Calcium is essential for the bone mineral accretion, which reaches peak in mid-adolescence. Accelerated muscular and skeletal development increases the demand for dietary calcium at this age. Inadequate calcium intake during this period can decrease the bone mineral mass with sometimes lifelong consequences in the form of increased risk of osteoporosis. Zinc is required for physical growth as well as sexual development, and deficiency can impair these processes **(Table 15.3.2)**.

NUTRITIONAL DISORDERS

Some of the important nutritional disorders seen in adolescents are as follows:

- Undernutrition
- Iron-deficiency anemia
- Obesity
- Eating disorders.

Adolescent period has its own behavioral complexities, which are closely linked with dietary intake. The growing teenager is breaking free from parental control, and this is reflected in the decision-making for food intake and accepting the norms and dietary guidelines. Dissatisfaction with body image, peer conformity, search for self-identity, and a busy schedule add to the nutritional problems. Some of the common characteristics of food habits of adolescents are as follows:

- Missing meals, especially breakfast
- Frequent out of home meals

Table 15.3.1: Dietary requirements for adolescents (Indian Council of Medical Research, 2010).

Gender	*Age (years)*	*Proteins (g)*	*Calories*	*Fat (g)*	*Calcium (mg)*	*Iron (mg)*	*Zinc (mg)*
Boys	10–12	39.9	2,190	35	800	21	9
Girls	10–12	40.4	2,010	35	800	27	9
Boys	13–15	54.3	2,750	45	800	32	11
Girls	13–15	51.9	2,330	40	800	28	11
Boys	16–17	61.5	3,020	50	800	28	12
Girls	16–17	55.5	2,440	35	800	26	12

Table 15.3.2: Recommended dietary allowances for micronutrients (Indian Council of Medical Research, 2011).

Gender	Age-group (years)	Vitamin A (mg/day)		Thiamin (mg/day)	Riboflavin (mg/day)	Niacin equivalent (mg/day)	Pyridoxine (mg/day)	Ascorbic acid (mg/day)	Dietary folate (mg/day)	Vitamin B_{12} (mg/day)	Magnesium (mg/day)	Zinc (mg/day)
		Retinol	Beta-carotene									
Boys	10–12	600	4,800	1.1	1.3	15	1.6	40	140	0.2–1.0	120	9
Girls	10–12			1.0	1.2	13	1.6				160	9
Boys	13–15			1.4	1.6	16	2.0	40	150		165	11
Girls	13–15			1.2	1.4	14	2.0				210	11
Boys	16–17			1.5	1.8	17	2.0	40	200		195	12
Girls	16–17			1.0	1.2	14	2.0				235	12

- Snacking, especially on calorie-dense fast foods
- Fad diets.

Excessive consumption of sugar can also be risk factor for future heart health. A recent report on the US adolescents concluded that usual intake of added sugar was significant risk for dyslipidemias (2015).

Some practical tips for optimum adolescent nutrition are as follows:

- Ensure balanced diet—adolescent thali.
- Morning breakfast is very vital, it is a brain tonic.
- Avoid empty-calorie foods, such as carbonated drinks.
- Iron-rich foods.
- Adolescent boy should eat as much as father eats (2,400 cal).
- Adolescent girl should eat a little more than what the mother eats (2,100 cal).
- Adolescent girls should take enough calcium-rich foods to increase bone density, which delays the onset of osteoporosis.
- Adolescents are fond of junk foods which are not supposed to be healthy.

The disadvantages include:

- Do not provide balanced nutrition.
- Unsafe/unhygienic.
- Additives and colors added to them which can be allergens as well.
- Repeated frying and refrying produces many free radicals and oxides, causing antioxidant deficiency and are carcinogenic.

Obesity

Adolescent obesity has been a cause for concern in the developed nations and also emerging as an important problem in the developing countries. It is likely to track into adulthood and can lead to related lifestyle disorders; hence, it is important to prevent and manage obesity at this age. Different criteria have been used to define obesity. BMI cutoffs are most frequently used in clinical setting, although addition of skinfold thickness is reported to make the assessment better. Obese adolescent needs a detailed dietary and clinical assessment, and usually, this is sufficient to rule out any significant pathological causes of obesity. Moderate-to-severe obesity can lead to a number of systemic and psychological disorders. Managing an obese teenager requires empathy as they usually have significant psychological problems. The first step is to motivate, as without motivation all modalities of treatment are likely to give poor results. Decreasing calorie intake along with increasing physical activity is the basis for management. Dietary and activity management are essential for other modalities of treatment, such as pharmacological interventions or bariatric surgery also.

Eating Disorders

Eating disorders refer to a group of conditions defined by abnormal eating habits that may involve either insufficient or excessive food intake leading to health problems. Some of the better known eating disorders are anorexia nervosa, bulimia nervosa, binge-eating disorder, and eating disorders not otherwise specified. These are common in the developed countries, especially among young girls or women. A combination of biological, psychological, and environmental factors plays a role in causation. The treatment involves behavioral therapy along with nutritional rehabilitation and pharmacotherapy.

BIBLIOGRAPHY

1. International Institute for Population Sciences (IIPS) and ICF. National Family Health Survey (NFHS-4), 2015-16, India:

Table 15.4.2: Preventive counseling for normative crises and life events.

Indication	***Focus of counseling***	***General principles in crisis management***
Normative crises	• Accepting one's body as it is and using the body effectively • Help form new and more mature relationship with age-mates of both sexes • Achieve gender appropriate social role • Achieve emotional independence from parents and other adults • Prepare oneself to have economic independence through an enjoyable and productive career, prepare for marriage and family life • Help to desire for and achieve socially responsible behavior • Assist to acquire a set of values and ethical system and develop an ideology as a guide to one's behavior	• Be nonjudgmental • Treat the adolescent's problems seriously and take all threats seriously • Do not try to talk the person out of it • Ask direct questions, such as "Have you been thinking of killing yourself?" • Communicate your concern and support, offer yourself as a caring listener until professional help can be arranged (e.g. in the case of imminent suicide) • Try to evaluate the seriousness of the risk in order to make the appropriate referral to a mental healthcare professional • Do not swear to secrecy, especially when there is a threat of suicide or homicide • Do not leave the person alone, if you feel the threat is immediate
Life events	• Help adolescent to realize the maladaptive response to the crisis (e.g. suicidal behavior for failing in board exam) • Assist one in crisis to identify the steps that lead to the crisis, identify the alternate steps that will not end in a crisis (e.g. failure in board exam) • Special attention on identifying the first step in the pathway that leads to the crisis and changes to the adaptive pathway, termination of counseling	

addition to appropriately using crises intervention to resolve the crises. The basic techniques of crisis intervention are summarized in **Table 15.4.2**.

Therapeutic Counseling

Indications for Psychotherapy in Primary Care

Knowledge of the indications of therapeutic counseling, in treating the emotional problems and psychiatric illness, is essential for offering adolescents with counseling options. The basic indications include those circumstances where the only intervention available is nonpharmacological (e.g. dissociative and somatoform disorders, attachment disorders). When an adolescent presents with stress-related physical symptoms or worsening of physical illness (e.g. worsening of asthma or diabetes with stress), counseling is required. When psychotropic medications are expected to interact with prescribed medication(s), and therefore, they have to be avoided, if intolerance for psychotropic adverse effects is noted or when potentiating of the psychotropic is required with combined interventions (e.g. psychotherapy for refractory symptoms in depression or for obsessive compulsive disorder), counseling has a significant role in minimizing or eliminating the symptoms among adolescents. Counseling for adolescents is prescribed when there is a high risk of deliberate self-harm (e.g. potential to overdose on psychotropic medication as with tricyclic antidepressants), medication abuse (e.g. prescription medications, such as psychostimulants being misused), and to improve treatment compliance or the illness has been controlled but the impairment of the illness persists in the patient (e.g. depression is treated with antidepressant but the child has school refusal as an impairment of the mood disorder). Therapeutic counseling for priority mental health disorders of adolescents recommended by the World Health Organization is presented in **Table 15.4.3**.

CONCLUSION

Psychotherapy has a principled tradition and a theoretical basis for their use. A number of techniques of proven effectiveness are available for helping adolescents with their normative crises, life event provoked difficulties, or mental illnesses. Primary-care pediatricians should be able to include simple counseling strategies in their therapeutic options for adolescents with mental health needs.

Existing literature readily supports to the evidence that various forms of counseling strategies are effective among adolescents with mental health needs. However, it should be noted that many of the current effectiveness evidence are a generalization of findings from the adult or childhood studies. It also seems that these therapies are acceptable and feasible in the primary-care settings in different cultural contexts.

Table 15.4.3: Therapeutic counseling for priority mental health disorders of adolescents as recommended by the World Health Organization (WHO)*.

Disorders	*Treatment modality as recommended by WHO*					
	Family therapy	*School intervention*	*Counseling*	*Specialized interventions*	*Others*	*CBT*
LD	–	–	Yes	Yes	–	Yes
ADHD	Yes	–	Yes	–	–	–
Tics	Yes	Yes	–	–	–	–
Depression	Yes	Yes	–	–	–	–
Psychoses	–	Yes	Yes	–	Yes	–
Schizophrenia	–	Yes	–	–	–	–

(ADHD: attention-deficit hyperactivity disorder; CBT: cognitive behavioral techniques; LD: learning disability)
*Because of the propensity of the illnesses of childhood to progress into adolescence, nonpharmacological intervention strategies for childhood disorders have also been included.

BIBLIOGRAPHY

1. Neinstein LS. Adolescent Health Care: A Practical Guide, 4th edition. Philadelphia, PA: Lippincott Williams and Wilkins; 2002. pp. 11-7.
2. Russell PS, Nair MK. Strengthening the Pediatricians Project 1: The need, content and process of a workshop to address the priority mental health disorders of adolescence in countries with low human resource for health. Asia Pac Fam Med. 2010;9:4.
3. Russell PS, Nair MK. Strengthening the Pediatricians Project 2: The effectiveness of a workshop to address the priority mental health disorders of adolescence in low-health related human resource countries. Asia Pac Fam Med. 2010;9:3.
4. Russell S, Russell PS, Kaur MS, et al. Priority mental health disorders of children and adolescents in primary-care pediatric settings in India 3: psychotherapy and other non-pharmacological interventions. Indian J Pediatr. 2012;79:S33-8.
5. Russell S, Subramanian B, Russell PS, et al. Psychopathology, traumatic life events, and coping skills among patients attending a primary-care adolescent clinic. Indian J Pediatr. 2012;79:S52-9.
6. Russell S, Subramanian B, Russell PS. Psychopathology and functional impairment among patients attending an adolescent health clinic: implications for healthcare model reform. Osteopath Med Prim Care. 2008;2:3.

15.5 Adolescent Mental Health

Paul SS Russell

INTRODUCTION

At present, we have the largest adolescent generation ever in the human history. Noncommunicable diseases among adolescents and mental health illnesses, in particular, have been documented to result in high levels of medical, social, and economic burden. Most of the adult mental health disorders have their onset during their childhood or adolescence. In the low- and middle-income countries, including India, with paucity as well as skewed distribution of resources for health, adolescents with mental health needs become doubly disadvantaged and often remain or perilously drift outside the safety of any healthcare system. An effective way to address the resource paucity is by enhancing the primary-care pediatrician (PCP) in the recognition, treatment, and when needed, referral of the adolescents to mental health specialists. This section will, therefore, brief the reader on the clinical skills of diagnosis, medical management, and referral protocols for the priority mental health disorders (PMHD) in PCP settings.

PRIORITY MENTAL HEALTH DISORDERS

Mental and behavioral disorders are common among adolescents in the community and in primary healthcare settings. Among the plethora of mental health illnesses the adolescents present with, the World Health Organization (WHO) has suggested the gatekeeping physicians to apply their resources, on a group of illnesses identified as the PMHD. PMHD have been targeted for identification and intervention based on their higher prevalence, propensity to progress into adulthood, enduring impairment and therapeutic potentials in the primary-care settings. Although during adolescence, WHO suggests to address depression and attempted suicide, as psychiatric disorders of childhood onset having a continuous course and will often continue into adolescence, other disorders, such as autism and attention-deficit hyperactivity disorder, will also have to be addressed but in decreasing priority. The epidemiology and their intervention strategies are mentioned in **Table 15.5.1**.

DIAGNOSTIC PRACTICE

Missed diagnosis and misdiagnosis often result in failure to involve adolescents in treatment and poor follow-up care. These diagnostic difficulties by PCP can be minimized in several ways. Firstly, it is important to maintain a high index of suspicion for PMHD, which are widely prevalent in primary-care settings. Secondly, the PCP should be enabled to clinically recognize the common overt, and if possible, the covert symptom presentations of PMHD. Thirdly, training the pediatrician in using a two-tier diagnostic approach might lessen the diagnostic errors. As an initial approach, the PCP should administer a general psychiatric screening questionnaires (self, parent, or clinician rated) routinely, or certainly, when a mental health need is suspected. The use of screening instruments has been documented to improve the case identification among those who are suffering from mental disorders, and clinicians support the use of screening instruments, as they are usually brief and easy-to-use in busy primary-care practice. As using only brief screening measures can result in both under or over recognition of the PMHD, it is a good practice to confirm the potential mental illness with diagnostic clinical criteria.

Among the screening measures available, the most favored instruments for use in primary-care settings are pediatric symptom checklist, the child and adolescent psychiatric screen, and child behavior checklist. It should, however, be noted that none of the above or other measures (scales, inventories, questionnaires) in the mental health field is diagnostic in nature, and only the clinical diagnostic criteria [e.g. International Classification of Diseases and diagnostic and statistical manual of mental disorders (DSM) systems] supported with extensive field trials have the diagnostic accuracy, reliability, and validity characteristics to act as diagnostic tools.

For the confirmatory assessment, using the DSM, fifth edition (DSM 5) is recommended. The difficulty in using these clinical criteria is that it needs an extensive degree of training to achieve high interrater reliability in diagnosing adolescent psychiatric disorders, and hence, in primary-care settings, untrained PCP may attain only low interrater reliability. But if DSM 5 can be used effectively, with training for PCP during their pediatric training or with follow-up workshops, then the advantages are the ability to confirm the primary diagnosis, identify comorbidities (as presence of comorbidity is a rule than an exception in child and adolescent psychiatry), quantify the impairments (in the areas of education, peers, and home),

Table 15.5.1: The epidemiology and management of priority mental health disorders.

Stage	*PMHD*	*Prevalence*	*Medication*	*Nonpharmacological*
Adolescence	Depression	0.1	Yes	Yes
	Psychoses*	–	Yes	Yes
	Mania*	–	Yes	Yes
	Conduct disorder	1.1	Yes	Yes
	OB syndromes*	–	Yes	Yes
Childhood	Tic	0.2	Yes	Yes
	Enuresis	6.2	Yes	Yes
	Anxiety disorder	4.1	Yes	Yes
Toddler	ID	2.3	No†	Yes
	Autism		No†	Yes
	ADHD	1.7	Yes	Yes

*No recent epidemiological data from India is available.

†Medication is prescribed only for targeted symptoms.

(ADHD: attention-deficit hyperactivity disorder; ID: intellectual disability; OB: organic brain; PMHD: priority mental health disorders)

and recognize the unhealthy psychosocial situations (such as unstable family background) to help formulate a multiaxial treatment approach, the norm in treating adolescent mental health issues. The various characteristics of these screening and confirmatory measures are summarized in **Table 15.5.2**.

MEDICATION USE

All PMHD, except the developmental disabilities (such as intellectual disability and autism), need pharmacological treatment and can be effectively treated in the primary-care setting. However, even adolescents with developmental disabilities will require medications if medication responsive symptom (such as self-injurious behaviors or stereotypic movements) is documented or a superimposed mental illness is diagnosed. The PCP can effectively treat all PMHD with a thorough knowledge in using five psychotropic medications at the appropriate dose and dosing schedules **(Table 15.5.3)**. Best psychopharmacologic treatment in this population requires an appreciation that adolescents have an increased disposition to comorbidities, awareness of pharmacokinetic and pharmacodynamic aspects of specific medications and medication classes, in particular the elimination half-life, developmental considerations, drug interactions, and adverse effects. In this context, it should also be noted that many of the psychotropic drugs prescribed for adolescents have not been tested for their use in well-controlled trials. Instead, from the evidences available with adults, a weight-based dosing is used to estimate the necessary dosage in this population.

Table 15.5.2: Screening and confirmatory instruments for priority mental health disorders.

Screening measures	*Number of PMHD addressed*	*Brevity*	*Age*	*Availability*	*Psychometric properties*
PSC	Not specific	35 items; 5–10 min	6–16 years	Available free of cost in public domain	Strong
CAPS	10/11 disorders except attachment disorders	85 items; 15–20 min	3–21 years	Available free of cost in public domain	Published data could not be located
CBCL	5/11 disorders	96 items; 15–20 min	5–14 years	Has to be purchased	Strong
Confirmatory measure	Number of PMHD addressed	Brevity	Age	Availability	Psychometric properties
ICD-10	All PMHD	Reference criteria	All ages	Has to be purchased	Strong
DSM-PC	All PMHD	Reference criteria	All ages	Has to be purchased	Strong

(CAPS: child and adolescent psychiatric screen; CBCL: child behavior checklist; DSM-PC: diagnostic and statistical manual for primary care; ICD-10: International Classification of Diseases-10; PMHD: priority mental health disorders; PSC: pediatric symptom checklist)

Table 15.5.3: Pharmacological treatment for the priority mental health disorders in primary-care pediatric setting.

Stages	*Disorders*	*Medications*	*Doses/day*	*Dosing/day*
Adolescence	Depression	Fluoxetine	10–20 mg	OD (breakfast)
	Psychoses	Risperidone	2–4 mg	OD–TID
	Mania	Risperidone ± sodium valproate	2–4 mg 20 mg/kg	OD–TID OD (dinner)
	Conduct disorder	Sodium valproate	20 mg/kg	OD (dinner)
	OB syndromes	Risperidone	0.25–1 mg	OD–TID
Childhood	Tic	Risperidone	0.25–2 mg	OD (dinner)
	Enuresis*	Imipramine/Vasopressin	According to the drug and route	OD (dinner)
	Anxiety disorder	Fluoxetine	10–40 mg	OD (breakfast)
Toddler	Autism	Risperidone	0.25–1 mg	OD–BD
	ADHD	Atomoxetine	1.2–1.8 mg/kg	OD–BD (breakfast, lunch)

*Enuresis is not a PMHD, but it is added in this schedule because of its high prevalence in primary-care settings.
(ADHD: attention-deficit hyperactivity disorder; BW: body weight; OB: organic brain; OD: one day; OD–BD: one day–twice a day; OD–TID: one day–three times a day)

REFERRAL PATTERN

Majority of the mental health problems are managed in primary care, and only a handful of adolescents are referred to expert mental healthcare providers. However, not all cases of PMHD are suited for treatment in a primary-care setting, and the PCP should be aware of the indications to refer an adolescent to a specialist adolescent psychiatric care.

If there is poor response to pharmacotherapy or failure to attain remission status (such as in refractory depression), or a rapidly deteriorating clinical picture, then the adolescents need to be referred to a specialist setting. Adolescents with comorbidities that significantly complicate treatment with the need for a complex regimen (such as depression with substance abuse) or multiple medications (such as depression with catatonic symptoms), disorders that require high doses of psychotropic medication (such as acute psychosis), and treatment that can result in significant side effects (such as monoamine oxidase inhibitors) should be referred. When the patient requires specialized psychotherapy as the only modality of treatment (such as conflict resolution in dissociative disorder) and when the adolescent needs a strong component of adjuvant psychotherapy (such as exposure and response prevention in obsessive compulsive disorder) or formal family support (such as empowering parents for conduct disorder), an appropriate referral is needed. Psychiatric disorders with significant impairment (such as school or occupational impairment), atypical presentation (such as atypical depression), cases with diagnostic uncertainties (such as the overactivity disorder with stereotypic movements), multiple axis I or multiaxial comorbidities, primary-care treatment failure in the past, those who had been in contact with specialist mental health care, need of mental health referral of parent, patients with homicidal or suicidal risk, adolescents with serious abuse, inability to maintain self-care or survival skill, and polysubstance abuse need referral to specialist adolescent psychiatric care.

In addition, it is known that despite the appropriate referral, many families are not effectively engaged in mental health services. To minimize this therapy attrition along the referral pathway, prior to the referral, the PCP has to, first, establish a good working relationship with a psychiatrist knowledgeable in current psychiatric diagnosis and pediatric psychopharmacology, and second, prepare the adolescent and his family to visit the mental health expert in a collaborative manner.

CONCLUSION

Priority mental health disorders affect a substantial number of adolescents. Making an accurate diagnosis, using appropriate psychotropic medications and proper referral when required, is an important part of the clinical practice of PCP.

BIBLIOGRAPHY

1. Nair MK, Russell PS. Adolescent health care in India: progressive, regressive or at the cross-roads? Indian J Pediatr. 2012;79:S1-5.
2. Patel V, Flisher AJ, Hetrick S, et al. Mental health of young people: a global public-health challenge. Lancet. 2007;369:1302-13.
3. Russell PS, Mammen P, Nair MK, et al. Priority mental health disorders of children and adolescents in primary-care pediatric setting in India 1: developing a child and adolescent mental health policy, program, and service model. Indian J Pediatr. 2012;79:S19-26.
4. Russell PS, Nair MK, Mammen P, et al. Priority mental health disorders of children and adolescents in primary-care pediatric settings in India 2: diagnosis, pharmacological treatment and referral. Indian J Pediatr. 2012;79:S27-32.
5. Russell PS, Tsheringla S, Nair MK, et al. Priority mental health disorders of children and adolescents in primary-care pediatric settings in India 4: training and capacity building. Indian J Pediatr. 2012;79:S39-44.
6. Russell S, Russell PS, Kaur MS, et al. Priority mental health disorders of children and adolescents in primary-care pediatric settings in India 3: psychotherapy and other non-pharmacological interventions. Indian J Pediatr. 2012;79:S33-8.
7. Srinath S, Girimaji SC, Gururaj G, et al. Epidemiological study of child and adolescent psychiatric disorders in urban and rural areas of Bangalore, India. Indian J Med Res. 2005;122(1):67-79.
8. World Health Organization: Caring for children and adolescents with mental disorders. Geneva: World Health Organization; 2003.

15.6 Adolescent Sexuality

MKC Nair

INTRODUCTION

Sexuality education, better termed "family life education," is important at all ages. It is more important if it is imparted during childhood and adolescence, but in a graded fashion and appropriate to the age. Many parents feel that knowing too much may lead to sexual misbehavior on the part of the youngsters. But, this is not true. Studies have shown that by offering sex education and correct scientific information, premature involvement in sex has been delayed as discussing the subject satiates curiosity and removes the compulsive motive to experiment. On the other hand, ignorant children are more prone to sexual abuse and sex-related crimes. Sex education should be targeted at individuals in the highest risk group, i.e. pubertal, prepubertal, and young adults. But before attempting to do so, we need to understand adolescent sexuality.

Sexuality encompasses the whole range of thoughts, feelings, fantasies, emotions, desires, and language along with action, as sexual behavior is only a part of it. Thus sexuality is an integrated part of every individual's personality and includes men, women as well as children. There is an energy that drives us to seek out love, contact and warmth, closeness that is expressed in our way to feel and to awake feelings as well as contact with each other. Our sexuality is expressed in the way we dress, the way we walk, and relate to people. It makes us feel alive and good about ourselves. Hence, sexual behavior is only a part of the whole sexuality of an individual.

CONCEPTS IN SEXUALITY

Sexual behavior of people finds many expressions, and it seems extremely difficult to classify behavior as normal or abnormal. However, it can be said that sexual behavior is inappropriate, when it is uncomfortable for the other person and has the intention of doing harm either physically or psychologically on self or others. Socialization and related processes may contribute to the development of sexuality in individuals. This may be quite influenced by the norms surrounding sexuality in the society. Those who were fortunate to have a healthy childhood environment do not consider sex as sin, do not approach it with guilt, or go through it as a traumatic experience but will only have positive concepts about sexuality. Sexual right is the freedom to be enjoyed by an individual to decide without any compulsion, when, where, how, and with whom sexual acts are to be performed or not.

DIMENSIONS OF SEXUALITY

We often tend to forget that sexuality has eight other dimensions apart from physical, yet we often focus only on the physical dimension. Dimensions of sexuality could be related to Maslow's hierarchy of needs theory as follows:

- *Physical*: Biological need
- *Legal*: Safety and security
- *Romantic*: Love and belonging
- *Social/cultural*: Acceptance
- *Aesthetic*: Self-esteem
- *Emotional*: Caring and affection
- *Existential*: Self-awareness
- *Psychological*: Self-actualization
- *Spiritual*: Transcendence.

DEVELOPMENT OF SEXUALITY

Sexuality Concepts in Boys versus Girls

Boys and girls develop gender-based differences in their sexual selves. Men are often bombarded with sexual information from childhood. Society's view that men are sexual by nature is in contrast with a women's sense of herself, in which her sexuality is usually kept private even from her partner.

Puberty

Puberty is the stage of physical maturation in which an individual becomes physiologically capable of sexual reproduction. The biological changes that occur during puberty are mainly indicated by the development of the sexual characteristics. Secondary sexual development in girls involves the enlargement of the ovaries, uterus, vagina, labia, and breasts and growth of pubic hair. Secondary sexual development in boys involves the enlargement of the testes, penis, and growth of pubic hair.

Concept of Virginity

The concept of virginity is an emotional issue with a lot of gender bias and an obsession for an intact female hymen. Hence, one's viewpoint may not be acceptable to all. A person who has never undergone sexual intercourse is considered a virgin, male or female. The customs and traditions of our society consider marriage as a religious ceremony conducted invoking blessings of God. To be or not to be a virgin is a personal choice, but the concept of keeping oneself for the one and only one person in your life can be a pleasant decision. However, much the younger generation may want to disagree, it is a fact that we tend to get more emotionally attached to the first person with whom we have physical or sexual relationship.

Female virginity is counted unnecessarily as the presence of a thin-skin membrane in the outer vagina, the hymen. But, there are situations in which this skin can be destroyed other than by sexual acts. For example, females engaged in heavy works, athletes, cyclists, dancers, vigorous exercises, swimming, bicycling, horse riding, use of tampons during menses (not recommended), and insertion of fingers or other objects into the vagina for self-stimulation that will lead to stretching or rupture of hymen well before the first intercourse.

Functions of Sexual Relation

- *Procreative:* Rewarding for those who want to have children.
- *Recreative:* Recreative for mere sexual pleasure.
- *Relational:* Relation ensures a rewarding partner relationship.

Sex is not just a means of procreation. Sex, after all, is the art of enhancing love. Human sexual arousal is a primitive physiological response that cannot be consciously willed. Every partner is different, and even the same partner has different preferences from time-to-time. Good sex involves finding out what the partner wants to happen before, during, and after lovemaking.

Genital Response

The biological function of the genital response in the male and female is to enable entry of the penis into the vagina, with the consequent deposition of semen in the vagina.

Genital Response in Boys

In the male, the principal response is erection of the penis, due to filling of the erectile tissue with blood. In addition to penile erection, the testes becomes somewhat enlarged, and the walls of the scrotum becomes thicker and tighter.

Genital Response in Girls

In the female, the principal response is vaginal. The lining of the vagina is normally moist. This results in part from fluid from the uterus and mucus secretion from the cervix, as well as from the vaginal wall. The cervical fluid varies in amount and consistency through the ovarian cycle, i.e. close to ovulation; there is marked increase in volume and has watery consistency. This facilitates entry of the sperm from the vagina into the uterus. Without sexual stimulation, the vagina is not sufficiently lubricated for comfortable entry of an erect penis. It is generally assumed that the sole function of the clitoris is to provide sexual pleasure for the woman as it contains large number of nerve endings.

Teaching an Adolescent about Sexuality

Sex education focuses, largely though not exclusively, on self-awareness, personal relationships, human sexual development, reproduction, and sexual behavior. Human sexuality is a function of the total personality, which includes reproductive system and processes, attitudes toward being a man or woman, and relationships among members of the same sex and the opposite sex. It embraces the biological, psychological, sociocultural, and ethical aspects of human sexual behavior. It helps people to understand their sexuality, learn to respect others as sexual beings, and to make responsible decisions about their behavior. Sex is considered to have an inseparable role in married life, and it makes the bond between the couple more strong and healthy. Sexual relationship involves respect, trust, and caring of the partner, perceiving the needs of the partner and feeling free to communicate desires and feelings.

BIBLIOGRAPHY

1. Bancroft JHJ. Human Sexuality and its Problems, 3rd edition. New York, NY, USA: Churchill Livingstone, Elsevier; 2009.
2. Nair MKC. Adolescent sexual and reproductive health. Indian Pediatr. 2004;41:7-13.
3. Nair MKC, Parthasarathy A (Eds). Sexual reproductive health of young people (10–19 years). New Delhi: Jaypee Brothers Medical Publishers (P) Ltd.; 2006.
4. Nair MKC, Russell PS, George B, et al. Adolescent Pediatrics. New Delhi: Noble Vision (Medical Book Publishers); 2017.
5. Savithri R, Mehra S, Kole SK, et al. Sexual behavior among adolescents and young people in India: Some emerging trends. Working Paper Series No. 3. New Delhi: MAMTA; 2003. RFSU, Supported by SIDA.

15.7 Common Health Problems in Adolescents

Sukanta Chatterjee

INTRODUCTION

Adolescence is the period of least organic diseases in human life span. Mental health and social health issues become important. The significant amount of growth and developmental maturation in this period makes the adolescents vulnerable to growth and nutritional disorders. The development of sexual instinct with yet to complete self-protective maturation leads to unwanted pregnancy and sexually transmitted infections. Tendency to explore and adaptation of risk-taking behavior increase the incidence of accidents or unintentional injuries. Problem of social adaptation leads to intentional injuries, such as suicide attempts and homicide. Abuse of substance, such as smoking, consumption of alcohol, etc., also starts at this age. Many controllable chronic diseases of adult life might be detected at this age, such as juvenile diabetes mellitus, bronchial asthma, and epilepsy. Acute infections of any system, although not specific for adolescents, commonly affect this population as well. This section deals with those health problems prevalent in adolescents excluding issues described in other sections, such as nutrition, sexuality, gynecology, mental health, and counseling.

Table 15.7.1 shows common adolescent problems presenting in a Teaching Medical College in Kolkata, India.

ACNE

Acne is a nodular cutaneous lesion consisting of multilobular sebaceous gland that drains its products into the follicular canal. More than 80% of adolescents and young adults are affected.

Etiopathogenesis

Abnormal keratinization at the lower infundibulum of the hair follicle causes plugging of the follicular duct. This

Table 15.7.1: Patient profile of adolescent health clinic, Medical College Kolkata, 2014 (n = 1,302).

	Male			*Female (m/um = married/unmarried)*		
Name of the disease/problems	***10–14 years***	***15–19 years***	***Total***	***10–14 years***	***15–19 years***	***Total***
Menstrual problem n = 508/1,302 (39%)				259 um	210 um, 39 m	508
RTI/STI (12%)	26	6	32	55	59 um, 9 m	123
Skin problem (10.5%)	59	24	83	43	11	54
Anemia (9%)			35			67
Learning issues (8%)	61	15	76	31	9	40
Growth problem (6.5%)			36			49
Seizure disorder (3.8%)			24			26
Asthma (3.7%)			28			20
Goiter (2%)			8			20
Vision problem (1.7%)			11			10
Depression (1.2%)			10			6
Autism (1%)			10			4
Prenatal case (1%)						14
ADHD (0.6%)			5			3

(ADHD: attention-deficit hyperactivity disorder; RTI: reproductive tract infection; STI: sexually transmitted infections)

leads to impaction and distention of the duct giving rise to open or closed comedones. At puberty, sebum secretion is increased by androgenic stimulation. *Propionibacterium acnes* hydrolyze sebum and secrete proinflammatory and chemotactic factors to attract neutrophils, which release lysosomal enzymes leading to rupture of the follicles causing inflammatory papules and pustules.

Clinical Features

Basic lesion of acne is comedone, which may be blackhead (open type) or whitehead (closed type). Subsequently, it may turn into papules, pustules, or cysts. Acne is distributed in areas having largest number of sebaceous glands, such as face, chest, back, and shoulder. It may be secondarily infected by scratching due to itch. Resolution occurs with dyspigmentation and indented or hypertrophic scar.

Treatment

Topical treatment alone may be indicated for mild-to-moderate comedonal lesions, superficial inflammatory (papular or pustular), and usually nonscarring lesions. In addition, systemic treatment may be indicated for moderate-to-severe (scarring or nonscarring) lesions or that in patients with persistent hyperpigmentation. Systemic treatment may need to be used alone in patients who are intolerant to topical treatment or in whom such treatment has failed. When antibiotics are used for the treatment of moderate-to-severe acne, the guideline recommends that topical therapy be used at the same time. Once a course of antibiotics is complete, patients should continue using topical treatments to manage their condition. Topical medications, such as retinoids and benzoyl peroxide, also may be combined with one another to create an effective treatment regimen. In addition, some female patients may see their acne improve with the use of oral contraceptives, which can be combined with other treatments.

- *Nonsurgical topical therapy*: The most commonly used are as follows:
  - Benzoyl peroxide gel, benzoyl peroxide gel—erythromycin, benzoyl peroxide gel—sulfur
  - Topical antibiotics: Tetracycline lotion; clindamycin lotion, gel; erythromycin lotion, swabs, gel; meclocycline cream; tretinoin, salicylic acid; α-hydroxy acid
  - Sulfur: Including Vleminckx solution
  - Resorcinol
  - Miscellaneous: Astringents, soaps, cleansers
- *Systemic therapy*: Most commonly used are as follows:
  - *Antibiotics*: Oral tetracycline, erythromycin, minocycline, trimethoprim-sulfamethoxazole
  - *Others*: Isotretinoin—only approved use is for severe, recalcitrant, cystic acne, refractory to conventional anti-acne measures, including systemic antibiotics. Because this medication carries a high risk of birth defects, females must take careful steps to prevent pregnancy while on isotretinoin

Hormonal treatments may include the oral contraceptives that exert their therapeutic effect by decreasing sebum production. Glucocorticoids will have anti-inflammatory action in addition to adrenal suppression of androgen production.

Other treatments may include the following: Dapsone, diet (in selected cases), ultraviolet light, superficial exfoliation, carbon dioxide-acetone slush, and sulfur-resorcinol combination.

Surgical Lesional Therapy

It includes the following: extraction of comedonal contents, drainage of superficial pustules and cysts, excision of sinus tracts and cysts, intralesional corticosteroids, cryotherapy, dermabrasion (scars), filling materials (scars), and surgical repairs (scars).

Follow-up examinations should be a part of the optimal management of patient's acne, specifically to gauge degree (or lack) of improvement, tolerance to medications, need to augment or attenuate treatment depending on clinical response, and employment of lesional therapy. Intervals between visits will vary, dependent on, the severity of the problem, the intensity of treatment, and the need for frequent visits for lesional therapy. In the early phase of treatment, more frequent follow-up visits are required than later when the condition has become less active. On average, the interval between visits will range from 1 week to 12 weeks, with a median of 4 weeks.

Approach to Treatment

General approach: An example of an initial approach to acne based upon the principles above is outlined below. Additional therapeutic options are reviewed in a table derived from the 2016 acne treatment guidelines from the American Academy of Dermatology.

- *Comedonal (noninflammatory) acne*
  - Topical retinoid (alternatives include azelaic acid and salicylic acid)
- *Mild papulopustular and mixed (comedonal and papulopustular) acne*
  - Topical antimicrobial (e.g. benzoyl peroxide alone or benzoyl peroxide ± topical antibiotic) and topical retinoid

    or
  - Benzoyl peroxide and topical antibiotic (for patients who cannot tolerate a retinoid or who require a simplified treatment regimen)

- *Moderate papulopustular and mixed acne*
  - Topical retinoid and oral antibiotic and topical benzoyl peroxide
- *Severe acne (e.g. nodular acne)*
  - Topical retinoid and oral antibiotic and topical benzoyl peroxide

    or

  - Oral isotretinoin monotherapy (see "oral isotretinoin" below and "oral isotretinoin therapy for acne vulgaris")

The oral hormonal therapy is an alternative to oral antibiotic therapy in postmenarche females with moderate-to-severe acne. Consistent adherence to acne therapy is critical for achieving clinical improvement. When recommending topical therapy, the clinician should design a regimen that is feasible for the patient. This should involve a discussion with the patient to ensure that each component of the treatment regimen is acceptable to the patient. We typically design regimens that require the patient to treat no more than once or twice daily.

A sample regimen for a patient with mild inflammatory facial acne who is using a topical retinoid, topical benzoyl peroxide, and topical clindamycin is as follows:

- *Morning*: Wash face with a gentle facial cleanser. Apply a thin layer of a fixed-dose combination of benzoyl peroxide/clindamycin gel to the entire face (An alternative regimen could require the patient to wash the face with a benzoyl peroxide cleanser, followed by application of a thin layer of topical clindamycin to the entire face).
- *Night*: Wash face with a gentle facial cleanser. Apply a thin layer of the topical retinoid to the entire face. Some patients may prefer the use of fixed-dose combination of products to simplify treatment. However, the cost of such treatments may be higher than single-active ingredient agents.

The selection of the delivery system for topical acne medications also may help to improve the likelihood of adherence to treatment. The choice depends upon the patient's skin type (dry vs oily) and preference. Some gels have a drying effect; patients with oily skin may prefer them. Creams and lotions tend to be moisturizing. Solutions are drying but they cover large areas more easily than other preparations, and foams are easy to apply to hair-bearing areas. Pledgets are single-use absorbent pads impregnated with medication. They are convenient to use and facilitate the spreading of medication over large areas.

Mild Acne

They are small papular lesions without cutaneous inflammatory erythema and tenderness. It is treated with topical agents, such as: (1) topical antibiotics e.g. clindamycin (1% solution, lotion, gel, foam; once or twice daily application), erythromycin (2% gel or liquid once daily), or sodium sulfacetamide, (2) benzoyl peroxide agents comedolytic and bactericidal (2.5%, 5%, 10% gel or wash once or twice daily). Side effects are irritation and pigmentary changes. Combinations of topical antibiotic and benzoyl peroxide are available, (3) topical retinoids prevent follicular hyperkeratosis. It is the mainstay for the treatment of comedonal acne. Gels are better on oily skin but may cause irritation due to alcohol base. Lowest strength preparations should be used initially, increasing concentration, if comedones persist. Application on dry skin may avoid irritation and erythema. Small amount (pea size) is sufficient to cover the entire face and apply only once at night. Preparations available are: (i) topical tretinoin e.g. 0.025%, 0.05%, 0.1% cream, gel, or liquid, and (ii) adapalene (0.1% gel or cream). Combinations of benzoyl peroxide + topical antibiotic and tretinoin are beneficial by synergistic action but they should be applied separately at different time of the day since benzoyl peroxide may deactivate tretinoin, and (4) other topical agents are salicylic acid: comedolytic, found in many over the counter creams, washes, solutions or azelaic acid: comedolytic, anti-inflammatory, and used twice daily for postinflammatory hyperpigmentation as 20% cream.

Moderate Acne

They are also known as inflammatory or nodular acne. It is treated with oral antibiotics to decrease inflammation and suppress *P. acnes* organisms a tetracycline (250–500 mg orally twice daily), erythromycin (250–500 mg orally twice daily), doxycycline (100 mg orally once or twice daily), and minocycline (50–100 mg orally twice daily). All of them carry a risk of photosensitivity except erythromycin. Antibiotics should be used for a minimum of 5–8 weeks before progress is evaluated. All antibiotics carry a risk of vulvovaginal candidiasis and risk of decreased efficacy of birth control pill. Oral contraceptives, e.g. *ortho*-tri-cyclen, may also be used.

Severe Nodulocystic Acne

This may be treated with isotretinoin (1 mg/kg/day orally, given as a 4–5-month course). Most important side effect involves teratogenicity.

Prevention

Diet and climate has little evidence to influence acne. Cleansing of skin is recommended. Greasy cosmetics and hair preparations should be avoided. Manipulation and squeezing of facial lesions leads to rupture of intact lesions and provokes a localized inflammatory reaction.

BREAST ENLARGEMENT

Breast enlargement as a small mass is often a presenting problem in preadolescents and also in boys during adolescence. Girls and boys have the potential of full breast development by appropriate stimulation. Circulating estradiol along with that produced in the breast tissue by aromatase enzyme activity stimulates proliferation and differentiation of parenchymal epithelium. Fibrocystic changes and fibroadenoma are the most common masses. In girls, it might start as a unilateral swelling at the onset of puberty (thelarche) around 7 years of age. In boys' benign breast enlargement or puberty gynecomastia is common and may last for 6 months to 2 years, but when it persists after achieving Tanner Stage V, surgical opinion is recommended. Obesity and hereditary factor may be responsible for the gynecomastia due to increased aromatase activity. Differential diagnosis includes normal variant, recreational drug abuse, testicular malignancy, chronic renal failure, and Klinefelter's syndrome.

Treatment

Normal variant does not require any treatment except reassurance and follow-up. Breast mass should not be squeezed. Specific etiology as mentioned above needs to be managed appropriately.

NOCTURNAL ENURESIS

Definition

Involuntary voiding of urine at night after 4–6 years is called nocturnal enuresis. Incidence: it is seen in 5% of 10 years old. Male-to-female ratio is 3:2 with a spontaneous resolution of 15% per year.

Etiology

It may be genetic, 15% in nonenuretic families, 44% and 77% when one or both parents, respectively, are enuretic. Stress, fear, insecurity, and psychological factors are common factors associated with it. Constipation, urinary tract infection (UTI) and worms, neurogenic bladder, and diabetes may contribute. Urinary tract anatomical anomaly is unlikely in the absence of daytime incontinence.

Diagnosis

Family history, primary or secondary enuresis, and presence of other medical conditions are noted, such as distended bladder or colon. Urinalysis and culture sensitivity are helpful investigations with renal ultrasonography and voiding cystourethrogram in the case of obstructive manifestations or previous UTI.

Treatment

Combined approach with supportive education, behavior modifications, and pharmacotherapy are important components of its treatment.

Supportive Education

- No punishment since bedwetting is not under conscious control.
- It is common and adolescents often get better of their own.
- Involve the adolescent in working toward a cure, praise for success, encouragement for lack of control and attach responsibility, such as change of bed clothes.
- Record keeping by calendar or star chart for success and lapse with agreed-on rewards for success.
- Bed-wetting alarm is good with 65–100% cure after 4–6 months.

Drugs

- Desmopressin (nasal spray or 0.2 mg tablet)—one spray in each nostril or one tab at bedtime initially and may be increased to two sprays each nostril or three tablets. If successful, continue for 3–6 months and then taper. Success rate is 75% with high relapse.
- Imipramine (25–75 mg at bedtime) has high success rate but with possibility of relapse on discontinuation. Side effects are anxiety, dry mouth, and sleep disturbance.

BIBLIOGRAPHY

1. Carlsen AR. Enuresis. In: Alario AJ, Brinkrant JD (Eds). Practical Guide to the Care of the Pediatric Patients, 2nd edition. Philadelphia, PA: Mosby, Elsevier; 2008. pp. 668-71.
2. Joseph G, Morelli JG. Acne. In: Kliegman RM, Behrman RE, Jenson HB, Stanton BF (Eds). Nelson Textbook of Pediatrics, 18th edition. Philadelphia, PA: Saunders, Elsevier; 2008. pp. 2759-64.
3. Somasundaram S, Ammini AC. Gynecomastia. In: Desai MP, Menon PSN, Bhatia V (Eds). Pediatric Endocrine Disorders, 3rd edition. Chennai: Orient Longman; 2014. pp. 159-62.
4. Zaenglein AL, Pathy AL, Schlosser BJ, et al. Guidelines of care for the management of acne vulgaris. J Am Acad Dermatol. 2016;74:945.

15.8 Adolescent Gynecology

Suneeta Mittal

INTRODUCTION

The transition from childhood to adolescence in girls is marked by various changes in physiology. As the physiology changes, various disorders may also manifest which are unique for this age. It is imperative that one should have a clear idea of the common diseases that adolescent girls may encounter in the process of reaching adulthood.

EPIDEMIOLOGY

India has the largest population of adolescents in the world with 243 million individuals aged 10–19 years. Girls below 19 years of age comprise one quarter of India's rapidly growing population. Adolescent gynecology is an emerging specialty, involving pediatrics, endocrinology, gynecology, pediatric surgery, dermatology, psychiatry, public health medicine, and genetics. The relatively common complaints in adolescents are dysmenorrhea, pelvic mass or pain, genital irritation, and amenorrhea with underlying uncommon etiologies, such as Müllerian anomalies, ovarian tumors, foreign bodies, labial hypertrophy, dermatopathies, genital ulcers, and imperforate hymen. Common problems observed in an adolescent gynecology clinic are discussed here.

POLYCYSTIC OVARIES SYNDROME

Definition

The Rotterdam criteria define polycystic ovaries syndrome (PCOS) when two of the three primary features are present: unexplained clinical or biochemical signs of hyperandrogenism, oligoanovulation, and/or a polycystic ovaries on sonography.

Prevalence

Prevalence of PCOS in Indian adolescents is 9.13%. The pathogenesis is unknown; however, both genetic and environmental factors play a role, resulting in disordered gonadotropins release, dysregulated steroidogenesis, ovarian and adrenal hyperandrogenism, and hyperinsulinism. It is important to appreciate that PCOS is a syndrome, not a disease, reflecting multiple potential etiologies and variable clinical presentations. Adolescent girls with PCOS may present with hirsutism, menstrual irregularities, obesity, acne, and/or signs of insulin resistance (IR), such as acanthosis nigricans. There may be no evidence of clinical and biochemical hyperandrogenism; ovarian volume and morphology may be of limited use. Hyperandrogenism and IR are more severe in obese adolescent with PCOS. Adolescents who have irregular menstrual cycles have higher serum androgens than those who have regular menstrual cycles.

Treatment

Treatment of PCOS is symptomatic; early intervention, counseling, lifestyle changes, and weight management may be preferable as first line in adolescents, because it targets both menstrual dysfunction and long-term associated morbidity. The use of combined oral contraceptives (COCs) is recommended as first-line treatment for adolescents who suffer from the menstrual and cutaneous symptoms of PCOS. Other therapeutic options for menstrual irregularities include progestin alone and the low-dose oral contraceptives containing estrogen and progesterone. The COCs containing drospirenone have a better outcome than with desogestrel containing pills. Adding spironolactone or cyproterone is sometimes required, if the hirsutism is severe. Metformin or myoinositol can be used in obese adolescents with PCOS as an adjunct to weight-control measures and to treat coexistent insulin-resistant metabolic abnormalities.

MENSTRUAL DISORDERS

Dysmenorrhea (33–67.2%) is common, and premenstrual syndrome (PMS) affects daily routine in 50–60% girls. If dysmenorrhea occurs early with menarche, Müllerian anomalies must be suspected. For primary dysmenorrhea, analgesics with fixed-dose combination of aceclofenac and drotaverine are a suitable, effective, and well-tolerated treatment option.

Menstrual cycles are often irregular in the first few months after menarche. Most cases of abnormal uterine bleeding (AUB) in adolescents are caused by anovulatory cycles during the first 12–18 months after menarche, which is related to immaturity of the hypothalamic-pituitary-ovarian axis. Other common causes include pregnancy, infection, the irregular use of hormonal contraceptives, stress (psychogenic or exercise induced), bleeding disorders, and endocrine disorders (e.g. hypothyroidism, PCOS). Once pregnancy has been excluded, it is helpful to determine whether the bleeding is cyclic (regular) or acyclic (irregular) in nature. The differential diagnosis varies accordingly. Blood dyscrasias and structural anomalies (e.g. polyps, fibroids) are common with cyclic bleeding. Bleeding disorders should be considered in all adolescents with AUB, who present with extremely heavy first menses, bleeding requiring blood transfusion and patients with refractory menorrhagia and concomitant anemia. Sexually transmitted infections (STIs) and pelvic inflammatory disease (PID) should be considered in all sexually active (or sexually abused) adolescents who complain of irregular, breakthrough, or postcoital bleeding.

Investigations should be done to establish the cause. If there is no obvious cause, the diagnosis is dysfunctional uterine bleeding (DUB) and is due to anovulation.

Mild DUB can usually be managed with iron supplementation and observation. Hormonal therapy is sometimes necessary for controlling moderate or severe DUB. Combined oral contraceptive pills (OCPs) or progesterone alone can be given. Red blood cell transfusion may be necessary for patients who are hemodynamically unstable, have extremely low hemoglobin concentrations, or have symptomatic anemia. Peripheral blood should be obtained from the patient for the evaluation of bleeding disorders, including von Willebrand disease, before the blood is transfused. Puberty menorrhagia can be severe, sometimes requiring blood transfusion. Anovulation or DUB is the most common cause but bleeding disorders, other medical and organic conditions must be ruled out. The treatment includes hematinics, tranexamic acid, and hormones. Tranexamic acid in 2 g/day dosage is an effective and safe option to control bleeding, while waiting for complete evaluation. But hormones are the mainstay of treatment in DUB. Such children need thorough gynecological examination and evaluation to arrive at a correct diagnosis.

PRIMARY AMENORRHEA

The common causes are hypothalamic amenorrhea, PCOS, hyperprolactinemia, Müllerian agenesis, and ovarian failure. A careful medical history and clinical examination, distinction between primary and secondary amenorrhea, together with the presence or absence of secondary sexual characteristics are essential. The presence or absence of uterus and ovaries is evaluated with transabdominal sonography. Other investigations include measurement of follicle-stimulating hormone, prolactin and androgen levels if acne or hirsutism is present. If Turner's syndrome or androgen insensitivity is suspected, a karyotype is done.

The analysis of 48 patients of primary amenorrhea in a tertiary hospital over 3 years showed 54.2% Müllerian anomalies, 22.9% hypogonadotropic hypogonadism, 16.6% hypergonadotropic hypogonadism, and 6.3% genital tuberculosis.

Surgical vaginoplasty is required for complete or partial Müllerian agenesis. Patients with Müllerian agenesis are counseled regarding opportunities for adoption or surrogacy. The administration of hormone treatment is remarkably beneficial for young women with primary or very premature ovarian failure resulting in restoration of menstrual cycles and the prevention of short-term and long-term hormonal imbalance consequences.

SEXUALLY TRANSMITTED INFECTIONS

In India, 26% girls are married before 15 years, and 54% before 18 years. Multiple partners, new partners, inconsistent use of condoms are well-known risk factors for acquiring STI among adolescents. Sexually transmitted diseases increase the rate of transmission of human immunodeficiency virus (HIV), and 50% of all HIV-positive new infections are in the age-group of 10–25 years.

The evaluation and treatment of STI in adolescents raises a number of unique issues, including consent for diagnosis and treatment, confidentiality, parental notification, and mandatory reporting of sexual abuse in unmarried girls. Sexual history should be taken, with appropriate counseling regarding risk-taking behaviors. Sexually active adolescents should be screened for gonorrhea and chlamydia. Symptomatic genital herpes and primary syphilis are important diagnostic considerations. PID is a common sequel of genital gonorrhea and chlamydia infections. Microscopic examination of vaginal fluid mixed with saline and with potassium hydroxide, and Gram stain is useful for the diagnosis of trichomoniasis, bacterial vaginosis, and candidiasis. Culture is used widely for the diagnosis of gonorrhea, chlamydia, and genital herpes. For treatment of STI, syndromic approach with single dose, observed therapy is preferable. Three bacterial STIs (chlamydia, gonorrhea, and syphilis) and one parasitic STI (trichomoniasis) are generally curable with existing, effective single-dose regimens of antibiotics. Syndromic management is simple, assures rapid, same-day treatment, and avoids expensive or unavailable diagnostic tests.

VULVOVAGINITIS AND UROLOGIC ISSUES

Vulvovaginitis is mainly nonspecific but is the most common gynecological problem (95–98%). Perineal pain, interlabial masses, urinary tract infections, and daytime incontinence are commonly seen. Improving hygiene, avoiding irritants, and keeping vulva dry are the basic principles of treatment.

ADOLESCENT ENDOMETRIOSIS

Endometriosis is a progressive disease that can cause chronic pelvic pain and infertility. The most immediate issue in adolescents is to relieve pain. Ultrasound will usually diagnose the condition when there are chocolate cysts. Usually, medical management is preferred in an adolescent but laparoscopy may be required in the case of large chocolate cysts or intractable pain.

ADOLESCENT CONTRACEPTION

There is an unmet need of contraception and misinformation requiring urgent intervention. Both married and unmarried adolescents may be in need for contraception, and depending on requirement, may be counseled regarding the use of COC pill and condoms. Dual protection against pregnancy and STI is important. Given the transience of many adolescent relationships and the high probability of multiple, sequential sexual partners prior to marriage, condom is the single best protective option for many adolescents. But it may be best to combine with an OCP, if possible. Emergency contraception as an emergency backup should also be available to young women.

TEENAGE PREGNANCY

Adolescent girls face considerable health risks during pregnancy and childbirth, accounting for 15% of the global burden of disease for maternal conditions and 13% of all maternal deaths. The risk of medical complications, such as high blood pressure, iron-deficiency anemia, and eclampsia, is greater among adolescent mothers. An underdeveloped pelvis can lead to obstructed labor and grave complications, such as vesicovaginal fistula, infant mortality, or maternal death. Teenage mothers also have a high risk of genital tract infection, preterm labor, and intrauterine growth restricted babies. Early booking, adequate prenatal care, and delivery by trained obstetrician can improve the obstetric and perinatal outcome in teenage pregnancies.

Pregnancy may be unwanted resulting in unsafe abortion. Girls from troubled family backgrounds are at 11 times more risk of unmarried teenage pregnancy than those from happy family circumstances, according to a new study in Kerala. As much as 64.5% of the unmarried pregnant girls or young women covered by the study came from "problem families." The problems included divorced or separated parents, polygamous families, parents with marital disharmony, mentally challenged parents, old and debilitated parents, and single parent with little other support.

PRACTICE GUIDELINES

- In the absence of functioning uterus, the usual age for vaginal reconstruction is 16–20 years or 6 months before the marriage is fixed. First operation has the best chance of success.
- Normal sexual development depends on normal karyotype, presence or absence of genes for testicular determination, and appropriate endocrinal milieu.
- Management of menorrhagia aims to find cause and institute appropriate treatment. Some adolescents require medical intervention for PMS.
- Hirsutism is a common disorder causing considerable psychological embarrassment. It may signify benign conditions, such as idiopathic hirsutism or PCOS and malignant neoplasms of ovaries or adrenals.
- Polycystic ovary syndrome may first manifest as persistent menstrual disorder, obesity, and/or hirsutism.
- Suspect endometriosis, if progressively severe dysmenorrhea is occurring for increasing number of days.
- Breast problems are common in young girls. About 1–5% have developmental defects and 5–10% present with benign breast disorders.
- Amenorrhea demands evaluation if there is no menstruation up to 15 years of age with normal puberty; up to 13 years in the case of delayed pubertal development and cessation of menstruation for three cycle lengths or 6 months. In the cases of normal uterus but delayed puberty, bone age assessment rules out constitutional delay.
- Tuberculosis in India is very common, and the aim is to diagnose and treat early to avoid long-term sequelae.

Practice Points or Tips

- A high degree of suspicion of sexual abuse to be kept in mind in all cases of genital tract trauma in young girls.
- Malnutrition is a major health problem, and 50% of adolescent girls are anemic in India.
- Imaging is an important adjuvant in the diagnosis of adolescent gynecologic disorders.

BIBLIOGRAPHY

1. Bhattacharya SM, Jha A. Prevalence and risk of metabolic syndrome in adolescent Indian girls with polycystic ovary syndrome using the 2009 "joint interim criteria". J Obstet Gynaecol Res. 2011;37(10):1303-7.
2. Formuso C, Stracquadanio M, Ciotta L. Myo-inositol vs. d-chiro inositol in PCOS treatment. Minerva Gynecol. 2015;67(4):321-5.
3. Iyengar K, Iyengar SD. Reproductive health on the groundmeeting of women's needs in Southern Rajasthan, India. Udaipur: Action Research Training for Health; 2000.
4. Levitt-Dayal M, Motihar R, Kanani S, et al. Adolescent girls in India choose a better future: an impact assessment of an educational programme. In: Bott S, Jejeebhoy S, Shah I, Puri C (Eds). Towards Adulthood: Exploring the Sexual and Reproductive Health of Adolescents in South Asia. Geneva: World Health Organization; 2003. pp. 187-9.
5. Moni SA, Nair MKC, Devi RS. Pregnancy among unmarried adolescents and young adults. J Obstet Gynaecol India. 2013;63(1):49-54.

6. Mukhopadhyay P, Chaudhuri RN, Paul B. Hospital-based perinatal outcomes and complications in teenage pregnancy in India. J Health Popul Nutr. 2010;28(5):494-500.
7. Nidhi R, Padmalatha V, Nagarathna R, et al. Prevalence of polycystic ovarian syndrome in Indian adolescents. J Pediatr Adolesc Gynecol. 2011;24(4):223-7.
8. Rotterdam ESHRE/ASRM-Sponsored PCOS Consensus Workshop Group. Revised 2003 consensus on diagnostic criteria and long-term health risks related to polycystic ovary syndrome. Fertil Steril. 2004;81(1):19-25.
9. Sagili H, Pramya N, Prabhu K, et al. Are teenage pregnancies at high risk? A comparison study in a developing country. Arch Gynecol Obstet. 2012;285(3):573-7.
10. Sharma A, Taneja DK, Sharma P, et al. Problems related to menstruation and their effect on daily routine of students of a medical college in Delhi, India. Asia Pac J Public Health. 2008;20(3):234-41.
11. Sharma P, Malhotra C, Taneja DK, et al. Problems related to menstruation amongst adolescent girls. Indian J Pediatr. 2008;75(2):125-9.

15.9 Adolescent-Friendly School Initiatives

Abraham K Paul

INTRODUCTION

Children and adolescents are the wealth of nation and future citizens of our country; hence, it is imperative that they be brought up in a healthy, stimulating, and safe environment. Such an environment will positively contribute to their physical, mental, cognitive, emotional, spiritual, and social development. Since children and adolescents spend a considerable period of time in schools and colleges, these places should definitely provide such a positive environment. There are certain issues that particularly pertain to adolescents as compared to their younger counterparts, which include emotional problems, high-risk behavior, sexual matters, unwanted peer influence, and mental health issues. A school that addresses all these issues may be considered an adolescent-friendly school. The following may be adopted by the schools to make it an adolescent-friendly school.

HEALTH CHECKUP AND MONITORING, LIFESTYLE DISEASE PREVENTION

A good health depends on a proper diet, a positive attitude, and exercise. The major killer disease, the coronary artery disease, and its risk factors, such as hypertension, diabetes, dyslipidemia, and obesity, have their origin in childhood. All children before admission to school or college should have weight, height, blood pressure (BP) check, and a general medical examination once in a year. Nutritional advice should be given to all children and adolescents by a professional on a regular basis. Discourage eating excess snacks, confectionaries, fast food, soft drinks, and fun drinks. Routine dental checkup and eye checkup should be compulsory. Lapsed immunization, if any, should be completed, and adolescent immunization schedule should be followed. Psychological, emotional, and social problems, if any, should be evaluated and necessary referrals made.

SAFE TRANSPORT TO AND FROM SCHOOL

Considering the risk-taking behavior peculiar to this age-group, strict monitoring of those using two-wheelers should be supervised for overspeeding and careless and rash driving. Use of helmet should be made compulsory. Safety measures for other modes of transport should also be enforced.

COUNSELING SERVICES

Teenagers experience stress on various situations related to education, psychological or emotional, physical and environmental or social problems. As part of a normal developmental process also adolescents experience adjustment problems with peers, parents, and sometimes teachers. Scholastic expectations from parents, examination stress, learning disabilities, attention-deficit disorders, all may require professional assessment, remedial measures, and counseling, and these services should be made available in the schools or colleges.

SAFE AND HEALTHY ENVIRONMENT

Schools or colleges and their neighborhood should be safe and healthy, free from environmental and sound pollution. Silent zone should be maintained near schools as per government rules. Since children and adolescents are particularly vulnerable to initiate use of tobacco, alcohol, and drugs at this age, their nonavailability near schools should be strictly ensured. Children with signs of depression, emotional problems, and low self-esteem should be closely monitored since they are at high risk for taking up tobacco and drug use.

GAMES PERIOD AND EXERCISE

Adolescence is a period, particularly prone to obesity. The hormonal changes, erratic dietary habits, lack of exercise, and sedentary habits make an adolescent highly susceptible to obesity. Decreasing caloric intake and increasing physical activity are the basis for prevention and management. Four games period per week must be made compulsory in schools and colleges. There should be adequate playground area (10 acres land for high schools). Provision of health club with equipment, such as treadmill, will motivate adolescents to a healthy lifestyle.

CLEAN AND HEALTHY EATING PLACE

Academic institutions with canteen should have clean kitchen and a clean place wherein children can bring in homemade food and eat. Outside vendors should not be allowed in the campus. Fast food, fried items, oily food, and aerated drinks should be discouraged in the canteen. Advertisements of aerated drinks should be prohibited in the canteen and neighborhood. Ensure that child labor is prohibited in the canteen and other workplaces.

FACILITIES FOR PERSONAL HYGIENE

Since children and adolescents spend about 5–6 hours in the schools, there should be adequate facilities for personal hygiene. Provision for adequate hygienic drinking water is a must to prevent waterborne diseases and to prevent urinary tract infection. Water requirement per person is more because of the excess physical activity peculiar to this age-group.

There should be minimum one urinal for 60 students and one latrine for every 100 students. Schools and colleges with more number of girls should have a proportionately higher number. There should be adequate supply of water in the toilets for maintaining genital hygiene and for washing hands. Sanitary napkins may be made available through school store or office. One may also consider napkin vending machines, and facility for disposing sanitary napkins should be made available. Toilets should be kept neat and clean so that children will not hesitate to make use of the facility.

CAREER GUIDANCE

Many adolescents require help and guidance to select a career of their interest and choice. A career guidance program will go a long way in building a secure future for him or her and the family.

MEDIA LITERACY

Apart from all the benefits of the television (TV), the ill effects of media cannot be overlooked. Many studies have shown constant watching of violent scenes on TV, and fantasy violence make children more aggressive in their behavior to others. Media is certainly the one factor contributing to early sexual behavior. Since teenagers tend to follow the behavior they observe in the media without seeing the known consequences, they may end up pregnant with human immunodeficiency virus (HIV) or with other sexually transmitted diseases. Considering all these, counseling on the appropriate use of TV and other media should be a part of the school or college program.

FAMILY LIFE EDUCATION

Regular classes on family life education consisting of classes on adolescent nutrition, personal hygiene, menstrual hygiene for girls, emotional support, awareness on one's own sexuality, HIV or acquired immunodeficiency syndrome, and substance abuse should be conducted in schools or colleges. Classes may be conducted once a month by a specialist.

ADOLESCENT HEALTH CARD AND IMMUNIZATION

Adolescent health card developed at Child Development Center, Thiruvananthapuram, may be issued to all children and adolescents on admission to school or college and relevant data, such as weight, height, BP, immunization status, body mass index, to be recorded. Health checkup as prescribed could be conducted by the school.

LIFE SKILL TRAINING: TEENAGE CLUBS

Life skill training should be conducted in school or college on a yearly basis or more often to prevent substance abuse, smoking, alcoholism, sexual contact, and adolescent pregnancy. It should also enable children and adolescents to deal actively with various demands of life.

Learning Problems

Learning problems are being increasingly recognized among school children. Early identification of scholastic backwardness is absolutely vital as early remediation and intervention has the best chance of favorable outcome.

Learning problems unidentified in early childhood may continue to manifest in later childhood and adolescence and should be recognized and interventional strategies instituted.

CONCLUSION

A school that addresses the issues, which particularly pertain to adolescents as compared to their younger counterparts, may be considered an adolescent-friendly school. The issues mainly include emotional problems, high-risk behavior, sexual matters, unwanted peer influence, and mental health issues. Regular health checkup and immunization also should be an integral part.

BIBLIOGRAPHY

1. Agarwal RK. Promoting adolescent friendly reproductive and sexual health services. Indian Pediatr. 2008;45(1):881-2.
2. Bansal CP. Adolescent friendly school initiative program under IAP Vision—2007 module.
3. Nair MKC, George B, Sharma PS, et al. Nutrition, health and psychological status of teenage girls. Journal of the Teenage Care and Premarital Counseling—Teens. Thiruvananthapuram, Kerala: UNICEF and Child Development Centre; 2003. pp. 8-9, 22-3.
4. Verma M, Chhatwal J. Common health problems in adolescents. In: Parthasarathy A, (Ed). IAP Textbook of Pediatrics, 3rd edition. New Delhi: Jaypee Brothers Medical Publishers; 2006. pp. 943-50.

Section 16

Rheumatology

16.1 Approach to a Child with Arthritis

Raju P Khubchandani

INTRODUCTION

- The common causes of articular disorders in children are wide and varied. The common causes of articular involvement in children are shown in **Box 16.1.1**.
- Arthritis too can be an emergency. It is imperative to identify those conditions whose early recognition is likely to influence management options and eventual outcome (e.g. acute bacterial arthritis).
- Not all musculoskeletal or limb pains necessarily indicate arthritis. Limb pains may arise from disease in bone or neurovascular structures. On the other hand, the absence of pain does not preclude arthritis since children below the age of 5 years seldom vocalize pain. Infants may present with mere irritability while toddlers may exhibit limb preference or a barely discernible limp.
- Several systemic diseases present with arthritis as a lead symptom (e.g. leukemia) and many rheumatologic diseases may have significant extra-articular manifestations [e.g. systemic-onset juvenile idiopathic arthritis (JIA)].

Box 16.1.1: Common causes of articular involvement in children.

- Avascular necrosis and other orthopedic conditions, dislocations, slipped capital epiphysis
- *Reactive*: Reiter arthritis, toxic synovitis of hip
- Trauma
- Hematological conditions: Leukemia, coagulopathies, hemoglobinopathies
- Rickets and other deficiencies: Scurvy
- *Infections and postinfectious disorders*:
  - *Bacterial*: Septic arthritis, infective endocarditis, tuberculosis, Lyme disease, brucellosis
  - *Viral*: Rubella, parvovirus, hepatitis viruses
  - Poststreptococcal arthritis, rheumatic fever
- *Tumors*:
  - *Benign*: Hemangioma, osteoid osteoma
  - *Malignant*: Bone tumors, neuroblastoma
- *Idiopathic*: juvenile idiopathic arthritis
- *Drugs*: Pyrazinamide, thiazides, MMR vaccine
- Ehler Danlos and other hypermobility syndromes and inherited metabolic disorders, e.g. mucopolysaccharidosis, Wilson disease
- Systemic connective tissue disorders and vasculitides
- Lupus, dermatomyositis, scleroderma, mixed connective tissue disease
- Henoch-Schönlein purpura, Kawasaki disease, polyarteritis and other vasculitides

(MMR: measles, mumps, and rubella)

- Several rheumatological conditions evolve over time (e.g. lupus, JIA) and, therefore, it is not always possible to give a diagnostic label to the child at first presentation. Indeed several diagnoses are established on follow-up.
- Several rheumatological conditions are essentially clinical diagnosis and/or diagnosis of exclusion. Investigations only help to rule out mimics or assess disease activity. Examples include JIA and Kawasaki disease (KD).

The rheumatology consult often begins even as the patient enters the clinic with observation of the gait and level of pain virtually written on the child's face. The Ask and Look approach **(Tables 16.1.1 and 16.1.2)** works extremely well with the first two components being often affected simultaneously while the child is comfortably seated on the couch or in the parents' lap.

MUSCULOSKELETAL EXAMINATION

Needless to say musculoskeletal examination is the most crucial part of the evaluation of the child with arthritis. The reader is advised to be familiarized with pGALS (pediatric Gait, Arms, Legs and Spine)—a simple short video, which illustrates the method of screening evaluation of the musculoskeletal system in children.

- *Articular versus periarticular involvement:* Pain on active and passive movement, swelling, instability, locking, crepitus or deformities suggests joint disorders. Periarticular pain occurs on active movement only and that too in certain planes **(Table 16.1.3)**.
- *Inflammatory versus mechanical disease*: Warmth, erythema, swelling and tenderness (the cardinal signs of inflammation) characterize inflammatory disease while mechanical diseases lack these features and often affect the overuse joints (ankle, knee, shoulder).
- *Disease active or inactive*: This may change therapeutic approaches. Although, it may be difficult, it is vital to decide whether limited joint range and persistent deformity indicate old, burnt out, inactive arthritis or whether there is ongoing inflammation present. Intra-articular effusion should always be taken to indicate active inflammation. The next most sensitive indicator of active arthritis is pain at the end of range of joint movement.
- *Pointers to chronicity*: Pigmentation over joints, presence of deformity, contractures and deformities are indicators.
- *Joint or joints (site/s) involved specific to certain disease*: There are certain joints typically involved in some

Table 16.1.1: Approach to a child with arthritis: Ask.

What	*Why (the list is illustrative and not complete)*
Age	Several age specific diseases, e.g. oJIA, KD (2–5 years), lupus and ERA (adolescent)
Sex	Several diseases with sex preference, e.g. oJIA, lupus (females) ankylosing spondylitis, ERA (males)
Length of history	Hours: trauma, hemophilia; Days: septic or reactive arthritis, Weeks: vasculitides, connective tissue disorders, indolent infections, Months: juvenile idiopathic arthritis, mechanical disorders, e.g. hypermobility, Years: pain syndromes, e.g. reflex sympathetic dystrophy, genetic disorders
Onset	Explosive and sudden: septic arthritis, transient synovitis of hip, gradual and insidious: connective tissue disorders
Time of worst symptoms	Morning stiffness or pain after rest (gelling): inflammatory disease, evening pains after physical activity improving with rest: mechanical pain, night pains: osteoid osteoma, malignancy
Pattern	Solitary: infections or tumors, Additive: reactive, migratory: rheumatic fever, intermittent: lupus, sickle, hemophilia
Constitutional features, e.g. fever, fatigue malaise	Presence usually suggests inflammatory pathology with the exception of most types of JIA. Absence is typical of noninflammatory or mechanical disorders
Associated symptoms	**Table 16.1.3**
Antecedent events or drugs	Trauma, recent viral or bacterial infections or recent dysentery recent immunization (MMR) reactive arthritis, drugs (pyrazinamide)
Known previous conditions	For example, sickle cell disease or hemophilia, structural heart disease (infective endocarditis and septic emboli, Down syndrome, Perthes disease)
Consanguinity	Autosomal recessive conditions sickle, periodic fever syndromes, bone dysplasias
Family history	Similar disease-genetic syndromes, spine/eye/joint disease: HLA-B27-related arthropathies, psoriasis: psoriatic arthritis

(JIA: juvenile idiopathic arthritis; KD: Kawasaki disease; oJIA: oligoarticular juvenile idiopathic arthritis; MMR: measles, mumps and rubella; ERA: enthesitis-related arthritis; HLA: human leukocytic antigen)

conditions, e.g. psoriasis and the distal interphalangeal joint, reactive arthritis and the large joints of the lower limb, temporomandibular joint involvement in polyarticular juvenile arthritis.

- *Number of joints involved (single, four or more)*: While the causes of polyarticular disease (greater than four joints) are plenty, oligoarticular involvement is seen only in a few conditions such as oligoarticular juvenile idiopathic arthritis (oJIA), psoriasis, sarcoid and leukemia.
- *Large/small joints or combination (size)*: Purely large joint involvement characterizes certain diseases such as rheumatic fever and the combination of large and small joint disease can change the diagnostic thought.
- *Symmetry of involvement*: While polyarticular juvenile arthritis, connective tissue diseases and vasculitides present with symmetric arthritis, oligoarticular juvenile arthritis, enthesitis-related arthritis (ERA) and infections are asymmetric in their presentation. Beware the remarkable symmetry of hereditary dysplasias.
- *Spine involvement (axial disease)*: The presence of cervical spine involvement is seen frequently in polyarticular and systemic-onset juvenile arthritis and sacroiliitis is an important feature of the spondyloarthropathies. On the other hand, some rheumatologic conditions seldom affect the spine, e.g. lupus and vasculitis.
- *Surrounding structures, e.g. enthesitis, skin nodules*: Enthesitis-related arthritis is a specific diagnostic entity

Table 16.1.2: Approach to a child with arthritis: Look.

What	*Why (the list is illustrative and not complete)*
General look	Toxic-septic arthritis, highly irritable-KD, comfortable when seated: JIA, la belle indifference: chronic pain syndromes
Gait and movements	May give a clue to the joints involved especially in uncooperative infants and toddlers
Deformities and limb length discrepancies	Juvenile idiopathic arthritis and hereditary dysplasias
Striking inspection features	Red-hot single swollen joint-septic arthritis. Alopecia-lupus, rashes: JIA, lupus, dermatomyositis, Henoch-Schönlein purpura, KD, High myopia, hypermetropia, dysmorphic facies: syndromes short or tall stature: syndromes, obesity: mechanical disorders, e.g. slipped capital femoral epiphysis. Also ***see* Table 16.1.1**
Detailed general and systemic examination	***See* Table 16.1.3**
Musculoskeletal examination	*See* text

(JIA: juvenile idiopathic arthritis; KD: Kawasaki disease)

Table 16.1.3: Extra-articular features that may be associated with arthritis.

Where	***What***	***Why***
Eye	• Nonpurulent conjunctivitis • Uveitis (acute anterior, painful, red eye) • Uveitis (insidious anterior, presents as visual loss) • Uveitis (posterior)	• KD • ERA • OJIA • Sarcoidosis
Mouth	• Painful cracked, bleeding lips and strawberry tongue • Mouth ulcer • Red gums at tooth line	• KD • SLE, BS, ERA, DMS, methotrexate • DMS
Head and neck	• Alopecia/hair loss	SLE
Skin	• Psoriasis • Periorbital rash (heliotrope) • Malar rash (photosensitive)	• Psoriatic arthritis • DMS • SLE
Hands	• Raynaud's phenomenon • Nail pitting, onycholysis • Nail fold infarct • Subcutaneous calcinosis • Digit infarction • Gottron's papules • Periungual desquamation	• DMS, SD • Psoriatic arthritis • CTD • DMS, SD • PAN • DMS • KD
Trunk and arms	• Macular rash • Erythema marginatum • Subcutaneous nodules • Urticaria	• SOJIA, SLE, KD, parvovirus rubella • ARF • ARF, RF+ve-JIA • CTD: Systemic vasculitides
Lower limbs and feet	• Livedo reticularis • Purpura • Erythema nodosum	• Vasculitides • HSP, SLE • Sarcoid, IBD, TB, systemic vasculitides, CTD
Muscles	• Wasting/contractures • Tender swollen • Proximal muscle weakness	• JIA • DMS • DMS
Hematological	• Lymphadenopathy • Petechiae • Pallor	• oJIA, SLE, malignancy, TB, KD • SLE, malignancy • SOJIA, SLE, malignancy, SCD
Gastrointestinal	• Dysphagia • Abdominal pain • Diarrhea • Malabsorption • Hepatic dysfunction • Organomegaly	• DMS, SD • PAN, SLE • Reactive arthritis, IBD • SD • Wilson's, SLE, hepatitis (B/C), SCD • OJIA, SLE, malignancy, SCD
Respiratory	• Upper airway disease • Pleural effusion/pleuritis	• Wegener's granulomatosis • SLE, SOJIA, ARF
Cardiovascular	• Pericarditis • Myocarditis • Valvular disease • Hypertension	• SLE, SOJIA, ARF • Polymyositis, ARF, SOJIA, amyloidosis • ARF, JAS, SLE,APS, hypermobility • PAN, SLE
Genitourinary	• Urethritis • Genital ulcers • Proteinuria • Renal failure/hematuria	• Reiter's, reactive arthritis • BS • SLE, drug, amyloidosis • SLE, NSAIDs, amyloidosis, systemic vasculitides
Neurological	• Fits, coma, psychosis • Chorea • Neuropathies • Headache	• SLE • SLE, ARF • PAN • SLE

(DMS: dermatomyositis; SLE: systemic lupus erythematosus; CTD: connective tissue disease; IBD: inflammatory bowel disease; ARF: acute rheumatic fever; PAN: polyarteritis nodosa; PsA: psoriatic arthritis; SD: scleroderma; KD: Kawasaki disease; ERA: enthesitis-related arthritis; NSAIDs: nonsteroidal anti-inflammatory drugs; HSP: Henoch-Schönlein purpura; SCD: specific carbohydrate diet; BS: Behçet syndrome; SOJIA: systemic-onset juvenile idiopathic arthritis; IBD: inflammatory bowel disease)

Source: Khubchandani R, D'Souza S. Initial evaluation of a child with arthritis—An algorithmic approach. Indian journal of pediatrics. 2002;69: 875-80. (With the kind permission of the editors) (*see* Chapter on Juvenile Idiopathic Arthritis) and the presence of subcutaneous nodules (rheumatoid nodules or nodules in rheumatic fever) may offer a clue.

PATTERN RECOGNITION

This final stage of clinical evaluation is easily the most important as the clinician attempts to collate the history and physical findings as if fitting several pieces of a jigsaw puzzle. For example:

- A pattern of scattered, asymmetric large and small oligoarticular or limited polyarthritis (especially distal interphalangeal joints) suggests juvenile psoriatic arthritis.
- Onset of polyarthritis in a teenage girl should suggest the possibility of systemic lupus erythematosus (SLE) or polyarticular JIA.
- Isolated hip involvement may be caused by toxic synovitis, Perthes disease, and slipped capital femoral epiphysis or less likely by chronic inflammatory arthritis.
- An older child or young adolescent male with low back pain may have ankylosing spondylitis but mechanical causes, infections or malignancy are more likely.
- Beware the toddler male with oligoarticular involvement and fever. He may have leukemia.

CONCLUSION

All the musculoskeletal or limb pains necessarily do not indicate arthritis. Limb pains may arise from disease in bone or neurovascular structures. On the other hand, the absence of pain does not preclude arthritis since children below the age of 5 years seldom specify and localize pain. Infants may present with irritability while toddlers may exhibit limb preference or a barely discernible limp. Many systemic diseases also present with arthritis. Musculoskeletal examination is the most crucial part of the evaluation of the child with arthritis.

BIBLIOGRAPHY

1. Khubchandani RP, D'Souza S. Initial evaluation of a child with arthritis—an algorithmic approach. Indian J Pediatr. 2002;69(10):875-80.

16.2 Juvenile Idiopathic Arthritis

Raju P Khubchandani, Prajakta Joshi

INTRODUCTION

Juvenile idiopathic arthritis (JIA), previously known as juvenile rheumatoid arthritis or juvenile chronic arthritis, is a group of diseases with arthritis of unknown cause (implying that other diseases have been excluded) characterized by age of onset below 16 years and duration of at least 6 weeks.

PREVALENCE

It is estimated that JIA affects up to 1 in 1,000 children worldwide and is the most common cause of autoimmune musculoskeletal disease in children. There is no particular geographic or racial predilection.

ETIOPATHOGENESIS

The pathogenesis of JIA is extremely complex and involves interplay of genetic predisposition and inflammatory mechanisms. The major players in the pathogenesis are T-cells, macrophages and B-cells. Cytokines are glycoproteins secreted from inflammatory cells such as activated T-cells and macrophages. They are essentially of two varieties, proinflammatory (IL-1, IL-6, TNF-alpha, IL-8) or anti-inflammatory (IL-4, IL-10, IL-1 receptor antagonist). Cytokines are instrumental in regulating the magnitude, nature and duration of the inflammatory response in arthritis. The inflammation resulting from the various interactions are responsible for the development of synovitis. This complex set of interactions elaborate the release of various metalloproteinase and other enzymes which cause the damage to the synovium and the adjacent tissues. The cytokines involved in the pathogenesis of JIA as a whole and in different subsets are still being investigated.

The group of disorders under the term JIA (with the exception of the systemic-onset variety) is considered as a group of disorders of adaptive immunity occurring as a result of yet unidentified environmental factors in genetically predisposed individuals. Familial clustering, the presence of autoantibodies such as rheumatoid factor and antinuclear antibodies (ANA) in distinct subgroups are seen and a small but definite proportion of patients develop second rheumatologic/immunologic conditions.

In contrast, the view emerging now is that the systemic-onset variety [systemic juvenile idiopathic arthritis (sJIA)] is an autoinflammatory syndrome, i.e. it is a disorder with abnormalities in the innateimmunity (cytokines like IL-1, IL-6 and IL-18, and neutrophils and monocytes/macrophages rather than lymphocytes play a major role in the pathogenesis of sJIA), distinguishing sJIA from other subtypes.

CLASSIFICATION

The updated classification scheme for JIA was presented by the International League of Associations for Rheumatology (ILAR) in 2001. It is based on mode of onset (presence of systemic findings), the number of joints affected and their progression, and the presence or absence of specific serologic findings **(Table 16.2.1).**

Table 16.2.1: Category, observed frequency* and diagnostic criteria.

Category	Criteria
Systemic arthritis (10–20%)	Fever of at least 2 weeks duration (daily for at least 3 days) and arthritis in one or more joints, plus one of the following: • Erythematous rash • Generalized lymph node enlargement • Hepatomegaly and/or splenomegaly • Serositis
Oligoarthritis (50–60%)	Arthritis affecting ≤ four joints during the first 6 months of the disease. If after 6 months more than four joints are involved the term extended oligoarthritis is used
• Polyarthritis (20–30%) • RF negative	Arthritis affecting ≥ five joints during the first 6 months of the disease with rheumatoid factor negative
• Polyarthritis (5–10%) • RF positive	Arthritis affecting ≥ five joints during the first 6 months of disease with rheumatoid factor positive on two occasions at least 3 months apart
Psoriatic arthritis (2–15%)	Arthritis and psoriasis or arthritis and at least two of the following: • Psoriasis in a first degree relative • Dactylitis • Nail pitting or onycholysis
Enthesitis-related arthritis (1–7%)	Arthritis and enthesitis** or arthritis or enthesitis with at least two of the following: • Presence/history of sacroiliac joint tenderness and/or inflammatory lumbosacral pain and HLA-B27 positive • Onset of arthritis in a male over 6 years of age • Acute (symptomatic) anterior uveitis • History of ankylosing spondylitis, enthesitis-related arthritis, sacroiliitis with inflammatory bowel disease or acute anterior uveitis in a first degree relative
Undifferentiated arthritis	Arthritis that fulfills criteria in no category or in two or more of the above categories

*The relative frequencies of the various subtypes stated above are based on Western literature. Scantily published Indian data shows that the oJIA is not as common as in the West and the majority of cases seen in India are the sJIA variety.

**Enthesitis is inflammation at the site where tendon, muscle or fascia inserts on bone.

(RF: rheumatoid factor; HLA: human leukocytic antigen)

CLINICAL FEATURES

Some of the varieties of JIA are very age and sex specific. While sJIA may involve any age or sex the oJIA and polyarticular juvenile idiopathic arthritis (pJIA)—particularly the former, dominantly affect females. Oligoarticular juvenile idiopathic arthritis is a disorder afflicting the 2–5 year age group while pJIA is usually seen in children over 10 years. Enthesitis-related arthritis is a disease of the adolescent male.

Clinical manifestations in JIA are variable. The onset is usually insidious with a history of trauma which often precipitates the doctor visit. Patients with pJIA or sJIA may experience constitutional features such as fatigue or anorexia but these symptoms are rare in oJIA. Fever and extra-articular features are usually absent or minimal in varieties other than sJIA in which lymphadenopathy, hepatosplenomegaly, classic evanescent rash and serositis are seen. Children with rheumatoid factor positive disease may have subcutaneous "rheumatoid nodules" on the forearm or legs. The arthritis leads to joint pain and the child's age will affect how they communicate pain and dysfunction, e.g. infants and toddlers may become irritable or simply use affected joints in a different way. They may stop using an affected limb (e.g. refusal to weight bear). Older children express pain on movement and report it to be aching in quality, of mild-to-moderate severity, appreciated by examination of the affected joints. Other common symptoms at presentation include morning stiffness and "gelling" after inactivity. Parents will often report their child to be "slow to get moving" in the morning or after a daytime nap with improvement after a period of time.

On examination, affected joints are usually warm and swollen with reduced range of motion, but not erythematous. Large joints are more commonly affected, with smaller joints affected in pJIA. Examination of a child with arthritis should always include the temporomandibular joints and cervical spine, as arthritis in these joints is often underappreciated. The reader is advised to get familiarized with musculoskeletal examination in the pediatric age group. The pGALS is a simple 3-minute procedure and a video clipping can be viewed on the internet.

DIAGNOSIS AND INVESTIGATIONS

The diagnosis of JIA is essentially clinical, and exclusion and investigations are largely performed to rule out mimics **(Table 16.2.2)**. A complete blood count may demonstrate anemia of chronic inflammation and the C-reactive protein (CRP) and erythrocyte sedimentation rate (ESR) may show mild to modest elevations which may be used to guide therapy. In sJIA anemia, polymorphonuclear leukocytosis and thrombocytosis are classically seen.

Rheumatoid factor (RF) should be performed in patients with polyarthritis as its presence helps to classify **(Table 16.2.1)** and prognosticate about severe erosive disease. The presence of a positive ANA identifies risk for the development of asymptomatic uveitis, particularly in those with oJIA, but should be performed in all children with JIA. Human leukocytic antigen (HLA)-B27 should be tested in children who present with signs and symptoms consistent with ERA **(Table 16.2.1)** and can indicate susceptibility to the development of axial arthritis in future years.

Plain X-rays may demonstrate effusions but erosions are rarely seen in childhood. Bedside ultrasonography is being increasingly used to evaluate joints at diagnosis and follow-up as a complement to clinical evaluation.

MANAGEMENT

Children with JIA are best managed in a specialist multidisciplinary setup. While drug therapy is a crucial part of management, the role of the physiotherapist, occupational therapist, child psychologist and social worker is immense in supporting the physician to achieve maximum possible success.

There is currently no cure for JIA. The primary goals of medical therapy are to eliminate active disease, to normalize joint function, to preserve normal growth and to prevent long-term joint damage. The drugs used more commonly in the present day management of JIA are shown in **Table 16.2.3**. Detailed pharmacology and usage are beyond the scope of this article.

The present day paradigm of care is toward early and aggressive management to capitalize on the window of opportunity that exists before erosive disease and deformity sets in. Thus in contrast to earlier days where NSAIDs formed the initial therapy with drugs being sequentially added to nonresponders, the approach today is to introduce disease-modifying antirheumatic drugs (DMARDs) early in the course of the disease using steroids as a bridge till they begin to take effect. TNF-α and IL-1 or IL-6 inhibitors which come under the heading of biologicals are being increasingly used in the West, sometimes as first-line agents but their prohibitive cost prevents their routine use in our setting. Autologous stem cell transplant has been used for the most refractory cases.

Certain precautions are to be followed before starting any immunosuppressives. Screening for latent tuberculosis, a Mantoux test and an X-ray chest are mandatory. Immunization status of the child should be checked in particular for varicella and if not immunized or infected should be vaccinated atleast 3–4 weeks prior to immunosuppresives, if a window of opportunity exists prior to starting treatment.

The ACR (American College of Rheumatology), 2011 recommendations have divided JIA into five treatment groups:

1. History of arthritis of four or fewer joints
2. History of arthritis of five or more joints
3. Active sacroiliac arthritis
4. Systemic arthritis with active systemic features (and without active arthritis)
5. Systemic arthritis with active arthritis (and without active systemic features).

Furthermore, each treatment group is stratified according to presence or absence of poor prognostic features (defined for each treatment group) and disease activity levels (includes laboratory parameters, parent/patient visual assessment score/PVAS and physician's global assessment score).

Detailed description is beyond the scope of the chapter. Please refer to reference no. 1 for further details.

The next few lines give the salient outline of care of the various subtypes of JIA.

- *Oligoarticular:* Nonsteroidal anti-inflammatory drugs may be used initially in select cases but repeated intra-articular steroids in affected joints are the mainstay of therapy.
- *Polyarticular:* Treatment is started with NSAIDs and DMARDs (methotrexate) and if needed, a low bridging dose of steroids. As methotrexate takes effect steroids and NSAIDs are withdrawn. Flares in individual joints are managed with intra-articular injections.

Table 16.2.2: Common mimics of juvenile idiopathic arthritis.

Oligoarticular disease	*Polyarticular disease*	*Systemic-onset disease*
• Chronic infections, e.g. tuberculosis • Reactive arthritis • Benign and malignant tumors • Acute leukemia • Inflammatory bowel disease	• Rheumatic fever • Skeletal dysplasias • Pain amplification syndromes • Hypermobility syndromes • Vitamin D deficiency • Vasculitides	• Infections with leukemoid reactions/exanthems • Systemic lupus erythematosus • Kawasaki disease

Table 16.2.3: Various agents used in the treatment of JIA in India.

A. NSAIDs					
Medication	***How supplied***	***Dose range***	***Interval***	***Major side effect***	***Laboratory monitoring***
Ibuprofen	• Liquid: 100 mg/5 mL • Tablets: 200, 400, 600, 800 mg	30–40 mg/kg/d	Tid	Gastrointestinal, renal, hepatic	Every 4–6 months
Naproxen	Tablets: 250, 275 500 mg	10–15 mg/kg/d	Bid	Same as ibuprofen + pseudoporphyria	Same as above
Indomethacin	Capsule: 25 mg, 75 mg (sustained release)	1–3 mg/kg/d	Tid	Renal toxicity, GI irritation	Same as above
Salicylates, e.g. Aspirin	Tablets: 325 mg	70–100 mg/kg/d	Qid	Gastrointestinal, renal, hepatic, tinnitus, caries, association with Reye's syndrome	Same as above
B. DMARDs					
Methotrexate	• Tablets: 2.5 mg • Parenteral: 25 mg/mL (IV, IM, SC) • Parenteral form may be used orally in young children	10–15 mg/m^2 or 0.3–1.0 mg/kg orally or subcutaneously. Start at the lowest dose, gradually increase till response	Weekly	• Gastrointestinal, hepatic, bone marrow suppression, acute pulmonary insufficiency immunosuppression, teratogenicity, alopecia • Incidence of most of above very low in children at doses used thereby making it a rather safe drug • The most common adverse effects in children are gastrointestinal and mouth ulcers	• *At onset:* As given above *plus* Renal function if history of kidney disease (excreted by kidneys) • *Follow-up:* CBC and LFT 4–8 weekly
Sulphasalazine	Tablets: 500 mg	40–60 mg/kg/d: Maximum: 2 g	Bid	Gastrointestinal, hepatic, rash, allergic reactions, Stevens-Johnson syndrome, bone marrow suppression, associated with Reye's syndrome. Contraindicated in G6PD deficiency	Q 3 months. CBC and LFT
Leflunomide	Tablets: 10 mg, 20 mg	• <20 kg: 10 mg alternate day • 20–40 kg: 10 mg daily • >40 kg: 20 mg daily	OD	Hepatotoxicity (more when combined with Methotrexate), nausea, diarrhea, alopecia, mild weight loss	CBC, ALT, AST, albumin 3 monthly
Thalidomide	Capsule: 50 mg, 100 mg	2.5–4 mg/kg/day	OD, preferably at bedtime	Drowsiness, tingling numbness, peripheral neuropathy (irreversible), hypothyroidism, hypoglycemia, stimulation of ACTH, prolactin	Enquire about tingling numbness, check deep tendon reflexes

Contd...

Contd...

C. Biologicals					
IVIG	IV	1–2 g/kg	Monthly	Allergic reactions, headache, risk of blood-borne disease	
Etanercept* (anti-TNF)	SC	0.4 mg/kg, Maximum 25 mg	Twice weekly	Irritation at injection site, increased frequency of infection	
Infliximab** (monoclonal antibody to TNF)	SC	3–10 mg/kg IV infusion	Every 4–8 weeks	Headache, dizziness, nasal and throat irritation. Irritation at injection site	
Anakinra (anti-IL1)	SC	100 mg	Daily	Fever, flu-like reactions, MAS	
Tocilizumab (anti-IL6)	IV	8–12 mg/kg	Fortnightly	Infusion reactions, rashes	

*Etanercept has not been studied in children younger than 4 years.
**Infliximab is usually used in conjunction with methotrexate to reduce the chances of developing antibodies against it.
(NSAIDs: nonsteroidal anti-inflammatory drugs; DMARDs: disease-modifying antirheumatic drugs; IV: intravenous; IM: intramuscular; SC: subcutaneous; ALT: alanine aminotransferase; AST: aspartate aminotransferase; CBC: complete blood count; LFT: liver function test; ACTH: adrenocorticotropic hormone; IVIG: intravenous immunoglobulin; TNF: tumor necrosis factor)

- *Systemic onset:* The systemic features are treated with NSAIDs and oral or intravenous steroids based on severity. The articular features are managed depending on the number of joints involved as cited above.

COMPLICATIONS

Uveitis

Anterior uveitis, which is often asymptomatic and therefore treacherous may lead to the "painless blind eye". The child with oJIA is most prone followed by those with pJIA and then sJIA. Antinuclear antibodies positivity identifies those at higher risk and ophthalmic monitoring periodically is mandatory. Guidelines exist for risk stratification and periodicity of monitoring which ranges from 3 monthly to annually. Affected cases are treated with topical steroids with resistant cases needing systemic methotrexate.

In contrast, the HLA-B27 positive child with ERA may develop symptomatic anterior uveitis—the "acute painful red eye", which may promptly be treated with topical steroids. Routine monitoring is not indicated.

Growth Issues and Deformities

Growth failure and short stature is seen particularly in sJIA, not only from chronic inflammation but also from the high or prolonged doses of steroids consumed. Local deformities may lead to significant loss of hand function or locomotion, consequent handicap and even loss of vocation. Bony overgrowth caused by hyperemia of the affected joints (classically the knee) can lead to limb length discrepancy. Complications of cervical spine involvement include bony ankylosis and atlantoaxial subluxation making neck extension and intubation difficult. Temporomandibular joint involvement may cause significant micrognathia and consequent malocclusion.

Macrophage Activation Syndrome

This dreaded life-threatening complication of sJIA is characterized by a change in the fever pattern with hectic spikes, a sick looking child with neurological alteration, abnormal liver function, coagulopathy, hypertriglyceridemia and hyperferritinemia. Prompt recognition and treatment with intravenous steroids with or without cyclosporine can be lifesaving.

Iatrogenic Issues

The drugs used in the management of JIA can have complications with long-term use. The nephropathy and gastropathy with prolonged NSAID usage or the osteoporosis, propensity to infections, growth retardation and subcapsular cataracts due to steroid usage are examples. Careful monitoring of all drugs is paramount. Since most of the drugs are immunosuppressive a careful watch for infections and attending to immunizations are important.

OUTCOME AND PROGNOSIS

In general, children diagnosed in this century are doing better than those toward the end of the last. This has been largely possible owing to the improved therapeutic armamentarium.

Since JIA is not one disease, the outcome and prognosis varies with the subtype. Children with oJIA have the best outcomes, as do children who are pJIA RF negative. The sJIA group, follows yet unpredictable variable course with one group of children having monocyclic disease, a second group with a polycyclic course and a third with a chronic continuous course.

KEY MESSAGES

- Juvenile idiopathic arthritis is the most common chronic inflammatory arthropathy of childhood and the etiology is as yet unknown.
- The International League of Associations for Rheumatology classification of 2001 recognizes seven subgroups of disease.
- The diagnosis of JIA is based mainly on clinical considerations and is one of exclusion.
- Investigations mainly help to rule out mimics or follow-up disease activity.
- Tests such as ANA, rheumatoid factor or HLA-B27 are not diagnostic tests and should not be recommended as an "arthritis panel". They are correctly used for classification or risk stratification.
- Multidisciplinary care is crucial for affected children.
- Significant advances in pharmacology coupled with a changed paradigm of care with an early aggressive approach have vastly improved the lives of these children.
- Uveitis, deformities, iatrogenic issues and the dreaded macrophage activation syndrome are complications which need to be watched for.

BIBLIOGRAPHY

1. Beukelman T, Patkar NM, Saag KG, et al. 2011-American College of Rheumatology recommendations for the treatment of juvenile idiopathic arthritis: initiation and safety monitoring of therapeutic agents for the treatment of arthritis and systemic features. Arthritis Care Res (Hoboken). 2011;63(4):465-82.
2. Prakken B, Albani S, Martini A. Juvenile idiopathic arthritis. Lancet. 2011;377(9783):2138-49.
3. Ravelli A, Martini A. Juvenile idiopathic arthritis. Lancet. 2007;369(9563):767-78.

16.3 Systemic Lupus Erythematosus

Surjit Singh

INTRODUCTION

Systemic lupus erythematosus (SLE) is the classic prototype of an autoimmune disease, where an immune dysregulation leads to formation of excess autoantibodies directed against self-antigens. Subsequent development of immune complexes and their deposition causes inflammatory damage of various organs chiefly the skin, kidneys, blood vessels and nervous system.

EPIDEMIOLOGY

Though SLE is distinctly uncommon in children, there is paucity of precise prevalence data. In adults, the female:male ratio is 9:1. Female preponderance is much less obvious in the prepubertal age group. SLE is uncommon in the first decade.

ETIOPATHOGENESIS

Exact etiology of SLE is not known. Several factors (including genetic, environmental, hormonal, B-cell and T-cell interactions, abnormal apoptosis) are believed to contribute to the development of immune dysregulation characteristic of this condition. As a result, autoantibodies are formed against DNA and other nuclear antigens, ribosomes, various tissue antigens, RBCs, WBCs and platelets. Several triggering factors (e.g. sunlight, infections and drugs) are believed to have a role in the initiation and perpetuation of the immune dysregulation. Damage to cells and tissues results from pathogenic autoantibodies and immune complexes. Antinuclear antibodies (ANA) are present in almost all patients with SLE and a negative result should warrant a review of the diagnosis. These are, however, not specific for SLE. Antibodies directed against double-stranded DNA (anti-dsDNA) are more specific than ANA and are especially raised in active lupus nephritis. Antibodies to histones are characteristic of drug-induced lupus.

CLINICAL FEATURES

Systemic lupus erythematosus is a multisystem disorder and children may present in many different ways depending on the organs involved. Further, the clinical presentation can be acute, subacute or chronic. Fever, arthritis, and rash are common clinical manifestations in children with lupus. Several organ systems (e.g. renal, hematological and nervous) may be involved at presentation or subsequently in the course of the disease. Diagnosis of SLE is based on a set of clinical and laboratory criteria **(Table 16.3.1)** which have been enumerated by the systemic lupus international collaborating clinics (SLICC). It must be noted that these are "classification", and not "diagnostic", criteria. For a given patient, the diagnosis of lupus remains essentially clinical and can be made even if the requisite number of criteria is not being fulfilled at that point of time.

The characteristic butterfly rash of lupus is distributed over the cheeks and nasal bridge and spares the nasolabial folds. Other mucocutaneous lesions include purpura, alopecia, photosensitive rash, palatal and various vasculitic ulcers **(Figs. 16.3.1 to 16.3.3)**. Arthritis is polyarticular, non-deforming and can involve both large and small joints; hepatosplenomegaly and lymphadenopathy are often present. Renal involvement is more common in children as compared to adults and occurs in 60–80% of patients. It remains an important cause of morbidity and mortality. Renal manifestations can vary from asymptomatic microscopic hematuria to edema, hypertension or rapidly progressive glomerulonephritis. Renal biopsy provides important information on the severity of kidney disease. Proliferative lupus nephritis (Class III and Class IV) represents the most aggressive forms of renal disease.

Neuropsychiatric manifestations in childhood lupus can be seen in more than 50% patients. Both central and peripheral nervous system may be involved and manifestations include headache, seizures, stroke, psychosis, transverse myelitis or peripheral neuropathy. Cardiac manifestations include myocarditis, valvular thickening, verrucous (Libman-Sacks) endocarditis, conduction defects and coronary artery disease.

Pulmonary manifestations (e.g. infiltrates, hemorrhage) can also occur and may be difficult to differentiate from infection. Several commonly used drugs (e.g. isoniazid, hydralazine, and some anticonvulsants) can result in a lupus like disease but renal and neurological involvement is unusual. Neonatal lupus may be seen in babies born to mothers with lupus and results from the transplacental passage of anti-Ro and anti-La antibodies. The clinical manifestations (rash, thrombocytopenia) are usually mild and self-limiting except

Table 16.3.1: The 2012 SLICC classification criteria for systemic lupus erythematosus.

Clinical	***Laboratory***
Acute cutaneous lupus	ANA
Chronic cutaneous lupus	Anti-DNA
Oral/nasal ulcers	Anti-Sm
Nonscarring alopecia	Antiphospholipid antibodies
Arthritis	Low complement (C3, C4, CH50)
Serositis	Direct Coombs' test
Renal	
Neurologic	
Hemolytic anemia	
Leukopenia	
Thrombocytopenia (<100,000/mm^3)	
For diagnosis: >4 criteria (at least 1 clinical and 1 laboratory) or biopsy proven lupus nephritis with ANA or Anti-dsDNA	

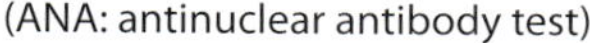
(ANA: antinuclear antibody test)

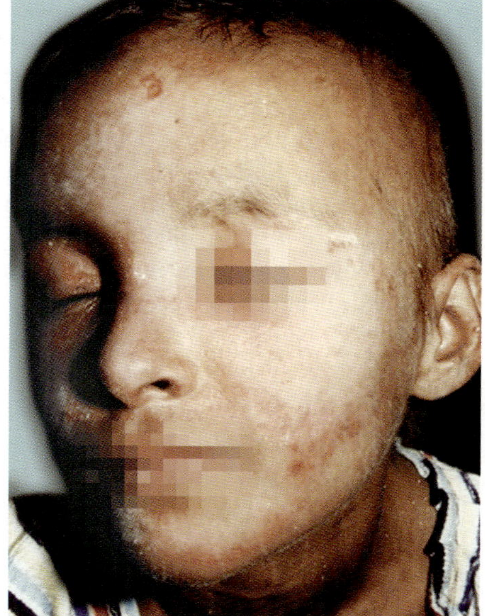

Fig. 16.3.1: Alopecia, photosensitive rash.

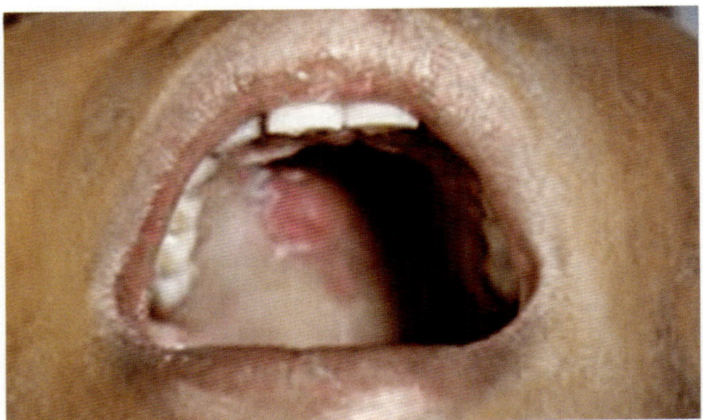

Fig. 16.3.2: Palatal ulcer.

for congenital heart block which is always permanent and may require urgent treatment with a pacemaker.

LABORATORY INVESTIGATIONS

Laboratory investigations that need to be carried out are determined by the clinical presentation of lupus.

Initial laboratory investigations include:

- Complete hemogram, erythrocyte sedimentation rate
- C-reactive protein assay
- Urea, creatinine, liver function tests and lipid profile
- Tuberculin test and chest radiograph
- Urine examination
- *Specific tests*: Antinuclear antibodies (ANA), anti-dsDNA, C3 and C4.

The C-reactive protein is usually not elevated in patients with lupus unless there is concomitant infection or serositis. Workup for antiphospholipid antibodies [immunoglobulin M (IgM) and IgG anticardiolipin antibodies, IgM and IgG anti-β2 glycoprotein I antibodies, lupus anticoagulant] is mandatory as more than a third of all children with lupus may have these antibodies. Complement fractions, C3 and C4, are usually reduced in active disease and can be used to detect disease flare. Other investigations like echocardiography and imaging studies are indicated based on clinical assessment of the patient.

COMPLICATIONS

Lupus in children can be a devastating disease and is often associated with several complications. These may result from the disease itself or may be a consequence of drugs (e.g. prednisolone, cyclophosphamide) used for therapy of lupus. Further, there is a high-risk for end-organ damage from ongoing disease activity. Long-term use of glucocorticoids predisposes the patient to the risk of infections, avascular necrosis of the femoral head, posterior subcapsular cataracts, glaucoma and osteoporosis. Use of cyclophosphamide may result in infertility and predispose to the development of malignancies later in life. Development of venous (and occasionally arterial) thrombosis is not uncommon in children with lupus. Pregnancy in lupus may be associated with increased risks of disease flare and thrombosis.

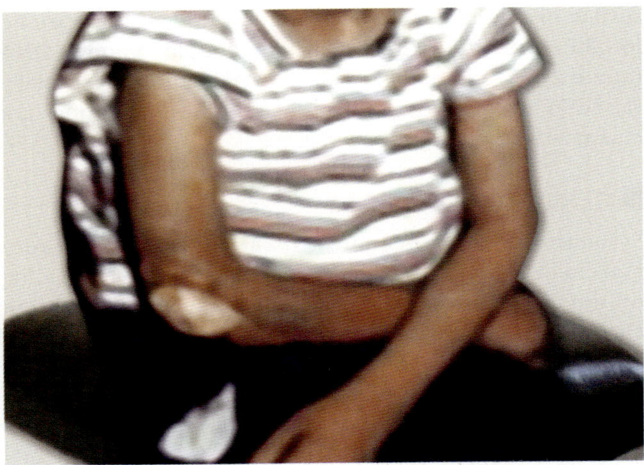

Fig. 16.3.3: Vasculitic ulcer on elbow.

TREATMENT

Lupus is a chronic disease and patients need to be on virtually life-long follow-up. Appropriate counseling is essential. Under ideal circumstances a pediatric rheumatologist should coordinate the treatment with inputs from relevant specialties such as hematology, nephrology and neurology. Daily hydroxychloroquine, given at night, forms the cornerstone of management of lupus and needs to be continued virtually indefinitely. All patients must be asked to use sunscreen lotions (SPF 15–20) three to four times in a day.

Skin manifestations without systemic involvement can be managed with hydroxychloroquine (5 mg/kg/day) alone. A short course of naproxen may suffice for arthritis. Low dose prednisolone (0.3–0.5 mg/kg/day for 4–6 weeks followed by slow tapering) usually suffices for milder manifestations of lupus.

More severe forms of the disease [especially that affecting kidneys, blood, central nervous system (CNS) or lung] would require high-dose prednisolone (1–2 mg/kg/day in divided doses) until disease activity is fully controlled (usually 4–6 weeks) and then slowly tapered to a small maintenance dose on alternate days for 4–6 months or longer.

Acutely ill and toxic patients may be treated with pulses of intravenous methylprednisolone (30 mg/kg/day for 3–5 days) and then switched to oral prednisolone. Patients with class III and class IV lupus nephritis, as also those with severe involvement of other vital organs, should receive intravenous pulses of cyclophosphamide in addition to high-dose steroid. Mycophenolate mofetil is now being increasingly used in several forms of lupus, including proliferative lupus nephritis. Rituximab is occasionally required for life-threatening lupus.

Children with lupus have an increased predisposition to infections and should be carefully monitored. Fever in a child with lupus needs prompt assessment and appropriate management. Children on long-term glucocorticoids must receive supplemental calcium and vitamin D.

Management of lupus in children requires experience and skill. The consequences of both undertreatment and overtreatment can be grave. Children, and especially adolescents, often default on the prescribed treatment regimen and need to be handled with tact and patience.

PROGNOSIS

Lupus in children in developing countries is associated with significant morbidity and mortality. There are many reasons for this. Lack of awareness about the disease, delays in diagnosis and inability to access appropriate medical care for intercurrent infections and disease activity have important bearing on long-term prognosis of this condition. Accurate clinical assessment of ongoing disease activity in children is often difficult and this may result in cumulative organ damage over time. Although, 5-year survival rates of childhood lupus are now upwards of 80–85% in the developed countries, the results are more modest in our setup.

CONCLUSION

Systemic lupus erythematosus is uncommon in children. But children may present in many different ways depending on the organs involved. It is a multisystem disorder and children may present in many different ways depending on the organs involved.

BIBLIOGRAPHY

1. Hari P, Bagga A, Mahajan P, et al. Outcome of lupus nephritis in Indian children. Lupus. 2009;18(4):348-54.
2. Hiraki LT, Benseler SM, Tyrrell PN, et al. Clinical and laboratory characteristic and long-term outcome of pediatric systemic lupus erythematosus. J Pediatr. 2008;152(4):550-6.
3. Hochberg MC. Updating the American College of Rheumatology revised criteria for the classification of systemic lupus erythematosus. Arthritis Rheum. 1997;40(9):1725.
4. Kumar A. Indian guidelines on the management of SLE. J Indian Rheumatol Assoc. 2002;10:80-96.
5. Marks SD, Tullus K. Modern therapeutic strategies for paediatric systemic lupus erythematosus and lupus nephritis. Acta Paediatr. 2010;99(7):967-74.
6. MedScape (2011). Pediatric Systemic Lupus Erythematosus. [Online] Available from: www.emedicine. Medscape. com/ article/1008066. [Accessed November, 2018].
7. Mondal R, Nandi M, Ganguli S, et al. Childhood lupus: experience from eastern India. Indian J Pediatr. 2010;77(8):889-91.
8. Singh S, Abujam B, Gupta A, et al. Childhood lupus nephritis in a developing country-24 years' single-center experience from North India. Lupus. 2015;24(6):641-7.

16.4 Approach to Vasculitis

Surjit Singh

INTRODUCTION

Vasculitic disorders are not uncommon in children but are frequently missed in clinical practice. These should be thought of whenever a child presents with a multisystemic disorder. These conditions can be classified according to the size of the vessel involved:

- Large vessel vasculitis (e.g. Takayasu arteritis)
- Medium-vessel vasculitis [e.g. Kawasaki disease (KD), polyarteritis nodosa (PAN)]
- Small vessel vasculitis (e.g. Henoch-Schönlein purpura, granulomatosis with polyangiitis)

Of these, Henoch-Schönlein purpura and Kawasaki disease are, by far, the most common conditions seen in pediatric practice. The classification criteria for the common types of childhood vasculitis are given in **Box 16.4.1**. Kawasaki disease is discussed in Chapter 16.5. Other common vasculitides are detailed here.

TAKAYASU ARTERITIS

This usually involves the aorta and its major branches. Four major patterns of involvement are recognized:

- *Type 1:* Branches from the aortic arch
- *Type IIa:* Ascending aorta, aortic arch and its branches

- *Type IIb:* Ascending aorta, aortic arch and its branches, thoracic descending aorta
- *Type III:* Thoracic descending aorta, abdominal aorta, and/or renal arteries
- *Type IV:* Abdominal aorta and/or renal arteries
- *Type V:* Combined features of Type IIb and IV.

The classification criteria for childhood Takayasu arteritis are given in **Box 16.4.1**. In India, many children with Takayasu arteritis may have a clinical association with tuberculosis and are frequently Mantoux positive. Takayasu arteritis must be excluded in children with renovascular hypertension.

Diagnosis can be confirmed by digital subtraction angiography. Computed tomography angiography and magnetic resonance angiography are being increasingly used for diagnosis of this condition. Treatment is based on long-term immunosuppression with prednisolone and oral weekly methotrexate. Mycophenolate mofetil is also of benefit. With angioplasty and appropriate stent placements, the long-term prognosis is now reasonable and 5-year survival rates above 90% have been reported from several centers.

Box 16.4.1: Diagnostic criteria for vasculitis in children.

Takayasu arteritis: Angiographic abnormalities (conventional, CT or MR) of the aorta or its main branches plus at least one of the following four features:

1. Decreased peripheral artery pulse(s) and/or claudication of extremities
2. Blood pressure difference greater than 10 mm Hg
3. Bruits over aorta and/or its major branches
4. Hypertension (based on childhood normative data)

Polyarteritis nodosa: A childhood illness characterized by the presence of either a biopsy showing small and midsize artery necrotizing vasculitis or angiographic abnormalities* (aneurysms or occlusions) plus at least two of the following:

- Skin involvement
- Myalgia or muscle tenderness
- Systemic hypertension (based on childhood normative data)
- Abnormal urine analysis and/or impaired renal function
- Mononeuropathy or polyneuropathy
- Testicular pain or tenderness
- Signs or symptoms suggesting vasculitis of any other major organ systems (gastrointestinal, cardiac, pulmonary or central nervous system)

Granulomatosis with polyangiitis (Wegener's granulomatosis):
Three of the following six features should be present:

1. Abnormal urinalysis
2. Granulomatous inflammation on biopsy
3. Nasal sinus inflammation
4. Subglottic, tracheal or endobronchial stenosis
5. Abnormal chest X-ray or CT scan
6. Positive C-ANCA staining

*Should include conventional angiography, if magnetic resonance angiography is negative
(C-ANCA: C-anti-neutrophil cytoplasmic antibody; CT: computed tomography)

POLYARTERITIS NODOSA

Polyarteritis nodosa (PAN) is distinctly uncommon in children and can be a very difficult condition to diagnose in pediatric practice, as the clinical manifestations can be extremely variable. Usual clinical features include fever, rash (typically *livedo reticularis*), hypertension, abdominal pain, joint pains and myalgia. Neurological involvement can take the form of seizures, encephalopathy and peripheral neuropathy. The latter can be very difficult to evaluate in young children. Clinical diagnosis is facilitated by angiography when aneurysms are demonstrable in the renal arteries or celiac axis. On histopathology, there is fibrinoid necrosis in medium sized arteries typically with segmental involvement. The diagnostic criteria for childhood PAN have been recently revised and are given in **Box 16.4.1**. Treatment consists of long-term immunosuppression, initially with prednisolone and cyclophosphamide, and followed by maintenance azathioprine.

HENOCH-SCHÖNLEIN PURPURA

See Chapter 10.5 on Renal Vasculitis and Lupus Nephritis**.**

GRANULOMATOSIS WITH POLYANGIITIS (WEGENER'S GRANULOMATOSIS)

Granulomatosis with polyangiitis (formerly Wegener's granulomatosis) is an uncommon disorder in pediatric practice in which there is involvement of the respiratory tract and kidneys. The diagnostic criteria are given in **Box 16.4.1**. The condition usually has an insidious onset and constitutional symptoms (e.g. fever/malaise), which are quite common. Laboratory diagnosis is based on detection of anti-neutrophil cytoplasmic antibodies (ANCAs), especially C-ANCA, which are virtually pathognomonic of the condition. Treatment with prednisolone and cyclophosphamide (followed by long-term azathioprine) results in long-term remissions.

BEHÇET DISEASE

Behçet disease is an unusual vasculitic disorder characterized by the following clinical manifestations:

- *Major features:* Aphthous stomatitis, genital ulceration, cutaneous manifestations and ocular disease.
- *Minor features:* Gastro intestinal disease, thrombophlebitis, arthritis, family history and neurological involvement. The disease is characterized by multiple relapses.

Major morbidity is because of the ocular and neurological manifestations. Behçet disease can be associated with arterial and venous thrombosis and these can, at times, be the presenting features of the condition. The pathergy test (i.e. cutaneous pustular reaction following needle pricks) is virtually pathognomonic in a clinical setting of the disease. Individuals with human leukocytic antigen B5 (B51) haplotype have an increased predisposition to this condition. Drug therapy involves use of colchicine and thalidomide.

BIBLIOGRAPHY

1. Cassidy JT, Petty RE. Textbook of Pediatric Rheumatology, 5th edition. Philadelphia: Elsevier Saunders; 2005.
2. Jain S, Sharma N, Singh S, Bali HK, Kumar L, Sharma BK. Takayasu arteritis in children and young Indians. Int J Cardiol. 2000;75(Suppl 1):S153-7.
3. Mahajan V, Singh S, Khullar M, et al. Serum and urine nitric oxide levels in children with Henoch-Schönlein purpura during activity and remission: a study from North India. Rheumatol Int. 2009;29(9):1069-72.
4. Ozen S, Ruperto N, Dillon MJ, et al. EULAR/PReS endorsed consensus criteria for the classification of childhood vasculitides. Ann Rheum Dis. 2006;65(7):936-41.
5. Singh S, Aulakh R. Kawasaki disease and Henoch-Schönlein purpura: changing trends at a tertiary care hospital in north India (1993–2008). Rheumatol Int. 2010;30(6):771-4.
6. Singh S, Bali HK, Salaria M, et al. Takayasu's arteritis in young children: a potentially treatable condition. Indian Pediatr. 1999;36(3):291-6.
7. Singh S, Das R. Clinical approach to vasculitides. Indian J Pediatr. 2002;69:881-8.
8. Singh S, Devidayal, Kumar L, et al. Severe Henoch-Schönlein nephritis: resolution with azathioprine and steroids. Rheumatol Int. 2002;22(4):133-7.

16.5 Kawasaki Disease

Surjit Singh

INTRODUCTION

Kawasaki disease (KD) is a common vasculitic disorder of young children. It is now the most common cause of acquired-heart disease amongst children in Japan, Europe, and North America. KD has been reported from all continents and is being increasingly recognized in developing countries like India and China. The epidemiology of KD shows two distinct patterns. Countries in the Far East (e.g. Japan, Korea and Taiwan) report incidence figures, which are not only the highest in the world, but have also shown a gradual increase over the last 2 decades. While Japan currently reports an incidence figure of 265/100,000 children below 5, comparable figures from Korea and Taiwan are 134 and 83, respectively. Western countries, on the other hand, report much lower incidence figures (4–25/100,000 children below 5), and the incidence seems to plateau over the last 2 decades.

The etiology of KD remains obscure though there is evidence in support of a genetic basis for this condition. Infection appears to act as a trigger in a genetically predisposed host. Siblings of affected children are at a significantly higher risk of developing KD compared with the general population. The basic pathology is a necrotizing inflammatory vasculitis with a striking predilection for the coronary arteries. All three layers of blood vessels are involved with destruction of the internal elastic lamina causing weakness and aneurysm formation and intimal proliferation leading to stenosis.

CLINICAL FEATURES

In the developed world, more than 80% of children with KD are below 5 years. In India, however, almost one-third of affected children are above 5 years. This could be a reflection of different genetic backgrounds but may also be due to the fact that infants with KD in India are still being missed or confused with viral exanthemata. The male:female ratio is 1.5:1.

The diagnosis is essentially clinical and is based on presence of fever of five or more days duration, accompanied by four of the five principal clinical criteria given in **Table 16.5.1**. The fever is usually high grade, persistent and does not respond to antimicrobials. It is often accompanied by

Table 16.5.1: Diagnostic criteria of Kawasaki disease.

- Fever lasting 5 days or more
- *Presence of at least four of the following five principal criteria:*
    1. Bilateral nonpurulent conjunctivitis
    2. Redness of the mucosa of oropharynx, strawberry tongue and dry fissured lips
    3. Changes in extremities, such as edema and erythema of hands and feet and later periungual desquamation which may also involve palms and soles
    4. Polymorphous nonvesicular rash
    5. Cervical lymphadenopathy of at least 1.5 cm in size usually unilateral
- Illness not explained by another known disease

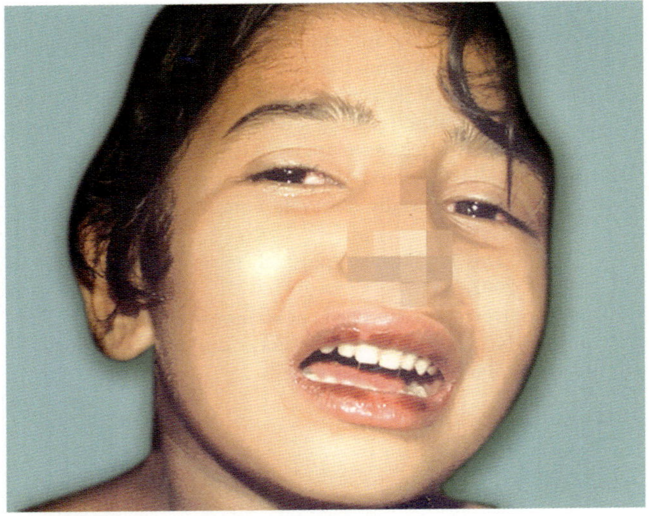

Fig. 16.5.1: Characteristic irritability of Kawasaki disease; also note the red lips and conjunctival injection.
Source: Dr A Santhosh Kumar.

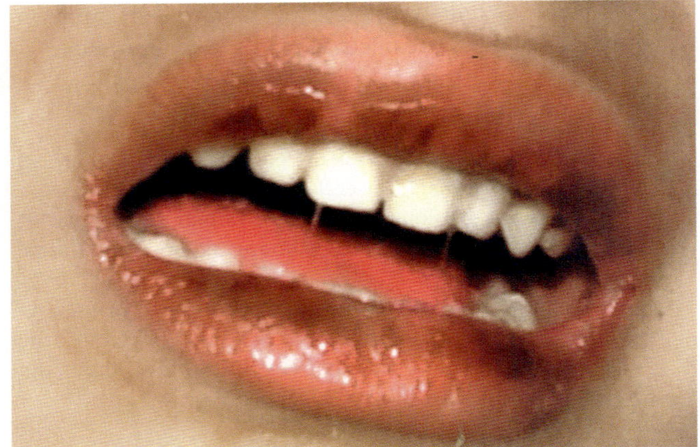

Fig. 16.5.2: Swollen and dry fissured lips; and strawberry tongue.
Source: Dr A Santhosh Kumar.

irritability **(Fig. 16.5.1)** and characteristic mucosal changes **(Figs. 16.5.1 and 16.5.2)**.

Kawasaki disease is a cascade of clinical findings, which appear sequentially over 10–14 days. Taken individually none of these clinical findings is pathognomonic of the disorder. It cannot be overemphasized that there is no gold standard for diagnosis of KD. While the criteria provide broad guidelines to the diagnosis of KD in a given child, it must be understood that their sensitivity and specificity remains to be ascertained. Too rigid an application of these criteria would undoubtedly result in high specificity, but this would be at the cost of sensitivity. Further, as KD is a cascade of evolving clinical findings all clinical features may not be present at a given point of time. As a result the clinical findings seen in the early phase of the disease may not be present later in the course. If the parents choose to seek another pediatrician during this time many of the clinical features may have already disappeared by the time they have obtained the second consultation. As a result an erroneous diagnosis of "incomplete KD" may be proffered when, in fact, the child may have sequentially had all the findings of classic KD.

Three distinct phases of KD can usually be recognized an acute phase of 10–14 days: characterized by high-grade fever, rash (often polymorphous but never vesicular), mucosal and acral skin changes, and lymphadenopathy; a subacute phase of 2–3 weeks: characterized by the characteristic periungual desquamation **(Fig. 16.5.3)** and thrombocytosis; a convalescent phase of 4–6 weeks: characterized by normalization of the raised acute phase reactants. Beau's lines over the nails are seen during this time.

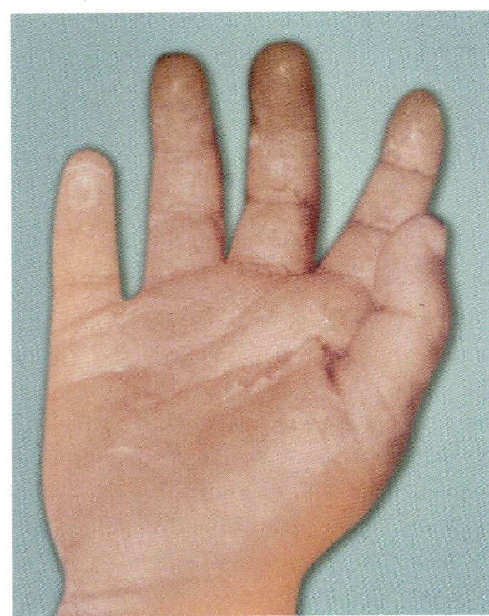

Fig. 16.5.3: Characteristic periungual desquamation of hand.

Kawasaki disease has several associated clinical features which are very suggestive of the disorder but do not find a mention in the diagnostic criteria. These include a perineal rash with perianal desquamation, reactivation of the Bacillus Calmette-Guérin scar (seen only in young infants), sterile pyuria and hydrops of the gallbladder. Arthritis is not uncommon and can occur both in the acute and subacute phases of the disease. Occasionally, it can be the presenting feature of KD and can result in diagnostic confusion.

Left untreated, KD can result in coronary artery abnormalities (CAA) in 15–25% patients. CAAs usually do not appear in the first week of illness and a normal echocardiographic examination early in the course of the

Box 16.5.1: Differential diagnosis of Kawasaki disease.

- Scarlet fever
- Drug reactions
- Stevens-Johnson syndrome
- Febrile viral exanthemata
- Toxic shock syndrome
- Staphylococcal scalded skin-syndrome

disease may be misleading. With appropriate treatment the risk of CAA can be brought down to 3–5%. Myocarditis is also a common accompaniment of KD and can, at times, present with congestive cardiac failure.

Box 16.5.1 lists some of the conditions, which are commonly considered in the differential diagnosis of KD.

INVESTIGATIONS

In the acute phase, a normocytic normochromic anemia and polymorphonuclear leukocytosis are frequently seen. Acute-phase reactants [erythrocyte sedimentation rate (ESR) and C-reactive protein (CRP)] are usually elevated. Thrombocytosis, however, becomes evident only after the first week of illness. Urine examination in children with KD may often reveal pus cells (sterile pyuria) and this laboratory finding can be mistaken for a urinary infection in a febrile child. A mild increase in transaminases is not unusual. Electrocardiography may show several nonspecific abnormalities decreased voltage, ST-T changes and, occasionally, transient conduction defects.

Echocardiography may reveal several "soft signs" (in the form of increased echogenicity of the coronary arteries, pericardial effusion, mild valvular regurgitation and, at times, a decreased ejection fraction) in addition to CAA, which may take the form of ectasia, or aneurysms. Echocardiography should be repeated in the subacute phase of KD and then on follow-up 6–8 weeks later. Coronary artery diameters should be assessed by age-based nomograms and the Z-scores calculated.

TREATMENT

Intravenous immunoglobulin (IVIG) 2 g/kg as a single infusion along with aspirin (initially 30–50 mg/kg during the acute phase followed by an antiplatelet dose of 3–5 mg/kg/day thereafter) is the standard of care for KD. IVIG should be administered preferably before day 10 of fever but can be given even later in the course, if fever is persisting or acute phase reactants are still elevated. With administration of IVIG, there is usually prompt defervescence of fever and resolution of other clinical signs. In a proportion of children (approximately 10–15%) with KD the fever may persist even after IVIG. The term "refractory KD" is used, if the fever persists (or reappears) 36 hours after completion of IVIG therapy. Children with refractory KD have a significantly higher risk of development of CAA and need prompt management. Therapeutic options include a second dose of IVIG (1–2 g/kg), pulse intravenous methylprednisolone (30 mg/kg for 1–3 days), or intravenous infliximab (5–8 mg/kg).

Low dose aspirin is usually continued till 6–8 weeks and may be stopped, if the follow-up echocardiography examination is normal. In children with persisting CAA, however, aspirin may have to be continued till the abnormality gets resolved. Children with giant aneurysms (defined as coronary artery Z-scores >10) need long-term anticoagulation along with aspirin.

PROGNOSIS

Kawasaki disease is not a one-time disease of childhood. Several children go on to develop significant cardiac sequelae. Recently, published long-term follow-up studies of children with KD and CAA have shown that while some coronary artery remodeling does occur, affected segments may develop stenosis and/or occlusion on healing and predispose the patient to cardiac ischemia in young adulthood.

CONCLUSION

Kawasaki disease is a common vasculitic disorder of young children and the most common cause of acquired-heart disease. Several children go on to develop significant cardiac sequelae. The diagnosis is mainly clinical. Early treatment provides good outcome.

ACKNOWLEDGMENT

This chapter was written by Dr Noel Narayanan in the previous editions of this book. His contribution is gratefully acknowledged.

BIBLIOGRAPHY

1. Burns JC. Kawasaki disease update. Indian J Pediatr. 2009; 76(1):71-6.
2. Narayanan SN, Ahamed MZ, Safia M. Cardiovascular involvement in Kawasaki disease. Indian Pediatr. 2005; 42(9):918-22.
3. Onouchi Y, Gunji T, Burns JC, et al. ITPKC functional polymorphism associated with Kawasaki disease susceptibility and formation of coronary artery aneurysm. Nat Genet. 2007;40(1):35-42.
4. Rowley AH, Shulman ST. Recent advances in the understanding and management of Kawasaki disease. Curr Infect Dis Rep. 2010;12(2):96-102.
5. Singh S, Aulakh R, Bhalla AK, et al. Is Kawasaki disease incidence rising in Chandigarh, North India? Arch Dis Child. 2011;96(2):137-40.
6. Singh S, Bansal A, Gupta A, et al. Kawasaki disease: a decade of experience from North India. Int Heart J. 2005;46:679-89.

anti-β_2 glycoprotein I (IgM and IgG) antibodies and the lupus anticoagulant test. Treatment is with long-term oral anticoagulation.

INTRAVENOUS IMMUNOGLOBULIN IN PEDIATRIC PRACTICE

Intravenous immunoglobulin (IVIG) is a powerful therapeutic tool and can be lifesaving therapy for several clinical conditions. It is prepared by fractionation of pooled plasma obtained from remunerated healthy donors and consists of normal intact polyspecific IgG. These donors are subjected to strict screening procedures and the quality of the end product essentially depends on the quality of this screening. Each batch of IVIG represents a donor pool of 4,000–10,000 individuals. Such large donor pools serve to ensure that the antibody repertoire is complete and representative of the population at large. Intravenous immunoglobulin preparations presently being marketed contain 90–95% monomeric IgG with only small amounts of IgA and IgM. The efficacy of IVIG depends essentially on the IgG subclass distribution of the given preparation. Some IVIG preparations do not contain the IgG3 subclass in adequate quantities.

It is the preferred treatment for several childhood conditions such as Kawasaki disease, autoimmune demyelinating polyradiculoneuropathy, and idiopathic thrombocytopenic purpura. The recommended dose is 2 g/kg given as a single infusion or 1 g/kg given over two consecutive days. IVIG is used as physiological replacement therapy in children with hypogammaglobulinemia, where the therapy has to continue lifelong. The recommended dose is 0.4–0.6 g/kg every 3–4 weeks. It has also been used in children with autoimmune hematological disorders (e.g. hemolytic anemia, neutropenia), severe myasthenia gravis and patients with life-threatening lupus.

Intravenous immunoglobulin should be administered under careful supervision as there is a risk of anaphylactoid reactions. The infusion must be started very slowly and the child monitored for any side-effects.

CONCLUSION

Proper clinical diagnoses supplemented by appropriate investigations are the mainstay in the diagnosis of rheumatological conditions. Intravenous immunoglobulin (IVIG) is a powerful therapeutic tool and can be lifesaving therapy for several clinical conditions.

BIBLIOGRAPHY

1. Ahluwalia J, Singh S, Garewal G. Antiphospholipid antibodies in children with systemic lupus erythematosus: a prospective study in Northern India. Rheumatol Int. 2005;25(7):530-5.
2. Ahluwalia J, Sreedharanunni S, Kumar N, et al. Thrombotic primary antiphospholipid syndrome: the profile of antibody positivity in patients from North India. Int J Rheum Dis. 2016;19(9):903-12.
3. Burnouf T, Radosevich M. Reducing the risk of infection from plasma products: specific preventative strategies. Blood Rev. 2000;14(2):94-110.
4. Cassidy JT, Petty RE. Textbook of Pediatric Rheumatology, 5th edition. Philadelphia: Elsevier Saunders; 2005.
5. Mahajan V, Singh S. Pediatric rheumatological disorders. In: Syngle A, Deodhar SD (Eds). Rheumatology: Principles and Practice. New Delhi: Jaypee Brothers Medical Publishers; 2010. pp. 325-33.
6. Parslow TG, Sittes DP, Terr AI, et al. Medical Immunology, 10th edition. New York: Lange Medical Books/McGraw-Hill Medical Publishing Division; 2001.
7. Singh S, Ahluwalia J, Naseem S, et al. Antiphospholipid antibodies in children with systemic lupus erythematosus: An 18 years of clinical experience. Arthrit Rheumat. 2010; 62(Suppl):S2.
8. Singh S, Bansal A. Twelve years' experience of juvenile dermatomyositis in North India. Rheumatol Int. 2006;26(6):510-5.
9. Singh S, Gupta MK, Ahluwalia J, et al. Neuropsychiatric manifestations and antiphospholipid antibodies in pediatric onset lupus: 14 years of experience from a tertiary care center of North India. Rheumatol Int. 2009;29(12):1455-61.
10. Singh S, Suri D, Aulakh R, et al. Mortality in children with juvenile dermatomyositis: two decades of experience from a single tertiary care centre in North India. Clin Rheumatol. 2014;33(11):1675-9.

16.7 Allergic Disorders

K Nagaraju

INTRODUCTION

The term *allergy* means "altered state of reactivity". The term *"atopy"* refers to an individual being prone to develop allergies because of a genetic state of hyper-responsiveness to allergens. *"Sensitization"* is the first allergic reaction in response to exposure to an allergen. Allergic disorders are increasing in all over the world and India is no exception. These disorders are chronic/recurrent and should be dealt with selective use of medications with no/lower side effects, parental education, and monitoring the patient. Evaluation includes detailed medical history and comprehensive physical examination of the allergic child along with appropriate diagnostic tests. Common allergic diseases are mentioned in **Table 16.7.1**. This chapter discusses in brief regarding allergic rhinitis, atopic dermatitis, urticaria, food allergy, and drug allergy. Bronchial asthma is dealt in detail in Chapter 8.10.

EPIDEMIOLOGY

Although, it is often remarked that everyone is allergic to something, in truth, only about 25–30% of the population is allergic to anything. The prevalence of allergic rhinitis symptoms in the International Study on Asthma and Allergies in Childhood (ISAAC) varied between 0.8 and 14.9% in 6–7 years old and between 1.4 and 39.7% in 13–14 years old children. Children with risk factors like family history go on to develop asthma and persistent rhinitis. About 75% of asthmatics have associated-allergic rhinitis, whereas 30–35% of allergic rhinitis patients have associated hyper-reactive airway disease.

Table 16.7.1: Common allergic disorders.

- *Gastrointestinal tract:* Food allergies
- *Skin:* Atopic dermatitis, urticaria/angioedema, contact dermatitis
- *Respiratory tract:* Allergic rhinitis, allergic rhinosinusitis, allergic asthma
- Generalized anaphylaxis
- *Ocular:* Allergic conjunctivitis
- *Others:* Insect sting allergy, drug allergy, latex allergy

The Atopic March

The atopic march refers to the characteristic evolution of allergic manifestations in a child with atopic tendencies with progression of age. According to this theory, food allergies and eczema precedes rhinitis and asthma in atopic individuals and may be a predictor of future respiratory allergy. However, unlike respiratory allergies, which tend to persist into adulthood, atopic eczema generally improves with age. Most of the food allergies will overgrow with age, however, nut and seafood allergies will persist throughout life.

Diagnosis of Allergic Disorders

A detailed history and thorough physical examination remains the cornerstone of diagnosing atopic disorders. In no other branch of medicine history proves so rewarding or investigations extremely futile as allergic disorders **(Tables 16.7.2 and 16.7.3; Figs. 16.7.1 and 16.7.2)**.

Table 16.7.2: Signs of allergy/atopy.

Face	Allergic shiners, allergic salute, allergic mannerisms, Dennie-Morgan folds, allergic line, allergic gape, long face syndrome
Eyes	Conjunctivitis, long silky eyelashes
Nose	Pale nasal mucosa, hypertrophied turbinates, nasal polyps hypernasality
Ears	Serous otitis media (glue ear)
Mouth	Cobblestone pharynx, throat clearing sounds (allergic cluck), dry lips
Neck	Lymphadenopathy
Skin	Flexural ulcers, urticarial rashes, dry skin, dermographism
Chest	Wheezing, accessory muscle use

Table 16.7.3: Clinical tips for diagnosis of allergic disorders.

- Persistent symptoms in a well-thriving child
- Pattern of exacerbations and remissions with diurnal and seasonal variations
- Family history of allergic disorders
- Clinical: Pale nasal mucosa with inferior turbinate hypertrophy
- Allergic salute, allergic shiners, flexural lesions and nasal crease

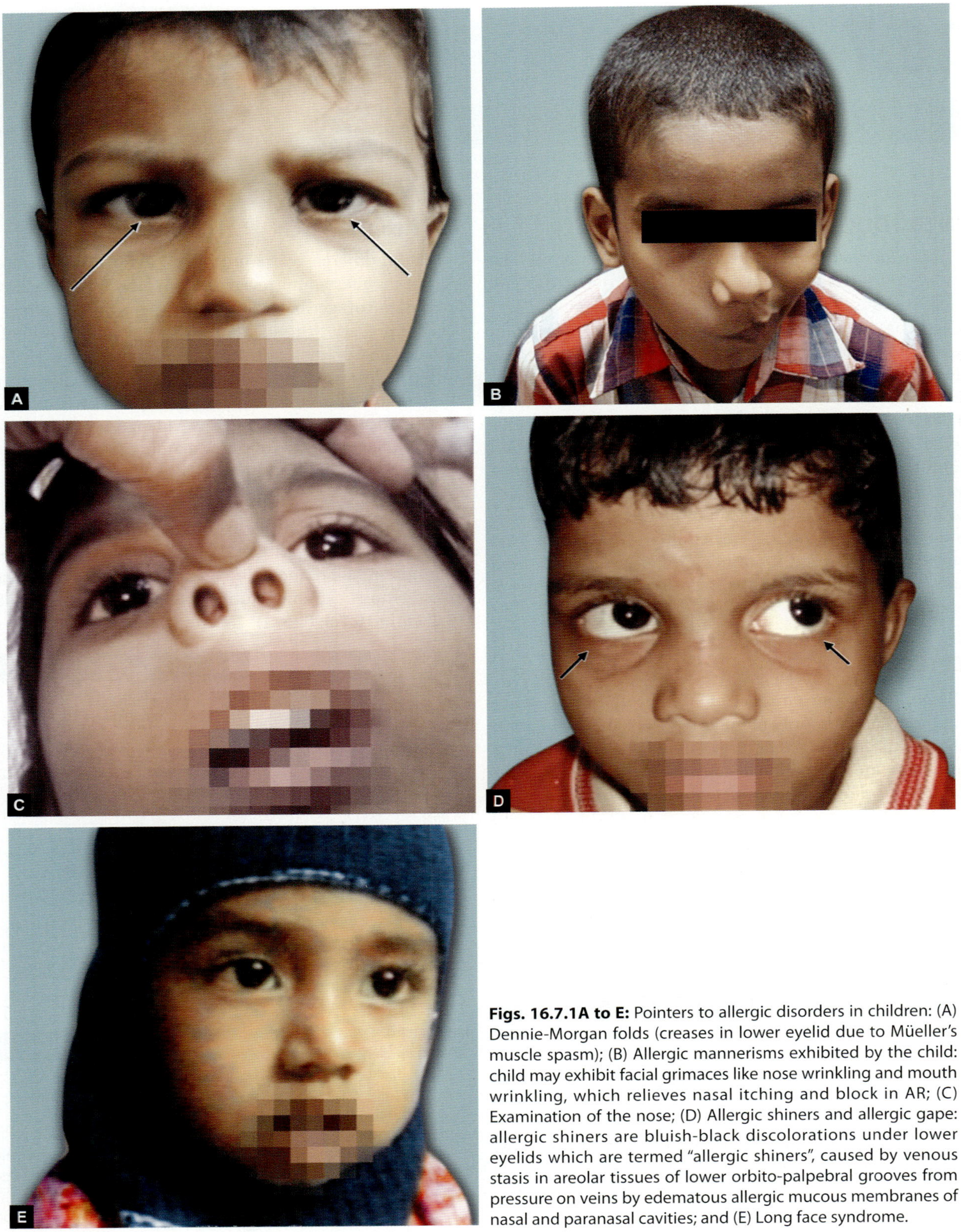

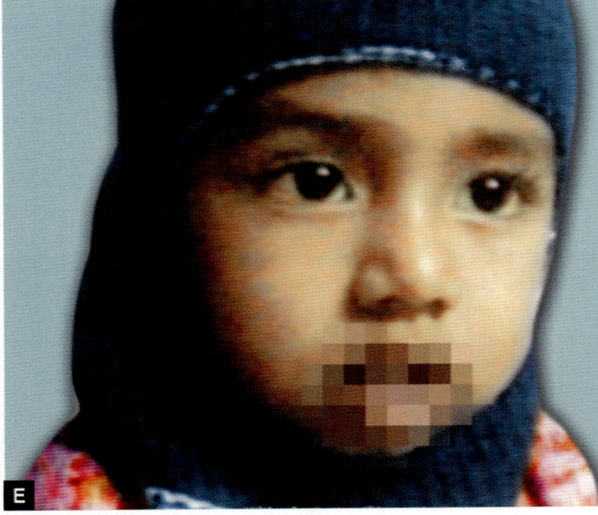

Figs. 16.7.1A to E: Pointers to allergic disorders in children: (A) Dennie-Morgan folds (creases in lower eyelid due to Müeller's muscle spasm); (B) Allergic mannerisms exhibited by the child: child may exhibit facial grimaces like nose wrinkling and mouth wrinkling, which relieves nasal itching and block in AR; (C) Examination of the nose; (D) Allergic shiners and allergic gape: allergic shiners are bluish-black discolorations under lower eyelids which are termed "allergic shiners", caused by venous stasis in areolar tissues of lower orbito-palpebral grooves from pressure on veins by edematous allergic mucous membranes of nasal and paranasal cavities; and (E) Long face syndrome.

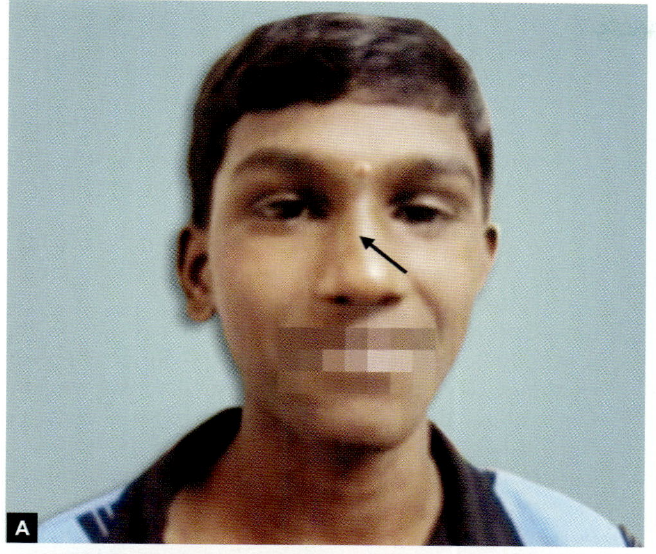

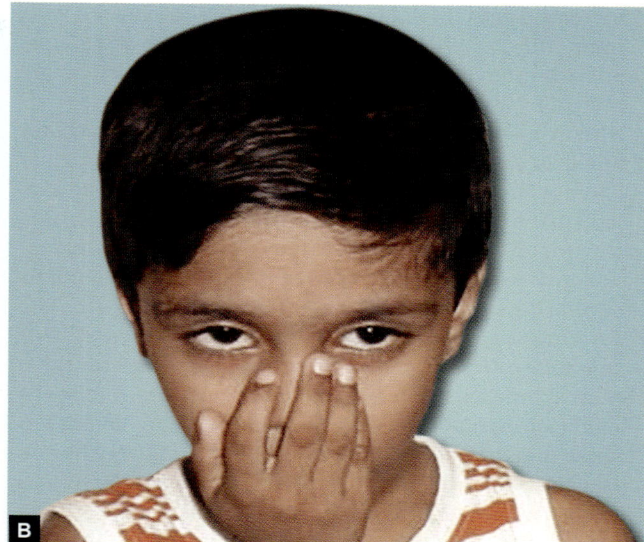

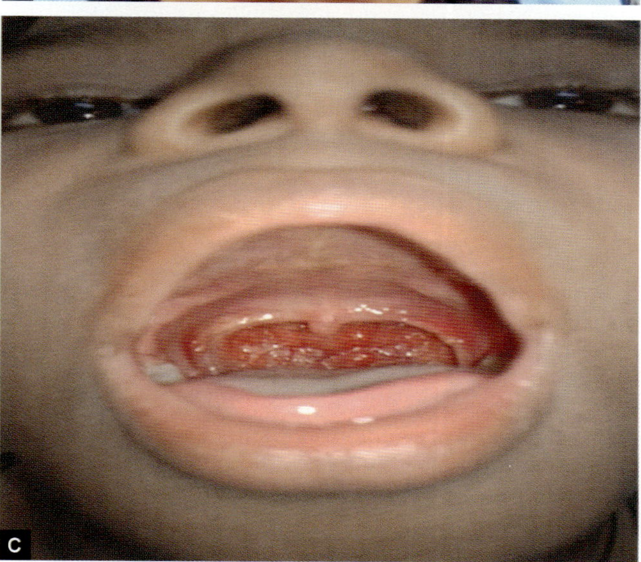

Figs. 16.7.2A to C: (A) Allergic nasal crease: Dark line between cartilaginous and bony septum due to constant edematous turbinate to relieve itching and free from septum pressing over the cartilaginous portion of the septum; (B) Allergic salute; and (C) Cobble stone pharynx.

The following histories are absolutely necessary while evaluating a child suspected to have allergy:

- Family history of allergy
- Number of episodes, frequency, duration, and severity
- Seasonal variations
- Potential triggers, if any
- Pets at home
- Stuffed animals/toys—exposing to the child
- Type of bed and furniture
- Smoking in the family
- Air-conditioner/s (AC) in the bedroom, if yes, how frequently is it cleaned?
- Individual events
- Response to medication.

Investigations

Clinical pointers mentioned in **Tables 16.7.2 and 16.7.3** should not be overlooked. However, the following investigations favor an allergic etiology:

- *Peripheral eosinophilia* (>450/mm^3)—not a specific marker for allergy. Other causes should be excluded.
- *Elevated eosinophils in nasal mucus smear* (>4% young children and >10 in adolescents) by Hansel stain indicate nasal allergy.
- *Total serum immunoglobulin E (IgE):* Four-fold increase of IgE for the age is considered as a nonspecific marker of allergy. It should be remembered that normal IgE level does not eliminate the possibility of allergic disease and nonallergic diseases may be associated with

increased serum IgE level. Raised IgE is implicated with many other conditions such as parasitic infestations, allergic bronchopulmonary aspergillosis (ABPA), fungal infections, Job syndrome, etc.

- *Allergy skin test (skin prick test)* is the most important ancillary test to know the sensitized allergen causing the allergy. The skin prick test results must be interpreted in light of the history and physical examination to determine the importance of a positive test. Main disadvantage of allergy skin testing is the need to withhold antihistamines several days prior to testing.
- *In vitro testing for specific IgE antibodies by ImmunoCAP or Immulite or Hycor method* is expensive and less sensitive than skin tests. Main advantages are no interference of medications and no risk of anaphylaxis. It can be used to know that the child has outgrown the food allergy or not. However, the clinical utility of these tests is limited and history with examination remains the diagnostic criteria for diagnosis of allergic disorders.
- *Component resolved diagnosis (CRD):* Component resolved diagnosis may decrease the need for provocative testing, improve recommendations for allergen avoidance has an important role in allergen immunotherapy (which antigen to choose for immunotherapy preparation), and helps to know cross-reactive antigens, pollen polysensitization, food allergy, latex allergy or anaphylaxis. While doing allergen components IgE testing, it is possible to create an allergen component IgE profile of each patient identifying the relevant allergen components from different allergenic sources.
- *Immuno-solid phase allergy chip (ISAC):* It is the most advanced *in vitro* diagnostic test for the simultaneous determination of specific IgE antibodies to 112 allergenic proteins present in more than 50 different allergens. It is a semiquantitative analysis that uses microchip technology.
- *Spirometry* measures the airway obstruction and reversibility after a bronchodilator (FEV_1 >12 (200 mL) of the baseline) indicates asthma. Similarly exercise-induced bronchospasm (8 minutes running or its equivalent) is helpful in the diagnosis of asthma (15% decrease of FEV_1). However, normal spirometry does not rule out asthma. Forced expiratory flow (FEF) between 25 and 75% of vital capacity is an early marker of bronchial involvement in patients with allergic rhinitis (AR).
- *Peak expiratory flow rate (PEFR)* measured by using Mini Wright peak flow meter is inexpensive and to be used in clinic setup for monitoring of asthma. Self-monitoring of peak expiratory flow (PEF) by patients is recommended for better asthma control.
- *Peak nasal inspiratory flow meter* used to detect the severity of nasal obstruction and can be used in nasal challenge testing.
- *Imaging* may be a useful modality to rule associated comorbid conditions.
  - *Chest radiograph* is indicated to exclude alternate diagnosis for asthma.
  - *X-ray of paranasal sinuses* is rarely required as 40% of allergic rhinitis patients have sinus abnormalities.
  - *CT scan of paranasal sinuses* is recommended only when maximum medical treatment has failed, when surgery is planned or when there are complications of sinusitis.
  - *X-ray neck lateral view for adenoids* is rarely correlates with the adenoidal size, may be indicated if they really add to the clinical diagnosis.
- *Nasal endoscopy* in allergic rhinitis patients is not routinely recommended. It can be done whenever anatomical abnormalities are suspected, for knowing the size of adenoids and the status of osteomeatal complex, with the help of an otolaryngologist.
- *Elevated tryptase* levels can help in anaphylaxis and also in systemic mastocytosis.
- *Patch testing:* Patch testing is used for delayed hypersensitivity reactions, e.g. contact dermatitis.
- *Newer modalities* such as eosinophil cationic protein, exhaled nitric oxide, and assays for histamine-releasing factor are useful tools to identify eosinophilic inflammation but are not routinely recommended.

Allergic Rhinitis

Clinical Features

Cardinal signs of allergic rhinitis (AR) include:

- Paroxysmal sneezing
- Nasal congestion
- Rhinorrhea
- Nasal itching.

Two or more of symptoms for more than 1 hour for most of days are suggestive of allergic rhinitis. Most of the children present with non-nasal symptoms such as itching in eyes, palate, throat and ears, lacrimation, and headache. Symptoms of allergic rhinitis are often ignored or mistakenly attributed to a respiratory infection. Physical examination **(Table 16.7.2)**, along with inspection of nasal cavity (may reveal pale or bluish, boggy nasal mucosa) will guide the diagnosis.

Treatment

The management of allergic disorders includes avoidance of offending allergens/irritants, pharmacotherapy and when indicated immunotherapy. Management of allergic diseases is summarized in **Flowchart 16.7.1**.

Avoidance of Allergen

This is the single most important step in the treatment of allergic disorders. The most important environmental measures include avoiding furred pets in bedroom, prevention of water stagnation, use of air-conditioners,

Flowchart 16.7.1: Algorithm for management of allergic diseases.

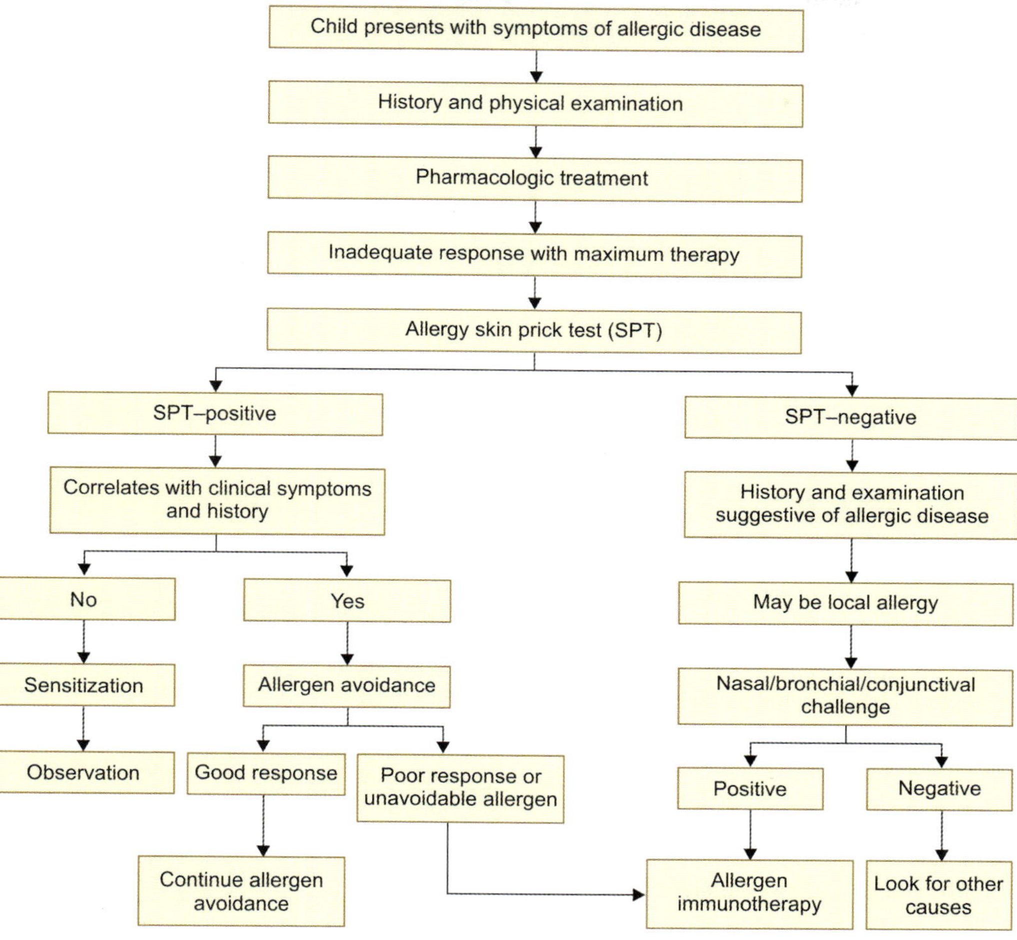

regular washing and sun drying of beddings and professional extermination **(Tables 16.7.3 and 16.7.4)**. Use of specialized high-efficiency particulate air filtered air cleaners reduces air-borne allergens.

Table 16.7.4: Allergen-control measures for house dust mite.

- Washing all walls and floors
- Removing carpets from bedrooms
- Replacing carpets with hard flooring
- Washing bedding on a hot cycle (55–60°C)
- Applying tannic acid
- Using vacuum cleaners for bedding
- Dust mite free bed/pillow covers

Pharmacotherapy

First-line pharmacotherapy includes second-generation antihistamines **(Table 16.7.5)**, mast cell stabilizers and adrenergic agents used as decongestants. Combining H_1 and H_3 antihistamine blockade provides the novel approach for the treatment of AR especially nasal congestion without the hypertensive liability of current adrenergic agonists. The second-line agents include inhaled intranasal steroids **(Table 16.7.6)**. Systemic glucocorticosteroids are useful during exacerbations. Newer agents used in the treatment of allergic disorders include olopatadine, lodoxamide and omalizumab. Recombinant soluble IL-4 receptor antagonists and monoclonal antibody against IL-5 are agents presently available.

If these modalities fail after an adequate trial period, it may be prudent to try allergen immunotherapy provided the provoking allergen is known. It is fundamental and imperative that a patient understands the premise of treatment plan before accepting and adhering to avoidance steps and medication regimens. Delivery systems for use in the nose must be demonstrated and, in turn, the patient's technique is to be observed in each visit.

Table 16.7.5: Second generation antihistamines and the dose.

Drug	Age-wise dose	Conditions requiring dose adjustment	Clinically relevant drug–drug interactions
Cetirizine	• *6 months to < 2 years*: 0.25 mg/kg • *2–5 years*: 2.5 mg OD • *6–11 years*: 5 mg OD • *>12 years*: 10 mg OD	Renal and hepatic impairment	Unlikely
Levocetirizine	• *6 months to 5 years*: 1.25 mg OD • *6–11 years*: 2.5 mg OD • *>12 years*: 5 mg OD	Renal and hepatic impairment	Unlikely
Fexofenadine	• *6 months to 2 years*: 15 mg BD • *2–12 years*: 30 mg BD • *>12 years*: 120 mg or 180 mg OD	Renal impairment	Unlikely
Loratadine	• *1–2 years*: 2.5 mg OD • *2–12 years*: 5 mg OD • *>12 years*: 10 mg OD	Hepatic impairment	Unlikely
Desloratadine	• *6–11 months*: 1 mg OD • *12 months to 5 years*: 1.25 mg OD • *6–11 years*: 2.5 mg OD • *>12 years*: 5 mg OD	Renal and hepatic impairment	Unlikely

Montelukast was found to improve nasal and bronchial symptoms. Montelukast is effective in allergic rhinitis associated with other comorbid conditions such as asthma, urticaria etc. The addition of an antihistamine to montelukast does not appear to have added benefits and FDA has not approved this combination.

Table 16.7.6: Intranasal steroids and the dose.

Drug	Age-wise dosing	Indication
• Budesonide • Each spray (64 μg)	• *6 to <12 years*: 1 spray/nostril BD • *>12 years*: 2 sprays/ nostril BD	Allergic rhinitis
• Fluticasone propionate • Each spray (50 μg)	• *4–11 years*: 1 spray/ nostril OD • *>12 years*: 2 sprays/ nostril OD	Allergic rhinitis
• Fluticasone furoate • Each spray (27.5 μg)	• *2–11 years*: 1 spray/ nostril OD • *≥12 years*: 2 sprays/ nostril OD	Allergic rhinitis
• Mometasone furoate • Each spray (50 μg)	• *2–11 years*: 1 spray/ nostril OD • *>12 years*: 2 sprays/ nostril OD	Allergic rhinitis and nasal polyps
• Ciclesonide • Each spray (50 μg)	• *>6 years*: 2 sprays/ nostril OD	Allergic rhinitis
• Triamcinolone • Each spray (50 μg)	• *>2 years*: 1 spray/ nostril OD	Allergic rhinitis

Decongestants

Intranasal decongestants are used in the treatment of nasal obstruction, in both allergic and non-allergic rhinitis and are effective in the short-term. A prolonged use (>10 days) of intranasal vasoconstrictors may lead to tachyphylaxis, a rebound swelling of the nasal mucosa and to "drug-induced rhinitis" (rhinitis medicamentosa).

Allergen-specific Immunotherapy

This is the practice of administering gradually increasing quantities of an allergen extract to an allergic subject to ameliorate the symptoms associated with the subsequent exposure to the causative allergen. There is good evidence that immunotherapy using inhalant allergens are clinically effective to treat respiratory allergies. It induces clinical and immunologic tolerance thereby preventing the progression and improving the quality of life. It also prevents progression to asthma from allergic rhinitis. Sublingual immunotherapy has gradually replaced the injection immunotherapy because of its safety profile. Hypoallergenic immunotherapy (Allergoid) is available now in India and reduces the side effects. Allergen-derived T-cell peptide epitope offer the possibilities of modulating the immune response to allergen with only minimal side effects. Recombinant allergens are designed to simultaneously retain the immunogenic/tolerogenic properties of the mild type allergens and to exhibit a strongly reduced allergenic activity and less risk of anaphylactic side effects.

New Modalities

The recent, recombinant, humanized, monoclonal anti-IgE antibody (omalizumab) forms complexes with free

IgE, blocking its interaction with mast cells and basophils and lowering free IgE levels in the circulation. However, this treatment modality is expensive and is not routinely recommended in our setup.

Atopic Dermatitis

Atopic dermatitis (AD) is a chronic skin disease characterized by itching, exudation, crusting and scaling. It has a chronic relapsing course. It first manifests in young infants has acute onset, later becomes chronic as disease progresses. Atopy is a common finding in these patients. However, non-IgE mediated inflammation is also seen. AD in infancy is a predictor for risk of development of allergic disorders in later life.

Epidemiology

True prevalence of atopic dermatitis is very difficult to define. However, this disease is alarmingly increasing all over the world especially in developed countries. In India, we do not have exact incidence.

Etiopathogenesis

AD is a product of complex interaction between various susceptibility genes, host environments, infectious agents, defects in skin barrier function, and immunologic responses.

Clinical Features

In infants: AD presents in infants with itchy oozing dermatitis on cheeks, and extensor aspects of forearms, usually from the third month onwards. Xerosis, itching of the scalp and sleep disturbance may also be seen. The diaper area is usually spared.

In children: Childhood AD involves flexures such as antecubital, popliteal fossa and neck. Erythematous patches, plaques, and lichenification may be seen. Evidence of secondary infection in the form of brown colored crusts is seen in some cases of AD. Skin is usually dry in most of the patients. Most children outgrow their lesions by 3 years of age **(Figs. 16.7.3A to D)**.

Diagnosis

Essential features (must be present):

- Pruritus
- Eczematous dermatitis (acute, subacute, or chronic)
- Typical morphology and age-specific patterns
- Chronic or relapsing history.

Important features (observed in most cases and providing support to diagnosis) include:

- Early age of onset
- Atopy
- Personal or family history
- IgE reactivity
- Xerosis.

Diagnosis of AD is made mainly by clinical evaluation.

Management

The aim of treatment is to maintain the epithelial integrity and to avoid contact with triggers **(Table 16.7.7)**.

- *Emollients* are used first.
- For difficult lesions, soft *topical steroids like hydrocortisone* are used.
- Newer drugs like tacrolimus and pimecrolimus (disease modifying agents) are used in severe cases.
- Ultraviolet (UV) therapy holds good promise but carries a theoretical risk of future cutaneous malignancies.
- Antihistamines, oral/topical antibiotics are used whenever there is itching, superadded bacterial infection accordingly.

Urticaria or Angioedema

Urticaria is a vascular reaction of the skin marked by the transient appearance of smooth, slightly elevated patches that are erythematous and that are often associated with severe pruritus. Angioedema is a condition when deep skin tissues are also affected.

Urticaria that lasts for less than 6 weeks is considered *acute*, whereas those that occur at least twice a week for >6 weeks are designated chronic. Chronic urticaria is common in children compared to acute urticaria. Chronic urticaria must be differentiated from recurrent episodes of acute urticaria.

Epidemiology

The prevalence of urticaria has been reported to be 2.1–6.7% in children and adolescents. A study in India recorded urticaria in 2.5% of children below 14 years of age.

Etiopathogenesis

Most acute urticarias in children are noted following viral infections, insect bites, and medications or related to food. Common foods causing urticaria are egg, seafood, nuts and soya. Persistent symptoms require investigations to identify the triggering allergen. Common causes of chronic urticaria are physical urticaria, aquagenic urticaria, cholinergic urticaria and pressure-induced urticaria. Recent data suggest that perhaps 25% of chronic idiopathic urticaria do have an underlying autoimmune etiology.

Clinical Features

Urticarial vasculitis should be looked for when clinically indicated. When urticaria is associated with angioedema,

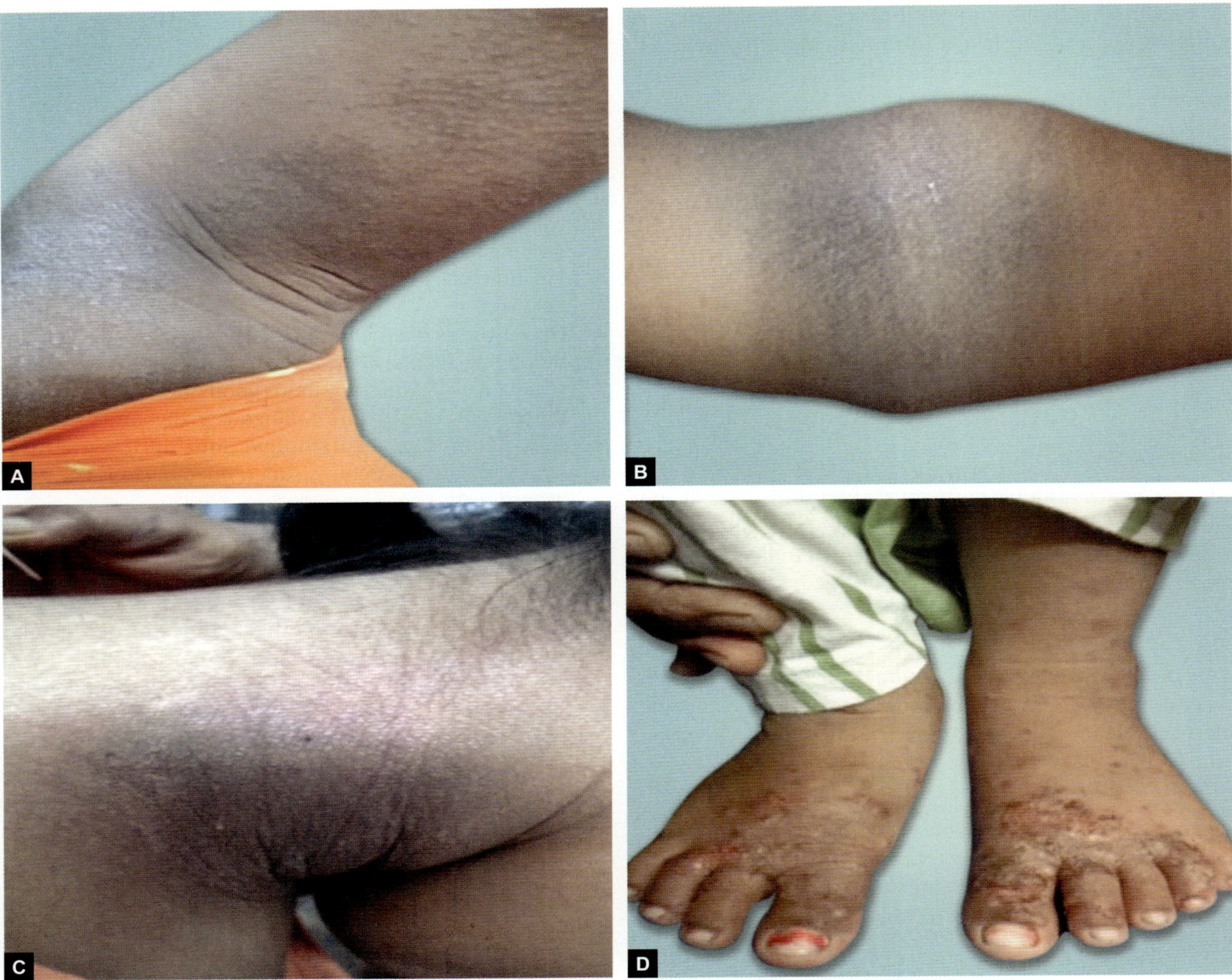

Figs. 16.7.3A to D: Clinical features of Atopic dermatitis: (A) Flexural dermatitis with lichenification in the axilla; (B) Flexural dermatitis wrist; (C) Lichenification with dermatitis in the nape of the neck; and (D) Eczema feet.

Table 16.7.7: Management of atopic dermatitis.

Mild disease	***Moderate-to-severe disease***
• *Acute treatment*: – Low potency corticosteroids twice daily for up to 3 days postclearance • *Basic management*: – *Skin care*: Liberal and frequent use of moisturizer – *Antiseptic*: Dilute bleach baths twice weekly or daily (for young children) – *Trigger avoidance*: Avoid common irritants and proven allergens	• *Acute treatment*: – Medium potency corticosteroids twice daily for up to 3 days postclearance – Add oral antibiotic in cases of secondary infection • *Maintenance topical calcineurin inhibitor*: – Pimecrolimus or tacrolimus (2–3 times/week or 1–2 time/day if patient is nonresponsive) • *Maintenance topical corticosteroids*: – Medium potency corticosteroids 1–2/weekly or – Low potency corticosteroids 1–2 daily

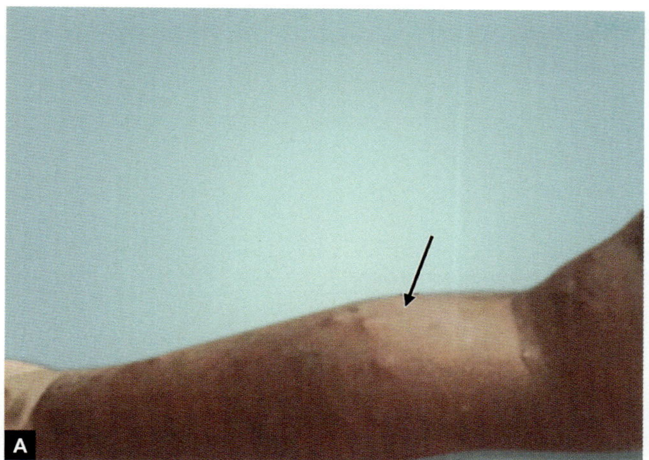

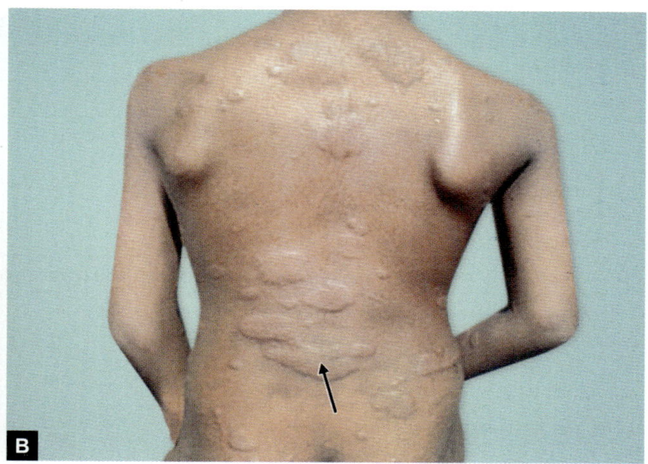

Figs. 16.7.4A and B: (A) Papular urticaria; (B) Giant urticaria.

abdominal pain, Raynaud's phenomenon or eye pain (scleritis), the diagnosis of urticarial vasculitis should be pursued. Low complement forms of vasculitis are usually associated with autoimmune disorders like SLE **(Figs. 16.7.4A and B)**.

Management

Antihistamines still are the cornerstone in the treatment of urticaria. If chronic urticaria does not respond to high doses of antihistamines, cyclosporine can be used. Cyclosporine therapy should be limited to 3 months or less for chronic urticarial **(Flowchart 16.7.2)**.

Flowchart 16.7.2: Management of urticaria

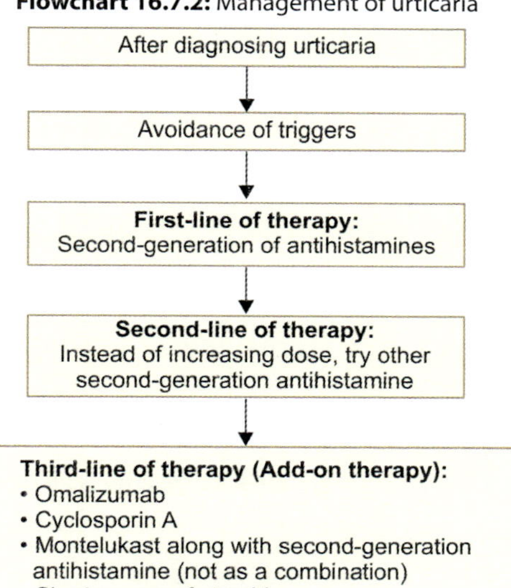

Food Allergy

Food allergy encompasses hypersensitivity reactions to food, which have an immunological mechanism (IgE-mediated and/or non-IgE-mediated). The conditions presenting as IgE-mediated, mixed or non-IgE-mediated and their common symptoms due to food allergies are described in **Table 16.7.8**. Food allergy may be suspected when a child or young person who has one or more of the signs and symptoms in **Table 16.7.9**. The management of food allergy is detailed in **Flowchart 16.7.3**.

Table 16.7.8: Immunological mechanism of food allergies.

IgE-mediated	*Mixed (IgE/non-IgE-mediated)*	*Non-IgE-mediated*
• Acute urticaria • Anaphylaxis • Food-induced asthma • Pollen food allergy syndrome	• Allergic eosinophilic esophagitis/ gastritis/ gastroenteritis • Atopic dermatitis	• Celiac disease • Heiner syndrome • Protein proctocolitis/ proctitis • Protein-induced enterocolitis syndrome

Drug Allergies

Drug hypersensitivity reactions (DHRs) are less commonly seen in children. Diagnosis of DHRs is mainly by detailed clinical history and *in-vivo* tests such as skin tests (prick test and intradermal test) and drug provocation tests.

Drug allergies classified into allergic and nonallergic. Allergic drug reactions are about 5–10% of adverse drug

Table 16.7.9: Manifestations of food allergies.

IgE-mediated	*Non-IgE-mediated*
1. Skin	
• Acute angioedema—most commonly of the lips, face and around the eyes • Acute urticaria—localized or generalized • Erythema • Pruritus	• Atopic eczema • Erythema • Pruritus
2. The respiratory system (usually in combination with one or more of the above symptoms and signs)	
• Lower respiratory tract symptoms (cough, chest tightness, wheezing or shortness of breath) • Upper respiratory tract symptoms [nasal itching, sneezing, rhinorrhea or congestion (with or without conjunctivitis)]	
3. The gastrointestinal system	
• Angioedema of the lips, tongue and palate • Colicky abdominal pain • Diarrhea • Nausea • Oral pruritus • Vomiting	• Angioedema of the lips, tongue and palate • Colicky abdominal pain • Diarrhea • Nausea • Oral pruritus • Vomiting
4. Other systems	
• Anaphylaxis (signs or symptoms of anaphylaxis or other systemic allergic reactions)	

Flowchart 16.7.3: Management of food allergy.

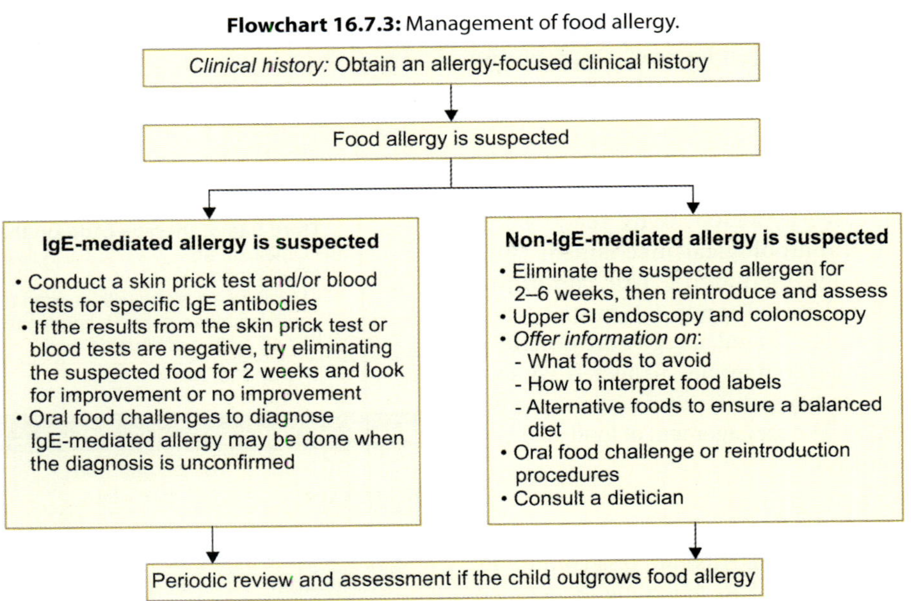

reactions (ADR). Though all four types of Gel and Coomb's reactions can occur, type 1 and type IV are common. Type 1 reactions are immediate and induced by specific IgE antibodies, which are produced against the hapten carrier conjugate of the drug, e.g. penicillin group of drugs, some of the anesthetic agents and insulin. Type IV is late reaction mediated by the T-cells, e.g. NSAIDs, radiocontrast medium and opioids. Treatment of drug allergy is to avoid the offending drug and use the alternative drug of similar efficacy. If we have to use the allergic drug compulsorily, we have to perform drug desensitization.

KEY MESSAGES

- An allergic reaction in the airways caused by the natural exposure to the allergens has been shown to lead an increase in inflammatory reaction.
- Allergens (inhalants and ingestants) are responsible for the development of allergic diseases such as allergic rhinitis, allergic asthma, atopic dermatitis/eczema and food allergy.
- The inhalant allergens include house dust mites, molds, pollen, animal dander and insects like cockroach.
- Food allergens usually cause skin symptoms, respiratory symptoms and gastrointestinal symptoms or anaphylaxis in severe cases. They are not a common cause of allergic asthma, however, cow's milk allergy along with some other food allergens may present as asthma.
- Treatment of drug allergy is to avoid the offending drug and use the alternative drug of similar efficacy
- Skin prick test (gold-standard) and *in vitro* specific IgE testing may be utilized for the diagnosis of allergic diseases.
- Treatment of allergic diseases includes allergen avoidance, pharmacotherapy, and allergen immunotherapy when indicated.
- Allergen immunotherapy is the only disease-modifying therapy for the treatment of allergic diseases.

BIBLIOGRAPHY

1. Berger WE. Allergic rhinitis in children: diagnosis and management strategies. Paediatr Drugs. 2004;6(4):233-50.
2. Brozek JL, Bousquet J, Baena-Cagnani CE, et al. Allergic rhinitis and its impact on asthma (ARIA) guidelines: 2010 revision. J Allergy Clin Immunol. 2010;126(3):466-76.
3. Brunetti L, Francavilla R, Miniello VL, et al. High prevalence of autoimmune urticaria in children with chronic urticaria. J Allergy Clin Immunol. 2004;114(4):922-7.
4. Burks AW, Tang M, Sicherer S, et al. ICON: Food allergy. J Allergy Clin Immunol. 2012;129(4):906-20.
5. Gaur SN, Kumar R, Singh AB, et al. Guidelines for practice of allergen immunotherapy in India: 2017-An update. Indian J Allergy Asthma Immunol 2017;31(1):3-33.
6. Jauregui I, Mullol J, Dávila I, et al. Allergic rhinitis and school performance. J Investig Allergol Clin Immunol. 2009;19 (Suppl 1):32-9.
7. Management of allergic rhinitis and its impact on asthma: A Pocket Guide. [online] Available from: www.whiar.org/docs/ARIA_PG_08_View_WM.pdf. [Accessed November, 2018].
8. Nagaraju K. Allergen Specific Immunotherapy, Allergic Disorders. Indian J Pract Pediatr. 2013;15(3):212-16.
9. Nagaraju K. Atopic dermatitis: In: Manual of Pediatric Allergy, 1st edition, New Delhi: Jaypee Brothers Medical Publishers (P) Ltd.; 2015. pp. 29-44.
10. Sampson HA, Aceves S, Bock SA, et al. Food allergy: a practice parameter update-2014. J Allergy Clin Immunol. 2014;134(5):1016-25.e43.
11. Weinberg EG. The atopic march current allergy and clinical immunology. 2005;18:4-5.

Section 17

Intensive Care and Emergencies

17.1 NICU and PICU Set-up in Tertiary Care Hospitals

Santosh T Soans, Maninder Dhaliwal

INTRODUCTION

The practice of pediatric and neonatal critical care medicine has established itself throughout India in the past few decades and has presently become an integral part of our health care system. In the year 1997, the intensive care group of the Indian Academy of Pediatrics (IAP) was formed and in 1998, the pediatric section of the Indian Society of Critical Care Medicine (ISCCM) was established. Subsequently, consensus guidelines were introduced by the joint chapters in 2002. The concept of level I, level II, level III pediatric intensive care units (PICUs) was established by the guidelines set forth in 2002, which will be adhered to in this chapter, with few recent international recommendations or suggestions. Neonatal intensive care units (NICU) in India have had a similar evolution. Recently there have been certain additions in the nomenclature and development of level IV NICU and new PICU levels by some international societies. In this chapter we will review, on how to set up NICU and PICUs in tertiary care hospitals in India in both private and public sector.

DEFINITION

Intensive Care

Intensive care, also known as critical care, is a multidisciplinary and interprofessional specialty dedicated to the comprehensive management of patients having, or at risk of developing acute, life-threatening organ dysfunction. Intensive care uses an array of technologies that provide support to failing organ systems, particularly the lungs, cardiovascular system, and kidneys.

Consultant Intensivist

The suggested definition of consultant intensivist is a physician who should have a postgraduate qualification in pediatrics and either:

- An additional qualification in intensive care such as Doctor of Medicine (DM), Diplomate of National Board (DNB) Post-Doctoral Fellowship, FNB Fellowship in National Board, Certificate Course of the IAP Intensive Care Chapter/IAP Neonatal Chapter/National Neonatology Forum, or qualifications from abroad such as the European Society of Paediatric and Neonatal Intensive Care (ESPNIC), American Board Certification, Australian or New Zealand Fellowship. It must be noted though that in India, government approved [Medical Council of India recognized (MCI)] degrees in pediatric and neonatal intensive care are: DM Neonatology, DM Pediatric Intensive Care, DNB Post-Doctoral Fellowship—Pediatric Intensive Care and FNB Fellowship National Board—Neonatology/Pediatric Intensive Care.
- In case of doctors neither of the above-mentioned qualifications or training, they should have extensive experience in pediatric or neonatal intensive care in India, quantified as at least 5 years' experience in the ICU (at least 50% time spent in the ICU). These are only suggestions.

LEVELS OF CARE IN NICU

Neonatal intensive care unit is usually located in proximity to delivery rooms. Though, in some hospitals with large volume maternity services or children's hospitals, the NICU may be located on a separate floor. In this case, a stabilization area must be provided within or adjacent to the delivery area where the infant can be stabilized before transfer to the NICU. But a newborn care corner is mandatory for all health facilities where deliveries take place. This is a space within the delivery room where immediate care is provided to all newborns. Levels of neonatal care vary from region to country, but a broad-based guideline was given by American Academy of Pediatrics (AAP), where an effort for defining neonatal care levels and their specifications was proposed **(Table 17.1.1)**.

The National Neonatology Forum (NNF) of India stratifies levels of neonatal care as:

- *Level I*: Basic resuscitation and healthy newborn care;
- *Level II*: Preterm care more than 32 weeks gestational age (subdivided into IIA: do not provide mechanical ventilation, and IIB: brief ventilation of <24 hours and continuous positive airway pressure support); and
- *Level III*: Extreme preterm care and complex critical care subdivided into:
    - *Level IIIA*: Conventional mechanical ventilation; and
    - *Level IIIB*: High frequency ventilation (HFOV), inhaled nitric oxide (INO) therapy.

Table 17.1.1: Care capabilities and provider needs at different levels of neonatal care centers.

Level	*Care specification*	*Personnel*
Level I or well-newborn nursery	• Provide neonatal resuscitation at every delivery • Postnatal care to stable term newborn infants • Stabilize and provide care to physiologically stable infants born between 35 weeks and 37 weeks gestation • Stabilize newborn infants who are ill and those born at less than 35 weeks gestation until transfer to a higher level of care	Pediatrician, family physician, registered nurse, other government approved health care workers
Level II or special care nursery	• Infants born at more than 32 weeks gestation and weighing more than 1,500 g who have physiologic immaturity concerns such as apnea of prematurity, inability to maintain body temperature, or are moderately ill with issues that are expected to resolve rapidly. • Need mechanical ventilation or CPAP for less than 24 hours • Are recovering from intensive care • Stabilize infants born before 32 weeks gestation and weighing less than 1,500 g until transfer to a higher neonatal intensive care level	Pediatrician, neonatologist, neonatal nurses are ideal
Level III NICU	Comprehensive care for infants with critical illness who are: • Born less than 32 weeks gestation and less than 1,500 g • Need sustained life support • Presence of high respiratory support including high frequency ventilation and inhaled nitric oxide • Availability of advanced imaging within center or nearby (computed tomography, MRI, and echocardiography)	Pediatric surgeon, and availability of other pediatric medical subspecialists, pediatric anesthesiologists and pediatric ophthalmologists (on visiting basis within close distance or as permanent staff)
Level IV or regional NICU	• Care for infants with complex congenital and acquired conditions and within center availability of surgery for such cases • Full range of medical subspecialist, surgical subspecialist, and pediatric anesthesiologist available within center • Facilitate high risk transport and provide outreach education	May or may not offer ECMO Pediatric surgical subspecialist on site

(CPAP: continuous positive airway pressure; ECMO: extracorporeal membrane oxygenation; MRI: magnetic resonance imaging; NICU: neonatal intensive care unit)

In India, nationwide creation of Newborn Care Corners (NBCC) at every point of child birth, newborn stabilization units (NBSUs) at First Referral Units (FRUs) and special newborn care units (SNCUs) at district hospitals was started way back in late 1990s. Guidelines and tool kits for standardized infrastructure, human resources, and services at each level have been developed and a system of reporting data on SNCUs is routinely done. SCNUs have been set up to provide quality level II newborn care services in several district hospitals in India. By 2015, there were 565 SNCUs, 1,904 NBSUs and 14,163 NBCCs operating in the country.

LEVELS OF CARE IN PICU

A level of PICU is mostly defined by the services it offers, beyond the immediate demands of individual patient care. There are pre-existing consensus guidelines for PICUs in India, published in 2002. There has been a sea of change since then internationally and therefore it is probably a time to have a relook into our guidelines and consider revising the same. We suggest few modifications to the 2002 guidelines. The criteria within each level may be regarded as suggested guidelines: specific criteria will vary with local resources, capabilities and different clinical needs; and for a PICU to be classified at a certain level, it should meet most, but not all, of the suggested criteria. The proposed levels in PICU and care specification are outlined in **Table 17.1.2**.

The classification of types of PICU must not be confused with the description of intensive care beds within a hospital. Level 4 PICU was previously suggested by the pediatric intensive care society, which included particularly unstable children requiring the most intensive interventions [such as extracorporeal membrane oxygenation (ECMO)] requiring an ideal nurse to patient ratio of 2:1. However the recent recommendations of the same society mention only up to 3 levels of PICU.

TYPES OF INTENSIVE CARE MODELS IN PICU AND NICU WITHIN TERTIARY CARE HOSPITAL

Based on the extent of involvement and supervision by pediatric intensivist or neonatologist, ICUs function on different models. This is more applicable for PICUs, rather than NICU. Some models are mentioned here.

Table 17.1.2: A proposed classification on levels of PICUs.

Specification	*Level 1*	*Level 2*	*Level 3*
Organ support	Capacity for oxygen therapy and noninvasive respiratory support	Basic invasive ventilation support, pharmacologic support of hemodynamic function, intermittent renal replacement therapy, parenteral nutrition	Advanced ventilator and hemodynamic support, continuous renal replacement therapy, ability for tracheostomy and other basic surgical procedures. Ability for isolation of patients needing contact or airborne precautions
Therapeutic component	Physiologic stabilization and short-term support of mild organ dysfunction	Basic support of failing organ function	Complex, comprehensive support and management of organ dysfunction
Monitoring component	Noninvasive or minimally invasive monitoring: transcutaneous oxygen saturation, urine output, blood pressure	Invasive monitoring of blood pressure and central venous pressures as dictated by patient status. Blood gas analyzer immediately available	Advanced hemodynamic monitoring (ultrasonography, etc.), advanced monitoring of pulmonary, cerebral, and other physiology as directed by clinical needs. Blood gas analyzer within ICU
Personnel	Physicians with experience in critical care in children or pediatrician	Pediatrician with ICU training or comparable experience present during day and available at night	Pediatrician with ICU training on call 24/7; immediate in-hospital availability of medical staff with PICU experience
Nurse to patient ratio	Higher than on ward; preferably 1:3	Appropriate to patient needs but no less than 1:3	Appropriate to patient needs and no less than 1:2. Ideal 1:1
Adjuvant medical staff	Variable access to other pediatric medical and surgical specialties in hospital (visiting basis)	Ready access to pediatric nephrologists, cardiologists, pediatric gastroenterologist and pediatric surgeon	Rapid access to full complement of pediatric medical and surgical consultant specialists

Note: A Level I/II PICU should have an established relationship with a Level II or a Level III PICU unit.
(ICU: intensive care unit; PICU: pediatric intensive care unit)

Open Intensive Care Unit Model/Low-Intensity Staffing

This is an ICU in which patients are admitted under the care of a primary attending pediatrician or surgeon, with the pediatric intensivist or neonatologist being available to provide their expertise in PICU or NICU. Intensivists may play a de facto primary role in the management of patients, but only within the discretion of the admitting physician, and have no overreaching authority over patient care, except in emergencies. The patient's primary physician determines the need for ICU admission and subsequent discharge, in consensus with the intensivist. Although the primary physician may have less expertise in PICU or NICU, he may have a longer association with the patient. For reasons such as the above-mentioned one, the hospital or parent may choose a primary physician, other than a neonatologist or pediatric intensivist to be mainly responsible for the patient care. This model may lead to greater variability in practice patterns depending on primary physicians and conflicting orders, misunderstanding, etc. among teams.

Closed Intensive Care Unit Model/High-Intensity Staffing

In a closed model ICU, all patients admitted to the PICU or NICU are cared for by an intensivist-led team that is responsible for making clinical decisions. The admissions and discharges are controlled by the on-site PICU or NICU physicians. It is believed that management by a team of pediatric intensivist or neonatologist provides patients with better care and is associated with improved outcomes with a more efficient use of PICU or NICU resources.

Intensivist Co-management

This involves an open ICU model in which all patients receive mandatory consultation from a pediatric intensivist or neonatologist. The pediatrician, or pediatric surgeon remains a co-attending consultant along with the intensivists collaborating in the management of all ICU patients.

Hybrid or Transitional Intensive Care Unit or Semiclosed Intensive Care Unit Model

Hybrid/transitional/semi-closed ICU is one in which pediatric intensivist or neonatologist provides direct patient care in collaboration with other "privileged" physicians, who are also allowed to write orders. Mainly surgical and cardiothoracic, cardiac intensive care units maintain this model.

Multiple Consultant Model

Multiple consultant model is one where multiple specialists are involved in the patient's care. Here, the intensivist may act as the team leader and coordinate between all consultants, providing an integrated approach to the patient and family. Patient may be admitted under any physician.

Mixed Intensive Care Unit Models

In practice, the above-mentioned models overlap to a considerable extent. The level of involvement of the intensivist may vary from daily rounds by an intensivist to the presence of a full-time, 24 × 7, intensivist in the PICU or NICU.

TYPE AND SIZE OF PICU

An institution may organize its pediatric intensive care beds into multiple units under separate management by single-discipline specialists (e.g. neurology ICU, liver ICU, surgical ICU, burns ICU). Although this may be functional in some hospitals, general multidisciplinary PICUs are common and largely successful. Thus, except for pediatric cardiac ICUs and neonatal ICUs, critically ill pediatric patients are admitted to the hospital's multidisciplinary ICU or PICU and are managed by intensive care specialists or pediatric intensive care specialists. PICUs with fewer than four beds are considered not to be cost-effective and are too small to provide adequate clinical experience for skills maintenance for medical and nursing staff. On the other hand, the emerging trend of very large PICUs can create major management problems. There is a suggestion that efficiency deteriorates once the number of critically ill patients per medical team exceeds 12. It is felt that a multispecialty hospital requires about 5% of beds for critical care, out of which 1–2% should be in ICU. The Indian consensus guidelines for PICU, published in 2002, divided the designing of PICUs into following subparts:

- Unit design
- Equipment
- Organization and staffing
- Ancillary support services; and
- Levels of PICU care and admission and discharge criteria.

The new suggested designing factors in PICU are mentioned briefly in **Table 17.1.3**.

Table 17.1.3: Key factors in designing pediatric intensive care units.

Variables	*Care specifications*
Room and bed area	At least 20 m^2 of floor area is required for each bed space in an open area (ward like PICU) exclusive of service areas and circulation space. Single room in PICU should be at least 25 m^2. There must be adequate access to the head of each bed. There should be at least 2.5 m traffic area beyond the bed area. In addition, there should be 100–150% extra space to accommodate nursing station, storage, patient movement area, equipment area, doctors' and nurses' rooms and toilet. Single rooms should have an optimal clearance of not less than 1.2 m at the head and the foot of the bed, and not less than 1.8 m on each side.
Partition between beds in open PICU	Patient privacy is desired while designing PICU. Standard curtains between beds with regular cleaning is not ideal but is widely practiced. Two rooms may be separated by unbreakable fixed or removable partisans, which may be aluminum, wood or fiber. Ideally cubicles should have sliding glass doors and windows to allow full visibility from nursing station.
Bed strength	Ideal 6–8 beds per unit. 1–5% of total hospital beds are usually suggested.
Central station	A central station should provide visibility to all patient areas. Adequate space for computer, printers, and central monitor is essential. Ample space for doctors to write on patient files and space for unit secretarial staff is essential. At least two telephone lines should be available. A cordless telephone instrument is desirable. If possible, a telephone line dedicated to incoming calls only to facilitate critical care transport requests is desirable.
Location	Should be separate from adult ICU ideally. PICU should be located near lift with easy access to emergency department, children's ward and operation theater. Easy access to radiology would be ideal. No thoroughfare can be provided through PICU. Emergency exit points in case of emergencies and disasters are a must.
Utilities per bed	*Special electric outlets*: Two, for ventilator and portable X-ray machines. All the outlets must be properly earthed and have earthing circuit breakers to protect against electrocution. *Utilities per bed* / *Level I PICU* / *Level II and III PICU*: Electric output: 12 / 16–18 Oxygen: 2 / 2–4 Vacuum: 2 / 2–3 Compressed air outlet: 1 / 2–3 Data outlet: 1 / 2–4
Temperature control	Adjustable between 22°C and 26°C, with air-exchanges of at least 6 per hour; of which 2 are of outdoor air. It is recommended that all air should be filtered to 99% efficiency down to 5 microns. Smoking should not be allowed in the ICU complex.

Utilities per bed	*Level I PICU*	*Level II and III PICU*
Electric output	12	16–18
Oxygen	2	2–4
Vacuum	2	2–3
Compressed air outlet	1	2–3
Data outlet	1	2–4

Contd...

Contd...

Variables	*Care specifications*
Illumination	Access to outside natural light is recommended. It should be bright enough to ensure adequate vision without eyestrain. Overhead lighting should be at least 20-foot candles. Recommended spot lighting for procedures should be shadow free 150-foot candles (fc) strength.
Noise	The international noise council recommends that the noise level in an ICU be under 45 dB in the daytime, 40 dB in the evening and 20 dB at night.
Beds	Beds should have ability to maneuver head end and foot end, with availability to accommodate air or water mattresses when needed, to prevent bedsores. All beds must have a railing to prevent accidental falls. Each bed should have an emergency alarm button. A cart at the bedside is important to hold personal belongings and required patient items.
Head end panel	Head wall panel or freestanding systems (power columns) hanging usually from the ceiling are both practiced.
Provision for RRT	Two beds ideally, should be specially designated for RRT (HD/CRRT) where outlets should be available for RO/ deiodinated water supply for HD machines in level II or III PICU.
Negative pressure isolation rooms	Isolation of patients infected or suspected to be infected with organisms spread via airborne droplet nuclei. In these rooms the windows do not open. They have greater exhaust than supply air volume. Pressure differential of 2.5 Pa is recommended. Clean to dirty airflow, i.e. direction of the airflow is from the outside adjacent space (i.e. corridor, anteroom) into the room.
Positive pressure isolation rooms	To provide protective environment for patients at highest risk of infection, e.g. neutropenia, post-transplant, etc. These rooms should have greater supply than exhaust air. Pressure differential of 2.5–8 Pa, preferably 8 Pa. Positive airflow relative to the corridor (i.e. airflows from the room to the outside adjacent space). HEPA filtration is required if air is returned.
Chairs number	Individual units should decide whether they want to allow the relative to sit by the side of the patient. Usually chair with safety belts are recommended for patients to sit out of bed during rehabilitation.
Hand hygiene	Every bed should have attached alcohol based antimicrobial instant hand wash solution source, which is used before caregiver (doctor/nurse/relative/paramedical) handles the patient. Water basin at all bedsides has not proven popular, but every room should have one washbasin. An operation room style sink with elbow or foot operated water supply system with running hot and cold-water supply with antiseptic soap solution should be there at a point easily accessible.
Storage	Storage areas should take up a total floor space of at least 10 m^2 per bed. They should have separate access remote from the patient area and be no farther than 30 m from the patient area. Two separate spaces for clean (15 m^2) and dirty (25 m^2) utility rooms with separate access are necessary. Other suggested area also includes bulk supplies (21 m^2), clinical equipment (30 m^2), X-ray or imaging equipment area (5 m^2), furniture store (15 m^2), gas cylinders (4 m^2).
Crash cart	A crash cart with emergency drugs and portable monitor or defibrillator should be readily accessible. Area should be marked for crash cart.
Other areas	Adequate arrangements for offices (consultation, counseling and changing rooms), doctor-on-call rooms (min 15 m^2), wash rooms (for both health care staff and patients) and seminar room (40 m^2) should be considered while designing PICU.
Biomedical waste	As per standard national and state guidelines.

(CRRT: continuous renal replacement therapy; HD: intermittent hemodialysis; ICU: intensive care unit; PICU: pediatric intensive care unit; RO: reverse osmosis; RRT: renal replacement therapy)

TYPE AND SIZE OF NICU

Operational guidelines for SNCU have been developed to provide detailed information about the design, infrastructure, equipment, manpower, data collection system, and newborn care protocols **(Table 17.1.4)**.

Level III facilities should be able to provide ongoing and sustained assisted ventilation for 24 hours or more, which may include conventional ventilation, HFOV, and INO. Level III NICUs are defined by having continuously available personnel (neonatologists, neonatal nurses, pediatric surgeon) and equipment to provide life support for as long as necessary. Facilities should have advanced respiratory support and advanced monitoring equipment, laboratory and radiological imaging facilities, nutrition and pharmacy support, ideally with neonatal expertise. Level III units should have the capability to perform major surgery on site or at a closely located institution.

CONCEPT OF HIGH-DEPENDENCY UNIT

A high-dependency unit (HDU) is a special equipped area within a hospital that provides intermediate level of care between pediatric or neonatal intensive care and the in-

Table 17.1.4: Newborn services at various levels of facilities in India: a brief outlook.

	NBCC: at all delivery points	*NBSU in FRUs/CHCs*	*SNCU in subdistrict/district*
Care specifications			
Care at birth	Resuscitation, provision of warmth, prevention of infection, early initiation of breastfeeding and weighing the newborn		
Care of normal newborn	Breastfeeding/feeding support		
Care of sick newborn	Identification and prompt referral of "at risk" and "sick" newborn	Management of low birth weight infants >1,800 g with no other complication, phototherapy for newborns with hyperbilirubinemia, management of newborn sepsis, stabilization and referral of sick newborns and those with very low birth weight (rooming in) and referral services	Managing of low birth weight infants <1,800 g, managing all sick newborns >1,800 g or those who have any complications from delivery like asphyxia, meconium aspiration (except those requiring mechanical ventilation and major surgical interventions), follow-up of all babies discharged from the unit and high risk newborns and referral services
Infrastructural specifications			
Beds	1	4	12–20
Area (sq feet)	20–30	200	Min 1,200 (100 sq ft/extra bed)
Location	Within labor room and OT	Close to the labor room	Vicinity of labor room
Civil work	None or minimum	Power supply, water supply, lighting, floor spaces and walls	Power supply, floor spaces, walls, water supply, lighting, and temperature
Personnel specifications			
Specialist	0	0	1
Doctors	1	1	3
Nurses	1	4	10
ANMs	1	—	—

(ANM: auxiliary nurse midwife; CHCs: community health centers; FRUs: first referral units; NBCC: newborn care corner; NBSU: newborn stabilization unit; OT: operation theater; SNCU: special newborn care unit) [NBCC, FRUs, and DHs (district hospitals)]

patient ward care, which is essentially managed by PICU or NICU staff. Although HDUs were traditionally located near specialty wards (like cardiac ward, newborn ward, etc.), they are now gradually being located within or immediately adjacent to a PICU or NICU complex; citing easy availability of trained PICU or NICU staff. The HDU usually provides noninvasive monitoring and clinical support for managing patients, who are at risk of developing acute (or acute-on-chronic) single organ dysfunction, particularly where the predicted risk of clinical deterioration is variable or unknown, where it acts as "step-up unit". Continuous monitoring is provided in these units to recognize early worsening, in recovering patients who were earlier in tertiary care level, where it acts as "step-down unit". Equipment should be readily available to manage short-term emergencies (e.g. need for intubation and mechanical ventilation). It is beneficial for both patients and doctors but benefit in overall outcomes is unknown. It is financially less burdening for patients in private setups to have HDUs.

EQUIPMENT AND MEDICATIONS

The type and quantity of equipment will vary with the level, size and subspecialty care of the PICU or NICU and it must be apt to the workload and skill of the unit. There must be a protocol in place for checking asepsis, safety, and quality of equipment. Regular education and in-service training (like simulation for intubation or securing airway, etc.) for medical and nursing staff must be available for the use of all available equipment, including troubleshooting in event of malfunction. There should also be a system in place for regular maintenance and service, cross checked and labeled by biomedical service providers of the hospital. A system of stock control in the unit should be in place to ensure consumables are always in adequate supply and have not crossed expiry date, usually checked by nursing team leader. The PICU or NICU director should have a major role in the purchase of new equipment to ensure it is appropriate for the activities of the unit.

FAMILY SUPPORT

For parents and relatives, a separate area of usually least 10 m^2 per eight-beds (which includes one chair per bed) might be considered, within PICU or NICU. To allow parents or relatives to sit beside patient during visiting time or throughout are individual units or institutes policies. Nursing mothers should be provided facility with bed as a sleep or rest cubicles and other relatives (usually one relative) may be provided with some overnight sleeping or lying down facility in the institute. Some institutions have their own guesthouses or dharmshalas or have provisions to provide same services which are located near hospital. There should be facilities like a water dispenser, and toilets near PICU or NICU. It is desirable to have separate entrances to the PICU or NICU for visitors and health care professionals. One or more separate areas for counseling or family communication are must.

STAFFING

The level of staffing depends on the type of hospital, and NICU/PICU units within tertiary hospital usually need large teams. It is crucial that there is clear and proper communication and collaboration among team members and a true multidisciplinary approach especially in such setups.

Team Leader

It is ideal to have a NICU or PICU team led by a pediatric intensivist or neonatologist (who spends >50% of his time in PICU or NICU). He should be a full timer particularly in tertiary care centers. He should be qualified and proficient to lead the team.

Resident Doctors (Only Medical Council of India Registered)

Postgraduates trainees in pediatrics, senior residents, fellows in pediatric intensive care/neonatology, DM residents constitute this section. Though need of postgraduate and graduate resident doctors per number of ICU patient has not been agreed in literature, however, it is understood and suggested that one doctor cannot take care of more than five patients who are critically sick on ventilator and/or undergoing invasive monitoring for multiorgan dysfunction (MODS). Therefore, it is only suggested that one postgraduate resident with one graduate resident may be good for a level III PICU or NICU of 10–14 beds where one-third of the patients may be falling into above mentioned sick group of patients.

Nursing Staff (Preferred Nursing Council of India Registered)

1:1 nurse to patient ratio for ventilated or MODS patients is desirable in tertiary level of neonatal or pediatric intensive care, but the ratio less than 1:2 is not acceptable in such critical patients (1 nurses for 2 such patients).

Allied Healthcare Staff

Access to physiotherapists, nutritionists, social workers, and other therapists should also be readily available **(Fig. 17.1.1)**. A dedicated ward clinical pharmacist, with experience in neonatal and pediatric medicine is invaluable, he will be a strong wall in checking of drug errors, etc. Respiratory therapists a concept well recognized abroad is slowly becoming standard of care in PICU or NICU in India. Technical support staff and biomedical department are necessary to service and repair equipment. Trained dietician in pediatric and neonatal medicine is an essential professional component of the team who can contribute significantly to outcome of patient. They must be trained in desired practices (like knowledge of various enteral nutritional balanced preparations—locally made or commercially available, etc.) and should be more inclined toward enteral feeding than total parenteral nutrition (TPN). Cleaning, class IV and security guards are also important to

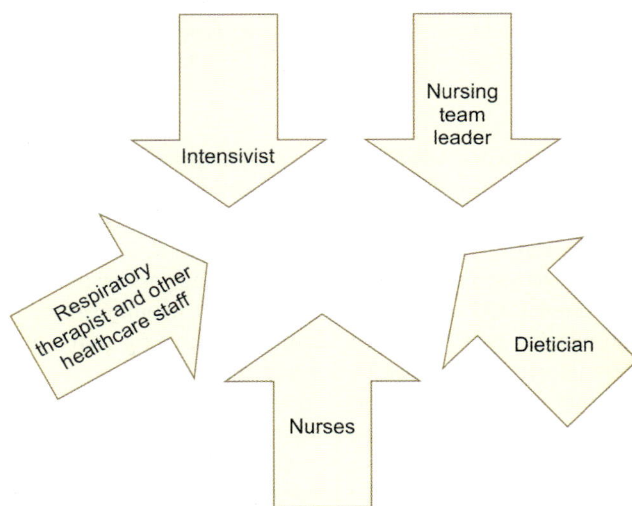

Fig. 17.1.1: Typical pediatric or neonatal intensive care unit team structure highlighting co-leading the team by an intensivist and nurse, thus incorporating high-reliability organization principles.

Box 17.1.1: Key factors in designing neonatal intensive care units.

Location of NICU:
- Proximity or controlled access to delivery and transport areas
- Controlled access for patient and staff safety

Space per bed:
- Minimum of 120 square feet per bed space, excluding sinks and aisles
- 165 square feet minimum for single-patient NICU rooms
- Adequate and easily accessible storage (30 square feet per bed) for supplies and equipment

Privacy:
- Minimum of 8 feet between beds, with provisions for family and speech privacy if needed

Headwall:
- Twenty accessible electrical outlets divided between normal and emergency power circuits
- Two to three each of compressed air, oxygen, and vacuum outlets, all simultaneously accessible
- Data transmission port-2

Handwashing station:
- Large sinks with hands-free controls within 20 feet of NICU bed (minimum sink size 61 x 41 x 25 cm)
- Appropriate provision for soap, towel dispensers, and color coded bins for trash, and biohazardous waste
- Handwashing instructions, pictorial and written, should be provided

Surfaces:
- *Floors:* Easily cleanable, durable, and glare free in-patient care areas
- *Walls:* Easily cleanable and durable; attractive visual accents and sound-absorbent materials can be used where they can be protected from damage
- *Ceilings:* Washable, highly sound-absorbent acoustical tile wherever feasible

Lighting:
- Ambient lighting levels adjustable through a range of 10–600 lux
- Light sources with suitable spectrum to permit accurate color rendering
- Procedure lighting capable of providing at least 2,000 lux at the bed surface, and adjustable in both location and intensity
- Day lighting for adult work areas, with appropriate shading and insulation

Acoustics:
- Noise control measures to maintain the combination of background and operation sound below a mean level of 45 dB

Heating, ventilation, and air conditioning:
- Ambient temperature of 22–26°C (72–78°F)
- Relative humidity of 30–60%
- Minimum of six air exchanges per hour with appropriate filtering; two changes should be with outside air

Family zone:
- Adequate and welcoming directional and informational signage
- Lounge, refreshments, restrooms, storage, library, telephones
- Overnight beds at least one per one patient bed. If outborn baby, provision for mother is a must
- Consultation/grieving room
- Lactation area (if sufficient privacy is not available at the bedside)
- Dedicated area at the bedside for infant care and work

Staff requirements:
- Lockers, changing room, restrooms, on-call rooms
- Adequate and comfortable charting or work area at each bedside
- Clerical or work areas away from, but easily accessible to, each bedside
- Office or desk space for all disciplines that routinely provide care

PICU or NICU particularly when they understand needs of ICU, its patients and relatives. They have a huge role to play in prevention of nosocomial infections, keeping PICU or NICU clean and restrict visitors. One person should also be responsible for observing protocols of infection control. Such person should act in close collaboration of infection control team of the hospital. **Box 17.1.1** enlists key requirements for a NICU.

OPERATIONAL POLICIES

There must be clearly defined policies for PICU or NICU admission, discharge, management, and referral of patients. Responsibilities must be delineated for all staff members and their job descriptions well-defined in tertiary care set ups. Policies for the care of patients in NICU or PICU

Table 17.2.1: Common toxic substances and their clinical manifestations.

Physical sign	***Poison***
Odors	
Bitter almonds	Cyanide
Acetone	Isopropyl alcohol, methanol, paraldehyde, salicylates
Alcohol	Ethanol
Oil of wintergreen	Methyl salicylate
Garlic	Organophosphates, arsenic, thallium
Eyes	
Miosis	Narcotics, OPC, mushrooms (muscarinic), clonidine, phenothiazines, barbiturates (late)
Mydriasis	Atropine, alcohol, cocaine, amphetamines, antihistamines, cyclic antidepressants, cyanide, carbon monoxide
Nystagmus	Phenytoin, barbiturates, ethanol, carbon monoxide
Lacrimation	OPC, irritant gas/vapors
Skin	
Dry, hot skin	Anticholinergics, botulism
Diaphoresis	OPC, Mushrooms (muscarinic), aspirin, cocaine
Erythema	Anticholinergics, boric acid, mercury
Oral cavity	
Salivation	OPC, corrosives, salicylates
Dry mouth	Anticholinergics, antihistamines, amphetamines
Burns	Corrosives, oxalate-containing plants
Gastrointestinal	
Cramps	OPC, arsenic
Diarrhea	Antibiotics, iron, boric acid
Constipation	Narcotics, botulism, codeine, lead
Hematemesis	Corrosives, iron, salicylates and aminophylline
Cardiovascular	
Tachycardia	Atropine, aspirin, amphetamines, cocaine, cyclic antidepressants, theophylline
Bradycardia	Digitalis, narcotics, mushrooms, clonidine, OPC, beta-blockers, calcium-channel blockers
Hypertension	Sympathomimetics, anticholinergics, MAO inhibitors
Hypotension	Phenothiazines, barbiturates, cyclic antidepressants, iron, beta-blockers, calcium-channel blockers
Respiratory	
Hypopnea/apnea	Alcohol, narcotics, barbiturates
Tachypnea	Amphetamines, aspirin, ethylene glycol, CO, cyanide
Pulmonary edema	Hydrocarbons, heroin, OPC
Neuromuscular	
Coma	Sedatives, narcotics, barbiturates, OPC, salicylates, cyanide, CO, lead, cyclic antidepressants
Hyperpyrexia	Anticholinergics, quinine, salicylates, phenothiazines, amphetamines, cocaine
Ataxia	Alcohol, antidepressants, barbiturates, anticholinergics, phenytoin, narcotics
Muscle fasciculation	OPC, theophylline
Paralysis	OPC, mercury, arsenic
Altered behavior	Anticholinergics, alcohol, camphor, amphetamines

(OPC: organophosphate compound; CO: carbon monoxide; MAO: monoamine oxidase)

Table 17.2.2: Products that are nontoxic when ingested in small quantities.

Abrasives	***Antacids (nonsalicylate containing)***	***Antibiotics, topical***
Antifungals (topical)	Ballpoint (ink pen)	Bathtub (floating toys)
Bath oil (unless aspirated)	Body conditioners	Bubble bath soap
Calamine lotion	Candles (beeswax/paraffin)	Caps (toy pistols/potassium chlorate)
Chalk (calcium carbonate)	Children toy cosmetics	Clay (modeling)
Oral contraceptives (without iron)	Corticosteroids, topical	Cosmetics
Crayons (marked as AP or CP, gel)	Dehumidifying packets (silica)	Deodorants, underarm
Fabric softeners	Fertilizers (insecticides, herbicides)	Detergents, hand/dish washing
Diaper rash creams/ointments	Fishbowl additives	Glow products
Glues and paste	Golf ball (core may cause mechanical injury)	Grease
Hand lotions and creams	Ink (black/blue-nonpermanent)	Incense
Indelible markers	Lipstick	Iodophil disinfectants (unless the individual is allergic)
Laxatives	Magazines	Lozenges (anesthetics)
Lubricating oils (unless aspirated)	Matches	Markers, porous tip
Modeling compound (Play-Doh)	Newspaper (chronic ingestion leads to lead poisoning)	Mineral oil (unless aspirated)
Paints, water colors	Pencil lead (graphite, coloring)	Paint, indoor latex, water-based
Plant food (no insecticides/herbicides)	Polaroid picture coating fluid	Petroleum jelly (Vaseline)
Rubber cement	Shampoo	Putty
Silica gel	Soap and soap products (non-caustic)	Shaving creams and lotions
Starch	Sun screen lotion	Spackles
Toothpaste (with/without fluoride)	Warfarin rodenticides (<0.5%) exclude superwarfarin	Sweetening agents (saccharin, aspartame)
Zinc oxide		Water color paints

Table 17.2.3: Common toxidromes.

Toxins	***Toxidrome***
Cholinergic (organophosphates, carbamates)	(Dumb-bells) diarrhea, diaphoresis, urination, miosis, bradycardia, bronchial secretions, emesis, lacrimation, lethargic, salivation
Anticholinergics (antihistamines, cyclic antidepressants, atropine, phenothiazines, scopolamine)	Hyperthermia (hot as a hare), flushed (red as a beet), dry skin (dry as a bone), dilated pupils (blind as a bat), delirium, hallucinations (mad as a hatter), tachycardia, urinary urgency and retention
Sympathomimetics (cocaine, ephedrine, pseudoephedrine)	Mydriasis, tachycardia, hypertension, hyperthermia, seizures
Opioids (heroin, morphine, codeine, methadone, fentanyl, hydrocodone)	Miosis, bradycardia, hypotension, hypoventilation, coma
Opioid withdrawal	Diarrhea, mydriasis, goose flesh, tachycardia, lacrimation, hypertension, yawning, cramps, hallucinations, seizures

fitting into any diagnosis or not responding in predicted manner; should be suspected of poisoning. Altered mental status, gastrointestinal (GI) complaints, cardiovascular compromise, seizures, and temperature-related disorders can all be toxin-related. Some are subtle, such as the flu-like symptoms seen with carbon monoxide poisoning, whereas cardiotoxins, such as digitalis, may mimic intrinsic heart disease.

GENERAL APPROACH TO A POISONED CHILD

The general approach to the diagnosis and management of the poisoned patient can be described using a two-pronged model as shown in **Flowchart 17.2.1**. In practice, the two prongs occur simultaneously. The left-sided prong begins with basic emergency medical, which should address the airway, breathing, and circulation (ABC). Focused therapy involves antidote administration when appropriate or aggressive supportive care tailored to the poison in question. Finally, when treating any poisoned patient it is prudent to consider early consultation with a toxicology service or regional poison center for further guidance (e.g. AIIMS, National Poison Centre, New Delhi).

Detoxification

Detoxification involves enhanced elimination of exposed toxin from body, avoidance of further systemic absorption and enhanced elimination of systemically absorbed toxin. The various methods of decontamination should be considered in poisoned child. The exact method used should be based on each individual clinical situation. Once a poisoning has been identified, various methods of enhanced elimination should be considered.

There are four modalities to remove a poison from the gastrointestinal tract (GIT):

1. Syrup of ipecac
2. Gastric lavage
3. Activated charcoal
4. Whole bowel irrigation.

Syrup of Ipecac

- Induces vomiting by both central and peripheral mechanisms
- Mean time of vomiting 15–30 minutes
- Removes 30–40% of ingested toxin
- Not indicated in less than 6 months of age due to poorly developed gagreflex

Flowchart 17.2.1: General approach to a poisoned child.

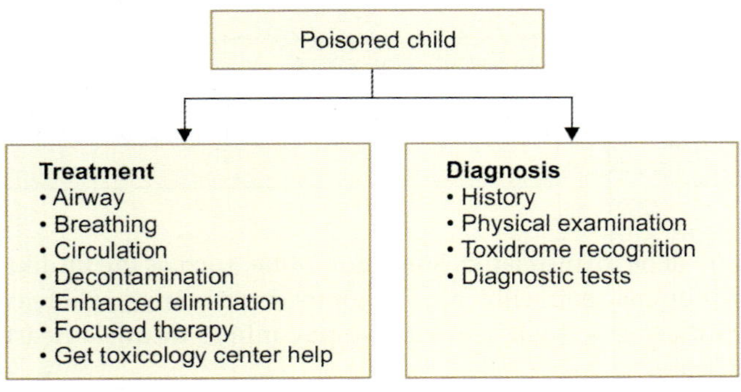

- Contraindicated in corrosives, hydrocarbons (HCs), sharp foreign bodies and low Glasgow Coma Scale (GCS).

Gastric Lavage

- Done in left lateral position
- 15 mL/kg cycles
- Contraindicated in HC poisoning
- May delay treatment with activated charcoal.

Activated Charcoal

- Wood, coconut, petroleum heated to 900°C with steam and CO_2 in activation process
- 1–2 g/kg
- Increased surface area to 1,600–1,800 m^2/g
- Multiple doses needed for digoxin, phenobarbitone, carbamazepine, and dapsone
- Ineffective in caustics, HCs, heavy metals, iron, ethanol, methanol, and ethylene glycol
- Contraindicated in ileus, intestinal obstruction.

Whole Bowel Irrigation

- Polyethylene glycol
- Useful in iron, sustained release theophylline, and heroin body packers
- 25–40 mL/kg/hour till rectal effluent is clear
- Contraindicated in perforation and ileus.

(*Note:* Details of other methods of enhanced elimination are beyond the scope of the chapter, interested reader may refer further recommended readings given at the end of this chapter).

Antidotal Therapy (Specific Detoxification)

Focused therapy involves antidote administration when appropriate or aggressive supportive care tailored to the poison in question. **Table 17.2.4** lists antidotes available for some common poisonings.

COMMONLY ENCOUNTERED POISONINGS

Hydrocarbon Poisoning

- *Classes of HCs:*
  - *Aliphatic/straight chain*: Acetone, butane, propane, isopropane
  - *Aromatic/cyclic structures*: Benzene, toluene, xylene
  - *Toxic/halogenated*: Carbon tetrachloride, trichloroethylene
  - *Petroleum distillates*: Kerosene, gasoline, furniture polish
- Aspirational potential of a HC is measured in saybolt universal seconds (SUS)
- *Clinical picture*: Chemical pneumonitis, acute respiratory distress syndrome (ARDS)
- Fatal dose 10–15 mL

Table 17.2.4: Antidotes.

Toxin	*Antidote*	*Dose and route*
Paracetamol	N-acetyl cysteine	140 mg/kg stat orally followed by 70 mg/kg Q 4h for 17 doses (in chronic poisoning only 12 doses). IV administration within 8–10 hours of ingestion, loading dose of 150 mg/kg infused over 15–60 minutes, followed by an initial maintenance dose of 50 mg/kg over 4 hours, followed by 100 mg/kg over 16 hours
Anticholinergics (atropine)	Physostigmine	0.02 mg/kg IV
Benzodiazepines	Flumazenil	0.01 mg/kg IV (maximum 3 mg)
Beta-blockers	Glucagon	0.15 mg/kg IV stat followed by 0.1 mg/kg/h
Calcium-channel blockers	Calcium chloride 10%	0.1–0.2 mL/kg IV
Calcium-channel blockers	Glucagon	0.15 mg/kg IV stat followed by 0.1 mg/kg/h
Carbamates	Atropine	0.1 mg/kg/dose (repeated till atropinization)
Organophosphates	Atropine	0.05 mg/kg/dose (repeated till atropinization)
	Pralidoxime	50 mg/kg IV stat followed by 25 mg/kg every 4 hourly
Cyanide	Amyl nitrite inhalation	
	3% sodium nitrite	0.15–0.3 mL/kg IV infusion (maximum 300 mg)
	Sodium thiosulfate	400 mg/kg (maximum 12.5 g)
Digoxin	Digibind (digoxin immune antibody fragment)	1 mL binds 0.6 mg digoxin
Methanol	10% ethanol	10 mL/kg IV stat followed by 1–2 mL/kg/h
Ethylene glycol	10% ethanol	10 mL/kg IV stat followed by 1–2 mL/kg/h
	Fomepizole	15 mg/kg/dose IV
Iron	Desferrioxamine	5–15 mg/kg/h IV infusion
Isoniazid	Pyridoxine	1 g ingested
Methemoglobinemia	Methylene blue	1–2 mg/kg/dose IV
Opioids	Naloxone	0.5–2 mg IV titrated to effect
Salicylates	Sodium bicarbonate	150 mEq + 40 mEq KCl in 1 L of 5% dextrose infused to maintain a urine output of 1–2 mL/kg/h and a urine pH of 7.5
Tricyclic antidepressants	Sodium bicarbonate	1–2 mEq/kg
Warfarin/superwarfarin	Vitamin K_1	0.5 mg/kg IV/SC/PO
	FFP	15 mL/kg/dose till PT normalizes
Botulism	Botulinum antitoxin	
Heparin	Protamine	
Type 1 antiarrhythmics	Sodium bicarbonate	1–2 mEq/kg

(FFP: fresh frozen plasma; PT: prothrombin time)

- Chest X-ray (CXR) to be done after 6–8 hours
- Usually gastric lavage is contraindicated, but due to low viscosity, good GIT absorption and high systemic toxicity, it is indicated in camphor, halogenated, aromatic, metal (heavy), and pesticides (CHAMP) poisoning
- Symptomatic management of chemical pneumonitis.

Anticholinergics

- *Datura stramonium*: Entire plant including nectar is toxic
- Thorn apple
- *Contains belladonna alkaloids*: Scopolamine, hyoscyamine, and atropine
- Mad as hatter, hot as hare, dry as bone, red as beet, and blind as beet
- *Fatal dose*: 4 mg
- *Fatal period*: 24 hours
- *Mode of action*: Antagonizes the muscarinic action of acetylcholine. Nicotinic receptors are much less sensitive.
- *Peripheral antimuscarinic effects*: Dry mouth and skin flushing, excessive thirst, blurred vision, loss of

accommodation reflex, hyperthermia, tachycardia, symmetrical pupillary dilatation, and urinary retention.

- *Central antimuscarinic effects*: CNS stimulation followed by depression, agitation, confusion, picking at clothes, auditory, visual, and tactile hallucinations.
- *Treatment*: Activated charcoal 1–2 g/kg
- *Specific antidote*: Physostigmine 0.02 mg/kg up to 2 mg maximum.

Opioids

The classification of opioids has been given in **Flowchart 17.2.2**.

- *Endogenous opioids*: Endorphin, enkephalin, and dysmorphine
- *Classic triad*: CNS depression, respiratory depression, and miosis
- *Clinical features:*
  - *Cyclic vomiting syndrome*: Bradycardia and orthostatic hypotension
  - *GI tract*: Ileus, constipation
  - *Respiratory system*: Bronchospasm (due to histamine release)
  - *Renal*: Urinary retention
  - *Genital*: Loss of libido
- *Withdrawal*: Mydriasis, piloerection, myalgias, cramps, hyperthermia, and muscle twitching
- *Specific antidote*: Naloxone, 0.5–2 mg IV titrated to effect
- *Other antidotes*: Nalorphine, levallorphan, and naltrexone.

Paracetamol Poisoning

- Primarily hepatotoxicity, but, renal tubular damage and hypoglycemic coma can also occur
- Congestion of ethanol is cytoprotective (due to competition of P-450 site)
- *Toxicity four stages*:
  - *Stage I*: First day, nausea and vomiting present—liver function test (LFT) and prothrombin time (PT) are normal.
  - *Stage II*: Second day, upper abdominal pain, hepatomegaly, and jaundice. Elevated bilirubin, serum glutamic oxaloacetic transaminase (SGOT), serum glutamic pyruvic transaminase (SGPT), and PT.
  - *Stage III*: 2–4 days, maximum liver dysfunction, acute renal failure. Liver biopsy shows centrilobular necrosis.
  - *Stage IV*: 4 days to 2 weeks, resolution of hepatic dysfunction.
- Lethal dose is more than 200 mg/kg or single dose of 7 g
- Diagnosis of hepatotoxicity is by Rumack–Matthew nomogram (not given in this chapter).
- Rumack–Matthew nomogram is not useful in poisoning with sustained release formulation, chronic poisoning and when paracetamol is ingested along with anticholinergics or opioids.
- *Specific antidote*: N-acetyl cysteine (NAC) 140 mg/kg stat orally followed by 70 mg/kg Q4h for 17 doses (in chronic poisoning only 12 doses). Intravenous administration within 8–10 hours of ingestion, loading dose of 150 mg/kg infused over 15–60 minutes, followed by an initial maintenance dose of 50 mg/kg over 4 hours, followed by 100 mg/kg over 16 hours.
- *Alternative antidotes*: Methionine and cysteine.
- *Contraindication to NAC*: Coma, vomiting, hepatic failure/encephalopathy, pretreatment with activated charcoal.
- *Poor prognostic factors*: pH less than 7.3.
  - Serum creatinine more than 300 µmol/L
  - Prothrombin time more than 100 seconds, encephalopathy grade III to IV
  - Factor VIII to factor V ratio more than 30
- Among all these factor VIII to factor V ratio more than 30 is the best prognostic indicator.

Flowchart 17.2.2: Classification of opioids.

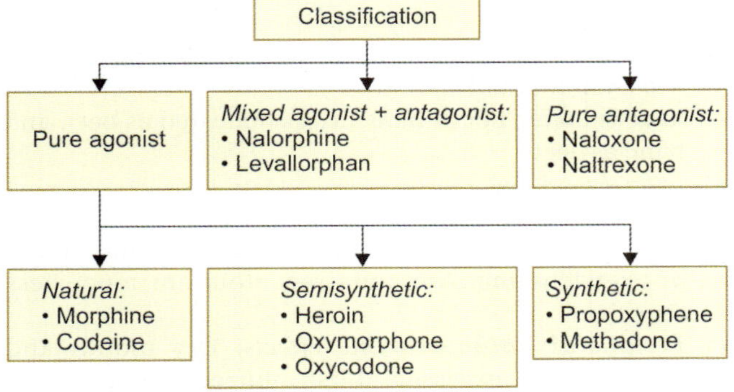

Iron Poisoning

- Acts as a metabolic poison
- Ferritin (iron storage protein) is abundant in the heart and liver and leads to tissue destruction
- *Mechanisms of toxicity:*
  - Direct corrosive effect
  - Electron sink mechanism
  - Free radical damage
  - Concentration-dependent coagulation disorder
- *Toxic dose:*
  - 20 mg/kg subtoxic
  - 20–60 mg/kg potentially lethal
  - Greater than 60 mg/kg lethal
- *Five stages:*
  - *Stage I (GIT)*: Local necrosis, hemorrhage, acidosis, and drowsiness.
  - *Stage II (apparent recovery)*: Iron accumulation continues in mitochondria.
  - *Stage III (circulatory failure)*: Shock, coagulopathy, acute tubular necrosis, and pulmonary hemorrhage.

- *Stage IV (hepatic necrosis)*: Increased bilirubin, SGPT, SGOT, and PT
- *Stage V (gastric scarring)*: Gastric outlet obstruction and intestinal obstruction
- Predisposes to infection with *Yersinia enterocolitica*, and *Listeria monocytogenes*
- *Serum level:*
  - *Less than 50 μg/dL*: No toxicity
  - *Greater than 50 μg/dL*: Toxicity manifests
  - *Greater than 350 μg/dL*: Toxicity evident, lethal
- *Initial management:*
  - Gastric lavage
  - Activated charcoal does not bind iron
  - Milk of magnesia 100 mL
- *Specific antidote*: Desferrioxamine, 1 g chelates 90 mg of iron. Winrose-color-urine when on treatment. Therapy to be continued till urine color is normal or serum iron less than 300 μg/dL.

Corrosive Poisoning

- *Alkalis*: Esophagus—liquefaction necrosis
- *Acids*: Stomach—coagulative necrosis
- Fibrosis starts in 3 weeks, followed by strictures
- Mortality 50%—in survivors 95% develop strictures

The early and late complications of corrosive poisoning have been listed in **Table 17.2.5**.

Table 17.2.5: Early and late complications of corrosive poisoning.

Early (<72 hours)	*Late (>72 hours)*
Esophageal perforation, mediastinitis	Esophageal stricture
Stomach perforation, peritonitis	Pyloric stenosis
Glottic edema	
Shock	

- Immediate upper GI endoscopy within 48 hours
- Not recommended now—neutralizing agents, vinegar for alkali, and sodium bicarbonate for acids (release CO_3, can cause distension and rupture)
- First aid—500 mL milk or water
  - Suck a piece of ice
- Oral prednisolone for 2–3 weeks
- *Management:*
  - Repeat barium studies after 3 weeks
  - Esophageal bougies—dilatation
  - Esophageal replacement with colon or jejunum.

Naphthalene Poisoning

- Moth balls contain 100% naphthalene
- Toxic metabolite—alpha-naphthol has hemolytic effect
- Most common presentation
- Pain abdomen, vomiting, diarrhea, jaundice, dark urine, pallor, and seizure
- Massive intravascular hemolysis in certain North Indian communities
- G6PD deficiency patients are more prone
- *Management:* Syrup of Ipecac, gastric lavage, and activated charcoal
  - May require exchange transfusion
  - Forced alkaline diuresis prevents acute renal failure by preventing
  - Precipitation of hemoglobin, in renal tubules
  - Methemoglobinemia may require methylene blue.

Organophosphorus Poisoning

- A list of organophosphorus substances is given in **Table 17.2.6**.
- *Mode of action*: Inhibition of acetylcholine esterase by irreversibly binding to it. Deactivate it by phosphorylation,

Table 17.2.6: Common organophosphorus substances.

Natural	*Organophosphorus*	*Organochlorine*	*Carbamates*	*Repellents*	*Synthetic pyrethroids*
Pyrethrum	Chlorthion	DDT	Carbaryl	Benzyl benzoate	Resmethrin
Nicotine	Fenthion	BHC	Dimetilan	Indalone	Bioresmethrin
Mineral oils	Malathion	Chlordane	Pyrolan	Diethyl-meta-toluamide	Pothrin
Rotenone	Parathion	Aldrin	Propoxur	Dimethyl phthalate	
Derris	• Methyl parathion • Fenitrothion • Dioxathion • Diazinon Dicapthon • Chlorpyrifos • Dichlorvos Trichlorfon • Abate Dimethoate • Gardena	• Dieldrin • Methoxychlor • Heptachlor • Toxaphene • Kepone • Mirex		Ethyl hexanediol	

17.3 Foreign Body

Pallab Chatterjee

INTRODUCTION

Foreign body (FB) in children is one of the most common emergencies faced by pediatricians in their day-to-day practice, and a potent medicolegal hazard if not handled efficiently in time. Children tend to introduce all kinds of material leading to foreign bodies in the airways, ears, and gastrointestinal tract (esophageal, abdominal, and rectal). Foreign bodies in the eyes (corneal, conjunctival, and intraorbital) and retained surgical foreign bodies are not so common.

FOREIGN BODIES IN THE AIRWAYS

Introduction

Nasal FBs are one of the most common in pediatrics and areusually easily removed in the outpatient department (OPD). Tracheobronchial FB can be a life-threatening event, particularly if the central airways are blocked leading to impaired ventilation and oxygenation.

Epidemiology

Nasal FBs are most commonly seen around 3 years of age and are usually asymptomatic or presents as a foul smelling unilateral nasal discharge. Seeds are the most common, followed by rubber and batteries; and more than half are usually in the right nostril.

Tracheobronchial FBs are a common cause of morbidity and mortality in young children accounting for around 1 death in 100,000 children less than 4 years of age. Foreign body aspiration (FBA) accounted for around 24% mortality in the early 20th century and is much less now, thanks to improved bronchoscopy techniques, instruments and expertise. Majority (80%) of FBAs occur in children less than 3 years, with the peak incidence being between 1 year and 2 years of age, as at this age most children can stand and explore their world by putting small things in the mouth, while they lack the molars necessary for adequate chewing. The presence of older siblings who tend to insert food in their mouth and the tendency to engage in various playful activities during feeding also increase the prevalence of FBAs at this age; while the small size of their airways makes them more vulnerable. In older children and adolescents, it is seen more commonly in neurologic disorders, altered sensorium and sedative or alcohol overdose. There is a male preponderance of approximately 2:1 on an average in various studies.

The features of foreign bodies that make them dangerous are round, smooth and slippery surface and compressibility. Vegetable foreign bodies, like groundnuts and Bengal gram (approximately 50%), other nuts, seeds (like watermelon seeds), popcorn, and other food items are commonly aspirated by toddlers, while older children and adolescents tend to aspirate nonfood items, like coins, button batteries, clips, pins, caps of pens, marbles, etc. Balloon-like materials (like gloves or condoms) are most commonly associated with fatal FBAs. Certain drugs like iron and potassium cause severe inflammation and stenosis by tending to dissolve in the airways, and hence early diagnosis and definitive treatment is essential.

Most of the aspirated foreign bodies tend to locate in the right lung (60%), of which 52% is in the bronchus intermedius; followed by the left lung (23%), trachea (13%), larynx (3%), and bilateral (2%). The laryngotracheal foreign bodies are usually large or irregular and are associated with increased mortality than those that lodge in the bronchi.

Presentation

Nasal FBs are usually a late presentation with around a third of the children presenting within 24 hours. Unilateral foul smelling nasal discharge is very typical of nasal FB.

Foreign body aspirations present within 24 hours of the episode in 50–75% of children. The signs and symptoms depend on the age of the child, nature of the FB, location and degree of blockage of the airways, and time elapsed. Only about half of the children present with a history of choking, which is defined as a sudden onset of cough, with or without dyspnea or cyanosis, in a previously healthy child.

If there is a complete airway obstruction or reflex laryngospasm following an acute choking episode, there can be immediate death due to suffocation. However, most children enter a temporary symptom-free period after the acute episode, which may last for seconds to minutes, followed by persistent symptoms in the form of unexplained dyspnea, recurrent wheeze and cough; or may come back later with suppurative complications like pneumonia (acute or recurrent), lung abscess and bronchiectasis. A minority can expectorate the foreign body FB after a bout of violent cough following the choking episode. The classic triad of cough, localized wheeze, and decreased breath sounds, present in about 57% of children, has a high specificity.

Signs and symptoms vary according to the site of the FB. In the central airways, they are usually life-threatening and present with stridor, difficulty in breathing, hoarseness and sometimes dysphagia (in case of large penetrating FBs). The FBs in the large bronchi present with cough, wheeze, dyspnea, cyanosis, and decreased breath sounds. FBs in the lower airways are usually the ones that present with a delayed diagnosis with fever and chest infiltrates on the X-ray that do not resolve or recur.

Management

In around 5% of children, the nasal FB can be dislodged spontaneously. Majority of nasal FBs can be removed in the OPD using a Magill forceps. However, old FBs with granulations and dangerous FBs like button batteries and penetrating FBs should be handled by a specialist in the operating room under general anesthesia.

In a life-threatening FBA where the child has a complete obstruction of the airway, dislodgement should be attempted. In infants below 1 year, five slaps on the back in the head low position with five chest thrusts; while in kids above 1 year, five abdominal thrusts (Heimlich maneuver), is recommended. After each such series the airway obstruction is to be reviewed. However, such procedures, including "blind finger-sweep", should be avoided in children who are able to cough or speak, as they may convert a partial obstruction to a complete obstruction.

If the FB is still not dislodged, a direct laryngoscopy and an attempt to removal by a Magill forceps should be done. If it is still not removed and the FB is above the vocal cords, a cricothyroidotomy should be done either surgically or with a needle. If the FB is below the vocal cords, the patient should be intubated intentionally to the right side to push the FB into the right main bronchus, and then to withdraw the ET tube and ventilate the left lung with the right side down, while proceeding for definitive removal by a rigid bronchoscopy under vision.

In cases of a suspected FBA and an asymptomatic child, a plain chest X-ray is performed, preferably in both inspiration and expiration (or left lateral decubitus if expiratory film is not possible). The usual findings are hyperinflation, atelectasis, mediastinal shift away from the FB and consolidation. Late manifestations include bronchiectatic changes and abscess. However, if this is normal (approximately in 30% of cases), and the suspicion is very high, a flexible bronchoscopy or a CT scan of the chest is performed, the former being more definitive **(Figs. 17.3.1 and 17.3.2)**. Once detected, the definitive management is usually removal with the help of a rigid bronchoscope. Though the American Thoracic Society recommends only rigid bronchoscopy, some centers with high expertise use the flexible bronchoscope for removal of FBs, the main advantages being avoidance of general anesthesia and the ability to reach deeper, with the disadvantage of dislodging the FB and leading to a further compromise.

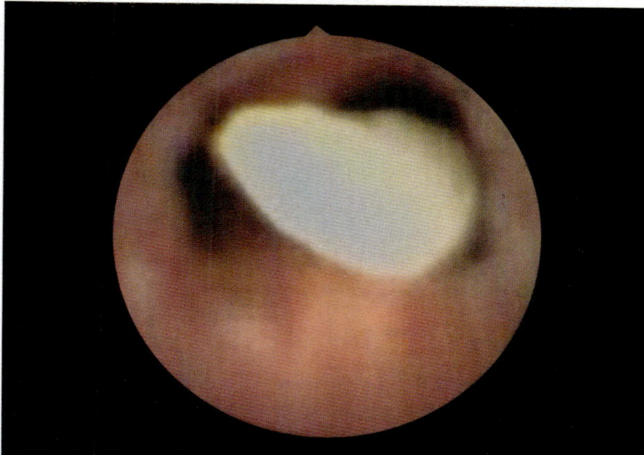

Fig. 17.3.1: Bronchoscopic view of a foreign body (shirt button) in the right main bronchus of a 3-year-old boy.

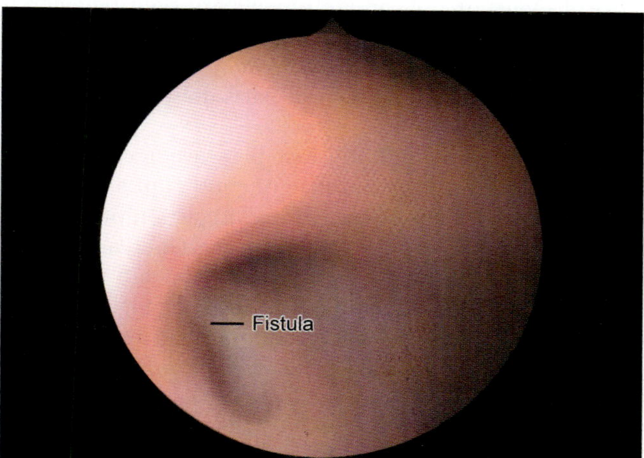

Fig. 17.3.2: Bronchoscopic view of an acquired tracheoesophageal fistula caused by aspirated button battery in an 18-month-old child.

In case of a prolonged retained FB, it may be difficult to remove it at one sitting and may require a second bronchoscopy after a course of antibiotics and steroids.

Prevention

The American Academy of Pediatrics suggests some guidance to be provided to all caregivers at 6 months of age regarding FBA. These include avoidance of marbles, balloons, coins, and toys with small parts; feeding of solid food in infants only by adults, and supervised feeding in older children sitting only in the upright position, and not during other activities like playing, running, crying or laughing; chewable medications after 3 years of age and hard round foods above 4 years of age. All child caregivers, teachers, and parents should take a course in basic life support.

FOREIGN BODIES IN THE GASTROINTESTINAL TRACT

Introduction

Ingested foreign bodies are the most common in children. However, they are usually not life-threatening and a majority tends to pass spontaneously.

Epidemiology

Most of ingestions of foreign objects are seen between 6 months to 3 years. Of these, only about 10% need endoscopic removal. The most common FBs ingested are coins, followed by button batteries, small toys or parts thereof, safety pins, marbles, magnets, etc.

Button batteries tend to cause pressure necrosis and a high risk of perforation because of contact of esophageal walls with both poles of the battery. Ingestion of magnets has increased in the recent times with their increased usage in various toys and household items. They are known to cause intestinal obstruction when they stick together from two different sites in the small intestine. Lead items present in certain household materials like toys, curtain weights, rifle pellets, etc. are known to cause lead toxicity and fatalities.

Foreign bodies in the gastrointestinal tract tend to get stuck in physiological narrow areas, like upper esophageal sphincter, at the level of the arch of the aorta and at the lower esophageal sphincter.

Presentation

In about half of the children, ingested FBs are asymptomatic and brought by parents or caregivers who have noticed the episode. Symptoms, when present, are according to the site of the FB. Esophageal FBs may be associated with dysphagia, drooling, stridor, wheeze, and retrosternal pain. More serious complications such as perforation into the trachea to cause a fistula, or into the mediastinum to cause pneumomediastinum, or into the aorta to cause severe gastrointestinal hemorrhage have also been reported.

Foreign bodies that reach the stomach are usually asymptomatic. However, occasionally FBs may lead to gastric outlet obstruction or distal obstruction mimicking appendicitis.

Management

Initial evaluation of swallowed FBs should be an X-ray of the neck, chest and abdomen. CT scan is done if the patient is symptomatic, or the FB is either long (>5 cm length) or large (>2 cm width) or sharp or is unknown.

In case of a blunt radiopaque object in the esophagus, watchful expectancy is advocated. Foreign bodies that are small and cross over into the stomach are most likely to pass out by 1–2 weeks. Hence, serial radiographs at weekly intervals are recommended. If it is still in the esophagus after 24 hours, or in the stomach by 4 weeks, or in case of other warning signs suggestive of obstruction or distress, retrieval by endoscopy is advocated. Urgent endoscopic removal is advised in cases of a long or sharp object, magnets, disk battery, and in cases of esophageal obstruction, airway compression or intestinal obstruction.

Of the various ingested FBs, disk batteries and magnet ingestions have increased in the recent times and they deserve special mention. Batteries can cause very early ulceration, and perforation by 8 hours, due either to the electrical discharge from the negative pole, release of various caustic substances or pressure necrosis. They can be differentiated from coins on the X-ray by their double-ring and scalloped edge. In an asymptomatic child, they should be removed as early as possible endoscopically. A symptomatic child usually signifies perforation and should be removed in the operation theater by a pediatric surgeon or a cardiothoracic surgeon, depending on whether there is bleeding. Multiple magnets have a higher risk of complications than single ones, and thus both AP and lateral views should be taken to differentiate multiple magnets sticking together leading to a misdiagnosis. Multiple magnets in the intestine may attract layers of the gut leading to obstruction, necrosis and perforation, fistula or volvulus. Magnetic or metallic objects (like buckles or buttons) should be kept away from the child and an attempt must be made for early removal.

Gastrointestinal FBs are usually removed by flexible endoscopy, while Magill forceps, rigid endoscopy or surgery may sometimes be used depending on the site and nature of the FB.

Prevention

Caregivers should be counseled about keeping small objects away from the reach of children. Battery compartment of household items and toys should preferably be secured with extra tapes.

FOREIGN BODIES IN THE EAR

Introduction

Commonly seen foreign bodies in the ear in children are in the external auditory canal and pinna.

Epidemiology

Most FBs in the external auditory canal are seen in children below the age of 6 years. Common objects are beads, seeds, stones, paper, small toy parts, button batteries, and insects. FBs in the pinna are from embedded earrings and are seen in older children and adolescents.

Presentation

Usually the caregiver gives a history of introduction of a FB being observed. Rarely children may present with decreased hearing or pain in the ears, unilateral purulent ear discharge incidentally found on otoscopy.

Management

Button batteries can cause extensive damage because of electrical discharges leading to damage to the skin, tympanic membrane and ossicles, and may even cause permanent deafness; and hence early removal is required. Live insects, like cockroaches, may cause severe discomfort and should be first killed with mineral oil and then removed. Penetrating foreign bodies such as pins, cotton ear buds, and pencil tips, etc. can damage the middle ear and need urgent ENT referral.

BIBLIOGRAPHY

1. Centers for Disease Control and Prevention. Nonfatal choking-related episodes among children—United States, 2001. MMWR. 2002;51:945-8.
2. Hitter A, Hullo E, Durand C, et al. Diagnostic Value of various investigations in children with suspected foreign body aspiration. Eur Ann Otorhinolaryngol. 2011;128:248-52.
3. Jatana KR, Litoritz T, Reilly JS, et al. Pediatric button battery injuries: 2013 task force update. Int J Ped Otolaryngol. 2013;77:1392-9.
4. Kramer TA, Riding KH, Salkeld LJ. Tracheobronchial and esophageal foreign bodies in the pediatric population. J Otolaryngol. 1986;15:355-8.

17.4 Cardiopulmonary Resuscitation

Sunil Dutt Sharma

INTRODUCTION

Sudden cardiac arrest is sudden stopping of "effective" heart beat or cardiac mechanical activity confirmed by the absence of signs of circulation, e.g. unresponsiveness, not breathing or gasping, and absent central pulses leading to cessation of nutrient flow causing progressive tissue ischemia and organ dysfunction. The stoppage can be complete (no electric activity) or abnormal electric activity (arrhythmia). Primary respiratory etiology and/or shock are the leading causes for cardiac arrest in children.

CARDIOPULMONARY RESUSCITATION

Components of cardiopulmonary resuscitation (CPR) include chest compression, airway, and breathing. Early and prompt recognition and action in prehospital setting is much better than heroic measures at intensive care units (ICUs) and earliest bystander CPR initiation [basic life support (BLS)] is a major outcome factor than doing advanced life support strategies (every minute delay shortens survival probability by 17%).

In-hospital pediatric cardiac arrests (IHCA) were reported to be 1.8–6%. Almost two-thirds of these cardiac arrest patients were initially successfully resuscitated (i.e. attained sustained ROSC (Return of Spontaneous Circulation—resumption of cardiac electrical rhythm with palpable central pulses). Out-of-hospital cardiac arrests (OHCA) have worse outcome than IHCA especially traumatic arrests and those associated with sudden infant death syndrome (SIDS).

For CPR the categorization of the victim is done as:

- Adults including adolescents (i.e. after the onset of puberty—signs include chest or underarm hairs in males and any breast development in females) and older
- Children (age 1 year to puberty); and
- Infants (age less than 1 year, excluding newborns).

Basic steps of CPR are:
- Scene safety and assessment
- Activation of emergency response system (ERS)
- Breathing and pulse check and recognition of cardiac arrest
- High-quality CPR
- Defibrillation with automated external defibrillator (AED) or manual defibrillator; and
- Continuation of high-quality CPR and postresuscitative care.

SCENE SAFETY AND ASSESSMENT

It is important for rescuer's safety, smooth conduction of BLS sequence and gathering of circumstantial evidence. For OHCA the victim should be shifted to safe place, e.g. in road traffic accident shift the victim to the side of the road and place should be hard enough for smooth and effective CPR. In IHCA victim should be on hard surface; and the surroundings should be dealt with caution, e.g. tubing, ventilators, and electricity wires, etc.

ACTIVATION OF EMERGENCY RESPONSE SYSTEM

Emergency response system varies depending upon setting and local protocols, e.g. in OHCA it can be 108 ambulances and in IHCA it can be blue code team, etc.

BREATHING AND PULSE CHECK AND RECOGNITION OF CARDIAC ARREST

Cardiac arrest basically means absence of signs of life, i.e. unresponsiveness, not breathing or gasping (look and listen), absent central pulses; and proceed for cardiac arrest as depicted in **Figure 17.4.1**. If breathing is labored, then airway opening can be done to align the airway structures by head tilt or chin lift **(Fig. 17.4.2A)**; use jaw thrust maneuver in cervical spine injury suspect **(Fig. 17.4.2B)**.

For pulse checking, do not delay for more than 10 seconds. Following are the sites of pulse check:
- *Adult:* Carotid;
- *Child:* Carotid/femoral—depending upon the size of the victim; and
- *Infant:* Brachial.

HIGH-QUALITY CARDIOPULMONARY RESUSCITATION

Basically, it means chest compression and ventilation in coordinated and defined way with minimum interruptions **(Tables 17.4.1 and 17.4.2)**.

When an adult, child or infant has a pulse but is not breathing effectively, rescuers should give breaths without chest compressions; this is rescue breathing. In infants and

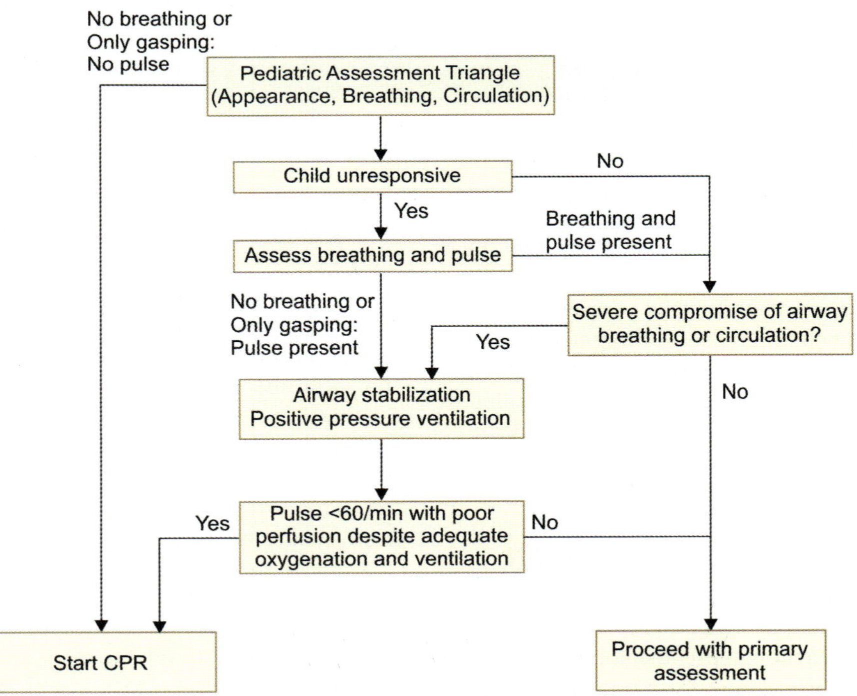

Fig. 17.4.1: Cardiac arrest protocol for HCP.

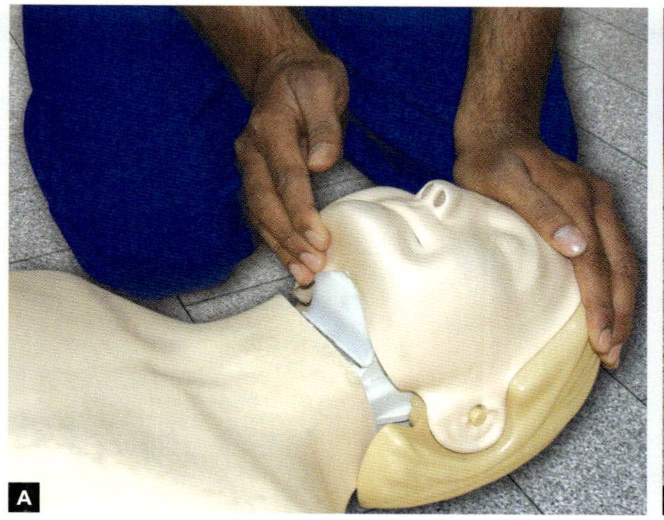

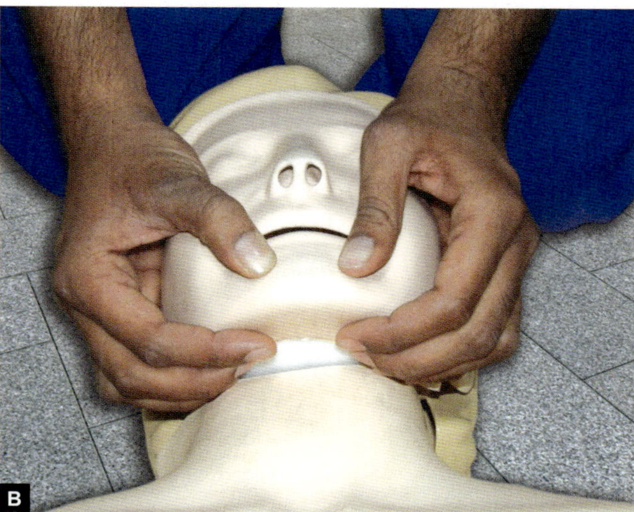

Figs. 17.4.2A and B: (A) Head tilt chin lift maneuver; (B) Jaw thrust maneuver.

Table 17.4.1: High-quality CPR steps.

Component	***Adults and adolescents***	***Children (age 1 year to puberty)***	***Infants (age less than 1 year; excluding newborns)***
Scene safety	Make sure the environment is safe for rescuers and victim		
Recognition of cardiac arrest	• Check for responsiveness • No breathing or only gasping (i.e. no normal breathing) • No definite pulse felt within 10 seconds • (breathing and pulse check can be performed simultaneously in less than 10 seconds)		
Activation of emergency response system	If you are alone with no mobile phone, leave the victim to activate the emergency response system and get the AED before beginning CPR. Otherwise, send someone and begin CPR immediately; use the AED as soon as it is available	*Witnessed collapse:* • Follow steps for adults and adolescents on the left *Unwitnessed collapse:* • Give 2 minutes of CPR • Leave the victim to activate the emergency response system and get the AED • Return to the child or infant and resume CPR; use the AED as soon as it is available	

(AED: automated external defibrillator; CPR: cardiopulmonary resuscitation)
Source: de Caen AR, Berg MD, Chameides L, et al. Pediatric Advanced Life Support Guidelines Update for Cardiopulmonary Resuscitation. Circulation. 2015;132(18 Suppl 2):S526-42.

children despite adequate oxygenation and ventilation if the pulse is 60 beats/min or less with signs of poor perfusion, start CPR. For giving rescue breaths we pinch nose in case of adult or adolescent and give it through mouth and in case of infants we can give it through mouth and nose both; barrier device can be used **(Table 17.4.3)**.

If we are using bag and mask for it; it should cover victim's mouth and nose completely without covering the eyes or overlapping the chin **(Figs. 17.4.3A and B)**. Breaths should be given, watching for chest rise and avoiding excessive ventilation. Switch roles with another rescuer every 5 cycles or about 2 minutes—taking less than 5 seconds to switch. In case of 15:2 ratios as used in 2 rescuers in child or infant, this switching would be every 10 cycles or about 2 minutes. Bag and mask ventilation are preferred in short transport distance.

Endotracheal intubation (ET) is done if bag and mask is ineffective, or trained person for ET insertion is there; other advantage is we can give medications through it.

Laryngeal mask airway is an alternative to bag-mask ventilation, both in OHCA and IHCA in case of prolonged resuscitation and when ET cannot be done due lack of

Table 17.4.2: Components of high-quality CPR.

Component	***Adults and adolescents***	***Children (age 1 year to puberty)***	***Infants (age less than 1 year; excluding newborns)***
Compression rate	100–120 beats/min		
Compression depth	At least 2 inches (5 cm)*	At least one-third AP diameter of chest About 2 inches (5 cm)	At least one-third AP diameter of chest about 1.5 inches (4 cm)
Hand placement	2 hands on the lower half of the sternum	2 hands or one hand (optional for very small child) on the lower half of the sternum	1 rescuer 2 fingers in the center of the chest, just below the nipple line 2 or more rescuer 2 thumb-encircling hands in the center of the chest, just below the nipple line
Chest recoil	Allow full recoil of chest after each compression, do not lean on the chest after each compression		
Minimizing interruptions	Limit interruption in the chest compression to less than 10 seconds		

*Compression depth should not be more than 2.4 inches (6 cm).
Source: de Caen AR, Berg MD, Chameides L, et al. Pediatric Advanced Life Support Guidelines Update for Cardiopulmonary Resuscitation. Circulation. 2015;132(18 Suppl 2):S526-42.
(AP: anterior-posterior; CPR: cardiopulmonary resuscitation)

Table 17.4.3: Rescue breathing.

Rescue breathing for adults	***Rescue breathing for infants and children***
Give 1 breath every 5 to 6 seconds (about 10–12 breaths per minute)	Give 1 breath every 3 to 5 seconds (about 12–20 breaths per minute)
• Give each breath in 1 second • Each breath should result in visible rise • Check the pulse about every 2 minutes	

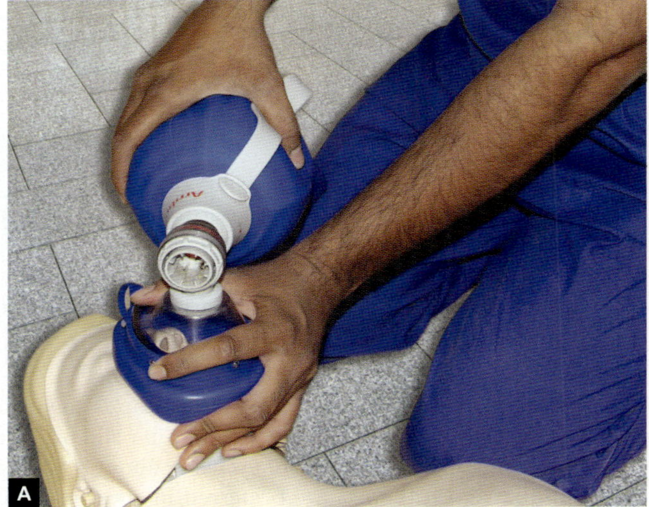
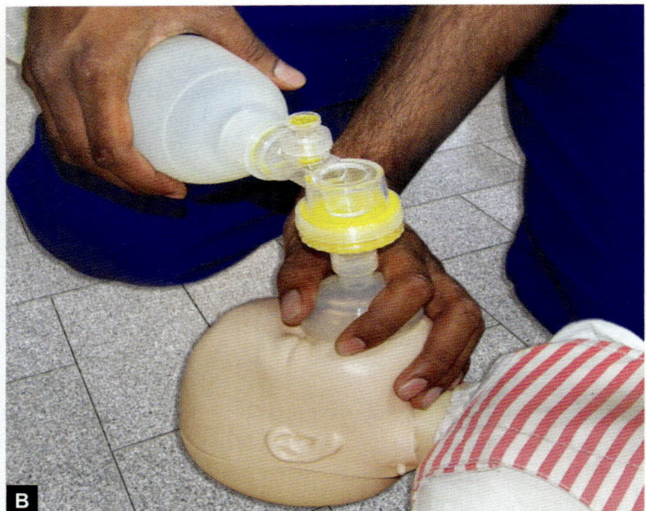

Figs. 17.4.3A and B: (A) Bag and mask ventilation adult; (B) Bag and mask ventilation in infant.

experienced provider. 100% oxygen should be given during early phase of resuscitation and later on when we have ROSC it can be tailored as per requirement (maintain saturation 92–94%).

Chest compressions with rescue breaths should be provided for infants and children in cardiac arrest. If bystanders are unwilling or unable to deliver rescue breaths it is recommended that rescuers should provide chest compressions for infants and children in cardiac arrest (C-A-B can be taken here rather than A-B-C sequence). For an OHCA, if rescuer is a lay person he or she may provide only chest compression till further help arrives or victim is shifted to health care facility; if rescuer is skilled and can provide rescue breaths he or she may coordinate it with CPR as 30:2 till further help or AED arrives (**Table 17.4.4** for compression ventilation ratio).

For chest compression in adults and adolescents, CPR is done with heel of both hands in mid of the chest just below the nipple line but above the xiphisternum **(Figs. 17.4.4A and B)**, in children single hand can be used **(Figs. 17.4.5A and B)**. For infants and lone rescuer 2 finger technique is used **(Fig. 17.4.6A)** and for 2 rescuers; thumb-encircling technique is used **(Fig. 17.4.6B)**. As per National Neonatology Forum (NNF) guidelines in newborns the compression and ventilation ratio should be 3:1 (90 and 30 compression and ventilation respectively in a minute).

The compression rate for 2-rescuer CPR is 100–120 beats/min until an advanced airway (e.g. laryngeal mask airway, supraglottic, or endotracheal tube) is in place; rescuers must pause compressions to provide breaths. When advanced airway is in place during 2-rescuer CPR, do not stop compression to give breaths. Give 1 breath every 6 seconds (10 breaths per minute) with self-inflatable bag, without any pause in compressions to deliver breaths **(Table 17.4.5)**.

Early vascular access has pivotal role during resuscitation from circulation point of view. The routes of delivery can be intravenous (IV), intraosseous and/or endotracheal routes. Veins close to heart must be selected and every time drugs should be followed by 5 mL saline infusion. In children if three successive venipunctures are failed or more than 90 seconds have elapsed (whichever is earlier) go for intraosseus route. Various sites used are proximal tibia (anteromedial surface, 2–3 cm below the tibia tuberosity), distal tibia (proximal to the medial malleolus) or distal femur (midline, 2–3 cm above

Table 17.4.4: Compression ventilation ratio.

Component	***Adults and adolescents***	***Children (age 1 year to puberty)***	***Infants (age less than 1 year; excluding newborns)***
Compression ventilation ratio without advanced airway	1 or 2 rescuers 30:2	1 rescuer 30:2 2 or more rescuers 15:2	
Compression ventilation ratio with advanced airway	Continuous compression at a rate of 100–120/min Give 1 breath every 6 seconds (10 breaths/min)		

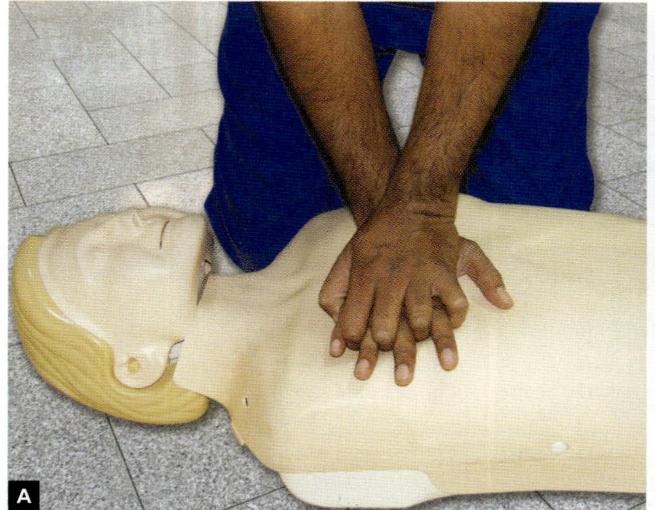

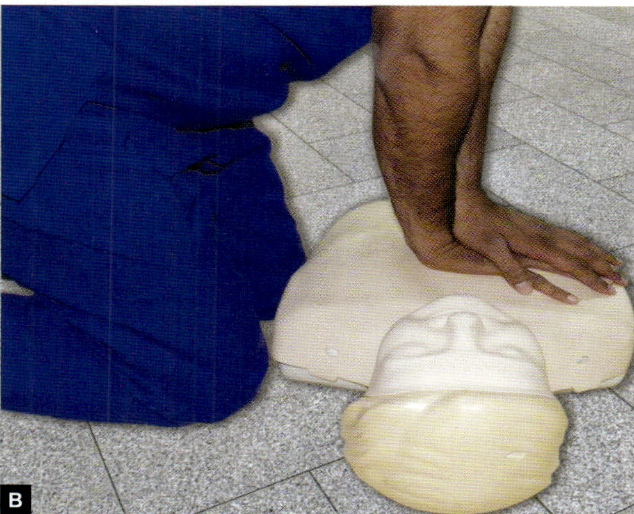

Figs. 17.4.4A and B: Chest compression in adult.

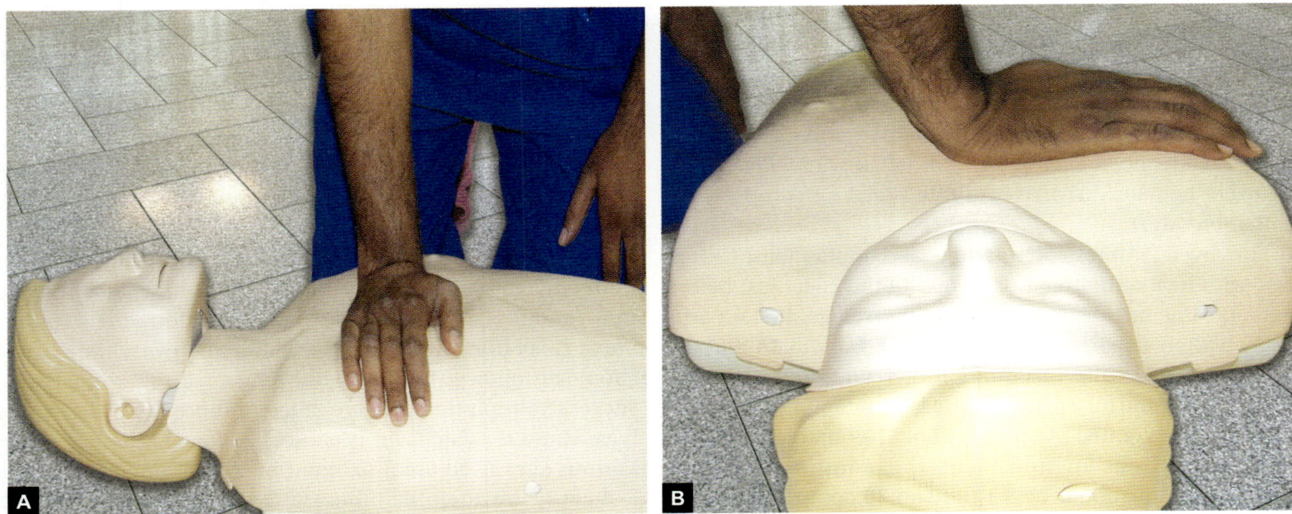

Figs. 17.4.5A and B: Chest compression in child.

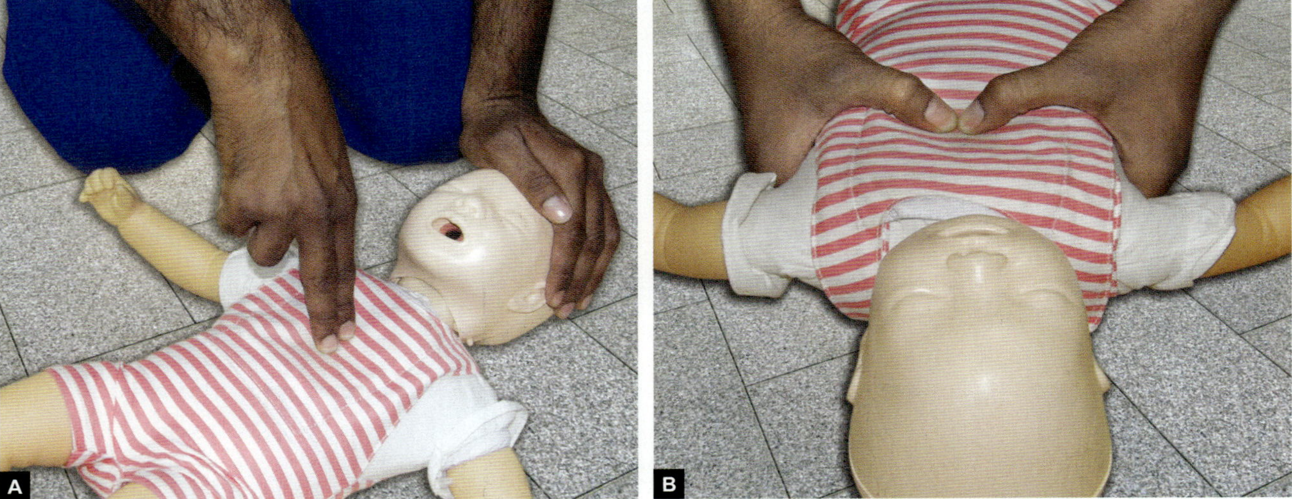

Figs. 17.4.6A and B: (A) Two finger technique of chest compression in infant; and (B) Thumb-encircling technique of chest compression in infant.

Table 17.4.5: CPR with an advanced airway.

Ventilation technique	*Compressions to breaths (adults)*	*Compressions to breaths (child and Infant)*
No advanced airway (mouth-to-mouth, mouth-to-mask, bag-mask)	30 compressions to 2 breaths Compression rate of 100–120 beats/minute	15 compressions to 2 breaths Compression rate of 100–120 beats/min
Advanced airway (endotracheal intubation, laryngeal mask airway, supraglottic)	Compression rate of 100–120 beats/min, without any pauses for breaths 1 breath every 6 seconds (10 breaths per minute)	Compression rate of 100–120 beats/min, without any pause for breaths 1 breath every 6 seconds (10 breaths per minute)

the external condyle). Endotracheal route is the last resort, ET dose of epinephrine is 10 times of the IV dose and for other drugs it is 2–3 times; during ET drugs instillation compressions should be withheld and should be followed by 5 mL normal saline (NS) and five rapid manual breaths. Drugs that can be given through ET route are LEAN (Lignocaine, Epinephrine, Atropine, and Naloxone).

DEFIBRILLATION

Although the rhythms during most IHCA (both in children and adults) are asystole and pulseless electrical activity (PEA); recent studies indicate that shockable rhythms such as ventricular fibrillation (VF) and ventricular tachycardia (VT) occur in 27% of IHCA at some time during the arrest and resuscitation.

Delivery of unsynchronized shock during a cardiac cycle to terminate the abnormal rhythms is defibrillation. For defibrillation we have AEDs and manual defibrillator. Generally, we have AEDs for outpatient CPR in view of portability; manual defibrillator is placed in hospitals and some of them have AED mode too. For children above 8 years, we can use adult dosage AED or manual defibrillator while in infants and child below 8 years of age manual defibrillator, or adult-dosage AED with pediatric dose attenuator or AED specially designed for these ages can be used depending upon availability. In absence of these standard nonattenuated adult-dosage AEDs should be used. AEDs have adult and pediatric pads separately; in manual defibrillator size is chosen as mentioned in manual either adult or child paddles, and some have smaller one for infants too. For position of pads in AEDs and paddles in manual defibrillators anterolateral position **(Fig. 17.4.7A)** is preferred (right pad/paddle position is below the right collar bone and on left side apply it slightly left to the nipple and electrode being in mid axillary line); in case it cannot be applied as such due to small size of the victim (infants or small children) anteroposterior position can be used (anteriorly over the precordium, and posteriorly behind the heart, in the right infrascapular or infrascapular region; **Fig. 17.4.7B**).

The pediatric dose for manual defibrillator is 2 J/kg. If unsuccessful, the subsequent doses should be increased to 4 J/kg (max 9 J/kg). Likelihood of survival decreases by 7–10% with each minute delay of defibrillation. Synchronized cardioversion is done for supraventricular tachycardia (SVT) or VT with pulses (smaller dose is used: 0.5–1 J/kg first dose and later on 1–2 J/kg). Pulseless VT (pVT) and VF are shockable rhythms apart from SVT and VT with pulses while asystole and PEA are nonshockable rhythms; defibrillation as such has no role in sinus tachycardia and bradycardia. For detailed use of defibrillator, we have to follow the instructions of the manufacturer.

In the in-hospital setting, the electrocardiogram (ECG) should guide for further resuscitative actions. For children without a pulse and in asystole or electromechanical dissociation (PEA), providers should continue rescue breathing and CPR, obtain vascular access, and give emergency IV epinephrine (**Fig. 17.4.8**; pulseless cardiac arrest). For continued asystole or PEA, epinephrine can be repeated every 3–5 minutes. At this stage revaluation of the patient in perspectives of history, physical examination supported by laboratory evaluation to find out the possible and correctible cause of cardiac arrest (such as the reversible Hs and Ts; **Table17.4.6**) should be carried out. CPR should be continued after epinephrine administration, to circulate the drug through the body. After 5 cycles of CPR, providers should

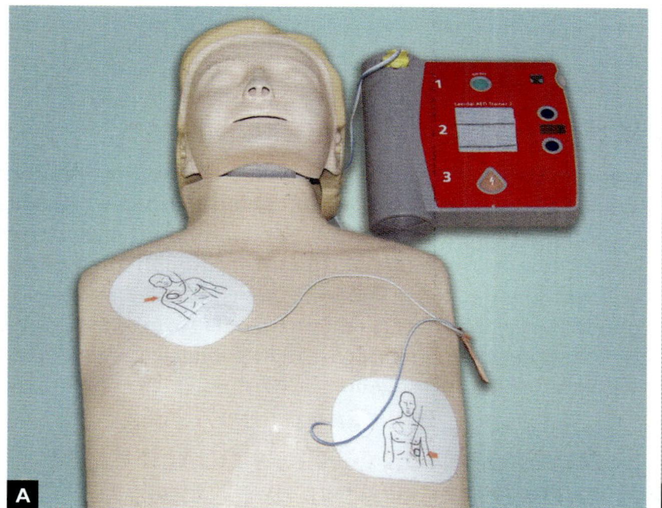

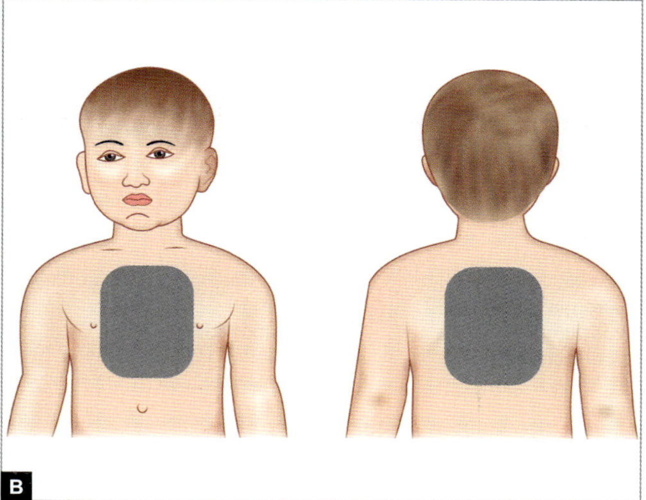

Figs. 17.4.7A and B: (A) AED application anterolateral in adults; and (B) AED pad application anteroposterior in infants or smaller child.

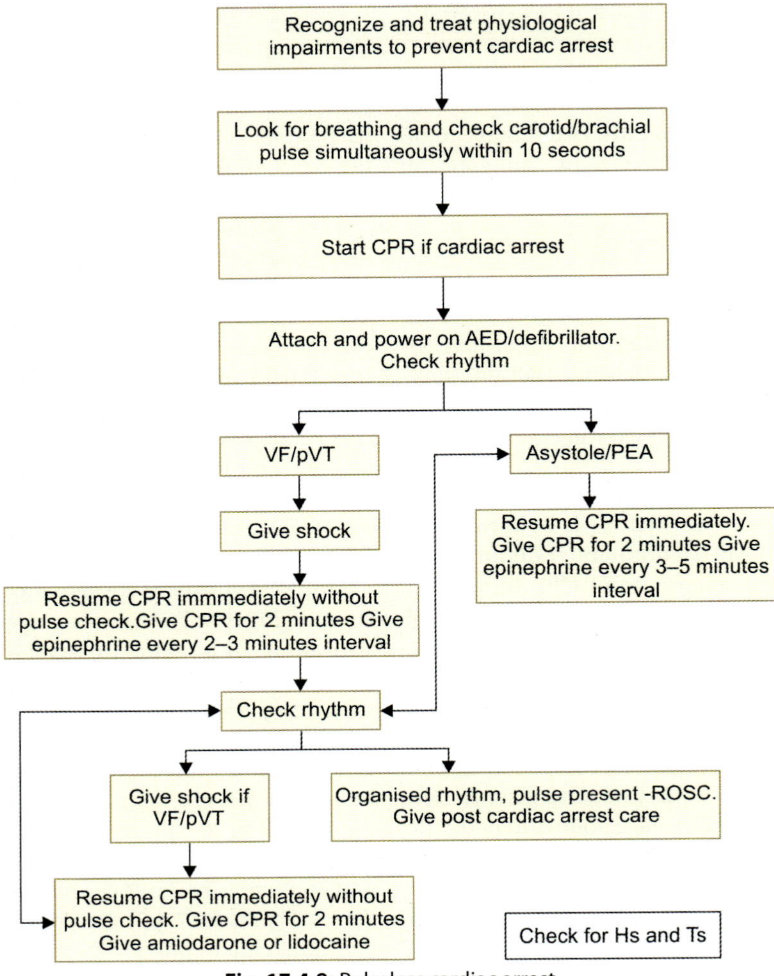

Fig. 17.4.8: Pulseless cardiac arrest.
Source: Pediatric Advanced Life Support Guidelines Update for Cardiopulmonary Resuscitation, Circulation 2015;132S:526-S542.

Table 17.4.6: Hs and Ts—identify and treat.

Hs	*Ts*
Hyperkalemia/hypokalemia Hypovolemia Hypotension Hypoxia Hydrogen ion (acidosis) Hypothermia Hyperthermia Hypervagal response Hypoglycemia	Toxins (drugs, poison) Tension pneumothorax Trauma Thromboembolism (coronary artery) Tamponade (cardiac) Prolonged QT interval Pulmonary hypertension

reassess the child for the presence of a pulse or a change in the ECG rhythm necessitating a different action depending on the findings. For refractory VF or VT, an IV antiarrhythmic, such as amiodarone or lidocaine, can be given **(Table 17.4.7)**.

DRUGS USED IN CARDIAC ARREST

Commonly used drugs, their doses and indications are discussed in **Table 17.4.7**. Vasopressin is a drug, which acts on V2 receptors and causes vasoconstriction; it increases blood flow to the heart and brain. Although vasopressin will not likely replace epinephrine as a first-line agent in pediatric cardiac arrest, preliminary data suggest that its use in conjunction with epinephrine in pediatric cardiac arrest deserves further investigation.

CONTINUATION OF HIGH-QUALITY CPR AND POSTRESUSCITATIVE CARE

Postarrest care emphasis after ROSC is to maintain normothermia, normocapnia, normoxemia and normoglycemia

Table 17.4.7: Drugs in cardiopulmonary resuscitation.

Drugs	***Indication/Remark***	***Dose***
Adenosine	SVT Monitor ECG/Give bolus as two syringe technique	mg/kg (maximum 6 mg) Repeat: 0.2 mg/kg (maximum 12 mg)
Atropine	Symptomatic bradycardia like AV block	IV/IO: 0.02 mg/kg ET: 0.03 mg/kg Repeat once if needed Minimum dose: 0.1 mg Minimum single dose: Child, 0.5 mg Adolescent, 1 mg
Epinephrine	Cardiac arrest as per algorithm	IV/IO route 0.1 mL/kg (0.01 mg/kg) of 1:10,000 (1 mL = 0.1 mg) solution followed by 5 mL NS push ET route 0.1 mL/kg (0.1 mg/kg) of 1:1000 (1 mL = 0.1 mg) solutions followed by 5 mL NS push
Amiodarone	VF or pVT refractory to defibrillation	IV/IO route 5 mg/kg bolus (maximum single dose 300 mg) followed by 5 mL normal saline flush. Can be repeated 2 times (i.e. total dose of 15 mg/kg) for refractory VF/pVT ET route: Not recommended
Lidocaine	VF or pVT refractory to defibrillation	IV/IO 1 mg/kg loading dose followed by maintenance 20–50 µg/kg/min as infusion. Repeat bolus if infusion is initiated >15 min of initial loading dose. ET route: 2–3 mg/kg
Magnesium sulfate	Torsades de pointes and hypomagnesemia	IV/IO 25–50 mg/kg bolus; maximum dose 2 g ET: Not recommended
Calcium, soda-bicarbonate and atropine are not routinely indicated in pulseless arrest except: • Calcium for hypocalcemia, hyperkalemia, hypermagnesemia, and calcium channel blocker overdose; • Sodium bicarbonate for hyperkalemia, tricyclic antidepressant dose; and • Atropine for symptomatic bradycardia like AV block that can progress to asystole.		

(CPR: cardiopulmonary resuscitation; ECG: electrocardiography; ET: endotracheal intubation; IV: intravenous; IO: intraosseous; NS: normal saline; pVT: pulseless ventricular tachycardia; VF: ventricular fibrillation)

and prevent ill-effects of ischemia or reperfusion injury in postcardiac arrest syndrome (PCAS) specially seen in brain, heart, kidney, etc. Myocardial dysfunction should be optimized with inotropic or vasoactive drugs; adequate sedation and analgesia should be given in accordance with validated scores.

For infants and children in OHCA either maintain normothermia (36–37.5°C) or 2 days of initial continuous hypothermia (32–34°C) followed by normothermia for 3–5 days; for IHCA no evidence is in favor of hypothermia.

Postarrest outcomes are better if pupillary reactivity is present at 12–24 hours after cardiac arrest, low lactate at first 12 hours and poor outcome if longer duration of cardiac arrest or in case of nonshockable rhythm, IHCA due to septic shock, long interval elapsed between cardiac arrest and CPR initiation, prehospital hypothermia, ice water drowning despite more than 30 minutes of cardiac arrest. Resuscitative efforts should be prolonged in case of drug overdose, severe prearrest hypothermia (e.g. near drowning in cold water), toxin exposure, and in presence of electrolyte abnormality; otherwise efforts are unlikely after 30 minutes of cumulative advance life support.

Make sure to search out for complications of CPR such as rib fractures, sternal fractures, hemopericardium, pneumothorax, laceration of abdominal viscera, etc.

BIBLIOGRAPHY

1. Babbs CF, Kern KB. Optimum compression to ventilation ratios in CPR under realistic, practical conditions: A physiological and mathematical analysis. Resuscitation. 2002;54(2):147-57.
2. Bobrow BJ, Clark LL, Ewy GA, et al. Minimally interrupted cardiac resuscitation by emergency medical services for out-of-hospital cardiac arrest. JAMA. 2008;299(10):1158-65.
3. de Caen AR, Berg MD, Chameides L, et al. Pediatric Advanced Life Support Guidelines Update for Cardiopulmonary Resuscitation. Circulation. 2015;132(18 Suppl 2):S526-42.
4. Doherty DR, Parshuram CS, Gaboury I, et al. Hypothermia therapy after pediatric cardiac arrest. Circulation. 2009;119(11):1492-500.
5. Hegenbarth MA, American Academy of Pediatrics Committee on Drugs. Preparing for pediatric emergencies: drugs to consider. Pediatrics. 2008;121(2):433-43.
6. Markenson D, Pyles L, Neish S, et al. Ventricular fibrillation and use of automated external defibrillators on children. Pediatrics. 2007;120(5):e1368-79.
7. Nadkarni VM, Larkin GL, Peberdy MA, et al. First documented rhythm and clinical outcome from in-hospital cardiac arrest among children and adults. JAMA. 2006;295(1):50-7.
8. Ogawa T, Akahane M, Koike S, et al. Outcomes of chest compression only CPR versus conventional CPR conducted by lay people in patients with out of hospital cardiopulmonary arrest witnessed by bystanders: nationwide population based observational study. BMJ. 2011;342:c7106.
9. Slonim AD, Patel KM, Ruttimann UE, et al. Cardiopulmonary resuscitation in pediatric intensive care units. Crit Care Med. 1997;25(12):1951-5.
10. Suominen P, Olkkola KT, Voipio V, et al. Utstein style reporting of in-hospital paediatric cardiopulmonary resuscitation. Resuscitation. 2000;45(1):17-25.

17.5 Shock

M Jayashree, Rajalakshmi Iyer

DEFINITION

Shock is a state of impaired tissue perfusion resulting in an imbalance between oxygen demand and supply. This causes widespread reduction in effective tissue perfusion, and insufficient or improper delivery and distribution of oxygen and nutrients, the end result of which is altered cellular and subcellular function leading to anaerobic metabolism, accumulation of lactic acid, and consequently, cellular damage, multiple organ dysfunction and finally cardiovascular collapse. Clinically, signs of hemodynamic instability such as tachycardia, impaired peripheral perfusion, hypotension and evidence of organ hypoperfusion characterize shock.

ETIOLOGIC CLASSIFICATION OF SHOCK

The patient with shock has abnormalities of either:

- Circulating blood volume
- The heart; or
- Blood flow distribution.

Accordingly, shock can be classified into the following groups:

- Hypovolemic (decreased circulating blood volume)
- Cardiogenic (impaired myocardial function)
- Distributive (inappropriate distribution of blood flow); and
- Obstructive [mechanical obstruction to cardiac output (CO)].

Several etiologies, which fall into these broad groups, are outlined in **Table 17.5.1**.

Pathophysiology of Shock

The primary pathophysiological event in shock, regardless of inciting etiology is tissue hypoperfusion, leading to tissue hypoxia, acidosis, and end-organ dysfunction.

The pathway to cardiovascular failure results from impairment of CO and systemic vascular resistance (SVR) or both. CO is the product of heart rate and stroke volume while stroke volume is determined by left ventricular filling pressure and myocardial contractility. SVR, on the other hand, represents the impedance to left ventricular ejection (afterload) as well as the tone of the peripheral vasculature. After adequate volume resuscitation, patients in hyperdynamic or warm shock are peripherally vasodilated with high CO (e.g. septic shock) whilst patients in a hypodynamic or cold shock (e.g.

Table 17.5.1: Causes of shock.

Hypovolemic
Fluid and electrolyte loss: • Diarrhea, vomiting • Excessive sweating • Pathologic renal loss *Blood loss*: • External—laceration • Internal—ruptured viscera, gastrointestinal (GI) bleed • Intracranial bleed (neonates) *Plasma loss*: • Burns • Leaky capillaries—sepsis, inflammation • Nephrotic syndrome • Third space loss—intestinal obstruction, peritonitis *Endocrine*: • Diabetes mellitus • Diabetes insipidus • Adrenal insufficiency
Cardiogenic
Myocardial insufficiency:* • Congestive heart failure (congenital, or acquired heart disease) • Cardiomyopathies—myocarditis • Arrhythmias • Hypothermia • Drugs, toxins
Obstructive
Outflow obstruction: • Cardiac tamponade • Pneumopericardium • Tension pneumothorax • Pulmonary embolism
Distributive
• Septic shock • Anaphylaxis • Drugs/toxin • Tissue injury • Prolonged hypoxia of ischemia

*Myocardial depressant effect of hypoglycemia, acidosis, hypoxia.

hypovolemic shock) present with increased vascular tone and low CO. Children with septic shock have a combination of vascular and myocardial failure unlike the adult septic shock which predominantly presents as vascular failure.

When CO is unable to meet the demands of the tissues, compensatory sympathetic activity produces selective vasoconstriction of the skin and splanchnic vessels to divert blood flow to vital organs, namely brain, heart and kidney.

Three pathophysiological concepts that need understanding especially in septic shock are as follows:

1. *Myocardial dysfunction*: It develops in nearly all patients with septic shock. This dysfunction peaks soon after the onset of sepsis and resolves within 7–10 days in survivors. Sepsis stimulates the release of inflammatory mediators that can compromise cardiac function. Dilatation of ventricles, reduced contractility and decreased ventricular compliance may be seen. Both systolic and diastolic dysfunctions are well described in septic shock. Diminished responsiveness of the myocardium to β1 agonists is secondary to down regulation of β1 receptors, uncoupling of receptors from adenylate cyclase or depressed generation of cyclic adenosine monophosphate (cAMP). The myocardium is dysfunctional despite an increase in CO during the hyperdynamic phase of sepsis.
2. *Mean arterial pressure (MAP)*: It is important to recognize that oxygen is not distributed uniformly to the body. Modulation of SVR in different vascular beds is one of the body's primary compensatory mechanisms to shunt blood preferentially to vital organs such as the heart and brain. In this way, an increase in SVR may maintain a normal blood pressure (BP) even in the face of inadequate oxygen delivery. Maintenance of an adequate MAP is fundamental to ensure adequate perfusion and organ function. When MAP falls below the autoregulatory range of an organ, blood flow decreases, resulting in tissue ischemia and organ failure. As the kidneys receive the second highest blood flow of any organ in the body, measurement of urine output (with the exception of patients with hyperosmolar states, like diabetic ketoacidosis, leading to osmotic diuresis) and creatinine clearance can be used as an indicator of adequate perfusion pressure.
3. *Oxygen delivery versus consumption*: Oxygen delivery is primarily dependent on CO. Enhancing CO by increasing preload and contractility or by decreasing afterload will thus increase oxygen delivery. Contrary to adults, oxygen delivery, not oxygen extraction, is the major determinant of oxygen consumption in children. Attainment of the therapeutic oxygen consumption goal of greater than 200 mL/min/m^2 has been found to be associated with improved outcome. In patients with septic shock, the concept of pathological oxygen utilization explains dependence of oxygen consumption on oxygen delivery even at supernormal oxygen delivery. The goal in such patients is therefore to increase oxygen delivery to avoid flow-dependent tissue hypoxia and not to overdo at supraphysiologic levels.

Hypovolemic Shock

Hypovolemic shock is the most common form of shock in children worldwide. It is usually caused by hemorrhage or dehydration. Relative hypovolemia may occur secondary to "third spacing" of fluids (extravascular fluid shifts) as it may be observed in children with burns, sepsis or dengue shock syndrome. Depending on the severity and rate of development of hypovolemia, the shock may appear abruptly or evolve gradually over several stages. Regardless of etiology, the final common pathway to circulatory insufficiency is diminished intravascular volume. This volume reduction results in decreased systemic venous return and ventricular filling pressure (preload), thereby decreasing the stroke volume. Children with hypovolemia due to fluid and electrolyte losses have both intravascular and interstitial depletion. Clinical findings include sunken eyes, depressed anterior fontanel, dry mucous membrane, poor skin turgor, delayed capillary refill, and cool extremities. On the other hand, patients with hypovolemia due to increased capillary permeability such as in burns or sepsis, have intravascular hypovolemia in the setting of interstitial euvolemia or hypervolemia. This clinically manifests as signs of decreased end-organ perfusion such as altered mentation, decreased urine output, and cool, but often turgid extremities. The classical signs of dehydration based on interstitial fluid depletion are absent. Once again, hypotension is a late finding and may not occur until intravascular volume has decreased by about 25%. This is the time when the compensatory mechanisms fail, and profound reduction of CO and fall of BP occur.

Cardiogenic Shock

Cardiogenic shock is commonly described as "pump failure". The common causes are myocarditis, dysrhythmias and drugs with a myocardial depressant action, acidosis, congenital heart lesions and sepsis. It can also result from obstruction to the outflow tract, e.g. coarctation of aorta or aortic stenosis or in states of increased afterload like hypertension. Cardiogenic shock will have low CO, hypotension and clinical signs of inadequate tissue perfusion. Typically intravascular volume is adequate or even increased, but cardiac dysfunction limits CO.

Distributive Shock

The most common cause of distributive shock is sepsis. The common denominator in this shock is leakage of intravascular fluid through capillary bed into interstitial space known as "third spacing" of fluids because of endothelial damage. Sepsis is a systemic disease caused by microorganisms or their products in the blood. Gram-negative bacilli cause the majority of cases of septic shock but it may be caused by Gram-positive, rickettsial, fungal, and viral infections. Early septic shock is known as "warm shock" or hyperdynamic phase as warm extremities, low SVR, characterized by high or normal cardiac CO, normal BP, and increased pulse pressure. Low SVR increases skin blood flow and causes bounding peripheral pulses. Therefore, despite high CO, shock and metabolic acidosis develop because blood flow is inappropriately distributed.

Adequate and early treatment at this stage may prevent progression. Cold extremities, high SVR, low CO, narrow pulse pressure and hypotension leading to hypoxia, acidosis and death characterize the later phase of "cold shock".

CLINICAL FEATURES AND STAGES OF SHOCK

Shock refers to dynamic state ranging from early, compensated shock to irreversible, terminal shock. Shock can progress over a span of few hours or occur over minutes, e.g. in hemorrhagic shock. The progression can be arbitrarily divided into three stages:

1. Compensated shock
2. Hypotensive shock
3. Irreversible or refractory shock.

Compensated Shock

Compensated shock refers to preserved vital organ functions secondary to effective compensatory mechanisms. BP is maintained although signs of inadequate tissue and organ perfusion are observed. The early physical signs are that of an exaggerated sympathetic response to stress. Tachycardia and signs of decreased peripheral perfusion namely cold, clammy skin, capillary refill time more than 2 seconds and difference between core and surface temperature of greater than equal 2°C are the most important clinical pointers to early shock. Tachypnea may be seen without evidence of an underlying pulmonary disease. BP is maintained within normal range during the early stages.

Septic shock in the early stages presents with fever, warm well perfused extremities, bounding pulses, and wide pulse pressure. A capillary refill time of 3 seconds or more denotes impaired skin perfusion. It is a valuable sign during assessment and monitoring.

Hypotensive Shock

In this stage, the BP and CO fall, as they cannot be sustained by the intense peripheral vasoconstriction. A cascade of anaerobic tissue metabolism and multiorgan dysfunction sets in. Patient presents with poor pulses, peripheral cyanosis, cold extremities, hypotension, and acidosis. Vital organ perfusion gets progressively compromised. Oliguria or anuria results from diminished renal perfusion. Diminished cerebral perfusion manifests in the form of lethargy, confusion, and disorientation. Rapid aggressive intervention is required to halt the progression to irreversible stage. **Table 17.5.2** summarizes the clinical features in shock syndrome.

Irreversible Stage

Irreversible stage of shock is a progressive reduction in CO, fall in BP and worsening metabolic acidosis, and multiorgan

Table 17.5.2: Clinical stages of shock and physical signs.

Clinical parameters	*Stage I (compensated)*	*Stage II (hypotensive)*	*Stage III (irreversible)*
Heart rate	Tachycardia	Marked tachycardia	Severe tachycardia, bradycardia
Respiration rate	Normal	Tachypnea	Tachypnea/apnea
Blood pressure	Normal	Hypotension	Severe hypotension
Pulse pressure	Normal	Low	Markedly low
Skin	Cool	Mottled	Cold and cyanotic
Mental status	Anxious	Obtunded	Coma
Urine	Normal	Oliguria	Anuria

failure. Delayed recognition or inadequate treatment can lead to refractory shock.

Difference between Pediatric and Adult Shock

The compensatory cardiovascular responses of a child with decreased preload, impaired myocardial contractility and alterations in vascular tone differ from those of an adult.

Cardiac output is the product of heart rate and stroke volume. Stroke volume in turn is determined by preload, afterload, and myocardial contractility. In children, CO is predominantly heart rate dependent owing to the lack of adequate ventricular muscle mass. Therefore, a child in shock maintains an adequate CO by mounting a tachycardic response. Stroke volume is determined by ventricular filling (preload), the impedance to ventricular ejection (afterload) and intrinsic pump function (myocardial contractility).

Children maintain adequate cardiac output by mounting a tachycardic response.

Children maximize SVR to maintain a normal BP, in the face of significant decrease in the CO. This increase due to peripheral vasoconstriction mediated by the sympathetic nervous system results in diversion or redistribution of blood flow from less vital organs such as skin, skeletal muscles, kidneys, and splanchnic organs, to more vital organs like the brain, heart, lungs, and adrenal glands. Therefore, BP will remain maintained till very late stages of shock and hence is a poor indicator of cardiovascular homeostasis in children. The evaluation of other hemodynamic variables like heart rate and end-organ perfusion, including capillary refill, the quality of the peripheral pulses, mentation, urine output, and acid-base status, is more reliable than BP in determining the adequacy of hemodynamic status in a child.

Presence of hypotension is not a must for diagnosis of shock in children.

COMPLICATIONS OF SHOCK

Myocardial depression, acute respiratory distress syndrome (ARDS), acute renal failure, and disseminated intravascular coagulation (DIC) are the most dreaded and life-threatening complications of shock.

DIAGNOSIS

Shock is a clinical diagnosis. Laboratory investigations are basically required to ascertain the etiology, and severity of organ dysfunction. The investigations that should be obtained in a patient with shock are shown in **Table 17.5.3**.

MANAGEMENT OF SHOCK

Two major priorities in treatment of septic shock are:

1. Rapid assessment of patient's disease process
2. Achievement of cardiopulmonary stability.

Table 17.5.3: Investigations in shock.

Cardiovascular system: • ECG • Chest X-ray • Echocardiogram	*Gastrointestinal:* • Stool occult blood • Gastric pH • Liver function test • Pancreatic functions
Respiratory system: • Blood gases arterial and mixed venous • Lung function tests	*Metabolic:* • Serum Na^+, K^+, Ca^+, Mg^{2+}, phosphorus • Blood glucose
Renal system: • Serum urea/creatinine • Urine Na^+/specific gravity/sediments • Urine protein/sugar	*Infection screen:* • Cultures: Blood, CSF, urine, stool, pus • Rapid diagnostic tests for tropical infections like dengue, malaria, scrub typhus, leptospirosis • Biomarkers like CRP/procalcitonin • USG to screen for deep seated foci of infection
Hematologic system: • Hematocrit, TLC, DLC • Coagulation parameters • Platelet counts	• Toxicology screen

(CRP: C-reactive protein; CSF: cerebrospinal fluid; DLC: differential leukocyte count ECG: electrocardiogram; TLC: total leukocyte count)

Irrespective of the etiology, the ABC's should guide the initial resuscitation and stabilization of all forms of shock. Stabilization of airway, provision of oxygen and establishment of vascular access are immediate goals followed by fluid resuscitation.

Oxygen Administration

Supplemental oxygen should be administered to all patients in shock in view of the impaired oxygen delivery to the tissues. Intubation for airway stabilization is indicated in children with shock having altered sensorium, increased work of breathing or respiratory failure.

Vascular Access

An immediate intravenous (IV) access has to be established. In children where IV access is difficult due to collapsed veins an intraosseous (IO) line must be established instead. Obtaining rapid vascular access with at least two wide bore peripheral venous lines is extremely crucial. Vascular access may be extremely difficult in children with shock, as they have collapsed veins. Since time is extremely crucial, pediatric advanced life support (PALS) guidelines recommend placement of an intra-asseus (IO) needle in infants and children for pushing fluids.

If peripheral access is not readily obtained, IO access should be established quickly in children.

Central venous access should be considered for children in fluid refractory shock as this access helps in infusion of vasoactive drugs and monitoring of mixed venous oxygen saturation ($ScVO_2$).

Fluid Therapy

The objective of fluid administration in shock is to rapidly restore effective circulating volume so as to re-establish vital organ perfusion. Optimization of circulating volume with help of fluids is the most important cornerstone of therapy in shock. Volume expansion should be achieved rapidly with a crystalloid solution, i.e. isotonic saline or Ringer's lactate given as 20 mL/kg IV while one is trying to assess the etiology. Response to fluid challenge includes an improvement in capillary refill, decreasing tachycardia, elevation of BP and maintenance of an adequate urine output (1 mL/kg/h). Subsequent choice of fluid may depend on the etiology, acid-base and electrolyte status, and oxygen delivery and coagulation parameters. The amount of fluid and the rapidity of administration depend on hemodynamic status, patient's response and the ongoing losses. Hypotensive patients require rapid fluid infusion using a pull push method. In patients with compensated shock, fluids can be given over 30–60 minutes. Caution during fluid administration is required for malnourished and anemic children. Children should be closely monitored for signs of fluid overload in the form of worsening tachypnea and or hepatomegaly.

Patients in hypovolemic and septic shock may require up to 40–60 mL/kg in first 1 hour to achieve therapeutic end points of perfusion and BP. Once a child is labeled as fluid refractory, further stabilization is achieved with vasoactive drugs as described below. Volume resuscitation beyond the first hour should be titrated to signs of improved perfusion, age, appropriate MAP, a mixed venous oxygen saturation (SVO_2) of greater than 70% and cardiac index greater than 3.3 L/min/m^2 [American College of Critical Care Medicine (ACCM) Practice Guidelines, 2017].

Colloids and blood products may be required in selective situations. Blood as volume expander should be given for traumatic hemorrhagic shock or bleeding due to coagulopathies. Even in these situations crystalloids are the first choice for volume expansion while blood is being arranged.

Dextrose containing solution should be avoided during shock resuscitation unless there is documented hypoglycemia. This is because dextrose-containing fluids cause hyperglycemia and osmotic diuresis, which can further aggravate shock.

The initial fluid for resuscitation should always be a crystalloid either isotonic saline or Ringer's lactate.

Cardiovascular Support

Following adequate intravascular volume repletion, continued presence of hypotension and/or poor perfusion warrants the consideration of vasoactive therapy, which should be goal directed. Vasoactive drug therapy in the treatment of shock aims to increase oxygen delivery or organ perfusion or both. Increasing MAP to a level that allows appropriate distribution of CO for adequate organ perfusion and hence oxygen delivery is one of the key functions of vasopressors.

Optimal preload is essential for all patients in shock before vasoactive therapy is contemplated.

The vasoactive agents used to support circulatory function may be classified as inotropes, vasopressors, vasodilators, and inodilators.

Inotropes increase myocardial contractility and often increase heart rate as well, e.g. dobutamine, mid-dose dopamine (5–10 μg/kg/min), low-dose epinephrine (0.05–0.3 μg/kg/min).

Vasopressors increase systemic and pulmonary vascular resistance and are therefore useful in patients with low SVR. If myocardial function is adequate, vasopressors will typically increase systemic and pulmonary artery pressures, e.g. norepinephrine, high-dose dopamine greater than 10 μg/kg/min, high-dose epinephrine (>0.3 μg/kg/min).

Vasodilators are designed to reduce systemic and pulmonary vascular resistance. Although vasodilators do not directly increase myocardial contractility, they reduce ventricular afterload, which often improves stroke volume and CO. Vasodilators are the only class of agents that can increase CO and simultaneously reduce myocardial oxygen demand, e.g. nitroglycerin, nitroprusside.

Inodilators (inotropes + vasodilator) improve cardiac contractility and reduce afterload, e.g. phosphodiesterase inhibitors like milrinone and amrinone.

How to Choose the Appropriate Drug?

The clinician must determine whether there is evidence of low CO with high cardiac filling pressure that requires inotropic support or if hypotension is accompanied by high CO that requires pressor support. Children with severe sepsis can present with low CO and high SVR (cold shock) or low CO and low SVR (warm shock). Accordingly in cold shock, inotropic support should be started in case of fluid refractory shock while a combination of inotrope together with a vasopressor is warranted in warm shock.

Generally β-adrenergic agents are chosen for support of cardiac contractility and α-adrenergic agonists for maintenance of perfusion pressure to maintain flow distribution to the tissues.

Adequate CO is more important than BP because adequate tissue oxygen delivery is the underlying goal. Adequate distribution of flow depends on an adequate pressure head.

When should One Consider Inotropic Therapy?

Patients with low CO (myocardial failure) despite adequate fluid resuscitation will require inotropes. Clinically, it will manifest as tachycardia, low BP, prolonged capillary refill and narrow pulse pressure. The CO can be improved with use of dobutamine (up to 20 μg/kg/min). If used in the presence of low BP, it is preferable to combine it with a vasopressor. Similarly, a patient with fluid refractory septic shock may need low-dose adrenaline (<0.3 mg/kg/min) for narrow pulse pressure and/or prolonged capillary refill for improving CO. Children with catecholamine resistant cold shock requiring inotrope can be treated with phosphodiesterase inhibitors like milrinone (0.3–0.7 μg/kg/min). Children with primary cardiogenic shock can be treated with inotropes at the first go.

When should One Use Vasopressors?

When an appropriate fluid challenge fails to restore adequate BP and organ perfusion in patients with high CO and low SVR (warm shock), vasopressor agents should be started. Clinically these children will have tachycardia, flush capillary refill, low to normal BP MAP and wide pulse pressure. Since children with septic shock more often have associated myocardial dysfunction as opposed to adults, it is preferable to combine inotropic agent with a vasopressor. Norepinephrine is first-line vasopressor in warm septic shock having low SVR while vasopressin is second-line agent in patients with catecholamine-resistant warm shock. However, its experience in children is limited.

When should One Consider Use of Vasodilators?

Vasodilators are drug of choice in shock with increased afterload. In situations where myocardial failure is associated with increased afterload, inodilators like milrinone having dual action of inotropy and afterload reduction can be considered. However, the prerequisite for using vasodilators is that patient should have adequate BP or perfusion pressure. Prostaglandin E1, a potent vasodilator is indicated in newborns with ductus dependent lesion presenting in cardiogenic shock due to ductus closure. Common conditions requiring inodilators are myocarditis, and dilated cardiomyopathy.

Therapeutic End Points of Shock

The therapeutic end points of shock resuscitation are:

- Capillary refill of less than 2 seconds
- Normal pulses with no difference between central and peripheral pulses
- Warm extremities
- Urine output greater than 1 mL/kg/h
- Normal mental status
- Decreased lactate
- Mixed SVO_2 greater than 70%.

Correction of Metabolic Derangements

Metabolic Acidosis

Poor tissue perfusion and resultant anaerobic metabolism leads to significant metabolic acidosis. Uncorrected acidosis can lead to further cellular damage and myocardial depression. Sodium bicarbonate as a rescue therapy for acidosis is indicated only in a desperate situation where imminent myocardial failure secondary to severe and persistent acidosis (pH is below 6.9–7) is suspected. In all other situations bicarbonate must be avoided and all attempts must be taken to correct the underlying shock. Overcorrection with sodium bicarbonate can be hazardous leading to paradoxic central nervous system (CNS) acidosis, coma, and death.

Calcium

Acute hemodynamic deterioration in various types of shock can lead to decrease in the ionized Ca^{++} level. This hypocalcemia leads to tachycardia, hypotension, alteration in sensorium, and motor nerve excitability. An IV infusion of 1–2 mL/kg of 10% calcium gluconate should be given when ionized Ca^{++} level falls below 0.8 mEq/L. Target calcium should be between 0.8 mEq/L and 1.2 mEq/L.

Hypoglycemia

Target blood glucose is between 80 mg/dL and 180 mg/dL. Hypoglycemia and hyperglycemia are independent risk factors of poor outcome.

Acute Kidney Injury

Adequate fluid replacement is necessary to prevent development of acute kidney injury (AKI). Dialysis will be indicated in case of hyperkalemia, refractory acidosis, and fluid overload. The current trend is toward early renal replacement therapy especially in septic shock as this helps in removal of noxious triggers too.

Hematologic Support

Hematocrit needs to be maintained between 35% and 45% with the help of transfusions during resuscitation of shock. However, in hemodynamically stable patients the current recommendations favor a restrictive transfusion trigger at 7 g/dL to prevent transfusion related complications like transfusion-related acute lung injury (TRALI), transfusion-associated circulatory overload (TACO) and other transfusion-related cytokine mediated multiorgan dysfunction. Bleeding, which complicates shock may need management with fresh frozen plasma (FFP), vitamin K, and platelet concentrates. However, it is important to remember that platelet transfusions are indicated only when counts are less than 5,000/mm^3 regardless of apparent bleeding. Higher platelet counts greater than 50,000/mm^3 is required when some surgical or invasive procedure is contemplated in a child. Similarly FFP is only indicated in select patients like those with active bleeding, before invasive procedures and to reverse warfarin effect.

Gastrointestinal Support

Prophylactic use of antacids and/or an H_2-receptor antagonist is recommended to prevent stress bleeds.

Nutritional Support

Shock leads to excessive catabolism; hence nutritional support is one of the important pillars in the management. Nasogastric feeding should start as soon as patient can accept enteral feeds.

Respiratory Support

Mechanical ventilation is indicated for acute respiratory failure, to improve oxygenation and to decrease work of breathing.

Antibiotic Therapy

Appropriate empiric antibiotics should be started in suspected septic shock. It should provide broad-spectrum coverage depending upon site of infection, local epidemiologic data and sensitivity pattern. An aminoglycoside (gentamicin or amikacin) and a third-generation cephalosporin (cefotaxime, ceftriaxone) should be used for suspected Gram-negative sepsis. Combination of cloxacillin and an aminoglycoside should be used if staphylococcal sepsis is suspected.

Adjunctive Therapies

Corticosteroids

The ACCM-PALS 2017 guidelines for pediatric septic shock recommend use of stress dose of steroids (hydrocortisone 50 mg/m^2 per 24 hours) in children once they are diagnosed to have catecholamine-resistant septic shock and in suspected or proven adrenal insufficiency. Pediatric data has shown high prevalence of adrenal insufficiency in children with septic shock especially catecholamine refractory shock.

Newer Inodilators

Levosimendan and enoximone are two new inodilators being investigated for use in cardiogenic shock. They possess inotropy as well as coronary and systemic vasodilatory properties. They increase myocyte sensitivity to calcium and mediate vasodilatation through activation of adenosine triphosphate (ATP)-dependent potassium channels in vascular smooth muscles.

Immunoglobulin

Intravenous immunoglobulin may be considered in children with suspected staphylococcal or streptococcal toxic shock syndrome.

Extracorporeal Membrane Oxygenation

After adequate treatment and correction of all possible reasons for refractory shock, [such as source control, drainage of pleural or pericardial effusions/pneumothorax, adrenal or thyroid hormone replacement (if indicated), ongoing blood loss], if end points of shock are not attained, one must consider veno-arterial extracorporeal membrane oxygenation (ECMO) where facilities are available. Although survival in pediatric septic shock on ECMO is around 50%, it has been shown to decrease vasoactive-inotropic requirement and hasten recovery of shock.

MONITORING OF SHOCK

The objectives of monitoring a patient with shock are:

- To assess the efficacy of the therapeutic interventions (e.g. response to fluid bolus or vasoactive therapy)
- To recognize complications and correct them; and
- To assess the degree of associated organ dysfunctions that will help in prognostication.

Monitoring involves careful and repeated examination of the child's physiological status, i.e. vital parameters like heart rate, pulse volume, respiratory rate, BP, MAP, temperature (skin and core) and capillary refill. In addition, patients need continuous EKG monitoring and a strict intake or output record.

Blood pressure by itself is not a reliable end point for resuscitation. Children normally have a lower BP than adults and can prevent fall in BP by vasoconstriction or by increasing heart rate. MAP is instead used as a surrogate of organ perfusion in shock. Mixed SVO_2 is dependent on CO, oxygen demand, and hemoglobin and arterial oxygen saturation. The normal value is greater than 70% in critically ill patients. If CO becomes inadequate then SVO_2 falls. Persistent low SVO_2 even though other end points of resuscitation have been corrected suggests more oxygen extraction and inadequate resuscitation. Central SVO_2 is being increasingly used as an alternative to SVO_2 as it correlates well with mixed venous saturation and can be obtained from a central venous catheter.

Another surrogate marker used to assess resolution of shock is serum lactate and its clearance. Although there are no established cut-offs, a serum lactate level more than 4 mmol/L is associated with higher mortality (studies have shown values ranging from 3.3 mmol/L to 5.5 mmol/L). A more clinically relevant approach is the reduction of lactate by more than 10% in the first 6 hours of resuscitation of shock, which has been shown to be associated with better outcome. However, these levels are not yet established as guidelines or targets in the treatment of pediatric septic shock.

Regardless of the vasoactive drug therapy used, increasing CO above physiologic levels is not recommended. Two recent prospective clinical trials in critically ill patients with sepsis have failed to demonstrate benefit from increasing oxygen level to supernormal levels. The goal of resuscitation should be to achieve adequate levels of oxygen delivery to avoid flow-dependent tissue hypoxia.

Invasive Hemodynamic Monitoring

The central venous pressure (CVP) which was being used as a measure of right ventricular function and the preload is no longer used in most set ups it has been found in studies to have a poor correlation with blood volume; being a static parameter it is a poor predictor of volume status. Furthermore it is unreliable measure for volume status in children with pulmonary hypertension, noncompliant right ventricle, poor right ventricular function, tricuspid regurgitation, pericardial tamponade and high positive end-expiratory pressure (PEEP).

The multilumen pulmonary artery catheters (Swan-Ganz catheter) may yield valuable information about pulmonary artery occlusion pressure (PAOP), pulmonary artery pressure, mixed venous saturation, CO, vascular resistance, oxygen delivery and consumption **(Flowchart 17.5.1)**. However, its

Flowchart 17.5.1: Practice guidelines: An algorithmic approach.

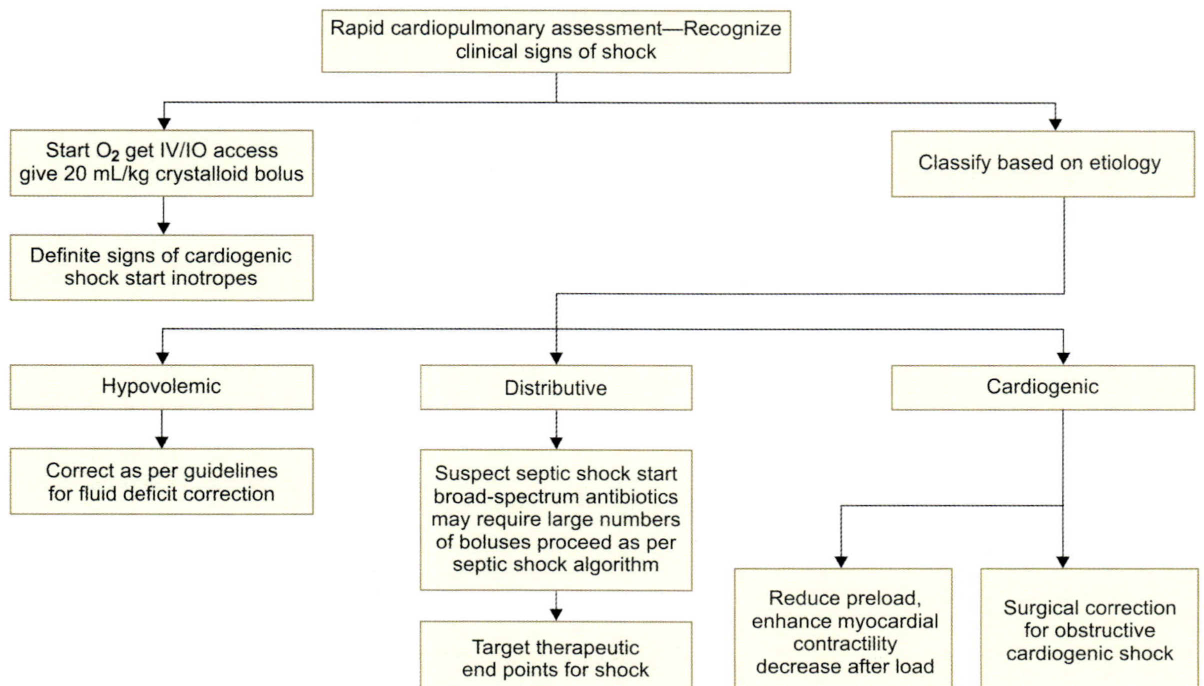

use has been abandoned in most of the units due to recent studies showing poor correlation of PAOP with volume status.

Noninvasive Hemodynamic Monitoring

Clinical determination of intravascular volume in critically ill children has its limitations. Clinicians have to walk a tight rope balancing between under filling and overfilling as both can be detrimental for sick patients. With the application of technologies like Doppler, ECHO and ultrasound, many dynamic indices of assessing fluid responsiveness have emerged and being studied in critically ill children. Important among them are pulse pressure variation (PPV) derived from analysis of arterial waveforms and stroke volume variation (SVV) derived from pulse contour analysis. Both have been shown to be highly predictive of fluid responsiveness. Inferior vena cava diameter (IVC collapsibility index) is another measure used to determine fluid responsiveness; a collapsed IVC indicative of volume depletion while a distended IVC suggests high right atrial pressure.

PROGNOSIS

Better outcome depends on early recognition and aggressive intervention in the stage of compensated shock. The mortality also depends on the etiology of shock; septic shock has mortality up to 50%. Hypothermia, decreased CO, decreased O_2, development of multiple organ dysfunctions are poor prognostic indicators in shock.

KEY MESSAGES

- Shock is a state of widespread tissue hypoperfusion resulting in an imbalance between oxygen supply and demand.
- Causes include hypovolemia, septic (distributive), cardiogenic, and obstructive.
- The diagnosis is clinical, based on a constellation of altered hemodynamic parameters like tachycardia, poor peripheral perfusion and evidence of organ hypoperfusion.
- Blood pressure is relatively preserved in early compensated shock due to sympathetic overactivity. Presence of hypotension is therefore not a must for diagnosis of shock.
- Hypotensive shock occurs when compensatory mechanisms have failed.
- Immediate treatment in all forms of shock irrespective of etiology involves stabilization of the ABCs (airway, breathing, circulation).
- Timely vascular access either peripheral IV or IO is crucial for fluid therapy.
- All patients of hypovolemic and septic shock should receive a crystalloid bolus of 20 mL/kg, rate of correction depends on underlying hemodynamic status, and ongoing losses.
- Subsequent requirement of fluids and vasoactive medications depend on therapeutic response and etiology of shock.
- Frequent monitoring of hemodynamic parameters by clinical, noninvasive and invasive methods is required to judge response to treatment and to recognize complications early.
- Vasoactive medications should be started only after patient is adequately volume depleted.
- Immediate broad-spectrum antibiotics preferably within an hour are indicated for suspected septic shock.

Obstructive cardiogenic shock may require an urgent echocardiography and surgical correction.

BIBLIOGRAPHY

1. Brierley J, Carcillo JA, Choong K, et al. Clinical practice parameters for hemodynamic support of pediatric and neonatal septic shock: 2007 update from the American College of Critical Care Medicine. Crit Care Med. 2009;37(2):666-88.
2. Choudhary R, Sitaraman S, Choudhary A. Lactate clearance as the predictor of outcome in pediatric septic shock. J Emerg Trauma Shock. 2017;10(2):55-9.
3. Davis AL, Carcillo JA, Aneja RK, et al. American College of Critical Care Medicine Clinical Practice Parameters for Hemodynamic Support of Pediatric and Neonatal Septic Shock. Crit Care Med. 2017;45(6):1061-93.
4. de Caen AR, Berg MD, Chameides L, et al. Part 12: pediatric advanced life support: 2015 American Heart Association Guidelines Update for Cardiopulmonary Resuscitation and Emergency Cardiovascular Care. Circulation. 2015;132(18 Suppl 2):S526-42.
5. Dellinger RP, Levy MM, Rhodes A, et al. Surviving sepsis campaign: International guidelines for management of severe sepsis and septic shock: 2008. Crit Care Med. 2008;36(1):296-327.
6. Levy MM, Fink MP, Marshall JC, et al. 2001 SCCM/ESICM/ACCP/ATS/SIS. International sepsis definitions conference. Crit Care Med. 2003;31(4):1250-6.
7. Lodha R, Oleti TP, Kabra SK. Management of septic shock. Indian J Pediatr. 2011;78(6):726-33.
8. Marik PE. Techniques for assessment of intravascular volume in critically ill patients. J Intensive Care Med. 2009;24(5):329-37.
9. Meyer S, Gortner L, McGuire W, et al. Vasopressin in catecholamine-refractory shock in children. Anaesthesia. 2008;63(3):228-34.
10. Singhi S, Khilnani P, Lodha R. Guidelines for treatment of septic shock in resource limited environments. J Pediatric Infectious Dis. 2009;4(2):173-92.

17.6 Respiratory Failure

Uday B Nadkarni

INTRODUCTION

Acute respiratory failure (ARF) remains an important cause of morbidity and mortality in children. It accounts for about 50% of pediatric intensive care unit (PICU) admissions and carries high mortality cardiac arrest in children frequently results from respiratory failure. Hence, early recognition of respiratory failure and timely intervention would help to prevent cardiorespiratory failure in majority of pediatric patients.

PATHOPHYSIOLOGY

Pediatric respiratory failure develops when the rate of exchange of gases in lungs and blood is unable to match body's metabolic demands. Respiratory failure develops when child's respiratory system loses the ability to provide sufficient oxygen to the blood leading to hypoxemia or when the child is unable to adequately ventilate leading to hypercarbia. Hypoxemia is defined as decreased level of oxygen in blood. A mismatch between ventilation and perfusion is the most common cause of hypoxemia.

Definition

Acute respiratory failure can be defined as the clinical state in which the respiratory system fails to meet the metabolic demands of the body for oxygenation and removal of carbon dioxide from the pulmonary circulation, thereby leading to arterial hypoxemia or hypercapnia or both.

Basic Mechanisms

- Poor availability of oxygen
- Alveolar hypoventilation
- Ventilation orperfusion mismatch
- Presence of a shunt (right to left)
- Limitation of diffusion.

Poor availability of oxygen: Low PO_2 of inspired air as occurring in high altitude.

Alveolar hypoventilation: This results in abnormal increase in PCO_2 leading to respiratory acidosis. Significant hypercapnia is always associated with hypoxemia unless the patient receives supplemental oxygen since increased alveolar CO_2 dilutes available O_2 in lungs.

Ventilation or perfusion (V/Q) mismatch: Most common reason is hypoxemia. V/Q mismatch results when gas exchange in different regions of the lungs is poor due to poor ventilation in relation to their blood flow and *vice-versa*. Hence, alveolar PaO_2 is low and alveolar $PaCO_2$ is high.

Presence of shunt: In a shunt situation, perfusion is maintained, however there is no ventilation. Thus, shunt can be considered as an extreme form of V/Q mismatching. This causes alveolar to arterial oxygen difference to increase.

Limitation of diffusion: Diffusion impairment may occur as a result of increased distance between alveoli and their associated capillaries as in interstitial edema or fibrosis and alveolar proteinosis.

TYPES OF RESPIRATORY FAILURE

- *Type I: Oxygenation Failure or Lung Failure*
  - It is always caused by venous admixture and is always manifested by elevated alveolar-arterial oxygen pressure difference $P(A-a)O_2$. Here, PaO_2 is less than 50 mm Hg and $PaCO_2$ is low or normal with patient breathing room air at sea level. Oxygenation failure is always a manifestation of pulmonary parenchymal disease.
- *Type II: Ventilatory Failure or Pump Failure*
  - The physiologic basis for pure ventilator failure is decreased minute ventilation and increased dead space ventilation or combination of both. PaO_2 is below the normal level and $PaCO_2$ more than 50 mm Hg with patient breathing room air at sea level.

ETIOLOGY

Predisposing Factors

The small size of the airways and the fewer alveoli in infants and children is the primary difference compared to older patients. In infants and children, collateral ventilation is not developed. Children have large tongue that fills oropharynx and the larynx is cephalad. Infants and young children have a narrow subglottic area hence small amount of subglottic edema can cause significant narrowing leading to upper airway obstruction. Infants and young children have relatively little cartilaginous support of the airways, which makes thoracic cage soft and compliant, ribs are positioned horizontally. Intercostals musculature and diaphragm are not fully developed.

Causes

Airway or Lung Dysfunction

- Central airway obstruction—croup, foreign body (FB), epiglottitis, retropharyngeal abscess, vascular ring, bacterial tracheitis, subglottic stenosis, laryngeal web, laryngomalacia
- Peripheral airway or parenchymal lung disease, bronchiolitis, acute severe asthma, pneumonia, drowning, lobar emphysema, acute respiratory distress syndrome (ARDS), cystic fibrosis and diaphragmatic hernia.

Respiratory pump dysfunction: May be associated with signs of decreased respiratory drive.

Decreased central nervous system (CNS) input: Head injury, meningitis, encephalitis, intracranial bleeding and ingestion of CNS depressant.

Peripheral nerve or neuromuscular junction: Polio, Guillain-Barré syndrome, spinal cord injury, botulism, organophosphorus poisoning, myasthenia gravis, flail chest and kyphoscoliosis.

Muscle weakness: Respiratory muscle fatigue, myopathies and muscular dystrophies.

Early recognition of impending respiratory failure is of paramount importance and is based primarily on clinical features. A good history and thorough clinical examination would arrive at early diagnosis of respiratory failure and its cause.

CLINICAL FEATURES

- *Increased respiratory drive:* Increased rate and depth of breathing, anxiety, breathlessness or dyspnea, retractions, prominent accessory muscles of respiration and nasal flaring.
- *Decreased respiratory drive:* Decreased rate and depth of breathing, lethargy, confusion and snoring.
- *Evidence of lung disease:* Wheezing (expiratory sound), crepitations (inspiratory sound), retractions—suprasternal, intercostal and subcostal.
- *Respiratory muscle weakness or fatigue:* Irregular or shallow breathing, paradoxical see-saw respirations, grunting.
- *Upper airway obstruction:* Stridor, drooling, absent breath sounds.
- *Secondary effects:* Tachycardia and hypertension due to increased circulatory catecholamines, peripheral vasoconstriction may develop secondary to respiratory acidosis or hypoxia. Gallop rhythm suggestive of myocardial dysfunction.

DIAGNOSIS

Clinical

- Respiratory rate more than 50 breaths/min (2 months to 1 year) and more than 40 breaths/min (1–12 years)
- State of consciousness—lethargy, confusion, agitation may be signs of hypoxemia and hypercarbia
- Decreased or absent breath sounds, inspiratory retractions, flaring of alae nasi
- Use of accessory muscles, apnea
- Cyanosis—fairly late and unreliable sign as it is influenced by skin perfusion and hemoglobin concentration.

Blood Gas Estimation (Arterial Blood Gas)

It provides information about oxygenation, ventilation and acid-base status:

- pH less than 7.25, PaO_2 less than 60 mm Hg and $PaCO_2$ more than 50 mm Hg or increasing at the rate of more than 5 mm Hg per hour is important to assess the extent of respiratory failure
- Other monitoring modalities are pulse oximetry, capnometry or capnography, transcutaneous O_2/CO_2 tension, lung volumes and airway graphic analysis **(Tables 17.6.1 and 17.6.2)**.

A complete blood count (CBC) may be helpful in detecting polycythemia suggestive of chronic hypoxia. Electrolyte abnormalities such as hypokalemia, hypocalcemia and

Table 17.6.1: Normal values of blood gases.

Age	*PaO_2*	*$PaCO_2$*
0–2 years	60–90 mm Hg	30–35 mm Hg
2 years and above	80–100 mm Hg	30–35 mm Hg

($PaCO_2$: partial pressure of arterial carbon dioxide; PaO_2: partial pressure of oxygen in arterial blood)

Table 17.6.2: Types of respiratory acid-base imbalance.

Types	*pH*	*$PaCO_2$*	*HCO_3^-*
Respiratory acidosis			
Uncompensated (acute)	↓	↑	N
Partially compensated (subacute)	↓	↑	↑
Compensated (chronic)	N	↑	↑
Respiratory alkalosis			
Uncompensated (acute)	↑	↓	N
Partially compensated (subacute)	↑	↓	N
Compensated (chronic)	N	↓	↓

($PaCO_2$: partial pressure of arterial carbon dioxide)

hypophosphatemia may impair muscle contraction. Alveolar-arterial oxygen difference is an index of efficiency of gas exchange by lungs.

Radiological Examination

Lateral and anteroposterior (AP) views of neck can reveal radiopaque foreign bodies (FBs) or soft tissue structures such as swollen epiglottis. Imaging studies also include plain X-ray chest, computed tomography (CT) or magnetic resonance imaging (MRI). Radioopacities due to vascular, pleural and interstitial lesions are defined better with CT and MRI.

Fluoroscopy is useful to evaluate movement of diaphragm and dynamic obstructive lesions of airways.

Bronchoalveolar Lavage, Lung Biopsy and Thoracocentesis

Bronchoalveolar lavage (BAL) is performed to identify specific infectious pathogen. It is indicated in critically-ill children to guide antimicrobial therapy.

Lung biopsy is indicated if BAL does not reveal a pathogen especially in immune compromised host. However, risk of invasive procedure as against yield in diagnosis should be kept in mind.

Thoracocentesis is done in pleural effusion to check whether pleural fluid is exudate or transudate.

Other Tests

Fiberoptic and rigid bronchoscopy are performed to assess air-ways for anatomic abnormalities or for FB removal.

GOALS OF TREATMENT

- Ensure adequate gas exchange and circulation [airway, breathing and circulations (ABCs) of cardiopulmonary resuscitation (CPR)]
- Eliminate triggering factor causing ARF
- Oxygen should be delivered to maintain arterial oxygen saturation more than 95% since hypoxemia is more dangerous than hypercarbia. Maintain blood pH at normal or near normal levels.
- If ventilation appears to be inadequate, breathing should be initiated with bag-mask system with added oxygen.
- Patient should be transferred immediately to referral facility after stabilization.

MANAGEMENT

Managing a case of respiratory failure is a challenging task, but if recognized early and treated promptly can prevent mortality and morbidity associated with it.

It consists of ABC approach of CPR which includes assessing and ensuring airway patency, breathing and circulation. It should commence within a half minute of cardiopulmonary arrest to avoid damage to vital organs. If CPR is instituted after 4 minutes have elapsed, there is a high possibility of hypoxic brain damage.

Airway Patency

Maintaining airway patency is the first step in the management of respiratory failure. It includes proper positioning of the patient, avoiding neck flexion, splinting the chest and clearing oropharyngeal secretions.

Indications for Endotracheal Intubation

- Cardiopulmonary failure or cardiopulmonary arrest
- Severe respiratory distress or respiratory muscle fatigue
- Loss of cough or gag reflex
- Need for ventilator support due to apnea or hypoventilation or excessive secretions
- Transportation of patient who has the potential for respiratory failure.

Tracheostomy

It is indicated in upper airway obstruction, excessive secretions causing blockage of endotracheal (ET) tube, prolonged ventilation and vocal cord paralysis.

Breathing

After the airway is opened, one must determine if the child is breathing. Look for rise and fall of the chest and abdomen.

Listen for exhaled air flow at the mouth. If spontaneous breathing is present, a patent airway must be maintained. If there is no breathing or ineffective breathing, patient should be placed in recovery position. Rescue breaths to be given by mouth to mouth breathing or bag and mask ventilation with added oxygen. If rescue breaths are ineffective and airway is obstructed, then one must resort to interventions such as ET intubation and tracheostomy.

Oxygen Therapy

A good clinical rule is to administer sufficient oxygen to keep PaO_2 in the range of 60–90 mm Hg unless higher values are warranted. Humidified oxygen may be administered through mask, nasal prongs, hood or tent. Limitation of simple mask is the attainment of only 35–55% concentration of oxygen at a flow rate of 6–10 L/min. Partial rebreathing and non-rebreathing masks can deliver 50–60% and 95% oxygen concentration respectively with a flow rate of 6–10 L/min. Nasal prongs are less restrictive and better tolerated and provide oxygen concentration of 25–45% with 1–6 L/min (low flow) of oxygen flow. Oxygen hoods can be used up to 12 months of age but require gas inflow rate of at least 10–12 L/min (high flow). High flow oxygen delivery also includes a venturi type device that places an adjustable aperture lateral to the stream of oxygen. It is necessary to monitor patients by pulse oximetry to keep the oxygen saturation more than 90%.

Continuous Positive Airway Pressure

Continuous positive airway pressure (CPAP) is used in lung diseases that cause severe oxygenation abnormalities. CPAP from 3 cm to 10 cm water is applied to increase lung volume and may also help to redistribute pulmonary edema fluid.

Noninvasive Positive Pressure Ventilation

Noninvasive positive pressure ventilation (NPPV) refers to assisted ventilation provided with nasal prongs or facemask. This therapy helps in decreasing work of breathing and provides adequate gas exchange.

Conventional Mechanical Ventilation

An infant or child whose respiratory failure persists despite oxygenation and establishment of an adequate tracheal airway needs ventilation. It is defined as a technique that incorporates a commercially available ventilator to improve either oxygenation or ventilation or both with oxygen-enriched air. This is instituted when all conservative modalities of treatment fail. It increases minute ventilation and decreases dead space. The objective of mechanical ventilation is to support the critically-ill patient by improving gas exchange in lungs, increasing lung volume to prevent or treat atelectasis and to relieve the patient of work of breathing.

Inverse Ratio Ventilation

During positive pressure ventilation, the inspiratory phase is prolonged in excess of expiratory phase. Useful in severe acute lung disease when conventional positive pressure ventilation fails.

Airway Pressure Release Ventilation

Airway pressure release ventilation (APRV) is a type of inverse ratio ventilation in which continuous gas flow is used. This allows patient to breathe spontaneously throughout the ventilator cycle.

Novel Therapies

A number of novel therapies such as high frequency oscillatory ventilation (HFOV), extracorporeal membrane oxygenation (ECMO), inhaled nitric oxide and perfluorocarbon liquid ventilation have been tried in an attempt to improve outcome in children with ARF which is refractory to traditional modalities.

High Frequency Oscillatory Ventilation

It combines small tidal volumes with frequencies of 15 Hz to minimize the barotrauma. This ventilation is very useful option where conventional mechanical ventilation fails to improve the patient's condition. High frequency oscillation also helps in decreasing iatrogenic morbidity such as barotrauma, volutrauma, etc. associated with conventional mechanical ventilation. It is useful strategy for treatment of air-leak syndrome and acute lung injury.

Inhaled Nitric Oxide

Nitric oxide (NO) is an endogenous free radical that mediates smooth muscle relaxation. It is delivered by means of its inhalation causing enhancement of pulmonary blood flow, which results in improving ventilation perfusion matching.

Extracorporeal Membrane Oxygenation

In extracorporeal membrane oxygenation (ECMO), blood is removed from the patient passed through an artificial membrane where gas exchange occurs and is returned to the body either by arterial or venous route. Survival rate varies from 60% to 85%.

KEY MESSAGES

- Acute respiratory failure (ARF) is an important cause of morbidity and mortality in children and accounts for about 50% of the admissions in pediatric intensive care unit.
- There are basic anatomical and functional differences in the airways of adults and children which account for high incidence of ARF in children.
- Respiratory failure can be either due to failure of oxygenation or pump failure.
- ARF is diagnosed on the basis of clinical features and arterial blood gas estimation.
- Early recognition of impending respiratory failure and appropriate timely intervention such as following ABCs of resuscitation improves ultimate outcome
- Maintaining airway patency and oxygenation remains the mainstay of therapy. If this fails, then one must resort to mechanical ventilation.
- Although mechanical ventilation is lifesaving, it is accompanied by trauma to airways.
- Amongst the newer modalities of managing ARF in children, high frequency oscillation (HFO) and nitric oxide inhalation are time-tested techniques and other options such as ECMO and liquid ventilation remain experimental in nature.

BIBLIOGRAPHY

1. Carroll L. Non-invasive ventilation for the treatment of acute lower respiratory tract diseases in children. Clin Pediatr Emerg Med. 2009;10:90-6.

2. ECC Committee, Subcommittees and Task Forces of the American Heart Association. 2005 American Heart Association Guidelines for Cardiopulmonary Resuscitation and Emergency Cardiovascular Care. Circulation. 2005;112(24):IV11-203.
3. Essouri S, Durand P, Chevrett L, Hass, et al. Physiological effects of non-invasive positive ventilation during acute moderate hypercapnic respiratory insufficiency in children. Intensive Care Med. 2008;34(12):2248-55.
4. Gupta P, Green JW, Tang X, et al. Comparison of high frequency oscillatory ventilation and conventional mechanical ventilation in pediatric respiratory failure. JAMA Pediatr. 2014;168(3):243-9.
5. Khilnani P. Mechanical ventilation in pediatrics. Indian J Pediatr. 1993;60(1):109-17.
6. Naiditch JA, Barsness KA, Rothstein DH. The utility of surgical lung biopsy in immunocompromised children. J Pediatr. 2013;162 (1):133-6.
7. Randolph AG. Management of acute lung injury and acute respiratory distress syndrome in children. Crit Care Med. 2009;37(8):2448-54.
8. Rettig JS, Smallwood CD, Walsh BK, et al. High-frequency oscillatory ventilation in pediatric acute lung injury: A multicenter international experience. Crit Care Med. 2015;43(12):2660-7.
9. Venkatraman ST. Mechanical ventilation and respiratory care. In: Fuhrman BP, Zimmerman JJ (Eds). Pediatric Critical Care, 3rd Edition. Philadelphia: Mosby Elsevier; 2006. pp. 683-719.
10. Zimmerman JJ, Akhtar SR, Caldwell E, et al. Incidence and outcomes of pediatric acute lung injury. Pediatrics. 2009;124(1):87-95.

17.7 Fluids, Electrolytes and Acid-base Disorders

Sunit Singhi

INTRODUCTION

The integrity of an organism depends on a stable water and electrolyte balance. Total body water (TBW) is about 75% body weight at birth, which gradually declines to 65% of body weight by 1 year of age. Almost all the reduction in TBW is contributed by loss of extracellular water (ECW) over time. Two principle compartments of TBW, the intracellular water (ICW) and the extracellular water spaces remain constant at 2:1 after infancy. The ECW compartment consists of the interstitial and intravascular spaces, which are separated in a 3:1 ratio. Thus, the intravascular space constitutes one-twelfth of the TBW.

Concentration of electrolytes in body fluids is shown in **Table 17.7.1**. Sodium and chloride are the principal electrolytes in the extracellular fluid (ECF) while potassium and phosphates are the principal electrolytes in the intracellular fluid (ICF). Electrolyte concentration of plasma is somewhat different from that of interstitial fluid.

A major determinant of movement of water between plasma and interstitial fluid, and interstitial fluid and ICF is osmolality. Water will flow from a region of low to high osmolality. Osmolality of the plasma can be calculated by the following formula:

Table 17.7.1: Electrolyte composition of body fluids.

Electrolytes	*Intracellular Fluid*	*Extracellular Fluid*	*Interstitial Fluid*
Cations (mEq/L)			
Na^+	9.0	140	147
K^+	158	4.5	4.0
Ca^+	3.0	5.0	2.5
Mg^+	30	2.0	1.0
Anions (mEq/L)			
Cl^-	4.0	103	114
HCO^-_3	10.0	25	30
Proteins	65	15	0
Phosphates	95	2.0	2.0
Organic acids	4.0	6.0	7.5
Sulfates	22	–	1.0

$$\text{Plasma osmolality} = 2 \times (\text{Serum Na}^+ \text{ in mEq/L}) + \frac{\text{Glucose (mg/dL)}}{18} + \frac{\text{Blood urea nitrogen (BUN) (mg/dL)}}{2.8}$$

Thirst is activated when extracellular fluid (ECF) water deficit is about 2.0%. It remains the major early defense mechanism against hypertonicity and dehydration. Kidneys regulate water balance and the osmolality of body fluids by controlling excretion of solutes and free water under the influence of antidiuretic hormone (ADH) and natriuretic peptides. Hypovolemia and hyperosmolarity are potent stimulus for ADH secretion.

REQUIREMENTS OF WATER AND ELECTROLYTES

Physiological requirements of fluids and electrolytes consist of the amount of water and electrolytes necessary to replace obligatory urinary and insensible water losses (ISWL), and the water required for metabolic activity. For every 100 kcals metabolized, a child requires approximately 110–115 mL of water, 3 mEq of sodium and 2.5 mEq of potassium **(Table 17.7.2)**. About 10–15 mL of water is produced in the body during oxidation of endogenous and exogenous carbohydrates, proteins and fats. Thus, for all practical purposes, 100 mL of fluid is sufficient to metabolize 100 kcals. **Table 17.7.3** shows maintenance requirements of fluids and electrolytes on the basis of body weight and surface area in a healthy child. Clinical conditions that affect water loss from the body or the total caloric expenditure require modification of normal requirement and it is given in **Tables 17.7.4 and 17.7.5.**

The fluid recommendations given in **Tables 17.7.4 and 17.7.5** can only serve as a rough guideline to initiate modified volume of maintenance of intravenous (IV) fluid in specific conditions but subsequent titration needs to be done based on ongoing volume status assessment, urine output measurement, fluid balance (positive or negative), and myocardial function. It is reasonable to use N/2 saline as maintenance fluid in all acutely ill hospitalized children.

Neonatal Period

Approximately, 70% of usual maintenance requirements are given during the first 2 days. It is gradually increased to 100% by 4–5 day. Low-birth weight infants require relatively more water. **Table 17.7.6** provides guidelines for fluid requirements in the neonate.

Sodium supplementation is started when cumulative weight loss from birth reaches greater than 6% of birth weight, after ensuring initial diuresis unless serum sodium falls to less than 130 mEq/L. Potassium supplementation usually not required till day 3 of life, and then to be started based on serum potassium level. Elemental calcium at the dose of 36–72 mg/kg/day (4–8 mL/kg/day of 10% calcium gluconate)

Table 17.7.2: Physiological losses of fluids and electrolytes.

	Losses per 100 kcals Metabolized Energy		
Source	***Water (mL)***	***Na^+ (mEq)***	***K^+ (mEq)***
Insensible losses			
Lungs	–15	0	0
Skin	–30	0.1	0.2
Stool losses	–10	0.1	0.2
Urinary losses	–55	3.0	2.0
Water for oxidation	+15		
Total for maintenance	100 mL	3.2 mEq	2.4 mEq

Table 17.7.3: Daily maintenance requirement of fluids and electrolytes (Holliday and Segar).

Requirements	***By Body Weight***	***By Surface Area***
Water		
Up to 10 kg	100 mL/kg	1,500 mL/m^2 (range 1,200–1,800 mL)
11–20 kg >20 kg	1,000 mL + 50 mL/kg for extra weight above 10 kg 1,500 mL + 20 mL/kg for extra weight above 20 kg	
Sodium	3–4 mEq/kg/day	40–60 mEq/m^2
Potassium	2–3 mEq/kg/day	30–40 mEq/m^2
Chloride	3–4 mEq/kg/day	–

Table 17.7.4: Factors increasing insensible water loss (ISWL).

Conditions Increasing Insensible Water Loss	***Change (%)***	***Volume Change (mL)***	***Modified Maintenance Fluid Volume to be Started Based on Body Surface Area (BSA)***
Prematurity	100–300	500–1,500/m^2	1,500 mL/m^2 + 500 mL/m^2
Radiant warmer	50–100	250–500/m^2	1,500 mL/m^2 + 250 mL/m^2
Phototherapy	25–50	125–250/m^2	1,500 mL/m^2 + 125 mL/m^2
Hyperventilation	20–30	100–150/m^2	1,500 mL/m^2 + 100 mL/m^2
Increased activity	5–25	25–125/m^2	1,500 mL/m^2 + 25 mL/m^2
Hyperthermia	12/°C	60/°C	1,500 mL/m^2 + 60 mL/°C

Table 17.7.5: Factors reducing insensible water loss.

Conditions Increasing Insensible Water Loss	***Change (%)***	***Volume Change (mL/ m²)***	***Modified Maintenance Fluid Volume to be Started Based on Body Surface Area (BSA) (mL/m²)***
Enclosed incubator	25–50	125–250	1,500–125
Humidified air	15–30	75–150	1,500–75
Sedation	5–25	25–125	1,500–25
Decreased activity	5–25	25–125	1,500–25
Hypothermia	5–15	25–75	1,500–25

Table 17.7.6: Neonatal fluid requirements (mL/kg/day).

Birth Weight	***Day 1***	***Day 2***	***Day 3***	***Day 4***	***Day 5***
<1,000 g	80–100	Advance fluids as per hydration status			
1,000–1,500 g	80	100	120	140	150
>1,500 g	60	80	100	120	140

would be initiated in all sick babies and babies less than 1,500 g from day 1 of life.

DEHYDRATION

Dehydration is net loss of body water. It is the most common imbalance of body water in infants and children. The most common causes are diarrhea, vomiting and excessive urinary losses (diabetes insipidus, osmotic diuresis, hyperglycemia and diuretic use).

Dehydration may be hypotonic, isotonic or hypertonic. In isotonic form, there is a proportionate loss of water and solutes from ECF. In hypotonic dehydration, the depletion of solutes (sodium, chloride) in ECF is much more than water. This leads to movement of water from ECF to ICF, causing a further contraction of ECF and shock. In hypertonic dehydration, there is an excessive loss of water proportionate to the solutes. This leads to movement of water from cells into the ECF causing intracellular dehydration.

The steps in the successful management of dehydration in infants and children include the following:

- Assessment of degree of dehydration
- Rapid restoration of intravascular volume
- Correction of total fluid deficit (rehydration therapy)
- Replacement of ongoing loses and nutritional support
- Provision of maintenance fluids and electrolytes
- Monitoring to prevent resurfacing of fluid deficit and dyselectrolytemia.

Assessment of Dehydration and Estimation of Volume Deficit

Clinical history and examination, remains the mainstay of assessment of dehydration **(Table 17.7.7)** though their reliability has been questioned. Tachycardia, decreased skin turgor, sunken eyes and fontanel, lethargic or impaired mental status and oliguria predict a more than 10% weight loss, though their reliability has been questioned. Signs and symptoms of shock are more conspicuous in hypotonic dehydration, while in hypertonic dehydration central nervous system (CNS) signs are more prominent.

Table 17.7.7: Severity of dehydration assessment.

Characteristics			
Infants	Mild 1–5%	Moderate 6–9%	Severe ≥10% (>15% shock)
Children	Mild 1–3%	Moderate 4–6%	Severe ≥7% (>9% shock)
Pulse	Normal	Tachycardia	Tachycardia, weak pulse
Systolic BP	Normal	Normal-low	Orthostatic to shock
Urine output	Decreased	Decreased	Oliguria
Buccal mucosa	Slightly dry	Dry	Parched
Anterior fontanel	Normal	Sunken	Markedly sunken
Eyes	Normal	Sunken	Markedly sunken
Skin turgor/ capillary refill	Normal	Decreased	Markedly decreased
Skin (<12 months age)	Normal	Cool	Cool, mottling, acrocyanosis

Note: In a malnourished child, subcutaneous tissue is markedly reduced. Reliance on sunken eyeball, fontanel and loss of skin turgor in these children may lead to overestimation of dehydration. On the other hand, in chubby children, dehydration may be underestimated. Thirst, dry mucosa, urine flow, metabolic acidosis and circulatory status, therefore are more reliable indicators of dehydration in these children.

Laboratory Investigations

Blood urea, serum creatinine, serum sodium level and measured osmolality may help in further categorizing the pattern of fluid and electrolyte deficits and to guide the fluid therapy.

Rapid Restoration of Intravascular Volume

Rapid expansion of intravascular volume is required to restore perfusion. This can be achieved by infusing 20–40 mL/kg 0.9% saline or Ringer's lactate solution over a 1-hour-period, followed by an additional 20–40 mL/kg if the circulation is not fully restored.

Correction of Total Fluid Deficit: Intravenous Rehydration Therapy

In severe dehydration and hypovolemia, after rapid volume restoration, IV rehydration therapy is initiated **(Table 17.7.8)**. If child can drink, he can be started on complete oral rehydration therapy after ensuring that child had passed urine and dehydration is isotonic.

Replacement of Ongoing Loses and Nutritional Support

If diarrhea continues after rehydration has been achieved, the ongoing loss can be replaced according to the stool frequency. For a large watery stool in small infants (<6 months) 50 mL/stool, larger infants (>6 months) 100 mL/stool and in older children 200 mL/stool should be replaced with close monitoring of the child.

ELECTROLYTE DISTURBANCES

Common electrolyte disorders in sick children include hyponatremia, hypernatremia, hypokalemia, hyperkalemia, hypocalcemia and hypomagnesemia.

Hyponatremia

Hyponatremia is defined as serum sodium concentration of less than 135 mEq/L. It can occur due to water retention, sodium loss or redistribution of sodium and water. Pseudohyponatremia refers to relatively low serum sodium due to the expansion of plasma volume in hyperglycemia and hyperlipidemia. Serum sodium concentration is decreased by 1.6 mEq/L for every 100 mg/dL rise of glucose concentration above 100 mg/dL.

Hyponatremia is a common occurrence in hospitalized sick children. The common causes in our experience are acute diarrhea, acute infectious disease namely pneumonia, meningitis and sepsis, heart failure, renal diseases and hepatic failure. Presence of hyponatremia generally indicates a serious illness and poor outcome.

Hyponatremia with Dehydration or Hypovolemia

This can occur due to excessive salt and water loss from gastrointestinal tract consequent to diarrhea and/or vomiting, or renal losses due to diuretic therapy, less commonly but often dramatically in congenital adrenal hyperplasia, adrenal insufficiency and cerebral salt wasting syndrome. In hyponatremia due to renal losses, urinary sodium is usually more than 20 mEq/L.

Dilutional Hyponatremia

Hyponatremia can occur in patients with congestive cardiac failure, nephrotic syndrome, or hepatic failure due to greater increase in the body water as compared to sodium content. The total body sodium in these patients is high and urinary sodium is often less than 5 mEq/L; there is relative excess of free water in conjunction with an underlying condition that impairs the ability to excrete free water.

Hyponatremia due to Syndrome of Inappropriate Antidiuretic Hormone Secretion

Hyponatremia due to syndrome of inappropriate antidiuretic hormone secretion (SIADH) requires fluid restriction to about two-thirds of the normal requirement. Furosemide (1–2 mg/kg) may be used in symptomatic patients with SIADH and in dilutional hyponatremia to remove excess water while administering hypertonic saline. The common causes are CNS disorders (infection, trauma, hypoxic ischemic encephalopathy, Guillain-Barré syndrome, cerebral malformations, and intracranial hemorrhage), pulmonary infections, cystic fibrosis, abdominal and cardiothoracic surgical procedures. Syndrome of inappropriate antidiuretic hormone (ADH) secretion has well-defined diagnostic criteria

Table 17.7.8: Recommended fluid therapy for intravenous rehydration.

Type of Fluid Therapy	*Solution*
Maintenance	5% dextrose in 0.45% saline with 20 mEq/L KCl over 24 hours
Isotonic dehydration	5% glucose in 0.45% saline with 20 mEq/L KCl given over 24 hours
Hypotonic dehydration	5% glucose in 0.9% saline with 20 mEq/L KCl given over 12 hours followed by 5% dextrose water in 0.45% saline with 20 mEq/L KCl given over the next 24 hours
Hypertonic dehydration	5% dextrose water in 0.2% saline containing 20 mEq/L KCl to be given over the number of days necessary to lower the Na^+ concentration by 10 mEq/day

Table 17.7.9: Difference between syndrome of inappropriate antidiuresis (SIADH) and cerebral salt-wasting syndrome (CSWS).

	SIADH	*CSWS*
Sodium	Low	Low
Body water	Increased	Decreased
Serum osmolality	<280 mOsm/L	Decreased
Urine osmolality	>500 mOsm/L	Increased
Urine to serum osmolality ratio	>1	>1
Urine output	Low	High
Urine Na concentration	Increased	Increased

and needs to be differentiated **(Table 17.7.9)** *from cerebral salt-wasting syndrome (CSWS) before initiating management.*

Clinical Features

Hyponatremia is often associated with state of extracellular hypoosmolality and a tendency for water to move into the cells. This movement of water in the brain, which is encased in a rigid cranium, is responsible for the most clinical manifestations of hyponatremia. These features include nausea, difficulty in concentrating, confusion, lethargy, agitation, headache, seizures, and in extreme cases brainstem herniation and death.

Hyponatremia can be acute or chronic: Chronic hyponatremia occurs when serum sodium falls slowly over a period of 48 hours. A patient with chronic hyponatremia will be less symptomatic. Acute hyponatremia occurs when serum sodium falls rapidly, in less than 48 hours. The brain does not have the opportunity to adjust to the change and brainstem herniation may occur.

Management of Hyponatremia

Treatment of acute symptomatic hyponatremia (with seizures or impaired consciousness) and serum sodium less than 120 mEq/L should be treated with IV infusion of 3% saline, 10 mL/kg at a rate of 1 mL/minute, to correct the sodium deficit by about 5 mEq/L. Rest of the correction should be achieved slowly by administration of saline (0.9% or 0.45%). The deficit may be calculated as follows:

$$\text{Sodium deficit} = 0.6 \times \text{body weight (kg)} \times (135 - \text{observed serum Na+})$$

Further correction should then proceed at an overall rate no greater than 0.5 mEq/L/hour or 12 mEq/L/day. Rapid correction may result in demyelination syndrome and cerebral pontine myelinolysis. In asymptomatic hyponatremia, sodium deficit is calculated as above but the correction is achieved over a period of 48–72 hours.

Management of syndrome of inappropriate ADH secretion: Initial aim is to correct the underlying cause. If serum sodium is below 120 mEq/L or is associated with CNS symptoms, 3% saline should be given along with furosemide (1–2 mg/kg IV). Isotonic saline or N/2 saline should never be given. Since blood volume is already expanded, fluid administration may lead to pulmonary edema and heart failure.

Management of cerebral salt-wasting syndrome: Cerebral salt-wasting syndrome has volume contraction and hyponatremia in the setting of polyuria and increased urine sodium losses. Treatment with high dose fludrocortisone (0.2–0.4 mg/day) has proven to be beneficial in some patients.

Since SIADH and cerebral salt wasting syndrome (CSWS) can occur in neurological illnesses, it is important to differentiate these two conditions **(Table 17.7.9)**.

Hypernatremia

Hypernatremia is defined as serum sodium concentration of more than 145 mEq/L. It represents a deficit of water with respect to body's sodium stores and can result from a net water loss (diarrhea, vomiting, diuresis and burns) or excessive sodium intake. It can, therefore, be associated with any state of hydration; dehydration, overhydration or normal hydration.

Hypernatremia with dehydration is common with acute diarrheal disease when water loss is more than the electrolyte losses and occasionally in patients with diabetes insipidus. Hyperventilation, fever and inadequate water intake are other factors contributory to hypernatremia. Sometimes, it may be iatrogenic due to excessive replacement of sodium in oral or IV fluids. It is commonly seen in newborn during hot summer months, especially with lactation failure.

Clinical Features

Signs of dehydration are minimal in hypernatremia as ECF is relatively preserved, skin turgor is maintained and it may feel rather doughy. Intracellular dehydration and severe hyperosmolality may cause cerebral damage with widespread cerebral hemorrhages, thromboses or subdural effusion. Hence, CNS symptoms are very prominent. Child is hyperirritable with high-pitched shrill cry. Seizures may also occur. Subsequently, progressive CNS depression may set in, leading to coma, pronounced metabolic acidosis and deep rapid breathing.

Treatment

If the child is in shock or severely dehydrated, he should receive a rapid intravenous infusion of ringer's lactate or saline (0.9%) to correct hypovolemia. The next step is to address the underlying cause.

In patients with hypernatremia that has developed over a period of hours, rapid correction (1 mEq/L/hour) is safe and improves prognosis. Slow correction is advisable in patients with hypernatremia of longer duration. The targeted fall should be 0.5 mEq/L per hour and 10 mEq/L per day. The goal is to bring serum sodium to 145 mEq/L. Peritoneal dialysis is indicated if serum sodium is 180 mEq/L or more.

If child develops convulsions during correction of hypernatremic dehydration, it is usually due to water intoxication. In such cases, 3–5 mL/kg of 3% saline or 20% mannitol should be given intravenously to reduce cerebral edema.

Disorders of Potassium Homeostasis

Normal values: Preterm up to 48 hours—3.0–6.0 mEq/L; term newborn: 3.7–5.9 mEq/L; infant: 4.1–5.3 mEq/L; child: 3.4–4.7 mEq/L; adult: 3.5–4.5 mEq/L.

Average potassium concentration in body fluids: Sweat: 4.5 mEq/L, stool water: 85–95 mEq/L. Potassium concentration falls with increasing stool volume. In severe cholera, stool potassium is less than 10 mEq/L, stomach: 10 mEq/L, biliary drainage, duodenal and ileal secretions: 5 mEq/L.

Hypokalemia

Hypokalemia is defined as a serum potassium level below 4.0 mEq/L. It occurs due to gastrointestinal (GI) losses (vomiting, diarrhea and gastric aspiration), urinary losses (prolonged use of diuretics, renal tubular acidosis, hyperaldosteronism, steroid therapy) hypomagnesemia, intracellular K^+ shift (alkalosis, therapy with β-agonists, insulin and diabetic ketoacidosis), protein-energy malnutrition, therapy with carbenicillin and in critically ill children.

Clinical Features

Potassium mainly affects bioelectric processes, including muscle contraction, nerve conduction and myocardial pacing. It can cause muscular weakness, hypotonia, diminished reflexes and paralytic ileus. Cardiac effects include various arrhythmias and electrocardiography (ECG) changes at serum potassium below 2.5 mEq/L. These include prominent U-wave, prolongation of QTc (>0.425 seconds), T-wave inversion and flattening or depression of ST segment, prolonged PR interval, sinoatrial block, and ventricular extra systole. ECG changes may not correlate with serum potassium level. Long-standing hypokalemia decreases the concentrating capacity of kidneys (hypokalemic nephropathy). Respiratory paralysis may occur in severe hypokalemia.

Treatment

- Identify and treat the underlying cause.
- Oral potassium supplementation (Syrup Potklor 15 mL = 20 mEq/L) or IV replacement (injection KCl 1 mL = 2 mEq). The concentration of potassium in IV fluid should not exceed 60 mEq/L
- Rapid correction.

Indication—serum potassium less than 2.5 mEq/L, symptomatic, ECG changes.

Around 100 mL of stock solution is made by adding 90 mL NS with 10 mL KCl. Infusing the stock solution at the rate 1.5 mL/kg/hour will deliver 0.33 mEq/kg/hour of potassium (10% KCl, 1 mL = 2 mEq) under cardiac monitoring. In severe life-threatening hypokalemia, the infusion is given with an infusion pump at a rate of 0.35–0.5 mEq/kg/hour till the ECG changes revert back to normal.

- Mg repletion, if Mg deficiency is present
- K^+ sparing diuretics can be added.

Potassium should be administered only when urinary flow is established.

Hyperkalemia

Hyperkalemia is defined as a serum potassium level of more than 5.5 mEq/L. It usually occurs due to impaired renal excretion (oliguria, acute renal failure, adrenal insufficiency and chronic renal failure), shift or release of K^+ into ECF as seen in metabolic acidosis, sepsis, acute hemolysis, acute rhabdomyolysis, and tumor lysis syndrome and tissue necrosis.

Clinical Features

Mild hyperkalemia is often asymptomatic. When severe, the effects are mainly seen on the cardiac and skeletal muscles. Muscular weakness and paresthesias, shock, bradycardia or cardiac arrhythmias may occur. Early ECG changes include prolonged PR, tall T waves, shortened QT interval and wide QRS complexes of decreased amplitude. In severe cases absent P waves, first degree heart block, sine wave (bizarre QRS complex), ventricular fibrillation and cardiac arrest may occur.

Management

The treatment modalities are as follows:

- Stop oral/IV potassium supplementation
- Check the drugs and stop those that can precipitate hyperkalemia
- Treat the underlying cause
- Hyperkalemia with ECG abnormality is an emergency. Use the measures outlined in **Table 17.7.10** for acute reduction in serum potassium.

Dialysis is recommended, if above measures are unsuccessful. Continuous venovenous hemofiltration (CVVH), hemodialysis, peritoneal dialyses are the different options available in the order of efficacy.

Hypocalcemia

Normal range of serum total calcium concentration is 8.5–10.2 mg/dL (2.1–2.5 mmol/L) and ionized calcium is 4.8–7.2 mg/dL (1.1–1.8 mmol/L). Although hypocalcemia is known to cause several signs and symptoms **(Table 17.7.11)**, it is often

Table 17.7.10: Treatment options for acute reduction in serum potassium.

Drug	*Dose*	*Onset of Action*	*Duration of Action*
Injection calcium gluconate 10%	100 mg/kg/dose (1 mL/kg/dose) IV over 5–10 minutes	1–3 minutes	30 minutes
Injection $NaHCO_3$	1–2 mEq/kg/dose IV over 5–10 minutes	10–30 minutes	2 hours
Glucose + insulin	0.5 g/kg (2 mL/kg of 25% D) 0.1 μ/kg regular insulin IV over 15–30 minutes	30 minutes	2–4 hours
Nebulized salbutamol	2.5 mg <25 kg; 5 mg >25 kg over 10 minutes		120 minutes
Sodium polystyrene resins*	0.5–1 g/kg orally/rectally	60–120 minutes	4–6 hours
Furosemide (restricted usage)	1–2 mg/kg IV/IM	15–30 minutes	4–6 hours

*Sodium polystyrene sulfonate (SPS) resin—mix each gram in 3–4 mL of water and mix with 10% dextrose and give as retention enema-retained for 15–30 minutes.

Table 17.7.11: Signs and symptoms of hypocalcemia.

- *Nervous system:* Fasciculations, muscle spasm, Chvostek's and Trousseau's signs, tetany, seizures
- *Pulmonary:* Bronchospasm
- *Cardiovascular:* Arrhythmias, hypertension or hypotension, congestive heart failure
- *Gastrointestinal:* Dysphagia, abdominal pain, biliary colic

a laboratory diagnosis because the clinical manifestations are minimal or absent.

Sepsis is often associated with hypocalcemia, mild degree of hypocalcemia (ionized calcium greater than 0.8 mmol/L or 3.2 mg/L) are usually asymptomatic. Symptomatic ionized hypocalcemia presents with neurological and cardiovascular features.

One should treat hypocalcemia if symptomatic or if the ionized calcium concentration is less than 0.8 mmol/L. The dose is 0.5–1.0 mL/kg of calcium-gluconate over 5–10 minutes followed by a continuous infusion 0.1–0.2 mL/kg hour (equal to 0.5–2 mg/kg/hour) over 2–4 hours. Thereafter, rate of elemental calcium should be maintained at a rate of 0.3–0.5 mg/kg/hour. Calcium chloride 10% solution, contains 1.36 mEq/mL or 27 mg/mL and calcium gluconate 10% solution, and has 0.45 mEq/mL or 9 mg/mL.

Hypomagnesemia and Hypermagnesemia

Magnesium is essential for maintenance of several cellular functions through its role in activation of adenosine triphosphate (ATP). Normal serum Mg^{++} concentration range between 1.5 mEq/L and 1.9 mEq/L. Hypomagnesemia can develop in a wide variety of clinical conditions such as protein energy malnutrition, malabsorption, hypoalbuminemia, sepsis, following prolonged GI suctioning, diarrhea, blood transfusion, aminoglycoside therapy, osmotic diuresis and use of diuretics, etc.

Hypomagnesemia is associated with prolonged PR interval, widened QRS-complex, ST segment depression and low amplitude T-wave on ECG. It may potentiate dysrhythmia due to hypocalcemia and digitalis toxicity. Refractory hypokalemia is a prominent feature of hypomagnesemia.

Hypermagnesemia produces tall peaked T-waves and narrow QRS complexes.

Treatment

Most patients with symptomatic magnesium depletion and normal renal function have an estimated deficit of 1–2 mEq/kg. About twice the estimated magnesium deficit is replaced at a rate of 1 mEq/kg for the first 24 hours and 0.5 mEq/kg/day for the next 3–5 days.

FLUID THERAPY IN SPECIAL SITUATIONS

Parenteral fluid therapy may be required in a wide variety of clinical situations to provide normal or adjusted maintenance fluid needs or to replace abnormal deficits as shown in **Table 17.7.12**.

Table 17.7.12: Clinical situations requiring parenteral fluid therapy.

- Maintenance fluids
  - In a comatose or sick child who is unable to take orally
- Adjusted maintenance fluids
  - Oliguria or anuria
  - Severe community-acquired pneumonia
  - Syndrome of inappropriate secretion of ADH
  - Raised ICP
  - Postoperative patient
  - Cardiac failure
  - Edema
- Maintenance plus deficit replacement and replenishment of concurrent losses of fluids:
  - Continuous gastrointestinal fluid losses (vomiting, diarrhea, nasogastric tube drainage and colostomy, etc.)
  - Burns
  - Diabetic ketoacidosis
  - Salicylate intoxication
  - Pyloric stenosis

(ADH: antidiuretic hormone; ICP: intracranial pressure)

Table 17.7.13: Average electrolyte contents of various gastrointestinal (GI) fluids (mmol/L).

GI fluids	H^+	Na^+	K^+	Cl^-	HCO_3^-
Gastric	80	40	20	150	0
Small bowel	0	130	20	120	30
Pancreatic	0	135	15	100	50

Gastrointestinal losses: Losses through nasogastric tube, ileostomy, and pancreatic fistula needs to be replaced volume for volume with a solution containing appropriate electrolytes in **Table 17.7.13**.

Increased intracranial pressure (ICP): Overhydration should be avoided, but fluid restriction as had been advocated in the past may be harmful. Close monitoring is required especially when osmotic diuretic such as mannitol is used.

Diabetic ketoacidosis: It is a hyperosmolar state and for all practical purposes most children would have an estimated fluid deficit between 8% and 10%. These patients have moderately low sodium, normal potassium and total body depletion of phosphate. Hypokalemia is a frequent occurrence once insulin therapy is started.

If in shock, patient needs fluids not insulin. Give one 20 mL/kg normal saline or ringer's lactate boluses in an hour till pulse volume returns to normal. Then give half of estimated deficit + insensible losses + ongoing losses as N/2 saline + 20 mEq/L KCl in the first 8 hours. It is followed up with half of estimated deficit + insensible losses as N/2 saline + 20 mEq/L of KCl for next 16 hours. Glucose is added when blood glucose drops down to 250 mg/dL. Accurate and frequent monitoring is essential.

Oliguria and Anuria

Fluid therapy whether oral or IV should be limited to 300–400 mL/m^2 (15–20 mL/kg or 30–40 mL/100 kcal) per day. Urinary water loss can be added to it every 4–6 hours. Non-urinary fluid losses are replaced by 10% glucose solution. Electrolytes are given only if these are being lost. Hyperkalemia or hypokalemia can occur and should be treated as discussed earlier. Patients with acute volume overload may require renal supportive therapy (peritoneal dialysis or continuous renal replacement therapy (CRRT)].

Fluid Overload

Fluid overload is common in critically ill children and is thought to contribute to oxygenation failure by increasing extravascular lung water (EVLW). Maintenance fluid calculated by Holliday-Segar formula may often overestimate the fluid requirement in acute illness state. Significant decrease in insensible water loss, altered neurohormonal response along with increased fluid administration contributes to fluid overload in this patient population.

While timely administration of fluids is lifesaving, positive fluid balance after hemodynamic stabilization is detrimental to organ function and negatively influences important outcomes in critically ill patients.

Fluid overload from intensive care unit admission is defined as a percentage equal to [fluid in (L)—fluid out (L)]/[ICU admit weight (kg)] × 100.

Management

If the child has greater than 10% of cumulative fluid overload, low dose furosemide infusion (0.1–0.4 mg/kg/hour) can be started for controlled diuresis. If the child remains unresponsive to diuretics and cumulative fluid overload increases beyond 20%, early initiation of renal replacement therapy should be strongly considered. Frequent (6–12 hourly) fluid balance calculation would help to make such decisions at the earliest. Though CRRT is the well-studied modality of renal replacement therapy in critically ill children, sustained low efficiency dialysis or peritoneal dialysis can be considered as alternatives in resource limited setting. Early initiation of renal replacement therapy may improve the prognosis in these children.

Near Drowning

Patients with clinical evidences of poor peripheral perfusion should receive volume expanders (saline, Ringer's lactate) at a rapid rate. Monitoring of the central venous pressure and acid-base values are mandatory to guide the initial therapy. Subsequent fluid and electrolyte therapy depends upon the status of serum electrolytes and complications such as cerebral edema.

ACID-BASE PHYSIOLOGY

Acid-base balance is an essential part of fluid and electrolyte management. Acid is a substance that tends to dissociate or give a hydrogen ion (proton donor) whereas base is a substance that tends to bind or associate a hydrogen ion (proton acceptor).

Normal pH of blood is 7.40 (range 7.35–7.45). As a rule of thumb, 1 mm Hg increase in $PaCO_2$ decreases pH by 0.01 and 1 mEq/L decrease in HCO_3 decreases pH by 0.02.

Disturbances in acid-base balance can occur due to primary respiratory or metabolic events. In general, if acidbase imbalance is predominantly metabolic in nature, changes in pH, HCO_3^- and $PaCO_2$ occur in the same direction (all are reduced or increased and the main alteration is in HCO_3^-). In contrast, if the disturbance is predominantly respiratory in origin, changes in HCO_3^- and arterial $PaCO_2$ are opposite to changes in pH and main alteration is in $PaCO_2$. The primary and compensatory changes always occur in the same direction.

Assessment and Identification of the Acid-base Disorder

Comprehensive History and Clinical Examination

- Information about patient's immediate environment—fraction of inspired oxygen (FiO_2), barometric pressure.
- Clinical information, including the history and physical examination with emphasis on patient's respiratory rate and vital signs, degree of respiratory effort, mental status and state of tissue perfusion.
- *Additional laboratory data*: Previous arterial blood gas (ABG) reports, electrolytes, blood sugar, blood urea nitrogen (BUN), hemoglobin or hematocrit, chest X-ray, pulmonary function tests (if available).

Identify the Disturbance

- *Assess pH*: High or low
  - *Low pH*: pH less than 7.38—acidemia
  - *High pH*: pH greater than 7.42—alkalemia
- Determine the primary acid-base disturbance **(Table 17.7.14)**
- Calculate the degree of compensation **(Table 17.7.15)**
- Calculate anion gap.

Calculate the Anion Gap

Anion gap = $Na^+ - [Cl^- + HCO_3]$. Normal anion gap ranges from 8 mEq/L to 16 mEq/L (12 ± 4) but it is variable in different laboratories. The patient may have high anion gap metabolic acidosis when the calculated anion gap is more than 16.

Metabolic Acidosis

Metabolic acidosis is a clinical disturbance characterized by decrease in plasma bicarbonate concentration and low $PaCO_2$ resulting from compensatory hyperventilation.

Causes

- *Normal anion gap acidosis*: Diarrhea, renal tubular acidosis, ureterosigmoidostomy, early stage of acute renal failure.
- *Increased anion gap acidosis*: Diabetic ketoacidosis, lactic acidosis, inborn errors of metabolism, salicylate poisoning, methanol poisoning, uremia and starvation.

Clinical Features

Manifestations of acidosis are related to the degree of acidosis. Worsening acidosis may produce hypotension, lethargy, stupor and progresses to coma. pH less than 7.2 is associated with increased risk of cardiac arrhythmias. Increased work of breathing (Kussmaul's breathing) may predispose to superimposed respiratory acidosis. Chronic acidemia results in osteopenia, muscle wasting, and growth retardation.

Table 17.7.14: Identification of the primary disturbance.

Primary Disorder	*pH*	*HCO_3*	*$PaCO_2$*	*Compensation*
Metabolic acidosis	Low	Low	N/low	Fall in $PaCO_2$, acidic urine
Metabolic alkalosis	High	High	N/high	Rise in $PaCO_2$, alkaline urine
Respiratory acidosis	Low	N/low	High	Acidic urine
Respiratory alkalosis	High	N/high	High	Alkaline urine

Examples:
1. pH 7.3, HCO_3 14 = Primary metabolic acidosis
2. pH 7.57, HCO_3 42, $PaCO_2$ 47 = Primary metabolic alkalosis
3. pH 7.57, HCO_3 18, $PaCO_2$ 18 = Primary respiratory alkalosis
4. pH 7.2, HCO_3 28, $PaCO_2$ 58 = Primary respiratory acidosis.

Table 17.7.15: Compensatory changes in $PaCO_2$ and HCO_3 in response to acidosis and alkalosis.

Primary Disorder	*Compensatory Change*	*Expected Compensation*
Metabolic acidosis fall in HCO_3	Fall in $PaCO_2$	$\Delta PaCO_2 = 1.2 \times \Delta HCO_3$
Metabolic alkalosis rise in HCO_3	Rise in $PaCO_2$	$\Delta PaCO_2 = 0.7 \times \Delta HCO_3$
Respiratory acidosis rise in $PaCO_2$	Rise in HCO_3	*Acute*: $\Delta HCO_3 = 0.1 \times \Delta PaCO_2$ *Chronic*: $\Delta HCO_3 = 0.3 \times \Delta PaCO_2$
Respiratory alkalosis fall in $PaCO_2$	Fall in HCO_3	*Acute*: $\Delta HCO_3 = 0.2 \times \Delta PaCO_2$ *Chronic*: $\Delta HCO_3 = 0.5 \times \Delta PaCO_2$

MANAGEMENT

- *Emergency measures*: Prevent further production of H^+ by ensuring a proper airway, adequate peripheral perfusion, oxygen delivery
- Treat underlying disorder if possible
- *Bicarbonate therapy*: Intravenous bicarbonate should be used very judiciously if the pH is less than 7.2 and/or HCO_3 less than 5 mEq/L aiming to raise pH to 7.2. $NaHCO_3$ needs to be diluted at 1:1 concentration for IV infusion and the amount of bicarbonate to be given = 0.3 × body weight × base deficit.

Disadvantages of $NaHCO_3$ therapy are hyperosmolality, hypernatremia, hypokalemia, decrease in ionized calcium, intracerebral acidosis, shift of oxygen dissociation curve resulting in worsening of tissue hypoxia and worsening of intracellular acidosis. Metabolic acidosis is a common occurrence in a patient with shock. Meticulous fluid therapy and successful treatment of shock automatically corrects acidosis.

Hemodialysis or peritoneal dialysis can be done to treat metabolic acidosis if severe or if associated with renal failure (uremic acidosis), or in poisonings.

Metabolic Alkalosis

Metabolic alkalosis is defined as HCO_3 greater than 28–30 mEq/L, usually with a rise in pH greater than 7.45.

Clinical Features

Symptoms are due to hypokalemia and decreased ionized calcium levels.

- *Mild metabolic alkalosis*: $HCO_3 < 36$ is asymptomatic
- *Moderate metabolic alkalosis*: HCO_3, 36–42 mEq/L can cause paresthesia, weakness, orthostatic hypotension, fatigue, muscle cramps, lethargy, hyporeflexia, muscular irritability.
- *Severe metabolic alkalosis*: $HCO_3 > 45–50$ mEq/L arrhythmias, tetany, seizures, delirium, stupor. Child may develop hypoventilation, which could result in hypoxemia, difficulty in weaning from ventilator, increased digoxin toxicity, worsening of hepatic encephalopathy.

Management

- *Chloride responsive*: Treating the underlying cause is the primary therapy. Correct the hydration status with intravenous 0.9% saline infusion at 10 mL/kg over 10–30 minutes and if there is coexisting hypokalemia, that needs to be corrected with KCl supplementation. In case of diuretic-induced metabolic alkalosis, stop the loop diuretic and it can be replaced by K sparing diuretics.
- *Chloride resistant metabolic alkalosis*: Treat the underlying cause and give potassium supplementation or potassium sparing diuretic.

Respiratory Acidosis

In respiratory acidosis there is decreased elimination of carbon dioxide from the body due to poor ventilation, which leads to accumulation of carbon dioxide. Acute respiratory acidosis is characterized by a primary rise in $PaCO_2$ above 45 mm Hg that remains at this high value up to 6–12 hours. Sustained elevation of $PaCO_2$ beyond 12 hours is defined as chronic respiratory acidosis.

Clinical Features

Signs and symptoms are related to the degree of hypercapnia. Child develops headache with either irritability or depression due to increase in ICP. There is impairment of consciousness varying from drowsiness to deep coma. Muscular tremors can occur. Tachycardia, flushing of skin or perspiration may be present. Blood pressure may be low with signs of shock. Ventricular fibrillations may occur.

Management

Treatment is directed at the underlying cause and improvement of alveolar gas exchange by assisted ventilation. Oxygen administration with high flow rates may help to wash out carbon dioxide. If hyperkalemia or ventricular fibrillation develops in a child with acute respiratory acidosis, sodium bicarbonate may be lifesaving. It should be administered after establishing ventilation.

Respiratory Alkalosis

It usually occurs due to hyperventilation; psychogenic or neurogenic. It may be one of the earliest signs of sepsis. Acute respiratory alkalosis last no longer than 6–12 hours. The compensatory response to this phase involves consumption of HCO_3 by body buffers. In the chronic phase renal suppression of H^+ ion excretion and chloride retention occurs.

Clinical Features

Usually there is hyperventilation with features of tetany as alkalosis decreases blood levels of ionized calcium.

Treatment

Breathing in a closed circuit would cause accumulation of carbon dioxide. The underlying condition should be treated. Sodium bicarbonate therapy is not indicated.

Mixed Acid-base Disorders

Mixed acid-base disturbances are conditions where more than one primary acid disturbance occurs. The four commonly encountered mixed acid-base disorders are: (1) respiratory acidosis + metabolic acidosis, (2) respiratory acidosis + metabolic alkalosis, (3) respiratory alkalosis + metabolic

Table 17.7.16: Recognition of type of disturbance in acid-base balance.

PaCO$_2$	***HCO$_3$ (mEq/L)***		
	<21	21–26	<21
>45	Combined metabolic acidosis plus respiratory acidosis	Respiratory acidosis	Mixed* metabolic plus respiratory acidosis
35–45	Metabolic acidosis	Normal	Metabolic alkalosis
<35	Mixed* metabolic acidosis plus respiratory alkalosis	Respiratory alkalosis	Combined respiratory alkalosis plus metabolic alkalosis

*pH reflects which mixed disorder is primary and which is secondary because compensation is never complete.

acidosis, and (4) respiratory alkalosis + metabolic alkalosis **(Table 17.7.16)**. The most serious acid-base disorders are of mixed type when respiratory and metabolic disturbances result in a pH change in the same direction.

MONITORING OF FLUID AND ELECTROLYTE THERAPY

During IV infusion in early resuscitation phase (0–2 hours) pulse rate, blood pressure, capillary refill time and sensorium should be monitored continuously and urine output, hourly. Subsequently recording intake and output, body weight to detect renal compensatory mechanisms or consequences due to fluid excess or deficit are the most important concerns. A chart should be maintained to record the relevant parameters at regular intervals.

Clinical parameters should be reviewed at least 6 hourly and laboratory tests every 12–24 hours to adjust intake of water and electrolytes accordingly. The young infant can concentrate urine to about 800 mOsm/L. During parenteral administration of fluids, it is best not to tax the kidneys to concentrate maximally, but provide enough fluids to achieve urine osmolality between 300 mOsm/L and 400 mOsm/L.

KEY MESSAGES

- Understanding that the body water compartments and their electrolyte composition are essential for effective fluid management.
- Current clinical evidence recommends the use of N/2 saline as maintenance fluid in all acutely ill hospitalized children.
- Clinical conditions that affect the amount of water loss or total caloric expenditure mandate the modification in the quantity of maintenance fluid.
- All children who are on parenteral fluid therapy require frequent Na, and urine output monitoring to titrate parenteral fluid and electrolyte administration.
- Signs and symptoms of shock are more conspicuous in hypotonic dehydration. Neurological signs are more prominent in hypertonic dehydration.
- Symptomatic hyponatremia requires immediate 3% saline administration at 5–10 mL/kg targeting the safe margin 120 mEq/L.
- Serum biochemical parameters along with serum and urine osmolality would help to differentiate SIADH, diabetes insipidus (DI) and CSWS as the clinical differentiation is often difficult.
- Hypomagnesemia needs to be looked for whenever there is refractory hypokalemia.
- Sodium bicarbonate therapy may not be useful in correcting high anion gap acidosis where correcting the primary cause would correct the acidosis.

BIBLIOGRAPHY

1. Adler SM, Verbalis JG. Disorders of body water homeostasis in critical illness. Endocrinol Metab Clin North Am. 2006;35(4):873-94.
2. Adrogue HJ, Madias NE. Hypernatremia. N Engl J Med. 2000;342(20):1493-9.
3. Emmett M. Anion-gap interpretation: the old and the new. Nat Clin Pract Nephrol. 2006;2(1):4-5.
4. Greenberg A. Hyperkalemia: Treatment options. Semin Nephrol. 1998;18(1):46-57.
5. Jayashree M, Singhi S. Diabetic ketoacidosis: Predictors of outcome in a pediatric intensive care unit of a developing country. Pediatr Crit Care Med. 2004;5(5):427-33.
6. Kurtz I, Nguyen MK. A simple quantitative approach to analyzing the generation of the dysnatremias. Clin Exp Nephrol. 2003;7(2):138-43.
7. Moritz ML, Ayus JC. Intravenous fluid management for the acutely ill child. Curr Opin Pediatr. 2011;23(2):186-93.
8. Singhi S, Jayashreee M. Free water excess is not the main cause for hyponatremia in critically ill children receiving conventional maintenance fluids. Indian Pediatr. 2009;46(7):577-83.
9. Singhi S, Singh J, Prasad R. Hypocalcaemia in a paediatric intensive care unit. J Trop Pediatr. 2003;49(5):298-302.
10. Singhi S. Hyponatremia in hospitalized critically ill children: current concepts. Indian J Pediatr. 2004;71(9):803-7.

17.8 Assisted Ventilation

Suchitra Ranjit

INTRODUCTION

Ventilation may be defined as the movement of air in and out of the lungs. Respiration is defined as the process of gas exchange within the lungs (external) or at the tissue level (internal). It may be spontaneous (patient breathing for himself) or assisted. Assisted ventilation involves an external device connected directly to the patient, which provides the movement of air into and out of the lung. This device may be a resuscitative bag or a mechanical ventilator.

ASSISTED VENTILATION

Mechanical ventilation may deliver a volume of gas to the patients' lungs in one of two ways.

Positive-pressure Ventilation

Positive-pressure ventilation (PPV) is applied directly to the airway which forces air down the airways and into the lungs.

Invasive versus Noninvasive Ventilation

- Invasive ventilation implies that PPV is applied directly to the patients' trachea via an endotracheal (ET) tube or tracheostomy.
- If the PPV is applied to the patients nose ± mouth via an interface (mask, prongs), the patient is said to be receiving noninvasive positive-pressure ventilation (NPPV) or simply, noninvasive ventilation (NIV).
  - Noninvasive positive pressure ventilation is generally applied to patients, who are not very sick and are alert with normal airway reflexes and hemodynamics.
  - This mode avoids many of the dreaded risks of invasive ventilation such as infections and barotrauma but needs careful patient selection to succeed.

Negative-pressure Ventilation

Negative pressure applied externally to the chest cage, which will change the pressure gradients so that gas flows from the relatively positive atmosphere to the relatively negative air spaces. Negative-pressure ventilators range from tank ventilators (iron lungs) to abdominal and thoracic cuirasses. Although these ventilators are more physiological and avoid many of the complications of endotracheal intubation and PPV, the apparatus is more cumbersome and, access to the patient is limited. Both techniques may be used in pediatric ventilation although PPV is more common by far.

BASIC TERMINOLOGY

Tidal volume (V_T): This is the volume of gas that flows in and out of the chest during quiet breathing. In adults, the normal tidal volume is 500 mL. In children, the tidal volume is 6–10 mL/kg. The current directive is to ventilate patients with low tidal volumes of about 6 mL/kg, which are considered to be lung protective.

Frequency/ventilatory rate: The rate that is initially set depends on the indications for ventilation and the physiologic norm for the patient's age.

Minute ventilation (MV): This is the product of the tidal volume and the ventilatory rate and is expressed in liters/minute (L/min).

Peak inspiratory pressure/pressure limit (PIP): This is the highest pressure during the inspiratory period and is expressed in cm H_2O. The PIP level is usually kept as low as possible since it has been implicated as one of the causes of barotrauma.

Positive end-expiratory pressure (PEEP): It is designed to keep alveoli from collapsing at the end of expiration. The technique is very useful when lungs are stiff and noncompliant and has become the mainstay of treatment of acute respiratory distress syndrome (ARDS), and pulmonary edema. Normal levels of PEEP (physiological PEEP) are 3–5 cm H_2O. Higher PEEP (10–15 cm H_2O or even greater) may be used with caution. Adverse effects of PEEP are ventilator-induced lung injury (VILI), fall in cardiac output, increased dead space leading to pCO_2 retention and increased intracranial tension. The optimal PEEP must be a balance between maintaining adequate oxygenation at safe levels of fractional inspired O_2 concentration (FiO_2) while avoiding overinflation and maintaining adequate tissue perfusion.

Inspiratory time and inspiratory: expiratory ratio (I:E ratio): The I:E ratio refers to the relationship between inspiratory time (I) and the expiratory time (E). The normal I:E ratio is usually 1:1.5 to 1:2. Adjustment of the inspiratory time is the primary method by which the I:E ratio is altered.

Fractional inspired O_2 concentration (FiO_2): It stands for fractional inspired oxygen concentration where 100% oxygen is represented as 1.0, oxygen in room air (21%) as 0.21 and so on.

Mean airway pressure (MAP): It is a measure of average positive pressure generated in the lung throughout the respiratory cycle. It is not a ventilator setting. MAP is critical factor in determining both oxygenation and the potential for barotraumas. It is determined by several factors including PIP, PEEP, inspiratory time, ventilator rate, and flow rate. Many ventilators have the ability to continuously monitor and display MAP allowing the clinician to see the effects of ventilatory adjustments on this value.

Sensitivity/trigger: This refers to the ease with which a ventilator can sense the patient's demand for a breath and is usually expressed as the amount of negative pressure (pressure trigger) or change in flow (flow trigger) that a patient must create in order for the ventilator to respond. Setting the sensitivity too high may increase the work of breathing (the patient must create a higher intrathoracic negative pressure in order to get assistance from the ventilator). Setting the sensitivity too low may lead to overtriggering and the potential for ventilator—patient dyssynchrony.

MODES OF VENTILATION

This may be broadly classified as:
- Controlled mechanical or mandatory ventilation (CMV)
- Assist mode—patient's effort is assisted by the ventilator
- Spontaneous mode—patient is predominantly breathing on his or her own with some support from the ventilator.

Controlled Mechanical Ventilation

In this mode, all breaths are initiated, sustained, and terminated by the ventilator with the patient taking no active role in the ventilatory cycle. In general, this mode is reserved for patients who have insufficient or absent ventilatory drive (either from the disease process or iatrogenically due to sedative or paralytic agents).
- CMV may be volume controlled where a preset tidal volume is delivered during a set inspiratory time at a set frequency and constant flow irrespective of the peak pressure generated. Here volume is guaranteed but pressure is variable depending on the lung mechanics.
- In pressure-controlled or pressure-limited time cycled CMV, the ventilator delivers a positive pressure up to a predetermined pressure limit of PIP above PEEP during a preset inspiratory time at a set frequency. Here, while the clinician has guarantee over the preset pressure, delivered volumes may be variable and depend on the mechanics of the patients lungs, airways, and ventilator circuit.

Assisted Modes

- *Assist-control ventilation*: This is essentially identical to the respective controlled modes except that the patient plays a significant role in initiating the breath. The patient performs only the triggering work, while the ventilator completes the remaining limiting and cycling work.
- *Intermittent mandatory ventilation (IMV) and synchronized intermittent mandatory ventilation (SIMV):*
  - Intermittent mandatory ventilation was developed as a method of partial ventilatory support to facilitate "liberation" or "weaning" from mechanical ventilation.
  - In this mode, the patient can breathe spontaneously while also receiving mandatory breaths. As the patient's respiratory function improves, the number of mandatory machine breaths may be decreased, until the patient is breathing unassisted on continuous positive airway pressure (CPAP).
  - For the spontaneous breaths, the ventilator simply acts as a source of humidified gas flow.
  - Unfortunately, there are two problems with this system:
    1. It is possible for the patient and the ventilator to inspire in series, thus "stacking" one breath on top of another, leading to high airway pressures;
    2. The workload of spontaneous breaths remains quite high—as the patient still has to inspire without assistance through an ET tube and ventilator circuit—a difficult prospect with normal lungs and a serious burden with an acute lung injury.
  - A variation of this mode, SIMV allows the mechanical breaths to be given on patient's demand. An inbuilt sensor that synchronizes the patient's spontaneous breaths up to the set rate solves the issue of breath stacking.
  - However, most neonatal ventilators deliver IMV, not SIMV as developing appropriate sensitivity and rapid response times to a tiny infant's efforts is technically more difficult.
  - The problem of excessive spontaneous effort is addressed by introducing an assisted spontaneous breathing mode—*pressure support (PS)* ventilation. PS is described in more detail in the following section.
  - The combination of SIMV-PS is sometimes used as a weaning mode in younger children.

Spontaneous Modes

Pressure Support Ventilation

- Here all the patient's sensed ventilatory efforts are supported (boosted) by the ventilator to various degrees determined by the operator. The patient's spontaneous inspiratory effort is sensed and gas flows until a preset pressure is reached which is actively sustained until the end of inspiration.

- The patient controls the breathing rate and the inspiratory and expiratory times (the I-time and E-time, respectively).
- Pressure support ventilation (PSV) has been shown to decrease inspiratory work, abolish diaphragmatic fatigue and has emerged as an important weaning mode, primarily as a standalone mode or in conjunction with SIMV.
- Weaning is facilitated since the level of pressure support may be adjusted from full to partial to none in a gradual fashion.

Continuous Positive Airway Pressure

- Continuous positive airway pressure (CPAP) is usually defined as positive pressure maintained in the airways throughout the respiratory cycle during spontaneous respiration.
- *Technical considerations of CPAP*: May devices have been developed to deliver CPAP. All work on the same principle, using a continuous gas flow, a valve to maintain positive pressure above the atmospheric pressure and a humidification device. CPAP is most commonly applied to the patient's airway via an ET tube. Other modes of application include face-mask, nasal prongs or nasopharyngeal tube.
- *Indications and applications of CPAP*: The primary indications are in acute lung injury, e.g. ARDS and hyaline membrane disease (HMD). Other conditions in which CPAP is useful include apnea, trachea-bronchomalacia, and weaning from mechanical ventilation.

CARE AND MONITORING OF THE VENTILATED PATIENT: CONSIDERATIONS

- Whenever mechanical ventilation is initiated, the caregiver has to undertake a serious responsibility since the potential for disastrous consequences of this life support technique is enormous. Close monitoring of the patient's condition is therefore essential.
- *Nutrition*: A ventilated child with an ET tube cannot be given direct oral feeds, since the tube interferes with normal swallowing, and are instead fed enterally via a nasogastric tube. The few patients in whom enteral feeding is also not possible because of ileus or abdominal pathology should receive parenteral nutrition. Whichever may be the route chosen, an attempt to meet calorie and protein requirements must be made, however, excessive carbohydrates should be avoided as it may result in increased CO_2 production.
- *Indications for sedation*: Intubation and ventilation are uncomfortable, painful and fear-provoking. Most patients receiving this therapy will require some form of sedation, which must be monitored using sedation scores, so that the lowest doses are used. The current trend is to avoid muscle relaxants as far as possible.

Prior to the use of medications to sedate the patient, it should be ensured that the ET tube is patent, in good position and well secured and the ventilator settings are appropriate and no complications (see following section) have occurred.

Monitoring of the Ventilated Patient

Clinical assessment may provide valuable information:

- Assess frequency and strength of spontaneous breathing
- Synchronization with the ventilator
- Chest wall excursion and frequency of air entry/exit
- Circulation—pulse, blood pressure (BP), systemic perfusion
- Abdominal distension, feed tolerance
- Neurobehavioral activity
- Readiness for weaning.

Radiological Assessment

Radiographs should be done at least once daily in the acute phase and whenever acute deterioration occurs. The following should be looked for:

- Position of ET tube and nasogastric tube
- Overall lung volume, evidence of hyperinflation
- Air leak syndromes—interstitial emphysema, pneumothorax, etc.
- Presence of atelectasis, pneumonia, pulmonary edema
- Heart size.

Laboratory Investigations

Arterial blood gas should be done within 20–30 minutes of initiating ventilation, after altering ventilatory settings and every 4–6 hours thereafter, unless there is a marked change in condition. After the acute phase has subsided, patients need gases infrequently, generally only in the event of change in condition. The goal should be to maintain PaO_2 60–90 mm Hg, PCO_2 35–45 mm Hg, and pH 7.35–7.45. These goals may vary markedly depending on the disease state (e.g., ARDS, intracranial hypertension, chronic respiratory disease).

Others: Complete blood counts, electrolytes, and renal function tests daily, culture of lower respiratory tract secretions when ventilator-associated pneumonia is suspected.

CAUSES OF DETERIORATION IN VENTILATED PATIENTS

Acute Deterioration

- **D**—displaced tube-in esophagus, or slipped down in right main bronchus
- **O**—obstructed tube

- **P**—pneumothorax, pneumopericardium
- **E**—equipment failure, disconnection.

Gradual Deterioration

- Partial tube occlusion
- Sepsis, pneumonia
- Myocardial dysfunction, pulmonary edema
- Biochemical—glucose, electrolyte disturbances, metabolic alkalosis.

COMPLICATIONS OF ASSISTED VENTILATION

Numerous complications may contribute to patient morbidity and mortality.

Related to Increased Airway Pressures and Lung Volume

- *Ventilator-induced lung injury (VILI):* It may be multifactorial ranging from *barotrauma, volutrauma, atelectrauma, and biotrauma*. End results may be in the form of pulmonary interstitial pneumonia, pneumothorax, pneumopericardium, pneumoperitoneum, and subcutaneous emphysema.
- Pulmonary parenchymal damage and chronic lung disease.
- Decreased cardiac filling and poor perfusion.
- Other organ dysfunction like renal, hepatic, and central nervous system (CNS).

Related to Endotracheal/Tracheostomy Tube

- Tracheal mucosal damage
- Sinusitis/middle ear infection (nasal ET tubes)
- Laryngeal edema, subglottic stenosis.

Nosocomial Infections

- Ventilator-associated pneumonias
- Ventilator-associated tracheobronchitis.

Mechanical Operational Problems

- Mechanical failure
- Alarm failure
- Inadequate humidification.

BIBLIOGRAPHY

1. Esteban A, Frutos F, Tobin MJ, et al. A comparison of four methods of weaning patients from mechanical ventilation. Spanish lung failure collaborative group. N Engl J Med. 1995;332(6):345-50.
2. Heulitt MJ, Wolf GK, Arnold JH. Mechanical ventilation. In: Nichols DG (Ed). Rogers Textbook of Pediatric Intensive Care, 4th edition. Philadelphia: Lippincott, Williams and Wilkins; 2008. pp. 508-31.
3. Heffner JE. Airway management in the critically ill patient. Crit Care Clin. 1990;6(3):533-50.
4. Martin LD, Bratton SL, Walker LK. Principles and practice of respiratory support and mechanical ventilation. In: Nichols DG (Ed). Rogers Textbook of Pediatric Intensive Care, 3rd edition. Baltimore: William and Wilkins; 1996. p. 265.

17.9 Monitoring in the Pediatric Intensive Care Unit

Bala Ramachandran

INTRODUCTION

Monitoring is an integral part of intensive care, not only to follow the progress of the patient, but also to detect deterioration early so that appropriate interventions can be instituted. Despite the availability of a variety of technological measures, the most important "monitor" continues to be a vigilant bedside nurse and physician.

Broadly speaking, monitoring can be invasive or noninvasive. The various systems that are commonly monitored include the cardiovascular, respiratory and neurological systems.

BASIC INTENSIVE CARE UNIT MONITORING

Most often, a multiparameter monitor is used to monitor the electrocardiogram (ECG), respiratory rate, pulse oximetry and noninvasive blood pressure. In addition, various options, such as invasive pressure, exhaled CO_2 and temperature, are available. The important factors in selection of a particular monitor include the parameters, cost, durability, availability and cost of spare parts and after sales service.

Noninvasive Blood Pressure

Noninvasive blood pressure uses an oscillometric technique to measure the blood pressure. Care must be taken to ensure that the correct size cuff is used. In addition, the measurement may not be accurate in patients with shock.

Pulse Oximetry

This is one of the most important modalities of monitoring in the pediatric intensive care unit (PICU). It uses a probe placed on the skin to measure the percentage of oxyhemoglobin. Pulse oximetry is invaluable in the care of seriously ill children. However, the user should be aware of its shortcomings. It may be inaccurate in patients with poor peripheral perfusion, such as hypotension or shock. Extremity movement, ambient light and abnormal hemoglobin like carboxyhemoglobin, also alters it.

Invasive Monitoring

Invasive hemodynamic monitoring is one of the mainstays of therapy in the PICU. It is used for diagnosis, surveillance and titrating response. It is especially important in patients who are hemodynamically unstable because invasive pressures have been shown to be higher than noninvasive pressures. Also invasive measurement allows continuous measurement, thereby allowing early detection of deterioration. The basic principle is that a catheter is inserted into a vessel and connected via a fluid filled noncompliant tubing system to a pressure transducer that converts the pressure into electrical signals, which are processed and displayed on the monitor. In addition to the actual pressure, valuable information can be obtained from the waveforms. One must be aware of the various factors that can affect the measurement. These include the position of the catheter, the presence of clots or air bubbles, and improper calibration or zeroing of the transducer.

Invasive monitoring is used most often to measure the arterial blood pressure. The catheter is commonly inserted into either a peripheral or the femoral artery. Catheters should not be inserted into end arteries, like the brachial artery, since a thrombus can lead to limb loss.

The same assembly is used to measure the central venous pressure. For this purpose, a catheter is inserted into a central vein, with its tip being positioned inside the thorax. The central venous catheter (CVC) is used for hemodynamic purposes. Again, the user should be aware of the various factors that can affect the central venous pressure.

A similar setup is used to noninvasively monitor the intra-abdominal pressure via an indwelling urinary catheter, allowing early detection of intra-abdominal hypertension.

A variety of newer techniques, such as PiCCO® and LiDCO™, are available. These use proprietary algorithms to measure and calculate various hemodynamic parameters, like cardiac output, systemic vascular resistance, etc. Another system, called PediaSat, continuously measures the central venous oxygen saturation via a special CVC.

Exhaled CO_2 Monitoring

This uses a sensor to measure the CO_2 in the exhaled gas and displays it either as a number (capnometry) or graphically (capnography). In addition to the numerical value, the shape of the waveform gives useful information about the pulmonary status. Exhaled CO_2 monitoring is extremely useful in that, as it can be used in conjunction with pulse oximetry, to noninvasively monitor both oxygenation and ventilation. This enables the number of blood gases required to be minimized, thereby reducing the cost of care.

Neurological Monitoring

Various techniques are available to monitor the neurological status in the PICU. These include intracranial pressure (ICP), electroencephalogram (EEG) and bispectral index (BIS).

Intracranial pressure monitoring is used in patients with head injuries and other conditions with elevated ICP. Various methods are available to monitor ICP. Most commonly, this is done with a fiberoptic intraparenchymal monitor. Alternatively, an intraventricular catheter connected to a transducer assembly can measure the ICP. This system has the advantage of allowing drainage of cerebrospinal fluid (CSF) and therefore has a therapeutic role as well.

Many patients in the PICU are admitted with seizures. In these, EEG monitoring is very useful since it allows immediate detection of seizure activity, especially nonconvulsive status epilepticus. The incorporation of a video camera allows continuous recording, so that abnormal movements often confused with seizures can be differentiated from true seizure activity.

Other forms of neurological monitoring include BIS, which measures the state of wakefulness with a forehead electrode and cerebral function monitoring.

Near infrared spectroscopy (NIRS) monitoring is a technique of measuring regional oxygenation using noninvasive sensors applied to the skin. It uses the principle that oxygenated and deoxygenated hemoglobin absorb light differently and determines the oxygenation of the tissue underneath the sensor. It is typically used by means a forehead sensor to determine cerebral oxygenation in patients undergoing cardiac surgery or those with impaired cerebral perfusion. Along with other modes of monitoring, it can give an early warning when oxygenation of the underlying brain is compromised.

Respiratory Monitoring

Both the multiparameter monitor and the ventilator provide basic monitoring of the respiratory rate. Most modern ventilators now allow monitoring of pulmonary graphics. A detailed discussion of this topic is beyond the scope of this chapter.

Other Methods of Monitoring

The use of bedside echocardiography is rapidly gaining acceptance. The initial learning curve is steep but, once trained, the technique allows rapid, repeated assessment of cardiac dysfunction, fluid accumulation in various serous cavities and pneumothorax.

Bedside noninvasive measurement of various hemodynamic parameters, especially cardiac output is now available through a variety of devices. They may be based on bioimpedance (ICON), respiratory derived cardiac output using partial CO_2 rebreathing (NICO and INNOCOR) and ultrasonic (USCOM). All have their limitations and should be used only by experienced personnel in conjunction with other methods.

BIBLIOGRAPHY

1. Hertzig JS, Evan JM, Scheckman KA. Principles of invasive monitoring. In: Zimmerman J, Fuhrman B (Eds). Pediatric Critical Care, 3rd edition. Philadelphia: Mosby Inc.; 2004. pp. 251-64.
2. Khilnani P, Irazzuta J. Monitoring in pediatric intensive care unit. In: Khilnani P (Ed). A Practical Approach to Pediatric Intensive Care. New Delhi: Jaypee Brothers Medical Publishers (P) Ltd.; 2004. pp. 45-53.
3. Scheeren TWL, Schober P, Schwarte LA. Monitoring tissue oxygenation by near infrared spectroscopy (NIRS): Background and current applications. J Clin Monit Comput. 2012;26(4):279-87.

17.10 Neurocritical Care

Soonu Udani

INTRODUCTION

Children with neurological problems account for 25–35% of admissions to pediatric intensive care units (PICUs). The most common reason for hospitalization for an acute neurological problem is an altered level of consciousness or coma. The potential causes of coma are numerous and central nervous system infections are the most common in children with nontraumatic coma. Regardless of the etiology, initial management of the comatose child involves immediate attention to sustain life and prevent secondary brain injury from hypoxia, hypercarbia, hypotension and other insults.

Box 17.10.1 gives a broad outline of the overall management and general care. Neuromuscular diseases will have issues mainly of ventilation where sensorium may be reasonably intact.

Coma is a state of altered consciousness with loss of both wakefulness and awareness of self and surroundings characterized by a state of sustained, pathologic, unarousability, unresponsiveness and absence of sleep wake cycles, which must last for at least 1 hour.

Box 17.10.1: Steps needed in the initial management.

- Airway, breathing, and circulation assessment and stabilization
- Assessment of depth coma: GCS score
- Identify and treat critical elevations in intracranial pressure
- Blood pressure management depends on considerations regarding underlying coma etiology
- Initial investigations
- Neurologic assessment
- Empirical anti-infective therapy if indicated (discussed elsewhere)
- Give specific antidotes if toxic exposures are known (discussed elsewhere)
- Imaging
- Seizure control
- Detailed history and examination
- Nursing care
- Further investigations and monitoring

(GCS: Glasgow coma scale)

ASSESSING LIFE-THREATENING AIRWAY PROBLEMS

Airway management is of paramount importance in comatose children as their protective reflexes are obtunded and they are more prone to aspiration. Even without direct trauma to the airway or respiratory system, disorders of breathing **(Table 17.10.1)** commonly accompany serious brain disorders. Abnormalities in respiratory rate and breathing pattern may indicate pathology that originates in the lungs, acidosis or nervous system dysfunction. Hypoxia and specifically a $PaO_2 < 60$ mm Hg are associated with reflex vasodilatation and increased cerebral blood flow, which will increase intracranial pressure (ICP). Hence, airway should be protected and adequate oxygenation should be ensured at the first suspicion of need. Indications for tracheal intubation are given in **Box 17.10.2**.

Rapid sequence intubation (RSI) should be performed in comatose children with due attention to cervical spine stabilization (jaw thrust not head up-chin lift). Thiopental or propofol can be used as inducing agents as they have a cerebroprotective effect, with a rapid uptake and rapid washout. Fluid loading needs to be exercised with caution if there is poor perfusion or hypotension. Midazolam with Fentanyl is a useful alternative especially in hypotensive patients. For paralysis, a nondepolarizing neuromuscular blocking agent (NMBA) like rocuronium (0.6–1.2 mg/kg) should be used. Lignocaine (1–2 mg/kg) should be administered 2–5 minutes before laryngoscopy. Correctly done, this is the safest method to prevent a surge in ICP and catecholamines during intubation. Assisted ventilation to maintain normoxia and normocarbia is then required along with continued sedation in such patients.

- Nondepolarizing neuromuscular blocking agents should never be used in neuromuscular diseases—myasthenia, Guillain-Barré syndrome (GBS), and snakebite.
- Common error: Deep coma, so no sedation required; Correct—all patients require proper RSI.

Table 17.10.1: Localization by respiratory pattern.

Pattern	Localization
Cheyne-Stokes	Bilateral cerebral hemispheres with intact brainstem, midbrain, upper pons. Metabolic (uremia, hypoxia, hypertensive)
Neurogenic hyperventilation	Midbrain, pons, raised intracranial pressure (ICP), acidosis, hypoxia
Apneustic	Mid or caudal pons, pontine infarction
Cluster breathing	Low pons/high medulla
Ataxic breathing	Medulla, pontine/cerebellar hemorrhage

Box 17.10.2: Indications for tracheal intubation.

- Loss of pharyngeal reflexes—risk of aspiration
- Apnea
- Cervical spine injury
- GCS < 10
- Decrease in GCS by > 2 irrespective of previous GCS
- Anisocoria
- Hypercarbia $PaCO_2 > 45$ mm Hg
- Hypoventilation from neuromuscular disease
- Need to control ventilation—even when the patient is hyperventilating—$PaCO_2 < 25$ mm Hg

Circulation

A drop in mean arterial pressure (MAP) will drop the cerebral perfusion pressure (CPP) and lead to secondary brain injury.

CPP = MAP–ICP is an important equation that needs to be remembered while dealing with a child with serious cerebral dysfunction. Hence, most therapies are focused on preventing rises in ICP and keeping MAP normal or high normal so that CPP stays in the range of 40 mm Hg in infants, 45–50 mm Hg in children, and > 50 mm Hg in 12 years and above.

Assessing the Level of Consciousness

This is the primary task performed when a child is first seen. A precise record of repeated examinations and assessments is essential. For consistence and interobserver accuracy, the Glasgow coma scale (GCS) with its pediatric modification is used **(Table 17.10.2)**.

Raised Intracranial Pressure

It is a fair assumption that any deeply comatose patient from whatever causes **(Box 17.10.3)** should be treated as having raised intracranial pressure (ICP) until proven otherwise. **Box 17.10.4** outlines the initial measures to reduce ICP. Cerebral edema may cause herniation syndromes (**Table 17.10.3**), which often herald deterioration and death unless ICP is lowered rapidly by medical or surgical means.

Initial and immediate management of critically raised ICP includes IV hyperosmolar therapy (mannitol or 3% saline) and temporary hyperventilation to achieve a $PaCO_2$ of 32–36 mm Hg. Excessive or prolonged hyperventilation may compromise cerebral perfusion, resulting in further hypoxic-ischemic injury.

While we may focus attention on ICP as a number easier to chase, CPP guided therapy may be a more physiological way to deliver substrate and preserve brain function. For this invasive arterial blood pressure, ICP and central lines would

Table 17.10.2: Level of consciousness—Glasgow coma scale: pediatric modification.

Eye opening	Spontaneous	Spontaneous	4
	To command	To sound	3
	To pain	To pain	2
	None	None	1
Verbal response	Oriented	Age-appropriate verbalization, orients to sound, fixes and follows, social smile	5
	Confused	Cries, but consolable	4
	Disoriented	Irritable, uncooperative, aware of environment	3
	Inappropriate words	Irritable, persistent cries, inconsistently consolable	
	Incomprehensible sounds	Inconsolable crying, unaware of environment or parents, restless, agitated	2
	None	None	1
Motor response	Obeys commands	Obeys commands, spontaneous movement	6
	Localizes pain	Localizes pain	5
	Withdraws	Withdraws	4
	Abnormal flexion to pain	Abnormal flexion to pain	3
	Abnormal extension	Abnormal extension	2
	None	None	1
Best total score			15
Usually a score of less than 12 corresponds to "coma". Children less than 2 years of age should receive full verbal score for crying after stimulation.			

Box 17.10.3: Causes of increased intracranial pressure in coma.

- Intracranial hemorrhage
- Space-occupying lesions
- Infection/inflammation and resulting edema
- Diffuse axonal injury in trauma
- Edema of infarction or contusion
- Hypertensive encephalopathy with posterior reversible edema syndrome (PRES)
- Hydrocephalus
- Posthypoxic-ischemic (Post-CPR, near drowning, inhalation injury)

Box 17.10.4: Initial measures to reduce intracranial pressure.

- Place head and neck in midline
- Elevate head end of the bed not more than 30°
- Minimize stimulation (suctioning and movement)
- Maintain normoxia (> 60 mm Hg) and normocarbia (32–36 mm Hg)
- Give normal maintenance isotonic IV fluids
- Maintain normal blood sugar and serum electrolytes
- Osmotic diuretics like mannitol (0.5–1 g/kg intravenously), or hypertonic saline 3% (5 mL/kg loading then 0.1–1 mL/kg/hour on a sliding scale) serum Na 150–155 mEq/L range
- Use controlled hyperventilation briefly if clinical signs of impending herniation appear

be needed as vasopressor support to keep mean arterial pressure high is commonly used. This could only be done with tertiary level ICU care.

Principles of Ventilation in Raised Intracranial Pressure

- Provide uniform ventilation with adequate and fixed tidal volume so as to have the least fluctuations in arterial carbon dioxide levels.
- PaO_2 > 60 mm Hg.
- $PaCO_2$ 35–39 mm Hg.
- Peak inspiratory pressure below 8 cm H_2O as far as possible.
- Central neurogenic hyperventilation may need to be overcome by sedation and paralysis to prevent the vasoconstricting effects of hypocapnia.
- Endotracheal suctioning is done only when required and should be preceded by lignocaine 1–2 mg/kg IV 2 minutes prior to suction.

Unlike a comatose child, the child with neuromuscular illness (e.g. Guillain-Barré syndrome, myasthenia gravis) will be awake after the initial period of adjustment. The chest wall has poor tone and is very compliant and VT needs to be adequate to maintain splinting and prevent atelectasis. Neuromuscular blocking agents must never be used in them as the weakness will be potentiated. Sedation and analgesia must be tailored to the level of anxiety and adaptability of the child and parents. Family interaction must be kept to a maximum.

Table 17.10.3: Herniation syndromes.

Uncal	Unilateral fixed dilated pupil
	Unilateral ptosis
	Minimal deviation of eyes on oculocephalic/ oculovestibular testing
	Hemiparesis
Diencephalic	Small or midpoint pupils reactive to light
	Full deviation of eyes on oculocephalic/ oculovestibular testing
	Flexor response to pain and/or decorticate posturing
	Hypertonia and/or hyperreflexia with extensor plantars
	Cheyne-Stokes respiration
Midbrain	Midpoint pupils, fixed to light
Upper pontine	Minimal deviation of eyes on oculocephalic/ oculovestibular testing
	Extensor response to pain and/or decerebrate posturing
	Hyperventilation
Lower pontine	Midpoint pupils, fixed to light
	No response on oculocephalic/oculovestibular testing
	No response to pain or flexion of legs only
	Flaccidity with extensor plantars
	Shallow or ataxic respiration
Medullary	Pupils dilated and fixed to light
	Slow, irregular, or gasping respiration
	Respiratory arrest with adequate cardiac output

Seizures

Seizures are common, be it trauma, febrile, nonfebrile, metabolic coma or febrile status. Around 12–25% of these may have obvious convulsive seizures and the rate of subclinical or nonconvulsive seizures or status epilepticus (NCSE) may be as high as 33–53% in some studies. These are detrimental in terms of brain metabolism and need urgent treatment and can only be diagnosed by monitoring EEG. In severe traumatic brain injury, prophylactic anticonvulsant therapy with phenytoin may be considered to reduce the incidence of early post-traumatic seizures.

Status epilepticus management protocol is shown in **Flowchart 17.10.1**.

GENERAL CARE

All neurocritically ill children should be cared in extremely controlled and well-monitored conditions. Gentle handling

Flowchart 17.10.1: Seizure algorithm.*

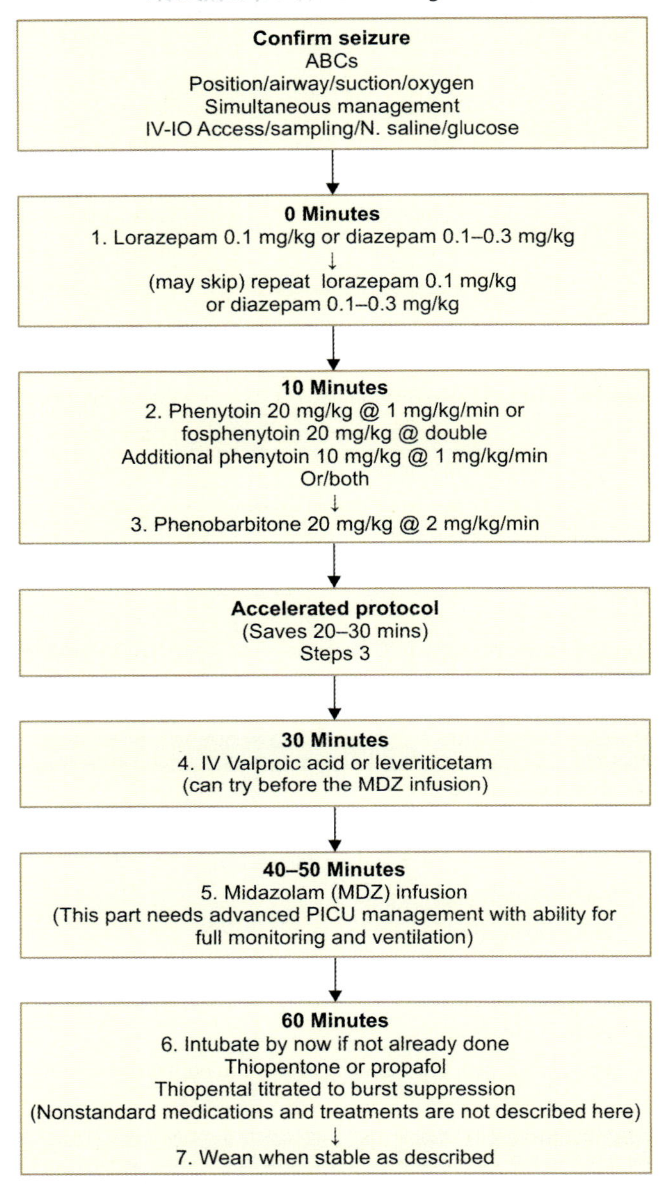

***Key messages:**
1. Prolonged status injuries the brain.
2. Attention to ABC simultaneously while treating seizures.
3. Accelerated protocol saves 30 minutes.
4. Early treatment aborts status faster and prevents BZD resistance.
5. Do not forget glucose and calcium.
6. Strict attention to hemodynamics especially in the stage of refractory status.
7. Get expert help as newer drugs and advanced treatments options may exist.
8. Treat within the facility's capabilities and transfer early.

and good protocolized nursing care is crucial. Following measures should be implemented:

- Around 30° head up unless shock contraindicates.
- Hourly pupil and GCS check and recording.
- Eye care with lubricant and closure to prevent exposure keratitis.
- Feeding at intervals to prevent hunger, gastric ulceration.
- Bladder and bowel care with soft stools to prevent pain and constipation.
- Suctioning with premedication with intravenous and endotracheal lignocaine.
- Prevention and prompt treatment of fever.
- Prompt recognition of seizures to further prevent rises in ICP.
- Bed sore and other pain check as pain can cause discomfort and raise ICP.
- Watching for development of autonomic dysfunction: sweating, tachy/bradycardia, swings in BP and temperature (in spinal injury, GBS, status epilepticus).
- Deep vein thrombosis prevention in older, heavier children.
- Steroids have no role in trauma or pyogenic meningitis.

First-line Investigations

Lumbar puncture is performed in every febrile patient with coma unless contraindicated. The contraindications include clinical features of raised ICP, focal signs, thrombocytopenia, local infection and shock. CT scan should be performed in all children with coma except those with a known cause of coma such as hypoglycemia and postictal state. CT head is abnormal in approximately 50% of cases and initial normal CT scan does not rule out an evolving lesion or raised intracranial pressure.

PROGNOSIS

In dealing with emergencies, it is best to leave prognostication for a later date and only deal with the condition of the child as it is seen, while explaining that things change from hour to hour for the first few days.

Brain Death Criteria

It often falls upon the intensivist to declare death and deal with the bereaved family. No ambiguity should exist in thought or speech when this announcement is made to the family of a child on life support. There is no turning back once this declaration is made **(Box 17.10.5)**.

Box 17.10.5: Criteria for brain death.

- Core temperature > 35°C
- Absence of reversible conditions causing coma (hypo- or hypernatremia, hypoglycemia, depressant drugs, etc.)
- Flaccid tone and absence of spontaneous or induced movements
- Apnea (complete absence of documented respiratory effort at $PaCO_2$ > 60 mm Hg
- Loss of all brainstem reflexes including mid position or fully dilated nonreacting pupils, no gag, cough or sucking reflex, absent corneal and oculovestibular reflexes
- Isoelectric electroencephalogram
- All of the above are repeated after 24 hours

These guidelines may vary slightly but remain the same in principle.

CONCLUSION

- A GCS in children of < 12 should be treated as raised ICP until proven otherwise.
- Spinal tap should be deferred until the patient is stable.
- ABCs should be a priority at all times: Hypoxia, hypercarbia and hypotension alone or in combination have devastating effects causing secondary brain injury.
- Isotonic maintenance fluids with glucose check at presentation.
- Fever, pain, seizures also contribute to secondary brain injury.
- Stepwise management of ICP is crucial to outcome.
- Appropriate investigations and treatment as per etiology.

BIBLIOGRAPHY

1. Markham C, Proctor EK, Pineda JA. Implementation strategies in pediatric neurocritical care. Curr Opin Pediatr. 2017;29(3):266-71.
2. Murphy SA, Bell MJ, Clark ME, et al. Pediatric Neurocritical Care: A Short Survey of Current Perceptions and Practices. Neurocrit Care. 2015;23(2):149-58.
3. Wainwright MS, Grimason M, Goldstein J, et al. Building a pediatric neurocritical care program: a multidisciplinary approach to clinical practice and education from the intensive care unit to the outpatient clinic. Semin Pediatr Neurol. 2014;21(4):248-54.

theater arrangements must be communicated in advance

- Safe movement of patient in and out of vehicle
- Ongoing monitoring of major organ systems during transport
- Prompt recognition and treatment of problems en route
- A transport care record should be maintained which should include the initial evaluation of the referring physician
- Treatment given during transport and any change in condition of the patient and condition of patient at the time of admission to the tertiary center apart from medications given en route must also be documented
- Safety of the patient as well as the personnel and adherence to the standard universal precautions including gloves, masks and hand washing or use of alcohol base hand rubs
- Use of restraints or stretcher belt for the patient should be always practiced. Most transport teams allow one family member to ride in front seat of the ambulance if possible
- Special considerations for air transport especially if uncompressed aircraft or helicopter—use 100% oxygen and pneumothorax must be drained if already there. If there is gastrointestinal distention or obstruction, a large bore nasogastric tube should be in place. As a general rule all drains should be kept open during air transport
- Tertiary hospital responsibility starts when transport team takes over the medical care at the referring institution.

Receiving Physician's Responsibilities

- After obtaining history, assess appropriateness of transport and dispatch team
- Document all information exchanged and record the timing of transport activation
- Advise and assist referring physician in initial stabilization of patient
- Maintain communication and provide additional recommendations as needed until transport team arrives at the receiving institution.

Pediatric transport teams are a unique service for critically ill children. Safe and timely transport saves lives. Transport can be safely and effectively performed if conducted by specially trained team, strongly supported by established protocols. The approach must be evidence based and goal directed. Legal issues can be avoided by proper communication, consents and adequate documentation of patient condition before transport, during transport and at the time of handover to the receiving institution. Some do's and don'ts are listed in **Table 17.11.3**.

Table 17.11.3: Do's and don'ts of transport.

• Do not transfer with an unstable airway
• Stabilize cervical spine
• If in doubt, intubate!
• Secure endotracheal tube
• End-tidal CO_2 ($EtCO_2$) monitoring with capnograph
• Secure all IV lines well
• Recognize tube dislodgment: $EtCO_2$ helps
• Keep the patient warm
• Repeated reassessment
• Move patient safely in and out of vehicle
• Do not give unrealistic expectation of referred hospital
• Do not sedate for "agitation" (unintubated)
• Do sedate if intubated

BIBLIOGRAPHY

1. Ajizian SJ, Nakagawa TA. Interfacility transport of the critically ill pediatric patient. Chest. 2007;132(4):1361-7.
2. Brink LW, Neuman B, Wynn J. Air transport. Pediatr Clin North Am. 1993;40(2):439-56.
3. Duke T. Transport of seriously ill children: a neglected global issue. Intensive Care Med. 2003;29(9):1414-6.
4. Johnson CM, Gonyea MT. Transport of the critically ill child. Mayo Clin Proc. 1993;68(10):982-7.
5. Khilnani P, Chhabra R. Transport of critically ill children: how to utilize resources in the developing world. Indian J Pediatr. 2008;75(6):591-8.
6. Orr RA, Felmet KA, Han Y, et al. Pediatric specialized transport teams are associated with improved outcomes. Pediatr. 2009;124(1):40-8.
7. Pon S, Notterman DA. The organization of a pediatric critical care transport program. Pediatr Clin North Am. 1993;40(2):241-61.
8. Pristas LR, Rausch T. Transport considerations for the critically ill child. Crit Care Nurs Q. 1997;20(1):72-80.
9. Reynolds M, Thomsen C, Black L, et al. The nuts and bolts of organizing and initiating a pediatric transport team. The Sutter memorial experience. Crit Care Clin. 1992;8(3):465-80.
10. Turner DA, Kleinman ME. The use of vasoactive agents via peripheral intravenous access during transport of critically ill infants and children. Pediatr Emerg Care. 2010;26(8):563-6.

Section 18

Pediatric Subspecialties

18.1 Common Behavioral Problems

Manju Mehta

INTRODUCTION

Parents often complain to the pediatrician that their child is very stubborn, does not listen to their commands, is very demanding and aggressive. School authorities may refer the child for recurrent abdominal pain. These are some examples of behavioral problems. It is important to identify these problems in the initial stages as they can be managed optimally to help the child grow normally and have balanced mental health.

DEFINITION

Behavioral problems in children are reported by parents and school teachers in the developmental period. These children are also termed as maladjusted or having emotional disturbance. They may manifest behaviors that deviate from normal behavior expected from a child of same age. These problems are related to inappropriate behaviors and feelings, unsatisfactory interpersonal relationships, school learning problem, unhappiness, physical symptoms or fears related to school or personal problems. They range from mild, short-lived periods of unacceptable behavior to more severe problems such as hyperactivity, conduct disorders and refusal to go to school. Behavioral problems may occasionally occur in any child but require to be managed by the specialist when they become frequent and disrupt school and/or family life. Children who are not able to process their behavior or lack of problem-solving skills can have trouble adjusting to a normal life and require medical and educational intervention.

PREVALENCE

Behavioral problems are very common in children, but serious disorders have been reported between 10% and 15% in different studies. With the changing sociocultural scenario behavior and emotional problems are on increase. These problems are seen in both genders, but certain problems like attention deficit hyperactivity disorder (ADHD) are more commonly seen in boys.

BEHAVIORAL AND EMOTIONAL PROBLEMS: CLASSIFICATION

Behavioral problems have a wide spectrum ranging from normal behavior, maladjustment to serious behavioral and emotional disorders. Some behavioral problems occur during the development period are transient and resolve on their own, whereas some become more complicated and need professional intervention. Criteria to label a child to be having a problem are discussed here.

Age

Certain behaviors are normal for an age, e.g. thumb sucking or enuresis in 2 years old child is normal but abnormal for 10 years old child.

Frequency

If a behavior occurs occasionally it is normal, but if it occurs very often, it is a matter of concern, e.g. a child has abdominal pain every morning before going to school.

Severity

Even a single episode of high intensity or severity requires professional attention, e.g. violent behavior, fainting, muteness, etc.

Effect on Development

Some behavior is persistent and has negative impact on growth of the child, e.g. poor concentration or hyperactivity causes decline in academic performance. One way to identify a problem in a child is if his behavior does not match the expectations within the family. If that behavior inhibits his ability to work in the classroom or interact with peers, or if he is constantly talking and disrupting other classmates and not focusing on his work, then you have an issue.

Behavioral problems can be global as well as culturally specific and ever-evolving. This affects their acceptance in the family as well as society further influencing treatment-seeking behavior, e.g. self-injury may warrant acceptance as abnormal behavior but not shyness.

Though, International Classification of Diseases and Related Health Problems (10th edition) (ICD-10) and Diagnostic and Statistical Manual of Mental Disorders (5th edition) (DSM-5) are used for classification of mental disorders in children, behavioral problems are classified as externalizing and internalizing. Externalizing behavioral problems include problems related to acting out like conduct problems, antisocial behavior, aggressiveness, inattention, hyperactivity, impulsiveness and addiction problems both drugs and internet and phone. Internalizing disorders include problems like anxiety, phobia, depression, somatic complaints, somatoform disorders and obsessive and compulsive disorders. Autism spectrum disorders and childhood onset psychosis are not included under behavioral problems, they are mental disorders.

Behavioral and emotional problems can also manifest as comorbidity with chronic physical problems like epilepsy, diabetes, nephrotic syndrome, etc. They also manifest with developmental problems like mental retardation, speech disorders and specific learning disability.

BEHAVIORAL PROBLEMS

Habit Disorders

In childhood, some habits are very persistent and cause concern to parents. These are tension-discharging phenomena such as head banging, body rocking, temper tantrums, breath holding spells, thumb sucking, nail-biting, teeth grinding (bruxism) and tics. The details are given in **Table 18.1.1**.

Conduct Disorder

Conduct disorder is defined by DSM-5 as severe repeated acts of aggression that can cause physical harms to themselves

Table 18.1.1: Habit disorders.

Problem behavior	*Meaning*	*Reason*	*Treatment*
Head banging	Rhythmic rocking and head banging in early life	Sensory stimulation or pleasure for the child who is otherwise uncared for or deprived of human touch or interaction	• Environment should be created in a way that child cannot get injured • Activities should be provided to the child, which can be comprehended by him and can engage him • Provide emotional security
Temper tantrum	• Disobedient, attention-attracting behavior on part of a child to get demands met, especially in social situations • Breath-holding spells	• The problem increases when child is recovering from an illness, fatigue or when the child is hungry. This occurs in children when parents fail to discipline a child or get manipulated by the child • Iron deficiency	• Firm, consistent parenting, early social skill training and professional intervention when severe • Role of iron supplementation
Thumb sucking	• Normal in infancy • Abnormal in preschool and above years	May start later after birth of a sibling or when in stress	• Record situation when thumb sucking is done • Occupy child in activity engaging his/her hands • Anxiety management skills • Behavioral reinforcement
Nail-biting	Common in girls and boys in middle and late childhood	It is often associated with anxiety and nervousness	Keeping the child busy and teaching anxiety management
Tics	• Repetitive movement of muscle groups that have no apparent useful function • Mostly muscles of face, neck, shoulders, trunk and hands are involved, e.g. lip smacking and grimacing, tongue thrusting, eye blinking, throat clearing • Unaccompanied by loss of consciousness • Not seen during sleep and can be controlled voluntarily for short periods of time	• Represent discharges of tension originating in emotional and physical states • Must be differentiated from involuntary movements	Combination of pharmacological and nonpharmacological treatment is effective
Teeth grinding or bruxism	• Voluntary grinding of teeth • It may create problems in dental occlusion	• Calcium deficiency • Stress mannerism • Release of tension originating in unexpressed anger or resentment	Helping the child to find ways to express that resentment may relieve the problem

and others and violate the basic rights of others or major age-appropriate societal norms or rules are violated. The persistent antisocial behavior of children and adolescents significantly, impairs their ability to function in the social or academic area. Such children are arrested as they get in conflict with law such as theft, attempt to murder, and sexual offences. The milder form is telling lies, running away from school or stealing. The rate is much higher among boys than girls.

There is evidence for two clusters of symptoms in conduct disorder:

1. Aggressiveness and
2. Delinquency.

Aggression may be directed toward people (e.g. peers) or animals (cruelty toward animals) or objects (destruction of property). Delinquency, on the other hand, includes antisocial behaviors such as lying, stealing, running away and truancy that do not primarily involve physical attack on others. The onset of these symptoms may be preceded by the presence of a difficult temperament and high level of physical aggression in preschool years.

While evaluating a child for conduct disorder, one must consider whether the reported behavior is appropriate developmentally for the age of presentation. Defiance and temper tantrums are often used by children between 1.5 years and 3 years of age when frustrated. This often resolves with time. Similarly, 2–4 years old often use lying as a method of playing with language. By observing the reactions of parents and caregivers, preschoolers learn about expectations for honesty in communication. Almost all children steal something at some point in their lives. It becomes a problem when it happens more than once or twice. Thus, certain behaviors become a symptom only when they occur at a greater frequency or persist beyond a developmentally appropriate age. Unlike the previous behaviors, however, truancy, runaway behavior, destruction of property (e.g. through fire-setting) and repeated aggression against animals or others are never developmentally appropriate.

Factors contributing to the development of conduct disorders are as follow:

- Parents who had conduct disorder, antisocial personality disorder or substance abuse disorders
- High testosterone levels
- Abusive, chaotic and neglectful family environments
- Exposure to marital conflict and physical aggression, maternal depression, large family size combined with lower socioeconomic status and early loss of either parent due to divorce.

Children with conduct disorders are often school dropouts, have specific learning disability. They may be abusing illegal substances.

Management of child with conduct disorder is described below:

- Pharmacological management for reducing aggression.
- These include individual therapy based on alliance building and behavioral principles.
- Family therapy designed to improve communication among family members and to elicit underlying conflicts is somewhat effective.
- Correctional schools can address the educational needs of juvenile delinquents.

Childhood conduct disorder often persists into adolescence and predicts antisocial behavior and alcohol or substance abuse in adulthood. In general, risk factors for poor prognosis are childhood onset (<10 years of age), high level aggression, low intelligence, early court involvement and peer rejection.

Bullying

Bullying is an intentional and unprovoked abuse of power by one or more adolescents. It causes mental distress and physical pain to the victim. Bullying is a serious problem plaguing school going adolescents, incidents of bullying among students in recent years have increased and newer methods of bullying are used. Bully victims have a higher risk for conduct problems and hyperactivity and are the most likely to have academic difficulties. Longitudinal studies have shown that adult violent criminals frequently have school records of bullying and other forms of aggressive behavior. When students are victimized, it may negatively affect their feelings of safety at school, reduce their willingness to attend school, and thereby lower their academic achievement. Even minor forms of victimizations, such as minor theft and being bullied, have been linked to these consequences and the effects of bullying may persist into adulthood and produce long term negative outcomes such as antisocial behavior, drug use and abuse, and criminal behavior. Consequences of bullying victimization can be categorized into four types:

1. Low psychological well being
2. Poor social adjustment
3. Psychological distress
4. Physical unwellness.

Adolescents who do not get emotional support at home may try to attract attention towards themselves in the classroom through bullying. In some cases, a child who is bullied sometimes ends up bullying others. Other factors such as teacher's indifference to the victims and poor disciplining by parents of bullies can also cause bullying. Some adolescents learn from their homes as their parents may encourage aggressive behaviors.

Oppositional Defiant Disorder

Oppositional defiant disorder is characterized by extreme demanding and aggressive behavior. Adolescent appropriate behaviors like increased peer group interaction, striving for independence and experimentation with risky behavior become exaggerated, severe and disruptive.

Oppositional defiant disorder is seen more often in boys. It involves temper tantrums, continuous arguing, defiance of rules, continual blaming of others and frequent use of obscene language. Adolescent has very good relationship with peers outside his immediate family. Treatment approaches are commonly employed including behavior therapy, family therapy and parent management training.

Substance Abuse

Substance abuse and alcohol are increasing like an epidemic in children and adolescents. The substances abused are inhalants—thinner, white fluid, cough syrups, smokeless tobacco (*pan masala*, *gutka*), opioids, *charas* and *ganja*. Twenty percent of children and adolescents start experimenting with alcohol and drugs by 11 years of age. Internet and phone addiction are also increasing these days. There are other psychosocial factors, which lead to addiction namely, change in lifestyle, low frustration, tolerance, easy availability of drugs and peer pressure. The clinical manifestation of substance use in children includes decline in academic performance, change in behavior, irritability, decreased interaction with family members, lying and stealing and changes in eating and sleeping behavior. These children can be assessed on detailed case history, mental status examination, tobacco and standardized psychological rating scales such as cut down, annoyed, guilty and eye opener (CAGE), teen addiction severity index and Fagerstrom test for nicotine dependence, cognitive behavior therapy and family therapy can help to control the craving and developing coping strategies. Parent training can be useful in phone addiction.

Enuresis

Enuresis (bed-wetting) is a very common problem in both boys and girls in developmental period. It is the involuntary voiding of urine not occasioned by a physical condition. The severity is determined by frequency of urination, and the quantity is not a diagnostic consideration. The child should have a mental age or chronological age of at least 5 years (DSM-5). The diagnosis of enuresis is made when urine is voided twice a week for at least three consecutive months or the bed-wetting causes significant distress to the child. While most patients have nocturnal bed-wetting, a diurnal (but during sleep) variety and a combined variety have also been described.

Enuresis is classified as persistent (primary) and regressive (secondary). In primary, the child has never been dry at night. About 75% belong to this category and is probably the result of inadequate or inappropriate toilet training (e.g. parents do not want to wake up the child in the middle of the sleep). The regressive type is often precipitated by stressful environmental events, such as birth of a sibling, marital conflict in parents or death of a family member. Bed-wetting in this case is transitory and prognosis is better. Methods to control enuresis are given in **Table 18.1.2**.

Encopresis (Soiling)

Encopresis refers to a condition of overt psychogenic soiling at inappropriate places at any age when bowel control should have been established. Encopresis is very embarrassing for the child as it leads to rejection by peer group; it also indicates a more serious emotional disturbance than enuresis. This condition was less common (around 1% of school age children), but now the problem is on increase due to early morning school timings. Some children try to postpone going to the toilet due to laziness, and then control is lost at the wrong place. Management is primarily with behavioral techniques.

Masturbation

Masturbation in children is a type of self-abuse. Children resort to this type of abuse as a means of self-pleasure. When children are lonely and insecure, they seek pleasure by self-stimulation. Though, this is a common problem in older children; yet sometimes a mother of 2–3 years old boy may report that the child rubs his genitalia against the bed repeatedly. Some children engage in this activity even in classroom. Masturbation can be one of the most embarrassing aspects of growing up, and parents feel very disturbed. Parents need to be counseled that masturbation has no physical or mental side effects until taken to an extreme. But the child goes through the fear of being caught with his pants down and brought to shame. And this fear leads to an extreme state of anxiety that would require proper counseling and therapy.

Gender Identity Disorder

Gender identity disorder (GID) manifests through a presence of strong and persistent cross-gender identification manifested by a desire to be of other sex, wearing clothes of other gender, e.g. girls dressing in boys' clothes, showing preference in

Table 18.1.2: Methods to control enuresis.

- Reward the child for dry night
- Once bed-wetting occurs, older children should be asked to wash their own clothes and soiled bedsheets
- Children should not be given any fluids after dinner
- Waking the child 1–2 hours after sleep to void urine again may help
- Punishment and humiliation by parents or siblings should be discouraged
- Stress and anxiety management for the child
- Tricyclic antidepressants

games and play of other sex. There is discomfort in one's own gender role. Both biological (hormones) and psychological factors can precipitate this behavior. In this problem, families with girl children may reinforce younger child to behave like a boy. In assessment, normal cross dressing in young age should be differentiated with persistent maladaptive behavior. In case family and child insist in corrective sex change operation, comprehensive psychological assessment is required.

Child Sexual Abuse

Victims of child sexual abuse can present with many problems such as shock, mutism, fearfulness and depressed mood. At times, some victims show high sexual arousal after once being sexually abused. Such sexually aroused children become problematic for their family members as they look at their younger siblings as a source of gratification of their increased sexual arousal. As a result, the problem of incest is commonly reported. For the management of such children, the same therapeutic approach is applied as in the post-traumatic stress disorder. Psychoeducational medical programs of both short-term and long-term types help effectively to the individual and the family members.

Pica

This disorder involves repeated or chronic ingestion of non-nutrient substances—plaster, charcoal, clay, toothpaste, paint and mud; the age of onset is usually 1–2 years. Although, tasting or mouthing of objects is normal in infants and toddlers, pica after the second year of life needs investigation. It is associated with mental retardation, iron deficiency, high frequency of maternal and paternal deprivation, family disorganization, poor supervision and low socioeconomic status. Children with pica are at increased risk for lead poisoning and parasitic infestations. Pica can be treated with a combination of education and guidance, family counseling and behavior modification and oral iron where appropriate.

Rumination Disorder

The main characteristic of this disorder is weight loss or failure to gain at the expected level because of repeated regurgitation of food without nausea or associated gastrointestinal illness. This rare condition occurs more commonly in boys and usually appears between 3 months and 14 months of age. It is potentially fatal in up to one-fourth of affected children. Behavioral treatment is directed toward positively reinforcing correct eating behavior and negatively reinforcing rumination. Parent counseling and family therapy are often necessary.

Sleep Disorders

A substantial portion of children struggles around bedtime due to difficulty in falling asleep. Many use special methods to help them fall asleep. Infants who show difficulty in establishing regular night time sleep patterns may also show general fussiness and irritability. In some household, night time is very hectic due to socializing, which causes lack of interest to sleep in children. Sleep difficulty may reflect parental strife or underlying anxiety disorder such as separation anxiety disorder. If there is conflict in parents, alcoholism, too many demands from parents on the child to excel, it can also lead to sleep problems. Children with ADHD also are reported to have sleep problems like difficulty in falling asleep, restless leg syndrome and parasomnias. Different types of parasomnias have also been described:

- Nightmares are common phenomena, occurring in the rapid eye movement (REM) phase of sleep. These occur more often in girls with affective or anxiety disorders
- Night terrors occur in the stage 4 of non-REM sleep. The child usually wakes with a scream, is confused, shows signs of intense autonomic activity (labored breathing, dilated pupils, sweating, tachycardia), and appears frightened. The patient often does not recall the incident on waking-up the next morning. They may be related to a specific developmental conflict or to a precipitating event.
- Sleepwalking or somnambulism occurs in stage 3 or 4 of non-REM sleep. There may be an associated history of enuresis or family history of sleepwalking. It is usually benign but temporal lobe epilepsy should be ruled out.
- Narcolepsy is characterized by frequent daytime naps, cataplexy, sleep paralysis and/or hypnagogic hallucinations. Polysomnographic studies, showing early onset of REM sleep following sleep onset, are required for definite diagnosis.

Some children talk in sleep about the things happened during the day. This is considered normal if it occurs occasionally and does not have impact on child's functional ability during the daytime. There are standardized rating scales to assess sleep disorders. For management, underlying cause should be assessed. Both pharmacotherapy and psychological interventions can be given.

EMOTIONAL DISORDERS

Anxiety Disorders

Anxiety fearfulness and worrying are regularly experienced as a part of normal development. When they become disabling to the point that they negatively affect social interactions and development, they are pathologic and warrant intervention. Separation anxiety disorder, social anxiety, overanxious (generalized anxiety) disorder, obsessive-compulsive disorder (OCD), phobias and post-traumatic stress disorder are all defined by occurrence of either diffuse or specific anxiety related to predictable situations. Of these, the former two are more specific in their onset at any age. The prevalence of anxiety disorders has been reported to be 6.8%.

About one-third of these children were overanxious, and another third had specific fears or phobias.

Separation Anxiety Disorder

The main characteristic of a child with separation anxiety disorder is excessive anxiety concerning separation from home or a primary caretaker. The antecedents of developmentally normal anxiety, initially present at 7–8 months of age as infants begin to differentiate from their primary caregivers.

The prevalence of this disorder has been estimated to be between 3% and 4%. There is a female predominance of 3:1. Children with separation anxiety disorder show intense anxiety to the point of panic when they are separated from their primary caretaker. They can have difficulties playing outside of home, staying with babysitters, going to school or even being alone in a part of their home. Physical symptoms (e.g. headache, abdominal pain, etc.) can occur when separation is about to occur (e.g. when going to school). Sleep disruption can occur with the child, requiring someone to stay with them till they fall asleep. They may also refuse to sleep alone. Children can worry about getting lost and never being reunited with parents. Fears about harm to the family may become exaggerated (e.g. fears of kidnappers/monsters coming into house).

Mothers of children with separation anxiety disorder very commonly have a history of psychiatric illness, especially an anxiety or a depressive disorder. Then, children can be managed by behavior therapy and family therapy.

Social Anxiety

Many teachers report the problem of excessive shyness and social anxiety among the primary school children. Children with social anxiety disorder display an excessive fear in interacting with strangers. They are overly concerned with the fear that they may do something embarrassing or humiliating, or others will think badly of them. These children constantly feel that they are being judged by others, which can lead to a great deal of self-consciousness. These children do not participate in classroom activities, which results in difficulties in integrating them into classroom environment. The management is primarily nonpharmacological. The children are given social skill training and anxiety management.

Overanxious Disorder

Children with this disorder have unrealistic worries about future events, the appropriateness of past behavior and concerns about competence. They frequently present with somatic complaints (e.g. sweating, palpitation, chest pain, difficulty in breathing, nausea, etc.) are markedly self-conscious, need large amounts of reassurance, and have trouble relaxing. These children may be managed with self-control measures like relaxation techniques—yoga and biofeedback.

Examination Anxiety

Many children before examination experience feeling of apprehension and anxiety. The anxiety begins with preparation period and becomes intense near examination. Children with this type of anxiety develop poor appetites, recurring abdominal pain, and headache and sleep disturbance. Mild cases of examination anxiety can be managed by psychological intervention. In severe cases, pharmacological treatment is required.

Phobias

Children with phobias are anxious only under specific conditions. They try to avoid specific objects or situations that automatically lead to anxiety (e.g. animals, closed or open spaces, heights, etc.). School phobias are commonly seen in children; in this, the child develops irrational fear to some aspects of school situations. The child is not able to attend school despite deep interest in studies. Though, anxiety is prominent, some children also have depressive feelings. Other complaints may be abdominal pain, vomiting, anorexia, headache and giddiness. The symptoms are usually intense or present during the school-going hours. Generally, the cause of school phobias is disturbed family relationships.

The first step of treatment is to help the child to attend school. Behavioral techniques (like graded exposure) are very effective in the management of school phobias. Parents should be given insight into the mechanism involved. Drugs may be considered when anxiety and depression are severe.

Somatoform Disorder

Somatoform disorder or conversion disorder is the most common disorder seen in child psychiatric clinics. It is the disturbance of voluntary motor or sensory system. Often, the symptoms are means to get primary and secondary gains. These patients commonly seek first consultation with the pediatrician as the symptoms are primarily physical such as pseudoseizures, aches and pains, hyperventilation, headache, vomiting and paralysis. The symptoms are variable, fluctuating, and usually do not follow any organic pathway. It occurs in both boys and girls, generally above the age of 8 years.

A variety of methods have been recommended for symptom removal such as reassurance, suggestions, behavioral modification (operant conditioning and aversive therapy), hypnosis, use of placebo and use of sedatives. Parent counseling is very important to decrease anxiety in parents and to modify their reinforcing behavior. A simple antecedent-behavior-consequence (ABC) chart may be maintained by the parents to understand the cause of the symptoms.

Recurrent Abdominal Pain

Among somatic complaints, recurrent abdominal pain is very common in young children, 80% of these have nonorganic cause for pain. The pain can occur before going to school before examination or under other stressors. These children are generally anxious, have poor coping skills and may have unrealistic high expectation in school performance. Parents also are very anxious and reinforce illness behavior in the child. Behavioral assessment helps in understanding cause, and parent's anxiety can be reduced.

Obsessive-compulsive Disorder

Children with OCD present with repetitive thoughts (obsessions) or repetitive rituals or movements (compulsions). Obsessions have been defined as intrusive thoughts, fears or images, which become imposed on the conscious mind repeatedly. The fear that some bad event might happen causes anxiety in the child. Compulsions are concerned with fears of contamination. The most common compulsions are "hand-washing" continuous checking of school words, mathematics or writing and repeated touching. The other fears are death of parent, sexual fears, moral worries about doing the right thing. This condition is treated with specialized behavioral techniques, e.g. thought stopping, graded exposure and response prevention. Often, drug treatment and behavior therapy are combined.

Depression

Depression has been on rise in children and adolescents; it presents with sadness, mood disturbance in children. It affects the child's ability to participate in relationship with parents and peers. The child is not able to enjoy activities, which he/she did earlier. It has impact on school performance also. Depressed school-aged children present with sad facial expressions, easy tears, irritability, social withdrawal, vegetative symptoms, anxiety and behavioral disturbances. They have lack of interest in activities liked earlier, there is decline in school performance and decrease in interaction with family members and friends. Delusions are uncommon in psychotically depressed prepubertal children. There is 2–4% increase in prevalence of depression with age. The prevalence of depressive disorders in childhood has been estimated to be 0.15–2.0%. Girls report significantly more depressive symptoms than boys. Depressive symptoms vary according to the age and developmental level.

CAUSES OF CHILDHOOD AND ADOLESCENT DISORDERS

Why a child behaves in an abnormal way will depend upon his/her biological and environmental factors, which include family, school and society in which he/she lives. Some behavioral problems can occur, whatever the family or home situation is. In some cases, however, stressful external events, such as moving home or divorce, may produce periods of behavioral problems. **Table 18.1.3** summarizes these factors.

ASSESSMENT OF BEHAVIORAL AND EMOTIONAL DISORDERS

Examination of the child consists of interviewing the child as well as his/her family. Often, a child's understanding of what troubles him/her may be at variance with the reports of his/her parents and teachers. Also, many behavior problems are situation-specific. For example, a child may have severe temper tantrums, only when he/she is with his/her mother or a child who is obedient at school may be destructive at home. Therefore, as a rule, information should be gathered from multiple sources (e.g. parents, peers, teachers, etc.). Child's

Table 18.1.3: Causes of behavioral and emotional problems.

	Psychosocial		
Biological	***Family***	***School***	***Culture***
• Genetic disposition • Fragile-X syndrome • Down syndrome • Brain damage • Intelligence • Temperament • Illness • Physical handicap • Fatigue • Malnutrition	• Attitudes of parents • Overprotection • Rejection • Child abuse • Discipline • Anxiety • Role model • Expectation • Time spent with child • Conflict • Parents • Family members • Alcoholism	• Stress • Self-esteem • Achievement • Peer group • Discipline • Social skills • Antisocial	• Media • Terrorism • Violence • Neighborhood • Ethnicity

behavior and cooperation may vary from time-to-time. A child may have his/her good days and bad days. A comprehensive assessment would therefore, require observing the child serially over several sessions.

Assessment for behavioral problems is carried out in the following steps:

Case History and Mental Status Examination

A detailed case history is taken from the time of conception to the present. This includes beginning of behavioral problem, development of the child, family history, family environment, child's temperament, school performance and interpersonal relationship.

The mental status examination refers to child's current abilities to understand his/her actions and interaction with the environment. The child is observed in a structured situation and standard questions are asked to assess his/her feelings and thoughts. Both case history and mental status examination are important in making diagnosis of the child.

Cognitive Assessment

On a standardized objective test, child's cognitive abilities are assessed. These include attention, concentration, verbal and performance intelligence, social maturity, adaptive behavior and memory. Attention and concentration can be assessed on digit span test, color/letter cancellation test. Verbal and performance tests of intelligence, Wechsler Intelligence Scale for Children (WISC), Malin's Intelligence Scale for Indian Children (MISIC) should be used to assess intelligence. In children less than 5 years of age, social maturity level referred as social quotient (SQ) can be assessed using Vineland Social Maturity Scale. The diagnoses of mental subnormality, specific learning disorders and developmental language disorders can be diagnosed based on these tests.

Projective Technique

Projective tests are unstructured stimulus material on which child's unconscious conflicts and thoughts are elicited. These tests are very useful in understanding the psychodynamic aspect of child's behavior and his/her interactions with family members. Some of the examples of these types of tests are Draw-a-Person Test, House-Tree-Person Test, in which a child is asked to draw a plain sheet of paper with his/her imagination. In Children's Apperception Test, child must make a story on the pictures given to him/her. They are very useful in understanding the psychopathology and planning treatment.

Rating Scales and Questionnaires

Rating scales and questionnaires are objective methods to assess psychopathology and personality of the child. Parents or teachers rate the rating scales. Self-rating scales are used for adolescents. The well-known checklists for children are:

- Child Behavior Checklist (CBCL)
- Conner's Rating Scale for assessment of ADHD, parent and teacher versions.

Examples of self-report instruments are:

- Child Depression Inventory (CDI),
- Strength and Difficulty Questionnaire (SDQ), and
- Perceived Competence Scale (PCS).

There are Indian standardized rating scales and norms available for the assessment. One example of the Indian rating scales is—Developmental Psychopathology Checklist for Children (Kapur, 1995).

Behavioral Assessment of a Child

Child's behavior is systematically observed and recorded, according to antecedents (situations), feeling, thought, behavior and consequences. Parent can be involved in this recording. Older children can do this on their own.

PREVENTION

Majority of behavioral problems in the child arise from a complex interaction between child and environmental characteristics, related to situational family stresses psychoeducation to parents and members of extended family if staying together can help in reducing anxiety in the child and to modify family environment. Pediatrician can help parents cope with troublesome behaviors through education and brief intervention techniques such as behavior modification. In addition, the pediatrician can help to promote "competence" by teaching parents how to interact with their children in more affectionately and cognitively stimulating ways. By providing parenting skills, high expectations from the child can be lowered, his/her needs and uniqueness can be appreciated. In this current situation, parents want the child to be perfect, strong, smart and quick. He/she may be humiliated for not living up to the expectations of the parents. Thus, parents should create an environment in the family to make the child comfortable and anxiety free. Providing parents with knowledge and helping the child to develop emotional regulation will help in preventing behavioral problems. Parents' own anxiety should be under control. The expectations from the child should be proportionate to the child's cognitive and physical ability.

PRACTICE GUIDELINES

National Institute for Health and Clinical Excellence (NICE), World Health Organization (WHO), American Academy of Child and Adolescent Psychiatry and Indian

Psychiatric Society (Child Psychiatry Section) have developed detailed practice guidelines. Details can be seen on www.iacap.org. According to these guidelines, the ultimate judgment regarding treatment must be made by the clinician, depending on the clinical evidence provided by the patient and his/her parents. The treatment will be carried out, according to the options and resources available. They have developed pocket cards for each disorder, which include key points, diagnosis and evaluation procedure, criteria for diagnosis and treatment algorithm.

PRACTICE POINTS/TIPS

Management should begin with an explanation to the parents of the diagnosis, its probable cause, the way in which the child can be helped and the likely outcome. It is important to reassure parents, as they play an important role in management of their children. Coping strategies and skill building can be done in play manner. As much as possible, sick role should not be given to the child.

Certain elements of standard pharmacological treatment require modification when treating disorders in the context of the developing body and brain. The potential for long-term adverse effects in children of psychotropic drugs on the development of brain and body is of critical concern. Indeed, there are at least two instances of age-related effects of drugs on biological development:

1. The slowing of body growth by psychostimulants (like methylphenidate).
2. The hepatotoxicity induced by valproate.

Due to these fears, the clinician will need to carefully consider if pharmacological treatments are required at all.

SUMMARY

Availability of parents in developing years of the child, consistent discipline style, understanding uniqueness of the child and ability in parent to control their negative emotions will help the child to have positive mental health.

BIBLIOGRAPHY

1. American Psychiatric Association. Diagnostic and Statistical Manual of Mental Disorders, 4th edition - Text Revision (DSM-IV-TR). Washington: American Psychiatric Publishing Inc.; 2000.
2. Bailey A, Philips W, Rutter M. Autism: towards an integration of clinical, genetic, neuropsychological, and neurobiological perspectives. J Child Psychol Psychiatry. 1996;37(1):89-126.
3. Conners CK. Conner's Rating Scales—revised technical manual. Toronto: Multi Health Systems; 1997.
4. Dhalla S, Kopec JA. The CAGE questionnaire for alcohol misuse: a review of reliability and validity studies. Clin Invest Med. 2007;30(1):33-41.
5. Harter S. The perceived competence scale for children. Child Dev. 1982;53(1):87-97.
6. Kaminer Y. The Teen Addiction Severity Index around the Globe: The Tower of Babel revisited. Subst Abus. 2008;29(3):89-94.
7. Kapur M. Psychological management of childhood problems. In: Kapur M (Ed). Mental Health of Indian Children. New Delhi: Sage Publications; 1995.
8. Machover K. Drawing of the human figure: a method of personality investigation. In: Anderson HH, Anderson GL (Eds). An Introduction to Projective Techniques. New York: Prentice Hall; 1951.
9. Mehta M, Pilania VM. Bullying in Indian School Going Adolescents. Indian J Pediatr. 2014;81(11):1143-4.
10. Peterson B S. Neuroimaging in child and adolescent neuropsychiatric disorders. J Am Acad Child Adolesc Psychiatry. 1995;34(12):1560-76.

18.2 Common Surgical Problems

Ketan Parikh

INGUINAL HERNIA AND HYDROCELE

It is the persistence of patency of the processus vaginalis through which the abdominal contents descend into the inguinoscrotal region.

Embryology

During the process of testicular descent antenatally, a tongue of peritoneal fold, the "processus vaginalis" envelops the testis traversing through the inguinal canal. Normally, its communication with the peritoneal cavity should seal off by birth. The persistence of this communication in a variable portion of its extent is termed "patent processus vaginalis" (PPV) **(Fig. 18.2.1)** and may lead to hernia/hydrocele or an encysted hydrocele of the cord.

Inguinal Hernia

- *Incidence:* 3–4% of children are affected but the incidence can rise to 30% in premature babies.
- Male: female ratio—6:1.
- *Presentation:* Any time after birth but most commonly around 1 year and thus the term "congenital" is a misnomer in most cases.
- *A swelling in the groin or the scrotum:*
  - Bilateral in a small number of cases.
  - Often a history of increase in the size of swelling on crying or any activity which increases intra-abdominal pressure.
  - The swelling is reducible unless incarcerated or strangulated.
- Palpation of the root of the scrotum after reduction gives a characteristic "silk glove" feeling.
- *Investigations:* No diagnostic investigations routinely recommended.
- *Ultrasonography (USG) (inguinal region):* USG may help to differentiate from a hydrocele; however, an intermittent hernia may be missed during imaging, especially in a sedated child.
- *Diagnostic laparoscopy to identify a PPV:* Recommended only in select situations **(Fig. 18.2.2)**.
- *Complications*: An inguinal hernia has a high chance of complications in the form of irreducibility, obstruction and strangulation.
  - Higher chance of complication in premature babies, (as high as 50% in the first 3 months); hence, they should be operated early.
  - On strangulation, the edematous and congested sac presses onto the testicular vessels causing a variable degree of testicular ischemia and resultant testicular dysfunction.
  - In most children, the contents of a hernia are bowel or ovary (in females) and thus strangulation can lead to intestinal gangrene and potentially fatal peritonitis or ovarian gangrene **(Figs. 18.2.3 and 18.2.4)**.
  - The overall surgical complication rate of an obstructed hernia is 10 times more than an unobstructed hernia.
  - *Apneic spells:* Premature babies with hernia are known to suffer apneic spells.

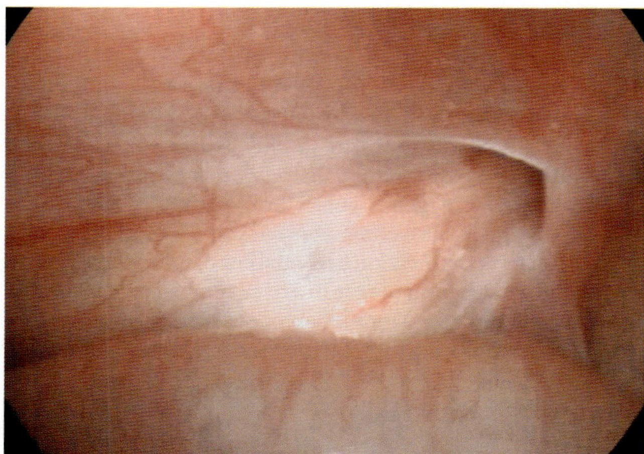

Fig. 18.2.2: A patent processus vaginalis as seen during laparoscopy.

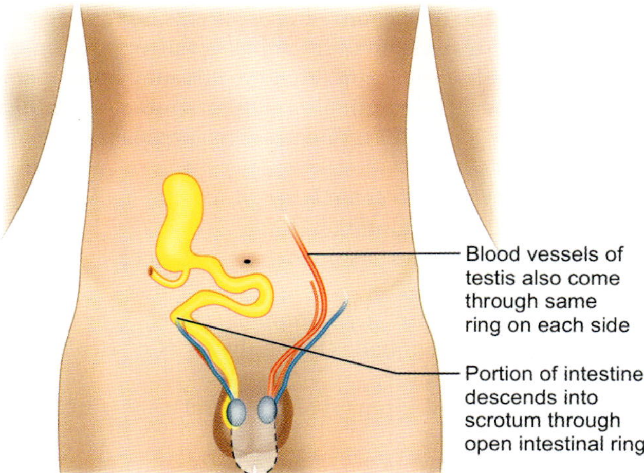

Fig. 18.2.1: Diagrammatic representation of intestines (yellow) passing through patent processus vaginalis.

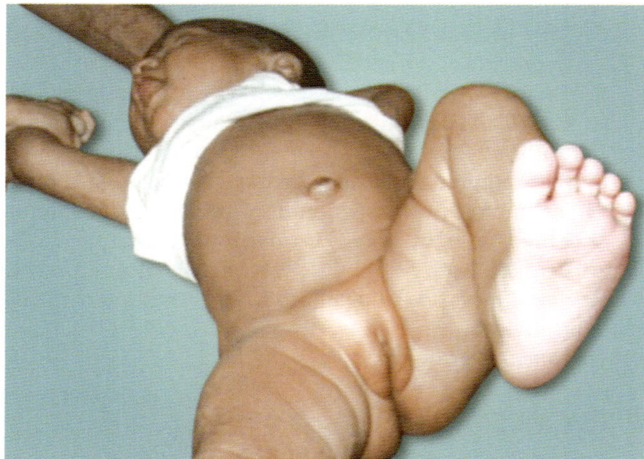

Fig. 18.2.3: Acute right groin swelling in a female child—strangulated hernia.

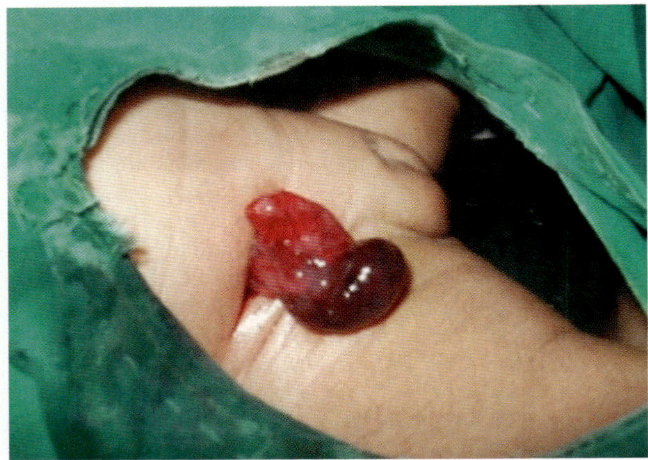

Fig. 18.2.4: Gangrenous ovary in a strangulated hernia.

- *Treatment*: Surgery (herniotomy) should be advised as soon as a hernia is diagnosed. Traditionally, performed through a small incision in the ipsilateral groin, the communication with the peritoneum is exposed, divided and ligated. In recent years, herniotomy is also being done by the laparoscopic approach. This modality offers significant magnification and enables the dissection of the vas and vessels from the sac in a relatively easier area (where there are less adhesions). Laparoscopy can also detect a contralateral PPV, which can be tackled simultaneously.

Congenital Hydrocele

Structurally, a hydrocele is a PPV where the communication with peritoneal cavity is very narrow, permitting only peritoneal fluid into the sac.

- *Clinical presentation:* An inguinoscrotal or a scrotal swelling:
  - May be restricted to the inguinal region (encysted hydrocele of the cord)
  - Diurnal variation in the size of swelling possible.
  - Usually, not easily reducible because of inverted ink-bottle effect.
- Unlike an inguinal hernia, a hydrocele has a high chance of resolution in the first 6 months of life. Since the contents are only fluid, a hydrocele is not prone to complications and thus surgery can be deferred till after infancy. However, in the event of a hernia, an early surgery needs to be advised.
- *Treatment*: Herniotomy.

KEY MESSAGES

- An inguinal hernia in a child needs to be operated at whichever age it is identified with minimal delay to avoid preventable complications.
- The parents must be warned to identify complications when first consulted for a swelling in the groin.

UNDESCENDED TESTES

Undescended testes (UDT) results from a failure of the testis to complete its normal descent into the scrotum.

Embryology and Incidence

Although the incidence of UDT is almost 3% in the term "neonate", it drops to only 0.8% at about 6 months. Most of this postnatal descent is complete by the 1st month in a term "neonate". The exact cause of non-descent is not always known.

Clinical Features

- The scrotum on the side of nondescent will be empty and less developed than the contralateral normal side and the testis is not palpable within it.
- The testis may be palpable in the inguinal region.

Various locations of UDT have been described, but clinically the most relevant is to differentiate a palpable gonad from an impalpable one. Careful clinical examination can identify an extra-abdominal gonad in most cases. Inability to palpate the testis along the path of descent would indicate either of these possibilities:

- *Retractile testis:* After a normal descent, the testis may get pulled up due to the hyperactive cremasteric reflex and may temporarily become intra-inguinal. It may become palpable by examining the child in a squatting position or by milking the testis down the inguinal canal. The scrotum is well-formed, and the testis can definitely be located in the scrotum in sleep. An ultrasound examination may misdiagnose these cases as UDT. In most cases, this condition does not require any medical/surgical treatment and only counseling of parents is required.
- An ectopic testis is one, which has got diverted from the normal path of descent. Such a testis may be palpable in the superficial inguinal pouch, prepubic or perineal locations. All these cases need surgical repositioning into the scrotal sac.
- *A nonpalpable testis could be:*
  - A high intra-abdominal UDT
  - An atrophied testis due to a vascular accident such as torsion
  - *Disorder of sex development (DSD):* Wherein the nonpalpable gonad is either dysgenetic/streak gonad or ovotestis/ovary
  - True nondevelopment of ipsilateral testis (rare).

INVESTIGATIONS

- *Imaging:* USG/computed tomography (CT)/magnetic resonance imaging (MRI)/radioisotope scanning where they may pick up testicular tissue, but the sensitivity and specificity do not justify their routine use.

- *Diagnostic laparoscopy:* It is the only reliable investigation in UDT. It enables identification of the site of the gonad, its gross structural configuration and also gives a clue to the need for a single/2-stage orchidopexy.

Complications of an Untreated UDT

- *Prone to infertility:* Intra-abdominal temperature, which is higher than the scrotal temperature, affects germ cell maturation and the fertility potential of the UDT. Ultramicroscopic changes in the seminiferous tubules have been conclusively documented beyond the age of 1 year in an UDT.
- *Prone to trauma:* In the inguinal region, the testis can get damaged due to blunt trauma.
- *Prone to torsion:* The UDT is significantly more prone to torsion and may present as an acute abdomen or as an enlarged tender mass in the groin.
- *Prone to tumor:* Undescended testes are approximately 50 times more prone to malignant change. The propensity may be decreased by early orchidopexy.
- *An accompanying inguinal hernia* on the ipsilateral side could develop its own complications as discussed above.

Treatment

- The testis is extremely unlikely to descend after 6 months of age.
- Efficacy of hormonal treatment has not been proved.
- Only surgical treatment has withstood the test of time universally.
- Desirable to complete therapy by the age of 1 year. Since there may be a need for a two-staged procedure in selected cases, a patient with UDT should undergo his first pediatric surgical assessment by 6 months of age and surgery between the ages of 6 months and 1 year.

Earlier surgery is indicated in case of:

- *Presence of an ipsilateral hernia:* Since the hernia needs surgery as early as possible, the orchidopexy should be combined with this surgery, may be done before 6 months of age in such cases.
- *Any other complication:* Since UDT has a high chance of undergoing torsion, the parents of a child with UDT need to be warned (during the period of observation before 6 months age) that in the event of an acute inflammation in the inguinal region, an urgent surgery may be warranted to derotate the torsion and bring the testis down into the scrotum.

Procedure

Surgery for UDT involves: Locating the testis, releasing the vascular pedicle from the retroperitoneal tissues to mobilize the testis up to the scrotum and securing the same in the ipsilateral scrotum.

Recent Advances

In a nonpalpable testis, laparoscopy has emerged as an important modality to locate the testis or confirm its atrophy or absence. It can also be used to mobilize the retroperitoneal vessels in UDT. Additionally, it helps effectively to stage the procedure in case of a high intra-abdominal testis with a short vascular supply.

KEY MESSAGES

- A patient with UDT should get his first pediatric surgical assessment latest by the age of 6 months.
- The testis should be brought down into the scrotum by the age of 1 year.
- In case of an ipsilateral hernia, an earlier surgery is necessary.

TESTICULAR TORSION

Testicular torsion signifies a twist of vascular pedicle of the testis. It can occur at any age including the neonatal age.

Clinical Features

- A history of sudden onset of pain in the scrotum with redness and swelling on that side.
- The testis itself is tender and swollen **(Fig. 18.2.5)**.
- In case of neonatal torsion, symptoms are much milder.

Differential Diagnosis

Cellulitis, epididymo-orchitis.

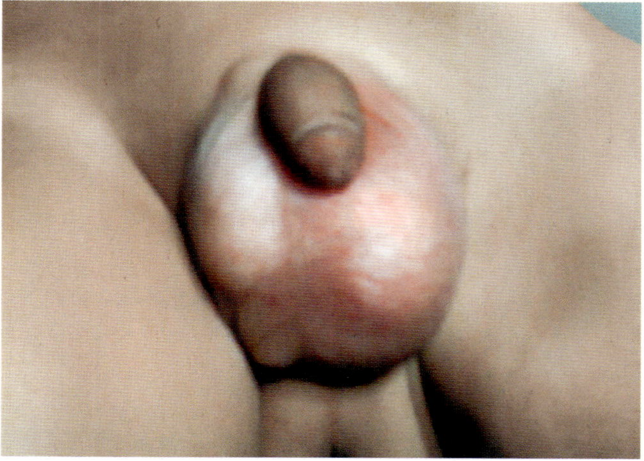

Fig. 18.2.5: Left testicular torsion.

patients, the prepuce is deficient ventrally, and the preputial skin gets concentrated onto the dorsum of the penis forming a cape like hood (dorsal hood). In many cases, there is also an accompanying ventral curvature of the penis (chordee) **(Fig. 18.2.10)**. Additionally, there may be a meatal stenosis leading to a very thin (needle point) stream of urine and straining.

A multifactorial genetic inheritance pattern has been documented in a few cases. The more severe varieties may also have penile shortening and a bifid scrotum. Some of these cases may also have disorders of sexual development **(Fig. 18.2.11)**.

Principles of Management

Meatal stenosis, if present, should be corrected at the earliest because it can lead to obstructive uropathy.

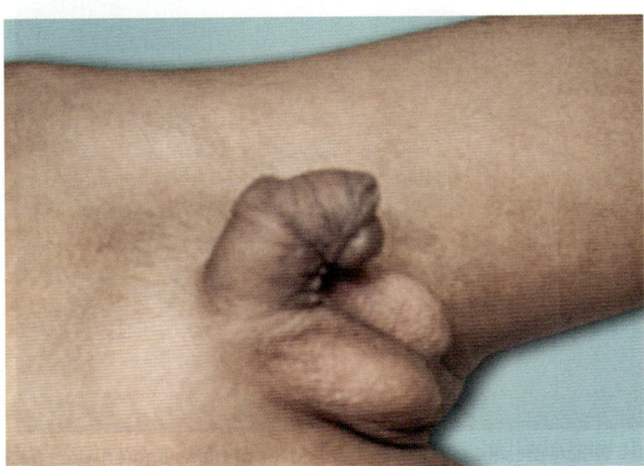

Fig. 18.2.10: Chordee in case of hypospadias.

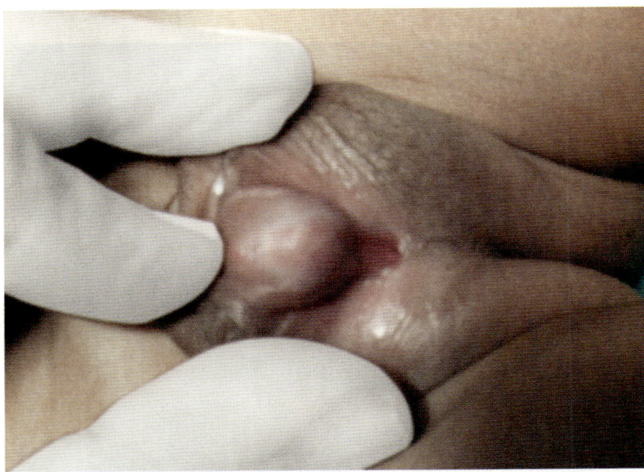

Fig. 18.2.11: Hypospadias with right undescended testes (UDT)—a case of true hermaphroditism.

- Distal hypospadias without chordee are compatible with a normal urinary and sexual function. Treatment in these cases is predominantly for cosmetic and psychological satisfaction.
- Proximal hypospadias may affect fertility.
- Correction of chordee must precede the urethroplasty either in two stages or as a combined single surgery.
- Tissue used for the urethral reconstruction should be hair-free skin or nonmucus secreting mucosa.
- *Timing of the repair:* All the stages of repair should be completed before the child is school-going. Generally speaking, surgery for proximal hypospadias between 6 months and 1 year, and the more severe varieties between 12 months and 24 months.
- *Epispadias:* In this much rare condition, the urethral opening is situated dorsally on the penis.

  The more proximal variety is associated with urinary incontinence.

UMBILICAL HERNIA

Umbilical hernia is the protrusion of the intra-abdominal contents through a weakness in the umbilical fascia into a skin-lined sac. Idiopathic in most cases, may rarely be associated with hypothyroidism, Trisomy 13 or 18 and Beckwith-Wiedemann syndrome.

- A variable protrusion of the umbilicus, which increases on crying or straining.
- Palpable defect in the umbilical ring.
- *Outcome*: Most hernias close spontaneously by the age of 2–3 years.
- *Surgery* is indicated for persistent hernia or in case of complications.
- *Complications*: Irreducibility, strangulation or fear of strangulation.

RECTAL POLYP

Rectal polyp is a benign adenomatous polyp, usually single.

- Common in the age group of 3–6 years.
- *Clinically presents as:*
  - Bleeding per rectum (PR)—fresh blood in drops at the time of defecation
  - Something coming out PR **(Fig. 18.2.12)**.
- Polyp may be felt on digital examination
- It needs to be removed surgically.

RECTAL PROLAPSE

Something coming out per rectum (PR) **(Fig. 18.2.13)**

- Bleeding may be associated
- *Predisposing factors*: Constipation, diarrhea, severe cough
- *Treatment*:
  - Of the predisposing factors.

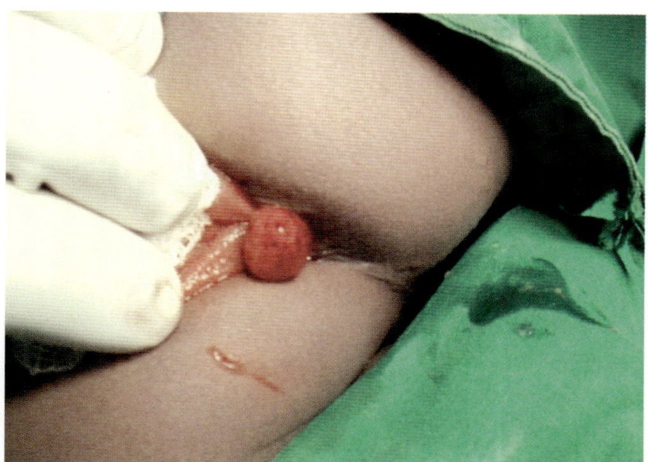

Fig. 18.2.12: Rectal polyp.

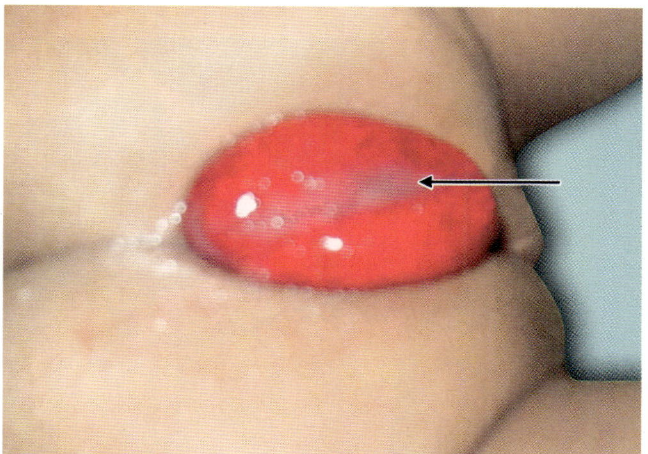

Fig. 18.2.13: Prolapse of rectum—arrow points to the lumen in the center of the prolapse to differentiate from a prolapsed polyp.

- Submucosal sclerosant injections—usually curative.
- Per-rectal/abdominal or laparoscopic surgery required in very rare cases.

CLEFT LIP AND PALATE

Embryology

The mouth and the lips are formed by a fusion of five processes of mesenchyme. Cleft lip and cleft palate result due to a variable failure of this fusion process **(Fig. 18.2.14)**. In 12% of the cases, the condition is familial.

Cleft Palate

- *Feeding:* Problems with sucking are dealt with by special teats or spoon feeding. However, in most cases, the Indian mother learns to place nipple to the side of mouth and the child manages to suck on the breast.
- *Speech:* Nasal twang is often seen even after successful repair.
- *Breathing:* A special mention must be made of the child with a cleft palate and a short mandible—Pierre Robin syndrome—these babies have a tendency of tongue fall and choking.
- *Infections:* Recurrent upper respiratory tract infection (URTI/URI) and middle ear infection due to the free communication between the oral and nasal cavities.

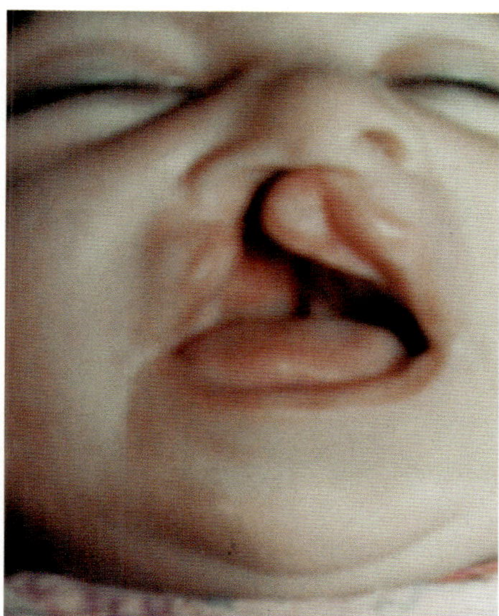

Fig. 18.2.14: Complete cleft of the lip and palate—unilateral.

Treatment

- Surgical correction of the lip—often advised early to protect parents from psychological trauma. Early repair also allows proper moulding of the alveolus for better long-term results.
- Classically—at 10 weeks, 10 lbs. weight and hemoglobin (Hb) of 10 g/dL; however, some centers repair the lip at birth.
- Repair of the palate between 9 months and 12 months.

BRANCHIAL FISTULA/SINUS

Remnants or anomalies of the branchial apparatus lead to congenital anomalies, e.g. branchial fistula, sinus or cyst in that order of frequency **(Fig. 18.2.15)**. Usually, the external opening of the fistula lies in the lower third of the neck near the anterior border of the sternomastoid muscle. The tract penetrates deeper and traverses within the bifurcation of the common carotid artery toward the tonsillar fossa.

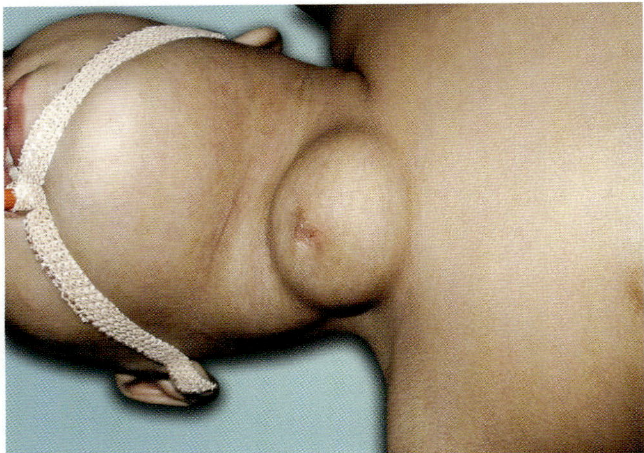

Fig. 18.2.15: Obstructed branchial sinus—the blocked opening is seen in the center of the swelling.

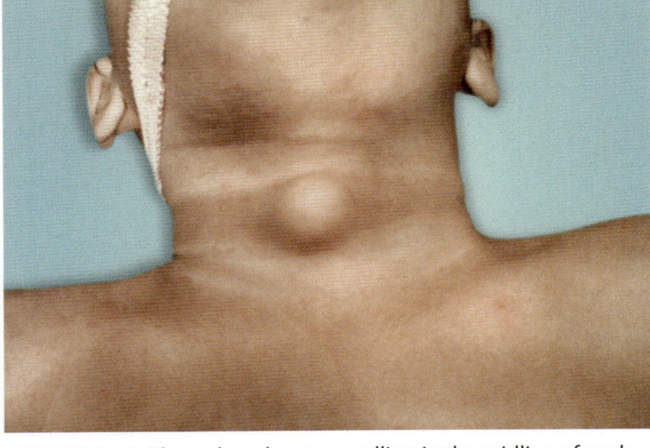

Fig. 18.2.16: Thyroglossal cyst—swelling in the midline of neck.

- The opening is often seen later in infancy—intermittent small quantities of mucoid discharge.
- There may be a small skin tag or a tiny cartilaginous tag near the opening.
- Secondary infection may lead to abscess formation. Fistulogram is routinely not recommended.

Complications

There is a high chance of secondary infection. In late cases, malignant transformation of the lining is also known.

Treatment

- If infected, antibiotics and surgical excision in the noninflamed stage
- Surgery—dissection of the entire tract through the carotid bifurcation up to the tonsillar fossa.

THYROGLOSSAL CYST

The thyroid gland develops from the base of the tongue where it descends to take its formal position. During its course of descent, small groups of cells may get sequestrated, which gradually form a cyst—thyroglossal cyst.

Epidemiology, Clinical Features, and Diagnosis

- About three times more common than branchial remnants in childhood.
- Asymptomatic mass in the midline of neck **(Fig. 18.2.16)**.
- Smooth, round, elastic and opaque.
- Moves with deglutition and protrusion of tongue.
- If infected—red and tender and if incised may form sinus.
- USG may be used for diagnosis.

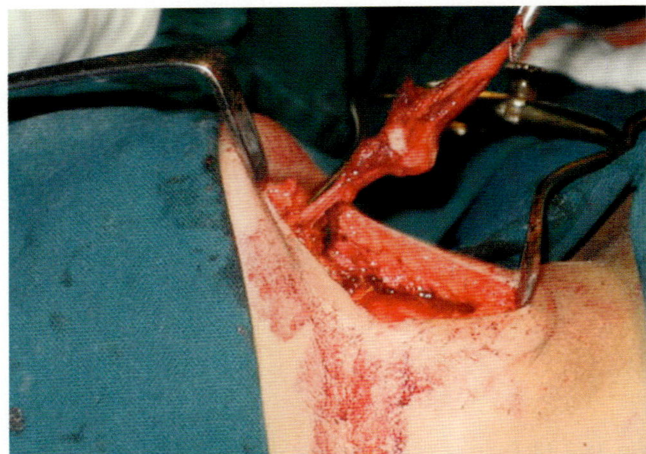

Fig. 18.2.17: Sistrunk's surgery for thyroglossal cyst. Note the excised hyoid bone along with the entire tract till the base of the tongue.

Treatment

Surgery—excision of the entire tract with body of hyoid bone (Sistrunk's operation) **(Fig. 18.2.17)**.

MECKEL'S DIVERTICULUM

This is the persistent proximal part of the vitello-intestinal duct. The diverticulum is present on the antimesenteric border of the terminal ileum **(Fig. 18.2.18)**.

The Rule of Two: Meckel's diverticulum is present in 2% of the population is situated 2 feet from the ileocecal junction, is 2-inch-long and is usually symptomatic before the age of 2 years.

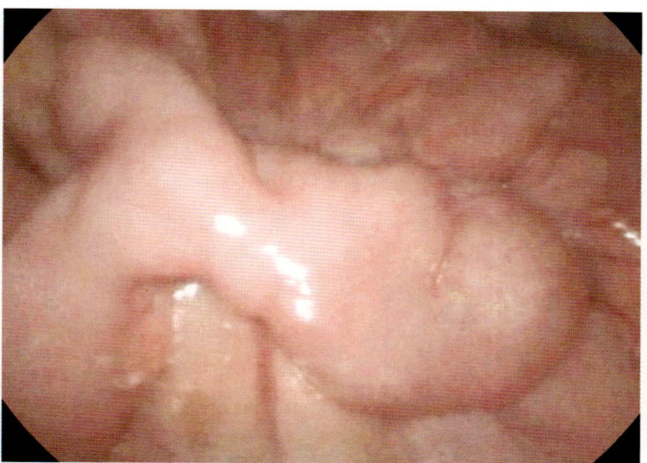

Fig. 18.2.18: Laparoscopic view of a Meckel's diverticulum.

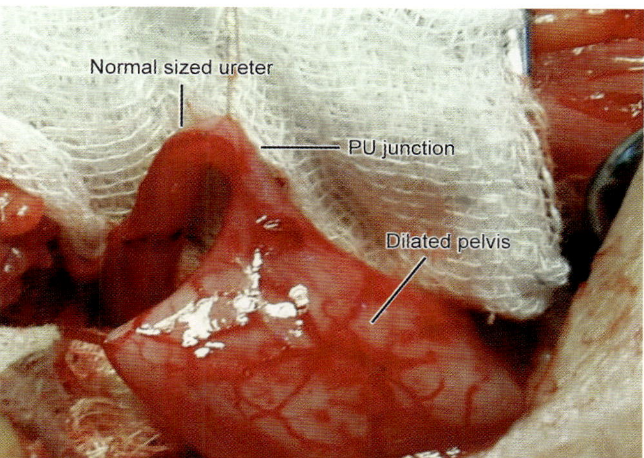

Fig. 18.2.19: Dilated pelvis of a hydronephrotic kidney.

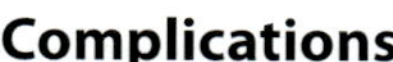

Complications

Meckel's diverticulum is symptomatic only if complications arise. These could be:

- *Bleeding:* It is usually painless and profuse. It is due to peptic ulceration in the surrounding ileal mucosa due to acid secretion from heterotopic gastric mucosa seen in some cases.
- *Intestinal obstruction:*
  - As a lead point of an intussusception
  - A band from the diverticulum to the umbilicus may cause internal herniation or volvulus.
- *Diverticulitis:* It produces symptoms and signs identical to appendicitis, but the prognosis is worse as the diverticulum is more prone to perforation and peritonitis.

Diagnosis

- Most commonly at abdominal exploration or laparoscopy on a clinical suspicion.
- A radionuclide scan may show the diverticulum as a hot spot only in case there is ectopic gastric mucosa—may be missed during active bleeding.
- Barium (Ba) study—rarely beneficial.

Treatment

Diverticulectomy—open or laparoscopic.

OBSTRUCTIVE UROPATHIES

Obstructive uropathy is a set of condition causing chronic, partial obstruction to the flow of urine anywhere distal to the renal calyces.

Common Sites of Obstruction

- The pelviureteric junction **(Fig. 18.2.19)**.
- The vesicoureteric junction.
- *The urethra:* Posterior and anterior urethral valves. Obstruction to the flow of urine could lead to:
  - Ballooning of calyces and thinning of the renal parenchyma. The renal function gradually deteriorates. High pressures in the antenatal period could cause renal dysplasia.
  - Infection further deteriorates renal function.

Clinical Features

- Antenatal detection
- Pain in the abdomen
- Recurrent urinary tract infection (UTI)
- Lump in the abdomen—kidney or palpable bladder
- Rarely hematuria
- Gastrointestinal symptoms such as nausea, vomiting and anorexia, especially in an infant
- Nonspecific symptoms such as failure to thrive, weakness and lethargy
- Poor urinary stream/straining at micturition/retention of urine in case of urethral valves.

Diagnostic and Evaluative Imaging

- *Abdominal ultrasonography:* It identifies the extent of pelvic and ureteric dilatation, bladder hypertrophy, urethral dilatation and postvoid residue besides any other anomalies.
- *Intravenous pyelography (IVP)—replaced by CT urography or MR urography:* Detailed anatomical delineation.
- A *micturating cystourethrogram (MCUG)* to look for vesicoureteric reflux (VUR) or urethral obstruction, which may mimic or present as a pelviureteric obstruction **(Fig. 18.2.20)**.
- *Isotope renogram:* To assess differential function and scarring (preferably done with an open indwelling bladder catheter).

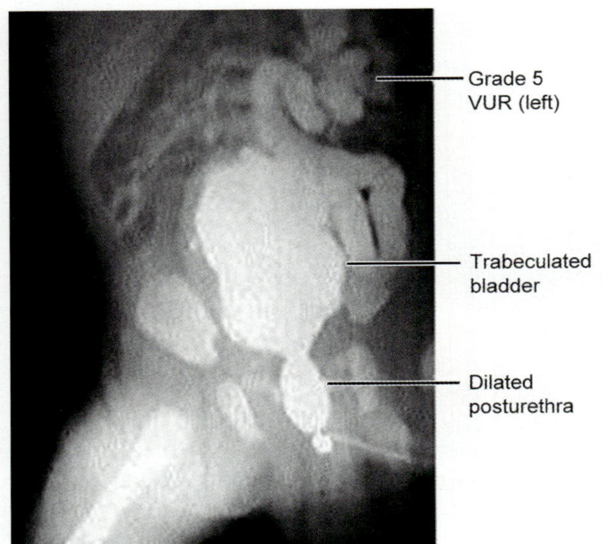

Fig. 18.2.20: Micturating cystourethrogram (MCU) showing grade 5 vesicoureteric reflux (VUR) on left side with trabeculated bladder, dilated posterior urethra with normal caliber distal urethra.

Complications

- Deterioration of renal function due to progressive renal dilatation.
- Pyonephrosis and septicemia in case of infection.

Pelviureteric Junction Obstruction

Pathology

- The obstruction is either due to an adynamic segment or an external compression commonly by an aberrant renal artery. The partial obstruction gets exacerbated during any diuretic period.

Management Principles

- *Antenatally:* Urgent antenatal consultation required, if there is oligohydramnios. In unilateral isolated hydronephrosis, an expectant line of management is usually followed.
- *Postnatal management*: Based on the differential renal function, size and progress of hydronephrosis.
- Spontaneous resolution known in infancy.
- Definite indications for surgery—deteriorating renal function/pain/infection/palpable mass—Anderson-Hynes pyeloplasty (open or laparoscopic).

Vesicoureteric Reflux

Vesicoureteric reflux is due to the failure of the normal valvular action at the vesicoureteric junction, which thus permits a variable quantity of urine to reflux back into the ureter and at times even in the renal pelvicalyceal system.

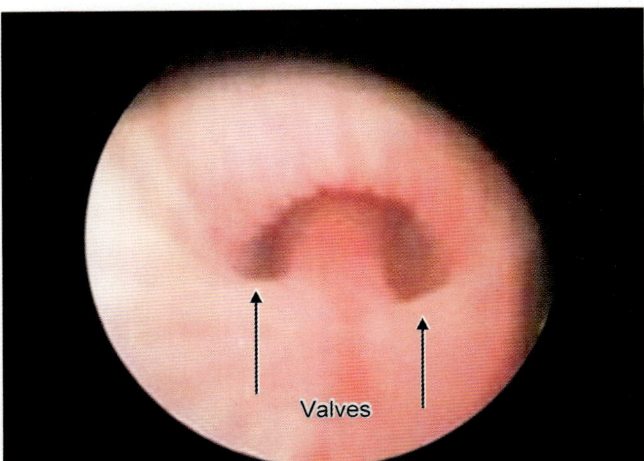

Fig. 18.2.21: Urethroscopic view of posterior urethral valve.

Vesicoureteric reflux may be either primary or secondary to high pressures in the bladder either in case of distal outflow obstruction or certain variants of neurogenic bladder.

Pathology

- Features of obstructive uropathy
- Renal damage could be significant in presence of active infection.

Management Principles

- Prevent and control of infection
- Monitor renal function
- Minor degrees of VUR can be self-limiting
- Treat primary cause of VUR, if possible, e.g. posterior urethral valves (PUV) or neurogenic bladder
- *Surgery (definitive treatment)*:
  - *STING procedure*: Endoscopic injection of dextranomer hyaluronic acid (Deflux)® at the vesicoureteric junction.
  - *Ureteric reimplantation*:
    - Transvesical
    - Extravesical
    - Laparoscopic.

Posterior Urethral Valves

They are thin curtain like membranes in the posterior urethra causing a partial obstruction to the flow of urine **(Fig. 18.2.21)**. Poor urine stream in a male child should make one suspect PUV.

Management Principles

- Essential to reduce back-pressure on bladder at the earliest
- Aggressive treatment of azotemia or sepsis, if present
- Strict asepsis during all urinary tract interventions including catheterizations.

Surgical Options
- Primary urethroscopic fulguration of valves
- *Diversion of urine*: Vesicostomy/ureterostomy/pyelostomy. Long-term follow up is essential to identify and treat renal malfunction.

Prognosis
- Poor in case of antenatal oligohydramnios
- Guarded in case of early uremia/sepsis
- Cautious in case of significant dilatation of ureters/pelvis
- Good in others.

KEY MESSAGES

- Obstructive uropathy or UTI may have insidious presentations.
- Need to identify the patients who will require urgent aggressive treatment.
- Obstruction may resolve or may be progressive.
- Long-term follow-up is essential.

NEONATAL SURGICAL EMERGENCIES

General Principles of Management

- *Nil by mouth (NBM):* When in doubt, keep the baby nil orally.
- Keep baby warm—in the hospital and during transport.
- Cover open wounds, e.g. exomphalos, meningomyelocele, etc.
- *Pass nasogastric tube (NGT) and always keep it open:* (No. 6 or higher), especially in case of vomiting or breathless child (pass NGT minimizes aerophagia and aspiration).
- Transport preferably in prone position.
- Recording passage of urine and meconium with its color and informing surgeon.
- *Supportive:* Antibiotics, intravenous (IV) fluids, monitoring of vitals.

NEONATAL EMERGENCIES: SPECIFIC CONDITIONS

Intestinal Obstruction

Intestinal obstruction is the failure of aboral progression of intestinal contents.

- *Dynamic obstruction:* It is due to a physical occlusion of a portion of bowel, which may arise either:
  - From outside the wall of the bowel as in compression due to bands, etc.
  - From within the wall, e.g. atresia, etc.
  - From within the lumen like inspissated meconium, etc.
- *Adynamic obstruction:* It is due to absence of peristalsis in the whole or a segment of the bowel.

  Clinically, the presentation is dependent on the level of obstruction, the severity of obstruction, the acuteness of obstruction, and the possibility of vascular compromise, if any.
- *Upper intestinal obstruction:* Early onset of vomiting and failure to tolerate feeds. Abdominal distension, if present, is confined to the upper abdomen. The baby may pass some normal colored meconium or pale colored meconium. Dehydration occurs early and is severe:
  - *Duodenal atresia:* The vomitus may be bilious or nonbilious. Antenatal hydramnios
  - Malrotation with midgut volvulus
- *Small intestinal obstruction:* It is characterized by abdominal distension, failure to pass meconium and later vomiting (invariably bilious):
  - Jejunal or ileal atresia
  - Meconium ileus
- *Large intestinal obstruction:* The earliest symptom is failure to pass meconium; other symptoms of intestinal obstruction follow. Abdominal distension is gross and generalized:
  - Hirschsprung disease
  - Anorectal malformations (ARM)
  - Meconium plug syndrome
  - Colonic atresias.

KEY MESSAGES

- Bilious vomiting or bilious gastric aspirate in a newborn is considered pathognomonic of intestinal obstruction.
- Higher the obstruction, more the dehydration.

INTESTINAL ATRESIA

Intestinal atresia is an obstruction of the intestine due to a complete occlusion of the lumen **(Fig. 18.2.22)**.

Clinical Features and Diagnosis

These are dependent on the site of atresia.

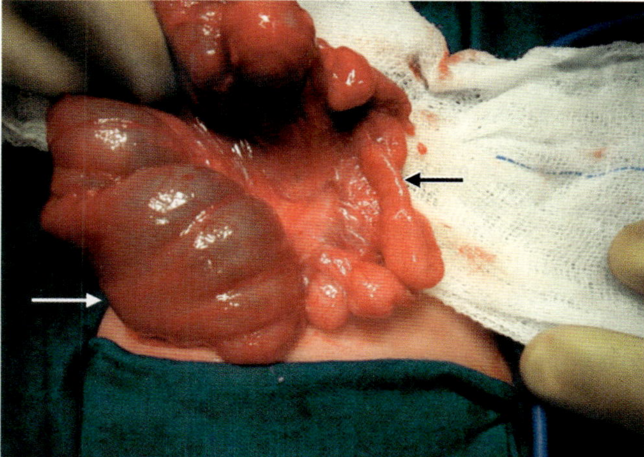

Fig. 18.2.22: Atresia showing complete block of the intestine.

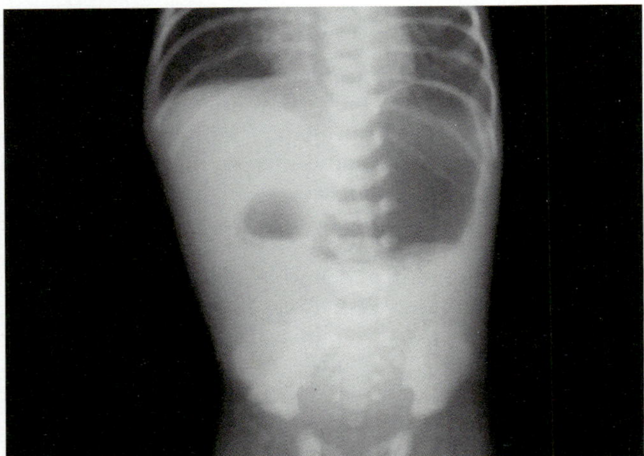

Fig. 18.2.23: An erect plain X-ray showing a double-bubble sign of a duodenal atresia.

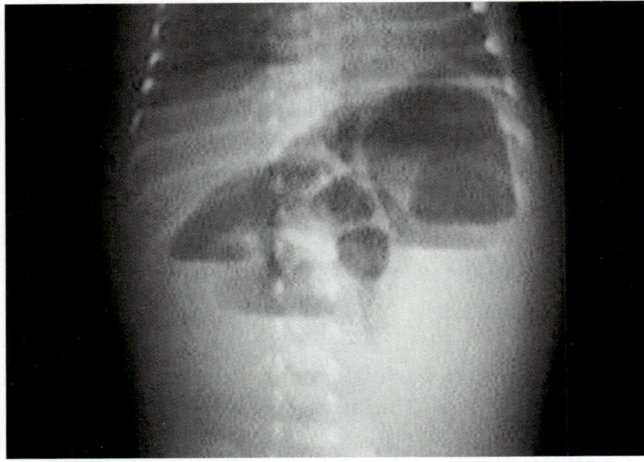

Fig. 18.2.24: An erect X-ray of abdomen showing fluid levels in the upper abdomen with a gasless lower abdomen suggesting a jejunal atresia.

Investigations

- *Double-bubble sign:* Duodenal atresia **(Fig. 18.2.23)**
- *Multiple fluid levels:* Jejunal or ileal atresia **(Fig. 18.2.24)**
- *Treatment:* Early surgery, after at least partial correction of dehydration
- *On laparotomy:* Resection and anastomosis or bypass of atretic segment **(Fig. 18.2.25)**.

Prognosis

- Fairly good in uncomplicated cases.
- Deteriorates, if treated late, low birthweight or premature, or presence of sepsis or other anomalies.
- Poor if multiple atresias or there is a large section of the bowel, which does not have a proper vascular supply (apple peel atresia)

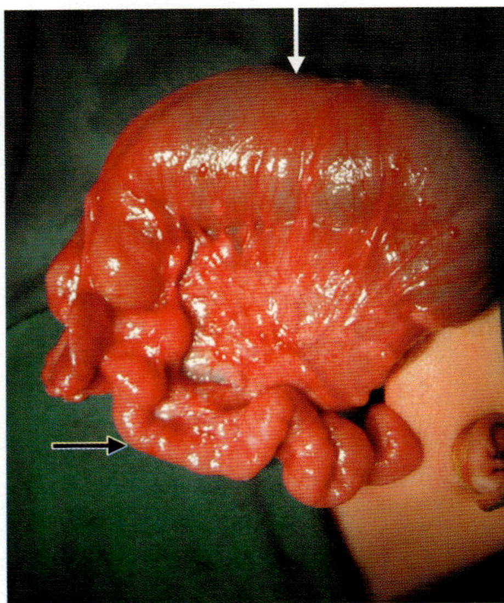

Fig. 18.2.25: Jejunal atresia—massively dilated jejunal loops (white arrow) and collapsed and small caliber distal small bowel (black arrow).

INTESTINAL MALROTATION

If the process of intestinal rotation is incomplete, then malrotation is said to have taken place.

Pathological Anatomy

- The duodenojejunal flexure is to the right of the midline and cecum adjacent on its left, and thus significantly narrowing the root of the mesentery; the ascending and transverse colon are mobile. Together these anomalies can lead to twisting of the intestine (volvulus neonatorum).
- Abnormal peritoneal bands [Ladd's bands **(Fig. 18.2.26)**] run from right peritoneal wall to the cecum over the third part of the duodenum compressing the duodenum.
- In case of volvulus neonatorum, the vascularity of entire midgut can suffer, leading to gangrene, if not corrected early.

Clinical Features

There is a sudden development of upper intestinal obstruction in an apparently normal child, who may have passed normal meconium earlier. If volvulus neonatorum sets in duodenal atresia with gangrene of the midgut (bleeding PR), there is progressive deterioration in the general condition with septicemia.

Diagnosis

- *An erect X-ray of abdomen:* A large stomach bubble or a double-bubble and may show few distal gas shadows. Multiple fluid levels are not seen in this variety of intestinal obstruction.

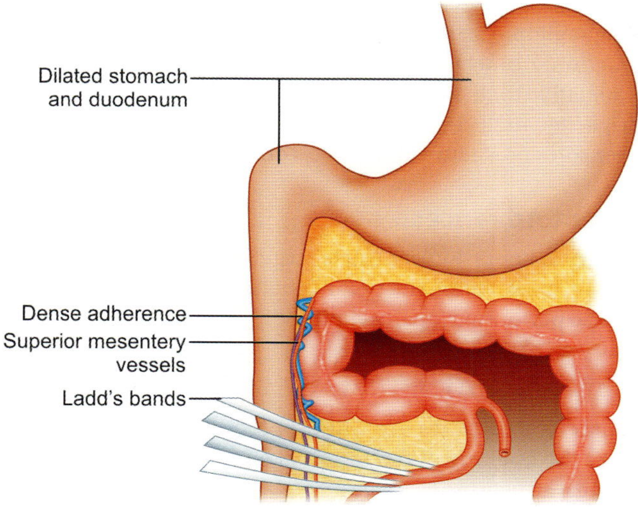

Fig. 18.2.26: Diagrammatic representation of the pathological anatomy in a malrotation—ileocecal region to the left with Ladd's bands crossing from the right abdominal wall toward the ileocecal region compressing the duodenum (which is entirely on right side). Note the narrow root of mesentery—a cause for midgut volvulus.

- *Barium studies:* Duodenum lies to the right of midline; alternatively, a barium enema would show the entire colon to the left of midline.
- Ultrasonography with Doppler can identify the abnormal lie of the superior mesenteric artery and bowel ischemia if any.

Treatment

- Resuscitation as required (high fluid requirement)
- *Exploratory laparotomy:* Ladd's bands released, and root of the mesentery widened to prevent further episodes of volvulus (Ladd's procedure)
- *Gangrenous bowel, if any:* Resection or exteriorization.

Prognosis

Good, if surgery done before gangrene sets in.

MECONIUM ILEUS

Introduction

The neonatal manifestation of cystic fibrosis—a condition affecting all the mucus secreting glands of the body, causing excessive viscidity of the mucus secretion. It is an autosomal recessive disease, which is common in Western countries. In recent years, incidence is increasing in India.

Pathology

The mucus secreted in the intestine is extremely sticky, like plasticine, leading to adherence of meconium to the intestinal mucosa, and thus choking up the lumen of the distal intestine, not allowing any contents to pass through.

Clinical Features

- Mid-intestinal obstruction
- Baby may pass some white chalky meconium
- Viscid meconium may be palpable as a doughy substance in the lower abdomen.

Diagnosis

- *Plain X-ray of the abdomen:* Dilated bowel but no fluid levels.
- *Gastrograffin or (conray/urograffin) enema:* Microcolon (a thin narrow segment of distal relatively unused bowel).

Treatment

The very high osmolarity of conray or gastrograffin enema causes dissolution of the inspissated mucus and may be curative. In case, the obstruction does not resolve after the use of conray, surgery will be required to relieve the obstruction.

HIRSCHSPRUNG DISEASE

Hirschsprung disease is a common condition characterized by congenital aganglionosis of a variable length of the colon extending proximally from the anorectal junction.

Physiology

Normal peristaltic activity involves a wave of relaxation preceding a wave of contraction. Parasympathetic innervation is essential for this wave of relaxation.

Pathological Anatomy

In Hirschsprung disease, the parasympathetic ganglia are absent from the Meissner's and Auerbach's plexuses of the affected bowel. The aganglionic bowel is normal in caliber but due to the absence of the peristaltic activity, the wave of relaxation is absent thus leading to a functional obstruction. The proximal bowel with normal ganglion undergoes massive dilatation and hypertrophy.

Etiology

Usually sporadic but occasionally the disease runs in families. Male:female ratio is 4:1.

Clinical Features

- *Presentation*—at birth or later.
- *Constipation* dating back to early infancy or a delay in passage of the first meconium beyond 24 hours of life.
- *Intestinal obstruction*—may be relieved by enemas.

- Rarely, attacks of foul smelling diarrhea interspersed with constipation may confuse the picture.
- In chronic cases, child fails to thrive and is malnourished.
- *Abdominal distension:* Usually marked, the transverse colon is often visible.
- *On rectal examination:* The rectum is felt to be empty, and on withdrawal of the examining finger, there is an explosive passage of flatus and feces.

Diagnosis

- A plain X-ray of the abdomen shows features of intestinal obstruction—large dilated colon loops.
- In newborns—pelvic region—gasless due to empty lower colon.
- *Ba enema [essential to do under screening or image intensifier television (IITV) control with limited quantity of Ba in saline]:* A cone shaped colon at the junction of the ganglionic and aganglionic segments **(Fig. 18.2.27).**
- *Anorectal manometry:* Anorectal manometry may strongly suggest the diagnosis of Hirschsprung's disease.
- The final confirmation is only with a full thickness biopsy of the rectal wall, which will show absence of ganglion cells in the rectal muscle wall.

Differential Diagnosis

Absence of soiling distinguishes it from habitual constipation, which usually presents after the age of 6–12 months.

Treatment

Conservative treatment involving repeated enemas/ suppositories, may help in overcoming an acute attack of intestinal obstruction and postpone the surgery. Definitive treatment is surgical. The principle of surgery is the removal of aganglionic segment of colon and ensuring that normal ganglionic bowel is anastomosed to the anal canal. This is usually done in stages. Various commonly performed surgeries include the modified Duhamel's procedure, Swenson's procedure and Soave's procedure.

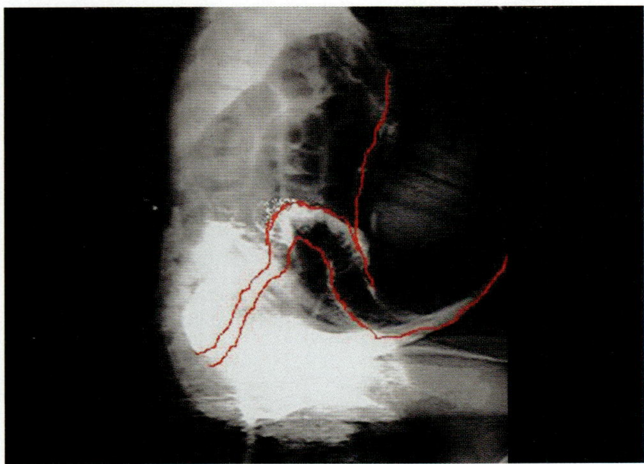

Fig. 18.2.27: Barium (Ba) enema (late view) in case of Hirschsprung disease. Note the normal caliber anorectal portion with a massively dilated sigmoid.

Recent Advances

Surgery is being done in single stage for the neonates, but its long-term results are still being debated. The main procedures may be performed laparoscopically.

ANORECTAL ANOMALIES

Anorectal anomalies are wide spectrum of anomalies that affect the opening of the terminal anorectum and adjacent perineal structures.

Incidence

Roughly 1 in 5,000 live births.

Pathological Anatomy

The anus does not open normally at the usual site. The opening may be severely stenotic or absent. In the latter case, the rectum ends as a blind pouch. There may be a fistulous communication from the rectal pouch to perineum or the urinary tract in the male or the genital structures in a female. The usual muscles of continence are present in the normal positions but since the terminal gastrointestinal tract (GIT) may not pass through them, they may be poorly developed.

Associated anomalies with this Group:

- *VATER association:* Vertebral, anorectal, tracheoesophageal and renal.
- *VACTERL association:* Vertebral, anorectal, cardiac, tracheoesophageal, renal and limb.
- Genitourinary anomalies, especially VUR are probably the most common association.

CLASSIFICATION

The classification centers around the relation of the terminal anorectum and the levator ani muscle.

- *Low variety:* The rectum passes through the levator funnel entirely. The continence muscles are well-developed **(Fig. 18.2.28)**.
- *Intermediate variety:* Rectum enters the levator funnel but does not pass through it entirely. There is frequently a fistula to the posterior urethra in the male, or the vestibule in the female. The continence muscles are developed.
- *High variety:* The anorectum does not pass through the levator, which is poorly developed—externally manifested as a flat perineum **(Fig. 18.2.29)**, and the fistula is to the

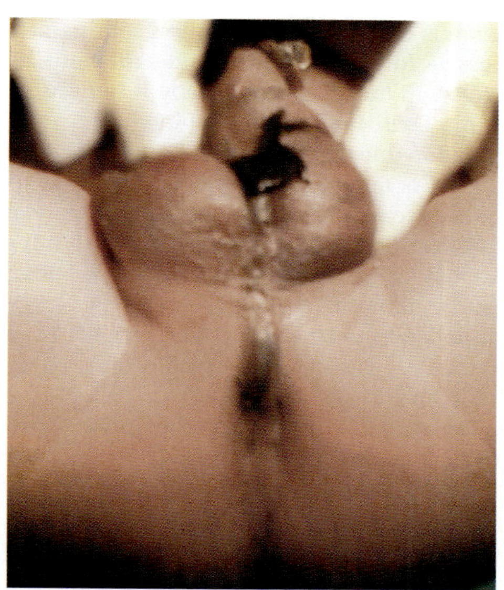

Fig. 18.2.28: Anorectal malformations (ARM)—cutaneous fistula opening on scrotal raphe (low variety).

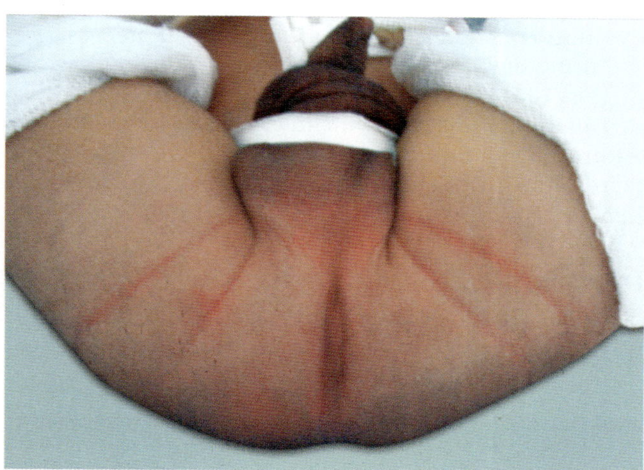

Fig. 18.2.29: Flat perineum as seen in a baby of high anorectal malformations (ARM).

urethra or bladder in male and there may be a cloacal anomaly in the female.

Clinically, most varieties of ARM should be identified at birth itself or may present as low-intestinal obstruction. In those with a wide external fistula, the presentation may be of recurrent constipation.

Investigations

Mainly directed at ascertaining the relationship of the anorectum with levator ani and the identification of a fistula if any.

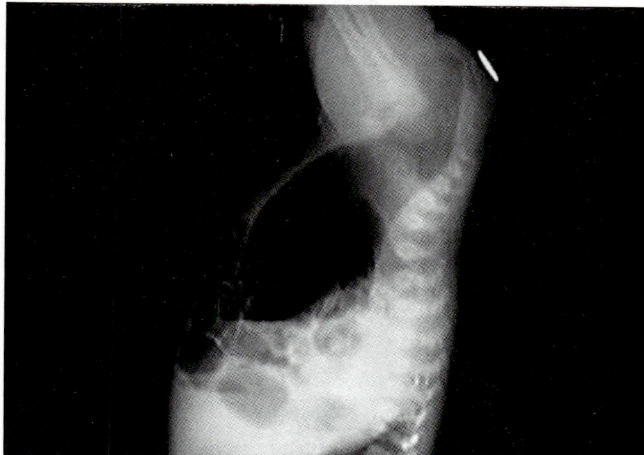

Fig. 18.2.30: Invertogram in case of low anorectal malformations (ARM).

Invertogram or a Lateral Prone Film

Figure 18.2.30: Assesses the level of air shadow in the blind rectal pouch with respect to bony landmarks. Since the swallowed air can take 24 hours to reach the rectum, this assessment is likely to be fallacious if done earlier. In patients with an open fistula, the same relationship can be ascertained by dye studies through the fistula.

Treatment

- *Low anomalies:* Since the rectum has already descended through the levator muscles, treated by a surgical exploration of the perineum at birth.
- *Intermediate or high anomaly:* An initial colostomy to relieve the intestinal obstruction. At a later stage, a definitive surgery—the most common being posterior sagittal anorectoplasty (PSARP). The colostomy is closed as the third stage of surgery.

INFANTILE HYPERTROPHIC PYLORIC STENOSIS

Incidence

- 1:300 children (Western literature); possibly much lower for Indian children.
- Mostly sporadic but few cases may run in families.
- The ratio of male:female is 5:1, especially first-born males.

Pathology

Musculature of the pyloric antrum is significantly hypertrophied; thus, the pylorus is thickened; pyloric canal is lengthened and narrowed. The olive-shaped pylorus becomes hard to feel when contracted. This hypertrophied pylorus is clinically palpable as a "pyloric tumor" **(Fig. 18.2.31)**. The stomach proximal to the obstruction is dilated and hypertrophied. Gastric mucosa in infancy produces a potent lipase, which hydrolyses milk to free fatty acids. The rancidity of the curdled milk gradually causes progressive mucosal edema and precipitates complete obstruction **(Fig. 18.2.32)**, and thus symptoms often delayed till 3–6 weeks.

Clinical Features

Usually, child is seen between 3 weeks and 6 weeks or any time between 1 week and 4 months.

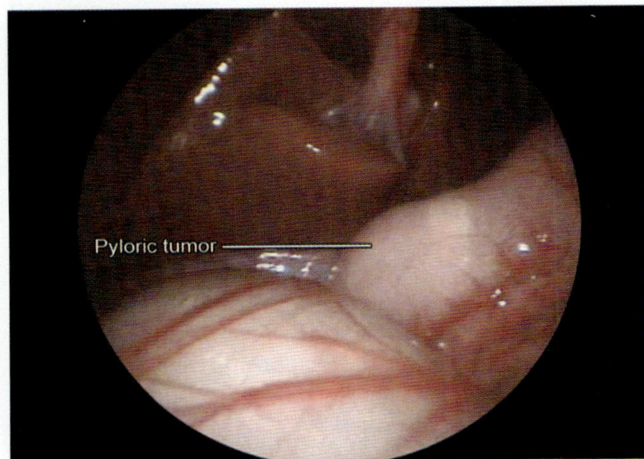

Fig. 18.2.31: Laparoscopic view of the hypertrophied pylorus in a case of infantile hypertrophic pyloric stenosis (IHPS).

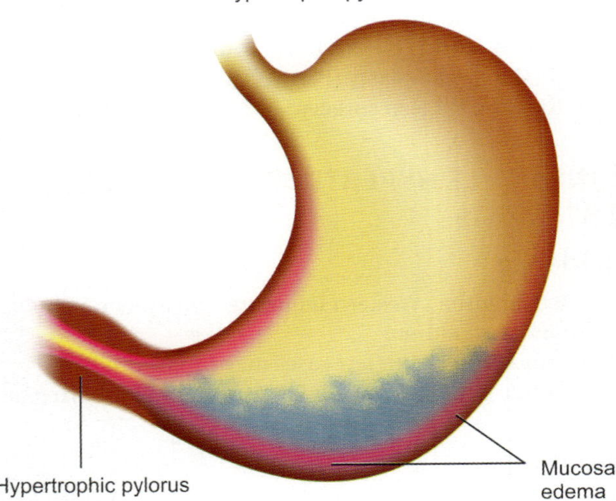

Fig. 18.2.32: Diagrammatic representation of the hypertrophy of the pylorus along with the mucosal edema precipitating the complete obstruction of the pyloric outlet.

- Vomiting is the most important presenting symptom—progressive, forcible, projectile and nonbilious, may come from nose. In most cases, the baby is hungry again after the vomit. There may be altered blood.
- Constipation due to poor intake.
- Weight loss or failure to gain weight.
- Jaundice—occasionally seen due to nutritional deficiencies.
- Facies is characteristic—alert, anxious and hungry look. Unlike a toxic or septicemic baby, these babies have a slow and shallow breathing due to alkalosis.
- Visible peristalsis on inspection (left to right). Examination must be done with the child comfortably placed in the mother's lap and in good light.
- Palpation of the "tumor" (palpable in 70% cases) is the diagnostic sign. It should be looked for with the left hand, sitting on the patients' left palpating below the right costal margin, underneath the liver border.

Specific Investigations

- *Serum electrolytes*: Hypokalemic, hypochloremic alkalosis.
- Ultrasonography shows the "tumor".
- Contrast studies with barium only if necessary—"string sign", large stomach, delayed emptying, gastritis **(Fig. 18.2.33)**.

Differential diagnosis includes almost any condition leading to nonbilious vomiting in children, especially gastroenteritis, septicemia, meningitis, intracranial hemorrhage and gastroesophageal reflux (GER).

Treatment

- *Nonsurgical treatment with prokinetics:* To be used only in case of strong contraindication to surgery as the treatment has erratic results and is too prolonged

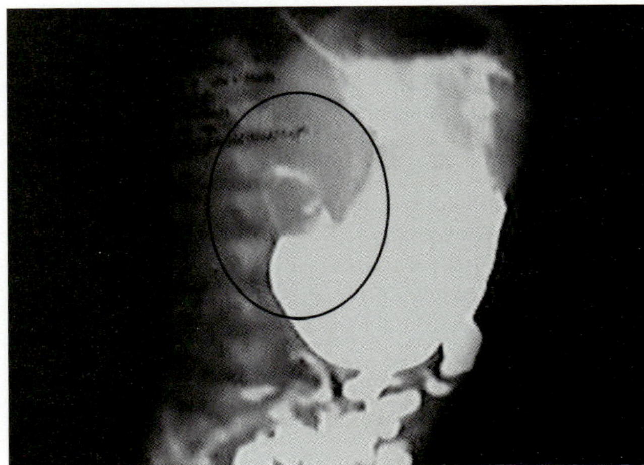

Fig. 18.2.33: String sign seen on barium (Ba) meal examination in case of infantile hypertrophic pyloric stenosis (IHPS).

- *Surgical treatment:* Treatment of choice.
  - *Preoperative*: Correct dehydration and electrolyte imbalance by:
    - *Rheolytic thrombectomy* (RT) aspirate and stomach wash with normal saline.
    - Administer 1/3 or 1/2 strength saline through NGT or IV.
  - *Operation*: Fredet-Ramstedt's pyloromyotomy—laparoscopic surgery possible.
  - *Results*: In experienced hands, results are excellent.

EXOMPHALOS OR OMPHALOCELE

It is the herniation of the abdominal contents through open umbilical ring into the base of umbilical cord. The contents are not covered by skin but a thin, translucent and avascular membrane consisting of peritoneum and amniotic membrane sandwiching a thin layer of Wharton's jelly. This sac, translucent at birth, gradually opacifies after a few hours.

The contents range from a small length of bowel to almost the entire bowel, stomach, liver, spleen, pancreas and bladder. **Table 18.2.1** lists the difference between an exomphalos major and an exomphalos minor **(Fig. 18.2.34)**, as they are of prognostic significance.

Table 18.2.1: Difference between exomphalos major and minor.

Exomphalos major	*Exomphalos minor*
Defect is more than 5 cm in diameter	Defect is less than 5 cm in diameter
Cord is attached to the base of sac	Cord is attached to the tip of sac
It may contain liver, stomach, etc.	It contains only bowel
Primary closure may not be possible	Primary repair is easy

Clinical Features

- Prenatal USG diagnosis, desirable and termination of pregnancy an option
- *Incidence*: 1:6,000 births
- Associated with many chromosomal defects and syndromes like exomphalos-macroglossia-gigantism (EMG) syndrome
- Multiorgan defects are common
  Complications: If left untreated—septicemia.

Treatment:
- Primary—prevent heat loss and infection.
- Attempt primary closure under general anesthesia (GA).
- If not possible—staged closure or silo method.

CONGENITAL DIAPHRAGMATIC HERNIA

The diaphragm is formed from different embryonal components, viz:
- The septum transversum.
- The pleuroperitoneal membranes.
- The dorsal esophageal mesentery and the body wall.

Failure of fusion of any one of these components can result in a defect in the diaphragm, which allows the abdominal viscera to herniate into the chest cavity **(Fig. 18.2.35)**. The most common variety is the "Bochdalek hernia", which involves the posterolateral part of the diaphragm. It is more common on the left side **(Fig. 18.2.36)**.

Pathophysiology

Pathophysiological events leading to respiratory distress in congenital diaphragmatic hernia (CDH):
- The shift of mediastinum during the antenatal period causes pressure on the contralateral developing lung

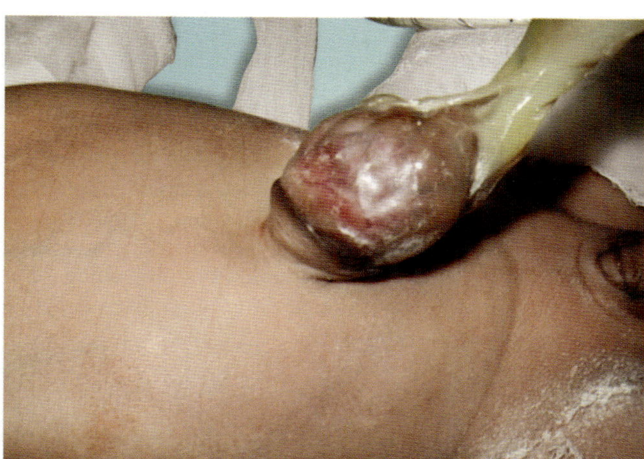

Fig. 18.2.34: Exomphalos minor.

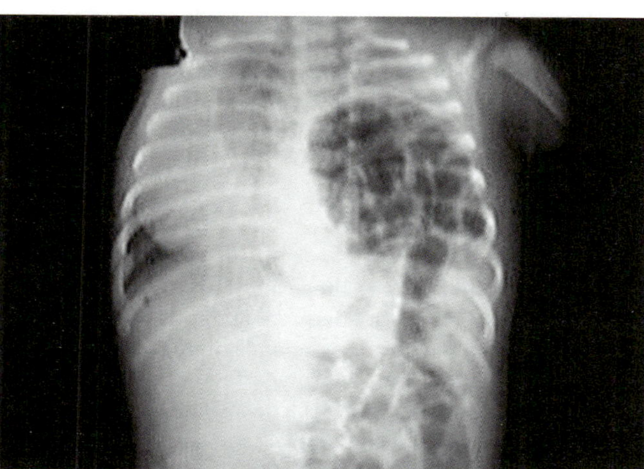

Fig. 18.2.35: Left-sided diaphragmatic hernia with marked mediastinal shift.

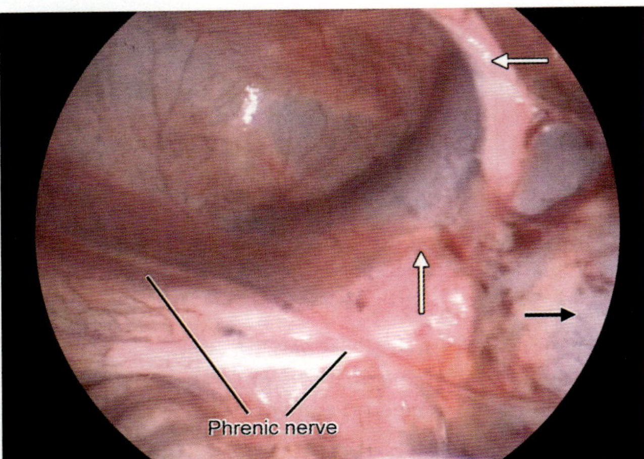

Fig. 18.2.36: Thoracoscopic view of diaphragmatic defect (white arrows) in a case of congenital diaphragmatic hernia (CDH). Black arrow shows the heart.

affecting its development also. This pulmonary hypoplasia limits the gaseous exchange in the available lung tissue.
- Pulmonary hypoplasia also affects the vascular component of the lung. Thus, there is an increased resistance in the pulmonary vasculature resulting in pulmonary hypertension. This may prevent closure of the ductus arteriosus, which may further lead to a persistent fetal circulation.
- The presence of abdominal contents in the chest causes pressure on the lung—this restricts lung expansion, which can be compounded by the gaseous distension of the bowel in a crying baby.
- The hypoplastic lung may not be able to handle normal inspiratory pressures and the resultant alveolar rupture may result in pneumothorax on the affected side or even on the other side.

The severity of symptoms and signs depends mainly on the status of lung development. A severely hypoplastic lung may not be compatible with life, whereas at the other extreme, some cases of CDH may be relatively asymptomatic for years and may present much later in childhood due to repeated chest infections.

Clinical Features

If antenatally diagnosed, these patients must preferably be born in hospitals with adequate facilities for immediate advanced neonatal care and neonatal surgical facilities.

Postnatally: In the severely affected baby, there is respiratory distress and cyanosis. The ipsilateral chest appears prominent with evidence of mediastinal shift. Breath sounds on the involved side are absent, occasionally peristaltic sounds can be heard due to displacement of viscera to the chest. In most cases, the abdomen is scaphoid. Heart sounds and apical impulse are on the right side.

Occasionally, patients present late with only recurrent lower respiratory tract infection (LRTI).

Investigations

- A chest X-ray is diagnostic. It shows loops of bowel in the chest cavity. There may be significant mediastinal shift or an associated pneumothorax. In right-sided Bochdalek hernia, liver is the main constituent of the chest cavity.
- In doubtful cases, an abdominal USG or CT scan of the chest is useful.
- Hypoxia and acidosis should be estimated by arterial blood gas analysis.

Treatment

Primary Management
- An NGT passed immediately to deflate the stomach and reduce aerophagia
- Intubation with an endotracheal tube at the earliest for a breathless child. If intubation is not possible, oxygen may be administered by an oxygen hood. Bag and mask ventilation is avoided for fear of increasing aerophagia.
- Ventilation ideally with a high frequency ventilator.
- Acidosis correction.
- In case of severe pulmonary hypertension, drugs to cause pulmonary vasodilatation.

Surgery
- Surgery is performed only after stabilizing the baby's condition as much as possible.
- Through a laparotomy, the defect in the diaphragm is identified, the herniated viscera are reposited in the abdomen, and the defect is repaired.
- Thoracoscopic surgery is being deployed in an increasing number of patients who are stable enough to tolerate the same.
- Very rarely, extracorporeal membrane oxygenation (ECMO) may be indicated in these patients.

KEY MESSAGES

- Antenatally diagnosed CDH patients should be delivered in a center with advanced neonatal care.
- Clinically, a strong suspicion should be made on seeing a breathless child with a scaphoid abdomen since other causes of breathlessness cause abdominal distension due to aerophagia.

TRACHEOESOPHAGEAL FISTULA

The trachea and esophagus are formed by splitting of the primitive foregut around the 4th week of intrauterine life. An abnormality during this process causes this anomaly.

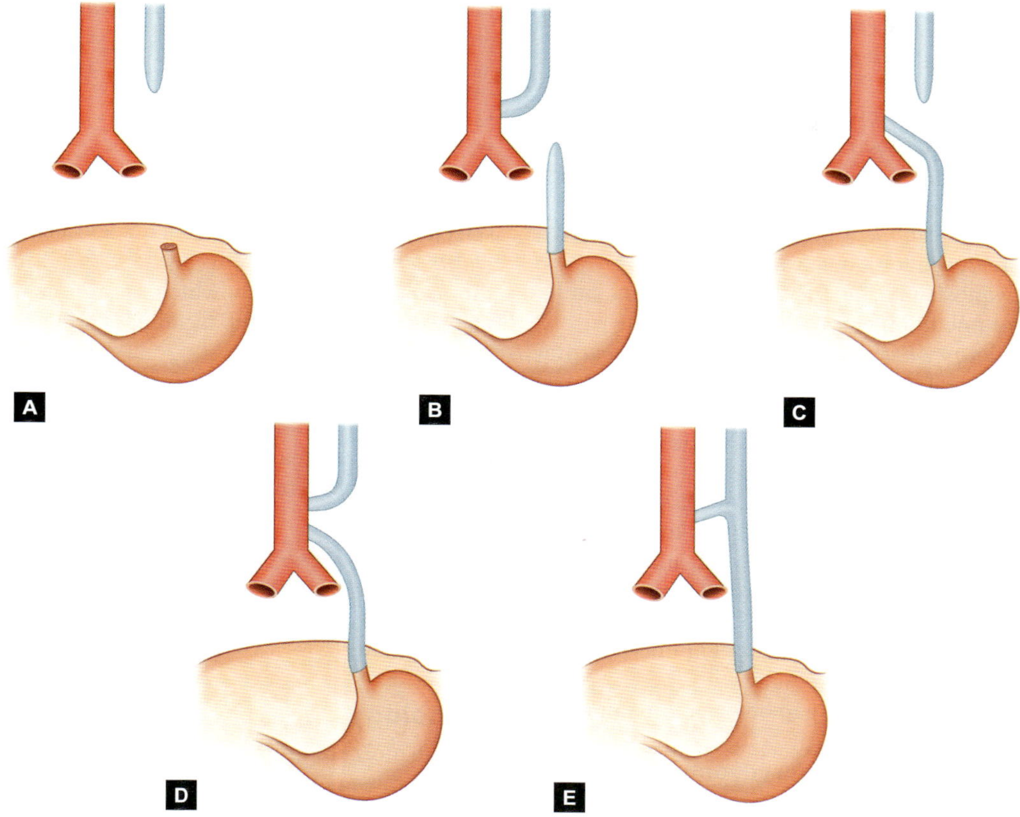

Figs. 18.2.37A to E: Different types of esophageal atresia. (A) Esophageal atresia without tracheoesophageal fistula; (B) Esophageal atresia with an upper pouch fistula; (C) Esophageal atresia with lower end fistula (the most common); (D) Esophageal atresia with fistula at both ends of the esophagus; and (E) H-type tracheoesophageal fistula.

Etiology

Whereas, the exact etiology is unknown, associated anomalies occur as a part of the vertebral, anorectal, tracheoesophageal and renal anomalies (VATER) association and vertebral, anorectal, cardiac, tracheoesophageal, renal and limb (VACTERL) association. Incidence ranges from 1:3,000 to 1:4,500 live births.

Five types of anomalies are recognizable **(Figs. 18.2.37A to E)**:

1. Esophageal atresia without tracheoesophageal fistula.
2. Esophageal atresia with an upper pouch fistula.
3. Esophageal atresia with lower end fistula (the most common).
4. Esophageal atresia with fistula at both ends of the esophagus.
5. H-type tracheoesophageal fistula **(Fig. 18.2.38)**.

In the most common variety **(Figs. 18.2.37C to 18.2.39)**, saliva collects in the upper pouch and may spill over in the trachea leading to aspiration pneumonia. Inspired air is partly shunted into the stomach through the fistula causing gaseous distension of the stomach.

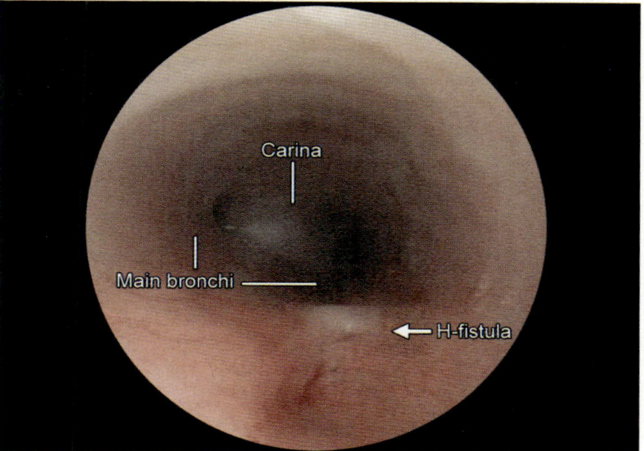

Fig. 18.2.38: Bronchoscopic view of H-type tracheoesophageal fistula.

The gastric distention leads to reflux of the acidic contents of the stomach through the trachea into the lungs causing chemical pneumonia.

Clinical Features

- *Antenatally*: There may be hydramnios, especially in pure atresia without fistula.
- *Frothing of saliva* is the most characteristic feature due to air bubbling through the collected salivary secretions in the pharynx.
- *Vomiting*—only if baby is inadvertently fed.
- *Abdominal distension* is a prominent feature except in type-A where the abdomen is scaphoid.
- *Cyanosis*: Cyanosis may be due to—concomitant cardiac anomalies or pneumonia.
- *Associated anomalies*: Vertebral, anorectal, cardiac, tracheoesophageal, renal and limb defects.
- A baby with an H-fistula usually presents late, with choking during feeds, excessive vomiting, gross aerophagia and recurrent pneumonia.
- *Diagnostic clinical test in all except the H-type fistula*: A stiff no. 10/12 rubber catheter or Ryle's tube is passed into the pharynx of the baby through mouth, and a characteristic resistance is felt as the catheter gets arrested in the atretic "upper pouch". A soft feeding tube or catheter may coil in the dilated upper pouch and miss the diagnosis. A lateral chest X-ray with the catheter in place will give an idea of the gap between the upper and the lower pouches.
- An H-fistula can be diagnosed only on detailed investigations.

Treatment

The therapy for esophageal atresia must consider the maturity and weight of the baby besides the presence if any of the lung infection and associated anomalies. Waterston's criteria are a guide to treatment.

Surgical Priorities

- Disconnection of fistula
- Prevention of salivary pooling
- Establish esophageal continuity.

Surgery is performed through a right thoracotomy. In selected cases, a staged approach is adopted.

Recent advances: The surgery is being done by the thoracoscopic approach, which minimizes the morbidity of an open thoracotomy and facilitates earlier recovery.

Prognosis

Depends on the weight, associated anomalies and the time elapsed before treatment can be started. If all factors are favorable, survival rates of over 80% can be achieved.

INTUSSUSCEPTION

Intussusception indicates the telescoping of one part of the intestine into another—common around 8–10 months of age **(Fig. 18.2.40)**.

Pathology

- The most common site—ileocecal region **(Fig. 18.2.41)**.
- The most common lead point—a hypertrophied Peyer's patch following a change in the bacterial flora during weaning or gastrointestinal infection or due to ingestion of infected respiratory secretions.
- Compression of the mesentery and venous congestion within the innermost layer of intussusception causes secretion of blood and mucus, characteristically labeled as red currant jelly stool. Further, vascular compromise may lead to gangrene of a portion of the bowel.

Clinical Features

- Classically a healthy, well-nourished child, less than 1 year of age.

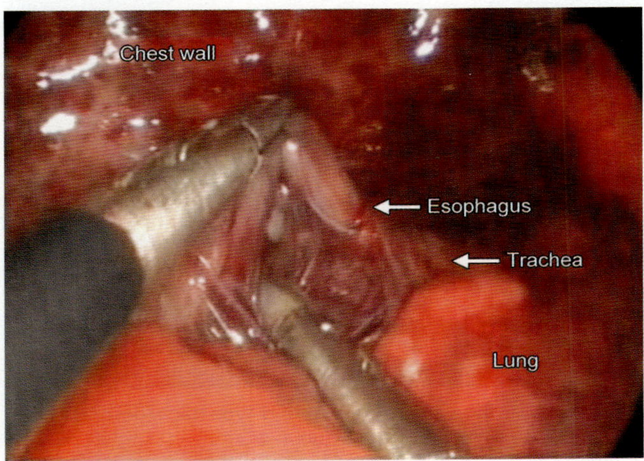

Fig. 18.2.39: Thoracoscopic view of lower esophagus arising from trachea in type "C" esophageal atresia case.

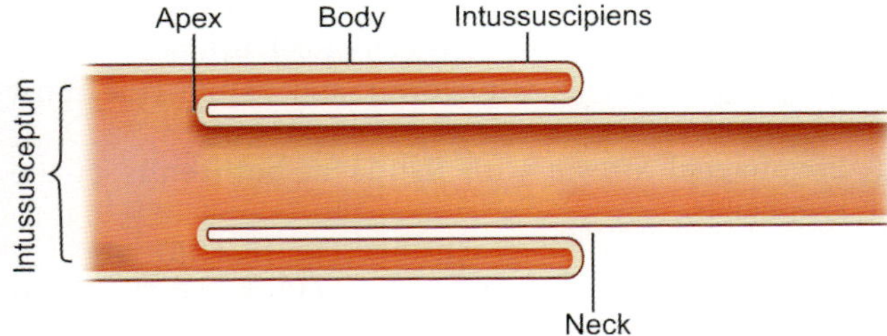

Fig. 18.2.40: Diagrammatic representation of intussusception and its parts.

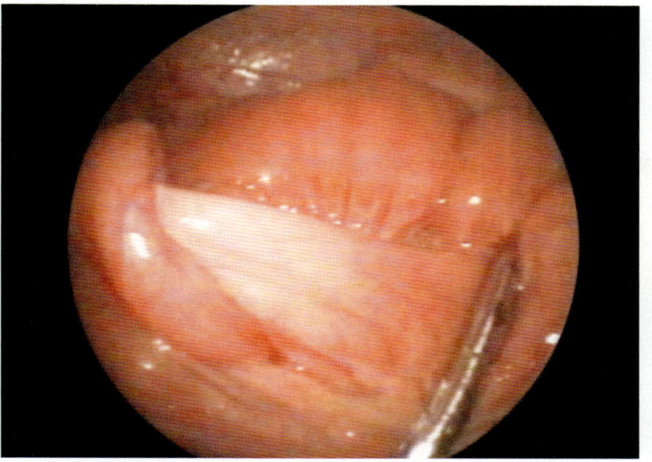

Fig. 18.2.41: Laparoscopic view of an intussusception.

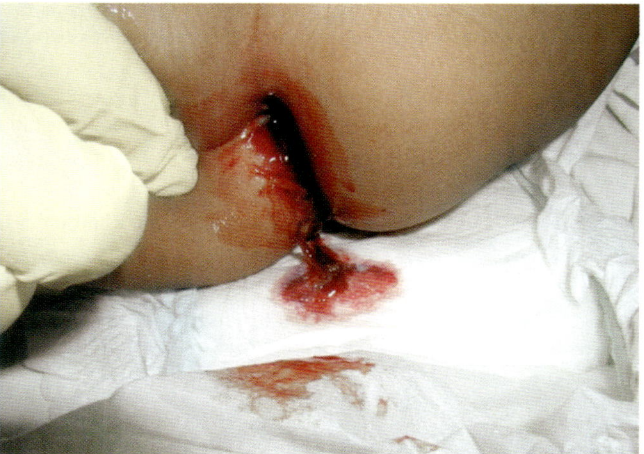

Fig. 18.2.42: Red currant jelly stools.
Courtesy: Dr A Vaidya.

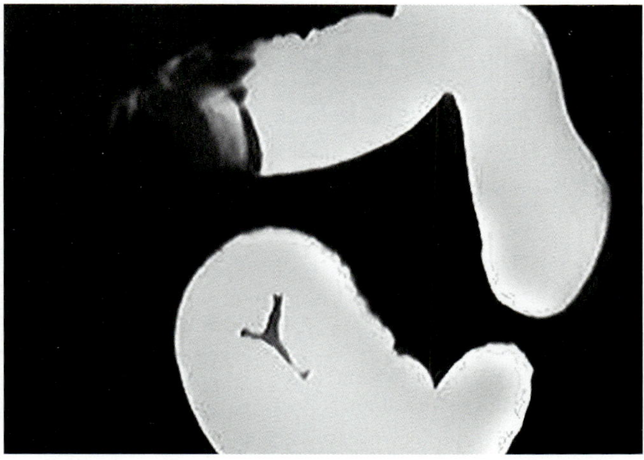

Fig. 18.2.43: Coil spring picture in a barium (Ba) enema for intussusception.

- There may be a prior history of a URTI/URI.
- Colic's pain occurs in short bursts with intermittent periods of remission.
- Vomiting—bilious only in late cases.
- Red currant jelly stools—usually with no fecal matter after one to two times (a differentiating feature from dysentery) **(Fig. 18.2.42)**.
- On abdominal palpation—intussusception may be felt as banana-shaped mass with its concavity toward the umbilicus. Occasionally, it can be felt PR.
- In late cases—features of septicemia and peritonitis.

Investigations

- Ultrasound of the abdomen can be diagnostic.
- Alternatively, a barium enema—the coiled spring sign or the claw sign **(Fig. 18.2.43)**.

Treatment

- If diagnosed within 24 hours of attack, hydrostatic reduction attempted by a pediatric surgeon (under USG or radiological control) with facilities for immediate surgery in case of complications.
- *If hydrostatic reduction fails or is contraindicated—exploratory laparotomy*: Operative reduction or if necessary, resection and anastomosis.
- The commonly seen pediatric surgical conditions and the treatment plan are summarized in **Table 18.2.2**.

Table 18.2.2: Common pediatric surgical conditions and their basic management plan.

Conditions	***Management plan***
Congenital inguinal hernia	• Operate early even at 1 week of age, if necessary • Fear of strangulation is the highest in newborn period
Tunica vaginal hydrocele/ encysted hydrocele of cord	No need for of urgency. Operate after 6 months of age but preferably before 2 years of age unless seen later
Phimosis	Usually after 2 years of age, rarely before 6 months of age. Preputioplasty—an alternative surgery
Paraphimosis	• Reduce as soon as possible (ASAP), plan early surgery • Emergency surgery if not reduced manually
Undescended testis	After 6 months of age and preferably before 1 year of age Earlier, if accompanied with hernia
Cleft lip	Usually around 3 months of age
Cleft palate	Usually between 9 months and 12 months of age
Tongue-tie	Preferably before 1 year of age
Branchial cyst and sinus	After 6 months of age
Cystic hygroma	After 3 months of age. Earlier if respiratory symptoms
Thyroglossal cyst and sinus	Usually after 6 months of age
Torticollis	After 1 year of age
Umbilical hernia	Usually after 2 years of age, any time earlier if history of recurrent irreducibility. Emergency in case of obstruction
Omphalocele	Primary or delayed primary depending on the size
Gastroschisis	At birth
Hypospadias	Usually after 6 months of age, may be after 1 year of age if severe chordee

BIBLIOGRAPHY

1. Belman AB. Hypospadias and chordee. In: Belman AB, King LR, Kramer SA (Eds). Clinical Pediatric Urology, 4th edition. London, UK: Martin Dunitz Ltd; 2002.
2. Gupta D, Carachi R. Pediatric Surgical Oncology, 1st edition. New York: McGraw-Hill; 2009.
3. Gupta DK, Sharma S, Azizkhan RG. Pediatric Surgery: Diagnosis and Management, 1st edition. New York: McGraw-Hill; 2010.
4. Hutson JM. Undescended testis, torsion and varicocele. In: Grosfeld JL, O'Neill JA, Coran AG, Fonkalsrud EW (Eds). Pediatric Surgery, 6th edition. Philadelphia: Mosby, Elsevier. 2006. pp. 1193-214.
5. Mattei P. Congenital diaphragmatic hernia. In: Mattei P (Ed). Fundamentals of Pediatric Surgery, 2nd edition. New York: Springer; 2011. pp. 535-42.
6. Puri P, Höllwarth ME. Pediatric Surgery: Diagnosis and Management, 2nd edition. Berlin, Heidelberg, Germany: Springer-Verlag; 2009. pp. 990-8.
7. Puri P. Newborn Surgery, 3rd edition. Oxford: Oxford University Press; 2003.
8. Rodgers BM, McGahren ED. Mediastinum and pleura. In: Oldham KT, Colombani PM, Foglia RP, Skinner MA (Eds). Principles and Practice of Pediatric Surgery. Philadelphia, USA: Lippincott Williams and Wilkins; 2005. pp. 929-49.
9. Sinha CK, Davenport M. Handbook of Pediatric Surgery, 1st edition. New York: Springer; 2010.
10. Smithers CJ, Fishman SJ. Vascular anomalies: lymphatic malformations. In: Holcomb GW III, Murphy JP, Ostlie DJ (Eds). Ashcraft's Pediatric Surgery, 5th edition. Philadelphia: Saunders Elsevier; 2010. pp. 989.

18.3 Common Orthopedic Conditions

Prakash P Kotwal

DEVELOPMENTAL DYSPLASIA OF THE HIP

The term developmental dysplasia of hip (DDH) is preferred to congenital dislocation of hip (CDH) as in many children the hip is normal at birth but develops subluxation or dislocation later. Its significance lies in its early diagnosis because neglect or delay in treatment can make the patient handicapped.

Diagnosis

Girls are affected 5-6 times more in comparison to boys. One or both hips may be affected. The diagnosis is difficult in the early years, and therefore, the condition has to be looked for.

In the Newborn

Asymmetrical skin folds may be seen on the inner aspect of thigh **(Fig. 18.3.1)**. Abduction of the hip joint may be limited. The clinical tests—*Barlow's* or *Ortolani's* test may help in the diagnosis. These tests are meant to dislocate or reduce the hip, respectively **(Figs. 18.3.2A and B)**.

In Older Children

The diagnosis may not be difficult as there is a limp and shortening in unilateral cases while widening of the perineum, marked lumbar lordosis and a characteristic waddling gait in bilateral cases.

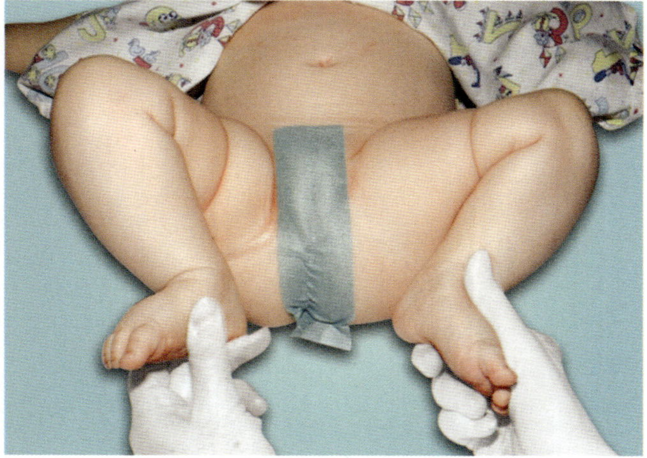

Fig. 18.3.1: Asymmetrical skin folds of thighs in developmental dysplasia of the hip.

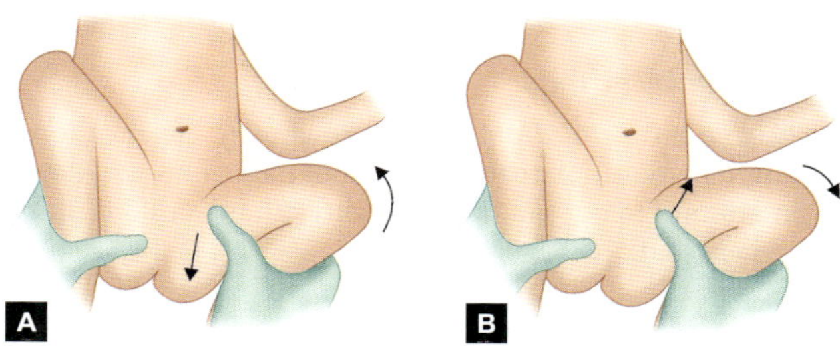

Figs. 18.3.2A and B: (A) Barlow's test; (B) Ortolani's test.

Investigations

A radiograph will confirm the diagnosis. However, arthrography and magnetic resonance imaging (MRI) are more useful as they show the cartilaginous parts of the joint.

Treatment

The treatment depends upon age of the patient. The prognosis is better when treated early. The dislocation is reduced by the following methods:

- Closed manipulation under general anesthesia and POP cast application
- Open reduction of the hip joint by surgery.

Additional surgical procedures may be required to reconstruct a shallow acetabulum or to correct excessive anteversion of the femoral neck.

CONGENITAL TALIPES EQUINOVARUS

Clubfoot or congenital talipes equinovarus (CTEV) is a deformity of the foot, in which the foot is turned inward **(Fig. 18.3.3)**. Though a congenital deformity, it may be part of a systemic disease such as arthrogryposis multiplex congenita (AMC), muscular dystrophy or *meningocele*, etc.

The clubfoot deformity consists of equinus (plantar flexion) at the ankle joint, inversion of the foot at the subtalar joint and adduction of the forefoot at the midtarsal joint. There is also medial rotation (torsion) of the tibia. The incidence of this condition is 1 in 1,000 live births.

Diagnosis

It may be a unilateral or bilateral deformity. The foot, calf and heel are smaller in size. The deformity cannot be passively corrected fully due to tightness of the soft tissues, particularly Tendo-Achilles.

In neglected clubfoot, callosities develop over the lateral border or the dorsum of the foot, as the child walks on it **(Fig. 18.3.4)**.

Principles of Treatment

The deformity is corrected fully and maintained up to the skeletal maturity to prevent recurrence. The treatment should start as early as possible.

Nonsurgical Methods

- *Passive manipulation*: In the newborn, the mother is taught to manipulate the child's foot passively everyday in an attempt to correct the deformity, till the child is about 6 weeks old.

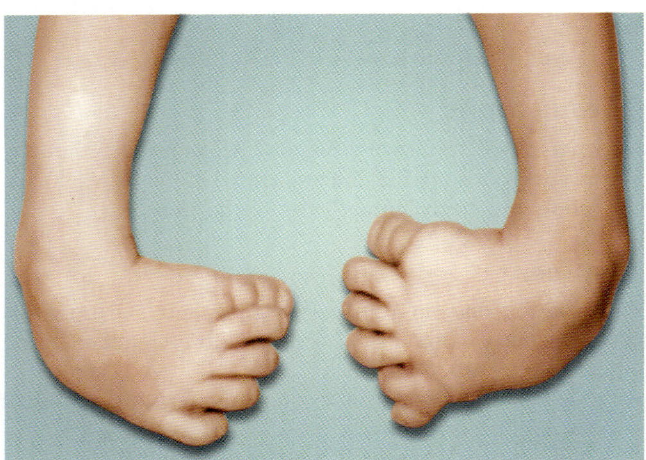

Fig. 18.3.3: Congenital talipes equinovarus (clinical photograph).

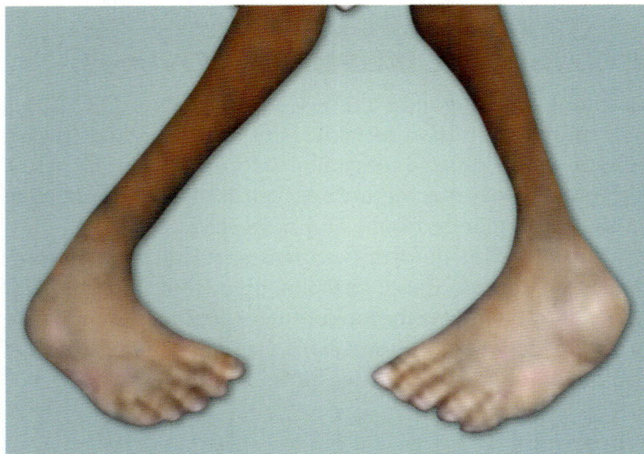

Fig. 18.3.4: Neglected clubfoot with callosities.

- *Plaster of Paris cast*: The deformity is corrected by passive manipulation and maintained in a plaster of Paris (POP) cast. The cast is changed every 2 weeks till the deformity is fully corrected or requires surgery. Splint or special shoes are given after correction.

Surgical Methods

In rigid clubfoot or in cases, where some residual deformity is left after conservative treatment, surgical treatment is resorted to which can be as follows:

- "Tendo-Achilles lengthening" and/or release of the contracted soft-tissue structures is done on the medial and posterior aspects of the foot and ankle.
- "Bony operations" are indicated after 4 years of age.

SPINA BIFIDA

In spina bifida, defective fusion of the posterior vertebral arch creates a neural tube defect resulting into protrusion of the contents of the spinal canal. It may present merely as a tuft of hair overlying the defect (spina bifida occulta) or as meningocele/myelomeningocele (cystica).

Treatment

Orthopedic surgeons have to work jointly with pediatric surgeons, urologists and neurosurgeons due to the complex problems.

CONGENITAL PSEUDARTHROSIS OF TIBIA

A rare condition where there is a defect or deformity in the tibia in its middle third. The X-ray picture is similar to that of a nonunion of a fracture **(Fig. 18.3.5)**. The treatment is essentially surgical.

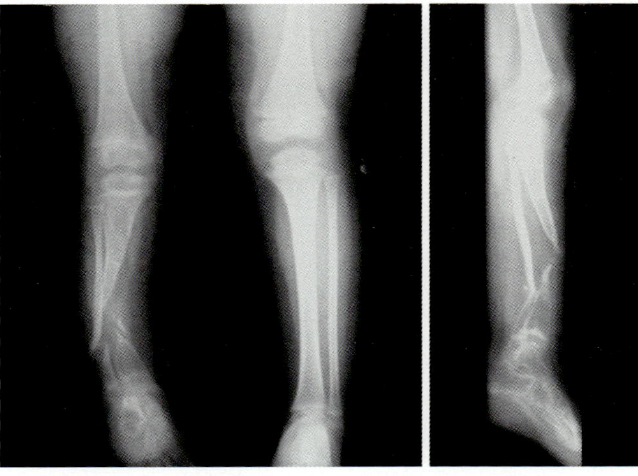

Fig. 18.3.5: Pseudarthrosis of right tibia—anteroposterior view (comparing with normal) and lateral view.

ACUTE OSTEOMYELITIS

Acute osteomyelitis is defined as acute infection of the bone marrow. The common organism responsible is *Staphylococcus aureus*. However, *Streptomyces albus, Streptococcus* and *Escherichia coli* are also known to cause it. *Clostridium welchii* are found in infections following a compound fracture.

Pathogenesis

Hematogenous osteomyelitis starts in the metaphysis of long bones. An abscess develops, which rapidly spreads to the medullary canal. The infection then comes under the periosteum lifting the latter from the bone, resulting in a subperiosteal abscess **(Fig. 18.3.6)** and cutting off the blood supply to the bone underneath. The bone becomes dead and develops into a sequestrum. In children, the periosteum can get lifted off easily resulting in a large diaphyseal sequestrum **(Fig. 18.3.7)**.

In situations, where the metaphysis is intracapsular, e.g. upper end of the femur, the abscess may burst open from the metaphysis directly into the hip joint and cause septic arthritis.

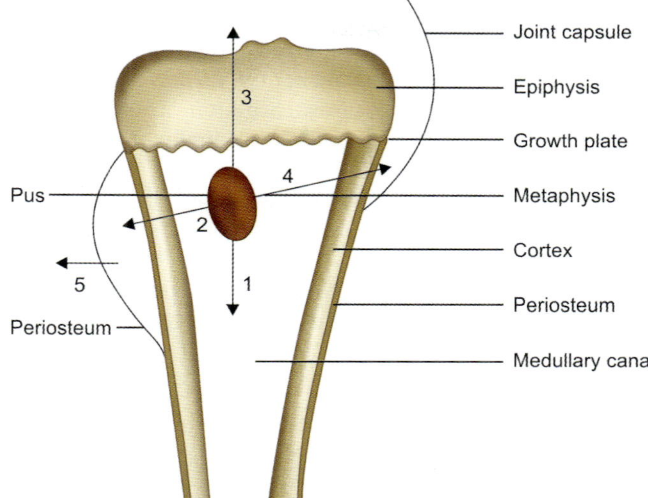

Fig. 18.3.6: Hematogenous (acute) osteomyelitis. Spread of pus from metaphysis to: (1) the medullary canal; (2) subperiosteal abscess. The pus has come out through the cortex and lifted the periosteum. The cortex underneath will lose its blood supply and become sequestrated; (3) directly into the joint (rarely); (4) the joint, since the metaphysis is intracapsular (note the attachment of the joint capsule); and (5) the muscular plane or outside through a sinus.

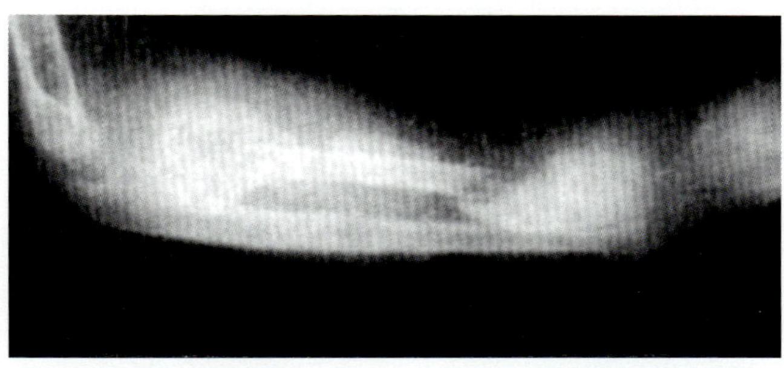

Fig. 18.3.7: Chronic osteomyelitis. Large diaphyseal sequestrum involving radius (radiograph).

Diagnosis

Early diagnosis is important and yet difficult since the radiograph may look normal in the initial period. The diagnosis is made essentially by clinical judgment. There may be a history of trauma to the affected part preceding the onset of symptoms. One may also find a primary focus of infection in the body, e.g. skin, throat, etc.

The child presents with high fever, headache, restlessness and dehydration; occasionally with signs of toxemia. The child resists movement of the limb and there is tenderness over the metaphysis.

The investigations are nonspecific and may not clinch the diagnosis. The investigations show: (1) raised local leukocyte count (up to 20,000) and a raised erythrocyte sedimentation rate (ESR), (2) blood culture may isolate the organism, (3) radiograph may show a periosteal reaction in the metaphysis, as late as 7–12 days, and (4) a technetium-99m bone scan may show an increased uptake.

Differential Diagnosis

Acute osteomyelitis has to be differentiated from pyogenic and other noninfective arthritis.

Treatment

The most important factor for a successful treatment is early diagnosis. At the first suspicion of acute osteomyelitis, the child should be admitted and investigated. A blood culture is sent and empirically intravenous chemotherapy using ampicillin and cloxacillin should be started. One may also add gentamicin to broaden the spectrum. The antibiotic is subsequently changed according to the culture and sensitivity report. The limb is immobilized in a POP cast. If there is no response to this treatment within 24 hours, surgical drainage of the abscess is carried out. Antibiotics are continued for a period of 6 weeks approximately.

CHRONIC OSTEOMYELITIS

Acute osteomyelitis, when treated inadequately, becomes chronic osteomyelitis. Sometimes, it may become chronic due to poor host defense mechanism.

Diagnosis

Chronic osteomyelitis is characterized by discharging sinuses, which are fixed to the underlying bone. Pain may occasionally be present during an acute exacerbation. There may be irregular thickening of the bone. Occasionally, the adjacent joint may be stiff due to secondary arthritis.

The radiograph may show a cavity in the bone containing a sequestrum, sometimes with a pathological fracture **(Fig. 18.3.8)**.

Chronic osteomyelitis should be differentiated from Ewing's sarcoma and tuberculous osteomyelitis.

Treatment

- Antibiotics are given according to the pus culture and sensitivity reports
- *Surgery*: Removal of the sequestrum (sequestrectomy) and the infected granulation tissue (curettage)
- Amputation may be indicated very rarely, when the sinus undergoes a malignant change or the patient develops amyloidosis.

Complications

- Stiffness of the adjacent joints
- Pathological fracture
- Deformity due to malunion of a pathological fracture
- Shortening, when the growth plate is damaged
- A long-standing discharging sinus may rarely cause squamous cell carcinoma
- Secondary amyloidosis.

Osteomyelitis in human immunodeficiency virus disease: The destruction of bone is much more extensive with little or no reparative new bone formation. Upper tibia and lower femur are usually involved. The disease is often bilateral, and septic arthritis is common.

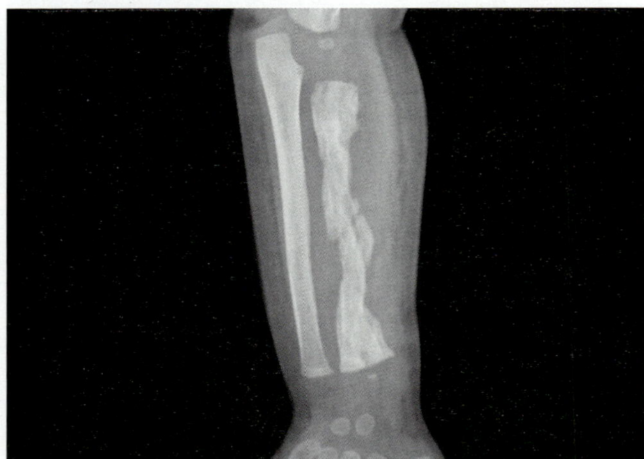

Fig. 18.3.8: Pathological fracture of humerus in chronic osteomyelitis.

PYOGENIC (SEPTIC) ARTHRITIS

Pyogenic organisms, mainly *Staphylococcus aureus*, cause it. However, Streptococci, Pneumococci, Gonococci, Meningococci and *E. coli* may infect the joint occasionally. In young children, *Haemophilus influenzae* has also been reported to be a common organism.

Acute pyogenic arthritis may also occur in acute infectious diseases such as enteric fever, influenza, pneumonia, etc.

Routes of Infection

The organisms gain entry through:

- Hematogenous route from a primary focus in the respiratory tract, genitourinary tract, intestinal tract, teeth, tonsils, etc. or umbilical cord sepsis.
- An infection in the bone, particularly when the metaphysis is intra-articular as in hip or shoulder.
- A puncture wound.

Diagnosis

Knee, hip, elbow and shoulder joints may be affected. The child presents with the symptoms and signs of acute inflammation, occasionally toxemia. Examination of the joint fluid may help in the diagnosis. The blood examination may show a raised leukocyte count and ESR, which is also present in most inflammatory conditions.

Differential Diagnosis

- Tuberculous arthritis
- Acute rheumatism
- Acute pyogenic osteomyelitis.

Treatment

Principles of Treatment

Early diagnosis, appropriate antibiotics and joint drainage can save the joint from complete destruction and disorganization.

ACUTE SEPTIC ARTHRITIS OF INFANCY (TOM SMITH ARTHRITIS)

Acute septic arthritis of infancy (Tom Smith arthritis), seen in infancy, is generally secondary to a neighboring bone lesion. The child presents with the signs and symptoms of acute inflammation, occasionally toxemia. In infants, the femoral head is cartilaginous and gets destroyed completely by the infection thereby, affecting the future function of the limb. The treatment in the acute stage is early drainage under proper antibiotic cover.

OSTEOARTICULAR TUBERCULOSIS

Tuberculosis of the bones and joints is almost always secondary to a primary focus somewhere in the body.

Tuberculous Osteomyelitis

It is a subacute infection commonly seen in small bones, such as metacarpals, metatarsals, phalanges **(Fig. 18.3.9)**, carpals and calcaneus, etc. The long bones are rarely affected. It presents as pain, swelling of the affected part and occasionally, a discharging sinus.

Tuberculous Infection of the Joint

Tuberculosis, synovial or osseous, may affect any joint; however, the commonly affected joints are hip **(Fig. 18.3.10A)**, knee and elbow. The shoulder, wrist and ankle joints are rarely affected.

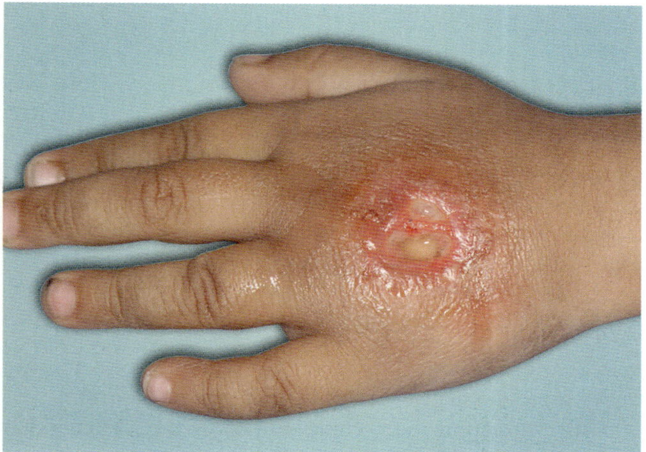

Fig. 18.3.9: Tuberculosis of phalanges.

Clinical Features

The patient usually presents with pain, swelling and restriction of movements of the affected joint. In advanced cases, there may be a discharging sinus and deformity of the joint.

Treatment

The treatment consists of following:

- Antituberculous drugs four drug regime (HRZE) is started initially for 4 months, followed by two drugs (HR) for a total period of 4–7 months
- Immobilization of the affected part in a plaster for about 4–6 weeks
- Surgery—curettage of the bony lesion with or without bone grafting
- The aim of treatment is to achieve a fixed or a mobile joint based on the condition of the joint. Surgical fusion (arthrodesis) achieves a painless fixed joint; whereas some sort of arthroplasty is done to get a mobile joint.

Tuberculosis of the Spine (Pott's Spine)

Tuberculosis commonly affects the thoracolumbar spine; however, it is also seen in the other regions of the spine.

Clinical Features

- *Pain*: Patients present with constitutional symptoms such as fever, cough, loss of appetite and weight, but generally pain in the back is the predominant symptom. It is usually the first indication of the disease, and is localized over the affected area of the spine. In tuberculosis of the dorsal spine, the patient may feel referred pain, called as "girdle pains", along the intercostal nerves, to the front of the chest.
- *Deformity*: Deformity of the spine kyphosis (**Fig. 18.3.10B**) results from destruction and collapse of the affected vertebra.

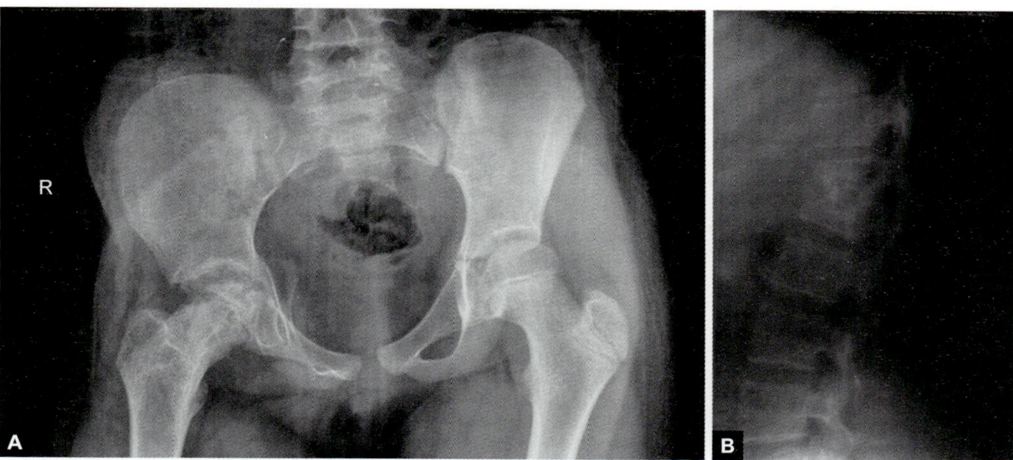

Figs. 18.3.10A and B: (A) X-ray picture showing tuberculosis of right hip joint; (B) Kyphotic deformity of the spine due to destruction and collapse of the affected vertebrae.

- *Abscess*: It is called "cold" abscess because it presents away from the site of activity of the disease, and therefore, does not present with the usual signs of inflammation over it. Clinically, the abscess can present as: (1) psoas abscess, (2) abscess in the lumbar triangle, (3) abscess over the side of the chest wall and occasionally, (4) an abscess in the gluteal region.
- *Paralysis*: Paraplegia is often the presenting symptom in patients with tuberculosis of the dorsal or dorsolumbar spine. This results from compression of the spinal cord due to abscess, granulation tissues, bony sequestrum or due to mechanical pressure caused by angulation of the vertebral column. Quadriplegia will result from tuberculosis in the cervical spine.

Treatment

- *Antituberculous drugs*: Given for a total period of 6–9 months.
- *Rest to the part*: Given by means of a POP jacket or a corset.
- *Drainage of the abscess*: A cold abscess may require aspiration or drainage.
  - *Decompression:* The cord compression is relieved by various procedures such as costotransversectomy, anterolateral decompression, radical operation or laminectomy.

PERTHES' DISEASE (LEGG-CALVÉ-PERTHES' DISEASE)

Perthes' disease, also known as coxa plana, is an avascular necrosis (AVN) of the head of femur resulting from interference with its blood supply. The femoral head subsequently reforms but results in deformation **(Fig. 18.3.11)**. It occurs between the ages of 3 years and 10 years, with 80% male preponderance. Usually unilateral, but may be bilateral (10%).

Clinical Features

Though the classical presentation is that of a painless limp, the child may present with a history of periodic attacks of limping with pain in the hip or referred pain to the knee. In early stages, there is limitation of movement with muscle spasm.

Plain X-ray clinches the diagnosis; however, MRI may be required occasionally.

Treatment

The aim of treatment is prevention of deformity of the femoral head by ensuring containment of the head within the acetabulum by surgical or nonsurgical methods.

In the early stage, the child is treated by skin traction to relieve pain and muscle spasm. When the muscle spasm is relieved, the child is allowed to walk with a weight-relieving caliper.

Surgery may be required to improve containment of the femoral head within the acetabulum.

PEDIATRIC BONE TUMORS

Osteosarcoma

Osteosarcoma is a highly malignant primary bone tumor that occurs between 10 years and 20 years of age. It is commonly seen in males, in the metaphysis of distal end of femur **(Fig. 18.3.12)**, proximal end of tibia and the proximal end of humerus.

Clinical Features

Pain is the initial and dominating symptom. After some weeks, a progressively increasing bone swelling appears.

On examination, the swelling is fusiform; the overlying skin is stretched and shiny with prominent veins. The swelling is

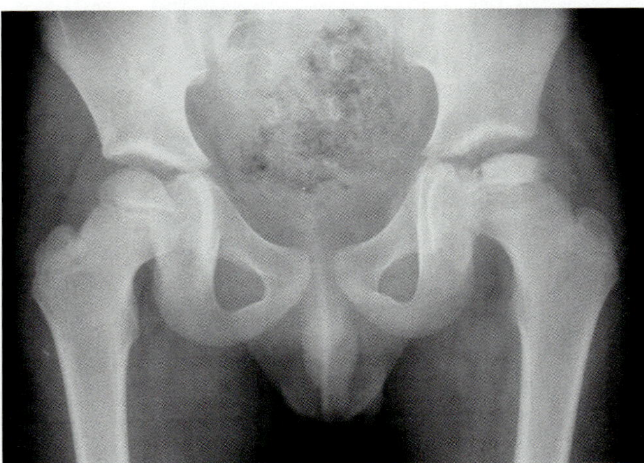

Fig. 18.3.11: Perthes' disease of the left hip.

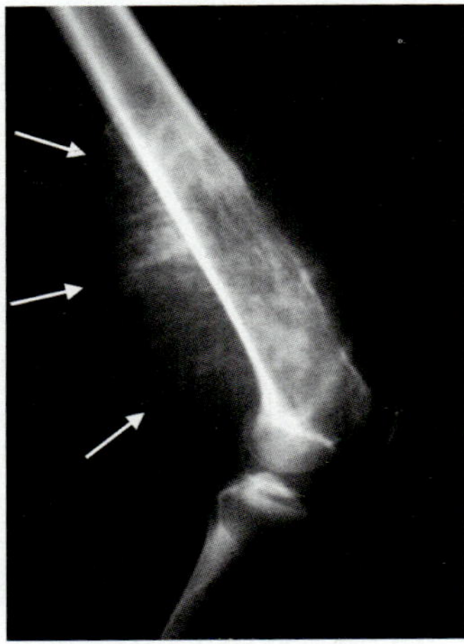

Fig. 18.3.12: Osteosarcoma of lower end of femur.

warm to touch, and has a variegated consistency. The patient's general health deteriorates with anemia, loss of weight and cachexia. Biopsy is mandatory to establish the diagnosis.

Treatment

Broadly speaking, the treatment of osteosarcoma is usually a combination of the following:

- *Surgery*: A limb saving surgery is done, after neoadjuvant chemotherapy, if the lesion is small. Amputation is indicated, if limb salvage is not feasible.
- Radiotherapy and chemotherapy are indicated for local control of the disease after incomplete surgical removal of the tumor and to control micrometastasis.

A regular follow-up every 3 months is mandatory to detect any recurrence or spread of the tumor.

Ewing's Tumor

It is an uncommon type of highly malignant bone tumor occurring commonly in males, in the age group of 10–20 years. It affects the diaphysis of long bones such as femur, tibia and humerus **(Fig. 18.3.13)**. It also occurs in flat bones like pelvis.

Clinical Features

The patient presents with gradually increasing pain, followed by swelling. The swelling is firm to soft in consistency with indefinite margins. There is usually fever, anemia and leukocytosis, and therefore, the condition often simulates subacute osteomyelitis. The swelling rapidly increases in size with involvement of soft tissues and the general condition deteriorates.

Treatment

Ewing's tumor is radiosensitive and is best treated by local resection combined with pre- and postoperative chemo- and radiotherapy. This regimen has increased the survival rate from 5% to 50%.

Amputation is indicated in locally advanced cases.

MISCELLANEOUS PROBLEMS

Transient Synovitis of the Hip

It is also called observation hip. It is a sterile inflammation and effusion, of unknown etiology, of the hip joint affecting children between 4 years and 8 years of age. The importance of this condition lies in the fact that it may precede other conditions such as septic arthritis of hip or Perthes' disease. The child, therefore, is kept under observation.

Clinical Features

The main complaints are pain in the groin and refusal to move the limb or walk. There is usually no fever. The movements of the hip are restricted, especially internal rotation. However, the child is otherwise comfortable when resting in bed with a pillow under the knee.

Treatment

The child is admitted for observation. Immobilization by skin traction to the limb may relieve muscle spasm and pain. The condition resolves spontaneously within a week's time.

Bow Legs (Genu Varum) and Knock-Knees (Genu Valgum)

Genu Valgum

Genu valgum denotes a malalignment in the frontal (coronal) plane, in which the part distal to the site of deformity deviates away from the midline **(Fig. 18.3.14)**. Unilateral genu valgum

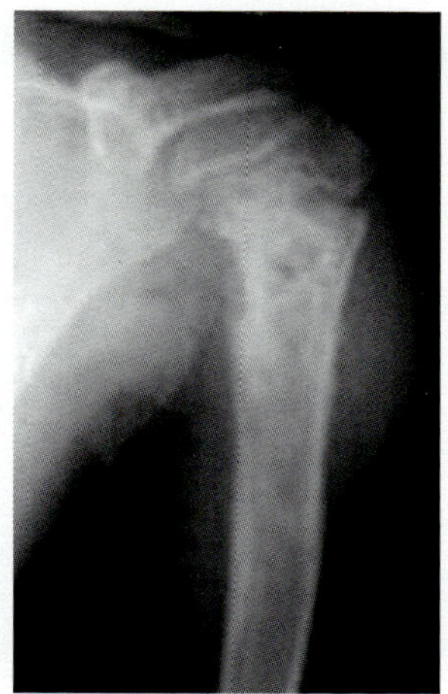

Fig. 18.3.13: Ewing's sarcoma.

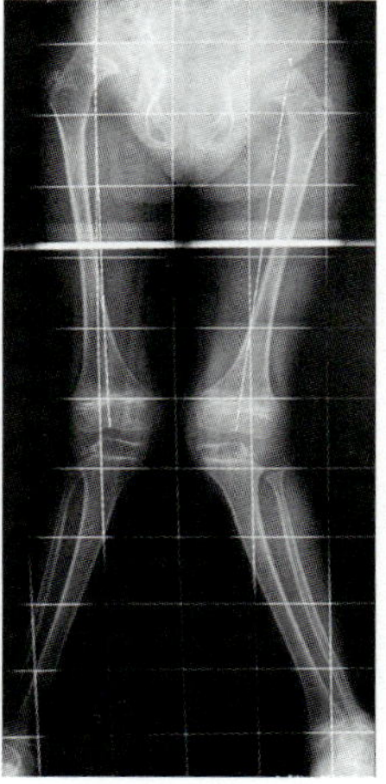

Fig. 18.3.14: Genu valgum.

may be caused by disturbance in the epiphyseal growth at the lower femur or upper tibia due to trauma or osteomyelitis. Bilateral genu valgum can be caused by endocrine or metabolic disorders, rickets and epiphyseal dysplasia or can be idiopathic.

Treatment: Genu valgum deformity can be ignored in the toddlers as it may get corrected spontaneously. However, if the distance between the two medial malleoli (intermalleolar distance) is more than 10 cm at the age of 10 years, it will need surgical correction.

Genu Varum

Genu varum or "bow legs" is the lateral curvature of leg involving either the tibia or femur or both **(Fig. 18.3.15)**. Mild genu varum is physiological up to 3 years of age and will get corrected spontaneously in the majority.

The other causes are: Rickets, post-traumatic or infective and idiopathic.

Treatment: A mild deformity can be treated by modifications in the shoes. Moderate-to-severe deformity needs surgical correction.

Flat Foot

Normally, the foot has longitudinal and transverse arches. The normal longitudinal arch is visible on the medial side of the foot **(Fig. 18.3.16)**. When this arch is less developed, it is called as flat foot **(Fig. 18.3.17)**.

Causes and Types of Flat Foot

- *Congenital vertical talus*: The talus bone is placed vertically in the foot, instead of being horizontal, which is normal. A radiograph will confirm the diagnosis. The treatment is difficult. Manipulation and serial plaster casts may be indicated in mild cases, whereas severe cases need surgery (**Fig. 18.3.18**).

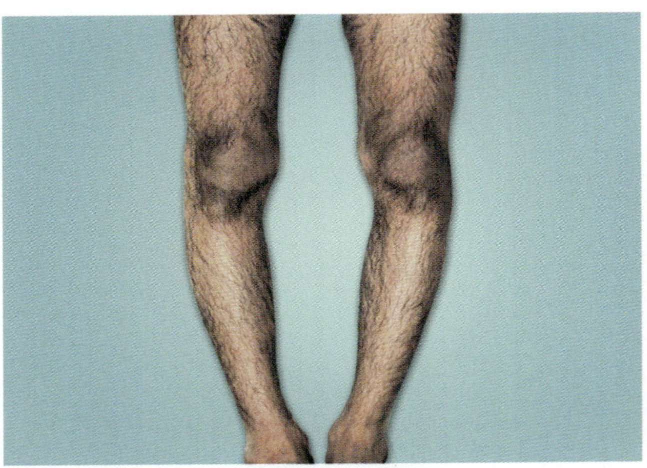

Fig. 18.3.15: Clinical photograph of genu varum of both knee joints.

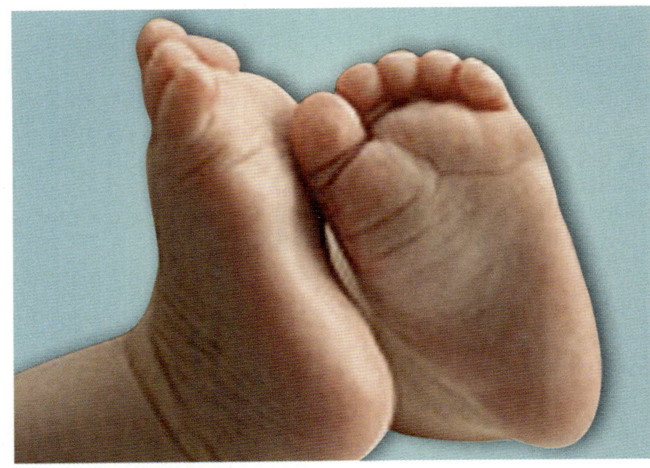

Fig. 18.3.16: Normal arch of the foot.

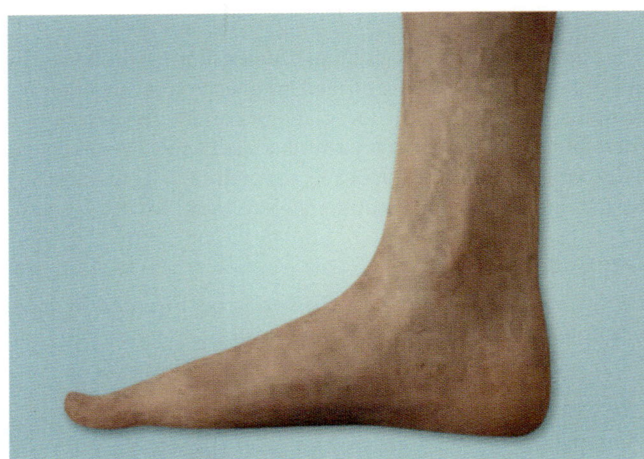

Fig. 18.3.17: Flat foot.

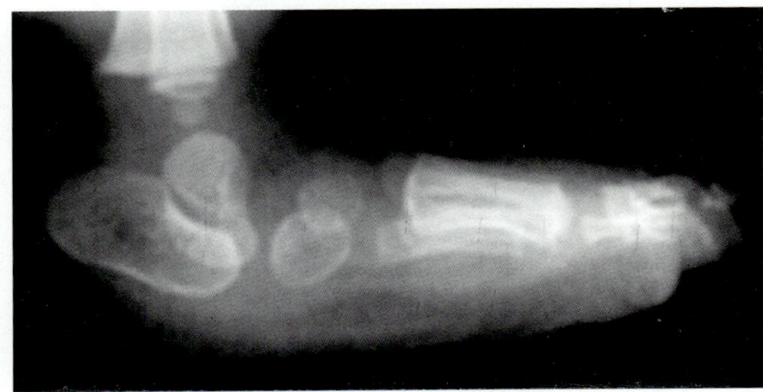

Fig. 18.3.18: Congenital vertical talus.

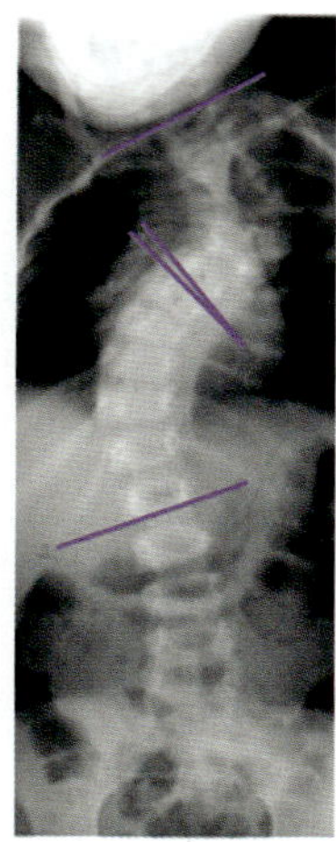

Fig. 18.3.19: Scoliosis.

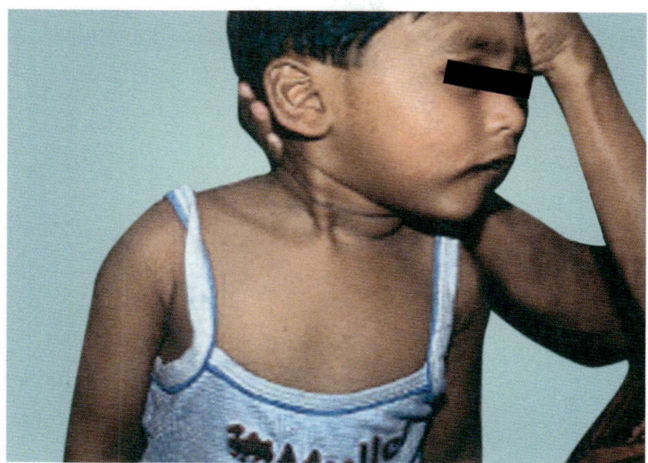

Fig. 18.3.20: Contracted sternocleidomastoid muscle on right side causing torticollis.

- *Physiological or infantile flat foot*: This is the most common type, in which the child has flat feet when he or she starts walking. But gradually, the arch develops within the next 2–3 years. In such a case, no specific treatment is required. However, an arch support inside the shoe and slight modification in the sole of the foot may be prescribed. In an older child, exercises for the intrinsic muscles of foot may be taught.

In severe cases, triple arthrodesis, i.e. fusion of the selected tarsal joints is indicated after skeletal maturity.

Scoliosis

Scoliosis is defined as lateral curvature of the spine **(Fig. 18.3.19)**. It can be congenital due to growth of only one-half of a vertebra (called as hemivertebra), idiopathic (the most common type) or paralytic. The treatment should be started as early as possible to prevent progression of the curve, and also to prevent cardiorespiratory complications as a result of severe deformity.

Torticollis

Torticollis results from contracture of the sternomastoid muscle on one side **(Fig. 18.3.20)**. Thickening of the muscle (sternomastoid tumor) occurs in infancy, replaced by fibrous tissue. The tight sternomastoid muscle exerts a pull on the head tilting it on the same side. If not treated early, it results in asymmetrical development of the face. Treatment is surgical release of the tight muscle.

18.4 Common Eye Problems

Upreet Dhaliwal, Payal Gupta

INTRODUCTION

Eye development is critical in the first few months of life; processes that interfere with development may seriously impact vision. It is recommended that children receive their first eye screening at birth, followed by an assessment at 6 months and thereafter, at every visit to the pediatrician **(Table 18.4.1)**.

The following children should be referred for ophthalmic evaluation as early as possible:

- Abnormal history (does not make eye contact or focus on and follow objects by 3 months of age, or reach for objects by 6 months of age)
- Abnormal appearance (redness of eyes or eyelids, watery or purulent discharge, white cornea, white pupil, asymmetric pupil size, swelling or drooping of eyelids, squint)

Table 18.4.1: Important milestones in the development of the pediatric eye.

	At birth	*1 month*	*2–3 months*	*6 months*	*1 year*	*3 years*
Visual acuity	Can see up to 3 months	Can see up to 4 months	Can see up to 8 months	6/12	6/9	6/6
Fixation reflex		Normal optokinetic, nystagmus		Well developed		
Convergence reflex		Starts		Well developed		
Binocularity			Starts	Well developed		
Pupillary reflex	Sluggish	Well developed				
Color vision	Black and white, and shades of gray				Full color	
Menace reflex		Present				

- Evidence of discomfort (excessive rubbing of eyes, avoids bright light, keeps one or both eyes closed most of the time).

VISUAL PROBLEMS

Refractive Errors

A refractive error is an optical defect in the eye that prevents light rays from focusing on the macula, thus preventing clear vision. Most children are hypermetropic at birth; however, the eyeball enlarges over time so that the eye becomes emmetropic; if the process of enlargement continues, older children will be myopic.

Refractive errors are due to an abnormality in axial length, curvature or index of the optical media. Thus, longer length, steeper curvature and higher index will cause rays of parallel light to focus sooner, in front of the retina, producing myopia. The reverse situation will cause hypermetropia where rays of parallel light are brought to focus behind the retina. Accommodation (increasing the curvature of the lens) shifts the focus anteriorly so that a clear image is formed on the retina. Constant accommodation in hypermetropes causes headaches, eyestrain and excessive convergence (convergent squint). Astigmatism results when the refractive power of the eye is different in different meridia and different foci are formed on the retina.

One should suspect refractive errors when children report difficulty in reading off the blackboard, eyestrain on near work and holding books close to the eyes. Check vision using Snellen chart; repeat using a pinhole. In refractive errors, vision improves with the pinhole since it prevents spherical aberrations by cutting off peripheral rays. A pinhole can easily be made by creating a hole (< 1 mm in diameter) at the center of an opaque disc of cardboard. Refractive errors are commonly treated using corrective lenses such as spectacles or contact lenses. Refractive surgery can also correct some refractive errors.

Amblyopia

Amblyopia (lazy eye) is a partial decrease of vision in the absence of anatomical/structural abnormality. It results when there is inadequate foveal stimulation and/or abnormal binocular interaction (different visual input from the two foveae) during the first 5 years of life when the visual system is still developing. When there is a difference in the quality of the image recorded by each eye, the brain disregards the blurred image; this results in the visual system developing more slowly for that eye.

Amblyopia may be due to uncorrected refractive errors, strabismus or due to visual deprivation (ptosis, surgical lid closure, bandaging, corneal opacity, cataract). In preverbal children, suspect poor vision in one eye when the child protests covering of one eye (the eye with better vision), shows fixation preference for one eye, has unilateral squint or eccentric fixation.

The four "Os" of amblyopia treatment are as follows:

1. *Optics:* Treat all conditions that prevent a clear foveal image from forming.
2. *Occlusion:* Occlude the better eye so that the amblyopic eye is forced to work (conventional occlusion). It should be alternated between the two eyes to prevent the occluded eye from developing amblyopia. The duration of occlusion and alternation depends on the age of the child and the severity of amblyopia. If older children resist occlusion, atropine is used to blur vision in the sound eye (penalization).
3. *Orthoptics:* Foveal stimulation exercises.
4. *Operation:* For strabismus or any media opacity-like cataract.

The endpoint of therapy is alternation of fixation or equal vision in both the eyes.

Color Vision Deficiency

Photosensitive pigments in the cones allow us to see colors. There are three types of cones, each containing a different pigment—red (erythrolabe), green (chlorolabe) or blue (cyanolabe); each preferentially absorbs only one part of the visible spectrum. Many millions of hues can be generated by stimulation of all three cones to varying degrees.

Genes contain the coding instructions for the three pigments; if the instructions are wrong, the wrong pigments are produced, and the abnormal cones will be sensitive to a different wavelength. A child that has difficulty in identifying colors by 3–4 years of age could be color blind. All children, especially boys, should have a routine color vision check once during a school health checkup.

Color blindness is most common for red and green colors. Inherited as an X-linked recessive genetic defect, it is seen in 10% of males and 0.4% of females. Blue color blindness, due to defect on chromosome-7, is seen in 5% of people. Color blindness may also be acquired in conditions that involve the cones or the visual pathway (chorioretinitis, diabetic retinopathy, optic neuritis, partial optic atrophy, migraine, stroke and cerebral trauma). Unlike congenital color blindness, the acquired forms may be unilateral, progressive or transient, and show no gender predisposition.

Screening tests (Ishihara pseudoisochromatic plates) are used to detect, if a color vision defect is present or not. More sophisticated tests (Farnsworth-Munsell 100-Hue test or Lantern test) are required, if the objective is to exactly classify the type and degree of defect. Persons with abnormal color vision cannot take up jobs dealing with public safety, and the driving of commercial vehicles, train engines or airplanes; children should be aware of this when they are considering future careers. There is no treatment for congenital color vision deficiency, although the use of filters can help differentiate colors in some instances.

Xerophthalmia

Xerophthalmia is a bilateral, dry, lusterless condition of the conjunctiva and cornea due to vitamin A deficiency. It occurs in malnourished children since they already have low stores of vitamin A; it may be precipitated by exanthematous febrile illness or persistent diarrhea. Children may report night blindness. Bitot's spots, conjunctival and corneal xerosis, corneal melting (keratomalacia) or corneal scars may be present.

The child should be referred to an ophthalmologist. Treatment comprises replacement of vitamin A, treatment of the precipitating condition, and taking care of the general health of the child and of the ocular condition. Keratomalacia requires emergency management to prevent corneal perforation. Corneal transplantation is the only treatment once corneal scars form.

INFECTIONS

Infective Conjunctivitis

Etiology

- *Bacterial*: *Staphylococcal spp., Haemophilus spp., Neisseria spp., Streptococcus spp.*, etc.
- *Viral*: Adenovirus, picornavirus, *Herpes simplex*
- *Fungal*: *Aspergillus, Candida*, etc.

Clinical Features

- Redness, itching and foreign body sensation
- Swollen lids
- Rarely, reduced vision (due to corneal involvement)
- Discharge helps in differentiating between viral (watery) and bacterial conjunctivitis (mucopurulent).
- Preauricular lymphadenopathy in viral conjunctivitis due to adenovirus or picornavirus.

Management

Etiological diagnosis is usually not necessary. Adenoviral conjunctivitis is very common and is highly contagious (epidemic keratoconjunctivitis). The pediatrician should advise frequent handwashing, separate towels, handkerchiefs, etc. to reduce the risk of spreading infection. There is no specific treatment; however, symptoms can be reduced with instillation of artificial tears, topical antihistamines or applying cold compresses. Bacterial conjunctivitis resolves spontaneously without specific treatment; however, topical, empirical antibacterial therapy results in earlier microbiological remission.

Ophthalmia Neonatorum

Etiology

The infection may be chlamydial, gonococcal or due to *Herpes simplex* virus. Conjunctivitis occurs due to infection acquired from the birth canal.

Clinical Features

- Watering and purulent discharge from both eyes in the first few days of life (**Fig. 18.4.1**).
- There may be an associated keratitis or uveitis
- In gonococcal infection, the local symptoms and signs are severe; there are systemic features such as fever, urethritis, arthritis, endocarditis, meningitis and septicemia.

Management

A conjunctival swab will help identify the organism, but treatment should begin at once. Wash eyes copiously with saline water frequently. Apply atropine eye ointment, if there is associated keratitis or uveitis (common in gonorrhea).

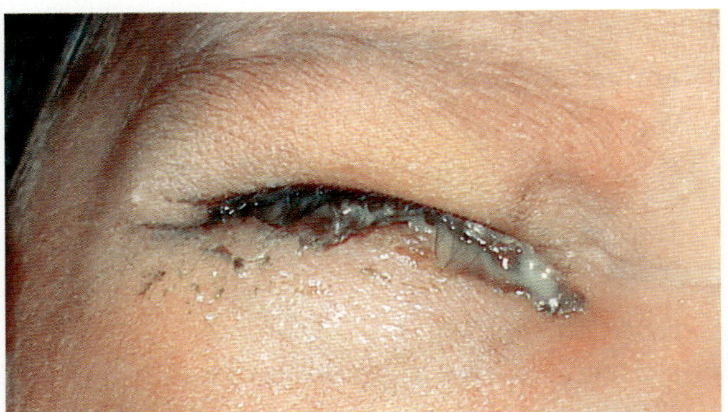

Fig. 18.4.1: Purulent conjunctivitis in a neonate (Ophthalmia neonatorum).

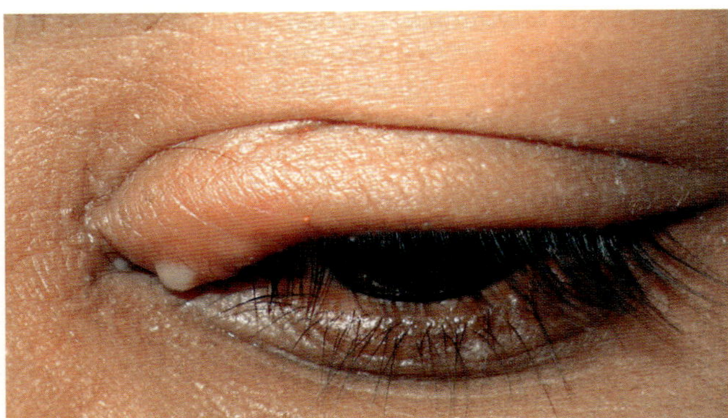

Fig. 18.4.2: Infective swelling in the upper eyelid in the region of the eyelashes (hordeolum externum).

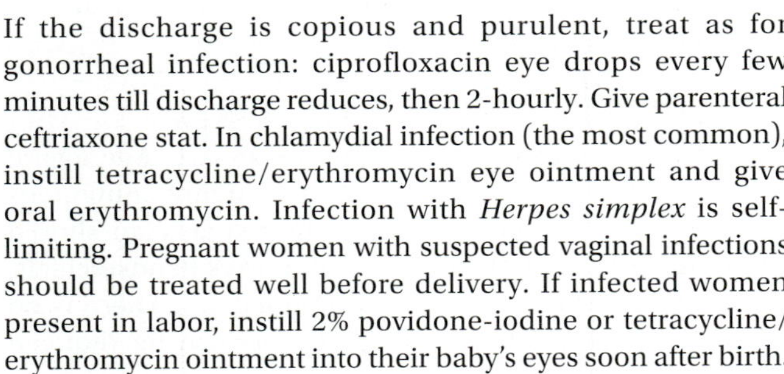

If the discharge is copious and purulent, treat as for gonorrheal infection: ciprofloxacin eye drops every few minutes till discharge reduces, then 2-hourly. Give parenteral ceftriaxone stat. In chlamydial infection (the most common), instill tetracycline/erythromycin eye ointment and give oral erythromycin. Infection with *Herpes simplex* is self-limiting. Pregnant women with suspected vaginal infections should be treated well before delivery. If infected women present in labor, instill 2% povidone-iodine or tetracycline/erythromycin ointment into their baby's eyes soon after birth.

Membranous Conjunctivitis

Etiology

Typically seen in diphtheritic infection; may occur in infections due to other bacteria when virulence is high, or host immunity is low.

Clinical Features

- Conjunctivitis with mucopurulent or blood-stained discharge
- Conjunctival membranes or pseudomembranes
- Symblepharon (adhesions between palpebral and bulbar conjunctiva)
- Keratitis
- Necrosis of conjunctiva.

In severe cases, membranes may also form on the conjunctiva when the infective organism is highly virulent, or the host immunity is low.

Management

Diphtheritic membranes are difficult to peel off; membranes that do peel off (pseudomembranes) should be removed as this reduces the infective load in the eye. Treatment is directed to both the local and systemic conditions; the child must be isolated and appropriate specific antimicrobial treatment should be given.

Corneal Ulcer

Etiology

Bacterial, fungal, viral or protozoal.

Clinical Features

- There may be a history of injury with vegetative material (plant leaf, twig, animal tail in fungal ulcer), fever (in viral ulcer) or abuse of steroid eye drops.
- The child presents with pain, redness of eye and blepharospasm
- Diminished vision due to corneal involvement or associated intraocular infection (endophthalmitis)
- The corneal epithelium is abraded and there may be slough resulting in loss of transparency
- There is mucopurulent (bacterial or fungal ulcer) or watery discharge (viral ulcer).

Management

When a corneal ulcer is suspected, refer urgently to an ophthalmologist. It is best to apply a sterile eye pad during the transfer, although one does not usually patch an eye with an infective ulcer unless it is very deep and could perforate.

Eyelid Infections

Acute Infections

Etiology: Usually caused by *Staphylococcal* species and include blepharitis, hordeolum externum (stye; due to blockage of the duct of glands associated with an eyelash follicle, i.e. Ziess gland; **Fig. 18.4.2**) and hordeolum internum (suppurative inflammation due to blockage of the duct of a meibomian gland).

Clinical Features

- In hordeola with painful swelling, there is blockage of the glands associated with an eyelash follicle (externum); **(*see* Fig. 18.4.2)** or meibomian gland (internum), along with staphylococcal infection.
- Blepharitis results in inflamed lid margin with ulceration and yellow crusts (ulcerative blepharitis) or dandruff-like flakes (squamous blepharitis)
- May be recurrent, if associated with uncorrected refractive errors or reduced immunity.

Management

Treat refractive errors and prescribe empirical local antibiotics. If a lid abscess forms, it must be drained under cover of systemic and topical antibiotics.

Chronic Inflammation (Chalazion)

Etiology: Blockage of the duct of a meibomian gland results in a granulomatous reaction to lipid content of the gland.

Clinical Features

- Painless mass in eyelid
- Free from skin; visible as a bluish discoloration on the conjunctival side.

Management: Chalazion may resolve on its own. If it is large or does not resolve, intralesional steroid injection may help or it may be incised, and its contents curetted under regional anesthesia.

Orbital Cellulitis

Etiology

This is a serious condition; infection of the soft tissue of the orbit usually derives from the adjacent ethmoidal sinus, or from preseptal (eyelid) cellulitis.

Clinical Features

- Painful proptosis
- Lid edema
- Restricted ocular movements
- The cornea may develop exposure keratitis
- Optic nerve function may be compromised due to increased orbital pressure
- Signs of regional infection
- There may be systemic signs suggestive of septicemia.

Management

The condition mandates an urgent ophthalmic consult, admission, and immediate local and systemic broad-spectrum antibiotic therapy. If an orbital abscess forms, it must be surgically drained.

ALLERGIC AND INFLAMMATORY CONDITIONS

Phlyctenular Keratoconjunctivitis

Etiology

An allergic response to protein from endogenous infections (*Staphylococcus*, mycobacteria, *Herpes simplex*, helminthiasis).

Clinical Features

- Itching, foreign body sensation and redness of eye
- One or more phlyctens (blisters) on the bulbar or palpebral conjunctiva, limbus or cornea
- The blisters ulcerate and heal by scarring, and are recurrent unless the endogenous infection is treated
- The patient complains of itching, foreign body sensation and redness of eye. Corneal lesions cause pain, photophobia and may affect vision

Management

Topical steroids, along with investigation and treatment of infectious causes elsewhere in the body. When there is local staphylococcal infection (conjunctivitis, blepharitis), give topical antibiotics followed later by topical steroids, if required.

Spring Catarrh

Etiology

An allergic conjunctivitis due to exogenous allergens such as pollen, animal hair, etc.

Clinical Features

- Seen mainly in the 1st decade of life, more often in boys
- It has seasonal recurrence (in the warm months, subsiding in winter); it usually subsides by puberty
- The child has itching and ropy mucoid discharge in both eyes
- In the bulbar form, there are gelatinous papillae around the limbus
- In the palpebral form, there are large papillae in the palpebral conjunctiva, giving a cobblestone appearance
- The two forms may coexist; the cornea may be involved too.

Management

We know that the allergen should be avoided. Just before the warm months, to delay onset of symptoms, start topical antihistamines and mast cell stabilizers. During symptomatic periods, give topical corticosteroids and cold compresses. Topical immunosuppressant (cyclosporine A) may be required in recalcitrant cases.

Anterior Uveitis

Etiology

Anterior uveitis in children is seen in a variety of systemic conditions; hence, the pediatrician may be the first to see these patients. Infectious causes include tuberculosis, *Herpes simplex, Herpes zoster* and mumps.

Noninfectious causes are more common; the strongest association is with juvenile idiopathic arthritis (JIA), where the child has no ocular symptoms and may progress to band-shaped keratopathy, cataract and glaucoma. Other non-infectious causes are spondyloarthropathies and sarcoidosis. A general medical history, physical examination and specific laboratory tests may elicit cause. Children with these conditions should be seen by an ophthalmologist, even if they have no ocular complaints.

Clinical Features

- Redness of eye from deep ciliary congestion (circumcorneal)
- Pain in the eye
- Blurred vision
- Associated systemic features depending on etiology.

Management

A complete examination of the eye and ocular adnexa is essential, including the cornea (herpes simplex keratitis), uvea (granulomatous or non-granulomatous uveitis), lacrimal glands and regional lymph nodes (sarcoidosis). A fundus examination is mandatory to detect cystoid macular edema in eyes with chronic uveitis and to rule out posterior uveitis. Topical cycloplegics, and topical or periocular corticosteroids are the mainstay of treatment.

DISORDERS OF NERVES AND MUSCLES

Squint

Squint (strabismus) is the condition when the axes of the two eyes are misaligned relative to each other. The misalignment may be horizontal or vertical resulting in esotropia (one eye is relatively convergent), exotropia (one eye is relatively divergent; **Fig. 18.4.3**) or hypertropia (one eye is directed upward relative to the other). In addition, deviations may be concomitant or incomitant. Concomitant deviations do not vary with the direction of gaze; incomitant deviations vary with the direction of gaze and are usually due to paralysis of an extraocular muscle.

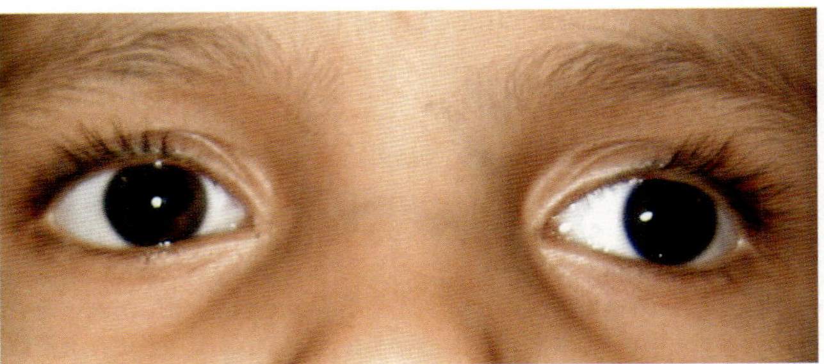

Fig. 18.4.3: Divergent squint (exotropia), left eye.
Source: Used with permission from Gupta P. Clinical Methods in Pediatrics, 2nd edition. New Delhi: CBS Publishers and Distributors; 2011.

Squint may be constant, being present throughout the day, or it may appear intermittently.

Etiology

Most squints develop sometime in the first 3 years of life. Newborn babies may squint occasionally, until their binocular reflexes develop; thus, any squint that presents or persists after the age of 3 months must be investigated.

In many cases, the cause is not known. In some, there is a strong family history (infantile esotropia). Squint may occur in uncorrected hypermetropia (excessive accommodation to see clearly causes excessive convergence, producing convergent squint); due to poor vision in one eye; or due to cerebral palsy, hydrocephalus or brain injury.

Clinical Features

- Misalignment of the visual axes relative to each other
- The fovea of each eye is focusing on a different object; thus, two different images reach the brain leading to confusion. The brain ignores the image coming from the deviated eye, leading eventually to strabismic amblyopia in that eye
- Binocular vision cannot develop so the child loses depth perception.

Management

Intermittent squint permits each fovea to receive adequate stimulation some of the time; hence treatment, though mandatory, is not emergent. Constant squint, however, needs early and aggressive treatment. If a refractive error is present, children should wear the spectacles constantly. In many cases, no other treatment is required. As the child grows, spectacle power is adjusted appropriately. If any squint remains despite spectacle correction, it can be corrected by muscle surgery.

A small number of children require surgery on the eye muscles to straighten the alignment. After surgery, it is usually necessary to continue spectacles, occlusion and exercise as advised by the ophthalmologist.

A false impression of squint (pseudostrabismus) may result from a flat, wide bridge of nose, or due to epicanthal folds so that the eyes look closer together than they really are. This appearance gradually disappears as the baby's nose bridge grows.

TUMOR AND TUMOR-LIKE CONDITIONS

Dermoid Cysts

Etiology

They represent surface ectoderm that got entrapped during bony fusion; thus, they overlie bony sutures.

Clinical Features

- These are painless, cystic masses usually found around the orbit at birth, near the medial or lateral part of the eyebrow.
- They are filled with sebaceous material including hair.
- They may leak after trauma; extruded sebaceous material produces inflammation and pain.
- Dermoids may be connected by a stalk to an intraorbital component.

Management

While periorbital dermoids are superficial, and thus simpler to remove surgically, orbital ones require an orbital approach.

Retinoblastoma

Retinoblastoma is the most common primary ocular malignancy of childhood. It has been already discussed in Chapter 12.6 Retinoblastoma.

WATERING FROM THE EYES

Congenital Dacryocystitis

Etiology

This is a result of incomplete canalization of the nasolacrimal duct, usually due to epithelial debris, membranes or valves in the duct.

Clinical Features

- Excessive unilateral or bilateral watering soon after birth
- The lacrimal sac may distend with accumulated secretions to form a palpable, cystic mass below the medial canthal tendon (mucocele)
- *Regurgitation test may be positive:* Pressure over the sac area (medial canthus) causes mucopus to regurgitate through the puncta into the conjunctival sac.

Management

The condition is amenable to conservative treatment with lacrimal sac massage several times a day for a few months, to push debris into the nose. Sustained pressure should be applied directly over the lacrimal sac, just under the medial canthal tendon, with the small finger of the parent's hand. The parent should be advised to ensure closure of the eyelids so that the puncta are always occluded during massage. In this way, the lacrimal sac does not empty into the conjunctival sac during massage, ensuring an adequate hydrostatic pressure to push debris into the nose. Empirical antibiotic eye drops are prescribed to prevent infection. If there is no relief after a month or two, the ophthalmologist will perform syringing and probing (under general anesthesia) to mechanically push the debris into the nose. Probing may be repeated two or three times; if it fails, surgery in the form of dacryocystorhinostomy is indicated.

Acute Dacryocystitis

Etiology

Bacterial overgrowth in congenital dacryocystitis may produce an acute condition.

Clinical Features

- Painful, erythematous swelling of the lacrimal sac
- The inflamed sac may rupture through the overlying skin resulting in fistula formation
- Infection may spread beyond the sac to produce preseptal cellulitis, or into the orbit (orbital cellulitis)
- More serious complications (cavernous sinus thrombosis, blindness and death) may supervene in immunocompromised individuals.

Management

The discharge should be cultured, and immediate broad-spectrum systemic antimicrobial therapy started. If an abscess forms, it should be drained. The condition should be reassessed 2–3 weeks after the acute condition subsides. Scarring from the acute event may prevent successful syringing and probing; dacryocystorhinostomy is usually indicated.

CATARACT AND GLAUCOMA

Pediatric Cataract

Cataract is a visually disabling opacity in the lens. It can occur at birth or develop later. Pediatricians play a vital role in diagnosing cataract since they are able to screen children for ocular abnormalities. Cataract can be diagnosed by noting a poor red reflex in the eye, or a white reflex in the pupil. All such children should be urgently referred to an ophthalmologist.

Etiology

The cause of cataract, in about a third of the cases, is obscure; a quarter shows autosomal-dominant inheritance. Bilateral cataracts can be due to infection during pregnancy (rubella, chickenpox, cytomegalovirus, herpes, syphilis and toxoplasmosis), galactosemia, diabetes, hypoglycemia, hypocalcemia, drugs (corticosteroids) and trisomy or myotonic dystrophy. Congenital unilateral cataract can be associated with ocular abnormalities such as posterior lenticonus and persistent hyperplastic primary vitreous. Ocular trauma is an important cause of unilateral cataract in older children **(Fig. 18.4.4)**; uveitis and retinoblastoma are other causes.

Clinical Features

- History of white reflex in pupil
- When cataract is visually significant and occurs in the first few months of life, there will be amblyopia (macula fails to develop fully), nystagmoid movements (fixation reflex fails to develop), and strabismus (binocularity fails to develop).

Management

Some types of cataracts are visually insignificant, and the child may only require refractive correction. Surgery is indicated, if the cataract is located centrally, or is large enough to block vision, and must be performed as soon as possible to prevent amblyopia.

To ensure optical correction, the convex power of the cataractous lens must be replaced by spectacles, contact lenses or intraocular lenses. Intraocular lenses are not implanted in children less than 2 years of age since the eyeball is yet to grow and the refractive power will change. Contact lenses or spectacles are used full time. If children are older than 2 years of age at the time of surgery, intraocular lenses are preferred. All children will need additional spectacle correction for near work as they get older. They will need intensive follow-up to manage refractive changes, amblyopia, squint, and possible complications of surgery such as glaucoma or retinal detachment, and after-cataract (inflammatory pupillary membranes or thickening of the posterior capsule after cataract surgery). If an after-cataract forms, the visual axis must be cleared using laser or surgery. If the cataract is a familial abnormality, all siblings and offsprings must be screened within 2 weeks of birth, and periodically thereafter for some years.

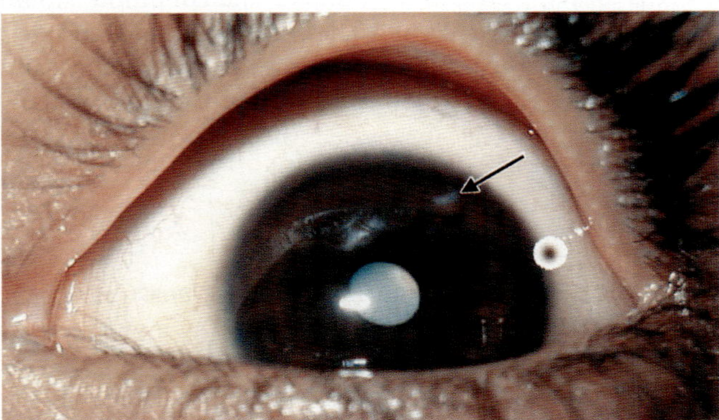

Fig. 18.4.4: Corneal opacity (arrow) and cataract after injury with bow and arrow.

Congenital Glaucoma

Primary developmental glaucoma (congenital glaucoma) results when elevated intraocular pressure occurs in the first 3 years of life. It is rare, its incidence being between 1:10,000 and 1:15,000 live births. It is bilateral in 75% of cases.

Etiology

The principal defect is a failure in cleavage of the anterior chamber angle during embryogenesis causing aqueous humor to accumulate in the eye.

Clinical Features

- The characteristic clinical picture is enlargement of the eyeball; the infant sclera is more elastic than the adult and stretches in response to elevated intraocular pressure. The enlarged eye resembles that of the ox, and the condition is called buphthalmos (ox eye).
- The presenting triad is watering, photophobia and blepharospasm; these result from the large edematous cornea.
- A horizontal corneal diameter greater than 12 mm is highly indicative of the disease.
- Optic disc cupping is seen early, increases rapidly and reverses to some extent with treatment.
- Glaucoma in childhood may be secondary to ocular developmental disorders such as aniridia (congenital absence of iris), or ectopia lentis (subluxation of lens). It may also be associated with systemic syndromes (Sturge-Weber syndrome, neurofibromatosis). Children with these disorders should be referred for periodic examination to an ophthalmologist.

Management

Examination under anesthesia is mandatory to rule out other conditions that mimic congenital glaucoma (megalocornea, keratitis, ophthalmia neonatorum, mucopolysaccharidosis). Large corneal diameters (vertical and horizontal), optic disc cupping, characteristic corneal edema and elevated intraocular pressure clinch the diagnosis. The mainstay of treatment is surgical. Pressure must be medically controlled before surgery. Even after successful control of glaucoma, the child needs treatment for refractive error induced in the enlarged eye and for amblyopia. Follow-up must be life-long, since the effect of surgery tends to diminish over time.

TRAUMA

Ocular injuries are the major cause of morbidity in children.

Etiology

Most injuries occur due to unsupervised play and are preventable. Usual modes of injury in children include stick, bow and arrow **(*see* Fig. 18.4.4)**, ball, stone, fist, *gilli-danda*, fireworks, scissors, knives, needles and other sharps.

Clinical Features

- The type of injury may be mechanical or chemical.
- Mechanical trauma may result in concussion or a sharp, lacerating injury.
- The eyelids, orbits or eyeball may be involved **(Figs. 18.4.5 to 18.4.7)**.
- Very often, there is a clear-cut history of injury; sometimes, particularly in preverbal children, no history is given.
- In suspected injury, like child abuse, even if there are no obvious ocular signs, refer for ophthalmic evaluation to rule out posterior segment trauma.
- Ocular injuries have potential to cause loss of vision **(Fig. 18.4.8)**.
- Eyelid and orbital injuries may result in disfigurement, causing psychosocial morbidity.

Management

Chemical injuries must be urgently managed at first presentation by thoroughly washing out all chemicals using any available inert solution; tap water, saline, Ringer's lactate may be used. Particulate material should be mechanically removed, and washing should continue for 15 minutes, before referral to an ophthalmic center. In mechanical trauma too, the child should be referred; however, if there is bleeding from the eyelid or eyeball, apply a sterile pad and bandage before transport.

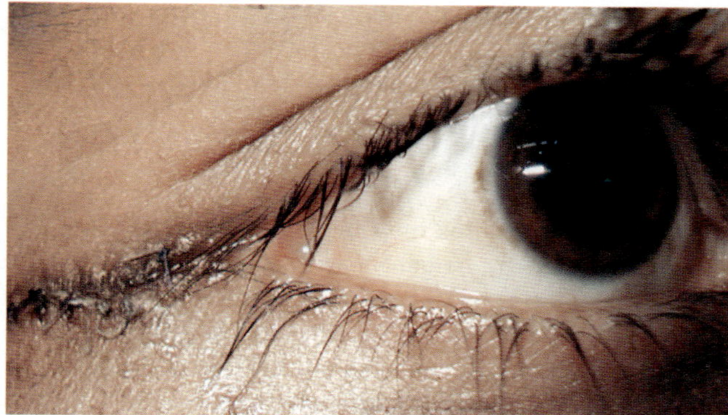

Fig. 18.4.5: Sutured laceration at lateral canthus after injury with a stick.

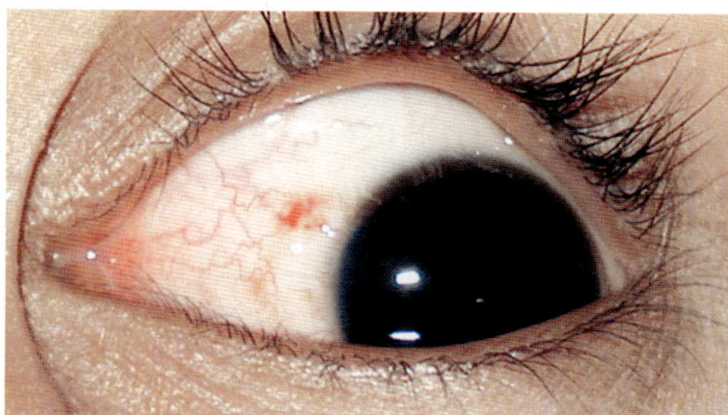

Fig. 18.4.6: Subconjunctival hemorrhage after injury with a pencil.

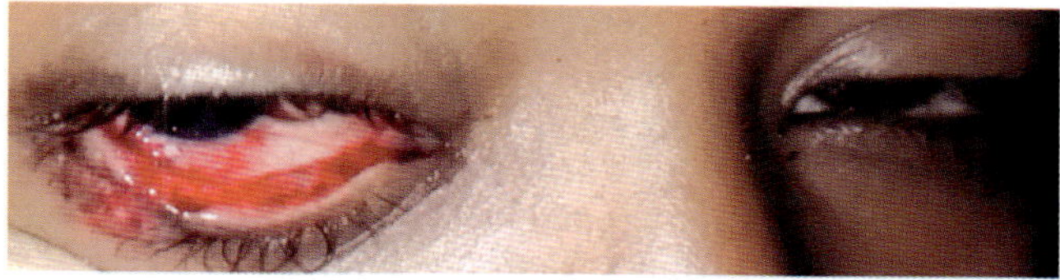

Fig. 18.4.7: Lid laceration with singeing of eyelashes after firecracker injury.

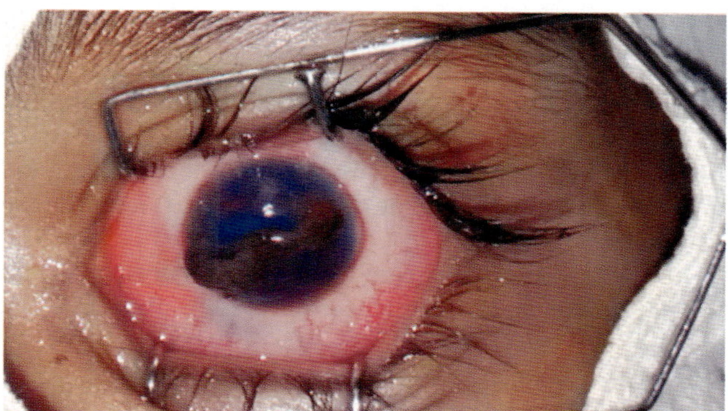

Fig. 18.4.8: Corneal perforation with iris prolapse following firecracker injury.

SUPERFICIAL FOREIGN BODY

Etiology

Particles of sand, wood, metal, or wing cases of insects or plant seeds, etc. may get blown into the eye and get impacted in the superficial layers (conjunctiva or cornea).

Clinical Features

- Sudden onset of foreign body sensation, with watering and redness.

- While conjunctivitis can also cause foreign body sensation, the pricking sensation of a foreign body is aggravated on eyeball movement in a particular direction, or on blinking.

Management

Corneal foreign bodies may be immediately visible; if it is not dislodged by irrigating with normal saline (under topical anesthesia), refer to an ophthalmologist. A foreign body on the bulbar or inferior palpebral conjunctiva may be removed using a sterile cotton swab stick; one in the superior palpebral conjunctiva can only be visualized and removed on everting the eyelid. If eversion is not possible, refer to an ophthalmologist. After removal, topical antibiotics should be prescribed for a few days to prevent infection. Corneal abrasion induced by the foreign body or by the process of its removal will necessitate padding and bandage.

RETINAL AND OPTIC NERVE DISORDERS

Optic Atrophy

Etiology

Optic atrophy is the endpoint of any disease process that causes retinal ganglion cell axons to degenerate.

In children, it can be hereditary (Leber-optic atrophy) or induced by retinal degeneration [retinitis pigmentosa (RP), retinopathy of prematurity (ROP)], orbital (compression by tumor or inflammation, traumatic neuropathy) or intracranial conditions (optic neuritis in meningitis or encephalitis).

Clinical Features

- Decreased visual acuity
- Scotomas in the visual field
- A relative afferent pupillary defect may be the only objective sign of optic atrophy
- Visual field defects on field testing.

Management

If unexplained optic atrophy is discovered during a routine checkup, the following investigations may assist in the diagnosis of cause: fundus examination, ultrasound of orbit, CT or MRI of orbit and brain, visual-evoked response, visual fields and color vision. All cranial nerves must be examined to rule out associated nerve involvement and to locate the site of lesion.

Since there is no treatment for the atrophy, it is important to detect and treat the underlying cause before atrophy sets in.

Papilledema

Papilledema is swelling of the optic nerve head due to elevated intracranial pressure. Elevated intracranial pressure raises the pressure in the subarachnoid space around the optic nerve, causing stasis of axoplasmic flow, build-up of toxic material and swelling.

Etiology

Causes of papilledema include malignant hypertension, central nervous system (CNS) space-occupying lesions, head injury, meningitis, encephalitis, venous sinus thrombosis, hydrocephalus, craniosynostosis and use of drugs such as tetracycline and corticosteroids.

Clinical Features

- It is usually bilateral and may develop over hours or weeks.
- Elevation of intracranial pressure in infancy, before the fontanels close, may not result in manifest papilledema.
- Symptoms specific to papilledema include transient obscurations of vision, constriction of visual field and decreased color perception.
- Vision may be normal until late in unresolved papilledema, when optic atrophy sets in.

Management

Investigative modalities include neuroimaging (CT scan, MRI) and venography for cause, and perimetry and fluorescein angiography to establish the diagnosis. Early detection, identification of cause and its appropriate treatment may be lifesaving.

Retinitis Pigmentosa

Etiology

Retinitis pigmentosa is a group of inherited disorders characterized by retinal pigment dystrophy. The worldwide prevalence is approximately 1 in 5,000. It can be associated with all types of inheritance, with autosomal dominant being the most common. It may also be associated with systemic disease, i.e. hearing loss (Usher syndrome).

Clinical Features

- Progressive night blindness (nyctalopia)
- Loss of peripheral vision (tunnel vision)
- Progression, sometimes up to complete blindness
- There may be loss of central vision
- It can present at infancy and up to the 3rd or 4th decade of life
- The characteristic triad seen in the retina includes bone spicules in the midperipheral retina, waxy optic disc pallor and retinal arteriolar attenuation
- Some patients develop cystoid macular edema, which reduces central vision as well.

Management

There are very few treatment options available; vitamin A, vitamin E, docosahexaenoic acid, acetazolamide (for macular edema) and lutein/zeaxanthin have been tried. Refraction and low-vision aids may help. Cataract surgery is done, if complicated cataract develops. Siblings and children of the affected individual should be screened. Gene therapy and transplantation of retinal pigment cells or stem cells is under experimentation.

Retinopathy of Prematurity

Etiology

Retinopathy of prematurity (ROP) is a fibrovascular proliferation in the retina of premature infants. Vascularization of the fetal retina reaches the periphery by 32–40 weeks of gestation. Thus, eyes of premature babies may have avascular peripheral retina. In response to hyperoxic conditions in the nursery, vasoconstriction occurs to protect the immature retina. When babies are removed from oxygen rich environments, the resultant relative hypoxia triggers angiogenic factors, which promote neovascularization at the junction of vascular and avascular retina. All babies less than 1,500 g birthweight or less than 32 weeks of gestational age at birth are at risk; other risk factors include hypoxic episodes, supplemental oxygen, sepsis, respiratory distress, hypercarbia and concurrent illness.

Clinical Features

- Retinal vascularization may proceed normally after removal from the oxygen rich environment with no adverse consequences.
- Progression of retinopathy may result in macular scarring or traction, and focal or total retinal detachment.
- Complications may arise with or without treatment and include myopia, astigmatism, cataract, amblyopia, strabismus, and phthisis bulbi (shrinking of severely affected eyes).
- Secondary glaucoma may be due to neovascularization of the angle or due to angle closure.

Management

All high-risk babies should have retinal screening examinations to detect ROP. The first eye examination should be performed at 27–28 weeks of gestational age, or at the 4th week of life. Follow-up examinations should continue till the retina is fully vascularized or signs of ROP develop. Treatment is in the form of laser or cryotherapy to prevent retinal detachment. Surgery is indicated, if the retina detaches; however, visual prognosis is very grave at this stage. Recently, intravitreal anti-VEGF injections have been studied for the treatment of ROP but no consensus building study to recommend the same is available. Treatment must, therefore, begin early in order to prevent retinal complications.

BIBLIOGRAPHY

1. Adams AJ, Verdon WA, Spivey BE. Color vision. In: Tasman W, Jaeger EA (Eds). Duane's Foundations of Clinical Ophthalmology, 15th edition. Philadelphia: Lippincott Williams and Wilkins; 2009.
2. Braverman R. Diagnosis and treatment of refractive errors in the pediatric population. Curr Opin Ophthalmol. 2007;18(5): 379-83.
3. Custer PL. Blepharoptosis. In: Yanoff M, Duker JS (Eds). Ophthalmology, 3rd edition. St. Louis: Mosby Elsevier; 2008.
4. Forbes BJ, Guo S. Update on the surgical management of pediatric cataracts. J Pediatr Ophthalmol Strabismus. 2006;43(3):143-51.
5. Goldstein HP, Scott AB. Ocular motility. In: Tasman W, Jaeger EA (Eds). Duane's Ophthalmology, 15th edition. Philadelphia: Lippincott Williams and Wilkins; 2009.
6. Rubenstein JB, Virasch V. Conjunctivitis: infectious and noninfectious. In: Yanoff M, Duker JS (Eds). Ophthalmology, 3rd edition. St. Louis: Mosby Elsevier; 2008.
7. World Health Organization (2003). Vitamin A supplementation. [online] Available from: www.who.int/vaccines/en/vitamina.html. [Accessed November, 2018].

18.5 Common Problems of Ear, Nose and Throat

Divya Prabhat

HEARING TESTS

Hearing tests are mandatory for the newborn in certain countries. As development of natural speech is all but over by the age of 3–5 years, the earlier an auditory disease is diagnosed, the better are the chances of helping a child to overcome hearing handicap and have a natural speech.

REFLEX TESTS

- *At birth*: Moro or startle reflex
- *3 months*: Blinking on response to sound
- *5 months*: Eyes turn toward sound
- *6 months*: Head turns toward sound.

BEHAVIORAL TESTS

- *7–18 months*: Distraction tests are performed. The child may be distracted from behind by various sounds
- *18–30 months*: Child's cooperation is sought. The child is given simple tasks to perform in response to certain sounds.

PERFORMANCE TESTS

These are done between the ages of 2 years and 5 years, where the child is asked verbally to perform tasks.

Beyond 5 years, pure-tone audiometry is done, which requires the child's response to different sounds.

SUBJECTIVE TESTS

- *Visual reinforcement audiometry (VRA)*: Here, a young child is conditioned to press a button when a sound is heard
- *Conditioned audiometry*: The child is taught to build a tower of bricks each time he or she hears the (test) sound.

OBJECTIVE TESTS

- *Otoacoustic emission (OAE) tests*: It tests the outer hair cells function of the cochlea and can be performed in the neonate.
- *Impedance audiometry*: Where a low frequency sound is introduced into a sealed external canal. The impedance to sound would be much greater, if the tympanic membrane is stiff (e.g. middle ear fluid) than when compliant. Various graphs obtained help us to diagnose Eustachian tube block, serous otitis media, ossicular discontinuity, otosclerosis, etc.
- *Brainstem auditory evoked responses (BERA)*: Electrical signals are picked-up by surface electrodes resulting from acoustic signs passing from the cochlear nerve to the brainstem.

DEAFNESS

Depending upon the site of diseases, the hearing loss or deafness is classified as follows:

- *Conductive deafness*: The disease affects the external or middle ear, i.e. involving the sound conducting mechanism of the ear, which is correctable
- *Sensorineural deafness*: The disease affects the perceiving apparatus, i.e. cochlear or VIII nerve or any area up to the brainstem.

Causes

A. *Prenatal*
- *Genetic:*
  - Waardenburg syndrome
  - Klippel-Feil syndrome
  - Pendred syndrome
- *Non-genetic:*
  - *Diseases during pregnancy:*
    - Toxemia
    - Diabetes mellitus
    - Nephritis
    - Measles and other viral infections
  - *Drugs taken during pregnancy:*
    - Streptomycin
    - Quinine
    - Salicylates

B. *Perinatal*
- Birth trauma—anoxia/hypoxia
- Hemolytic disease—kernicterus
- Prematurity.

C. *Postnatal*
- *Genetic:*
  - Otosclerosis
  - Familial perceptive deafness

- *Non-genetic:*
  - Infectious diseases, e.g. measles, mumps, etc.
  - Trauma
  - Otitis media
- Ototoxic drugs.

Management

Conductive deafness is fully corrected by either medical or surgical treatment. Sensorineural deafness is managed by using a hearing aid, which amplifies the basic sound. Children with sensorineural loss not benefitting with a hearing aid are candidates for a cochlear implant, which is done as early as 10 months of age.

FOREIGN BODY IN THE EAR

The types of foreign bodies that are found in the external canal may be living (e.g. maggots or insects) or non-living (e.g. stones, beads or hygroscopic foreign bodies such as pea, bean, etc.). Symptoms include pain, irritation, noise and cough.

Management

- Living foreign bodies are killed by borospirit drops and then syringed out.
- Non-living foreign bodies are removed with wax hook.
- Forceps should never be used for removal as they push the foreign body dangerously further in.
- Impacted hygroscopic foreign bodies may be removed after using glycerin drops, which would shrink the foreign body
- General anesthesia may be required for the above procedure in a non-cooperative child or for impacted foreign bodies.

ACUTE SUPPURATIVE OTITIS MEDIA

Acute suppurative otitis media (ASOM) is nearly always a sequel to an upper respiratory tract infection, which is seen commonly during childhood. In infants, the Eustachian tube is relatively short, wide and horizontal, thus allowing easy access of milk and vomitus in the middle ear. Thus, feeding while lying down, vomiting or forcible nose blowing in older children may lead to acute otitis media.

Etiology

Organisms reach the middle ear:
- Via the Eustachian tube following nasopharyngitis, rhinitis, sinusitis, pharyngitis, etc.
- Through a perforated tympanic membrane due to a previous disease, trauma or tympanotomy
- Rarely by blood-borne infections.

Investigations

- Ear discharge for culture and antibiotic sensitivity
- X-ray mastoid to detect the destruction of the mastoid air cells
- Hearing test to detect the hearing loss.

Treatment

Local

- *Aural toilet* is maintained by sucking out the ear discharge
- *Borospirit* eardrops are used only after a perforation occurs. Eardrops are not recommended before a perforation as they are unable to disinfect the middle ear, and they may obscure the otoscopic picture.

Systemic

- Antibiotic therapy is the most important form of treatment and must be used in all stages of the disease.
- Nasal decongestant drops are used to improve drainage of the exudate via the Eustachian tube.
- Antihistamines are given to decongest the middle ear, Eustachian tube and paranasal sinus mucosa.
- Analgesics to relieve pain.

Surgical

Myringotomy may be done only in cases of severe earache with a bulging drum or when impending intracranial complications are present with an inadequate drainage.

CHRONIC OTITIS MEDIA

Types

- *Tubotympanic disease (safe type)* occurs as a residual effect of ASOM
- *Atticoantral disease (unsafe type)* is associated with a cholesteatoma, which is a three-dimensional epidermal and connective tissue structure in the form of a sac that has the capacity for progressive and independent growth at the expense of the underlying bone **(Fig. 18.5.1)**.

The characteristic of each type is given in **Table 18.5.1**.

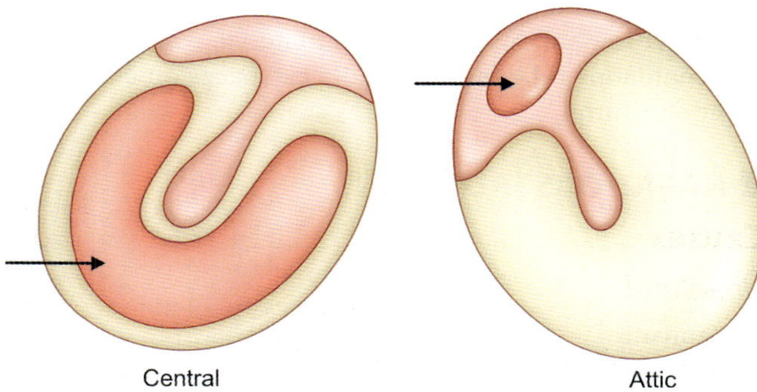

Fig. 18.5.1: Different types of perforation (shaded).

Table 18.5.1: Clinical features of chronic otitis media.

Clinical features	*Safe ear*	*Unsafe ear*
Type of disease	Tubotympanic	Atticoantral
Perforation site	Central	Attic
Granulations	Absent	Common
Discharge	Copious, mucoid and non-foul smelling	Scanty, purulent and foul smelling
Bleeding	Never	Sometimes
Respiratory tract infection	Increase in the amount of discharge	Not affected
Audiogram	Conductive hearing loss	Mixed hearing loss
X-ray mastoid	Sclerotic	Sclerotic with destruction
Complications (fatal)	Nil	Common
Treatment	Tympanoplasty	Mastoidectomy

SEROUS OTITIS MEDIA

Serous otitis media is characterized by the presence of nonpurulent fluid in the middle ear, also known as "glue ear".

Etiology

Malfunction of the Eustachian tube is the underlying cause.

Clinical Features

- Deafness—which is of mild conductive type
- Fullness—with sensation of fluid moving in the ear
- Air-bubbles or fluid may be seen on otoscopic examination.

Treatment

- Valsalva's inflation to improve Eustachian tube function
- Local decongestant nasal drops as well as antihistaminics for the same
- Myringotomy may be required, if no response to medical line of treatment
- Grommet insertion when recurrence is seen after a myringotomy.

Grommet

Grommet is a hollow tube of inert material, which is placed as a ventilating tube for the middle earspaces on either side of the eardrum.

NASAL OBSTRUCTION

Causes

Unilateral

- Sinusitis
- Foreign body
- Antrochoanal polyp
- Deviated nasal septum
- Rhinolith
- Unilateral choanal atresia
- Meningocele/encephalocele
- Rhinosporidiosis.

Bilateral

- Allergic rhinitis
- Ethmoidal polyp
- Adenoids
- Sinusitis
- Angiofibroma
- Septal abscess
- Atrophic rhinitis.

NASAL POLYPS

Nasal polyp is prolapsed edematous respiratory mucosa (**Fig. 18.5.2**).

Types

Antrochoanal Polyp

Antrochoanal polyp arises from the maxillary sinus, enters the nasal cavity through the natural ostia of the sinus and also passes backwards into the posterior choanae.

Ethmoidal Polyp

Ethmoidal polyp arises from the mucosa of the ethmoidal sinuses and by the effect of gravity occupies the anterior choanae.

Clinical features of nasal polyps are given in **Table 18.5.2**.

EPISTAXIS

Epistaxis is bleeding from the nose.

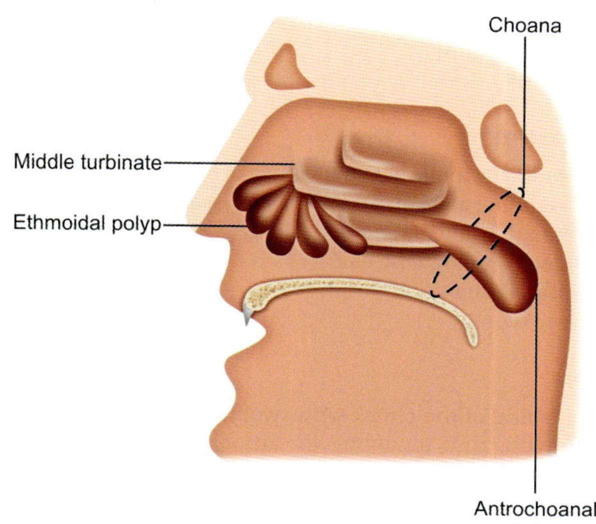

Fig. 18.5.2: Nasal polyps.

Table 18.5.2: Clinical features of nasal polyps.

	Antrochoanal	*Ethmoidal*
Number	Single	Multiple
Side	Unilateral	Bilateral
Etiology	Infective/allergy	Allergic
Source	Maxillary sinus	Ethmoid sinus
Age	Small children	Young adults
Type	Triradiate polyp	Single attachment
Direction	Grow toward posterior choanae	Toward anterior choanae
Recurrence	Rare	Common
Operation	Polypectomy with FESS	Polypectomy with FESS

(FESS: functional endoscopic sinus surgery)

Causes

Local

- *Congenital:*
  - Osler-Weber-Rendu disease (hereditary hemorrhagic telangiectasia)
- *Traumatic:*
  - *Breach in mucosal continuity:*
    - Fractures of nose
    - Operations, e.g. submucosal resection (SMR), polypectomy, etc.
    - Nose picking
  - *Barotrauma:*
    - Nose blowing
    - High altitudes
- *Inflammatory:*
  - *Acute:*
    - Nonspecific rhinitis, e.g. coryza
    - Specific rhinitis, e.g. diphtheria, adenoiditis, sinusitis, etc.
  - *Chronic:*
    - Nonspecific, e.g. atrophic rhinitis
    - Specific, e.g. scleroma, rhinosporidiosis, chronic sinusitis, etc.
    - Midline nasal granuloma
- *Neoplastic:*
  - *Benign:*
    - Angiomatous polyp
    - Papilloma
    - Nasopharyngeal angiofibroma
  - *Malignant:*
    - Carcinoma
    - Sarcoma of the sinuses/nasopharynx
  - *Miscellaneous:*
    - Foreign body
    - Rhinolith
    - Nasal parasites.

Systemic

- *Cardiovascular system:*
  - Rheumatic heart disease
  - Pulmonary hypertension
  - Infective endocarditis
- *Blood disorders:*
  - Christmas disease
  - Hemophilia
  - Purpura
  - Aplastic anemia
- *Drugs:*
  - Salicylates
  - Quinine
- Renal failure
- Hepatic failure
- Septicemia.

Investigations

- Vital parameters—for evaluation of shock
- Hemoglobin—anemia
- Coagulation tests—bleeding disorders
- Computed tomography scan—sinusitis, fractures, tumors
- Biopsy—malignancy.

Management

- *Immediate:*
  - Pressure—by compression of the nose between the thumb and the first two fingers **(Fig. 18.5.3)**
  - Ice cold packs—applied on the bridge of the nose, which may stop the bleeding by reflex vasoconstriction

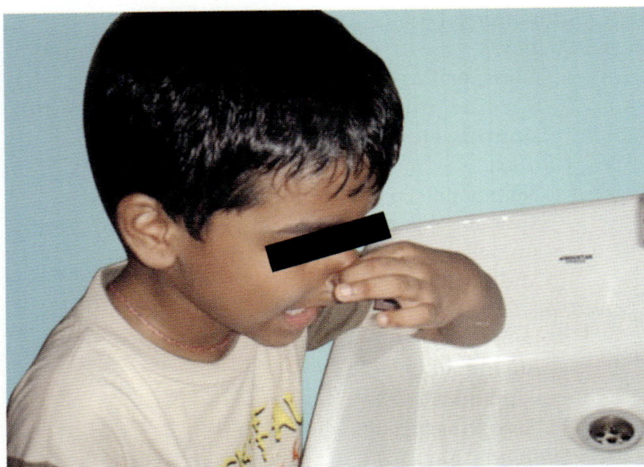

Fig. 18.5.3: Pinching the nostrils.

- Trotter's method, where the child is made to sit upright and incline forward with mouth open and pinched (self) nostrils, then asked to breathe out quietly spitting out all the blood from pharynx
- Assessment of blood loss and vital parameters checked. Treatment of shock and hypovolemia
- *Measures to control bleeding:*
  - Cautery (chemical or electro)
  - Anterior nasal packing
  - Posterior nasal packing
  - Foley's catheter (postnasal)
  - Surgical ligation of the vessels (last resort)
- *General measures:*
  - *Sedation*: This reduces restlessness of the patient and allays anxiety
  - Hematinics and multivitamins to improve the hemoglobin
  - Antibiotics are required along with packing to prevent infections.

SINUSITIS

Etiology

- *Age*: It affects children above 5 years of age, but infants are liable to suffer from acute ethmoiditis
- *Sex*: It affects both equally
- Acute rhinitis causes spread of infection to the sinuses via their natural ostia from the nasal cavities
- Pharyngeal infections, especially tonsillitis, act as a focus of infection
- Dental infections
- Swimming and diving lead to water penetrating into the sinuses
- *Trauma may be due to:*
  - Contusion of the sinuses
  - Compound fracture of one of the sinuses
  - Foreign bodies
  - Barotrauma
- General health if poor, precipitates sinusitis.

Symptoms

- Headache, malaise and fever
- Loss of normal vocal resonance
- Pain around the various sinuses
- Referred pain in the ear
- Nasal discharge
- Nose block.

Signs

- Flushing of the cheek with swelling in case of maxillary sinusitis and involving the upper eyelid in frontal or ethmoid sinusitis
- Tenderness is elicited at the canine fossa in maxillary sinusitis and above the medial canthus in frontal sinusitis
- Anterior rhinoscopy reveals redness and mucosal congestion. Pus may be seen trickling from the middle meatus area.

Investigations

- Bacteriological examination is required, if sinusitis does not respond to antibiotic treatment.
  - *Radiology:* Water's and Caldwell's view/CT scan of paranasal sinuses (PNS)
    - Mucosal thickening
    - Opacity of sinuses
    - An air-fluid level
- Nasal sinus endoscopy.

Treatment

- Prevention by improving general condition of the child. Lowering of resistance affects the mucosal blanket integrity as well as the ciliary action
- *Medical:*
  - *Antibiotics*: Appropriate for the infectious agent
  - Local decongestants are used
  - Analgesics and anti-inflammatory drugs
  - Antihistaminics
  - *Steam inhalation*: For clearing out the secretions
- *Surgical:*
  - After the acute phase is over
  - Correction of a deviated septum—Septoplasty
  - Antral puncture (rarely done nowadays)
  - Functional endoscopic sinus surgery (FESS) to restore the normal physiological mucociliary clearance of the sinuses via its natural ostia.

ACUTE TONSILLITIS

It is a triad of sore throat, fever and malaise lasting for a period of 5 days and usually responds to treatment dramatically.

Etiology

- *Age*: More common between 2 years and 5 years
- *Sex*: Both are equally affected
- *Organisms*: *Streptococcus, Staphylococcus* only and viruses like adenovirus, rhinovirus and *Enterovirus*
- *Predisposing factors:*
    - Ingestion of cold foods
    - Contact with infected children
    - Polluted and ill-ventilated environment
    - Pre-existing upper respiratory tract infection
    - Sinusitis
    - Lowered general resistance.

Symptoms

- Throat pain
- Fever
- Malaise and headache
- Neck swelling
- Earache (referred).

Signs

- Tachycardia and fever
- Tonsils are enlarged and congested
- Pharynx is often inflamed
- Tender and enlarged jugulodigastric lymph nodes (bilateral).

Complications

Local

- Chronic tonsillitis
- Quinsy (peritonsillar abscess)
- Parapharyngeal abscess
- Suppurative cervical lymphadenitis
- Acute otitis media.

Systemic

- Rheumatic fever
- Acute glomerulonephritis
- Sydenham's chorea
- Infective endocarditis.

Treatment

- Bed rest
- Plenty of fluids and soft solid foods
- Analgesics to reduce fever and throat pain
- Antibiotics
- Gargles
- Tonsillectomy for chronic tonsillitis.

ADENOIDS

Adenoids are enlarged hypertrophied nasopharyngeal tonsils.

Clinical Features

- *Due to nasal obstruction*: Mouth breathing, nasal discharge and voice becomes nasal (rhinolalia clausa)
- *Due to Eustachian tube blockage*: Earache, deafness, secretory otitis media and later chronic suppurative otitis media (CSOM)
- *Due to mouth breathing*: Dribbling of saliva, noisy breathing at night, high arched palate and chronic pharyngitis
- *General*: Mental backwardness and lethargy.

Diagnosis

- *Adenoid facies* **(Fig. 18.5.4)**:
    - Open mouth
    - Pinched nostrils
    - Nasal discharge
    - Narrow maxillary arch
    - Crowded protruding teeth
    - Vacant facial expression
- X-ray lateral skull reveals the enlarged adenoids
- Nasal endoscopy to visualize the adenoids
- Examination under general anesthesia to visualize or palpate adenoids.

Management

Medical

- Antibiotics
- Antihistaminics
- Local steroid nasal sprays
- Improvement of general condition.

Surgical

- Adenoidectomy
- Grommet insertion for treatment of deafness
- Nasal sinus endoscopy for sinusitis.

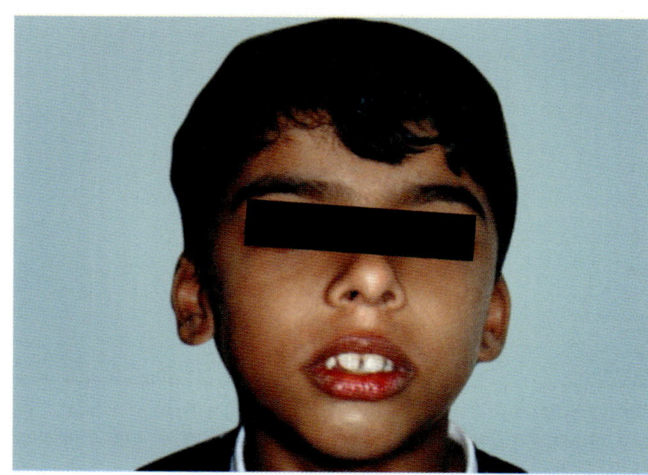

Fig. 18.5.4: Adenoid facies.

TRACHEOBRONCHIAL FOREIGN BODIES

These foreign bodies may lead to a life-threatening situation due to obstruction in the respiratory passage. The absence of a definite history of foreign body aspiration, changing clinical signs as the disease evolves, may mimic various other clinical conditions and thus making the diagnosis a difficult challenge in children.

Symptoms

- Cough
- Fever
- Breathlessness
- Stridor.

Signs

- Tachycardia
- Tachypnea
- Indrawing of the chest
- Cyanosis.

Investigations

- Radiograph of chest shows either obstructive emphysema or collapse or mediastinal shift or the foreign body itself (metallic) or may even be normal **(Figs. 18.5.5 and 18.5.6)**.
- Virtual bronchoscopy scan may be required in some cases.

Types

Foreign bodies are divided into various types, according to the airflow pattern:

- *Bypass of air*: Foreign bodies like a button, ring or bead, which have an opening within itself, allow passage of air to either side. Therefore, the child is never breathless, and the radiograph shows no abnormal findings other than the foreign body (if radiopaque)
- *One-way airway obstruction*: Metallic and other nonorganic foreign bodies lead to a unidirectional obstruction in the airway. Inspiration leads to passage of air distal to the foreign body. However, on expiration, it leads to entrapment of air distal to the foreign body. This airway pattern leads to obstructive emphysema, and therefore, the radiographic findings and breathlessness **(Fig. 18.5.7)**.
- *Total airway obstruction*: Vegetable foreign bodies like a pea or groundnut swell up in the bronchus due to their hygroscopic nature. The increase in size of foreign body causes impaction of the foreign body onto the bronchial wall. This leads to a collapse of the lung segment distal to the foreign body and compensatory emphysema of the other one.

Management

- Bronchoscopy (rigid or flexible) for removal of the foreign body
- Tracheostomy (very rare), only as an absolute emergency.

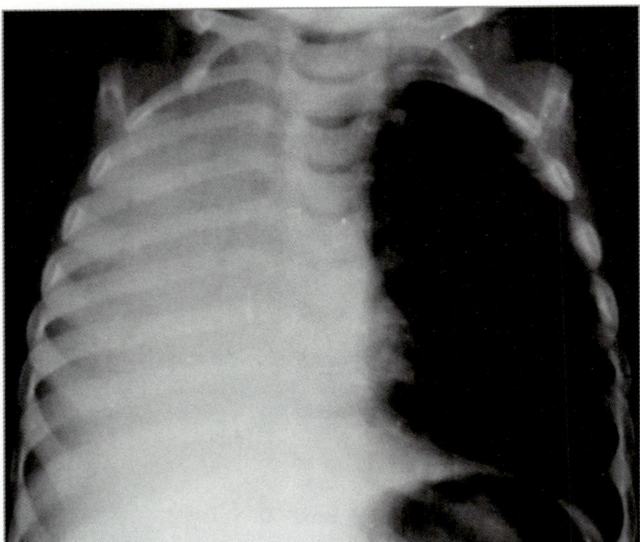

Fig. 18.5.5: Complete collapse of the lung (R) with mediastinal shift and emphysema of the lung (L). Foreign body *(supari)* was removed from the main bronchus (R).

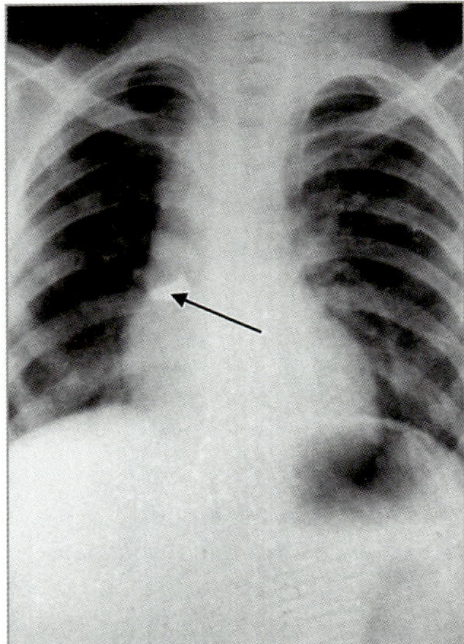

Fig. 18.5.6: Radiopaque foreign body seen in the (R) bronchus (arrow).

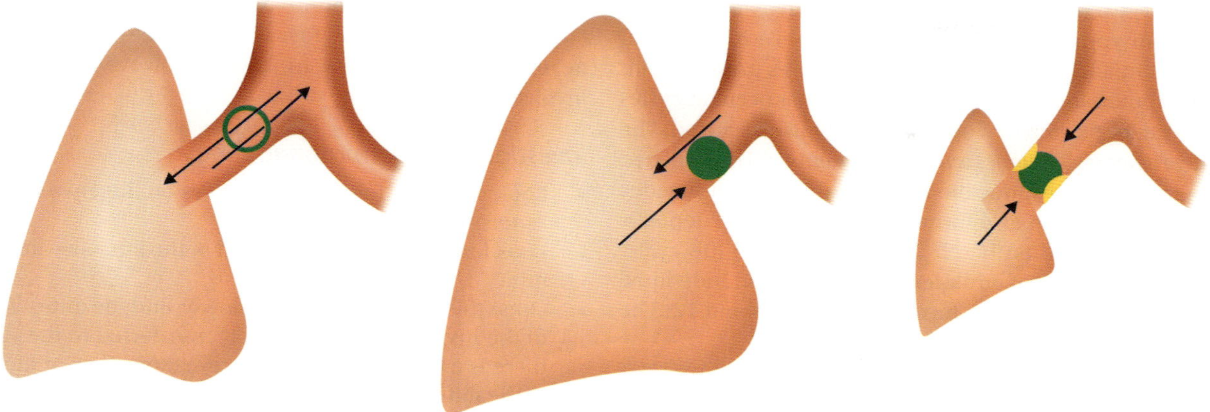

Fig. 18.5.7: X-ray findings with different types of foreign bodies.

BIBLIOGRAPHY

1. Blanc F, Ayache D, Calmels MN, et al. Management of otitis media with effusion in children. Eur Ann Otorhinolaryngol Head Neck Dis. 2018:S1879-7296(18)30066-8.
2. Choffor-Nchinda E, Atanga LC, Nansseu JR, et al. Effectiveness of amoxicillin alone in the treatment of uncomplicated acute otitis media: A systematic review protocol. BMJ Open. 2018;8(6):e021133.
3. Isaacson G. Pediatric tonsillectomy: An evidence-based approach. Otolaryngol Clin North Am. 2014;47(5):673-90.
4. Ivanovska V, Hek K, Mantel-Teeuwisse AK, et al. Age-Specific Antibiotic Prescribing and Adherence to Guidelines in Pediatric Patients in Primary Care. Pediatr Infect Dis J. 2018;37(3):218-23.
5. McCullough AR, Pollack AJ, Plejdrup Hansen M, et al. Antibiotics for acute respiratory infections in general practice: comparison of prescribing rates with guideline recommendations. Med J Aust. 2017;207(2):65-9.
6. Piltcher OB, Kosugi EM, Sakano E, et al. How to avoid the inappropriate use of antibiotics in upper respiratory tract infections? A position statement from an expert panel. Braz J Otorhinolaryngol. 2018;84(3):265-79.
7. Record S. Practice Guideline: Epistaxis in Children. J Pediatr Health Care. 2015;29(5):484-8.
8. Simon F, Haggard M, Rosenfeld RM, et al. International consensus (ICON) on management of otitis media with effusion in children. Eur Ann Otorhinolaryngol Head Neck Dis. 2018;135(1S):S33-9.
9. Tanner R, Harney MS. The initial management of epistaxis. Ir Med J. 2015;108(4):123-4.

18.6 Common Skin Diseases

Jayakar Thomas, Parimalam Kumar

INTRODUCTION

Dermatological problems are seen by pediatricians every day and comprise of around one-quarter of a busy outpatient clinic. Most children and adolescents present with skin disorders that can be easily diagnosed and treated. This chapter presents a brief account of some such skin conditions.

INFECTIONS AND INFESTATIONS

Parasitic Infestations

Scabies

Definition/Description: Scabies is a skin infestation by the mite, *Sarcoptes scabiei*, which is usually transmitted by skin-to-skin contact and causes generalized intractable pruritus, with frequent secondary bacterial infection.

Epidemiology/Etiology: Scabies affects all ages but is most common in young adults who often acquire it by sexual contact. In infants and young children, scabies presents with different clinical features. Epidemics of scabies occur in cycles every 15 years. Nosocomial outbreaks have also occurred. The causative agent is *Sarcoptes scabiei var. hominis*. The fertilized female parasite is responsible for the infestation; it invades the stratum corneum and forms burrows where it deposits its eggs. The eggs then hatch and continue the life cycle. The average number of adult female mites on an individual suffering from the common form of scabies is about 12. The incubation period is 14 days.

Clinical evaluation: Nocturnal, severe pruritus is commonly present. In children contracting the infection for the first time, pruritus develops 1 month after infestation. In subsequent infestations, itching develops within a few days (children already sensitized to the mite and its products).

The eruption is usually polymorphic consisting of small pointed papules, papulopustules, scratching marks (excoriations), sometimes vesicles, and urticarial lesions. The characteristic burrows are usually present in small numbers. The burrows are grayish-brown, curved or S-shaped, slightly elevated ridges, about 5 mm in length. The point of entry of the mite, the most superficial part of the burrow, has a slightly scaly appearance, and at the distal end, there may be a tiny vesicle, adjacent to which is the female mite.

Secondary pyogenic infection may complicate neglected scabies **(Fig. 18.6.1)**. At times, this may mask the original disease; therefore, scabies should always be suspected in cases presenting with extensive pyoderma. The lesions of scabies show a characteristic distribution: webs and sides of the fingers, anterior and ulnar sides of the wrist, anterior axillary fold, anterior abdominal wall and around umbilicus, the waist, lower parts of the buttocks, inner thighs, ankles, cubital, and popliteal fossae. The face and palms are never affected in adults. In infants, however, they may be involved.

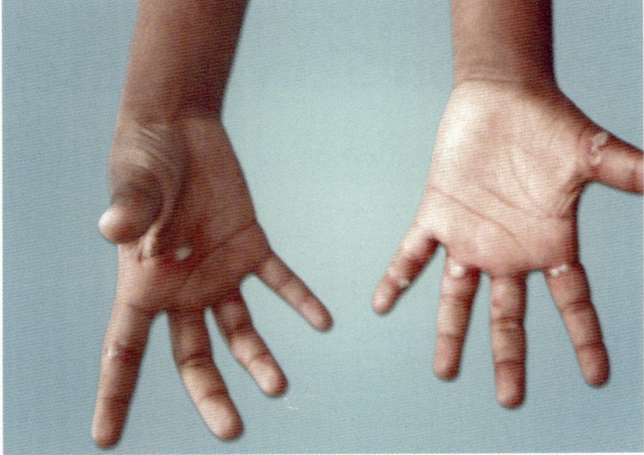

Fig. 18.6.1: Infected scabies of the hands. Note the vesicular lesions with pustules.

Investigations/Dermatopathology

- Look with lens for typical burrows on finger webs, flexor aspects of wrists and penis
- Look for "dark point" at the end of the burrow—this is the mite
- Open this part of the burrow slowly, and the mite will stick to the needle and can be easily transferred to the slide. If there is a nodule, biopsy may reveal portions of the body of the mite in the corneal layer.

Treatment

- All individuals in the house are preferably treated simultaneously. Clothes and bedsheets should be washed or dry-cleaned. The antiscabetic preparation should be applied from neck to toes. Any of the following may be used:
  - Permethrin 2.5–5% dermal cream, single application washed off after 8–12 hours. A second application may be indicated a week later if symptoms do not improve
  - Sulfur precipitate ointment 3–5% applied daily after a hot bath for three to four successive nights.
- Gamma benzene hexachloride is applied after a hot bath; the same clothing is retained for 48 hours and then a further bath is taken, and the clothing and bedsheets are changed. It must not be prescribed to infants or pregnant women or children with history of seizures.
- Benzyl benzoate emulsion 25–33% applied to the whole body except the head for three successive nights.
- Crotamiton 10% has an antipruritic effect in addition to its scabicidal action. The patient should take a hot bath and dry himself/herself carefully on a towel. Crotamiton should then be applied daily for 2 days followed by a bath on the 3rd day
- An oral antihistamine may be prescribed for itching
- Children should also receive systemic antibiotics if there is secondary bacterial infection (honey-colored crusts or tender erythema surrounding the lesions)
- Oral ivermectin 3–6 mg as a single dose is found to be very effective as a scabicide and larvicide. It is best suited for treatment of groups of children, as in boarding schools.

Pediculosis Capitis

Definition/Description: Pediculosis capitis is an infestation of the scalp by the head louse, which feeds on the scalp and neck and deposits its eggs on the hair.

Epidemiology/Etiology: *Pediculus humanus var capitis* is the causative agent. Pediculosis capitis is more common among school children, especially girls, but all ages may be affected. It does not respect any social class.

Unlike *P. humanus corporis* (the body louse), the head louse is not a vector of infectious diseases. Transmission occurs via shared hats, caps, brushes, and combs, and by direct head-to-head contact. Epidemics may occur in schools.

Clinical evaluation: Head lice may be identified with the naked eye or using a hand lens. Most patients have a population of less than ten head lice. Nits, the parasite's eggs, appear as oval grayish-white egg capsules (1 mm long) firmly cemented to the hairs. They vary in number from only a few to thousands. Head lice deposit nits on the hair shaft as it emerges from the hair follicle. So, with recent infestations, nits are seen near the scalp but with long-standing infestations; nits may be 10–15 cm from the scalp. As scalp hair grows 0.5 mm daily, the presence of nits 15 cm from the scalp surface indicates that the infestation is approximately 9-month-old. New viable eggs have a creamy-yellow color; empty eggshells are white.

Excoriations, crusts, and secondary impetiginized lesions are commonly seen and may extend onto neck, forehead, face and ears, and mask the presence of lice and nits **(Fig. 18.6.2)**. In extreme cases, the scalp becomes a confluent, purulent mass of matted hair, lice, nits, crusts, and purulent discharge, so-called plica polonica.

Papular urticaria may be seen on the neck as a reaction to louse bites.

Sites of predilection: Head lice are nearly always confined to the scalp. The occipital and postauricular regions are favorite sites. Head lice may rarely infest the beard or other hairy sites.

Treatment: One of the following preparations may be used:

- Carbaryl 0.5% (lotion-shampoo) or malathion 0.5% (lotion-shampoo): The lotion is applied to the scalp for a 12 hours period followed by shampooing with shampoo containing the same pediculocide. Repeat after 10 days. Unlike carbaryl, malathion has been shown to possess a residual protective effect against reinfection that lasts for about 6 weeks.
- Pyrethroids, e.g. tetramethrin 0.3% combined with piperonyl butoxide 3% applied for 1 hour and better left overnight. Repeat on the second day.
- Permethrin 1% rinse (a synthetic pyrethroid) applied to scalp and washed off after 10 minutes. It is a highly efficacious agent, and is much better than gamma benzene hexachloride.
- Gamma benzene hexachloride is applied to the scalp and left for 12 hours, followed by shampooing. Treatment may need to be repeated. It should not be used on pregnant or nursing women. Carbaryl and malathion, the acetyl cholinesterase inhibiting pediculocides, have replaced gamma benzene hexachloride following evidence of the emergence of resistance to organ chlorines.
- Oral cotrimoxazole.
- Ivermectol 3–12 mg stat.
- Remaining nits may be removed using a fine-tooth comb. Patients should be re-evaluated 1 week or 2 weeks after the last pediculocide application; retreatment may be necessary if lice are found or eggs are observed at the hair-skin junction. Affected family members and contacts should be treated. Combs and brushes should be washed.
- Secondary bacterial infection should be treated with appropriate doses of systemic antibiotics, e.g. erythromycin or cloxacillin, before the application of any pediculocide.

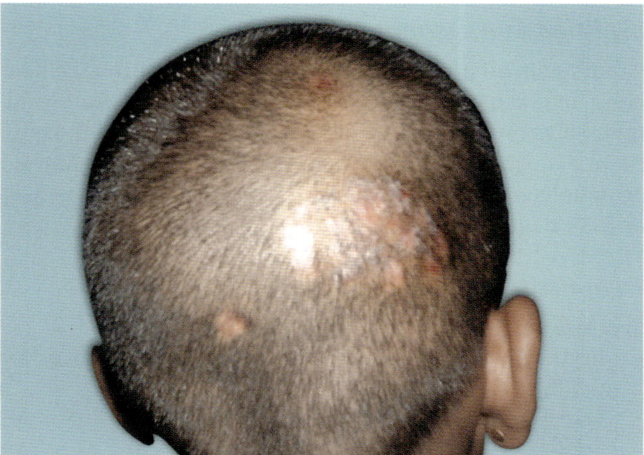

Fig. 18.6.2: Infected pediculosis capitis. Note lymph node behind the right ear.

PAPULAR URTICARIA

Definition/Description

Papular urticaria is a reaction pattern to insect bites most commonly affecting children. Crops of very itchy red bumps, 0.2–2 cm in diameter, appear every few days. Sometimes each spot develops a fluid-filled blister. It is sometimes called "insect bite allergy." In infants, it is given the name *Strophulus infantum* and in the more chronic states, called lichen urticatus. It is thought to be an allergic reaction to insects in the environment. Often after a few years, the child becomes desensitized to these insects and the reaction dies down. The most common identified causes are mosquitoes. It can be nearly impossible to work out, what a patient is reacting to. There have been reports of allergy to bird mites, carpet beetles, caterpillars, and insects that live in masonry disturbed by renovation. Quite often, there exists an atopic background.

Clinical Evaluation

They are most often on the legs and other uncovered areas such as forearms and face but sometimes they are scattered in

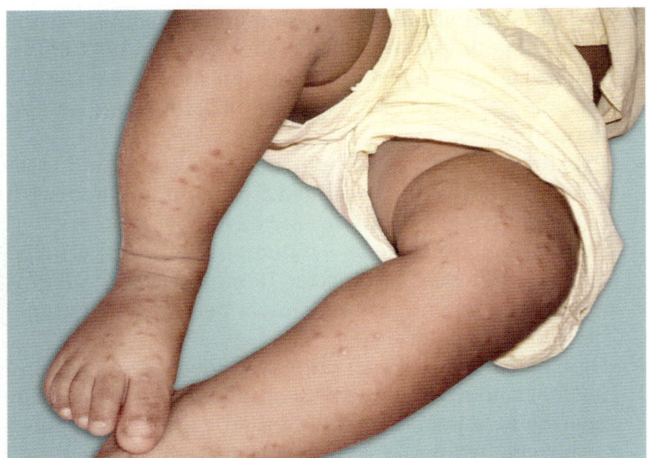

Fig. 18.6.3: Papular urticaria—lesions over legs of the infant.

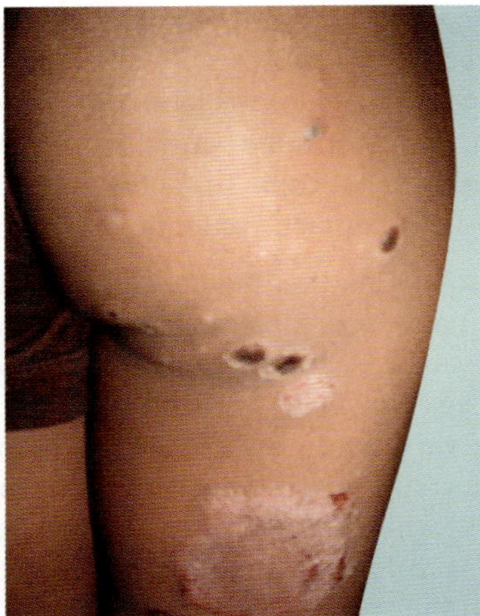

Fig. 18.6.4: Impetigo over the back of right thigh. Note circinate lesions that may be mistaken for ringworm infection.

small groups all over the body. The lesions are erythematous weals. It is difficult not to scratch the spots, which become crusted and may get infected—they are then purulent and sore. Sometimes one new spot provokes all the old ones to come up again and itch intensely **(Fig. 18.6.3)**. The spots seem to remain for a few days to a few weeks and can leave persistent marks or scars, especially if they have been scratched deeply. Recurrence is the hallmark and itching is very disturbing. It can be a marker of atopy.

Treatment

This is directed essentially toward prevention. All measures possible such as nets, covered clothing, and repellents may prove futile. Treatment is then aimed at topical antipruritics (crotamiton), oral antihistamines, and antibiotics if needed. Counseling forms a major portion of management with the parents be reassured of the disorder's self-limiting course.

BACTERIAL INFECTIONS

Impetigo Contagiosa

Definition/Description

Impetigo is a contagious acute pyogenic infection, which is at first vesicular and later crusted. It is a superficial infection of the upper layers of the epidermis and may be caused by *Staphylococcus aureus*, by Group A beta-hemolytic streptococci or by both.

Epidemiology/Etiology

Impetigo predominantly affects infants, preschool children, and young adults during hot humid seasons. Predisposing factors include crowded living conditions, poor hygiene, and neglected minor trauma. "Impetiginization" also occurs on lesions of eczema, scabies, and pediculosis capitis (itchy conditions). It is important to obtain cultures of household and other close contacts, and those who are positive should be treated.

Clinical Evaluation

The early lesions are thin-walled vesicles that rupture quickly leaving red wet erosions, or dry up forming gummy, golden-yellow/reddish-brown crusts. The crusts eventually separate and leave erythema that fades without scarring.

The lesions are scattered and discrete, 1–3 cm in diameter, round or oval and show central healing **(Fig. 18.6.4)**. There may be also some large confluent lesions. Satellite lesions may result from autoinoculation. The regional lymph nodes may be enlarged and tender. The face is the common site, but lesions also occur on the scalp, arms, legs, and buttocks.

Investigations/Dermatopathology

Gram's stain of early vesicle shows Gram-positive intracellular cocci, in chains or clusters. Use of a moistened culture swab to dissolve crusts may be necessary to isolate the pathogens. Biopsy is usually not necessary, but if done, it will show an acantholytic cleft in the stratum granulosum with leukocytes and cocci (subcorneal pustule).

Treatment

Systemic antibiotics:

- Erythromycin (30–50 mg/kg/day) in divided doses for 5–7 days
- Cloxacillin (25–50 mg/kg/day) in divided doses for 5–7 days
- Systemic treatment is required even when only a few localized lesions are present. This helps in combating

colonization of anterior nares or nearby apparently healthy skin by staphylococci. Such colonization may lead to relapses or treatment failure if topical antibiotics are used alone. The use of systemic antibiotics is also essential in cases caused by streptococci to prevent possible renal complications.

Removal of the crusts: This is done using warm olive oil or potassium permanganate 1/8,000 compresses. Removal of the crusts permits delivery of a sufficient concentration of topically applied antibiotics to the site of the lesion. Solutions such as potassium permanganate are not suitable for hairy areas like the scalp. Topically mupirocin 2% ointment/sisomicin 1% cream/fusidic acid 2% cream/gentamycin 0.1% cream or any other suitable topical antibiotic is useful. A cream is preferred to an ointment. The antibiotic should be applied three to four times daily.

Bullous Impetigo

Definition/Description

Bullous impetigo (staphylococcal impetigo, impetigo neonatorum) occurs as scattered thin-walled bullae arising in normal skin and containing clear yellow or slightly turbid fluid without surrounding erythema.

Epidemiology/Etiology

Bullous impetigo occurs mainly in the newborn, infants, and young children, but may occasionally affect adults. It may occur in epidemic form in infant nurseries. Phage Group II staphylococci, which produce an extracellular exotoxin, is the causative agent. Phage Group II staphylococci also produce, besides bullous impetigo, a rare exfoliative disease, the staphylococcal scalded skin syndrome (SSSS).

Clinical Evaluation

Vesicles that rapidly progress to large, thin-roofed, flaccid bullae with little or no surrounding erythema characterize the condition. The contents of the bullae are clear at first; later, they may be turbid. After rupture, erosions and brownish crusts form. Central healing and peripheral extension may give rise to circinate lesions **(Fig. 18.6.5)**.

The lesions are scattered and discrete, and occur on the trunk, face, intertriginous sites, and hands.

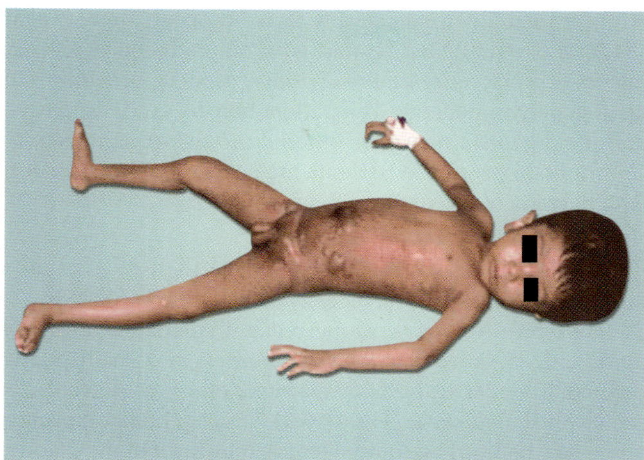

Fig. 18.6.5: Bullous impetigo of staphylococcal origin. Early diagnosis will prevent the development of "staphylococcal scalded skin syndrome."

Investigations/Dermatopathology

- Gram's stain of early vesicle shows Gram-positive cocci, extracellular and within polymorphonuclear leukocytes
- Culture reveals *S. aureus*.

Treatment

- Sparkling cleanliness with local and general hygiene is the hallmark of management. Mupirocin 2% ointment is effective treatment for some cases of bullous impetigo and should be applied to the lesions and nostrils. Fusidic acid 2% cream can also be used. Standard treatment, however, is the administration of systemic antibiotic:
    - Cloxacillin (25–50 mg/kg/day in four divided doses for 10 days) or alternatively, and if *S. aureus* is sensitive, erythromycin (30–50 mg/kg/day in four divided doses for 10 days).

Cellulitis

Definition/Description

Cellulitis is an acute, spreading infection of dermal and subcutaneous tissues, characterized by red, hot, tender area of skin, often at the site of bacterial entry, caused most frequently by Group A β-hemolytic streptococci or *S. aureus*.

Epidemiology/Etiology

Cellulitis affects children less than 3-year-old and older individuals. The most common organisms are Group A β-hemolytic *Streptococcus pyogenes* and *S. aureus*. In children, the common organisms include *Haemophilus influenzae*, Group A streptococci, and *S. aureus*.

Risk factors include diabetes mellitus, hematologic malignancies, IV drug use, chronic lymphedema, immune-compromise, and pre-existing dermatosis (e.g. tinea pedis).

Clinical Evaluation

The incubation period is few days. A prodrome occurs less often than commonly thought. Patients may have malaise and anorexia; fever and chills can develop rapidly before cellulitis is apparent clinically. Higher fever (38.5°C) and chills are usually associated with streptococci; lower fever (37.5°C) is usually associated with staphylococci. Ask for history of previous treatment of prior episode(s) of cellulitis in an area of lymphedema. The patient may be an IV drug user, and the organism may have entered through drug injection. Immunocompromized patients are susceptible to infection with bacteria of low pathogenicity.

Skin Findings

Entry sites: Breaks in skin, ulcers, and chronic dermatosis.

The typical lesion is a plaque: red, hot, edematous, and very tender area of skin of varying sizes; borders are usually poorly defined, irregular and slightly elevated; bluish-purple color is seen with *H. influenzae* **(Fig. 18.6.6)**. Vesicles, bullae, erosions, abscesses, hemorrhage, and necrosis may form in the plaque. Lymphangitis may occur. Cellulitis may also occur on the trunk at operative wound sites. In children, the cheek, periorbital area, head, and neck are the most common sites, and *H. influenzae* is usually the causative organism. On the extremities, cellulitis is usually caused by *S. aureus* and Group A streptococci.

The regional lymph nodes can be enlarged and tender.

Investigations/Dermatopathology

- *Laboratory examination of blood:* White blood cell count and ESR may be elevated
- *Cultures:* Material for culture is obtained from primary lesion, aspirate or biopsy of leading edge of inflammation, and blood. Cultures are positive in only one-quarter of cases. Fungal and mycobacterial cultures are indicated in atypical cases.

Treatment

- Supportive measures include rest, immobilization, elevation, moist heat, and analgesics.
- Given that most cases are caused by Group A β-hemolytic streptococci and/or *S. aureus*, initial therapy is best directed at both organisms.
- *For mild early cellulitis:* If staphylococci are suspected or if agent is not known, use oral cloxacillin 0.5–1 g every 6 hours. The alternative in penicillin-allergic patients is oral erythromycin 0.5 g every 6 hours.
- For more severe infections, use penicillin 100,000–200,000 units/kg body weight + cloxacillin 2 g 25–50 mg/kg tid IV. Ampicillin 25 mg/kg IV every 4 hours may be also used. The alternative in penicillin-allergic patients is vancomycin 10–15 mg/kg tid IV. Subsequent antibiotic therapy is modified, according to response and cultured bacteria.

Erysipelas

Definition/Description

A superficial cellulitis with marked lymphatic vessel involvement is caused by Group A (or rarely Group C or G) β-hemolytic streptococci. An interdigital fungal infection of the foot may provide a nidus for infection. The legs are the most frequent anatomic location.

Clinical Evaluation

The lesion is well-demarcated, shiny, red, edematous, indurated, and tender; vesicles and bullae sometimes develop **(Fig. 18.6.7)**. The face (often bilaterally), arms, and legs are the most common sites, although not in that order. Patches of peripheral redness and regional lymphadenopathy occasionally occur. High fever, chills, and malaise are common. Erysipelas may be recurrent and may result in chronic lymphedema. The characteristic appearance suggests the diagnosis. The causative organism is difficult to culture

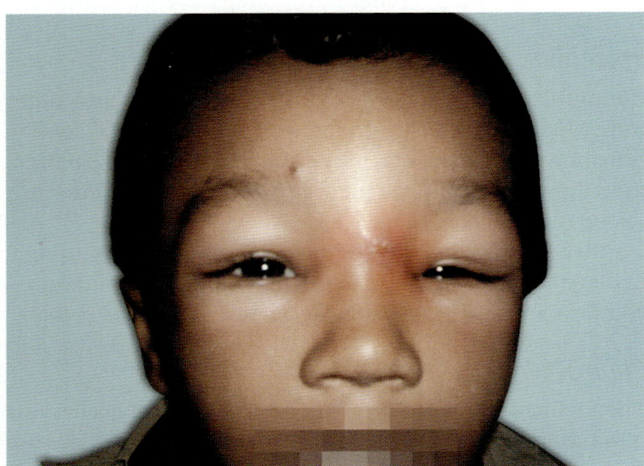

Fig. 18.6.6: Cellulitis following furuncles on the forehead. Note ill-defined borders.

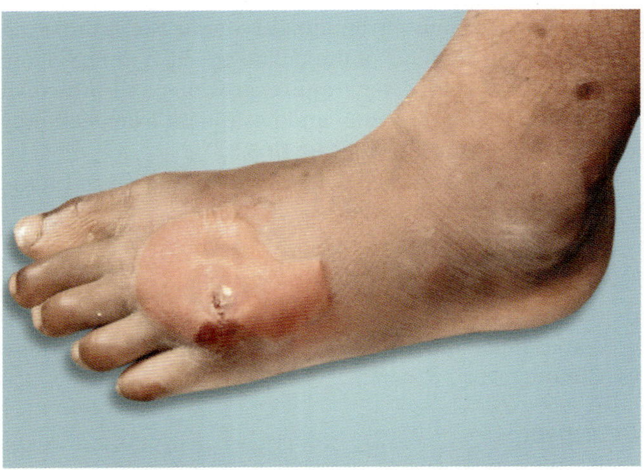

Fig. 18.6.7: Erysipelas with blistering on the dorsum of left foot. Note the well-defined border.

from the lesion but may occasionally be cultured from blood. Staining bacteria by direct immunofluorescence may also identify the causative organism, but the diagnosis is usually based on the clinical morphology. Erysipelas of the face must be differentiated from herpes zoster, angioneurotic edema, and contact dermatitis.

Treatment

Mild or limited episodes of erysipelas usually respond to oral penicillin, cephalosporins or erythromycin. More extensive and severe cases require hospitalization and IV antibiotics. Bed rest, limb elevation, cold packs, and analgesics add to the child's comfort and speed resolution of the illness. Long-term administration of oral penicillin may be warranted to prevent recurrences in selected cases.

Table 18.6.1 lists down the difference between cellulitis and erysipelas as they are of prognostic significance.

Table 18.6.1: Cellulitis versus erysipelas.

	Cellulitis	***Erysipelas***
Etiology	Group A β-hemolytic streptococci, Staphylococcus aureus, Haemophilus influenzae	Group A (C or G) β-hemolytic streptococci
Fever	Low/high	High
Margin	Poorly-defined	Defined
Blister	In the plaque	Advancing margin
Lymphatic	Usually involved	Markedly involved
Recurrence	Less frequent	More frequent
Treatment	May need surgical intervention	Appropriate medical
Long-term penicillin	No need	In selected cases

Furuncles and Carbuncles

Definition/Description

A furuncle, also called acute deep folliculitis and boil, is an acute, deep-seated, red, hot, very tender, inflammatory nodule that evolves from a staphylococcal folliculitis. A carbuncle is a conglomerate of multiple coalescing furuncles.

Epidemiology/Etiology

Furuncles occur in children, adolescents and young adults. They are more common in boys. Carbuncles occur predominantly in men, and usually in middle or old age.

Predisposing factors include chronic staphylococcal carrier state in nares or perineum, friction of collars or belts, obesity, excessive sweating, bactericidal defects [e.g. in chronic granulomatosis, defects in chemotaxis, hyperimmunoglobulin E (IgE) syndrome], malnutrition, and diabetes mellitus. Furuncles and carbuncles may also complicate scabies, pediculosis, or abrasions.

Clinical Evaluation

A furuncle appears as a bright-red, tender, indurated, round, follicular nodule evolving into a fluctuant abscess, with central suppuration and necrotic plug **(Fig. 18.6.8)**. The abscess may rupture discharging purulent, necrotic debris, and forming an ulcer with an erythematous halo. The ulcer then heals leaving a scar. There may be an isolated single lesion, or few, scattered, discrete lesions. The lesions occur only where there are hair follicles and in areas subject to friction and sweating, e.g. nose, neck, face, axillae, and buttocks.

A carbuncle is a conglomerate of multiple coalescing furuncles with separate "heads". In the initial stage of the infection, it appears as a red, tender, hard, dome-shaped nodule, rapidly increasing in size to reach a diameter of 3–10 cm or more. Suppuration begins after 5–7 days and pus is discharged from the multiple follicular orifices. Necrosis of the intervening skin leaves a yellow slough surmounting a crater form nodule. In some cases, the necrosis develops more acutely without a preliminary follicular discharge, and the entire central core of the lesion is shed, to leave a deep ulcer with a purulent floor.

Investigations/Dermatopathology

- Blood culture should be done in the cases with fever and/or constitutional symptoms before beginning treatment. If blood culture is positive, then IV antibiotics are necessary.
- Incision and drainage of abscess for Gram's stain, culture, and antibiotic sensitivity studies may be needed.
- If the condition is recurrent, diabetes mellitus must be ruled out.

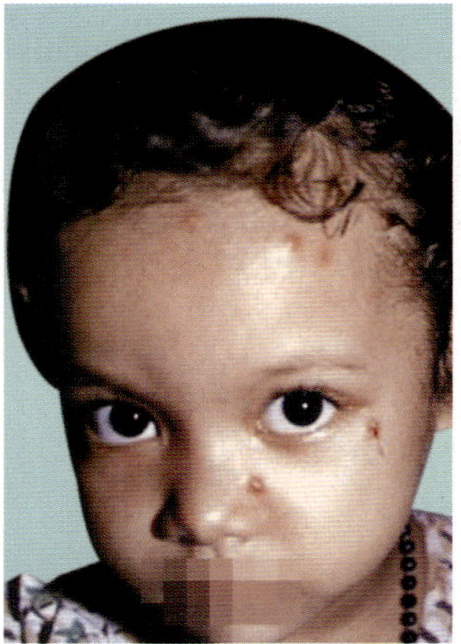

Fig. 18.6.8: Multiple furunculosis.

Table 18.6.2: Furuncles versus carbuncles.

Furuncles	*Carbuncles*
Single deep follicle	Multiple coalescing furuncles
Children, adolescents	Middle old age
Bright-red, tender, indurated, round, follicular nodule	Conglomerate of multiple coalescing furuncles, with separate "heads"
Diabetes less common	Diabetes more common

Treatment

Warm compresses and systemic antibiotics may arrest early furuncles. Cloxacillin, erythromycin or a cephalosporin should be given orally, according to the severity of the condition.

When the furuncle has become localized, showing definite fluctuation, a free incision with drainage should be done without delay and the cavity should be packed with iodoform or Vaseline gauze.

In furuncles of the external auditory canal, irrigations and early incisions should not be attempted. An antibiotic ointment (mupirocin) should be applied locally, and the patient should also receive systemic antibiotics. Heat should be applied to the auricle and the side of the face. Nasal furuncles should be treated in the early stages by the application of hot saline solution compresses inside and outside the nostril, until softening occurs. They should not be incised but steamed. Antibiotics should be given internally and applied locally. On the upper lip and nose, great care must be exercised, and immediate energetic treatment instituted because of the dangers of sinus thrombosis, meningitis, and septicemia developing from boils on these parts. Incision should not be made, and trauma must be prevented using an adequate dressing; local and systemic treatment should be prescribed. Adequate doses of systemic antibiotics are essential.

Recurrent furunculosis may be difficult to control. This may be related to persistent staphylococci in the nares, perineum, and body folds. Effective control can sometimes be obtained with frequent showers (hot baths) with povidone iodine soap and antibacterial ointments (mupirocin) applied daily to the inside of the nares.

The difference between furuncles and carbuncles are described in **Table 18.6.2**.

VIRAL INFECTIONS

Herpes Simplex

Etiology

Herpes simplex virus (HSV) is caused by HSV-1, HSV-2 [genital (sexual)] following exposure of abraded skin or mucosal surfaces to the virus. After inoculation, the virus travels to the sensory ganglion, where it replicates and establishes latency. Recurrence occurs when the virus subsequently migrates along the peripheral sensory nerve. Lifelong latency and periodic recurrences are hallmarks of the disease.

Incubation period: 3–7 days.

Clinical Features

Grouped vesicles on erythematous-base followed by erosions and healing. Lymphadenopathy and systemic complaints are common during primary infection. Abrupt onset of illness, fever, listlessness or irritability, inability to eat and/or drink, gingivitis (with markedly swollen, erythematous, and occasionally bleeding gums), increased drooling in infants due to pain on swallowing, vesicular lesions on the tongue, buccal mucosa and palate with extension, at times, to the lips and face. (These may rupture and coalesce to form large, ulcerated areas.) Tender submandibular or cervical adenopathy are features of primary infection.

Herpes labialis, gingivostomatitis, whitlow, keratoconjunctivitis are caused by HSV-1. Whereas herpes progenitalis, herpetic vulvovaginitis, and severe form of herpes encephalitis are caused by HSV-2. Genital herpes infections should arouse suspicion of child abuse. Lifelong latency and periodic recurrences are hallmarks of HSV infection. Ultraviolet light, stress, hormonal changes, immunosuppression, and infections precipitate reactivation. Disseminated infection with multiorgan involvement occurs when host immunity can no longer contain the viral replication, which is seen in neonates and immune-compromised children. Kaposi varicelliform eruption is a form of disseminated *Herpes virus* infection occurring in diseases such as seborrheic dermatitis, atopic eczema.

- *Investigations:* Tzanck smear prepared from a fresh uninfected vesicle will show multinucleate giant cells. Serology and other tests are required in disseminated lesions
- *Differential diagnosis:* Neonatal sepsis, aphthosis
- *Treatment:* Acyclovir oral or parenteral according to severity. Kaposi varicelliform eruption is managed as a dermatological emergency.

Pityriasis Rosea

Definition/Description

Pityriasis rosea is a benign, self-limited, exanthematous, maculopapular, red, scaling (Greek pityron, "bran") eruption that occurs largely on the trunk.

Epidemiology/Etiology

Pityriasis rosea affects 2% of dermatological outpatients. Most patients are 10–35 years old. The condition occurs more commonly in spring and autumn, and one attack usually gives long-lasting immunity. For these reasons, an infectious (viral) etiology is strongly suspected though not yet proven.

Clinical Evaluation

- *Herald patch:* (80% of patients) 2–5 cm, bright red with fine scaling. It usually occurs on the lower trunk or thighs but may appear anywhere. In abortive pityriasis rosea, the condition is limited to the herald patch and does not proceed beyond **(Figs. 18.6.9 and 18.6.10)**.
- *Exanthem:* Fine, dull-pink or tawny, scaling, macules, and papules with typical marginal collarette of thin scales. The lesions are oval, scattered, discrete, and predominantly macular. They are usually confined to trunk and proximal aspects of the limbs (vest and pants distribution), but an inverted type of pityriasis rosea (on face and extremities) is also known. The long axes of the lesions follow the lines of cleavage in a "Christmas tree" distribution.

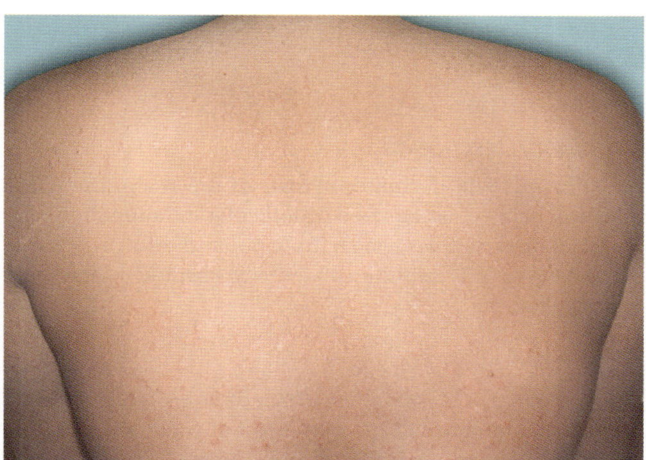

Fig. 18.6.9: Erythematous rash over the back consisting of scaly papules—pityriasis rosea.

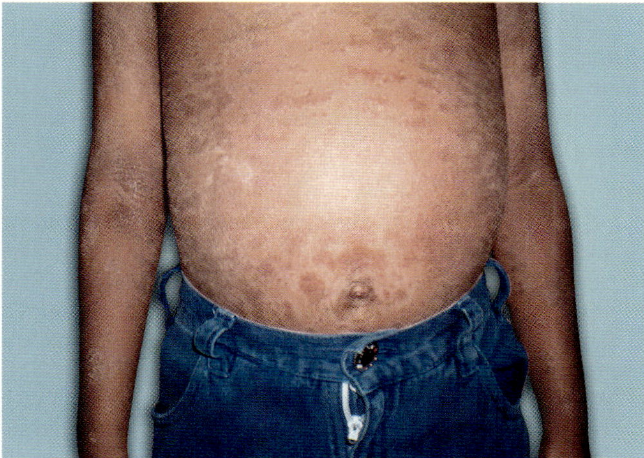

Fig. 18.6.10: Extensive lesions of pityriasis rosea—front of trunk showing scaly patches.

Treatment

Symptomatic: Avoid irritant woolen cloths, hot baths, and soap. A mild corticosteroid cream and an oral antihistamine may help. Pruritus may be controlled by ultraviolet-B (UV-B) treatment if this is begun in the 1st week of the eruption. The protocol is five consecutive exposures starting with 80% of the minimum erythema dose and increasing 20% each exposure.

Molluscum Contagiosum

Definition/Description

Molluscum contagiosum is due to infection with a poxvirus. The incubation period ranges from 14 days to 6 months.

Epidemiology/Etiology

Molluscum contagiosum occurs in both children and adults and is highly contagious. It is more common in males than in females. Infection may be acquired through direct contact, or indirectly through fomites and towels.

Clinical Evaluation

There is a variable number of small (usually 2–4 mm in size but may rarely grow slowly reaching a diameter of 10 mm), discrete, waxy, and pearly-white to skin-colored, hemispherical papules with smooth surface and umbilicated center. The papules are sessile and never pedunculated **(Fig. 18.6.11)**. On squeezing of fully developed lesions, a white curd-like substance can be expressed. In occasional instances,

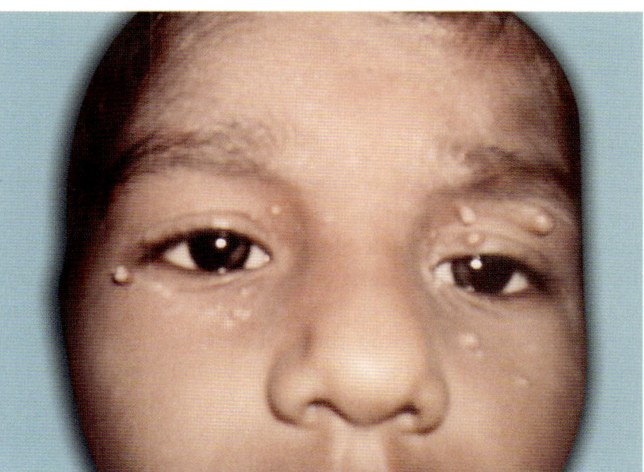

Fig. 18.6.11: Molluscum contagiosum. Note the pearly dome-shaped papules with central umbilication.

a papule of molluscum contagiosum appears markedly inflamed. Ultimately, the lesions involute spontaneously. During involution, there may be mild inflammation and tenderness.

The sites of predilection include the face and eyelids, neck, forearms, trunk (particularly around the axillae), anogenital area, and thighs.

Investigations/Dermatopathology

Direct microscopic examination of Giemsa-stained central semisolid core (obtained by pointed scalpel without local anesthesia) reveals "molluscum bodies" (inclusion bodies).

Treatment

- Cryotherapy using liquid nitrogen (10–15 seconds)
- Simple mechanical methods suh as expression of the contents of the papule by squeezing it with forceps held parallel to the skin surface, superficial curettage, or shaving off the lesions with a sharpened wooden spatula, followed by application of a silver nitrate stick, phenol or strong iodine solution
- Light electrocautery.

Viral Warts

Definition/Description

Viral warts are common, contagious, epithelial tumors caused by at least 60 types of human papillomavirus (HPV).

Epidemiology/Etiology

Warts may appear at any age but are most frequent in older children and uncommon in the elderly. It may be single or multiple and may develop by autoinoculation. Appearance and size depend on the location and on the degree of irritation and trauma. The course may be variable. Complete regression after many months is usual, but it may persist for years and may recur at the same or different sites.

Clinical Evaluation

Common warts (verrucae vulgaris) are sharply demarcated, rough-surfaced, round or irregular, firm and light-gray, yellow, brown or grayish-black nodules, and 2–10 mm in diameter. They appear most often on sites subject to trauma (e.g. fingers, elbows, knees, face) but may spread elsewhere. Periungual warts (around the nail plate) are common, as are plantar warts (on the sole of foot, which are flattened by pressure and surrounded by cornified epithelium). They may be exquisitely tender and can be distinguished from corns and calluses by their tendency to pinpoint bleeding when the surface is pared away. Mosaic warts are plaques formed by the coalescence of myriad smaller, closely set plantar warts.

Treatment

Treatment depends on lesion location, type, extent and duration and the patient's age, immune status, and desire to have the lesions treated. Most common warts disappear spontaneously within 2 years or with simple nonscarring treatment (e.g. a flexible collodion solution containing 17% salicylic acid and 17% lactic acid applied daily, after gentle peeling, by the patient or parent), or the physician may freeze the wart (avoiding the surrounding skin) for 15–30 seconds with liquid nitrogen. This procedure is often curative but may need to be repeated in 2–3 weeks. Electrodesiccation with curettage is satisfactory for one or a few lesions, but it may cause scarring. Laser surgery may be useful but may cause scarring. Recurrent or new warts occur in about 35% of patients within 1 year of treatment, so methods that scar should be avoided as much as possible.

FUNGAL INFECTIONS

Tinea Capitis

Definition/Description

Tinea capitis is a dermatophytosis of the scalp, the acute infection being characterized by follicular inflammation with painful, boggy nodules, which drain pus and result in scarring alopecia (kerion), and the subacute to chronic infection by scaling patches.

Epidemiology/Etiology

Tinea capitis affects children mainly; adults are rarely affected. Favus (inflammatory form) may affect any age. All the three major agents, namely: (1) *Epidermophyton*, (2) *Trichophyton*, and (3) *Microsporum* cause tinea capitis; although, the last two are more common.

Clinical Evaluation

History

Duration of lesions: Weeks to months. Symptoms include loss of hair and pain, and tenderness in inflammatory type (kerion).

Types

- *"Gray patch" scaly ringworm:* Well-defined, round or oval patch covered with small grayish-white scales. The scales tend to be more densely arranged around the openings of the hair follicles. The hairs in the affected area are broken-off into small stumps. Some hairs are not involved since the causative dermatophyte affects only anagen hair (85%) and spares telogen hair (15%). In most cases, the lesions are single or few, but multiple patches may be present rarely. Resolution is not followed by scar formation. Caused by *Microsporum audouini* and *Microsporum canis*.

- *"Black dot" ringworm:* Round or oval patch studded with black dots. The black dots represent the upper ends of infected hairs broken-off just at the point of their emergence from the scalp. More than one patch may be present. Caused by *Trichophyton tonsurans* and *Trichophyton violaceum.*
- *Kerion (Greek, "honeycomb"):* Boggy, elevated, purulent, inflamed nodules, and plaques that are painful and drain seropus **(Fig. 18.6.12)**. Hairs do not break off but fall out and can be pulled easily without pain (i.e. loose). Kerion heals with scarring alopecia. Caused mainly by dermatophytes of animal origin.
- *Favus:* The lesion shows the so-called sulfur cups or scutula. These are dry, yellowish, saucer-shaped, adherent crusts surrounding the openings of hair follicles. A patch of favus is formed of many sulfur cups, some of which may coalesce forming larger areas of crusting with no specific appearance. The hairs in the involved area are not broken-off and some of them are coarse, lusterless, and erect (coconut hairs). Favus runs a slowly progressive course, and may involve the whole scalp in neglected cases, with formation of scars that eventually end in permanent cicatricial alopecia.
- *Systemic findings:* Regional lymphadenopathy may be present, especially in chronic and superinfected cases.

Investigations/Dermatopathology

- *Examination of scalp under Wood's lamp:*
  - Examination of scalp with filtered ultraviolet (Wood's lamp) reveals bright-green hair shafts in scalp infections caused by *Microsporum audouini* and *Microsporum canis* (ectothrix). *Trichophyton schoenleinii* (favus) fluorescence is grayish-green.
- *Trichophyton tonsurans* (endothrix), however, does not exhibit any fluorescence.

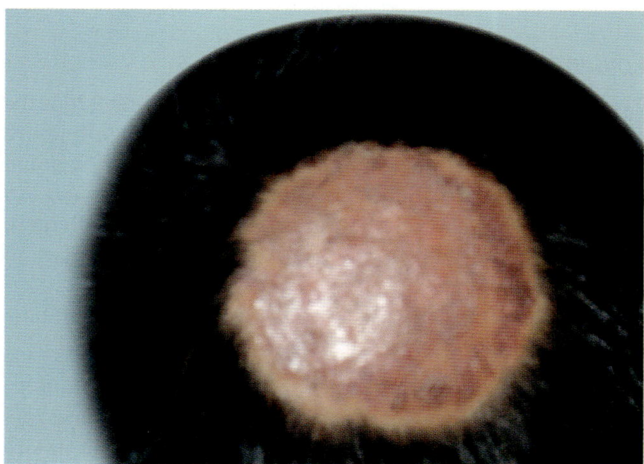

Fig. 18.6.12: Inflammatory type of tinea capitis—kerion.

- *Direct microscopic examination with 10% potassium hydroxide (KOH):*
  - Spores can be seen invading the hair shaft (*Trichophyton tonsurans* and *Trichophyton violaceum*).

Treatment

- Where possible, infected hair should be clipped away to reduce the infectivity of the child
- *Oral griseofulvin (ultramicrosize):*
  - Dose: 10–12.5 mg/kg body weight/day (maximum: 750–1,000 mg/day). Griseofulvin should be taken after meals for better absorption
- *"Gray patch" scaly ringworm:* 125 mg bid for 1 month or 2 months
- *"Black dot" ringworm:* Longer treatment and higher doses are required and should be continued 2 weeks after Wood's lamp, KOH examination, and cultures are negative
- *Kerion:* 250 mg bid for 1 month or 2 months; antibiotics may be needed if there is accompanying bacterial infection. Careful removal of crusts using wet compresses should not be neglected. Kerion should never be incised!
- *Favus:* Griseofulvin should be given for 10 weeks.

Itraconazole may be used instead of griseofulvin for treating certain infections, e.g. those due to *Trichophyton tonsurans*, although it appears to be less effective in infections caused by *Microsporum canis.*

Topical antifungal preparations may be used as an adjunct to oral therapy, e.g. clotrimazole cream, econazole cream, miconazole cream, etc. Ketoconazole shampoo can be used to prevent spread in the early phases of therapy.

Pityriasis Versicolor

Definition/Description

Pityriasis versicolor is a chronic, asymptomatic, superficial fungus infection of the trunk, characterized by white or brown scaly macules.

Synonym: Tinea versicolor.

Epidemiology/Etiology

Pityriasis versicolor is caused by *Malassezia furfur*, the pathogenic mycelial phase of the normal flora yeast *Pityrosporum orbiculare.* It is considered noncontagious by many authorities. It is more common in adolescents and young adults.

Predisposing factors: Climatic factors appear to be important, as the disease is far more common in the tropics and in the summer in temperate climates. High levels of cortisol appear to increase susceptibility—both in Cushing's syndrome and with prolonged administration of corticosteroids (topical or systemic).

Clinical Evaluation

Skin lesions consist of sharply-marginated, scattered, discrete, round or oval macules, with fine branny scaling (pityriasis = bran-like). The scales can be easily scraped-off with the edge of a glass microscope slide. The macules vary in color from brown of varying intensities and hues to white, hence the term versicolor. They range in size from 1 cm to very large confluent areas more than 30 cm **(Figs. 18.6.13 and 18.6.14)**.

Sites of predilection: Upper trunk, upper arms, neck, abdomen, axillae, groins, thighs, and genitalia. The face is rarely affected.

Investigations/Dermatopathology

Direct microscopic examination of scales prepared with KOH or Parker Quink ink/KOH technique reveals spherical, thick-walled yeasts, and coarse mycelium often fragmented to short filaments. These short hyphae and round cells are commonly referred to as "spaghetti and meatballs."

Wood's lamp examination shows faint-yellow fluorescence of scales.

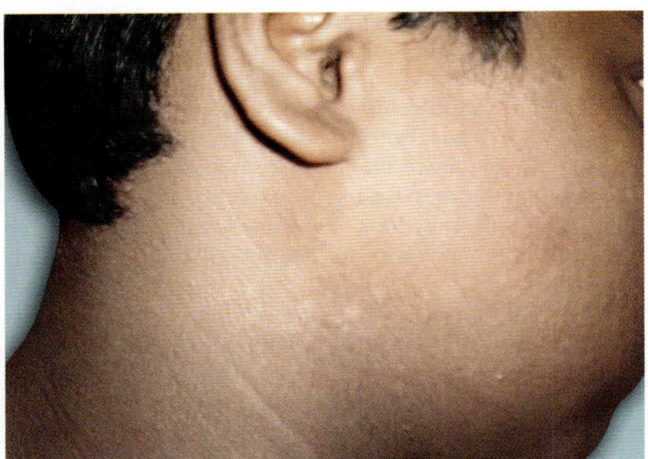

Fig. 18.6.13: Scaly hypopigmented patches of pityriasis versicolor over the sides of the neck.

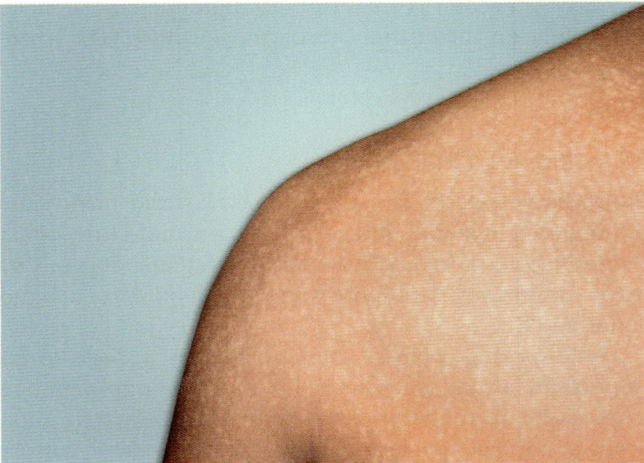

Fig. 18.6.14: Confetti-like patches of pityriasis versicolor over the back.

Treatment

- *Topical agents:*
  - Short applications of selenium sulfide (2.5%, to be washed off in 30 minutes) for 12 nights. Repeat every 2 weeks
  - Sodium thiosulfate (25%) solution in water applied once or twice daily
  - Miconazole cream
  - Topical ketoconazole (2%) either as shampoo or cream.
- *Systemic therapy:*
  - Ketoconazole 200 mg orally daily with breakfast for 10 days. It can cause on rare occasions liver cell damage.

Relapses are very common, whatever the primary treatment, and it is better to retreat each episode rather than resort to long-term suppressive therapy. Patients should be warned that repigmentation may take several months, as otherwise they will often report treatment failure even when the organisms have been destroyed, simply because the hypopigmentation persists.

DERMATITIS AND ECZEMAS

Atopic Dermatitis

Definition/Description

Atopic dermatitis is an acute, subacute, but usually chronic pruritic inflammation of the epidermis and dermis, often occurring in association with a personal or family history of hay fever, asthma, allergic rhinitis or atopic dermatitis.

Epidemiology/Etiology

The onset of atopic dermatitis is usually in the first 2 months of life and by 1st year in 60% of patients. It is slightly more common in boys than girls. Over two-thirds have personal or family history of allergic rhinitis, hay fever or asthma. An allergic workup is rarely helpful in uncovering an allergen. It is also considered by many to be related, at least in part, to emotional stress.

Clinical Evaluation

Skin lesions include erythema, papules, scaling, excoriations, and crusting. Xerosis or dry skin is the hallmark of atopic dermatitis. Lichenification occurs with time. Lesions are usually confluent and ill-defined.

Atopic dermatitis passes in three different phases:

1. *Infantile eczema:* Infantile eczema (age: 2 months to 2 years) affects the cheeks and may extend to the forehead. The lesion is an erythematous, edematous patch covered with vesicles. Eventually, it becomes exudative and crusted. Itching may interfere with sleep. There is no lichenification **(Fig. 18.6.15)**.
2. Childhood phase (Besnier's prurigo—age: 5–12 years). The flexural surfaces of the limbs and neck are affected. The lesions consist of itchy papules and lichenified plaques.
3. Adulthood phase (disseminated neurodermatitis in adults). The flexures are the most commonly involved sites; the front and sides of the neck, and the eyelids may also be affected. Pruritus is severe. The lesions consist of chronic lichenified papules becoming confluent to form poorly defined reddish-brown plaques. There is no oozing (chronic).

Special Features

- Atopic dermatitis patients tend to develop generalized infections, especially herpes simplex. Superimposed staphylococcal infection is also frequent
- White dermographism on stroking involved skin and/or delayed blanch to cholinergic agents
- Bilateral cataracts occur in up to 10% in the more severe cases; the peak incidence is between 15 years and 25 years of age
- Ichthyosis vulgaris and keratosis pilaris are present in 10% of children
- Periorbital pigmentation, infraorbital fold in eyelids (Dennie-Morgan sign), and loss of lateral portions of eyebrows (Hertoghe's sign) may be present in some.

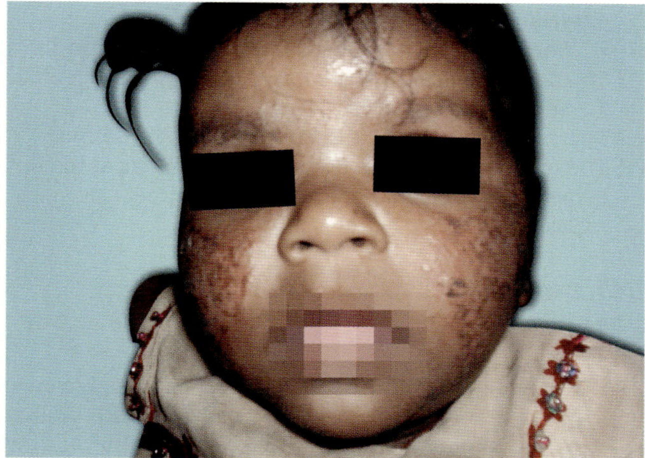

Fig. 18.6.15: Eczematous reaction on the face of an infant—atopic dermatitis.

Investigations/Dermatopathology

Changes are seen in the epidermis and dermis. There are varying degrees of acanthosis with rare intraepidermal intercellular edema (spongiosis). The dermal infiltrate is comprised of lymphocytes, monocytes, and mast cells with few or no eosinophils.

Treatment

General:

- The most important aspect of the management of a child with atopic eczema is sympathetic explanation of the nature of condition to the parents
- Education of the patient to avoid rubbing and scratching is most important
- Topical preparations are valuable but are useless if the patient continues to scratch and rub the plaques. Topical antipruritic (menthol/camphor) lotions are helpful in controlling the pruritus
- Warn parents of the special problems with herpes simplex and frequency of superimposed staphylococcal infection, for which oral erythromycin or cloxacillin is indicated. Acyclovir is indicated if HSV is suspected.

Specific:

- H1-antihistamines are probably useful in reducing itching
- Hydration (oiled baths) followed by application of unscented emollients (e.g. hydrated petrolatum) is a basic daily treatment needed to prevent xerosis. Soap showers are permissible to wash the body folds, but soap should not be used on the other parts of the skin surface
- Topical anti-inflammatory agents such as corticosteroids, hydroxyquinoline preparations and tar are the mainstays of treatment. Of these, corticosteroids are the most readily accepted by the patient
- Systemic corticosteroids should be avoided, except in rare instances for only short courses.

Seborrheic Dermatitis

Definition/Description

Seborrheic dermatitis is a very common chronic dermatosis characterized by dull or yellowish-red, sharply marginated lesions covered with greasy looking scales. It occurs in skin areas with a rich supply of sebaceous glands such as the face and scalp, and in the body folds, and presternal and interscapular regions. Dandruff (visible desquamation from the scalp surface) appears to be the precursor of seborrheic dermatitis, as it may progress through redness, irritation and increased scaling of the scalp to frank seborrheic dermatitis.

Epidemiology/Etiology

- *Affected age groups include:*
  - *Infancy* (confined to the 1st months of life): The sebaceous glands are active at birth, but when stimulation by maternal androgen ceases, they become inactive for 9–12 years
- *Puberty:* Most patients are between 18 years and 40 years of age; occasionally, cases are seen in old age.

At all ages, the condition is more common in males than in females.

Clinical Evaluation

Seborrheic dermatitis causes considerable itchiness. It also gives rise to soreness and much discomfort when it is exudative and affects the major flexures. The severity and course of seborrheic eruptions are very variable, but all show a tendency to chronicity and recurrence.

There are several morphological variants, which in the adult form occur in various combinations and degrees of severity.

Infantile Variants (Fig. 18.6.16)

- Cradle cap (scalp)
- Lesions on the trunk (including flexures and napkin area)
- *Leiner's disease (nonfamilial and familial C5 dysfunction):* Erythroderma appearing during the 1st few weeks of life, failure to thrive, and diarrhea.
- Dandruff is usually the earliest manifestation of seborrheic dermatitis. At a later stage, perifollicular redness and scaling gradually extend to form sharply marginated patches that may remain discrete or coalesce to involve the greater part of the scalp and extend beyond the frontal hairline as the "corona seborrheica." In chronic cases, there may be some degree of hair loss.

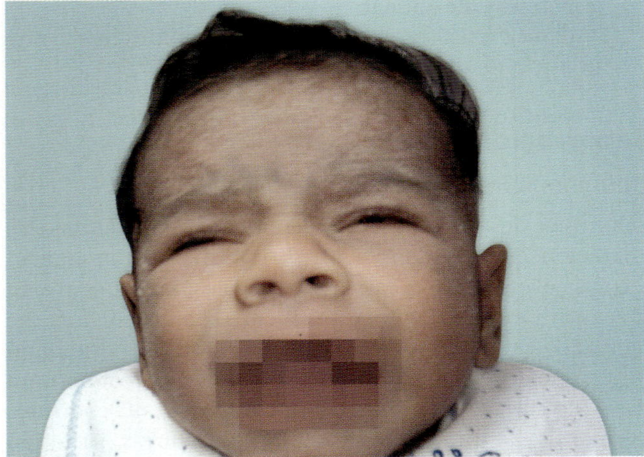

Fig. 18.6.16: Diffuse scaling over the scalp, forehead, and face of an infant—seborrheic dermatitis.

Behind the ears, there may be redness and greasy scaling, and a crusted fissure often develops in the fold. Adherent masses of sticky scale and crusts may extend into the adjacent scalp. Both sides of the pinna, the periauricular region and sides of the neck may be involved. Otitis externa, irritable, and intractable, may accompany seborrheic dermatitis on other sites, or may occur alone.

On the face, seborrheic dermatitis characteristically involves the medial side of the eyebrows, glabella, and nasolabial folds. Areas of erythema and scaling occur, usually associated with scalp involvement. Blepharitis is common. The margins of lids are red and covered by small white scales. Yellow crusts may form and separate to leave small ulcers, healing to form scars, with destruction of lash follicles. Episodic variation in intensity is common, often being precipitated by tiredness, stress, or sunlight exposure.

A superficial form of seborrheic dermatitis of the chin is common in young boys in the early stages of growing a beard but is cured when the beard is shaved off.

In the flexures, notably in the axillae, the groins and the anogenital and submammary regions, and the umbilicus, seborrheic dermatitis presents as an intertrigo with diffuse, sharply marginated erythema, and greasy scaling. A crusted fissure develops in the folds, and with sweating, secondary infection and inappropriate treatment, a weeping dermatitis may extend far beyond them. In both sexes, the genitalia may be involved, and the lesions show the usual range from minimal erythema and scaling to severe crusted dermatitis; chronic, thickened, dull-red, scaly patches of the psoriasiform variety may develop later.

Investigations/Dermatopathology

- The histopathology is not diagnostic, but generally shows features of both psoriasis and chronic dermatitis. Changes are seen mainly in the epidermis and include:
  - Focal parakeratosis with few pyknotic neutrophils, moderate acanthosis, and spongiosis (intercellular edema) are noted.
- There is also nonspecific inflammation of the dermis
- The most characteristic feature is neutrophils at the tips of the dilated follicular openings, which appear as crusts/scales.

Treatment

- *Topical therapy:*
  - *Scalp:*
    - Removal of crusts with 2–3% salicylic acid in olive oil is very helpful, especially in infants and children
    - Shampoos containing selenium sulfide or zinc pyrithione or tar, and more recently, ketoconazole-containing shampoos

- Topical vioform-hydrocortisone lotion or betamethasone lotion following one of these medicated shampoos, for more severe cases. In very severe involvement, for short periods only, clobetasol propionate 0.05% scalp application is excellent.
- *Face:* This is a difficult therapeutic problem.

- Topical nonsteroidal creams such as ketoconazole have been largely disappointing. Using the "foam" from a ketoconazole shampoo on the paranasal areas is very effective.
- Hydrocortisone acetate cream, 1% or 2.5% bid with or without vioform is helpful in some. Avoid prolonged fluorinated corticosteroids because of side effects (telangiectasia, erythema, and perioral dermatitis) that can occur, even with hydrocortisone acetate.
- Ketoconazole creams and 3% sulfur and 2% salicylic acid in oil-in-water emulsion-type base are alternatives to topical corticosteroids or can be used in combination for chronic resistant lesions, especially on the face and chest.
- Controlled, randomized, double-blind studies have established oral ketoconazole as an effective treatment for seborrheic dermatitis. It must be noted that seborrheic dermatitis is not an approved indication for oral ketoconazole, and it is rarely used in this disease for prolonged periods, largely because of the potential side effects, especially hepatotoxicity. Oral ketoconazole in high doses (400 mg) has been shown to lower serum testosterone levels.

Napkin Dermatitis

Definition/Description

Napkin dermatitis is an inflammatory disorder characterized by the development of erythema, papules, and sometimes vesiculation with scaling affecting the napkin or diaper area of usually infants.

Epidemiology/Etiology

Napkin dermatitis, also known as diaper rash or nappy rash, is very common. Some babies seem to get sore bottoms very easily, others very rarely, but they all grow out of it when they stop wearing nappies. Factors associated with the etiology include:

- *Irritant contact dermatitis:* Urine and feces will cause a rash on any skin left in contact for long enough. Sometimes ammonia is formed and burns the skin
- Infection with bacteria and *Candida* yeasts
- *Other skin disorders:* Psoriasis and atopic dermatitis can affect the napkin area. The nappies themselves are not responsible. Washing powder or nappy cleanser is not either if the nappies have been thoroughly rinsed to remove them.

Clinical Evaluation

The disease is characterized by the development of erythema in its early stages. This may be followed by the formation of vesicles that rupture to ooze out serous discharge. The lesions resolve with scaling. Areas affected are the convexities such as the prominences of the pubis, thighs, and buttocks. The classical "tide mark dermatitis" refers to the erythematous border sparing the depths of the flexures **(Fig. 18.6.17)**. Rarely violaceous nodules may be a presentation—the infantile gluteal granuloma—suggesting candidal reaction.

Treatment

Topical antibiotics, antifungals, and mild steroids, alone or in combination are found useful. Helpful tips to parents include—use disposable nappies if possible:

- If you use cloth nappies, use nappy liners to keep the skin dry and make sure the nappies are rinsed and dried well after washing
- Change the nappies frequently—do not leave your baby in a wet or dirty nappy
- Wash the baby's bottom at every change. Use warm water to remove all urine and bowel motions. Soap might sting if a rash is present; use aqueous cream or bath oil instead. Pat dry carefully
- Moisturize dry skin at every nappy change. Dimethicone (silicone) barrier creams can also help
- Apply prescription creams according to directions. Strong steroid creams should not be applied to a baby's bottom.

Acne Vulgaris

Definition/Description

Acne is a common chronic inflammation of the pilosebaceous units that affects many adolescents during puberty. The skin

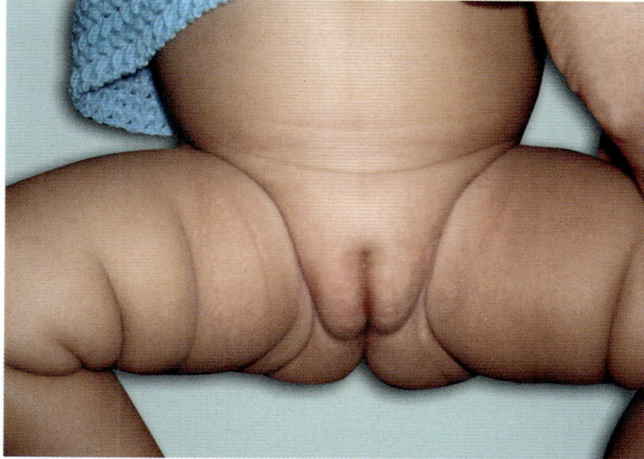

Fig. 18.6.17: Erythema over the convexities and classically sparing the depth of the intertriginous areas—a case of Napkin's dermatitis.

eruptions primarily appear on the face, upper back and/or chest and manifest as comedones, papules, nodules, cysts or papulopustules, often but not always, followed by pitted or hypertrophic scars.

Epidemiology/Etiology

Acne starts at the age of 10–17 years in females and 14–19 years in males, but it may appear first at 25 years of age. It is usually more severe in males than females but may persist in women till the age of 35 years.

Multiple factors—genetic, exposure to acnegenic mineral oils, and dioxin, some drugs such as lithium, hydantoin and systemic corticosteroids, endocrine factors (androgens), emotional stress (school, social problems), pressure on skin by leaning face on hands, are known to exacerbate acne. Acne is not caused by chocolate or fatty foods, or in fact, by any kind of food apart from iodine-containing products.

Clinical Evaluation

Skin lesions include:

- *Comedones:* Open (blackheads) or closed (whiteheads) **(Fig. 18.6.18)**
- *Papules:* With (red) or without inflammation
- *Nodules:* Noduloulcerative lesions, or cysts 2–5 cm in diameter
- *Scars:* Atrophic depressed (often pitted) or hypertrophic (keloid) scars.

Seborrhea of the face and scalp is often present. Acne lesions are round; nodules may coalesce forming linear mounds. The lesions may be isolated and single (e.g. nodule) or scattered and discrete (e.g. papules, cysts, nodules). The sites of predilection include the face, neck, upper arms, and trunk.

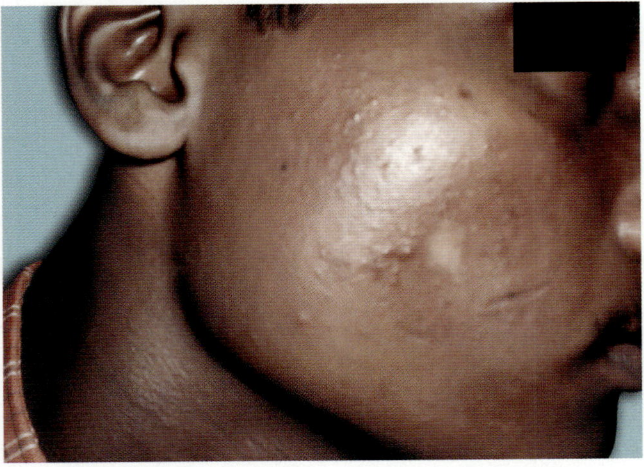

Fig. 18.6.18: Early acne vulgaris with comedones and papules.

Treatment

- *For mild acne:*
  - Topical antibiotics (clindamycin, erythromycin)
  - Benzoyl peroxide gels (2–5%)
  - Topical retinoids (vitamin A acid) are effective but require detailed instructions and gradual increases in concentration. Improvement occurs over a period of 2–5 months and may take even longer for noninflamed comedones. For most patients, start with tretinoin 0.01% gel and increase after 1 month to 0.025%, applied nightly after washing with a mild soap. Topical antibiotics are applied during the day.
- *For severe forms:*
  - Oral tetracyclines added to the above—minocycline, 50–100 mg bid, i.e. could be tapered to 50 mg/day
  - In females only, severe acne can be controlled with high doses of oral estrogens combined with progesterone. However, cerebrovascular disorders are a serious risk
  - Oral 13-cis-retinoic acid is highly effective for cystic acne. This treatment requires experience. As retinoids are teratogenic in pregnant females, it is necessary that female patients have a pretreatment pregnancy test and they must be on oral contraceptives at least 1 month prior to beginning treatment, throughout treatment and for 2 months after treatment is discontinued. Furthermore, a patient must have a negative serum pregnancy test within the 2 weeks prior to beginning treatment.

Dosage: 0.5–1 mg/kg/day with meals for a 15–20-week course, which is usually adequate. About 30% of patients require two 4-month courses with a 2-month rest period in between. Careful monitoring is necessary during therapy, especially in patients with elevated serum triglycerides before therapy is begun.

Urticaria and Angioedema

Definition/Description

Urticaria and angioedema are composed of transient weals (at times spelt as wheals—edematous papules and plaques, usually pruritic) and of larger edematous areas that involve the dermis and subcutaneous tissue (angioedema). Urticaria and/or angioedema may be acute or chronic recurrent. There are some syndromes with angioedema in which urticarial weals are rarely present (e.g. hereditary angioedema).

Epidemiology/Etiology

Angioedema and urticaria can be classified as IgE-mediated, hypocomplementemic, or related to physical stimuli (water, cold, sunlight, and pressure) or idiosyncratic. The syndrome, angioedema-urticaria-eosinophilia syndrome, is related to action of the eosinophil major basic protein.

General types include acute urticaria (<6 weeks), often IgE-dependent with atopic background and chronic urticaria: (>6 weeks), rarely IgE-dependent; the etiology is unknown in 80–90%; often emotional stress seems to be an exacerbating factor. Intolerance to salicylates may be present.

Clinical Evaluation

The duration of lesions is hours. Skin symptoms include pruritus, pain on walking (in foot involvement), flushing, burning, and wheezing (in cholinergic urticaria). Constitutional symptoms may be present in the form of fever in serum sickness and in the angioedema-urticaria-eosinophilia syndrome. In angioedema, hoarseness, stridor, and dyspnea also occur. Patients may have arthralgia (serum sickness, necrotizing vasculitis, and hepatitis).

Skin lesions consist of:

- *Transient pruritic papular weals:* Many small (a size of 1–2 mm is typical in cholinergic urticaria)
- *Weals:* Small (1 cm) to large (8 cm), edematous plaques
- *Angioedema:* Skin-colored enlargement of portion of the face (eyelids, lips, and tongue) or extremity **(Fig. 18.6.19)**.

Investigations/Dermatopathology

Changes are observed in the dermis, and include edema of the dermis or subcutaneous tissue, dilatation of venules and mast cell degranulation. In necrotizing vasculitis, biopsy is diagnostic. In angioedema-urticaria-eosinophilia syndrome, major basic protein is present outside the eosinophils around blood vessels and collagen bundles. There is dermal edema, a perivascular lymphocytic infiltration and diffuse eosinophilic in infiltration.

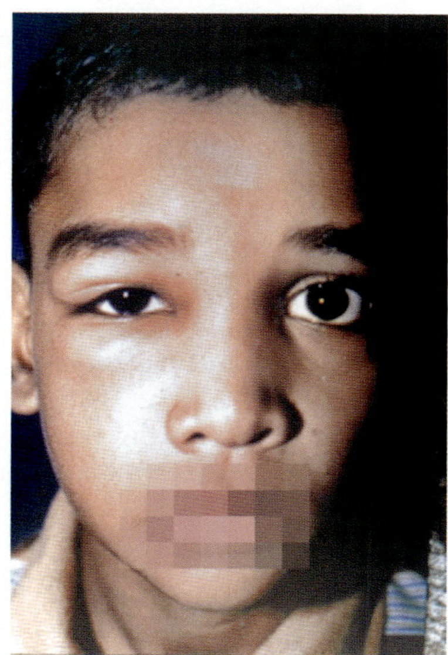

Fig. 18.6.19: A case of angioedema.

General laboratory tests:

- *Serologic tests:*
  - Search for hepatitis-associated antigen
  - Assessment of the complement system
  - Assessment of specific IgE antibodies by radioallergosorbent test (RAST).
- *Hematologic tests:*
  - Erythrocyte sedimentation rate is often elevated in persistent urticaria (necrotizing vasculitis), and there may be hypocomplementemia
  - Transient eosinophilia is observed in urticaria from reactions to foods and drugs
  - High levels of eosinophilia are present in the angioedema-urticaria-eosinophilia syndrome.
- *Special examinations:*
  - Screening for functional C1 esterase inhibitor
  - Ultrasonography for early diagnosis of bowel involvement; if abdominal pain is present; this may indicate edema of the bowel.

Treatment

Try to prevent attacks by elimination of etiologic chemicals or drugs: aspirin and food additives, especially in chronic recurrent urticaria. Detection of the cause and its elimination is the most important step in the treatment but is rarely successful. The cause can be known from careful history taking rather than from laboratory investigations or skin testing.

Antihistamines are effective in controlling symptoms if given in the proper dose; H_1 blockers, e.g. hydroxyzine, cetirizine, levocetirizine; and if they fail, H_1 and H_2 blockers (e.g. doxepin).

Prednisolone is indicated for angioedema-urticaria-eosinophilia syndrome.

Danazol is indicated as long-term therapy for hereditary angioedema; whole plasma or C1 esterase inhibitor may be used in the acute attack.

Emergency cases: Emergency treatment should start with injection of adrenaline subcutaneously. Hydrocortisone IV should follow but not before adrenaline.

Erythema Multiforme

Definition/Description

Erythema multiforme is a reaction of the skin to different causes as viral infections (commonly herpes simplex), bacterial, mycotic or parasitic infections, drugs or systemic diseases (rheumatic fever, systemic lupus erythematosus, etc.). This reaction pattern of blood vessels in the dermis with secondary epidermal changes is exhibited clinically as characteristic erythematous iris-shaped papules and vesiculobullous lesions typically involving the extremities (especially the palms and soles) and the mucous membranes. The characteristic lesions are also known as target lesions. The eruption begins rapidly with varying degrees of constitutional symptoms. It is distributed bilaterally and symmetrically in a centrifugal pattern. Stevens-Johnson syndrome is a severe bullous form of erythema multiforme; the mucous membranes are severely involved, and there are severe general constitutional symptoms.

Epidemiology/Etiology

- *Age and sex*: Patients are usually 20–30 under the age of 20 years. Erythema multiforme is more frequent in males than in females.
- *Causes*:
  - *Drugs:* Sulfonamides, phenytoin, barbiturates, phenylbutazone and penicillin
  - *Infection:* Especially following herpes simplex, mycoplasma
  - *Idiopathic:* In more than 50% of cases, no cause can be detected.

Clinical Evaluation

The duration of lesions is several days; lesions develop over 10 days or more. Patients may have a history of prior episode of erythema multiforme. Skin lesions may be pruritic or painful. Mouth lesions are painful and tender. Constitutional symptoms may be present in the form of fever, weakness, and malaise.

Skin lesions consist of:

- Macules (48 hours) evolving to papules, 1–2 cm; lesions may appear for 2 weeks
- Vesicles and bullae (in the center of papule forming the so-called iris or target lesions)
- Lesions are dull-red. Iris or target lesions are typical (see above). Lesions may be localized to the hands or generalized **(Fig. 18.6.20)**. They are usually bilateral and often symmetrical. The sites of predilection include the dorsa of hands, palms, soles, forearms, feet, elbows, and knees; the penis (50%) and vulva may be also involved
- *Mucous membranes:* Lesions may occur in the mouth and on the lips (99%) **(Fig. 18.6.21)**
- *Other organs:* Pulmonary manifestations may be present; the eyes may be affected with corneal ulcers and anterior uveitis.

Investigations/Dermatopathology

Changes are observed in the epidermis and dermis. An inflammatory process is seen characterized by perivascular mononuclear infiltrate, and edema of the upper dermis; in lesions with bulla formation, there is eosinophilic necrosis of keratinocytes with subepidermal bulla formation.

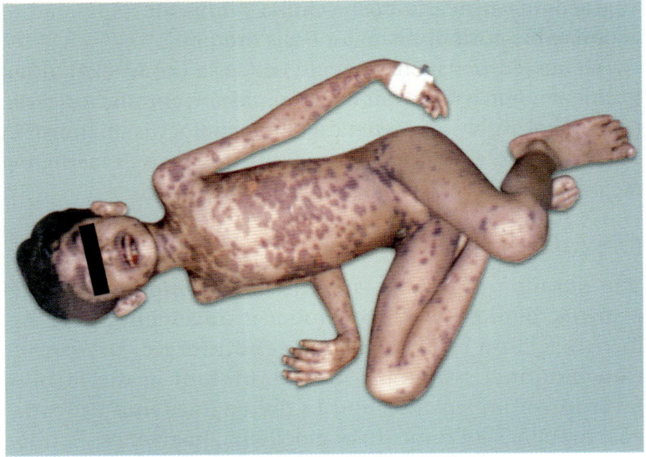

Fig. 18.6.20: Acutely ill child with erythema multiforme.

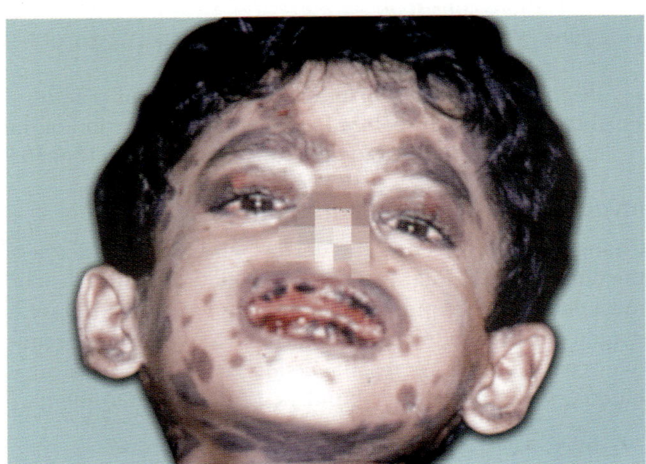

Fig. 18.6.21: Involvement of oral and conjunctival mucosae in erythema multiforme.

All attempts must be made to rule out occult viral, fungal and bacterial infections.

Treatment

Symptomatic: In severely ill patients, systemic corticosteroids are usually given (prednisolone 50–80 mg daily in divided doses, quickly tapered), but their effectiveness has not been established by controlled studies.

Control of herpes simplex using oral acyclovir may prevent development of recurrent erythema multiforme.

Toxic Epidermal Necrolysis

Definition/Description

Toxic epidermal necrolysis (TEN) is a cutaneous drug-induced or idiopathic reaction pattern characterized by tenderness and erythema of skin and mucosa, followed by extensive cutaneous and mucosal exfoliation. It is potentially life-threatening due to multisystem involvement. Patients become severely dehydrated and protein-depleted. They require intensive care and are best managed in a manner like burns patients.

Synonym: Lyell's syndrome.

Epidemiology/Etiology

Age and sex: Patients are usually adults more than 40 years old; the disease affects both sexes equally (some studies have reported a higher incidence in middle-aged and elderly women).

Clinical Evaluation

Ask about history of drug intake. Toxic epidermal necrolysis occurs within days of ingestion of the offending drug (when a drug is the cause); a newly added drug is most suspected. A prodrome occurs in most patients and consists of mild-to-moderate skin tenderness, fever, malaise, headache, conjunctival burning or itching, myalgias, arthralgias, nausea and vomiting, and/or diarrhea. Skin symptoms are present in the form of marked tenderness of rash, pain, pruritus, and paresthesia. Patients are usually mentally alert but are in distress due to severe pain. Acute renal failure and erosions in lower respiratory tract and gut may complicate the condition.

Skin findings: The prodromal rash is described as morbilliform or erythema multiforme-like. A tender erythema is initially observed. Small blisters then form, becoming irregularly confluent. The entire thickness of the epidermis becomes necrotic and shears off in large sheets, but large blisters only rarely form. Epidermal sloughing may be generalized, resulting in large denuded areas resembling a second-degree thermal burn. The idiopathic form is usually not preceded by rash but starts with erythema, which is rapidly followed by sloughing and denudation. The initial erythema affects the face and extremities, becoming confluent over a few hours or days. Denudation is most pronounced over pressure points. Scalp, palms, and soles may be less severely involved or spared, but nails may be shed. Nikolsky's sign is usually positive **(Figs. 18.6.22 and 18.6.23)**.

Mucous membranes are also severely affected; look for erythema and sloughing of lips, buccal mucosa, conjunctiva, genital, and anal skin.

The diagnosis is based on clinical findings and confirmed by biopsy.

Investigations/Dermatopathology

A biopsy will confirm the clinical diagnosis. Early findings include vacuolization/necrosis of basal keratinocytes and individual cell necrosis throughout the epidermis. Late lesions show necrosis of the entire epidermis with formation of subepidermal split above the basement membrane. Little or no inflammatory infiltrate is seen in the dermis.

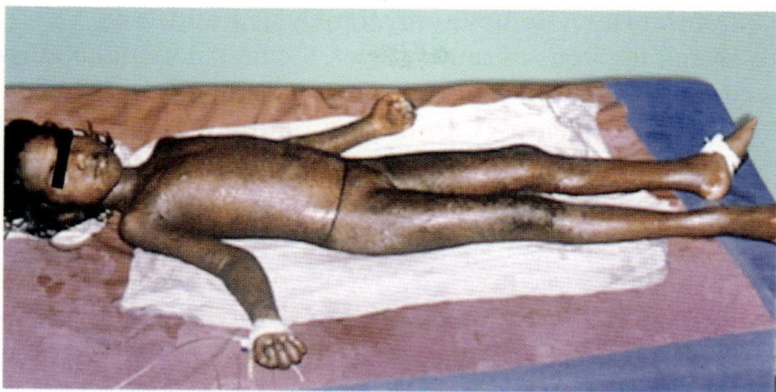

Fig. 18.6.22: Toxic epidermal necrolysis—note positive Nikolsky's sign.

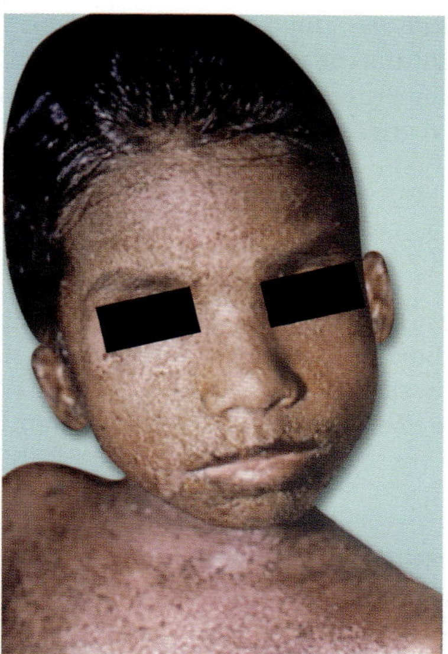

Fig. 18.6.23: The child seen in Fig. 18.6.22 with peeling of skin over face and neck.

Treatment

- Treat as a thermal burn patient in a burn unit of a hospital. Silver sulphadiazine is extremely effective but must be used with caution over large areas for fear of absorption and resultant neutropenia. The role of corticosteroids is controversial. There is general agreement that corticosteroids should not be used in TEN that has progressed to involve 20% or more of body surface. But it is still unproven whether they may arrest the progression of TEN if given in the first 24–48 hours.
- *Intravenous fluid replacement:* Water, electrolytes, albumin, and plasma

- *Debridement:* Remove only frankly necrotic tissue
- Watch for signs of sepsis (fever, hypotension and change in mental status)
- *Conjunctival care:* Erythromycin ointment
- Frequent suctioning is needed in oropharyngeal involvement to prevent aspiration pneumonitis
- Avoid re-exposure to offending drug.

PAPULOSQUAMOUS DISORDERS

Acrodermatitis Enteropathica

Definition/Description

Acrodermatitis enteropathica is a genetic disorder of zinc absorption, presenting in infancy, characterized by a triad of acral dermatitis (face, hands, feet, and anogenital), alopecia, and diarrhea; nearly identical clinical findings occur in older individuals with acquired zinc deficiency due either to dietary deficiency or failure of intestinal absorption.

Epidemiology/Etiology

- *Age:*
  - *Acrodermatitis enteropathica:* In infants bottle-fed with bovine milk, days to few weeks. In breast-fed infants, soon after weaning
  - *Acquired zinc deficiency:* Older children.

Etiology

- *Acrodermatitis enteropathica:* Autosomal recessive trait resulting in failure to absorb zinc.
- *Acquired zinc deficiency:*
  - Secondary to reduced dietary intake of zinc
  - Malabsorption (regional enteritis, following intestinal bypass surgery for obesity)
  - Increased urinary loss (nephrotic syndrome)
  - Prolonged parenteral nutrition without supplemental zinc
  - *Predisposition for acquired zinc deficiency:* Pregnancy, growing child or adolescent.

Clinical Evaluation

Skin, mucous membrane, and hair are involved. The skin lesions often become secondarily infected with *Candida albicans* and *S. aureus*. The lesions are initially pink, and later, brightly erythematous. They are initially confined to the face (particularly perioral), scalp, and anogenital area. Later, the hands and feet, flexural regions, and trunk become involved. There is impaired wound healing.

General examination: Patients are irritable with depressed mood. Infants and children have growth failure **(Figs. 18.6.24 and 18.6.25)**.

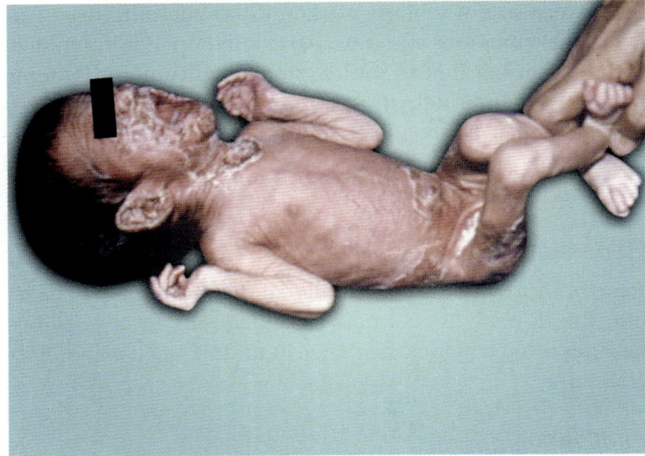

Fig. 18.6.24: Acrodermatitis enteropathica. Note acral lesions and scanty hair.

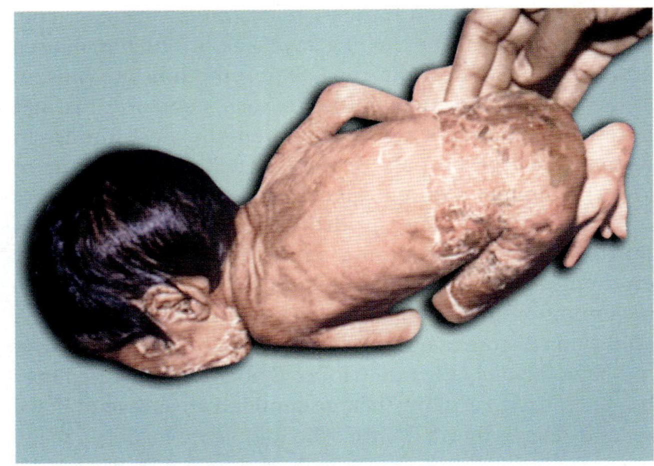

Fig. 18.6.25: Posterior aspect of child seen in the figure.

Investigations/Dermatopathology

- *Complete blood count:* Reveals anemia
- *Chemistry:* Serum/plasma zinc levels are low
- *Urine:* Urinary zinc excretion is reduced
- *Dermatopathology:* Intraepidermal clefts and blisters are observed with acantholysis.

Treatment

Dietary or IV supplementation with zinc salts with 2–3 times, the recommended daily allowances restores normal zinc status in days to weeks. Oral zinc in a dosage of 10 mg/kg of elemental zinc is as effective as parenteral administration and needs to be continued for at least 6 months.

BULLOUS DISORDERS

Epidermolysis Bullosa

Definition/Description

Epidermolysis bullosa (EB) are a group of dermatoses characterized by easy bullae formation on mild mechanical pressure, and hence, the name *mechanobullous disorders.* The dreaded complications are bleeding, infection, and scarring.

Epidemiology/Etiology

All forms of EB are genetic and most present at birth. There is no gender predilection. Most babies have impaired quality of life due to the psychological effects of easy blistering and scarring.

Clinical Evaluation

Several clinical types and subtypes have been described. Five of them need to be known **(Fig. 18.6.26)**.

Treatment

Treatment of EB is essentially supportive. Sterile dressings and topical antibiotics (2% mupirocin) form the mainstay of therapy. Cutaneous infections unresponsive to topical antibiotics will need systemic antibiotics (cloxacillin). Nutritional support is essential in the form of soft flexible intragastric feeding in selected children. Attempts of intermittent esophageal dilatation may be fruitful. Apparently, the management of severe forms of EB demands optimal care from the combined efforts of parents, pediatricians, and dermatologists. Genetic counseling plays an important role.

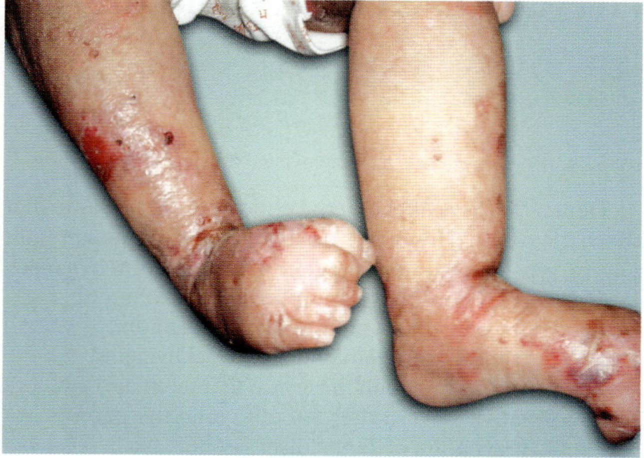

Fig. 18.6.26: Epidermolysis bullosa in an infant. Note the blistering and scarring over the lower limbs.

Staphylococcal Scalded Skin Syndrome

Definition/Description

Staphylococcal scalded skin syndrome is a toxin-mediated epidermolytic disease characterized by erythema and widespread detachment of the superficial layers of the epidermis, resembling the effects of scalding. It occurs mainly in newborns and infants under 2 years of age. Severity ranges from a localized form, bullous impetigo, to a generalized form with extensive epidermolysis and desquamation.

Synonyms: Pemphigus neonatorum, Ritter's disease.

Epidemiology/Etiology

- *Age:* Staphylococcal scalded skin syndrome occurs mainly in infants and young children. Adults with immunosuppression or renal insufficiency are subject to SSSS.
- *Etiology: S. aureus* of phase Group II, mostly Type 71.

Clinical Evaluation

- A low-grade fever may be present. The child is irritable.
- *Skin findings:*
  - *Bullous impetigo:* Lesions are often clustered in an intertriginous area and consist of intact flaccid, purulent bullae. Rupture of the bullae results in moist red and/or crusted erosive lesions.
  - *Generalized staphylococcal scalded skin syndrome:* It is a very tender, ill-defined erythema occurs initially. With epidermolysis, the epidermis appears wrinkled. The unroofed epidermis forms erosions with red, moist base. Initially, lesions are present on the face (periorificially), neck, axillae and groins, becoming more widespread in 24–48 hours. The initial erythema and later sloughing of the epidermis are most pronounced periorificially on the face, and in the flexural areas and pressure points: on the neck, axillae, groins, antecubital area, and back.
- *Scarlatiniform syndrome:* Presentation is like scarlet fever but without pharyngitis, tonsillitis, and strawberry tongue Nikolsky's sign (gentle lateral pressure causes shearing off superficial epidermis) is positive **(Fig. 18.6.27)**.
- *Mucous membranes:* Usually uninvolved.

Investigations/Dermatopathology

- *Gram's stain:*
  - *Bullous impetigo:* Findings include pus in bullae and clumps of Gram-positive cocci within polymorphonuclear leukocytes (PMNL).
  - *Generalized staphylococcal scalded skin syndrome:* Gram-positive cocci are only observed at colonized site, not in the areas of epidermolysis.
- *Bacterial culture:*
  - *Bullous impetigo: S. aureus* is isolated.

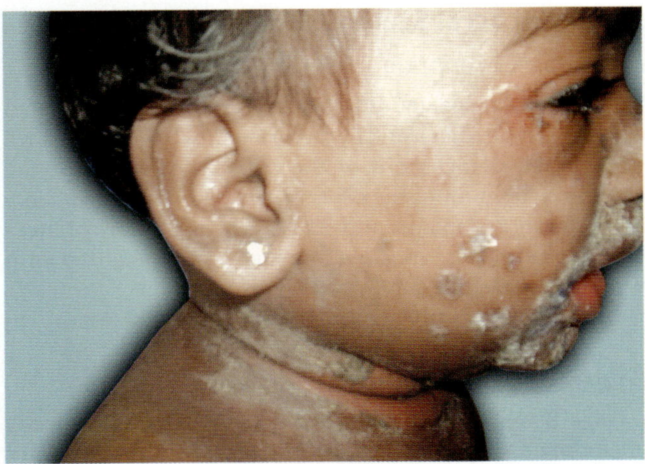

Fig. 18.6.27: Staphylococcal scalded skin syndrome—exfoliation and erythema over face and neck.

- *Generalized staphylococcal scalded skin syndrome: S. aureus* is only present in colonized site of infection, i.e. umbilical stump, conjunctiva or external ear canal; culture of sloughing skin or bullae usually yields no pathogens.

Treatment

For a newborn, hospitalization and treatment with IV cloxacillin, 200 mg/kg body weight/day in divided every 4 hours, are preferable. Hospitalize infants with extensive sloughing of skin or if parental compliance to treatment is questioned. With reliable home care and mild involvement, cloxacillin, 30–50 mg/kg body weight/day, can be given orally. Topical care includes baths or compresses, and mupirocin or bacitracin, or silver sulfadiazine/ointment.

BIBLIOGRAPHY

1. Bhave SY. Adolescent Health: Case Scenarios, 1st edition. New Delhi: Byword Books Private Limited; 2011.
2. Bhave SY. Bhave's Textbook of Adolescent Medicine, 1st edition. New Delhi: Jaypee Brothers Medical Publishers (P) Ltd.; 2006.
3. Gowrishankar NC, Lakshmi S, Ravikumar T, et al. Management Update for Common Pediatric Problems, 1st edition. New Delhi: Jaypee Brothers Medical Publishers (P) Ltd.; 2004.
4. Irvine AD, Hoeger PH, Yan AC. Harper's Textbook of Pediatric Dermatology, 3rd edition. London: Blackwell Publishing Ltd.; 2011.
5. Jones SL. Pediatric Dermatology. London: Oxford University Press; 2010.
6. Paller AS, Mancini AJ. Hurwitz Clinical Pediatric Dermatology: A Textbook of Skin Disorders of Childhood and Adolescence, 4th edition. Toronto: Elsevier Saunders; 2010.
7. Parthasarathy A. Partha's Fundamentals of Pediatrics, 1st edition. New Delhi: Jaypee Brothers Medical Publishers (P) Ltd.; 2007.
8. Thappa DM. Clinical Pediatric Dermatology, 1st edition. India: Elsevier Publishers; 2009.
9. Thomas J. Atopic dermatitis. In: Thomas J (Ed). Pediatric Dermatology Ward Rounds, 1st edition. New Delhi: Jaypee Brothers Medical Publishers (P) Ltd.; 2007. pp. 17-9.

18.7 Common Dental Problems

PK Baskar

INTRODUCTION

Dental diseases affecting the child may or may not be symptomatic. Further, certain physiological changes like eruption of a tooth may be associated with inflammation. Pediatricians should equip themselves to differentiate the physiological changes from pathological lesions.

Involving the parents in the prevention, treatment, and recurrence is particularly important in pediatric practice. Prevention of dental diseases should start from educating the pregnant mother.

Dental diseases affecting the child are not the same that affect the adult. The target organs are the same as teeth, gingiva, etc. but the etiopathogenesis are different because:

- The primary dentition is morphologically different.
- Food habits are different from that of the adult.
- Poorer control over maintenance of oral hygiene.

The pediatrician should be aware that teeth and jaws are in the formative stages. They should guide the parents not only in the prevention of dental diseases, but also in ensuring ideal and optimal growth of the dentition, both primary and permanent.

DENTITION

The primary dentition comprises 20 teeth—four incisors, two canines and four molars in each jaw.

The permanent dentition comprises 32 teeth—four incisors, two canines, four premolars and six molars in each jaw.

They are represented as follows with two digits for easy reference.

- *Primary dentition:*

55	54	53	52	51	61	62	63	64	65
85	84	83	82	81	71	72	73	74	75

- *Permanent dentition:*

18	17	16	15	14	13	12	11	21	22	23	24	25	26	27	28
48	47	46	45	44	43	42	41	31	32	33	34	35	36	37	38

The primary **(Box 18.7.1 and Fig. 18.7.1)** and permanent **(Box 18.7.2 and Fig. 18.7.2)** dentitions have distinct morphological characteristics, which identify them as incisors, canines, and molars.

DEVELOPMENT OF TEETH

The teeth are derived from highly specialized cells of ectodermal and mesodermal origin. Ectodermal cells perform special functions such as enamel formation, odontoblastic stimulation and determination of the shape of the crown and root. These cells disappear after performing their functions. Mesodermal cells persist throughout their life and form dentine, pulpal tissue, cementum, periodontal membrane and alveolar bone.

Each tooth, in achieving morphologic and functional maturity, through a well-defined and characteristic lifecycle is composed of many stages.

These stages of development are:

- Growth
- Calcification
- Eruption
- Attrition
- Resorption and exfoliation.

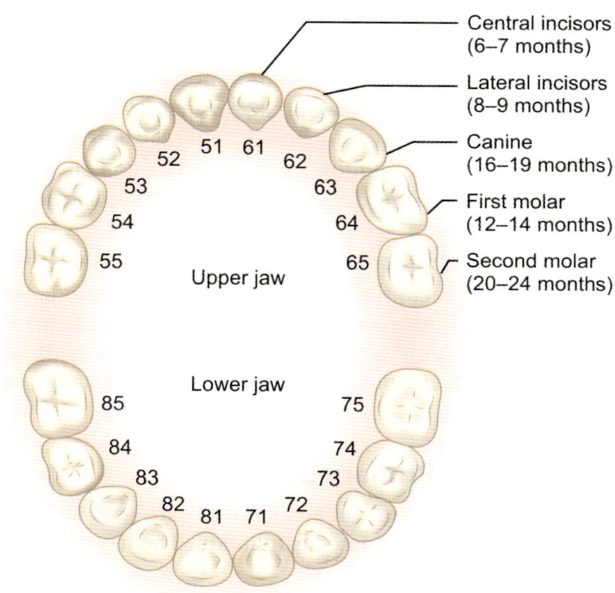

Fig. 18.7.1: Eruption sequence—primary dentition.

Box 18.7.1: Primary dentition.

- *Eruption sequence:*
  - Central incisors (6–7 months)
  - Lateral incisors (8–9 months)
  - Canine (16–18 months)
  - First molar (12–14 months)
  - Second molar (20–24 months)
- *Completion of enamel formation:*
  - Central incisors (1½ months)
  - Lateral incisors (2½ months)
  - Canine (9 months)
  - First molar (6 months)
  - Second molar (11 months)
  - Central incisor (6–7 months)
  - Lateral incisor (8–9 months)
  - Canine (16–19 months)
  - First molar (12–14 months)
  - Upper jaw second molar (20–24 months)

Box 18.7.2: Permanent dentition.

- *Eruption sequence:*
  - Central incisors (7–8 years)
  - Lateral incisors (8–9 years)
  - Canine (11–12 years)
  - First premolar (10–11 years)
  - Second premolar (10–12 years)
  - First molar (6–7 years)
  - Second molar (12–13 years)
- *Completion of enamel formation:*
  - Central incisors (4–5 years)
  - Lateral incisors (4–5 years)
  - Canine (6–7 years)
  - First premolar (5–6 years)
  - Second premolar (6–7 years)
  - First molar (2½–3½ years)
  - Second molar (7–8 years)
  - Lateral incisor (8–9 years)
  - Canine (9–12 years)
  - First premolar (10–11 years)
  - Second premolar (10–12 years)
  - First molar (6–7 years)
  - Second molar (12–13 years)

Diagnosis of Dental Caries

A sharp probe can be used to examine the tooth under good illumination to detect the presence of dental caries. Occlusal caries can be detected best by mouth mirror and explorer even at the early stages where radiograph cannot detect. The radiograph is sometimes useful for a complete oral examination by the dentist. The interproximal lesion appears as a small radiolucent area of the enamel. Opaque discoloration in the enamel is usually the earliest evidence of dental caries.

There may not be any pain even when dental caries has involved enamel. The enamel caries can be there for several months but when the caries extents into the dentine, it spreads very fast and reaches the pulp, which becomes very painful. Hence, periodical dental check-up with proper illumination with a sharp explorer and mouth mirror will help to detect dental caries, which can be filled with metal or any other restorative resins.

It must also be understood that the enamel is incapable of regeneration. Hence, there is a need for a foreign material to repair the decayed enamel. However, remineralization in the enamel has been found to be possible with topical fluorides and suitable diet rich in calcium and phosphorus.

Management of Dental Caries

- *Reduction in the intake of freely fermentable carbohydrates*: Frequency of eating and eating between meals has a direct bearing on the incidence of dental caries, particularly in children. The incidence is more when there is more sugar intake.
- Topical application of fluorides is very useful.
- Discouraging sweets help.
- Plaque control can be achieved by tooth brushing, flushing, scaling and antiseptic mouthwashes.
- *Water fluoridation*: It is important to understand that fluoride incorporation is beneficial only at the time of calcification of the tooth. There is evidence pointing to considerable tooth decay inhibition when the community water supply having fluoride in the drinking water is approximately 1 ppm, marked inhibition of dental caries without producing significant mottling of the enamel is seen.
- *Diet*: Feeding during sleep should be discouraged. During sleep, salivary flow is diminished, and swallowing reflex is absent. Hence, stagnation of milk is possible. The clearance of milk can be encouraged by intake of water.
- It has been observed that incidence of dental caries is high whenever bottle-feeding is preferred to breastfeed. Further breast-feeding also helps in proper development of orofacial structures. Drinking more soft drinks causes increased susceptibility to dental caries. High-protein diets, fats, phosphates and detergent diets have been found to be cariostatic. Sucrose, sweets, chocolates, jams, and ice cream are found to be cariogenic.
- *Detergents diet*: Any food that sticks to the teeth favors caries activity. Hence, such foods should be avoided. Detergent diets play a useful role in the prevention of dental caries. It serves two functions: (1) the fibrous content helps in better blood circulation in the gingival and (2) it removes all the food debris and plaque between teeth and gums and leaves the mouth clean. It has been observed that cheese and peanuts inhibit caries activity. Almonds and groundnuts are rich source of calcium and phosphorus. Among dry fruits, apricots, figs, and dates also provide rich source of calcium and phosphorus.
- *Pit and fissure sealants*: This is a very important treatment procedure, which protects susceptible surfaces. With improved utilization of this underutilized preventive measure, significant economic and health benefit can be realized.
- *Restoration of the decayed tooth*: The first step is to prevent further progression of the lesion. Gross superficial excavation of the caries and filling the cavity with zinc oxide—eugenol will temporarily arrest the caries process and prevent its rapid progression to the deeper tissues. Further, it helps in the sterilization of the cavity walls. These cavities can be later filled by permanent filling material. Dental amalgam has been studied extensively for safety and it has withstood the test of time, there is still a place for dental amalgam.
- A new method of treating dental caries that involves neither drill water, nor electricity called atraumatic restorative treatment (ART) consists of manually cleaning dental cavities with hand instrument and filling them with an adhesive fluoride releasing material.
- *Atraumatic restorative technique*: The ART is a procedure based on removing carious tooth structure using hand instrument alone and restoring the cavity with an adhesive restorative material. At present, the restorative material of choice is glass ionomer cement.

ACUTE GINGIVAL DISEASES

Acute Herpetic Gingivostomatitis

Acute herpetic gingivostomatitis is an infection of the oral cavity caused by a specific virus. Secondary bacterial infection complicates the clinical picture. This is caused by the herpes simplex virus (HSV). The condition usually occurs during and immediately after an episode of febrile disease such as pneumonia, influenza or typhoid. It also tends to occur during periods of anxiety, strain or exhaustion and during menstruation.

Clinical Features

This condition appears as a diffuse, erythematous, shiny involvement of the gingiva and the adjacent oral mucosa with edema and gingival bleeding. In the initial stage, it is characterized by the presence of discrete spherical gray vesicles, which may occur on gingiva, the labial and buccal mucosa, soft palate, pharynx, sublingual mucosa and tongue. After 24 hours, the vesicles rupture and form painful small ulcers with a red, elevated halo-like margin and a depressed yellowish-gray white central portion. Course of the disease is limited to 7–10 days, the diffuse erythema and edema persist for several days. Scarring does not occur; localized form consists of numerous pinpoint vesicles. The vesicles rupture and form painful ulcerations.

The disease is accompanied by generalized soreness of the oral cavity, which interferes with eating and drinking. The ruptured vesicles are the focal sites of pain and sensitivity to touch, thermal changes, and foods such as condiments and fruit juices. In infants, the disease is marked by irritability and refusal to take food. Herpetic involvements of lips or face with vesicles and surface scab formation may be present. Cervical adenitis, fever as high as 101°F and generalized malaise are common. Treatment is only supportive and symptomatic. Antibiotic therapy is of considerable aid in the prevention of secondary infection.

Oral Candidiasis

Candidiasis is a disease caused by infection with a yeast-like fungus, *Candida albicans*; although, other species may also be involved. This microorganism is relatively a common inhabitant of the oral cavity, gastrointestinal tract and vagina of clinically unaffected persons. This disease is said to be the most opportunistic infection in the world.

Acute pseudomembranous candidiasis is one of the more common forms of the disease. It may occur at any age but is especially prone to occur in the debilitated or the chronically ill, or in infants. The oral lesions are characterized by the appearance of soft, white slightly elevated plaques most frequently occurring on the buccal mucosa and tongue, but also seen on the palate, gingival and floor of the mouth. The plaques resemble milk, curd consist chiefly of tangled masses of fungal hyphae with intermingled desquamated epithelium, keratin, fibrin, necrotic debris, leukocytes and bacteria. The white plaque can be wiped away with a gauze leaving a normal appearing mucosa or an erythematous area. Chronic hyperplastic candidiasis is often spoken of as the leukoplakia type of candidiasis. The oral lesions consist of firm, white persistent plaques, usually on the lips, tongue and cheeks. These lesions persist for many years.

Clinical Features

The two types of candidiasis are:
1. Mucocutaneous candidiasis.
2. Systemic candidiasis.

The mucocutaneous form includes oral or oropharyngeal forms. The systemic form involves chiefly the eyes, kidneys and skin through hematogenous spread.

Treatment

Specific antifungal agents such as nystatin has been beneficial in the treatment, suspensions of nystatin, held in contact with the oral lesion have been successfully used in even chronic or severe cases of the disease. Painting the lesion with gentian violet is an older but effective treatment.

Acute Necrotizing Ulcerative Gingivitis

Acute necrotizing ulcerative gingivitis (ANUG) is an inflammatory destructive disease of the gingiva commonly known as Vincent infection. Spirochetal organism and fusiform bacilli termed Borrelia are always found in the disease.

Clinical Features

A well-defined punched-out, crater-like depressions at the crest of the interdental papillae is always seen. The surface of this gingival crater is covered by grayish, pseudomembranous slough, demarcated from the remainder of the gingival mucosa by a pronounced linear erythema.

The other salient features are constant radiating, gnawing pain that is intensified by eating spicy or hot foods, metallic taste, pasty saliva and hypersalivation.

Halitosis is always present much to the annoyance of the child and others, which is often very penchant.

Local lymphadenopathy and a slight elevation in temperature are common. However, in severe cases, high fever, increased pulse rate, leukocytosis, loss of appetite and general lassitude are also seen.

Management

The treatment consists of:
- Local treatment for alleviation of the acute inflammation should be started immediately.
- Systemic—appropriate supportive treatment to correct malnutrition and suitable antibiotics.

MALOCCLUSION

While dental caries has been regarded as the major dental disease throughout the world affecting the child, malocclusion is only next. Malocclusion may involve four tissue systems:
1. Teeth
2. Bones
3. Muscle
4. Nerves

The teeth are irregular, jaw relationship may be good and muscle and nerve function normal. Teeth may be regular in their alignment, but an abnormal jaw relationship may exist so that the teeth do not meet properly during function.

Habits

Impact of Pediatric Oral Habits

Oral habits can manifest in variety of activities, which may or may not be a concern to the child or parents. They include digit sucking, mentalis habits, lip wetting, lip sucking, abnormal swallowing, tongue thrusting, posture habits and self-mutilation. Assessment of such habits should be identified immediately to avoid long-term effect on the craniofacial complex and dentition.

Role of Pacifiers

Pacifiers can cause malocclusion of the anterior teeth and posterior cross bites, depending on the frequency, strength and duration of the pacifier use. Anterior open bite and maxillary construction are often seen with pacifier use.

Epidemiology

The most prevalent type of malocclusion in the primary dentition is anterior open bite, secondary to pernicious habits. In the mixed dentitions, crowding is the most common type of malocclusion. There is no difference in the incidence of malocclusions according to sex. It is interesting to note that the primary dentition usually has good occlusal relationship, particularly in breastfed children. Malocclusion may develop later when the primary teeth are shed, and permanent teeth erupt.

Diagnosis

- *Spacing*: Loss of contact between the teeth occurs when arch length is more compared to total width of the teeth or when the teeth moves out of arch alignment.
- *Crowding*: When arch length is less compared to total width of the teeth, crowding occurs.
- *Overjet*: This is the horizontal distance between the palatal surface of upper incisors and the labial surface of lower incisors when teeth are in occlusion.
- *Overbite*: This is the vertical distance covered by the upper incisors over the lower incisors when teeth are in occlusion.
- *Crossbite*: Normally, lower teeth are slightly overlapped by the upper teeth but if the lower teeth are positioned outside the upper arch when teeth are in contact, then it is crossbite, which can be anterior or posterior.
- *Open bite*: It can be anterior or posterior with space present between the incisal and cuspal edges of the upper and lower teeth during occlusion.
- *Lip incompetence*: Lips do not contact each other during the rest position.
- *Rotation*: Teeth are rotated.

Treatment

Treatment planning is based on:

- Case history
- Clinical examination
- Plaster study casts
- Radiographs—periapical, bitewing and panoramic
- Facial photographs.

Treatment should also include:

- Correction of abnormal pressure habits, if any
- Extraction of retained primary teeth
- Extraction of supernumerary teeth, depending on the merits of each patient.

The cause of malocclusion should be identified, and wherever possible, should be eradicated before starting the treatment. Otherwise, the treatment can be incomplete, and moreover, there can be relapse of the malocclusion. This is particularly more relevant when there is a pernicious habit existing. The treatment for malocclusion is usually simple when treatment is given in time. Most malocclusion responds well to removable appliances. However, fixed appliance gives more effective result for severe malocclusion.

BIBLIOGRAPHY

1. Ahiropoulos V. Fluoride content of bottled waters available in Northern Greece. Int J Paediatr Dent. 2006;16(2):111-6.
2. Balappanavar AY, Nagesh L, Ankola AV, et al. Antimicrobial efficacy of various disinfection solutions in reducing the contamination of toothbrush—a comparative study. Oral Health Prev Dent. 2009;7(2):137-45.
3. Bottled Water Industry in India. [online] Available from: www.gits4u.com/water/water16.htm. [Accessed November, 2018].
4. Brown D. Amalgam use in pregnant women. Br Dent J. 1998;184(11):524-5.
5. Carlisle D. Feeding babies with cleft lip and palate. Nurse Times. 1998;94(4):59-60.
6. Feigel RJ. The use of pit and fissure sealants. Pediatr Dent. 2002;24(5):415-22.
7. Gupta H, Gupta P. Fruit drinks how healthy and safe? Indian Pediatr. 2008;45(3):215-7.
8. Osborne JW, Summitt JB, Robert HW. The use of dental amalgam in pediatric dentistry: review of the literature. Pediatr Dent. 2002;24(5):439-47.
9. Qin M, Liu H. Clinical evaluation of a flowable resins composite and flowable components for preventive resin restorations. Oper Dent. 2005;30(5):580-7.
10. Roos EH, Donly KJ. In vivo dental plaque pH variation with regular and diet soft drinks. Pediatr Dent. 2002;24(4):350-3.

18.8 Pediatric Radiology

Arun Kumar Gupta, Manisha Jana

INTRODUCTION

Over the last several decades, pediatric radiology has not only emerged in the forefront, but has established itself as a definite subspecialty. A pediatric radiologist should not only have knowledge of general radiology, embryology and basic pediatrics, but should also be acutely aware of the indications, technicalities of various procedures and should be radiation conscious. Although, problem-oriented approach is ideal; in this chapter, an organ-oriented approach is used to present the essentials.

IMAGING TECHNIQUES

Conventional radiology, i.e. plain radiography and contrast studies (e.g. barium studies, excretory urography and contrast studies for the lower genitourinary tract) still remain the mainstay of pediatric radiology. However, with the introduction of ultrasound (US), computed tomography (CT) and magnetic resonance imaging (MRI), the diagnostic algorithm in several diseases has changed dramatically. Role of important imaging modalities is discussed under each organ system.

CHEST

Imaging Techniques

Conventional radiographs are still the most frequently carried out procedures. Proper immobilization is essential. Radiograph is taken in supine anteroposterior (AP) for children less than 3 years of age and in erect posteroanterior (PA) for older children. CT is the next best cost-effective imaging technique for complete chest evaluation. MRI and magnetic resonance angiography (MRA) are now increasingly used for assessing relationship of mediastinal vessels to mediastinal masses or for primary vascular diseases such as aortoarteritis, coarctation, etc. Sonography has a limited role in chest diseases due to reflection of ultrasound beam by air. However, for pleural diseases, mediastinal or pulmonary lesions abutting the chest wall and for cardiac and major vessel evaluation, sonography is a quick and easy technique, which can be carried out even at bedside.

Normal Chest X-ray

Usually, only a frontal chest radiograph (AP or PA) is taken. If any abnormality is detected or in patients with high index of suspicion, appropriate lateral radiograph is also taken.

Interpretation

Patient rotation and quality of exposure are first checked because improper patient position or exposure can be disastrous. Next, the film is read either from out-to-in or vice versa. Carefully examine in a sequence, always comparing with the opposite side for soft tissues, bones under review (ribs, clavicles, scapulae, humeri, etc.); aeration of each lung in the upper, mid and lower-thirds as well as medial-mid and outer-thirds; vascularity in each of these zones; tracheal position, diaphragm position and shape; costophrenic angles; mediastinal silhouette on each side; cardiac size and shape; retrocardiac space; position, size and density of each hilum; and last but not the least, look under the diaphragms for free air and dilated loops.

Lateral radiograph is usually taken to localize a lesion already detected on the frontal films, for evaluation of the hilar nodes and for assessing the position of diaphragm.

In a case with suspected free pleural effusion, a lateral decubitus view film is required with the affected side lower and closer to the film cassette.

- *Normal thymus*: An anterior mediastinal soft tissue "mass" is a common finding on conventional chest radiograph **(Figs. 18.8.1A and B)** in normal children up to the age of 3 years and is due to normal thymus. Several radiographic signs are helpful to identify it as normal thymus, e.g. *wave sign*; *sail sign*; change in shape during respiration and shrinking under the stress of steroid therapy (which reverts to the original size on stoppage of steroid).

Pathological Conditions

Discussions on important neonatal chest conditions such as hyaline membrane disease, transient tachypnea of the newborn and meconium aspiration are beyond the scope of this chapter.

- *Developmental anomalies*:
  - Agenesis of a lung is an extremely uncommon clinical entity. Completely opaque hemithorax on a frontal chest radiograph and absent pulmonary artery or main bronchus on the pulmonary angiogram or bronchogram, respectively, confirms the diagnosis.
  - Persistence of pleuroperitoneal canal results in herniation of intestinal loops into the chest cavity. Clinically, the baby presents with respiratory distress.

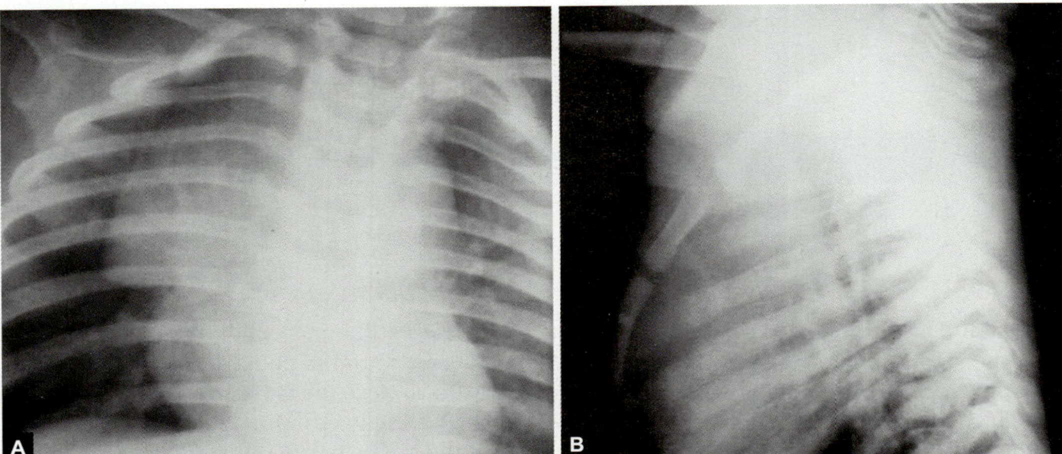

Figs. 18.8.1A and B: Normal (A) frontal and (B) lateral chest radiographs. Note a large right anterior "mediastinal mass" due to normal thymus (sail sign). Correlation with clinical information is mandatory before assigning a pathological label.

- *Foreign body inhalation*: One of the most important, noninfective causes of acute respiratory distress in children is inhalation of foreign body, which could be either radiolucent (in about 90%) or radiopaque (in 10%) **(Figs. 18.8.2 A and B)**. Radiographic findings depend upon several factors. Collapse **(Fig. 18.8.2 C)**, hyperlucent enlarged lobe (or lung) due to ball valve type of block or consolidation may be seen. In a suspected case of radiolucent foreign body inhalation and with equivocal chest radiographic findings, deep expiratory film may be very useful for the correct diagnosis.
- *Bacterial pneumonia:* It is most commonly caused by *Streptococcus pneumonia, Haemophilus influenzae* and *Staphylococcus aureus.*
  - About 50% of staphylococcal pneumonia cases are complicated by pneumatoceles **(Fig. 18.8.3)**.
  - Staphylococcal or pneumococcal pneumonia may produce a round-shaped pneumonia termed as round pneumonia, which may mimic hydatid cyst or metastatic lesion.
  - Abscess **(Figs. 18.8.4A to C)** is not an uncommon complication.
  - Empyema is another important complication necessitating imaging and many a times surgical intervention.
- *Viral infection*: Unlike bacterial infections, which result in airspace disease, viral infections tend to affect predominantly the airways. The resultant radiologic picture is bilateral hyperinflation with perihilar striations **(Fig. 18.8.5)**, the latter due to peribronchial thickening (cuffing). Radiograph may even appear normal. Pathologic-cum-clinical term used to describe this condition is bronchiolitis or "bronchitis". Thus, in a child presenting with acute respiratory distress but with very subtle radiologic changes, one should suspect this clinical entity.
- *Pulmonary tuberculosis* is one of the most commonly seen chest conditions in India. A wide spectrum of radiologic findings is observed in these children.
  - Primary complex **(Figs. 18.8.6A and B)** consists of the pulmonary parenchymal focus, draining lymphatics (rarely seen on chest radiograph) and mediastinal nodal enlargement.
  - As the infection becomes progressive, then radiological changes of postprimary tuberculosis are seen. Findings may include only nodal enlargement, pleural effusion **(Fig. 18.8.7)**, lobar or segmental consolidation; pneumonic consolidation with air bronchogram **(Figs. 18.8.8A to C)** and pulmonary cavitations.
  - Lymphatic or venous seeding in lungs produces miliary tuberculosis.
  - Following healing, by chemotherapy or by development of body immunity chest radiograph may become either completely normal or residual changes like calcified nodes, pulmonary scar, pleural thickening or loss of volume may be seen.
- *Bronchiectasis* is another common clinical problem, which usually follows infection by tuberculosis, viral or bacterial pneumonias. After the chest radiographs, thin section, high-resolution CT is the imaging modality of choice to detect subtle bronchiectasis. Bronchograms are rarely, if ever, used nowadays.
- On a chest radiograph; round, soft tissue density, either single or multiple is most commonly due to hydatid cyst in our country. CT would readily show its content to be fluid. If the lesion is abutting the chest wall or diaphragm, then ultrasound can also be used for characterizing the soft-tissue mass.

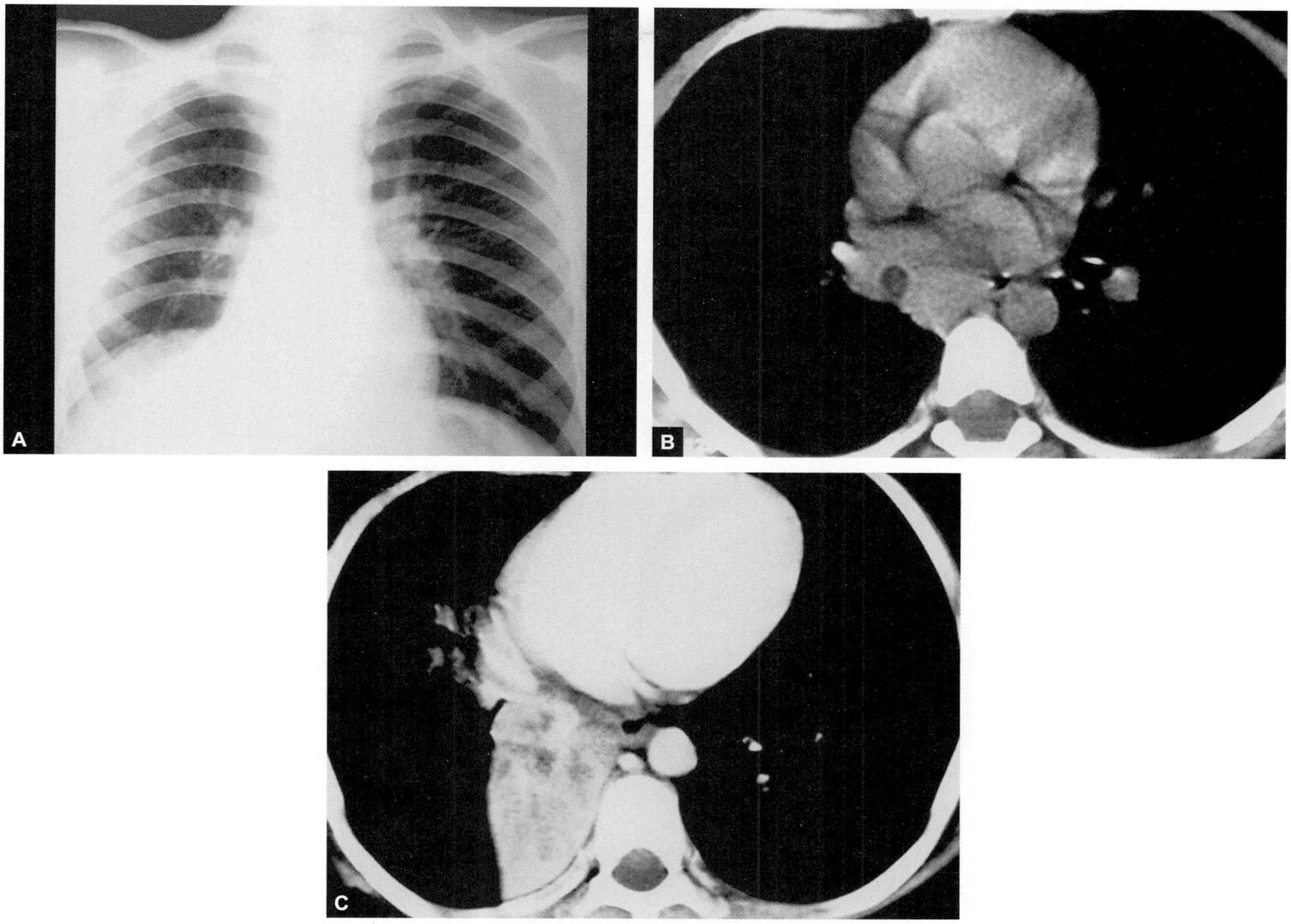

Figs. 18.8.2A to C: Foreign body inhalation. (A) Radiograph showing collapse right lower lobe; (B) Computed tomography (CT) mediastinal window is showing intraluminal foreign body in right lower lobe bronchus; (C) Collapse right lower lobe.

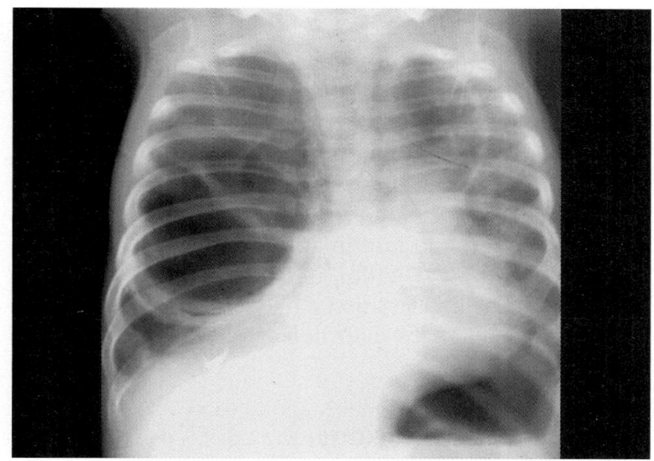

Fig. 18.8.3: Staphylococcal pneumonia with pneumatoceles.

- *Primary lung tumors* are rare in children. Metastatic lung disease is much more common and is usually from a Wilms tumor.
- *Mediastinum* is divided into three compartments: (1) anterior, (2) middle, and (3) posterior. It is important to remember that the radiological division of the mediastinum is different from the anatomical division. Masses can arise from any one of the structures normally present in these compartments:
    - Germ cell tumor is an anterior mediastinal malignant tumor.
    - Lymph nodes, bronchogenic cyst, pericardial tumors and hiatus hernia are important masses of middle mediastinum.
    - Neurogenic tumors predominate in the posterior mediastinum.

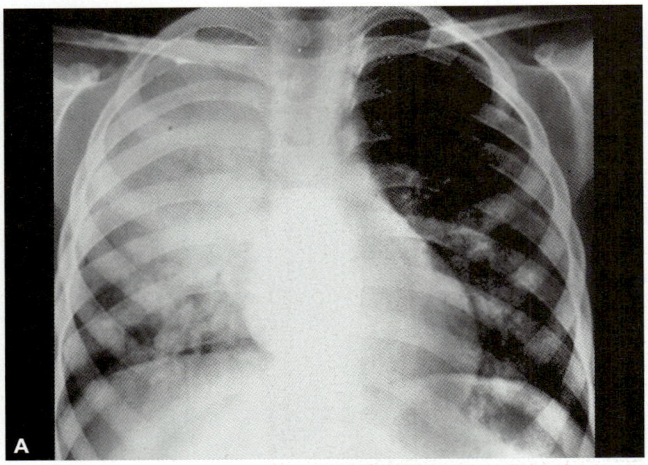

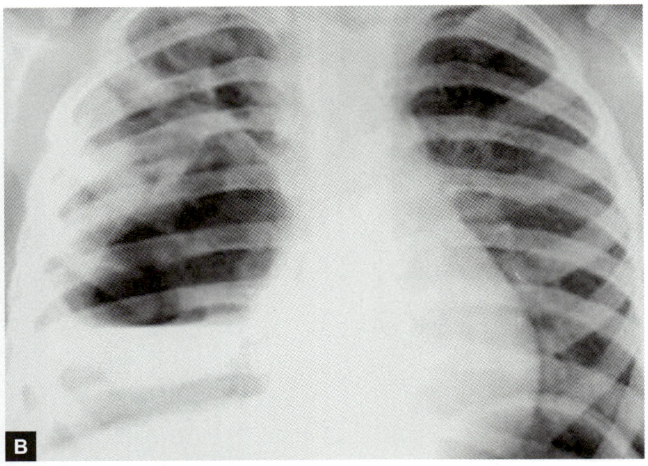

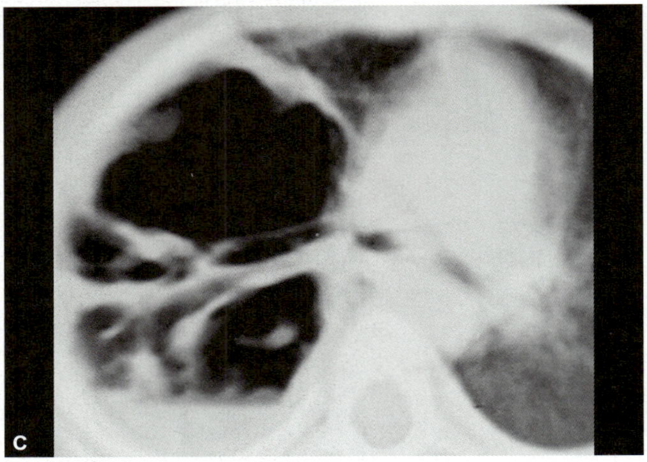

Figs. 18.8.4A to C: Lung abscess in evolution—(A and B) initially, consolidation which progressed to a huge lung abscess with a large air-fluid level; (C) The finding is confirmed on computed tomography (CT).

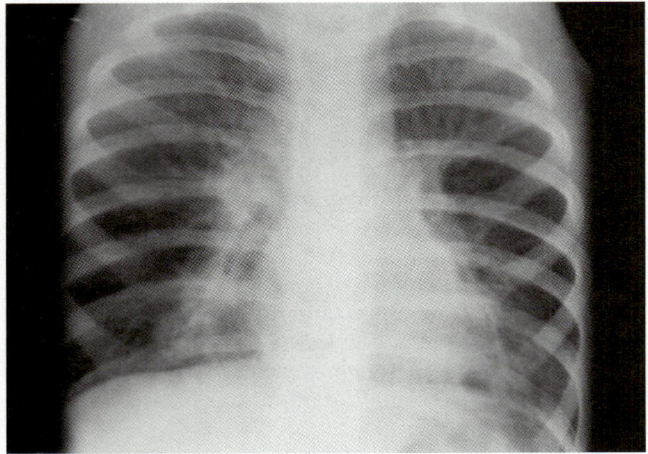

Fig. 18.8.5: Viral pneumonia, bronchiolitis; bilateral, generalized hyperinflation with minimal flattening of both domes. Note minimal perihilar striations, better appreciated on the left side due to peribronchial soft-tissue thickening.

SKELETAL SYSTEM

Imaging Techniques

Conventional radiographs still remain the mainstay for the evaluation of musculoskeletal diseases. CT and MRI provide detailed soft tissue, articular and bony imaging, and are thus helpful, especially for examination of masses regarding their content, extent and degree of vascular and marrow involvement. MRI is superior to CT due to its better soft tissue resolution and multiplanar capability. Sonography has a role in the evaluation of congenital dislocation of hip, hip effusion and soft tissue masses. Scintigraphy is the primary modality in the detection of metastatic disease and osteomyelitis.

Pathological Conditions

Before interpreting abnormality, one must have knowledge about the normal development of bone, parts of different

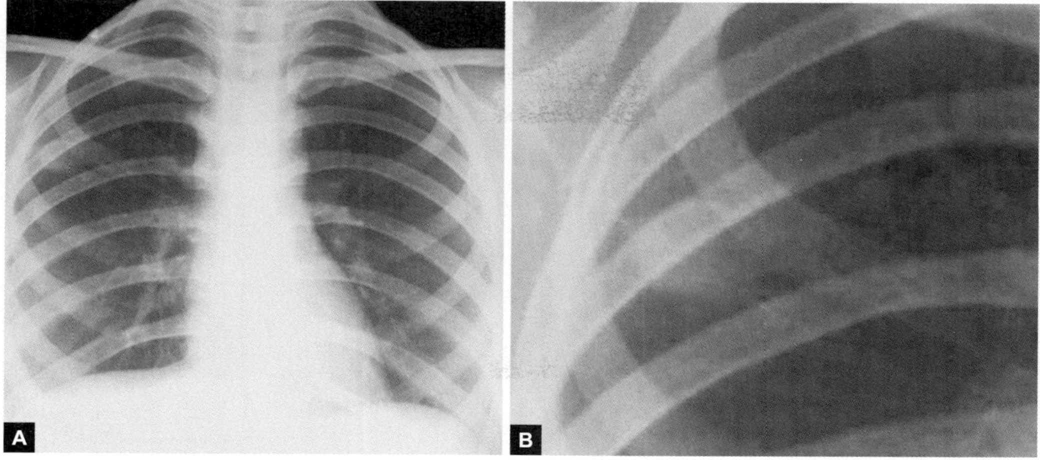

Figs. 18.8.6A and B: Primary pulmonary complex—consolidation just above the minor fissure.

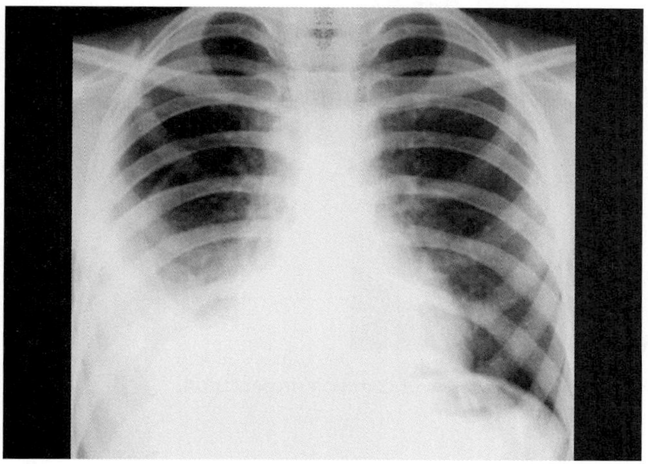

Fig. 18.8.7: Free pleural effusion on the right side, running along the lateral chest wall.

areas of skeletal system and several normal variants, which may mimic abnormalities:

- *Rickets* is still a relatively common clinical problem in India. Vitamin D deficiency results in failure of normal mineralization of the growing cartilage into bone. Classic radiographic findings are found in the most rapidly growing ends of bone, and include generalized osteopenia, disappearance of zone of provisional calcification, cupping with fraying and irregularity of the metaphyseal ends and perpendicular striations extending from the metaphyseal end toward epiphysis (**Figs. 18.8.9A and B**). Enlargement of the anterior ends of ribs (rachitic rosary) and lower ends of radius and ulna may also be noted.
- *Thalassemia major (homozygous form):* Radiographic changes are at times dramatic **(Figs. 18.8.10A to C)** and are the result of marrow hyperplasia.
- *Congenital syphilis* is caused by transplacental spread. Bone lesions may appear even up to 2 months later. Hallmark of this condition is metaphysitis **(Figs. 18.8.11A to C)**, i.e. a metaphyseal lucent band located directly beneath a dense band in the subphyseal region. Focal destructive bony lesions in diaphysis, periostitis and pathological fracture may also occur.
- *Skeletal tuberculosis* is still prevalent in India. Tuberculosis may affect any part of the skeletal system. In the spine, it typically affects the vertebral body. Partial collapse produces para- (and/or pre-) vertebral abscess and short angle gibbus. Long bone tuberculosis may be isolated or affect an adjacent joint. A high index of suspicion, chest radiograph, biochemical and hematological findings, family history and positive tuberculin test—all help in establishing the diagnosis in an equivocal case.
- *Developmental dysplasia of hip (congenital dislocation of hip)* is a common clinical problem. Following a thorough clinical examination, ultrasound is usually the first screening modality to confirm the diagnosis. On plain radiographs, several lines have been described to identify cases with subtle dislocation. Nowadays, three-dimensional CT (3D-CT) and 3D-MRI have shown promising results for in-depth evaluation of this entity.
- *Osteogenic sarcoma* is the most common primary malignant bone tumor between 10 years and 25 years of age and is usually located in the metaphysis of a long bone, especially around the knee. Typically, the tumor matrix is ossified and its metastases to lungs may also be ossified.

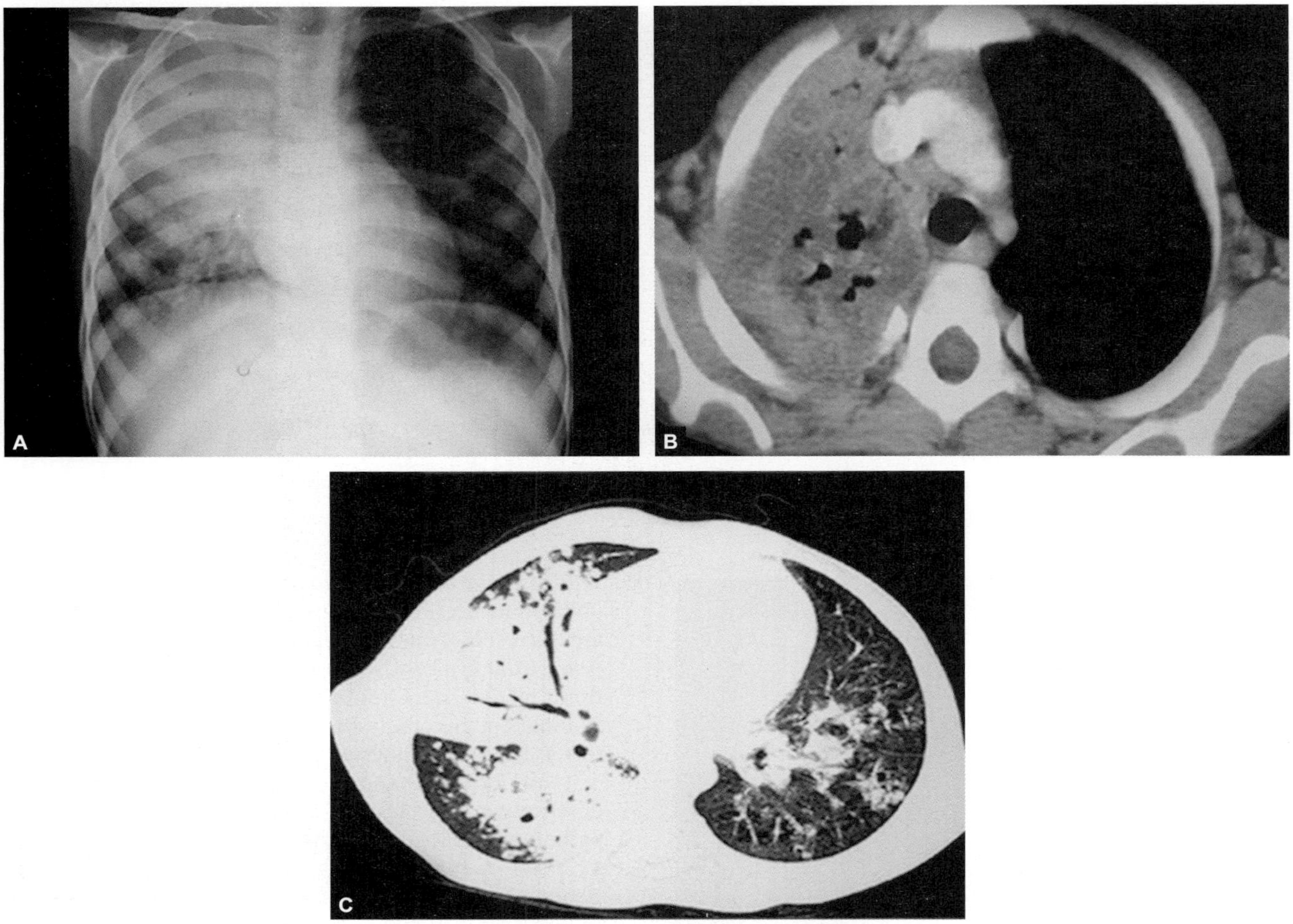

Figs. 18.8.8A to C: Primary progressive type of pulmonary tuberculosis—an uncommon presentation.

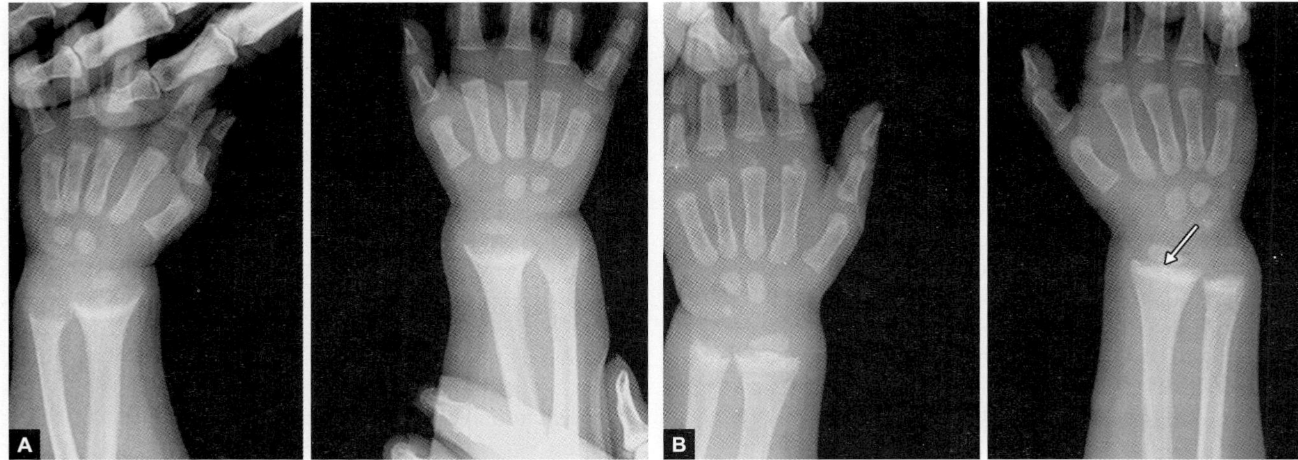

Figs. 18.8.9A and B: Rickets—primarily a metaphyseal disease. Note cupping of metaphyseal ends of both radius and ulna, widened physis, perpendicular striations extending from metaphysis into physis toward the epiphysis. (A) Generalized osteopenia is seen in the background; (B) Post-treatment radiographs show healing.

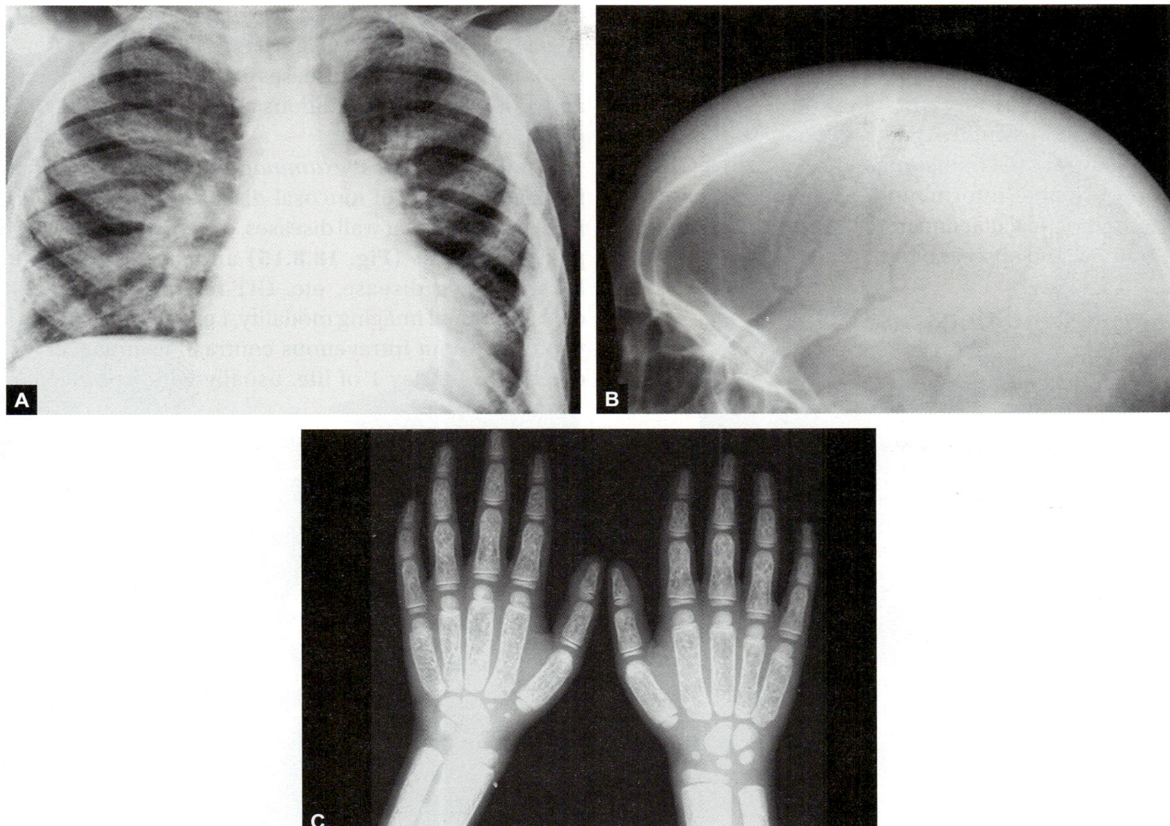

Figs. 18.8.10A to C: Thalassemia major—chest X-ray (CXR) showing marked expansion of the ribs. (A) Striking "hair-on-end" appearance in the skull; (B) Osteoporosis, widening of medullary spaces of all the bones of hands with coarse trabecular pattern, loss of lateral concavity of small bones of hand and molding abnormality of distal ends of long bones; (C) Radiographic changes reflect marked degree of marrow proliferation.

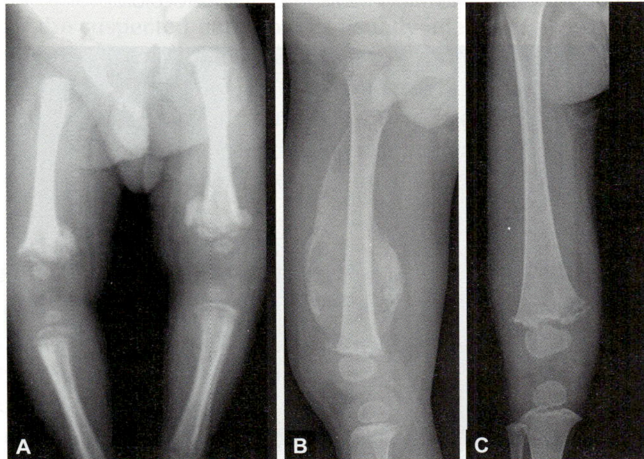

Figs. 18.8.11A to C: Congenital syphilis, both lower limbs anteroposterior (AP) view. (A) Characteristic metaphyseal changes (metaphysitis) and periostitis seen in all the long bones. Epiphysis is normal; (B and C) important differential diagnosis is scurvy, which is characterized by osteopenia with subperiosteal hemorrhage lifting the periosteum and metaphyseal changes.

- *Metastatic disease affecting the skeletal system* is common in the pediatric age group. Commonly, it is due to a round cell tumor—acute lymphoblastic leukemia, neuroblastoma, lymphoma, rhabdomyosarcoma or Ewing's sarcoma. Skeletal survey shows generalized demineralization, "moth-eaten" osteolytic lesions diffusely involving all the bones, metaphyseal lucent bands, and periosteal new bone formation with loss of focal areas of cortical line due to tumor invasion.

Assessment of Skeletal Maturity

Radiology of skeletal system would be incomplete without a few words on the methodology for skeletal maturity assessment or bone age assessment. Earlier method of observing the appearance and fusion of ossification centers is an obsolete technique; even though in India, it is still the only method used in most hospitals. More accurate methods are by using an atlas either by Greulich-Pyle or Tanner-Whitehouse 3 (TW3) method. The latter is, at present, the most accurate method for assessment of skeletal maturity in a child.

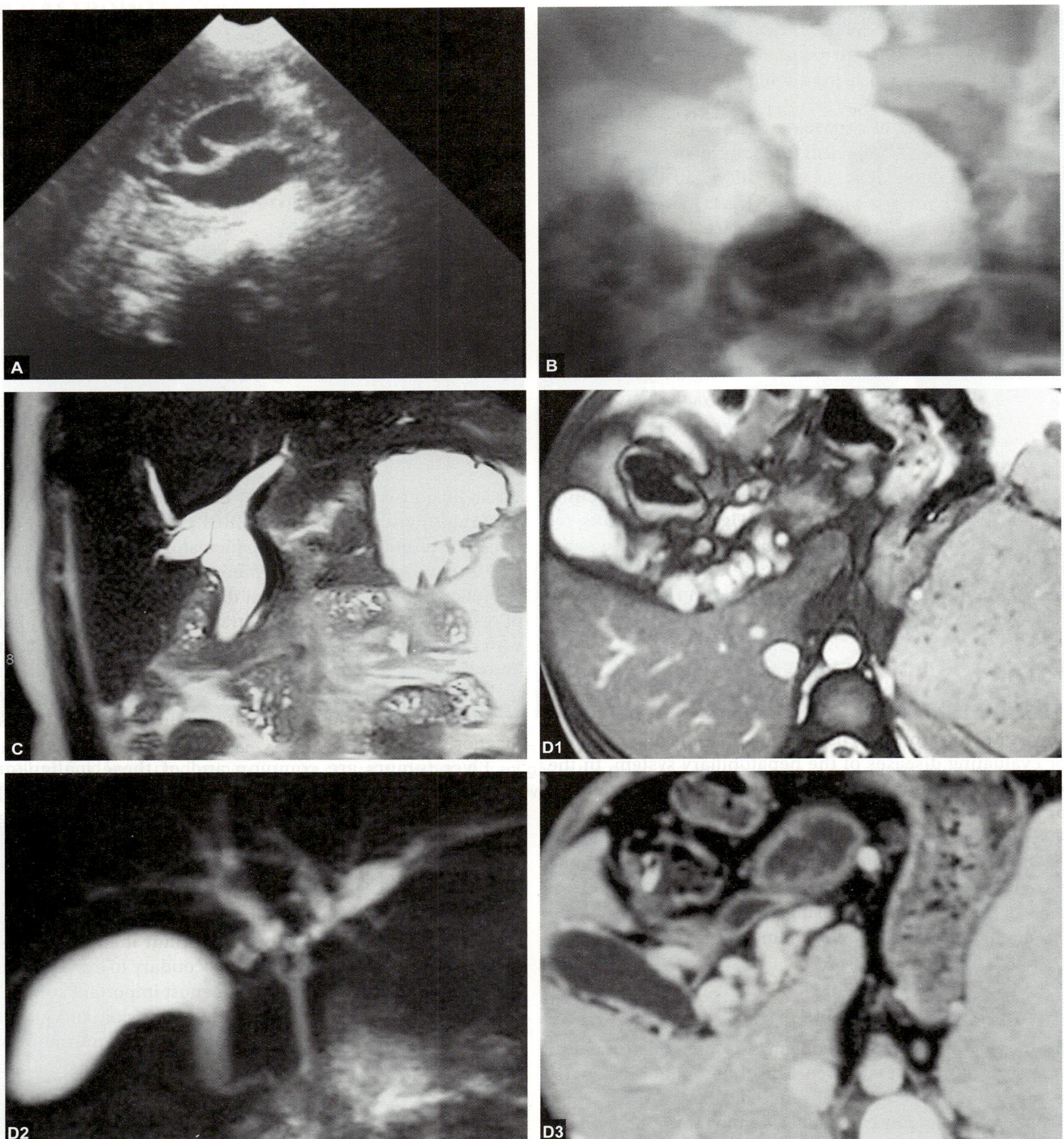

Figs. 18.8.17A to D3

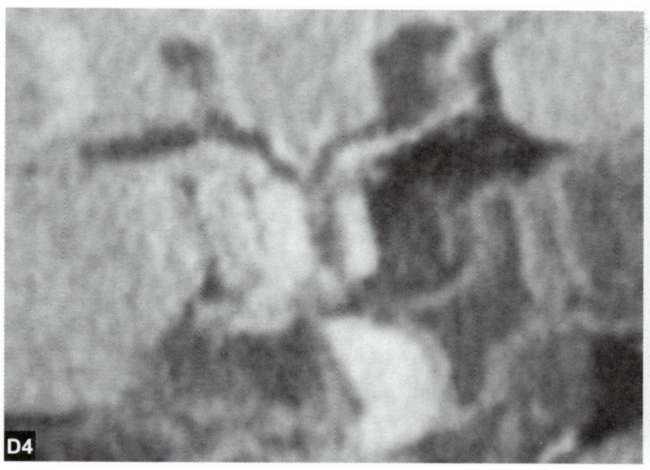

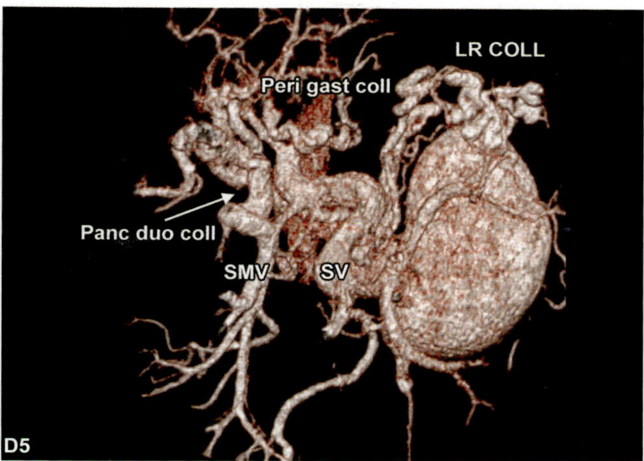

Figs. 18.8.17D4 and D5

Figs. 18.8.17A to D: (A and B) Huge, extrahepatic, cystic choledochal cyst on ultrasound; and on endoscopic retrograde cholangiopancreatography (ERCP); note the slightly dilated right main bile duct entering the cyst on ultrasound. Gallbladder should be documented separate from the cyst; (C and D) Magnetic resonance cholangiopancreatography (MRCP) images elegantly documenting the choledochal cystportal biliopathy: magnetic resonance imaging (MRI) axial (D1), and coronal (D2), computed tomography (CT) axial (D3), and coronal (D4) images showing portal cavernoma causing biliary dilatation. Three-dimensional CT (3D-CT) (D5) showing exquisite detail of the portosplenic axis and the collaterals developed.
(LR COLL: lienorenal collateral; SV: splenic vein)

However, it needs to be supplemented by a functional study. Nowadays, renal scintigraphy is preferred due to its low radiation dose, higher sensitivity and more objective assessment of renal function. Excretory urography is required when complex anatomical details need to be clarified or in patients with ureteric disease. CT or MRI is added in the workup of a case of tumor or trauma. For examination of the lower urinary tract, sonography for bladder and contrast examination for urethral evaluation are usually adequate.

Pathological Conditions

Hydronephrosis is one of the most important and common problems encountered in pediatric practice. Sonography and contrast study not only diagnose it reliably, but also provide a clue to its possible cause, e.g. pelviureteric junction (PUJ) obstruction **(Fig. 18.8.18)**, calculus, etc. and it can also delineate an associated hydroureter, if present.

Several congenital anomalies can be seen, e.g. horseshoe kidney, crossed ectopia, low lying kidney, etc.

Of the solid renal masses, Wilms' tumor is the most common. On cross-sectional imaging, it is seen as a solid tumor with variegated enhancement due to areas of necrosis. In 10%, it may be bilateral. For staging purposes, CT or MRI may be done in addition to sonography.

Bladder tumors are relatively rare in children, and of these, a malignant tumor, rhabdomyosarcoma, is the most common. On the cystogram phase of a contrast study, characteristic lobulated filling defects are seen from the bladder base. This appearance gives it the name of "sarcoma botryoides".

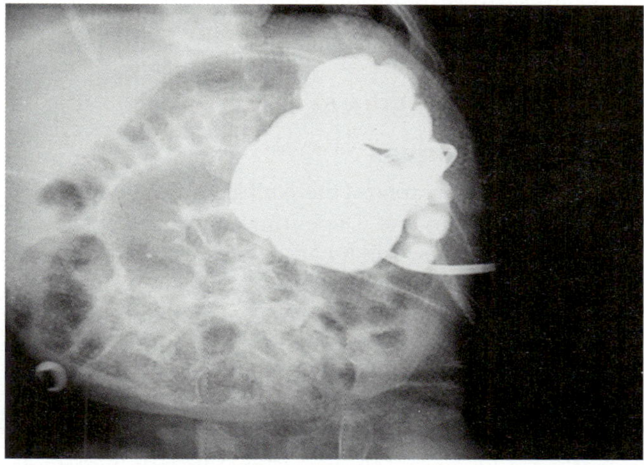

Fig. 18.8.18: Nephrostogram of left kidney shows dilated, rounded renal pelvis with caliectasis, a case of pelviureteric junction (PUJ) obstruction. Ureter is not opacified even on delayed images.

Vesicoureteric reflex (VUR) is one of the most important causes for urinary tract infection. Voiding cystourethrography (VCUG), either using contrast or an isotope, is required to diagnose it **(Figs. 18.8.19A and B)**. The latter is reported to be more accurate. Nowadays, even sonocystography is used in certain clinical situations to diagnose VUR with the added advantage of lack of ionizing radiation.

The most common cause for urinary outflow obstruction in a male child is posterior urethral valve (PUV). Micturating

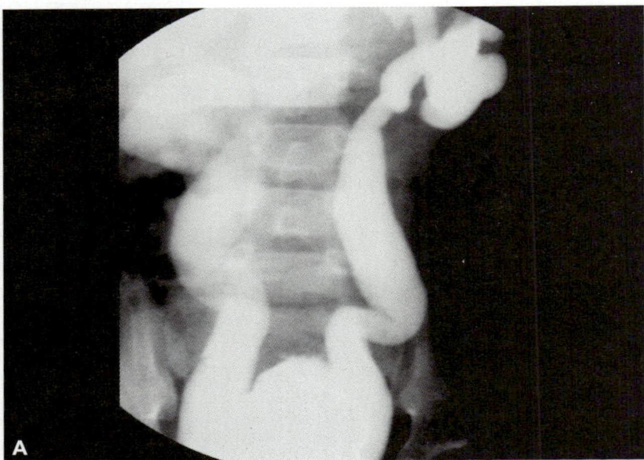

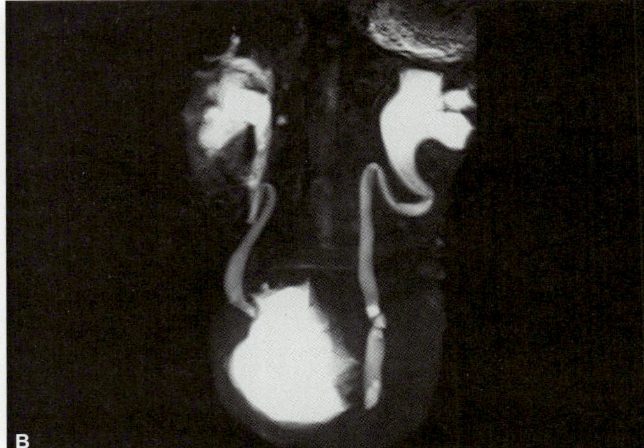

Figs.18.8.19A and B: (A) Micturating cystourethrography (MCU). Vesicoureteric reflux (VUR) on both sides. Urinary bladder shows trabeculation and sacculations due to neurogenic dysfunction (neurogenic bladder); (B) Same information could be seen on magnetic resonance (MR) urography.

cystourethrography (MCU) is mandatory for its diagnosis **(Fig. 18.8.20)**. Backpressure changes in the bladder and associated VUR are common. Magnetic resonance urography has been tried to be useful for demonstrating VUR. Moreover, it is free of radiation.

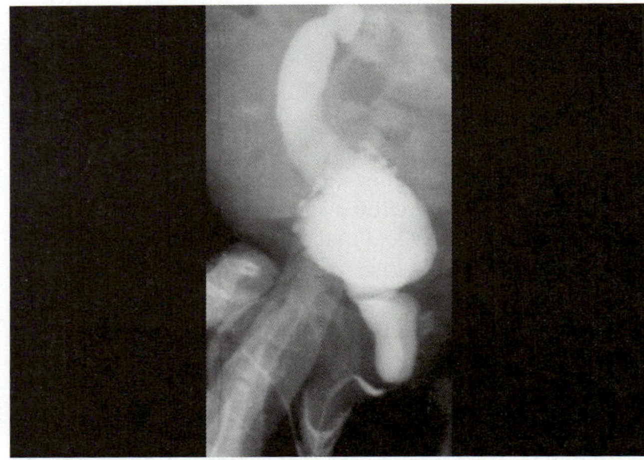

Fig. 18.8.20: Micturating cystourethrography (MCU) shows marked dilatation of posterior urethra, thin urinary stream and narrowing at the junction of posterior and anterior urethra due to posterior urethral valves. Also note gross vesicoureteric reflux (VUR) on the right side.

CRANIAL AND SPINAL IMAGING

Imaging Techniques

Conventional radiographs of the skull should include at least frontal and lateral view. Depending upon the suspected clinical disease, more views can be taken, e.g. for sinuses, atlantoaxial junction, pituitary fossa, etc. Plain X-rays of the spine are routinely done in all cases of spinal dysraphism, scoliosis, back pain, etc.

Transfontanel cranial US has a role to play, only if the anterior fontanel is open. Diagnosis of hydrocephalus, intracranial bleed, congenital malformations and tumors of the brain can be made. However, US has its own limitations. CT is the most cost-effective technique for cranial imaging. For posterior fossa, brainstem and white matter diseases, however, MRI is far superior to CT.

For the evaluation of spine and its contents, MRI is the modality of choice. But if it is not available, then myelogram with nonionic media followed by postmyelo-CT should be routinely done.

Pathological Conditions

The term craniosynostosis denotes premature fusion of cranial sutures. Depending upon the pattern of sutural closure, the shape of the head varies, and different names are used to describe them, e.g. brachycephaly (fused coronal sutures) and scaphocephaly (sagittal sutures fusion). Besides the plain radiographs, CT and nowadays 3D-CT, is the investigation of choice to assess the sutural status. Growing fracture at times may mimic a widened suture **(Fig. 18.8.21)**.

Intracranial calcification **(Figs. 18.8.22A to C)** could be seen in postinfectious states, e.g. cytomegalovirus (CMV), toxoplasma infection, tuberculous meningitis; in brain tumors, hypoparathyroidism and/or in dysplastic brain tissue. Cytomegalovirus produces periventricular calcifications

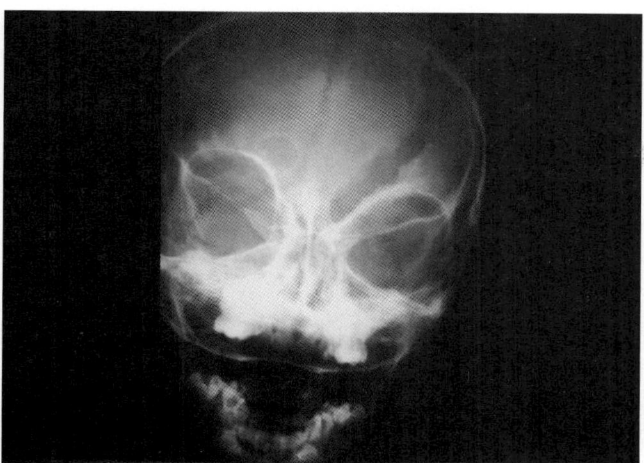

Fig. 18.8.21: Growing fracture—frontal radiograph of face and skull showing a linear oriented lytic lesion with beveled margins in left frontal bone.

(a "calcified mold of the ventricles") whereas, toxoplasmosis produces diffuse cerebral calcification. Bilateral basal ganglia calcifications have been reported in acquired immunodeficiency syndrome (AIDS) encephalopathy also. CT is essential for anatomical localization.

Skull vault may be affected in several diseases, e.g. histiocytosis **(Figs. 18.8.23A and B)**; neuroblastoma metastases **(Fig. 18.8.24)**, hematological and metabolic diseases and various skeletal dysplasias.

Infectious conditions, like brain abscess **(Fig. 18.8.25)**, tuberculomas **(Fig. 18.8.26)** and neurocysticercosis (NCC) **(Figs. 18.8.27A and B)** are readily diagnosed with CT and MRI.

Hydrocephalus, one of the most common causes of a large head in children, is readily diagnosed on any one of the cross-sectional imaging modalities **(Fig. 18.8.28)**. Similarly, other intracranial pathologic lesions can be imaged.

Spinal dysraphism **(Figs. 18.8.29A to C)** is the most common congenital abnormality affecting the spine. It is

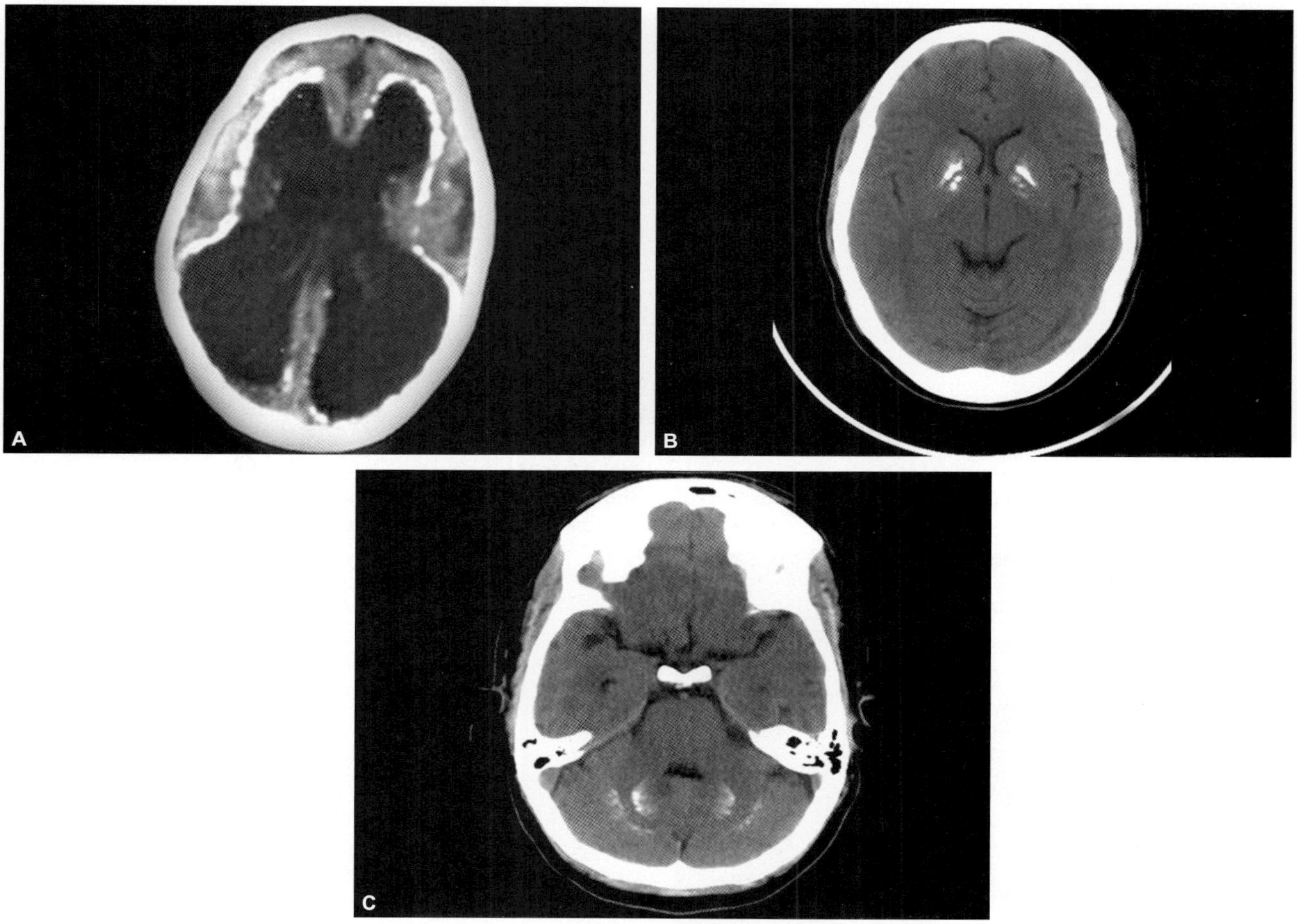

Figs. 18.8.22A to C: Intracranial calcification—(A) Noncontrast computed tomography (NCCT) axial sections showing periventricular calcification in congenital cytomegalovirus (CMV) infection; (B and C) Axial NCCT images showing intracranial calcifications in the bilateral basal ganglia's and cerebellar hemispheres—typical presentation of calcification in hypoparathyroidism.

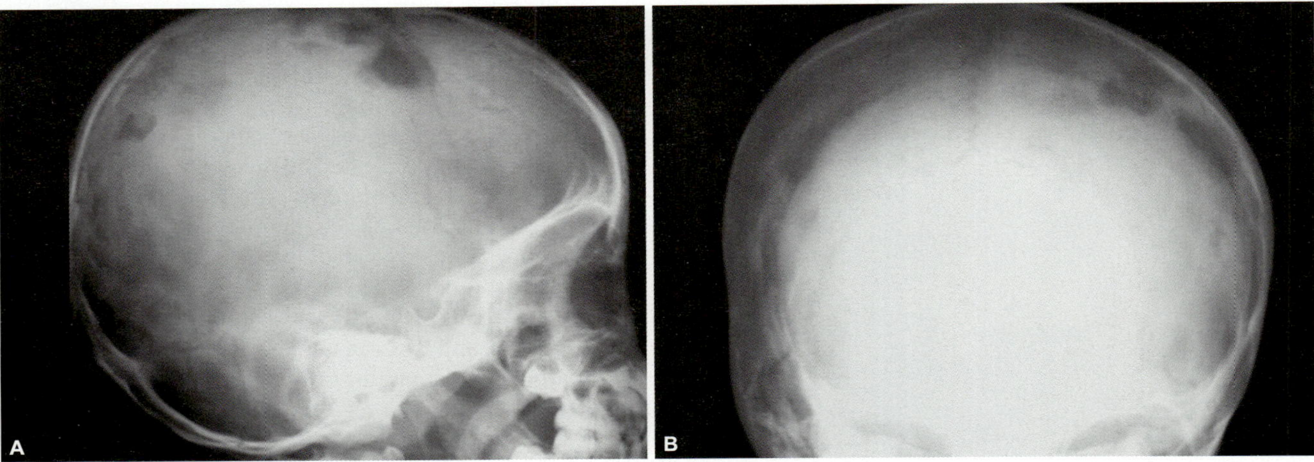

Figs. 18.8.23A and B: Skull X-rays—multiple, large "geographic" type bone destruction, characteristic of histiocytosis. These type of bone lesions indicate relatively slow growing pathology.

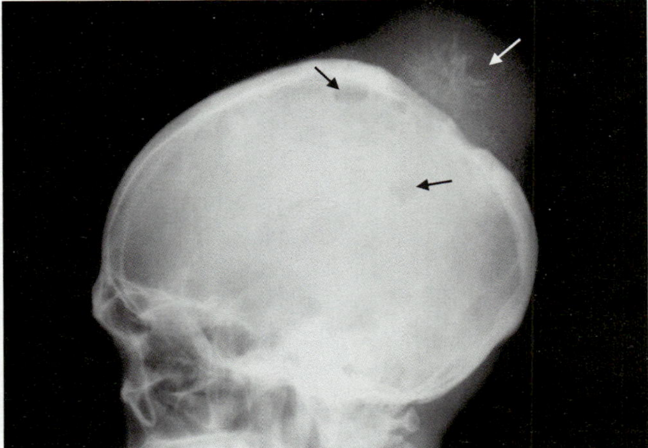

Fig. 18.8.24: Skull lateral view—multiple lytic lesions with sunray type of periosteal reaction in a case of neuroblastoma with skull metastases.

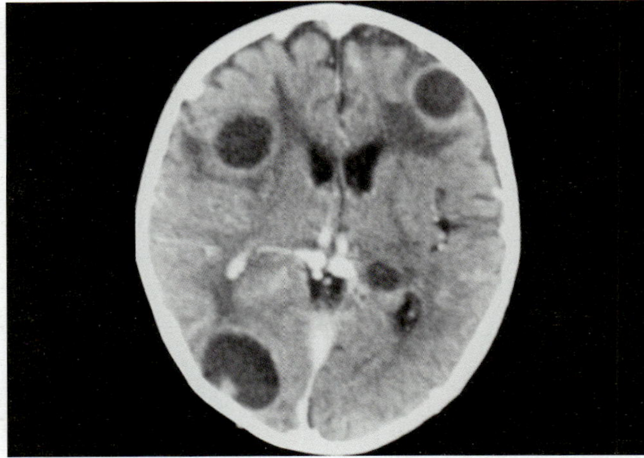

Fig. 18.8.25: Brain abscess—axial computed tomography (CT) showing multiple ring enhancing lesions in bilateral frontal and right occipital lobes with perilesional edema.

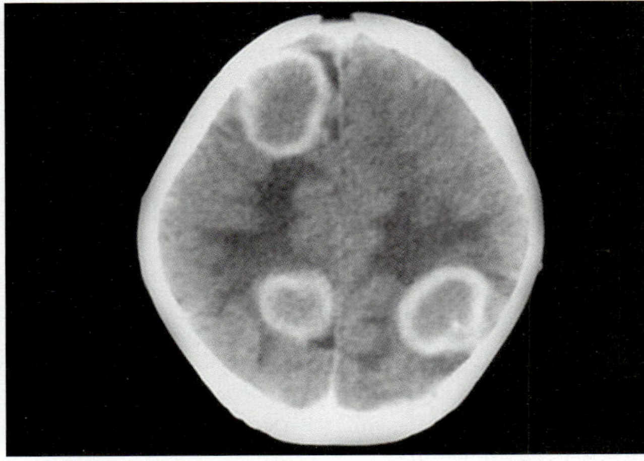

Fig. 18.8.26: Tuberculomas—contrast-enhanced CT (CECT) axial sections showing multiple ring enhancing lesions with hypodense centers and perilesional edema in bilateral high parietal lobes.

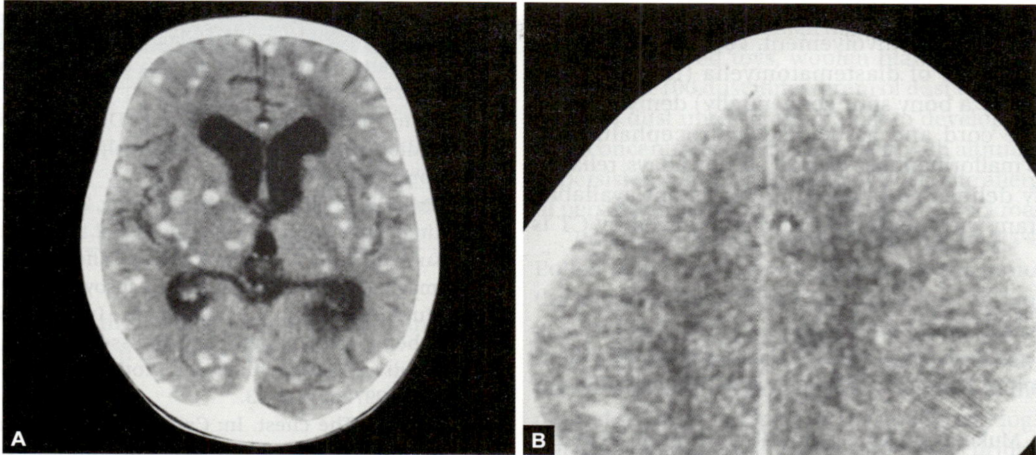

Figs. 18.8.27A and B: Neurocysticercosis (NCC)—multiple hyperdense lesions in brain suggestive of NCCS; note the eccentric scolex.

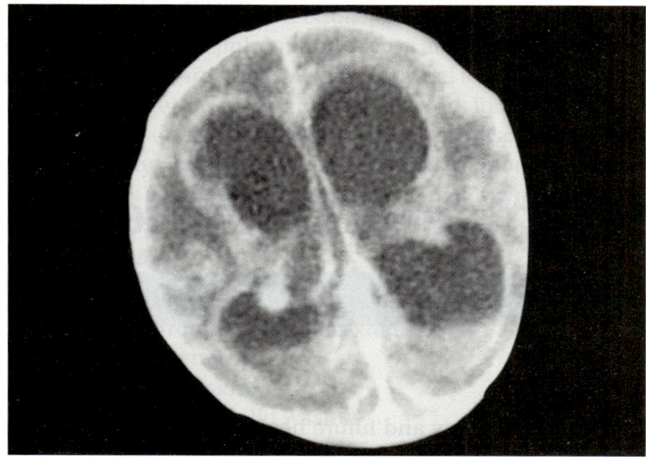

Fig. 18.8.28: Hydrocephalus with ventriculitis—axial CT showing dilated ventricles with enhancing ventricular margin and periventricular ooze.

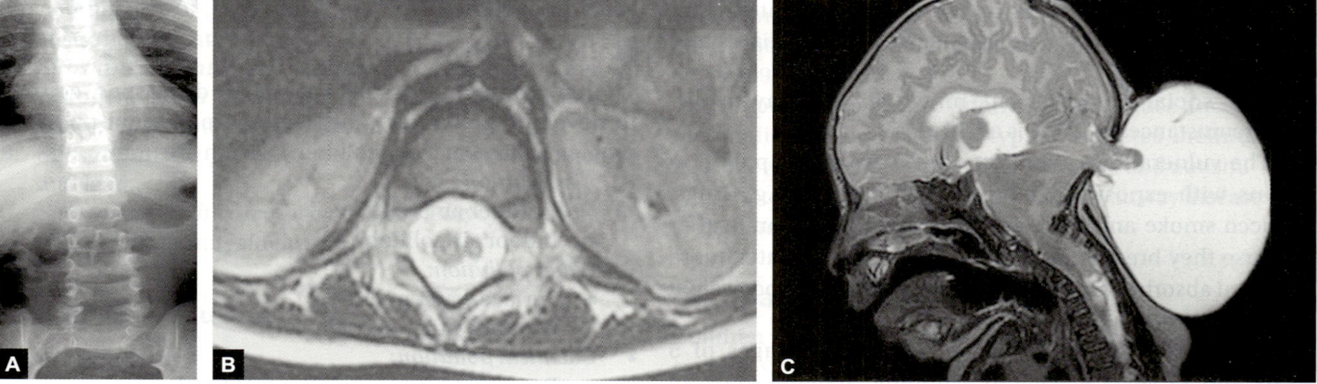

Figs. 18.8.29A to C: Diastematomyelia—radiograph showing bony septum in the spinal canal at L2 level with spina bifida from L3 onward (A) T2-weighted (T2W) axial magnetic resonance imaging (MRI) images; (B) Splitting of the cord into two; (C) Chiari III malformation—sagittal T2W MRI showing herniation of tonsil and brainstem (Chiari II) with occipital meningoencephalocele.

- Storm water run-off
- Industrial discharges
- Cross-media contamination, movement of pollution
- From air to water
- Pesticides and fertilizers drifting during the rainy season

Sources of Ground Water Pollution

- Industrial waste pits, discharge of effluents on land
- Septic tanks
- Oil well
- Chemicals in ground water.

Health Hazards of Water Pollution

Several constituents of ground water contamination due to industrial clusters are reported to be caused by electroplating units, tanneries, dyeing, printing units, distilleries and paper mills. The heavy metal and toxic compounds present in the effluent may pose considerable health risks to the population using such contaminated water.

- *Waterborne diseases*: Water contaminated by fecal matter and urine may produce gastroenteritis, dysentery, amebiasis, cholera, typhoid, paratyphoid and viral hepatitis. Gastroenteritis is the second biggest killer of the children under the age of 5 years. It has been noted that about 69% of people equate visual cleanliness with safe water. However, even today, around 80% of the rural population and 60% of the urban slum population practice open defecation.
- *Water-related vector borne disease*: Examples of diseases transmitted by the bite of mosquitoes are malaria, dengue fever, Japanese encephalitis and filarial disease.
- *Water-based disease*: Examples of diseases transmitted by aquatic invertebrate animals and stagnant water contaminated by rat urine are leptospirosis, guinea worm and schistosomiasis. The incidence of leptospirosis is increasing in urban slum areas, especially during the rainy season.
- *Water-based chemical diseases*: The major chemicals that enter and contaminate the water are fluoride, arsenic, nitrites, mercury and lead. Their effects are described in **Table 18.9.3**.

Waterborne diseases spread more rapidly in urban communities, where the density of population is more with no or poor access to water. The World Health Organization (WHO) guidelines for good potable water is the *Escherichia coli* count should be less than 10 microbes/100 mL and a higher count always indicates fecal contamination.

Public Health Education to Prevent Water Pollution

- Education of public about use of safe drinking water, toilet hygiene

Table 18.9.3: Chemicals contaminating water and their effects.

Chemical	*Mechanism*	*Ill effects*
Fluoride	Affects 6 million children less than 14 years	• Dental fluorosis
	Drinking water with more than 1 mg fluoride/L	• Skeletal fluorosis • Nonskeletal fluorosis
Arsenic (As)	Ingesting water with arsenic content more than 0.01 mg/L over a period of 5–15 years	• Skin rashes, hyperkeratosis • Cancer of lung, bladder, kidneys
Mercury	All mercury in India imported, used in equipment, batteries and thermometers	• *Major health effects:* Psychological, GIT cramps, colitis
	Poisoning occurs by ingestion and inhalation	• Persistent cough, emphysema, asthma, sinusitis • Excessive perspiration • Alzheimer's disease, Parkinson's disease, autism also reported
Nitrites	Seepage from septic tank, pit latrines and organic manures into ground water	• Ingestion of water with more than 45 mg/L of nitrites—"blue baby syndrome", methemoglobinemia • Chronic ingestion and cancer
Lead	Ingestion of water from lead pipes, food containers, paint and insecticides	• Lead level more than 10 µg/dL in blood: Progressive GIT, hematologic, peripheral and central nervous system involvement
	Inhalation of polluted air from leaded petrol, battery storage, crystal glass, ceramic glazes, enamel jewelry, plastic and rubber stabilizers, surma, vermillion	• Anorexia, abdominal pain, vomiting • Anemia, blue line in gums • Headache, seizures, altered sensorium • Peripheral neuropathy • Behavioral disturbances • Lower IQ, poor school performance

(GIT: gastrointestinal tract; IQ: intelligence quotient)

- Use of water filters
- Prevention of waste production and pollution
- Prevention of waste from various sources entering water protecting the source of water
- Water storage at home should be covered
- Avoid using dirty hands or implements to fetch water
- Drinking water can be purified by chlorination, boiling, slow sand filters and solar disinfection.

CHEMICAL POLLUTION

Persistent Organic Pollutants

They are man-made organic pollutants and are the most dangerous and hazardous compounds synthesized. They include pesticides, industrial chemicals, chemicals used in consumer products and byproducts of certain manufacturing and combustion process. They have long half-lives and hence persist in the environment for years or decades. They bio-accumulate and penetrate the food chain thus, polluting and exposing all living things.

They disperse universally and travel in air, water currents and in living organisms. Most POPs are lipophilic and remain in fat tissue, not well-metabolized or excreted, even small doses ingested daily accumulate to measurable amounts over time. They are endocrine disruptors, mimic, modify or block the actions of naturally occurring hormones as listed in **Table 18.9.4**. Prenatal exposure of pesticides negatively affects fetal growth like smaller head circumference and shorter birth length.

The major sources of human exposure are food, soil, indoor environment, toys and other objects, air and leaching from medical products. The important organic chlorine pesticides developed after dichlorodiphenyltrichloroethane (DDT) and widely used after World War II include—aldrin, dieldrin, endrin, chlordane, heptachlor, indane and pentachlorophenol. They helped a great deal in agriculture, which helped the world economy. Once adverse effects due to their persistence and accumulation in the environment became known, most uses were discontinued.

Plastics and Pollution

Plastics are the mostly used material in our day-to-day life. They are light, thermo and chemical resistant, low cost, strong and tough. Annual usage of plastic bags in the world is 500 trillion tons. Asia contributes 80% of total plastic leakage to ocean and 4 lakh marine mammals perish annually.

Plastics are made of two compounds:

1. *Polymers or resins—Bulk of plastics such as*
   - Polyvinyl chloride (PVC)
   - Polycarbonate (PC)
   - High density polyethylene (HDPE)
   - Polypropylene (PD).
2. *Plasticizers (Additive):*
   - Phthalates to give more flexibility
   - Bisphenol A (BPA) to give more rigidity.

Table 18.9.5 lists the sources of phthalates and bisphenols and their effects in the environment.

Table 18.9.4: Hormonal effect of persistent organic pollutants.

Persistent organic pollutants	*Hormonal ill effect*
DDT, dieldrin, endosulfan, methoxychlor PCBs—alkylphenols, phthalates, mycotoxins, phytoestrogens	Estrogenic
Dioxins, PCBs, phytoestrogens	Anti-estrogenic
DPT, vinclozolin	Anti-androgenic
PCBs, dioxins	Anti-thyroid
PCBs, DDT	Anti-progestins

(DDT: dichlorodiphenyltrichlorethane; PCBs: polychlorinated biphenyls; DPT: diphtheria, pertussis and tetanus)

Table 18.9.5: Impact of Plasticizers.

Phthalates	*Bisphenols A (BPA)*
• They migrate to the surface of plastics • They either evaporate or leach into the surroundings • They are the most abundant industrial pollutants of the environment	They are used for production of polycarbonate hand plastic and to make resins to line the metal and beverage cans with heat they leach from the source to adjacent materials—water, food from the lining of the cans
Source: Food packaging, food contamination, plastic toys, medical tubings, wall coverings, tablecloths, upholstery, deodorants, insecticides, nail polish, adhesives	*Source:* Food and beverage cans, gel capsules cosmetics, flame retardants
Route of exposure: Phthalate leach out from the above products high concentration when they are heated	*Route of exposure*: • By inhalation • Ingestion • Skin absorption • Blood by intravenous route by tubings • Transplacental, from maternal bisphenol A

Diseases from Plastics

- These are endocrine disrupting chemicals with effects in fetal and early postnatal development of male reproductive tract abnormalities such as—undescended testes and hypospadias, and decrease fertility
- Changes in immune system and inflammatory changes
- Acts as an antagonist for thyroid hormone
- Behavioral changes
- Early puberty
- Adult-onset diabetes mellitus
- Cancer.

Safety Measures for Plastic Use

Figure 18.9.8 shows the safety codes for use of plastics in industry. Safety testing of new chemicals before they are put into market seems ideal, but the long-term hazards of new chemicals until after they have been released into the environment, will not be known.

Do's and Don'ts of Plastics

These are listed in **Table 18.9.6**.

NOISE POLLUTION

Noise is known to affect 800 million people globally. The major chronic effect of noise-induced hearing loss is the result of cumulative effect of the magnitude of sound and the duration of exposure. India is known to have the largest deaf population in the world and noise pollution is known to be one of the significant causes.

Noise may be broadly classified as:

- *Industrial noise*: This includes noise from machines in factories, industries and mills. Significant among them are noise from mechanical saws and pneumatic drills.
- *Transport noise*: This includes road, railway and air traffic noise.
- *Community noise*: This includes noise from musical instruments, indiscriminate use of amplifiers and other gadgets in commercial establishments.

Psychological and physical effects of different decibel levels are given in **Table 18.9.7**.

The acceptable noise level in residential areas is given in **Table 18.9.8**.

The background noise level has increased over the last few decades. The noise level appears to double every decade.

Remedial Measures

- Effective noise control programs in industries and use of protective aids.
- Plantation of trees near schools, hospitals, public offices and libraries to reduce noise by 6–10 dB.
- Residential zones planned away from main roads, factories, airport and railways.
- Perforated plywood and other porous material to be used for office floors or ceilings.
- Implementation of noise control regulation by automobiles, social and religious functions and prayer halls.

RADIATION HAZARDS

Radiation is the emission of energy (as electromagnetic waves) or particle matter from unstable atoms. Some types of radiation are harmful to life while others such as heat energy and light radiating from the skin, are beneficial.

Source of Radioactive Substances

Natural sources of ionizing radiation are the most common and include cosmic rays from space and radioactive minerals. In source areas, the gas radon found in soil, rocks, building materials and granite stone are highly radioactive. Still we have to find out the level of uranium in water and its ill effects.

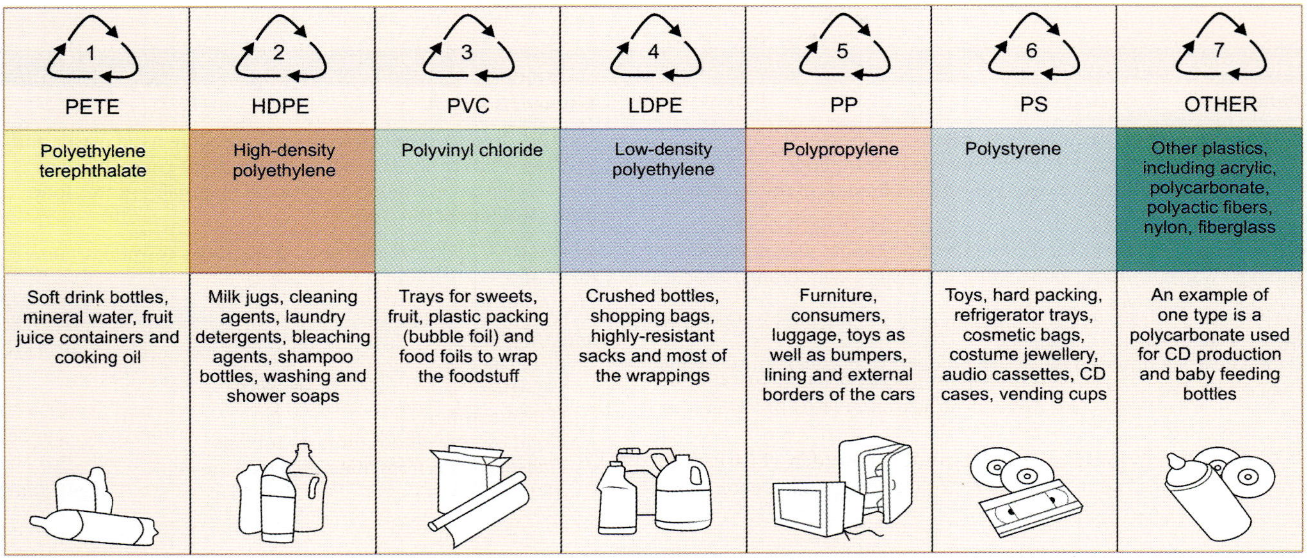

1 PETE	2 HDPE	3 PVC	4 LDPE	5 PP	6 PS	7 OTHER
Polyethylene terephthalate	High-density polyethylene	Polyvinyl chloride	Low-density polyethylene	Polypropylene	Polystyrene	Other plastics, including acrylic, polycarbonate, polyactic fibers, nylon, fiberglass
Soft drink bottles, mineral water, fruit juice containers and cooking oil	Milk jugs, cleaning agents, laundry detergents, bleaching agents, shampoo bottles, washing and shower soaps	Trays for sweets, fruit, plastic packing (bubble foil) and food foils to wrap the foodstuff	Crushed bottles, shopping bags, highly-resistant sacks and most of the wrappings	Furniture, consumers, luggage, toys as well as bumpers, lining and external borders of the cars	Toys, hard packing, refrigerator trays, cosmetic bags, costume jewellery, audio cassettes, CD cases, vending cups	An example of one type is a polycarbonate used for CD production and baby feeding bottles

Fig. 18.9.8: The safety codes for use of plastics.

Table 18.9.6: Do's and Don'ts of Plastics.

Do's	*Don'ts*
• Look at recycling code on the bottom of the product to find out the plastic type • Use plastic code 1, 2, 4, and 5 which are considered as safer • Use No. 7 also if it is labeled as "Bio based or greenware" • Use alternatives—glass, steel cups • Buy phthalate-free toys • Wooden furniture is always better	Avoid plastic code 3, 6, 7 (Bisphenol A) Avoid microwaving the food and drinks in plastics Avoid dishwashers Avoid clear plastic bottles Avoid boiling plastic bottles

Table 18.9.7: Psychological and physical effects of different decibel (dB) levels.

135 dB	Painful
110 dB	Discomfort
88 dB	Hearing impairment on prolonged exposure
80 dB	Annoying
65 dB	Intrusive

Table 18.9.8: The acceptable noise level in residential areas.

City area	45–55 dB
Rural area	25–30 dB
Urban residential	35–40 dB
Suburban areas	30–40 dB
Urban business	40–45 dB
Industrial area	50–60 dB
Music theater	30–35 dB
Hospitals	30–35 dB
Restaurants	50–55 dB
Public offices	50–60 dB

Artificial sources of ionizing radiation include X-ray machines, radioactive isotopes used in diagnosis, and treatment and nuclear reactors. Radiation hazards to health depend on the dose, duration of exposure and organs exposed.

The ill effects of ionizing radiation are listed in **Table 18.9.9**.

Table 18.9.9: Ill effects of ionizing radiation.

Dose exposure (REM)	*Adverse effects on health*
0–10	• None to premature aging • Mild malnutrition of offspring • Genetic and teratogenic effects
10–50	• Premature aging • Genetic and teratogenic effects • Radiation sickness • Transient effects in lymphocytes and neutrophils
50–150	• Acute radiation sickness • Burns • Abortion, stillbirths • Decreased leukocytes • Tumors
150–250	• Gastrointestinal (GI) symptoms • Fetal or embryonic death • Serious infections, death
250–600	• Gastrointestinal symptoms • Loss of hair • Bleeding from gastrointestinal, renal and nasal sites • Marked destruction of bone marrow leading to death
600–1,000	• Destruction of GI • Respiratory, hemopoietic, endocrine spleen and genital problems • Bleeding diathesis and death

(REM: radiation equivalent of mean)

BIBLIOGRAPHY

1. Childhood Lead Poisoning. Geneva, Switzerland: World Health Organization; 2010. pp. 13.
2. Etzel RA, Balk SJ. Pediatric Environmental Health, 2nd edition. Elk Grove Village, Illinois: American Academy of Pediatrics; 2003. pp. 721.
3. Indrayan A, Bachani D, Pandey A, et al. Burden of Disease in India. New Delhi: National Commission on Macroeconomics and Health; 2005.
4. Paramesh H, Cherian E. Tobacco smoke as an indoor pollutant on children health. 5th International Conference on Environment and Health Proceedings, Bengaluru; 2010. pp. 43-4.
5. Paramesh H. Air pollution and allergic airway diseases: Social determinants and sustainability in the control and prevention, Indian J Pediatr. Available at https://doi.org/10.1007/s12098-017-2538- 2018
6. Paramesh H. Asthma and the environment. Indian J Pediatr. 2006;73:S51-5.
7. Paramesh H. Asthma in children: seasonal variation. Int J Environment and Health. 2008;2(3/4):410-6.
8. Paramesh H. Epidemiology of asthma in India. Indian J Pediatr. 2002;69(4):309-12.
9. Paramesh H. Impact of air pollution and global warming on human health: an urgent need to mitigate by stake-holders. MOJ Research Review. 2018;1(6):262-267.
10. Paramesh H. Indoor air pollution and child health. In: Sachdeva A (Ed). Pediatric and Adolescent Environmental Health. IAP Presidential Action Plan. 2004. pp. 76-8.
11. Persistent Organic Pollutants: Impact on Child Health. Geneva, Switzerland: World Health Organization Press; 2010.
12. Ratageri VH, Paramesh H. Environmental health of children: time to translate knowledge into action; editorial. Indian Pediatr. Available at https://doi.org/10.1007/s12098-018-2629-9
13. State of Environment Report and Action Plan. Government of Karnataka and World Bank; 2003. pp. 217-26.

Section 19

Community Pediatrics

19.1 Vital Statistics

Joseph L Mathew

INTRODUCTION

Vital statistics are systemically collected and compiled data about vital events of life like birth and death. Sometimes these include information about additional events such as marriage, divorce, and adoption. These sociodemographic data directly and indirectly reflect the health profile of a community. They can also reflect the adequacy of health services such as family planning, maternal and reproductive health, and immunization programs in a community. The data are also the basis for projections on population growth and time trends. They are also used for the construction of life tables.

A vital statistics system is formally defined as the process of (1) collection of information on the frequency of occurrence of specified and defined vital events, characteristics of the events, and the person(s) concerned and (2) the compilation, processing, analysis, and evaluation of the data in conventional statistical formats.

Vital statistics are usually collected and compiled by government agencies, which record the births and deaths within a given jurisdiction. In India, the main sources for vital statistics data are from (1) the population census, (2) civil registration system (CRS) records of vital events, (3) sample registration system (SRS), (4) demographic surveys conducted by the National Sample Surveys Organization (NSSO), and (5) health surveys such as the National Family Health Survey (NFHS) and District Level Household Surveys (DLHS).

SAMPLE REGISTRATION SYSTEM

The registration of Births and Deaths Act (1969) made the registration of births and deaths compulsory instead of voluntary. This improved data collection significantly. In order to make it even more robust, the office of the Registrar General, India, initiated the nationwide SRS. The SRS in India is widely recognized as the world's single largest demographic survey. It covers nearly 1.5 million households with a total population over 7 million, spread over almost all districts in India. The SRS in India is unique in many respects; the most noteworthy being a system of dual recording. One component is the "field investigation" which is the continuous enumeration of births and deaths in the sample area by an enumerator. This is complemented by an independent 6 monthly retrospective survey by a supervisor. The data obtained independently through the two sources are then matched. Unmatched or partially matched events are reverified and confirmed. This quality-control step ensures reliability of the data collected. The SRS sampling frame is revised every 10 years. **Figure 19.1.1** presents the number of sampling units at different time periods. These data are generally updated once every 10 years.

Since 1999, the SRS also includes the "survey of causes of deaths (rural)." This uses the "postdeath verbal autopsy" technique to estimate the most probable cause of death. Specially trained professionals then verify and assign the final cause of death. **Table 19.1.1** summarizes the main components of SRS in India.

The current SRS report published in September 2014 includes data on various fertility and mortality indicators, viz. crude birth rate, crude death rate, and infant mortality rate (IMR). Data are presented for the whole country as well as states—separately for rural and urban areas. More recently, the sex ratio at birth and the sex ratio in the age-group 0–4 years have been included. From 2008 onward, the report also presents estimates of under-five mortality for India and some of the larger states.

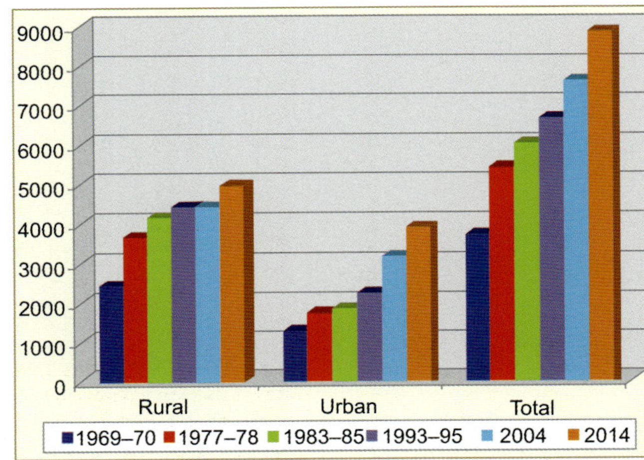

Fig. 19.1.1: Sample sets used for sample registration system (SRS) data collection since its inception.

Table 19.1.1: Steps of the sample registration system (SRS) data collection and compilation process.	
SRS step	***Purpose***
Baseline survey of sample units	To assess the resident population of the sample areas
Continuous (longitudinal) enumeration of vital events by an enumerator	To collect the primary data for the sample
Independent retrospective half-yearly surveys for recording births and deaths by a supervisor	To update house lists, household schedule, and list of women in the reproductive age-group (and pregnancy status)
Matching of events recorded during prospective continuous enumeration and retrospective half-yearly survey	Quality control measures to check reliability of data
Field verification of unmatched and partially matched events	To ensure completeness of data
Filling of verbal autopsy forms for finalized deaths	To assign causes of death

The vital statistics data collected are represented as indicators that convert the absolute numbers to rates. These are useful for comparing data from different areas and time frames. **Table 19.1.2** summarizes the key vital statistics indicators and the calculation for these.

Table 19.1.3 shows selected current vital statistics data for India, with a focus on data relevant to the pediatric age-group. It should be recognized that national data is the average of a wide range of data; the variations between rural and urban areas and data from different states are not reflected in the national average. It is encouraging that most indicators associated with mortality have shown a tremendous decline over time, and continue to decline in recent years also. This is evident in **Figure 19.1.2**. It is also important to note that the data represent the mean across the whole country. This sometimes masks the disparity between different states, regions, socioeconomic groups, etc. As an example, the average IMR of 34 masks the four-fold difference between Kerala with IMR of 10 and Odisha with IMR of 44. Even the mean IMR of 44 for a state masks the differences between the

Table 19.1.2: Key vital statistics indicators.	
Vital statistics indicator	***Calculation***
Crude birth rate (CBR)	(Number of live births during the year/mid-year population) × 1,000
Crude death rate (CDR)	(Number of deaths during the year/mid-year population) × 1,000
Age-specific mortality rate (ASMR)	(Number of deaths in a particular age-group/mid-year population of the same age-group) × 1,000
Under-five mortality rate	The probability that a child born in a specific year or time period will die before reaching the age of 5 years, subject to current age-specific mortality rates
Infant mortality rate (IMR)	(Number of infant deaths during the year/number of live births during the year) × 1,000
Neonatal mortality rate (NMR)	(Number of infant deaths of less than 28 days during the year/number of live births during the year) × 1,000
Early neonatal mortality rate	(Number of infant deaths of less than 7 days during the year/number of live births during the year) × 1,000
Late neonatal mortality rate	(Number of infant deaths of 7 days to less than 28 days during the year/number of live births during the year) × 1,000
Postneonatal mortality rate (PNMR)	(Number of infant deaths between 28 days and 1 year during the year/number of live births during the year) × 1,000
Perinatal mortality rate (PMR)	(Number of stillbirths and infant deaths of less than 7 days during the year/number of live births and stillbirths during the year) × 1,000
Stillbirth rate	(Number of stillbirths during the year/number of live births and stillbirths during the year) × 1,000
General fertility rate (GFR)	(Number of live births in a year/mid-year female population in the age-group 15–49 years) × 1,000
Age-specific fertility rate (ASFR)	(Number of live births in a particular age-group/mid-year female population of the same age-group) × 1,000
Total fertility rate (TFR)	5 × (sum of ASFR for the age groups, 15–19, 20–24, 25–29 etc.)/1,000. The average number of children a woman would have when she passed through her reproductive years bearing children at the same rates as the women now in each age group. It is calculated by summing the age specific fertility rates for all ages. If 5 years age-groups are used, then ASFR is multiplied by 5
Age-specific marital fertility rate (ASMFR)	(Number of live births in a particular age-group)/(mid-year married female population of the same age-group) × 1,000

Contd...

$$NMR = \frac{\text{Number of deaths in neonates aged less than 28 days in an year}}{\text{Total number of live births in the same year}} \times 1000$$

Stillbirth rate (SBR) is the number of stillborn infants (after 28 weeks of gestation) related to total number of births (both live and stillborn) during the same period.

$$SBR = \frac{\text{Number of stillborn infants in an year}}{\text{Total number of births in the same year}} \times 1000$$

Of the approximately 4.2 million global infant deaths occurring annually in year 2016, 2.6 million can be ascribed to the neonatal period with 98% of them in developing countries. Almost 65% of the estimated 2.6 million neonatal deaths occur in the early neonatal period, i.e., first 7 days following birth. Neonatal deaths contribute to 46% of all childhood deaths and more than 50% of infant mortality. Hence, priority should be given to perinatal and neonatal mortality in order to decrease infant mortality.

India accounts for 18% (25.6 million) of global births and 27% (0.7 million) of global newborn deaths. India has seen a substantial reduction in IMR and NMR in recent decades. Since the early 1970s, the IMR declined from 140 per 1,000 live births to 34 (SRS, 2017). The NMR has declined from 72 per 1,000 live births in 1972 to 24 in 2016 (SRS statistical report, 2016)—a reduction of almost 40%. The reduction in NMR is probably due to three reasons:

1. A major decline in neonatal tetanus (NNT) due to a successful maternal tetanus toxoid (TT) immunization program
2. A gradual increase in institutional deliveries and skilled attendance, and
3. Birth spacing leading to indirect benefits for neonatal survival.

However, the process of NMR decline has slowed down in recent years **(Table 19.2.2)**.

Infections, asphyxia, and prematurity are the leading causes of neonatal deaths all over the world. A similar pattern is seen in India where they contribute to 13%, 25%, and 33% of the total neonatal deaths, respectively. It is noteworthy that most of these deaths can be prevented by better community level maternal newborn care and care at the health facilities.

The NMR varies widely from as low as 6 in the State of Kerala to as high as 32 in the State of Odisha and Madhya Pradesh. Other States accounting for high burden of neonatal deaths include Uttar Pradesh, Uttarakhand, and Rajasthan.

Perinatal Mortality Rate

Perinatal mortality rate (PMR) refers to death of the fetus/newborn after 22 weeks of pregnancy, during birth, or within 7 days after delivery per 1,000 total births in a year (WHO, 1997). However, Government of India is using a cut-off of 28 weeks for calculation of PMR in India.

Table 19.2.2: Comparative rural/urban mortality indicators, 2015–2016, India.

Indicator	*Combined*	*Rural*	*Urban*	*Maximum*	*Minimum*
Crude death rate (2016)*	6.4	6.9	5.4	7.8 (Odisha)	4 (Delhi)
Infant mortality rate (2016)*	34	38	23	47 (MP)	10 (Kerala)
Percentage of infant/total deaths*	10.9	12.2	7.4	17.9 (MP)	2 (Kerala)
Percentage of neonatal deaths/infant deaths	68.8	70.7	60.4	79.1 (Uttarakhand)	53.4 (Assam)
Percentage of early neonatal to infant deaths*	53.2	54.8	45.8	62.9 (Uttarakhand)	40.5 (Kerala)
Neonatal mortality rate*	24	27	14	32 (Odisha, MP)	6 (Kerala)
Early neonatal mortality rate (NMR)*	18	21	11	24 (MP, Odisha, Uttarakhand)	4 (Kerala)
Late NMR*	6	6	3	–	–
Perinatal mortality rate*	23	26	14	37 (Odisha)	10 (Kerala)
Stillbirth rate*	4	5	3	24 (HP)	0 (Jharkhand)

*SRS statistical report, 2016.

$$\text{PNMR} = \frac{\text{Number of stillbirths + neonatal deaths during the first week of life in an year}}{\text{Total number of births in the same year}} \times 1000$$

More than 5.5 million perinatal deaths occur each year worldwide; 3 million of these happen during late pregnancy and birth (stillbirths), while 2.5 million newborns die in the first week (early neonatal mortality).

Perinatal deaths are more likely in the developing countries than in the developed world, where only 2% of the estimated perinatal deaths occur. Africa has the highest PMR of 56 per 1,000 total births (WHO, 2000 estimates) where almost 25% of the births occur. Perinatal mortality in these areas results from poor nutritional status of women, insufficient prevention of pregnancy-related complications, and even undersupervised deliveries. Some of these causes are rooted in the social, cultural, and economic structure of the society. Mortality indicators related to child health in India are summarized in **Table 19.2.2**.

What is RMNCH+A Approach

As per the latest data and trends, India has reaffirmed its commitment to make every effort toward achieving the millennium development goals 4 and 5, at the global platform. However, a more cohesive approach is required to manage child and maternal health care issues to reach the desired targets at the earliest. It has been realized that essential interventions to improve the health of women and children need to take place at all levels in the health system, that is, from the home to the community level and through all the health facilities. RMNCH+A (reproductive, maternal, neonatal child health plus adolescent) approach has been launched to provide the health secretaries, mission directors and program managers at national and state level a vision and understanding of the comprehensive approach to improving child survival and safe motherhood and attaining millennium development goals 4 and 5, to which India is sincerely committed. The key concept of this approach is "continuum of care" beginning from adolescent girl to pregnant women and child health care. This approach essentially looks to address the major causes of mortality among women and children as well as the delays in accessing and utilizing health care and services. The health of an adolescent girl impacts pregnancy while the health of a pregnant woman impacts the health of the newborn and the child.

The "plus" in the strategic approach denotes

- The inclusion of adolescence as a distinct "life stage" in the overall strategy
- Linking of maternal and child health to reproductive health and other components [like family planning, adolescent health, human immunodeficiency virus (HIV), gender and preconception and prenatal diagnostic techniques (PC&PNDT)], and
- Linking of community and facility-based care as well as referrals between various levels of health care system to create a continuous care pathway and to bring an additive/synergistic effect in terms of overall outcomes and impact.

Table 19.2.3 shows the mode of implementation of RMNCH+A.

Coverage Targets for Key RMNCH+A Interventions for 2017

- Increase facilities equipped for perinatal care (designated as "delivery points") by 100%.
- Increase proportion of all births in government and accredited private institutions at annual rate of 5.6% from the baseline of 61% (SRS, 2010).
- Increase proportion of pregnant women receiving antenatal care at annual rate of 6% from the baseline of 53% (CES, 2009).
- Increase proportion of mothers and newborns receiving postnatal care at annual rate of 7.5% from the baseline of 45% (CES, 2009).
- Increase proportion of deliveries conducted by skilled birth attendants at annual rate of 2% from the baseline of 76% (CES, 2009).
- Increase exclusive breastfeeding rates at annual rate of 9.6% from the baseline of 36% (CES, 2009).
- Reduce prevalence of under-5 children who are underweight at annual rate of 5.5% from the baseline of 45% (NFHS 3).
- Increase coverage of three doses of combined diphtheria-tetanus-pertussis (DTP3) at annual rate of 3.5% from the baseline of 7% (CES, 2009).
- Increase ORS use in under-5 children with diarrhea at annual rate of 7.2% from the baseline of 43% (CES, 2009).
- Reduce unmet need for family planning methods among eligible couples, married and unmarried, at annual rate of 8.8% from the baseline of 21% (DLHS 3).
- Increase met need for modern family planning methods among eligible couples at annual rate of 4.5% from the baseline of 47% (DLHS 3).
- Reduce anemia in adolescent girls and boys (15–19 years) at annual rate of 6% from the baseline of 56% and 30%, respectively (NFHS 3).
- Decrease the proportion of total fertility contributed by adolescents (15–19 years) at annual rate of 3.8% per year from the baseline of 16% (NFHS 3).
- Raise child sex ratio in the 0–6 years age group at annual rate of 0.6% per year from the baseline of 914 (Census 2011).

Table 19.2.3: Mode of implementation of RMNCH+A approach.

Reproductive care	***Pregnancy and child birth care***	***Newborn and childcare***	
Clinical			
• Comprehensive abortion care • Reproductive tract infections (RTI)/ sexually transmitted infections (STI) case management • Postpartum intrauterine contraceptive device and sterilization; interval IUCD procedures • Adolescent friendly health services	• Skilled obstetric care and immediate newborn care and resuscitation • Emergency obstetric care • Preventing parent to child transmission (PPTCT) of human immunodeficiency virus • Postpartum sterilization	• Essential newborn care • Care of sick newborn (Special newborn care units • (SNCU), newborn stabilization units (NBSU)) • Facility-based care of childhood illnesses (IMNCI) • Care of children with severe acute malnutrition (NRC) • Immunization	
Reproductive health care	***Antenatal care***	***Postnatal care***	***Child health care***
Outreach/subcenter			
• Family planning (including IUCD insertion, oral contraceptive pill and condoms) • Prevention and management of STIs • Peri-conception folic acid • supplementation	• Full antenatal care package • PPTCT	• Early detection and management of illnesses in mother and newborn • Immunization	• First level assessment and care for newborn and childhood illnesses • Immunization • Micronutrient supplementation
Family and community			
• Weekly iron and folic acid (IFA) supplementation • Information and counseling on sexual reproductive health and family planning • Community based promotion and delivery of contraceptives • Menstrual hygiene	• Counseling and preparation for newborn care, breastfeeding, birth preparedness • Demand generation for pregnancy care and institutional delivery Janani Suraksha Yojana (JSY), Janani Shishu Suraksha Yojana (JSSY)	• Home-based newborn care and prompt referral home based newborn care (HBNC) scheme • Antibiotic for suspected case of newborn sepsis • Infant and young child feeding (IYCE), including exclusive breastfeeding and complementary feeding • Child health screening and early intervention services (0–18 years) • Early childhood development • Danger sign recognition and care-seeking for illness • Use of oral rehydration salts and zinc in case of diarrhea	
Intersectoral: Water, sanitation, hygiene, nutrition, education, empowerment			
Adolescence/pre-pregnancy	Pregnancy → Birth	Newborn/postnatal	Childhood

(RMNCH+A: reproductive, maternal, neonatal child health plus adolescent)

BIBLIOGRAPHY

1. A strategic approach to reproductive, maternal, newborn, child and adolescent health (RMNCH+A) in India, for healthy mother and child. New Delhi: Ministry of Health and Family Welfare, Government of India; 2013.
2. Census of India (2016). Sample Registration System Report 2016. [online] Available from: http://www.censusindia.gov.in/vital_statistics/SRS_Reports_2016. [Accessed November, 2018].
3. Census of India (2017). Sample Registration System Bulletin 2017. [online] Available from: http://censusindia.gov.in. [Accessed November, 2018].
4. Public Health Foundation of India (2014). State of India's Newborns 2014. [online] Available from: http://www.newbornwhocc.org/SOIN_PRINTED%2014-9-2014.pdf. [Accessed November, 2018].
5. UNICEF (2017). Levels and Trends in Child Mortality Report, 2017. New York: UNICEF; 2017.
6. UNICEF (2017). The State of the World's Children 2017, UNICEF. [online] Available from: http://www.data.unicef.org. [Accessed November, 2018].
7. World Health Organization (2007). Neonatal and Perinatal Mortality. Country, Regional and Global Estimates. [online] Available from: http://whqlibdoc.who.int/publications/2007/9789241596145_eng.pdf. [Accessed November, 2018].

19.3 Primary Health, National Health Policy 2017, and Child Health

Piyush Gupta, Swati Kalra

PRIMARY HEALTHCARE IN INDIA

Primary healthcare is essential healthcare based on practical, scientifically sound, and socially acceptable methods and technology made universally accessible to individuals and families in the community through their full participation and at a cost that the community and country can afford to maintain at every stage of their development in the spirit of self-reliance and self-determination.

Healthcare system in India consists of many components and levels. So far, the interaction between these components of the system has been very poor. Despite the three tiers of healthcare facilities, there are no well-organized referral linkages between the primary, secondary, and tertiary care institutions in the same locality. The major effort should be on strengthening the first link between the people and health system, i.e. the primary health center (PHC) services.

HISTORICAL PERSPECTIVES

Healthcare system in India has undergone major changes over the past 60 years beginning with the introduction of PHCs in each community development block in the year 1952, progressing to the adoption of national norms of population coverage during the sixth and seventh five-year plan period. During the eighth and ninth plans, the emphasis was mainly on consolidation of the existing health infrastructure rather than expansion. The focus during the 10th plan was on reorganization and restructuring the existing government healthcare system at the primary, secondary, and tertiary care levels with appropriate referral linkages using information technology tools; improvement in the quality of care; exploring alternative systems of healthcare; improving medical education and research; and building up a fully functional, accurate health management information system (HMIS). However, none of these goals could be fully achieved.

Eleventh five-year plan came up with National Rural Health Mission (NRHM) (2005–2012) which aimed for an overhaul of the existing PHC system, by promoting policies that strengthen public healthcare management and service delivery with the support of accredited social health activist (ASHA) workers, village health plans, district health plans, and decentralization of services. The NRHM led to a significant strengthening of public health systems with engagement of around 900,000 community health volunteers, the ASHAs, who aided in bringing the community closer to public services, improving utilization of services, and health-seeking behaviors. However, much of the increase in service delivery was related to select reproductive and child health services and the national disease control programs affecting only few indicators. There is still a felt need for strengthening health systems for providing comprehensive care by means of higher levels of investment and human resources.

ACHIEVEMENTS IN CHILD HEALTH

Despite all the advances in health, education, and agriculture sectors as well as vast improvements in the country's economy, India figures in the list of countries that have made insufficient progress toward meeting the Millennium Development Goals as suggested by review of child health indicators.

Overview of mortality indicators showed that under-5 mortality rate (U5MR) declined from 126 in 1990 to 41 in 2016 as per sample registration system (SRS), 2017 data, which is almost a reduction by two-third. India has also witnessed a substantial reduction in infant mortality rate (IMR) and neonatal mortality rate (NMR) in recent decades. Since the early 1970s, the IMR declined from 140 per 1,000 live births to 34 (SRS, 2017), but this is highly variable within the country as well. Despite this, India accounts for 27% (0.7 million) of global newborn deaths.

With respect to nutritional status, India has been able to reduce proportion of under-weight children below 5 years of age to 29.4% in 2013 from the estimated 52% in 1990. However, it has the largest numbers of under-five children who are moderately or severely stunted, accounting for 38% of the global burden.

India is currently experiencing a rapid health transition with the emergence of epidemic of noncommunicable diseases (NCDs) under the background of unfinished agenda of addressing infectious diseases and nutritional deficiencies. Overall, communicable diseases contribute 28% of the entire disease burden, while NCDs 60% and injuries at 12% now constitute the bulk of the country's disease burden.

India's progress on communicable disease control is mixed. Polio has been eliminated along with maternal and neonatal tetanus. Leprosy, though significantly reduced, is stagnant at current levels of new infective cases and disabilities. Kala-azar and lymphatic filariasis are expected to decline below the threshold. There has been a decline in AIDS cases from a 0.41% prevalence rate in 2001 to 0.27% in 2011 but this still leaves about 21 lakh persons living with HIV, about 1.16 lakh new cases and 1.48 lakh deaths in 2011. The emergence of multidrug resistant tuberculosis cases has been posing serious challenges. In malaria, there has been a significant decline, but the challenges of resistant strains and of sustaining the gains still remain. Viral encephalitis, dengue, and Chikungunya are on the rise, particularly in urban areas.

The Tanahashi framework for systemic bottlenecks analysis identified six key bottlenecks under the NRHM:

1. Limited availability of skilled human resources
2. Low coverage in marginalized communities with low skilled staff posting
3. Inadequate supportive supervision of front line workers
4. Low quality of training and skill building
5. Lack of focus on quality of services
6. Insufficient IEC on key family practices.

Some of these elements are addressed in the new National Health Policy.

NATIONAL HEALTH POLICY, 2017

To overcome the limitations and pitfalls of the previous health strategies, Government of India has released the new National Health Policy in 2017. This policy has been conceptualized after keeping in mind the changes in healthcare sectors including the growing burden because of NCDs and some infectious diseases, emergence of a robust healthcare industry, growing incidence of catastrophic expenditure due to healthcare costs, and a rising economic growth.

The primary aim of the National Health Policy 2017 is to inform, clarify, strengthen, and prioritize the role of the Government in shaping health systems in all its dimensions - investments in health, organization of healthcare services, prevention of diseases and promotion of good health through cross sectoral actions, access to technologies, developing human resources, encouraging medical pluralism, building knowledge base, developing better financial protection strategies, strengthening regulation, and health assurance.

The goal of this policy would be attainment of the highest possible level of health and wellbeing for all at all ages, through a preventive and promotive healthcare orientation in all developmental policies, and universal access to good quality healthcare services without anyone having to face financial hardship consequently. This would be achieved through increasing access, improving quality, and lowering the cost of healthcare delivery.

The policy recognizes the pivotal importance of Sustainable Development Goals (SDGs). Development of "Health and Wellness Centers," at primary healthcare level to provide the larger package of comprehensive primary healthcare; emphasis on investment and action in school health—by incorporating health education as part of the curriculum, promoting hygiene and safe health practices within the school environs; promotion of healthy living and prevention strategies from AYUSH systems; and Yoga at the workplace, in the schools and in the community; are some of newer ideas for health promotion at primary level that have a special appeal and acceptability in the Indian context.

Various Child health programs are supported by the National Health Policy 2017 like RMNCH+A services to improve maternal and child survival, child and adolescent health program, interventions to address malnutrition and micronutrient deficiencies, universal immunization with special focus in Mission Indradhanush and Integrated Disease Surveillance program for communicable diseases. Some of these programs are further discussed in detail in *Chapter 19.5*.

KEY TO IMPROVE CHILD SURVIVAL

Availability of child health services is a must at all levels of healthcare. Essential newborn care is the first step toward establishing an effective chain to reduce infant mortality and increase the national output. Promotion of breastfeeding in the community essentially protects the children from their two biggest enemies—infection and malnutrition. Organization, planning, and execution of immunization services are the cardinal preventive measures for control of many life-threatening or disabling communicable illnesses. Growth monitoring is the fundamental tool for early detection of childhood morbidities. Management of common neonatal and childhood illnesses in an integrated manner is the final solution to reduce morbidity and mortality in this age-group. Adolescents have their special needs, which should be recognized and tackled.

Parents should be enlisted as partners in their children's health. They should understand ways of promoting good health, recognizing illness, and taking appropriate action, wherever essential. Appropriate counseling and guidance should be provided to them regarding the problem, care, possible complications, and prognosis in acute life-threatening illnesses, chronic ailments, genetic and metabolic afflictions, infectious diseases, and nutrition-related disorders.

BIBLIOGRAPHY

1. Census of India (2017). Sample Registration System Bulletin 2017. [online] Available from: http://censusindia.gov.in. [Accessed November, 2018].

2. National Health Policy (2017). [online] Available from: http://cdsco.nic.in/writereaddata/National-Health-Policy.pdf [Accessed November, 2018].
3. National Health Policy (2017). Situation Analyses, Backdrop to National Health Policy, 2017. [online] Available from: https://mohfw.gov.in/sites/default/files/71275472221489753307.pdf [Accessed November, 2018].
4. UNICEF (2013). Improving Child Nutrition. The achievable imperative for global progress. New York: United Nations Children's Fund (UNICEF); 2013. [online] Available from: www.unicef.org/publications/index.html. [Accessed November, 2018].
5. World Health Organization. Non-communicable Diseases (NCD) Country Profiles. Geneva: WHO; 2014. pp. 91.

19.4 Integrated Management of Neonatal and Childhood Illnesses

Shashi N Vani

INTRODUCTION

Despite introducing several effective healthcare interventions for past three decades and more, every year nearly 11 million children die globally before reaching age of 5 years. Majority of them die due to a few common illnesses for which we have the knowledge and the capability to prevent or treat. These children mostly from poor and deprived families are denied these benefits and unnecessarily succumb to death.

In response to this challenge, World Health Organization (WHO) and United Nation Children's Fund (UNICEF) designed a fresh strategy named Integrated Management of Neonatal and Childhood Illness (IMNCI) in the early 1990s for the developing countries of the world to provide effective and affordable interventions to reduce childhood morbidity and mortality and also to improve child health and development. Both preventive and curative healthcare interventions have been included in IMNCI.

BACKGROUND

Nearly 70% of deaths in under 5 years children are caused due to a very few common illnesses like acute respiratory infections (ARIs) (mostly bacterial pneumonia), diarrhea, measles, malaria, and malnutrition or a combinations of these conditions. Malnutrition and anemia may not be the direct cause of death, but these are compounding factors with other common childhood illnesses and worsen the condition. Every day millions of parents seek healthcare for their children, majority of whom suffer because of these few common childhood illnesses. They visit various hospitals, health centers, dispensaries, private practitioners, and traditional healers adding to the burden of the healthcare providers who are not trained to assess, classify, and decide the further approach of management rationally and start early treatment appropriately. They do not have adequate diagnostic and therapeutic facilities, adequate supply of basic but essential drugs or the training for offering quality care. Very often lack of time and awareness regarding parent counseling and preventive and promotive healthcare services like nutrition advice and immunization are lacking.

Many sick children never reach a healthcare facility due to lack of awareness of the parents or nonavailability of services nearer their homes or sheer poverty. There are many inequities in the health care of these children from deprived families.

During the past three decades or so many successful interventions such as oral rehydration salts (ORS) for diarrheal disease, rational use of antibiotic for pneumonia and other ARIs, early use of antimalarials, immunizations under expanded program on immunization/universal immunization program (EPI/UIP), anemia control program, vitamin A supplement program, etc. have been incorporated in national health programs as vertical programs and have helped in bringing down the childhood mortality to some extent. But, for further reduction of infant and under-5 mortality, a different strategy was needed and in this background, WHO and UNICEF conceived IMNCI approach. It is not a new program. It is an effective strategy or a different approach integrating all the vertical healthcare programs aiming for the holistic care of the young children up to 5 years

Table 19.4.1: Triage.

Assess for emergency signs (in all cases)			*Treat*: • Check for head/neck trauma before treating child (do not move neck if cervical spine injury possible) • Give appropriate treatment for +ve emergency signs • Call for help • Draw blood for glucose, malaria smear, Hb
Airway and breathing	• Not breathing or gasping or • Central cyanosis or • Severe respiratory distress	→ Any sign positive	• Manage airway • Provide baby life support (not breathing/gasping) • Give oxygen • Make sure child is warm
Circulation	*Cold extremities with:* • Capillary refill longer than 3 seconds and • Weak and fast pulse	If positive check for severe acute malnutrition	• If the child has any bleeding, apply pressure to stop the bleeding. Do not use a tourniquet • Give oxygen • Make sure child is warm* • Insert intravenous (IV) and begin giving fluids rapidly • If not able to insert peripheral I/V, insert an umbilical or intraosseous line
			If severe acute malnutrition (age ≥2 months) *If lethargic or unconscious:* • Insert IV line and give glucose and fluids *If not lethargic or unconscious:* • Give glucose orally or by nasogastric (NG) tube • Proceed immediately to full assessment and treatment
Coma convulsing	• Coma, or • Convulsing (now)	→ If coma or convulsing	• Manage airway • Position the child • Check and correct hypoglycemia • If convulsions continue give IV calcium in young infants • If convulsions continue, give anticonvulsants
Severe dehydration (only in cases with diarrhea)	*Diarrhea plus any two of these:* • Lethargy • Sunken eyes • Very slow skin pinch	→ Diarrhea plus two signs positive check for severe acute malnutrition	• Make sure child is warm* • Insert IV line and begin giving fluids rapidly following plan C If severe acute malnutrition (age ≥ 2 months) • Do not start IV immediately • Proceed immediately to full assessment and treatment
*Check treatment, if baby is cold to touch, rewarm			
If there are no emergency signs look for priority signs these children need prompt assessment and treatment			
• Tiny baby (<2 months) • Bleeding • Pallor (severe) • Malnutrition; visible severe wasting		• Respiratory distress (RR > 60/mm) • Trauma or other urgent surgical condition • Referral (urgent) • Edema of both feet	• Temperature <36.5°C or >38.5°C • Restless, continuously irritable or lethargy • Poisoning • Burns (major)

Nonurgent: Proceed with assessment and further treatment according to child's priority.
Note: If a child has trauma or other surgical problems, get surgical help or follow surgical guidelines.

Missing Areas in Integrated Management of Neonatal and Childhood Illness

- Antenatal care/birth preparedness
- Skilled birth attendance
- Management of important problems like asthma, tuberculosis (TB), etc.

Role of Private Practitioners in Integrated Management of Neonatal and Childhood Illness

Depending on the scope of practice, private practitioners can adapt IMNCI approach in their clinic works. It will definitely improve their quality of care and rationalize the use of drugs and investigations. In many areas, the community members prefer to take treatment from family physicians/private practitioners than from public health facilities for several reasons. The community health workers also refer their cases to local private doctors. If the private doctor adopts the same IMNCI approach there will be definitely a better continuum of care benefiting the patient and community at large. Unlike many other health care interventions where training is given to doctors in public service alone, IMNCI training is available for family physicians also.

If properly implemented and supported by strengthening the health system assuring quality training to all the functionaries, ensuring regular adequate supplies, good supervision and monitoring and community-based service like good counseling, behavior change, and communication, IMNCI in India has a great potential to achieve its main goal of reducing newborn and under-5 mortality in children within a short time and come closer to millennium development goals.

BIBLIOGRAPHY

1. National Institute of Health and Family Welfare (2009–2010). Status report of state institutes of health and family welfare (IMNCI State Institute of Health and Family Welfare), Jaipur. [online] Available from: http://www.nihfw.org/pdf/Status%20report%20of%20SIHFWs.pdf. [Accessed October, 2015].
2. Patwari A, Raina N. Integrated Management of Neonatal and Childhood Illnesses: A robust strategy. Indian Pediatr. 2002;69(1):41-8.
3. World Health Organization. Integrated Management of Neonatal and Childhood Illnesses (IMNCI): A guidebook for private practitioners. New Delhi: WHO/Department of Child and Adolescent Health, 2002.
4. World Health Organization. Students Handbook IMNCI (Integrated Management of Neonatal and Childhood Illnesses). New Delhi: WHO/Department of Child and Adolescent Health and Development and the Ministry of Health and Family Welfare, Government of India; 2003.

19.5 National Health Mission

RK Agarwal, Deepti Agrawal

INTRODUCTION

The National Health Mission (NHM) is India's flagship health sector program to revitalize rural and urban health sectors. The NHM envisages universal access to equitable, affordable, and quality health care services that are accountable and responsive to people's needs. The main programmatic components include health system strengthening in rural and urban areas, reproductive-maternal-newborn-child and adolescent health (RMNCH+A) services and control of communicable and noncommunicable diseases. NHM encompasses two submissions, the National Rural Health Mission (NRHM) and the National Urban Health Mission (NUHM).

National Rural Health Mission was launched in April 12, 2005 to address the health needs of the underserved rural population especially women, children, and vulnerable sections of the society and to provide affordable, accessible, and quality healthcare. Under the NRHM, the empowered action group States (Bihar, Chhattisgarh, Jharkhand, Madhya Pradesh, Odisha, Rajasthan, Uttarakhand, and Uttar Pradesh) as well as North Eastern States, Jammu and Kashmir, and Himachal Pradesh have been given special focus. The thrust of the mission is on establishing a fully functional, community owned, decentralized health delivery system with intersectoral convergence at all levels, to ensure simultaneous action on a wide range of determinants of health such as water, sanitation, education, nutrition, social, and gender equality.

National Urban Health Mission was launched in May 2013 in order to improve the health status of the urban population particularly urban poor and other vulnerable sections by facilitating their access to quality primary healthcare. NUHM covers all State capitals, district headquarters, and other cities/towns with a population of 50,000 and above (as per census 2011) in a phased manner. Cities and towns with population below 50,000 are covered under NRHM.

VISION AND OBJECTIVES

Vision

The vision of NHM is "attainment of universal access to equitable, affordable, and quality healthcare services, accountable and responsive to people's needs, with effective inter-sectoral convergent action to address the wider social determinants of health."

Objectives

- Reduction in infant mortality rate (IMR) and maternal mortality rate (MMR)
- Population stabilization, gender, and demographic balance
- Achieve universal access to public health services like women's health, child health, water, sanitation and hygiene, immunization, and nutrition
- Promotion of healthy lifestyles
- Prevention and control of communicable and noncommunicable diseases, including locally endemic diseases
- Access to integrated comprehensive primary healthcare
- Revitalization of local health traditions and mainstream AYUSH.

KEY FEATURES

NHM envisions building of an integrated network of primary, secondary and a substantial part of tertiary care, providing a continuum from community level to the district hospital, with robust referral linkages. To address issues of access and continuum of care, the plan is to prioritize the creation/ upgradation of a set of interconnected facilities based on "time to care and caseloads." The endeavor is to ensure that primary services are available within 30 minutes of any habitation and secondary services including cesarean section and blood transfusion are available within 2 hours of any habitation, with an assured referral transport system connecting the two.

NHM is the primary vehicle to move toward Universal Health Coverage (UHC). UHC means that all people receive the quality, essential health services they need, without being exposed to financial hardship. India has charted a path that depends largely on provision of affordable, quality healthcare by the public health system as its main form of social protection, with supplementation from the private sector to close gaps in service provision.

UHC through NHM aims to reduce out of pocket expenditure on health care, eliminating catastrophic health expenditures and providing social protection to the poor against the rising costs of health care, through cashless services delivered by public health care facilities. The government has already taken steps toward provision of free maternal, and child health services, including newborn care, immunization, adolescent health, and family planning. Free diagnostic and treatment services are provided for major communicable and a selected range of noncommunicable diseases. These are being further expanded and strengthened.

Health outcome indicators from various states and districts show that the progress is uneven across the country. Even states that are performing relatively well have pockets where the women and children are relatively disadvantaged in terms of the health status. Therefore, populations in certain geographical locations (like the hilly and remote places, tribal areas and desert) and those disadvantaged in terms of social and economic status (like the scheduled castes and tribes, poor) need special focus and differential planning to ensure that they are not left out from receiving the benefits from the investments made in the public health system. Also, because they suffer the highest burden of mortality and morbidity, maximum gains in reducing ill health and improving survival will come from reaching these groups and achieving greater coverage of health interventions amongst them. NHM provides for differential financial investments and technical support to cities, districts and states with higher proportions of vulnerable population groups, urban poor and destitute, and with difficult geographical terrain have to face special challenges to meet health goals.

NHM also addresses shortages of skilled workers in remote, rural areas, and other underserved pockets through appropriate monetary and nonmonetary incentives.

NHM continues to mainstream AYUSH (Department of Ayurveda, Yoga and Naturopathy, Unani, Siddha and Homeopathy), to enhance choice of services for users and to revitalize local healthcare traditions.

INSTITUTIONAL MECHANISMS

National Level

At national level, there is a Mission Steering Group (MSG) under the chairmanship of Union Minister of Health and Family Welfare, which provides policy direction to NHM. There is an Empowered Program Committee (EPC) headed by Secretary, Department of Health and Family Welfare, which scrutinizes all financial proposals before approval by MSG.

The NHM is headed by a Mission Director, of the rank of Additional Secretary, supported by a team of joint secretaries. The mission handles not just the day-to-day administrative affairs of the mission but is responsible for planning, implementing, and monitoring mission activities.

State Level

There is a State Health Mission with the State Health Society, headed by the Mission Director. It is further supported by the State Program Management Unit (SPMU).

District Level

At district level, the mission operates under the District Health Mission (DHM)/City Health Mission (CHM) with District Health Society (DHS). District Collector/District Magistrate is the Chairperson and Chief Medical Officer is the Chief Executive Officer (CEO) of the DHS. DHS is responsible for planning and managing all programs in the district.

PROGRAMS UNDER NATIONAL HEALTH MISSION

The key programs under NHM are RMNCH+A services and disease control programs. An overview of these programs is presented in **Tables 19.5.1 and 19.5.2**, respectively.

Reproductive, Maternal, Newborn, Child, and Adolescent Health Services

RMNCH+A approach launched in 2013 essentially looks to address the major causes of mortality among women and children as well as the delays in accessing and utilizing health care and services. The RMNCH+A strategic approach

Table 19.5.1: Reproductive, maternal, newborn, child and adolescent health (RMNCH+A) services under National Health Mission.

Domain	***Key provisions***
RMNCH+A services	
Maternal health	Increase coverage and quality of antenatal and postnatal care, increase access to skilled birth attendance, institutional delivery; basic and comprehensive emergency obstetric care through strengthening of health facilities
Access to safe abortion services	Improve access to comprehensive abortion care, including postabortion contraceptive counseling and services; expand the network of facilities providing medical termination of pregnancy (MTP) services
Newborn care	Provision of home-based newborn care through Accredited Social Health Activists (ASHAs); essential newborn care and resuscitation at all delivery points (through newborn care corner/NBCC). Facility-based care for sick newborns through the establishment of newborn stabilization units (NBSU) and special newborn care units (SNCU) at first referral units (FRU) and DH, respectively
Child care	Provision of community care for acute respiratory infections, diarrhea, and fevers, first contact curative care, or referral as appropriate. Institutional care for sick children, management of severely malnourished children at nutrition rehabilitation centers (NRC); promotion of infant and young child feeding (IYCF) practices and micronutrient supplementation
Universal immunization	Sustaining pulse polio campaigns and achieving over 80% routine immunization in all districts; introduction of new and underutilized vaccines; improved cold chain management; adequate number of vaccination sessions and sites, and logistics arrangements to reach all such sites especially in remote areas.
Child health screening and early intervention services	Early detection of 4Ds: birth defects, diseases, deficiencies, and development delays including disability and provide comprehensive care at appropriate levels of health facilities
Adolescent health	Iron and folic acid (IFA) supplementation, facility-based adolescent health services, community-based health promotion activities, information and counseling on sexual and reproductive health (including menstrual hygiene), substance abuse, mental health, noncommunicable diseases, injuries and violence including domestic violence
Family planning	Prioritize postpartum and postabortion contraception; promote spacing methods, especially intrauterine contraceptive devices (IUCDs); distribution of contraceptives at the doorstep through ASHAs. In high fertility states: promotion of healthy spacing after marriage and between the births by engaging ASHAs as the motivator and counselor
Addressing the declining sex ratio	Stricter enforcement of the preconception and prenatal diagnostic techniques (PCPNDT) act, improved monitoring and sensitization of the medical community, greater role for civil society action in addressing son preference, addressing neglect of the girl child in illness care, observing sex ratios in hospital admissions for illness in children, and providing proactive support for girl children through the ASHA and anganwadi system

Table 19.5.2: Disease Control Program under National Health Mission.

Program	***Key provisions***
Control of communicable diseases	
National Vector Borne Diseases Control Program (NVBDCP)	Prevention and control of vector bore diseases viz. malaria, Japanese encephalitis (JE), dengue, chikungunya, kala-azar, and lymphatic filariasis
Revised National Tuberculosis Control Program (RNTCP)	Prevention, control and treatment of tuberculosis
National Leprosy Control Program (NLEP)	Diagnosis and treatment [multi-drug treatment (MDT)] of leprosy patients
Integrated Disease Surveillance Program (IDSP)	Prevention and control of outbreaks of communicable diseases
Control of noncommunicable diseases	
National Program for Prevention and Control of Cancer, Diabetes, Cardiovascular Diseases, and Stroke (NPCDCS)	Specialized management of diabetes, cardiovascular disease (CVD), stroke, and cancer
National Program for the Control of Blindness (NPCB)	Providing screening for detection and management of diabetic retinopathy, refractory defects, and glaucoma
National Mental Health Program (NMHP)	Providing services for early detection and treatment of mental illness in the community
National Program for the Health Care of the Elderly (NPHCE)	Specialized accessible healthcare for elderly
National Program for the Prevention and Control of Deafness (NPPCD)	Prevention of avoidable hearing loss and early detection and treatment of ear problems
National Tobacco Control Program (NTCP)	Spread awareness and better implementation of tobacco control
National Oral Health Program (NOHP)	Promotive and preventive oral health care at primary and secondary level
National Program for Prevention and Control of Fluorosis (NPPCF)	Surveillance, management, and health education for prevention and control of fluorosis
National Iodine Deficiency Disease Control Program (NIDDCP)	To check iodine deficiency-related health problems
National Organ Transplant Program (NOTP)	Promotion of organ donation from deceased persons, retrieval, storage, and transplant of organs

provides an understanding of "continuum of care" to ensure equal focus on various life stages. There is additional focus on adolescence as a distinct "life stage." It also aims to strengthen the referral linkages between community and facility-based health services and between the various levels of health system (primary, secondary, and tertiary). The RMNCH+A appropriately directs the states to focus their efforts on the most vulnerable population and disadvantaged groups. It also emphasizes on the need to reinforce efforts in those poor performing districts that have already been identified as the high priority districts (HPDs).

Key RMNCH+A Initiatives

Janani Suraksha Yojana (JSY): It is a demand promotion scheme launched in April 2005 to reduce maternal mortality among pregnant women by encouraging them to deliver in government health facilities. Under the scheme, cash assistance is provided to eligible pregnant women for giving birth in a government health facility. It has brought about a surge in institutional deliveries since its launch.

Janani Shishu Suraksha Karyakram (JSSK): Launched on 1st June, 2011, entitles all pregnant women delivering in public health institutions to absolutely free and no expense delivery, including cesarean section. This marks a shift to an entitlement-based approach. The free entitlements include free drugs and consumables, free diagnostics, free diet during stay in the health institutions, free provision of blood, free transport from home to health institution, between health institutions in case of referrals and drop back home and exemption from all kinds of user charges. Similar entitlements are available for all sick infants (up to 1 year of age) accessing public health institutions.

Pradhanmantri Surakshit Matritva Abhiyan (PMSMA): Under the PMSMA, on the 9th of every month, pregnant women are given free health check-up including blood pressure, sugar level, hemoglobin test, blood test, etc. and the required treatment in all government medical facilities. Private sector gynecologists are encouraged to voluntarily participate and provide antenatal check-up (ANC) services in these public health facilities.

Facility-based newborn care: A continuum of newborn care has been established with the launch of home-based and facility-based newborn care components ensuring that every newborn receives essential care right from the time of birth and first 48 hours at the health facility and then at home during the first 42 days of life. Newborn care corners (NBCCs) are established at delivery points to provide essential newborn care at birth, while special newborn care units (SNCUs) at district hospital/medical college and newborn stabilization units (NBSUs) at first referral units (FRUs) provide care for sick newborns.

Mother and child tracking system: It is a web-based name-based tracking system, designed to capture information on and track all pregnant women and children (0–5 years) so that they receive "full complement" of maternal and child health services.

Mother and Child Health Wings (MCH wings): These are 100/50/30-bedded buildings sanctioned in public health facilities (district hospitals/district women's hospitals/sub-district hospitals/community health centers) to overcome the constraints of increasing caseloads and institutional deliveries at these facilities. These are envisaged as integrated facilities for advanced, optimal quality obstetric, and newborn care.

National Iron Plus Initiative: It aims at prevention and control of iron deficiency anemia. Besides pregnant women and lactating mothers, it aims to provide iron and folic acid (IFA) supplementation for children, adolescents, and women in reproductive age group. Weekly iron and folic acid supplementation (WIFS) for adolescents is an important strategy under this initiative.

Mission Indradhanush: To strengthen and invigorate the Universal Immunization Program (UIP) and achieve full immunization coverage for all children at a rapid pace, Mission Indradhanush was launched in December 2014. Mission Indradhanush ensures that all children under the age of 2 years and pregnant women are fully immunized with all available vaccines.

Kayakalp: This initiative has been launched to promote cleanliness, hygiene, and infection control practices in public health facilities. Under this initiative public healthcare facilities shall be appraised and such public healthcare facilities that show exemplary performance meeting standards of protocols of cleanliness, hygiene and infection control receive awards and commendation.

Free drugs and free diagnostic services: Extremely high out of pocket expenditure on health care due to high cost of drugs and diagnostics have proved to be a deterrent in provision of accessible and affordable healthcare for all. Under the NHM, states are required to notify policy for provision of free essential drugs and/or diagnostics to all patients accessing public health facilities, create a robust procurement, logistics and supply chain system, have essential drug list/diagnostic list depending, standard treatment guidelines and audit prescription to ensure rational use of drugs.

National Ambulance Services (NAS): Under NHM, States/UTs have provided the facility where people can dial 108 or 102 telephone number for calling an ambulance. Dial 108 is predominantly an emergency response system, primarily designed to attend to patients of critical care, trauma, and accident victims, etc. Dial 102 services consist of basic patient transport. JSSK entitlements, e.g., free transport from home to facility, interfacility transfer in case of referral and drop back for mother and children are the key focus of 102 service. The ambulance service can be accessed through a toll-free call to a call center.

Daksh Skill Labs: Skills Labs are established for competency-based training and skill enhancement of healthcare providers for RMNCH+A services, both in-service and preservice training. Skills Labs provide competency-based training through repetitive skills practice, simulation of clinical scenarios, and training under the supervision of a qualified trainer.

Dakshata Program: It is the capacity building program for service providers in labor room best practices during labor, delivery, and postpartum period.

Rashtriya Bal Swasthya Karyakram (RBSK): It was launched in February 2013 and provides for child health screening and early intervention services through early detection and management of 4 Ds, i.e., defects at birth, diseases, deficiencies, and development delays including disability in the age group of 0–18 years. This will be made possible by screening of the new born at public health facilities and at home, regular health screening of pre-school children up to 6 years of age in anganwadis and regular health checkup for children 6–18 years of age studying in Government and Government-aided schools. Children diagnosed with any of the 30 specified illnesses would receive follow-up referral support and treatment including surgical interventions at tertiary level free-of-cost under this program.

Rashtriya Kishor Swasthya Karyakram (RKSK): It was launched in January 2014 to reach out to 253 million adolescents in the country. This initiative broadens the focus of the adolescent health program beyond reproductive and sexual health and brings in focus on life skills, nutrition, injuries, and violence (including gender-based violence), noncommunicable diseases, mental health, and substance misuse.

National quality assurance framework for health facilities: To improve quality of healthcare in over 31,000 public health facilities and provide a clear roadmap to states, quality

19.6 National Health Programs Related to Child Health

Pukhraj Bafna

INTRODUCTION

Several measures have been undertaken by the Government of India to improve the health of the people after independence under the Constitution of India. The subject of health facilities, their planning, establishment and administration falls under the purview of respective governments of states of the union. Government of India has introduced national health programs from time to time, which are either centrally, partially sponsored or completely funded by the center. To improve the health of the people prominent measures launched by the central government are National Health Programs for the control/eradication of the communicable diseases, improvement of environmental sanitation, raising the standard of nutrition, control of population, and improving rural health.

Pediatrics is the first clinical subject to link itself to preventive medicine. There is no other discipline as comprehensive as pediatrics that teaches the value of preventive medicine.

According to changing health scenario new programs are being added and existing ones are modified. The important national programs are listed in **Table 19.6.1**.

NATIONAL RURAL HEALTH MISSION

The Government of India launched *National Rural Health Mission (NRHM)* on April 5, 2005 for a period of 7 years (2005–2012), and recently extended it up to year 2017 recognizing the importance of health in the process of economic and social development and to improve the quality of life of its citizens. This mission seeks to improve rural health care delivery system.

The main aim of NRHM is to provide accessible, affordable, accountable, effective, and reliable primary healthcare and bridging the gap in rural healthcare through creation of a cadre of "Accredited Social Health Activist (ASHA)".

NATIONAL HEALTH MISSION

National Health Mission (NHM) was approved by Ministry of Health and Family Welfare in May 2013. The main programmatic components include health system strengthening in rural and urban areas; *Reproductive-Maternal-Newborn-Child and Adolescent Health (RMNCH+A);* and control of communicable and noncommunicable diseases. This approach brings focus on integrated packages of service for different stages of life like adolescents as a critical life stage and linkage between child survival, maternal health, and family planning efforts.

Recently, new initiatives have been launched under NHM. *Rashtriya Bal Swasthya Karyakram* (RBSK) was launched to provide comprehensive healthcare and improve the quality of life of children through early detection of birth defects, diseases, deficiencies and developmental delays including disability. Another initiative, *Rashtriya Kishore Swasthya Karyakram* (RKSK) was launched to comprehensively address the health needs of the 253 million adolescents, accounting for over 21% of the country's population, by bringing in several new dimensions like mental health, nutrition, substance misuse, injuries and violence, and noncommunicable diseases. In addition, to these initiatives the weekly iron folic acid supplementation program (WIFS) was launched to address adolescent anemia.

INDIA NEWBORN ACTION PLAN

In India, Newborn Action Plan (INAP) developed in response to the global "Every Newborn Action Plan (ENAP)" was launched in June 2014. The goal is to attain "single digit neonatal mortality rate by 2030" and single digit stillbirth rate by 2030. The INAP will be implemented within the existing RMNCH+A framework.

MATERNAL AND CHILD HEALTH PROGRAMS

Maternal and child health (MCH) refers to the promotive, preventive, curative, and rehabilitative health care for mothers and children, which includes maternal health, child health, family planning, school health, handicapped children, adolescence, and health aspects of care of children in special settings like day care. The ultimate objective of MCH services is lifelong health.

Objectives of Maternal and Child Health Programs

- Reductions of maternal, perinatal, infant, and childhood mortality and morbidity

Table 19.6.1: National Health Programs.

National programs related to mother and child care	
1.	Maternal and Child Health Program (MCH)
2.	Integrated Child Development Services Scheme (ICDS)
3.	Child Survival and Safe Motherhood Program (CSSM)
4.	Reproductive and Child Health Program (RCH)
5.	Integrated Management of Neonatal and Childhood Illnesses (IMNCI)
6.	National Health Mission (NHM)
7.	Reproductive Maternal Newborn Child and Adolescent Health (RMNCH+A)
8.	India Newborn Action Plan (INAP)
9.	Rashtriya Bal Swasthya Karyakram (RBSK)
10.	Rashtriya Kishor Swasthya Karyakram (RKSK)
National programs related to control of communicable diseases	
1.	Universal Immunization Program (UIP)
2.	Mission Indradhanush (MID)
3.	Acute Respiratory Infection Control Program (ARI)
4.	Diarrheal Disease Control Program (CDD)
5.	Revised National Tuberculosis Control Program (RNTCP)
6.	Leprosy Eradication Program (LEP)
7.	Malaria and other arthropod—borne disease control program (NMEP)
8.	National Filaria Control Program (NFCP)
9.	National Guinea Worm Control Program (NGWCP)
10.	Acquired Immune Deficiency Syndrome (AIDS) and Sexually Transmitted Disease (STD) Control Program (AIDS and STDCP).
National programs related to control of nutritional deficiencies and disorders	
1.	Nutritional programs
2.	Mid-day meal program
3.	Anemia prophylaxis program
4.	Vitamin A deficiency control program
5.	National iodine deficiency disorder control program (NIDDCP)
National programs related to control of noncommunicable diseases	
1.	National school health program
2.	Cancer control program
3.	National mental health program
4.	Drug deaddiction program
5.	National diabetes control program
6.	National program for control of blindness

- Promotion of reproductive health
- Promotion of physical and psychological development of the child and adolescent within the family.

Details of Services Rendered in Maternal and Child Health Programs

These services are mainly handled by multipurpose health workers. Their job is to:

- Record occurrence of pregnancy in their work area on the basis of history of missed periods and
- Screen women identified as pregnant for any of the under mentioned "risk" factors.
  - Age less than 17 years or over 35 years
  - Height less than 145 cm
  - Weight less than 40 kg or more than 70 kg
  - History of bleeding in previous pregnancy
  - History of stillbirths
  - History of cesarean section as indicated by scar in lower mid-abdomen
- Identify women with moderate to severe anemia
- Administration of two doses of tetanus toxoid
- Provide iron and folic acid tablets to pregnant women for a period of 180 days.

The "at risk" pregnancies identified by above-mentioned criteria make the basis of 80% of total morbidity and mortality.

Antenatal Care

The primary aim of antenatal care is to achieve at the end of a pregnancy, a healthy mother and healthy baby. Ideally this care should begin soon after conception and continue throughout pregnancy. For all pregnant women the package of antenatal care comprises of:

- Anemia screening
- Eclampsia and pre-eclampsia detection
- Multiple pregnancy screening
- Hemoglobin estimation
- Blood pressure recording
- Fundal height measurement.

The pregnant mothers are given advice on diet generally consumed by them. Breast examination is done to exclude retracted nipples. The expectant mothers are advised about the personal hygiene, other necessary warnings and articles needed at the time of labor and after labor on arrival of newborn. They are also advised regarding spacing.

Intranatal Care

The aims of good intranatal care are:

- Thorough asepsis
- Delivery with minimum injury to the infant and mother
- Readiness to deal with complications like prolonged labor, ante partum hemorrhage, convulsions, malpresentations, prolapse of the cord, etc.

- Care of the newborn at delivery—resuscitation, care of the cord, care of the eyes, etc.

The mothers are advised regarding breast-feeding, immunization, family planning, and general hygiene. The health care of the delivered woman continues to be supervised by the health worker at the subcenter or at her home under the supervision of health visitor or female multipurpose worker. Initial health-care of the newborn baby is also under taken by these health workers.

Care of Children

The following activities are conducted by female multipurpose health worker under the supervision of the medical officer at primary health center.

- Monitoring of growth of children to detect weight gain or malnutrition
- Immunization against vaccine preventable diseases
- Treatment of common illness as per the integrated management of neonatal and childhood illnesses (IMNCI) guidelines
- Referral of cases to health institutions
- Implement National Health Programs
- Impart health and nutrition education to community.

It is necessary to identify and register "at risk" children and give them special intensive care because these "at risk" babies contribute so largely to perinatal, neonatal, and infant motility. The basic criteria for identifying these "at risk" babies are listed in **Table 19.6.2**.

Implementation of Maternal and Child Health Programs

The MCH services are essentially delivered through the staff members of the primary health centers and sub-centers comprising of medical officers, health assistants (female and male), and multipurpose female health workers, also called as auxiliary nurse midwives (ANM) and multipurpose male health workers. Traditional Birth Attendants (TBAs) and village health nurses guide and support the services. In Integrated Child Development Services (ICDS) blocks, "anganwadi" workers also help in various MCH programs tasks.

MCH clinics/immunization clinics are conducted on one or more fixed days in a month in a sub-center, which is for every 5,000 population in rural area and 3,000 population in urban area. Home visits are also done by health workers. Medical officer of primary health care (PHC) is the leader of the team where curative services, MCH and other preventive and promotive services are conducted. The community health centers (CHC) are upgraded PHCs where some additional health care services like anesthesia, dentistry, and pathology are available.

In selected district under child survival and safe motherhood (CSSM) program approximately with 5 lakhs population one first referral unit (FRU) is created with provision of a surgeon, an obstetrician, a pediatrician, and an anesthetist along with facilities for blood transfusion and operations. Other complicated cases are either sent to district hospitals or nearest teaching hospital attached to medical college.

Table 19.6.2: Children "at risk".

1.	Birth weight less than 2.5 kg
2.	Twins
3.	Birth order five and more
4.	Artificial feeding
5.	Weight below 70% of the expected weight (i.e., II and III degrees of malnutrition)
6.	Failure to gain weight during three successive months
7.	Children with PEM, diarrhea
8.	Working mothers/single parent

(PEM: protein-energy malnutrition)

INTEGRATED CHILD DEVELOPMENT SERVICE SCHEME

Integrated child development service scheme was launched in 1975 in pursuance of the national policy for children in 33 community development blocks. The network consists of 5,659 projects in rural and urban slum pockets.

ICDS scheme represents one of the world's largest and most unique programs for early childhood development, breaking the vicious cycle of malnutrition, morbidity, reduced learning capacity, and mortality.

The beneficiaries are children below 6 years, pregnant and lactating women, women in the age group of 15–45 years, and adolescent girls in selected blocks.

Objectives of Integrated Child Development Service

- Improve the nutritional and health status of preschool children in the age group of 0–6 years.
- Lay the foundation of proper psychological development of the child.
- Reduce the incidence of mortality, morbidity, malnutrition, and also school dropout.
- Achieve effective co-ordination of policy and implementation amongst the various departments to promote child development and
- Enhance the capability of the mother to look after the normal health and nutritional needs of the child through proper nutrition and health education.

Delivery of Services

- *Supplementary nutrition*: The target group for supplementary nutrition is children below 6 years and nursing and expectant mothers from low-income group.
- *Immunization*: Children are immunized against six preventable diseases and pregnant mothers are given immunization against tetanus.
- *Health checkup*: Here ICDS provides:
  - Antenatal care of expectant mothers
  - Postnatal care of nursing mothers and care of newborns
  - Care of children under 6 years of age which consists of:
    - Record of weight and height from time to time
    - Watch over developmental mile stones
    - Immunization
    - General checkup every 3–6 months
    - Treatment of prevalent diseases
    - Deworming
    - Prophylaxis against vitamin A deficiency and anemia
    - Referral of serious cases to hospital
    - Maintenance of health records.
  - *Nutrition and health education*: To all women in the age group of 15–45 with priority to pregnant and nursing mothers, nutrition and health education is imparted by "anganwadi workers"
  - *Referral services*
  - *Nonformal preschool education.*

Administration

The administrative unit of an ICDS project is a community development block in rural areas, the tribal development block in tribal areas, and a group of slums in urban areas. The focal point for the delivery of ICDS is the trained local women known as "anganwadi worker (AWW)".

An "anganwadi" is established for a population of 1,000 in rural and urban areas and 700 in tribal areas. For a population of 100,000 in a community development block 100 anganwadi workers are employed on a part time basis, supervised by 4–5 female supervisors (*Mukhya Sevika*). A child development project officer (CDPO) is the overall in-charge of ICDS work in CD block.

At present, there are two schemes for adolescent girls, i.e. "Kishori Shakti Yojana" and "Nutrition Program for Adolescent Girls." These programs are implemented through the administrative setup of ICDS scheme at the state, district, block, and anganwadi center level.

Two more schemes are being implemented at the ICDS level: (1) Rajiv Gandhi Scheme for empowerment of adolescent girls—"SABLA" for 11–18 years of age; and (2) Indira Gandhi Matritva Sahyog Yojana (IGMSY). During the year 2009–10, about 6,705 ICDS projects and 1.15 million anganwadi centers/mini *anganwadi* centers were functional in the country. About 71.8 million children and 15.6 million pregnant and lactating mothers (total 87.5 million) are getting the benefit of ICDS scheme.

The impact of program on the lives of children is evident in several important areas like increased birth rate, reduced incidence of malnutrition, increased immunization coverage, and a reduced infant and child mortality rate in areas covered by the ICDS.

REPRODUCTIVE AND CHILD HEALTH PROGRAM

In 1997, the National Family Welfare Program has been renamed as Reproductive and Child Health (RCH) program. RCH has been defined as "People have the ability to reproduce and regulate their fertility, women are able to go through pregnancy and child birth safely, the outcome of pregnancy is successful in terms of maternal and infant survival and well-being, and couples are able to have sexual relations free of fear of unwanted pregnancy and of contracting sexually transmitted diseases."

Components

Components of RCH program are listed in **Table 19.6.3**.

- RCH integrates all interventions of fertility regulation, maternal, and child health with reproductive health for both men and women.
- Services provided in RCH are client oriented, demand driven, high quality and based on need of community through decentralized participatory planning and target-free approach.
- RCH program envisages upgradation of level of care. Comprehensive emergency obstetric and newborn care is provided at sub-district levels, which are FRUs. RCH facilities at PHCs are also upgraded.
- Services of obstetric care, medical termination of pregnancy (MTP), and intrauterine device (IUD) insertion in PHCs level are improved.
- Specialist facilities for sexually transmitted diseases (STDs) and reproductive tract infections (RTIs) are available in all district hospitals and a good number of sub-district level hospitals.
- Special program is taken up for urban slums, tribal population and adolescence, the vulnerable group of population.

CHILD SURVIVAL AND SAFE MOTHERHOOD PROGRAM

This program, which started in 1992, had the following components:

- Early registration of pregnancy
- To provide minimum three antenatal check-ups

Table 19.6.3: Components of Reproductive and Child Health (RCH) Program.

1.	Population stabilization
2.	Maternal health (essential obstetric care)
3.	Reproductive tract and sexually transmitted infection control program (HIV/AIDS and Cancer of Reproductive system)
4.	Newborn and child health through IMNCI (including diarrheal disease control program, respiratory infection control program, breastfeeding, baby friendly hospitals initiatives, immunization etc.)
5.	Prevention and control of anemia
6.	Prevention and control of vitamin A deficiency
7.	Universal immunization program
8.	Polio eradication: Pulse Polio Program
9.	Adolescent health (sexuality development, adolescence education, and vocational component)
10.	Tribal health
11.	Urban health
12.	Effective family planning (ensuring informed choice, counseling, gender equality and greater male participation)
13.	Prevention, detection and management of genetic and environmental disorders
14.	Prevention and management of infertility and other reproductive disorders
15.	Reproductive health care of elderly persons

(AIDS: acquired immune deficiency syndrome; HIV: human immunodeficiency virus; IMNCI: integrated management of neonatal and childhood illnesses)

- Universal coverage of all pregnant women with TT immunization
- Advice on food, nutrition, and rest
- Detection of high risk pregnancy and prompt referral
- Clean and safe deliveries by trained personnel
- Birth spacing
- Promotion of all institutional deliveries

These services have been integrated in RCH program and the major interventions are:

- Essential obstetric care
- Emergency obstetric care
- 24-hour delivery services at PHCs/CHCs
- Medical termination of pregnancy
- Control of RTI and STD
- *Immunization*: In 1992, the universal immunization program (UIP) became a part of CSSM program and RCH program in 1997. It will continue to provide vaccines for polio, tetanus, diphtheria, tetanus toxoids and pertussis (DPT), diphtheria and tetanus toxoids (DT), measles and tuberculosis. *India was certified as Polio-free country on March 27, 2014.* Pentavalent vaccine (DPT+ Hep B+ Hib) has been expended to all States by April 2015.

Mission Indradhanush: Launched on December 25, 2014 to cover children who are either unvaccinated or partly vaccinated against seven vaccine preventable diseases. The goal is to vaccinate children under 5 by 2020.

- *Essential newborn care*: The main components of essential newborn care are resuscitation of newborn with asphyxia, prevention of hypothermia, prevention of infection, exclusive breastfeeding, and referral of sick newborn.
- *Diarrhea disease control*: India is the first country in the world to introduce low osmolarity [oral rehydration solution (ORS)]. Zinc is being added as an adjunct to ORS for the management of diarrhea. The incidence of diarrhea reduced by provision of safe drinking water.
- *Acute respiratory disease control*: Management of acute respiratory infections (ARI) and prevention of deaths due to pneumonia is now an integral part of RCH program. Peripheral health workers are trained to recognize and treat pneumonia.
- *Prevention and control of vitamin A deficiency in children*: Under this program doses of vitamin A are given to all children under 5 years of age. The first dose (1 lakh units) at 9 months of age, second dose, and subsequent doses after 9 months (200,000 units each) given at 6 months intervals up to 5 years of age. It covers subclinical deficiency of vitamin A.
- *Prevention and control of anemia in children*: To manage anemia, infants from the age of 6 months to 5 years are to receive iron supplements in liquid formulation in doses of 20 mg elemental iron and 100 µg folic acid for 100 days in a year. Children 6–10 years of age will receive 30 mg of elemental iron and 250 µg folic acid for 100 days in a year. Children above this age group would receive iron supplement in the adult dose.

REPRODUCTIVE AND CHILD HEALTH PHASE II

RCH phase II began from April 1, 2005. Under RCH II more flexibility has been given to the states for planning their own interventions for achieving the goals. The major strategies under the second phase of RCH are:

- Essential obstetric care
- Emergency obstetric care
- Strengthening referral system.

Child Health Components

- *Nutrition rehabilitation centers (NRCs)*: NRCs are being setup in the health facilities for inpatient management of severely malnourished children, with counseling of mothers on proper feeding.
- *IMNCI*: IMNCI strategy is one of the main interventions under the RCH II/NRHM.

- *Preservice IMNCI*: It is included in the curriculum of medical colleges of the country.
- *Facility-based IMNCI* (F-IMNCI): This is to empower the health personnel with the skill to manage newborn and childhood illnesses at the country level.
- *Sick newborn care units* (SNCU): As of January 2010 about 267 SNCUs, 1,772 FRUs providing newborn care services and 5,892 PHCs with newborn care corners are operational in India.
- *Home-based newborn care*: It has been developed for the use of ASHA in some of the States.
- *Navjat Shishu Suraksha Karyakram (NSSK)*: Aimed to train health personnel in basic newborn care and resuscitation.

NUTRITION PROGRAMS

Nutrition affects growth and development of a child. Malnutrition is by far the most important single cause of illness and death globally. Malnutrition is a multifaceted problem. Underprivileged section of the society like rural, tribal, and urban slums are worst affected by malnutrition particularly pregnant and lactating women and children are at higher risk. In the community the under nutrition leads to various diseases commonly as:

- Protein energy malnutrition
- Nutritional anemia
- Nutritional blindness
- Iodine deficiency disorders
- Deficiency of vitamins and trace element.

There is definite correlation between nutrition, immunity, and infection and the vicious cycle goes on. Malnutrition alters immunocompetence and increases the risk of infection. The nutrition plays a crucial role in the reproduction of poverty from one generation to the next. The cost of under nutrition in terms of development and productivity are enormous. Government of India has initiated several large-scale supplementary feeding programs aimed at overcoming specific deficiency diseases through various ministries to combat malnutrition as described in **Table 19.6.4**.

A number of programs were implemented in the past from time to time with some success. Some of these are mentioned below:

Table 19.6.4: Nutrition programs in India.

Program	*Ministry*
Vitamin A Prophylaxis Program	Ministry of Health and Family Welfare
Prophylaxis Against Nutritional Anemia	Ministry of Health and Family Welfare
Iodine Deficiency Disorders Control Program	Ministry of Health and Family Welfare
Special Nutrition Program	Ministry of Social Justice and Empowerment
Balwadi Nutrition Program	Ministry of Social Justice and Empowerment
ICDS Program	Ministry of Social Justice and Empowerment
Mid-day Meal Program	Ministry of Education
Mid-day Meal Scheme	Ministry of Human Resources Development

Special Nutrition Program

This program was launched in India in 1970–71. Special nutrition program (SNP) provided supplementary feeding of about 300 calories and 10 g of proteins to children below 6 years of age per day; about 500 calories and 25 g of proteins to expectant and nursing mothers and 600 calories and 20 g of proteins in severely malnourished children for 6 days a week. Vitamin A, iron, and folic acid tablets were also supplied in the last trimester of pregnancy. Nowadays majority of beneficiaries and funds of SNP have been shared by ICDS program. Some of the other major nutritional programs are:

- Tamil Nadu Integrated Nutrition Project (TINP)
- Wheat-based supplementary nutrition program
- World food program
- Applied nutrition program (ANP).

MID-DAY MEAL PROGRAM

The mid-day meal program (MDMP) is also known as "School Lunch Program" or "Noon meal program". It was started in 1961 throughout the country. This national program of nutritional support to primary education formally launched in 1995 and revised in 2004 was aimed at improving:

- School attendance
- Reduce dropouts and
- A beneficial impact on children's nutrition.

Priority is given to children belonging to backward classes, scheduled castes, and scheduled tribe families coming from under privileged backgrounds.

The mid-day meal scheme runs through central assistance provided by Government of India to states by way of free supply of food grain at the rate of 100 g per student per day to provide a cooked mid-day hot meal with minimum 300 calories and 8–12 g of protein content to all children in class I to V for 200 school days or equivalent precooked food or through the supply of 5 kg of wheat/rice per month per child in a family for 10 months. To be eligible the beneficiary has to attend school for 20 days in a month.

Some broad principles should be kept in mind while formulating mid-day meals for school children, like:

- The meal should be a supplement and not a substitute to the home diet.

- The meal should supply at least one-third of the total energy requirement and half of the protein need
- The cost of the meal should be reasonably low
- No complicated cooking process should be involved, it should be easily prepared in the schools
- To reduce the cost of the meal locally available foods should be used as far as possible
- To avoid monotony the menu should be changed frequently.

The major hurdles in the implementation of mid-day meal scheme are frequent interruptions in the supply of raw materials, low budget allocation per beneficiary, lack of effective monitoring and supervision, and wrong identification of beneficiaries. Studies have shown that in the long run we can hope to improve the nutritional status of our children only through improvement in the economic conditions of the community to a level at which families can afford balanced diets; sponsored feeding programs cannot be the permanent answer to the problem.

SCHOOL HEALTH SERVICES

School health services are comprehensive care of the health and well-being of children throughout the school years. It is an economical and powerful means of raising community health. It started in India in 1909 at Baroda in an under developed state because of shortage of resources and insufficient facilities.

The school health committee setup by the Government of India in 1960 recommended that school health service should be an integral part of the general health services which are, largely administered through primary health centers in rural areas.

Health problems of school children vary from one place to another, which mostly includes malnutrition; infectious diseases; intestinal parasites; disease of skin, eye, and ear dental caries. Objectives and components of school health services are listed in **Table 19.6.5**.

School health programs have beneficial impact on students, family, nation, and all people at large. It is the most efficient and cost effective way to improve students' health and their academic performance. Carefully designed and implemented comprehensive health education program can prevent many adverse behaviors like tobacco use, drug abuse, unhealthy dietary practices, unsafe sexual behavior, and physical inactivity. It is also an efficient means of improving pupils' health, life skills, and self-esteem in behavior.

Table 19.6.5: Objectives and components of school health services.

Objectives
Promotion of positive health: • Prevention of diseases • Early diagnosis, treatment, and follow-up • Awakening health consciousness in children • Provision of healthful environment
Components
The different aspects of school health service vary according to local priorities and are manifold, as follows: • Health appraisal of school children and school personnel: regular periodic medical examination; daily morning inspection; health card of students • Remedial measures and follow-up • Prevention of communicable diseases including immunization program • *Healthful school environment*: The location, site, structure, classrooms, furniture, doors and windows, color, lighting, water supply, eating facilities and lavatory arrangements of the school are the parts of environment in which the school child grows and develops. A healthful school environment is necessary for the best emotional, social, and personal health of the student • Nutritional services • *First aid in emergency care*: A fully equipped first aid post should be provided in every school according to regulations of St John Ambulance Association of India • *Mental health*: It is increasingly realized that there is need for counselors and psychologists in schools for guidance of students • Dental care • Eye care • *Health education*: This can cover personal hygiene, environmental health, and family life education. • *Maintenance of school health records*: This will have cumulative information on health aspects of school children and will be useful in evaluating school health programs providing a useful link between home school and community

REVISED NATIONAL TUBERCULOSIS CONTROL PROGRAM

National Tuberculosis Program (NTP) has been in operation since 1962 but Government of India, World Health Organization (WHO) and World Bank together reviewed the NTP in 1992 and a revised strategy for NTP was evolved in a phased manner as Pilot Phase I, Pilot Phase II (approved for a period of 5 years from October 2006 to September 2011), and Pilot Phase III with the salient features of:

- Achievement of at least 85% cure rate of infectious cases through supervised short course chemotherapy involving peripheral health functionaries.
- Augmentation of case finding activities through quality sputum microscopy to detect at least 70% estimated cases.
- *Involvement of NGOs*: Information, education and communication, and improved operational research.

Pediatric Tuberculosis

To address the concern expressed by pediatric experts about the diagnosis and treatment practices for pediatric patients under Revised National Tuberculosis Control Program (RNTCP), in 2003 a consultation of national (Indian Academy of Pediatrics) and international experts on pediatrics and tuberculosis (TB) culminated in national workshop on the "Management of pediatric TB under RNTCP". This workshop resulted in modification of the existing RNTCP guidelines for the diagnosis and treatment of pediatric patients. A major recommendation was that the drugs for pediatric TB cases under RNTCP should be supplied in patient-wise boxes (PWBs). Now, treatment will be based on child's body weight with two generic pediatric PWBs-one for the 6–10 kg weight band and second for the 11–17 kg weight band. Children weighing less than 6 kg will be treated with loose anti-TB drugs. This is to be a global "first" for the RNTCP, as no other directly observed treatment short-course (DOTS) program in the world has such PWDs for the treatment of children with TB. Children have also been identified as a high-risk group. The administration of Bacille Calmette-Guérin (BCG) as an essential component of the universal program of immunization to all newborns and infants up to 9 months of age is important.

NATIONAL LEPROSY ERADICATION PROGRAM

The National Leprosy Control Program (NLCP) has been operation since 1955 as a centrally added scheme to achieve control of leprosy through early detection of cases. During 2007–08, special activities in the form of block and urban leprosy awareness campaigns, providing treatment to newly detected leprosy cases was carried out along with screening of preschool children and youth. All the antileprosy drugs are supplied free of cost to the patients from central government funds.

District leprosy societies have been formed in every district. Rehabilitation of leprosy patients included physical, social, and vocational rehabilitation, where voluntary organizations are playing a major role. The stigma of leprosy as a punishment for past sins is deeply rooted in the Indian psyche. The prejudices and misconceptions of the public as well as sufferers are corrected through health education.

Recently, WHO has announced *enhanced global strategy* for further reducing the disease burden due to leprosy (2011–2015).

NATIONAL MALARIA CONTROL PROGRAM

National Malaria Control Program (NMCP) has been launched in 1958. Since then the program has undergone many changes. A strategic action plan for malaria control in India 2007–2012 has been developed by "Directorate of National Vector Borne Disease Control Program". According to the revised drug policy, there is no scope of presumptive treatment in malaria control. New drug policy in 2013 is another milestone of malaria control activity in India.

India is predominantly characterized by unstable malaria transmission, which is seasonal. The childhood deaths result mainly from cerebral malaria and anemia, which are higher in rural and remote areas. Malaria still continues to pose a major public health threat in India particularly due to *P. falciparum*. PHC is the focal point of all antimalarial activities, which includes epidemiological surveillance, lab examination of blood smear of fever cases, administration of chloroquine to all fever patients, spraying and antilarval operations, radical treatment of malaria positive cases and improvement of the environment.

Malaria control is now incorporated into the health service delivery programs under the umbrella of NRHM, which has been elaborated elsewhere in this book.

NATIONAL FILARIA CONTROL PROGRAM

National Filaria Control Program (NFCP) has been in operation since 1955. The activities were mainly confined to urban areas but now have been extended to rural areas since 1994, managed by the district malaria team and the PHC staff. The current strategy of filariasis control is based on chemotherapy and vector control. In India, the National Health Policy (2002) goal is to "Eliminate Lymphatic Filariasis (ELF) by 2015."

NATIONAL AIDS AND SEXUALLY TRANSMITTED DISEASE CONTROL PROGRAM

National AIDS control program was launched in India in 1987. The Ministry of Health and Family Welfare has set up "National AIDS Control Organization (NACO)" as a separate wing to implement and closely monitor the various components of the program. The aim of the program is:

- To prevent further transmission of HIV
- To decrease morbidity and mortality associated with HIV infection
- To minimize the socioeconomic impact resulting from HIV infection.

The Government of India has initiated programs of prevention and raising awareness under NACP-I (1992–1999) and NACP-II (1999–2000) and now the third National Program Implementation Plan (NACP-III, 2007–2012). The primary goal of NACP-III is to halt and reverse the epidemic in India over the next 5 years for prevention, care, support, and treatment to be achieved through these four stages:

1. Prevention of new infection in high-risk groups and general population.
2. Providing greater care, support, and treatment to a large number of people living with HIV/AIDS.
3. Strengthening the infrastructure system and human resources at the district, state, and national levels.
4. Strengthening a nationwide strategic information management system.

India Developed the Fourth National Program Implementation Plan (NACP-IV) for 5 Years (2012–2017)

Voluntary Counseling and Testing (VCT) is a key entry point for a range of intervention in HIV prevention and care like preventing HIV transmission from mother to child during child birth, referrals for STD treatment, condom promotion, care and support for treatment of opportunistic infections, management of HIV-TB coinfection and more recently for referrals to designated medical center for antiretroviral therapy (ART). VCT is a noncoercive, confidential, and cost-effective approach that provides information, education, and communication to motivate behavior change in HIV-positive individuals.

In 2006–07, voluntary counseling, testing and prevention of parent to child transmission (PPTCT) services were merged to form integrated counseling and testing centers (ICTCs) to expand the coverage.

National pediatric AIDS initiative: NACO launched national pediatric AIDS initiative on 30th November 2006. A guideline for pediatric ART including diagnosis of HIV in children has been developed.

School AIDS education program: This is one of the important activities of NACP focusing toward student youth to raise awareness level and develop a safe and responsible life style. A training module called "Learning for Life" has been prepared and distributed to all the States.

SEXUALLY TRANSMITTED DISEASE CONTROL PROGRAM

Early diagnosis and treatment of STD is now recognized as one of the major strategies to control spread of HIV infections. Most of the recently recognized STDs are now referred to as second generation STDs. The diagnosis and treatment of STD based on syndromic approach (simplified STD treatment) is being introduced at PHC level. The control of STD may be considered under the following heads:

- Initial planning
- Intervention strategies
- Support components
- Monitoring and evaluation.

NATIONAL IODINE DEFICIENCY DISORDER CONTROL PROGRAM

Realizing the magnitude of the problem, the Government of India launched a fully centrally assisted National Goiter Control Program (NGCP) in 1962 which was renamed as National Iodine Deficiency Disorder Control Program (NIDDCP) with a view to cover a wide spectrum of iodine deficiency disorders like mental and physical retardation, deaf mutism, cretinism, still births, abortion, etc. The NIDDCP has three components:

1. Initial survey to identify endemic areas
2. Supply of iodized salt to the identified areas
3. Resurvey after 5 years of continuous supply of iodized salt to assess impact of the measures.

NATIONAL MENTAL HEALTH PROGRAM

The Government of India has launched the National Mental Health Program (NMHP) in 1982, keeping in view the heavy burden of mental illness in the community and the absolute inadequacy of mental health care infrastructure in the country. The objectives of NMHP are:

- Provision of mental health services at district level
- Improvement of facilities in mental hospitals
- Training of trainers of PHC personnel in mental health
- Program for substance use disorders.

NATIONAL CANCER CONTROL PROGRAM

The cancer control program was launched in 1975–76 as a central sector project. It was renamed as National Cancer Control Program (NCCP) in 1985 and revised in 2004. The objectives of NCCP are:

- Primary prevention of cancers by health education
- Secondary prevention by early detection and diagnosis of common cancers such as cancer of cervix, mouth, breast and tobacco-related cancers by screening/self-examination methods.
- Tertiary prevention by strengthening of existing cancer treatment facilities including palliative care in terminal stage.

DRUG DEADDICTION PROGRAM

Globally, "drug culture" is fast making inroads into the lives of young people from all walks of life. The Government of India is signatory to several conventions aimed against spread of narcotic drugs. A Narcotics Co-ordination Committee of secretaries was set up in March 1994, which took important decisions regarding establishment of deaddiction centers. Subsequently an expert committee was set up by Government of India, which recommended the establishment of a National Drug Abuse Monitoring and Information System. The deaddiction centers provide treatment to patients and carry out other functions as envisaged by the expert committee.

NATIONAL DIABETES CONTROL PROGRAM

Diabetes has emerged as a major public health problem in India. The premature morbidity and mortality in most productive phase of life is posing a serious challenge to Indian society and economy. The pilot program interventions, launched on 4th January in 2008 in seven states, have been grouped in three components:

1. Health promotion for the general population.
2. Disease prevention for high-risk group.
3. Assessment of prevalence of risk factors.

NATIONAL PROGRAM FOR CONTROL OF BLINDNESS

India was the first country in the world to launch national level blindness control program. The national program for control of visual impairment and blindness was launched in 1976 as cent percent centrally sponsored which incorporated the earlier Trachoma Control Program (1963). The program was decentralized in 1994–95 with formation of District Blindness Control Society (DBCS) in each district of the country. The objectives of the program are:

- To reduce the backlog of blindness through identification and treatment of blind
- To develop eye care facilities in every district
- To develop human resources for eye care services
- To improve quality of service delivery
- To secure participation of voluntary organizations in eye care
- To enhance community awareness on eye care.

Strategies

The strategy evolved in this program include: developing institutional capacity; developing human resource for eye care; strengthening service delivery; and promoting outreach activities and public awareness. Targets for 11th 5-year plan include development of pediatric ophthalmology units and besides other activities.

Vision 2020: The "Right to Sight" is a global initiative to reduce avoidable (preventable and curable) blindness by the year 2020. India is also committed to this initiative.

BIBLIOGRAPHY

1. Chauhan LS, Arora VK. Management of Pediatric Tuberculosis under the revised national tuberculosis program (Meeting held on 6th and 7th August 2003). Consensus statement. Indian J Pediatr. 2004;71:341-3.
2. Dua AS. Programs for the control of leprosy, tuberculosis and malaria in National Commission on Macroeconomic and Health burden of disease in India. New Delhi: Ministry of Health and Family Welfare, Government of India; 2005.
3. Government of India (2013). A strategic approach to RMNCH+A in India, January 2013, Ministry of Health and Family Welfare, New Delhi.
4. Government of India (2013). National AIDS Control Programme Phase IV (2012-2017). New Delhi: Ministry of Health and Family Welfare; 2017.
5. Government of India (2013). Operational Guidelines, Rashtriya Bal Swasthya Karyakram (RBSK). New Delhi: Ministry of Health and Family Welfare; 2013.
6. Government of India. Statement on National Health Policy. New Delhi: Ministry of Health and Family Welfare; 1983.
7. Park K. Text book of Preventive and Social Medicine, 21st edition. Jabalpur: Banarsidas Bhanot; 2015.
8. United States Agency for International Development. MCHIP (2014), RMNCH+A Strategy. Washington: USAID; 2014.
9. Walia BNS, Vani SN. National Health Programs. IAP Textbook of Pediatrics, 3rd edition. New Delhi: Jaypee Brothers Medical Publishers (P) Ltd.; 2006. pp. 155-81.
10. WHO. The World Health Report 2006. Working Together for Health. Geneva: WHO; 2006.

19.7 Rights of the Child

Swati Y Bhave, Chhaya S Prasad

INTRODUCTION

The United Nations (UN) Convention on the Rights of the Child (UNCRC) is a guiding instrument for implementing all rights for all children up to the age of 18 years. There are other important documents related to child rights. The national policy for children states that children are supreme assets of India and we have to provide them with the four basic rights:

1. Right to survival
2. Right to development
3. Right to good health and education, and
4. Protection from abuse and exploitation and most importantly, to participate in the decisions that have an impact on their own lives.

Every child has a right to a formal identity, including birth registration, the right to nationality, and the right to be cared for by their parents. Health workers, teachers, police personnel, social workers and others who work with children should be well equipped with the skills and ability to identify and also have the authority to respond to child abuse in any form. Media has a unique role to play in ensuring that the rights of children are respected and that violators are brought to justice. India was amongst the 61 countries who first signed the child rights and child protection (CRC) on January 26, 1990, the opening day of the UN general assembly session, India ratified the CRC in 1992.

The development index of a country depends on the quality of the human resources. Children are the future of this country and thus there is a greater responsibility on part of the state to ensure a proper development of children of this country and to provide adequate safe environment.

CHILD RIGHTS IN INDIA

With more than a third of its population below the age of 18 years, India has the largest child population in the world. India has made some significant commitments toward ensuring the basic rights of children. Several constitutional provisions protect children in India. Various 5-year plans of India have progressively added more schemes for welfare and protection of child. Despite these laws, policies and commitments, the actual situation for India's children *vis-à-vis* health, education, early childhood care and protection is still not satisfactory.

Who is a Child?

The UN Convention on the Rights of the Child, 1989 (Article I) defined the child as below 18 years of age. There are various definitions of child in various laws in India:

- Constitution of India, Article 24: Any one below the age of 14 years.
- For obtaining medical care in a government health facility, a child is defined as one who is less than 12 years of age.
- During the initial census of India, persons below the age of 14 years were defined as children and most of the government programs on children are still targeted for the age-group below 14 years.
- The legal definition of child varies from 7 years to 18 years of age as evident from the various laws in India, but after the introduction of the Juvenile Justice Care and Protection of Children Act, for all practical purposes, a child is considered as a person below 18 years.

Laws for Protection of Child Rights

- *Criminal Law (Indian Penal Code, 1860)*: Nothing is an offence, which is done by a child under 7 years of age (section 82). Nothing is an offence, which is done by a child above 7 years of age under 12, who has not attained sufficient maturity of understanding to judge the nature and consequence of his conduct on that occasion (section 83).
- *Family Law (Child Marriage Restraint Act, 1929)*: "Child" means a person who, if a male, has not completed 21 years of age, and if a female, has not completed 18 years of age.
- *Labour Laws (Apprentice Act, 1951), Factories Act, 1948*: It states that a person shall not be qualified to be engaged as a worker unless he/she is not less than 14 years of age.
- *The Child Labour (Prohibition and Regulation) Act, 1986:* "Child" means a person who has not completed his 14 years of age.
- *Mines (Amendment) Act, 1983:* No person below 18 years of age shall be allowed to work in any mine or part thereof.
- *The Child Labour (Prohibition and Regulation) Act, 1986*: Prohibit Employment of children below 14 years in hazardous occupations and processes and also regulating the working conditions of children in other employment. In the last 5 years, the number of hazardous "occupations" listed in the schedule of the act has increased from 7 to 13 and "processes" from 18 to 57. The notice for prohibiting employment of children as domestic servants and in tea shops and *dhabas*, etc. is with effect from 10th October, 2006.
- *Factories Act, 1948:* No child who has not completed his 14 years shall be required or allowed to work in any factory.

Special Provisions for Children According to the Indian Constitution

- *Article 21(a)* of the Constitution states that all children between the ages of 6 and 14 should be provided with free and compulsory education.
- To ensure that children are not abandoned by their parents/guardians, *Section 317 of IPC,* provides imprisonment extending up to 7 years for whoever exposes or leaves their child in any place with the intention of wholly abandoning the child.
- *Section 363 of IPC* provides the punishment extending up to 7 years and fine for the offense of kidnaping any child from India or from lawful guardianship.
- *Section 369 of IPC* provides punishment for up to 7 years for whoever kidnaps or abducts any child under the age of 10 years with the intention of taking dishonestly any movable property.
- *Section 363A of IPC* asserts that kidnapping or maiming a minor for purposes of begging is a criminal offense under IPC and the offender is liable to imprisonment of up to 10 years.

The Juvenile Justice (Care and Protection of Children) Act, 2000

This is a comprehensive legislation to provide justice and opportunities to children of India for their growth and development. "Juvenile" or "child" means a person who has not completed 18 years of age, the Act is based upon the provisions of the Indian Constitution and four broad rights of the UN convention on the rights of the child including right to survival, protection, development, and participation. The Act came into force with effect from 1st April, 2001.

The Act calls for establishment of the Juvenile Justice Boards (JJBs) for adjudication and disposition of matters related to juveniles; and Child Welfare Committees (CWC) to take care of children in need of care and protection.

Certain amendments have been effected in the Act recently. One of the important amendments includes the definition of adoption and that no juvenile in conflict with law can be placed under imprisonment for any term, which may extend to imprisonment for life. The Act has, therefore, been made more child-friendly to protect children from exploitation and violence as provided in the World Fit for Children (WFFC) targets.

CHILDLINE

This is a national helpline for children in distress. It is India's first 24-hour service for children. It operates through a national toll free number 1098 and responds to the urgent and emergency needs of children such as medical assistance, shelter, protection from abuse and exploitation, assistance in child missing cases, repatriation, sponsorship, etc.

Aims and Objectives of Convergence of Child Helpline Services Provided by Various Departments

- To have a structured approach to respond appropriately to a child in need of care and protection.
- To understand the importance of networking with other organizations working for child protection and child wellbeing.
- To understand the Helpline protocol.

LEGISLATION FOR RIGHTS OF CHILDREN IN INDIA

National Charter for Children, 2003

This covers the following:

- To secure for every child its inherent right to be a child and enjoy a healthy and happy childhood
- Survival, life, and liberty
- Protection from economic exploitation and all forms of abuse
- Protection of the girl child
- Care, protection, welfare of children of marginalized, and disadvantaged communities and
- Ensuring child-friendly procedures.

Other important aspects addressed are:

- Promoting high standards of health and nutrition
- Assuring basic minimum needs and security—play and leisure, early childhood care for survival, growth and development, free and compulsory primary education, protection from economic exploitation and all forms of abuse, protection of the girl child, empowering adolescents, equality, freedom of expression, freedom to seek and receive information, freedom of association and peaceful assembly, and
- Strengthening family ensuring child-friendly procedures.

All matters and procedures relating to children, viz. judicial, administrative, educational or social, should be child-friendly. All procedures laid down under the juvenile justice system for children in conflict with law and for children in need of special care and protection shall also be child-friendly.

National Plan of Action for Children, 2005

This covers all rights to all children up to the age of 18 years. The action plan includes the following:

- System of identification, investigation, reporting, follow-up, and referral of children at risk
- Care, protection, and developmental programs for all children
- Child beggars
- Facilitate convergence with related ministries
- Rehabilitate all children in need of care and protection
- Professional counseling services
- Children affected by disasters
- Developmental and protective services to children of sex workers and prisoners
- Children are not used in armed conflict, and
- Prevent the use of children, including adolescents.

The guiding principles of the National Plan of Action for Children, 2005 are:

- To regard the child as an asset and a person with human rights
- To address issues of discrimination emanating from biases of gender, class, caste, race, religion, and legal status in order to ensure equality
- To accord utmost priority to the most disadvantaged, poorest of the poor and least served child in all policy and programmatic interventions
- To recognize the diverse stages and settings of childhood, and address the needs of each, providing to all children the entitlements that fulfill their rights and meet their needs in each situation.

National Initiative for Protection of Children

The National Initiative for Child Protection (NICP) is a campaign initiated by Ministry of Social Justice and

Empowerment which aims to place child's rights on every agenda through partnership with allied systems for child protection and promotion of child's rights. The allied systems are police, health-care system, justice (juvenile) system, education system, transport system, labor department, media, department of telecommunications, corporate sector, elected representatives, and all of us. The NICP will be implemented at district levels through state governments. It will design a curriculum that will be incorporated into the various training programs of academic institutions of the allied systems.

The Commissions for Protection of Child Rights Act, 2006

India has a National Commission for Protection of Child Rights (NCPCR) and Child Courts. There are also commissions at state level. This ensures speedy trial of offences against children or of violation of child rights and matters connected thereto.

The aims of this commission are to spread awareness of child rights; review all the laws and other documents for children; setup a mechanism to hear complaints about violation of child rights; undertake and promote research in the field of child rights; and examine the situation of children. The powers of the commission are similar to a Civil Court under Civil Procedure Code (CPC) and they can forward a matter to a magistrate to be tried under Criminal Procedure Code (CrPC).

The National Commission for Children, 2007

The NCPCR was set up in March 2007 under an Act of Parliament. The commission's mandate is to ensure that all laws, policies, programs, and administrative mechanisms followed in India are in consonance with the child.

Right to Free and Compulsory Education, 2010

The law came into effect in the whole of India except the state of Jammu and Kashmir from 1st April, 2010. This also includes children with disabilities. Subsequently, the 86th Constitutional Amendment Act, 2002 has inserted a new Article 21(8), which provides for free and compulsory education to children of the age-group of 6–14 years being a right to education. The same amendment act provides for amendment of the Article 45 as directive principle of the state policy to provide provision for Early Childhood Care and Protection Bill up to the age of 6 years. It also made a fundamental duty of parents and guardians under new Article 51(a) to provide opportunities for education to children between the ages of 6 and 14 years.

PROTECTION OF ABUSED CHILDREN

Abuse and neglect are forms of maltreatment of a child. Abuse can occur by inflicting harm, or by failing to act to prevent harm. Children may be abused in a family or in an institutional or community setting; by those known to them or, more rarely, by a stranger. They may be abused by an adult or adults or another child or children.

The political will and professional commitment, particularly from the health sector and the Government of India is the most vital in reducing the suffering from abuse and violence in children and providing adequate safe environment for potential growth.

POCSO ACT, 2012

The responsibility of supporting children who have been sexually abused should be embraced by the whole community, but it is the professionals that work in this field who play an important role in enabling the healing process.

The NCPCR Guidelines are therefore aimed at various professionals involved in providing services to the child and other affected persons including his/her family. Their objective is to foster better response mechanisms involving coordination amongst these professionals, so as to result in the evolution of a multisectoral, multidisciplinary approach that will go a long way in achieving the objectives of the Protection of Children from Sexual Offences Act (POCSO Act), 2012.

The POCSO Act, 2012 was formulated in order to effectively address sexual abuse and sexual exploitation of children. The POCSO Act, 2012 received the President's assent on 19th June 2012 and was notified in the Gazette of India on 20th June, 2012.

The POCSO Act should be read by all physicians in details as it is now mandatory to report sexual abuse cases. Please refer to Chapter 19.10 Sexual Abuse and POCSO Act for details.

Mandatory Reporting

When a doctor has reason to suspect that a child has been or is being sexually abused, he/she is required to report this to the appropriate authorities (i.e., the police or the relevant person within his/her organization who will then have to report it to the police). Failure to do this would result in imprisonment of up to 6 months, with or without fine.

The Act says that no person shall incur any liability, whether civil or criminal for giving the information in good faith.

Role of Medical Professionals in the Context of the POCSO Act, 2012

Doctors have a dual role to play in terms of the POCSO Act, 2012. They are in a position to detect that a child has been or is being abused [for example, if they come across a child with a sexually transmitted disease (STD)]; they are also often the first point of reference in confirming that a child has indeed been the victim of sexual abuse.

Children with Special Needs

The Act reminds the professionals' needs to recognize that the child may have also some degree of cognitive disability: intellectual disability, mental illness, developmental disabilities, traumatic brain injury, etc. Note however that not all developmental disabilities affect cognitive ability (e.g., cerebral palsy may result in physical rather than mental impairment).

CHILDREN'S COURT

These have been established for speedy trial of offences against children or of violation of child's rights. In each district the court of sessions appoints a special public prosecutor.

Integrated Child Protection Scheme, 2006

This is a centrally-sponsored scheme run by the Ministry of Women and Child Development. The aim of Integrated Child Protection Scheme (ICPS) is based on the cardinal principles of "protection of child rights" and "best interests of the child." It covers (1) punitive measure against perpetrators of abuse and crimes and (2) rehabilitation for all children in need of care and protection. The target groups are children in need of care and protection; children in conflict with the law; children in contact with law; and any other vulnerable child.

Integrated Child Protection Scheme brings together multiple existing child protection schemes of the ministry under one comprehensive umbrella, and integrates additional interventions for protecting children and preventing harm.

The ICPS also promises to provide a powerful platform to promote government partnerships with civil society actors and international organizations.

The scheme plans to setup a child protection data management system to formulate and implement effective intervention strategies and monitor their outcomes.

BIBLIOGRAPHY

1. Agarwal K, Dalwai S, Galagali P, et al. Recommendations on recognition and response to child abuse and neglect in the Indian setting. Indian Pediatr. 2010;47(6):493-504.
2. Childline India Foundation (2000). Juvenile Justice Care and Protection of Children Act in India. [online] Available from: http://www.childlineindia.org.in/Juvenile-Justice-Care-and-Protection-of-Children-Act-2000.htm. [Accessed November, 2018].
3. Infochange India (2005). Child rights in India and status of children in India. [online] Available from: http://infochangeindia.org/agenda/child-rights-in-india/status-of-children-in-india.html. [Accessed November, 2018].
4. Resource Book for Commissions for Protection of Child Rights - Developed by National Commission for Protection of Child Rights with support from UNICEF, India, 1st edition. Published in December, 2016.
5. Resource Book. First National Conference on Child Abuse for Multidisciplinary Professionals (COCAMP 2004). Chennai: Indian Council for Child Welfare, Tamil Nadu and Sri Ramchandra Medical College and Research Institute; 2004.
6. Shagun (2009). Bare Act of Right to Education Act, 2009 and Model Rules under the Right to Education Act, 2009. [online] Available from: http://ssashagun.nic.in/docs/RTI_Model_Rules.pdf. [Accessed November, 2018].
7. Shagun (2011). Sarva Shiksha Abhiyan, framework for Implementation, published in 2011. [online] Available from: http://ssashagun.nic.in/docs/SSA-Frame-work.pdf. [Accessed November, 2018].
8. Study on Child Abuse, India (2007). Ministry of Women and Child Development, Government of India, Delhi, 2007. [online] Available from: http://wcd.nic.in/childabuse.pdf. [Accessed November, 2018].
9. The Integrated Child Protection Scheme (ICPS). Ministry of Women and Child Development, Govt. of India. [online] Available from: http://wcd.nic.in/icpsmon/home1.aspx. [Accessed November, 2018].
10. UNICEF (2005). Convention on Rights of the Child. [online] Available from: http://www.unicef.org/crc/index_30229.html. [Accessed November, 2018].

Contd...

Feature/ Parenting style	***Authoritarian***	***Permissive/Indulgent***	***Authoritative***	***Neglectful***
Opinionated	Yes	Nil	Not opinionated but explains possible opinions that can be formed by certain behaviors	Not applicable
Care of children	Care is complete, all acts of service done in a methodical but in an impersonal manner. Attempt to self-care is not encouraged. Dependency is seen as obedience and subordination	Very good with personal attention to begin with to the level of not allowing the child to self-learn skills; later years with scare that the child might scold the parents for lapses	Very good with personal attention, involving children in inculcation of habits of self-care very early in life, generation of independence and preparation of the children to survive without the support of parents is practiced	Care is not adequate and children usually fend for themselves with breach in self-care and hygiene
Appreciation and encouragement	Rarely offered	Offered more than necessary as the parents are scared at consequences if not offered	Offered in right doses at right occasions	Not offered as the parents are rarely aware of accomplishments
Criticism	Liberal and frequent	Nil	Yes, but with explanations and ways to rectify	Rarely take note of deviance in behaviors or actions
Outcome in children	Submissive or rebellious, lack of self-control and self-esteem and self-confidence as they have been controlled always. Performance anxiety is high and accomplishments are less	Self-driven, anxious at outcomes as they have not been exposed to challenges appropriately with guidance from parents; Self-esteem low with reduced confidence at new activities	Self-motivated, self-disciplined, self-confident, children with high self-esteem and frequent success in many tasks	Feel that they lack direction or may latch on to people to receive direction, which may be right or wrong
Children's perception about the parents	Strict, controlling parents who gave no space for growth	Ineffective parents who offered no guidance and direction	Excellent parents who were available always but at the same time encouraged independence	Nonavailable parents who were totally away in mind, body, and actions

for prolonged periods of time. This style is annoying as it is difficult to understand the persons' thoughts.

- Assertive style of communication is by far the best style used by authoritative parents who express their intent with firmness. This style entertains mutual respect and helps in effective parenting.

THE ROLE OF THE FAMILY CONTEXT IN THE DEVELOPMENT OF EMOTION REGULATION

Emotion regulation consists of internal and external processes involved in initiating, maintaining, and modulating the occurrence, intensity, and expression of emotions. Emotional regulation helps in the socialization process that happens from infancy to adulthood by modulating ones expression of emotions by understanding the actual emotions, with respect to tone, intensity, and dynamics like duration of the emotional experience **(Flowchart 19.8.1)**.

- *Internal processes* would be child-specific factors like temperament of the child, child's responsiveness or reactivity to external cues, stage of development, individual thoughts about emotions, and the associated physiological responses to each of the emotion.
- *External processes* would depend on the emotional climate of the family and on the specific characteristics of the parents and the parent figures. Emotional climate of the family is further determined by the status of the marital relationship, parenting styles practiced, attachment patterns established, emotional coaching by parents like "When you are angry take a deep breath etc.", emotional expressivity of parents, social referencing like adapting the responses of significant others at similar situation,

Flowchart 19.8.1: Factors determining the emotional regulation of the children in the family context.

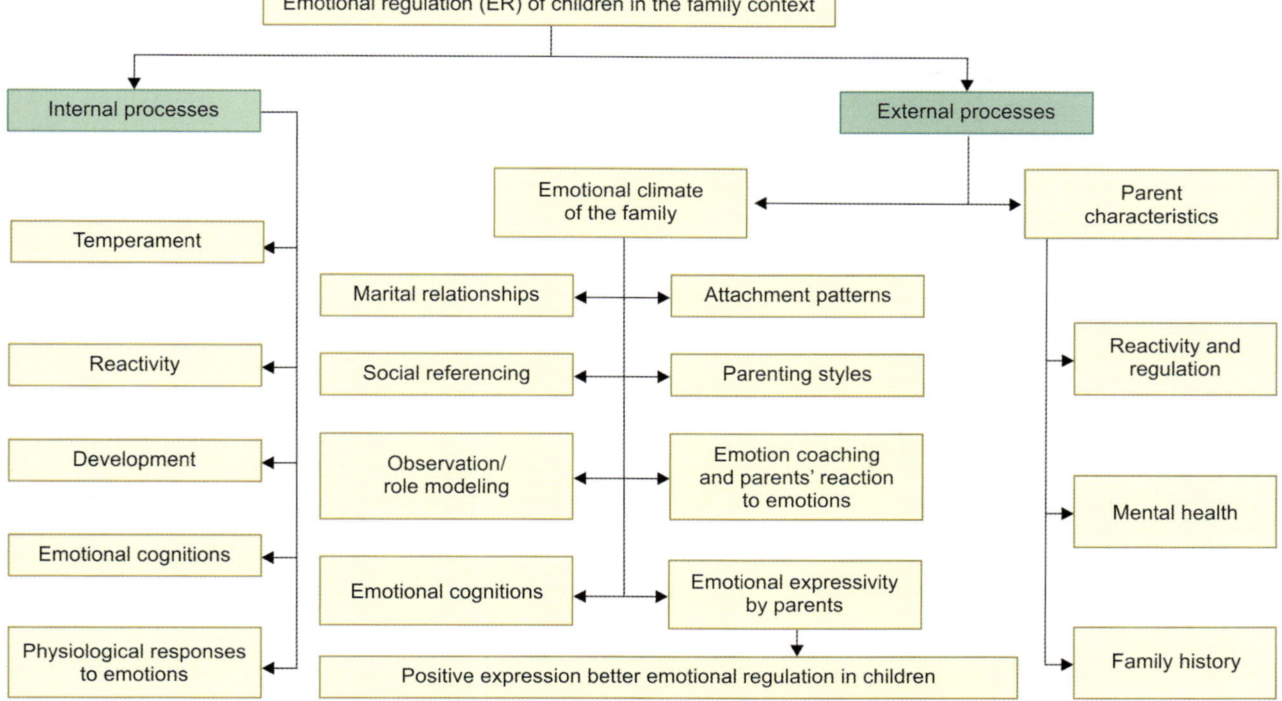

parental role modeling, the predominant emotional state in the family, etc.

INFLUENCE OF PARENTING STYLES

Parent-specific factors are related to the mental health of the parents and the kind of emotional regulation they have imbibed from their parents. With increasing age the dependency on parents for emotional regulation comes down but the influence of peer group intensifies.

Influence of parenting styles and parenting practices on certain aspects of growth and development in children and adolescents are being studied extensively. The previous endorsement of authoritarian parenting to inculcate certain qualities and habits in children is being replaced by new understanding that are encouraging parents to practice authoritative parenting styles.

Eating Practices

In a study on the influence of parenting styles and the consumption of fruits and vegetables by preschoolers, authoritative parenting style emerged as a better style in ensuring cooperation. This has been attributed to the utilization of teachable moments by parents to give information on the benefits of consumption of fruits and vegetables, practical methods like role modeling by both parents, firmness in maintaining discipline with respect to eating schedules, restriction of availability of junk foods within the household, and limiting accessibility to the same outside the home and enhancement in the availability of fruits and vegetables at all times of the day.

Similarly children with overweight and obesity are less common in families with authoritative parents.

Physical Activity

Though studies on the influence of parenting style on physical activity are not many, the knowledge gained has been quiet different. Children's participation in sports, acquisition of skills in a game and excelling in the tournaments has been more commonly associated with permissive style of parenting. Logistic support to continue sports activities is higher in households with permissive parents.

Externalizing Behaviors

Externalizing behaviors like usage of aggression and violence is more common in families with authoritarian style as the children learn by observing parents. It is also widely seen in children brought up by permissive parents because the parents might have failed to establish their role in disciplining between 2 and 6 years when the externalizing behaviors begin and reduce respectively. Authoritative parents are quiet clear about establishing their role and achieving cooperation from children as they practice methods of differential reinforcement, which reduces the negative behaviors.

MINDFUL PARENTING

Being mindful as a parent means that the parent should have the knowledge of

- Who they are
- What is their expectation from the child
- Whether the expectation is age and developmentally appropriate for the child
- Where this expectation comes from
- Whether it is from what they received as a kid from their own parents
- What is the deep-seated emotion surrounding the expectation
- Whether it is fear, sadness, worry, anxiety or pain about being incapable of teaching the child the best
- Whether the underlying emotion is disappointment with the child which gets expressed as anger
- What is the need of the child at that moment
- Whether the need is physical like sleep or hunger, emotional like being sad or frustrated at lack of skills or social like wanting a hug of appreciation and kiss of nurturance
- What is the predominant emotion of the child
- Whether the child is doing something due to ignorance
- What can be the ways used to help the child
- What words to use to convey the same to the child in a way the child feels helped and not judged or ridiculed or criticized
- When is the best time to explain to the child
- Willful expression of love and compassion in a manner that is needed and understood by the child.

Mindfulness in all actions that an adult carries out would help the adult to respond to any situation keeping in mind their deep-seated emotion and not react with emotions that surface. Imparting this to parents at every meeting with the pediatrician is likely to help parents inculcate empathy for the child and feel fulfilled as being an effective parent.

PARENTING PROGRAMS

Inculcation of authoritative parenting skills in parents is gradually being adapted in the developing world based on the evidence generated by the developed world. Indian Academy of Pediatrics has also created the Happy Parenting Program in 2010 where a self-training module titled, "Stepping Stones–Paediatricians' Recipe for Happy Parenting" along with a CD containing slides for introspective learning have been posted to all its members who are now equipped to train the parents.

RESEARCH OPTIONS IN THE INDIAN CONTEXT

As of now the parenting styles practiced in India are diverse and in multiple combinations as the parenting responsibility is not limited to biological parents only. The recent generations of parents who are evolving from a collectivistic society to individualistic practices are usually not consistent with the parenting style. Hence, knowledge about the parenting received and the styles being practiced can be accessed from various groups of urban, semi-urban, rural parents by using qualitative research methods and then arrive at new hypotheses for further research.

CONCLUSION

Parenting is a science that is based on human development, temperament, and interpersonal relationships. Use of warm, responsive, firm authoritative parenting style with mindfulness helps in bringing up children as healthy, self-confident, self-reliant, and independent adults. Pediatricians can start introducing parenting principles during well baby visits when parents are usually receptive. Parenting programs can be included as a primary prevention activity to prevent behavior disorders in children.

BIBLIOGRAPHY

1. Berge JM, Wall M, Neumark-Sztainer D, et al. Parenting style and family meals: Cross-sectional and 5-year longitudinal associations. J Am Diet Assoc. 2010;110(7):1036-42.
2. Buschgens CJ, van Aken MA, Swinkels SH, et al. Externalizing behaviors in preadolescents: Familial risk to externalizing behaviors and perceived parenting styles. Eur Child Adolesc Psychiatry. 2010;19:567-75.
3. Chang L, Schwartz D, Dodge KA, et al. Harsh parenting in relation to child emotion regulation and aggression. J Fam Psychol. 2003;17(4):598-606.
4. Darling N. Parenting style and its correlates. [online] Available from: http://www.kidneeds.com/diagnostic_categories/articles/parentcorrelates.pdf. [Accessed November, 2018].
5. Lahey BB, Van Hulle CA, Keenan K, et al. Temperament and parenting during the first year of life predict future child conduct problems. J Abnorm Child Psychol. 2008;36(8):1139-58.
6. Morris AS, Silk JS, Steinberg L, et al. The role of the family context in the development of emotion regulation. Soc Dev. 2007;16(2):361-88.
7. O'Connor TM, Hughes SO, Watson KB, et al. Parenting practices are associated with fruit and vegetable consumption in pre-school children. Public Health Nutr. 2010;13(1):91-101.
8. Spijkers W, Jansen DE, de Meer G, et al. Effectiveness of a parenting programme in a public health setting: A randomized controlled trial of the positive parenting programme (Triple P) level 3 versus care as usual provided by the preventive child healthcare. BMC Public Health. 2010;10:131.
9. Ugra D, Yamuna S. Stepping Stones: Paediatricians' Recipe for Happy Parenting. Mumbai: Indian Academy of Paediatrics; 2010.

19.9 Child Abuse and Neglect

Meenakshi N Mehta

INTRODUCTION

We are guilty of many errors and many faults
But our worst crime is abandoning the children
Neglecting the fountain of life
Many of the things we need can wait
The ***child*** *cannot.*
Right now is the time his bones are being formed
His blood is being made and
His senses are being developed
To him we cannot answer
"Tomorrow" His name is "Today".

—Gabriela Mistral, Nobel Laureate Poet, Chile

Children are the principle assets of any country and their future well-being to become healthy, educated, and economically independent citizens depends on their families, society and the government.

India is home to nearly 19% of the world's children. More than a one-third of the country's population, i.e. around 440 million is below 18 years of age. Constituting more than 40% of the total population of 132 million (2017), each year around one half of all deaths are attributed to under nutrition translating into loss of 3 million young lives. In 2018, the under 5 mortality rate (U5MR) is 43, infant mortality rate (IMR) is 34 and 36% are underweight (UW). The immunization coverage was 62% for all basic vaccines (2015–16). The proportion of population with access to drinking water and rural sanitation coverage in 2016–17 was 89.60% and 63.68%, respectively.

India has a double jeopardy. On one hand there is advancing economy, improving technology, new medical interventions, and research in health care and rapid transportation, yet on the other hand the child population faces many problems. Thus, a sizeable number of children are underprivileged, deprived of their basic rights to survival, shelter, health, nutrition, education, protection, and social status. Those from poorer families with denied opportunities for daily survival are vulnerable to exploitation and abuse; they are forced to work in a variety of sectors organized or unorganized to support their families and themselves. Unknowingly quite a few resort to antisocial activities. Childhood is too often lost in a period of insecurity and deprivation. According to one assumption 40% of these cohort children are in need of care and protection.

Furthermore, children in all societies in the process of their normal upbringing are often neglected, maltreated, abused intentionally or unknowingly by their parents and caretakers as well. Child abuse—physical, sexual or emotional is a significant community problem of enormous gravity and unconscionable crime. The norms of child rearing differ culturally with wide differences between conservative and advanced societies. Child abuse, although an old phenomenon, has been the subject of serious societal concern in recent years. Although earlier known in economically advantaged nations, now it has spread globally, more so in disadvantaged and endangered communities engulfing thousands of children, resulting in street children, refugees, children in armed conflicts, orphans of acquired immune deficiency syndrome (AIDS), professional sex workers, disabled children and those trapped in trafficking, sale and kidnapping. Child abuse is a worldwide social and public health problem with no social, racial or ethnic bounds and exerts a multitude of short and long-term effects on children.

The convention on Rights of the Child was adopted by UN General Assembly in 1990. It has been ratified by 191 countries including India. Child rights, like other human rights, are globally applicable. However, the needs and the problems of children are very different in South Asian countries, as indeed in many developing countries, than those in high-income countries in Europe, USA and other regions. There are great disparities in socioeconomic and educational status within a country. A small variable proportion of population enjoys affluence where the families are not constrained by finances in taking care of their children. The majority, however belong to low economic status, limited education and inadequate access to whatever societal support is available. This is worsened if the family size is large. Poor, illiterate parents often cannot take adequate care of their children and moreover may not seek, or may be denied, benefits of various government sponsored child welfare programs. Despite various constitutional provisions, legislations and policies India has failed in the commitment to look after the basic rights of her children. Child rights must be prioritized, problems to be identified and appropriate actions to be undertaken to address them.

DEFINITION AND NOMENCLATURE

Since the first term "battered baby syndrome" given by Henry Kempe for chronic repetitive injuries due to abuse, the definition of child abuse and neglect (CAN) has been broadened to include any problem resulting from lack of reasonable care and protection of child and adolescents by their parents, guardians or caretakers. "Child abuse," "child neglect," "child maltreatment," "physical abuse," "child battering," "Silverman's syndrome," "illegitimate child syndrome," "parental dysfunction" and most recently "nonaccidental injury" (NAI) are terms often used interchangeably. The distinction in child abuse and child neglect is probably the element of deliberateness in the former. WHO has defined "child abuse" as a violation of basic human rights of a child, constituting all forms of physical, emotional ill treatment, neglect or negligent treatment, commercial or other exploitation, resulting in actual harm or potential harm to the child's health, survival, development or dignity in the context of a relationship of responsibility, trust or power **(Table 19.9.1)**.

Although the exact etiology of child abuse is not known, it is thought to be due to interaction of three primary factors as shown in **Tables 19.9.2 and 19.9.3**.

Various forms of child exploitation are shown in **Table 19.9.4**.

Table 19.9.1: Forms of child abuse and neglect.

Physical	Cuts, bruises, hematoma, fracture, head injury, visceral injury, burns, ophthalmic injury, blunt trauma, injury due to slapping, pushing, squeezing, kicking, shaking, "shaken baby syndrome" **(Fig. 19.9.1)**
Nutritional	Failure to thrive, marasmus, stunting, deprivation of varying severity
Sexual	Rape, incest, fondling, pornography, prostitution, involvement in sex-related activities, exhibitionism, coercion and female feticide and infanticide, neglect of girl child and female discrimination—deprivation from food, education, clothing, entertainment, love and social status and early girl child marriage
Behavioral	Wariness of adult contact, aggressiveness/ withdrawal, apprehension when other children or adults cry/shout, prefers to stay away from home as much as possible, excessive compliance, attaching readily to strangers, frequent absenteeism and unwillingness to go to school, not reporting injury to parents or giving inappropriate explanation of an injury
Emotional	Humiliation, depression, extremely low self-esteem, passive, withdrawn, tearful, apathetic, aggressive or demanding behavior, constant high anxiety, poor social and interpersonal skills, persistent habit disorders such as sucking, biting, or rocking, self-destructive behavior, and unexplained academic delays, comparison with siblings/other children, girl child neglect/ discrimination
Nonaccidental poisoning	Opium
Abandonment/ desertion	Newborns, infants, children deserted
Substance abuse	Drugs which alleviate mood or create illusions, happiness, e.g. cocaine, marijuana, etc. and alcohol and allied substances
Medical neglect	By the professionals and health care personnel dealing with the medical management of the child and if neglected could be potentially fatal

DIAGNOSIS

- *When to suspect child abuse*: Child abuse is not an obvious diagnosis at initial consultation. One should suspect child abuse, in all cases of injuries at uncommon distribution sites or having unusual pattern: suspected if the child victims and the parents' history is at variance or if the features do not match with known conditions/disease/ disorder.
- Clinical manifestations are bizarre and often symmetrical. Child is drowsy, unconscious or emotionally scared. He/ she is too shocked to reveal anything. Importantly, the injuries are more serious/grievous than expected from the given history.

Effects of Child Abuse and Neglect

Child abuse can have severe and deleterious short- and long-term effects on cognitive, socioeconomic, and behavioral development **(Tables 19.9.5)**.

PROVISIONS FOR SAFEGUARD/CHILD PROTECTION IN INDIA

The Indian constitution contains provisions for safe-guarding the interests of children and protecting them against cruelty and exploitation. The provisions are detailed in the various articles: 15[3], 39[1], 39[e and f], 24, 45. Indian Penal Code (IPC) sections 363a, 365, 366, 366a, 366b, 370, 372, 373, 376 and national policies namely "the National Policy for Children, 1974, "the National Policy on Education 1986,"the Child Labor Policy, 1987," "the National Decadal Plan of Action for Girl Child, 1991–2000," "the National Initiative for Child Protection (NICP)" through the allied system, "the National Charter for Children, 2003 and various acts such as Juvenile Justice Act, 1986, Child Marriage Restrain Act [amendment]. All deal with comprehensive welfare of children of India, right from survival and development, health and health services,

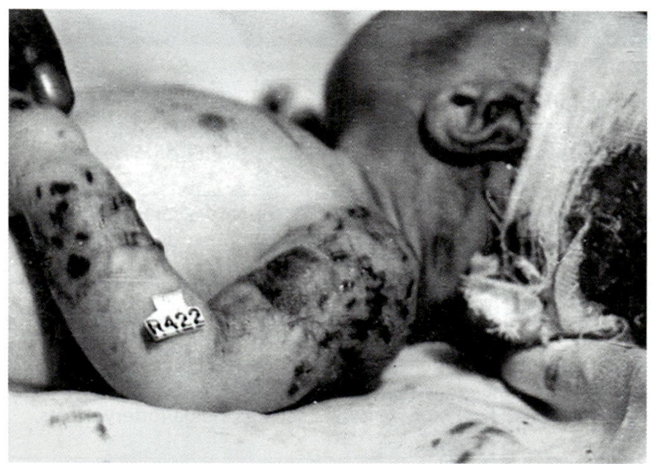

Fig. 19.9.1: Severely-injured child found by police with multiple injuries of left upper limb, neck, and scalp.

Table 19.9.2: Factors affecting child abuse and neglect (CAN).

Sociocultural factors	
Family norms	Values and norms of discipline and physical punishment
Family structure	Number of members in the family, joint/ nuclear family, socioeconomic status
Family and situational stresses	Poverty, illiteracy, unemployment, alcohol abuse, isolation, poor housing, caste system and landlessness
Parent-child relationship	Punitive child rearing style, excess/unwanted children, role reversal
Economic	Lack of economic opportunities, rural urban migration
Child producing stresses	
Disabled	Mentally retarded, physically handicapped, disabled, deformed, chronically ill
Behavior	Hyperactive and behaviorally different, strong willed
Difficult	Temperamental
Types	Too many children, girls, premature infants, foster child, boys twice more common than girls to be victims of physical abuse
Parent producing stresses	
Psychological	Low self-esteem, depression, character disorder, psychiatric illness
Past experiences	Unhappy childhood experiences, neglected/ abused as a child, emotionally deprived
Addictions	Parental substance abuse
Sex of the child	Disappointment over the sex of the child
Child rearing	Ignorance of child rearing, unrealistic expectations
Familial violence	Violence among adult family members

Table 19.9.3: Predictions—known to correlate and precipitate child abuse.

The parents	
Age	Young mother, age less than 18 years
Own experiences	Abused/experienced family disruption in their childhood
Anxiety	Lack of family support, unreasonably fearful of caring for their child
Expectations	Have unreasonable expectations of their child and treat him/her as much older child
Temperament	Poor impulse control
Rigid discipline	May be generally rigid/authoritarian, e.g. incidence of abuses more than in some strict religious groups and families of military personnel
Aggressive parent	Usually the father may be aggressively psychopathic and assault others within/without his family, psychiatrically ill
The child	
Unwanted	Unwanted, denial of pregnancy, request for abortion, adoption
After birth attachment	Separated from mother at birth, because of prematurity, maternal illness, preventing/ interrupting initial attachment with mother
Emotional	Disappointing because of defect/disability, child of opposite sex other than wanted
Temperament	Hyperactive by day, troublesome/cries at night
Demanding	Difficult because of illness
Different	Different from rest of the family
Gender	Girls three times more likely than boys to be victims
Social	
Basic	Crisis in housing, disconnection of services, lack of safe water, hygiene, sanitation, unhealthy environment
Unemployment	Loss of work, unemployment increases abuse by fathers
Economic	Poverty and economic crisis
Loneliness	Loneliness/isolation of mothers when partners have left/working away from home
Marital crisis	Marital crisis, new liaisons, step children, unwanted pregnancy
Traditional practices	Harmful practice—child marriages, caste system, child forced to work/earn to support family, girl child discrimination, *devadasi* tradition

nutrition, education, sexual, social status, protection, to prevention and rehabilitation from exploitation, abuse, cruelty, work/labor and justice, social security, drug abuse,

For the comprehensive childcare adequate funds both from the family and community and the government are essential. Global evidence states that, unless a country expends at least 5% of its GDP on health with Government expenditure contributing to a major part, fundamental healthcare needs are hard to meet. The Government spending on healthcare in India is pathetically only 1.15% of GDP. Ironically, the portion that trickles down for Child Health Services further reduces at each level. Apart from existing schemes like Integrated Child Development Scheme (ICDS), Integrated Child Protection Scheme (ICPS) and Sarva Shiksha Abhiyaan (SSA), there are additional schemes for children with disabilities, girl children and more related to other child welfare issues.

In view of the alarming state of children's health, legislation for "right to health" for children should be advocated. While the state is the primary duty-bearer for the delivery of health care (which is the child's right) the civil society, professionals, nongovernmental organizations and all concerned citizens, i.e. we the parents/guardians must also share this responsibility.

BIBLIOGRAPHY

1. CANCL News. Child Abuse and Child Labour (IAP). New Delhi: CANCL News; 2015.
2. CANCL News. Child Abuse, Neglect and Child Labour (IAP). New Delhi: Child Sexual Abuse and Convergence. CANCL News; 2018.
3. Foreman DM. Detecting fabricated or induced illness in children. BMJ. 2005;331(2):978-9.
4. Indian Institute for Population Sciences (IIPS) and MoHFW. (2017). National Family Health Survey-4. Available from http://rchips.org/nfhs/pdf/NFHS4/India.pdf. [Assessed November, 2018].
5. Kacker L. Child Protection Scenario in India. Ministry of Women and Child Development, Government of India. New Delhi: CANCL News; 2008. pp. 30-2.
6. Kanth AK. Legal and judicial implications of child abuse in India-Global to national perspective. Pediatr Today. 2008;12(3):101-13.
7. Mehta MN, Prabhu SV, Mistry HN. Types of physical health problems in working children. In: Naidu US, Kapadia K (Eds). Child Labor and Health. Bombay: Tata Institute of Social Sciences; 1982. pp. 138-49.
8. Mehta MN. Abuse of abandoned children in India. ICCW News Bull. 1990;37:3-7.
9. Mehta MN. Child abuse and neglect. In: Banerjee SR (Ed). Community and Social Pediatrics. New Delhi: Jaypee Brothers Medical Publishers (P) Ltd.; 1995. pp. 157-74.
10. Mehta MN. Sexual abuse in children. Pediatr Today. 2008;12(3):121-6.

19.10 Sexual Abuse and POCSO Act

Kiran Aggarwal

SEXUAL ABUSE

Child sexual abuse (CSA) is a universal problem with grave life-long outcomes. In 1999, World Health Organization (WHO) formulated a Consultation on Child Abuse Prevention, which defined CSA as "the involvement of a child in sexual activity that he or she does not fully comprehend, is unable to give informed consent to, or for which the child is not developmentally prepared and cannot give consent, or that violates the laws or social taboos of society." CSA is evidenced by this activity between a child and an adult or another child who by age or development is in a relationship of responsibility, trust or power, the activity being intended to gratify or satisfy the needs of the other person. This may include but is not limited to the inducement or coercion of a child to engage in any unlawful sexual activity; the exploitative use of a child in prostitution or other unlawful sexual practices; the exploitative use of children in pornographic performance and materials.

After the enactment of the new law "Protection of Child against Sexual Offences (POCSO) Act 2012" the concept and management of CSA in India has changed a lot safeguarding the best interest of the child in every respect at each step including rehabilitation, compensation and all legal procedures. This law gives a set of guidelines for all the stakeholders to perform their role, as even the maintaining silence to allow sexual abuse to happen to the child is a crime and punishable offence under the law of the land; there is mandatory reporting under the Act.

EPIDEMIOLOGY

Child sexual abuse implies initiation of any kind of sexual act (physical, verbal, visual or online), or a nonsexual act aiming towards a child with an intention for sexual gratification is sexual abuse. The abuser can be of any age; gender and socioeconomic class, at times can be a family member. Sexual abuse may not be necessarily penetration, but use of force, causing pain, or just even touching. Most sexual abusers know the child (even the family) they abuse.

Worldwide reports have indicated boys are equally abused as girls and have suggested that protective shield should be provided not only to the girls but also to the boys right from the day they are born. Children can be sexually abused even by their lawful male guardians; CSA can take place inside or outside homes. Play schools and places where children are left by their parents for baby-sitting are the most vulnerable places.

Boys if get sexually abused by an adult or an older child usually keep it to themselves, may blame themselves under feeling of guilt. But when they grow up and gain some physical strength, may experiment the same act on younger powerless boys; their marital relationship may suffer; they may become abusive husbands leading to domestic violence or even may abuse their own children to repeat the cycle of abuse.

Children may sexually abuse a child younger to them to experiment, this is CSA as well but in such cases the older child/juvenile offender will be tried as per JJ act 2015 (revised in 2016) that gives complete innocence to a child under 7 years; for those between 7 years and 12 years court has to assess the mental ability and intention of the child. The child rights activist noble Laureate Kailash Satyarthy called for all political parties to unite for the cause with 90,000 cases of POCSO pending in the court (NCRB 2016 report).

INDIAN SCENARIO

In a nation-wide survey on child abuse across 13 states of India report released in 2007 by Ministry of Women and Child Development, Government of India (MWCD, GOI) in which 12447 children participated, more than half (53.22 %) were subjected to one or more forms of sexual abuse (52.94% were boys and 47.06 girls). The age wise distribution showed abuse started at 5 years, gained momentum 10 years onwards, peaking at 12 to 15 years. In 9 states out of 13 reported higher percentage of sexual abuse in boys as compared to girls; Delhi reporting a figure of 65.64% boys; children at work faced the highest at 61.61%. Out of the total children interviewed 20.90% were subjected to severe form including sexual assault (57.30% were boys and 42.70% were girls). Preadolescent to adolescent children seemed to be more atrisk of suffering severe form. It was also disturbing to note that age, those between 6 to 10 years also face severe form of sexual abuse. Assam, Delhi, Andhra Pradesh and Bihar reported maximum sexual abuse (Source: Child abuse study India 2007, MWCD, GOI).

According to the NCRB data for 2016, incidents of rape of children have spiked alarmingly compared to 2015. It is for the first time that such a sharp increase in sexual assaults on children has been registered. The NCRB data shows that while in 2015, 10,854 cases of rape under Section 376 of the IPC and under sections 4 and 6 of the POCSO Act were registered across the country, 2016 saw 19,765 such cases being registered. Uttar Pradesh and Tamil Nadu have registered very high increases in comparison to 2015 (Source: NCRB report 2016). It must be noted that the NCRB figures merely reflect the number of crimes registered by the police. These may or may not reflect the actual situation on the ground.

WHO MAY GET ABUSED?

All children are at the risk of being abused despite of their social, economic, religious, cultural or educational background. However, some children are more at risk than the others **(Box 19.10.1)**.

EARLY WARNING SIGNS OF SEXUAL ABUSE

Warning signs of sexual abuse are important as they help suspect and identify the victims. Some of these are listed in **Box 19.10.2**.

IMPORTANT TERMINOLOGIES

Incest: The term incest means a forbidden sexual relationship between close relatives in a family, e.g. between brother and sister or parent and child.

Commercial Sexual Exploitation of Children (CSEC): The main forms of CSEC are child prostitution (including child sex tourism), child sexual abuse images and trafficking of children for sexual purposes.

Box 19.10.1: Children more at risk of child abuse.

- Children with disabilities
- Children from lower socioeconomic backgrounds, especially if coupled with lack of adult supervision
- Children with low self-esteem
- Children who are questioning their sexuality
- Children who are isolated and have limited peer support/friend circle
- Children who have an unhealthy or dysfunctional home atmosphere, e.g. children from families that do not give the child enough love and attention at home

Box 19.10.2: Early warning signs of sexual abuse.

- Child has nightmares or other sleep problems without an explanation
- Seems distracted or distant at odd times
- Has a sudden change in eating habits—refuses to eat or losses or drastically increases appetite
- Writes, draws, plays or dreams of sexual or frightening images
- Develops new or unusual fear of certain people or places
- Suddenly has money, toys or other gifts without reason
- Thinks of self or body as repulsive, dirty or bad
- Exhibits adult-like sexual behaviors, language and knowledge
- Self-injury (cutting, burning)
- Inadequate personal hygiene
- Drug and alcohol abuse
- Suicide attempts
- Fear of intimacy or closeness
- Compulsive eating or dieting

Source: NCPCR User Handbook on POCSO Act 2012.

Child Sex Tourism: Child sex tourism is the sexual exploitation of children by a person or persons who travel from their home district or home country in order to have sexual contact with children.

Pedophile: The pedophile manifests an exclusive sexual inclination for prepubescent children.

Online Sexual Abuse/Cyber-stalking: Online abuse is any type of abuse that happens on the web, through social networks. Children may feel as if they cannot escape from online abuse—abusers can contact them at any time of the day or night. Children being sold online for live sexual abuse online.

WHY CHILDREN DO NOT DISCLOSE ABUSE?

There are many reasons children do not disclose being sexually abused **(Box 19.10.3)**.

PATTERN OF EVENTS

The delay between the initial happening and the subsequent disclosure of the abuse varies, depending on a number of factors such as the age and the gender, relationship with the perpetrator, severity of the abuse, developmental and cognitive variables, and likely consequences of the disclosure. Consequently, CSA is significantly underreported. When victims do report, they often do so years after the abuse occurred making the subject all the more difficult to deal with. The "child sexual abuse accommodation syndrome", propounded by Summit (1983), proposes that children's responses to CSA comprise of five stages:

1. Secrecy.
2. Helplessness.
3. Entrapment and accommodation.
4. Delayed and unconvincing disclosure.
5. Recantation.

Box 19.10.3: Why children do not disclose abuse?

- Fear, disbelief.
- May feel a sense of guilt that it is 'their own fault' that the abuse occurred
- Every time a child talks about the incident of abuse they may be revisiting the trauma
- Children are afraid that the person who groomed and abused them will stop loving them or get in trouble because of them
- The child may have been manipulated by the offender into believing that their relationship is normal as a result child does not realize of being abused
- Fear of retaliation and further abuse also forces a child to keep silent
- Generally, children are not encouraged to talk about their feelings and when they do, adults do not listen or believe
- Very young children may not have the verbal skills to communicate about the abuse or may not understand that the actions of the perpetrator are abusive, particularly if the sexual abuse is inflicted as a game or play

Source: NCPCR User Handbook on POCSO Act 2012.

The typical pattern of events is as follows: The child is forced to keep the sexual abuse a secret and initially feels trapped and helpless. These feelings of helplessness and the child's fear that no one will believe the disclosure of abuse leading to accommodative behavior. If the child does disclose, failure of family and professionals to protect and support the child adequately, augment the child's distress and may lead to retraction of disclosure.

HOW CHILDHOOD GETS AFFECTED?

Childhood sexual abuse violates the basic rights of children: CSA robs children of their innocence and sense of control affecting their holistic development and wellbeing. The dynamics of being manipulated by someone they trusted, and a loss of control over the situation can lead them to lifelong implications.

They are not prepared developmentally for sexual activity: The natural course of their emotional and sexual development gets restricted, when abuse comes from one giving them care and safety. It breaks the attachment patterns and leaves them in a confused mental state; some other forms of abuse like neglect, emotional and even physical abuse may be associated with it. Most survivors of CSA are found with higher levels of anxiety, guilt, immunity-related health problems, issues related to identity, sexuality, self-esteem, and relationship related issues in future life.

Children are not prepared to cope with repeated sexual stimulation: Even a three to four year old, who is unable to know the sexual activity is wrong, may develop problems while trying to cope up with the overstimulation.

The abuse should stop, problem should be identified and the child should be rehabilitated with professional help.

In absence of the help, the long-term emotional damage of sexual abuse can be very damaging to the child.

PREVENTION

By the parents: Tell the children that if someone making advances to touch your body inappropriately or do things to make you feel uncomfortable, funny or hurting say NO to that person and tell me right away. Teaching children that respect does not mean to blindly obey adults. For example, do not tell children to always do everything the teacher or baby-sitter tells you to do.

By Culture of Zero Tolerance Policy on Child Safety: There are no proper prevention mechanisms in place to address the issue of child protection, nor we have empathetic understanding and intervention plans with adequately backing by sustained investment on child safety. "Child protection in India cannot be ensured with just having legislations and formal guidelines. We as a country need to commit in creating a culture of zero tolerance policy on child abuse considering all children are at risk with gaps in infrastructure, processes and systems as well as people.

PROTECTION OF CHILDREN FROM SEXUAL OFFENCES (POCSO) ACT, 2012

In order to effectively address the heinous crimes of sexual abuse and sexual exploitation of children through less ambiguous and more stringent legal provisions, the MWCD, GOI championed the introduction of the Protection of Children from Sexual Offences (POCSO) Act, 2012 that has revolutionary provisions in the management of CSA.

The Act was enacted by the Government of India to provide an extremely strong legal framework for the protection of children from Sexual offences, while safeguarding the interest of the child at every stage of the judicial process by incorporating child-friendly mechanisms for reporting, recording of evidence, investigation and speedy trial of offences through designated special courts and offenders are brought to justice.

WHY IS THE POCSO ACT IMPORTANT FOR THE MEDICAL PROFESSIONALS?

Medical professionals while dealing with adolescents for their healthcare may come across several medicolegal, ethical and confidentiality issues closely linked with Juvenile justice act 2015 (revised in 2016) and POCSO act that too has linkages with the JJ act. One such example is dealing with consensual sex under 18 years and teen pregnancies resulting in demand for medical termination of pregnancy (MTP) by teens under 18 years unaccompanied by their parents at health facilities, since inception of POCSO Act from 14th November 2012 law of the land refuses to recognize consensual sex in persons below 18 years. MTP in a teen below 18 years would require parent's signature. Medical professionals while dealing with teen pregnancies and MTPs are liable to get punished if they do not follow mandatory reporting to police under POCSO Act 2012. They should make the adolescents aware of law of the land on understanding of consensual sex under 18.

Under Section 19 of the POCSO Act, "Reporting of sexual offences" by any person including the child has been made mandatory. Section 21 of the Act provides punishment for failure to report or record a child sexual abuse case. However, a child cannot be punished for failure to report {S.21 (2)}.

The National Commission for Protection of Child Rights (NCPCR) has been mandated to monitor the implementation of POCSO Act 2012. NCPCR has come out with an excellent user manual in the form of a Handbook on POCSO Act for Practical Application (NCPCR User Handbook on POCSO Act 2012) and a helpline 9868235077 for reporting directly and Suraksha POCSO e-box (by a click away on www.ncpcr.gov.in).

Objectives

- To protect all children irrespective of their gender from the offences of sexual assault, sexual harassment and pornography.
- To establish special courts for speedy trial of such offences, keeping their best interest and well-being in mind throughout the investigations with child-friendly procedures.
- Mandatory reporting of a child sexual abuse case under section 19.
- Punish the offender as per graded severity of the crime.

Definitions of Sexual Offences

Child [Section 2(D)]: Any person below the age of 18 years.

Sexual Assault (Section 7): All acts of physical nature without penetration.

Penetrative Sexual assault (Section 3): Manipulating the body of the child so as to cause penetration with sexual intent. Offences of sexual assault if committed by a person in a position of power, authority and trust or in certain circumstances are called and punished as aggravated sexual assault (Section 9).

Sexual harassment (Section 11): A person is said to commit sexual harassment upon a child when such person with sexual intent:

1. By uttering word or making sound or gesture or exhibiting any object or part of body with the sexual intention to the child.
2. Making a child exhibit his/her body or any part of his/her body with sexual intent.

3. Repeatedly or constantly followings or watching or contacting a child either directly or through electronic, digital or any other means.
4. Threatening to use in any form of media, a real or fabricated depiction through electronic, film or digital or any other mode, of any part of the body of the child or the involvement of the child in a sexual act.

Pornography: Showing any object to a child in any form or media for pornographic purposes. It also includes constantly following or watching the child either directly or through digital or any other means and also showing any object to the child in any form or enticing the child for pornographic purposes.

Provisions of the Act

The act applies to all the persons below 18 years of age, is gender-neutral (means the victim and accused can be male, female or a third gender). Any person (including a child) can be prosecuted for engaging in a sexual act with a child, irrespective of whether the latter consented to it (age of consent for sex has been increased from earlier 16 to 18 years under the POCSO Act) and punishes (as per graded severity and provisions in the law without discrimination) them as sexual offenders, the burden of proof is solely on the accused, it safeguards the rights and dignity of the child at every stage of the legal process by strictly following child friendly procedures by all stakeholders.

Act gives set guidelines to the media for reporting and other stakeholders to be careful and behave on child's issues of identity, dignity, not to make child revisit the crime by questioning repeatedly and prohibits from making the child come face to face with the accused and direct questioning by the defence lawyer at any point of time at the trial in the special court.

Police can be punished if refused to lodge FIR in case of a sexual crime (even if it may turn false on investigation). Statement of the child can be recorded preferably by a lady rank of sub-inspector (not to be in uniform) not at the police station but the place of choice of the child who cannot be retained at the police station in the night in any case, has to inform CWC and the special court within 24 hours of the reporting and inform CWC if the child has been assessed as in need of care and protection (unsafe home as abuser within the family/shared home, without parent and home) specifically, has to get medical examination done within 24 hours of reporting as per rule no 5, has to make sure forensic sample collection to reach the forensic lab in time, has to make sure child does not come in contact with the accused during the entire process of investigation.

The special court shall create a child friendly atmosphere and permit frequent breaks to the child during trial, shall ensure child is not called repeatedly to testify in court, shall not permit aggressive questioning or character assassination of the child and ensure the dignity is maintained and proceedings are done under the camera. Speedy trials are expected under the Act.

- Act gives provisions for compensation to the child.
- Emergency care will not be refused to the victim in any health care facility.
- Consent of the child is required if child is more than 12 years and parental consent if child is less than 12 years.

Note: Genital examination may not be required routinely in all the cases of sexual offence if history is taken thoroughly.

In case of sexual offender is a person under 18 years of age (age determination done by all possible means) the child/juvenile will be produced before the JJ board, JJ board will have to follow all the guidelines given under JJ act 2015 (revised in 2016).

Processes to be followed are outlined in **Flowchart 19.10.1**.

Emergency Medical Care and Counseling

The child victim who is in need of urgent medical care and protection, SJPU/local police shall within 24 hours of receiving information about the crime, arrange to take such child to the nearest hospital or medical care facility for emergency medical care {Rule 5 (1)}. The medical examination of child shall be conducted whether FIR or complaint is registered or not, by a women doctor, if the victim is a girl. In case parent is not available for any reason, medical examination of child shall be conducted in the presence of a women nominated by the head of the medical institution (Section 27).

ROLE OF MEDICAL PROFESSIONALS

In many cases of sexual offences parents and caregivers prefer to take their children to a nearest hospital or a clinic even before they go to the police. A medical professional and hospital's response is key to the child's immediate well-being and long term recovery **(Flowchart 19.10.2)**. The evidence collected in the course of medical examination of victims of sexual assault is core in most investigations in POCSO cases.

- Rule 5 of the POCSO Rules, 2012 states that emergency medical care is to be provided by any medical facility private or public. Sexual assault is, therefore, a medical emergency.
- Regarding medical examination, ensure that the child does not feel threatened or scared during the process of a medical examination.
- In case the parents/guardians or the child does not want the medical examination to be conducted, can refuse the same. The doctor has to document informed refusal. However, the doctor has to provide medical treatment to the victim if he/she is in need of it.
- The child/parents must get a copy of the medical certificate free of cost.

Flowchart 19.10.1: Procedures under POCSO Act.

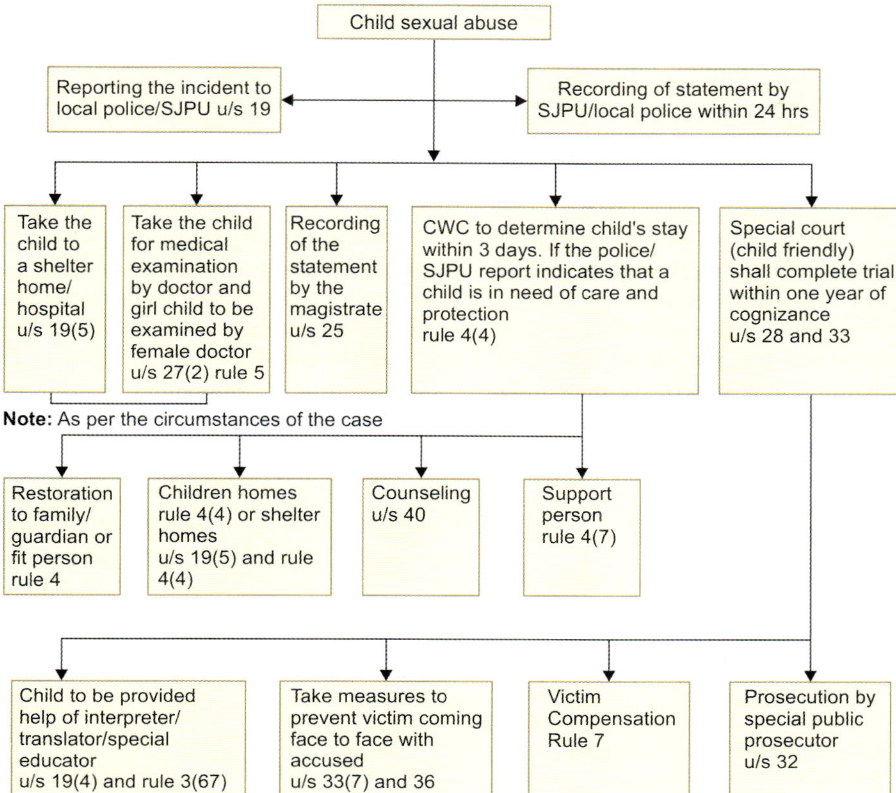

Source: Procedure under POCSO Act 2012; NCPCR User Handbook on POCSO Act 2012.

Flowchart 19.10.2: Procedures for medical professionals.

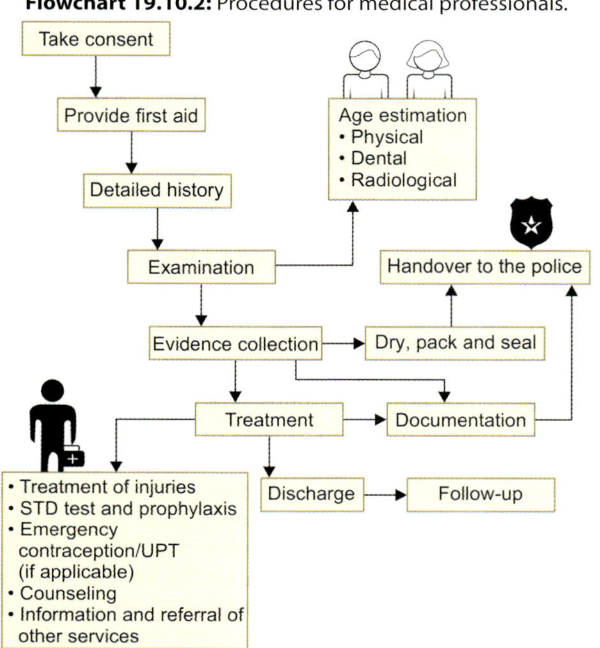

Source: Procedure under POCSO Act 2012; NCPCR User Handbook on POCSO Act 2012 (CEHAT Safe Kil, www.cehat.org).

Note: Medical examination is to be conducted as per the provisions of Section 27 of the POCSO Act, 2012 and Section 164A of the CrPC, 1973.

Taking Medical History

The doctor has to take a detailed medical history of the child's experience before beginning the examination of the child. The history should be obtained in a facilitating, nonjudgmental and empathetic manner. It is important for the doctor to remember that child sexual abuse is often a diagnosis based on medical history, rather than on physical findings. The medical history will guide the physical examination. Its objective is not to obtain information for forensic purposes but for treatment and diagnosis and to ensure the safety of the child too.

Interviewing Techniques

- The interview should begin by assessing the child's competence. This can be done by asking questions unrelated to the abuse, such as favorite colors, school activities, and likes and dislikes. The interview should not have an investigative tone. Relevant questions need to be asked to obtain a detailed pediatric history.

19.11 Child Labor

SR Banerjee

INTRODUCTION

The problem of child labor continues to pose a challenge before the nation. The Indian government has been taking various proactive measures to tackle this problem. However, considering the magnitude and extent of this problem and that it is essentially a socioeconomic problem inextricably linked to poverty and illiteracy, it requires concerted efforts from all sections of the society to make a dent in the problem. Child labor in India is a human rights issue for the whole world. It is a serious and extensive problem, with many children under the age of 14 years working in the carpet making factories, glass blowing units and making fireworks with bare little hands. According to the statistics given by the Indian government, there are 20 million child laborers in the country, while other agencies claimed that it is 50 million. Any working child, who is under the age specified by law is designated as a child laborer. The word "work" means full-time commercial work to sustain self or add to the family income. Any child, who is employed in activities to feed self- and family, is being subjected to "child labor."

DEFINITION

It is not a simple task to define the notion of "child," "child work" and "child labor." The problem is compounded by differences in social and cultural perceptions. It is also not easy to draw a distinction between work and labor. The dictionary meaning of "workers" is an employee especially in manual or industrial work, while a laborer is one, who, for wages does work that requires strength or patience rather than skill or training. In many situations, these two words are synonymous.

According to Child Labor (Prohibition and Regulation) act, 1986, a "child" is a person who has not completed 14 years of age. As per the 1983 report of the director general of International Labor Organization (ILO), child labor includes children prematurely leading adult lives, working long hours for low wages, under conditions damaging to their health and to physical and mental development.

The United Nations Children's Fund (UNICEF) has given a comprehensive formulation in its attempt to define child labor:

1. Starting full-time work at too early an age
2. Working too long within or outside the family so that the children are unable to attend the school
3. Work resulting in excessive physical, social and psychological strain upon the child
4. Work and life on the street is dangerous and unhealthy
5. Inadequate remuneration for working outside the family
6. Too much responsibility at too early an age
7. Work that does not facilitate the psychological and social developments, and
8. Work that inhibits the child's self-esteem as in bonded labor and prostitution.

In conclusion, a simple workable definition of child labor is any work within or outside the family that threatens health and mental development of the child by denying him or her both fundamental as well as non-fundamental rights.

CAUSES OF CHILD LABOR

Absence of compulsory education at the primary level, parental ignorance regarding the ill effects of child labor, the ineffective implementation of child labor laws, non-availability and non-accessibility of schools, boring and impractical school curriculum and cheap child labor (CCL) are some other factors which encourage child labor. For the immature minds and bodies, it is difficult to understand the exploitation of child labor in the absence of adult guidance. The figure translates into 13.2% of all children between ages 10 years and 14 years being subjected to child labor. Out of 12.6 million children in hazardous occupations, India has the highest number of laborers in the world less than 14 years of age. Although the constitution of India guarantees free and compulsory education to children between the ages of 6 and 14 years and prohibits employment of children younger than 14 years in hazardous environments, child labor is present in almost all sectors of the economy.

MAJOR FORMS OF CHILD LABOR AND DETERMINANTS OF ITS PATTERN

Two types of workers are classified, namely, main and marginal. Main workers are those who are engaged in a full-time economic activity and marginal workers are those who are part-time workers.

Many children work in their families as helpers in different household chores, caring for younger siblings. It has been observed that this sort of work discourages school attendance.

Rural children are often involved in nondomestic work, which is agricultural in nature and quite a good proportion of them are involved in work, which is generally seasonal. In cities, on the other hand, children are found to work in market places and almost in every street corner. They are engaged in a variety of working situations such as vendors, waiters in restaurants, helpers in all kinds of shops, private houses, in industries such as carpet weaving, *saree*-embroidery, brassware, precious stone polishing, leather tannery, *beedi* (handmade cigarettes) making, bangle manufacturing, glass industry, brick field, match and fire industries, construction sites, garages, gas station, fishing, mines, handloom industries, lock industry and rag-picking.

Girls at a fairly early age are recruited to the profession of prostitution. Children involved in gainful employment sometimes are bonded laborers in the backward areas of some developing countries. Progenies of single parent households are more likely to join the labor force at an early age. Another factor is the birth order of child, the first child having the highest probability of being gainfully employed. Moreover, during the last few decades, in developing societies, the mortality rates have declined markedly, which has resulted in the survival of a larger number of children. The proportion of children under 14 years of age as compared to 15–19 years of age-groups is higher among the poor. Thus, poor families are left with only young children as potential workers.

To summarize, children are engaged in various activities such as visible, invisible, formal, informal, paid or unpaid. Boys are usually engaged in relatively larger number of occupations than girls. Types of work for urban children are classified here:

- *Within the family:*
  - Domestic house tasks; cooking, child care, fetching water, cleaning utensils, washing clothes, etc.
  - Handicrafts and cottage industries, weaving, leather work, wood work, etc.
  - Within the family but outside home; domestic service, construction work, mining, i.e. quarry mines; informal economy, i.e. laundry, recycling rubbish.
- *Outside the family:*
  - Bonded labor
  - Apprentices
  - Skilled traders; carpets, embroidery, brassware works, gem polishing, etc.
  - Industries/unskilled occupations, mines, etc.
    - Commercial shops, restaurants and hotels
    - Begging.

HEALTH HAZARDS FOR WORKING CHILDREN

Chronic starvation and unhealthy environment does contribute to ill health in all children, whether working or otherwise. Also many children start working at a very early age and do hazardous work for 12–15 hours a day without any holiday. Several occupations may not be hazardous by themselves but the environment makes them such. These environmental factors include lack of ventilation, dust, gases, fumes, odors, poor lighting, noise, humidity, crowding, vibrations and ionizing radiations. All the children are in the process of growing and attaining their full physical stature and therefore, their growth is likely to be affected, resulting in stunting. This has been proved in several studies. Children, who started working early in life suffered from deterioration in their nutritional status but such impact was not seen for those children, who started work after the age of 11 years. Health effects of labor on children also vary according to the type of work situation. Children, who are engaged in their own household jobs or family-based industries, may have no direct adverse health effects. On the other hand, bonded and wage child workers may have greater effects on health because of the exploitative and unregulated nature of work, in which children are exposed more to health hazards, heavier workload and physical and mental abuse. Most of the poor child workers go to work without adequate food, clothing and proper shelter. They ultimately become victims of a wide range of diseases like diarrhea, general weakness and various viral and bacterial infections.

Other potential common psychological problems include habit disorders; personality disorders such as timidity, irritability, sensitiveness, temper tantrums, obstinacy, day-dreaming, negativity, fear, jealousy, inferiority complex; psychoneurotic disorders such as nervousness, tremors, headache, pain, hyperventilation syndrome, masturbation, etc. Antisocial behavior such as stealing, sexual offences, premarital sex; depressive psychosis and anxiety neurosis; drug abuse, and psychosexual problems.

OCCUPATIONAL HEALTH HAZARDS

Any occupation which allows the working children to come in contact with harmful substances like chemicals, as in the balloon and lock industry or fire in glass industry, match and fireworks, or cotton puff and dust as in power loom industry is termed intrinsically hazardous, which may have an adverse effect on physical and psychological development of children. Various occupational health hazards are depicted in **Table 19.11.1**.

EXPLOITATION OF CHILD LABOR

Child labor is economically unsound, psychologically disastrous, physically as well as morally harmful and precludes the full enfoldment of a child's potentialities. It also deprives them of education, training and skills, which are essential pre-requisites of earning power and economic

Table 19.11.1: Occupational health hazards in children.

Occupation	***Disease/disability***
Balloon factories	Pneumonia, bronchopneumonia, breathlessness and even heart failure
Match and firework	Breathing problems, severe burns, muscle fatigue from lifting heavy loads, deformities due to long hours of work in one position
Lock industry	Tuberculosis and respiratory tract diseases, asthma, acute breathlessness, acid burns, acute headache
Glass industry	Heat strokes, conjunctivitis, tuberculosis (TB) and burns, life span reduced by a third due to heat and dust
Slate industry	Silicosis, TB, pneumoconiosis
Power loom industry	Byssinosis, fibrosis of lung tissue and TB
Beedi industry	*Nicotine poisoning*: Nausea, headache blackouts and muscle fatigue, loss of eye sight
Brass industry	Additional burns and TB
Zari industry	Eye diseases, postural deformities and spinal problems
Domestic workers shop bays, etc.	Overwork physical and sexual abuse, drug addiction, isolation from society
Carpet industry	Poisoning from coloring agents, lung diseases from fiber dust

(*Source*: Health for the Millions. New Delhi: Voluntary Health Association of India; 1989.)

development. Sexual abuse is a common problem faced by girl children who work as a contract labor. The working girls in sleazy "B" and "C" grade hotels, lodging house, restaurants and also in domestic houses are exposed to physical assaults and sexual abuses by their employers and customers.

INITIATIVE AGAINST CHILD LABOR

Abolition of child labor is not possible from developing countries in the near future. However, the improvement in condition of work and work environment should be seriously considered. Child labor (prohibition and regulation) act, 1986 was enacted to replace the employment of children act, 1938. This act is the culmination of the process of consideration that the government has been giving to this pervasive problem figuring in the economic and social landscape in the country. This law is aimed to identify processes and industries, which are hazardous, with a view to ban child labor in these sectors and to regulate the condition of work in nonhazardous industries. The implementation of this act depends largely on labor inspectors. However, it has been found that there are not enough inspectors and most are easily threatened and bribed. Thus, in this view, the future action program is set out under the following three heads: (1) The legislative action plan, (2) focusing of general development program for benefiting child labor, wherever possible and (3) project based plan of action in areas of high concentration of child labor engaged in wage/quasi-wage employment.

NATIONAL CHILD LABOR POLICY

The National Child Labor Policy (NCLP) was formulated in 1987 and 10 industries were selected for remedial action. The NCLP aims to revitalize and coordinate employment generating the asset-building antipoverty programs in the designated areas, to strengthen the labor law enforcement machinery and to provide the children with better facilities for education, nutrition and health. However, the NCLP can only cover, at best, 30,000 children, a minute fraction of the total 44 million working children in India.

BIBLIOGRAPHY

1. Banerjee SR. Agricultural child labor in West Bengal. Indian Pediatr. 1993;30(12):1425-8.
2. Banerjee SR. Child Labor in India. London: Antislavery Society; 1979.
3. Banerjee SR. Child labor. In: Gupta S (Ed). Recent Advances in Pediatrics. New Delhi: Jaypee Brothers Medical Publishers (P) Ltd; 1992. pp. 134-6.
4. Banerjee SR. Child labor. In: Banerjee SR (Ed). Community and Social Pediatrics. New Delhi: Jaypee Brothers Medical Publishers (P) Ltd; 1995. pp. 364-83.
5. Banerjee SR. Child labor in suburban areas of Calcutta, West Bengal. Indian Pediatr. 1991;28(9):1039-44.
6. Banerjee SR. Female working children. Indian Pediatr. 1990;27(11):1153-8.
7. Banerjee SR. Occupational health hazards of working children. J Indian Med Assoc. 1995;93(1):22-4.
8. Mendelievich E. Children at work. Geneva: International Labor Office; 1980.
9. Pinto GJ. Child labor. New Delhi: United Nations Children's Fund; 1987.
10. Rodgers G, Standing G. Economic roles of Children in Low-income Countries. Geneva: International Labor Organization;

19.12 Adoption and Care of Orphans

RD Potdar

DEFINITION

Adoption is essentially a social process by which the reciprocal need of childless parents and an orphan (or parent-deprived) child is satisfied. Legally it may be defined as "transfer of rights and responsibilities concerning the child from biological or birth parents to the adoptive parents irrevocably."

Adoption is also an instrument through which one can ensure the following important children's rights accepted by the United Nations (UN) convention of rights of children and the world community at large. These are:

- Inherent right to life survival and development
- Right to name and nationality
- Child's interest being always a primary consideration
- Special protection from physical harm and neglect
- No discrimination through universal brotherhood
- Social security through education, employment and earning
- Special attention to disabled children.

Considering the above definition and objectives, adoptions could be divided into various types such as intrafamily adoptions, single parent adoptions, adoption of older children, adoption of disabled or "special needs" children and inter-country adoptions.

Whatever the type, it is always prudent not to do it secretly (by feigning pregnancy) but do it properly within the law of the country. Since the emotional, psychological, social and legal consequences of adoption are far-reaching in nature it must be conducted in a very open and supportive environment. Parents should be strongly advised not to arrange private or secret adoptions through hospitals and medical practitioners directly. Adoption must always be done through an institute, which has been recognized as a "fit person institute" by the central government. In every states of India, there are many orphanages and adoption agencies recognized in this manner.

LAWS

In India, two laws govern the process of adoption. First, "the Hindu Adoption and Maintenance Act 1956" governs all Hindus adopting children and the second, "the Guardians and Wards Act of 1890" governing adoptions by parents, who are not Hindus by religion. In inter-country adoptions children are given for adoption under the "the Guardians and Wards Act of 1890" in foster care till they are finally adopted according to the law of the country of adoptive parents.

Every doctor should be conversant with the process of adoption, be able to and should advise any prospective adoptive parents on all aspects of adoption. The doctor can help in all the following standard steps of adoption process always using sympathy and empathy at all stages.

MAKING UP A DECISION TO ADOPT

"Childless couples, who are involuntarily childless have a desire for parenthood combined with complex set of emotions ranging from guilt of infertility to apprehensions to fears related to the social status, family acceptance and reactions of decision to adopt, unforeseen elements of taking home a child borne by parents not known and their own capabilities regarding coping with a new challenge in life.

PREPARATION FOR ADOPTION

Preparation for adoption, mentally, physically, procedure and document-wise: The ideal age difference between at least one parent and the baby to be adopted should be not more than 40 years so that they have enough time and physical strength on their side to look after the baby till the baby becomes a young adult and legally a major. Parents should be equipped with the following documents, *viz.* marriage certificate, proof of age, income certificate and bank balance and property certificates (if any), doctor's certificate regarding their health and also their infertility status, references and photographs when they go to apply for adoption of a baby to "Specialized Adoption Agencies (SAAs) recognized by State Governments, preferably registered with CARA (Central Adoption Resource Authority Ministry of Women and Child Development Government of India (Free Toll No.: 1800-11-1311, E-mail: carahdesk.wcd@]nic.in).

Failure to do adoption not according to the above and through unrecognized unregistered health facilities such as maternity homes, institutions, individuals, agents, etc. will amount to illegal adoption, making such persons unintentionally become part of child trafficking network and exposure to legal ramifications.

Preadoption Counseling and Home Study Preparation

This is mandatorily done by the social worker of the agency and consists of social and family background of both parents, current marital and family relationships, attitudes and motivation toward infertility, childlessness and adoption, anxieties regarding child's illegitimacy, social and genetic background, sharing the fact of adoption with family and the child, parenting experience, aspirations and financial capabilities, recommendations of their friends and referees. The purpose of this procedure is to protect the rights of the Child to the maximum before the irrevocable adoption takes place.

Choosing a Child, Medical Screening and Certifying the "Fit for Adoption" Report

While it is true that "choosing" can imply a bias of an arbitrary and discriminatory selection or rejection, in the Indian context it should be left to the social worker to place a child, who is near compatible to adoptive parents in looks, color of the eyes and complexion and their specific requests if any. This is likely to ensure better adjustment and integration of the baby in the new family and society.

While doing the medical screening for fitness the doctor should remember that this baby should be examined and certified fit, normal or otherwise in the context of the situational background that the baby may have suffered physical, nutritional and emotional deprivation in the recent past. Due consideration needs to be given to the fact that child has been living in an environment where not a single foster mother, but multiple mothers have looked after the baby and the confusion of identity may have led to a pseudo-retardation of social development.

Clinical examination consists of identification data, anthropometry, systemic examination, detection of any gross deficiency disorders and overt or covert anomalies and their correctability potential, clinical clues to metabolic disorders if observed and physical and mental milestones evaluation. Standard investigations which are expected to be done are hemogram, urinalysis, tuberculin test, X-ray chest, stool examination for parasites, tests for venereal disease research laboratory (VDRL), human immunodeficiency virus (HIV), hepatitis B, toxoplasmosis, other infections rubella, cytomegalovirus and herpes (TORCH) titers and any other indicated tests with special reference to hypothyroidism, hemolytic anemia, chromosomal anomalies, and metabolic screening tests for intellectual disability like phenylketonuria, galactosemia, aminoaciduria, etc.

The entire exercise should be a balanced one to ensure welfare and maintain interest of both the baby and the adoptive parents with a benefit of doubt given to child (than adoptive parents) since the child is totally dependent on the caregivers.

MEDICAL CARE OF THE ORPHANS AND ADOPTED BABIES

Vast majority of orphans, who go for adoption after 1 month of age and those who were not abandoned immediately after a hospital delivery are highly vulnerable to sepsis, malnutrition, frequent attacks of acute respiratory and gastrointestinal and skin infections. They may be frankly marasmic and lack immunity increasing the incidence of morbidity and mortality amongst them. In the management of sick orphans three actions are of utmost importance. First is immunization against hepatitis B in addition to current standard schedule; second is the urgency of action when even slightly sick and the third is early use of higher antibiotics even if it may appear an irrational and expensive proposition. By introducing simple inputs such as IV fluids, oxygen therapy and higher antibiotic therapy in the orphanage itself prior to transferring to a higher center a large number of such sick babies can be saved. Apart from this the care of orphans and adopted babies should be like any other normal baby.

In postadoption care, in addition to problems of general health and standard immunization schedule, an extra vigil should be kept on feeding and sleep patterns, motor development pattern, speech and language development which may appear delayed for some time initially. Advice of patience and perseverance is usually very rewarding in most cases. However, the experience of workers in *adoption shows that tender (one) mother care* usually prevents/allays such problems in an overwhelming manner than any other action.

FOLLOW-UP AND POSTADOPTION COUNSELING

Follow-up after adoption is necessary for advice and care in the following crisis situations, which are likely to arise in some of the babies:

- *Sudden change* crises, where the baby (and parents) may take long-time to cope with the unexpected change in environment, climate, living conditions, language, noise level, food styles and surrounding strange faces resulting in different types of reactions like anxiety, rejection or aggression or any combinations of these.
- *Behavior crisis* is likely to manifest after first few years and may be as a result of pampering and overprotection (or even a covert rejection) by one or both parents and other family members. There may be a considerable delay in detection and management of likely behavior problems due to the unwillingness of the parents to seek interventions by adopting an attitude of "keeping all in the family". Such problems may become worse in adolescence if not tackled earlier.

- *Communication and identity crisis* may come up at any age if the child's sense of security is not well ensured by the parents and immediate family members. This problem is more likely to come up in inter-country adoptions because of the obvious difference in skin color.
- *Crisis of assimilation* is likely to occur in inter-country adoptions in a small number of cases where the young adults may face discrimination in getting jobs, married, etc.

Every doctor must be aware of these problems and be able to either counsel the family himself or convince and refer them to the appropriate agencies.

TELLING THE CHILD THAT HE/SHE IS AN ADOPTED CHILD, ENCOURAGING, INSISTING AND HELPING THE PARENTS

Encouraging, insisting and helping the parents to tell the child about his or her adoption is the most vital postadoption follow-up action. Every child who is adopted must be told that he or she is adopted by the parents themselves, howsoever it may appear difficult for them. When a child comes to know the fact from sources other than his parents, it can lead to a severe trauma (of betrayal or breach of trust) that it might even ruin relations between the parents and the child forever totally defeating the very objective for which the adoption was undertaken in the first place. Later the age of the child, when the trauma happens, worse are the consequences for the parents. It is therefore necessary and appropriate to encourage all adoptive parents to tell the child as early in life as possible when the child can comprehend the concept of biological and adoptive parenthood. *If done between the ages of 6 years and 10 years most children take it into their stride and future problems can be averted.*

Golden rules of child adoption are summarized in **Box 19.12.1.**

Box 19.12.1: Golden rules of adoption.

- The primary responsibility for providing care and protection to children shall be that of his/her family
- Adoption shall be resorted to for the rehabilitation of the children, who are orphan, abandoned or surrendered through such mechanism as may be prescribed
- In keeping with the provisions of the various guidelines for adoption issued from time to time, by the state government, or the central adoption resource agency and notified by the central government, children may be given in adoption by a court after satisfying itself regarding the investigations having been carried out, as are required for giving such children in adoption
- The state government shall recognize one or more of its institutions or voluntary organizations in each district as specialized adoption agencies in such manner as may be prescribed for the placement of orphan, abandoned or surrendered children for adoption in accordance with the guidelines notified under sub-section (3)
- Provided that the children's homes and the institutions run by the state government or a voluntary organization for children in need of care and protection, who are orphan, abandoned or surrendered, shall ensure that these children are declared fit for adoption by the committee and all such cases shall be referred to the adoption agency in that district for placement of such children in adoption in accordance with the guidelines notified under sub-section (3) till the 2 months period for reconsideration by the parent is over in the case of surrendered children, and without his consent in the case of a child who can understand and express his consent
- The court may allow a child to be given in adoption: (1) to a person irrespective of marital status, (2) to parents to adopt a child of same sex irrespective of the number of living biological sons or daughters or (3) to childless couples

BIBLIOGRAPHY

1. CARA (2016). Role of Judiciary and Court Procedure for Adoption. [online] cara.nic.in/PDF/Role%20of%20Judiciary.pdf. [Accessed November, 2018].
2. Ministry of Women and Child Development (2017). Adoption Regulations 2017. [online] Available from: www.wcd.nic.in/acts/adoption-regulations-2017. [Accessed November, 2018].

19.13 Prevention and Control of Injuries

K Nedunchelian

INTRODUCTION

Injuries are important cause of preventable morbidity and mortality among children and adolescents of developed as well as developing countries. The World Health Organization (WHO) and United Nations Children's Fund Report (2008) draws global attention on the five leading causes of death related to child injury—road traffic injuries, drowning, poisoning, burns and falls—and set out what could be done to prevent these injuries. Yet there is not much of focus on the issue of childhood and adolescent injuries and its prevention, especially in under developed and developing countries.

DEFINITIONS/CLASSIFICATIONS

Term "accident" represents an incident occurring by chance that cannot be predicted and prevented, whereas "injury" represents an event occurring at predictable circumstance among individuals who are at high risk. The term "injury" is preferable in the sense that it promotes awareness program as it leads to proper planning of prevention and possibility of injury control. Injury control comprises "primary prevention" attempting prevention of injuries, as well as "secondary" and "tertiary" prevention, representing trauma care and rehabilitation respectively. Instead of just trying to attribute it to accident proneness of children, physical and social environment of children at which injury occurred are to be considered. Injuries can be "unintentional (road traffic injuries, falls, burns, poisoning, and drowning)" or "intentional" (interpersonal violence/homicide, self-inflicted injuries/suicides and war). Also classified based on the place of injury: domestic injuries, injuries at public places and the settings of injuries: recreational injuries and occupational injuries (including industrial and agricultural injuries). Our focus here is going to be mainly on the prevention and control of injuries arising out of accidents due to unnatural causes and not those due to natural disasters.

EPIDEMIOLOGY

Those who are injured was observed to be on decline since 2015. Accidents reduced in 2017 by 3.3% and injuries by 4.8% when compared to 2016. Whereas mortality reduced by just 1.9%. Accidents attributable to unnatural causes (falls, poisoning, traffic accidents, etc.) were 97.5% and natural causes (lightning, heat stroke, flood, landslide, etc.) were 2.5%.

RISK FACTORS

Age

Injuries occur at a particular age when a child or an adolescent encounter a new task or hazard against which they may not have the skills to handle. In view of exploratory nature of toddlers, they are at high risk for injuries especially burns, drowning, and fall. They do not know that medications can be poisonous, or some houseplants are not to be consumed. Many parents expect young school-aged children to walk home from school, the playground, or the local store, tasks for which most children are not developmentally ready. Young school-aged children are at-risk for pedestrian injuries, bicycle-related injuries, motor vehicle occupant injuries, burns, and drowning. The lack of skills and experience lead to particularly motor vehicle injuries, drowning, burns and risk of intentional trauma among teenagers. Alcohol and other drugs often add to these limitations. Work-related injuries are associated with child labor.

Age also determines the severity of injury and long-term disability. For example, outcome of head injuries among young children is poor when compared to adolescents or adults.

Sex

Males have higher rates of injury than females. Variation in exposure to risk, greater risk-taking behavior, combined with greater frequency of alcohol use, may lead to the disproportionately high rate of motor vehicle crashes among teenage males and not due to developmental difference between the sexes.

Children with psychiatric problems, especially those with attention deficit-hyperactivity disorder (ADHD) are at more risk for injuries.

Ethnicity

Risk for injury is primarily related to poverty, educational status and presence of hazardous environments, rather than to race alone.

Socioeconomic Status and Environment

Mortality from fire, motor vehicle crashes and drowning are higher among poor children. Other factors are single-parent families, teenage mothers, multiple care providers, family stress and multiple siblings, which are primarily due to poverty rather than independent risk factors. Poor children are exposed to more hazards in their living environments, in the form of poor housing, which is less likely to be protected by smoke detectors, etc. The roads are more likely to be major thoroughfares. Neighborhoods experience higher levels of violence and they are more likely to be victims of assault.

Rural versus Urban Status

Unplanned urbanization with slums and informal urban settlements lead to high risks of injury for children especially in developing world. Injury rates are higher in rural and homicide in urban areas. Case fatality from injury is generally twice as high in rural areas than in urban areas, due to increased severity of some injuries (such as motor vehicle crashes occurring at higher speeds) and poor access to emergency medical and definitive trauma care services. Agricultural injuries are confined to rural areas.

Those prone for injury are more likely to be unsupervised, having families in disharmony and hazardous environments conducive for injuries.

STRATEGIES TO PREVENT AND CONTROL INJURIES

Children have the right to have a safe environment and protection from injuries. Many developed nations have been able to bring down child deaths related to injuries drastically over the decades by adopting multisectoral, multipronged approaches to child injury prevention. The approach should aim to reduce the

1. Risk of new injuries
2. Severity of injuries occurred, and
3. Frequency and severity of injury-related disability.

Following are the strategies suggested in general:

- *Promotion of awareness:* "Passive intervention" is for entire population, irrespective of individual's involvement, whereas "active intervention" requires behavior change of parents and children. Community education is an active intervention, whereas product and environment modification are passive interventions.
- *Education to parents:* Behavior modification is the most important step toward injury control. Focus should be specific, e.g. use of car seat restraints, helmets, use of smoke detectors, etc. This will be successful than very vague general instructions.
- *Modification of product designs:* More useful than repeated attempts on behavior change among the parents or children. Lowering the water heater temperature, installing smoke detectors, and using child-resistant caps for containers with medicines and household products are examples of effective product modifications. Many interventions require both active and passive measures. Seat belts provide passive protection when used, but behavior change is required to use it regularly.
- *Modification of the social and physical environment:* Greater effort is required when compared to individual product modification, but very effective in controlling injuries. Safe roadway traffic and speed limits are examples of such interventions. Changes in the social environment through legislation is needed sometimes, such as laws mandating child seat restraint and use of seat belt, bicycle helmet and stream lining motor vehicle licensing laws, etc.
- *Campaigns* combining two or more of these approaches have been particularly effective in controlling injuries.

All these can be achieved in the following ways:

- Health-promoting initiatives in schools can incorporate injury prevention and safety promotion.
- Child-injury prevention can be taken up by "healthy cities" programs.

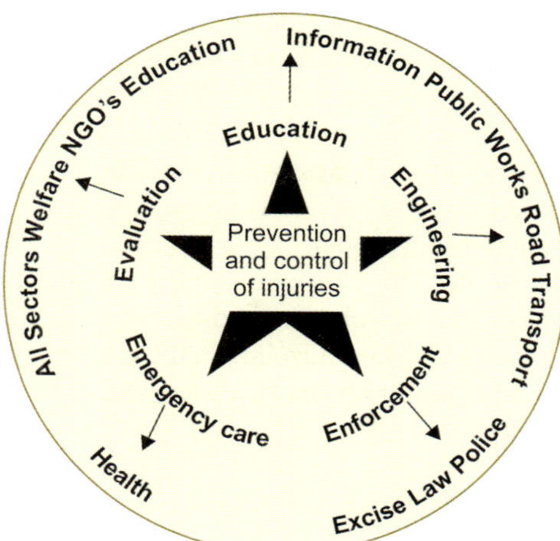

Fig.19.13.1: An intersectoral approach to injury prevention and control.

Source: Strategic Plan for Injury Prevention and Control in South-East Asia. WHO Project: ICP. New Delhi: WHO, Regional Office for South East Asia; 2002.

- Community-based approaches to child injury prevention can work well and
- Education, skills development and behavior change, etc. directed toward, child injury prevention needs to be integrated with other health promotion campaigns designed to change child and adolescent behavior as well as public in general. An intersectoral approach to injury prevention and control has been suggested by the World Health Organization **(Fig. 19.13.1)**.

INDIVIDUAL TYPES OF INJURIES

Falls

Falls form most of the injuries among children. Mostly falls are from vehicles, walkers, staircase and while on play, etc. Prevention is by redesigning the furniture and other products, raising the level of railing of staircase, window guards, and playground with energy absorbent materials like sand, rubberized surface or coir mats.

Road Traffic Injuries

Traffic accidents are the major contributors of accidental deaths of unnatural cause and constitute the leading cause of serious and fatal injuries among all age groups. Injury can be to the occupant, driver or both.

Occupants-related Issues

Injuries to passenger vehicle occupants are the predominant cause of motor vehicle death among children and adolescents, except for the 5–9-year-old group, in whom pedestrian injuries are common.

Infants or children weighing less than 10 kg should be placed in the rear seat facing backward. Toddlers and children can be placed in the rear seat in a forward-facing toddler seat. Children in the back of uncovered vehicles, face the possibility of being thrown out leading to head injury and those in covered trucks carbon monoxide poisoning if exhaust system is not proper.

The safest place for children is in the rear seat, properly restrained for their age and size. Educational and legislative interventions for children traveling in the rear seat are found to be successful. Audio visual aids can be shown to parents in waiting rooms.

Driver-related Issue

These are twice more among teenagers when compared to elder drivers; five to ten folds more likely to encounter fatal crash while driving at night compared with driving during the day. The difficulty of driving at night combined with the inexperience of teenagers appears to be a deadly combination. The inexperience in driving and driving in a drunken state is more dangerous.

Pedestrian Injuries

Mostly injuries occur during the day, with a peak in the after-school period. Risk is more with factors like heavy traffic, high speed, absence of play space near home, household crowding and low socioeconomic status.

Young children are more prone since poor ability to judge distance and speed of vehicle and easily distracted by playmates or environmental factors. Other factors are poor socioeconomic status, low educational status, living in mobile homes, etc.

Bicycle Injuries

Head trauma is the leading cause for mortality. Education programs to be organized by physicians and service organizations in promoting the use of bicycle helmets to children. Separate bicycle path is an ideal option.

Prevention of road traffic injuries is by multifaceted approach. Younger children should never cross streets alone until 10 years of age. Select streets with little traffic. Following legislation and police enforcement will be useful:

1. Measures to slow the speed of traffic, especially around schools, residential areas, play areas
2. To route traffic away from schools and residential areas
3. Networks of "one way streets"
4. Proper placement of transit or school bus stops, sidewalks in urban and sub-urban areas
5. Edge stripping in rural areas to delineate the edge of the road
6. Strictly implementing parking rules.

Burns

Flame burns resulting from ignition of clothing is common followed by household fire injuries, especially among small children. Using nonflammable fabrics will minimize this. Scalds from hot liquids and foods are most common in children less than 5 years. Avoid taking hot drinks while holding an infant, keeping children away from pots, cooking stove and use of child-resistant lighters are few steps to avoid scalds and burns.

Fireworks-related injuries are usually seasonal, where supervision by adults while children use fireworks is mandatory. Smoking constitutes half of the household fires. The combination of smoking and alcohol use will increase risk for injury and mortality. Enforce laws on smoke alarms. Smoke detectors are inexpensive, at the same time effective method of preventing majority of these deaths. Sometimes burns result from fire setting (exploratory play) by children or adolescents. Burns following exposure to corrosives, especially acids and electric shock should be kept in mind. To treat patients with burns and scalds, a greater number of dedicated burns centers to be established to have the best outcome for these patients.

Drowning

It is common among older children and adolescents during swimming or boating; and children less than 5 years of age, as they do not know the consequence of getting into the water and do not call for help, they are more prone to submersion injury. Four-sided fencing of pools, personal flotation device and not allowing toddlers unattended at swimming pool/bath tub will prevent drowning. When intoxicated with alcohol risk is many folds. Ensure immediate resuscitation in case of submersion injuries.

Suffocation

It is more common in infants and toddlers due to food, nuts, parts of toys, etc. getting aspirated into the airway or smothering accidentally by pillow, bed sheet and strangulation while playing with swings.

Poisoning

Poisoning with common household substances is a subject by itself (Please refer to Chapter 17.2 Common Poisonings in Childhood for a detailed description). The prevention can be by keeping the poisonous substances out of reach of children, stored in proper containers with child-resistant caps, package of drugs in non-lethal quantities with appropriate label, etc. Legislate for child-resistant packaging of medicines and poisons. Establish poison control centers to guide, supervise and manage poisoning related issues.

Sports

The health benefits of physical activity cannot be under estimated. Children especially adolescents who participate in sports and recreational activities are exposed to various injury risks.

Homicide

Homicide may be observed in "infantile" and "adolescent" groups. The earlier group may be subjected to "child abuse" by caretakers and the later to firearm injuries from peers or otherwise.

MANAGEMENT

Management consists of preventing further injury, transport, maintenance of vitals, and advanced management of the injury. Emergency treatment may need to be instituted immediately in case of respiratory or cardiovascular compromise. Following transfer to a trauma care center, accurate evaluation of the injuries and appropriate management are essential. "Post-traumatic stress disorder" among parents and children who survived near fatal injuries is yet another important issue, which should be addressed to.

BIBLIOGRAPHY

1. Chapman JI, Walker DM. Emergency medical services applicable for children/Principles applicable to the developing world–Injuries. In: Kliegman RM, Stanton BF, St. Geme III JW, Schor NF, Behrman RE (Eds). Nelson's Textbook of Pediatrics, First South Asia Edition. New Delhi: Reed Elsevier India Pvt. Ltd.; 2016. pp. 385-6.
2. Harvey A, Towner E, Peden M, et al. Injury prevention and the attainment of child and adolescent health. Bull World Heal Organ. 2009;87:390-4.
3. The National Crime Records Bureau (NCRB). Accidental deaths and suicides in India 2015. New Delhi: Ministry of Home Affairs, Government of India; 2016.
4. World report on child injury prevention. Geneva: World Health Organization and United Nations Children's Fund; 2008.

Section 20

Pediatric Procedures

20.1 Common Procedures in Pediatric Practice

Baldev S Prajapati

INTRODUCTION

It is very essential for every medical student and practicing pediatrician to learn performing common pediatric procedures. The procedures are best learnt by observation, performing the procedure under supervision and repetitive performances. It should be practical, methodological and safe for both patients as well as for the individual who performs the procedure.

GENERAL CONSIDERATIONS

Healthcare Counseling

Healthcare counseling (HCC) is a relatively new concept that amalgamates human biology, human psychology and medical sociology principles, and applies the same in real-time clinical situations. HCC is especially important for the child population as the pediatricians need to partner the parenting responsibilities in different illness care settings covering the period from newborn to adolescence.

Explain to the parents in detail regarding the procedure including its indications, technique of the procedure, possible complications, etc. If the child is older and able to understand, talk to him also in simple language. By this, cooperation is available from parents as well as the child. It decreases the anxiety of all and the procedure can be performed smoothly.

An informed consent is a must for all the procedures. In certain procedures such as lumbar puncture, pleural and pericardial tapping, liver biopsy, renal biopsy, exchange transfusion, bone marrow aspiration and biopsy, it is prudent to get signed consent along with HCC to avoid medicolegal problems.

Procedure Room and Lighting

Separate procedure room is desirable. It should have good daylight and should be well-illuminated and well-equipped. All the equipment and drugs to perform the procedure as well as to manage any emergency if it arises should be made available.

Containers

It is very important to confirm that proper containers are available for collection and transferring the specimens.

Identification of the Patient

It should be a routine to identify the child before performing the procedure. It should be confirmed with hospital staff as well as the parents that you are dealing with the correct child.

Sedation

Children are afraid of procedures and their reactions in the form of crying and struggling and frightened appearance increases the parental anxiety. It affects the performance of the person who is performing the procedure. It results in increased rate of failure and complications related to procedure. In this situation, sedation to the child may help. Promethazine 1 mg/kg/dose or triclofos sodium 20 mg/kg/dose by oral route will suffice in most of the cases. Diazepam, ketamine and general anesthesia are other options as per indications.

Restraint

Physical restraint of the frightened child may be essential for the successful outcome of any practical procedure. The child may be wrapped with a blanket taking care to prevent aspiration or airway obstruction. The help of the person who is assisting is very crucial in deciding the outcome of the procedure.

Anesthesia

Local anesthesia may be achieved by infiltrating tissues around the site with 0.5–2% lignocaine. The maximum dosage of 1% lignocaine that can be infiltrated is 0.3 mL/kg. An alternative is to apply lignocaine cream to small area of the skin 60 minutes prior to performing the procedure, protected by adhesive dressing. Sedation or general anesthesia may be needed in certain cases.

Asepsis

The physician should scrub hands and forearm using an effective cleaning agent like 4% chlorhexidine or hexachlorophene before undertaking any procedure. Wearing of sterile gloves by the doctor is very important both for his and the patient's safety. The site of the patient's skin is then cleaned with 70% isopropyl alcohol and the surface is allowed to dry, the surface is then again washed three times with 10% povidone-iodine or 0.5% chlorhexidine gluconate in 70% isopropyl alcohol. It should be cleaned in a circular fashion from the center outwards.

INTRAMUSCULAR INJECTION

Common Sites

Muscles commonly used for intramuscular (IM) injection are vastus lateralis, deltoid and gluteus medius. Children do not have well-developed gluteus medius and therefore, it is not the site of preference for IM injections. It has been documented that some vaccines like hepatitis B and antirabies vaccines administered at gluteal region produce very poor antibody response.

The vastus lateralis (anterolateral aspect of thigh) is the preferred site in infants. The site in vastus lateralis is the middlethird of the area between the greater trochanter and lateral femoral condyle **(Fig. 20.1.1)**.

In case of deltoid, the site for injection is midway between acromion process and deltoid insertion, which is 3–5 cm below the acromion process. This site may be used in children above 5 years and adults. The quantity of drug should be less than 5 mL. Only watery injections with less viscosity should be injected at deltoid region.

Technique (WHO Technique)

- The site of injection should be exposed well.
- For anterolateral aspect of thigh, the child may be laid supine or be held in mother's lap. For deltoid, child may be held in mother's lap or may sit.
- The muscle selected for injection should be relaxed.
- The skin over injection site should be cleaned with spirit. A circular motion of swab is used, proceeding from puncture site and extending outward for 5 cm. Let the spirit evaporate and skin become dry otherwise spirit entering into tissues is painful.
- The syringe is filled with the medicine.
- In children, usually 23G needles with 25 mm length are used for IM injections.
- Stretch the skin flat and push the needle down at 90° **(Fig. 20.1.2)**.
- Aspiration before injecting the vaccine is not required.
- Inject the vaccine at the rate of 1 mL per 10 seconds.
- The needle is withdrawn and injection site is pressed for few seconds. Do not rub the injection site.
- Needle should be withdrawn smoothly with steady movement.
- Discard the needle and syringe as per standard guidelines.

Alternative to WHO technique, Advisory Committee on Immunization Practices (ACIP) technique may be used. It is also called bunching technique. In this technique, bunch the muscle and direct needle inferiorly along long axis of leg at an angle of 45°. It stabilizes leg and increases the muscle mass.

SUBCUTANEOUS INJECTION

Drugs or vaccines are injected subcutaneously when slow absorption and long duration of action are desired. Another indication of subcutaneous (SC) injection route is a coagulopathy, which makes IM injection hazardous, for fear of development of intramuscular hematoma. Insulin and heparin like drugs as well as measles, mumps, rubella (MMR), varicella vaccines are given by SC route.

Technique

- Common sites are arm, anterior abdominal wall and thigh. Atrophic and infected areas are avoided.

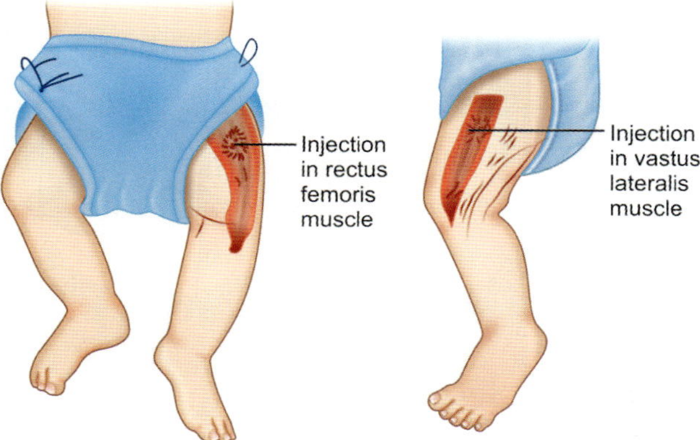

Fig. 20.1.1: Site for intramuscular injections (IM) in an infant.
Source: Prajapati BS. Essential Procedures in Pediatrics, 1st edition. New Delhi: Jaypee Brothers Medical Publishers (P) Ltd; 2003.

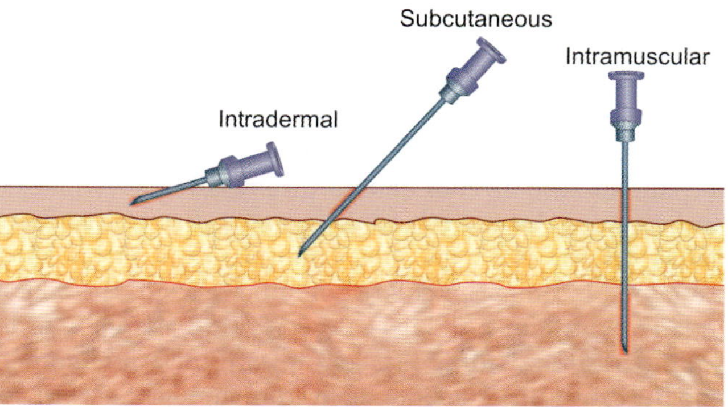

Fig. 20.1.2: The position of the needle during different ways of administering injections.
Source: Wechter EH, Philips J, Holaday B. Nursing Care of Children, 10th edition. Philadelphia: JB Lippincott Co; 1985.

- The skin is cleaned and disinfected with spirit.
- 26G needle with 13 mm length is commonly used for SC injection.
- The skin is raised into a fold with thumb and index finger of the left hand.
- The midpoint of the fold is pierced with the needle held at 45° with its surface. The tip of the needle is advanced into the subcutaneous tissue **(Fig. 20.1.2)**.
- Aspiration is not required.
- Drugs or vaccine is injected, needle is withdrawn and site is pressed for few minutes.

INTRADERMAL INJECTION

Indications for intradermal (ID) injection are Bacillus Calmette-Guérin (BCG) vaccination, Mantoux test, skin tests for allergy, test for sensitization of certain drugs like penicillin. Antirabies vaccine also can be given by ID route.

Technique

- Ventral (volar) aspect of forearm is commonly used for ID injection.
- Skin is cleaned with sterile water.
- A measured amount of antigen (usually 0.1 mL) is drawn into the syringe.
- 26G or 27G needle with 1/4 to 1/2 inch (6.35–12.7 mm) length needle is used for ID injection.
- The skin is held taut between thumb and index finger of the left hand. The syringe is held at an angle of 10–15° with the skin. Needle is inserted for about 2 mm, so that entire needle bevel penetrates the skin and the injected solution raises a small bleb of about 5 mm in diameter. The development of perifollicular puckering (peau d'orange) indicates successful ID injection **(Fig. 20.1.2)**.
- The needle is withdrawn.
- The site is circled and it is recorded in patient's chart.
- The reaction is observed in defined time.

RECTAL ADMINISTRATION OF DRUGS

It is a safe and easy way of administering drugs. The human rectum represents a body cavity in which drugs can be easily introduced and retained. The absorption of the drugs is well through this route. Rectal administration of drugs is indicated in patients who are not able to take orally due to nausea and vomiting, having convulsions, uncooperative children, before surgery, etc. If the child can understand, it should be explained to him. The child should be relaxed. He is kept in lateral position with knees flexed toward abdomen or in supine position with legs taken upward toward abdomen and the drug is inserted into the rectum through anal orifice, and buttocks are held firmly to prevent expulsion of the drug. Paracetamol, diazepam, midazolam, paraldehyde, glycerine, bisacodyl, diclofenac sodium, steroids, neomycin, artesunate and many more drugs can be administered through rectal route. When rectal preparations are not available, some liquid preparations like injection diazepam may be given per rectum. For this purpose, a lubricated tube is inserted into the rectum to a distance of about 5 cm and then the medication is administered through it using a syringe. The buttocks are held together for a couple of minutes. Local irritation and ulcerations in rectum may develop as complication of this procedure, if done repeatedly.

PERIPHERAL INTRAVENOUS ACCESS

Peripheral intravenous access is one of the mainstays of modern medicine. It allows blood sampling, administration of medicines, fluids, nutrients, blood and blood products. Intracaths and scalp vein needles are commonly used for this purpose. Various sites for venous access are as follows in order to preference **(Fig. 20.1.3)**:

- Veins on dorsum of hand.
- Superficial radial vein on radial aspect of wrist.
- Superficial veins over volar aspect of forearm.
- Basilic vein and median cubital vein over antecubital fossa.
- Superficial veins over dorsum of foot and long saphenous vein on medial aspect of leg above the ankle.
- Veins of scalp in newborns and infants.
- External jugular vein.

Straight, large and easily accessible peripheral veins in healthy subcutaneous tissues are ideal for venous access. Veins of the upper extremities are preferred because there are many potential sites and more comfortable to the patient. The distal and superficial veins are preferred as complications are more, following extravasation and thrombophlebitis in proximal and deep veins. When the veins are not visible, they can be palpated at common sites and can be accessed.

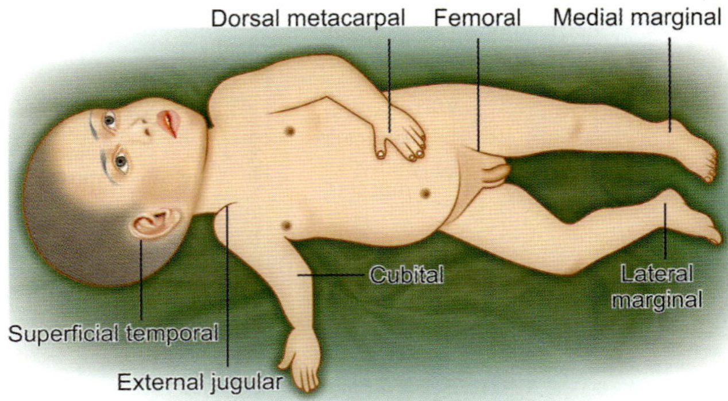

Fig. 20.1.3: Common sites for venipuncture.
Source: Prajapati BS. Essential Procedures in Pediatrics, 1st edition. New Delhi: Jaypee Brothers Medical Publishers (P) Ltd; 2003.

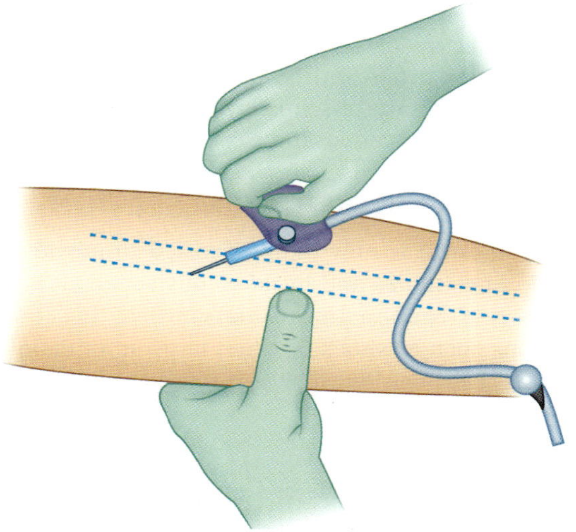

Fig. 20.1.4: Technique of venipuncture with scalp vein needle. *Source:* Prajapati BS. Essential Procedures in Pediatrics, 1st edition. New Delhi: Jaypee Brothers Medical Publishers (P) Ltd; 2003.

Scalp vein needle is a hollow needle with butterfly plastic handle and a plastic tube, at the other end of which, a syringe or infusion set can be attached. It is useful for venous sampling of blood and short-term use of intravenous route **(Fig. 20.1.4)**. Vein is counter punctured very easily on movement of the limb.

Intracaths are plastic catheters over a hollow metallic needle. The metallic needle just projects beyond the tip of plastic catheter. The metallic needle is to provide stiffness during insertion into the vein, after which it is withdrawn. The plastic catheter is then advanced further gently so that vein is not counter punctured. The plastic catheter is well tolerated. Intracaths and scalp vein needles are available in various sizes from 26G to 16G. In children commonly, we use 26G–21G depending on age of the child and requirement.

Technique

- A tourniquet is placed over the limb, 3–4 cm proximal to the site selected for venipuncture, taking care not to pinch the skin of the child. The pressure should be such that it occludes venous flow but allows arterial blood flow.
- Tapping sharply over the vein causes mechanical reflex dilatation of the vascular walls. It should be light otherwise pain will cause vasoconstriction.
- Active or passive pumping of extremity enhances blood flow and distends veins.
- A warm moist towel may be applied to the site for several minutes. It causes venous dilatation.
- Aseptic precautions are mandatory.
- The methylated spirit is applied over 4–5 cm area at planned site. Let it dry.

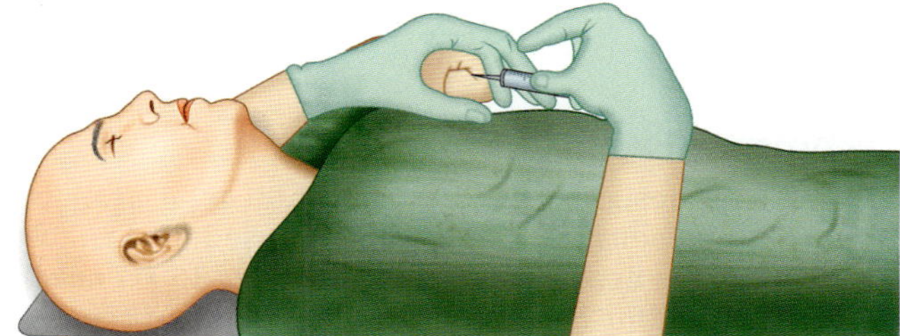

Fig. 20.1.5: For inserting the intravenous (IV) cannula on the dorsum of the hand. The hand may be held flexed at the wrist to occlude venous return and make the veins prominent.

- The skin is pulled taut distally to stabilize the vein with a nondominant hand. It is punctured by the needle bevel. up at 15–30° angle parallel to the vein **(Fig. 20.1.5)**. After the entry into the subcutaneous tissue, the needle is aligned parallel to the skin surface and along the long axis of the vein. Its tip is depressed a little and is advanced until it penetrates the vein. Then, it is made parallel to the vein again and advanced until it is passed fully into the vein. Blood is collected if indicated and then the intravenous (IV) set is attached to it.
- The tourniquet is removed and the infusion is started by releasing the clamp on the tubing. A hub of the cannula and IV set are secured to the skin with the adhesive plaster.
- For flushing the cannula, normal saline should be used and not the distilled water. Distilled water causes pain at IV site and it also causes hemolysis.
- If venipuncture is performed only for collection of blood, pull the needle gently after collecting the required sample and apply steady pressure at the site with a piece of spirit swab for few minutes.

INTRAOSSEOUS INFUSION

Peripheral percutaneous venous access is the fastest method of obtaining vascular access in children. However, during life threatening emergencies, rapid access to venous compartment through peripheral or central venous route is occasionally difficult or an impossible procedure for a pediatrician to perform. Small peripheral vessels in children often collapse during shock and efforts at setting up an IV line in a peripheral vein may fail. When IV access cannot be established within three attempts or 90 seconds time, intraosseous route should be used as per the recommendations.

Common Sites

- Anteromedial surface of the proximal tibia, one or two finger breadths distal to tibial tuberosity to avoid damage to epiphyseal growth plate.
- 2–3 cm above the lateral condyle of the femur in the midline.

- Medial surface of the distal tibia proximal to the medial malleolus.

Technique (Fig. 20.1.6)

- Specially designed needles, Jamshidi type available for intraosseous infusion should be used, if available. Hypodermic needle can also be used. 20–16 FG needle can be used for children below 18 months of age, and 16–12 FG for older children.
- Identify the site of placement.
- Patient's leg should be restrained, a small sand bag is placed behind the knee.
- The use of local anesthesia is optional, but usually recommended as it may be more painful once the child is resuscitated.
- Aseptic precautions are must.
- Insert the needle perpendicular to the skin and advance to the periosteum and then with a screwing motion penetrate into the marrow. A distinct "give way" sensation indicates that your needle is in marrow. Confirm that the needle is firmly embedded in the bone.
- Insertion of needle to a depth of 1 cm is usually adequate as the distance from skin through the cortex is rarely more than 1 cm in infants and children.
- The needle should maintain erect posture without support.
- Trocar is removed and correct position is verified by aspiration of marrow and easy flushing with 5–10 mL of normal saline without signs of extravasation.
- The needle should be secured and apply sterile dressing over the site.
- It should be watched for local complications like extravasation and infection.
- As soon as the peripheral IV route is established, intraosseus needle should be removed.
- Emergency drugs and fluids can be administered via intraosseous route, essentially the same dosage and rates as given by intravenous route.

VENOUS CUTDOWN (VENESECTION)

Venous cutdown is now rarely resorted to in the present scenario of cannulas and intraosseous access. It is mainly useful when routine intravenous access has failed in conditions such as shock or when large amounts of fluids have to be given for a long time as in total parenteral nutrition.

Sites

- *Lower limb*: Most preferred site is saphenous vein near ankle.
- *Upper limb*: Median cubital or basilic vein in front of elbow.
- Cephalic vein at the wrist at anatomical snuff box.
- External jugular vein in the neck.

Technique (Fig. 20.1.7)

- Get all the instruments ready.
- Prepare the part aseptically. Then it is draped with sterile towels.
- 0.5% Xylocaine is infiltrated subcutaneously at the site of incision. In emergency, local anesthesia can be skipped.
- A 1–2 cm long transverse incision is made 1.5 cm above and in front of medial malleolus over the saphenous vein.
- The vein is exposed by blunt dissection, opening the blades of mosquito forceps parallel to the vein.

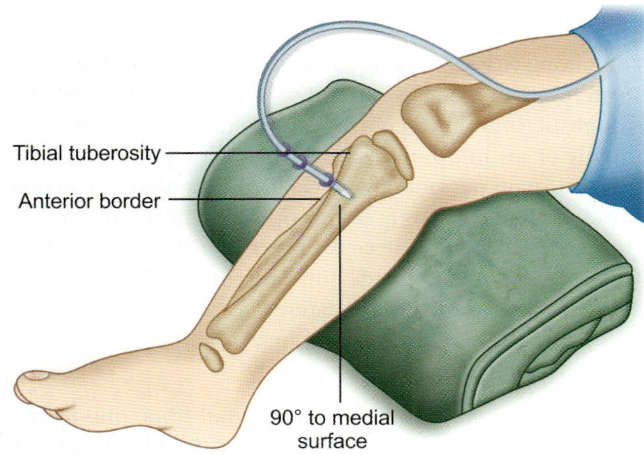

Fig. 20.1.6: Intraosseous cannulation technique.
Source: Chameides L. Textbook of Pediatrics Advanced Life Support. American Heart Association—American Academy of Pediatrics; 1988.

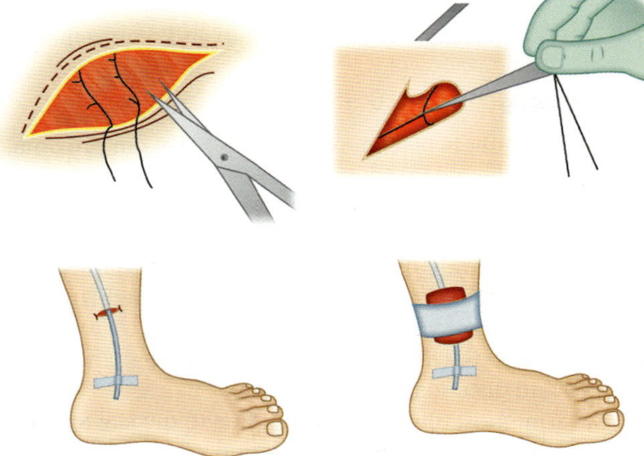

Fig. 20.1.7: Venous cut down.
Source: Prajapati BS. Essential Procedures in Pediatrics, 1st edition. New Delhi: Jaypee Brothers Medical Publishers (P) Ltd.; 2003.

- Pass the tip of mosquito artery forceps beneath the vein and elevate at least 1 cm above the vein.
- Pass two silk ligatures under the vein.
- Separate the proximal and distal ligatures for full length of exposed vein.
- Tie the distal ligature and hold the ends with mosquito forceps.
- With venesection scissors put "v" shaped cut on anterior wall of the vein at middle of the exposed part.
- Introduce polyethylene tube of suitable size proximally through the cut in the vein till the free flow of blood is obtained.
- Cannula is fixed by tying proximal ligature on the vein with cannula in vein.
- Ends of proximal and distal ligatures are trimmed.
- Wound is sutured by silk sutures in a way so that cannula or tube does not get kinked or obstructed.
- Dressing is applied and remaining part of the tube is properly fixed with dressing.
- IV drip is connected to the venesection needle.

Complications

- Wound infections
- Thrombophlebitis
- Deep vein thrombosis
- Air embolism
- Injury to adjacent nerves and vessels.

As alternate route is possible, earliest venesection tube should be removed.

EXTERNAL JUGULAR VEIN PUNCTURE

The external jugular vein is formed below the ear and behind the angle of mandible, passes downwards and obliquely backward across the surface of sternocleidomastoid muscle and ends in subclavian vein lateral to anterior scalene muscle.

Technique (Figs. 20.1.8 and 20.1.9)

- Place the patient in supine. Both the shoulders should touch the table and head is rotated fully to one side and extended partly over the end of the table so as to extend the vein. Making the child cry makes the vein prominent.
- Restraining the child properly is very important.
- Clean the overlying skin.
- Use proper size of the cannula. Keep the cannula in the direction of the vein with the point aimed toward the same shoulder.
- Make the venipuncture midway between the angle of mandible and midclavicular line.
- Proceed as described for veins of extremities.
- After removing the needle, apply constant pressure at puncture site for 5 minutes while the child is sitting.

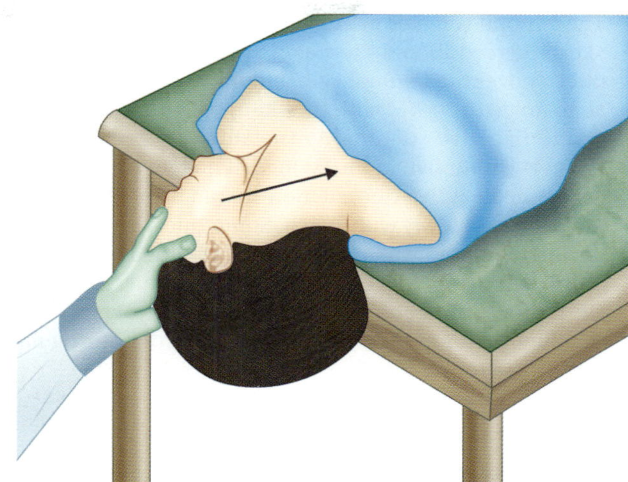

Fig. 20.1.8: Position for jugular vein (both internal and external) puncture. The arrow shows the direction of insertion of the needle for external jugular vein puncture.
Source: Silver HK, Kempe CH, Bruyn HB. Handbook of Pediatrics, 13th edition. Singapore: Lange-Maruzen Asia Publications; 1980.

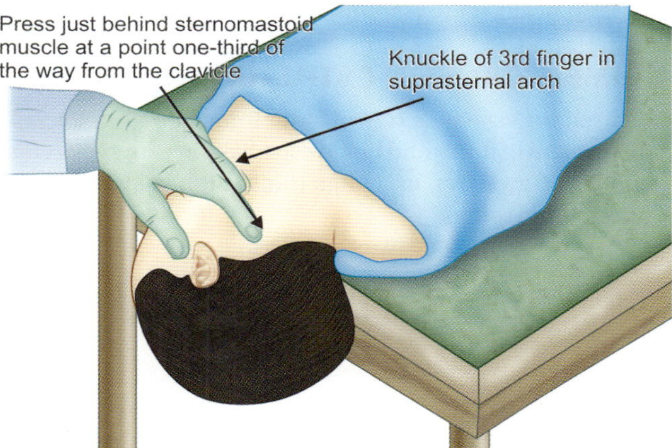

Fig. 20.1.9: Internal jugular vein puncture technique.
Source: Silver HK, Kempe CH, Bruyn HB. Handbook of Pediatrics, 13th edition. Singapore: Lange-Maruzen Asia Publications; 1980.

FEMORAL VEIN PUNCTURE

In view of the risks of femoral venipuncture, it should be used as a last resort for collection of blood samples in neonates and infants.

Technique

- Restraining the infant in frog leg position.
- Clean the inguinal area properly. The part is cleaned properly with spirit—iodine-spirit.
- The femoral artery is located just below the midpoint of inguinal ligament.

- The femoral vein lies medial to the artery.
- Skin is pierced about 1–2 cm as below the inguinal ligament directly over the femoral vein and the needle is advanced at an angle of 30–45° with the skin while maintaining the gentle negative suction. As the vein is punctured, the blood is withdrawn in the syringe. If no blood is obtained while needle is inserted, suction should be maintained as the needle is slowly withdrawn. Sometimes needle passes through both the walls of the vein and blood is obtained only when the needle is being withdrawn.
- On removal of needle, apply firm pressure over the site of puncture for at least 3–5 minutes to avoid oozing and hematoma formation.

Precautions

- As far as possible avoid this procedure.
- Strict asepsis is must as there is potential risk of septic arthritis and osteomyelitis.
- Be careful regarding piercing the femoral artery, which can be identified by bright red color of blood as jet flow of it. If artery is pierced inadvertently, remove the needle and apply pressure for a long time and check the limb periodically for pulsations, color and warmth.

UMBILICAL VEIN CATHETERIZATION

It is used for exchange transfusion. It may be used for rapid replacement of fluids and blood especially in extreme preterm neonates. Nowadays, exchange transfusion is also preferred by peripheral route.

The umbilical vein spirals through the cord and is at 12 o'clock position at the level of the abdominal wall. Here, it turns cephalad and runs slightly toward right to enter the porta hepatis. It continues with left portal vein, communicates with left hepatic vein and then with inferior vena cava. The umbilical vein is much wider than umbilical arteries.

Technique

- The child should be in supine position with gentle restraining. A padded crucifix splint is used to restrain the baby.
- Sterilize and drape the skin around the umbilical stump.
- The cord is then cut cleanly about 2 cm above the umbilicus and umbilical vein is located at 12 o'clock position. The blood clot in the vein is expressed or pulled out by fine forceps **(Figs. 20.1.10A and B)**.
- Mark the catheter for the correct distance to be inserted, which is about 20% of the crown heel length.
- The catheter is passed into the vein slowly and gently, giving caudal traction on the cord stump till free flow of blood is obtained.
- Flush the catheter with heparinized saline.
- The free end of the catheter should be strapped to the abdominal wall.

Special Points

- If the cord is dried up, it can be excised flush with the umbilicus, which can expose the orifice of the umbilical vein at 12 o'clock position. This can be gently dilated with Hagar's dilator and then catheterized.

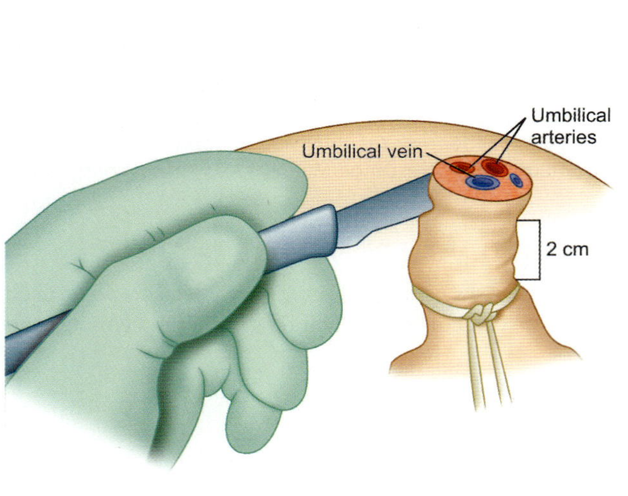

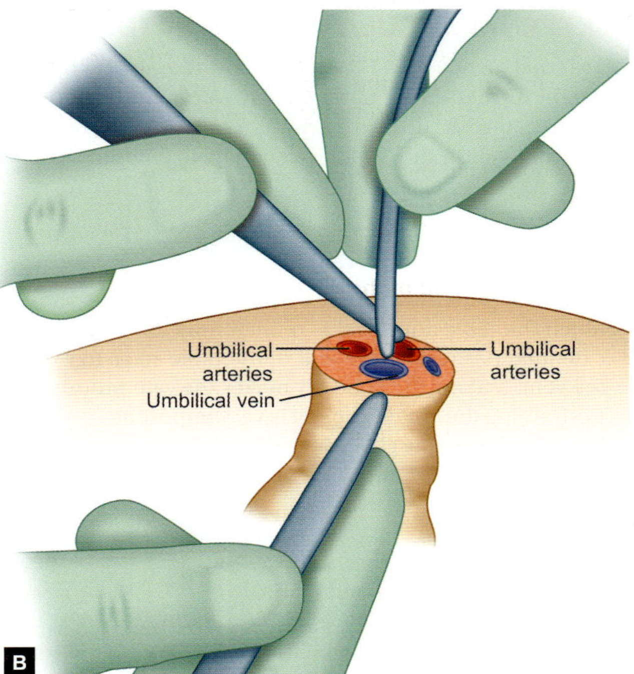

Figs. 20.1.10A and B: (A) Cutting the umbilical cord for vessel catheterization; (B) Insertion of umbilical catheter in umbilical vein.
Source: Prajapati BS. Essential Procedures in Pediatrics, 1st edition. New Delhi: Jaypee Brothers Medical Publishers (P) Ltd; 2003.

- If both these methods fail, supraumbilical cut down will become necessary.
- Remove the umbilical vein catheter within 24–48 hours.
- The catheter tip should be advanced up to thoracic portion of the inferior vena cava.
- While passing the catheter, the resistance is felt at the ductus venosus. The catheter should be passed 1–2 cm beyond this point.

Complications

- Infection
- Vessel perforation
- Thrombosis of portal vein and portal hypertension in the future
- Liver infarction
- Liver abscess
- Necrotizing enterocolitis
- Cardiac arrhythmias.

UMBILICAL ARTERY CATHETERIZATION

It is used for periodic monitoring of arterial blood gases and for constant monitoring of blood pressure in a neonate. There are two umbilical arteries and the lumen appears patent.

Technique

- Prepare the umbilical stump as for venous catheterization.
- Identify the artery and insert the catheter gently in the caudal direction, pulling the umbilical stump superiorly.
- Position the tip of the catheter at either high (in the lower thoracic aorta above the diaphragm between T4 and T11 vertebre) or low position (in the abdominal aorta opposite L4 vertebra).
- Keep observing the color of the lower limbs during the procedure.
- Fix the catheter in place using purse string sutures at the place.
- Strap the free end of the catheter to the abdominal wall after filling it with heparinized saline and closing the end with a rubber stopper.
- Every time before sampling, remove the heparinized saline in the syringe along with same blood, then collect the sample and reinfuse the previously collected blood to the child.

Complications

- Vessel perforation
- Thromboembolism
- Air embolism
- Hypertension
- Necrotizing enterocolitis
- Infarction of distal extremities
- Renal infarction.

RADIAL ARTERY CATHETERIZATION

It is very useful and frequently used for repeated sampling of arterial blood and for continuous arterial pressure monitoring. The radial artery is easily accessible at the wrist in the groove between the tendon of the flexor carpi radialis medially and the distal radius laterally.

Before puncturing the radial artery, carry out the Allen test to assess the ulnar collateral circulation.

Allen Test (Figs. 20.1.11A to D)

- Make the patient's hands warm to make pulsations easily demonstrable.
- Have the patient open and close the hand held out in front and then clinch the first tightly closed.
- Occlude both radial and ulnar arteries for 30 seconds. Have the patient open the hand. Hand becomes pale due to occlusion of radial and ulnar arteries.
- Release the pressure over the ulnar artery and observe the open hand for return of normal pink color. Return of normal color within 6 seconds indicates patency of the ulnar artery and an intact arch with good collateral circulation.
- Delay of appearance of normal color from 10 seconds to 15 seconds indicates slow filling of the ulnar artery and collaterals.
- Persistent blanching for more than 15 seconds indicates an incomplete arch or poor collaterals.
- Same test can be performed to check patency of radial artery.
- If ulnar collateral circulation is good, radial artery puncture can be performed.

Technique (Figs. 20.1.12A and B)

Patient's hand should be supported and dorsiflexed at the wrist approximately 60° with both hands and lower forearm

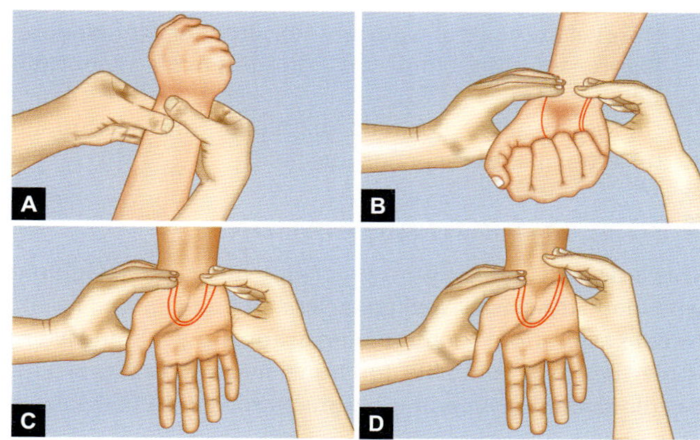

Figs. 20.1.11A to D: Allen test.
Source: Prajapati BS. Essential Procedures in Pediatrics, 1st edition. New Delhi: Jaypee Brothers Medical Publishers (P) Ltd; 2003.

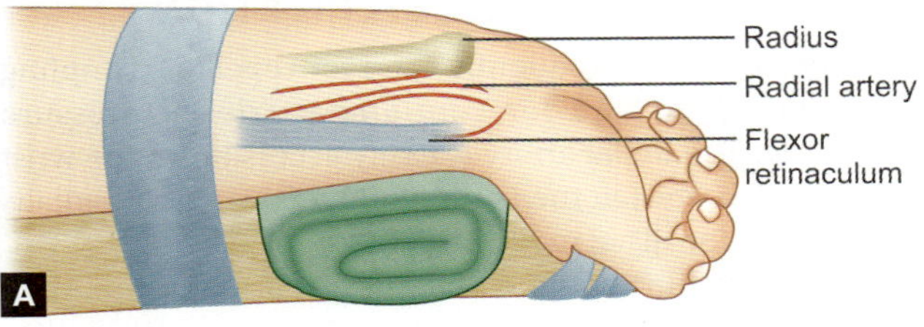

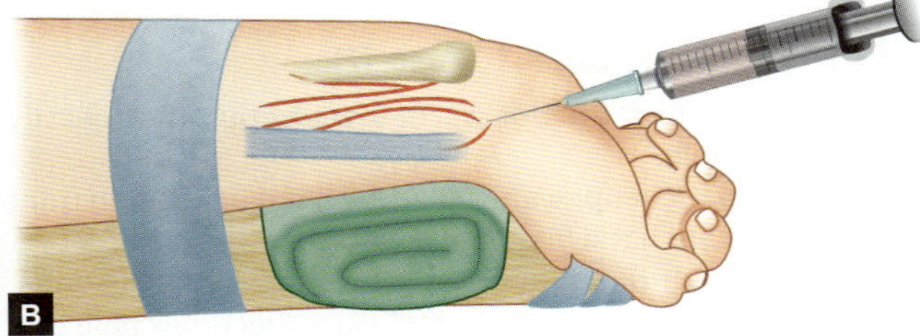

Figs. 20.1.12A and B: Radial artery—(A) Anatomy; (B) Catheterization technique.

secured to a board. A roll of gauze behind the wrist will maintain dorsiflexion.

- Locate the radial artery just proximal to head of radius.
- Clean the area and observe the absolutely aseptic precautions.
- Infiltrate the skin with local anesthetic agent.
- Insert the catheter needle at about 30° angle to the surface of the skin and advance the catheter and needle stylet into the artery until blood appears in hub of the needle.
- Remove the needle and attach the hub of the catheter to the connecting tubing.
- Secure the catheter at the place with silk sutures.
- Fix the wrist in a neutral position to the board. It is essential as flexion at wrist can disturb the arterial line.
- Cover the insertion site with sterile dressing.

Special Points

- Do not perform the procedure if Allen's test is delayed.
- Observe the color of palm periodically after cannulation.
- Before sampling blood, flush the line with 2% normal saline.
- Do not infuse medications and blood products through the arterial line except flushing fluid.

BONE MARROW ASPIRATION

This is a very common ward procedure indicated in children with blood dyscrasias, malignancies and undiagnosed fevers. Needle aspiration, trephine biopsy and surgical biopsy are three methods available for bone marrow examination. Needle aspiration is commonly practiced in most of the cases

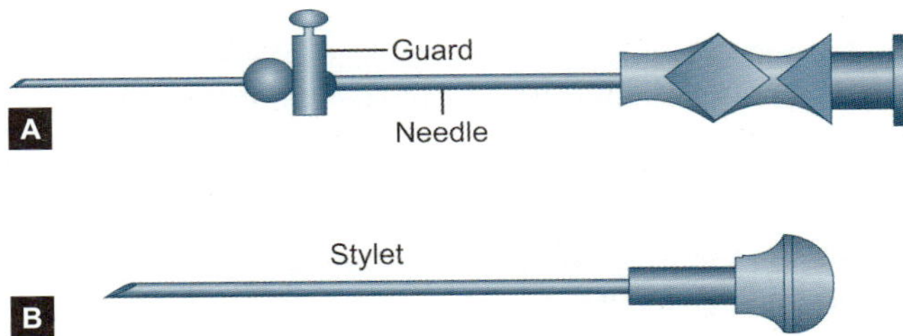

Figs. 20.1.13A and B: Bone marrow aspiration needle.
Source: Prajapati BS. Essential Procedures in Pediatrics, 1st edition. New Delhi: Jaypee Brothers Medical Publishers (P) Ltd; 2003.

in children. It should be done with caution when a defect in clotting mechanism is suspected.

Common Sites

- *Iliac crest*: This is the most preferred site in children. It is performed at 1 cm below the posterior iliac crest.
- *Tibia*: At the upper end of tibia, just below tibial tuberosity on its medial aspect.
- *Sternum*: It should be used in children beyond 7–8 years of age. Manubrium sterni can be used 1 cm above sternomanubrial angle, slightly to one side of the midline.
- Rarely, lumbar spinous processes may be used.

Technique

- Atropine should be given as premedication.
- Aseptic and antiseptic precautions are must during the whole procedure.
- Local infiltration of 1% lignocaine from skin to periosteum. In some irritable children, general anesthesia is desirable for successful outcome of the procedure.
- The needle for bone marrow aspiration should be stout and made of hard stainless steel. It is about 7–8 cm long with a well-fitting stylet and an adjustable guard **(Figs. 20.1.13A and B)**. The point of needle and edge of bevel should be sharp. The Sahan and Klima needles are most commonly used needles. Some people prefer to use stout hypodermic needles so that these can be disposed after use and complications of reuse of the needle can be avoided.
- The needle with the guard adjusted 0.5–1 cm from the tip of the needle is introduced into the iliac crest or sternum with screwing or boring movements keeping the needle vertical. The force required varies but needs to be considerable. Sudden giving in of resistance indicates entry of the needle into the bone marrow. Leave the needle and if it remains steady, it indicates that the needle is in the bone marrow.

- The stylet is withdrawn and marrow is aspirated with the syringe. About 0.2 mL of marrow is aspirated. This procedure is performed swiftly to obtain only bone marrow particles as slow sluggish aspiration causes dilution of marrow with blood.
- To prevent dilution of marrow with blood, aspirate material only till it appears beyond nozzle of syringe. It is sufficient material for examination. Aspiration beyond it increases the chances of marrow dilution.
- The needle is withdrawn and smear is prepared with marrow. With good material and well-prepared smear marrow, particles can be seen by naked eyes.
- Press the site for 5 minutes. Apply tincture of benzoin seal at puncture site.
- Along with smears of bone marrow, smears from peripheral blood should be prepared and sent for examination.

Complications

- Local pain and hematoma
- Injury to mediastinal structures in case of aspiration at sternum
- Infection
- Dry tap.

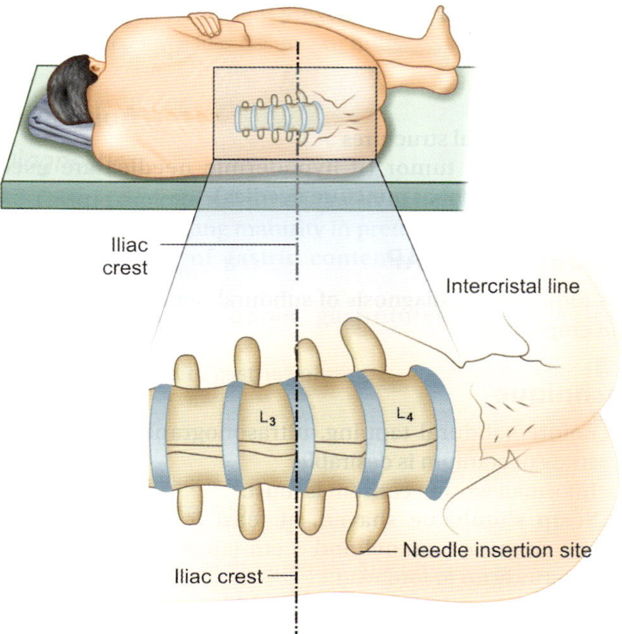

Fig. 20.1.14: Position for lumbar puncture.
Source: Prajapati BS. Essential Procedures in Pediatrics, 1st edition. New Delhi: Jaypee Brothers Medical Publishers (P) Ltd; 2003.

LUMBAR PUNCTURE

This procedure is performed to obtain cerebrospinal fluid (CSF) sample for analysis in diagnosing infections and other disorders of central nervous system. It is also used for monitoring CSF pressure, intrathecal drug administration and removing CSF in some cases of hydrocephalus.

Contraindications

- Marked raised intracranial pressure (ICP) with closed fontanel because of the risk of herniation of brain substance through foramen magnum. Papilledema is a marker of raised ICP
- Local infection
- Cardiovascular and respiratory instability.

Technique

- Informed written consent is must.
- The patient is placed on his side at the edge of the table or bed with the knee drawn up toward abdomen and the head flexed to get maximum flexion of the spine **(Fig. 20.1.14)**. If the child is newborn or child has respiratory problem, child should be firmly fixed at shoulders and buttocks only without flexing neck and drawing up knees. In infants, sitting position allows easier identification of the midline. An experienced assistant has a vital role in positioning, restraining and comforting the patient.
- Aseptic and antiseptic precautions are must.
- Routinely, local anesthesia is not used. But in older children those are irritable; local anesthesia may be useful for performing the procedure smoothly.
- Site of puncture is defined by palpating the iliac crest, which corresponds to L3–L4. Hold the needle between index and middle fingers. In children, instead of lumbar puncture needle with stylet, simple hypodermic needle is commonly used. This should be avoided.
- Gently introduce the needle in midline at above mentioned space, needle being directed toward umbilicus. Entry into the subarachnoid space is indicated by giving the way sensation and free flow of CSF.
- Collect the CSF 0.5 cc in ethylenediaminetetra acetic acid (EDTA) bulb for cell count and 1 cc in plain bulb for biochemistry. It should also be collected in sterile bulb for culture.

CSF for cell count should be examined at the earliest, usually within 30 minutes.

- Remove the needle and apply firm pressure for few minutes.
- Apply tincture benzoin seal at puncture site.
- In a case of raised intracranial pressure, head should be kept little down to prevent herniation of brain through foramen magnum.
- Monitor the patient for sometime after the procedure for pulse and respiration.

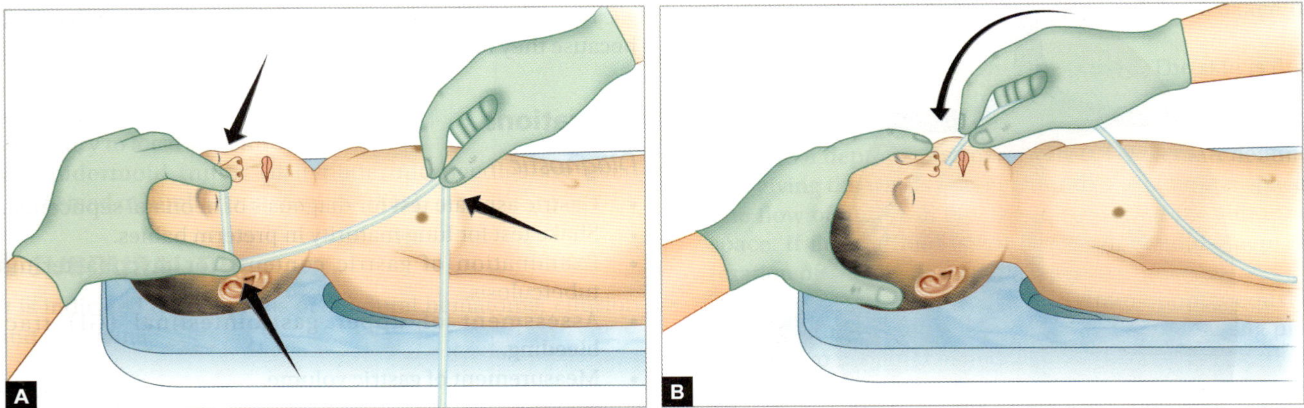

Figs. 20.1.17A and B: Method of inserting a nasogastric tube in a child.

Source: World Health Organization. Management of the child with a serious infection or severe malnutrition: guidelines for care at the first-referral level in Developing Countries Department of Child and Adolescent Health and Development, World Health Organization. Geneva; 2000.

  - Air is injected into the tube while epigastric area is auscultated. A sound is heard if the tube is in the stomach.
  - Placing a tube in a glass of water and escape of air bubbles in the water indicate that the tube lies in the trachea.
  - Placement of a radiopaque tube can be assessed by radiography.
- The tube is fixed with a tape in a butterfly fashion around the tube or with vertical tapping over the nose and the tube. The tapping is done in such a way that the tube rests in the middle of the nasal lumen and not directly in contact with mucosa. It is not taped over the forehead as it may cause pressure necrosis of the nose.
- The feed or drug should be allowed to go in the tube by gravity method. It should not be pushed by piston. The tube should be flushed with water periodically.
- While removing the tube, pinch the tube end to prevent spilling of the contents into the trachea.

Complications

- Pulmonary aspiration
- Esophageal perforation
- Gastric perforation
- Nasal necrosis
- Esophageal stricture.

Instead of nasogastric tubing, nowadays orogastric tubing is preferred to avoid certain complications.

GASTRIC LAVAGE

It is useful in removing the poisonous substance from the stomach. In corrosives and hydrocarbons ingestion, gastric lavage is contraindicated. In corrosives, passing the tube may cause perforation. Since passing the gastric tube is likely to induce vomiting, it increases the risk of aspiration of hydrocarbons into the trachea and lungs, which causes pneumonia.

After passing the tube in the stomach as described in nasogastric tube insertion, lavage of the stomach using aliquots of normal saline is done in cases of poisoning. It is continued till the color of the lavage is normal.

ABDOMINAL PARACENTESIS

Abdominal paracentesis is performed for diagnostic purpose in case of ascites, peritonitis and hemorrhage. In huge ascites, it is also done to relieve discomfort and respiratory embarrassment. In some situations, drugs may be instilled in peritoneal cavity such as malignancies.

Technique

- The patient should be placed in supine position. If the patient is not comfortable in supine position, reclining or upright position may be used.
- Site for paracentesis is selected in midline, midway between umbilicus and pubic symphysis or in an iliac fossa lateral to the rectus abdominis.
- The needle should never be advanced through a surgical scar because it can penetrate bowel adherent to the under surface of the scar, or lacerate an omental or mesenteric vessel.
- Informed written consent should be taken.
- Aseptic and antiseptic measures must be taken.
- Injection atropine as premedication.
- One percent lignocaine is infiltrated under skin and into the deeper structures at the site selected for paracentesis. Wait for few minutes for full effect of anesthetic agent.

- The hypodermic needle 20 FG is attached to 20 mL syringe. It is passed into the peritoneal cavity perpendicular to the skin. As the needle enters the peritoneal cavity, it gives the way and ascitic fluid starts to drain through the needle.
- In a case of tense ascites, needle should be passed obliquely or skin should be retracted caudald before insertion of the needle to produce a Z track effect on withdrawing the needle so that needle tract after paracentesis gets sealed properly and persistent drainage can be prevented after removal of the needle.
- After removal of fluid, 10–15 mL for diagnostic purpose, the needle is withdrawn and a seal of tincture benzoin is applied locally.
- If the paracentesis is for therapeutic purpose, the needle should be connected with IV set and regulator of IV set is adjusted in such a way that ascitic fluid is drained slowly. One liter of fluid may be drained over a period of 2–3 hours.
- The patient should be watched following the procedure.

Complications

- Intestinal perforation or laceration
- Peritonitis
- Post paracentesis shock
- Electrolyte imbalance
- Hypoproteinemia
- Perforation of urinary bladder
- Pneumoperitoneum

LIVER BIOPSY

Nowadays, liver biopsy is done under the ultrasound guidance rather than blind biopsy.

Indications

- Chronic hepatitis
- Undiagnosed hepatomegaly
- Neonatal hepatitis
- Cirrhosis of liver
- Fever of unknown origin

Contraindications

- Bleeding tendency
- Massive and tense ascites
- Severe portal hypertension

Prerequisites

- Bleeding time, clotting time, platelet count and prothrombin time
- Ultrasound (USG) study of liver
- *Premedication*: Atropine 0.01 mg/kg IM 30 minutes before the procedure.

Technique

- Vim-Silverman needle, Menghini's needle and Tru-cut needles are used for liver biopsy. Tru-cut needle is disposable, easy to operate and has more success rate, so it is common in use.
- Informed written consent is a must.
- Patient is kept in supine position, near the edge of the bed or table with the right arm under the head and left arm by the side.
- Preparation of the local area.
- Aseptic and antiseptic precautions are must.
- One percent lignocaine is infiltrated in the skin, intercostal muscles and Glisson's capsule. Wait for some time for good effect of the anesthetic agent. Some children may require sedation or general anesthesia.
- The Tru-cut needle is introduced under ultrasound guidance into the liver substance with the inner needle retracted. The latter is then advanced, holding the outer cutting sheath steady. The outer sheath is then advanced to cut the liver in the biopsy notch. The whole apparatus is then withdrawn together quickly. The entire sequence should take only few seconds.
- The Vim-Silverman needle has trocar and bifid needle to cut the liver tissue. In Menghini's needle, the cut piece of liver is sucked into the syringe applied with negative pressure.
- On removal of the needle, the puncture site is sealed with tincture of benzoin.

THORACOCENTESIS (INTERCOSTAL DRAINAGE)

Thoracocentesis refers to temporary insertion of a needle or a catheter into the pleural space for removal of fluid or air from the pleural cavity. The fluid is collected for diagnostic purpose and in some situations it is done for therapeutic purpose to remove fluid or air, which is in large quantity and causes respiratory embarrassment. Drugs can also be instilled in the pleural cavity by this procedure, if it is indicated, such as in a case of malignancy.

Technique

- Written consent is must.
- *Injection*: Atropine as premedication.
- Site of insertion of needle can be decided by chest X-ray, dull note on percussion and ultrasound study of thorax. Best way to perform the procedure is under ultrasound guidance.
- It should be performed in sitting position of the patient. Patient can lean forward on the table of suitable height with head resting on his forearms **(Fig. 20.1.18)**.
- Strict aseptic and antiseptic measures should be taken.
- One percent lignocaine is infiltrated at the upper border of the rib below the space chosen. Anesthetizing wide

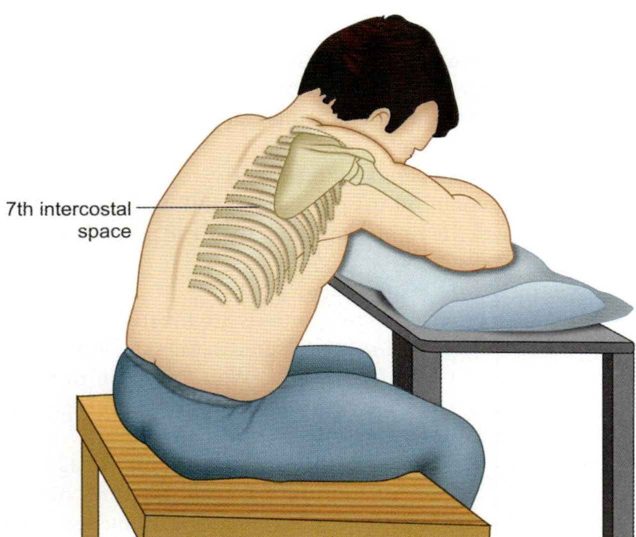

Fig. 20.1.18: Another position for doing thoracocentesis.
Source: Johnson KB. The Harriet Lane Handbook—a manual for pediatric house officers, 13th edition. New Delhi: Jaypee Brothers Medical Publishers (P) Ltd; 1993.

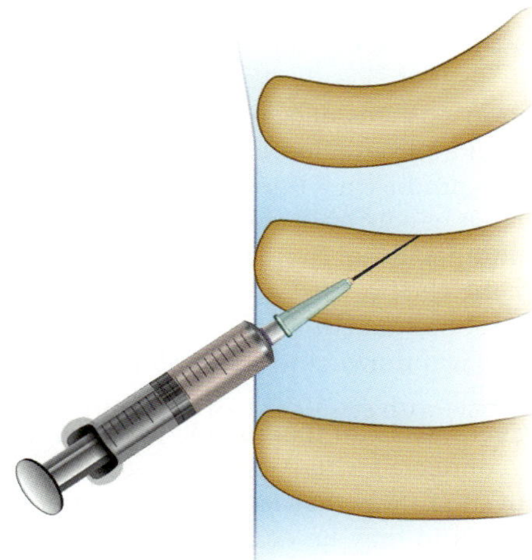

Fig. 20.1.19: Site of needle for pleural fluid aspiration.
Source: Prajapati BS. Essential Procedures in Pediatrics, 1st edition. New Delhi: Jaypee Brothers Medical Publishers (P) Ltd; 2003.

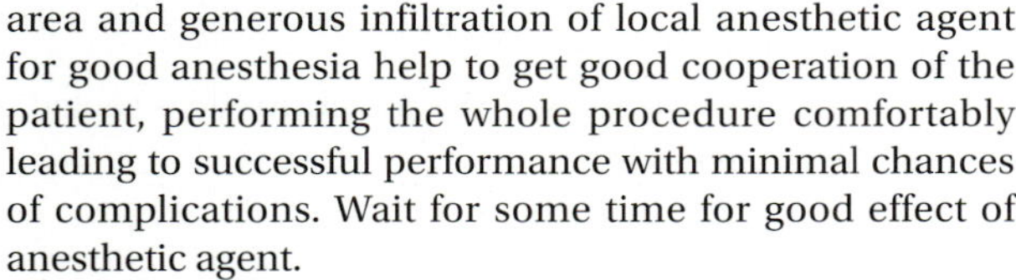

area and generous infiltration of local anesthetic agent for good anesthesia help to get good cooperation of the patient, performing the whole procedure comfortably leading to successful performance with minimal chances of complications. Wait for some time for good effect of anesthetic agent.

- A wide bore needle is connected on one side of the three-way stopcock and opposite to it a syringe is attached. Three-way stopcock is arranged in such a way that there is a single track between the needle, stopcock and syringe.
- The needle is inserted into the chest in the same manner as for the anesthetic needle, finding the intercostal space and stepping over the lower rib with care, thereby preventing damage to underlying structures **(Fig. 20.1.19)**. Slight suction is applied to the syringe so that the fluid is aspirated in the syringe immediately as the needle enters the pleural space.
- Fluid should be withdrawn slowly and steadily.
- A forceps should be attached to the needle at the skin level, which helps to prevent excessively deep insertion of the needle into the thorax.
- The fluid is aspirated in the syringe and then three-way stop cock is turned to connect the syringe with the outlet, which is attached to IV set.
- Collect the fluid in EDTA and plain tubes. It is also collected for culture. Smear should be prepared for Gram's stain and Ziehl-Neelsen stain.
- The three-way tap is now turned again to connect the syringe with the needle and the pleural space, a further aspiration is carried out. It is expelled into the drainage bag by turning the three-way tap. The drainage bag or bottle should be placed well below the level of the patient's chest.
- As fluid is removed, the lung expands and this often makes the patient to cough.
- The needle is withdrawn and puncture site is covered with a benzoin seal. A sterile gauze is put over it and adhesive tape is applied.

Complications

- Pneumothorax
- Hemothorax
- Infection
- Unilateral pulmonary edema
- Hypoproteinemia.

ENDOTRACHEAL INTUBATION

Endotracheal intubation is a procedure, which every pediatrician and one working in intensive care units must be well conversant with. The critically ill patient often requires endotracheal intubation. It secures patent airway. It is a pre-requisite for mechanical ventilation. Endotracheal suction can most efficiently be done through an endotracheal tube. It is indicated when bag and mask resuscitation fails in a case of an asphyxiated newborn.

Indications

- *In neonatal asphyxia*:
  - Bag and mask resuscitation fails.

- Apparently, stillborn baby after adequate suctioning of upper airways.
- Infants with diaphragmatic hernia.
- Meconium aspiration.

- Cardiorespiratory arrest due to any cause.
- Central nervous system depression in a case of head injury or comatose child.
- Diseases of peripheral nervous system, poliomyelitis, Guillain-Barré syndrome, tetanus, organophosphorus poisoning, etc.
- Administration of general anesthesia.

Equipment

- Laryngoscope—with straight blade for neonates
- Endotracheal tubes (ET) for various sizes with stylet

Weight/age	*Endotracheal tubes size (ID in mm)*
< 1,000 g	2.5
1,000–2,000 g	3.0
2,000–3,000 g	3.5
> 3,000 g	4.0
1–5 years	4–5
5–12 years	5–6.5

Approximately size of ET, internal diameter (ID) in mm = Age (years) + 16/4.

Technique

- The patient is placed in a supine position. The operator stands beyond the patient's head. Patient's neck is slightly extended with the head in midline.
- Clear the oropharynx with gentle suctioning.
- Empty the stomach.
- Hold the handle of laryngoscope in left hand with thumb and first three fingers; stabilize the hand with fifth finger resting on patient's cheek. The blade should be pointing away from oneself.
- Open the baby's mouth and push the tongue left with the back of right forefinger and steady the head with the rest of right hand.
- While visualizing insert the blade midline until the tip is between base of tongue and epiglottis within the vallecula **(Figs. 20.1.20A and B)**.
- If the infant is making respiratory effort, free flow of oxygen with an oxygen tubing held close to the infant's mouth and nose is to be provided during intubation.
- Open the mouth further by pulling on laryngoscope handle, simultaneously tilt the blade tip upward slightly to elevate epiglottis and visualize the glottis. Use base of the tongue as pivot rather than maxilla.
- Suction is needed.
- Have the assistant to palpate suprasternal notch with index finger, applying gentle pressure, if desired.

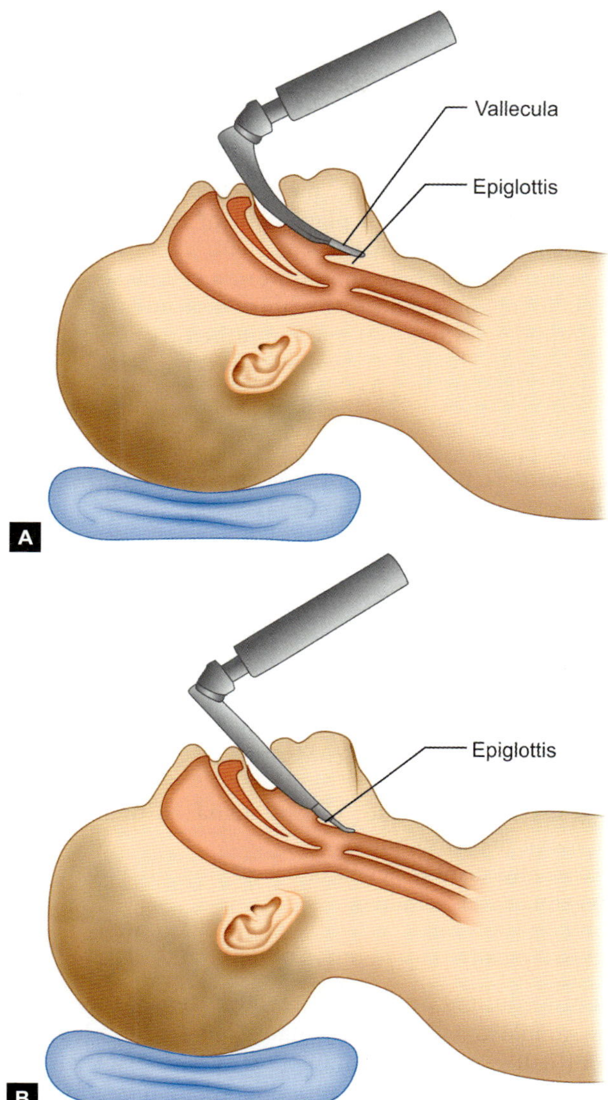

Figs. 20.1.20A and B: Position of laryngoscope blade when using (A) Curved blade, it is in the vallecula; (B) Straight blade, it is over the epiglottis.
Source: Prajapati BS. Essential Procedures in Pediatrics, 1st edition. New Delhi: Jaypee Brothers Medical Publishers (P) Ltd; 2003.

- Hold the tube with concave curve anterior and pass it down to right side of the mouth, outside the blade, along with maintaining visualization.
- As the patient inspires, pass the tube through cords 2 cm into trachea or until immediately after tip passes under assistant's finger in suprasternal notch.
- The tube is then held firmly at the lips with the right hand, and the laryngoscope and stylet are carefully removed.
- Initially, confirmation of the tube placement is accomplished by attaching a resuscitation bag with the

connector and ventilating the infant. With correctly placed tube, the air entry is heard on both sides of the chest, breath sounds are of equal intensity and air is not heard entering the stomach. While listening to the breath sounds, the stethoscope is to be placed at approximately the nipple line.
- Note the centimeter marks on the tube at the level of upper lips and then secure the tube to the infant's face.
- Final confirmation of placement of the tube can be obtained by chest film, if it is needed.
- Attempts to intubate should not exceed 30 seconds. If you are unable to intubate within 30 seconds, abort and continue with bag and mask and then try again after a few minutes. Repeated attempts may cause serious glottic edema and bleeding.
- Intubation is not a matter of prestige. If you are unable to do so, please ask for help.
- ET route is also used for administration of some drugs such as epinephrine, atropine, naloxone, etc.

Complications

- Hypoxia.
- Bradycardia.
- Apnea.
- Pneumothorax.
- Injury and lacerations to tongue, gums, pharynx, epiglottis, trachea, vocal cords, etc.
- Infections.
- Postextubation stridor can be managed by nebulized epinephrine or steroids.

Some physicians prefer nasotracheal intubation when long-term ventilation is required.

SUPRAPUBIC BLADDER ASPIRATION

This procedure is performed to collect noncontaminated urine sample in neonates and infants. It is a safe and reliable way of collecting urine samples. It is easy, especially in neonates, as bladder is an intra-abdominal organ in these patients unlike a pelvic organ in older children and adults.

Technique

- The infant is placed on a flat surface in supine position.
- The assistant stands opposite the operator and immobilizes the infant by grasping the thorax with one hand and thighs and hips with the other.
- Make sure that the bladder is full.
- Local part is cleaned. Aseptic and antiseptic measures are a must.
- A 10 cc disposable syringe with 22 FG, 4–5 cm long needle is taken.
- The pubic symphysis is located with one finger and the needle is inserted 2 cm above the symphysis in the midline with syringe held at 10–20° angles from perpendicular **(Fig. 20.1.21)**.

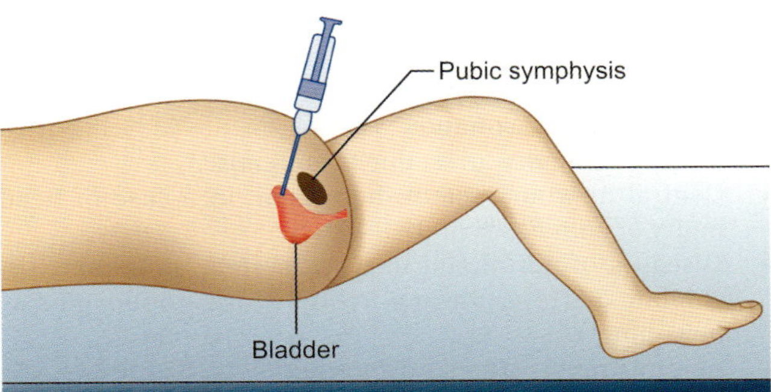

Fig. 20.1.21: Suprapubic bladder puncture technique.
Source: Prajapati BS. Essential Procedures in Pediatrics, 1st edition. New Delhi: Jaypee Brothers Medical Publishers (P) Ltd; 2003.

- With a single steady motion, the needle is inserted until a perceptive change in resistance is felt as the needle enters the bladder.
- Light aspiration is applied to aspirate the urine specimen.
- After removal of needle, a seal of tincture benzoin is applied at puncture site.

PERITONEAL DIALYSIS

Dialysis involves the use of semipermeable membranes that permit the simultaneous passage of smaller molecular weight solutes and water while retarding or inhibiting the movement of large sized particles. The basic principle controlling the transmembrane movement of solute and water are similar whether the membrane is artificial (hemodialysis) or natural (peritoneal dialysis).

Indications

- Blood urea more than 300 mg/dL.
- Serum hyperkalemia—K^+ more than 6.5 mEq/L not responding to medical line of treatment.
- Severe acidosis.
- Pulmonary edema.
- Acute left ventricular failure.
- Drug intoxications such as barbiturates, salicylates, etc.
- Life-threatening electrolyte imbalance.

Contraindications

- Peritonitis.
- Abdominal adhesions.
- Laparotomy done.
- Pleuroperitoneal communication.

Technique (Fig. 20.1.22)

- Informed written consent.
- Aseptic and antiseptic measures are must.

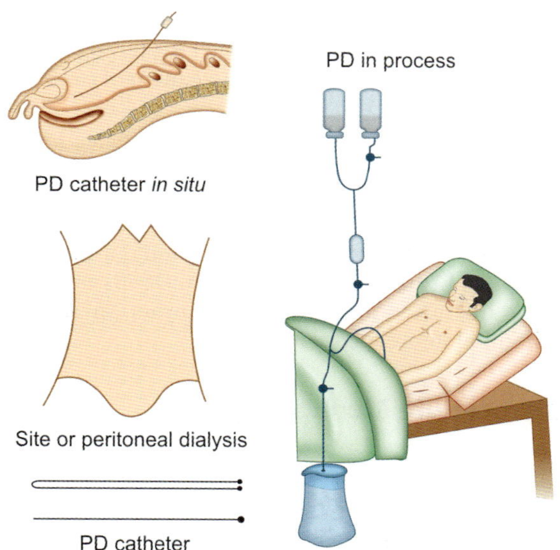

Fig. 20.1.22: Peritoneal dialysis (PD).
Source: Prajapati BS. Essential Procedures in Pediatrics, 1st edition. New Delhi: Jaypee Brothers Medical Publishers (P) Ltd; 2003.

- Injection atropine 0.01 mg/kg IM 30 minutes before the procedure as the premedication.
- Sedation, if required.
- Proper restraining
- Bladder is emptied by its own or catheterization, if it is necessary.
- Abdominal wall is prepared, painting spirit—Betadine spirit. Towel draping.
- The catheter is usually placed in the midline few centimeters below the umbilicus.

If midline insertion is not possible, the catheter can be inserted in the flank area, outside the line of inferior epigastric artery.

- The site is anesthetized by injecting 1% lignocaine up to peritoneum.
- If there is no ascites, distend the abdomen with 10 mL/kg dialysate solution using 17–20 FG angiocath or needle.
- Needle is withdrawn and a knife blade is used to enlarge the puncture wound in the skin.
- If ascites is present, a very small penetrating incision is made in the skin and the trocar with catheter is stabilized with the fingers of one hand on the skin while the other hand introduces the trocar through the abdominal wall with an alternating drilling motion.
- Penetration up to peritoneum is detected by a definite sensation of giving the way and also by the appearance of fluid in the catheter when trocar is removed.
- On reaching the peritoneal cavity and before removing the trocar, the catheter is gradually advanced in the peritoneal cavity in right or left paracolic gutter and trocar is gradually withdrawn.
- When the catheter is sufficiently introduced in the peritoneal cavity, trocar is removed totally. All the fenestrations on the catheter must be within the peritoneal cavity to avoid subcutaneous fluid infiltration in the abdominal wall. In neonates and infants, IV catheters or simple feeding tube can be used.
- The catheter should be stabilized with adhesive plaster.
- The catheter is connected with the administration tubing through small connector, and dialysis fluid is flown.
- Because hyperkalemia is often present, potassium-free fluid is used for the first three–six cycles.
- Time of input of dialysis fluid will be about 10–15 minutes. The fluid is kept in the peritoneal cavity for about 30 minutes. Time for output of dialysis fluid will be about 15–20 minutes. Each cycle will take about an hour. First few cycles should be of half an hour (rapid cycles).
- Record the weight of the patient prior to the procedure and every 12 hours.
- Total duration of dialysis is about 40 hours depending on the clinical and biochemical parameters.
- Warm the dialysate to body temperature.
- Infuse it by gravity flow.
- Each cycle should be of 30–50 mL/kg.
- Blood sugar, blood urea, serum creatinine, serum electrolytes and serum proteins should be checked 12 hourly.
- In the presence of fluid overload, use hypertonic dialysate.
- Tip of the catheter should be sent for culture.
- Close the site of dialysis by sterile bandage.
- Peritoneal dialysis related problems such as pain in abdomen, diarrhea, dyspnea, bleeding and fluid delivery should be sorted out appropriately.

Complications

- Pain may be due to over distention, peritonitis, etc.
- Bleeding.
- Dialysate leak.
- Outflow obstruction.
- Peritonitis.
- Metabolic complications.
- Thrombosis.
- Pulmonary complications.

RENAL BIOPSY

Indications

- Steroid-resistant nephrotic syndrome.
- Asymptomatic proteinuria.
- Glomerulonephritis associated with conditions such as systemic lupus erythematosus, Henoch-Schönlein purpura, etc.
- Rapidly progressive glomerulonephritis.

Contraindications

- Bleeding diathesis.
- Solitary functioning kidney.
- Ectopic/horseshoe-shaped kidney.
- Severe uncontrolled hypertension.

Prerequisites

- Bleeding time, clotting time, partial thromboplastin time (PTT) or activated partial thromboplastin time (APTT) and platelets count.
- Blood grouping and cross-matching.
- Hypertension and uremia should be controlled.
- Informed written consent is a must.

Technique

- Atropine 0.01 mg/kg IM before 30 minutes of the procedure.
- The patient is placed in the prone position on a firm bed. A pillow is placed under patient's abdomen. This compresses and fixes the kidneys to the posterior abdominal wall, bringing the kidneys closer to the skin and limiting possible ballottement of the kidney by the biopsy needle.
- Ultrasonography is commonly used to mark the location of kidneys and point of entry of the needle into the kidney perpendicular to the skin surface and to obtain depth of tissue from skin surface. Usually, lower pole of left kidney is selected for biopsy.
- The area is prepared and local anesthesia is given. Irritable children may need general anesthesia.
- A 23-gauge exploring lumbar puncture needle is passed downwards and obliquely toward the lower pole of the kidney. A needle can be felt going through different structures and renal capsule. Experienced person feels 'give-in' feeling up on penetration of capsule of kidney.
- The patient is asked to take slow deep breathings. If the needle is in the kidney, a characteristic pendular movement is seen with respiration, the hub of needle swings through a wide arch, moving toward head during inspiration and toward buttock during expiration. If the needle is not in the kidney tissue, it is slightly advanced until it penetrates kidneys and moves characteristically on breathing. The depth of the kidney below the skin is measured on the stem of the needle.
- A small nick is made over anesthetized area with a scalpel.
- Franklin modified Vim-Silverman needle and Tru-cut needle are commonly used in the practice. Tru-cut needle is easy to use and having less failure rate. Therefore, Tru-cut needle is preferred nowadays.
- Tru-cut needle is one-piece apparatus with a length of 11.4 cm or 15 cm. The needle with cannula covering the obturator is advanced in the kidney to desired length in a direction perpendicular to skin surface.
- The patient is asked to hold the breath in deep inspiration.
- The obturator is advanced by firm tap on the handle. The specimen is cut by downward movement of cannula over obturator.
- Entire assembly is removed.
- The patient is asked to breathe normally.
- Firm pressure is applied over biopsy site for few minutes and the site is sealed with tincture benzoin. Two good cores of tissue (8–10 mm long) are needed for adequate histological examination. One is immediately fixed in buffered formalin and other in saline (for immunofluorescence study).

Postprocedure Management

- The patient is asked to remain in prone position for 2 hours and in bed for 24 hours.
- Monitoring temperature, pulse, respiratory rate (RR) and blood pressure (BP) 1 hourly for 6 hours and then 4 hourly for 24 hours.
- Urine should be collected in separate bottles during each voiding and should be checked for hematuria.
- Patient is asked to take ample liquids orally.
- Diuretics may be given in case of oliguria to flush any clot in the passage.
- If no frank hematuria and vitals are normal, patient can be discharged after 24 hours with instructions not to do exertion for a week.

Complications

- Hematuria.
- Perinephric hematoma.
- AV fistula.

PERICARDIOCENTESIS

Pericardiocentesis is a procedure for removal of fluid from pericardial cavity for diagnostic purpose or to relieve cardiac tamponade. It is occasionally a life-saving procedure. It is a risky procedure. It should be performed only by skilled person under continuous cardiac monitoring. Echocardiographic diagnosis is must before performing the procedure. It gives idea regarding amount of fluid and also helps to determine the anatomical approach.

Prerequisites

- Echocardiographic diagnosis.
- Coagulation profile.
- Resuscitation kit including defibrillator.
- Cardiac monitor.
- IV line.
- Premedication with injection atropine 0.01 mg/kg IM 30 minutes before the procedure.

Technique

- Informed written consent should be taken.
- Sedation may be required in some patients. If possible, it should be avoided.
- Child should be seated leaning backward at approximately 60° and carefully restrained.
- The best site is xiphocostal angle. The other sites are fourth, fifth or sixth intercostal spaces 1-2 cm medial to the border of cardiac dullness on percussion.
- Aseptic and antiseptic precautions are must.
- One percent xylocaine is infiltrated in the skin at left xiphocostal angle, 3-4 cm below left costal margin. The needle is advanced initially perpendicular to the skin surface and after traversing the soft tissue under the rib cage, its tip is pointed to the left shoulder. While advancing the needle in the deeper structures, if it reaches to pericardial cavity, the pericardial fluid is withdrawn in the syringe. Local anesthetic agent should not be injected in the pericardial cavity.
- The pericardiocentesis needle is passed along the same path until the fluid is obtained. The distance from skin to the pericardium is less than 5 cm in a child. A distinct "give" or "pop" is felt when the pericardium is punctured. Pericardial fluid can then be aspirated.
- Getting the fluid confirms the position of needle into the pericardial cavity. Normal saline can be injected under two-dimensional (2D) echo monitoring, which shows bubbles of saline.
- If the blood or bloody fluid is withdrawn, it is vital to determine if cardiac chamber or coronary artery has been punctured. Still uremia and malignant diseases can give rise to hemorrhagic pericardial effusion. Blood obtained from heart or coronary vessel clots immediately.
- Fluid is sent for appropriate examinations.
- The needle is withdrawn and benzoin seal is done at puncture site.
- Postprocedure monitoring of heart rate, RR and BP should be done. 2D echo may be performed to study postpericardiocentesis condition.

Complications

- Hemopericardium
- Arrhythmias
- Vasovagal reactions
- Infection
- Pneumothorax
- Air embolism
- Perforation of an abdominal viscus, commonly stomach
- Cardiac arrest and death.

FINE-NEEDLE ASPIRATION BIOPSY

Fine-needle aspiration biopsy (FNAB) is very useful for cytological and bacteriological evaluation of a mass or a lymph node. It is minimally invasive and requires no sedation.

It aids in tissue diagnosis and in determining the course of management.

Requirements

- 1^2 1.5^2 20-25 FG needles. 22 FG 1^2 long is the most commonly used size of needle.
- 10-20 mL plastic disposable syringes.
- Clean glass slides.
- 70-90% ethanol for routine wet fixation.
- Containers for culture media whenever needed.

Technique

- Sterilize the area.
- Anesthesia is usually not required, local anesthetic agent may be used in uncooperative and irritable children.
- Immobilize the lump to be biopsied between your thumb and finger with one hand.
- Hold the syringe in the other hand and insert needle into the assigned area, perpendicular to the skin surface and position the needle within the target tissue.
- Pull the syringe plunger to apply negative pressure.
- While maintaining suction, make several passes through the mass or node.
- Release the negative pressure while needle remains in the target tissue.
- Withdraw the needle.
- Detach the needle, draw 2-3 mL air into the syringe, reattach the needle and blow the aspirates on to the slide.
- Apply the pressure over the puncture site with cotton swab for 5 minutes.
- Deep biopsies can be done with assistance of radiological imaging techniques like ultrasound.

The following situations can give unsatisfactory yield during FNAB:

- When needle misses the lesion tangentially.
- When central area is cystic, necrotic or hemorrhagic and devoid of diagnostic material.
- When there is a small malignant lesion close to a dominant benign mass.
- When the target tissue is fibrosclerotic and poor in cells.

BIBLIOGRAPHY

1. Chameides L. Vascular access. In: Textbook of Pediatric Advanced Life Support. American Heart Association. American Academy of Pediatrics; 1988. pp. 37-46.
2. Koebke J, McFarland E, Mein M. Venipuncture Procedures. In: Slockbower JM, Blumenfeld TA (Eds). Collection and Handling of Laboratory Specimens—a Practical Guide. Philadelphia: JB Lippincott Co; 1983. pp. 3-45.

3. Laing IA, Doyle E. Practical procedures. In: Campbell AGM, Mclntosh N (Eds). Forfar and Arneil's Textbook of Pediatrics, 5th edition. New York: Churchill Livingstone; 1998. pp. 1829-47.
4. Nair MK, Leena ML, Ajithkumar K. Concept of health care counseling for pediatricians. Indian Pediatr. 2016;53(11): 961-3.
5. Prabha S. Renal biopsy in children. In: Nammalwar BR, Vijayakumar M (Eds). Principles and Practice Of Pediatric Nephrology, 2nd edition. New Delhi: Jaypee Brothers Medical Publishers (P) Ltd; 1991. pp. 85-9.
6. Prajapati BS. Essential Procedures In: Pediatrics, 1st edition. New Delhi: Jaypee Brothers Medical Publishers (P) Ltd; 2003.
7. Silver HK, Kempe CH, Bruyn HB. Pediatric procedures. In: Handbook of Pediatrics, 13th edition. Singapore: Lange-Maruzen Asia; 1980.pp.629-44.
8. Singh M. Procedures. In: Singh M (Ed). Care of the Newborn, 4th edition. New Delhi: Sagar Publications. 1991. pp. 340-67.
9. Singhi S. Procedures in pediatric intensive care. In: Sachdev HPS, Puri RK, Bagga A, Choudhury P (Eds). Principles of Pediatric and Neonatal Emergencies, 1st edition. New Delhi: Jaypee Brothers Medical Publishers (P) Ltd. 1999. pp. 364-72.
10. Subramanyam L, Thangavelu S, Somu N. Pathophysiology of pleural fluid collection and management of empyema. In: Somu N, Subramanyam L (Eds). Essentials of Pediatric Pulmonology, 2nd edition. Siva and Co: Madras. 1996. pp. 142-9.

20.2 Physiotherapy and Rehabilitation

Somu Sivabalan, Suresh Kumar S

PHYSIOTHERAPY OR PHYSICAL THERAPY

Physiotherapy or physical therapy aims at physical treatment and management of any disease or condition thereby enabling people to reach their maximum potential. Physiotherapists or physical therapists are healthcare professionals who diagnose and treat individuals of all ages with illness or injuries that limit their ability to mobilize and perform functional activities unlike their normal peers.

Physical therapy aims at providing treatment techniques, which promote mobility, reduce pain, restore function, and prevent disability. In addition, by developing fitness and wellness-oriented programs they device strategies to prevent immobility even before it occurs. In the elderly, physiotherapy helps them to have a healthy and active lifestyle by maintaining or restoring maximum movement and functional ability throughout their lifespan.

REHABILITATION

Rehabilitation means to restore good condition, operability, and capacity to lead a productive life through therapy and education. Pediatric rehabilitation assists in early detection and in the management of a variety of injuries, disorders, and diseases that affects the muscles, bones and joints of infants, children, and adolescents. Optimization of function is brought about by a combination of medications prescribed by the pediatrician and usage of physical modalities. These include physical training with therapeutic exercise, movement and activity modification, adaptive equipment and assistive devices, orthotics (braces), and prosthetics, in turn helping the child to regain independence and in leading a near normal life.

The rehabilitation team consists of physiotherapists, occupational therapists, speech and language pathologists, psychologists, social workers, special educator, prosthetists, and orthotists headed by a doctor.

Aims of Rehabilitation

- To improve child's gross and fine motor skills
- Balance and coordination
- Improve strength and endurance
- Help in cognitive and sensory processing and integration
- Promote mobility
- Manage pain.

Goals, Outcome, and Intervention

- Primary prevention of disability through education and treatment.
- Secondary prevention of disabilities such as contractures or deformities, or improvement of the same.
- Attain maximum functional goals expected by the child and his/her family.

- Improve the lung function and aid in the clearance of secretions.
- To help the children in leading a near normal life with their disability and to integrate them with the society.
- Provide appropriate wheelchairs, orthotics and prosthetics, and modify architectural barriers.

Evaluation

It is the most important component to assess the extent and severity of involvement and also to device management strategies for a particular patient. The evaluation includes:

- Observation
- Measurement of limb length
- Assess muscle power using manual muscle power grading
- Measure the active and passive range of motion using goniometer
- Grade spasticity by modified Ashworth scale
- Examine for persistence of abnormal reflexes
- Posture and gait observation
- Assess child's abilities and disabilities.

Indications for Rehabilitation

Rehabilitation medicine plays an important role in the following conditions:

- Neurological conditions such as cerebral palsy, autism, developmental delay, spina bifida, muscular dystrophies, poliomyelitis, infantile hemiplegia, and peripheral nerve lesions
- Orthopedic conditions such as congenital talipes equinovarus, congenital dislocation of hip, torticollis, and post-traumatic stiffness
- Genetic and chromosomal anomalies with motor involvement
- Cardiovascular diseases—mostly involves postoperative care
- Respiratory disorders—chronic obstructive pulmonary disease (COPD), bronchiectasis, chronic restrictive pulmonary diseases (CRPD), which include chest deformities and neuromuscular disorders
- Postoperatively—after an abdominal surgery or urosurgery to train the bladder and bowel muscles
- Athletes—for prevention and rehabilitation of sports injuries.

Methods of Intervention

To optimize function through the combined use of:

- Medications
- Physical modalities, e.g. warming or cooling the soft tissues
- Physical training with therapeutic exercise, movement, and activity modification
- Adaptive equipment and assistive device, orthotics (braces), and prosthesis.

Physical Modalities

There are various methods of warming or cooling the soft tissues.

Warming the Soft Tissues

The sources of heat may be:

- Paraffin wax
- Heat pad
- Moist hot packs
- Interferential therapy (IFT)
- Transcutaneous electrical nerve stimulation (TENS)
- Ultrasound therapy.

The modality of choice in an individual depends on the objective of the treatment, the part to be treated, depth of the lesion, state of the cutaneous nerve supply, and the underlying pathology.

In pediatric age group, paraffin wax and heating pad are safer. Ultrasound given at the epiphysis end may damage the growth plates. In peripheral nerve lesions such as Erb's palsy and facial palsy, electrical stimulation is indicated and is later followed by tendon transfer surgery.

Ice Therapy or Cooling the Soft Tissues

It is the local or generalized application of cold for therapeutics and prevention. It results in alternating periods of vasoconstriction and vasodilatation, thereby reducing the nerve conductivity, relieving muscle spasm and spasticity. It helps in relieving pain, reducing swelling, spasticity, and hematoma formation.

Cold therapy can be applied by ice cold towels, as an ice pack or by immersion in an ice-filled bath depending upon the comfort of the patient.

Physical Training

Exercises may be in the form of:

- Active/passive exercises
- Stretching
- Strengthening exercises
- Endurance exercises
- Coordination exercises
- Posture correction
- Gait training.

Rehabilitation Strategies in Common Disorders

Newborn

Early intervention supports the needs of infants and toddlers with developmental delay and disabilities. Comprehensive care enhances the development of physical, cognitive, communication, social, and emotional development in infants and toddlers. This also encloses the initiation of adaptive approach among family members, to enhance their capacity to meet the special needs of their children.

Any child at the earliest of age, with obvious developmental delay or who has been found to lag in development as compared to his/her peers, requires proper assessment to device an early and appropriate intervention plan. Physiotherapy and occupational therapy are of prime importance in early intervention. They can act as service coordinators to coordinate among other specialists and therapists for collaborative care.

Assessment of High-risk Children

There are various development assessment scales currently used according to the child's age:

- *Movement assessment of infant (MAI):* From 0 months to 12 months of age
- *Alberta infant motor scale (AIMS):* From 0 months to 18 months of age
- *Test of infant motor performance (TIMP):* From 34 weeks postconception age to 4 months post-term.

At the community level, our own Trivandrum Developmental Screening Chart (TDSC) can be utilized. It has been designed in such a way that it takes only around 5 minutes to complete. TDSC (0–6 years) is a simple, reliable and valid screening tool for use in the community to identify children between 0 year and 6 years with developmental delay, enabling early intervention practices.

The BSID-III current version (Bayley Scales of Infant Development) is a standard series of measurements, originally developed by psychologist Nancy Bayley, who used it primarily to assess the motor (fine and gross), language (receptive and expressive), and cognitive development of infants and toddlers, less than 3 years of age.

Physiotherapy helps children to achieve meaningful sustained activity. In the initial stages the aim is to, at the least, take care of their day-to-day needs. The ultimate goal is to achieve normal or near normal motor skills as their peers.

Physiotherapy also integrates family members and care providers to:

- Understand and meet the child's needs
- Find resources in their community that are suited to meet their needs
- Create opportunities for the child to develop motor abilities
- Provide transition of the child to preschool or other facilities
- Provide inclusive education in normal schools
- Help families to make decisions on adaptive equipment when and if needed by the child
- Improve the overall well-being and quality of both the children and their family.

Neuromuscular Conditions

Poliomyelitis:

- *Acute phase*: Rest and positioning with splint
- *Recovery phase*: Passive exercise, active assisted, and strengthening exercises
- *Residual phase*: Continue exercise and application of orthotics.

Cerebral palsy: Multidisciplinary rehabilitative approach should be initiated at the earliest to get the maximum outcome. The different technique includes neurodevelopment therapy, Rood's approach, and motor relearning theory. The treatment is tailor-made to the child's need and presentation (spastic, hypotonic, athetoid or mixed type).

The aims are:

- Reduce spasticity
- Inhibition of abnormal reflexes
- Sensory integration
- Prevention of deformity/contractures
- Treatment of associated problems such as hearing, visual, and feeding problems.

These are achieved by:

- Proper positioning
- Active/passive movements
- Facilitating the development of delayed/missing milestones
- Standing training
- Gait training with or without supports such as ankle-foot orthosis, knee-ankle-foot orthosis, walkers, crutch, etc.
- Stretching and resting splint to relieve spasticity, postbotulinum toxin injection for spastic muscles.

Muscular dystrophy: This is a genetic disorder characterized by progressive muscle weakness. Though many types of dystrophies are reported, the Duchenne dystrophy seems quite common. The management includes passive exercise, proper muscular positioning of the weak joints with splints, stretching, chest physiotherapy, and customized wheel chair to prevent the worsening of the spinal deformity.

Erb's Palsy: This is a nerve injury sustained during birth, affecting the C5-C6 spinal nerves or the whole of the upper trunk of brachial plexus due to traction injury. The upper extremity is adducted, internally rotated, elbow extended, and forearm pronated. In some babies, nerve recovery occurs on its own. Often, early physiotherapy is required to prevent contractures and regain motor power. However, if the child has not achieved improvement between 6 months and 9 months of age nerve graft or nerve decompression is indicated.

Torticollis: It is commonly known as twisted neck. The head is typically tilted with a lateral bent to the side of the affected muscle. Birth trauma or intrauterine malpositioning is considered to cause damage to the sternocleidomastoid muscle in the neck. This results in a shortening or excessive contraction of the sternocleidomastoid muscle, often with limited range of motion in both rotation and lateral bending. The general stretching of the sternocleidomastoid muscle and positioning will help.

Spina bifida: This is a neural tube defect resulting in vertebral and/or spinal cord malformation. Management includes:
- Teaching parents proper positioning and handling of the child
- Educating about the anesthetic skin and potential for sustaining anesthetic ulcers
- Passive stretching exercise to prevent contractures
- Providing appropriate splints.

Post-traumatic muscle stiffness: The physiotherapy plan is divided into two phases, i.e. during immobilization and during mobilization.
- *During immobilization:*
  - Reduce edema and prevent the formation of adhesions—limb elevation and isometric exercises
  - Avoid undue stress—proper positioning is recommended
  - Maintain circulation—active movement of extremities
  - Maintain range of joint movements—range of movement (ROM) exercises
  - Maintain function—exercises to unaffected limb and parts
  - Training to use frames, crutches, etc.
- *During mobilization:*
  - To reduce swelling—limb elevation and active movement
  - Maintain joint range—ROM exercises
  - Strengthen muscles—strengthening exercises and isometric contractions are taught.

Orthopedic Conditions

Congenital talipes equinovarus: It is also known as clubfoot. This deformity is characterized by plantar flexion at ankle joint, inversion at subtalar joint, and forefoot adduction. Management includes passive stretching, retaining in corrected position by adhesive strapping, night splints, gait training, and corrective shoes.

Congenital dislocation of hip: In congenital dislocation of hip, there is dysplasia of acetabulum and femoral head and dislocation of femoral head. Management is divided into two phases:
1. *Immobilization phase*:
   - Active movement of all joints of lower limb including hip
   - Splinting
   - Isometric exercises
2. *Mobilization phase:*
   - Mobilization exercises
   - Passive adduction
   - Muscle-strengthening exercises
   - Gait training
   - Weight bearing and weight transfers.

Dysplasia: This disorder originates from the abnormal organization of cells into tissues leading to abnormal tissue differentiation, e.g. osteogenesis imperfecta. The management includes:
- Instruction to parents about positioning and handling
- Supported sitting in stroller and wheelchairs
- Encourage developmental activities
- Stretching exercises
- Ambulation with assistive orthotics devices.

Pediatric flatfoot: Flatfoot is common in both children and adults. When this deformity occurs in children, it is referred to as pediatric flatfoot. Although there are various forms of flatfoot, they all share one characteristic—partial or total collapse of the arch.

Pediatric flatfoot can be classified as symptomatic or asymptomatic. Symptomatic flatfeet exhibit symptoms, such as pain and limitation of activity, while asymptomatic flatfeet show no symptoms. These classifications can assist the foot and ankle surgeon in determining an appropriate treatment plan.

Symptoms: Flatfoot can be apparent at birth or it may not show up until years later. Most children with flatfoot have no symptoms, but some have one or more of the following symptoms:
- Pain, tenderness or cramping pain in the foot, leg, and knee
- Outward tilting of the heel
- Awkwardness or changes in walking
- Difficulty with shoes
- Reduced energy when participating in physical activities
- Voluntary withdrawal from physical activities.

Nonsurgical treatment: If a child has no symptoms, treatment is often not required. Instead, the condition will be observed and reevaluated periodically by the pediatrician.
- *Activity modifications*: The child needs to temporarily decrease activities that bring pain as well as avoid prolonged walking or standing.
- *Orthotic devices*: The foot and ankle surgeon can provide custom orthotic devices that fit inside the shoe to support the structure of the foot and improve function.
- *Physiotherapy*: Stretching exercises, supervised by the foot and ankle surgeon or a physical therapist, provide relief in some cases of flatfoot.
- *Shoe modifications*: Footwear modifications include inbuilt medial arches in the shoes to address the navicular drop.

Trigger finger: Pediatric trigger finger, also known as congenital trigger finger, is a condition affecting the flexor tendon of the finger or thumb. Symptoms occur when there is a size mismatch between the tendon and the sheath that surrounds the tendon. This causes a locking or catching of the finger with attempted bending of the finger with associated pain, which is referred to as "triggering". In pediatric trigger finger, there is often a nodule (a benign thickening of the tendon) that catches on the overlying sheath, causing the finger or thumb to trigger. This is diagnosed based on history and clinical examination with the finding of triggering of the digit and with a palpable nodule at the base of the finger. Physiotherapy management includes massage and stretching and/or splinting to keep the finger straight. Trigger thumb is more likely to be successfully treated with nonsurgical techniques than trigger finger.

Sports Injuries

Increasingly common in pediatrics due to faulty training, musculotendinous imbalance, and anatomical misalignment; includes flatfeet, immature structures, improper footwear, and playing surface.

Types of injuries:
- Stress fractures
- Tendonitis and bursitis
- *Joint disorders*:
  - Subluxation
  - Dislocation
  - Ligament injuries.

Management in general includes rest, ice compression, strapping/taping, and anti-inflammatory drugs. This has to be followed by muscle strengthening exercise, proper training, and education to the child as well as the parents. Surgical correction may be required, if conservative treatment fails.

Pulmonology

Chest physiotherapy: It is an airway-clearance technique that combines manual percussion of the chest wall by the caregiver, strategic positioning of the patient for mucus drainage with cough and breathing techniques. It is useful for individuals with copious mucus or thick secretions, those with weak respiratory mechanics or those with ineffective cough. Chest physiotherapy consists of various manipulative procedures such as the following:
- *Positioning (postural drainage)*: Placing the patient in varying positions for optimal gravity drainage of secretions to increase the expansion and prevent occlusion of that individual segment.
- *Percussion (chest percussion, vibration, and thoracic squeezing)*: In conjunction with postural drainage; to hasten clearing of secretion from the tracheobronchial tree.
- *Airway clearing technique:* To facilitate clearance of lower airway secretions through the upper airways by cough stimulation, huffing, flutter, cough assist devices, and/or tracheal stimulation.

Breathing exercise: It is an integral part of chest physiotherapy. It plays a significant role in airway clearance and parenchymal expansion by improving the efficiency of respiratory muscles. Diaphragmatic, costal, and apical breathing techniques are for the different segments of the lungs.

"Cough-assisted devices" are used to help clear the lungs and airways of secretions. Although limited evidence exists regarding the efficacy of secretion clearance strategies, many patients with impaired airway clearance seem to benefit from the use of secretion clearance devices. Adequate hydration, physical activity, bronchodilators, controlled breathing, and postural drainage in addition help.

"Cough-assisted" is a handheld device that combines the benefits of both positive expiratory pressure (PEP) therapy and airway vibrations to mobilize pulmonary secretions. The physiologic rationale is that by exhaling against resistance we slow down our expiratory phase of breathing. This slower exhalation against resistance or positive pressure generates a backpressure, which in-turn splints or stents open the more peripheral airways and lessens airway collapse distally. This facilitates mobilization of secretions from distal or peripheral airways to the larger more central airways. However, the patient or individual must be able to generate adequate air flow to use this device.

Cough insufflator-exsufflator: A cough assist machine helps to clear secretions in the lungs and bronchioles by using a combination of positive and negative air pressure, by simulating a cough. With correct usage the device may decrease the risk of chest infections, such as pneumonia due to stagnant secretions that invites a secondary infection.

Single valve Ambu bag: In restrictive lung disease due to thoracic cage-skeletal anomalies or neuromuscular disease, a single valve Ambu bag is useful in removing the secretions. "Air/breath stacking method" facilitates to breathe in more air, as the bag is squeezed a second time. This should fill the airways further and the patient is asked to hold as long as possible this air, which then is breathed out as cough. This helps in removing secretions from the lungs, which further improves the ventilation, and prevents/clears atelectasis and assist in cough.

Burns

In burns, there is coagulative necrosis of tissue and skin loss. It may be caused due to heat, flame, chemical, electricity or radiations. The main aim and treatment line of rehabilitation are to:

- Prevent respiratory complications—chest physiotherapy
- Prevent contractures and deformities—splinting and positioning
- Maintain range of motion and muscle strength—exercises
- Reduce scar contracture—soft tissue release techniques by passive stretching or surgical correction.

Cardiovascular Disorders

In older children who are to undergo cardiothoracic surgery, a preoperative preparation and continued postoperative care should be given.

- *Preoperatively, activities which are to be carried out postoperatively are taught:*
  - Breathing exercises with emphasis on deep breathing
  - Incentive spirometry to aid lung expansion
  - Instructions to effectively cough and splinting techniques
  - Postural drainage to remove accumulated secretions
  - Lower extremity exercises to maintain circulation and prevent deep vein thrombosis (DVT).
- *On postoperative days, the emphasis is on the following activities*:
  - Promote relaxation and relieve pain
  - Positioning in bed
  - Maintain ventilation through deep breathing exercises and incentive spirometry
  - Assist in secretion removal—begin with deep effective coughing
  - Prevent DVT—lower limb exercises
  - Maintain range of motion—ROM exercises
  - Correct postural defects—positioning and postural training
  - Improve exercise tolerance—graded exercise program.

Augmented Bladder

Bladder augmentation also called augmentation cystoplasty, and is a surgical procedure used in children who lack adequate bladder capacity or detrusor compliance. Physiotherapy by means of TENS and exercise to improve the bladder and bowel muscles will help.

Posture

Posture is the position in which you hold your body and limbs when standing, sitting or lying down. Good posture is one, which puts the least strain on our back, and should be maintained while doing any activity. Poor posture is commonly diagnosed in children and is more frequent in boys. A significant portion of children with poor posture is found between 7 years and 11 years of age.

The most frequently detected defects are protruding scapulae and increased lumbar lordosis. Children with poor posture more frequently present with headache and pain in the cervical and lumbar region. On an average, children spend 4 hours per week performing sports activities and 14 hours per week watching TV/VCR and playing video games. Children with limited sports activities have a significantly higher risk of developing poor posture, than children performing sports. Regular exercises such as running, walking, cycling, and playing a variety of sports will help the back to become strong.

Management

This includes maintaining the normal spinal curvature and shoulder bracing exercises.

Tips for Proper Posture

- *Standing up*: To have good posture when you are standing, you need to practice. Stand in front of the mirror.
  - Hold your head up and chin in, and look straight ahead
  - Put your shoulders back
  - Tuck your tummy in
  - Keep your knees straight
  - Take a deep breath and relax your shoulders
  - Keep your chest forward
  - Standing for a long time is tiring, so try to rest one foot at a time a bit higher up than the other, like on a step, or a stool
  - Slumping sideways into your hip is not good posture and can strain your back muscles. Try to move about rather than standing in one position for too long.
- *Sitting down:*
  - When you sit, try to keep your back straight
  - Put your back against the backrest of the chair
  - Your knees should make a right angle
  - Feet flat on floor
  - Do not cross your legs.
- *Working on the computer*:
  - If you are working on a computer, then your chair should be moved to fit you
  - Do not lean forward. Sit back and stretch your arms out to the keyboard
  - Bring your chair up close to the keyboard so that you can rest your arms on the chair or desk. Keep your shoulders relaxed. Sitting-like this is the least stressful posture for your back
  - If you are playing computer or video games, be aware that your shoulders may be hunching up as you get more excited
  - You need to rest and move around every 30 minutes to let your body relax
  - Try bending back a few times to stretch your muscles and help them relax.

- *Lifting things*:
  - Never lift alone anything that is an awkward shape or is more than a quarter of your body weight
  - Always bend your knees and straighten your legs as you lift. This way your leg muscles are doing the work and not your back muscles
  - Use a trolley if you have to move something heavy
  - To lift something, put your feet apart, hold the object close to your body and keep your arms bent. This way you are using your arm muscles and not pulling on your shoulder and back muscles
  - Never lift anything higher than your waist
  - Bend your legs and hips, tighten your tummy muscles, and use your leg muscles to help you lower the object down again.
- *Lying down:*
  - Even when we are lying down or sleeping, look after your posture by:
  - Keep the natural curves in your back
  - Lie on your side with your knees bent
  - Lie with your head on one soft pillow so that your spine is in a natural position.

Assistive Devices

When there is imbalance in the muscle tissues, assistive devices shall be advised for the ambulation and for support when there is injury or inflammation.

The following are the different assistive devices:

- Hip-knee-ankle-foot orthosis **(Fig. 20.2.1A)**
- Knee-ankle-foot-orthosis **(Fig. 20.2.1B)**
- Ankle-foot orthosis **(Fig. 20.2.1C)**
- Taylor's brace **(Fig. 20.2.2A)**
- Elbow crutches **(Fig. 20.2.2B)**
- Axillary crutches **(Fig. 20.2.2C)**.

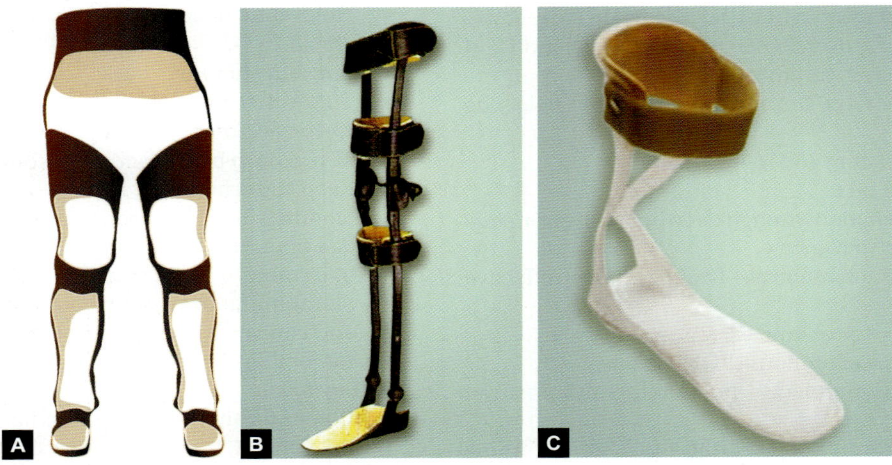

Figs. 20.2.1A to C: (A) Hip-knee-ankle-foot orthosis; (B) Knee-ankle-foot orthosis; and (C) Ankle-foot orthosis..

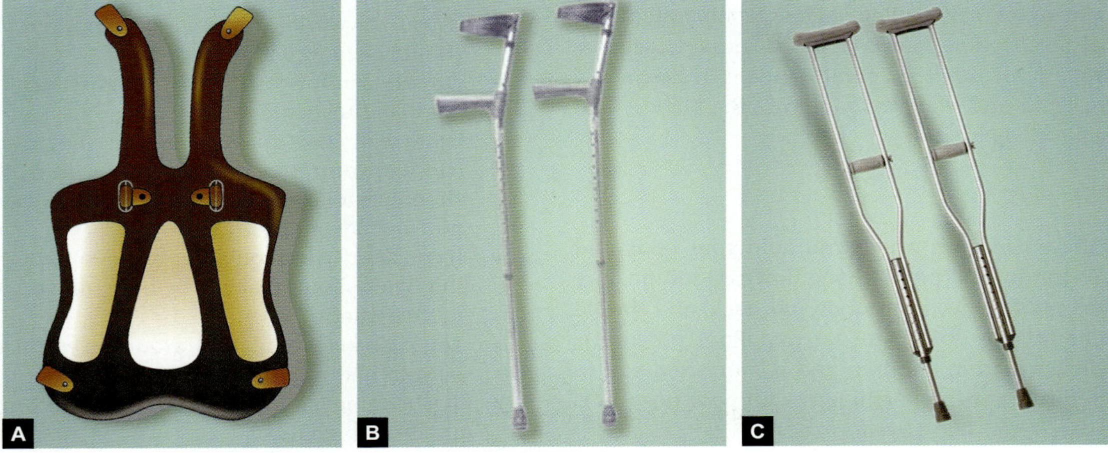

Figs. 20.2.2A to C: (A) Taylor's brace; (B) Elbow crutches; and (C) Axillary crutches.

Overall, physical therapy is concerned with identifying motor impairment and maximizing their movement potential, whereas rehabilitation aims to enhance and restore functional ability, improve their quality of life in those with physical impairments or disabilities due to any neuroskeleto-muscular problems.

BIBLIOGRAPHY

1. American physical Therapy Association. Guide to Physical Therapist Practice, 2nd edition. Alexandria VA: APTA; 2001.
2. American Thoracic Society. Secretion clearance devices. [online] Available from: http://www.thoracic.org/members/assemblies/assemblies/pr/resources/secretionclearance-devices.*pdf#page=1&zoom=auto,-9,792* [Accessed November 2018].
3. Bandy W, Sanders BW, Sanders B. Therapeutic Exercise Techniques for Intervention. Philadelphia: Lippincott William and Wilkins; 2001.
4. Behrens B, Michlovitz S. Physical Agents: Theory and Practice, 2nd edition. Philadelphia: FA Davis; 2005.
5. Byrne EM, Campbell SK. Physical therapy observation and assessment in the neonatal intensive care unit. Phys Occup Ther Pediatr. 2013;33(1):39-74.
6. Homnick DN. Mechanical insufflation-exsufflation for airway mucus clearance. Respir Care. 2007;52(10):1296-305.
7. Huber F, Wells C. Therapeutic Exercise Treatment Planning for Progression. St Louis: Saunders Elsevier; 2006.
8. Kisner C, Colby L. Therapeutic Exercise Foundation and Techniques, 4th edition. Philadelphia: FA Davis Co; 2002.
9. O'Sullivan S, Schmitz T. Physical Rehabilitation Laboratory Manual Focus on Functional Training. Philadelphia: FA Davis Co; 1999.
10. Nair MKC, Nair GS, George B, et al. Development and validation of Trivandrum Development Screening Chart for children aged 0-6 years [TDSC (0-6)]. Indian J Pediatr. 2013;80 (Suppl 2):S248-55.

Section 21

Pediatric Therapeutics

21.1 Basics of Pediatric Therapeutics

Sandeep B Bavdekar

INTRODUCTION

It is usually believed that every illness should be treated. This principle of therapeutic enthusiasm is clearly appropriate in severe and life-threatening illnesses. It, however, does not apply to all clinical situations. Infants, children, and adolescents have intrinsic recuperative capacities. Therefore, therapeutic intervention may not be required in many conditions. It should be borne in mind that drug therapy is not synonymous with good healthcare. Drug therapy in children differs from that in adults for several reasons. Their abilities to metabolize drugs mature over the years and their capacity to excrete drugs reach adult levels by late infancy. Before initiating drug therapy, the treating doctor should undertake the following steps.

STEPS IN INITIATION OF THERAPY

Reach an Initial Working Diagnosis

Reaching an initial working diagnosis based on history, examination, laboratory findings, and epidemiological considerations is the first step in starting treatment. A critically ill child would require immediate therapy aimed at stabilization of vital signs without waiting for results of investigations. In such serious and life-threatening conditions, therapy can be initiated taking into consideration the patient's age, likely etiological agent and the pattern of resistance likely to be encountered. The treatment can be changed subsequently based on results of investigations and response to therapy.

Define Therapeutic Objectives

Once having reached a working diagnosis, the next step is to specify what intends to be achieved through therapy and when. Depending upon the patient's condition and the possible diagnosis, it could include relief of symptoms, prevention of complications, eradication of cause or etiological agents or reversal of metabolic abnormalities, etc. For example, when a patient presents with fever and burning micturition and is diagnosed to have urinary tract infection, therapeutic objectives would include symptomatic relief (relief of pain during micturition and control of fever), eradication of infectious agent (with the help of appropriate anti-microbial therapy), steps to prevent further attacks of urinary tract infection, and preservation of renal function. Defining therapeutic objectives helps the doctor prescribe minimum number of appropriate drugs and provides a benchmark for the assessment of success of therapy.

Assess Effectiveness of Therapies

There is hardly any therapeutic regimen that is completely effective in all cases. Efficacy is dependent on several factors, which include patient's own defenses, drug's pharmacokinetic properties, and stage of illness. The treating doctor should be aware of the comparative efficacy of various therapeutic interventions. If the initial response is good, the treatment can be continued irrespective of microbiological studies. At the same time, drug resistance to conventional drugs is not uncommon. This has been encountered, for example, in certain illnesses such as typhoid fever, urinary tract infection, and malaria.

Assess Risk to the Patient

Every drug has adverse effects. No drug is completely innocuous. The risk to patient increases when multiple pharmacological agents are used. The physician should be aware of drug interactions and should anticipate them. Every new drug will have its potential adverse effects not known at the time of introduction.

Plan Strategies to Ensure Compliance

A patient will not derive benefits from therapy, if the drug is not properly administered. The physician must explain to the parents the importance of administering drug and the symptoms would help to control or the manifestations that it might ameliorate and when this is expected to happen and the importance of completing the course. The focus is on the active drug substance while determining dose, clinical effects and adverse effects. However, issues such as nonpalatability or presence of unpleasant smells may influence compliance. It should also be remembered that the sense of smell and taste are well-developed right from the neonatal period. Hence, the doctor should be familiar with the available preparations, their flavors, and unpleasant characteristics. Frequency of administration either as a single dose, twice daily, or thrice daily will depend on the drugs prescribed, based on the half-life of these drugs.

Consider Costs Involved

For many families, expenses involved including travel expenses, cost of drugs, expenses for diagnostic tests, and professional fees, if any, are some of the important factors determining compliance. Where oral medications are sufficient to treat an illness; parenteral drugs must be avoided. Generic drugs are generally less expensive. When time-honored cheaper but effective medications are available, one should not push the parents to buy more expensive drugs.

Enquire about Previous Experience

Another consideration in choosing a drug is to know what has failed with this patient in the past. This includes questions about hypersensitivity, adverse reaction, noncompliance, and noneffectiveness. If a preparation is taken by child with least degree of fuss, it could also mean that the preparation is acceptable to the child in terms of smell, taste, and flavor.

SPECIAL ASPECTS OF PEDIATRIC PHARMACOLOGY

Children develop and grow, and their response to drug therapy is conditioned by age, size, and stage of development. Physiological processes that influence pharmacokinetic variables in children change significantly during the first few months. Pharmacodynamic differences between pediatric and other patients are probably small.

Drug Absorption

Gastrointestinal Absorption

Drug absorption in infants and children follows the same principles as in adults. The patient and drug characteristics that affect absorption of a drug from the gastrointestinal tract are, in turn, influenced by several factors. These include age of the child, lower secretion of gastric acid, lower concentration of gastrointestinal enzymes, prolonged gastric emptying, and slower peristalsis in the first few days of life, which may affect absorption of drugs from the gastrointestinal tract. For example, plasma concentrations after oral administration of paracetamol and phenytoin have been shown to be lower in infants than those in older children and adults. Delayed development of gastrointestinal flora and its metabolic abilities can influence the absorption of certain drugs like digoxin.

Parenteral Routes of Absorption

Physiological and physiochemical factors affect the rate and extent of logical drug absorption from parenteral sites. The primary means of extravascular drug administration in infants and children, other than the oral route, is the intramuscular route. Blood flow to and from the injection site should be adequate to ensure absorption into the systemic circulation. Premature babies have very little muscle mass and children in whom perfusion is diminished; the drug may remain in the muscle and be absorbed very slowly.

Drug Distribution

Knowledge about drug distribution is important while designing an optimal dosage regimen. The distribution characteristics of drugs differ markedly amongst term infants, premature babies, and children as compared with adults. These differences are a result of much important age-dependent variables. These include the following:

- *Composition and size of body water compartments:* Neonates have a higher percentage of their body weight in the form of water (70–75%) as compared to adults (50–60%). Similarly, the extracellular water compartment accounts for 40% of the body weight in neonates compared to 20% in adults. The volume of extracellular water compartment is important in determining the concentration of drugs at receptor sites.
- *Protein-binding*: Albumin, alpha-glycoprotein, and lipoprotein are the most important circulating proteins responsible for drug-binding in plasma. The concentration of most of these proteins is low in infancy. These factors will influence the resultant balance between free and bound drug concentrations and hence have an affect on drug distribution.
- *Membrane permeability:* Permeability of membrane has an influence on the distribution of the drugs.

Drug Metabolism

Liver is the primary organ for drug metabolism and different hepatic enzyme systems mature at different ages. The cytochrome P-450 monooxygenase system appears to mature rapidly, with metabolic activity like adults being achieved by 6 months of age. In contrast, glucuronide formation reaches adult values at 3–4 years of life. Although infants are regularly characterized as being slow metabolizers of drugs, some drugs (for example, theophylline, phenytoin, and phenobarbitone) are more rapidly metabolized by infants than adults. There are qualitative differences, too. A drug may be preferentially metabolized by one pathway during the neonatal period (e.g. theophylline) as compared to adulthood. All these have practical implications. While determining dosages of drugs that undergo hepatic biotransformation, sequence of maturation of process of drug metabolism must be considered. The drugs that are metabolized at a rapid rate are required to be administered in higher dose.

Thus, theophylline is administered at much higher dose and frequency during infancy than in adulthood.

Drug Excretion

Kidney is the main organ that excretes drugs. Drugs are also excreted through the gastrointestinal tract; biliary tract, respiratory tract, and sweat glands, but these are important routes of excretion only for a miniscule minority of drugs. The excretion of drugs in the urine is dependent upon glomerular filtration rate (GFR), renal blood flow (RBF), and rate of active tubular secretion, which, in turn, are dependent on age and maturity. For example, a full-term baby's GFR and RBF are about 30% of the adult values. In premature neonates, these renal capabilities are at 15% or less of the adult values. The renal excretory capacity improves quickly and is equivalent to that of adults by about 9–12 months of age.

Drug Dosages

Because of the differences in pharmacokinetics in infants and children enumerated above, simple proportionate reduction in the adult dose is not adequate to determine a safe and effective pediatric dose. Formulae or rules providing calculations based on age or weight of the child are mere approximations. The most reliable pediatric dose information, wherein the dose is given in terms of weight or surface area, is usually that provided by the manufacturer in the package insert, in the Pharmacopoeia or in Pediatric Textbooks.

METHODS OF DRUG DELIVERY AND PEDIATRIC FORMULATIONS

Oral Administration

Depending on age, various drug forms like drops, suspensions, dry syrups (powder to be mixed with water before use), dispersible tablets, tablets, and capsules are used for oral administration in children. Suspension containing sorbitol base or alcohol base provides uniform drug amount even without shaking but there may be objections on religious or moral grounds for use of alcohol as a base. Syrupy suspensions contain undissolved particles of drug and these may not be evenly distributed throughout the vehicle. Therefore, the bottle should be shaken prior to administration of each drug dose. Proper measurement of the drug dose administered is necessary in terms of mL and not in terms of teaspoonful. The parents should be advised to use calibrated medicine cups or syringe (without needle) for measuring and administering correct doses. Advent of dispersible tablets has simplified administration of oral medicines. As these tablets can be dissolved in small volume of water, their administration is easier. Children over 8–12 years can be taught to take medicines in tablets or capsule form. This avoids inaccurate measurement, minimizes spills, and bypasses bad taste.

Parenteral Administration

This may have to be resorted to in serious illnesses, when only parenteral form of drug is available or when compliance must be ensured. Local application to skin and mucous membranes is mainly used for treating local ailments. Drugs administered by subcutaneous route are slowly absorbed. The drug behaves as if it is in a reservoir as the subcutaneous tissue has limited blood supply. Intramuscular injections should be administered in the anterolateral aspect of the thigh rather than in the gluteal muscles. This avoids the risk of injury to the sciatic nerve and the possibility of a part of the dose getting injected in the subcutaneous fat that is abundant in the buttocks. After 5 years of age, when deltoid mass is generally well-developed that site can be used for intramuscular administration.

Intravenous (IV) administration of drugs to children requires certain special considerations. Some drugs must be administered as IV push so that the drug is placed in the circulation with a minimum delay. This is an important factor when rapid onset of action is essential (e.g. adrenaline for treatment of anaphylaxis and adenosine for managing supraventricular tachycardia). This method should, however, be resorted to only by individuals familiar with acute toxicities of medications. The route carries the risk of sudden cardiac or respiratory collapse, severe anaphylaxis due to sudden antigen-antibody reaction, and local venous thrombosis, if the drug damages the vascular wall (e.g. crystalline penicillin and cloxacillin). Some drugs are required to be administered over a longer period to avoid acute toxicities or vessel wall irritation. The volume of fluid that can be administered to neonates and young infants or to children with renal failure or congestive cardiac failure is restricted. Hence, novel methods of IV administration are used in pediatrics. IV piggyback (IVPB) route is used to infuse drugs over a period of 1–2 hours. This is a common way for administering antimicrobial agents in children.

The dose of medication is injected into volumetric chamber inserted between the IV bag and the device controlling the rate of administration. The method is simple, does not require costly equipment like syringe pump, and as the medication is diluted in existing IV fluid, no extra fluid is administered. The syringe pump method is the gold standard for administration of drugs intravenously as there is absolute control over drug delivery. But this is not necessary for many medications. The syringe pumps are expensive and entail administration of extra amounts of fluid. The retrograde system is a simpler method mainly used in neonates, as it does not require injection of additional fluids.

There are only limited indications for administration of drugs through sublingual, intrathecal, and intraperitoneal routes. For example, sublingual administration is used for control of severe hypertension with nifedipine, and intrathecal route is used for administering methotrexate in the treatment of childhood leukemia. Antidiuretic hormone (ADH) is administered with the help of a nasal spray for the control of nocturnal enuresis and diabetes insipidus in selected patients. Use of pulmonary absorption of aerosolized drugs has revolutionized the management of childhood asthma. Beta-agonists and steroids are administered through this route. Advantages of this route of administration include almost instantaneous absorption of the drug into the blood, avoidance of hepatic first-pass loss, and direct delivery of the drug at the desired site of action and lesser chance of developing systemic toxicity on prolonged use. The cumbersomeness of method of administration that could come in the way of its use in young children has been overcome by using spacer devices or rotahalers.

Drugs and Breastfeeding

When a mother is on medications, many drugs appear in the breast milk. One must be aware of the side effects of these medications on the neonate (e.g. chloramphenicol and phenobarbitone). When a nursing mother needs medications, the physician must keep in mind the safety profile of the drugs that need to be administered.

PRACTICAL HINTS WHILE PRESCRIBING DRUGS FOR CHILDREN

In addition to the usual considerations, it is worthwhile emphasizing the following points that need to be considered while prescribing medications for children:

- Prescribe drugs only when necessary keeping in mind the risks, benefits, and costs involved. Review therapy as and when additional information becomes available.
- Do not rush to use the latest drug in the market, unless there is a compelling reason to do so.
- Prescribe minimum number of appropriate, inexpensive drugs of good quality, one is familiar with. Do not succumb to pressures of prescribing newly marketed drugs unless a clear indication exists.
- Prescriptions should be easily legible. It should include the date of prescription, patient details (name, age, and sex), drug details (name, formulation, composition, dose and frequency of administration, and duration for which it needs to be taken), and doctor's details (including name, signature, registration number, and contact details). It is a good idea to write the names of the drugs in capitals and write the generic name of the drugs.
- To ensure compliance, explain to parents the nature of the disease and the likely benefits to be obtained from the therapy. Give clear instruction, preferably in writing to avoid misinterpretation, including the need to complete a given course even if child appears to be asymptomatic.
- Prescribe doses at a frequency as advised in product insert or as per standard pediatric texts.
- Prescribe medications for a complete course in appropriate formulations, e.g. drops for neonates, liquid preparations or dispersible tablets for infants and young children, and tablets and capsules for children older than 8–12 years.
- Direct parents to discard all remaining doses to protect the child from accidental poisoning or improper self-medication later.
- Explain the adverse effects of the drug, if any, to the parents, especially when long-term treatment is suggested. Whenever necessary, explain the need for periodical clinical and/or laboratory monitoring when on long-term drug therapy for epilepsy, tuberculosis, renal diseases, etc. to assess the response and prevent serious side effects. Ask the parent to report any worsening, unexplained event, or adverse effect immediately.
- Drug combinations must be used with caution, unless the drugs are in the specified dose requirements (e.g. sulfonamide plus trimethoprim, amoxicillin and clavulanic acid, sulfonamide plus pyrimethamine, isoniazid, and rifampicin). Avoid fancy but inappropriate combinations such as metronidazole plus nalidixic acid or norfloxacin, ampicillin and cloxacillin, etc.
- Drug interactions between two drugs can happen, if administered simultaneously, e.g. penicillin and aminoglycoside in the same syringe.
- Be conversant with the ongoing developments and progress in the fields of therapeutics and drug development. Prescribe drugs in a judicious manner to ensure that children do not remain therapeutic orphans and at the same time their safety is not sacrificed while prescribing newer drugs.

BIBLIOGRAPHY

1. deVaries TPGM, Henning RH, Hogerzeil HV, Fresle DA. Guide to Good Prescribing, Geneva: World Health Organization; 2000.
2. Loebstein R, Vohra S, Koren G. Drug therapy in pediatric patients. In: Carruthers SG, Hoffman BB, Melman KL, Nierenburg DW (Eds). Melmon and Morrelli's Clinical Pharmacology: Basic Principles in Therapeutics, 4th edition. New York: McGraw Hill Medical Publishing Division; 2000. pp. 1143-9.

21.2 Adverse Drug Reactions, Drug Interactions, and Therapeutic Drug Monitoring

Archana Kher, PSN Menon

ADVERSE DRUG REACTIONS

Introduction

Children constitute a vulnerable group since new drugs get released into the market without adequate trials in children due to ethical reasons, the exceptions being oncology and vaccines. Only a careful postmarketing surveillance detects adverse drug reactions (ADRs) occurring in children. Measures should be undertaken to improve detection and reporting of ADRs by all healthcare professionals.

Definitions

Adverse drug reaction (ADR) generally refers to any unwanted consequence/s of administration of a drug during or following the course of therapy. These unpleasant effects occur at *doses intended for therapeutic (prophylactic or diagnostic) effect* and necessitate reduction of the dose or withdrawal of the drug or predict a hazard from future administration.

The Joint Commission on the Accreditation of Healthcare Organizations (JCAHO) defines an ADR as "an undesired effect of a medication that either increases toxicity, decreases desired therapeutic effect, or both".

World Health Organization (WHO) defines ADR as "a response, which is noxious and unintended, and which occurs at doses normally used in humans for the prophylaxis, diagnosis or therapy of disease, or for the modification of physiological function".

Intolerance denotes a low threshold to the normal pharmacological action of a drug.

An *idiosyncratic reaction* is an inherent qualitative abnormal reaction to a drug.

Harmful reactions due to drug overdose (poisoning), drug abuse, and therapeutic errors are excluded from ADRs.

Epidemiology

The ADRs can cause severe morbidity and even death. They are responsible for nearly 7% of admissions and about 60% of reported ADRs could be avoided. ADRs are the seventh most common cause of death. In clinical practice, antibiotics, anticonvulsants, and antitubercular drugs cause most reported ADRs. A retrospective cohort study of 1,087 ADRs was analyzed from 1995 to 2004. The incidence was 1.6%, with low-level severity 89%, and high-level severity 11%. Antibiotics induced mild reactions; anticonvulsants and antineoplastic agents caused severe reactions. The reported incidence of ADRs in children is around 9.5% accounting for 2.1% of hospital admissions and 39% were life-threatening. In general, it appears that ADRs are underreported; especially in children and current rates represent only 10–15% of the true rate.

Classification

The administration of a drug may result in the development of side effects, untoward effects, toxic effects, or allergic and idiosyncratic effects. ADRs could be either local (irritation, necrosis, and thrombophlebitis) or systemic. They are classified as follows:

- *Type A ADR*: These are also known as augmented, attenuated, or quantitative ADR. They comprise a hyper-response to the main action of the drug, e.g. insulin-induced hypoglycemia. In general, they are dose-dependent and preventable by slow introduction of low dosages. Hypotension by beta-blockers and nonsteroidal anti-inflammatory drugs (NSAID)-induced gastric ulcers are other examples.
- *Type B ADR*: They are bizarre or qualitative ADRs manifesting as unpredictable or unexpected effects. The exact mechanisms are unknown and they are unrelated to the dose of the drug. They may be serious and often fatal. Examples include halothane-induced hepatitis and chloramphenicol-induced aplastic anemia.
- *Type C ADR*: The effect is time- and dose-related as in analgesic nephropathy. It is often due to continuous drug use, and may be irrevocable, unanticipated, or even unpredictable. Tardive dyskinesia caused by antipsychotic drugs, and dementia following anticholinergic agents are examples of type C ADRs.
- *Type D ADR*: The ADR is time-related event as in carcinogenesis. It may be delayed, and may occur even after cessation of treatment, e.g. corneal opacities after

thioridazine, ophthalmopathy following chloroquine, retroperitoneal fibrosis following ergot alkaloids, analgesics, and methyldopa.

- *Type E ADR:* These include the end-of-dose or withdrawal reactions. They occur typically with antidepressant drugs. Other examples include seizures on alcohol or benzodiazepine withdrawal, hypertension in an opiate abstainer, and first dose hypotension caused by alpha-blockers (prazosin) or angiotensin-converting enzyme (ACE) inhibitors.
- *Type F ADR:* These include failure of therapy or ineffective therapy, e.g. augmented hypertension because of inefficient control.

Common Manifestations of Adverse Drug Reactions

The commonly reported ADRs include the following:

- *Dermal reactions:* Erythema multiforme, fixed drug eruptions, and Stevens–Johnson syndrome
- *Gastrointestinal symptoms:* Nausea, vomiting, and diarrhea
- *Hepatic:* Elevated enzymes and liver cell failure
- *Neurological manifestations:* Tremors, dystonia, and impaired cognitive function
- *Hematological effects:* Neutropenia and aplastic anemia
- *Anaphylaxis:* Commonly due to penicillin and vaccines.

There are several reasons for the excessive number of ADRs. These include:

- There is a general tendency to prescribe a large number of drugs for a specific disease or group of symptoms in children and there is unwanted polypharmacy
- The ever-increasing number of new drugs in the market, which have not undergone proper pre- and postmarketing surveillance
- The lack of a formal system for monitoring ADRs.

Special Issues Related to Adverse Drug Reaction in Children

Children warrant different attention as they have special issues, when ADRs are detected. Many complaints like poor attention span and visual impairments may go unnoticed. Their growth potential may get affected with steroids. Children are more vulnerable to dermal reactions. Our pediatric population represents a wide variety of ethnic and sociocultural groups and may therefore react to drugs in a different manner. Infections are widely prevalent in Indian children; therefore it is worth identifying ADRs to drugs used to treat endemic infectious diseases. Over 50% children are malnourished and malnutrition affects drug kinetics. This should be given due consideration while prescribing antitubercular drugs. Very often children are not necessarily treated by pediatricians and irrational multiple drug prescriptions are commonly given. Ayurvedic and homeopathic medicines are additionally prescribed and drug interactions (DIs) may go unnoticed. Ciprofloxacin is not recommended for routine use in children and the reported incidence of ADR is 3.1%, but it is used for resistant enteric fever. Additives, coloring agents, sugars, and flavorings used in medications induce urticaria and asthma; they are often not mentioned on the labels.

Causes of Adverse Drug Reactions

Non-Drug Factors

Factors such as age, drug allergy, and genetic predisposition are intrinsic to the patient. Extrinsic factors like the prescriber and environment influence ADRs. In neonates and infants, the drug distribution is affected by lower proportion of fat and higher proportion of water. The blood-brain barrier is more permeable. The enzyme systems are immature, conjugation is impaired and elimination by the kidney is lowered. Drugs such as gentamicin and digoxin have a prolonged half-life. Older children metabolize drugs more rapidly than adults. Heritable conditions like methemoglobinemia and glucose-6-phosphate dehydrogenase (G6PD) deficiency may precipitate ADRs.

Drug Factors

These factors include the choice of drug and DIs. Side effects of drugs are undesired but are an inevitable part of the pharmacological action of the drug at therapeutic doses, e.g. drowsiness with phenobarbitone. Secondary effects occur due to indirect consequences of a primary drug action, e.g. diuretic-induced hypokalemia leading to digoxin intolerance. A high dose of a drug can cause toxicity, e.g. eighth cranial nerve damage with gentamicin. Incorrect technique of administration of drugs can cause adverse reactions.

Allergic reactions to drugs result from an interaction of the drug or metabolite with patient and disease and reexposure may cause severe reactions. Most drugs are simple chemicals and act as incomplete antigens or haptens. Test dose alone at times will be inadequate to rule out any ADR. One must be cautious while using a drug first time, when there is a positive family history of drug allergy. Reactions include rashes, angioedema, serum sickness, anaphylaxis, and asthma.

The reactions can be classified by the time of onset as:

- *Immediate,* which typically begin within 30 minutes of administering the drug.
- *Accelerated,* which are immunoglobulin E (IgE)-mediated begin in 2–72 hours after the drug use.
- *Late* reactions occur 72 or more hours later, are often unrelated to IgE-mediated mechanisms.

Drugs and the Fetus

Drugs such as thalidomide and anticancer drugs affect cell division, protein synthesis, or deoxyribonucleic acid (DNA) synthesis, and can be teratogenic. Indirect action may result from drugs acting on the placenta or on the uterus (e.g. vasoconstrictors cause fetal anoxia by reducing blood supply). Lipid-soluble drugs easily pass into the fetus; drug metabolites persist due to immature excretory processes.

Pharmacovigilance: Detection and Monitoring of Adverse Drug Reaction

Adverse drug reaction monitoring is generally referred to as pharmacovigilance. WHO defines pharmacovigilance as the science and activities related to the detection, assessment, understanding and prevention of adverse effects, or any other drug-related problems. Pharmacovigilance took a firm grip on clinical practice following the thalidomide tragedy. WHO started the pharmacovigilance programs in 1968. The Uppsala Monitoring Centre (UMC) in Sweden is the collaborating WHO center for this global initiative. The main function of UMC is communication of safety signals recognized through analysis of global data of ADR.

A formal and official ADR monitoring system was started in India in the year 1986. Detection and reporting of ADR is a professional responsibility. The National Pharmacovigilance Programme of India (PvPI) was started in 2010, the aim being to collate, analyze, and archive data on adverse events and ADRs in children. This is a three tier system with peripheral centers, 5 regional centers and 2 zonal centers at KEM Hospital, Mumbai and AIIMS, New Delhi. The National Pharmacovigilance Center is at the Central Drugs Standard Control Organization, New Delhi.

Indian Pharmacopoeia Commission (IPC), functions as the National Coordination Centre (NCC) for the PvPI since April 2011 under the aegis of Ministry of Health and Family Welfare, Government of India. Currently over 250 ADR monitoring centers (AMCs) are functioning in various healthcare institutions:

- Medical colleges and hospitals
- Medical or central or autonomous institutes
- Private hospitals
- Corporate hospitals.

The major functions of NCC are to collect, collate, and analyze ADRs data as per a standard procedure. The *Individual Case Safety Reports* (ICSRs) are collected in the standard suspected ADR reporting form, which consists of four sections, i.e. (1) patient's information, (2) suspected adverse reaction, (3) suspected medication(s), and (4) reporter's information. They are analyzed and reported to the NCC to arrive at an inference to recommend regulatory interventions to Central Drugs Standard Control Organization (CDSCO). NCC also communicates risks to healthcare professionals and the public through PvPI newsletters. AMCs have been setup under NCC to collect the ADRs from patients. The main objective of setting-up the AMCs is to identify rare ADRs that could not be found through clinical trial programmes. NCC provides the logistic support and manpower to AMCs for their smooth functioning and reporting of ADRs. Despite all efforts, the underreporting of ADR is a mammoth and daunting challenge for PvPI.

Reporting Adverse Drug Reaction

Suspected ADR reporting forms for healthcare professionals and consumers are available on the website of IPC to report ADR. The consumer reporting forms are made available in 10 major vernacular languages (Hindi, Tamil, Telugu, Kannada, Bengali, Gujarati, Assamese, Marathi, Oriya, and Malayalam) to remove the language barrier in ADR reporting. ADRs can be also reported via PvPI helpline number (1800-180-3024) on weekdays from 9:00 am to 5:30 pm. The mobile Android application for ADR reporting has also been made available to the public.

DRUG INTERACTIONS

Drug interactions (DI) refer to the interface of a drug, food, or nutrient in the action of another drug. DI result from the use of two or more drugs, this may lead to an enhanced or diminished effect. The effect may be desired or undesired, beneficial, or harmful. A study was conducted in a Brazilian hospital in children, where four or more drugs were used and the data revealed 5.6% DI, 1.9% interaction or prescription, and 0.5% incompatibility or prescription. DI represents 3.5% of all preventable ADRs; also contributes to emergency room visits and hospital admissions. Pediatric patients have immature systems of eliminating drugs, extended half-life of drugs, and therefore behave differently. DI is important in the following situations:

- Drugs that have a small therapeutic index or exhibit zero order kinetics
- Drugs that are enzyme inducers or inhibitors
- Drugs used for the same disorder, e.g. theophylline and salbutamol increase the risk for cardiac arrhythmias, use of beta-blockers, and calcium channel blockers
- Long-term use of any drugs
- Presence of comorbid conditions and multiorgan failure
- Use of multiple drugs.

Drug interactions are of two types:

1. *Pharmacokinetic interaction*: These are easy to detect and quantify. They are related to the absorption, metabolism, distribution, and excretion of the drug. They can occur outside the body or in the body. Drug incompatibilities may occur before administering when the drugs are mixed, e.g. dopamine with bicarbonate is not compatible, and phenytoin precipitates in dextrose solution. Intravenous solutions must be checked for visible changes such as turbidity, color, and precipitates. Use of correct vehicle and appropriate pH of the infusion is essential.

Concomitant administration of aminoglycosides and beta-lactam antibiotics leads to loss of their effectiveness due to chemical inactivation; it is therefore important to monitor serum levels of aminoglycosides and allow an interval of 1–2 hours between the injections. The use of phenobarbitone and valproic acid leads to elevated levels of phenobarbitone and reduced efficacy of valproic acid through enzyme induction. The absorption and protein binding of drugs are different; when drugs are combined they may be ineffective or their metabolites could be toxic. Few interactions occur through competition at drug transporters.

2. *Pharmacodynamic interaction*: Effects such as synergism and antagonism occur at the action sites of the drugs. They may be mediated through receptors, transport processes, or electrolyte levels, e.g. potassium depletion enhances digoxin effect. Synergism results, when there is summation or addition with two drugs having the same effect. Potentiation also occurs when one drug increases the action of another, e.g. trimethoprim and sulfonamides. The effect is seen on the target organ.

Drugs are metabolized by cytochrome P450 system and many polymorphisms are known in the populations. The differences in the drug metabolism can be genetically determined. In clinical practice, drug-disease and drug-food interactions are evident.

Therapeutic Drug Monitoring

If a drug has a narrow therapeutic range, samples are taken to allow the dose to be adjusted so that the concentration remains between a minimum value for efficacy and a maximum value for safety. This is called "therapeutic drug monitoring (TDM)". It has been widely used to adjust dosages of antiepileptic drugs such as phenytoin. Although TDM is usually restricted to monitoring of drug concentrations, similar monitoring schemes that aim to maintain effects in a desirable range between upper and lower limits are also common. Examples include testing capillary blood glucose levels during insulin therapy in diabetics and testing blood clotting time during warfarin or anticoagulant therapy.

Monitoring is often advocated as a way of avoiding or mitigating the harm from ADRs. Monitoring for ADRs by repeated laboratory testing probably started with the observation that the antibiotic chloramphenicol could cause bone-marrow toxicity of two types, one occurring at high dosage and is reversible, and the other of which could occur at any therapeutic dosage and generally results in fatal aplastic anemia.

Therapeutic drug monitoring is unlikely to be cost-effective as a monitoring scheme for a rare adverse reaction of little consequence, but very cost-effective to introduce one for a common and serious adverse reaction, assuming the other criteria are fulfilled.

Therapeutic drug monitoring was introduced in India in late 1980s. TDM involves tailoring a dose regimen to an individual patient by maintaining plasma or blood concentration within the therapeutic range. Automation has made it possible to develop assays but proper interpretation is required. Genetic variation in metabolism, elimination rates, disease states, pregnancy, nutritional deficiencies, and interactions with other drugs gives rise to a wide range of plasma levels in patients administered the same dose. Ayurvedic, Homeopathic, and Unani medicines are often taken together with allopathic medicines. Experimental studies showed that *shankhapushpi* had both pharmacokinetic and pharmacodynamic interactions with phenytoin and phenytoin levels dropped. Drug levels can be altered with a hypoproteinemic state, and conditions such as acquired immune deficiency syndrome (AIDS), which lead to low levels of antituberculosis (TB) drugs. Nutritional deficiencies also affect drug pharmacokinetics. TDM is useful in drugs with a narrow therapeutic index, those that are highly protein-bound or liable to interact or when the metabolites are very toxic.

During estimation of drug level, the actual time that the sample was obtained is important. The levels can be determined anytime during dosing interval for drug with a long half-life, e.g. phenobarbitone. For drugs that have a short half-life, peak, and trough concentrations must be measured at specific times. Concentrations measured during the distribution phase are variable and do not correlate with usual therapeutic range. Ideally, plasma drug samples should be procured after four half-lives of the drug. Peak concentrations are observed within 1–2 hour after oral administration of a drug; to ensure proper absorption levels must be measured before the next dose (trough).

Patients with chronic renal or liver disease, prolonged therapy with anticonvulsant drugs, need TDM to avoid undertreatment and adverse events. Patients on theophylline can have increased plasma levels and toxicity when given with erythromycin. Cisapride, when given with theophylline can induce cardiac arrhythmias. TDM can help to identify noncompliant patients. Quality of products (drug content and bioavailability) is important especially for drugs with a narrow margin of safety for which TDM is relevant. The TDM service can be used to provide an important early indication of substandard drugs.

The most common indication for TDM of anticonvulsants, carbamazepine, valproic acid, and phenytoin, has been nonresponse to a standard dose of drug. This allows differentiation between noncompliance, need for a higher dose, and true drug resistance requiring change over to second drug. Other common indications include suspected drug toxicity, dose adjustment in pregnancy, and DIs (especially common with anti-TB drugs). TDM of antimycobacterial drugs offers the clinician a chance to ensure that the patient achieves a serum concentration above the minimum inhibitory concentration (MIC). The Madras Tuberculosis Center in South India has developed a urine test to identify noncompliance with isoniazid therapy.

Therapeutic drug monitoring can also be used as a useful research tool. In developing countries, TDM is important, where there are spurious poor quality drugs are available, drug legislation is inadequate and self-medication is easily practiced. With good prescribing practices and appropriate use of drug monitoring therapeutic concentrations can be achieved in over 70% patients. Accuracy of drug assays, laboratory variability in reporting, and poor access to the tests are the limitations. A lot of information in clinical pharmacology and therapeutics is available on the Internet for reference, e.g. *www.ascpt.org*.

PRACTICE POINTS

- Do not prescribe a drug unless there is a clear indication for its use.
- Ask the child or parents, if he or she had previous allergy or idiosyncrasy to any drug or formulation before prescribing.
- Probe whether the child is already on other drugs—including self-medication, health supplements, and alternative therapies as DIs may occur.
- Genetic factors and diseases of liver and kidney may alter the metabolism and excretion of drugs requiring a change in dosage.
- Prescribe as few drugs as possible and avoid polypharmacy.
- Give clear instructions on how to administer the drugs to children.
- Use familiar drugs as far as possible. Be alert to adverse or unexpected effects, whenever a new drug is used.
- Be aware that excipients may be responsible for the ADR. If the ADR is minor, consider prescribing an alternate formulation before altogether abandoning the drug.
- Warn the child and family that serious ADRs are likely to occur.

BIBLIOGRAPHY

1. Amale PN, Deshpande SA, Nakhate YD, et al. Pharmacovigilance process in India: An overview. J Pharmacovigilance. 2018;6(2):259.
2. Gawade SP. Overview of monitoring of therapeutic drugs. Indian J Pharm Pract. 2016;9(3):152-6.
3. Kalaiselvan V, Kumar P, Mishra P, et al. System of adverse drug reactions reporting: What, where, how, and whom to report? Indian J Crit Care Med. 2015;19(9):564-6
4. Kalaiselvan V, Thota P, Singh A. Current status of adverse drug reactions monitoring centres under pharmacovigilance programme of India. Indian J Pharm Pract. 2014;7(3):19-22.
5. Kang JS, Lee MH. Overview of therapeutic drug monitoring. Korean J Intern Med. 2009;24(1):1-10.
6. Le J, Nguyen T, Law AV, et al. Adverse drug reactions among children over a 10-year period. Pediatrics. 2006;118(2):555-62.
7. Mahajan MM, Thatte UM, Gogtay NJ, et al. An analysis of completeness and quality of adverse drug reaction reports at an adverse drug reaction monitoring centre in Western India. Perspect Clin Res. 2018;9(3):123-6.
8. Patel KJ, Kedia MS, Bajpai D, et al. Evaluation of the prevalence and economic burden of ADRs presenting to the medical emergency department of a tertiary referral centre: a prospective study. BMC Clinical Pharmacol. 2007;7:8.
9. Sharma G, Kumar R, Singh J, et al. Pharmacovigilance in India and its impact in patient management. Curr Trends Diagn Treat. 2017;1(1):27-33.
10. Uday Kumar P, Adhikari P, Periera P. A prospective analysis of ADRs in a South Indian Hospital. Online J Health Allied Sci. 2009;3:12.

21.3 Antiviral Agents

P Ramachandran

INTRODUCTION

Viral infections range from subclinical or mild with a self-limiting course to a life-threatening problem. Compared to antibiotics antiviral drugs were developed much later, in 1950s. The first antiherpetic drug, idoxyuridine was synthesized in 1959.

As the viruses closely integrate with the cellular function, there is a risk of collateral damage to cell function by antiviral agents. The challenge was to develop such molecules, which will target the infecting virus without damaging the cells. The other problem encountered in the development of antivirals is the difficulty in confirming viral infections with objective laboratory investigations such as culture to determine the efficacy of drugs. Advent of molecular diagnostic tests and their availability at affordable cost have helped in choosing appropriate antivirals and also in monitoring the response to treatment. Success of therapy will hinge on collecting appropriate specimens before initiating therapy, assessing the age and the immune status of the child and the function of various organ systems. Drug doses depend on age and suitable modifications may be required depending on renal or liver function. The decision for treatment, preventive therapy, and its duration also will be based on whether the child is immunologically competent or not. Immunocompromised children are susceptible to common viruses and develop severe local or disseminated disease. These viruses include herpes group of viruses such as cytomegalovirus (CMV), Epstein-Barr virus (EBV) and varicella-zoster virus (VZV).

MODE OF ACTION

The commonly targeted sites of action for antiviral agents are at the—(1) viral entry, absorption, penetration, and uncoating (amantadine and rimantadine), (2) transcription or replication of the viral genome (acyclovir, valacyclovir, cidofovir, famciclovir, penciclovir, foscarnet, ganciclovir, valganciclovir, ribavirin, and trifluridine), (3) viral protein synthesis [interferons (IFNs)], and (4) viral assembly or release (oseltamivir, zanamivir, and IFNs). Antiviral agents exhibit their effect maximally during viral replication inside the cells. They may not eliminate the viruses, which are dormant or not replicating actively.

Antiviral resistance is an emerging problem, which can be attributed to high degree of mutation and prolonged and repeated courses of therapy as seen in immunocompromised children.

CLASSIFICATION OF ANTIVIRAL AGENTS

- *Nucleoside or nucleotide analogs:* These agents are structurally similar to the naturally occurring nucleosides or nucleotides. When incorporated into the nucleic acid of the virus, they inhibit viral deoxyribonucleic acid (DNA) polymerase and block further addition of nucleotide resulting in chain termination. Their efficacy and toxicity are based on their selective incorporation into viral nucleic acid in preference to host cell DNA. They are the ones mainly effective against viruses under herpes virus family.
- *Neuraminidase inhibitors:* These drugs target a viral specific enzyme (neuraminidase) as in influenza virus that helps in the deaggregation and release of newly formed virus from the host cells.
- *Interferons:* These are naturally occurring components of cellular immunity used against viral infections. Currently, these are used in conjunction with other antiviral agents for hepatitis B and C infections.

Table 21.3.1: Antiviral agents.

Viral infection	***Antivirals***
Herpes (HSV, VZV, and CMV)	Acyclovir, famciclovir, valacyclovir, ganciclovir, valganciclovir, cidofovir, and foscarnet
Influenza	Oseltamivir, zanamivir, ribavirin, amantadine, and rimantadine
RSV	Ribavirin, RSV immune globulin, and palivizumab
Hepatitis B	Lamivudine (3TC), emtricitabine (FTC), adefovir, tenofovir, entecavir, and interferon (IFN)
Hepatitis C	Peg IFN, ribavirin, sofosbuvir, ledipasvir, and sofosbuvir (Harvoni)
HIV	More than 20 approved drugs

(CMV: cytomegalovirus; HIV: human immunodeficiency virus; HSV: herpes simplex virus; RSV: respiratory syncytial virus; VZV: varicella-zoster virus)

Antiviral drugs commonly used in practice are against herpes viruses, influenza virus, and hepatitis viruses **(Table 21.3.1)**. Antiviral therapy of human immunodeficiency virus (HIV) is discussed separately.

ANTIVIRAL AGENTS AGAINST HERPES VIRUS INFECTIONS

The important herpes viruses are herpes simplex virus (HSV), VZV, EBV, and CMV. The antivirals effective for herpes viruses predominantly are nucleoside analogs causing inhibition of DNA polymerase of the virus **(Table 21.3.2)**. The important drugs in this group are acyclovir, valganciclovir, ganciclovir, foscarnet, and cidofovir. Some of the prodrugs of these antivirals have better absorption and are orally effective, making them suitable for use in specific situations. For example, valacyclovir is the L-valyl ester of acyclovir and three times more bioavailable than is acyclovir.

Acyclovir

Acyclovir is most active against HSV1, HSV2 (two-fold less susceptible than HSV1), and also effective against VZV (requires higher dose). Acyclovir is an analog of guanosine and selectively inhibits HSV and VZV replication. The drug is converted to acyclovir monophosphate by virus-encoded thymidine kinase, a reaction that does not occur to any significant extent in uninfected cells. Subsequent phosphorylation steps are catalyzed by cellular enzymes resulting in high concentrations of acyclovir triphosphate

Table 21.3.2: Drugs active against herpes viruses.

Drug	*Composition*	*Active component*	*Active against*	*Route of admin*	*Side effects*
Acyclovir	Acyclic nucleoside	Triphosphate	HSV and VZV	Oral, IV, and topical	Renal, neuro, and hematol
Valacyclovir	Prodrug of acyclovir	Triphosphate	HSV and VZV	Oral	Renal, neuro, and hematol
Penciclovir	Acyclic nucleoside	Triphosphate	HSV	Topical	Local irritation
Famciclovir	Prodrug of penciclovir	Triphosphate	HSV and VZV	Oral	Gastrointestinal
Ganciclovir	Acyclic nucleoside	Triphosphate	CMV, HSV and VZV	IV-Oral	Hematol
Valganciclovir	Prodrug of ganciclovir	Triphosphate	CMV	Oral	Hematol
Foscarnet	Pyrophosphate analog	Drug itself	HSV and CMV (resistant to first line drugs)	IV	Renal and metabolic
Cidofovir	Nucleotide analog	Diphosphate	CMV, HSV and HPV	IV	Renal and ocular
Trifluridine	Nucleoside analog	Triphosphate	HSV keratitis	Topical	Ocular
Idoxiuridine	Nucleoside analog	Triphosphate	HSV keratitis	Topical	Ocular

All of the above inhibit viral DNA polymerase except foscarnet, which inhibits viral DNA polymerase and reverse transcriptase.
(CMV: cytomegalovirus; DNA: deoxyribonucleic acid; HSV: herpes simplex virus; HPV: Human papilloma virus; VZV: IV; intravenous varicella-zoster virus)

Table 21.3.3: Acyclovir for neonatal HSV infection.

Clinical situation	*Acyclovir dose*	*Duration of treatment*
Skin, eye and mucous membrane (SEM) disease	IV acyclovir 60 mg/kg/day in three divided doses	14 days
CNS disease	IV acyclovir 60 mg/kg/day in three divided doses	21 days (if HSV PCR positive in CSF at the end of treatment, continue treatment till it becomes negative)
Disseminated disease	IV acyclovir 60 mg/kg/day in three divided doses	21 days
Suppressive treatment (in SEM, CNS and disseminated disease)	300 mg/m^2/ dose three times daily	6 months (monitor neutrophil count)

(CNS: central nervous system; CSF: cerebrospinal fluid; HSV: herpes simplex virus; IV: intravenous; PCR: polymerase chain reaction)

in infected cells. Acyclovir triphosphate inhibits viral DNA synthesis by inactivating viral DNA polymerase resulting in restriction of further DNA chain elongation. Viral DNA polymerase has a much higher affinity for acyclovir triphosphate than does cellular DNA polymerase, resulting in little interference of the function of uninfected cells. This relatively selective mechanism of antiviral action provides a uniquely high therapeutic index.

Acyclovir does not have an effective action against CMV, EBV, and also ribonucleic acid (RNA) viruses such as influenza, which lack thymidine kinase, thereby limiting its usefulness in these infections.

Clinical Situations for Acyclovir Use in HSV Infections

Neonatal HSV infection ***(Table 21.3.3)****:* In all types of neonatal HSV infections, acyclovir is indicated in parenteral form. This is followed by suppressive therapy for 6 months to optimize neurological outcome and to prevent recurrences.

- *Herpes simplex virus encephalitis*: In both suspected or confirmed HSV encephalitis, intravenous (IV) acyclovir is administered for 3 weeks followed by confirmation of virological clearance by repeat cerebrospinal fluid (CSF) examination **(Table 21.3.4)**.
- Mucocutaneous infection.

Varicella Infection

In healthy, immunocompetent children with chickenpox without any complication, treatment with acyclovir is not routinely recommended as varicella is associated with low rates of morbidity and mortality. For most children, supportive care alone is sufficient.

The beneficial clinical effects of oral acyclovir are—decrease in (1) the number of days in which new lesions

Table 21.3.4: Acyclovir dose for herpes simplex infection in children.

Type of HSV infection	*Acyclovir dose*
HSV encephalitis > 4 months age	IV acyclovir 10–20 mg/kg per dose 8 hourly for 21 days
Mucocutaneous infection (Immune competent)	Acyclovir oral 20 mg/kg per dose 4 times daily for 5–7 days
Mucocutaneous infection (Immune compromised)	Acyclovir IV 5–10 mg/kg per dose 8 hourly for 7 days

(HSV: herpes simplex virus; IV: intravenous)

appear, (2) the duration of fever by 24 hours, (3) the severity of cutaneous and systemic signs and symptoms, and (4) the time to total crusting of lesions by 2 days, when acyclovir is administered within 24 hour of onset of rash. Oral acyclovir is well tolerated.

When there is an increased risk of complications as in adolescents, children with chronic skin or respiratory conditions, children on oral or inhaled steroids including those on short-term therapy, and secondary cases from household exposure, acyclovir therapy is recommended. Oral acyclovir in a dose of 20 mg/kg dose (maximum of 800 mg) four times daily for 5 days is administered. Treatment should be initiated within 72 hour of onset of rash preferably within 24 hour to prevent severe disease. Acyclovir administration does not interfere with the induction of immunity against VZV. An alternative is valacyclovir, approved for use in children more than 2 years of age, administered in a dose of 20 mg/kg dose thrice daily for 5 days. It is absorbed better than acyclovir **(Table 21.3.5)**.

Immunocompromised Children and Children with Severe Varicella (Pneumonia, Encephalitis, Severe Thrombocytopenia, and Severe Hepatitis)

In these children, IV acyclovir therapy is initiated at the earliest, preferably within 72 hour of onset of rash with the aim of preventing progression and dissemination. It is given in a dose of 20 mg/kg/dose diluted in 5% dextrose as slow IV infusion over 1 h; given 8 hourly for 7–14 days **(Table 21.3.5)**. Rapid infusion may result in renal damage due to crystalluria. Adequate hydration should be ensured. A switch to oral acyclovir therapy can be considered, when the patient is afebrile and new lesion formation has ceased. When feasible, the dosage of immunosuppressive medications should be temporarily reduced. Infection can relapse in immunocompromised children requiring multiple courses of acyclovir therapy.

Resistance to acyclovir is rare, but can occur in children with HIV infection and other immunodeficiency disorders. Such resistant infections may require second-line drugs such as IV foscarnet in a dose of 40 mg/kg/dose 8 hourly for 3 weeks. VZV isolates resistant to both acyclovir and foscarnet have been encountered infrequently. Cidofovir is the drug of choice for dually-resistant VZV. These second-line drugs are associated with increased toxicity.

Table 21.3.5: Acyclovir in varicella zoster virus infection.

Clinical situation	*Acyclovir dose and duration*
VZV infection in immunocompetent child	Oral acyclovir 20 mg/kg/dose four times daily for 5 days (maximum 800 mg per dose) Oral valacyclovir (approved for children > 2 years of age) 20 mg/kg/dose three times daily for 5 days (Maximum 1 g per dose)
VZV infection in immunocompromised child and children with severe varicella (pneumonia, encephalitis, severe thrombocytopenia, and severe hepatitis)	10–20 mg/kg/dose IV acyclovir 8 hourly usually for 7–14 days

(IV: intravenous; VZV: varicella-zoster virus)

Cytomegalovirus Infection

Ganciclovir

Ganciclovir has a uniquely potent action against CMV. It is used for:

- Newborns congenitally infected with CMV with central nervous system (CNS) involvement
- Preemptive therapy in immunocompromised patients with virologic markers of active infection predictive of CMV disease
- Prophylaxis of high-risk patients, such as those who are CMV seropositive or who have received transplants from CMV-seropositive donors
- Immunocompromised individuals with invasive CMV disease, including pneumonia, colitis, esophagitis, myocarditis, encephalitis, persistent fever and leukopenia syndrome, and viral sepsis syndrome

It is administered in two phases, induction and maintenance **(Table 21.3.6)**.

In newborns with congenital CMV infection involving CNS, IV ganciclovir is recommended for 6 weeks. Monitoring has to done for neutropenia. Granulocyte colony-stimulating factor (GCSF) can be administered whenever required to improve neutropenia. For babies who can take orally, valganciclovir is an alternative.

Valganciclovir

It is a prodrug of ganciclovir and has a similar spectrum of action including potent action against CMV. It can be administered orally with a high bioavailability. Treatment of newborns with symptomatic congenital CMV infection can be done with oral valganciclovir (15–18 mg/kg/dose every 12 hour) continued

Table 21.3.10: Prophylactic agents in viral infections.

Human immunoglobulin	• Prevention of hepatitis A • Treatment of B19 parvovirus infection in immunodeficient individuals
CMV immunoglobulin	• Prophylaxis of CMV in solid organ and hematopoietic stem cell transplant recipients • Treatment of CMV pneumonia in combination with ganciclovir
Hepatitis B immunoglobulin	Prophylaxis of hepatitis B infection especially in newborns born to HBsAg positive mothers
Rabies immunoglobulin	Postexposure prophylaxis for rabies
RSV immunoglobulin	Prevention of complications of RSV infection in young infants
Palivizumab (humanized RSV monoclonal antibody with anti RSV activity)	Prevention of complications of RSV infection in young infants
Varicella-zoster immune globulin	Prevention of varicella infection in high-risk newborns and Immunocompromised children

(CMV: cytomegalovirus; HBsAg: hepatitis B surface antigen; RSV: respiratory syncytial virus)

BIBLIOGRAPHY

1. Balistreri WF, Murray KF, Rosenthal P, et al. The Safety and Effectiveness of Ledipasvir-Sofosbuvir in Adolescents 12-17 years Old with Hepatitis C virus Genotype 1 infection. Hepatology. 2017;66(2):371-8.
2. Gnann Jr JW. Antiviral therapy of varicella-zoster virus infections. In: Arvin A, Campadelli-Fiume G, Mocarski E, Moore PS, Roizman B, Whitley R, Yamanishi K (Eds). Human Herpesviruses: Biology, Therapy, and Immunoprophylaxis. Cambridge, UK: Cambridge University Press; 2007.
3. Hall CB. Respiratory syncytial virus and parainfluenza virus. N Engl J Med. 2001;344:1917-28.
4. Hammer SM. Antiviral Agents. [online] Available from: http://www.columbia.edu/itc/hs/medical/pathophys/id/2005/MID40-HammerAntiviralsColor.pdf [Accessed December, 2018].
5. Jonas MM, Lok AS, McMahon BJ, et al. Antiviral therapy management of chronic hepatitis B infection in children: a systematic review and meta-analysis. Hepatology. 2016;63(1):307-18.
6. Marshall AC, Koch WC. Antivirals for cytomegalovirus infection in neonates and infants: focus on pharmacokinetics, formulations, dosing and adverse events. Pediatr Drugs. 20009;11(5):309-21.
7. Ministry of Health and Family Welfare. Ministry of Health & Family Welfare Seasonal Influenza A (H1N1) Guidelines on Categorization of Seasonal Influenza A H1N1 Cases During Screening for Home Isolation, Testing, Treatment and Hospitalization. [online] Available from: https://www.mohfw.gov.in/media/disease-alerts/Seasonal-Influenza/technical-guidelines [Accessed December, 2018].
8. Muthuri SG, Venkatesan S, Myles PR, et al. Effectiveness of neuraminidase inhibitors in reducing mortality in patients admitted to hospital with influenza A H1N1pdm09 virus infection: a meta-analysis of individual participant data. Lancet Respir Med. 2014;2:395-404.
9. Stronati M, Lombardi G, Garofoli F, et al. Pharmacokinetics, pharmacodynamics and clinical use of valganciclovir in newborns with symptomatic congenital cytomegalovirus infection. Curr Drug Metab. 2012;14(2):208-15.
10. WHO. WHO Guidelines for Pharmacological Management of Pandemic Influenza A (H1N1) 2009 and other Influenza Viruses. Revised February 2010. Geneva: World Health Organization; 2012.

21.4 Antifungal Therapy

Pooja Dewan, Anjali Tomar

INTRODUCTION

Fungi are nonmotile eukaryotic organisms that include microorganisms such as yeasts and molds. Fungi are characterized by the presence of chitin in their cell walls, which distinguishes them from plants and animals. Fungi are ubiquitous in the environment, being found outdoors in soil and on plants and trees as well as on many indoor surfaces and on human skin. Fungi thrive and proliferate well in warm and moist environment. Fungal infections are also more prevalent in warm, moist areas of the body, like the oral cavity, vaginal, and skin folds. Sweaty clothes and shoes can enhance fungus growth on the skin. Fungi are transmitted from person to person or from objects and surfaces to a person. Also, an individual can transfer fungi to other parts of the body by touching.

RISK FACTORS FOR FUNGAL INFECTIONS

With the widespread use of antibiotics, there has been a steady increase in the incidence of serious secondary fungal infections. Fungi are also dreaded cause of opportunistic infections in immunocompromised hosts [people living with human immunodeficiency virus (PLHIV), acquired and congenital immunodeficiencies], those receiving chemotherapy, those undergoing transplantation, and those receiving immunosuppressive medications. Older individuals are particularly susceptible to fungal infections. Patients with diabetes are also vulnerable to fungal infections.

FUNGAL INFECTIONS IN HUMANS

Millions of species of fungi have been reported. Most of the fungi are pathogenic in plants. About 400 species of fungi are pathogenic in animals and about 50 species are pathogenic in humans. The infections caused by fungi in animals are called "mycoses". Fungi cause a spectrum of diseases in humans ranging from comparatively innocuous superficial skin diseases to invasive life-threatening infections. The type of fungal disease can be classified depending upon the site of infection, route of acquisition of infection, and virulence of fungal infection.

- *Classification based on site*: Superficial, cutaneous, subcutaneous, or systemic (deep)
- *Classification based on route of acquisition*: Endogenous or exogenous. Endogenous infection involves colonization by a commensal specie, or reactivation of a past infection. Exogenous fungi may enter through air or mucocutaneous contact, blood, or gastrointestinal tract
- *Classification based on virulence*: Primary pathogens can establish infections in normal hosts. Opportunistic pathogens cause disease in immunocompromised hosts.

Table 21.4.1 enlists the mycoses encountered in humans with possible fungal etiologic organisms.

CLASSIFICATION OF ANTIFUNGAL DRUGS

With the emergence of invasive fungal illnesses, the market for antifungal drugs has expanded in the recent years. **Table 21.4.2** depicts the antifungal drugs available. However, not all these drugs are approved for use in children and neonates.

SITE OF ACTION OF ANTIFUNGAL DRUGS

Antifungals can be grouped into various classes based on their site of action (***see* Fig. 21.4.1**):

- *Interference with fungal cell membrane function*: Polyenes (alter permeability of cell membranes by binding irreversibly)
- *Interference with fungal cell membrane synthesis*: Azoles (inhibit biosynthesis of ergosterol)
- *Interference with cell wall function*: Caspofungin
- *Interference with nucleic acid synthesis*: 5-fluorocytosine
- *Disruption of microtubular function in cells and inhibiting cell division*: Griseofulvin.

Table 21.4.1: Mycoses encountered in humans.

Type of mycoses	*Disease (etiological agent)*
Superficial	• Black piedra (*Piedraia hortae*) • White piedra (*Trichosporon beigelii*) • Pityriasis versicolor (*Malassezia furfur*) • Tinea nigra (*Phaeoannellomyces werneckii*).
Cutaneous	• *Dermatophytoses: Tinea capitis, T. barbarae, T. corporis, T. cruris, T. unguium, T. pedis* (*Epidermophyton, Microsporum*, and *Trichophyton*) • Dermatomycoses (cutaneous infections due to other genera fungi, the most common of which are *Candida* spp).
Subcutaneous	Chromoblastomycosis (*Fonsecaea pedrosoi, Fonsecaea compacta, Cladosporium carrionii*, and *Phialophora verrucosa*), mycetoma (*Pseudallescheria boydii* and *Nocardia brasiliensis*), and sporotrichosis (*Sporothrix schenckii*)
Systemic (primary infections)	Coccidioidomycosis (*Coccidioides immitis*), Histoplasmosis (*Histoplasma capsulatum*), Blastomycosis (*Blastomyces dermatitidis*), and *Paracoccidioides brasiliensis*.
Systemic (Opportunistic infections)	Cryptococcosis (*Cryptococcus neoformans*), Candidiasis (*Candida* spp.), Aspergillosis (*Aspergillus* spp.), penicilliosis (*Penicillium marneffei*), zygomucormycosis (*Rhizopus spp., Mucor spp.*), trichosporonosis (*Trichosporon beigelii*), and fusariosis (*Fusarium* spp.)

Table 21.4.2: Classes of antifungal drugs.

Polyene macrolides: • Amphotericin B deoxycholate • Amphotericin B lipid complex (ABLC) • Amphotericin B colloidal dispersion (ABCD) • Liposomal amphotericin B (LAMB) • Nystatin
Echinocandins: • Caspofungin • Micafungin • Anidulafungin
Heterocyclic benzofuran: Griseofulvin
Antimetabolites: Flucytosine
Azoles: • *Imidazoles:* – *Topical:* ▪ Clotrimazole ▪ Econazole ▪ Miconazole ▪ Oxiconazole – *Systemic:* ▪ Ketoconazole • *Triazoles* – *Systemic:* ▪ Fluconazole ▪ Itraconazole ▪ Voriconazole ▪ Posaconazole ▪ Isavuconazole
Allylamine: Terbinafine
Other topical agents: • Tolnaftate • Undecylenic acid • Benzoic acid • Ciclopirox olamine • Quiniodochlor

POLYENE ANTIBIOTICS

Polyene antimycotics are derived from *Streptomyces* bacteria. They bind irreversibly to ergosterol in the fungal cell membrane and alter the permeability of the fungal cell membranes leading to metabolic disruption and cell death. Additionally, polyenes act by immune activation leading to oxidation-dependent activation of macrophages.

Amphotericin B

The most important polyene antimycotic is amphotericin B (AMB), a heptaene macrolide containing seven conjugated double bonds in the transposition and 3-amino-3,6-dideoxymannose connected to the main ring by a glycosidic bond. The conventional AMB is AMB deoxycholate and is used by intravenous route. The other preparations of AMB with better safety parameters include AMB lipid complex (ABLC), AMB colloidal dispersion (ABCD), and liposomal AMB (LAMB).

- *Mechanism of action*: Antifungal activity depends upon its binding to a sterol moiety, primarily ergosterol in the membrane of the fungi. This leads to formation of pores in the fungal membrane and increased permeability and leakage of a variety of small molecules.
- *Pharmacology*: The gastrointestinal absorption of AMB is negligible. Pharmacokinetics of AMB differs according to the formulation. LAMB has the highest plasma concentration at therapeutic doses. Conventional AMB is released from its complex with deoxycholate in the blood stream. AMB that remains in the plasma gets bound to B lipoprotein. Concentration of AMB in the fluids from inflamed pleura, peritoneum, synovium, and aqueous humor is approximately two-thirds of the trough concentration in plasma. Penetration into cerebrospinal fluid (CSF), vitreous humor, and normal amniotic fluid is poor. About 60% of AMB gets metabolized in liver. Excretion occurs in urine and bile.

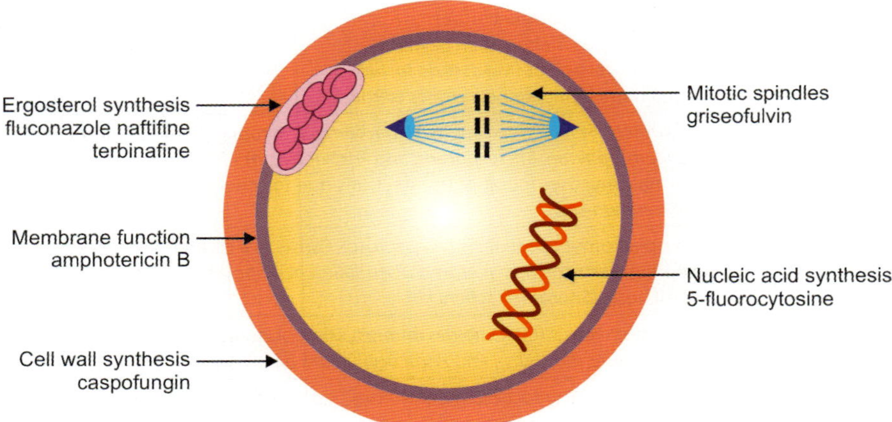

Fig. 21.4.1: Site and mechanism of action of common antifungal drugs.

- *Antifungal spectrum*: AMB is a broad-spectrum antifungal active against most invasive fungal infections as well as leishmaniasis and *Naegleria*. It is effective against *Candida spp., Cryptococcus neoformans, Blastomyces dermatitidis, Histoplasma capsulatum, Sporothrix schenckii, Aspergillus spp., Penicillium marneffei, Paracoccidioides brasiliensis, Coccidioides spp., Rhizopus spp.,* and *Mucor spp.* AMB is useful for treating children with febrile neutropenia who do not improve with antibacterial therapy and have an underlying risk for invasive fungal infections. AMB is currently the drug of choice for the treatment of systemic infections caused by *Aspergillus* and *Candida* spp.
- *Dosage and side effects:* **Table 21.4.3** shows the recommended dosages for AMB in children and common side effects.
- *Indications in Children*: Amphotericin B is useful in invasive fungal infections like candidiasis and cryptococcal meningitis. It is also recommended in mucormycosis and refractory invasive aspergillosis. See **Table 21.4.3**, AMB can attain good CSF concentration in neonates due to immature blood-brain barrier. Neonates can tolerate AMB better than older children. For cryptococcal meningitis, AMB is given with flucytosine. The duration of therapy is 10–12 weeks after CSF cultures are clear.

AZOLES

Azoles act by inhibiting the cytochrome P-450-dependent lanosterol 14-α-demethylase (CYP51), which inhibits lanosterol synthesis. This leads to increased cell membrane permeability, impairs membrane-associated oxidative enzymes, and leads to intracellular phospholipid accumulation and cell death. Since azoles act by inhibiting cytochrome P-450-dependent enzymes are metabolized by cytochrome P-450

Table 21.4.3: Therapeutic doses and side effects of common antimycotic drugs.

Antifungal drug	*Route of administration*	*Dose in neonates*	*Dose in infants*	*Dose in older children*	*Side effects*	*Indications*
Amphotericin B deoxycholate	Intravenous	0.5–1 mg/kg/day IV infusion q 24 h; dose in preterm is 0.5 mg/kg/day and in term neonates is 1 mg/kg/day	0.7–1 mg/kg/day IV infusion q 24 h	0.7–1 mg/kg/day IV infusion q 24 h	Anorexia, chills, diarrhea, fever, headache, hypokalemia, hypomagnesemia, hypotension, malaise, pain at injection site, azotemia, renal function abnormalities, vomiting, agranulocytosis, and bone marrow suppression *Renal dose adjustment*: *CrCl <10 mL/min*: 0.5–0.7 mg/kg IV q24–48 h	Invasive aspergillosis, cryptococcal meningitis
ABLC	Intravenous	2.5–5 mg/kg/day q24 h	–	5 mg/kg/day q24 h	Less infusion related toxicity and lesser nephrotoxicity than AMB deoxycholate; rest of side effect profile is similar as AMB deoxycholate	Invasive aspergillosis, cryptococcal meningitis
ABCD	Intravenous	–	3–4 mg/kg/day q24h	3–4 mg/kg/day q24h	Less infusion related toxicity and lesser nephrotoxicity than AMB deoxycholate; rest of side effect profile is similar as AMB deoxycholate	Invasive aspergillosis, cryptococcal meningitis

Contd...

Contd…

Antifungal drug	***Route of administration***	***Dose in neonates***	***Dose in infants***	***Dose in older children***	***Side effects***	***Indications***
LAMB	Intravenous	3–5 mg/kg/day q24h	3–5 mg/kg/ day q24h	3–5 mg/kg/ day q24h	Less infusion-related toxicity and lesser nephrotoxicity than AMB deoxycholate; rest of side effect profile is similar as AMB deoxycholate	Invasive aspergillosis, cryptococcal meningitis
Fluconazole	Intravenous, oral	25 mg/kg loading dose; 12 mg/ kg/day q24h maintenance dose	12 mg/kg/day q24h	6–12 mg/kg/ day q24h	Vomiting, diarrhea, transaminitis, stomach ache, chills, and tachycardia	Candidiasis, blastomycosis, coccidiodomycosis, cryptococcosis, histoplasmosis, dermatophytosis, and pityriasis versicolor
Itraconazole	Oral; should be taken with food	–	–	5–10 mg/kg/ day q12h	Nausea, vomiting, constipation, headache, dizziness, abnormal liver function tests, swelling, and weight gain	Trichophyton and *Microsporum tinea capitis* infections, Onychomycosis
Posaconazole	Intravenous, oral; should be taken 1 h before meals	–	–	200–400 mg/ dose q6–12h	Fatigue, dry mouth, nausea, diarrhea, vomiting, and hypokalemia	Oral thrush, candidemia, invasive aspergillosis, prophylaxis of invasive aspergillus and *Candida* infections in high-risk, severely immunocompromised patients
Voriconazole	Intravenous, oral; should be taken 20 min after a meal	4–6 mg/kg q 12h loading dose, 2–3 mg/kg q12h maintenance dose	4–6 mg/kg q12h loading dose, 2–3 mg/kg q12h maintenance dose	7–9 mg/kg q12h loading dose, 5–6 mg/kg q12h maintenance dose	Blurred vision, nausea, vomiting, hepatotoxicity, cardiac arrhythmias, swelling in hands and feet, and photosensitivity	Esophageal candidiasis, invasive aspergillosis, Candidemia, Scedosporiosis and Fusariosis
Ketoconazole	Intravenous, oral, and topical	–	–	3–6 mg/kg/ day	Nausea, vomiting, stomach pain, diarrhea, dizziness, photosensitivity, and QT prolongation on ECG	Blastomycosis, coccidioidomycosis, histoplasmosis, chromomycosis, and paracoccidioidomycosis; not useful for onychomycois
Caspofungin	Intravenous	25 mg/m^2/ day (safety not established)	50 mg/m^2/ day	70 mg/m^2/ day loading dose; 50 mg/m^2/day maintenance dose	Fever, anaphylaxis, hepatotoxic, diarrhea, vomiting, shivering, rash, and hypokalemia	Candidemia, invasive aspergillosis, empirical therapy for presumed fungal infections in febrile, neutropenic patients
Micafungin	Intravenous	–	2–4 mg/kg/ day	2–4 mg/ kg/day (*Prophylaxis*: 1 mg/kg/day)	Hepatotoxic, stomach ache, nausea, vomiting, weight gain, flushing, and rash	Candidemia, invasive aspergillosis, empirical therapy for presumed fungal infections in febrile, neutropenic patients, Prophylaxis of *Candida* Infections in HSCT Recipients

Contd…

Contd...

Antifungal drug	***Route of administration***	***Dose in neonates***	***Dose in infants***	***Dose in older children***	***Side effects***	***Indications***
Anidulafungin	Intravenous	1.5 mg/kg/day	1.5–3 mg/kg/day	1.5–3 mg/kg/day loading dose; 0.75–1.5 mg/kg/day maintenance dose	Flushing, diarrhea, nausea, vomiting, headache, and constipation	Candidemia, esophageal candidiasis
Flucytosine (5-fluorocytosine (5-FC)	Oral and intravenous	80–160 mg/kg/day q6h PO	50–150 mg/kg/day q6h PO	50–150 mg/kg/day q6h PO	Confusion, headache, dizziness, phototoxicity, sedation, psychosis, bone marrow suppression, nausea, and vomiting	Serious *Candida* infections and cryptococcosis
Griseofulvin	Oral; should be given with milk, eggs, and fatty foods	–	–	*Microsized*: 10–20 mg/kg/day q12–24h *Ultra-microsized*: 10–15 mg/kg/day q12–24h	Headache, nausea, vomiting, diarrhea, photosensitivity, peripheral neuritis, lethargy, mental confusion, and leucopenia	Dermatophytosis, Athlete's foot, ringworm
Terbinafine	Oral and topical	–	–	*≥4 years:* • *<25 kg*: 125 mg/day • *25–35 kg*: 187.5 mg/day • *>35 kg*: 250 mg/day	Gastrointestinal distress, headache, hepatotoxicity, severe neutropenia, and Stevens-Johnson syndrome	Dermatophytosis, Onychomycosis, Pityriasis versicolor, mucosal and cutaneous candidiasis

(ABCD: amphotericin B colloidal dispersion; ABLC: amphotericin B lipid complex; AMB: amphotericin B, LAMB: liposomal amphotericin B)

isoenzymes, several drugs, which either induce or interact with these cytochrome-dependent enzymes interact with azoles. Astemizole, cisapride, pimozide, quinidine, halofantrine, terfenadine, and ergot alkaloids are contraindicated with azoles as they can lead to azole toxicity. Rifabutin, phenytoin, omeprazole, benzodiazepines, nevirapine, and efavirenz need to monitor as coadministration with azoles can lead to therapeutic failure. Compared to polyenes, azoles take much longer time to begin action. Several fungal are resistant to azoles inherently such as *Candida krusei* is resistant to fluconazole and itraconazole.

Fluconazole

Fluconazole is a first-generation triazole antifungal drug used for treating candidiasis, blastomycosis, coccidioidomycosis, cryptococcosis, histoplasmosis, dermatophytosis, and pityriasis versicolor. Fluconazole is particularly active against *Candida albicans* and *C. neoformans*. It is also used to prevent candidiasis in those who are at high risk such as following organ transplantation, low birth weight babies, and those with neutropenia. Fluconazole is, however, ineffective against *C. krusei* and *Candida glabrata*.

- *Pharmacokinetics*: Fluconazole is almost completely absorbed within 2 hour following oral intake unaffected by gastric acids. It follows zero order kinetics. Only 10% of elimination is due to metabolism, the rest of the drug is excreted in urine and sweat.
- *Dosage and side effects:* **Table 21.4.3** shows the recommended dose for fluconazole and the expected side effects with its use.

Itraconazole

Itraconazole is a triazole antifungal drug most active against *Aspergillus* spp. and has greater activity than fluconazole against resistant strains of *Candida spp.* other than *C. albicans.* The safety of itraconazole in children less than 18 years and neonates has not been established. Yet, itraconazole is recommended for use in children (not neonates) as salvage or compassionate therapy. Children with cystic fibrosis and allogeneic bone marrow transplant are given itraconazole 5 mg/kg twice daily for prophylaxis against fungal infections. Gastric acid affects the absorption, and hence therapeutic drug monitoring is recommended with a target trough level of 0.5 µg/mL.

Posaconazole

It is a triazole antifungal drug especially active against *Mucor*. Its antifungal spectrum includes *Candida spp.*, *Aspergillus spp.*, and *Zygomycetes spp.* Oral administration of posaconazole taken with a high-fat meal increases it bioavailability. The safety and efficacy in children less than 13 years need to be established.

Voriconazole

It is a triazole antifungal with a structure related to that of fluconazole and a spectrum of activity comparable to that of itraconazole. It is effective in treatment of invasive aspergillosis and refractory infections of *Scedosporium apiospermum* and *Fusarium spp.* and empirical therapy in febrile neutropenic patients.

- *Pharmacokinetics*: Voriconazole metabolism follows saturable kinetics. Therefore, increased dosage of voriconazole a disproportionate increase is seen in its drug levels. A variable elimination half-life (from 6 hours to 24 hours) is seen depending on the dosage of voriconazole given. It is well absorbed. However, fatty meal decreases its absorption. Voriconazole is extensively metabolized in the liver.
- *Antifungal spectrum*: Voriconazole has fungicidal action against the various *Aspergillus* spp. most active especially against *Aspergillus fumigatus*. It is fungistatic against all *Candida* spp. Voriconazole exhibits better potency than fluconazole or itraconazole for most *Candida* isolates studied. Since it can be given orally, it is emerging as a popular choice for empirical antifungal therapy in febrile neutropenic patients when compared to AMB, which must be administered intravenously.
- *Adverse effects*: Common side effects include visual disturbances, fever, rash, hepatic abnormalities, nausea, vomiting, abdominal pain, and headache.

ECHINOCANDINS

This newer category of antifungal drugs acts by inhibiting the synthesis of glucan in the cell wall. Caspofungin, micafungin, and anidulafungin are semisynthetic echinocandin derivatives with clinical implications.

- *Antifungal spectrum:* Echinocandins are fungicidal against most species of *Candida* (including strains that are fluconazole resistant), but not against *Cryptococcus, Trichosporon*, and *Rhodotorula*. They display synergistic activity with AMB and additive activity with fluconazole against *Candida spp.* Echinocandins are fungistatic against *Aspergillus* and are also partly active against dimorphic fungi (*Blastomyces* and *Histoplasma*). These have some activity against the spores of the fungus *Pneumocystis jirovecii*, formerly known as *Pneumocystis carinii*. Caspofungin is used in the treatment of febrile neutropenia and as salvage therapy for the treatment of invasive aspergillosis. Micafungin is used as prophylaxis against *Candida* infections in hematopoietic stem cell transplantation patients.
- *Pharmacokinetics:* Due to the large molecular weight, echinocandins have poor oral bioavailability and are administered by intravenous infusion. In the plasma, they are 97% bound to albumin. They are metabolized slowly by N-acetylation as well as spontaneous degradation and have a longer half-life in plasma. Due to the larger size, echinocandins are also poorly concentrated in CSF, eyes, and urine.
- *Dosage and side effects*: **Table 21.4.3** shows the common side effects and doses for echinocandins.

HETEROCYCLIC BENZOFURAN

Griseofulvin

Griseofulvin is an antifungal agent derived from mold *Penicillium griseofulvum* that is used to treat fungal infection of skin and nails.

- *Mechanism of action:* It causes disruption of the mitotic spindle by interacting with polymerized microtubules. Multinucleated and stunted fungal hyphae result from its action. The effect of the drug is like that of colchicine and vinca alkaloids but its binding sites on the microtubular protein are distinct.
- *Pharmacology:* Griseofulvin has very low water solubility, which leads to its irregular absorption from the gastrointestinal tract. To improve its bioavailability, microsized, and ultramicrosized preparations are available. It gets deposited in keratin precursor cells of skin, hair, and nails; it gets concentrated and persists in tinea infected cells and due to its fungistatic activity, the newly formed keratin is not invaded by the fungus. As the fungus-containing keratin is shed, it is replaced by normal tissue. Griseofulvin is metabolized by methylation and excreted in urine. Its plasma half-life is about 1 day, but it persists for weeks in skin and keratin.
- *Antifungal spectrum:* It is active against most dermatophytes including *Epidermophyton, Trichophyton,*

Microsporum, etc. but not against *Candida* and other fungi-causing deep mycosis.

- *Dose and side effects:* **Table 21.4.3** shows the recommended dosages in children and the common side effects.
- *Indications in children:* It is mainly used to treat ringworm (*Tinea*) infections. In adolescents and young adults, it is also used to treat athlete's Foot (epidermophytosis involving the skin and nails of the foot).

ALLYLAMINES

Terbinafine

Terbinafine is a synthetic allylamine and is a fungistatic agent. It is structurally similar to the topical agent naftifine.

- *Mechanism of action:* It is a noncompetitive inhibitor of squalene epoxidase, which is an early step enzyme in ergosterol biosynthesis by fungi. Accumulation of squalene within the fungal cells is responsible for its action.
- *Pharmacology:* Terbinafine is well absorbed but bioavailability is decreased to about 40% because of first pass metabolism in the liver. It is lipophilic, strongly plasma-protein bound and concentrated in sebum, stratum corneum, and nail plates. It is excreted in urine (80%) and feces (20%).
- *Antifungal spectrum:* It is used to treat dermatophytosis and onychomycosis and activity is also seen against *Candida* species and *Malassezia furfur*.
- *Dose and side effects:* **Table 21.4.3** shows the recommended dosages in children and the common side effects.
- *Indications in children:* It is mainly used to treat *Tinea cruris, T. corporis, T. capitis* and *T. pedis*, pityriasis versicolor, and onychomycosis. It is less effective against cutaneous and mucosal candidiasis.

FEW IMPORTANT TOPICAL ANTIFUNGALS

Ketoconazole

It is a broad-spectrum antifungal drug, useful in both dermatophytosis and deep mycosis. It is effective in blastomycosis, histoplasmosis, coccidioidomycosis, paracoccidioidomycosis, ringworm, tinea versicolor, chronic mucocutaneous candidiasis, etc.

Clotrimazole

It is effective in topical treatment of tinea infections such as ringworm, athlete's foot, otomycosis, oral, cutaneous, and vaginal candidiasis. It is particularly favored for vaginitis because of long-lasting residual effect after once daily application. It is well-tolerated by most patients, but local irritation and stinging and burning sensation occur in some patients.

Miconazole

It is used for tinea, pityriasis versicolor, otomycosis, cutaneous, and vulvovaginal candidiasis. It is highly efficacious. Adverse effects from topical application to vagina include burning, itching, irritation and infrequently pelvic cramps headache, and hives.

BIBLIOGRAPHY

1. Bennett JE. Antifungal agents. In: Brunton LL, Hilal-Dandan R (Eds). Goodman and Gilman's Manual of Pharmacology and Therapeutics, 13th edition. New York, NY: McGraw-Hill; 2013.
2. Ghannoum MA, Rice LB. Antifungal agents: mode of action, mechanisms of resistance, and correlation of these mechanisms with bacterial resistance. Clin Microbiol Rev. 1999;12(4):501-17.
3. Greer ND. Voriconazole: the newest triazole antifungal agent. Proc (Bayl Univ Med Cent). 2003;16(2):241-8.
4. Hardman JG, Limbird LE, Gilman AG. Goodman & Gilman's The Pharmacological Basis of Therapeutics. 12th edition. New York: McGraw-Hill; 2011.
5. Katzung BG. Basic and Clinical Pharmacology. 11th edition. New York: McGraw-Hill; 2015.
6. Rang HP, Ritter JM, Flower RJ, Henderson G. Rang and Dale's Pharmacology, 8th edition. London: Elsevier; 2015.
7. Ribes JA, Vanover-Sams CL, Baker DJ. Zygomycetes in Human Disease. Clinical Microbiology Reviews. 2000;13(2): 236-301.
8. Tripathi KD. Essentials of Medical Pharmacology, 7th edition. Delhi: Jaypee Brothers Medical Publishers; 2013.
9. Walsh TJ, Dixon DM. Spectrum of Mycoses. In: Baron S (Ed). Medical Microbiology, 4th Edition. Galveston, Texas; University of Texas Medical Branch at Galveston, Department of Microbiology and Immunology; 1996.

21.5 Rational Drug Therapy

Arun Phatak

INTRODUCTION

The word "rational" means something sensible, based on reasoning. After about 8 years of experience in the field of clinical medicine, the practicing pediatrician is expected to base the case management on accepted scientific principles and practice guidelines. A pediatrician largely depends on the use of drugs for treating the patients and should use them judiciously. Previous chapters have discussed how the drug therapy of children differs from that of adults.

Unfortunately, irrational use of drugs is not uncommon, and it is observed at all levels. Irrationality in drug therapy is observed mainly in four areas:

1. Drugs not indicated
2. Improper choice
3. Inappropriate use
4. Inadequate patient counseling

UNNECESSARY DRUGS

This is the most commonly occurring irrationality. The so-called "tonics", cough mixtures, and antibiotics are the most misused drugs. Very few drug combinations are rational. When preparations of drug combinations are used, the child often receives some unnecessary drugs. Combinations of paracetamol-ibuprofen or paracetamol-antihistamine-decongestant are often prescribed. As far as possible, preparations containing only one drug should be prescribed and when the proprietary preparation contains multiple drugs, the ingredients and their individual amounts should be checked. Most of the combination drugs are irrational with faulty proportion of doses.

WRONG CHOICE OF DRUGS

This is most frequent while prescribing antibiotics. One must have the basic idea of pathogens responsible for that infection and their likely sensitivities before selecting an antibiotic. The drug should not only be effective but also should be affordable and acceptable. When two or more drugs are likely to be equally effective, one that is well known to us, cheap, and can be orally administered would be preferable. Even when injections are needed in the acute state, a drug that can be given parenterally as well as orally would be preferable—as the child stabilizes one can switch over to oral administration. Often the latest arrival in the market is prescribed without knowing its short-term and long-term adverse effects. A known, familiar drug is preferable to an unknown drug.

INAPPROPRIATE DOSE AND ROUTE

In children, the dose of the drugs is calculated by weight or surface area and the dose may be different for neonates, infants, and older children. The doses for parenteral and for oral administration may be different. Also, the doses of certain drugs need readjustment, if there is renal or hepatic impairment. A high dose given inadvertently can be catastrophic. It is better to check the dose from the formulary if one is not sure. After calculating the dose required, it must be translated to the nearest measurable volume or number of tablets according to the strength of the available product—some products are available in varying strengths. For instance, paracetamol and amoxicillin are available as 125 mg or 250 mg per 5 mL of syrups. Paracetamol drops may contain 50 mg/mL, 100 mg/mL, or 125 mg/mL. It is, therefore, necessary to make sure that the patient gets what was intended. The recommended frequency of dosing should be followed so that optimal blood levels are maintained.

One should switch over from parenteral to oral route, if possible, as the child stabilizes. This reduces not only the duration of hospital stay and the visits to outpatients but also reduces the complications of injections. In case of antibiotics, if the one being used cannot be administered orally, another belonging to the same or different group that is effective can be given—guided by the culture report (or the probable-likely-infective organism).

INAPPROPRIATE PRESCRIPTION WRITING AND COUNSELING

The prescription should be written in the standard format **(Box 21.5.1)**. Several pediatricians in big cities have started giving computerized prescriptions but the majority still writes them by hand and legibility is very important. Doctor's handwriting is notorious for its illegibility and there is nothing to be proud of it. Writing the prescription legibly does not require lot of effort. Many drugs have similar syntax and

Box 21.5.1: Standard format for prescriptions.

- Doctor's name, qualification, address, and registration number
- Patient's name, age, sex, weight, and date
- Names of the drugs (if necessary with the pharmaceutical name) with the recommended strengths, forms, and amount to be bought
- Clear instructions about the dose, frequency, and duration of medication, preferably in a language understood by the parents
- Explanation (at least verbally) of the common side effects and their significance (black stools after iron therapy, "red" urine after rifampicin).

pronunciations and serious mistakes have occurred because a wrong medicine was dispensed by the chemist who could not read the prescription correctly. Indeed, in January 2014, The Executive Committee of the Medical Council of India approved a draft resolution that doctors should use capital letters while writing prescriptions.

Counseling the parents about administrations of the different medicines is another very important aspect of prescribing drugs. Many doctors indicate symbolically how the different drugs are to be taken and it can be quite confusing. It is better to write the instructions in the language understood by the parents. Many of the patients are illiterate and need to be explained and demonstrated how dry syrups are to be prepared, and how the various quantities of the different drugs are to be measured.

A rare type of irrationality occurs, when a drug that was necessary is not used either due to oversight or due to ignorance.

REASONS FOR IRRATIONAL BEHAVIOR

Ignorance

Medicine is a continuously expanding and improving science and its practitioner must commit to continuous updating and life-long learning. Every year new drugs are introduced in the market. One must know the basic pharmacology of the drug (and not go by what the medical representative said) before using the drug. Prescribing information (product insert) provided with the proprietary medicine may be useful, especially as guidance for the administration of the new drug.

Lack of Conviction

The pediatrician starting his private practice fears that "what is preached cannot be practiced". Although the circumstances, work conditions, and the patient profile in the medical college hospital are different from those encountered in private practice, in both circumstances, the pharmacology of the drugs is the same.

Inappropriate Peer Model

Many times, a young doctor fresh in practice looks at the senior "established" peers as role models and tries to imitate their prescribing behavior without scrutinizing the rationality. In scientific matters, it is not the person but the scientific facts that are important.

Undue Pressures

The young pediatrician is anxious to establish oneself. He feels that curing the patient quickly will increase his clientele and tries to treat every possible cause of the illness simultaneously (polytherapy). Many patients demand medicines even when they are not necessary (e.g. antibiotics when the child has diarrhea, viral upper respiratory infection or tonics and vitamins for "debility"). Some demand injections or intravenous drips under the impression that they bring quick cure. A doctor should not succumb to such demands but spend some time in counseling the parents about the nature of the disease and its management.

Life Goals and Ambitions

The practice of medicine is a profession and not a business. Our main objective, while earning a decent and comfortable life, must always be the total care of the patient. The pharmaceutical industry is a big business with an objective of earning as great a profit as possible. Some of them give rich gifts and other enticements to doctors and lure them into writing their products. In the interest of the child and his family, the pediatrician must be vigilant and avoid the trap.

EVIDENCE-BASED CLINICAL PRACTICE

Till a few decades ago, patients equated doctors to God and accepted whatever that was advised without any question. The doctor had clinical freedom and the treatment was often guided by one's experience. Now, the time has changed. Clinical freedom is considered as "at best a cloak for ignorance and at worst an excuse for quackery". A doctor is accountable and should be able to justify the management. The clinical practice must be evidence based.

The evidence comes from published and unpublished research papers and reports. One cannot take everything published in print and on electronic media as gospel truth. There are evidences and evidences. Some are of high quality and reliable, others are of low quality and unreliable. A simple hierarchy for the quality of the evidence may be put down by the type of the paper as:

- Meta-analysis or systematic reviews of randomized clinical trials (RCTs)
- Randomized clinical trials

- Other controlled clinical trials
- Observational studies (cohort and case control)
- Case studies, anecdotal and personal opinion

Apart from its type, the paper needs to be scrutinized for its methodology and validity of the results.

Most of the professional bodies issue guidelines/recommendations for the management of common diseases and disorders. They are usually based on high-quality evidence. When high-quality evidence is not available, the guidelines represent the consensus opinion of the experts in the field. As a rule, these guidelines should be followed in clinical practice. However, under some circumstances, it may not be possible to follow the guidelines or recommendations. The necessary medicines or equipment or skills may not be available locally or the recommended drugs or management may be unacceptable or unaffordable to the patient. One then must try to do the best with what is available and possible.

It is said that "half of what we have learned today will in 10 years be shown to be wrong—and no one knows which half". So, the practicing doctor must commit to continuous updating and life-long learning.

THE ROAD TO LIFE-LONG LEARNING

Books give the basic information about drugs and therapy, but the information is likely to be 5–10 years old. Yet it is better to possess the latest edition of the standard textbook as a ready reference to start off.

Papers published in journals (especially the online issues) give more recent information, but the original papers need critical appraisal. There is an explosive increase in the medical information over the last few decades. The National Library in the United States of America accesses some 11 million papers every year from about 4,300 journals, of which only 10–15% are of lasting value. Searching and appraising papers is a time-consuming and laborious work that is out of bounds for the busy clinician.

Systematic reviews and practice guidelines can be accessed on various websites **(Box 21.5.2)**. The official journals of professional bodies also publish updated practice guidelines and recommendations and these are available on their websites as well.

Box 21.5.2: Some useful websites.

- *www.cochrane.org*
- *www.evidence.nhs.uk*
- *www.clinicalevidence.com*
- *www.nice.org.uk*
- *www.sign.ac.uk*
- *www.tripdatabase.com*

TIPS FOR RATIONALIZING THE CLINICAL PRACTICE

- Make a list of common diseases and disorders that are seen in your practice.
- Read through the guidelines and textbooks and select the essential drugs that you want to use.
- Know the basic pharmacology of the selected drugs.
- Consider the availability and cost of the various proprietary preparations.
- Keep a basic record of the age group, gender, disease/disorder, and the drugs used and at the end of the year audit your own prescription behavior.
- If you have deviated from the current standard recommendations, consider the reasons and correct yourself, if the deviation was not justifiable.

BIBLIOGRAPHY

1. Feldman W (Ed). Evidence-based Pediatrics. Indian Reprint. Bengaluru: Panther Publishers Private Limited; 2001.
2. Greenhalgh T. How to Read a Paper: The Basics of Evidence-Based Medicine, 3rd edition. London: Oxford Blackwell Publishing Ltd; 2006.
3. Strauss SE, Richardson WS, Glasziou P, et al. In: How to Read a Paper: The Basics of Evidence-Based Medicine, 3rd edition. Edinburgh: Elsevier Churchill Livingstone; 2005.
4. World Health Organization. (1990). The Use of Essential Drugs. WHO Technical Report Series 796. [online] Available from: http://apps.who.int/iris/bitstream/10665/39338/1/WHO_TRS_796.pdf. [Accessed November, 2015].

21.6 Drugs Licensed for Use in Neonates, Children, and Adolescents

Jeeson C Unni, PSN Menon

A

Abacavir: *Dosage:*
Human immunodeficiency virus (HIV) infection in combination with at least two other antiretroviral medicines, by mouth, adolescent: 300 mg twice daily; 3 months–16 years, 8 mg/kg twice daily (maximum, 600 mg daily). For adolescents, the initiation of antiretroviral therapy is recommended in any patient: with a history of an AIDS-defining infection; with a CD4 less than 350/mm^3; who has HIV-associated nephropathy; or who is being treated for hepatitis B (HBV) infection. For children, the initiation of antiretroviral therapy is recommended in any symptomatic patient.

For asymptomatic or mildly symptomatic children ≥5 years: The initiation of antiretroviral therapy is recommended for patients with HIV-RNA more than or equal to 100,000 copies/mL and CD4 less than 350/mm^3. 1–5 years, the initiation of antiretroviral therapy is recommended for patients with HIV-RNA more than or equal to 100,000 copies/mL and CD4 <25%.

For infants, the initiation of antiretroviral therapy is recommended in any infant regardless of clinical status, CD4 percentage, or viral load.

Abciximab: *Dosage:*
Kawasaki disease: 0.25 mg/kg intravenous bolus, followed by 0.125 µg/kg/min infusion for 12 hours. Platelet counts and coagulation time must be monitored. Preferably used by specialist experienced in its use.

Acetazolamide: *Dosage:*
Epilepsy: As adjunct—starting dose up to 12 years, 2.5 mg/kg and 12–18 years, 250 mg 2–3 times daily and increase every 4–5 days to maintenance dose of 5–7 mg/kg/dose 2–3 times daily up to 750 mg/day in <12 years old and 1 g/day in 12–18 years old. The intravenous (IV) bolus dose is 6–7 mg/kg 2–3 times daily in <12 years and 250 mg 2–4 times in 12–18 years.

Edema: Oral or IV starting dose—up to 12 years, 2.5 mg/kg and 12–18 years, 250 mg 2–3 times daily.

Raised intracranial pressure: Oral/IV—8 mg/kg thrice daily and gradually increased.

Hydrocephalus: Due to communicating *intraventricular hemorrhage* (IVH)—neonates 25 mg/kg/24 hour.

Glaucoma: Oral/IV—5 mg/kg in <12 years and 250 mg in 12–18 years 2–4 times daily to a maximum of 750 mg/day in <12 years and 1 g/day in 12–18 years. If creatinine clearance is 10–20 mL/min/1.73 m^2, reduce to twice daily and if <10 years avoid.

Acetylcysteine: *Dosage:*
Paracetamol poisoning: Initial IV infusion over 15 minutes (<12 years, 150 mg/kg in 100 mL; 12–18 years, 150 mg/kg in 200 mL) followed by IV infusion over 4 hours (<12 years, 50 mg/kg in 250 mL; 12–18 years, 50 mg/kg in 500 mL) and then IV infusion over 16 hours (<12 years, 100 mg/kg in 500 mL; 12–18 years, 100 mg/kg in 1,000 mL).

Meconium ileus: 20% injection given orally diluted 1:4 at 1–2 mL in newborn.

Mucolytic: As 10% solution for inhalation—infants 2–4 mL 3–4 times, children 6–10 mL 3–4 times, and adolescents 10 mL 3–4 times.

Acitretin: *Dosage:* Maximum duration of continuous treatment is 6 months. Given orally in 12–18 years old at 500 µg as single dose daily. Occasionally up to 1 mg/kg needed (maximum 35 mg daily for short periods).

Activated Charcoal: *Dosage:* Dose related more to dose of poison (10 times weight of poison is given) than age/weight of child. If amount of toxin unknown, either give as single dose within 1 hour of ingestion of poison or as multiple doses 4th hourly till toxicity abates or side effects of charcoal become evident—by weight 1 g/kg or by age 25–50 g in 2–12 years old.

Acyclovir: *Dosage:*
Herpes simplex: Oral 1 month–2 years, 100 mg; 2–18 years, 200 mg 5 times daily for 5–7 days start within 72 hours of onset for best results. IV infusion—neonate of 3 months, 20 mg/kg 8 hourly for 14 days; 3 months–12 years, 250 mg/m^2 8 hourly for 5 days. Double the dose, if immunocompromised or when treating herpes encephalitis.

Encephalitis: Give IV for 21 days; confirm cerebrospinal fluid (CSF) is negative for *Herpes simplex virus* (HSV) before stopping. To avoid excessive dose in obese—IV dose calculated on the basis of ideal weight for height. Treatment of initial infection—reduces severity and duration but no effect on frequency of subsequent recurrent infections. Adolescent, 400 mg tid; child, 10–20 mg/kg/dose qid × 7–10 days.

Episodic therapy for recurrent genital herpes: Adolescent, 800 mg tid × 2 days. Herpes simplex prophylaxis in the immunocompromised—oral 1 month–2 years, 100–200 mg 4 times daily; 2–18 years, 200–400 mg 4 times daily.

Herpes simplex suppression: Oral—12–18 years, 400 mg twice daily or 200 mg 4 times daily. Increased to 400 mg thrice daily, if recurrences occur on standard suppressive therapy or for suppression of genital herpes during late pregnancy (from 36 weeks gestation). Therapy interrupted every 6–12 months to reassess recurrence frequency—consider restarting after two or more recurrences.

Local treatment of Herpes simplex infections: Eye—apply 1 cm ointment 5 times daily (continue for at least 3 days after complete healing). Skin—apply to lesions every 4 hours (5 times daily) for 5–10 days, starting at first sign of attack.

Chickenpox and Herpes zoster: Neonates—regardless of immune status/use of any immunoglobulins, give IV (risk of severe disease). Oral not recommended as absorption is variable. Healthy child, 1 month–12 years—no treatment. Adolescent—treat within 24 hours. Immunocompromised and those at special risk (severe CVS/respiratory disease/chronic skin disorder)—10 days with at least 7 days of parenteral treatment.

Prophylactic acyclovir should be considered for neonates whose mothers develop chickenpox 4 days before to 2 days after delivery. Oral—1 month–2 years, 200 mg; 2–6 years, 400 mg; 6–12 years, 800 mg 4 times daily for 5 days; 12–18 years, 800 mg 5 times daily for 7 days.

Herpes zoster in the immunocompromised: Continue for 2 days after crusting of lesions. IV infusion—neonate 3 months, 10–20 mg/kg 8th hourly for at least 7 days; 3 months–12 years, 250 mg/m^2; 12–18 years, 5 mg/kg 8th hourly for 5 days. At all ages—double dose in encephalitis or immunocompromised (given for 10–14 days in encephalitis, possibly longer if also immunocompromised). To avoid excessive dose in obese—IV dose calculated on the basis of ideal weight for height.

Prophylaxis of chickenpox after delivery: IV infusion–Neonate 10 mg/kg 8 hourly; continued until serological tests confirm absence of virus. Attenuation of chickenpox, if varicella zoster (VZ) immunoglobulin not indicated—oral, 1 month–18 years, 10 mg/kg 4 times daily for 7 days starting 1 week after exposure.

Adalimumab: *Dosage:* With methotrexate or alone if methotrexate inappropriate: Subcutaneously, child 13–17 years, 40 mg alternate week; review treatment if no response in 12 weeks.

Adapalene: *Dosage*:
Topical: Wash and dry affected area and apply a thin film before bedtime. Assess for improvement after 3 months treatment.

Adenosine: *Dosage:* Up to 12 years, 0.05 mg/kg IV push and then increase bolus doses by 0.05 mg/kg every 2 minutes till clinical response occurs or a maximum dose of either 0.3 mg/kg or 12 mg. And 12–18 years, 3 mg IV bolus, increase after 2 minutes to 6 mg and to 12 mg, if supraventricular tachycardia (SVT) not controlled after another 2 minutes.

Adrenaline (Epinephrine): *Dosage:*
Cardiac arrest or profound bradycardia, asystole, ventricular fibrillation, or pulseless electrical activity—IV: 10 μg/kg (0.01 mg/kg). *Initial Dose*: Intraosseous: 10 μg/kg (0.01 mg/kg); *endotracheal*: 100 μg/kg (0.10 mg/kg)–10 μg/kg = 0.01 mL/kg of 1:10,000 dilution.

Note: 100 μg/kg = 0.1 mL/kg of 1:1,000 dilution. If administered through an endotracheal tube, follow the dose with saline flush or dilute in isotonic saline flush (1–5 mL) based on patient's weight.

Note: Subsequent doses—given every 3–5 minutes—IV: 100 μg/kg (0.1 mg/kg); *intraosseous*: 100 μg/kg (0.1 mg/kg); *endotracheal*: 100 μg/kg (0.1 mg/kg).

Note: For subsequent doses of epinephrine, a dosage up to 200 μg/kg (0.2 mg/kg) may be given.

Anaphylaxis—subcutaneous (SC): 10 μg/kg per dose (maximum 3 doses); IV: 10 μg/kg per dose: 10 μg/kg = 0.01 mL/kg of 1:1,000 dilution or 0.1 mL/kg of a 1:10,000 dilution. Repeat the SC dose every 20 minutes while attempting IV access.

Note: Some anaphylactic reactions, e.g. latex allergy, require large doses of epinephrine. A continuous infusion of epinephrine may be necessary.

Continued shock after volume resuscitation—IV infusion: 0.1–3.0 μg/kg/min. Start at lowest dose and titrate for desired clinical effect.

Note: Preparation of infusion solution: 0.6 mg × body weight (kg) diluted to 100 mL. Infuse at 1 mL/h = 0.1 μg/kg/min using a constant infusion pump.

Note: Extravasation can result in tissue necrosis injuries.

Status asthmaticus, bronchospasm—SC: 10 μg/kg per dose—10 μg/kg = 0.01 mL/kg of 1:1,000 dilution. Maximum single dose, 300 μg (0.3 mL of 1:1,000 dilution).

Note: Repeat SC dose every 20 minutes, if needed for clinical effect. Total of three doses.

Laryngotracheobronchitis: Racemic epinephrine, 2.25% inhalation solution. *Dosage:* Body weight 0–20 kg—0.25 mL in 2 mL with normal saline administered by nebulizer; 20–40 kg—0.50 mL in 2 mL with normal saline administered by nebulizer; more than 40 kg: 0.75 mL in 2 mL with normal saline administered by nebulizer.

Note: L-epinephrine: An equal volume of 1% L-epinephrine (1:100) is approximately equivalent in biologic activity to 2.25% racemic epinephrine; one can be substituted for the other in equal volumes for inhalation.

Note: Alternatively, 5 mL of 1:1,000 L-epinephrine is equivalent to 0.5 mL of 1:100.

Agalsidase Beta: *Dosage*:
Intravenous 16–18 years, 1 mg/kg once in 2 weeks.

Albendazole: *Dosage:*
Whipworm, trichuriasis, pinworm, threadworm, hookworm, roundworm, ascariasis: <2 years, 200 mg; >2 years, 400 mg. Single dose may be repeated after 2–3 weeks for pinworm, threadworm.

Ankylostomiasis: 400 mg single dose.

Strongyloidosis (*Strongyloides stercoralis*): 2–12 years, 400 mg daily once for 3 days. May repeat after 3 weeks, if necessary. 400 mg twice daily for 3 days, repeated after 3 weeks. More effective than mebendazole.

Enterobiasis: 100–200 mg single dose, repeated after 4 weeks.

Trichinosis: 2–12 years, 400 mg daily once for 5 days. Repeat if necessary.

Tapeworm: 400 mg daily once for 3 days.

Neurocysticercosis: Albendazole is used in dose of 15 mg/kg for 3–4 weeks. A short course of 8 days is also found to be effective depending upon location of cyst. 7.5 mg/kg up to maximum of 400 mg twice daily for 14–28 days. Take with food, repeat if necessary. Under steroid and anticonvulsant and in readiness for shunting for raised intracranial pressure.

Hydatid disease, echinococcosis: 15 mg/kg daily for 4 weeks. In hydatid disease, a large dose of mebendazole is required (400–600 mg 3 times a day for 21–30 days). This large dose may cause bone marrow aplasia and hence albendazole is a preferred drug nowadays for hydatid disease. Repeat the dose after 14 days, if required for next such three doses.

Cutaneous larva migrans: Less than 2 years, 10 mg/kg twice daily for 5 days; 2–12 years, 400 mg daily once for 5 days.

Toxocariasis: 2–12 years, 10 mg/kg up to maximum of 400 mg; 12–18 years, 400 mg, twice daily for 5 days. Steroid cover in symptomatic cases, especially if there is ocular involvement. Albendazole 400 mg bid for 5 days is also used for all the ages. Therapy may be adjunct with corticosteroid, if inflammatory symptoms with ocular involvement.

Filariasis: It has adjuvant value to diethylcarbamazine (DEC) or ivermectin in lymphatic filariasis. A single dose in combination has been used in mass programs.

Alemtuzumab: *Dosage*: One study used initial infusions with a low dose of 0.06 mg/kg (maximum 3 mg); increased over 5 days—6 mg/kg (maximum 30 mg) over 2 hours, 5 times per week for 1 week, then 3 times per week for 3 additional weeks.

Alendronate: *Dosage*: Experience of the use of bisphosphonates in children is limited and expert advice should be sought. Their use is only justified when the potential benefits outweigh any risk. 5 mg/day or 35 mg/week for less than 30 kg, 10 mg/day or 70 mg/week for = 30 kg—mean dosage; 0.37 ± 0.069 mg/kg/day.

Alendronic Acid (Sodium alendronate): *Dosage*: Experience with bisphosphonates in children is limited; expert advice required and use only in specialist centers experienced in its use.

Alfentanil: *Dosage:* Used only by trained anesthetist/interventionist, as assisted ventilation is required. Initially 20–50 mg/kg followed by 15 µg/kg both as IV bolus over 30 seconds. Alternatively, loading dose 50–100 µg/kg IV over 10 minutes followed by IV infusion at 500 ng–1 µg/kg/min.

Alginate: *Dosage:*
Management of gastroesophageal reflux disease:

Oral:
Neonate (body-weight up to 4.5 kg): 1 dose as required, to be mixed with feeds (or water, for breastfed infants); maximum 6 doses per day.

Neonate (body-weight 4.5 kg and above): 2 doses as required, to be mixed with feeds (or water, for breast-fed infants); maximum 12 doses per day.

Child 1–23 months (body-weight up to 4.5 kg): 1 dose as required, to be mixed with feeds (or water, for breastfed infants); maximum 6 doses per day.

Child 1–23 months (body-weight 4.5 kg and above): 2 doses as required, to be mixed with feeds (or water, for breastfed infants); maximum 12 doses per day.

Alimemazine Tartrate (Trimeprazine tartrate): *Dosage:*
Urticaria and/or pruritus: Orally, 6/12–2 years, 250 µg/kg (maximum 2.5 mg) 3–4 times daily; 2–5 years, 2.5 mg 3–4 times daily; 5–12 years, 5 mg 3–4 times daily; 12–18 years, 10 mg 2–3 times daily, in severe cases up to maximum 100 mg daily.

Premedication: Orally—2–7 years, up to 2 mg/kg 1–2 hours before procedure.

Allopurinol: *Dosage*:
Hyperuricemia due to tumor lysis syndrome: IV/oral—100 mg/m^2 3 times daily to be commenced 24 hours before starting cytotoxic drugs.

Glycogen storage disease and methyl malonic acidemia: 10–15 mg/kg (maximum 400 g) as single daily dose, if serum uric acid more than 0.36 mmol/L.

Phosphoribosyl pyrophosphatase (PRPP) synthetase superactivity and Lesch-Nyhan syndrome: 10–20 mg/kg (maximum 400 mg) daily once at minimum dose to maintain normal uric acid levels.

Adenine phosphoribosyl transferase (APRT) deficiency: 10 mg/kg (maximum 400 mg).

Alfacalcidol (1 Alpha-Hydroxycholecalciferol, Alfacalcidol): *Dosage*: 30–60 ng/kg/day

Alprazolam: *Dosage*: *Anxiety*: Orally for 12–18 years old, 200–500 µg 3 times daily (maximum 4 mg/day in divided doses)—use minimum effective dose.

Panic disorder: Orally for 12–18 years old—500 µg 3 times daily, increase once in 4 days to maximum of 10 mg/day in divided doses.

Aluminum Chloride: *Dosage:*
Hyperhidrosis: Apply 1–2 mL of aluminum chloride hexahydrate in the affected areas (armpits, palms, legs) only at night. This can be washed off in the morning. This has to be applied initially for every night in the 1st week and once the sweating comes down this can be brought down to thrice weekly and then to twice weekly and weekly. Eventually, the patient can be maintained with a weekly dosage.

Bromhidrosis and prevention of tinea pedis: Apply powder to the dry affected skin areas.

Aluminum Hydroxide: *Dosage*: *Antacid*: 4% w/w 6–12 years, 5 mL 3 times daily; 12–18 years, 5–10 mL 4 times daily and as required between meals and at bed time.

Hyperphosphatemia: Oral—1 month–1 year, 2.5–5 mL 3–4 times daily; 1–5 years, 5–10 mL 3–4 times daily; 5–12 years, 10–20 mL 3–4 times daily—dose may be increased or decreased as required within the ranges given. 12–18 years—tablet 840 mg 1–3 tablets 4–5 times daily.

Amantadine: *Dosage*:
Influenza A virus infection: Oral—children more than or equal to 10 years, 5 mg/kg/day PO in two divided doses, not to exceed 200 mg/day (100 mg PO twice daily in children who weigh ≥ 40 kg). Children less than 10 years, 5 mg/kg/day PO (up to 150 mg/day) in two divided doses.

Primary influenza prophylaxis (influenza virus type A only): Oral—adolescents, 200 mg/day PO as a single dose or two divided doses; begin as soon as possible after initial exposure and continue for at least 10 days after exposure. Begin as soon as possible after initial exposure and continue for at least 10 days after exposure.

HIV-infected adolescents, and children ≥10 years: As an alternative to influenza vaccination amantadine 100 mg PO twice daily be considered for primary prophylaxis during outbreaks of influenza A. Monitor these patients closely. Children ≥10 years, 5 mg/kg/day PO in two divided doses; begin as soon as possible after initial exposure and continue for at least 10 days after exposure. Do not exceed 200 mg/day. Children less than 10 years, 5 mg/kg/day PO (up to 150 mg/day) given in two divided doses; begin as soon as possible after initial exposure and continue for at least 10 days after exposure.

In all above-mentioned scenarios, prophylaxis may be continued for up to 90 days for repeated or suspected exposures, if influenza virus vaccine is unavailable. If used with the influenza virus vaccine, continue amantadine for 2–3 weeks until vaccine protection develops.

Amikacin: *Dosage*: Many dose regimens exist depending on target concentration aimed for and patient groups treated. The doses mentioned are accepted initial doses and dose adjustments done depending on serum levels. *See "Aminoglycosides".*

Newborn: Loading dose of 10 mg/kg then 7.5 mg/kg every 12 hours IV—<35 weeks up to 14 days 10 mg/kg once daily and >14 days 10 mg/kg loading dose followed by 7.5 mg/kg/dose two times daily; More than 35 weeks <14 days 15 mg/kg as single dose daily and >14 days 10 mg/kg loading dose followed by 7.5 mg/kg/dose two times daily. Extended interval dose regimen by slow intravenous injection or intravenous infusion—15 mg/kg every 24 hours.

Children (1 month–18 years): IV/IM 7.5 mg/kg/dose 2 times daily up to maximum of 500 mg/dose. Child >12 years with life-threatening infection, 1.5 g/day in three divided doses for up to 10 days may be given. Aim for 1 hour postdose (peak) of 15–30 mg/L.

Once daily dose regimen (not for endocarditis or meningitis): Child 1 month–18 years, initially 15 mg/kg, then adjusted according to serum amikacin concentration.

Amiloride: *Dosage*: Oral
Prophylaxis of drug-induced hypokalemia: <12 years, 100–200 µg/kg and >12 years, 5–10 mg twice daily.

Nephrogenic diabetes insipidus: Along with hydrochlorothiazide 100 µg/kg 3 times daily.

Aminoglycosides: *Dosage*: Many dose regimens exist for aminoglycosides depending on target concentration aimed for and patient groups treated. The dose regimens shown here are generally accepted initial doses and dose adjustments should be made in the light of serum concentration measurement.

Gentamicin: Neonates IV/IM <7 days 1,200–2,000 g 2.5 mg/kg once in 12–18 hours and >2,000 g 2.5 mg/kg once in 12 hours; >7 days 1,200–2,000 g 2.5 mg/kg once in 8–12 hours and >2,000 g 2.5 mg/kg once in 8 hours.

Child 1 month–11 years: 2.5 mg/kg every 8 hours, to be given in a multiple daily dose regimen, intravenous injection to be administered over at least 3 minutes;

12–17 years: 2 mg/kg every 8 hours, to be given in a multiple daily dose regimen, intravenous injection to be administered over at least 3 minutes.

Plasma levels done after 3–4 doses to achieve predose level of less than 2 mg/L and 1 hour postdose peak of 5 mg/L. Alternatively 5–7.5 mg/kg/24 hours IV once daily. Plasma levels done 18–24 hours after 1st dose to achieve predose level of <1 mg/L and 1 hour postdose peak of 16–20 mg/L. Intrathecal/ventricular-preservative free preparation: newborn 1 mg/24-hour; children 1–2 mg/24-hour; 16–18 years.

Netilmicin:
Newborn: IV 3 mg/dose 12 hourly. Increase to 8 hourly after 1 week age postnatal. Monitor after 3rd dose for 1 hour postdose peak of 8–12 mg/L and a trough of less than 3 mg/L. Prolong dose interval in *patent ductus arteriosus* (PDA), prolonged hypoxia, and indomethacin therapy. Children: IV/IM less than 12 years, 7.5 mg/kg/day and more than 12 years, 6 mg/kg/day in three divided doses or 1 month–18 years, 7.5 mg/kg as single dose daily. Intraperitoneal 7.5–10 mg/L in peritoneal dialysis fluid. See heading "*Netilmicin*" for more details.

Tobramycin:
Newborn: IV less than 32 weeks, 4–5 mg/kg 36 hourly and more than 32 weeks, 4–5 mg/kg once in 24 hours. PDA, prolonged hypoxia, indomethacin treatment necessitate increased dose intervals. Child—IV/IM 2.5 mg/kg/dose three times daily or 7 mg/kg as single daily dose. Intraventricular—newborn 1 mg/day, child 1–2 mg/day, adolescent 2–4 mg/day. See heading "Tobramycin" for more details.

Amikacin:
Children (1 month–18 years): IV/IM 7.5 mg/kg/dose two times daily up to maximum of 500 mg/dose. Child >12 years with life-threatening infection: 1.5 g/day in three divided doses for up to 10 days may be given. See heading "Amikacin" for more details.

Aminophylline: *Dosage*:
Neonatal apnea: IV 6 mg/kg (loading) followed 24 hours later by maintenance of 2.5 mg/kg IV twice daily (long half-life and so continuous infusion not required). Give slowly over 20 minutes (undiluted or diluted in NaCl 0.9% or glucose 5%). Monitor theophylline level, if possible, therapeutic range 8–12 mg/L.

Bronchial asthma and bronchospasm of anaphylaxis: IV loading dose of 5 mg/kg (maximum 500 mg) over 20–30 minutes, if no theophylline given in prior 24 hours followed by IV infusion at 0.5 mg/kg/hour in 6 weeks–6 months, 0.7 mg/kg/hour in 5 months–1 year, 1 mg/kg/hour in 1–12 years, and 0.7 mg/kg/hour in >12 years. Oral dose of 6 mg/kg for 1 week and then 12 mg/kg 3–12 years and 100–200 mg initially and then 200–450 mg in >12 years given two times daily.

Diuresis in ICU: IV over 20–30 minutes 2–4 mg/kg (up to 6 mg/kg in critically ill) 30 minutes before IV furosemide.

Amiodarone Hydrochloride: *Dosage*: Given under the direct supervision of cardiologist. The minimum effective dose used at all times. Oral loading dose of 5 mg/kg (maximum 200 mg) 2–3 times daily for 5 days followed by maintenance dose of 5 mg/kg (maximum 200 mg) once daily. IV loading dose of 5 mg/kg (in rare cases up to maximum of 15 mg/kg may be given) slowly over 30 minutes followed by maintenance continuous infusion at 5–15 μg/kg/min (maximum 1.2 g in 24 hours). Central line preferred.

In cardiopulmonary resuscitation (CPR) for shock resistant ventricular fibrillation and pulseless tachycardia: rapid IV bolus of 5 mg/kg may be given.

Amiodarone has a long duration of action and may exert effect for weeks or months after discontinuing. Since it is metabolized in liver, its dose must be adjusted in hepatic dysfunction.

Amisulpride: *Dosage*:
Acute psychotic episode (under specialist supervision): By mouth—child 15–18 years, 200–400 mg twice daily adjusted according to response; maximum 1.2 g daily.

Predominantly negative symptoms (under specialist supervision): By mouth—child 15–18 years, 50–300 mg daily.

Renal impairment: Halve dose if estimated glomerular filtration rate 30–60 mL/min/1.73 m^2; use one-third dose if estimated glomerular filtration rate 10–30 mL/min/1.73 m^2; no information available, if estimated glomerular filtration rate is less than 10 mL/min/1.73 m^2.

Amitriptyline: *Dosage*:
Nocturnal enuresis: 6–12 years, 10–25 mg; 12–18 years, 25–50 mg at bedtime daily for up to 3 months. Review before deciding on need for further courses.

Depression: >12 years, 25 mg 2–3 times or 50 mg at bedtime, initially at lower dose and increased, if tolerated/required. Usual maintenance—50–150 mg/day.

Neuralgic pain: 30 mg bedtime; increased, if required/tolerated up to 150 mg/day.

Idiopathic musculoskeletal pain syndromes: 10–50 mg bedtime, starting at lower dose.

Amlodipine: *Dosage:*
Oral: 100–200 µg/kg daily once increased, if required to maximum of 10 mg (6–15 kg 1.25 mg, 15–25 kg 2.5 mg, > 25 kg 5 mg).

Amodiaquine: *Dosage*:
PO: Usually taken in combination with another medicine for malaria. The dose is 10 mg/kg/day (range 7.5–15 mg/kg/day). One tablet contains 150 mg amodiaquine base. The dosage should be adjusted in accordance with the patient's age as listed in the following Table.

Age	Number of tablets per day		
	Day 1	Day 2	Day 3
1–6 years	1	1	1
7–13 years	2	2	2
Over 13 years	4	4	4

Amorolfine: *Dosage*:
Cream—apply once daily after cleansing in the evening for at least 2–3 weeks (up to 6 weeks for foot mycosis) continuing for 3–5 days after lesion has healed.

Nail lacquer—apply to infected nails 1–2 times weekly after filing and cleaning; allow drying (approximately 3 minutes). Treat finger nails for 6 months; toe nails for 9–12 months. Review 3 monthly.

Amoxicillin: *Dosage*: Oral 20–50 mg/kg/day in two or three divided doses. Higher dose of 80–90 mg/kg in acute suppurative otitis media (Maximum of 500 mg 2–3 times daily).

In uncomplicated gonorrhea—3 g with 1 g probenecid.

Amphotericin: *Dosage: Children:* 2.5–5 mg/kg intravenous (IV) infused over 1–2 hours once a day. May use higher doses of 7.5–10 mg/kg/24 hours, if indicated and tolerated.

Renal impairment: No dose reduction is generally required in pre-existing renal failure. Dose reduction may be advisable, if amphotericin is suspected of causing nephrotoxicity. Lipid complex formulations should also be considered in such situations. In renal dialysis patients, administration of amphotericin should commence only when dialysis is completed.

Ampicillin: *Dosage:* Neonate—50 mg/kg/dose for <7 days 12 hourly, 7–21 days 8 hourly, >21 days 6 hourly. 100 mg/kg/dose for suspected meningitis and Group B Streptococcal infection. *Children*: Oral 1 month–2 years 12.5 mg/kg/dose, 2–12 years 250 mg/dose, and 12–18 years 500 mg/dose; IV/IM 25 mg/kg/dose (maximum 1 g/dose); IV infusion 100 mg/kg/dose (maximum 3 g/dose)—all given 4 times daily.

Antiperspirants: *Dosage:* Preparations containing aluminum chloride hexahydrate are among the most effective. Aluminum chloride hexahydrate concentrations of 10–15% are recommended for excessive sweating of the underarms. For the hands or feet, higher concentrations are needed—usually around 30%. Apply on dry skin at bedtime when sweating is minimal. Use the antiperspirant every night until sweating is reduced. Once that is achieved, reduce frequency of application.

Antiscorpion venom serum: *Dosage:* The usual mode of administration of scorpion antivenin IP is either by IM or IV route. Generally, 10 mL of the reconstituted scorpion antivenin IP is sufficient for the treatment. However, if the patient continues to show clinical signs of envenomation for more than 3 hours or if the signs aggravate further, 10 mL of the antiserum may be administered by the IV route. In very rare cases, further 10 mL will have to be given.

Antisnake venom polyvalent: *Dosage:* Prior to administering the snake antivenin, it is obligatory to observe precautions and carry out sensitivity test. The usual mode of administration to snake antivenin is either by IM or IV route. The actual dose of snake antivenin, to be administered to the patient varies according to site of bite, severity of bite, age, and physical status, degree of envenomation, involvement of systematic organs and time factor of initiation of treatment.

A suitable dosage schedule recommended 100 mL given over 30–60 minutes by IV route (avoid bolus administration which may rapidly activate the compliment system and result in severe reaction). The 50 mL to be repeated, after 30 minutes of the initial dose, if active bleeding persists. This may be followed by 100 mL given by slow IV route over 24 hours to counteract the venom absorbed into the circulation from the site of bite, which act as a depot. This is especially so for krait, cobra, Russell's viper bites. Echis carinatus bites require less than 50 mL of the initial dose.

Some centers use for minimal envenomation: 20–40 mL; moderate envenomation: 50–90 mL; severe envenomation: 100–150 mL; if systemic symptoms increase in severity or new manifestations appear, administer an additional 10–50 mL.

Sea snake and pit viper specific antivenin is not available. However, due to paraspecificity of venom and antivenin same polyvalent antivenin is recommended. No more test dose is indicated.

Intramuscular adrenaline is given before administering the antisnake venin as prophylaxis.

Note: Local tourniquet should not be released unless full dose of antisnake venin is administered.

Arginine: *Dosage:*
Carbamyl phosphate synthetase (CPS) and ornithine carbamyl transferase (OCT) deficiency—oral 25–35 mg/kg 3–4 times

daily, IV 200 mg once given over 1½ hours, IV continuous infusion 200 mg/kg/24 hour.

Citrullinemia and argininosuccinic aciduria (ASA)— oral 100–175 mg/kg 3–4 times daily up to 700 mg/day, IV 600 mg once given over 1½ hour, IV continuous infusion 600 mg/kg/24 hours (25 mg/kg/hour).

Growth hormone stimulation test: IV infusion 500 mg/kg as single dose over 30 minutes.

Argipressin (arginine vasopressin, vasopressin): *Dosage:* A continuous infusion administered when no alternative measures available and discontinued at earliest. Treatment should not normally continue for more than 72 hours. Monitor carefully. IV over 20–30 minutes—birth–18 years 0.3 units/kg. *Continuous infusion:* 0.3 units/kg/hour or 0.0003–0.006 units/kg/minutes (maximum 1 unit/kg/hour).

Aripiprazole: *Dosage:* Oral—15–18 years, 2 mg once daily, increased to 5 mg once daily after 2 days, then further increased to 10 mg once daily after a further 2 days; further increased if necessary in steps of 5 mg to maximum 30 mg daily. Start with small doses in severe renal impairment because of increased cerebral sensitivity.

Artemisinin and its derivatives: *Dosage:* Expert advice should be sought for optimum treatment including choice of preparation and dosage.

Artesunate + Lumefantrine: *Dosage:* Treatment of uncomplicated *Plasmodium falciparum* and other *Plasmodium* malaria— Oral: Infant or child 5–14 kg initially 1 tablet followed by 5 further doses of 1 tablet each at 8, 24, 36, 48, and 60 hours (total 6 tablets over 60 hours); 15–24 kg initially two tablets followed by five further doses of two tablets each at 8, 24, 36, 48, and 60 hours (total 12 tablets over 60 hours); 25–34 kg initially three tablets followed by five further doses of three tablets each at 8, 24, 36, 48, and 60 hours (total 18 tablets over 60 hours); over 34 kg initially 4 tablets followed by five further doses of four tablets each at 8, 24, 36, 48, and 60 hours (total 24 tablets over 60 hours).

Renal impairment—severe: caution; monitor electrocardiogram (ECG) and plasma potassium.

Hepatic impairment—severe: caution; monitor ECG and plasma potassium.

Nondispersible tablets may be crushed. If the dose is vomited within 1 hour of taking, the dose should be repeated.

Asparaginase: *Dosage:* Always consult the current treatment protocol for details of dosage and scheduling. As part of combination therapy—6,000 units/m^2, 3 times/week for 3 weeks. High-dose IM therapy 25,000 units/m^2/dose weekly once for doses. IV therapy 1,000 units/kg/24 hours for 10 days; or 200 units/kg/24 hour for 28 days.

Aspirin: *Dosage:*

Fever—10–15 mg/kg/dose 4–6 times daily (maximum 4 g/day). Anti-inflammatory, analgesic dose—80–100 mg/kg/day.

Kawasaki disease—25 mg/kg/dose 4 times daily for 14 days followed by 5 mg/kg once daily for 6–8 weeks. If no evidence of coronary lesions discontinue.

Antiplatelet dose—3–5 mg/kg/day, given as a single dose (maximum 75 mg).

Rheumatic fever—25 mg/kg/dose for 4 doses/day for 2–3 weeks. Then 60 mg/kg/day for total period of 9–12 weeks.

Aspirin resistance, as seen in adults is prevalent in children also; 26% in one study.

Atazanavir: *Dosage:* Oral with low-dose ritonavir. 6–18 years 16–20 kg 150 mg OD; 20–40 kg 200 mg OD; >40 kg 300 mg OD.

Atenolol: *Dosage:* 0.5–2 mg/kg once daily. Adjust according to pulse and blood pressure (BP). May be given two times daily up to maximum of 100 mg/24 hour.

Renal failure—No dose adjustment is required in patients with a creatinine clearance for more than 35 mL/minute/1.73 m^2. If creatinine clearance 10–35 mL/minute/1.73 m^2 give 50% dose, less than 10 mL/minute/1.73 mm^2 give 30–50% dose and adjust according to response. In hemodialysis and continuous ambulatory peritoneal dialysis (CAPD) give 30–50% of dose and adjust according to response.

Atomoxetine: *Dosage:* Children and adolescents may be started at 0.5 mg/kg/day and dose may be increased after a minimum of 3 days to a target dose of 1.2 mg/kg/day, given once daily or in two divided doses in the morning and late afternoon. No additional benefit is seen in doses more than 1.2 mg/kg/day. Do not exceed 1.4 mg/kg/day or 100 mg/day.

Atorvastatin: *Dosage:* Hyperlipidemia including familial hypercholesterolemia—By mouth—Child 10–18 years initially 10 mg once daily, increased if necessary at intervals of at least 4 weeks to usual maximum 20 mg once daily (maximum 80 mg once daily in homozygous familial hypercholesterolemia.

Note: Reduced dose required (maximum 10 mg daily) with concomitant ciclosporin, or tipranavir combined with ritonavir-seek specialist advice.

Atracurium besylate: *Dosage:* Single IV bolus dose—neonate 300–500 µg/kg; 1 month–18 years 300–600 µg/kg. Continuous IV infusion: neonate 300–400 µg/kg/hour; 1 month–18 years 300–600 µg/kg/hour.

Atropine sulfate: *Dosage:*

Premedication—Neonates (never give IM) 15 µg/kg and children: subcutaneous (SC)/IM 1 month–12 years 20 µg/kg

of 200 mg 3 times daily but experience in children is limited; refer to an expert.

Biotin: *Dosage:* Oral/IV bolus—initially single dose of 5–10 mg followed by maintenance of 10–50 mg daily once.

Bisacodyl: Dosage:

Constipation—Orally, <10 years 5 mg, >10 years 5–10 mg daily bedtime (maximum 15–20 mg). Rectal suppositories <10 years 5 mg, >10 years 5–10 mg daily once in the morning.

Preparation for surgery, labor, or radiological investigation—Orally, <10 years 5 mg and >10 years 5–10 mg at bedtime for 2 days prior to procedure and rectally, if necessary, 1 hour before procedure.

Bleomycin: *Dosage:* 10–20 units/m^2/dose IV, IM or 0.25–0.50 mg/kg SC 1–2 times/week in combination regimens. Always consult the current treatment protocol for details of dosage and scheduling.

Botulinum A toxin-hemagglutinin complex: *Dosage:* Only those who have been trained in its use should administer this drug. It can be an effective tool for reducing muscle tone in the appropriately selected patient. The "ideal" patient is the one who has hypertonia that interferes with function, is expected to develop fixed contractures, and requires treatment of only a few muscles at any given time. The effect is seen within days—a couple of weeks and lasts for 3–8 months. Use 23–26 gauge needles and administer on 2 sites of each muscle (used mainly for gastrocnemius muscles) up to a total dose of 4 units/kg. If more than one muscle group needs to be injected at the same time, this total dose is divided between these muscles. Dose may be repeated when clinical effect diminishes but not within 2 months of previous injection.

Blepharospasm—Initially, 1.25–2.5 U injected into the medial and lateral orbicularis oculi of the upper lid and the lateral orbicularis oculi of the lower lid. Subsequently, the dose may be increased up to twofold. Initial dose should not exceed 25 U per eye. Total dose should not exceed 100 U every 12 weeks.

Hemifacial spasm—Treat as for unilateral blepharospasm (as above). Inject other affected facial muscles as needed.

Cervical dystonia—Inject using a 25, 27 or 30 gauge needle (for superficial muscles) or 22 gauge (deeper musculature). Tailor dosing to individual patient based on the head and neck position, location of pain, muscle hypertrophy, body weight and response. Do not inject sternocleidomastoid muscle bilaterally. Maximum total dose usually not more than 200 U.

Hyperhidrosis of the axillae—Inject using a 30 gauge needle. Inject 50 U intradermally to each axilla, evenly distributed in multiple sites 1–2 cm apart.

Pediatric cerebral palsy—Inject using a 23–26 gauge needle into the medial and lateral heads of the affected gastrocnemius muscle. *Recommended total dose:* 4 U/kg. Divide dose between two limbs, if injected on same occasion. Repeat dose not more frequently than every 2 months.

Focal spasticity associated with infantile hemiplegia—Inject using a 25, 27, or 30 gauge needle (superficial muscles) or longer needle for deeper musculature. Multiple injection sites may facilitate more uniform contact with the innervation areas of the muscle, especially in larger muscles. Tailor dose and number of sites based on size, number and location of muscles involved the severity of spasticity, and the presence of local muscle weakness.

Budesonide: *Dosage:*
Prophylaxis and management of bronchopulmonary dysplasia (BPD)—For ventilated babies, 400 μg/kg inhaled two times daily. For nonventilated babies 500 μg two times daily inhaled with nebulizer. May be increased to 1 mg, 2 times daily in babies more than 2.5 kg with severe symptoms.

Asthma prophylaxis—Aerosol 1 month–12 years 50–400 μg, 12–18 years 200–400 μg and Turbohaler in 6–18 year olds 100–400 μg twice daily to be used regularly. Can use up to 800 μg/day in severe asthmatics. Nebulizer in 3 month–12 years 250–500 μg and 12–18 years 500 μg–1 mg 2 times daily—higher doses may be used.

Croup—1 month–18 years 2 mg with nebulizer when required.

Bumetanide: *Dosage:* Oral 1 month–12 years, 0.015–0.05 mg/kg/dose (maximum 2 mg); 12–18 years 1–2 mg 1–4 times daily. IV bolus—12–18 years 1–2 mg repeated after 20 minutes, if required. IV infusion over 30–60 minutes—1 month–12 years 0.025–0.050 mg/kg; 12–18 years, 1–5 mg.

Bupivacaine hydrochloride: *Dosage:*

Caudal block—Children 1–3.7 mg/kg; adolescent 15–30 mL of 0.25% or 0.5%.

Epidural block—Children 1.25 mg/kg/dose; adolescent 10–20 mL of 0.25–0.5%.

Peripheral nerve block—5 mL of 0.25% (12.5 mg) or 0.5% (25 mg); maximum 400 mg/24 hour.

Sympathetic nerve block—20–50 mL of 0.25% (no epinephrine).

The dosage of bupivacaine will depend upon the site of injection and the procedure used. Expert advice should be obtained. Epidural administration should be carried out by, or under the supervision of, a consultant anesthetist.

Bupropion: *Dosage:* Orally 150–300 mg (usually 150 mg) once in the morning.

Buspirone hydrochloride: *Dosage:* Orally 2–12 years, 5 mg and 12–18 years, 5–10 mg 2–3 times daily (maximum dose in adolescent 45 mg in divided doses).

C

Caffeine citrate: *Dosage:* Birth–3 months, IV/oral loading dose, 20 mg/kg followed by maintenance dose 24 hours later at 5–10 mg/kg/day once or twice daily.

Calamine lotion: *Dosage:* Apply to external affected area as needed.

Calcipotriol: Dosage: All preparations—apply to affected area morning and evening. Do not apply to face. Wash hands after use to avoid inadvertent transfer to other body areas. Cream or ointment: Weekly maximum to be applied—6–12 years, 50 g; adolescents >12 years, 75 g; adults, 100 g. Scalp solution: weekly maximum to be applied—adults, 60 mL. When used with the cream or ointment, weekly maximum of total calcipotriol 5 mg.

Calcitonin (Salmon/Salcatonin): *Dosage:* There is very limited experience of use in children; dose depends on the condition being treated.

Calcitriol (1,25-dihydroxycholecalciferol): *Dosage:* Premature 0.05 µg/kg/24 hours IV or 1 µg/24 hours orally; children 0.01–0.08 µg/kg/24 hours; adolescent 0.25–1 µg/24 hours.

Calcium (Oral supplements): *Dosage:* Orally—birth–4 years 0.25 mmol/kg/dose; 5–12 years 0.2 mmol/kg/dose; 12–18 years 10 mmol/dose–4 times daily.

Calcium carbonate: Dosage: 50–75 mg/kg/day in 2–3 divided doses and adjusted according to plasma phosphate and calcium levels.

Calcium folinate (Folinic acid): *Dosage:* Oral/IV 15 mg once daily. See methotrexate monograph for folate rescue.

Calcium gluconate: *Dosage:*

Hypocalcemia—Urgent correction—2 mL/kg of 10% solution IV bolus over 5–10 minute (0.3 mL/kg/dose), followed by oral maintenance. If IV maintenance desired for a few days, be careful to avoid extravasation and administer 10% solution at 0.1 mL/kg/hour in neonates, 0.2 mL/kg/hour up to 2 years and 40 mL/24 hour in 2–18 years.

Cardiopulmonary resuscitation—0.3 mL/kg of 10% solution as single IV bolus.

Parenteral nutrition regimen—Approximate doses to maintain normal serum calcium-1 mmol/kg in neonates, 0.2–1 mmol/kg up to 2 years, 0.2 mmol/ kg in 2–12 years and 5–10 mmol/24 hour continuous IV over 12–24 hour.

Hyperkalemia—1–2 mL/kg intravenously.

Calcium polystyrene sulfonate (Ion exchange resin): *Dosage:* Rectally and orally 125–250 mg/kg 4 times daily. Not given orally in neonates. Must monitor electrolytes.

Captopril: *Dosage:* IAP Working group on management of congenital heart disease in India: The starting dose is 0.1 mg/kg/dose; it is gradually increased to 0.5–1 mg/kg/dose three times a day (increase after every 4–5 doses). Maximum dose is 2 mg/kg/dose. BP and renal parameters should be monitored when uptitrating the dose. Captopril is the preferred angiotensin-converting enzyme inhibitors (ACEI) in young infants, requires dosing every 6–8 hours.

Carbamazepine: *Dosage:* Children <6 years (use in neonates limited) initially 5 mg/kg/day in 1–2 divided doses; increase by 5 mg/kg/day every 5–7 days till response obtained or toxicity develops or serum levels attained. 6–12 year initially 10 mg/kg in 2–4 divided doses; increase by 100 mg or 5 mg/kg/day weekly till effect obtained (usually 800–1,200 mg/24 hour). 12–18 years initially 200 mg twice daily; increase by 200 mg/day once in a week till effect obtained (usually 1.6–2.4 g/day in 3–4 divided doses).

Carbamyl glutamate: *Dosage:* Orally 12.5–25 mg/kg/dose four times daily.

Carbapenems: Dosage:

Meropenem—Newborn, 40 mg/kg/day in two divided doses for <7 days and in 3 divided doses >7 days. Double dose in meningitis and severe infection.

Children—UTI, gynecological infections, skin and soft tissue infection—30 mg/kg in 3 divided doses (maximum 500 mg/dose).

Pneumonia, peritonitis, neutropenia, septicemia—60 mg/kg/day in 3 divided doses (maximum 1 g/dose).

Meningitis and life-threatening infections—120 mg/kg/day in three divided doses (maximum 2 g/dose).

In renal impairment—CrCl (mL/min/1.73 m^2) 25–50—give full dose but at 12 hours intervals, 10–25–50% dose at 12 hours intervals <10–50% dose at 24 hours interval. See Meropenem also below.

Imipenem with cilastin—Newborn IV 20 mg/kg/dose in the frequency—less than 7 days, 7–21 days and more than 21 days at 2 times, 3 times and 4 times daily, respectively.

Children—IV <3 months 80 mg/kg/day, 3 month–12 year 60 mg/kg/day, 12–18 years 2 g/day in four divided doses (maximum/dose <12 years 500 >12 year 1 g). See imipenem with cilastin below also.

Carbaryl: Dosage: Topical—gently rub into dry hair and scalp until all the hair is fully soaked. Allow the hair to dry naturally away from heat or sun in a well-ventilated room. After 12 hours wash in ordinary shampoo and remove dead lice and eggs with comb while the hair is still wet. Repeat after 1 week, if lice are still present.

Carbimazole: Dosage: Orally up to 12 year 250 µg/kg/dose and 12–18 year 10 mg thrice daily (maximum 40 mg). Give until euthyroid and then taper to once daily dose barely enough to sustain normal thyroid function.

Carboplatin: Dosage: Always consult the current treatment protocol for details of dosage and scheduling. Total cumulative doses vary with protocol. An increasing number of protocols employ doses based on glomerular filtration rate (GFR) (e.g. UKCCSG GC2, MMT 98) or Ethylene diaminetetra-acetic acid (EDTA) half-life (e.g. UKCCSF CNS 2000-01).

Children: Solid tumor—300–600 mg/m^2 IV once in 4 weeks.

Brain tumor—175 mg/m^2 IV once a week for 4 weeks.

Adolescent: 360 mg/m^2 IV once in 4 week.

Carnitine (Levocarnitine): *Dosage:* Premature—8–16 mg/kg/24 hour IV infusion; Children—Orally, 50–100 mg/kg/24 hour in 2–3 divided doses or IV 50 mg/kg/dose 4th–6th hourly (maximum 300 mg/kg/24 hour); adolescent 0.33–1 g/dose 2–3 times daily orally.

Carvedilol: Dosage: Oral—0.1 mg/kg/day in two divided doses increase at 1–2 weekly interval to 1 mg/kg/day with a maximum of 2l mg/kg/day. *Patients with hepatic impairment:* not recommended for patients with clinically evident hepatic impairment. *Patients with renal impairment:* No dosage adjustments are needed. Intermittent hemodialysis: Due to its high degree of plasma protein-binding, carvedilol is not likely to be significantly removed by hemodialysis. No supplemental dosage is needed.

Cefaclor: *Dosage:* Orally <1 year 62.5 mg, 1–5 year 125 mg, 6–18 years 250 mg/dose three times daily. Dose doubled in severe infection with susceptible organisms. *See* Cephalosporins below.

Cefadroxil: *Dosage:* Children—Orally 30 mg/kg/24 hours in two divided doses (maximum 2 g/day); adolescent 250–500 mg 8th–12th hourly. *See* Cephalosporins below.

Cefdinir: *Dosage:* 14 mg/kg/day in two divided doses. See Cephalosporins below.

Cefepime: Dosage: Neonates less than 14 days 30 mg/kg/dose twice daily IV/IM. Neonates more than 14 days 50 mg/kg/dose twice daily IV/IM. Children IV 50 mg/kg every 8 hour (maximum 2 g/dose). Intraperitoneal 15 mg/kg/dose. In peritoneal dialysis associated with peritonitis 1,000 mg/24 hours. However, not yet licensed for use in children less than 12 years in UK and US. *See* Cephalosporins below.

Cefixime: *Dosage:* 8 mg/kg/24 hours in 1–2 divided doses; adolescent: 400 mg/24 hours in 1–2 divided doses. *See* Cephalosporins below.

Cefoperazone: *Dosage:* 50–200 mg/kg/day in two or more divided doses (maximum in adolescent 1–2 g IM/IV 12 hourly).

Cefotaxime: *Dosage*: Newborn (severe infections such as meningitis) 50 mg/kg/dose—less than 7 day 2 times, 7–21 day 3 times, 21–30 days 3–4 times. 1 month–12 years 50 mg/kg/dose and 12–18 years 1–3 g 2 times daily. Dosage adjustment in renal impairment. Due to extrarenal elimination, it is only necessary to reduce dose in severe renal impairment (creatinine clearance <10 mL/minute/1.73 m^2). A normal single dose should be given as a loading dose then the daily dose should be halved without a change in frequency.

Cefpodoxime: *Dosage:* 9 mg/kg/day in two divided doses (maximum single dose—200 mg). The dose frequency should be reduced in renal impairment. Creatinine clearance 10–40 mL and less than 10 mL/min/1.73 m^2—frequency of dosing once in 24 hours and once in 48 hours, respectively. See Cephalosporins below.

Ceftazidime: *Dosage:* Neonates <7 days and >7 days <1,200 g 100 mg/kg/24 hour in 2 divided doses IV/IM, >7 days >1,200 g 150 mg/kg/day divided 8 hourly IM/IV. Children 150 mg/kg/24 hour divided 8 hourly. Maximum 6 g/day. Single dose >1 g to be given IV only.

Dose adjustment in renal failure—In mild impairment give a dose every 12 hours, in moderate impairment (creatinine clearance 10–50 mL/minute/1.73 m^2) give a dose once daily and in severe impairment (creatinine clearance <10 mL/minute/1.73 m^2) give 50% of dose once daily. Levels may be monitored, if clinically indicated.

In hemodialysis: The appropriate maintenance dose should be repeated after dialysis. In *peritoneal dialysis:* 125–250 mg may be added to 2l of dialysis fluid, and given in addition to the IV dose.

Ceftriaxone: *Dosage:* Neonates 50–75 mg/kg once daily IM/IV. Infuse over 10–30 minutes. Avoid in premature, acidotic or hyperbilirubinemic neonates. Children 50–75 mg/kg once daily IV/IM.

Meningitis—loading dose 75 mg/kg followed by 80–100 mg/kg/24 hour once or divided 12 hourly. Maximum 4 g/day.

In severe renal failure—reduce dose to a maximum of 2 g or 50 mg/kg. No dose adjustment required in hepatic impairment, if both hepatic and severe renal impairment monitor serum concentrations. In patients undergoing dialysis no supplemental dose required but serum concentration monitoring advisable.

Cefuroxime: *Dosage:* Infections due to sensitive gram-positive and gram-negative bacteria—Orally (as cefuroxime axetil)—3 months–2 years 10 mg/kg (maximum 125 mg) twice daily; 2–12 years 15 mg/kg (maximum 250 mg) twice daily; 12–18 years 250 mg twice daily; double the dose for severe lower respiratory tract infections; 125 mg twice daily in lower UTI. IV, IV infusion, IM—<7 days age—25 mg/kg 12 hourly; 7–21 days age 25 mg/kg 8 hourly; 21–28 days age—25 mg/kg 6th hourly; severe infection in neonates give IV at double these doses. 1 month–18 years 20 mg/kg (maximum 750 mg) 8 hourly; increase to 50–60 mg/kg (maximum 1.5 g) 6–8 hourly in severe infection and cystic fibrosis. See Cephalosporins below.

Lyme disease—Orally—3 months–12 years 15 mg/kg (maximum 500 mg) BD for 14–21 days (for 28 days in Lyme arthritis); 12–18 years 500 mg BD for 14–21 days (for 28 days in Lyme arthritis).

Surgical prophylaxis—IV—1 month–18 years 50 mg/kg (maximum 1.5 g) up to 30 min before procedure; up to 3 more doses of 30 mg/kg (maximum 750 mg) may be given IM/IV 8 hourly for high-risk procedures.

Cephalexin: Dosage: Children 25–100 mg/kg/24 hour in 3–4 divided doses; adolescent 250–500 mg 4 times daily (maximum 4 g/24 hour. Reduce dose in severe renal impairment (creatinine clearance <10 mL/minute/1.73 m^2) by reducing dose frequency. Removed by dialysis thus an additional dose may be required after dialysis. *See* Cephalosporins below.

Cephalosporins: *Dosage:*

1st generation cephalosporins.
Dose:
Cephalexin—children 25–100 mg/kg/24 hour in 3–4 divided doses and 12–18 years 250–500 mg 4 times daily (maximum 4 g/day). See above for more details.

Cefadroxil—children 30 mg/ kg/24 hour in two divided doses maximum 2 g/day) and in 12–18 years 250–500 mg 8th–12th hourly. See above for more details.

2nd generation cephalosporins.
Dose:
Cefuroxime—neonates, 40–100 mg/kg/day IM/IV given 12 hourly; children 200–400 mg/kg/day 8 hourly IM/IV and 20–30 mg/kg/day 3 times a day orally. Maximum dose not to exceed 1.5 g/dose IV or 6 g/24 hour. See above for more details.

Cefaclor—Orally less than 1 year 62.5 mg, 1–5 years 125 mg, 6–18 years 250 mg/dose 3 times daily. Dose doubled in severe infection with susceptible organisms. See above for more details.

3rd generation cephalosporins.
Dose:
Cefixime—Children, 8 mg/kg/24 hour in 1–2 divided doses. *In adolescent:* 400 mg/24 hour in 1–2 divided doses. *See* above for more details.

Cefpodoxime—Children—9 mg/kg/24 hour in two divided doses (maximum single dose—200 mg. *In adolescent:* 200 mg 2 times daily. *See* above for more details.

Cefdinir—Children—7 mg/kg/dose 2 times daily. 12–18 year—300 mg/dose 2 times daily. 4th generation cephalosporins. See above for more details.

Cefpirome—Children 12–18 year IV injection or infusion 1 g 12th hourly and increased to 2 g 12th hourly in severe infections and infections in immunocompromized children.

Cefepime—Children IV 50 mg/kg every 8 hour (maximum 2 g/dose). See above for more details.

Cetirizine: *Dosage:* 2–6 years 5 mg and 6–18 years 10 mg as single or 2 divided doses. In renal impairment give 50% of above dose.

Chenodeoxycholic acid: *Dosage:* Cerebrotendinous xanthomatosis 5 mg/kg/dose 3 times daily;

Bile acid synthesis defects initially 5 mg/kg/dose 3 times daily then 2.5 mg/kg 3 times daily; Others 7 mg/kg/ dose in 1 or divided doses.

Chloral hydrate: *Dosage:*

Sedation for procedures—<12 years 25–50 mg/kg 12–18 year 1–2 g 45–60 minutes prior to procedure (maximum single dose 100 mg/kg);

Long-term sedation—20–30 mg/kg/dose 4 times daily.

Night sedation—<12 year 30–50 mg/kg, 12–18 year 500 mg–1 g single dose at bedtime.

Chlorambucil: *Dosage:* Hodgkin disease and non-Hodgkin lymphoma—consult the current treatment protocol for details of dosage and scheduling.

Systemic amyloidosis and severe juvenile idiopathic arthritis (JIA)—*All ages:* 100–120 µg/kg orally once daily.

Chloramphenicol: *Dosage:* Neonates <14 days 12.5 mg/kg/dose twice daily; >14 days 12.5 mg/kg/dose 2–4 times daily—monitor levels. Children 50 mg/kg/day (maximum 1 g/day) 4 divided doses—double dose for meningitis, septicemia).

Ear drops—2–3 drops 2–3 times daily. Eye ointment may be used in the ear.

Eye drops—1 drop 4–6 times daily (1–2 hourly in severe infections). In addition, a small amount of ointment may be applied at bedtime.

Eye ointment—apply 4 times daily (1–2 hourly in severe infections). Continue treatment till 48 hours after the eye is clinically normal.

Chlorhexidine gluconate: *Dosage:*

Dental gel—1 inch of gel brushed around the teeth and gums once or twice daily for 1 minute. For gingivitis, apply for 1 month.

Mouth wash —0.12%: 15 mL for 30 seconds twice daily. Mouth wash 0.2%: 10 mL for 1 minute twice daily.

Oral spray—up to 12 actuations to be used twice daily, morning, and night. For the prevention of gingivitis, use for 1 month. In aphthous ulceration and oral infections use for 48 hours after the infection has cleared.

Postoral surgery or trauma—on the advice of the supervising clinician.

Chloroquine: *Dosage:* Doses expressed as chloroquine base–

Malaria prophylaxis—1 month–12 year 5 mg/kg, 12–18 years 300 mg once weekly. Start 1 week before entering and 4 weeks after leaving endemic area.

Malaria treatment—(*P. vivax, P. ovale, and sensitive P. falciparum*) Oral/IV—1 month–12 years—Initially, 10 mg/kg followed by 5 mg/kg 6–8 hours later, and then daily once for 2 days. 12–18 years Initially, 600 mg followed by 300 mg 6–8 hours later and then daily once for 2 days.

Chlorothiazide: *Dosage:* 20–40 mg/kg/day in two divided doses oral; 2–8 mg/kg twice a day IV.

Chlorpheniramine: *Dosage:* Oral less than 2 years 1 mg 2 times (maximum 2 mg), 2–5 year 1–2 mg 3 times (maximum 6 mg), 6–12 years 2–4 mg 3–4 times (maximum 12 mg), 12–18 years 4 mg 4–6 times daily (maximum 24 mg) IM/IV/SC less than 1 year 250 µg/kg; 1–5 year 2.5–5 mg, 6–12 year 5–10 mg, 12–18 year 10–20 mg once. Repeated up to 4 times daily (maximum 49 mg in adults).

Chlorpromazine: *Dosage:*

Withdrawal symptoms in baby born to drug abuser—Orally, 1 mg/kg/day 3 times or orally/IV 500–750 µg/kg/dose 4 times (Maximum 6 mg/kg/day)—dose-doubled, if withdrawal is severe.

Children with schizophrenia, violent behavior, agitation—less than 6 years 500 µg/kg/dose 4 times daily (maximum 40 mg/day); 6–12 years 10 mg/dose (maximum 75 mg/day) and 12–18 years 25 mg/dose 4 times daily (maximum 300 mg/day).

Intractable hiccup—6–12 year 10 mg/dose 1–3 times daily; 12–18 years 25–50 mg/dose 3–4 times daily.

Nausea and vomiting of terminal illness—2–12 years 500 µg/kg/dose (maximum 40 mg/day; 12–18 years 10–25 mg/dose (maximum 75 mg/day)-4 times daily.

Cholecalciferol (Vitamin D3): *Dosage:* Orally for less than 6 months 3,000 units, 6 months–12 years 6,000 units and 12–18 years 10,000 units. Check biochemistry after 6 weeks therapy. Stop once serum alkaline phosphatase (ALP) and parathyroid hormone (PTH) are normal.

Routine supplementation—400 IU/day.

Rickets—IM 5,000–50,000 IU daily or 1 single dose of 3–600,000 units once in 3 weeks.

Cholestipol hydrochloride: *Dosage: Oral:* 12–18 years initially 5 g once daily. May be increased at intervals of 1 month to a maximum of 30 g daily in 1–2 divided doses.

Cholestyramine: *Dosage:* Cholesterol reduction—Oral 240 mg/kg/24 hour in 3 divided doses. 12–18 years 1 sachet (4 g) start at 1 daily and usually require 4 times daily but up to 9 sachet/day in adults according to cholesterol levels.

Cholestatic pruritus—Oral less than 6 year half sachet (2 g), 6–12 years 1 sachet (4 g) and 12–18 year 1–2 sachet once daily.

Diarrhea in ileal resection, Crohn's disease, vagotomy, radiation—same as for cholesterol reduction but alternate treatment to be instituted, if no response in 3 days.

Choline salicylate: *Dosage:* Children more than 4 months: Apply quarter of an inch of gel to the dried area of affected oral mucosa, no more frequently than once every 3 hours to a maximum of 6 applications in 24 hours. >12 years: Apply half an inch of gel with massage not more often than every 3 hours.

Ciclesonide: Dosage: Ciclesonide is administered once daily as MDI in doses of 80–640 mg depending on the clinical severity and response.

Ciclopirox (Topical antifungal): *Dosage:* Apply once a day with an applicator brush to all affected nails and immediately adjacent skin. Daily applications should be made over the previous coat and removed every seven days. Up to 48 weeks of daily applications, weekly trimming by the patient, and monthly professional removal of the unattached, infected nail, is needed.

Cimetidine: *Dosage:* Oral/IV <1 month 5 mg/kg/dose and <12 years 5–10 mg/kg/dose 4 times daily; 12–18 years 400 mg/dose 2–4 times/day.

Cinnarizine: *Dosage:*

Vestibular disorders—Oral—5–12 years, 15 mg 3 times daily, 12–18 years, 30 mg 3 times daily.

Motion sickness—Oral—5–12 years, 15 mg 2 hours before travel then 7.5 mg 8th hourly during journey, if necessary, 12–18 years, 30 mg 2 hours before travel then 15 mg 8th hourly during journey, if necessary.

Ciprofibrate: *Dosage: Oral:* 2–4 mg/kg (maximum 200 mg) has been used in adolescents but experience in children is limited; refer to an expert.

Ciprofloxacin: *Dosage:* Neonates 10 mg/kg 12 hourly orally or IV; children 15–30 mg/kg/24 hour in 2 divided doses oral or IV (Maximum single dose IV 400 mg and oral 750 mg). Dose adjustment in renal or liver failure: In severe impairment (creatinine clearance <20 mL/minute/1.73 m^2), total daily dosage may be reduced by half, although monitoring serum levels provides the most reliable basis for dose adjustment. No adjustment in impaired hepatic function. See Quinolones below also.

Corneal ulcers—apply throughout the day and night. 1st day—2 drops every 15 min for 6 hour followed by 2 drops every 30 min for the rest of the day. 2nd day—2 drops every hour and from 3rd day to 14th day—2 drops 4th hourly.

Superficial infections of eye—1–2 drops 4 times daily till 48 hours after the eye is clinically normal (use for maximum of 21 days).

Cisapride: *Dosage:* Orally birth–12 years 0.15–0.3 mg/kg/dose; 12–18 years 10 mg/dose 3–4 times daily. Doses to be given 15–30 min before meals.

Cisplatin: *Dosage:* 37–75 mg/m^2 once in 2–3 weeks or 50–150 mg/m^2 once in 21–28 days given over 4–6 hours. *Renal failure:* Creatinine clearance 10–50 mL/minute–75% of dose and if less than 10 mL/minute 50% of dose. Always consult the current treatment protocol for details of dosage and scheduling.

Citalopram: *Dosage:* 12–18 years 20 mg in the morning increased to maximum of 60 mg.

Citrulline: *Dosage:* Birth–18 years 42.5 mg/kg/dose 4 times daily.

Clarithromycin: *Dosage: See* lincosamines and streptogramins as well. Oral 15 mg/kg/24 hour in 2 divided doses up to maximum of 500 mg twice daily for 5–10 days.

H. pylori—1–2 years 125 mg, 2–6 years 250 mg, 6–9 years 375 mg, 9–12 years 500 mg, and 12–18 years 1 g/day in 2 divided doses along with amoxicillin and omeprazole or amoxicillin and lansoprazole or metronidazole and omeprazole.

CAP and pharyngitis in children due to *Chlamydophila pneumoniae*, *Mycoplasma pneumoniae*, or *Streptococcus pneumoniae*—give for 10 days.

Bacterial endocarditis prophylaxis—15 mg/kg (single dose maximum 500 mg) 30–60 minutes before procedure in children and adolescents allergic to penicillin.

Treatment and post-exposure pertussis prophylaxis—For postexposure prophylaxis, administer to close contacts within 3 weeks of exposure, especially in high-risk patients (e.g. women in 3rd trimester, infants <12 months). Oral dosage: Infants >6 months and children: 15 mg/kg/day up to maximum of 500 mg twice daily for 7 days. Not used in neonates.

Patients with renal impairment—CrCl >60 mL/minute: no dosage adjustment needed. CrCl 30–60 mL/minute: No dosage adjustment needed except in patients receiving concurrent ritonavir. In these patients, reduce the recommended clarithromycin dose by 50%. CrCl less than 30 mL/minute: Reduce recommended dose by 50%. In patients receiving ritonavir, decrease the recommended clarithromycin dose by 75%.

Clindamycin: See lincosamines and streptogramins also. *Dosage:* Neonates—<7 days <2,000 g 10 mg/kg/day divided 12 hourly IV/IM; less than 7 days more than 2,000 g 15 mg/kg/day divided 8 hourly IV/IM; more than 7 days less than 1,200 g 10 mg/kg/day divided 12 hourly IV/IM; 1200–2000 g 15 mg/kg/day divided 8 hourly, more than 2,000 g 20 mg/kg/day divided 8 hourly IV/IM. Children 10–40 mg/kg/day divided 8 hourly IV/IM or orally. 12–18 years 150–300 mg up to maximum of 450 mg/dose 4 times daily.

Falciparum malaria (alternate therapy)—with 20 mg/kg/day for 5 days.

Acne—topical application as thin film 2 times daily with lotion and once with gel.

Dose adjusted in hepatic failure—Dose-reduced and liver function monitored. Not readily removed by dialysis or peritoneal dialysis.

Clobazam: *Dosage:* Initially orally less than 12 years 125 µg/kg/dose, 12–18 years 10 mg/dose 2 times daily followed by maintenance of 250 µg/dose (maximum 500 µg)/dose in less than 12 years and 10–15 (maximum 30) mg/dose in 2 doses.

Clobetasone: *Dosage:* Apply thin layer 2–3 times daily on affected area for a maximum of 2 weeks.

Clofazimine: *Dosage:*

Multibacillary leprosy—(in combination with dapsone and rifampicin), by mouth; Adolescent: 50 mg once daily and 300 mg once a month; Child 10–14 years, 50 mg on alternate days and 150 mg once a month; Children less than 10 years: 1 mg/kg PO once daily plus an additional 6 mg/kg PO once per month in combination with dapsone and rifampin; continue treatment for 12 months.

Type 2 lepra reaction (erythema nodosum leprosum)—by mouth, adolescent, and child, 200–300 mg daily in 2 or 3 divided doses for a maximum of 3 months; 4–6 weeks treatment may be required before any effect is seen.

Clomiphene: *Dosage:* 100 mg daily once–roughly at the same time each day.

Clomipramine: *Dosage:* Start with 25 mg/day and gradually increase up to 250 mg/day according to response usually as single dose at bedtime (may give in divided doses).

Clonazepam: *Dosage:* 1 month–12 years—start with 25 μg/kg (0.25 mg <5 year and 0.5 mg 6–12 years) as single bedtime dose and increasing every 4 days over 2–4 weeks to maintenance of 80 μg/kg/dose (0.1–0.3 mg less than 1 year, 0.3–1 mg 1–5 years, and 1–2 mg 6–12 years) 3 times daily. 12–18 years—start with 1 mg bedtime to maintenance of 1–2.5 mg/dose 3 times daily.

Clonidine: *Dosage:*

Hyperactivity and Tourette syndrome—Oral initially 0.05 mg/24 hour once daily increase by 0.05 mg once in 5–7 days up to maximum of 0.4 mg/kg/day in 3–4 divided doses.

Hypertension—Oral 5–10 μg/kg/day in 2–4 divided doses (maximum 0.9 mg/kg/day); IV 2–6 μg/kg as single dose.

Sedation, pain and narcotic withdrawal—Oral initial test dose 1 μg/kg, monitoring for hypotension and escalate in steps of 1–3–5 μg/kg/day if required, 3 times daily (maximum 5 μg/kg 4 times daily).

Growth hormone stimulation test—Oral 150 μg/m^2 as single dose.

Clopidogrel: *Dosage:* 0.2 mg/kg/day is sufficient to achieve platelet inhibition level similar to that in adults taking the standard dose of 75 mg/day. The 80% of children would also be taking aspirin. When appropriate, tablets were rounded to the nearest one half, one-third, or one-fourth tablet.

Clotrimazole: *Dosage:* Apply 2–3 times daily continuing for 14 days after lesions have healed.

Oral thrush—10–20 drops gently apply to buccal mucosa (covering all lesions) 4 times daily for 5–7 days.

Vaginal candidiasis—Apply 2% vaginal gel 5 g deep into vagina at bedtime for 6 consecutive nights (not to be used during menstruation). Or alternatively—100 mg vaginal pessaries for 6 days, 200 mg for 3 days or 500 mg single dose at bedtime.

Scalp seborrhea—Apply to liquid with selenium to scalp, massage gently, leave for 5 minutes and then rinse well with water 2–3 times/week.

Otomycosis—Instill 4–5 drops in ear 3–4 times daily till 2 weeks after infection subsides.

Cloxacillin: *Dosage:* Newborn IV/oral <7 days 50–100 mg/kg/day in 2 divided doses; 7–21 days 75–150 mg/kg/day in 3 divided doses, >21 days 100–200 mg/kg/day in 4 divided doses. May be increased to 100 mg/kg/dose in severe infection (meningitis, cerebral abscess, *S. osteitis*). Oral used only for minor infections. Children-IV/IM 50–100 mg/kg/day in 4 divided doses (maximum single dose 1 g-may be doubled in severe infection). Oral >1 year 250 mg/day, 1–5 years 500 mg/day, 5–18 year 1 g in 4 divided doses. Doses may be doubled in severe infection. In renal failure—if creatinine clearance is less than 10 mL/minute/1.73 m^2, increase dosage interval to 8th hourly.

Clozapine: *Dosage:* Oral 12–18 years initial dose on 1st day given as inpatient 12.5 mg/dose 1–2 times daily and from 2nd day 25 mg/dose 1–2 times daily and if tolerated gradually increased in steps of 25–50 mg over 14–21 day to maintenance dose of 300 mg/day in divided doses (maximum 900 mg/day if necessary).

Coal tar: *Dosage:*

Topical—Bath 60–90 mL of a 5–20% solution or 15–25 mL of 30% solution is added to bath water. Soak for 5–20 minutes, and then pat dry. Use once daily to once every 3 days. *Shampoo*—apply 2 times in a week for 1st 2 weeks and then once weekly or more often, if needed. Skin—apply to affected areas 1–4 times daily. Decrease frequency to 2–3 times/week once condition is controlled.

Atopic dermatitis—2–5% coal tar cream once daily or every other day to reduce inflammation.

Scalp psoriasis—Tar oil bath or coal tar solution may be applied sparingly to lesions 3–12 hours before each shampoo.

Psoriasis of body, arms and legs—apply at bedtime. If thick scales are present, use a product containing salicylic acid and apply several times during the day.

Coamoxiclav (Amoxicillin and clavulanic acid): *Dosage:* Dosed on amoxicillin content. *Neonates*—30 mg/kg/day in 2 divided doses. Children 20–45 mg/kg in 2–3 divided doses. Higher doses of 80 mg/kg/day may be required in otitis media.

Administration— Oral: Give at the start of a meal. Dispersible tablets should be stirred into a little water before taking. IV: Reconstitute a 600 mg vial with 10 mL Water for injections (final volume 10.5 mL) and a 1.2 g vial with 20 mL (final volume 20.9 mL). Give by slow IV injection (over 3–4 minutes, within 20 minutes of reconstitution) or infuse over 30–40 minutes and complete infusion within 4 hours of reconstitution. For infusion the reconstituted injection can be diluted to 5 times its volume in NaCl 0.9%. Do not infuse in glucose solutions, as coamoxiclav is less stable in infusions containing glucose.

Cocareldopa: *Dosage:*

Metabolic disorders—start with 250–500 μg/kg/dose of levodopa 4 times daily. Increase every 4–5 days to maintenance of 2.5–3 mg/kg/dose of levodopa. Review dose every 3–6 months in early childhood and adjust if needed according to weight and cerebrospinal fluid (CSF) amine metabolic concentration.

Dystonia—3 month–18 years start with 250 μg–1 mg/kg/dose of levodopa 2–3 times daily and increase every 2–3 days.

Codeine phosphate: *Dosage:* Children—Pain 0.5–1 mg/kg/dose 4–6 hourly (maximum 60 mg/dose) and for dry cough 1–1.5 mg/kg/24 hour divided 4–6 hourly.

Adolescent: Pain 15–60 mg/dose 4–6 hourly and for cough 10–20 mg/dose 4–6 hourly (maximum 120 mg/24 hour).

Colchicine: *Dosage:* Children—Prophylaxis of Mediterranean fever —Less than 5 years 0.5 mg/24 hour and more than 5 years 1–1.5 mg/24 hour in 2–3 divided doses.

Colestipol hydrochloride: *Dosage:* Oral: 12–18 years initially 5 g once daily. May be increased at intervals of 1 month to a maximum of 30 g daily in 1–2 divided doses.

Colistin: *Dosage:* Nebulized along with oral ciprofloxacin for *Pseudomonas* lung infection in cystic fibrosis—less than 1 year 500,000 units, 1–10 years 1 million units, more than 10 years 2 million units 2 times daily. IV for early *Pseudomonas* infections not cleared by ciprofloxacin and nebulized colistin or moderate or severe infection or multiresistant strains along with aminoglycoside where other regimens fail (IV preparation not available in India).

Coloxyl: *Dosage: Oral:* Up to 6 months—10 drops three times daily. 6 to 18 months: 15 drops three times daily.

Cophenotrope (Diphenoxylate + atropine): *Dosage:* Oral 2–4 years ½ tab, 4–12 years 1 tablet, 13–16 years 2 tablets, 16–18 years initially 4 tablets followed by 2 tablets-3–4 times daily. Avoid in treatment of diarrhea in children.

Copper histidine: *Dosage: Dosage* tailored to individual patient requirements. SC 50–150 µg elemental copper/kg daily once; IM 200 µg elemental copper, increase monthly to maximum of 1 g daily once.

Corticosteroids (Topical): *Dosage:* Initial treatment, certainly in infants less than 12 months, should always be with the weakest topical steroid, hydrocortisone. Apply sparingly to the affected areas once or twice a day.

Corticotropin (Corticotrophin, Adrenocorticotropic hormone, ACTH): Dosage: IM/SC 1 month–18 years, 20–80 units once daily. Duration and frequency of doses depend on individual child. *See* Tetracosactide also.

Cotrimoxazole: Dosage: children—Orally 6–20 mg TMP/kg/24 hour divided 12 hourly (Maximum 160 mg TMP 12 hourly).

P. carinii pneumonia: Oral/IV15–20 mg TMP/kg/24 hour divided 12 hourly.

P. carinii prophylaxis: Orally 5 mg TMP/kg/24 hour or 3 times/week.

The use of cotrimoxazole is not generally recommended under 6 weeks of age, but some neonatologists feel that there is no specific reason for this caution other than the risk of hemolytic anemia in babies with G6PD deficiency and the risk of kernicterus because sulfamethoxazole competes for the protein binding sites usually available to bilirubin in babies with jaundice. If cotrimoxazole is used in newborn infants it is given in the same dosage as for 6 weeks–5 months but trimethoprim on its own is now usually preferred to cotrimoxazole.

Crotamiton: *Dosage: Topical:* After patient has a warm bath and dried well, the preparation should be rubbed into the entire body surface excluding face and scalp. The application should be repeated once daily preferably in the evening for a total of 3–5 days. Children <3 years of age should not apply crotamiton more than once a day.

Cyclizine: *Dosage:* Children—6–12 years orally 25 mg/dose up to 3 times/24 hour as required and *Older:* Adolescents 50 mg up to 4–6 hourly 30 min before travel (maximum 200 mg/24 hour; IM 50 mg 4–6 times.

Cyclopentolate: *Dosage:* 1–2 drops or as required. Its effect lasts 24 hours.

Cyclophosphamide: *Dosage:* Children—Induction IV 40–50 mg/kg (1.5–1.8 g/m^2) in divided doses over 2–5 days; Orally 1–5 mg/kg/24 hour followed by maintenance IV 10–15 mg/kg (350–550 mg/m^2) once in 7–10 days or 3–5 mg/kg twice in a week.

Systemic lupus erythematosus—500–750 mg/m^2/month.

Juvenile rheumatoid arthritis or vasculitis—IV 10 mg/kg once in 2 weeks.

Bone marrow transplant conditioning—IV 50 mg/kg/24 hour for 3–4 days.

Nephrotic syndrome—Orally 2–3 mg/kg/24 hour-up to 12 weeks. In steroid dependent normal saline (NS), use with alternate day prednisolone. Dose not to exceed a dose of 166 mg/kg.

Immune thrombocytopenic purpura (ITP)—1–2 mg/kg/day orally. Response occurs in 2–10 weeks. Adjust doses for:

Renal failure—CrCl 25–50 mL/minute give half dose and if less than 25 mL/minute avoid.

Decreased bone marrow function—give 33–50% of dose.

Cycloserine: *Dosage:* Tuberculosis—Oral—10–20 mg/kg/ day in 2 divided doses. Maximum 1 g/day. Adolescent—250–500 mg twice daily for 2 weeks and then increased to 500 mg–1 g in divided doses.

Cyclosporin: Dosage:

Juvenile idiopathic arthritis, collagen disease, vasculitis, uveitis—orally 1–2 mg/kg per dose 2 times daily increased gradually up to 3 mg/kg/dose twice daily.

Organ transplant— Orally 5-7 mg/kg/dose 2 times daily starting 12 hours before transplant and continued for 1-2 weeks postoperatively gradually reducing to maintenance dose of 1-3 mg/kg/dose 2 times daily. OR 1.5-4 mg/kg/dose 2 times daily when given with other immunosuppressants as part of triple or quadruple regime.

Bone marrow transplant—6-7.5 mg/kg/dose 2 times daily starting on day prior to transplant.

Psoriasis/atopic dermatitis—1.25 mg/kg/dose 2 times daily—increased, if no response, after 2 weeks for dermatitis and 4 weeks for psoriasis till 2.5 mg/kg/dose 2 times daily.

Severe ulcerative colitis—Orally, 3-4 mg/kg 2 times daily.

Crohn's disease—2.5-4.5 mg/kg/dose 2 times daily.

Steroid resistant nephrotic syndrome—4-6 mg/kg/day in 2 divided doses. Monitor trough levels of cyclosporine to adjust dose.

Cyproheptadine: *Dosage:* Pruritus and urticaria—0.25 mg/kg/day or 8 mg/m^2 body surface area in 2-3 divided doses, or by age—2-6 years: 2 mg orally 2-3 times a day, not to exceed 12 mg/day; 7-14 years: 4 mg orally 2-3 times a day, not to exceed 16 mg/day.

Anorexia—More than 13 years: 2 mg orally 4 times a day. May be increased gradually over a 3 week period to 8 mg 4 times a day. Maximum dose is 32 mg/day.

Migraine—4 mg orally two to three times a day.

Hepatic failure—Not studied. Since cyproheptadine is primarily metabolized by the liver, caution is advised when it is administered to patients with impaired hepatic function.

Cyproterone acetate: *Dosage:* Seek expert advice on use in McCune-Albright Syndrome or testotoxicosis. 1 tablet daily for 21 days starting on first day of menstrual cycle and repeated after a 7 day interval, usually for several months.

Cytarabine (Cytosine arabinoside, ara-C, arabinosyl-cytosine): *Dosage:* Doses depend on individual protocols. Typically Induction—IV 100-200 mg/m^2/24 hour for 5-10 days or until remission followed by maintenance 70-200 mg/m^2/24 hour for 2-5 days/month. Always consult the current treatment protocols for details of dosage and scheduling. Maximum intrathecal dose is 30 mg. Consider dosage reductions when liver function is poor.

D

Dacarbazine: *Dosage:* Always consult the current treatment protocol for details of dosage and scheduling.

Children:

Solid tumors—200-470 mg/m^2/24 hour over 5 days once in 21-28 days;

Neuroblastoma—800-900 mg/m^2 on day 1 of combination therapy once in 3-4 weeks.

Hodgkin disease—375 mg/kg/m^2 on day 1 and 15 of combination therapy and repeat once in 28 days.

Dactinomycin (Actinomycin D): *Dosage:* Always consult the current treatment protocol for details of dosage and scheduling. Children more than 6 months age—15 µg/kg/24 hour or 400-600 µg/m^2/24 hour for 5 days; repeated once in 3-6 week.

Dalteparin sodium: See Heparin also. *Dosage: Thromboembolic disease*:

Treatment—SC 200 units/kg/24 hour in 2 divided doses in less than 12 years and as single dose in 12-18 years not to exceed 18,000 units/24 hour

Prophylaxis—SC 100 units/kg up to 12 years and 2,500-5,000 units as single dose in 12-18 years.

Dantrolene: Dosage:

Spasticity—>5 years 500 µg/kg/day once daily and increase once in 7 days in increments of 500 µg/kg/dose till response achieved and in 12-18 years 25 mg daily once and increased gradually till response.

Malignant hyperthermia—IV bolus of 1 mg/kg as single dose repeated as required at 5-10 minutes intervals to maximum cumulative dose of 10 mg/kg.

Dapsone: *Dosage*: *Leprosy*—Oral 1-2 mg/kg/day as single dose in combination with rifampicin.

Blistering skin conditions—Start at 500 µg/kg/day and increase or decrease as necessary in 12.5 mg increments.

Daunorubicin: *Dosage*: Always consult the current treatment protocol for details of dosage and scheduling. *Children*—remission induction in acute lymphoblastic leukemia (ALL) (combination therapy) 25-45 mg/m^2 on day 1 of every week for 4 cycles (maximum total dose 300 mg/m^2).

Deferasirox: *Dosage*: Start with 20 mg/kg orally once daily calculated to nearest whole tab. Adjust dose in increments of 5-10 mg/kg every 3-6 months based on ferritin levels (maximum 30 mg/kg/day since there is limited experience at higher doses.

Deferiprone: *Dosage*: Oral—more than 6 years 25 mg/kg/dose rounded to the nearest 250 mg dose 3 times daily (maximum 100 mg/ kg/day).

Deflazacort: *Dosage*: Oral 1 month-12 years 250 µg-1.5 mg/kg; 12-18 years 2-18 mg once daily. Up to 2.4 mg/kg may be used. 2 days dose could be taken as single dose on alternate days.

Desferrioxamine mesylate: *Dosage*:

Acute iron poisoning—Oral (injection given orally through NG tube as very bitter) 1 month–12 years 5 g and 12–18 years 5–10 g in 50–100 mL water. IM 1 month–12 years 1 g and 12–18 years 2 g repeated 8 hourly if necessary. IV continuous infusion—initially 15 mg/kg/ hour reducing after 4–6 hours as indicated so that total maximum dose does not exceed 80 mg/kg/day. Continue until serum iron is less than total iron binding capacity (TIBC).

Pathological iron overload—IV or SC infusion using pump over 8–12 hours—1 month–12 year 20 mg/kg and 12–18 years 500 mg at least 6 days in a week. Maintenance doses proportional to iron excretion rate. Not to exceed 50 mg/kg/dose.

Monitoring—Ferritin levels may be used to monitor the ideal dose of deferoxamine (DFO) for a given patient, by using the "therapeutic index" (T1):1 = mean daily dose (mg/kg)/serum ferritin (mg/L). The mean daily dose of DFO is calculated by multiplying the dose administered in each treatment by the total number of doses administered per week, divided by 7 (the no. of days in a week). The target is to maintain T1 under 0.025 at all times. IV infusion over 24 hours for high dose therapy, if cardiac damage due to iron overload is present-up to 180 mg/kg in 1 month–12 years.

Aluminum overload in dialysis patients—IV infusion at 5 mg/kg once weekly via fistula over last hour of hemodialysis or hemofiltration for 3 months. Reassess aluminum levels 4–8 weeks after completing course. Give IV, IM, SC or IP prior to last exchange of the day for continuous ambulatory peritoneal dialysis (CAPD) or continuous cycling peritoneal dialysis (CCPD).

Desloratadine: *Dosage*: Oral 2–5 years 1.25 mg; 6–11 years 2.5 mg; 12–18 years 5 mg once daily.

Desmopressin: *Dosage*:

Nocturnal enuresis—Intranasal in children more than 5 years 20 µg once at night half dose in each nostril for 3 months and then reassess by stopping for 1 week. Increase if necessary to 40 µg (20 µg in each nostril).

Assessment of ADH secretion—Intranasal 1–5 µg as single dose. Infants with congenital antidiuretic hormone (ADH) deficiency are very sensitive to desmopressin and dose may need to be reduced to 1/10th of mentioned dose.

Test dose for suspected diabetes insipidus—Intranasal 1 month–2 years 5–10 µg, 2–12 years 10–20 µg, and 12–18 years 20 µg. Restrict fluid input to maximum 1.5 times the urine volume from start of hydration phase to the test. Please refer to an expert for testing.

Established diabetes insipidus—Birth—1 month 1.25–5 µg, 1 month–2 years 2.5–5 µg, 2–12 years 5–20 µg, 12–18 years 10–20 µg 1–2 times daily. Individual dose titration required.

Mild-to-moderate hemophilia A and Von Willebrandt disease—Intranasal more than 1 year 4 µg/kg as single dose preoperatively—2 hours before procedures. IV more than 1 year 300 ng/kg diluted in 30–50 mL of 0.9% NaCl over 20 minutes, immediately before surgery—repeated after 12 hours, if there is no tachycardia.

Aspirin-induced platelet dysfunction—0.3 g/kg diluted in saline IV, or 150 g intranasally by metered dose spray. Adolescents may be given 300 g intranasally.

Dexamethasone: *Dosage*:

Croup—Oral 150 µg/kg/dose twice a day or 600 µg/kg as single daily dose up to maximum of 12 mg/day.

Antiemetic with chemotherapy—IV/oral per dose less than 1 year 250 µg–1 mg, 1–5 years 1–2 mg, 6–12 years 2–4 mg, and 12–18 years 4 mg thrice daily until 48 hours after chemotherapy.

Headache of increased intracranial tension (ICT)—IV/oral 250 µg/kg/dose 2 times daily for 5 days and then reduce the dose to 62.5–125 µg/kg/dose twice daily.

Brain tumor edema—IV/oral 125–500 µg/kg/dose 2 times daily.

Replacement—IV/oral 250–500 µg/m^2/dose 2 times daily.

Fetal lung maturation—Given to mother IM 12 mg repeated once after 24 hours and orally 6 mg twice daily for 4 doses.

Bronchopulmonary dysplasia—250 µg/kg IV/oral twice daily for 3 days, course repeated once every 10 days until baby is no longer oxygen dependent or 500 µg/kg once daily for 3 days and tapered over 6 weeks to 100 µg/kg on alternate day during the last week.

Post-intubation laryngeal edema—200 µg/kg IV/oral 8th hourly for three doses starting 4 hours before extubation.

Cerebral edema—Initially less than 35 kg 20 mg and more than 35 kg 24 mg, followed by 1–3rd day 4 mg q3h (<35 kg) and 4 mg q2h (>35 kg), 4th day 4 mg q6h (<35 kg) and 4 mg q4h (>35 kg), 5–8th day 2 mg q6h (<35 kg) and 4 mg q6h (>35 kg), and thereafter taper.

Eye drops—1 drop 4–6 hourly. Severe conditions—apply hourly till condition improves and then reduce to 4–6 hourly.

Eye ointment—Small amount into conjunctival sac 3–4 times daily or only at bedtime along with drops during daytime.

Congenital adrenal hyperplasia—0.25–0.5 mg once daily. The drug should be used only after epiphyseal fusion so as to avoid adverse effects on growth.

Dexamphetamine sulfate: *Dosage*: Oral initially 3–5 years 2.5 mg, >6 years 5–10 mg 1–2 times daily. Increase if required <6 years 2.5 mg a day at weekly intervals (maximum 20 mg/day)

doses, 6–12 years 40–150 mg/24 hours, more than 12 years 50–400 mg/24 hours.

Domperidone: *Dosage*:

Gastroesophageal reflux and gastric stasis—Oral 1 month–12 years 200–400 µg/kg/dose 3–4 times daily before food and at night. Not often used less than 2 years.

Radiotherapy/chemotherapy induced vomiting—Oral 1 month–12 years 200–400 µg/kg as single dose. Could give once in 4–8 hours.

Dopamine hydrochloride: *Dosage*: Continuous low dose IV infusion for renal effect 2–5 µg/kg/min IV infusion in newborn—start at 3 µg/kg/min and increase as clinically indicated to maximum of 20 µg/kg/min IV infusion; 1 month–18 years 5–20 µg/kg/min. Continuous low-dose IV infusion exerts effect on dopaminergic receptors which are present in renal, splanchnic, and coronary vascular beds producing vasodilatation. These effects are not antagonized by beta-blockers. The increased renal blood flow results in diuresis and natriuresis. At higher doses, 5–10 µg/kg/min, it is a pure β-agonist, producing positive inotropic effect on the heart. At doses of >10 µg/kg/min, it exerts α-agonistic action, resulting in vasoconstriction. The usual starting dose is 5 µg/kg/min; increased gradually, if required, up to a maximum of 20 µg/kg/min.

Dothiepin (Dosulepin hydrochloride): *Dosage*: Oral 12–18 years 50–75 mg at bedtime or in divided doses. Increase gradually as needed up to 150 mg/day. In hospital setting maximum 225 mg/day may be used.

Doxapram: *Dosage*: IV loading dose 2.5 mg/kg over 5–10 minutes IV infusion 300 µg/kg/hour (maximum 1.5 mg/kg/hour-side effects, if infused for >36 hours). Oral 6 mg/kg per dose 4 times daily after an IV dose.

Doxorubicin hydrochloride: *Dosage*: Always consult the current treatment protocol for details of dosage and scheduling. Children—35–75 mg/m^2/dose repeat every 21 days; or 20–30 mg/m^2 repeat every week; or 60–90 mg/m^2 given as continuous infusion over 96 hours once in 3–4 weeks.

Hepatic impairment—Reduce dose. If bilirubin 1.2–3 mg reduce by 50% and if bilirubin >3 mg reduce dose by 75%.

Doxycycline: *Dosage*:

Amebiasis, actinomycosis, brucellosis—>8 years age—*IV:* 45 kg or less: *Initial dose:* 4.4 mg/kg IV on the first day, given in 1 or 2 infusions; *Maintenance dose:* 2.2–4.4 mg/kg IV per day, given in 1 or 2 infusions, depending on the severity of the infection. >45 kg: Initial dose: 200 mg IV on the first day, given in 1 or 2 infusions. *Maintenance dose:* 100–200 mg IV per day, depending on the severity of the infection; 200 mg may be given in 1 or 2 infusions.

Oral: 45 kg or less: *Initial dose:* 4.4 mg/kg orally on the first day, given in two divided doses. *Maintenance dose:* 2.2 mg/kg orally per day, given once a day or in two divided doses.

More severe infections: Up to 4.4 mg/kg orally per day. More than 45 kg: Initial dose: 200 mg orally on the first day, given in two or four divided doses; *Maintenance dose:* 100 mg orally per day, given once a day or in two divided doses; *More severe infections:* 100 mg orally every 12 hours.

Acne—Initial dose: 100 mg orally twice a day for 3–6 weeks or until improvement occurs. *Maintenance dose:* 50–150 mg orally once a day.

Cholera—Single dose of 4 mg/kg (maximum 200 mg).

Multidrug resistant P. falciparum (resistant to both chloroquine and sulfadoxine-pyrimethamine)—with Quinine at 3.5 mg/kg once a day for 7 days.

Malaria prophylaxis-Short-term chemoprophylaxis (less than 6 weeks): 100 mg daily in adults and 1.5 mg/kg body weight for children more than 8-year-old. The drug should be started 2 days before travel and continued for 4 weeks after leaving the malarious area.

Uncomplicated urethral, endocervical, or rectal infections due to C. trachomatis—100 mg orally twice a day for 7 days.

Uncomplicated gonorrhea—100 mg orally twice a day for 7 days.

Periodontitis—20 mg orally twice a day for up to 9 months.

Plague—8 years or older: <45 kg: 2.2 mg/kg IV twice a day (maximum 200 mg/day); 45 kg or more: 100 mg IV twice a day. Duration of therapy: 10 days (or until 2 days after fever subsides).

Mycoplasma pneumonia—100 mg orally or IV every 12 hours for 10 to 21 days.

Rocky Mountain spotted fever, relapsing fever, or typhus—100 mg orally or IV twice a day for 7 days.

Trachoma—100 mg orally twice a day for 7 days.

Tularemia—100 mg orally or IV twice a day for 14 to 21 days.

Anthrax postexposure prophylaxis—<45 kg: 2.2 mg/kg orally or IV twice a day; 45 kg or more: 100 mg orally or IV twice a day. Total duration of therapy: 60 days after exposure.

Uncomplicated urethral, endocervical, or rectal infections due to C. trachomatis—8 years or older: 100 mg orally twice a day for 7 days.

E

Econazole: *Dosage*: Apply 2–3 times daily continuing for 14 days after lesions have healed.

Edrophonium chloride: *Dosage*:

Myasthenia gravis-for diagnosis—IV Birth–12 years 20 µg/kg followed 30 seconds later (if no adverse reaction noted) by remaining dose of 80 µg/kg; 12–18 years 2 mg and then 8 mg.

Cholinergic drug—To differentiate between under/overdosing—IV given 1 hour after cholinergic 1 month–12 years 20 µg/kg and 12–18 years 2 mg. In underdosing muscle strength increases transiently and in overdosing muscle strength decreases transiently.

Nondepolarizing muscular blockade antagonist—IV 1 month–18 years 500–700 µg/kg slowly over several minutes along with 7 µg/kg of atropine.

Efavirenz: *Dosage*: Children less than 3 years: There are no pharmacokinetic data available on the appropriate dose of efavirenz in children less than 3 years.

Treatment of HIV infection—Children PO ≥ to 3 years, 32.5–39.9 kg: 400 mg, 25–32.4 kg: 350 mg, 20–24.9 kg: 300 mg, 15–19.9 kg: 250 mg, 10–14.9 kg: 200 mg, ≥ 40 kg: 600 mg PO once daily at bedtime. For children who can swallow capsules combine efavirenz with either: (1) zidovudine plus lamivudine, emtricitabine, or didanosine or (2) didanosine plus lamivudine or emtricitabine. Adolescents >40 kg: 600 mg PO once daily at bedtime. Combine efavirenz with lamivudine or emtricitabine plus either zidovudine or tenofovir.

HIV postexposure prophylaxis—The Centers for Disease Control and Prevention (CDC) recommends that efavirenz once daily at bedtime (or nelfinavir, indinavir, or abacavir) be added to the basic 2-drug regimen in situations where exposure is associated with an increased risk of HIV transmission (e.g. severe percutaneous exposure (e.g. large-bore hollow needle, deep puncture, visible blood on device, or needle used in patient's artery or vein) from a Class 1 or 2 HIV+ source; or a large volume exposure to mucous membranes or nonintact skin exposures from a Class 2 HIV+ source; or if the source person's virus is known or suspected to be resistant to one or more antiretrovirals. In all cases, therapy should be initiated as soon as possible and continued for 4 weeks. Although animal studies suggest postexposure prophylaxis started >24–36 hours following exposure is substantially less effective, the interval after which no benefit is derived for humans is undefined. Therefore, if appropriate for the exposure, prophylaxis should be started even when the interval following exposure is >36 hours. The dose is the same as for treatment of HIV given above.

Patients with hepatic impairment—Dosing in patients with hepatic impairment has not been studied. Patients with renal impairment: No dosage adjustment is required.

Emollients: *Dosage*: All ages—Apply on affected areas as needed to prevent skin from drying out. 250–500 g required weekly for generalized dry skin in child.

Enalapril: *Dosage*: Neonate—Oral 0.1 mg/kg/24 hours in 1–2 doses (maximum 0.4 mg/kg/24 hours); IV 5–10 µg/kg/dose every 8–24 hours. 1 month–12 years—Oral 0.1–0.5 mg/kg/24 hours in 1–2 doses; IV 5–10 µg/kg/dose every 8–24 hours. 12–18 years. Oral 2.5–5 mg/24 hours and titrate to maximum 40 mg/24 hours in two divided doses; IV 0.625–1.25 mg/dose 4 times daily (maximum 20 mg/24 hours).

Antiproteinuric—Infant and child: 0.1–0.6 mg/kg/24 hours PO, increase PRN over 2 weeks, up to 5 mg/24 hours in 2–4 divided doses. IV: 0.005–0.01 mg/kg/dose 3–4 times/day, administer over 5 minutes, up to 5.0 mg 6th hourly may be tolerated for up to 36 hours. Onset of action within 15 minutes.

Enoxaparin: *Dosage*: *See Heparin also.*

Thromboembolic disease Prophylaxis—SC less than 2 months 1.5 mg/kg/day and more than 2 months 1 mg/kg/day in two divided doses (maximum 40 mg/day).

Treatment—<2 months 3 mg/kg/day and >2 months 2 mg/kg/day in two divided doses.

Ephedrine hydrochloride: *Dosage*: Intranasal 1–2 drops in each nostril 3–4 times daily (15 minutes before feeds) for maximum of 7 days.

Epirubicin hydrochloride: *Dosage*: Always consult current treatment protocols for details of dosage and scheduling.

Epoprostenol (Prostacyclin): *Dosage*: Neonate—IV infusion 20 ng/kg/min (maximum 40 ng/kg/min)—monitor for systemic hypotension. Children IV infusion 2 ng/kg/min (maximum 40 ng/kg/min)—monitor for systemic hypotension.

Ergocalciferol (Calciferol, vitamin D2): *Dosage*: Oral >6 months 3,000 units, 6 months–12 years 6,000 units and 12–18 years 10,000 units as single dose.

Erythromycin: *Dosage*: See *Lincosamines and Streptogramins as well.*

General indications: Neonates—Orally/IV—<7 days age 20 mg/kg/day 2 times daily; >7 days <1,200 g 20 mg/kg/day 2 times daily; more than 7 days more than 1,200 g 30 mg/kg/day 3–4 times daily. *Children:* Orally—30–50 mg/kg/day in 3–4 divided doses maximum 250 mg 4 times daily may be given. *12–18 years*—250–500 mg 4 times daily. IV—1 month–18 years 12.5 mg/kg/dose 4 times daily or as a continuous infusion. Maximum dose—4 g/day. Replace by oral dosage as soon as possible.

Special indications: Topical (acne vulgaris)—Wash and apply twice daily directly to the affected area.

Secondary prevention of rheumatic fever—When child is sensitive to penicillin—oral 20 mg/kg/ day maximum 500 mg twice daily (Contraindicated in liver disorder).

Chlamydia trachomatis pneumonia in infants and neonates—Oral—50 mg/kg/day (erythromycin base) in four divided doses for 14 days.

Ophthalmia neonatorum caused by Chlamydia trachomatis—Neonates—Oral-50 mg/kg/day in four divided doses for 14 days. If chlamydial conjunctivitis recurs after discontinuing therapy, the erythromycin dosage regimen should be repeated.

Group A beta-hemolytic streptococcal (GAS) pharyngitis (primary rheumatic fever prophylaxis as an alternative to penicillin in children allergic to penicillin)—40 mg/kg/day in four divided doses × 10 days.

Uncomplicated urethral, endocervical, or rectal gonorrhea, penicillinase—producing. Neisseria gonorrhoeae, or for gonorrhea during pregnancy—Adolescent: 500 mg PO 4 times per day for 7 days.

Treatment and postexposure pertussis prophylaxis—For postexposure prophylaxis, administer to close contacts within 3 weeks of exposure, especially in high-risk patients (e.g. women in 3rd trimester, infants < 12 months). *Oral dosage:* Infants, children, and adolescents: 40–50 mg/kg/day PO (maximum 2 g/day) in four divided doses for 14 days. For neonates: Azithromycin is the preferred. If azithromycin is unavailable, erythromycin 40–50 mg/kg/day PO in 4 divided doses may be used. Monitor for infantile hypertrophic pyloric stenosis.

Pneumococcal prophylaxis—1 month–2 years 250 mg/day, 2–8 years 500 mg/day, more than 9 years 1 g/day in two divided doses.

Gastric stasis—Oral/IV—1 month–18 years—3 mg/kg 4 times daily.

Erythropoietin (Recombinant human epoetin): *Dosage*: Start at 50–300 U/kg/dose thrice per week. For children receiving hemodialysis up to 450 U/kg/dose 2–3 times per week; 25–100 units/kg SC/IV 3 times in a week. Monitor the hemoglobin (Hb) at least twice weekly after drug initiation until the Hb stabilizes. In addition, monitor the Hb twice weekly for 2–6 weeks following any dosage adjustment. Any clinically significant change in Hb or hematocrit (HCT) following a dosage adjustment of epoetin-alfa may take 2–6 weeks. Reduce dose by approximately 25% if rise in Hb concentration exceeds 2 g/dL over 4 weeks or if Hb concentration exceeds 12 g/dL; if Hb concentration continues to rise, despite dose reduction, suspend treatment until Hb concentration decreases and then restart at a dose approximately 25% lower than the previous dose.

Epoetin-alfa and Epoetin-zeta—Symptomatic anemia associated with chronic renal failure (CRF) in children on hemodialysis—injection over 1–5 minutes—Child 1 month–18 years—initially 50 units/kg 3 times weekly adjusted according to response in steps of 25 units/kg 3 times weekly at intervals of at least 4 weeks; maintenance dose—less than 10 kg usually 75–150 units/kg 3 times weekly, 10–30 kg usually 60–150 units/kg 3 times weekly, more than 30 kg usually 30–100 units/kg 3 times weekly.

Esomeprazole: *Dosage*:

NSAID-associated duodenal ulcer |NSAID-associated gastric ulcer—Oral: Child (body-weight up to 30 kg): 0.5–1 mg/kg once daily (max. per dose 15 mg once daily), doses to be taken in the morning; Child (body-weight 30 kg and above): 15–30 mg once daily, doses to be taken in the morning

Gastroesophageal reflux disease—Oral: Child (body-weight up to 30 kg): 0.5–1 mg/kg once daily (max. per dose 15 mg once daily), doses to be taken in the morning; Child (body-weight 30 kg and above): 15–30 mg once daily, doses to be taken in the morning

Acid-related dyspepsia—Oral: Child (body-weight up to 30 kg): 0.5–1 mg/kg once daily (max. per dose 15 mg once daily), doses to be taken in the morning; Child (body-weight 30 kg and above): 15–30 mg once daily, doses to be taken in the morning

Fat malabsorption despite pancreatic enzyme replacement therapy in cystic fibrosis—Oral: Child (body-weight up to 30 kg): 0.5–1 mg/kg once daily (max. per dose 15 mg once daily), doses to be taken in the morning; Child (body-weight 30 kg and above): 15–30 mg once daily, doses to be taken in the morning.

Patients with hepatic impairment: No dosage adjustment is recommended for mild-to-moderate hepatic impairment. However, in patients with severe hepatic insufficiency, do not exceed 20 mg/day.

Patients with renal impairment: No dosage adjustment is necessary.

Intermittent hemodialysis: No dosage adjustment is necessary. Due to high-protein binding, esomeprazole is not expected to be removed by hemodialysis.

Etanercept: *Dosage*: All patients should have their varicella antibody status measured before commencing treatment. Siblings should be considered for varicella immunization prior to commencement of treatment of the patient. Patients in contact with varicella should be considered for treatment with varicella zoster immunoglobulin (VZIG), if their varicella titers are negative. Patients with a significant exposure to varicella should have their etanercept therapy temporarily discontinued. SC more than 4 years 400 µg/kg twice weekly at 72–96 hours interval (maximum 25 mg/dose).

Ethambutol: *Dosage*: *Tuberculosis—Daily regimen*–20 mg/kg as single morning dose (Range 15–25 mg/kg; maximum dose 1,500 mg/day); *Intermittent regimen*—30 mg/kg (Range 25–30 mg/kg).

Ethinyl estradiol: *Dosage*:

Induction of puberty—12–18 years 2 µg daily once. Increase every 6 months 5, 10 and then 20 µg. Add progestogen after 18–24 months. Maintenance 20 µg combined with progestogen.

Prevention of tall stature—Oral 20–50 µg before 12 years age.

Priming for growth hormone test in girls with bone age more than 10 years—Oral 100 μg as single dose for 3 days prior to test (diethylstilbestrol 1 mg twice is alternative for boys and girls).

Ethionamide: *Dosage*: *Tuberculosis*—Oral—15–20 mg/kg/day in two divided doses. Maximum 1 g/day.

Ethosuximide: *Dosage*: Oral—Start with 5 m/kg in 2–12 years old and 250 mg in older children. Increase at 2.5 mg/kg/dose taking 2–3 weeks to reach maintenance of 10–20 mg/kg/dose in 2–12 years old and 500–750 g/dose (maximum 1 g) 2 times daily.

Etoposide: *Dosage*: Always consult current protocol for dosage and scheduling.

Etoricoxib: *Dosage*: Only for 16–18 years age, orally—

Osteoarthritis: 30 mg once daily, increased ifnecessary to 60 mg once daily

Rheumatoid arthritis and ankylosing spondylitis: 90 mg once daily

Acute gout: 120 mg once daily for maximum 8 days.

Hepatic impairment: Maximum 60 mg daily in mild impairment; maximum 60 mg on alternate days or 30 mg once daily in moderate impairment.

Renal impairment: Avoid if estimated glomerular filtration rate less than 30 mL/min/1.73 m^2.

Extended spectrum penicillins (Ampicillin/amoxicillin): *Dosage:* Dose—Orally 20–40 mg/kg/day in 2–3 divided doses. Higher dose of 80 mg/kg/day may be required for otitis media (Maximum of 500 mg 2–3 times daily).

In streptococcal tonsillitis: 750 mg once daily

In uncomplicated gonorrhea: 3 g with 1 g probenecid are recommended.

F

Factor IX: *Dosage*: Dose should always be tailored to clinical effectiveness in each individual. The number of units needed and the duration of treatment depend on the condition being treated. *Dosage:* The 20–25 units/kg/dose up to once daily. In Factor VIII inhibitor patients 75–100 units/kg/dose up to 6 hourly.

Factor VIII: *Dosage*: The dose and dosing schedule for factor VIII must be calculated and adjusted according to the needs of the individual patient, taking into account the patient's body weight, the degree of factor VIII deficiency, the site and extent of the bleeding, the titer of inhibitors, the factor VIII level desired and the clinical condition. The required dosage may be estimated using the following formula as a guide: Number of factor VIII units required = Body weight (kg) × desired increase (International units) in factor VIII × 0.5 (% of normal).

Famotidine: *Dosage*: Infants and children: Less than 16 years—Oral/IV.

Peptic ulcer—0.5 mg/kg/day at bedtime or in two divided doses (maximum 40 mg/day).

Gastroesophageal reflux disease (GERD): 1 mg/kg/day in 2 divided doses (maximum 80 mg/day). IV—20 mg 12th hourly.

16–18 years: Oral. *Duodenal/gastric ulcer:* 20 mg/day at bedtime or 10 mg twice daily for 4–8 weeks—maximum 40 mg/day.

Hypersecretory conditions: 20 mg 6 hourly and may gradually increase up to 160 mg 6 hourly.

Esophagitis: 20–40 mg twice daily for up to 12 weeks.

GERD—20 twice daily for up to 6 wks. IV—20 mg 12th hourly.

Dose adjustment in renal impairment—Creatinine Cl 10–50 mL/min: Administer normal dose once daily or 50% of dose at normal dose interval. Creatinine Cl less than 10 mL/min administer normal dose once in 36–48 hours.

Felbamate: *Dosage*:

Children 2–14 years with Lennox-Gastaut syndrome: Adjunct therapy—initially 15 mg/kg/day in 3–4 divided doses and to increase in 15 mg/kg/day increments at weekly intervals till response is obtained; maximum 45 mg/kg/day or 3,600 mg/day whichever is less.

Children >14 year: Adjunct therapy—initially 1,200 mg/day in 3–4 divided doses and increase daily dose by 1,200 mg once every week to maximum of 3,600 mg/day.

Conversion to monotherapy—Initially 1,200 mg/day in 3–4 divided doses and from week 2 increase daily dose by 1,200 mg once every week to maximum of 3,600 mg/day. Decrease dose of other anticonvulsants by 1/3rd original dose when felbamate is started and at week 2, when felbamate dose is increased. Continue to reduce other anticonvulsants as clinically indicated.

Fenofibrate: *Dosage*: Experience in children is limited; refer to an expert.

Fentanyl: *Dosage*:

For pain relief—Neonates and infants—IV 1–4 μg/kg/dose, repeat every 2–4 hours or continuous infusion 0.5–5 μg/kg/hour. 1–12 year IM/IV 1–3 μg/kg/dose, repeat every 30–60 minutes or continuous infusion 1–5 μg/kg/hour. 12–18 year 0.5–1 μg/kg/dose, repeat every 30–60 minutes.

Anesthesia—IV/IM 2–50 μg/kg.

Fexofenadine hydrochloride: *Dosage*:

Seasonal allergic rhinitis—Tabs >6 years, suspension 2–11 years, Dose—2–11 years 30 mg, 12–18 years 60 mg 2 times daily/120 mg daily once.

Chronic idiopathic urticaria: Tabs >6 years, suspension 6 months–11 years. Oral 6 months–2 years–15 mg, 2–11 years 30 mg twice daily and 12–18 years—180 mg once daily.

For pediatric patients with decreased renal function, the recommended starting dose of fexofenadine is 30 mg once daily for patients 2–11 years of age and 15 mg once daily for patients 6 months to less than 2 years of age. The pharmacokinetics of fexofenadine in subjects with hepatic disease does not differ substantially from that observed in healthy subjects.

Flecainide acetate: *Dosage*:

Supraventricular arrhythmias—By mouth using modified-release medicines. Child 12–17 years: 200 mg daily.

Resistant re-entry supraventricular tachycardia, ventricular ectopic beats or ventricular tachycardia, arrhythmias associated with accessory conduction pathways (e.g. Wolff-Parkinson-White syndrome), paroxysmal atrial fibrillation—by mouth using immediate-release medicines. *Neonate:* 2 mg/kg 2–3 times a day, adjusted according to response, also adjust dose according to plasma flecainide concentration. *Child 1 month–11 years:* 2 mg/kg 2–3 times a day, adjusted according to response, also adjust dose according to plasma-flecainide concentration; maximum 8 mg/kg per day; maximum 300 mg per day. *Child 12–17 years:* Initially 50–100 mg twice daily; increased, if necessary up to 300 mg daily, maximum 400 mg daily for ventricular arrhythmias in heavily built children.

Fluconazole: *Dosage*:

Newborn—Systemic candidiasis and cryptococcosis—Oral/IV 6–12 mg/kg every 72 hours in less than 14 day, every 48 hours in 14–28 day and every 24 hours in more than 28 days old.

Mucosal candidiasis—3 mg/kg in same intervals.

Children—Mucosal candidiasis—Oral/IV loading dose 6 mg/kg followed by 3 mg/kg once daily for 7–14 days.

Systemic candidiasis and cryptococcosis—6–12 mg/kg daily once (maximum 400 mg)-dose dependent on severity of infection.

Prophylaxis of fungal infection in immunocompromised—3–12 mg/kg once daily (maximum 400 mg) dose dependent on extent and duration of neutropenia.

Flucytosine: *Dosage*: Newborn—IV/oral 100 mg/kg/day less than 7 days and 100–200 mg/kg/day more than 7 days in four divided doses. Children IV/oral 200 mg/kg/day (100–140 mg/kg/day if organism sensitive) in 4 divided doses. *In renal impairment*—CrCl in mL/min/1.73 m^2—20–40 50% daily dose in two divided doses; 10–20, 25% of daily dose once daily; < 10 50 mg/kg as single dose and adjust dose according to serum levels.

Fludrocortisone acetate: *Dosage*:

Adrenal insufficiency—Oral replacement therapy—50–200 µg once daily according to potassium and/or plasma renin activity levels. Higher doses are usually required in the neonatal period (Start with 100 µg once daily and increase up to 200 µg daily).

Sweat test—3 mg/m^2 single dose on two consecutive days prior to sweat test.

Cerebral salt wasting—Start with 100 µg daily and increase up to 200–300 µg according to response.

Flumazenil: *Dosage*: Dosage description—IV bolus over 15 seconds <12 years 10 µg/kg (maximum 200 µg) and >12 years 200 µg as single dose, repeated every minute to maximum total dose of 40 µg/kg. IV infusion <12 years 2–10 µg/kg/hour (maximum 400 µg dose/hour) and more than 12 years 100–400 µg/kg/hour.

Flunarizine: *Dosage*: Oral 3–12 years 5 mg and more than 12 years 10 mg daily once. Dose reduction required in liver impairment.

Flunisolide: *Dosage*: Intranasal 5–12 years 1 spray in each nostril up to 3 times daily and 12–18 years 2 sprays in each nostril up to 2–3 times daily.

Fluoride (Sodium fluoride, stannous fluoride): *Dosage*: *Oral drops and tablets—(*where water fluoride centration <0.3 ppm/300 µg/L) 6 month–3 years 250 µg F/day, 3–6 years 500 µg F/day, >6 years 1 mg F/day. Doses are expressed as fluoride ion (F). If water fluoride concentration 0.3–0.7 ppm use ½ dose in more than 3 years old and no fluoride required in <3 years old.

Gel—(for children > 3 years old) Applied with toothbrush over all surfaces of tooth after normal cleansing with toothpaste. Then gently rubbed over tooth surface for 1 minute before spitted out excess. No food/drink for 30 minutes after use for best effect.

Fluoxetine: *Dosage*:

Depression—Oral 6–18 years 10 mg once daily, gradually increase over 3 weeks to 20 mg once daily.

Bulimia—Oral 12–18 years 60 mg once daily.

Obsessive compulsive disorder (OCD) and anxiety—Oral 6–8 years 10 mg and 8–18 years 20 mg once daily. Gradually increase by 10–20 mg increments once in 2 weeks, if required (maximum 60 mg/day).

Idiopathic musculoskeletal pain—8–12 years 10 mg and 12–18 years 20 mg once daily.

Fluticasone propionate: *Dosage*: Inhaled—2–4 years 50–100 µg, 4–16 years 50–200 µg, >16 years 100 µg–1 mg 2 times daily. Starting dose appropriate for severity of disease adjusted to attain control and then reduced to minimal effective dose according to individual response.

Nebulized—1 mg 2 times daily for acute exacerbation of asthma.

Intranasal—4–12 years 50 µg (1 spray) in each nostril, 100 µg (2 sprays) in each nostril twice daily for allergic rhinitis.

Skin ointment/cream: Treatment of alopecia areata, atopic dermatitis, discoid lupus erythematosus, eczema (including hyperkeratotic eczema, nummular eczema, and severe eczematous conditions of the hands or feet), generalized exfoliative dermatitis, cutaneous lichen planus, lichen simplex chronicus, lichen striatus, nodular prurigo, pompholyx (dyshidrosis), pemphigus, polymorphous light eruption, psoriasis, seborrheic dermatitis, severe contact dermatitis, and xerosis.

Note: Occlusive dressings may be required for chronic or severe cases of lichen simplex chronicus, psoriasis, eczema, atopic dermatitis, or chronic hand eczema. More potent topical corticosteroids and/or occlusive dressings may be necessary for the treatment of discoid lupus erythematosus, lichen planus, granuloma annulare, psoriatic plaques, and psoriasis of the palms, soles, elbows, or knees.

Adolescents: 0.005% ointment or 0.05% cream applied sparingly to the affected area twice daily. Each treatment course may continue for up to 4 weeks. In the treatment of psoriasis, studies suggest that patients respond preferentially to the 0.005% ointment. In the treatment of eczema, fluticasone cream 0.05% applied once daily is as effective as twice daily application.

Children and infants 3 months of age or more: Fluticasone cream 0.05% applied sparingly to the affected area once daily or twice daily. Only fluticasone cream 0.05% has been approved for the treatment of atopic dermatitis in this population. In clinical trials, the 0.05% cream has been applied once daily to children for the treatment of atopic dermatitis for up to 4 weeks.

Fluticasone/Salmeterol: *Dosage*: Aerosol inhaler starting with 125 µg and taper to 50 µg of fluticasone and double dose of dry powder inhaler.

Fluvoxamine maleate: *Dosage*: Oral 6–18 years—25–50 mg after food twice daily or 12–18 years 100 mg once daily—increasing to maximum doses of 300 mg/day needs to be under expert supervision as Indian children tolerate lesser doses than in the West.

Folic acid: *Dosage*:

Supplementation in folate deficiency in child; cofactor in metabolic disorders, e.g. homocystinuria—Birth—12 years 250 µg/kg and 12–18 years 5–10 mg, once daily for 6 months if cause correctable and lifelong if uncorrectable.

Megaloblastic anemia due to folate deficiency—Oral newborn—1 mg, <1 year 500 µg/kg, 1–18 years 5 mg daily once for 4 months.

Hemolytic anemias—Oral <12 years 2.5 mg and 12–18 year 10 mg once daily.

To limit methotrexate associated side effects when it is used for juvenile idiopathic arthritis (JIA)—Oral 2–18 years—1 mg once daily. Dose may be omitted on day methotrexate is given. May be given 5 mg weekly or twice weekly.

Newborn infant (birth to 1 month): Preterm babies fed heat-treated human milk may benefit from a 500 µg supplement once a week unless a suitable breast milk fortifier is used. Supplementation has no impact on the risk of anemia developing in other term or preterm breast or formula fed babies.

Formaldehyde: *Dosage*: Lotion—Apply topically at night as a soak. *Gel:* Apply twice daily directly to the wart and cover with plaster. Remove the outer dead layers with an emery board or pumice stone as the treatment progresses.

Formoterol fumarate: *Dosage*: Aerosol inhaler/turbohaler >6 years 6–12 µg 1–2 times daily; dry powder inhaler–12 µg 1–2 times daily. For regular prophylactic use, increase up to 24 µg twice in a day in severe obstruction.

Foscarnet sodium: *Dosage*:

Cytomegalovirus (CMV) disease—Retinitis (Ganciclovir-resistant/ immunocompromised patient)—IV infusion—1 month–18 years induction 60 mg/kg Q8H for 2–3 weeks, then maintenance 60 mg/kg daily, increased to 90–120 mg/kg, if tolerated; if disease progresses on maintenance dose, repeat induction regimen.

Mucocutaneous Herpes simplex infection—(acyclovir-resistant or in immunocompromised patient)—IV infusion—1 month–18 years—40 mg/kg Q8H for 2–3 weeks or until lesions heal.

Fosphenytoin: *Dosage*:

Generalized, convulsive status epilepticus or acute tonic clonic seizures—IV: Avoid IM for status epilepticus since therapeutic concentrations are not reached as fast as with the IV route. The full antiepileptic effect of phenytoin is not immediate; IV benzodiazepines (e.g. lorazepam or diazepam) should be given initially or concurrently.

Adolescents: In patients with unknown, undetectable, or low (i.e. ≤10 µg/mL) phenytoin concentrations, the usual loading dose of fosphenytoin is 15–20 mg PE/kg IV, not to exceed 150 mg PE/min IV rate. If seizures are not terminated after the initial loading dose, consider additional anticonvulsants. Some experts give an additional dose of 5–10 mg PE/kg IV if the initial loading dose fails to terminate seizures; maximum total loading dose 30 mg PE/kg. The initial maintenance dose is 4–6 mg PE/kg/day IV or IM, divided into two or more doses.

Children less than 12 years and infants: In patients with unknown, undetectable, or low (i.e. ≤10 µg/mL) phenytoin concentrations, the usual loading dose of fosphenytoin is 15–20 mg PE/kg IV, not to exceed 3 mg PE/kg/min (max: 150 mg PE/min) IV rate. If seizures are not terminated after the initial loading dose, consider additional anticonvulsants.

Intrathecal—1 month–4 years 5 mg, 4–15 years 10 mg and more than 15 years 20 mg once daily. Children with enlarged ventricles need higher doses. Adjust dose according to CSF levels aiming for a trough level of less than 10 mg/L.

Teicoplanin—*Newborn*—Loading 16 mg/kg and 24 hours later start maintenance 8 mg/kg/day as single dose; *Children*—10 mg/kg/dose 2 times daily × 3 doses and then once daily in same dose for severe infection and 6 mg/kg/day once for mod infection. Orally for *pseudomembranous colitis* 10 mg/kg/dose 2 times daily. May be given intraventricular and intraperitoneal. *See Teicoplanin below also.*

Glycopyrrolate (Glycopyrronium bromide): *Dosage*:

Premedication and intraoperative use—IM/IV more than 1 month 4–8 µg/kg as single dose (maximum 200 µg. Larger dose greater and prolonged antisialogogue effect).

Antagonism of neostigmine muscarinic effect—IV more than 1 month 10 µg/kg as single dose with 50 µg/kg neostigmine to reverse residual nondepolarizing neuromuscular block.

Controlling upper airway secretions—Oral 40–100 µg/kg/dose 3–4 times daily (oral dose is 10 times parenteral dose).

GM-CSF (Molgramostim): *Dosage*: Newborn—very limited studies–IV infusion over 2 hours 5 µg/kg as single dose.

Cytotoxic chemotherapy—SC 5–10 µg/kg starting 24 hours after last dose of chemotherapy and continue for 7–10 days.

Bone marrow transplant—IV infusion over 4–6 hours 10 µg/kg starting 24 hours the day after bone marrow transplant (BMT) and continue daily once till absolute neutrophil count is more than 1×10^9/L. Maximum duration of therapy 30 days.

Adjunct to ganciclovir therapy—SC 5 µg/kg daily once. After 5th dose to adjust dose to maintain desirable absolute neutrophil count.

Gonadotropin-releasing hormone (GnRH; LH-RH): *Dosage*: IV/SC 2.5 µg/kg (maximum 100 µg) as single dose.

Goserelin: *Dosage*: 3.6 mg every 4 weeks or 10.8 mg every 12 weeks. Injections may need to be given more frequently (e.g. every 3 weeks or every 10 weeks), if patients show signs of failure of hormone suppression.

Granisetron: *Dosage*: Oral—1 month–12 years—20 µg/kg/dose to a maximum of 1 mg; 12–18 years–1 mg administered 1–2 times with the first dose given 1 hour prior to starting chemotherapy. IV—1 month–12 years—40 µg/kg/dose to a maximum of 3 mg; 12–18 years—3 mg as a single dose just before administering chemotherapy. The one more dose may be given within a 24 hours period.

Griseofulvin: *Dosage*: 1 month–12 years 10 mg/kg and 12–18 years 500 mg once daily.

Growth Hormone: *See Somatropin.*

H

Haemophilus influenzae **type b vaccine (Hib):** *Dosage*: Given at 6–8, 10–12, and 14–16 weeks of age. Children 13–48 months and older children with asplenia who have not received the vaccine need receive only one dose to develop immunity.

Haloperidol: *Dosage*:

Schizophrenia, mania, and tic disorders including Tourette syndrome—2–12 years 25–50 µg/kg/day (maximum 10 mg/day) and 12–18 years 0.5–30 mg/day (maximum 60 mg/day) in two divided doses.

Intractable hiccup—12–18 years 1.5 mg 3 times daily. Adjust according to response. Nausea—12–18 years 0.5–2 mg 2–3 times daily.

Halothane: *Dosage*: *Induction of anesthesia*—inhaled through calibrated vaporizer—1/12 to 18 years—start with 0.5% and increase gradually as required to 2–5% mixed with O_2 or N_2O–O_2. Maintain with 0.5–2% halothane mixed with O_2, O_2-air or N_2O–O_2.

Heparin [Low molecular weight heparin (LMWH)]: *Dosage*: Majority of data in children is with enoxaparin. Other LMWHs are reviparin, dalteparin, and tinzaparin. Dose of enoxaparin is 1.5 mg/kg 12 hourly for less than 2 months (<5 kg) and 1 mg 12 hourly for older infants and children. For preterm babies a higher dose, up to 1.5–2 mg/kg 12 hourly, may be required.

Heparin (Standard or unfractionated): *Dosage*:

Thromboembolic disease and ECMO—50 units/kg IV bolus and 15–35 units/kg/hour continuous IV infusion maintenance dose [adjust to target activated partial thromboplastin time (aPTT) or heparin level].

Catheter patency—0.5–1 unit/mL as heparin lock. An IV bolus dose of 75–100 units/kg of heparin results in a therapeutic aPTT in 90% of children. Maintenance dose (as IV infusion) less than 2 months of age 28 units/kg/hour 2 month–1 year 25 units/kg/hour more than 1 year 20 units/kg/hour. Older children 18 units/kg/hour (same dose as for adults). Dosage in catheterization lab: 50–100 units/kg bolus IV or through arterial sheath.

Monitoring—Heparin dosing monograms have been validated in children. Many physicians use anti-Xa levels for infants or in critically ill children as aPTT may not be very predictive. In relatively stable infants and in older children, aPTT is used for monitoring as it is more easily performed and is widely available. If aPTT is less than 60 seconds, dose of heparin should be increased by 10% every 4–6 hours till aPTT is over 60 seconds. If aPTT exceeds 85 seconds, heparin dose should be decreased and if aPTT is more than 95 seconds, the heparin infusion should be stopped.

Hepatitis A and Hepatitis B vaccine (Combined): *Dosage*:

Primary vaccination schedule—This consists of three doses, the second being administered 1 month after the first dose and the third 6 months after the first dose (a dose in 0.5 mL of the pediatric preparation for children 1–15 years and 1 mL of the adult preparation for those >16 years). Once initiated, the primary course of vaccination should be completed with the same preparation.

Booster dose—There is increasing evidence that once a satisfactory serological response had been attained after hepatitis B vaccine, no boosters are necessary. Booster vaccination with the combined vaccine can be recommended from 5 years after initiation of the primary course. If the monovalent vaccines are used as boosters they can be administered 5 years after initiation of the primary course for hepatitis B and 10 years after initiation of the primary course for hepatitis A.

Hepatitis A vaccine: *Dosage*:

Primary vaccination schedule—This consists of two doses, the second being administered 6 months–1 year after the first dose (a dose is 0.5 mL of the pediatric preparation for children 1–15 years. An adult preparation is for those >16 years). Once initiated, the primary course of vaccination should be completed with the same preparation.

Hepatitis B immunoglobulin (HBIG): *Dosage*: Baby to be given 200 IU or 40 IU/kg of HBIG immediately after birth. Accelerated course of Hepatitis B vaccine to be started on opposite arm—0.1 month, 2 months, and 1 year doses given.

Other postexposure prophylaxis—Treatment depends on immunization status and whether exposure is significant, e.g. percutaneous needle prick, bite, mucocutaneous exposure to blood, unprotected sexual intercourse, etc.

Hepatitis B vaccine: *Dosage*: Either given at 6–8, 10–12, and 14–16 weeks of age (if HbsAg negativity of mother is certain) or 0, 4–6 weeks, and 14 weeks or 0, 4–6 weeks and 6 months.

Postexposure prophylaxis might require four doses 0, 1 month, 1 months, and 1 year (accelerated) or 0, 7, and 21 days and 1 year (super accelerated).

Human albumin solution: *Dosage*:

In hypovolemic shock 10–20 mL/kg bolus as rapidly as possible. Repeat as necessary. In trauma, these requirements may increase up to 40 mL/kg. At this level, replacement with whole blood should be considered.

Nephrotic syndrome—500 mg–1 g/kg over 4 hours with IV furosemide.

Human chorionic gonadotropin (hCG): *Dosage*:

Short stimulation test—IM 1,500–2,000 units daily once for 3 days (Testosterone and androgen profile at base line and on 4th day).

Prolonged simulation test—IM 1,500–2,000 units twice weekly for 3 weeks (Testosterone and androgen profile at base line and 4–6 days after final dose).

Hypogonadotropic hypogonadism—IM 1,000–2,000 units twice weekly in addition to testosterone.

Prepubertal cryptorchidism—1,000–2,000 units/m^2/dose 3 times a week for 3 weeks or 500 units 3 times a week for 4–6 weeks.

Human cytomegalovirus (CMV) immunoglobulin: *Dosage*: Doses of CMV immunoglobulin G need to be individualized to suit the patient. Typical dosage regimens are shown below.

Prophylaxis—200 mg/kg pretransplant; 100 mg/kg on days 7, 21, 42, and 63.

Treatment—200 mg/kg on days 1 and 7, given with appropriate antiviral therapy.

Human normal immunoglobulin (HNIG): *Dosage*:

Measles and poliomyelitis—IM less than 1 year 250 mg, 1–2 years 500 mg, 3 years or more 750 mg;

Hepatitis A— Less than 10 years 250 mg more than 10 years 500 mg;

Rubella in pregnancy—750 mg.

Human papillomavirus vaccine, quadrivalent (HPV vaccine, quadrivalent): *Dosage*: *General information on immunization against human papilloma virus (HPV)*—The vaccine can be given to females with abnormal Pap tests, a positive hybrid capture II high-risk test, or genital warts. Data from clinical trials do not indicate that the vaccine will have any therapeutic effect on existing Pap test abnormalities, HPV infection, or genital warts. However, the vaccine should be given to these patients as it will provide protection against infection with vaccine HPV types not already acquired. Lactating females and females who are immunocompromised can receive the HPV vaccine.

Females 9–12 years—Routine vaccination with 3 doses of the quadrivalent HPV vaccine is recommended for all females 11–12 years of age. The vaccination series can be initiated in females as young as 9 years of age.

Females 13–18 years—Catch-up vaccination is recommended for females 13–18 years old who have not been vaccinated previously or who have not completed the full series. Ideally, the vaccine should be administered prior to exposure to HPV through sexual contact.

The vaccine is not indicated for the treatment of HPV infection; cervical neoplasia; or cervical, vulvar, and vaginal precancers and lesions including genital warts.

The vaccine is not indicated for use in males.

Although it is recommend for immunocompromised females, the human papillomavirus vaccine, quadrivalent may not elicit an effective immune response in patients with immunosuppression such as people with acquired immunodeficiency syndrome (AIDS) or other clinical manifestations of human immunodeficiency virus (HIV) infection. As with other vaccines, concomitant use of immunosuppressive therapies including irradiation, antimetabolites, alkylating agents, cytotoxic drugs, and high-dose corticosteroid therapy may reduce the immune responses.

Intramuscular dosage—Female children, adolescents and adults aged 9–26 years: 0.5 mL/dose IM. Give the first dose at an elected date, the second dose 2 months after the first, and the third dose 6 months after the first dose.

Hyaluronidase: *Dosage*: Infants and children—

IV extravasation—SC or intradermal—reconstitute 150 unit vial of lyophilized powder in 1 mL NS; dilute 0.1 mL of this solution with 0.9 mL of NS to prepare a 15 unit/mL solution—with a 25 or 26 gauge needle, five 0.2 mL injections are made SC or intradermally into the extravasation site at the leading edge, changing the needle after each injection. In older adolescents, 150 units of hyaluronidase may be added to the vehicle containing the drug given IM or SC to increase its absorption and dispersion.

Hypodermoclysis—SC 15 units added to each 100 mL of IV fluid administered. In premature infants and neonates, the volume of a single clysis should not exceed 25 mL/kg and the rate of administration should not exceed 2 mL/min. In children less than 3 years and in more than 3 years up to adolescents the volume of a single clysis should not exceed 200 mL and maintenance IV fluid volume, respectively.

Hydralazine: *Dosage*: Oral less than 12 years 0.75 mg/kg/day in 2–3 divided doses and 12–18 years 50 mg in two divided doses. Increase if needed to maximum dose of 7.5 mg/kg/day or 200 mg/day. IV bolus over 20 min—less than 12 years 100–500 μg/kg and more than 12 years 5–10 mg as single dose. May be repeated up to 4–6 times daily. IV infusion—less than 12 years 12.5–50 μg/kg/hour and more than 12 years 3–5 mg/hour. In hepatic and renal impairment start with small doses or increase interval between doses.

Hydrochlorothiazide: *Dosage*: Neonates and infants—Oral 2–4 mg/kg/24 hours in two divided doses; more than 6 months–12 years 2 mg/kg/24 hour in two divided doses; 12–18 years 12.5–100 mg/24 hours.

Nephrogenic diabetes insipidus—Oral less than 12 years 3 mg/kg and more than 12 years 37.5–75 mg/day in three divided doses.

Hydrocortisone: *Dosage*: *Adrenocortical insufficiency—Adrenocortical crisis*—50 mg/m^2/day stat followed by 100 mg/m^2/day in four divided doses. Reduce to 75 mg/m^2/day on day 2 and 50 mg/m^2/day on day 3. Maintenance dose 8–15 mg/m^2/day.

Hydrocortisone 1%: *Dosage*:

Corticosteroid-responsive dermatoses—Topical: Nonprescription hydrocortisone preparations should not be used in children less than 2 years of age unless directed and supervised by a clinician. Children more than 2 years of age: Apply appropriate cream, lotion, ointment, or solution sparingly 1–4 times daily.

Oral lesions—Apply a small amount of paste to the lesion 2 or 3 times daily after meals and at bedtime. If substantial regeneration or repair of oral tissues does not occur after 7 days, further investigate etiology of the lesions.

Ulcerative colitis and anorectal disorders—Retention enema—adjunctive treatment of ulcerative colitis: 100 mg nightly. Some clinicians recommend 100 mg twice daily followed by 100 mg nightly when improvement occurs. Usually given for 21 days or until clinical and proctologic remissions are achieved.

Lie on the left side during and for 30 minutes after administration to distribute drug throughout the left colon. Retain for around 1 hour, preferably all night. Symptoms may improve in 3–5 days, followed by proctologic improvement. Discontinue if clinical or proctologic improvement does not occur within 2–3 weeks. Proctologic remission may require 2–3 months of therapy. Following treatment for more than 21 days, gradually withdraw use; give every other night for 2–3 weeks, then discontinue.

Rectal (as Foam)—Ulcerative proctitis of the distal rectum—90 mg (1 applicatorful of a 10% aerosol foam suspension) 1 or 2 times daily for 2–3 weeks. Then, if necessary, every other day until clinical and proctologic improvement. Symptoms may improve within 5–7 days.

Rectal (as Suppository)—Adjunctive treatment of ulcerative colitis of the rectum and other inflammatory conditions of the anorectum: 25 mg in the morning and at night for 2 weeks. *Severe proctitis:* 25 mg 3 times daily or 50 mg twice daily.

Hydrocortisone and gentamicin: *Dosage*: Ear—2–4 drops 3–4 times daily and at night. Alternatively, wicks medicated with the drops may be placed in the ear or mastoid cavity.

Hydrocortisone, neomycin and polymyxin: *Dosage*: Ear—Place 3 drops into the ear 3–4 times daily.

Hydroxocobalamin (Vitamin B_{12}): *Dosage*:

Vitamin B_{12} deficiency—IM 250 μg–1 mg 3 times weekly for 2 weeks followed by 250 μg once weekly till blood counts are normal and then 1 mg once in 2–3 months as maintenance dose.

Hydroxocobalamin-responsive inborn errors of metabolism—IM initially 1 mg daily for 5 days and assess response. If responsive continue maintenance at 1 mg once or twice a week. Oral up to 10 mg once or twice weekly. Oral may be started as soon as response to IM is confirmed but some patients do not respond to oral administration.

Hydroxychloroquine: *Dosage*: Oral 5–6.5 mg/kg (maximum 400 mg) once daily. Adjusted according to plasma levels in severe renal and hepatic impairment.

Hydroxyethyl starches: *Dosage*: Use in children is probably best restricted to an intensive care setting. Consult a consultant intensivist for dosage details. Has been tried in controlled trial in pediatric cardiac surgery. Administration is by IV infusion.

Hydroxytryptophan: *Dosage*: Given orally at a starting dose of 250–500 µg/kg 4 times daily and increased according to patient response, weight and CSF amine metabolic concentration up to maintenance dose of 2–2.5 mg/kg 4 times daily.

Hydroxyurea (Hydroxycarbamide): *Dosage*:

Sickle cell disease—(To reduce frequency of painful crises and the need for blood transfusions in children with recurrent moderate to severe painful crises)—10–20 mg/kg/day and doses titrated as tolerated. Increase at 5 mg/kg/day every 12 weeks according to response (maximum 35 mg/kg/ day).

Malignant glioma, astrocytoma, medulloblastoma, and primitive neuroectodermal tumors—1,500–3,000 mg/m2 orally as a single dose administered every 4–6 weeks—given in combination with other chemotherapeutic agents.

Acute myelogenous leukemia (AML)—For WBC over 1 L/mm^3, 50–75 mg/kg/day orally will cause a rapid decline in the WBC. Once the child is beyond the critical stage, conventional antileukemia therapy may be given. Dosage needs to be modified depending on clinical response and the degree of hepatic and renal impairment, but no quantitative recommendations are available. Safety and efficacy have not been established for use in children and adolescents but doses up to 3,000 mg/m^2 have been given orally for malignant glioma (off label).

Hydroxyzine: *Dosage*:

Pruritus—Oral 6 months–6 years 5–15 mg; 7–12 years 10–15 mg and 12–18 years 25 mg at bedtime. Increase if required to maximum dose of 50 mg/day in 6 months–6 years, 50–100 mg/day in 7–12 years and 100 mg/day in 12–18 years in 3–4 divided doses.

Anxiety—Oral 12–18 years 50–100 mg/dose 4 times daily. In renal impairment dose needs to be reduced by half.

Hyoscine butylbromide: *Dosage*: Oral 5–12 years 10 mg/dose and 12–18 years 20 mg/dose 3–4 times daily. IM/IV less than 6 years 5 mg/dose, 6–12 years 5–10 mg/dose and more than 12 years 20 mg/dose 3–4 times daily.

Hyoscine hydrobromide: *Dosage*: Oral 2–12 years 10 µg/kg and 12–18 years 300 µg 4 times daily.

I

Ibuprofen: *Dosage*:

Pain/fever—5–10 mg/kg/dose 3–4 times daily (maximum 20 mg/kg/day up to 2.4 g/day).

Juvenile idiopathic arthritis and other rheumatic disorders—30–50 mg/kg/24 hours in 3–4 divided doses—higher doses in systemic JIA.

Closure of patent ductus arteriosus (PDA) in newborn (IV preparation)—Dose as ibuprofen base and given at 24 hours interval—1st dose 10 mg/kg, 2nd and 3rd dose 5 mg/kg. If PDA dose not close 48 hours after last dose or reopens, a 2nd course of 3 doses may be given.

Idarubicin: *Dosage*: Maximal lifetime dose = 137.5 mg/m^2. Lower dose by 25% if severe mucositis develops or if serum bilirubin more than 2 mg/dL; lower dose by 50% if bilirubin more than 2.5 mg/dL; do not give if bilirubin more than 5 mg/dL.

Ifosfamide: *Dosage*: Always consult the current treatment protocol for details of dosage and scheduling. Children IV—1,200–1,800 mg/m^2/24 hours for 5 days every 21–28 days; or 5 g/m^2 as single IV infusion.

Iloprost: *Dosage*: 12–18 years IV infusion start with 0.5 ng/kg/min over 6 hours daily once for 3–5 consecutive days followed by maintenance dose of 1–2 ng/kg/min/day.

Imatinib mesylate: *Dosage*: 260 mg and 350 mg/m^2 equivalent to the adult dose of 400 mg chronic phase and 600 mg/day accelerated/blast phase crisis respectively. Dose adjustment for hepatotoxicity: If elevation in bilirubin more than 3 times upper limit of normal or in liver enzymes more than 5 times upper limit of normal then stop imatinib. When bilirubin levels have returned to less than 1.5 times upper limit of normal and transaminases levels to less than 2.5 times upper limit of normal, treatment of imatinib can be continued at a reduced daily dose.

Imiglucerase: *Dosage*: IV infusion—Gaucher disease type I disease 60 units/kg and type III disease 120 units/kg given every 2 weeks.

Imipenem with cilastatin: *Dosage*: Newborn IV 20 mg/kg/dose in the frequency—less than 7 days, 7–21, days and more than 21 days at 2 times, 3 times, and 4 times daily respectively. Children—IV less than 3 months, 80 mg/kg/day, 3 month–12 years 60 mg/kg/day, 12–18 years 2 g/day in four divided doses (maximum/dose <12 years 500 >12 years 1 g). Children—IV less than 3 months 80 mg/kg/day, 3 months–12 years, 60 mg/kg/day, 12–18 years 2 g/day in four divided doses (maximum dose <12 years 500 >12 years 1 g). *See Carbapenems also.*

Imipramine hydrochloride: *Dosage*:

Nocturnal enuresis—6–12 years 25 mg and 12–18 years 25–75 mg ½ hour before bedtime. Maximum period of treatment 3 months. Review before giving further courses.

Hyperactivity—6–12 year 25–75 mg; 12–17 years 50–75 mg once daily. Start at lower doses. Doses more than 1.5 mg/kg given in two divided doses.

Depression—12–18 years 25 mg/dose 1–3 times daily. Increase up to 150–200 mg/day and maintained till improvement noted. Usual maintenance—50–150/day.

Neuropathic pain—Start at 0.2–0.4 mg/kg and gradually increase to 1–3 mg/kg at bedtime.

Immunoglobulin (intravenous): *Dosage*: Total dose for immunomodulation is 2 g/kg divided over 2–5 days or 1 g/kg for 2 days to be given as IV infusion. May stop if the platelet counts are normal after the 2nd dose. Repeated if symptoms warrant and not according to platelet count. Can be repeated every 3–6 weeks.

Kawasaki syndrome—IV infusion 2 g/kg given over 8–12 hours period. The treatment should be given within 10 days of onset of illness, preferably within 7 days (Class I). If active inflammation persists beyond 10 days in the form of persistent fever, raised ESR and C reactive protein, or presence of coronary aneurysms, IVIg can be given (Class IIa). IVIg is not indicated in Kawasaki after 10 days if there are no signs of ongoing inflammation or coronary aneurysms (Class III). IVIg is also indicated in incomplete Kawasaki disease with echocardiographic demonstration of coronary aneurysms (Class I) or with normal echo (Class IIb). In nonresponders or partial responders, a second course of IVIg may be given after 48 hours.

Immunodeficiency syndromes—IV infusion 400 mg/kg once in 3 weeks. Dose depends on severity, infection frequency, and serum IgG.

Intractable epilepsy—IV infusion 400 mg/kg once in 3 weeks for three doses. If 75% reduction achieved, continue therapy for 9–12 months and review.

JIA—IV infusion 1 g/kg once daily for 2 days. Repeat if clinically needed.

Guillain-Barré syndrome—400 mg/kg once daily for 3–5 days depending on severity and rate to recover.

Myocarditis—2 g/kg, however it is generally given over 2 days as the volume of fluid is too much in the presence of ventricular dysfunction.

Inactivated poliomyelitis vaccine (IPV): *Dosage*: IM or deep SC: 0.5 mL. Each dose of 0.5 mL replaces a single dose of oral polio vaccine (OPV). A basic course consists of three injections at monthly intervals. OPV and IPV are interchangeable and the same schedule should be followed whichever vaccine is used. It is not necessary to use the same vaccine throughout the course.

Indian Academy of Pediatrics (IAP) Recommendations on use of IPV for the individual practice by its members—Option 1: At birth: Zero dose OPV 6 weeks: OPV + IPV 10 weeks: OPV + IPV 14 weeks: OPV + IPV 18 weeks: 15–18 months: OPV + IPV 5 years: OPV, OPV at all NIDs and sNIDs.

Option 2: At birth: Zero dose OPV 6 weeks: OPV only 10 weeks: OPV + IPV 14 weeks: OPV only 18 weeks: IPV only 15–18 months: OPV + IPV 5 years: OPV. If child has received OPV primary series—2 primary doses of IPV at 8 weeks interval Booster of IPV, 6–12 months after the second primary dose; OPV at 5 years and OPV at all NIDs and sNIDs.

Immunocompromised child—OPV is C/I in immunocompromised child and contacts. Three primary doses of IPV at 6, 10, 14 weeks or 2 primary doses of IPV at 8 and 10 weeks;1st booster of IPV at 15–18 months and 2nd booster of IPV at 5 years.

Indomethacin: *Dosage*:

Pain/inflammation in rheumatic disease and nephrogenic diabetes insipidus—Oral 1–2 mg/kg in two divided doses.

Closure of PDA in newborn—IV over 20–30 minutes 100–200 µg/kg as a single dose followed by two doses 100 µg/kg at 24-hour intervals; if residual patency is noted, 100 µg/kg × 3 more doses 24 hourly. Monitor for adequate urine output.

Infliximab: *Dosage*: *Severe active Crohn's disease*—IV infusion 5 mg/kg single dose over 2 hours. If recurrence occurs readminister within 14 weeks after 1st dose. Beyond this point chances of delayed hypersensitivity are high.

Influenza vaccine (inactivated): *Dosage*: More than 6 months–those receiving it for first time will need a 2nd dose after 4 weeks. Vaccine given yearly for those at continuing risk.

Insulin: *Dosage*: Dosage should be adjusted according to response. Dose may need to be increased as patients reach the pubertal growth spurt. Usual dose of insulin is 0.7 unit/kg/day in prepubertal children and 1.0 unit/kg/day in midpuberty and 1.2 unit/kg/day by the end of puberty.

At the time of diagnosis, larger doses are required up to 2.0 units/kg/day or higher for a few days to enable restoration of body glycogen, protein, and fat stores by increased caloric intake.

This period rapidly ends within 7–10 days when the child enters the "honeymoon period" with some residual b-cell function. Exogenous insulin dose will then reduce up to 0.5 units/kg/day or even lower. The honeymoon period ends in a few months and this will manifest itself by increased insulin requirements triggered by wider fluctuations of blood glucose levels.

The optimal insulin dose can be arrived at only by frequent home blood sugar monitoring and insulin adjustment by the parents with help from the diabetes team.

Insulin regimens: Although the new insulin preparations are very effective, in the Indian scenario, these insulins should be recommended with care, depending on the family's financial status. In general, a combination of short (regular) and intermediate acting (NPH) insulins is recommended. Insulin analogs both short-acting and long-acting are also available. Insulin is preferably given in a basal-bolus regime with along-acting insulin or insulin analog in the evening along with short acting insulin or insulin analog given before each major meal of the day. The old two doses (split-mix regime) is not preferred.

The insulin doses can be refined and adjusted according to the blood sugar profiles obtained subsequently by home blood glucose monitoring using a glucometer or continuous glucose monitoring through a device. Intensive therapy improves glycogenic control toward normal, and diminishes the risk of complications.

IV in diabetic emergencies—Neonate 0.01–0.1 units/kg/hour adjusted according to blood glucose concentration. 1 month–18 years 0.025–0.1 units/kg/hour adjusted according to blood glucose concentration.

Hyperkalemia: 5–10 units in 25–50 g dextrose (e.g. 500 mL 5% dextrose with 10 units insulin; 500 mL push then 100–250 mL/hour).

Interferon alfa: *Dosage*: SC less than 12 years 3 million units/m^2; more than 12 years 3–10 million units/m^2 usually 3 times/week (daily for hemangioma) for 4–6 months.

Interferon gamma-1b (immune interferon): *Dosage*: SC surface area less than 0.5 m^2 1.5 µg/kg/dose and surface area more than 0.5 m^2 50 µg/kg/dose 3 times in a week. Avoid in children less than 6 months.

Intralipid 10%/Intralipid 20%: *Dosage*: The ability to eliminate intralipid 10%/20% should govern the dosage and infusion rate. 1 g triglycerides corresponds to 10 mL intralipid, 10% or 5 mL intralipid 20%.

Neonates and Infants: The recommended dosage range in neonates and infants is 0.5–4 g triglycerides/kg body weight/day. The rate of infusion should not exceed 0.17 g triglycerides/kg body weight/hour (4 g in 24 hours). In prematures and low birth weight neonates. Intralipid 10%/20% should preferably be infused continuously over 24 hours. The initial dosage should be 0.5–1 g/kg body weight/day followed by a successive increase by 0.5–1 g/kg body weight/day up to 2 g/kg body weight/day.

Only with close monitoring of serum triglyceride concentration, liver tests, and oxygen saturation may the dosage be increased to 4 g/kg body weight/day.

The rates given are maximum rates and no attempt should be made to exceed this in order to compensate for missed doses. The ability to eliminate fat should be tested regularly in neonates and infants. Measuring serum triglyceride levels is the only reliable method.

Essential fatty acid deficiency (EFAD)—To prevent or correct essential fatty acid deficiency, 4–8% of the nonprotein energy should be supplied as intralipid 10%/20% to provide sufficient amounts of linoleic and linolenic acid. When EFAD is associated with stress, the amount of intralipid 10%/20% needed to correct the deficiency may be substantially increased.

Adolescent: The recommended maximum dosage is 3 g triglycerides/kg body weight/day. Within this upper limit, intralipid 10%/20% can be given to contribute up to 70% of the energy requirements, also in patients with highly increased energy requirements. The infusion rate for intralipid 10%/20% should not exceed 500 mL in 5 hours. The ability to eliminate fat should be closely monitored in patients with conditions mentioned under contraindications and warnings and in patients given intralipid 10%/20% for more than 1 week. This is done by collecting a blood sample after a fat-free clearance period of 5–6 hours. Blood cells are then separated from plasma by centrifugation. If the plasma is opalescent, the infusion should be postponed. The sensitivity of this method is such that hypertriglyceridemia can pass undetected. Therefore, it is recommended that serum triglyceride concentrations should be measured in patients who are likely to have impaired fat tolerance.

Iodine: *Dosage*:

Thyrotoxicosis—neonatal—1 drop 3 times daily.

Thyrotoxicosis (preoperative)—0.1–0.3 mL 3 times daily.

Ipratropium bromide: *Dosage*: Inhaled 20–120 µg 4 times daily dry powder inhaler 40 µg (1 cap) 3–4 times daily. Nebulized newborn 25 µg/kg, less than 1 year 62.5 µg, 1–5 years 125–250 µg, 5–12 years 250–500 µg, and 12–18 years 500 µg every 20–30 minutes in first 2 hour and then tapered according to response.

Iron: *Dosage*: All mg doses are expressed as elemental iron.

Newborn infant (birth to 1 month) for prophylaxis of iron deficiency in low birth weight and breastfed babies—5–6 mg of elemental iron once daily.

Children treatment of iron deficiency anemia—3 months–12 years 5–6 mg/kg in two divided doses and 12–18 years 180 mg of elemental iron in three divided doses.

Chronic kidney disease: Iron dextran IV, IM: Total replacement dose of iron dextran (mL) = 0.0476 × lean body wt (kg) × [desired Hb (g/dL)–measured Hb (g/dL)] + 1 mL per 5 kg lean body weight (up to maximum of 14 mL). Maximum daily (IM) dose: less than 5 kg: 0.5 mL (25 mg), 5–10 kg: 1 mL (50 mg), more than 10 kg: 2 mL (100 mg) IM: use "Z-track" technique. Test dose: 25 mg (12.5 mg for infants) IV over 5 minutes or IM. May initiate treatment dose 1 hour after test dose. IV: Dilute in NS at a maximum concentration of 50 mg/mL and infuse over 1–6 hour at a maximum rate of 50 mg/min.

Iron saccharate (doses in elemental iron): Test dose: Children less than 14 kg: 1.5 mg/kg IV, more than 14 kg: 20 mg IV. Usual dose: 3 mg/kg IV thrice a week. Test dose to be given before 1st therapeutic dose; wait for 15 and remaining portion of initial dose may be given if no adverse reactions. Undiluted solution, slow IV (20 mg/min) and extend the arm after the injection or give into venous limb of the dialyzer. IV infusion: Dilute in NS to a concentration of 1 mg/mL. Infuse 100 mg dose over at least 15 minutes.

Iron sucrose: 1 mg/kg/dialysis adequate for correcting ferritin levels and 0.3 mg/kg/dialysis for maintaining ferritin levels between 193 and 250 μg/L. Should be administered during the last hour of each dialysis at a frequency of 3 times a week. A 10 mg test dose prior to total dose should be given. May administer drug undiluted over 2–5 minutes; or as an infusion, dilute each 100 mg with a maximum of 100 mL NS and infuse over at least 15 minutes.

Ferric gluconate IV: Iron deficiency anemia in patients undergoing chronic hemodialysis who are receiving supplemental erythropoietin therapy (most require 8 doses at 8 sequential dialysis treatments to achieve a favorable response). Child = 6 years: 1.5 mg/kg elemental Fe (0.12 mL/kg) IV; maximum dose: 125 mg elemental Fe/dose. Dilute dose in 25 mL NS and infuse over 1 hour.

Iron chloride injection: *Dosage*: 1 mL/kg as part of a balanced parenteral nutrition (PN) regimen.

Isoniazid (INH): *Dosage*:

Tuberculosis—Daily regimen—10 mg/kg as single morning dose (Range 10–15 mg/kg; maximum dose 300 mg/day);

Intermittent regimen—15 mg/kg (Range 12–17 mg/kg).

INH prophylaxis in doses of 10 mg/kg/day for 6 months:

a. All asymptomatic contacts (under 6 years of age) of a smear positive case, after ruling out active disease and irrespective of their Bacillus Calmette-Guérin (BCG), tuberculin skin test (TST), or nutritional status.
b. All HIV infected children who either had a known exposure to an infectious TB case or are TST positive (>5 mm induration) but have no active TB disease.
c. All TST positive children who are receiving immunosuppressive therapy (e.g. Children with nephrotic syndrome, acute leukemia, etc.).
d. A child born to mother who was diagnosed to have TB in pregnancy should receive prophylaxis for 6 months, provided congenital TB has been ruled out. BCG vaccination can be given at birth even if INH chemoprophylaxis is planned

Isoproterenol (Isoprinosine): *Dosage*: ECG monitoring required during administration—IV infusion as HCL salt—newborn 20–300 ng/kg/min, less than 12 years 20 ng–1 μg/kg/min and 12–18 years 1–4 μg/min.

Isotretinoin: *Dosage*: Oral 0.5 mg/kg daily once for 4 weeks and if response is good continue for further 8–12 weeks; if response poor, give up to 1 mg/kg for 8–12 weeks. If intolerant, reduce to 0.1–0.2 mg/kg/day. Topical apply 1–2 times daily over affected area.

Ispaghula husk: *Dosage*: Child 2–12 years 1 level 5 mL spoonful in water once or twice daily, preferably at mealtimes. Child 12–18 years 2 level 5 mL spoonful in water once or twice daily, preferably at mealtimes.

Itraconazole: *Dosage*: Oral less than12 years 3–5 mg/kg and 12–18 years 100 mg once daily for 15 days in tenia corporis, tenia cruris, and oropharyngeal candidiasis and 30 days for tenia pedis and tinea manuum.

Aspergillosis—allergic bronchopulmonary—3–5 mg/kg in two divided doses.

Ivermectin: *Dosage*: 5–18 years 0.15 mg/kg as single dose to repeat every 6–8 months.

Strongyloidosis—5–18 years 0.2 mg/kg for 2 days as single dose and repeat every 6–12 months if necessary.

Filariasis—Ivermectin has no lethal effects against adult worms and therefore it is to be given in dose of 150 μg/kg once a year for 10 years. If symptoms recur, then dose is given every 3 months instead of once a year. Ivermectin is also effective against lymphatic filaria caused by *W. bancrofti*. In endemic areas, for mass treatments single dose of albendazole 400 mg + Ivermectin 200 mg/kg every 12 months is highly effective in controlling filaria. Its effect is more sustained than diethylcarbamazine for elimination of microfilaria from skin and ocular tissues. Ivermectin is not used against filaria caused by Loa loa due to risk of encephalopathy (in Loa loa diethylcarbamazine and albendazole are first and second line drug of choice).

Scabies and pediculosis—Recently single dose of ivermectin (200 μg/kg) has been found to be highly effective in treatment of scabies and head lice. Ivermectin is typically helpful in treatment of crusted scabies found in patient with immunosuppression (e.g. HIV and leukemia, etc.). It is used to prevent and cure the outbreak of scabies in institution.

J

Japanese encephalitis vaccine (inactivated): *Dosage*: 2-dose schedule for those residing in endemic areas.

JEEV—Minimum age: 1 year. *Primary immunization schedule:* Two doses of 0.25 mL each administered intramuscularly on days 0 and 28 for children aged between 1 and 3 years; two doses of 0.5 mL for children more than 3 years. Need of boosters still undetermined.

JENVAC—Minimum age: 1 year. *Primary immunization schedule:* Two doses of 0.5 mL each administered intramuscularly at 4 weeks interval. Need of boosters still undetermined.

Catch-up vaccination: All susceptible children up to 15 years should be administered during disease outbreak/ahead of anticipated outbreak in campaigns.

Live attenuated, cell culture-derived SA-14-14-2. Minimum age: 8 months; two dose schedule, first dose at 9 months along with measles vaccine and second at 16 to 18 months along with DTP booster. Used in NIV for all children at 1 ½ years age in endemic districts as a single dose.

K

Ketamine: *Dosage*:

Anesthesia - induction and maintenance—Intermittent IV less than 12 years 1–2 mg/kg and 12–18 years 1–4.5 mg/kg as induction followed by maintenance as required—usually ½ induction dose or as IV infusion. IV infusion, induce with 0.5–2 mg/kg followed by maintenance newborn 0.5 mg/kg/hour and 1 month–18 years 0.6–2.7 mg/kg/hour.

Neuropathic pain for palliative care—0.1–0.2 mg/kg/hour (maximum 1.5 mg/kg/hour) will suffice IM 4 mg/kg for diagnostic/pain causing procedures.

Ketoconazole: *Dosage*:

Pityriasis versicolor—Use daily for a maximum of 5 days.

Seborrheic dermatitis and dandruff—use twice weekly for 2–4 weeks.

Candidiasis, candiduria, or chromomycosis—Oral: *Adolescent*: 200 mg PO once daily. Serious infection may require 400 mg PO once daily. Children more than or equal to 2 years of age: 3.3–6.6 mg/kg PO once daily. Children less than 2 years of age: Safety and efficacy have not been established.

Oropharyngeal candidiasis (thrush) in HIV-infected children—Oral: Children: 3–7 mg/kg/day for 5–49 days till cured.

Vulvovaginal candidiasis—Nonpregnant adolescent females: 200–600 mg PO once daily for 3–6 days. For recurrent vulvovaginal candidiasis, topical or oral therapy daily for 2 weeks, then 6 months of therapy that could include ketoconazole 100 mg PO every day. Not recommended in pregnancy.

Tinea capitis, tinea corporis, tinea cruris, tinea pedis, tinea manuum, tinea unguium (onychomycosis) caused by Trichophyton sp., Microsporum sp. or Epidermophyton sp., and tinea versicolor—Adolescent: 200 mg PO once daily. Serious infection may require 400 mg PO once daily. Children more than or equal to 2 years of age: 3.3–6.6 mg/kg PO once daily.

Ketotifen: *Dosage*: Adolescents: 1–2 mg once daily with food. Initial treatment is 0.5–1 mg at night. Children: Over 2 years: 1 mg once daily with food. Not recommended for children below 2 years.

L

Labetalol: *Dosage*: Oral—1 month—12 years 1–2 mg/kg 3–4 times a day; 12–18 years initially 50–100 mg twice daily increased if required at intervals of 3–14 days to usual dose of 200–400 mg twice daily (3–4 divided doses if higher); maximum 2.4 g daily. IV–1 month–12 years 250–500 μg/kg as a single dose, maximum 20 mg; 12–18 years 50 mg over at least 1 minute, repeated after 5 minutes if necessary, maximum total dose 200 mg.

Lactitol monohydrate: *Dosage*: Administer oral once daily along with evening meals—the dose may also be given in the morning if that is more convenient.

Constipation—2–6 years age—10 mL; more than 6 years 10–15 mL.

Prevention of hepatic encephalopathy—30 mL once in the evening.

Acute phase of hepatic encephalopathy—45–90 mL divided into three doses along with main meals.

Lactulose: *Dosage*:

Constipation-initial dose less than 1 year 5 mL, 1–5 years 10 mL, 5–10 years 20 mL, more than 12 years 30 mL in two divided doses. Then adjust according to response.

Hepatic encephalopathy—Initially 30–50 mL/dose 3 times daily. Then adjust to produce 2–3 soft stools/day.

Lamivudine: *Dosage*: Adolescents (weight ≥ 40 kg): 300 mg/day. Safe and effective use has not been established in adolescent less than 40 kg and in children. *Patients with renal impairment:* CrCl less than or equal to 50 mL/min: Lamivudine requires dose adjustment in the presence of renal insufficiency.

Lamotrigine: *Dosage*:

Monotherapy and as adjunct in focal seizures; primary and secondary generalized tonic-clonic seizures (GTCS); Lennox—Gastaut syndrome—oral—along with valproate-2–12 years-initially 50 μg/kg for 2 weeks (if <13 kg–mg A/D for weeks) followed by 300 μg/kg for next 2 weeks; then increase by 300 μg/kg once in 1–2 weeks up to 1–5 mg/kg/day in 1–2 divided doses (maintenance)—maximum 100 mg/dose. 12–18 years initially 25 mg on A/D for 2 weeks followed by 25 mg/day for next 2 weeks; then increase by 25 mg once in 1–2 weeks up to 100–200 mg/day in 1–2 divided doses (maintenance).

Adjunct in seizures (with enzyme inducing drugs) without valproate—2–12 years—initially 300 μg/kg/day two divided doses for 2 weeks followed by 600 μg/kg two divided doses for next 2 weeks; then increase by 1.2 kg (max) every 1–2 weeks up to 2.5–5 mg/kg (maximum 200 mg/dose) BD. 12–18 years initially 50 mg OD for 2 weeks followed by 50 mg BD for next 2 weeks; then increase by maximum 100 mg every 1–2 weeks up to 100–200 mg BD (maintenance-occasionally up to 700 mg required).

Adjunct in seizures (without enzyme inducing drugs) without valproate—2–12 years--initially 300 μg/kg/day 1–2 divided doses for 2 weeks followed by 600 μg/kg 1–2 divided doses for next 2 weeks; then increase by 600 μg/kg (max.) every 1–2 weeks up to 1–10 mg/kg/day (maximum 200 mg/day) in divided doses. 12–18 years—initially 25 mg OD for 2 weeks followed by 50 mg OD for next 2 weeks; then increase by maximum 100 mg every 1–2 weeks up to 100–200 mg/day in 1–2 divided doses (maintenance).

Monotherapy of seizures—12–18 year—initially 25 mg OD for 2 weeks followed by 50 mg OD for next 2 weeks; then increase by maximum100 mg every 1–2 weeks up to 100–200 mg/day in 1–2 divided doses (maintenance-occasionally up to 500 mg required).

Monotherapy of atypical absence seizures—2–12 years—initially 300 µg/kg/day two divided doses for 2 weeks followed by 600 µg/kg two divided doses for next 2 weeks; then increase by maximum 600 µg/kg every 1–2 weeks up to 1–10 mg/kg/day in 1–2 divided doses (maintenance-occasionally up to 15 mg/kg/day required).

Note: All dose titrations should be repeated if restarting after interval of more than 5 days.

Lansoprazole: *Dosage*: *GERD, acid-related dyspepsia, duodenal, and benign gastric ulcer including those following NSAID therapy*—Children less than 30 kg—0.5–1 mg/kg (maximum 15 mg) once daily; Children more than 30 kg—15 to 30 mg once daily for 8 to 12 weeks.

Leuprorelin acetate (Leuprolide): *Dosage*: 3.75 mg every 4 weeks or 11.25 mg depot preparation every 12 weeks. Injections may need to be given more frequently (e.g. every 3 weeks or every 10 weeks) if patients show signs of failure of hormone suppression.

Levamisole: *Dosage*:

Roundworm (ascariasis)—Less than 12 years 2.5–3 mg/kg and 12–18 year 150 mg as single dose.

Hookworm (ankylostomiasis)—Less than 12 years 2.5 mg/kg and 12–18 years 150 mg as single dose. Repeat after 7 days if severe infection. Adults 300 mg for 1–2 days.

Nephrotic syndrome—2.5 mg/kg on alternate days for 12–18 months.

Levetiracetam: *Dosage*: Oral—16–18 years old—initiated at 500 mg twice daily. The dose may be titrated based on patient response with 500 mg/day increments every 2 weeks, up to 1,500 mg/day (maximum 3 g/day).

When levetiracetam is withdrawn, it should be tapered slowly over 2–4 weeks to prevent withdrawal seizures.

In adolescents with moderate to severe renal impairment, reduce dose by half and give twice daily. Hemodialysis removes approximately 50% of a levetiracetam dose in one 4 hours session. Those undergoing hemodialysis should therefore receive a supplemental dose of half their standard maintenance dose after dialysis.

No dosage adjustment is needed in presence of hepatic impairment. But, if hepatic impairment is associated with renal impairment with CrCl less than 70 mL/min/1.73 m^2, half the usual dose is recommended.

Levobupivacaine hydrochloride: *Dosage*:

All doses for older adolescent—Epidural anesthesia during surgery—10–20 mL (50–150 mg) of 0.5%–0.75% levobupivacaine as an epidural infusion.

Ophthalmic anesthesia: Regional dosage—5–15 mL (37.5–112.5 mg) of 0.75% levobupivacaine.

Peripheral nerve block anesthesia including brachial plexus nerve block: Regional dosage—30 mL (75–150 mg) or 0.4 mL/kg (1–2 mg/ kg) of 0.25–0.5% levobupivacaine.

Levocetirizine: *Dosage*: Orally in the evening as hydrochloride-6–11 years 2.5 mg once daily (maximum dose; more than 12 years: 5 mg once daily (maximum dose-2.5 mg may suffice in some children).

Levonorgestrel: *Dosage:* Oral: 30 µg.

Levothyroxine (thyroxine) sodium: *Dosage*: Oral—Initial dose—newborn: 15 µg/kg/day, later infancy: 6–8 µg/kg/day, preschool 5–6 µg/kg/day, older children: 4–5 µg/kg/day, adolescents 2–3: 50–100 µg/kg/day.

The goal of therapy is to maintain the total thyroxine (TT4) in the upper normal range of 10–15 µg/dL and normalize elevated TSH. Adjust dose to correct free thyroxine (FT4) to more than 20 pmol/L and TSH to less than 1–3 mU/L within 4 weeks of therapy.

Monitoring has to be done: 2 weeks after starting treatment, every 2 weeks till normalization of TSH, every 1–3 months till 1 year of age, every 2–4 months from 1–3 years of age, every 3–12 months till growth is completed and 4–6 weeks after any change in dose.

Clinical evaluation and growth monitoring at each visit also are equally important.

It is preferable to monitor TT4 levels to FT4 levels. FT4 is preferred in special circumstances like pregnancy or inappropriately elevated TSH, and to cross check central hypothyroidism if T4 level is borderline as TSH will not be useful.

Lignocaine: *Dosage*:

Antiarrhythmic—Loading dose IV bolus less than 12 years 0.5 mg–1 mg/kg and 12–18 years 50–100 mg (50 mg for thin build or those with severely impaired circulation) followed by maintenance dose IV infusion with ECG monitoring less than 12 years 0.6–3 mg/kg/hour and 12–18 years start with 4 mg/min for 30 minutes then 2 mg/kg for 2 hour then 1 mg/min for the rest of the day. Lower concentration further if continued beyond 24 hours.

Ventricular fibrillation or pulseless tachycardia—IV less than 12 years 1 mg/kg repeat every 5 minutes to maximum of 3 mg/kg and 12–18 years 50–100 mg.

Local anesthetic—Local infiltration less than 12 years 3 mg/kg and 12–18 years up to 200 mg—not more frequently than once in 4 hours. Intraurethral 3–4 mg/kg prior to catheterization.

Lincosamines and Streptogramins: *Dosage*:

Clindamycin—Neonates—Less than 7 days, less than 2,000 g 10 mg/kg/day divided 12 hourly IV/IM; less than 7 days, more than

2,000 g 15 mg/kg/day divided 8 hourly IV/IM; more than 7 days, less than 1,200 g 10 mg/kg/day divided 12 hourly IV/IM; more than 7 days, 1,200–2,000 g 15 mg/kg/day divided 8 hourly IV/IM; more than 7 days, more than 2,000 g 20 mg/kg/day divided 8 hourly IV/IM; children 10–40 mg/kg/day divided 8 hourly IV/IM or orally; 12–18 years 150–300 mg up to maximum of 450 mg/dose 4 times daily.

Falciparum malaria (alternate therapy)—20 mg/kg/day for 5 days.

Quinupristin with dalfopristin—IV into central vein—1 month–18 years 7.5 mg/kg 8th hourly 7 days in skin and soft tissue infection, 10 days in hospital acquired pneumonia; duration for *E. faecium* infection depends on site of infection.

Linezolid: *Dosage*: IV infusion over 30–120 min-*Preterm neonates less than 7 days old (gestational age < 34 weeks):* 10 mg/kg 12th hourly for 14–28 days—10 mg/kg 8th hourly in those with a suboptimal clinical response; *Neonates, infants, and children less than 12 years*: 10 mg/kg 8th hourly for 14–28 days.

Linezolid is not recommended for empiric treatment of acute CNS infections.

Children exhibit variability in drug clearance and systemic exposure.

Those with ventriculoperitoneal (VP) shunts achieve variable CSF therapeutic concentrations; more than or equal to 12 years: 600 mg 12th hourly for 14–28 days. May give aztreonam or aminoglycosides concurrently if indicated. *Oral*: Adolescents and children more than or equal to 12 years: 600 mg 12 hourly for 10–14 days. Term neonates, infants, and children less than 12 years: 10 mg/kg 8 hourly for 10–14 days. Preterm neonates less than 7 days old (gestational age < 34 weeks): 10 mg/kg 12 hourly for 10–14 days—10 mg/kg 8 hourly in those with a suboptimal clinical response.

Liquid paraffin: *Dosage*: Oral 3–12 years 0.5–1 mL/kg and 12–18 years 10–30 mL once daily.

Lisinopril: *Dosage*: *Hypertension*—Oral

Adolescent: Initially, 10 mg PO once daily. The usual dosage range is 20–40 mg PO once daily. Lower dosage may be necessary in patients with renal impairment and in those receiving diuretics. In patients with a creatinine clearance of less than 30 mL/min, initiate therapy with 5 mg PO once daily. Maximum daily dose is 80 mg/day.

Children more than or equal to 6 years: Starting dosage is 0.07 mg/kg PO once daily (up to 5 mg/day). Adjust dosage based on blood pressure response. Doses more than 0.61 mg/kg/day PO or more than 40 mg/day have not been studied in pediatric patients. Lisinopril is not recommended in children with glomerular filtration rate less than 30 mL/min/1.73 m^2.

Children less than 6 years: Not recommended.

The doses for heart failure in children are not defined.

Lisinopril is removed by hemodialysis. For patients receiving dialysis, the initial recommended dosage is 2.5 mg PO once daily. Maximum 40 mg/day. Hemodialysis removal of lisinopril is not problematic in most hypertensive patients and may help avoid intradialytic hypotension. However, in patients who experience intradialytic hypertension, dialyzable angiotensin converting enzyme inhibitors (ACE-I) ought to be changed to either an angiotensin receptor blocking (ARB) or a nondialyzable ACE-I (i.e., fosinopril). Dosing should be daily; however, as a result of its longer half-life because of its predominant renal excretion, lisinopril has demonstrated good blood pressure control with thrice weekly administration following hemodialysis. For noncompliant patients, directly observed lisinopril administration immediately following hemodialysis may be a good therapeutic option.

Lithium: *Dosage*: Oral 12–18 years 200–800 mg/dose 3 times daily. Higher dose with citrate—citrate 509 mg = 200 mg carbonate. Maintain plasma level of 0.4–1 mmol/L 12 hours after last dose. Monitor once in 3 months.

Loperamide: *Dosage*:

Chronic diarrhea, e.g. short bowel syndrome—Less than 1 year 0.2 mg/kg 30 minute before feeds (up to 2 mg/kg/day may be required); 1–12 year 0.1–0.2 mg/kg/dose and 12–18 years 2–4 mg 3–4 times daily.

Acute diarrhea—Not recommended in children. 12–18 year—may be used—start with 4 mg and then give 2 mg after each loose stool up to 6–8 mg/day (maximum 16 mg/day). Not given for more than 5 days.

Loratadine: *Dosage*: Oral less than 6 years 5 mg, more than 6 year 10 mg once daily.

Lorazepam: *Dosage*:

Antiemetic—IV 0.4–0.8 mg/kg/dose 6 hourly as needed.

Anxiety/sedation—Neonates 0.1–0.4 mg/kg/dose 6 hourly as needed. Children 0.05–0.1 mg/kg/dose 4–8 hourly, adolescents orally 1–10 mg/24 hour in 2–3 divided doses.

Status epilepticus—Neonates IV 0.05–0.2 mg/kg/dose over 2–5 minutes; may repeat in 10–15 minutes, children 0.1 mg/kg loading over 2–5 minutes and if required, another 0.05 mg/kg bolus in 10–15 minutes; adolescent 0.07 mg/kg/dose over 2–5 minutes and may repeat after 10–15 minutes.

Losartan potassium: *Dosage*: *Hypertension*—

Adolescents: initially, 50 mg PO once daily, unless the patient is volume-depleted. The maintenance dosage range is 25–100 mg/day PO, given in 1–2 divided doses. Maximal effects generally occur within 3–6 weeks.

The addition of a diuretic has a greater effect on lowering blood pressure than increasing the losartan dosage beyond 50 mg/day. The addition of hydrochlorothiazide 12.5 mg to losartan 50 mg daily results in an additional 50% reduction in diastolic and systolic BP.

A modest reduction in blood pressure (up to 3 mm Hg) is achieved by increasing the daily dose of losartan from 50 to 100 mg.

When volume-depletion is suspected (e.g. patients taking diuretics), initiate therapy with 25 mg PO once daily.

Children more than equal to 6 years: The usual recommended starting dose is 0.7 mg/kg PO once daily (up to 50 mg/day). Individualize dosage to attain blood pressure goals. Doses more than 1.4 mg/kg/day (or > 100 mg/day) PO have not been studied.

Losartan can be prepared extemporaneously as an oral suspension.

Children less than 6 years: Not recommended.

Chronic congestive cardiac failure—75 to 1.4 mg/kg/day.

Other drugs in this group are Candesartan, Valsartan. Studies in children are in progress, primarily for treatment of hypertension.

M

Macrolides: *Dosage*:

Erythromycin: Dose—Neonates—Orally less than 7 days age 20 mg/kg/day 2 times daily; more than 7 days less than 1,200 g 20 mg/kg/day 2 times daily; more than 7 days more than 1,200 g 30 mg/kg/day 3 times daily. Children: 30–50 mg/kg/day in 3–4 divided doses.

Pneumococcal prophylaxis—1 month–2 years 250 mg/day, 2–8 years 500 mg/day, >9 years 1 g/day in two divided doses.

Clarithromycin: Dose-Oral 15 mg/kg/24 hour in two divided doses up to a maximum of 500 mg twice daily.

H. pylori—1–2 years 125 mg, 2–6 years 250 mg, 6–9 years 375 mg, 9–12 years 500 mg, and 12–18 years 1 g/day in two divided doses along amoxicillin and omeprazole or metronidazole and omeprazole.

Azithromycin: Dose—Children-6 months–12 years 10 mg/kg once daily for 3 days up to a maximum of 200 mg/dose in 3–7 years, 300 mg/dose in 8–11 years 400 mg/dose in 12–14 years and 500 mg/dose in more than 14 years.

Continued treatment may be required to prevent relapse of *cryptosporidiosis.*

For STD caused by *Chlamydia trachomatis* in 12–18 years 1g as single dose.

Magnesium glycerophosphate: *Dosage*—Oral <12 years 0.6 mmol/kg/day; 12–18 years 12–24 mmol/day in 3 divided doses.

Magnesium salts: *Dosage*—5–10 mL bedtime daily, reducing dose gradually until constipation is relieved.

Magnesium sulfate: *Dosage*—

Neonatal hypocalcemia—IM 100 mg/kg/dose two doses will suffice. A third dose is required in some babies.

Hypomagnesemia in newborn—IM/IV 1 dose of 100 mg/kg. Repeat more than 6–12 hour if needed.

Persistent pulmonary hypertension in newborn—IV loading dose 200 mg/kg followed by IV infusion maintenance 20–75 mg/kg/hour to maintain plasma magnesium between 3.5 mmol/L and 5.5 mmol/L. Can be given for 2–5 days.

Child—slow IV over 10 minutes less than 1 year 50 mg/kg 12–18 years 1 g (4 mmol)—may be repeated once in 12 hours.

Malathion: *Dosage*: Topical—Medical supervision is required for children less than 6 months of age.

Scabies— Apply to whole body excluding head and neck, allow to dry, wash off after 24 hours. Children less than 2 years should have a thin film applied to scalp, face and ears, avoiding eyes, and mouth. If hands or any other part are washed the treatment must be reapplied.

Head lice—Rub liquid gently into dry hair until all hair is thoroughly moistened. Comb and allow to dry naturally, away from heat or sunshine. A contact time of 12 hours or overnight is recommended. Repeat after 7 days only if live lice are found again.

Mannitol: *Dosage*: A test dose may be given to assess renal function—200 mg/kg (maximum 12.5 g) over 3–5 minutes to produce urine output of 1 mL/kg/hour for 1–3 hours. Then follow-up with specific treatment as follows:

Cerebral and ocular edema—IV over 30 minutes 0.5–1 g/kg initially followed by maintenance of 0.25–0.5 g/kg every 4–6 hours as required.

Peripheral edema and ascites—IV infusion over 2–6 hours 1–2 g/kg.

Measles vaccine: *Dosage*: 1 single dose amp. SC at 9 completed months of age. In case of an outbreak, however, the vaccine may be given to infants as young as 6 months with a recommendation for an additional MMR/Measles at 12–15 months. Commonly used strain is the Edmonston Zagreb strain grown in human diploic cell culture. Other strains used are Schwarz, Moraten and Edmonston B.

Mebendazole: *Dosage*: Oral more than 6 months 100 mg as single dose for all members of the family, may be repeated after 2 weeks.

All other susceptible worm infestations—100 mg 2 times daily for 3 consecutive days. Better than albendazole for Trichuris infestation.

Hydatid disease—200–400 mg bid or tid for 3–4 weeks, less effective than albendazole. Reduction in dose for hepatic impairment.

Mebeverine hydrochloride: *Dosage*—Oral—3–4 years 75 mg/day, 4–8 years 150 mg/day, 9–10 years 300/day and more than 10 years 450 mg/day in three divided doses 10–20 minutes before meals.

Mefenamic acid: *Dosage*: *Adolescents:* 250–500 mg thrice daily, preferably after food. *Children:* 9.5 mg–25 mg/kg/day in divided doses. Except for JIP (Still's disease) therapy should not exceed 7 days. Mefenamic acid should be used with extreme caution in children younger than 14 years old; safety and effectiveness in these children have not been confirmed.

Mefloquine: *Dosage*: *Antimalarial treatment*—Oral 15 mg/kg followed by 10 mg/kg 8–12 hours later (maximum 1.25 g).

Prophylaxis—Oral 1st dose 1 week before entering malarious area (may be started earlier to make sure drug is tolerated) and given weekly on same day for 6 weeks and continued for 4 weeks after return from malarious area. 3 month–3 years 6–16 kg 62.5 mg (1/4th tab), 4–7 years 16–25 kg 125 mg (½ tab), 8–12 years 25–45 kg 187.5 mg (3/4th tab) and more than 13 years more than 45 kg 250 mg (1 tab).

Meglumine antimoniate and sodium stibogluconate: *Dosage*: Intramuscular doses are expressed in terms of the equivalent amount of pentavalent antimony (Sb5+).

Visceral leishmaniasis—Injection of 20 mg of Sb5+/kg IM daily for a minute of 20 days. Treatment should be continued until no parasites are detected in consecutive splenic aspirates taken at 14-day intervals. Patients who relapse following the first course of treatment should be retreated immediately using the same daily dosage.

Cutaneous leishmaniasis except L. aethiopica—Local therapy: Injection of 1–3 mL into the base of the lesion, repeated once or twice if no response is apparent, at intervals of 1 to 2 days. *Systemic therapy:* 10–20 mg Sb5+/kg IM daily until a few days after clinical cure and slit-skin smears are negative. Relapse is unusual.

L. braziliensis therapy—Injection of 20 mg Sb5+/kg IM daily until lesion is healed and for at least 4 weeks. Relapse is usually associated with inadequate dosage or interrupted treatment. Should relapse occur following a full course of treatment, pentamidine should be used.

Mucocutaneous leishmaniasis (L. braziliensis)—Injection of 20 mg Sb5+/kg daily IM until slit-skin smears are negative and for at least 4 weeks. In the event of toxicity or inadequate response, 10–15 mg Sb5+/kg should be administered every 12 hours for the same period. Patients who relapse should be retreated for at least twice as long. Those who are unresponsive should receive amphotericin B or pentamidine.

Diffuse cutaneous leishmaniasis (L. amazonensis)—Injection of 20 mg Sb5+/kg daily IM for several months after clinical improvement occurs. Relapse must be expected until immunity develops.

Melatonin: *Dosage*: Oral 2–3 mg 20–30 minutes before bedtime. May be increased to 4–6 mg if benefit not achieved in 1–2 weeks. Maximum of 10 mg tried. If still no response in 2 weeks, drug is stopped.

Meloxicam: *Dosage*: Oral/rectal 12–18 years less than 50 kg 7.5 mg and more than 50 kg 15 mg once daily. In renal failure, dose of 7.5 mg not to be exceeded.

Melphalan: *Dosage*: Always consult the current treatment protocol for details of dosage and scheduling. IV 10–35 mg/m^2/dose once in 21–28 days. High dose: 140–220 mg/m^2 before bone marrow transplant. Oral 4–20 mg/m^2/day for up to 21 days.

Meningococcal A and C polysaccharide vaccine: *Dosage*: IM or deep SC: 0.5 mL of reconstituted vaccine.

Meningococcal A, C, W135 and Y polysaccharide vaccine: *Dosage*: Deep SC or IM: 0.5 mL of reconstituted vaccine.

Meningococcal C conjugate vaccine: *Dosage*: IM or deep SC–0.5 mL. Number of doses depends on age of recipient. When given as primary immunization—3 doses at 4 week intervals starting at 6–8 weeks, if started after 16 weeks age—2 doses at 4 weeks intervals and if started more than 1 year age—only 1 dose is required.

Meningococcal quadrivalent conjugate vaccine (MCV4): *Dosage*: 0.5 mL IM (licensed at present for 2 years and above). Adolescents—if primary at 11–12 years ages with booster at age 16 years if primary dose at age 11 or 12 years; at age 16 through 18 years if primary dose at age 13 through 15 years; no booster needed if primary dose on or after age 16 years.

Mepacrine hydrochloride: *Dosage*: Oral 100 mg 1–2 times daily.

Mercaptamine (cysteamine): *Dosage*: Oral initially less than 12 years 2–3 mg/kg/dose and more than 12 years 100 mg 4 times daily followed by maintenance of 12.5 mg/kg/dose and more than 12 years 500 mg 4 times daily. Eye—1 drop in each eye 4–6 times daily.

Mercaptopurine: *Dosage*: Always consult the current treatment protocol for details of dosage and scheduling. The dosage should be carefully adjusted according to blood counts.

Leukemia/lymphoma/T-NHL: Oral induction 2.5- 5 mg/kg once daily followed by maintenance of 1.5–2.5 mg/ kg/day.

Inflammatory bowel disease: 2–18 years 1–1.5 mg/kg once daily. (maximum initially 50 mg/day may be increased up to 75 mg/day).

Meropenem: *Dosage* Newborn: 40 mg/kg/day in 2 divided doses <7 days and in 3 divided doses >7 days. Double dose in meningitis and severe infection. See Carbapenems also.

Children—*UTI, gynecological, skin and soft tissue infection:* 30 mg/kg in 3 divided doses (maximum 500 mg/dose).

Pneumonia, peritonitis, neutropenia, septicemia: 60 mg/kg/day in 3 divided doses (maximum 1 g/dose).

Meningitis and life-threatening infections: 120 mg/kg/day in 3 divided doses (maximum 2 g/dose).

In renal impairment: CrCl (mL/min/1.73 m^2) 25–50, give full dose but at 12 hours intervals, 10–25 give 50% dose at 12 hours intervals < 10–50% dose at 24 hours interval.

Mesalazine [5-aminosalicylic acid (5-ASA)]: *Dosage*: Acute cases 15–20 mg/kg/dose 3 times daily followed by maintenance of 10 mg/kg/dose 2–3 times daily.

Mupirocin: *Dosage*: Apply topical cream to affected area 3 times daily for up to 10 days; nasal ointment apply to the inner surface of each nostril 2–3 times a day for 5–7 days; apply ointment to affected area 2–3 times daily for up to 10 days.

Mycophenolate mofetil: *Dosage*: Given along with cyclosporine or tacrolimus and steroids.

Renal: Oral 600 mg/m^2/dose 2 times daily—first dose within 72 hours after transplant (maximum 2 g/day).

Liver: Oral 10 mg/kg/dose 2 times daily increasing to 20 mg/ kg/dose 2 times daily—first dose within 72 hours after transplant (maximum 1 g/day).

N

Nalidixic acid: *Dosage*:

Urinary tract infection (UTI) due to susceptible organisms—Oral: Adolescents: 1 g suspension or tablet PO every 6 hours for 1 to 2 weeks. Maintenance dose of 500 mg PO every 6 hours. Children and infants ≥ 3 months: The recommended total daily dosage for initial therapy is 55 mg/kg/day PO, administered in four equally divided doses. For prolonged therapy, the total daily dose may be reduced to 33 mg/kg/day PO.

Urinary tract infection (UTI) prophylaxis in children: Oral: Children and infants ≥2 months to 2 years: A dose of 30 mg/kg/day PO in two divided doses has been recommended. *Maximum dosage limits*: Adolescents: 4 g/day PO. Children and infants ≥3 months: 55 mg/kg/day PO. Infants <3 months: Safe and effective use has not been established.

Patients with hepatic impairment: Exercise caution when using nalidixic acid in patients with liver disease, however, no specific dosage adjustments are indicated.

Patients with renal impairment: Decrease the dose by half in patients with a Cr Cl less than or equal to 20 mL/min.

Naloxone: *Dosage*: Newborn infant—Do not administer to newborns whose mother is suspected of narcotic abuse as a withdrawal syndrome may be precipitated. Ensure establishment and maintenance of adequate ventilation before administering naloxone. Specifically indicated for reversal of respiratory depression on newborn of mother who has received narcotics within 4 hours of delivery. IM preferred because it affords more prolonged effect. 0.1 mg/ kg may be repeated after 3–4 min. In older children with suspected narcotic depression same dose (maximum 2 mg) may be given IV. Repeat doses to maintain opioid reverse. If no response seen after 2 doses, diagnosis of opioid toxicity must be reviewed.

Naproxen: *Dosage*: Oral 10–20 mg/kg in 2 divided doses (maximum 1 g/day). In severe cases up to 15 mg/kg may be used for a few weeks.

Nedocromil: *Dosage*:

Asthma prophylaxis: Nedocromil sodium is intended for regular maintenance treatment and should not be used for relief of symptoms in an acute asthmatic attack. For maintenance therapy in the treatment of mild to moderate chronic asthma: Oral inhalation dosage (metered dose inhaler): Adolescents and children ≥ 6 years: 2 sprays (1.75 mg/spray) inhaled orally 4 times per day. Dosage may be reduced to 2–3 times per day once desired clinical response obtained. Safe and effective use has not been established in children < 6 years.

Prevention of exercise-induced bronchospasm: Oral inhalation dosage (metered dose inhaler): Adolescents and children >12 years: A dose of 2 sprays (1.75 mg/spray) inhaled orally 10–15 minutes prior to exercise.

Allergic conjunctivitis: Ophthalmic dosage: Adolescents and children >3 years: 1–2 drops in each eye twice daily at regular intervals. Maximum dosage limits: Adolescents: Dependent on route of administration and indication for therapy; 8 sprays (14 mg)/day via MDI. Children >6 years: Dependent on route of administration and indication for therapy; 8 sprays (14 mg)/day via MDI. Children < 6 years: Dependent on route of administration and indication for therapy.

Neomycin sulfate: *Dosage*: Adolescents: 0.25–1 g four times. Children: 12.5 mg/kg/dose oral in diarrhea and 3 g/m^2/day q 6 hours. Oral in hepatic coma.

Eye drops: Superficial eye infection—1 drop 2–4 times daily, severe infection 1 drop every 15–20 min initially then reducing frequency as infection gets controlled.

Eye ointment: 3–4 times daily. Treatment to continue till 2 days after condition is cured.

Neostigmine: *Dosage*:

Newborn myasthenia gravis: Oral 1–2 mg initially ½ hour before feed followed by 1–5 mg/dose (adjusted according to response) 6 times daily. IM 0.1 mg initially followed by 0.05–0.25 mg IM or SC (2–3 mg IM/SC is equal to 30 mg orally).

Reversal of nondepolarizing neuromuscular blockade: IV bolus over 1 min–80 µg/kg with 20 µg/kg of atropine (for drugs other than atracurium) and 50 µg/kg with 20 µg/kg of atropine (for atracurium).

Children myasthenia gravis: Oral 1 month–5 years 7.5 mg/dose, 6–12 years 15 mg/dose and 12–18 years 15–30 mg/dose repeated at suitable intervals according to response. IM 1 month–12 years 0.2–0.5 mg and 12–18 years 1–2.5 mg repeated at suitable intervals.

Nesiritide (hBNP; human B-type natriuretic peptide): *Dosage*: Infusions starting at 0.01 µg/kg/min and up titrated to a maximum of 0.03 µg/kg/min. Calculate the required bolus volume based on the patient's weight as follows: bolus volume (in mL) = 0.33 × patient weight (kg). Then withdraw the appropriate bolus volume from the nesiritide infusion bag, and inject it over about 60 seconds through an IV port in the tubing. Immediately following the administration of the IV bolus, infuse nesiritide solution at a flow rate of 0.1 mL/kg/ hour. The calculation for the infusion flow rate (mL/

hour) = 0.1 × patient weight (kg). This will deliver the initial recommended nesiritide maintenance infusion rate of 0.01 µg/kg/min. Nesiritide is generally administered at a fixed IV infusion rate. Due to a long onset and offset of action, nesiritide should be titrated upward no more frequently than every 3 hours. Do not titrate infusion rate at frequent intervals as is done with other IV agents that have a significantly shorter half-life (e.g. dobutamine, dopamine, nitroglycerin, nitroprusside).

Netilmicin: *Dosage*: Newborn IV 3 mg/dose 12 hourly. Increase to 8 hourly after 1 week age postnatal. Monitor after 3rd dose for 1 hour postdose peak of 8–12 mg/L and a trough of <3 mg/L. Prolong dose interval in PDA, prolonged hypoxia and indomethacin therapy. Children–IV/IM <12 years 7.5 mg/kg/day and > 12 years 6 mg/kg/day in 3 divided doses or 1 month–18 years 7.5 mg/kg as single dose daily. Intraperitoneal 7.5–10 mg/L in peritoneal dialysis fluid. See Aminoglycosides also.

Nevirapine: *Dosage*:

Treatment of HIV infection in combination with other antiretroviral agents: For adolescents, the initiation of ART is recommended in any patient: with a history of an AIDS-defining infection; with a CD4 less than 350/mm^3; who is pregnant; who has HIV-associated nephropathy; or who is being treated for hepatitis B (HBV) infection. For children, the initiation of ART is recommended in any symptomatic patient. For asymptomatic or mildly symptomatic children ≥ 5 years, the initiation of ART is recommended for patients with HIV RNA ≥ 100,000 copies/mL and CD4 less than 350/mm^3. For asymptomatic or mildly symptomatic children 1–5 years, the initiation of ART is recommended for patients with HIV RNA ≥ 100,000 copies/mL and CD4 less than 25%. For infants, the initiation of ART is recommended in any infant regardless of clinical status, CD4 percentage, or viral load.

Adolescents: 200 mg PO once daily for the first 14 days, then 200 mg PO twice daily. If mild to moderate rash with constitutional symptoms is observed during the first 14 days of therapy, do not increase the dose until the rash has resolved; if the rash does not resolve by treatment day 28, discontinue nevirapine and use an alternative treatment regimen. Permanently discontinue treatment if severe hepatotoxicity, severe cutaneous reactions, or hypersensitivity reactions occur. Adolescents in early puberty (Tanner I-II) should be dosed using pediatric schedules.

Neonates ≥ 15 days old, infants, and children: 150 mg/m^2 (not to exceed 400 mg) PO once daily for the first 14 days, then 150 mg/m^2 (not to exceed 400 mg) twice daily. Alternatively, the following volume recommendations per dose of nevirapine 50 mg/5 mL oral suspension, based on body surface area can be used: > 1.25 m^2, 20 mL; 1.08–1.25 m^2, 17.5 mL; 0.92–1.08 m^2, 15 mL; 0.75–0.92 m^2, 12.5 mL; 0.58–0.75 m^2, 10 mL; 0.42–0.58 m^2, 7.5 mL; 0.25–0.42 m^2, 5 mL; 0.12–0.25 m^2, 2.5 mL; and 0.06–0.12 m^2, 1.25 mL. Same rules as for adolescent in case of rash or appearance of indication for discontinuation of therapy.

Neonates < 15 days old: Dosing information is unavailable. (HIV) prophylaxis—to prevent perinatal transmission of HIV to neonates born to HIV-infected women in labor who have had no prior antiretroviral therapy: Oral dosage (nevirapine single agent): *Pregnant females—intrapartum:* The addition of single-dose maternal/infant nevirapine to an ongoing highly active combination antiretroviral therapy regimen does not provide additional efficacy in reducing perinatal transmission and may result in nevirapine resistance in the mother, and is therefore not recommended. In patients who are not receiving any antiretroviral treatment prior to labor, administer 200 mg PO as a single dose at the onset of labor.

Neonates ≥34 weeks gestation: The CDC recommends 2 mg/kg PO as a single dose 48–72 hours after birth. If the mother received nevirapine less than 1 hour prior to delivery, the infant should be given 2 mg/kg PO as soon as possible after birth and again at 48–72 hours. Oral dosage (nevirapine and zidovudine combination): *Pregnant females–intrapartum:* Due to synergistic inhibition of HIV with the combination *in vitro*, the following regimen has been suggested: nevirapine 200 mg PO as a single dose at the onset of labor plus zidovudine (2 mg/kg IV bolus followed by 1 mg/kg/hour IV continuous infusion until delivery). During or immediately after intrapartum treatment with nevirapine and zidovudine, consider initiation of maternal zidovudine and lamivudine, continuing for 3–7 days, to potentially reduce development of nevirapine resistance.

Neonates >34 weeks gestation: Due to synergistic inhibition of HIV with the combination *in vitro*, the following regimen has been suggested: nevirapine 2 mg/kg PO as a single oral dose at age 48–72 hours plus zidovudine (2 mg/kg PO every 6 hours for 6 weeks).

Maximum dosage limits: Adolescents: 400 mg/day PO. Children: 300 mg/m^2, up to 400 mg per day PO. Infants: 300 mg/m^2, up to 400 mg per day PO. Neonates ≥ 15 days old: 300 mg/m^2, up to 400 mg per day PO. Neonates < 15 days old: Safe and effective use not established.

Nicardipine: *Dosage*: Continuous IV infusion initially 500 mg/kg/min followed by maintenance infusion of 1–3 µg/kg/min.

Niclosamide: *Dosage*:

*Tenia solium (pork) Tenia saginata (beef), Diphyllobothrium latum (fish:)*Oral < 2 years 500 mg, 2–6 years 1 g, > 7 years 2 g once daily. Give the dose in 2 divided doses one before breakfast and the rest 1 hour later.

Hymenolepis nana (dwarf tapeworm): Oral single dose on first day followed by ½ that dose daily once for the next 6 days.

Initial day dose for <2, 2–6 and 7–18 years are 500 mg, 1 g and 2 g, respectively. No purgative is needed.

Nifedipine: *Dosage*:

Hypertensive crisis/angina: Sublingual/oral pierce the capsule and pour contents sublingually/into mouth—250–500 µg/kg as single dose.

Hypertension/ angina: < 12 years 0.2–0.3 mg/kg/dose and 12–18 years 5–20 mg/kg/dose 3 times daily (maximum 3 mg/ kg/day).

Raynaud's phenomenon: 2–18 years 2.5–10 mg 2–4 times daily. Start with low dose at bedtime and gradually increase to avoid postural hypotension.

Nimesulide: *Dosage*: 5 mg/kg/day in 2 or 3 divided doses. *The drug is banned for use in children below 12 years by The Drug Controller General of India (DCGI) after the subcommittee of the government's chief advisory body—the Drug Technical Advisory Board (DTAB) recommended for the same.*

Nitazoxanide: *Dosage*: *Amebiasis, Giardiasis, Cryptosporidiosis and Helminthiasis:* 12–47 months–100 mg 12 hourly for 3 days; 4–11 years–200 mg 12 hourly for 3 days; adolescents—500 mg 12 hourly for 3 days.

Nitrazepam: *Dosage*: Oral initially 0.25 mg/kg in 2 divided doses followed by maintenance of 0.5 mg/kg in 2 divided doses (maximum 1 mg/ kg/day). Total daily dose may be given in 3 divided doses. Achieve target maintenance dose in 2–3 weeks. Dosage reduction required for renal and hepatic impairment.

Nitric oxide: *Dosage*: Delivered along with oxygen through the ventilator circuit in a dose of 5–80 ppm. >33 weeks gestation: start at 20 ppm. If this produces a raise in post ductal pO2 of at least 3kPa (while ventilator parameters remain unchanged), reduce the dose after an hour to the lowest dose capable of producing a sustained response. <33 weeks gestation: start with a dose of 5 ppm and consider increasing in stages to a maximum of 40 ppm. If this produces no response, return to 5 ppm and give this for 12 hours. If still no response—stop. Tailing off: always try to use the lowest effective dose; failure to do so may result in increasing dependency. Try to reduce the dose further every 12 hours. Drop the concentration by 10% every 3 minutes but reverse any reduction that causes the arterial saturation to drop by more than 2%. Nitric oxide should not be used for long-term, as it results in methemoglobinemia. BP, pulmonary artery pressure, and arterial oxygen saturation should be monitored during therapy with nitric oxide.

Nitrofurantoin: *Dosage*: Contraindicated in infants less than 3 months age.

UTI treatment: 3 months–12 years 5–7 mg/kg/ day and in 12–18 years 200–400 mg/day in 4 divided doses.

UTI prophylaxis: 1–2.5 mg/kg/day in at bedtime or in 2 divided doses (maximum 100 mg/24 hours).

Nitroglycerine (Glyceryl trinitrate): *Dosage*: IV infusion—The initial dose is 0.5 µg/kg/min IV, it is up titrated depending on the response, to a maximum of 10 µg/kg/min. Monitor BP and heart rate. Tolerance may develop.

Nitrous oxide: *Dosage*: Inhalation: nitrous oxide is administered with oxygen to avoid the hypoxia which would otherwise occur. Doses may be self-regulated in most cases by the use of a face-mask connected through a demand valve to the cylinder. The valve is operated by the act of inhalation by the patient and closes when the patient ceases to inhale. This will generally only be possible with children aged about 5 years and over. It should be administered only by personnel trained in its use. Dose adjustments are not necessary in renal or hepatic disease.

Noradrenaline (Norepinephrine): *Dosage*: IV infusion 0.3–2 µg/kg/min. Monitor ECG and hemodynamic parameters.

Norethisterone: *Dosage*:

Induction of sexual maturity: Oral: 5 mg once daily for the last 7 days of a 28 day cycle. (Norethisterone is added after 1½–2 years of estrogen therapy or when breakthrough bleeding occurs to regularize menstrual cycles by adding progesterone in last 7 days of the cycle).

Postponement of menstruation: Oral: 5 mg three times a day, starting 3 days before the expected onset of menstruation.

Nortriptyline: *Dosage*:

Nocturnal enuresis: Oral > 6 years 20–25 kg 10 mg, 25–35 kg 10–20 mg, > 35 kg 25–35 mg once daily (bedtime). Maximum duration of treatment 3 months. Review before further courses are given.

Depression: Oral 12–18 years 30–100 mg once daily at night or in divided doses. Use low dose initially and increased if required up to 100 mg.

NTBC [2-(2-nitro-4-trifluoro-methylbenzoyl)-1,3 cyclohexanedione] (nitisinone): *Dosage*: Oral 0.5–0.75 mg/ kg as single dose initially. May require up to 2 mg/kg/day. Daily dose may be given in 2 divided doses.

Nystatin: *Dosage*: Newborn—Treatment and prophylaxis against oral candidiasis—1 mL 3–4 times daily. Children—Intestinal and oral candida 1 mL 3–4 times daily; oral candida in immunocompromised 1 mL 4–6 times, esophageal/ intestinal candida 5 mL or 1 tab 4–6 times daily.

O

Octreotide: *Dosage*:

Varices: IV infusion 1 µg/kg/hour initially may be increased to 3 µg/kg/hour till bleeding is controlled. Then taper over 24 hours to avoid rebound bleeding.

Hyperinsulinemia: SC 1 µg/kg 4 hourly initially and increased up to 40 µg/kg/24 hours depending on response. No change in dose required for renal impairment.

Ofloxacin: *Dosage*: See Quinolones also.

Eye drops: >1 year 1 drop 2–4 hourly for 1st 48 hours and then 4 times daily till 2 days after healing is achieved (maximum 10 days).

Ear drops: Otitis external—1–12 years 5 drops and 12–18 years 10 drops to affected ear(s) 2 times daily for 10 days.

Chronic suppurative otitis media (CSOM): >12 years 10 drops to affected ear(s) 2 times daily for 14 days.

Acute otitis media (AOM) with perforation or with tympanostomy tubes: 1–12 years—5 drops to affected ear(s) 2 times daily for 10 days. IV and oral—10–15 mg/kg/day in a single dose or divided twice daily.

Systemic use: it is replaced by levofloxacin which is an S—isomer of ofloxacin and has less side effects.

Olanzapine: *Dosage*: 12–18 years 5–20 mg once daily. Usual dose is 10 mg daily.

Olopatadine: *Dosage*: *Allergic conjunctivitis, including ocular pruritus:* Adolescents, and Children >3 years: 1 drop in each affected eye two times per day at an interval of 6–8 hours (this is the maximum dosage allowed) Children <3 years: Safety and efficacy have not been established. No dosage adjustment is necessary for ocular administration in patients with renal or hepatic impairment.

Olsalazine: *Dosage*: Oral—Adolescents and children (2–18 years): 30 mg/kg/day (not exceeding 3 g/day), in two or 3 divided doses. May initiate with 500 mg twice daily and increase over 1 week up to a maximum of 3 g/day (a single dose not exceeding 1 g). Maintenance dose is 250–500 mg 2 times daily. Olsalazine should be used cautiously in patients with pre-existing renal impairment or renal disease due to possibility of renal tubular damage. Monitoring BUN, serum creatinine and urinalysis.

Omeprazole: *Dosage*: Oral <12 years initially 0.7 mg/kg and increased to 3 mg/kg/day and 12–18 years 20–40 mg initially as single dose and at higher doses in 2 divided doses.

H. pylori: Oral 1–12 years 1–2 mg/kg rounded to nearest 10 mg and maximum 40 mg and in 12–18 years 40 mg as single dose for 14 days with amoxicillin and clarithromycin or amoxicillin and metronidazole or clarithromycin and metronidazole.

Ondansetron: *Dosage*:

Nausea and vomiting—chemotherapy induced: IV < 12 year 5 mg/m2 and 12–18 years 8 mg as single dose just before chemotherapy and repeated 8–12 hourly during therapy and for 24 hours after. Oral following initial IV dosing to get control—<12 years 4 mg and 12–18 years 8 mg 2–3 times daily for up to 5 days after a course of chemotherapy.

Postoperative nausea and vomiting: IV slow infusion 2- 12 year 0.1 mg/kg (maximum 4 mg) and 12–18 years 4 mg.

Pruritus: Oral 2–12 year 2–4 mg/dose and 12–18 year 4- 8 mg/dose 2 times daily.

Palliative for nausea/vomiting and pruritus: IV/SC 5 mg/m^2 continuous over 24 hours.

Oral rehydration salts (ORS): *Dosage*: *Fluid and electrolyte loss in diarrhea:* By mouth—1 month–1 year 1–1½ times usual feed volume; 1–12 years 200 mL after every loose motion; 12–18 years 200–400 mL after every loose motion.

Orlistat: *Dosage*: Orally—12–18 year–120 mg immediately before, during or 1 hour after each main meal (maximum 3 times/day); specialist advice required for treating for more than 12 weeks. If meal is missed or if meal contains no fat, the dose may be omitted.

Oseltamivir: *Dosage*:

Prevention of influenza: Oral—13–18 years—75 mg once daily for at least 7 days after exposure or for up to 6 weeks during an epidemic.

Treatment of influenza: Oral—for children above 1 year age—up to 16 kg–30 mg, 16–23 kg–45 mg, 23–40 kg–60 mg and >40 kg–75 mg every 12 hours for 5 days.

Oxandrolone: *Dosage*: Oral—1.25–2.5 mg once daily, generally for about 3–6 months, but has been used occasionally for up to 1 year; evidence suggests using doses as low as 625 µg for Turner syndrome, in combination with growth hormone, seek expert advice before prescribing.

Oxcarbazepine: *Dosage*: Oral—6–12 years 8–10 mg/kg/day in 2 divided doses—increase by 5 mg/kg/dose twice daily weekly till maximum of 30 mg/kg/dose for adjunctive therapy and 46 mg/kg/day for monotherapy. 12–18 years 8–10 mg/kg/day (maximum initial dose 300 mg/dose) in 2 divided doses. Increase over 2–4 weeks to 1200 mg/24 hours in 2 divided doses (maximum 2400 mg/24 hour).

Oxybutynin: *Dosage*: Oral 2–5 years—0.2 mg/kg/dose PO Q 8 hourly, 5–12 years 2.5–5 mg and 12–18 years 5 mg 2–3 times daily (maximum in 12–18 years 5 mg 4 times daily).

Oxygen: *Dosage*: Dependent on condition. In some conditions (e.g. bronchopulmonary dysplasia), very low flow rates (e.g. 0.1 L/minute) may maintain oxygen saturation.

Oxymetazoline hydrochloride: *Dosage*: 1 drop in each nostril twice daily or when required.

Oxytetracycline: *Dosage*:

Acne: Oral 12–18 years 250–500 mg/dose 12 hourly.

Infections: 250–500 mg/dose 6 hourly.

P

Palivizumab: *Dosage*: 15 mg/kg once monthly, starting just prior to the beginning of the RSV season, for a total of 5 doses. Not used in India as of now.

Pamidronate disodium: *Dosage*: Experience of the use of bisphosphonates in children is limited and expert advice should be sought. Their use is only justified when the potential benefits outweigh any risk. *Children:* 1 mg/kg/ 24 hours for three consecutive days once in 3 months or 10–40 mg/m^2 over 5–8 hours once a month. Dose adjusted according to serum calcium levels.

Pancreatin: *Dosage*: Dose varies widely and should be tailored to each individual patient according to symptoms, stool type and abdominal findings; should not exceed 10,000 lipase units/kg body weight per day.

Pancuronium bromide: *Dosage*: Newborn—IV loading 0.1 mg/kg followed by maintenance IV 0.05 mg/kg/dose 4–6 times daily as needed. Children—IV 1 month –18 years 0.06–0.1 mg/kg initially followed by 0.01–0.02 mg/kg as required.

Paracetamol: *Dosage*: Oral or suppository < 12 years 15 mg/kg/dose every 4–6 hourly; 12–18 years 325–650 mg every 4–6 hourly.

Paraldehyde: *Dosage*: Rectal < 12 years 0.4 mL/kg and 12–18 years 5–10 mL diluted in equal volume of olive or sunflower oil before administration. IM Newborn 0.2 mL/kg; 1 month–12 years 0.1–0.15 mL/kg and 12–18 years 5–10 mL as single dose. Deep IM with Z injection (maximum 1 mL [newborn] and 5 mL [older children] per site).

Paromomycin sulfate: *Dosage*:

Amebiasis: A symptomatic cyst passers (intraluminal infections)—Oral—25–35 mg/kg daily, in 3 divided doses, given for 5–10 days (usually 7 days).

Symptomatic intestinal amebiasis or extraintestinal disease (including amebic liver abscess): Oral—25–35 mg/kg daily, in 3 divided doses, given for 5–10 days (usually 7 days). Used as follow up after initial treatment with a tissue amebicide (oral metronidazole or oral tinidazole).

Cestode (Tapeworm) infections—Diphyllobothrium latum (Fish Tapeworm), Dipylidium caninum (Dog and Cat Tapeworm), Taenia saginata (Beef Tapeworm), or T. solium (Pork Tapeworm) Infections: Oral—11 mg/kg every 15 minutes for 4 doses.

Hymenolepis nana (Dwarf Tapeworm) infections: Oral—45 mg/kg daily, given as a single daily dose, for 5–7 days.

Cryptosporidiosis: Oral—25–35 mg/kg daily in 2–4 divided doses for HIV-infected children or adolescents. Maximum dosage is 500 mg 4 times daily in children.

Dientamoeba fragilis infections: Oral–25–35 mg/kg daily, in 3 divided doses, given for 7 days.

Giardiasis: Oral—25–35 mg/kg daily, in 3 divided doses given for 7 days.

Leishmaniasis: Cutaneous Leishmaniasis—Topical—Apply topically (as a preparation containing paromomycin 15% and methylbenzethonium chloride 12% in white petrolatum) twice daily for 10–20 days. If effective, clinical healing of lesions usually is complete within several weeks to a month after topical paromomycin treatment is completed. In patients with recurrent disease (*Leishmania recidivans*), more prolonged topical treatment (e.g. twice daily for about 3 months) may eliminate the protozoa from cutaneous lesions.

Visceral leishmaniasis (kala-azar): IM–11–20 mg/kg daily for 10–21 days.

Paroxetine: *Dosage*:

Obsessive compulsive disorder (OCD): Oral—12–18 years 20 mg (maximum 60 mg) once daily in the morning. Increase weekly by 10 mg/day to maximum dose.

Panic disorder: Oral—12–18 years 12.5 mg/day. Higher doses under supervision of specialist. (maximum 40 mg) once daily in the morning. Increase weekly by 10 mg/day to maximum dose.

Idiopathic musculoskeletal pain: Oral 8–12 years 10 mg and 12–18 years 20 mg once daily.

PAS (Para-aminosalicylic acid): *Dosage*: *Tuberculosis*—Oral—150 mg/kg/day in 2–3 divided doses. Maximum 12 g/day.

Penicillamine: *Dosage*: Full blood count (FBC), platelet count and urinalysis should be performed prior to treatment with penicillamine. Urinalysis and FBC should be carried out monthly during treatment. Caution should be exercised in patients with renal insufficiency, and modification of the dosage may be necessary. Renal function should be assessed monthly. An immediate blood count should be carried out if neutropenia or thrombocytopenia is suspected due to symptoms such as a sore throat, glossitis, buccal ulceration, easy bruising or bleeding. If any abnormal results are found, treatment should be withheld and discussed with the clinician responsible for the child's care. Severe dyspepsia or taste disturbances may necessitate dosage reduction.

Wilson disease: Adjust dose to maintain urinary copper excretion > 1 mg/24 hour. Orally 20 mg/kg/24 hours in 2–4 divided doses (maximum 1 g/24 hours).

Lead intoxication: Orally 30–40 mg/kg/24 hours in 2–3 divided doses (maximum 1.5 g/24 hours).

Juvenile idiopathic arthritis: 3 mg/kg/24 hours in 2 divided doses; increasing once every 3 months by 3 mg/kg/24 hours up to maximum of 10 mg/kg/24 hours.

Systemic sclerosis: Oral < 12 years 2.5–5 mg/kg/day in 2 divided doses increased 4 weekly to maximum of 15–20 mg/kg/day and 12–18 years 125–250 mg/day increased slowly to 250–375 mg in 2 divided doses.

Penicillinase-resistant penicillins (Flucloxacillin/Cloxacillin): *Dosage*: Dose—Newborn—IV or orally <7days 50–100 mg/ kg/day in 2 divided doses; 7–21 days 75–150 mg/kg/day in 3 divided doses; >21 days 100–200 mg/kg/day in 4 divided doses. Children—IV/IM 50–100 mg/kg/day in 4 divided doses (maximum single dose 1 g may be doubled in severe infection). Oral <1 year 250 mg/day, 1–5 years 500 mg/day, 5–18 years 1 g in 4 divided doses. Doses may be doubled in severe infection.

Penicillins (Benzylpenicillin/Penicillin G): *Dosage*: Given IV. In newborn—25 mg (approximately 40,000 units)/kg/dose 2 times daily up to 7 days of age and 3 times daily thereafter. Dose is doubled in meningitis. In children 25 mg/kg/dose 4 times daily. Double dose is given in meningitis 6 times daily to a maximum single dose of 2.4 g (approximately 40 L units) and a maximum daily dose of 14.4 g (approximately 2.3 crore units).

Pentazocine: *Dosage*: Adolescents: Inj. 30–60 mg IM or 30 mg IV. May be repeated 3–4 hourly. Doses in excess of 30 mg IV or 60 mg SC or IM not recommended. Maximum daily dose: 360 mg in labor. 30 mg IM or 20 mg IV 2–3 hourly. Max: 2–3 doses. Tab: 25–100 mg repeated when necessary maximum 600 mg daily. Children: Not for children below 12 years.

Permethrin: *Dosage*:

Scabies (dermal cream): Single topical application of up to: 1 tube for children >12 years. Half a tube for children aged 6–12 years. A quarter of a tube for children aged 1–5 years. An eighth of a tube for children aged 2 months–1 year. Medical supervision required for children <2 years of age. If necessary, a second application may be given not less than 7 days after the initial application. Apply to whole body excluding head. Wash off after 8–12 hours. Children <2 years old should also have the cream applied to the face, neck, scalp and ears. If hands or any part are washed, the treatment must be reapplied.

Pediculosis—Head lice (cream rinse): Apply to clean damp hair, leave on for 10 minutes, rinse and dry. Not affected by chlorine in swimming pools.

Pethidine hydrochloride (controlled drug): *Dosage*: SC/IM Newborn 0.5–1 mg/kg, <12 years 0.5–2 mg/kg, 12–18 years 25–100 mg as single dose-repeated if required once in 4- 6 hours. IV bolus <12 years 0.5 mg—1 mg/kg and 12–18 years 25–50 mg repeated if required once in 4–6 hours. IV infusion loading dose of 1 mg/kg followed by 0.1–0.4 mg/kg/hour—ventilated babies may require higher doses. Newborn and infants are prone to respiratory depression. Avoid in severe renal impairment, sickle cell crisis and prolonged infusions as accumulation of metabolite norpethidine can cause seizures. May precipitate coma in children with liver disease.

Phenobarbitone (phenobarbital): *Dosage*:

Anticonvulsant: Loading dose 15–20 mg/kg; Orally, IV or IM; then maintenance newborn 3–4 mg/kg/24 hours oral or IV in 2 divided doses or as single daily dose, children 5–6 mg/kg/24 hours oral or IV in 2 divided doses or as single daily dose and in adolescents 1–3 mg/kg/24 hours oral or IV in 2 divided doses or as single daily dose.

Sedation: children 2 mg/kg/dose.

Hyperbilirubinemia: Newborn 5–8 mg/kg/day orally for 2–7 days. Not widely used as phototherapy usually suffices.

Phenoxybenzamine hydrochloride: *Dosage*: Oral 1–2 mg/kg/24 hours in 2 divided doses. IV infusion 1 mg/kg bolus given IV over 30 min followed by 0.5–1 mg/kg/day infusion.

Phenoxymethylpenicillin (Penicillin V): *Dosage*: Oral 250 mg/day, 1–5 years 500 mg/day, 6–12 years 1 g/day and 12–18 years 2 g/day (severe infection 3 g/day) in 4 divided doses.

Pneumococcal infection prophylaxis: Half the above daily dose in 2 divided doses.

Rheumatic fever prophylaxis: 500 mg/day in 2 divided doses.

Phenytoin: *Dosage*:

Status epilepticus: Loading dose— neonate 15–20 mg/kg IV (not to exceed 0.5 mg/kg/min) and in children and adolescents 15–18 mg/kg IV (not to exceed 1–3 mg/kg/min).

Antiepileptic: Oral/IV newborn 5 mg/kg/24 hours once daily or in 2 divided doses, < 6 years 8–10 mg/kg/24 hours, 7–9 years 6–8 mg/kg/24 hours once daily or in 2 divided doses, 10–16 years 6–7 mg/kg/24 hours once daily or in 2 divided doses, >16 years 300–600 mg/24 hours once daily or in 2 divided doses.

Arrhythmias: loading dose 1.25 mg/kg IV once in 5 min until desired effect or total dose 15 mg/kg. Maintenance children 8–10 mg/kg/day in 2–3 divided doses and in adolescents 250 mg 3–4 times daily.

Pholcodine: *Dosage*: Oral 1 month to 6 years 2 mg/dose, 6–12 years 2.5 mg/dose, 12–18 years 5–10 mg/dose 3–4 times daily.

Phosphates: *Dosage*:

Hypercalcemia: Oral: newborn 1 mmol/kg, <5 years up to 48 mmol, > 5 years up to 96 mmol.

Hypophosphatemia: Oral: newborn 1 mmol/kg, <5 year up to 36–48 mmol, > 5 year up to 64–96 mmol. May be given in 3 divided doses in hypophosphatemic rickets. IV newborn 1 mmol/kg, <2 years 0.7 mmol/kg, > 2 years 0.4 mmol/kg.

Phosphocysteamine: *Dosage*: Oral >2 years 6 mg/kg 4 times daily. Increase every 2–3 weeks by 25 mg/kg/day up to maintenance of 125 mg/kg/day.

Pimozide: *Dosage*:

Schizophrenia: Oral 12–18 years 1–20 mg usually once daily but may be given in divided doses.

Tourette syndrome: Oral 2–12 years 1–4 mg, 12–18 years 2–10 mg usually once daily but may be given in divided doses. Do annual ECG to monitor QT interval.

Piperacillin with Tazobactam: *Dosage*: Newborn IV 90 mg/kg/dose 3 times daily. Children IV 90 mg/kg/dose 4 times daily (maximum single dose 4.5 g).

Piperazine: *Dosage*:

Round worm: 4 g once daily for 2 days— Children 0.75 g/year, maximum 4 g. Because of its capacity to relax worms mainly useful for intestinal obstruction caused by round worms.

Enterobiasis: 50 mg/kg OD for 7 days consecutively or 75 mg/kg single dose.

Piracetam: *Dosage*: *Learning difficulties:* 3g/day in 3 divided doses for 1 school year. Children: 50 mg/kg in 3 divided doses.

Once the desired result has been obtained reduce the initial dose by half up to 6–8 weeks.

Piroxicam: *Dosage*: Oral < 15 kg 5 mg, 16–25 kg 10 mg, 26–45 kg 15 mg and >46 kg 20 mg once daily.

Pizotifen: *Dosage*: 5–18 years start with 500 µg at night and increase gradually up to 1.5 mg daily in divided doses; maximum single dose (at night)–1 mg.

Pneumococcal conjugate vaccine: *Dosage*: Deep SC or IM injection: 0.5 mL. The number of doses for a primary course depends on the age of the child. For routine immunization 3 doses at 1 month interval from 6 weeks of age, if given below 6 months age, 2 doses at 1 month interval if given between 6 month and 1 year and 1 dose if given after 1 year with a booster at 1½ years age. For these high-risk groups, three doses at monthly intervals for children <2 years old and two doses at a month apart for those of >2 years. The course should then be followed by a single dose of the plain polysaccharide vaccine to increase the breadth of cover. This should be administered at >2 years with a min interval of 8 weeks after the conjugate vaccine.

Pneumococcal polysaccharide vaccine: *Dosage*: Deep SC or IM: 0.5 mL as single dose. Booster doses of the plain polysaccharide vaccine are not normally recommended and should certainly not take place within 3 years of the first dose as marked local reactions can occur. As the vaccine could be used in conjunction with the conjugate vaccine in children, one must ensure an 8 weeks gap between the last conjugate pneumococcal vaccine and the polysaccharide vaccine.

Podophyllum: *Dosage*: Topical: applied twice weekly. Leave on affected area for not more than 6 hours then wash off. Protect surrounding area with soft paraffin. Continue applying till eradication of wart or a maximum of 6 weeks.

Poliomyelitis vaccine, live oral (OPV): *Dosage*: Oral: 3 drops (0.135 mL). The primary course is usually given at birth, 8, 12 and 16 and 20 weeks of age. This is followed by a booster at 1½ years and 4½ years age. Given on National immunization days to all children < 5 years age for poliomyelitis eradication.

Polyethylene glycol 3350: *Dosage*: Polyethylene glycol 3350 powder—1 sachet or 1 heap tablespoon once daily—mix with a liquid and give orally once a day as needed for up to 2 weeks. It may take 2 to 4 days for polyethylene glycol 3350 to produce a bowel movement.

Potassium chloride: *Dosage*:

Potassium supplementation: Oral/IV 0.5–1 mmol/kg 2 times daily or 0.5–1 mEq/kg 2 times daily.

Acute hypokalemia: 0.08–0.2 mmol/kg/hour or mEq/kg/hour. Check dose carefully as overdose could be fatal. Recheck potassium levels after 3 hours. 1 g KCl = 13.4 mmol or 13.4 mEq.

Potassium permanganate: *Dosage*: Cleansing and deodorizing suppurating eczematous reactions and wounds. For wet dressings or baths, use approximately 0.01% (1 in 10,000) solution; or 1 granule dissolved in 300 mL (2 ½ glasses) of water.

Povidone-iodine: *Dosage*: *Antiseptic paint:* apply twice daily. *Dry powder:* use for minor wounds and infections. *Ointment:* Apply once or twice daily for up to 14 days. *Shampoo:* use as shampoo twice weekly until improvement noted then once weekly. *Skin cleanser:* retain on infected skin for 3–5 minutes before rinsing. Repeat twice daily. *Solutions, tinctures and scrub:* use undiluted for skin disinfection.

Pralidoxime: *Dosage*: Adolescents: Following resuscitation measures, and 2–4 mg atropine inj., 1–2 g IM or IV as 5% solution over 5–10 minutes or infusion in 100 mL sodium chloride over 15–30 minutes. Repeat therapy if required. Children: 20– 40 mg/kg once daily.

Pravastatin sodium: *Dosage*: Oral 2–12 years: 5 mg, 12–18 years: 10 mg once daily. Increase if needed over 6–12 weeks.

Praziquantel: *Dosage*:

Schistosomiasis hematobium (S. mansoni): Oral 4–18 years 40 mg/kg/day as single dose or in 2 divided doses with food for 1 day.

S. japonicum: Oral 4–18 years 60 mg/kg/day in 3 divided doses with food for 1 day.

Liver fluke: Oral 4–18 years 60 mg/kg/day in 2 divided doses with food for 3 days.

Lung fluke (Paragonimus westermani): Oral 4–18 years 75 mg/kg/day in 3 divided doses with food for 3 days.

Intestinal fluke (Fasciolopsis buski): Oral 4–18 years 75 mg/kg/day in 3 divided doses with food for 1 day.

Beef, pork and fish tapeworm: Oral 4–18 years 10–20 mg/kg/day as single dose with light breakfast for 1 day.

Dwarf tapeworm: Oral 4–18 years 25 mg/kg/day as single dose with light breakfast for 1 day.

Neurocysticercosis: Oral 4–18 year 50 mg/kg/day in 3 divided doses with food for 15– 21 days. Give steroids to reduce severity of adverse reactions.

Echinococcosis: Oral 4–18 years 40 mg/kg/day once in a week with food in combination with albendazole as adjunct to surgery and for inoperable cysts. No dosage adjustment for renal failure and hepatic failure.

Prazosin: *Dosage*:

Hypertension: Oral 1 month to 12 years 10–15 µg/kg/dose 2–4 times daily (maximum 0.5 mg/kg/ day) and 12–18 year 0.5 mg/dose 2–3 times daily (maximum 20 mg/day).

Congestive cardiac failure: Oral 1 month–12 years 0.5 µg/kg/dose, 2 times daily (maximum 0.1 mg/kg/day) and 12-18 years, 0.5 mg/dose 2-4 times daily (maximum 20 mg/day).

Prednisolone: *Dosage*:

Acute asthma: Oral 1-2 mg/kg in 2-3 divided doses (maximum 40 mg/day) for 1-5 days and stop without tapering if the episode is controlled.

Croup requiring intubation: Oral 2 mg/kg/day in 2 divided doses soon after intubation and continued for 24 hours after extubation.

Nephrotic syndrome: Oral initially for 4-6 weeks, 60 mg/m^2 (maximum 80 mg/day) in 2-3 divided doses as single morning dose and after proteinuria is absent for 3 days, maintenance for 4-8 weeks of then followed by 40 mg/m^2 (maximum 60 mg) as single morning dose on alternate days for 6 weeks. Then taper and stop. Repeat for relapses.

Autoimmune hepatitis: 2 mg/kg (maximum 40 mg) once daily.

Inflammatory bowel disease: 1-2 mg/kg (maximum 60 mg/day)—taper and stop over a few weeks

JIA, connective tissue disorder, vasculitis: Up to 2 mg/kg single morning dose or alternate day at lowest dose that controls disease. Avoid if possible as weaning would be difficult.

Ulcerative colitis, Crohn's disease: Rectal (enema) at bedtime for 2-4 weeks and continued, if response is good.

Infantile spasms and intractable seizures: 2 mg/kg/day higher doses in infantile spasms.

Chemotherapy regimens: Follow doses recommended for given protocol.

Transplant programs: Each unit has its own protocol.

Adrenal insufficiency including congenital adrenal hyperplasia: 2.5-5 mg/m^2 in two divided doses.

Thyroid storm: 1-2 mg/kg/day in two divided doses for 2 weeks.

Hypercalcemia due to vitamin D excess: 2 mg/kg/day in two divided doses for 4-6 weeks.

ITP: A course of prednisolone 2 mg/kg is given in divided doses. For patients with mucus membrane hemorrhage or extremely low platelet counts, higher doses—4 to 8 mg/kg/day have also been tried. It is gradually tapered off. If there is no response or if the platelets fall again when steroids are discontinued, a repeat 4 week course should be given for 4 weeks or so. Prolonged corticosteroid therapy is not indicated, even if platelet count remains low as it may depress the bone marrow.

Prilocaine hydrochloride: *Dosage*: Children <10 years 1 mL, > 10 years 1-2 mL.

Primaquine: *Dosage*: Oral 1-12 years 0.25 mg/kg/day and 12-18 years 15 mg once daily for 14 days.

For G6PD patients: 1-12 years 0.5-0.75 mg/kg and 12-18 years 30 mg once in a week for 8 weeks.

Primidone: *Dosage*: Oral—<2 years initially 125 mg daily at bedtime, increased by 125 mg every 3 days according to response; usual maintenance, 125-250 mg twice daily; 2-5 years initially 125 mg daily at bedtime, increased by 125 mg every 3 days according to response; usual maintenance, 250-375 mg twice daily; 5-9 years initially 125 mg daily at bedtime, increased by 125 mg every 3 days according to response; usual maintenance, 375-500 mg twice a day; 9-18 years initially 125 mg daily at bedtime, increased by 125 mg every 3 days to 250 mg twice daily, then increased.

Hepatic impairment: Reduce dose, may precipitate coma.

Renal-impairment: Refer phenobarbitone (phenobarbital).

Procarbazine: *Dosage*: Always consult the current treatment protocol for details of dosage and scheduling.

Hodgkin disease: Oral 1.5-3 mg/kg/24 hours (50-100 mg/m^2) once daily for 14 days per 28 day cycle.

Bone marrow transplant preparation: 12.5 mg/kg/dose.

Neuroblastoma and medulloblastoma: 100-200 mg/m^2/dose as part of protocol.

Prochlorperazine: *Dosage*: Oral/rectal > 1 year 0.1-0.25 mg/kg/dose 2-3 times daily. IM 0.1-0.15 mg/kg/24 hours divided in 2-3 doses.

Procyclidine: *Dosage*: Oral 7-12 years 4 mg/kg/day and 12-18 years 7.5 mg/kg/day in 3 divided doses.

Proguanil: *Dosage*: Oral 0-12 weeks < 6 kg 25 mg 1/4th tab; 12 weeks to 11 months 6-10 kg 50 mg ½ tab; 1-3 years 10-16 kg 75 mg 3/4th tab; 4-7 years 16-24 kg 100 mg 1 tab; 8-12 years 25-44 kg 150 mg 1½ tab; >13 years >45 kg 200 mg 2 tab. To be given once daily starting 1 week before entering endemic area and continue till 4 weeks after return.

Promethazine hydrochloride: *Dosage*:

Symptomatic relief of allergy: Oral < 1 year 2.5-5 mg, 1-6 years 5-10 mg, 6-12 years 10-15 mg and 12-18 years 10-20 mg 2-3 times daily.

Vomiting and nausea: Oral 1 mg/kg/24 hours in 4 divided doses.

Sedation: Oral 1-2 mg/kg as single dose.

Sedation in ICU: Slow IV/Oral/deep IM <12 year 2-4 mg/kg/day and > 12 years 100-200 mg in 4 divided doses. Start with lower dose and increase gradually depending on response. May use along with chloral hydrate.

Propafenone hydrochloride: *Dosage*: Oral 10-20 mg/kg/day in 2 divided doses; starting at lower dose. IV bolus followed by IV infusion 0.2 mg/kg slowly over 10 min repeated every 15 min up to maximum 2 mg/kg followed by IV infusion with ECG monitoring of 4 µg/kg/min increasing to 8 µg/kg/min (if required). 20-30% of this total dose if hepatic function is impaired.

Propantheline bromide: *Dosage*: Oral < 12 years 0.9–1.2 mg/kg/day in 3-4 divided doses (maximum 3 mg/kg/day larger doses in enuresis) and > 12 year 15 mg before meals and 20 mg at bedtime.

Propofol: *Dosage*: Sedation—IV 1.5–3 mg/kg/dose over 1–2 min.

Continuous sedation (mechanical ventilation): 5.5 mg/ kg for 30 min, increase to 6 mg/kg for 30 min, increase to 8 mg/kg for 1 hour, increase to 10 mg/kg for 1 hour, increase to final infusion rate of 12.5 mg/kg/ hour.

Induction of general anesthesia: 1.5–2.5 mg/kg (larger doses in children < 8 years) and maintain anesthesia with 9–15 mg/kg/hour.

Propranolol: *Dosage*:

Hypertension: Oral newborn 0.25–0.5 mg/kg, < 12 year 0.25–1 mg/kg 3 times daily and >12 years 80–160 mg 2 times daily. Maximum in newborn 2 mg/kg/day and in children increase weekly as required to usual dose 1–5 mg/kg/day.

Migraine prophylaxis and essential tremor: Oral 2–12 years 20 mg/dose and 12–18 years 20–40 mg/dose 2–3 times daily.

Dysarrhythmias: Oral <12 year 0.25–0.5 mg/dose and > 12 years 10–40 mg/dose 3–4 times daily. IV bolus—< 12 years 25–50 μg/kg and > 12 years 1 mg/kg as single dose slowly over 5 min with ECG monitoring. Repeat dose as required up to 4 times daily.

Hyperthyroidism and neonatal thyrotoxicosis: Oral 0.25–0.75 mg/kg/dose 3 times daily. Increase according to response. May require 1 mg/kg/dose 3 times daily.

Tetralogy of Fallot: Oral < 12 years 0.25–1 mg/kg/ dose 2 times daily in newborn and 3–4 times in > 1 month age. IV bolus up to 0.1 mg/kg over 5 min under ECG control 2 times daily in newborn and 4 times in > 1 month age.

Hypertrophic obstructive cardiomyopathy: Oral < 12 years 0.25–1 mg/kg/ dose and > 12 years 10–40 mg/dose 3–4 times daily (8 mg/kg/ day in 4 divided doses).

Propylthiouracil (PTU): *Dosage*: Oral < 1 year 2.5 mg/kg/dose, 1–4 years 25 mg/dose, 5–12 years 50 mg/dose and 12–18 year 100 mg/dose 3 times daily. Dose gradually tapered after child is euthyroid.

Protamine sulfate: *Dosage*: All ages: 1 mg (0.1 mL) for each 100 units mucous heparin (or low molecular weight heparin (LMWH) or 80 units lung heparin given at last dose, maximum dose 50 mg. Administer within 15 minutes. If the delay is longer, less protamine is required, as heparin is rapidly excreted (after 30 minutes give approximately half dose).

Pseudoephedrine hydrochloride: *Dosage*: Oral (not used in newborn) 1 month to 2 years 7.5 mg/dose, 2–12 years 15–30 mg/dose and 12–18 years 60 mg/dose 3 times daily.

Psoralen: *Dosage*: Adults: Tab: 0.6–0.7 mg/kg body wt. daily.

Pyrantel Pamoate: *Dosage*: 11 mg/kg/day as single dose. Repeat after two weeks (Maximum1 g). In heavy hookworm infestation give for two successive days.

Pyrazinamide: *Dosage*:

Tuberculosis—Daily regimen: Oral children 35 mg/kg/day (Range 30–40 mg/kg/24 hours) as single dose or in 2 divided doses (maximum 2 g/day) for the first 2 months of the standard 6 months regimen. 12–18 years <50 kg 1.5 g/day and > 50 kg 2 g/day as single dose or in 2 divided doses (maximum 2 g/day) for the first 2 months of the standard 6 months regimen.

Intermittent regimen: 35 mg/kg/ day (Range 30–40 mg/kg/day).

Pyridostigmine bromide: *Dosage*: Oral initially 1.5 mg/kg/dose (maximum newborn 10 mg, 1 month to 2 years 30 mg and 2–12 years 60 mg) and in 12–18 years 30–120 mg. The dose is increased in increments of 25–50% daily till maximum improvement is obtained and given in divided doses at suitable intervals. Usual total daily dose <12 years is 30–360 mg and > 12 year 300 mg–1.2 g.

Pyridoxine (Vitamin B_6): *Dosage*:

Metabolic indications: 50–250 mg/dose 1–2 times daily. Higher doses in partially responsive cases and for Wilson disease.

Pyridoxine dependent seizures: Newborn—Oral try test dose of 50–100 mg 1–2 times daily for 2 days and if responsive, maintenance of 25–100 mg 2 times daily lifelong. Increased dose may be required with intercurrent illness and with growth. IV bolus/IM 50–100 mg as test dose; may give for 2 days and then change to oral. If seizures persist, commence conventional anticonvulsant therapy. Children 20–50 mg 1–2 times daily— up to 500 mg twice daily may be required. IV bolus-1 month–12 years 25–100 mg as test dose for 2 days and then change to oral.

Pyrimethamine: *Dosage*:

Toxoplasmosis in pregnancy: if Toxoplasma infection is diagnosed in early pregnancy and the fetus is not infected, spiramycin is given (see spiramycin monograph). If the fetus is found to be infected, then pyrimethamine 50 mg once daily, sulfadiazine 1 g 3 times daily and calcium folinate (folinic acid) 15 mg 3 times per week are given until delivery.

Toxoplasmosis in infants: Pyrimethamine along with sulfadiazine (50 mg/kg 2 times daily) and calcium folinate (folinic acid) (15 mg/kg three times in a week) are given for 12 months. Pyrimethamine is started with loading dose of 1 mg/kg/dose 2 times daily for 2 days, then 1 mg/kg/dose once daily for 6 months followed by 1 mg/kg/dose thrice in a week for 6 months. Prednisolone at 0.5/kg/dose 2 times daily is also given until signs of CNS inflammation (CSF protein > 10 g/L) or active chorioretinitis have settled and then tapered.

Ocular toxoplasmosis, reactivation of toxoplasmosis during HIV infection and toxoplasmosis in immunocompromised child with protracted or incapacitating illness: 2 mg/kg loading dose for 2 days followed by 1 mg/kg in < 12 years and 25–100 mg in 12–18 years olds for 6 weeks to prevent relapse in HIV patients followed by maintenance of a quarter to half of starting dose indefinitely.

Pyrimethamine with sulfadoxine: *Dosage*: Oral 2 month–4 years ½ tab, 5–6 years 1 tab, 7–9 years 1½ tab, 10–14 years 2 tabs and > 14 years 3 tabs as a single dose after quinine therapy.

Pyritinol: *Dosage*: Children: 100–200 mg daily according to age. Continue therapy for several weeks. Infants: 2.5–5 mL 1–3 times daily.

Q

Quinidine: *Dosage*: Adolescents: 200–400 mg 3–4 times daily. Initially give test dose. Children: 2 mg/kg test dose to exclude idiosyncrasy. PO: 30 mg/kg/24 hours in divided doses every 4–6 hours.

Quinine: *Dosage*: Oral—birth–12 years 30 mg/kg/day (sulfate) and 12–18 years 1.8 g/day (sulfate) in 3 divided doses for 7 days. IV infusion over 4 hours initial loading dose of 20 mg/kg (maximum 1.4 g), then 10 mg/kg (maximum 0.7 g) every 12 hours for 48 hours and then maintenance of 5–7 mg/kg once in 8 hours if IV is needed after 48 hours. As soon as possible change to oral.

Quinolones: *Dosage*:

Ciprofloxacin: Neonates–10 mg/kg 12 hourly orally or IV; Children 15–30 mg/kg in 2 divided doses oral/IV (maximum single dose IV 400 mg and oral 750 mg).

Ofloxacin: Oral: Adolescents 200–800 mg/day. Not recommended for children less than 12 years age. IV: Adolescents 200 mg infusion over 30 min 2 times daily. May be increased to 400 mg twice in severe infections.

R

Rabies immunoglobulin, human (HRIG): *Dosage*: 20 IU/kg IM and infiltration: half infiltrated around wound with the rest IM. Give at a different site to the vaccine.

Rabies vaccine: *Dosage*:

Pre-exposure: 1 mL on days 0, 7 and 28. Two doses 4 weeks apart may be adequate in those not expecting to handle animals if postexposure treatment will be readily available. In this case, if exposure continues, a further dose after 6–12 months will be necessary. Boosters may be given every 2–3 years if there is continuing risk and postexposure treatment is not readily available. After 2–3 boosters, expert advice should be sought before giving more.

Postexposure: When an individual has been exposed via a break in the skin or contamination of a mucosal surface to a potentially rabid animal, consideration should be given to postexposure treatment. Advice should always be sought before starting treatment. Unimmunized/incompletely immunized (received < 3 doses or had intradermal)—low-risk 1 mL on 0, 3, 7, 14 and 30 day and in high-risk 1 mL on 0, 3, 7, 14 and 30 day plus rabies immunoglobulin. Fully immunized individual- 1 mL on 0, 3 and 7 day.

Ramipril: *Dosage*: Oral—Children-1.5 mg/m^2/24 h once daily. Adolescents—2.5 mg once daily. Adjust dosage to achieve proper blood pressure response, up to maximum of 20 mg/day. But more studies are required in children before it is used in pediatrics.

Ranitidine: *Dosage*: Newborn—Oral/IV 1 mg/kg 3 times daily (studies with oral treatment in newborn are limited) and IV infusion 30–60 µg/kg/hour (maximum 3 mg/kg/day). Child: Oral 6 months to 12 years 2–4 mg/kg/dose (maximum 150 mg) 12–18 years 150 mg/dose 2 times daily. Up to 9 mg/kg may be used. IV bolus 1 mg/kg 2–4 times daily IV infusion 125–250 µg/kg/hour. Reduce dose to 50% in severe renal failure.

Riboflavin (Vitamin B_2): *Dosage*: Oral 50 mg once daily. May give in frequent smaller doses. Doses up to 300–400 mg/day have been used.

Rifampicin: *Dosage*:

Tuberculosis in combination with other drugs: Oral 10 mg/kg (maximum 600 mg/day) as single morning dose.

Meningococcal infection prophylaxis and staphylococcal infections: Oral < 5 years 5 mg/kg/dose and > 1 year 10 mg/kg/dose (maximum 600 mg/dose) 2 times daily for 2 days for meningococcal infection prophylaxis and for 10–14 days for staphylococcal infections.

H. influenzae prophylaxis: Oral <3 months 10 mg/kg and >3 months 20 mg/kg/dose (maximum 600 mg/dose) once daily for 4 days.

Cholestasis—pruritus: 5–10 mg/kg (maximum 600 mg) once daily.

Dose adjustment in liver failure. Avoid altogether, or reduce doses for tuberculosis and prophylaxis to 8 mg/kg daily.

Risperidone: *Dosage*:

Aggressive behavior, Tourette syndrome: Oral 0.5–2 mg once daily or in 2 divided doses.

Schizophrenia: Oral 0.5–2 mg once daily or in 2 divided doses.

Ritonavir: *Dosage*:

Low dose ritonavir to increase effect of atazanavir: Oral-6–18 years <20 kg 80–100 mg OD; > 20 kg 100 mg OD.

Low dose ritonavir to increase effect of darunavir: Oral-6–18 years 20–30 kg 50 mg BD; 30–40 kg 60 mg BD; >40 kg 100 mg BD.

Low dose ritonavir to increase effect of fosamprenavir: Oral—6–18 years 25–33 kg 3 mg/kg twice daily; >33 kg 100 mg BD.

Low dose ritonavir to increase effect of saquinavir: Oral-6–18 years 100 mg BD.

Low dose ritonavir to increase effect of tipranavir: Oral-2–12 year 150 mg/m^2 (maximum 200 mg) BD; 12–18 years 200 mg BD.

Rituximab: *Dosage*: IV-to check protocols for dosage. 375 mg/m^2 as a 5 hours infusion once weekly for 4 to 8 weeks is a useful guide.

Rotavirus vaccine: *Dosage*:

Live attenuated human rotavirus vaccine: Oral—2 doses of 1 mL each. First dose at > 6 weeks, separated by an interval of at least 4 weeks.

Live pentavalent reassortment vaccine (human and bovine strains): 3 doses of 2 mL each given orally starting at 6–12 weeks, with subsequent doses at 4–10 weeks intervals—3rd dose latest by 32 weeks age.

Live attenuated Indian neonatal strain 116E: 3 doses 0.5 mL 6, 10 and 14 weeks first dose of all vaccines no later than at the age of 15 weeks. All the doses should be completed within 32 weeks of age. The vaccines may be administered to preterm infants according to their age in weeks since birth and infants with controlled gastroesophageal reflux disease. Immunization should not be initiated in infants 15 weeks or older because of insufficient safety data for vaccines use in older children.

Dose reduction is not necessary in renal or hepatic impairment.

Roxithromycin: *Dosage*: Adolescents: 150 mg twice daily at least 15 minutes before meals. *Children*: 5–8 mg/kg/day in two divided doses for not more than 10 days.

Rubella vaccine, live: *Dosage*: IM or deep SC: 0.5 mL. Booster doses of single antigen rubella vaccine are not recommended.

S

Salbutamol: *Dosage*: Oral—1 month–2 years 0.3–0.4 mg/kg/day; > 2 years 0.3–0.7 mg/kg/day. Aerosol inhaler up to 100–200 µg single dose on demand. Nebulizer solution 1.25–2.5 mg 1–2 hourly initially and then 4–6 hourly.

Salicylic acid: *Dosage*: Topical: remove dead skin by gentle rubbing with pumice stone or emery board before applying daily.

Salmeterol: *Dosage*: <4 years 25 µg, 4–12 years 50 µg and 12–18 years 50–100 µg 2 times daily as preventor.

Selenium sulfide: *Dosage*: Use as shampoo twice weekly for 2 weeks then once weekly for 2 weeks then as necessary.

Senna: *Dosage*: Oral tabs 6–12 years 1–2 tabs, 12–18 years 2–4 tabs. Liquid < 2 years 0.5 mg/kg 2–6 years 2.5–5 mL, 6–12 years 5–10 mL, 12–18 years 10–20 mL.

Serratiopeptidase: *Dosage*: 5–10 mg thrice a day after meals to be swallowed whole without chewing.

Sertraline: *Dosage*: Oral 6–12 years 25 mg, 12–18 years 50 mg once daily.

Sildenafil: *Dosage*: 0.5–5 mg/kg/day in 3 or 4 divided doses. Dose reduction is required in renal and hepatic disease.

Silver sulfadiazine (sulfadiazine): *Dosage*:

Burns: After cleaning the wound apply over all affected areas to a depth of 3–5 mm, using a sterile gloved hand or sterile spatula. Where necessary, reapply to any area from which it has been removed by patient activity. Reapply at least every 24 hours or more frequently if the volume of exudates is large.

Hand burns: Apply to the burn and enclose the whole hand in a clear plastic bag or glove, which is then closed at the wrist. The patient should be encouraged to move the hand and fingers and the dressing should be changed when an excessive amount of exudates has accumulated in the bag.

Leg ulcers/pressure sores: The cavity of the ulcer should be filled with cream to a depth of at least 3–5 mm, followed by application of an absorbent pad or dressing, with further application of pressure bandaging as appropriate. Dressings should be changed daily, but if less exudates every 48 hours may be sufficient.

Finger-tip injuries: Hemostasis of the injury should be achieved prior to the application of a 3–5 mm layer of cream, and then the finger covered with a finger dressing or the finger of a plastic glove. Dressings should be changed every 2–3 days. In all cases, use the contents of the tube or pot on one person only. Discard 50 g tubes 7 days after opening. Discard 250 g and 500 g pots 24 hours after opening.

Silymarin: *Dosage*: 70–140 mg bid/tid.

Simvastatin: *Dosage*: 5–10 years: 5 mg at night increased at 4 week intervals to 20 mg per night if required. Reduced dose required with concomitant cyclosporine, danazol, fibrates, amiodarone, diltiazem or verapamil—seek specialized advice.

Sodium benzoate: *Dosage*:

Hyperammonemia: Oral 250 mg/kg/day in 4 divided doses; IV 250 mg/kg as single infusion over 90 minutes.

Nonketotic hyperglycinemia: Newborn 250 mg/ kg/day in 4 divided doses; > 1 month 500 mg/kg/day in 4 divided doses.

Sodium bicarbonate: *Dosage*:

Renal tubular acidosis: Oral 2 years 1–2 mmol/kg/day >2 years 70 mmol/m^2/day.

Renal hyperkalemia: IV 1 mmol/kg/day.

Cardiopulmonary resuscitation: 1 mL/kg of 8.4% solution initially followed by 0.5 mL/kg 8.4% if needed.

Sodium chloride: *Dosage*: IV: 2–4 mmol/kg/24 hours in continuous IV infusion. Oral: 2–4 mmol/kg/24 hours in two to four divided doses.

Note:
1. Adjust dose according to clinical requirements for sodium.
2. Higher doses may be required in very premature infants because of significant renal loss of electrolytes.

Sodium chloride drops: *Dosage*: 0.9% given as nasal drops or spray may relieve nasal congestion by helping to liquefy mucous secretions in children with rhinitis. In infants, 1-2 drops of sodium chloride 0.9% solution in each nostril before feeds will help relieve congestion and allow more effective suckling.

Sodium cromoglycate:

Prophylaxis of asthma—by inhalation of aerosol: Child 5-17 years: Initially 10 mg 4 times a day, additional dose may also be taken before exercise, increased if necessary to 10 mg 6-8 times a day; maintenance 5 mg 4 times a day, 5 mg is equivalent to 1 puff.

Food allergy (in conjunction with dietary restriction): Oral: Child 2-13 years: Initially 100 mg 4 times a day for 2-3 weeks, then increased if necessary up to 40 mg/kg daily, then reduced according to response to be taken before meals. Child 14-17 years: Initially 200 mg 4 times a day for 2-3 weeks, then increased if necessary up to 40 mg/kg daily, then reduced according to response to be taken before meals.

Sodium nitrite: *Dosage*: 3% inj. (30 mg/mL) in water for injection—give IV over 5-20 min 1 month to 18 years 4-10 mg/kg (maximum 300 mg) or 0.13-0.33 mL/kg (maximum 10 mL) followed immediately by 25% inj. (250 mg/mL) sodium thiosulfate in water for injection given 400 mg/kg (maximum 12.5 g) or 1.6 mL/kg (maximum of 50 mL) over 15 min.

Recommended dose of both drugs vary with hemoglobin levels of the child. If Hb level is known—Sodium nitrite 3% soln. and sodium thiosulfate 25% soln. Hb 8 g/dL—Sodium nitrite 6.6 mg/kg (0.22 mL/kg); sodium thiosulfate 1.1 mL/kg. Hb 10 g/dL—Sodium nitrite 8.7 mg/kg (0.27 mL/kg); sodium thiosulphate 1.35 mL/kg. Hb 12 g/dL—Sodium nitrite 10 mg/kg (0.33 mL/kg); sodium thiosulphate 1.65 mL/kg. Hb 14 g/dL— Sodium nitrite 11.6 mg/kg (0.39 mL/kg); sodium thiosulfate 1.95 mL/kg.

If Hb is not known: Sodium nitrite 10 mg/kg (0.33 mL/kg); sodium thiosulfate 1.6 mL/kg-400 mg/kg IV repeated every 30-60 min to maximum of 50 mL.

Sodium nitroprusside: *Dosage*: Advisable to start with a low dose—IV infusion 500 mg/kg/min, increased in increments of 200 mg/kg/min according to improvement in symptoms, status of BP, filling pressures, to maximum of 10 µg/kg/min. In general, invasive monitoring of blood pressure is recommended when sodium nitroprusside infusion is being administered. Pediatric data on sodium nitroprusside is not available, however, due to its potent action on blood pressure, it is preferable to have invasive pressure monitoring in children also.

Sodium perborate: *Dosage*: For oral hygiene measures, 1 sachet to be dissolved in 30 mL water 3 times daily after meals. As a bleaching agent, a small quantity of granules to be mixed to a thick paste with a few drops of 30 vols hydrogen peroxide.

Sodium phenylbutyrate: *Dosage*: Oral 250 mg/kg/day in 4 divided doses; IV 250 mg/kg over 50 min; IV infusion 250-600 mg/kg/day as continuous infusion.

Sodium picosulfate: *Dosage*: 2-5 years 2.5 mL, 5-19 years 2.5-5 mL, >10 years 5-15 mL as single dose at bedtime.

Sodium stibogluconate: *Dosage*: IV/IM 1 month-18 years-20 mg/kg (maximum 850 mg) daily once for 20-30 days. Total daily dose may be given in 2 divided doses 12 hours apart.

Sodium thiosulfate: *Dosage*: 25% Inj. (250 mg/mL) in water for injection given 400 mg/kg (maximum 12.5 g) or 1.6 mL/kg (maximum of 50 mL) over 15 min. It is given after IV sodium nitrite.

Recommended dose of both drugs vary with hemoglobin levels of the child. If Hb level is known—Sodium nitrite 3% soln. and sodium thiosulfate 25% soln. Hb 8 g/dL—Sodium nitrite 6.6 mg/kg (0.22 mL/kg); sodium thiosulfate 1.1 mL/kg. Hb 10 g/dL—Sodium nitrite 8.7 mg/kg (0.27 mL/kg); sodium thiosulfate 1.35 mL/kg. Hb 12 g/dL—Sodium nitrite 10 mg/kg (0.33 mL/kg); sodium thiosulfate 1.65 mL/kg. Hb 14 g/dL—Sodium nitrite 11.6 mg/kg (0.39 mL/kg); sodium thiosulfate 1.95 mL/kg.

If Hb is not known: Sodium nitrite 10 mg/kg (0.33 mL/kg); sodium thiosulfate 1.6 mL/kg-400 mg/kg IV repeated every 30-60 min to maximum of 50 mL.

Sodium valproate: *Dosage*: Oral start with 10-15 mg/kg/day in 2 divided doses and maintain at 12.5-15 mg/kg/day. Even doses of 30-40 mg/kg/day have been used in infantile spasms.

Somatropin (Growth hormone): *Dosage*: SC

Growth hormone deficiency: 25-35 µg/kg once daily.

Turner syndrome: 50 µg/kg once daily.

Chronic renal failure: 50 µg/ kg once daily.

Prader-Willi syndrome: 70 µg/kg once daily.

Noonan syndrome: 35 µg/kg once daily.

Intra-uterine growth retardation (IUGR): 70 µg/kg once daily.

Sotalol: *Dosage*: Oral <12 years 1-4 mg/kg/dose (maximum 8 mg/kg/day or 40-80 mg) and 12-18 years 40 mg/dose (maximum 80-160 mg) 2 times daily. According to Shi J et al. body surface area is the better predictor for sotalol dosing; the recommended dose is 30-70 mg/m2/day.

Spiramycin: *Dosage*: Pregnant women with suspected or confirmed toxoplasma infection: 1.5 g (4.5 million international units) orally twice daily until term if the fetus is not infected.

Spironolactone: *Dosage*: Oral 1–3 mg/kg/day in 2 divided doses. In resistant ascites, up to 9 mg/kg/day have been given with careful serum potassium monitoring.

Hirsutism: Start with 50 mg in 2 divided doses, gradually increasing to 100 mg; maximum up to 200 mg daily can be given.

Stilbestrol: *Dosage*: Oral: 1 mg twice a day, for 2 days before the test.

Streptokinase: *Dosage*: The optimal dose for pediatric patients is not known. IV infusion over 30 min initially 2000 units/kg (<12 years) and 2.5 lakh units (12–18 years) followed by continuous infusion of 500–2000 units/kg/hour (<12 years) and 1 lakh unit/ hour (12–18 years) till vascular flow returns or maximum of 3 days. Local therapy may be better for catheter induced thrombosis, if the catheter is already *in situ*. Monitor Fibrinogen, TCT, PT, and a PTT.

Streptomycin: *Dosage*: *Tuberculosis*—IM-*Daily regimen*-15 mg/kg as single morning dose (Range 15–20 mg/kg; maximum dose 1g/day); *Intermittent regimen*-15 mg/kg (Range: 15–20 mg/kg).

Sucralfate: *Dosage*: Oral <2 years 250 mg; 1–12 years 500 mg; 12–18 years 1 g 4–6 times daily.

Sulfasalazine (Sulphasalazine): *Dosage*:

JIA: Oral 10 mg/ kg/day 1st week, 20 mg/kg/day 2nd week, 40 mg/kg/day 3rd week, 40–50 mg/kg/day maintenance (maximum 2 g/day <12 and 3 g/day 12–18 year.

Ulcerative colitis/Crohn disease: <12 year 10–15 mg/kg/dose 4–6 times daily (maximum 50 mg/ kg/day) and 12–18 years 1–2 g/kg/dose 4 times daily and half dose as maintenance. May be used as rectal suppository and enema if these preparations are available.

Sulfadiazine: *Dosage*: <12 years 100–200 mg/kg/day and 12–18 years 4–6 g/day in 4 div doses.

Sumatriptan: *Dosage*: Oral 6–10 years 25 mg; 10–12 years 50 mg; 12–18 years 50–100 mg as single dose. May be repeated if migraine recurs (maximum 300 mg/day. If there is no response, do not repeat for same attack. SC >10 years 6 mg single dose. May repeat once not less than 1 hour later for a recurrence (maximum 12 mg/day). If there is no response, do not repeat for same attack.

Surfactants (Natural): *Dosage*:

Survanta: Intratracheal 100 mg/kg or 4 mL/kg over 4 min; repeat after 8–12 hours if necessary. If birth weight is <1250 g, give first dose within 15 min of birth.

Curosurf: Intratracheal 100 mg/kg or 1.25 mL/kg over 4 min; repeat after 12 hours if necessary. If birth weight is <1250 g, give first dose within 15 min of birth.

Surfactants (Synthetic): *Dosage*: 67.5 mg/kg or 5 mL/kg.

Suxamethonium chloride: *Dosage*: Newborn—for 5–10 minutes muscular paralysis 2 mg/kg IV; for full neuromuscular blockade 3 mg/kg IV; IM 4 mg/kg provides 10–30 min muscle paralysis after 2–3 min delay. Children IV <12 years 1–2 mg/kg; 12–18 years 1 mg/kg; IM <1 year up to 4–5 mg/kg; >1 year up to 4 mg.

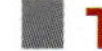

T

Tacalcitol: *Dosage*: 12–18 years apply sparingly at bedtime.

Tacrolimus: *Dosage*:

Liver transplant renal transplant: IV/ oral.

Atopic dermatitis: 2–16 years 0.03% for 3 weeks and then once till clearance, > 16 years 0.1% twice 3 weeks, then 0.03% twice, then once till clearance.

Teicoplanin: *Dosage*: Newborn-loading 16 mg/kg and 24 hours later start maintenance 8 mg/kg/day as single dose; children 10 mg/kg/dose 2 times daily × 3 doses and then once daily in same dose for severe infection and 6 mg/kg/day once for moderate infection. Orally for pseudomembranous colitis 10 mg/kg/dose 2 times daily. May be given intraventricular and intraperitoneal.

Terbinafine: *Dosage*: Topical 1–2 times daily 1–2 weeks, Oral 3–6 mg/kg 4–5 weeks.

Terbutaline: *Dosage*: Oral <7 years 0.25 mg/kg/day in 3 divided doses; 7–12 years 2.5 mg/dose and 12–18 years 2.5–5 mg/dose 3 times daily. Aerosol inhaler 250–500 µg/ dose 4–6 times daily. Turbohaler 500 µg/dose 4 times daily. Nebulizer 1 month to 5 years 2.5–5 mg, 5–12 years 5 mg and 12–18 years 10 mg per dose up to 8 times daily. SC/IM/slow IV 2–12 years 10 µg/kg/dose (maximum 300 µg/dose) 12–18 years 250–500 µg/dose of nebulizer not available. IV loading dose of 2–4 µg/kg followed by IV infusion of 1–10 µg/kg/ hour.

Testosterone and esters: *Dosage*:

Androgen replacement: Orally: Testosterone undecanoate starting dose 40 mg alternate days, increasing slowly up to 120 mg daily.

Delayed puberty: Dose/dose schedule depends on the product. An example is given but expert advice should be sought from a pediatric endocrinologist. IM injection: 1 mL by deep IM injection every month for 3 doses.

Priming: IM injection: 1 mL by deep IM injection 3–5 days before the test of growth hormone secretion.

Tetanus immunoglobulin (human): *Dosage*:

Prevention: A single dose of 250 international units. If there is a risk of heavy contamination or following burns, or more than 24 hours have elapsed since injury, 500 international units should be given.

Treatment of tetanus: 150 IU/kg IM in multiple sites or by IV infusion.

Tetanus toxoid and reduced dose diphtheria: *Dosage*: Contains Tetanus toxoid 5 LF units and 2 LF units of diphtheria toxoid. 0.5 mL deep IM on anterolateral thigh for children above 7 years age and routinely at 10 and 16 years (Td to replace TT boosters at 10 and 16 year).

Tetanus vaccine (Adsorbed): *Dosage*: IM/deep SC 0.5 mL.

Tetracosactide (Tetracosactrin, Cosyntropin, Synacthen): *Dosage*: *See* Corticotropin also.

Infantile spasm: 1 month—2 years 500 µg IM as depot injection.

Standard dose test: IV/IM (not depot preparation) <6 months 62.5 µg, 6 month to 2 years 125 µg and 2–18 years 250 µg.

Tetracycline: *Dosage*:

Acne: Topical application 2 times daily for maximum 10–12 weeks. May be repeated after 12 weeks interval.

Aphthous ulceration: Local mouth wash with contents of 250 mg cap of tetracycline in water 3–4 times daily for 2–3 min each time (do not swallow) for 3 days.

Tetrahydrobiopterin: *Dosage*: Oral 1–3 mg/kg once daily. Some require up to 5–20 mg/kg/day.

THAM (Trometamol, Tris-hydroxymethyl-amino-methane): *Dosage*: Dose in mL of 0.3M solution = weight (kg) × base deficit, or 1–2 mEq/kg/dose. Blood gases should be checked before, during and after administration. Only half the base deficit should be corrected initially. Blood gases should be checked before further correction.

Theophylline: *Dosage*: Oral >6 months 5 mg/kg/dose 3–4 times daily—adjust according to response and plasma levels. Sustained release preparations 8–12 years 10 mg/kg/dose and 12–18 years 8 mg/kg/dose (maximum 500 mg/dose).

Thiabendazole: *Dosage*:

Cutaneous larva migrans: 25 mg/kg (maximum 1.5 g), 2 times daily for 2 days. Repeat for 2 days if active lesions persist 2 days after completion of 1st course. 10–15% suspension is applied topically to lesions 4–6 times per day for 2–5 consecutive days.

Dracunculiasis (Guinea worm): 1–2 visible worms: 25 mg/kg (maximum 1.5 g), 2 times daily for 1 day; 3–9 visible worms: 50 mg/kg (maximum 1.5 g), 2 times daily for 1 day; >9 visible worms: 50 mg/kg (maximum 1.5 g), 2 times daily for 1 day, repeat once after 5–8 days.

Trichinosis: 25 mg/kg (maximum 1.5 g), 2 times daily for 2–4 days-up to 7 days if required.

Strongyloidosis: 25 mg/kg (maximum 1.5 g), 2 times daily for 2 days. For disseminated infection, 5–7 day course may be given.

Toxocariasis (Visceral larva migrans): Efficacy is limited. A course of 25 mg/kg (maximum 1.5 g), 2 times daily for 7 days may be tried.

Trichuriasis and hookworm: 25 mg/kg (maximum 1.5 g), 2 times daily for 2 days. Thiabendazole is not usually first-line therapy for pinworm; other agents are better tolerated and more effective. However, if pinworm infection occurs concurrently with any of the other listed indications for thiabendazole, thiabendazole therapy alone is usually adequate for most patients. May repeat the course after 1 week.

There is limited study of its use in infants and children with weight of <13 kg for any of the indications mentioned.

Patients with renal impairment: Dosage should be modified depending on clinical response and degree of renal impairment, but no quantitative recommendations are available.

Thiamine (Vitamin B1): *Dosage*:

Congenital lactic acidosis: Oral 100–300 mg once daily.

MSUD: Oral 10–300 mg once daily. A trial for 3 weeks in newly diagnosed MSUD to determine thiamine responsiveness.

Thioguanine: *Dosage*: Always consult the current treatment protocol for details of dosage and scheduling.

Thiopental (Thiopentone) sodium: *Dosage*: IV bolus 4 mg/kg maximum 10 mg/kg (facilities for ventilation must) followed in ventilated babies only with IV infusion 2.5 mg/kg/hour (newborn) and 2–8 mg/kg/ hour (1 month–18 years). Reduce dose in hepatic disease.

Thiotepa: *Dosage*: Children—IV 25–65 mg/m^2 every 3–4 week; high dose 300 mg/m^2/24 hours for 3 doses. Always consult the current treatment protocol for details of dosage and scheduling.

Thyroxine: *Dosage*: Oral; newborn: 15 µg/kg/d, later infancy: 6–8 µg/kg/d, Preschool 5–6 µg/kg/d, Older children: 4—5 µg/kg/d, Adolescents 2—3: 50–100 µg/kg/d. See Levothyroxine for details.

Tiagabine: *Dosage*: Doses are for patients receiving enzyme-induced antiepileptic drugs. Lower doses and slower titration may be required when used in patients not receiving enzyme-induced antiepileptic drugs. Children 12–18 years— initially 4 mg once daily for 1 week, then 8 mg/day given in 2 divided doses for 1 week, then increase weekly by 4–8 mg/ day once (given in 2–4 divided doses, preferably thrice in a day) to a maximum of 32 mg/day or till response is obtained. Doses >32 mg/day have been used in some adolescents for short periods of time.

Tinidazole: *Dosage*: Oral—1 month to 12 years 50–60 mg/kg and 12–12 years 2 g–single dose for *Trichomonas vaginitis* and amebiasis, 3 days for amebiasis and colitis and 5 days for liver abscess.

Tissue plasminogen activator (tPA): *Dosage*: Neonates—0.1–0.5 mg/kg/hour for 3 to 10 hours—use ultrasound assessment to monitor effect before considering 2nd course of treatment. Children—0.1–0.6 mg/kg/hour for 6 hours (maximum 100 mg total daily dose)—use ultrasound assessment to monitor effect before considering 2nd course of treatment. Adults 100 mg infused as 60 mg in first hour, 20 mg in 2nd hour and 20 mg in 3rd hour. Initiate heparin concurrently to avoid thrombosis and thrombotic emboli. Monitoring: D-dimer, fibrinogen, bleeding time.

Tobramycin: *Dosage*: Newborn—IV <32 weeks 4–5 mg/kg 36 hourly and > 32 weeks 4–5 mg/kg once in 24 hour. See Aminoglycosides.

PDA, prolonged hypoxia, indomethacin treatment necessitate increased dose intervals. Extended interval dose regimen by intravenous injection over 3–5 minutes or by intravenous infusion—Neonate less than 32 weeks postmenstrual age 4–5 mg/kg every 36 hours; Neonate 32 weeks and over postmenstrual age 4–5 mg/kg every 24 hours. Child–IV/IM 2.5 mg/kg/dose 3 times daily or 7 mg/kg as single daily dose. Once daily dose regimen by intravenous infusion—Child 1 month–18 years-initially 7 mg/kg, then adjusted according to serum tobramycin concentration.

Pseudomonal lung infection in cystic fibrosis: Child 1 month–18 years—8- 10 mg/kg/daily in 3 divided doses. Once daily dose regimen by intravenous infusion over 30 minutes—Child 1 month–18 years—initially 10 mg/kg (maximum 660 mg), then adjusted according to serum-tobramycin concentration.

Chronic pulmonary Pseudomonas aeruginosa infection in patients with cystic fibrosis: By inhalation of nebulized solution—Child 6–18 years 300 mg every 12 hours for 28 days, subsequent courses repeated after 28 days interval without tobramycin nebulizer solution.

Intraventricular: Newborn 1 mg/day, child 1–2 mg/day, adolescent 2–4 mg/day.

Eye drops: 1 drop 2 hourly and then reduce frequency as infection is controlled. To continue till 2 days after healing.

Tolazoline: *Dosage*: Newborn—IV bolus 1 mg/kg as single dose. Best result when blood pH > 7.2. IV infusion 0.2 mg/kg/ hour.

Tolnaftate: *Dosage*: Apply evenly to affected area and rub gently 2–3 times daily.

Tolterodine: *Dosage*: Oral 2–18 years 1 mg once daily may increase up to 2 mg twice daily according to response. Usually effective within 4 weeks.

Topiramate: *Dosage*:

Antiepileptic: Oral initially 0.5 mg/kg (1 month- 12 years) and 25 mg (12–18 years) followed by maintenance of 2–4.5 mg/kg (1 month–12 years) and 100–200 mg (12–18 years). Doses up to 6 mg/kg twice daily have been used. Use starting dose for 2 weeks then increase dose every 2 weeks taking at least 6 weeks to reach maintenance dose. Use with caution in renal failure, titrating dose and intervals between dose adjustments to efficacy and side-effects. Supplemental doses required after dialysis.

Migraine prophylaxis: 16–18 years—initially 25 mg bedtime for 1 week, increase weekly by 25 mg/day; a dose of 50–100 mg daily in 2 divided doses would suffice (maximum 200 mg/day).

Torsemide: *Dosage*: On a weight-to-weight basis torsemide is twice as potent as furosemide, and provides a longer duration of action at lower urinary concentrations allows for a 24 hours dosage interval and avoids the paradoxical antidiuresis seen with furosemide.

Dosage: *Edema associated with congestive heart failure or CRF:* Oral or Intravenous dosage: Adolescent: Initially, 10–20 mg PO or IV once daily. If needed, titrate by doubling the dose up to 200 mg PO or IV to achieve a satisfactory diuretic response. The safe use of a single dose ≥ 200 mg has not been evaluated.

Adjunctive treatment of ascites (e.g. due to hepatic cirrhosis) either alone or in combination with spironolactone or amiloride: Oral or intravenous dosage: Adolescent: initially, 5–10 mg PO or IV once daily. If needed, titrate upward by doubling the dose up to 40 mg PO or IV to achieve a satisfactory diuretic response. Doses ≥ 40 mg have not been evaluated in patients with hepatic cirrhosis. Chronic use in hepatic disease has not been evaluated.

Hypertension: Oral dosage: Adolescent: Initially, 5 mg PO once daily. May increase to 10 mg PO once daily if the desired reduction in blood pressure is not achieved in 4–6 weeks, if this dose is insufficient an additional antihypertensive agent should be added to the regimen.

Patients with hepatic impairment: No dosage adjustment is needed; see the dosage for the treatment of ascites. Diuretics should be used with caution in patients with hepatic disease since minor alterations of fluid and electrolyte balance may precipitate hepatic coma.

Patients with renal impairment: No dosage adjustment is needed; however, high doses may be effective in patients with end-stage renal disease.

Intermittent hemodialysis: Torsemide is not removed by hemodialysis; no dosage adjustment is needed.

Torsemide can be safely used, and appears to be effective for treatment of heart failure in children (Archives of Disease in Childhood 2008;93:768–71). Future clinical trials are warranted to verify the results of this study.

Tranexamic acid: *Dosage*: Oral 25 mg/kg/dose 3 times daily. *Menorrhagia*—1–1.5 g/dose 3–4 times daily for 3–4 days (maximum 4 g/day). Initiate treatment after heavy bleeding starts.

Tretinoin: *Dosage*: Topical: Apply 1–2 times daily thinly. The skin should be thoroughly washed first. Cream is recommended for dry or fair skin, gel for oily or dark skin.

Triamcinolone: *Dosage*: Intra-articular—> 1 year 1 mg/kg for large joints (maximum 40 mg), 0.5 mg/kg for small joints (maximum 20 mg but maximum 10 mg for finger and toe joints).

Triclofos sodium: Dosage: Oral 30–50 mg/kg as single dose. Doses up to 100 mg/kg used for level 4 sedation required prior to doing procedures. Most used in children < 12 years—chloral hydrate preferred > 12 years.

Trientine dihydrochloride: *Dosage*: Oral > 2 years initially 300–750 mg/dose 2 times daily to a maximum of 1.5 g/day (<12 years) and 2 g (>12 years).

Trifluoperazine: *Dosage*:

Schizophrenia and severe behavior disorders: 3–5 years 1 mg/day in div doses; 6–12 years 2–5 mg in div. doses as required; 12–18 years start with 5 mg 2 times daily and increased by 5 mg/week up to 15–20 mg/day.

Severe anxiety disorder—Oral—3–5 years up to 1 mg/day; 6–12 years up to 4 mg/day; 12–18 years 4 mg/day and increased if required up to 6 mg/day.

Vomiting not responding to other medication: Oral—3–5 years up to 1 mg/day in divided doses; 6–12 years up to 4 mg/day in divided doses; 12–18 years 2–4 mg/day in divided doses (maximum 6 mg).

Trihexyphenidyl (Benzhexol): *Dosage*:

Extrapyramidal symptoms and dystonia: 2 mg as single or divided doses.

Antispasmodic: Initial dose of 0.5 mg in < 7 years and 2 mg > 7 years and increased by 0.5–2 mg/day every 10 days till response and given in 3–4 divided doses.

Trimipramine: *Dosage*: Oral 6–12 years 50–100 mg and 12–18 years 75–300 mg at bedtime.

Tryptophan (L-Tryptophan): *Dosage*: 100 mg/kg in 3 divided doses.

Tuberculin purified protein derivative (PPD): *Dosage*: 10 TU 1:1000 solution 0.1 mL intradermal on right forearm.

Typhoid vaccine (polysaccharide): *Dosage*: 0.5 mL IM or deep SC.

Typhoid Vi capsular polysaccharide tetanus toxoid conjugate vaccine: *Dosage*: Single dose 0.5 mL at 9–12 months age and a booster during the second year of life. Catch up vaccination recommended throughout adolescent period (up to 18 years).

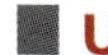

U

Urea cream: *Dosage*: Topical: wash affected area, rinse off all traces of sap and apply sparingly twice daily.

Urokinase: *Dosage*:

Thromboembolic disease: Loading dose of 4400 IU/kg in 15 mL solution over 10 min followed by IV infusion 4400 IU/kg/hour over 6–12 hours.

Blocked arteriovenous shunts, IV cannulas/central lines: 5000 IU/ kg directly into the catheter and clamp off and retain for 2–4 hours. If not cleared, instill 10,000 IU and clamp. Monitor with fibrinogen, TCT, PT, a PTT estimations.

Ursodeoxycholic acid: *Dosage*: Oral 5–10 mg/kg/dose 2–3 times daily (maximum 45 mg/kg/day).

Cystic fibrosis: 10 mg/kg/dose 2 times daily.

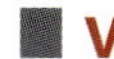

V

Valacyclovir: *Dosage*:

Heart transplant: 4 months to 16 years-total dose (mg) = [7 × BSA × CrCl] PO qd until 100 days post-transplant; Start: within 10 days of transplant; Max: 900 mg/day; Info: round calculated dose to nearest 25 mg increment; solution preferred, but may use tabs if calculated dose within 10% of available tab strength; give with food.

Kidney transplant: 4 months–16 years—total dose (mg) = [7 × BSA × CrCl] PO qid until 100 days post-transplant; Start: within 10 days of transplant; Max: 900 mg/day; Info: round calculated dose to nearest 25 mg increment; solution preferred, but may use tabs if calculated dose within 10% of avail. Tab strength; give with food. *Renal impairment:* dose adjustment required. Hepatic dosing: not defined.

Vancomycin: *Dosage*: Newborn—IV 15 mg/kg/dose <28 weeks once daily, 29–35 weeks twice daily and > 35 weeks 3 times daily. Intrathecal all newborn 2.5–5 mg once daily. Child IV 15 mg/kg loading dose followed by 10 mg/kg/dose 4 times daily. (maximum 2 g/day). Intrathecal 1 month–4 years 5 mg, 4–15 years 10 mg and > 15 years 20 mg once daily. Children with enlarged ventricles need higher doses. Adjust dose according to CSF levels aiming for a trough level of <10 mg/L. See also Glycopeptides also.

Varicella-zoster immunoglobulin (VZIG): *Dosage*: IM 0–5 years 250 mg (1 vial), 6–10 years 500 mg (2 vials), 11–14 years 750 mg (3 vials), >15 years 1 g (4 vials).

Varicella-zoster vaccine, live: *Dosage*: SC 1–12 years single dose of 0.5 mL if immunocompetent, otherwise 2 doses at least 6 weeks apart. >13 years 0.5 mL 2 doses at least 6 weeks apart.

Vasopressin: *Dosage*: By continuous intravenous infusion (may also be infused directly into superior mesenteric artery—Child 1 month–18 years—initially 0.3 U/kg (maximum 20 U) over 20–30 min then 0.3 units/kg/hour, adjusted according to response (maximum 1 U/kg/ hour); if bleeding stops, continue at same dose for 12 hours, then withdraw gradually over 24–48 hours; maximum duration of treatment 72 hours.

Vecuronium bromide: *Dosage*: IV bolus—80–100 μg/kg as single dose and adjust dose and interval as required. IV infusion 1 month–18 years 50–80 μg/kg/ hour.

Verapamil hydrochloride: *Dosage*: Oral newborn 1–2 mg/kg/dose, 1 month–2 years 20 mg/dose and 2–18 years 40–120 mg/dose 3 times daily. Slow IV bolus newborn–1 year 100–200 μg/kg (maximum 2 mg), >1 year 100–300 μg/kg (maximum 5 mg) as single dose with ECG monitoring. May repeat after 30 min usually lower doses suffice.

Vigabatrin: *Dosage*: Oral < 12 years 15–20 mg/kg/dose >12 years 1 g/dose 2 times daily as initial dose followed by maintenance of <12 year 30–40 mg/kg/dose, >12 years 1–1.5 g/dose 2 times daily. Increase to maintenance dose over 2–3 weeks except for infantile spasms when the maintenance dose should be reached in 5–7 days. Reduce dose in impaired renal function.

Vinblastine sulfate: *Dosage*: Hodgkin lymphoma in children—IV 2.5- 6 mg/m^2/24 hours 1–2/week for 3–6 weeks (maximum 12.5 mg/m^2/week). Always consult the current treatment protocol for details of dosage and scheduling. Maximum single dose 10 mg. A 50% dose reduction has been suggested in patients with serum bilirubin >50 mmol/L.

Vincristine sulfate: *Dosage*: Children <10 kg 0.05 mg/kg once a week, >10 kg 1–2 mg/m^2 once a week. Always consult the current treatment protocol for details of dosage and scheduling. Maximum dose in adults is 2 mg weekly. Small infants may be unexpectedly sensitive to vincristine. Dosage reductions may be necessary if toxicity is unacceptable. An increase in the severity of side-effects may be seen in patients with liver disease sufficient to decrease biliary excretion. A 50% dosage reduction is recommended in patients with a serum bilirubin level >50 mmol/L.

Vitamin A (Retinol): *Dosage*: Oral <1 year 500 IU and > 1 year 10,000 IU daily. *Prophylaxis of vitamin A deficiency* 1 lakh IU once in 6 months as a National Program.

Vitamin B complex: *Dosage:* Infants—5 mL daily. 1–12 years—5 mL twice daily. 12–18 years—5 mL thrice daily. Therapeutic-Infants-5 mL thrice daily. 1–12 years—10 mL thrice daily. 12–18 years—10–15 mL thrice daily.

Vitamin C (Ascorbic acid): *Dosage*:

Scurvy: Oral initially 500 mg then 100 mg/day for 1 week then 50 mg/day for prophylaxis.

Metabolic indications: 200–400 mg/day.

Transient tyrosinemia: 50–200 mg/day for 1–2 weeks.

Hawkinsuria, Tyrosinuria III: Up to 1 g daily for several weeks until symptoms subside.

Vitamin E (Alpha tocopheryl acetate): *Dosage*: Oral < 1 year 50 mg, 1–12 years 100 mg and 12–18 years 200 mg once daily.

Prophylaxis of vitamin E deficiency in newborn: Oral: 0.25 mL (29 mg) daily for all premature infants.

Therapy of symptomatic deficiency/prevention of RLF, BPD, IVH: Oral: 75–100 mg daily in three or four divided doses.

Note:
1. 1 mg of d-alpha tocopheryl acetate is equivalent in activity to 1.36 I.U. of vitamin E.
2. Folic acid status is also important in hemolytic anemia.

Vitamin K: *Dosage*:

Prophylaxis: In all newborn term babies 1 mg IM and 0.5 mg IM for preterm (birth weight <1,500 g). It may be given to patients on long-term broad-spectrum antibiotics. Oral dose is 5 mg daily.

Other indication for Vitamin K prophylaxis is neonatal cholestasis: Neonates and babies: biliary atresia and liver disease. 1 mg daily by mouth. At risk babies (those at increased risk of hemorrhagic disease, e.g. birth asphyxia, bleeding problems, maternal liver disease or mother receiving anticonvulsant or anti-tuberculosis drugs) may be given 1 mg IV repeated 8th hourly if necessary.

In bleeding disorders:
1. Asymptomatic patients with mild abnormal coagulation, where vitamin K deficiency is presumed, vitamin K may be given *SC*. Dose is 1–5 mg.
2. Bleeding in a patient due to vitamin K deficiency*:* Should be given 2–10 mg of vitamin K SC/IV. IM administration of vitamin K should be avoided as it causes pain, hematoma, and swelling. If bleeding is severe then fresh frozen plasma (FFP) may be given in the dose of 10–20 mL/kg.
3. Patients with life-threatening hemorrhage or intracranial bleed should be given systemic (intravenous) vitamin *K*—5–20 mg. Along with it prothrombin complex concentrates (not available in India) may be given in a dose of 50 units/kg. Immediate benefit may be derived from administration of FFP.

Vitamins A and D: *Dosage*: Infants 0–6 months: 2.5 mL of emulsion daily, orally. 6 months—adults: 5 mL of emulsion of 1 capsule daily, orally.

W

Warfarin: *Dosage*: *Newborn infant (birth to 1 month):* There is very little experience of the use of warfarin in the neonatal period. Always seek expert advice before starting anticoagulation. Initial loading dose is 0.2 mg/kg.

Infants: < 1 year usually need higher maintenance dose compared to older children. The dosage schedule is as per INR value. Average dose of warfarin in infants and young children is 0.33 mg/kg/ day to achieve an INR of 2.0–3.0. For teenagers, the dose is 0.09 mg/kg/day and for adults, 0.04–0.08 mg/kg/day.

Monitoring: Frequent dose adjustments warrant close supervision of INR. Vitamin K antagonists have extensive cross-reactivity with several commonly used drugs and dietary agents. Certain "point-of-care" monitors are commercially available, which are considered reliable and acceptable for checking INR in home setting. These are somewhat similar to "glucometers". INR level is affected by cumulative dose of warfarin taken over the last 5–7 days, so testing INR just after a day of change in dose is not useful.

Dosing of Warfarin: Loading dose (Day 1). 0.2 mg/kg (maximum 10 mg); 0.1 mg/kg in presence of hepatic dysfunction. Days 2–4. INR 1.1–1.3, repeat loading dose. INR 1.4–1.9, give 50% of initial loading dose. INR 2.0– 3.0, give 50% of initial loading dose. INR 3.1–3.5, give 25% of initial loading dose. INR > 3.5, hold until < 3.5, restart at 50% of previous dose. *Maintenance dose (*day 5 and beyond)—INR 1.1–1.4, increase dose by 20% of previous dose. INR 1.5–1.9, increase dose by 10% of previous dose. INR 2.0–3.0, no chance. INR 3.1–3.5, decrease dose by 10% of previous dose. INR > 3.5, hold until < 3.5, restart at 20% of previous dose. INR: international normalized ratio.

X

Xylometazoline hydrochloride: *Dosage*: Intranasal 3 months–12 years 1–2 drops 1–2 times of 0.05% and 12–18 years 0.1% 2–3 drops or 1 spray 2–3 times daily.

Y

Yellow fever vaccine, live: *Dosage*: Deep SC: 0.5 mL repeated every 10 years while still at risk.

Z

Zafirlukast: *Dosage*: 5–11 years–10 mg PO bid; Info: give 1 hour before or 2 hours after meals; >12 years 20 mg PO bid; Info: give 1 hour before or 2 hours after meals. *Renal impairment*-no dosing adjustment. *Hepatic impairment:* caution advised

Zidovudine (Azidothymidine or AZT): *Dosage*: *Newborn*—Prevention of fetomaternal transmission, Oral 2 mg/kg/dose 4 times daily started within 12 hours of birth and continued for 6 weeks. IV 1.5 mg/kg/dose 4 times daily. *Child:* Oral 180 mg/m^2 2 times daily (maximum 250 mg/dose). IV 120 mg/m^2 4 times daily.

Zileuton: *Dosage*: *Asthma,* maintenance >12 years–600 mg PO qid; Max: 2400 mg/day. *Renal impairment*-no dosing adjustment. Hepatic impairment: active hepatic disease/ baseline LFTs >3 times upper normal limit: contraindicated. Monitoring parameters—ALT at baseline, monthly × 3 months, then once in 2–3 months through 1st year of treatment, then continue periodically.

Zinc (Sulfate, Acetate or Gluconate): *Dosage*: As zinc base.

Acute fluid diarrhea: < 6 months 10 mg/day as single dose, > 6 months 20 mg/day as single dose for 14 days.

Acrodermatitis enteropathica: Oral 0.5 mg–1 mg/kg/dose 2 times daily.

Wilson's disease: Oral 2–12 years 25–37.5 mg/dose 12–18 years 50 mg/dose 2–4 times daily. Do not give at same time as penicillamine.

Zinc deficiency: Oral newborn 1 mg/kg once daily, 10–30 kg 22.5 mg once or twice daily. > 30 kg 45 mg 1–3 times daily. Adjust according to response.

Zinc Sulfate injection: *Dosage*: 2–5 mmol/kg depending on age and deficiency state.

Zonisamide: *Dosage*: 4–8 mg/kg/day should be administered once or twice daily, using 25 mg, 50 mg or 100 mg capsules. Given orally and can be taken with or without food.

Zopiclone: *Dosage*: Oral 12–18 years 3.75 mg once daily at bedtime.

21.7 Safe Injection Practices

S Sachidananda Kamath, Jaydeep Choudhury, A Parthasarathy

INTRODUCTION

Safe injection practice means that it does no harm to the recipient, does not expose the health worker to any avoidable risks, and does not result in waste that is dangerous to the community. The concept of safe injection has gained much importance in recent years in view of the increased incidence of various blood-borne infections.

According to World Health Organization (WHO), more than 12 billion injections are administered each year all over the world. Thus, injections are one of the most common healthcare procedures practiced all over the world. Of the vast majority of injections, about 95% are given as curative. Many of these "curative" injections may be unnecessary, ineffective, or inappropriate. Immunization accounts for around 3% of all injections. It is estimated that at least 50% of this are unsafe, posing serious health risks to recipients, health workers, and the public. Reducing unnecessary injections is one way to improve the safety of injections.

Patients sometimes tend to prefer injections because they believe them to be stronger and faster medications. They also nurture a belief that doctors regard injections to be the best treatment. In turn, doctors overprescribe injections. These misconception and misunderstanding can be avoided to a large extent. The doctors have to lead better communication between patients and providers can clarify these issues.

Unsafe injection practices are a powerful engine to transmit blood-borne pathogens, including hepatitis B virus (HBV), hepatitis C virus (HCV), and human immunodeficiency virus (HIV). Because infection with these viruses initially presents no symptoms, it is a silent epidemic. However, the consequences of this are increasingly recognized.

- *Hepatitis B virus*: HBV is highly infectious and causes the highest number of infections in developing and transitional countries. About 21.7 million people become infected each year, representing 33% of new HBV infections worldwide.
- *Hepatitis C virus*: Unsafe injections are the most common cause of HCV infection in developing and transitional countries, causing 2 million new infections each year and accounting for 42% of cases.
- *Human immunodeficiency virus*: Globally, nearly 2% of all new HIV infections are caused by unsafe injections. In South Asia, up to 9% of new cases may be caused in this way. Such proportions can no longer be ignored.

Hepatitis B virus, HCV, and HIV cause chronic infections that lead to disease, disability, and death a number of years after the unsafe injection. Those infected with HBV in childhood will typically present with chronic liver disease by the age of 30 years, at the prime of their life. This has a dramatic effect on national economies.

CONDITIONS CAUSING RISK: STEPS RELATED TO INJECTION GIVING

Unsafe injection practices are often viewed as a chronic problem with no easy solution. However, safe and appropriate use of injections can be achieved by adopting a three-part strategy.

Changing Behavior of Healthcare Workers and Patients

Thirty years into the HIV pandemic, knowledge of HIV among patients and healthcare workers (HCWs) in some countries has driven consumer demand for safe injection equipment and irreversibly improved injection practices. With growing knowledge of HCV and HBV, similar patterns of consumer demand for safe injections should emerge. HIV prevention programs can be expanded to include injection safety components.

Ensuring Availability of Equipment and Supplies

Simply increasing the availability of safe injection equipment can stimulate demand and improve practices. Because the cost of safe disposable syringes is low (about INR 2–5 per unit), patients are usually compliant to pay for safety once they personalize the risks.

Managing Waste Safely and Appropriately

As waste disposal is frequently not an integral part of health planning, unsafe waste management is common. However, when it is appropriately planned, significant results ensue. National healthcare waste management strategies require a national policy to manage healthcare waste, a comprehensive system for implementation, improved awareness, and training of health workers at all levels, as well as the selection of appropriate options for the local solutions.

SPECIFICS OF SAFE INJECTION PRACTICES

Medical treatment is intended to save life and improve health, and all health workers have a responsibility to prevent transmission of healthcare-associated infections. Adherence to safe injection practices and related infection control is part of that responsibility—it protects patients and health workers **(Table 21.7.1)**.

Injection is defined as a skin piercing event performed by a syringe and a needle to introduce a vaccine or a curative substance into a patient by various routes such as intravenous (IV), intramuscular (IM), subcutaneous (SC), intradermal (ID), etc.

What is a Safe Injection?

A safe injection, phlebotomy (drawing blood), lancet procedure, or IV device insertion is one that:

- Does not harm the recipient
- Does not expose the provider to any avoidable risk
- Does not result in any waste that is dangerous for other people.

Do's and Don'ts of Injection Safety

- Do carry out hand hygiene (use soap and water or alcohol rub), and wash carefully, including wrists and spaces between the fingers, for at least 30 seconds.
- Do use one pair of nonsterile gloves per procedure or patient.
- Do use a single-use device for blood sampling and drawing.
- Do disinfect the skin at the venipuncture site.
- Do discard the used device (a needle and syringe is a single unit) immediately into a robust sharps container where recapping of a needle is unavoidable. Do use the one-hand scoop technique.
- Do seal the sharps container with a tamper-proof lid.
- Do place laboratory sample tubes in a sturdy rack before injecting into the rubber stopper.
- Do immediately report any incident or accident linked to a needle or sharp injury, and seek assistance; start post-exposure prophylaxis (PEP) as soon as possible, following protocols.
- Do not forget to clean your hands.
- Do not use the same pair of gloves for more than one patient.
- Do not wash gloves for reuse.
- Do not use a syringe, needle, or lancet for more than one patient.
- Do not recap a needle using both hands.
- Do not touch the puncture site after disinfecting it.
- Do not leave an unprotected needle lying outside the sharps container.
- Do not overfill or decant a sharps container.
- Do not inject into a laboratory tube while holding it with the other hand.
- Do not delay PEP after exposure to potentially contaminated material; beyond 72 hours, PEP is not effective.

The essential steps for safe injection practices are:

- Clean work space for injection preparations (free from any blood contamination).
- Appropriately done hand hygiene (described further). Hand hygiene is a general term that applies to hand washing, antiseptic hand wash, antiseptic hand rub, or surgical hand antisepsis. It is the best and easiest way to prevent the spread of microorganisms.

Hand hygiene should be carried out as indicated in **Figure 21.7.1**, either with soap and running water (if hands are visibly soiled) or with alcohol rub (if hands appear clean).

Practical Guidance on Hand Hygiene

Perform Hand Hygiene Before

- Starting an injection session (i.e. preparing injection material and giving injections).

Table 21.7.1: Things to be kept in mind for patients and health workers.

Patients or clients	*Health workers who give injections or collect blood*	*Community or other health workers*

• Unnecessary injections
• Reuse of injection equipment
• Nonsterile or reprocessed syringes and needles
• Poor hand hygiene
• Cross-contamination through:
  – Poor hand hygiene
  – Medication vials
• Improper injection technique or site
• Sharps in hospital linen or other unexpected places
	• Unnecessary injections
	• Two-handed recapping of needles
	• Manipulation of used sharps
	• Lack of sharps box within arm's reach
	• Poor positioning of patient
	• Poor phlebotomy technique
	• Two-handed transfer of blood
	• Unsafe transport of blood
	• Poor hand hygiene
	• Nonsegregated sharps waste
		• Increased waste from unnecessary injections
		• Unsafe disposal of sharps waste:
		  – Outside safety boxes
		  – Mixed with hospital linen
		  – In nonsecure disposal sites
		• Lack of protective clothing (boots, gloves, etc.) for waste handlers
		• Reuse of needles or syringes

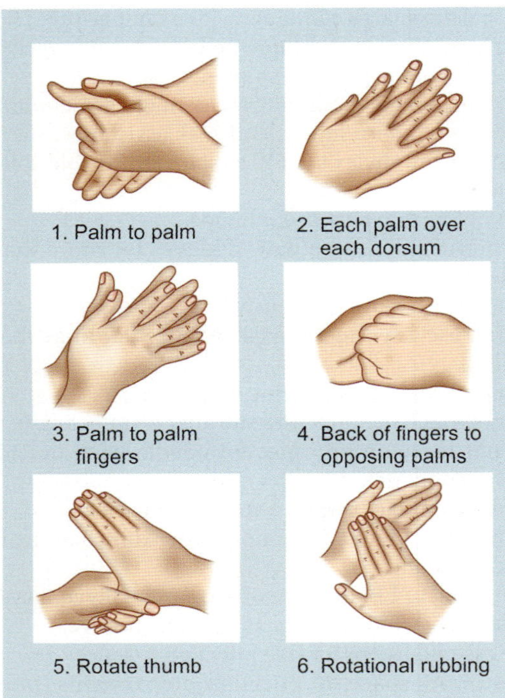

Fig. 21.7.1: Six steps of hand washing.

- Coming into direct contact with patients for health care-related procedures.
- Putting on gloves (first make sure hands are dry).

Perform Hand Hygiene After

- An injection session
- Any direct contact with patients
- Removing gloves. You may need to perform hand hygiene between injections, depending on the setting and whether there was contact with soil, blood, or body fluids. Avoid giving injections if your skin integrity is compromised by local infection or other skin conditions (e.g. weeping dermatitis, skin lesions, or cuts), and cover any small cuts.

Injection Site Preparation

- Apply a 60–70% alcohol-based solution (isopropyl alcohol or ethanol) on a single-use swab or cotton-wool ball. Do not use methanol or methyl alcohol, as these are not safe for human use.
- Wipe the area from the center of the injection site working outward, without going over the same area.
- Apply the solution for 30 seconds then allow it to dry completely.
- Do not presoak cotton wool in a container—these become highly contaminated with hand and environmental bacteria.

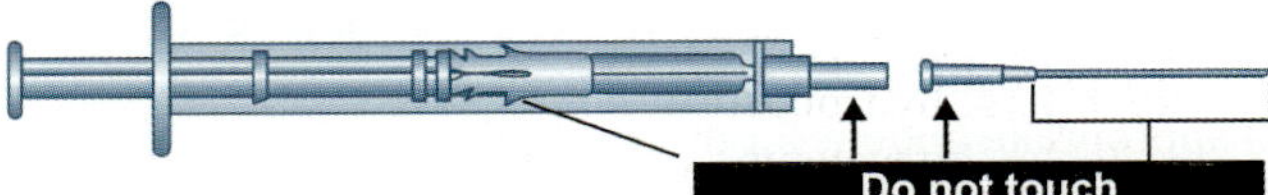

Fig. 21.7.2: Prevention of contamination of injection equipment.

- Do not use alcohol skin disinfection for administration of vaccinations.

Preventing Injection Equipment from Contamination

- Contamination of injection equipment should be prevented by not touching certain parts as shown in **Figure 21.7.2**.
- The used needles and syringes should be disposed as per biomedical waste management (BWM) rules.

RATIONAL INJECTION THERAPY

People may have different perceptions and meanings regarding the term "rational drug use". However, the conference of experts on the rational use of drugs, convened by the WHO in Nairobi in 1985 defined that "Rational use of drugs requires that patients receive medications appropriate to their clinical needs, in doses that meet their own individual requirements for an adequate period of time, at the lowest cost to them and their community".

A review of essential drug lists and management guidelines of common illnesses shows that injections are recommended only for acute care (emergency setting) and immunization. The reasons given for injection over use are that patients and health workers believe injections are more effective, act fast, and course of management is short.

These are wrong notions. There is need to promote rational injection therapy among all prescribers. It can be achieved through following steps:

- Defining effective and safe protocols
- Promoting minimal essential injection practices
- Promoting rational drug/injection therapy
- Reduction in procurement of injectable drugs at health facilities
- Encouraging prescription auditing at all health facilities, public as well as private sectors
- Continuing medical education for health workers
- Community awareness regarding harmful effects of injections.

BEST INJECTION TECHNIQUES

General Principles

- Give injections only when indicated.
- Emergency equipment should be kept ready to use in emergency situations like anaphylactic reactions—oxygen

bag and mask, laryngoscope and endotracheal tubes, as well as emergency drugs such as adrenaline, volume expanders, hydrocortisone, and dopamine should be available. Intravenous cannula, syringes, and needles are also essential.
- Check the appropriate drug or vaccine and its date.
- Make sure that vial or ampoule contains right medication, its appropriate concentration, and doses.
- The drug or vaccine should be kept sterile during the procedure.
- Clean the injection site properly.
- Use disposable or sterile needle and syringe, preferable with reuse prevention feature.
- Do not touch the parts of needle and syringe in which come in contact with injectable drug and body.
- If you accidentally touch these parts, discard the syringe-needle.
- Take care to avoid air bubble in the syringe or bulb.
- While injecting take care to prevent needle stick injury (NSI) (report immediately if you get injured—this is for your own safety).
- Used needles and syringes should be disposed as per standard guidelines.
- Observe the child for 15 minutes, after giving injection.
- Talk to the parents regarding drug or vaccine given by injection, necessary precautions, possible adverse reactions, and necessary remedial measures in case of adverse reactions.
- Guide them to give information to medical person in case of major problems.

Important Points

- Do not allow the needle to touch any contaminated surface.
- Do not reuse a syringe, even if the needle is changed.
- Do not touch the diaphragm after disinfection with the 60–70% alcohol (isopropyl alcohol or ethanol).
- Do not enter several multidose vials with the same needle and syringe.
- Do not re-enter a vial with a needle or syringe used on a patient if that vial will be used to withdraw medication again (whether it is for the same patient or for another patient).
- Do not use bags or bottles of IV solution as a common source of supply for multiple patients (except in pharmacies using laminar flow cabinets).

Intramuscular Injection

Common Sites

Muscles commonly used for IM injections are:
- Vastus lateralis
- Deltoid
- Gluteus medius

Children do not have well-developed gluteus medius and therefore injections should not be given in gluteal region.

The vastus lateralis (anterolateral aspect of thigh) is preferred site in infants. The specific site in vastus lateralis is the middle third of the area between the greater trochanter and lateral femoral condyle.

In case of deltoid, the site for injection is midway between acromion process and deltoid insertion; it comes to 3–5 cm below the acromion process. This site may be used in children above 5 years and adults. The quantity of drug should be less than 5 mL. Only watery injections with less viscosity should be injected at deltoid region.

Technique (World Health Organization Technique)

- The site of injection should be exposed well.
- For anterolateral aspect of thigh, the child may be laid supine or be held in mother's lap.
- For deltoid, child may be held in mother's lap or may sit.
- The muscle selected for injection should be relaxed.
- The skin over injection site should be cleaned with spirit. A circular motion of swab is used proceeding from puncture site and extending outward for 5 cm.
- Let the spirit evaporate and skin become dry, otherwise spirit entering into tissues is painful.
- The syringe is filled with the medicine.
- In children, usually 23G needle with 25 mm length is used for IM injections.
- Stretch the skin flat and push the needle down at 90° **(Figs. 21.7.3 to 21.7.6)**
- Aspiration before injecting the vaccine is not required.
- Inject the vaccine at the rate of 1 mL per 10 seconds.
- The needle is withdrawn and injection site is pressed for few seconds.
- Do not rub the injection site.
- Needle should be withdrawn smoothly with steady movement.
- Discard the needle and syringe as per standard guidelines.

Alternative to WHO technique, Advisory Committee on Immunization Practices (ACIP) technique may be used.

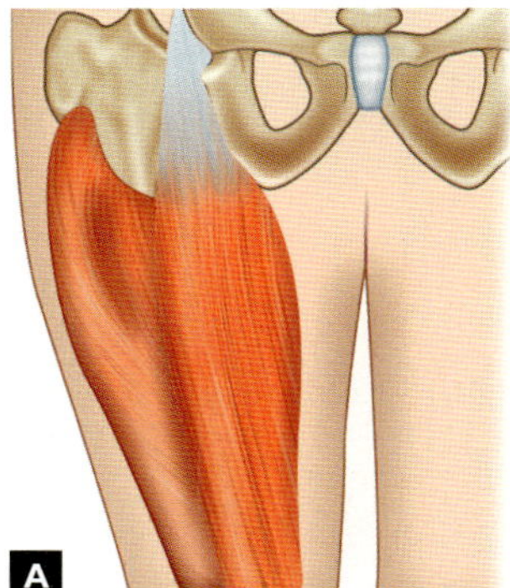

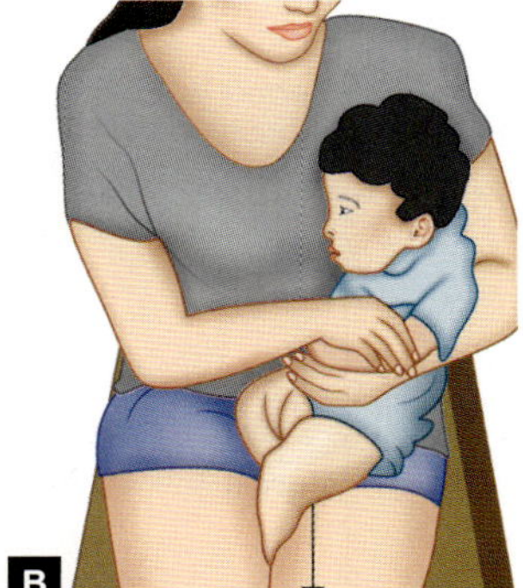

Figs. 21.7.3A and B: Positioning of the child for intramuscular (IM) injection (vastus lateralis).

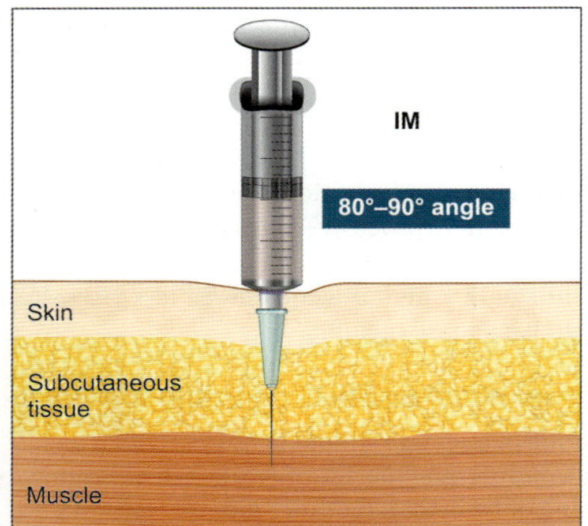

Fig. 21.7.4: Technique for intramuscular (IM) injection.

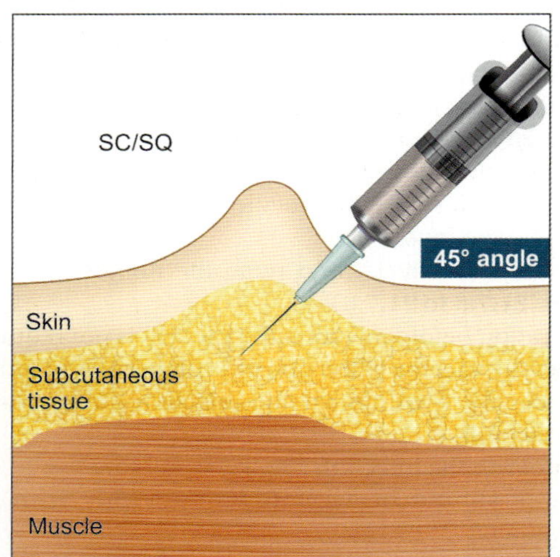

Fig. 21.7.5: Technique for subcutaneous (SC/SQ) injection.

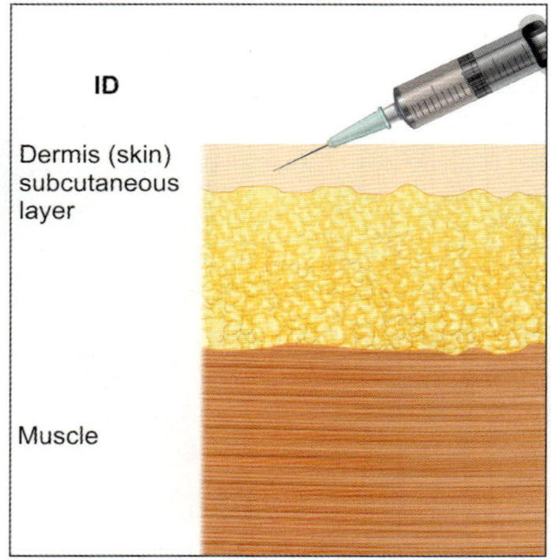

Fig. 21.7.6: Technique for intradermal (ID) injection.

It is also called bunching technique. In this technique, bunch the muscle and direct needle inferiorly along long axis of leg at an angle of 45°. It stabilizes leg and increases the muscle mass.

Subcutaneous Injection

Drugs or vaccines are injected subcutaneously when slow absorption and long duration of action are desired. Another indication of SC route is a coagulopathy, which makes IM injection hazardous, for fear of development of IM hematoma. Insulin and heparin-like drugs as well as measles, varicella, measles, mumps, and rubella (MMR), etc. vaccines are given by SC route.

Technique

- Common sites are arm, thigh, or sometimes anterior abdominal wall. Atrophic and injected areas should be avoided.
- The skin is cleaned and disinfected with spirit.
- 26G needle with 13 mm length is commonly used for SC injection.
- The skin is raised into a fold with thumb and index finger of the left hand.
- The midpoint of the fold is pierced with the needle held at 45° with its surface.
- The tip of the needle is advanced into the SC tissue.
- Aspiration is not required.
- Drugs or vaccine is injected; needle is withdrawn and site is pressed for few minutes.

Intradermal Injection

Indications for ID injections are:

- BCG vaccination
- Rabies vaccine
- Mantoux test
- Skin tests for allergy
- Test for sensitization of certain drugs like penicillin, etc.

Technique

- Ventral (volar) aspect of forearm is commonly used for ID injection.
- Skin is cleaned with spirit or clean water.
- A measured amount of antigen (usually 0.1 mL) is drawn into the syringe.
- 26 or 27G needle with 1/4–1/2 inch (6.35–12.7 mm) length needle is used for ID injection.
- The skin is held taut between thumb and index finger of the left hand. The syringe is held at an angle of 10–15° with the skin.
- Needle is inserted for about 2 mm, so that entire needle bevel penetrates the skin and the injected solution raises a small bleb of about 5 mm in diameter. The development

of perifollicular puckering (Peau d'orange) indicates successful ID injection.

- The needle is withdrawn.
- The site is circled and it is recorded in patient's chart.
- The reaction is observed in defined time.

NEEDLE STICK INJURY AND POSTEXPOSURE PROPHYLAXIS

Needle Stick Injuries

Needle stick injuries can be defined as an accidental exposure through needles, which may occur before, during, or after the process of injection giving. It might place healthcare professional or worker (HCP/HCW) at risk of blood-borne infections like hepatitis B, hepatitis C, or HIV and many others. Globally, NSIs are the most common source of occupational exposures to blood and the primary cause of blood-borne infections of HCWs. The two most common causes of NSIs are two handed recapping and the unsafe collection and disposal of sharps waste.

Determinants of Needle Stick Injuries

- Overuse of injections and unnecessary sharps.
- *Lack of supplies*: Disposable syringes, safer needle devices, and sharps-disposal containers.
- Lack of access to and failure to use sharps containers immediately after injection.
- Inadequate or short staffing.
- Recapping of needles after use.
- Lack of engineering controls such as safer needle devices.
- Passing instruments from hand to hand in the operating suite.
- Lack of awareness of hazard and lack of training.

Determinants of Transmission of Infection

The risks of transmission of infection from an infected patient to the HCW following an NSI are hepatitis B, 3–10%; hepatitis C, 3%; and HIV, 0.3%.

Immediate Management of Needle Stick Injuries

The exposure site should be cleaned immediately. This is the most important part of PEP. Puncture wounds and other cutaneous injury sites should be copiously washed with soap and water. Exposed oral and nasal mucous membranes should be vigorously flushed with water. Eyes should be irrigated with clean water or saline. There is no evidence that antiseptics for wound care reduce the risk of blood-borne pathogen transmission. The use of bleach or other caustic agents that cause local tissue trauma is not recommended.

Postexposure Prophylaxis for Hepatitis B

- If the exposed person is vaccinated and his serum antibody titer is more than 10 IU/mL, no further treatment is required.
- If antibody titer is less than 10 IU/mL and the exposed person is HbsAg negative or the source is unknown, then one course of three doses of vaccine is repeated and then antibody titer is rechecked.
- If the exposed person is HbsAg positive, then both hepatitis B vaccine is repeated and hepatitis B immune globulin (HBIg) is given within hours of exposure.
- If the exposed person is not vaccinated, then vaccination series is started within 7 days.

Flowchart 21.7.1 shows management following exposure to hepatitis B positive patient.

Management of Exposure to Hepatitis C Virus

The following are recommendations for follow-up of occupational HCV exposures:

- For the source, perform anti-HCV
- For the person exposed to HCV positive source:
  - Perform baseline testing for anti-HCV and alanine aminotransferase (ALT) activity
  - Perform follow-up testing at 4–6 months for anti-HCV and ALT activity
  - If earlier diagnosis of HCV infection is desired, testing for HCV RNA may be performed at 4–6 weeks
- Confirm all anti-HCV results reported positive by enzyme immunoassay, using supplement anti-HCV testing
- Immunoglobulins and antiviral agents are not recommended.

Flowchart 21.7.1: Management of healthcare professional or worker (HCP/HCW) exposed to hepatitis B injection.

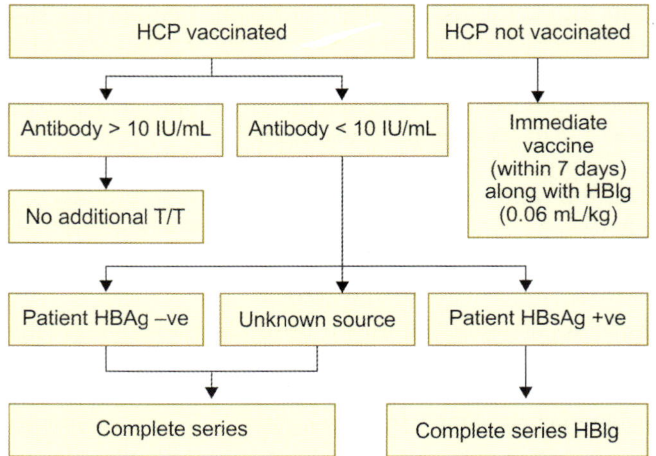

(HBIg: hepatitis B immune globulin; HBsAg: hepatitis B surface antigen; T/T: treatment)

Recommendations for Postexposure Prophylaxis for Human Immunodeficiency Virus

- Indian Academy of Pediatrics (IAP) endorses the National AIDS Control Organization (NACO) guidelines. These should be implemented all over the India
- If any exposed person reports with NSI to emergency services in a public health facility, it is recommended that immediate care, free testing, and free PEP medicines should be provided
- A nodal contact person should be in place in all facilities with 24 hours access to deal with immediate management of NSIs/other exposures
- Healthcare workers should ensure that a startup pack of PEP medication is available in their place of work.

DISPOSAL OF INJECTION WASTE (SYRINGES AND NEEDLES)

Biomedical waste (BMW) management is a process starting from the point of use of a device till its final disposal. It is not only an issue of technology but also requires lot of changes in the way we think. Healthcare waste is hazardous both to the HCP, patients and public at large.

Government of India under the provision of Environmental Act, 1988 notified the BMW Rules in 1988, which regulates the disposal of all biomedical waste with an objective to ensure safety of health and environment. All healthcare facilities are required to segregate, disinfect, transport, and dispose of the biomedical waste in an environmental-friendly manner. Biomedical waste shall not be mixed with other wastes.

As per the Schedule-I, Rule 5 of BMW Rules, sharp wastes are classified in Category 4, which says, sharp wastes means needles, syringes, scalpel blades, glass, etc. that may cause puncture and cuts. This includes both used and unused sharps, which should be treated. As per Schedule-II, color coding of the container for disposal sharps is a must. Blue/white translucent colored puncture-proof container has to be used and disposed as per the schedule.

Section 4 of the Act has given policy statement. The following steps should be followed: minimization, segregation, handling, storage of hospital waste, and disposal.

Sharp Waste Minimization

As far as possible, minimize the use of sharps. Emphasize the rational use of injections in the treatment of illness. The use of disposable syringes and needles has increased considerably, generating potentially infectious waste with limited options for treatment and disposal. The use of plastic disposables should be limited as far as possible because plastics are nondegradable and more likely to cause reuse.

Segregation of Sharps

Sharps should be segregated at source. The clinical staff is responsible for segregating the waste at source. Blue/white translucent puncture-proof containers should be placed at strategic and easily accessible locations. Needles should not be recapped, removed, and transported by hand. Sharps should be disinfected. Hub-cutters or needle and syringe destroyer should be used at the site of generation to reduce the bulk, to disinfect, and to prevent reusing.

Handling

Sharps containers should be picked-up and carried by the handle provided. They should not be supported at the bottom. Sharp containers should not be carried on back and should not be dropped or thrown. Containers should be labeled. Vehicles used to transport sharp containers should be authorized.

Containers

Sharps decontaminating units (SDUs) for syringes and needles are made of plastic and are puncture-proof; they can be foot operated with an inner-perforated container with secured handles. They should be filled one third with 1% hypochlorite solution (refer to the recent central pollution board guidelines). Sharps in inner containers after treatment with hypochlorite solution should be transferred to puncture-proof containers for shredding. They should be labeled as sharps only.

Mutilation/Destruction/Shredding

Types of waste required to be mutilated are needles, syringes, plastic disposables, etc. Shredders are equipment to cut the waste into small pieces to reduce the volume. They must have safety provisions to prevent contamination. They must be placed in a separate room. Waste must be properly disinfected before feeding into shredder.

Treatment and Disposal

It is necessary to treat certain waste before disposal to prevent hazards to human health and environment. Immediately after use, syringes with needles should be dropped into sharp decontaminating unit (SDU), so that both parts are completely immersed in disinfectant. When SDU is one-third full, after contact time of 30 minutes the inner perforated container contents are drained into puncture-proof containers for shredding. Heat disinfection, encapsulation, smelting, burial, incineration are modes for disposal of sharp wastes in mass.

The education and awareness of HCW and public is important. The general public coming to hospital and in the community should know the medical risks of hospital waste so that they keep away from risks and also to demand the proper care, services from the hospital.

NEWER TECHNOLOGIES

Technology plays a supportive role in enhancing the quality of patient care in our day-to-day working. This has over a period of time helped healthcare professionals to deliver services effectively and efficiently. Most of the technological advances have happened as a response to the demands of the health-care provider. These technologies for ease of understanding can be divided into three different kinds: autodisable (AD) syringes, prefilled AD devices, and HCW safety devices.

Autodisable Syringes

These are disposable syringes that lock once the medication has been injected and hence physically cannot be reused; these syringes prevent reuse and they present the lowest risk of patient-to-patient transmission of blood-borne pathogens. These are available as prefixed 0.5 mL syringes and are presently available for immunization only.

Syringe with different mechanisms are commercially available. These can be broadly divided into two types of AD mechanisms:

Active Mechanism

- Requires the user to "actively" disable the syringe/device after use
- Disadvantage—chances of reuse if mechanism is not activated.

Passive Mechanism

- The device is disabled as soon as the drug is fully injected out. The user has no control over the mechanism
- No chance of reuse as user has no control over mechanism. WHO-United Nations Children's Fund-United Nations Population Fund joint statement issued in 1999 on the use of AD syringes in immunization services has urged countries to use only AD syringes for immunization after 2003. It is also recommended that in the curative sector also, injection devices with reuse prevention mechanisms should be used **(Fig. 21.7.7)**.

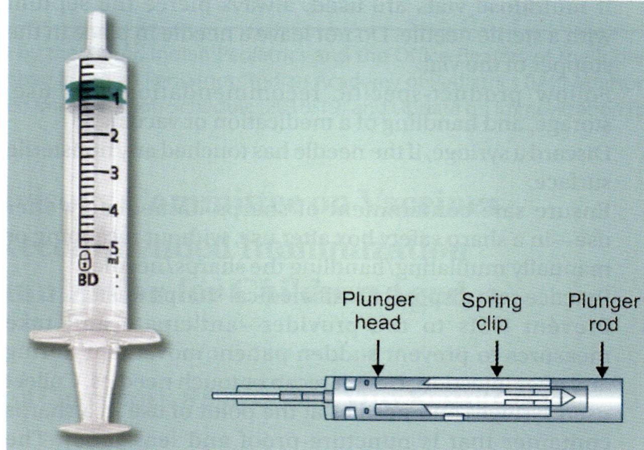

Fig. 21.7.7: Autodisable syringe.

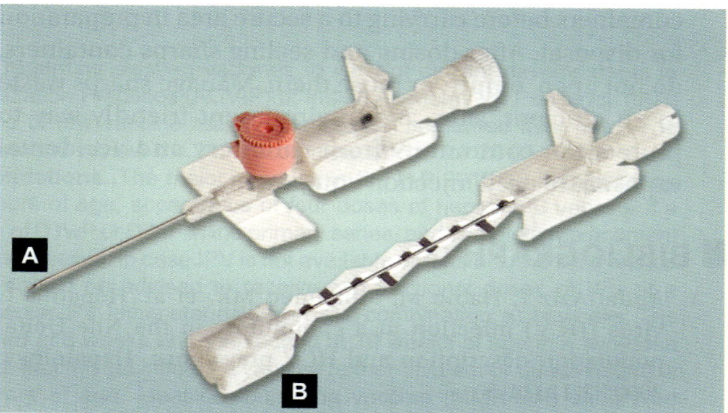

Figs. 21.7.8A and B: Safety cannula and needle shield.

Prefilled Vaccine Devices or Pouch and Needle Devices (Figs. 21.7.8A and B)

Prefilled vaccine devices or pouch and needle devices were also developed by PATH and are used by the pharmaceutical companies and vaccine manufacturers to fill vaccines into them and supply. They combine the benefit of prefilled device with that of AD technologies. Minimally trained volunteers can use them. Several vaccines are now available with this technology.

Healthcare Worker's Safety Devices

With the identification of the spread of blood-borne pathogens due to NSIs stick injuries and a Needle Stick Safety and Prevention Act passed in the United States in 2000, the trend, globally, is shifting toward use of safety engineered products. Now, a range of products, which help prevent accidental NSIs are available. These products are now widely available in India.

LEARNING POINTS

- Keep hands clean before giving injections.
- Always use "sterile injection equipment". Always use sterile syringe and needle for each injection and to reconstitute each unit of medication.
- Prevent contamination of injection equipment and medicines.
- Prepare each injection in a clean designated area where blood or body fluid contamination is unlikely.
- Clean skin prior to injection with water and wait for it to dry. Do not use cotton balls stored wet in a container.

TABLE I Key Updates and Major Changes in Recommendations for IAP Immunization Timetable, 2018-2019

Hepatitis B vaccine

- One dose of hepatitis B vaccine within 24 hours of birth.
- In case of use of a combination vaccines a total of four doses of hepatitis B vaccine are justified.

DTwP, DTaP and combination vaccines

- DTwP or DTaP can be offered in primary series.

Polio vaccines

- Ideally IPV should replace OPV as early as possible.
- Three doses of intramuscular IPV in primary series is the best option.
- Two doses of intramuscular IPV instead of three for primary series if started at 8 weeks, with an interval of 8 weeks between two doses is an alternative.
- In case IPV is not available or feasible, the child should be offered three doses of bOPV. In such cases, the child should be referred for two fractional doses of IPV at a Government facility at 6 and 14 weeks or at least one dose of intramuscular IPV, either standalone or as a combination vaccine, at 14 weeks of age.

Rota virus vaccine

- In case of Rotavirus vaccine, RV1 can be used in 6, 10 weeks schedule.

Influenza vaccine

- Inactivated influenza vaccine (either trivalent or quadrivalent) is recommended routinely to all children below 5 years of age starting from 6 months of age annually (2-4 weeks before influenza season).

Measles-containing vaccines

- Measles-containing vaccine (MMR/MR) should be administered after 9 months of age.
- MR vaccine as part of the national campaign is to be administered irrespective of previous vaccination.

Typhoid vaccines

- Single dose of any of Typhoid conjugate vaccine (TCV 25 mg) is recommended from 6 months onwards and can be administered with MMR also.
- Booster dose of Typhoid conjugate vaccine not recommended in subsequent years.

Rabies vaccines

- ACVIP IAP endorses administration of a 4-dose schedule of Rabies vaccine recommended by WHO 2018 for Post-exposure prophylaxis.
- ACVIP also endorses administration of Rabies monoclonal antibody as an alternative to Rabies immunoglobulin for category-III bites.

ACVIP: Advisory Committee on Vaccines and Immunization Practices; IAP: Indian Academy of Pediatrics; IPV: Injectable polio vaccine; OPV: Oral polio vaccine; bOPV: bivalent oral polio vaccine; MR: Measles-Rubella vaccine; MMR: Measles-Mumps-Rubella vaccine.

HBsAg report of the mother is not known or reported incorrectly, or in case of infants born to HBsAg positive mothers, this dose becomes a very important safety net [3].

Four doses of hepatitis B vaccine may be administered for programmatic reasons (*e.g.*, 3 doses of hepatitis B-containing combination vaccine or monovalent HBV after a single monovalent dose at birth [2].

Diptheria, Tetanus and Pertussis Vaccines (DTwP and DTaP)

Long-term efficacy over 10 years has been observed to be superior with whole cell pertussis vaccine (wP) [4]. Recent outbreaks of pertussis in various developed countries have sparked a debate on the effectiveness of acellular pertussis (aP) vaccines. However, none of these countries are planning to revert back to whole-cell pertussis vaccines as that can result in an increase in the prevalence of the disease due to poor acceptance of a vaccine that is much more reactogenic [5]. Though the reasons for this resurgence are complex and vary from place to place, the lesser duration of protection and decreased impact on transmission of the disease by acellular pertussis vaccines appears to be crucial [6]. Waning of immunity has been reported with whole cell and acellular vaccines over a period of time. Current evidence suggests that the efficacy of both aP and wP vaccines in preventing pertussis in the first year is equivalent. After the first year, the immunity wanes more rapidly with the aP vaccines and the impact on transmission by aP vaccines is also inferior to wP vaccines [7-9]. WHO clearly mentions that countries currently using the wP vaccine in their national programs should continue

	Birth	6 weeks	10 weeks	14 weeks	6 months	9 months	12 months	13 months	15 months	16–18 months	2–3 years	4–6 years	9–14 years	15–18 years
BCG	BCG													
Hepatitis B	HB 1	HB 2	HB 3	HB* 4										
Polio	OPV 0	IPV** 1	IPV** 2	IPV** 3						IPV*** B1				
DTwP/DTaP		DTP 1	DTP 2	DTP 3						DTP B1		DTP B2		
HiB		HiB 1	HiB 2	HiB 3						HIB B1				
Pneumococcal		PCV 1	PCV 2	PCV 3					PCV B1				PCV	
Rotavirus		Rota 1	Rota 2	Rota 3****										
MMR						MMR 1			MMR 2			MMR3/MMRV		
Varicella									Varicella 1			Varicella 2		
Hepatitis A							Hep A1			Hep A2*****				
Typhoid					TCV[#]									
Influenza							Influenza (yearly)******							
Meningococcal						MCV 1	MCV 2				MCV			
JE							JE 1	JE 2						
Tdap													Tdap	Td
HPV[##]													HPV 1 and 2	HPV 1,2,3
Cholera									Cholera 1 and 2					

Range of recommended age for all children

Range of recommended age for high-risk children/area

Range of recommended age for catch-up immunization

Not recommended

*Fourth dose of Hepatitis B permissible for combination vaccines only

**In case IPV is not available or feasible, the child should be offered bOPV (3 doses). In such cases, give two fractional doses of IPV at 6 weeks and 14 weeks

***b-OPV, if IPV booster (standalone or combination) not feasible

****Third dose not required for RV 1. Catcth-up up to 1 year of age in UIP schedule

*****Live attenuated Hepatitis A vaccine: Single dose only

******Begin influenza vaccination after 6 months of age, about 2–4 weeks before season; give 2 doses at the interval of 4 weeks during first year and then single dose yearly till 5 years of age

[#]TCV: typhoid conjugate vaccine; [##]HPV: human papilloma virus

Meningococcal vaccine (MCV): 9 months through 23 months: 2 doses, at least 3 months apart; 2 years through 55 years: single dose only

Japanese encephalitis (JE): For individuals living in endemic areas and for travelers to JE endemic areas provided their expected stay is for a minimum period of 4 weeks

HPV: 2 doses at 6 months interval 9–14 years age; 3 doses (at 0, 1–2 and 6 months) 15 years or older and immunocompromised

Cholera vaccine: Two doses 2 weeks apart for >1 year old; for individuals living in high endemic areas and traveling to areas where risk of transmission is very high

Fig. 1: IAP-ACVIP Recommended immunization schedule for children aged 0-18 years (2018-19).

the same for the primary series [10,11], while those using the aP vaccine should continue the same and consider additional boosters and strategies like immunization of mothers in case of pertussis resurgence [10]. The duration of protection for both the aP and wP vaccines after the three primary doses and a booster dose at least after a year varies from 6-12 years [11]. A German study reported acellular pertussis vaccine being quite efficacious (88.7%) (95% CI, 76.6% to 94.6%) [12].

Number of Components

In a couple of systematic reviews, it was concluded that multi-component acellular pertussis vaccines are more efficacious than the single- or two-component vaccines [13,14]. However, effectiveness studies of long-term usage of two-component acellular pertussis vaccines in Sweden [15] and Japan [16], and the mono-component vaccine in Denmark showed high effectiveness in prevention of pertussis. Thus the higher efficacy for the multi-component vaccine as demonstrated in the trials should be cautiously interpreted, and at present the evidence is insufficient to conclude categorically that the effectiveness of the aP vaccines is related to the number of components alone [10].

IAP ACVIP Recommendation on Pertussis-containing Vaccines

The primary series should be completed with three doses of either wP or aP vaccines, irrespective of the number of components. wP vaccine is definitely superior to aP vaccine in terms of immunogenicity and duration of protection but more reactogenic. In view of parental anxiety and concerns for its reactogenicity, aP vaccine can also be administered even in the primary series. The primary aim is to increase the vaccination coverage with either of the vaccines.

Polio Vaccines

The elimination of circulating wild poliovirus from our country and the decline worldwide in the number of cases is the proof of efficacy of Oral polio vaccine (OPV). At the beginning of 2013, 126 countries using OPV exclusively, decided to introduce Injectable polio vaccine (IPV), at least one dose, in their National Immunization Schedule. This was part of WHO's Endgame Plan to withdraw type-2 polio virus and prepare for 'the switch' from trivalent OPV (tOPV) to bivalent OPV (bOPV) in April 2016 [17,18]. However, IPV introduction in these countries has increased the global IPV demand, to over 200 million in 2016 from 80 million in 2013 [17,18]. The attempt to meet the global requirements for IPV by rapidly increasing the IPV production has led to multiple challenges, resulting in a shortage worldwide. Intradermal IPV administration with fractional doses of IPV (fIPV) (0.1 mL or one-fifth of a full dose) offers potential cost reduction and allows immunization of a larger number of persons with a given vaccine supply [19]. Two fractional doses administered *via* the intradermal (ID) route offer higher immunogenicity compared to one full intramuscular (IM) dose of IPV [20-23]. As a result, a two-dose fIPV schedule has been strongly recommended to countries that are endemic and the those with high risk of importation of wild polio virus [24].

Private medical practitioners have irregular and inadequate access to standalone IPV, and are thus compelled to administer combination vaccines, and thus are not able to follow the Indian government schedule, which consists of fIPV and standalone IPV. It is not feasible for pediatricians in private settings to refer all children to government facilities for the same. In addition, the recent controversy of the contamination of OPV with type-2 Poliovirus has resulted in the awareness of vaccine-derived paralytic poliomyelitis (VDPP) amongst public. In this background, there is a need to recommend a regimen containing IPV as combination vaccine in the private settings.

IAP ACVIP Recommendations

- Birth dose of OPV is a must.
- Extra doses of OPV on all Supplementary immunization activities should continue.
- No child should leave the health facility without polio immunization (IPV or OPV), if indicated by the schedule.
- bOPV should be continued in place of IPV, only if IPV is not feasible, with a minimum of 3 doses at 6,10,14 weeks of age.
- Minimum age of administration of IPV is 6 weeks with the best option being 3 doses of IM IPV in 6-10-14 weeks schedule. This can be as a combination vaccine, in view of non-availability of standalone IM IPV.
- Two doses of IM IPV, instead of 3 doses can be administered provided the primary series is started at 8 weeks with the minimum interval between them being 8 weeks.
- In case IPV is not available or feasible, the child should be offered 3 doses of bOPV in a 6-10-14 weeks schedule. In such cases, the child should be advised to receive two fractional doses of IPV at a Government facility at 6 and 14 weeks of age or at least one dose of IM IPV either standalone or as a part of combination vaccine at 14 weeks.

Rotavirus Vaccines

A review of studies from 38 populations found that all

rotavirus gastroenteritis events (RVGE) occurred in 1%, 3%, 6%, 8%, 10%, 22% and 32% children by age 6, 9, 13, 15, 17, 26 and 32 weeks, respectively. Mortality was mostly related to RVGE events occurring before 32 weeks of age [25]. The highest risk of mortality was noted in the children having earliest exposure to rotavirus, living in poor rural households, and having lowest level of vaccine coverage [26]. It is ideal if immunization schedule is completed early in developing countries where natural infection might occur early [27].

Infants in developing countries may be at risk of developing RVGE at an earlier age than those in developed countries. They also tend to have a higher risk of mortality coupled with the risk of lower vaccine coverage. No observational study has compared different ages at first dose. A schedule of two doses at 10 and 14 weeks may result in incomplete course of vaccination, especially in developing countries because of restriction of upper age limit for rotavirus vaccine administration. Such children would remain immunologically susceptible to get rotavirus infection. Early administration of the first dose of rotavirus vaccine as soon as possible after 6 weeks of age has been recommended by WHO recently [27]. Administration of RV1 or RV5 vaccine at 6 weeks has also been recommended and approved even in developed countries [28].

Two randomized controlled trials reported data on severe rotavirus gastroenteritis with up to one year follow-up, and directly compared children who received the first dose of RV1 at age 6 weeks *vs* 10 to 11 weeks. No statistically significant difference in efficacy was found between these two schedules [29]. The South Africa and Malawi RV1 trial [30] reported similar efficacy of vaccination schedules beginning at 6 weeks or 10 to 11 weeks against severe RVGE during the second year follow-up using only the Malawi cohort. Indirect comparisons based on stratification of RV1 and RV5 trials using different schedules showed no impact on mortality for different ages at first dose.

Considering these factors, ACVIP recommends RV1 in a schedule of 6 and 10 weeks. The recommendations for the schedule of other vaccines remain the same.

Currently the following live oral rotavirus vaccines are available in India: (*i*) Human monovalent live vaccine (RV1); (*ii*) Human bovine pentavalent live vaccine (RV5); (*iii*) Indian neonatal rotavirus live vaccine, 116 E; (*iv*) Bovine Rotavirus Vaccine – Pentavalent (BRV-PV). BRV-PV is a recently introduced pentavalent rotavirus vaccine that contains serotypes G1, G2, G3, G4, and G9 obtained from Bovine (UK) X Human Rotavirus Reassortant strains. It is a thermostable vaccine and can be stored below 24 ^{0}C till the duration of the shelf life of 30 months. This vaccine remains stable for 36 months at temperature below 25 ^{0}C, for 18 months between 37 ^{0}C and 40 ^{0}C, and a short-term exposure at 55 ^{0}C [31].

IAP ACVIP Recommendation on Rotavirus Vaccines

Any of the available rotavirus vaccines may be routinely administered as per the manufacturer's recommendations. All the available vaccines have been demonstrated to be safe and immunogenic.

- Minimum age: 6 weeks for all available brands
- Only two doses of RV-1 are recommended at 6 and 10 weeks
- If any dose in series was RV-5 or RV-116E or vaccine product is unknown for any dose in the series, a total of three doses of RV vaccine should be administered.

Recommendations on the age limit for the first dose and the last dose (16 and 32 weeks) should continue in spite of recommendation for increase in the age limit as per recent NIP guidelines.

TYPHOID VACCINE

Considering the continuation of significant burden of typhoid fever, widespread prevalence of antibiotic-resistant strains of *S. typhi* and availability of favorable evidence on the efficacy, effectiveness, immunogenicity, safety, and cost-effectiveness of typhoid vaccines, WHO recommends use of typhoid vaccines in national programs for the control of typhoid fever [32,33]. Typhoid conjugate vaccine (TCV) is preferred at all ages as it has improved immunological properties, can be used in younger children, and is expected to provide longer duration of protection. A meta-analysis summarized that typhoid cases across the age groups; 14% to 29% in <5 years, 30% to 44% in 5-9 years and 28% to 52% in 10-14 years [34]. It has been observed that more than one-fourth of all cases occur in children aged below 4 years, with approximately 30% of cases in children aged below 2 years, and 10% in children aged below 1 year [35]. Based on this, WHO has recommended TCV for infants and children from 6 months of age as a 0.5 mL single dose [36], and the same is endorsed by ACVIP.

Booster Doses/Revaccination

The need for revaccination with TCV is currently unclear [36]. The protection with TCV may last for up to 5 years after the administration of one dose, and natural boosting may occur in endemic areas [37]. The evidence concerning the need for booster vaccination is lacking currently. Until more data is generated or available, the ACVIP recommends only a single dose of TCV from 6 months onwards. If a child has received Typhoid polysachharide vaccine, it is recommended to offer one dose of TCV at least 4 weeks following the receipt of polysaccharide vaccine.

Currently, three products of TCV are licensed in India. Two of them contain 25 μg of purified Vi PS of *S. typhi*, and one of them containing 5 μg purified Vi PS of *S. typhi*. The WHO position paper in 2018 has remarked that the body of evidence for the 5 μg vaccine is very limited.

IAP ACVIP Recommendation on Typhoid Vaccines

Primary schedule

- A single dose of TCV 25 μg is recommended from the age of 6 months onwards routinely.
- An interval of at least 4 weeks is not mandatory between TCV and measles-containing vaccine when it is offered at age of 9 months or beyond.
- For a child who has received only Typhoid polysaccharide vaccine, a single dose of TCV is recommended at least 4 weeks following the receipt of polysaccharide vaccine. Routine booster for TCV at 2 years is not recommended as of now.

Measles, Mumps and Rubella (MMR/MR) Vaccines

Standalone measles vaccine is now not available for regular use. Measles-containing vaccine (MMR/MR) should be administered after 9 months of age (270 days). MR (Measles-Rubella) vaccine is currently not available in the private sector. Hence in view of morbidity following mumps infection, it has been recommended that MMR is administered instead of MR at 9 months, 15 months, and 4-6 years [38], or as two doses at 12 to 15 months of age with the second dose between 4 to 6 years of age. [39]. Additional dose of MR vaccine during MR campaign for children 9 months to 15 years, irrespective of previous vaccination status is to be administered, keeping in mind the need to support national programs.

Influenza Vaccine

A meta-analysis and systematic review evaluating studies published between 1995 to 2010 estimated that children under 5 years of age had 90 million (95% CI 49-162 million) new influenza episodes, 20 million (95% CI 13-32 million) cases of acute lower respiratory infections (ALRI) where influenza was associated, and 1 million (95% CI 1-2 million) cases of severe ALRI (associated with influenza). This resulted in 28,000-111,500 deaths attributed to influenza, with 99% of them from developing countries [40]. Another study estimated that globally 160,000-450,000 children below 5 years of age die in hospitals each year due to all-cause ALRI [41].

A systematic literature review described that during the peak rainy season, influenza accounted for 20-42% of monthly acute medical illness hospitalizations in India [42]. This suggests that influenza is a substantial contributor to severe respiratory illness and hospitalization. The findings from the studies also show that influenza circulation and influenza-associated hospitalization are major public health concerns in India. There is poor uptake of the influenza vaccine in India. IAP position paper on influenza in 2013 stated the while it may not be practical to recommend routine influenza vaccination to everyone in India, the vaccination for high-risk groups such as the elderly, children below 5 years, medical practitioners and pregnant women should be seriously considered [43]. Influenza incidence in children below 5 years of age from developing countries is three times higher than those from developed countries, with a 15-fold higher case-fatality [41].

Health utilization surveys conducted in two rural sites (Ballabgarh, Haryana and Vadu, Maharashtra) in 2010-2012 reported adjusted all-age incidence rates of influenza-associated hospitalization as 3.8-5.4 per 10,000 in Ballabgarh and 20.3-51.6 per 10,000 in Vadu [44]. The age-specific influenza-associated hospitalization rates varied from year to year. In 2010, these rates were highest among persons aged <1 year, in 2011 among patients >59 years of age, and in 2012 in children 1-4 years in Ballabhgarh. Whereas in Vadu, in 2010, these rates were highest among persons aged 1-4 years, in 2011 in children <1 year, and in 2012 in children 5-14 years. Influenza viruses were found throughout the year and the peaks coincided with peaks in rain fall at both the sites.

The Influenza Serotype-B is reported almost round the year in India. A multi-site influenza study in India found that 27.8% isolates were Influenza A (H1N1) virus, 29.8% were type A (H3N2), and 42.3% isolates were type B [45]. A global influenza study found that during seasons, out of all influenza B isolates, Victoria and Yamagata lineages predominated or co-circulated (>20% of total detections), and this accounted for 64% and 36% of seasons respectively. The vaccine virus mismatch was found in 25% of the seasons [46].

With the available data, there is enough reason to believe that the magnitude of the problem is much higher in developing countries (including India) *vis-a-vis* developed countries. India lies within the northern hemisphere. Some parts of the country experience a distinct tropical environment because of its location close to the equator. These areas have a southern hemisphere seasonality with almost round-the-year circulation of influenza viruses peaking during monsoon. Northern parts of India experience another peak during winters similar to northern hemisphere pattern. There is continuous influenza activity across the nation, with seasonal peaks during monsoon and winter, and an ever increasing number of influenza-like illnesses affecting a large number of children who can transmit the disease to their peers and adult counterparts.

In view of influenza activity round the year with seasonal peaks, high morbidity and mortality in high-risk groups, including children below 5 years, paucity of facilities for laboratory diagnosis, high transmission rate, substantial socioeconomic burden, limitations of oseltamivir, availability of moderately efficacious vaccine, it would be justifiable to use Influenza vaccine routinely in the high-risk group of children below age of 5 years.

Vaccine Strains

FDA recommended the following combinations for 2018-19 influenza vaccines.

- Trivalent vaccines-to have (*i*) an A/Michigan/45/2015 (H1N1)pdm09-like virus, (*ii*) an A/Singapore/INFIMH-16-0019/2016 (H3N2)-like virus; and (*iii*) a B/Colorado/06/2017-like virus (Victoria lineage).
- Quadrivalent vaccines to contain the above three, and a B/Phuket/3073/2013-like virus (Yamagata lineage) [47].

IAP ACVIP Recommendations

ACVIP recommends that quadrivalent/trivalent inactivated influenza vaccine should be routinely offered annually to all children between 6 months to 5 years of age. The latest available influenza vaccine can be administered after 6 months of age, 2-4 weeks prior to the influenza season: two doses at the interval of one month in the first year, and one dose annually before the influenza season up to 5 years of age.

Rabies Vaccine

Recent data indicate that duration and number of doses for post-exposure prophylaxis (PEP) and pre-exposure prophylaxis (PrEP) regimens can be shortened. ACVIP endorses the new schedule suggested by WHO in 2018 [48].

Pre-exposure prophylaxis (Pre-EP) is recommended in the following two situations.

- Children exposed to pets in home.
- Children identified to have a higher risk of being bitten by dogs.

WHO recommends a "1-site vaccine administration on days 0 and 7 for intramuscular administration" [48].

For post-exposure prophylaxis, recently the WHO [48] has recommended a new 4-dose schedule of either of the following: (*i*) 1-site intramuscular administration of vaccine on days 0, 3, 7 and between day 14-28, or (*ii*) 2-sites intramuscular administration on days 0 and 1-site on days 7, 21 (intramuscular).

Rabies Human Monoclonal Antibody (RHMAB)

Access to Rabies immunoglobulin (RIG) is limited resulting in high rabies mortality. RHMAB is a completely human IgG1 monoclonal antibody that binds to the ectodomain of the G glycoprotein produced by recombinant technology. It has been demonstrated to neutralize 25 different isolates of wild-type or street isolates of rabies virus. A recent study found that it is not inferior to Human rabies immunoglobulin (HRIG) in producing rabies virus neutralizing antibody in 200 subjects with WHO category-III suspected rabies exposures. The study subjects received either RMHAB or HRIG (1:1 ratio) in wounds, and intramuscularly wherever necessary, on day-0. All these patients also received five doses of rabies vaccine intramuscularly on 0, 3, 7, 14 and 28 days [49].

This newly introduced monoclonal antibody has emerged as a safe and potent alternative to rabies immunoglobulin. The WHO position paper on Rabies in 2018 has also suggested encouragement of use of this product, if available, instead of RIG. The comparative advantages include easy availability, standardized production quality, possibly greater effectiveness, no requirement of animals in its production, and less adverse events.

In view of the irregular availability and high cost of Rabies immunoglobin (RIG), ACVIP endorses the use of RHMAB as an alternative to RIG – human or equine – along with rabies vaccines in all category-III bites. RHMAB is licensed in India (as Rabisheild, Serum Institute of India; 40 IU/mL) since 2017. The recommended dose is 3.33 IU/kg body weight, preferably at the time of the first vaccine dose. However, this may also be administered up to the 7th day after the first dose of vaccine is given. If the calculated dose is insufficient (to infiltrate all the wounds), it should be diluted in sterile normal saline to get a volume that is enough to be infiltrated around all the wounds.

Funding: None. Indian Academy of Pediatrics provided the consultative meetings' expenses.

Competing interest: Representatives of a few vaccine manufacturing companies also presented their data in the consultative meetings. None stated for authors.

References

1. Vashishtha VM, Choudhury P, Kalra A, Bose A, Thacker N, Yewale VN, *et al.* Indian Academy of Pediatrics (IAP) recommended immunization schedule for children aged 0

Index

Page numbers followed by *b* refer to box, *f* refer to figure, *fc* refer to flowchart, and *t* refer to table.

A

B

D

F

I

J

M

N

O

P

Q

R

S

T

W

X

Y

 Z